DRUG INFORMATION HANDBOOK for ONCOLOGY

A Complete Guide to Combination Chemotherapy Regimens

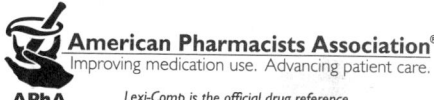

American Pharmacists Association®
Improving medication use. Advancing patient care.

APhA

*Lexi-Comp is the official drug reference
for the American Pharmacists Association.*

8th Edition

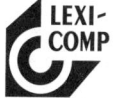

LEXI-COMP

DRUG INFORMATION HANDBOOK for ONCOLOGY

A Complete Guide to Combination Chemotherapy Regimens

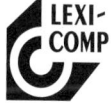

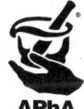

NOTICE

This data is intended to serve the user as a handy reference and not as a complete drug information resource. It does not include information on every therapeutic agent available. The publication covers more than 280 commonly used drugs and is specifically designed to present important aspects of drug data in a more concise format than is typically found in medical literature or product material supplied by manufacturers.

The nature of drug information is that it is constantly evolving because of ongoing research and clinical experience and is often subject to interpretation. While great care has been taken to ensure the accuracy of the information and recommendations presented, the reader is advised that the authors, editors, reviewers, contributors, and publishers cannot be responsible for the continued currency of the information or for any errors, omissions, or the application of this information, or for any consequences arising therefrom. Therefore, the author(s) and/or the publisher shall have no liability to any person or entity with regard to claims, loss, or damage caused, or alleged to be caused, directly or indirectly, by the use of information contained herein. Because of the dynamic nature of drug information, readers are advised that decisions regarding drug therapy must be based on the independent judgment of the clinician, changing information about a drug (eg, as reflected in the literature and manufacturer's most current product information), and changing medical practices. Therefore, this data is designed to be used in conjunction with other necessary information and is not designed to be solely relied upon by any user. The user of this data hereby and forever releases the authors and publishers of this data from any and all liability of any kind that might arise out of the use of this data. The editors are not responsible for any inaccuracy of quotation or for any false or misleading implication that may arise due to the text or formulas as used or due to the quotation of revisions no longer official.

Certain of the authors, editors, and contributors have written this book in their private capacities. No official support or endorsement by any federal or state agency or pharmaceutical company is intended or inferred.

The publishers have made every effort to trace any third party copyright holders, if any, for borrowed material. If they have inadvertently overlooked any, they will be pleased to make the necessary arrangements at the first opportunity.

If you have any suggestions or questions regarding any information presented in this data, please contact our drug information pharmacists at (330) 650-6506.

This manual was produced using Lexi-Comp's Information Management System™ (LIMS) — A complete publishing service of Lexi-Comp, Inc.

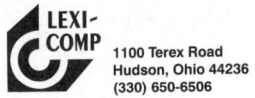

LEXI-COMP
1100 Terex Road
Hudson, Ohio 44236
(330) 650-6506

ISBN 978-1-59195-277-0

TABLE OF CONTENTS

ONCOLOGY EDITORIAL ADVISORY PANEL

EDITORIAL ADVISORY PANEL

3

4

Julie A. Golembiewski, PharmD
Clinical Associate Professor
Colleges of Pharmacy and Medicine
Clinical Pharmacist, Anesthesia/Pain
University of Illinois
Chicago, Illinois

Jeffrey P. Gonzales, PharmD, BCPS
*Critical Care Clinical
Pharmacy Specialist*
University of Maryland Medical Center
Baltimore, Maryland

**Roland Grad, MDCM, MSc,
CCFP, FCFP**
Department of Family Medicine
McGill University
Montreal, Quebec, Canada

Larry D. Gray, PhD, ABMM
Director, Clinical Microbiology
TriHealth Laboratories
Bethesda and Good Samaritan
Hospitals
Cincinnati, Ohio

Tracy Hagemann, PharmD
Associate Professor
College of Pharmacy
The University of Oklahoma
Oklahoma City, Oklahoma

Martin D. Higbee, PharmD
Associate Professor
Department of Pharmacy Practice
and Science
The University of Arizona
Tucson, Arizona

Edward Horn, PharmD, BCPS
Clinical Specialist, Transplant Surgery
Allegheny General Hospital
Pittsburgh, Pennsylvania

Jane Hurlburt Hodding, PharmD
*Executive Director, Inpatient Pharmacy
Services and Clinical
Nutrition Services*
Long Beach Memorial Medical Center
and Miller Children's Hospital
Long Beach, California

Mark T. Holdsworth, PharmD, BCOP
*Associate Professor of
Pharmacy & Pediatrics
Pharmacy Practice Area Head*
College of Pharmacy
The University of New Mexico
Albuquerque, New Mexico

Collin A. Hovinga, PharmD
*Assistant Professor of Pharmacy
and Pediatrics*
College of Pharmacy
University of Tennessee Health
Science Center
Memphis, Tennessee

Darrell T. Hulisz, PharmD
Department of Family Medicine
Case Western Reserve University
Cleveland, Ohio

Michael A. Kahn, DDS
Professor and Chairman
Department of Oral and
Maxillofacial Pathology
Tufts University School of
Dental Medicine
Boston, Massachusetts

Jeannette Kaiser, MT, MBA
Medical Technologist
Akron General Medical Center
Akron, Ohio

**Polly E. Kintzel, PharmD, BCPS,
BCOP**
Clinical Pharmacy Specialist-Oncology
Spectrum Health
Grand Rapids, Michigan

Daren Knoell, PharmD
*Associate Professor of Pharmacy
Practice and Internal Medicine*
Davis Heart and Lung
Research Institute
The Ohio State University
Columbus, Ohio

Sandra Knowles, RPh, BScPhm
Drug Safety Pharmacist
Sunnybrook and Women's
College HSC
Toronto, Ontario

**Jill M. Kolesar, PharmD, FCCP,
BCPS**
Associate Professor
School of Pharmacy
Associate Professor
University of Wisconsin Paul P.
Carbone Comprehensive
Cancer Center
University of Wisconsin
Madison, Wisconsin

Susie H. Park, PharmD, BCPP
Assistant Professor of Clinical Pharmacy
University of Southern Cormia
Los Angeles, California

Alpa Patel, PharmD
Antimicrobial Clinical Pharmacist
University of Louisville Hospital
Louisville, Kentucky

Deidre Payne, PharmD
Assistant Professor, Department of Pharmacy Practice
Hampton University School of Pharmacy
Hampton, Virginia

Gayle Pearson, BSPharm, MSA
Drug Information Pharmacist
Peter Lougheed Centre,
Alberta Health Services
Calgary, Alberta, Canada

James Reissig, PharmD
Assistant Director, Clinical Services
Akron General Medical Center
Akron, Ohio

A.J. (Fred) Remillard, PharmD
Assistant Dean, Research and Graduate Affairs
College of Pharmacy and Nutrition
University of Saskatchewan
Saskatoon, Saskatchewan

Curtis M. Rimmermann, MD, MBA, FACC
Gus P. Karos Chair, Clinical Cardiovascular Medicine
Department of Cardiovascular Medicine
Cleveland Clinic Foundation
Cleveland, Ohio

P. David Rogers, PharmD, PhD, FCCP
Professor and Associate Dean for Translational Research
University of Tennessee College of Pharmacy
Memphis, Tennessee

Martha Sajatovic, MD
Professor of Psychiatry
Case Western Reserve University
Cleveland, Ohio
Department of Psychiatry
University Hospitals of Cleveland
Cleveland, Ohio

Jennifer K. Sekeres, PharmD, BCPS
Infectious Diseases Clinical Specialist
The Cleveland Clinic Foundation
Cleveland, Ohio

Todd P. Semla, MS, PharmD, BCPS, FCCP, AGSF
Clinical Pharmacy Specialist
Department of Veterans Affairs
Pharmacy Benefits Management Services
Associate Professor, Clinical
Department of Medicine and Psychiatry and Behavioral Health
Feinberg School of Medicine
Northwestern University
Chicago, Illinois

Joseph Snoke, RPh, BCPS
Manager
Core Pharmacology Group
Lexi-Comp, Inc
Hudson, Ohio

Joni Lombardi Stahura, BS, PharmD, RPh
Pharmacotherapy Specialist
Lexi-Comp, Inc
Hudson, Ohio

Stephen Marc Stout, PharmD, MS, BCPS
Pharmacotherapy Specialist
Lexi-Comp, Inc
Hudson, Ohio

Dan Streetman, PharmD, RPh
Pharmacotherapy Specialist
Lexi-Comp, Inc
Hudson, Ohio

Darcie-Ann Streetman, PharmD, RPh
Clinical Pharmacist
University of Michigan Health System
Ann Arbor, Michigan

PREFACE

The *Drug Information Handbook for Oncology* was designed to meet the needs of all oncology professionals involved in prescribing, preparing, and administering therapy. Presented in a concise and uniform format, this book contains monographs with information pertaining to both antineoplastic agents and ancillary or supportive care medications. This handbook serves as a portable quick reference while providing comprehensive oncology-related drug information. Organized like a dictionary for ease-of-use, a drug monograph can be quickly located by generic name.

The Chemotherapy Regimen section provides a comprehensive presentation of cancer chemotherapy regimens. The regimens are listed alphabetically by regimen name (acronym). An index lists regimens by indication. In addition, a special Combination Chemotherapy Regimen field in each drug monograph will link you to the applicable regimens.

A special topics section addresses issues regarding Cancer Treatment-Related Complications (eg, fertility and cancer therapy, management of nausea and vomiting, management of infections); Cancer-Related Topics (eg, hypercalcemia, pain); Hematopoietic Stem Cell Transplantation; Drug Development, Approval, and Distribution; Investigational Drug Service; and Safe Handling of Hazardous Drugs.

The appendix section includes information related to common toxicity criteria, conversions, renal function, and adult reference values. A pharmacologic category index provides a practical approach to categorizing drugs by their respective therapeutic classification.

We know you will find this handbook to be a valuable source of information and we welcome comments or suggestions to further improve future editions.

USE OF THE DRUG INFORMATION HANDBOOK FOR ONCOLOGY

The *Drug Information Handbook for Oncology* is divided into five sections.

The first section is a compilation of introductory text pertinent to the use of this book.

The drug information section of the handbook, in which all drugs are listed alphabetically, details information pertinent to each drug. Extensive cross-referencing is provided by U.S. brand names, Canadian brand names, and index terms.

The Chemotherapy Regimen section provides a comprehensive presentation of cancer chemotherapy regimens. The regimens are listed alphabetically by regimen name (acronym). An index lists regimens by indications. In addition, a special Combination Chemotherapy Regimen field in each drug monograph will link you to the applicable regimens.

The Special Topics section contains important cancer-related issues (ie, chronic pain management, hematopoietic stem cell transplantation, and safe handling of hazardous drugs). These issues are discussed in detail.

The fifth section is an appendix section.

The last section of this handbook is an index listing drugs in their unique pharmacologic category.

Alphabetical Listing of Drugs

Drug information is presented in a consistent format and provides the following:

Generic Name	U.S. adopted name
Pronunciation Guide	Phonetic pronunciation
Medication Safety Issues	In an effort to promote the safe use of medications, this field is intended to highlight possible sources of medication errors such as look-alike/sound-alike drugs or highly concentrated formulations which require vigilance on the part of healthcare professionals. In addition, medications which have been associated with severe consequences in the event of a medication error are also identified in this field.
Related Information	Cross-reference to other pertinent drug information found elsewhere in this handbook
U.S. Brand Names	Trade names (manufacturer-specific) found in the United States. The symbol [DSC] appears after trade names that have been recently discontinued.
Index Terms	Includes names or accepted abbreviations of the generic drug; may include common brand names no longer available; this field is used to create cross-references to monographs
Generic Available	Specifies whether a generic equivalent is available
Canadian Brand Names	Trade names found in Canada
Pharmacologic Category	Unique systematic classification of medications

Use	Information pertaining to appropriate FDA-approved indications of the drug
Unlabeled/Investigational Use	Information pertaining to non-FDA approved and investigational indications of the drug
Restrictions	The controlled substance classification from the Drug Enforcement Agency (DEA). U.S. schedules are I-V. Schedules vary by country and sometimes state (ie, Massachusetts uses I-VI). May also include restricted availability information.
Pregnancy Risk Factor	Five categories established by the FDA to indicate the potential of a systemically absorbed drug for causing birth defects
Lactation	Information describing characteristics of using the drug while breast-feeding
Labeled Contraindications	Information pertaining to inappropriate use of the drug
Warnings/Precautions	Precautionary considerations, hazardous conditions related to use of the drug, and disease states or patient populations in which the drug should be cautiously used. Boxed warnings, when present, are clearly identified and are adapted from the FDA approved labeling. Consult the product labeling for the exact black box warning through the manufacturer's or the FDA website.
Adverse Reactions	Side effects are grouped by percentage of incidence (if known) and/or body system
Drug Interactions	
Metabolism/Transport Effects	If a drug has demonstrated involvement with cytochrome P450 enzymes, or other metabolism or transport proteins, this field will identify the drug as an inhibitor, inducer, or substrate of the specific enzyme(s) (eg, CYP1A2 or UGT1A1). CYP450 isoenzymes are identified as substrates (minor or major), inhibitors (weak, moderate, or strong), and inducers (weak or strong).
Avoid Concomitant Use	Designates drug combinations which should not be used concomitantly, due to an unacceptable risk:benefit assessment. Frequently, the concurrent use of the agents is explicitly prohibited or contraindicated by the product labeling.
Increased Effect/Toxicity	Drug combinations that result in a increased or toxic therapeutic effect between the drug listed in the monograph and other drugs or drug classes.
Decreased Effect	Drug combinations that result in a decreased therapeutic effect between the drug listed in the monograph and other drugs or drug classes.
Ethanol/Nutrition/Herb Interactions	Information regarding potential interactions with food, nutritionals, herbal products, vitamins, or ethanol
Storage/Stability	Information regarding storage of product. Provides the time and conditions for which a solution or mixture will maintain full potency. For example, some solutions may require refrigeration after reconstitution while stored at room temperature prior to preparation.
Reconstitution	Includes comments on solution choice with time or conditions for the mixture to maintain full potency before administration
Compatibility	Whether drug is compatible, Y-site compatible, or incompatible with other drugs
Mechanism of Action	How the drug works in the body to elicit a response

◄ Pharmacodynamics/ Kinetics — The magnitude of a drug's effect depends on the drug concentration at the site of action. The pharmacodynamics are expressed in terms of onset of action and duration of action. Pharmacokinetics are expressed in terms of absorption, distribution (including appearance in breast milk and crossing of the placenta), protein binding, metabolism, bioavailability, half-life, time to peak serum concentration, and elimination.

Dosage — The amount of the drug to be typically given or taken during therapy for children and adults; also includes any dosing adjustment for renal impairment or hepatic failure

Combination Regimens — List of combination chemotherapy regimens in which the drug is a component

Administration — Information regarding the recommended final concentrations, rates of administration for parenteral drugs, or other guidelines when giving the medication

Monitoring Parameters — Suggested monitoring parameters are listed

Test Interactions — Listing of assay interferences when relevant; (B) = Blood; (S) = Serum; (U) = Urine

Dietary Considerations — Specific dietary modifications and/or restrictions

Additional Information — Pertinent information about specific brands

Emetic Potential — Likelihood that the drug will cause nausea or vomiting

Vesicant — Indicates whether the drug is considered to be a vesicant and likely to cause significant morbidity if the infusion infiltrates soft tissues

High Dose Considerations — Special information regarding high dose chemotherapy use, such as transplantation of autologous or allogeneic bone marrow or peripheral blood cells to facilitate hematopoietic recovery after myeloablative chemotherapy (autologous, allogeneic), and replace a diseased hematopoietic system (allogeneic)

  Comments — Additional information

  High Dose — Chemotherapy doses 1.5- to 30-fold greater than standard dosages. Nonhematologic adverse reactions are dose-limiting.

  Unique Toxicities — Nonhematologic adverse reactions that occur commonly with, or are unique to, high-dose chemotherapy administration

  Product Availability — This field is utilized to provide availability information on products that have been approved by the FDA, but not yet available for use. Estimates for when a product may be available are included when this information is known. This field may also be used to provide any unique or critical drug availability issues (eg, drug shortage of a critical drug).

  Dosage Forms — Information with regard to form, strength, and availability of the drug. **Note:** Additional formulation information (eg, excipients, preservatives) is included when available. Please consult product labeling for further information.

  Extemporaneous Preparations — Directions for preparing oral or rectal suppositories or liquid formulations from solid drug products. May include stability information and references.

  References — Recommended for additional information

Chemotherapy Regimens

The Chemotherapy Regimen section provides a comprehensive presentation of cancer chemotherapy regimens. The regimens are listed alphabetically by regimen name (acronym). An index lists regimens by indications. In addition, a special Combination Chemotherapy Regimen field in each drug monograph will link you to the applicable regimens.

Special Topics

Important cancer-related issues (ie, managing infections, chronic pain management, hospice (end of life) care, palliative care medicine, hematopoietic stem cell transplantation, safe handling of hazardous drugs) are discussed in detail.

Appendix

The appendix offers a compilation of tables, guidelines, nomograms, algorithms, and conversion information which can often be helpful when considering patient care.

Pharmacologic Category Index

This index provides a useful listing of drugs by their pharmacologic classification.

FDA PREGNANCY CATEGORIES

Throughout this book there is a field labeled Pregnancy Risk Factor and the letter A, B, C, D, or X immediately following which signifies a category. The FDA has established these five categories to indicate the potential of a systemically absorbed drug for causing birth defects. The key differentiation among the categories rests upon the reliability of documentation and the risk:benefit ratio. Pregnancy Category X is particularly notable in that if any data exists that may implicate a drug as a teratogen and the risk:benefit ratio is clearly negative, the drug is contraindicated during pregnancy.

These categories are summarized as follows:

A   Controlled studies in pregnant women fail to demonstrate a risk to the fetus in the first trimester with no evidence of risk in later trimesters. The possibility of fetal harm appears remote.

B   Either animal-reproduction studies have not demonstrated a fetal risk but there are no controlled studies in pregnant women, or animal-reproduction studies have shown an adverse effect (other than a decrease in fertility) that was not confirmed in controlled studies in women in the first trimester and there is no evidence of a risk in later trimesters.

C   Either studies in animals have revealed adverse effects on the fetus (teratogenic or embryocidal effects or other) and there are no controlled studies in women, or studies in women and animals are not available. Drugs should be given only if the potential benefits justify the potential risk to the fetus.

D   There is positive evidence of human fetal risk, but the benefits from use in pregnant women may be acceptable despite the risk (eg, if the drug is needed in a life-threatening situation or for a serious disease for which safer drugs cannot be used or are ineffective).

X   Studies in animals or human beings have demonstrated fetal abnormalities or there is evidence of fetal risk based on human experience, or both, and the risk of the use of the drug in pregnant women clearly outweighs any possible benefit. The drug is contraindicated in women who are or may become pregnant.

REDUCING ONCOLOGY PRESCRIBING ERRORS

Prescribing errors account for the majority of reported medication errors and fatal chemotherapy errors resulting from poor prescribing habits and misinterpretation have been well-publicized in the media. Due to a narrow therapeutic index and often complex prescribing, communication of antineoplastic medication orders and prescriptions are associated with a high level of risk. Strategies have been identified to maximize the safety of the chemotherapy prescribing process as well as treatment protocols or plans used by the oncology team. Firstly, facilities providing chemotherapy should establish and ensure that members of the oncology team have appropriate education, competency, and credentialing to care for patients receiving antineoplastic therapy. Secondly, and fundamental to most safety strategies, is the standardization of the prescribing and documentation process through established policies and procedures which should be followed by all healthcare professional involved. The use of collaboratively developed preprinted order forms or predefined computer generated ordersets for approved protocols or treatment plans is one method to facilitate standardization. However, additional safe practices should be considered.

MEDICATION NAMES

Chemotherapy agents are highly susceptible to sound-alike/look-alike confusion (eg, fluorouracil / flucytosine / fluocinonide, leucovorin / Leukine® / Alkeran® / Leukeran®) so particular precaution should be heeded to ensure correct drug identified by those interpreting the order.

- Use full generic names including descriptive terms, (eg, liposomal). Brand names should be reserved for products when they assist in further identifying the correct product (eg, combination product or liposomal vs nonliposomal formulation).

- Use full study name and/or protocol number with investigational antineoplastic treatments.

- Avoid abbreviated medication names, (eg, CTX, HN_2, VCR, or generalized generic terms [eg, "platinum" which can create confusion between cisplatin, carboplatin, and oxaliplatin]).

- Avoid investigational names for medications **with FDA approval** (eg, VP-16, FK-506, CBDCA).

- Utilize TALLman lettering (eg, DAUNOrubicin / DOXOrubicin, VinBLAStine / VinCRIStine).

- Omit the use of numbers within a medication name (eg, fluorouracil is correct, 5-fluorouracil is **incorrect**; mercaptopurine is correct, 6-mercapto-purine is **incorrect**).

- Avoid abbreviated names or acronyms for multidrug regimens, (eg, MOPP, ICE, ProMACE).

DOSE AND DURATION

- Include variables used for dosage calculations on the chemotherapy orders to allow for necessary double-checks, (eg, height [centimeters], weight [kilograms], BSA, laboratory test results or creatinine clearance). It is recommended that organizations standardize equations used for BSA and creatinine clearance calculations and situations when dosing should be based on actual or ideal body weight.

- Provide supporting references and/or rationale when doses vary from a standard regimen or are prescribed as flat doses to allow for necessary double-checks.

- Provide complete dosing information including calculated dose with reduction noted with rationale, total volume and solution to administer dose (if applicable), route of administration, rate or number of hours or days that dose is to be administered, which specific days dose is to be administered and total dose per treatment course, cycle or cumulative lifetime (if applicable). In some situations, clearly defining when to initiate therapy (Day 0 or Day 1) may be necessary for clarity.

  Example: Patient = 1.8 m^2
  Drug "X" 50 mg/m^2/day I.V. push for 3 days = 90 mg I.V. push on Days 3, 4, and 5
  (Total Dose Drug "X" per cycle = 150 mg/m^2 = 270 mg)

- Always use a leading zero for numbers less than 1 (0.5 mg is correct and .5 mg is **incorrect**) and never use a trailing zero for whole numbers (2 mg is correct and 2.0 mg is **incorrect**).

- For doses that are greater than 1,000 dosing units, use properly placed commas to prevent 10-fold errors (100,000 units is correct and 100000 units is **incorrect**).

- Avoid dangerous, error-prone abbreviations (eg, regardless of letter-case: U, IU, QD, QOD, µg, cc, @).

- Establish dosing and administration constraints including maximum single doses, maximum doses within specified time limits and acceptable routes of administration.

ORDERING PROCESS FEATURES

- Do not permit or accept verbal orders for chemotherapy, except for discontinuation of treatment.

- Do not permit or accept "STAT" orders for chemotherapy.

- Use redundant checks and verifications at different points of the chemo-therapy medication use process, (eg, prescribing, dispensing, administration).

- Individuals verifying orders that contain calculations should independently perform their own calculations, rather than checking another's mathematical work.

REFERENCES

American Society of Clinical Oncology, "ASCO/ONS Standards for Safe Chemotherapy Administration: Public Comment Version, January, 27th, 2009 - Draft." Available at: http://www.asco.org/ASCO/Downloads/Cancer%20Policy%20and%20Clinical%20Affairs/Quality%20of%20Care/Chemotherapy%20safety%20standards%20public%20comment%20final%20for%20web%2012809.pdf

ASHP Council on Professional Affairs, "ASHP Guidelines on Preventing Medication Errors With Antineoplastic Agents," *Am J Health Syst Pharm*, 2002, 59(17):1648-68.

To Err is Human: Building a Safer Health System, Kohn LT, Corrigan JM, and Donaldson MS, eds, Washington, D.C.: National Academy Press, 2000.

ALPHABETICAL LISTING OF DRUGS

- ◆ **Abbott-43818** *see* Leuprolide *on page* 702
- ◆ **ABCD** *see* Amphotericin B Cholesteryl Sulfate Complex *on page* 62
- ◆ **Abelcet®** *see* Amphotericin B (Lipid Complex) *on page* 71
- ◆ **ABI-007** *see* Paclitaxel (Protein Bound) *on page* 904
- ◆ **ABLC** *see* Amphotericin B (Lipid Complex) *on page* 71
- ◆ **Abraxane®** *see* Paclitaxel (Protein Bound) *on page* 904
- ◆ **Abraxane® For Injectable Suspension (Can)** *see* Paclitaxel *on page* 898
- ◆ **ABX-EGF** *see* Panitumumab *on page* 919
- ◆ **Acetoxymethylprogesterone** *see* MedroxyPROGESTERone *on page* 739
- ◆ **Aciclovir** *see* Acyclovir *on page* 18
- ◆ **Aclasta® (Can)** *see* Zoledronic Acid *on page* 1199
- ◆ **4-(9-Acridinylamino) Methanesulfon-m-Anisidide** *see* Amsacrine *on page* 79
- ◆ **Acridinyl Anisidide** *see* Amsacrine *on page* 79
- ◆ **ACT-D** *see* DACTINomycin *on page* 299
- ◆ **Actinomycin** *see* DACTINomycin *on page* 299
- ◆ **Actinomycin D** *see* DACTINomycin *on page* 299
- ◆ **Actinomycin CI** *see* DACTINomycin *on page* 299
- ◆ **Actiq®** *see* FentaNYL *on page* 458
- ◆ **Activase®** *see* Alteplase *on page* 41
- ◆ **Activase® rt-PA (Can)** *see* Alteplase *on page* 41
- ◆ **ACV** *see* Acyclovir *on page* 18
- ◆ **Acycloguanosine** *see* Acyclovir *on page* 18

Acyclovir (ay SYE kloe veer)

Medication Safety Issues

Sound-alike/look-alike issues:

Acyclovir may be confused with ganciclovir, Retrovir®, valACYclovir

Zovirax® may be confused with Valtrex®, Zithromax®, Zostrix®, Zyloprim®, Zyvox®

International issues:

Opthavir® [Mexico] may be confused with Optivar® which is a brand name for azelastine in the U.S.

Related Information

Management of Drug Extravasations *on page* 1447

U.S. Brand Names Zovirax®

Index Terms Aciclovir; ACV; Acycloguanosine

Generic Available Yes: Excludes cream, ointment

Canadian Brand Names Apo-Acyclovir®; Gen-Acyclovir; Mylan-Acyclovir; Novo-Acyclovir; Nu-Acyclovir; ratio-Acyclovir; Zovirax®

Pharmacologic Category Antiviral Agent; Antiviral Agent, Topical

Use Treatment of genital herpes simplex virus (HSV), herpes labialis (cold sores), herpes zoster (shingles), HSV encephalitis, neonatal HSV, mucocutaneous HSV in immunocompromised patients, varicella-zoster (chickenpox)

Unlabeled/Investigational Use Prevention of HSV reactivation in HIV-positive patients; prevention of HSV reactivation in hematopoietic stem cell transplant (HSCT); prevention of HSV reactivation during periods of neutropenia in patients with cancer; prevention of varicella zoster virus

(VZV) reactivation in allogenic HSCT; prevention of CMV reactivation in low-risk allogeneic HSCT; treatment of disseminated HSV or VZV in immunocompromised patients with cancer; empiric treatment of suspected encephalitis in immunocompromised patients with cancer

Pregnancy Risk Factor B

Lactation Enters breast milk/use with caution (AAP rates "compatible")

Labeled Contraindications Hypersensitivity to acyclovir, valacyclovir, or any component of the formulation

Warnings/Precautions Use with caution in immunocompromised patients; thrombocytopenic purpura/hemolytic uremic syndrome (TTP/HUS) has been reported. Use caution in the elderly, pre-existing renal disease (may require dosage modification), or in those receiving other nephrotoxic drugs. Renal failure (sometimes fatal) has been reported. Maintain adequate hydration during oral or intravenous therapy. Use I.V. preparation with caution in patients with underlying neurologic abnormalities, serious hepatic or electrolyte abnormalities, or substantial hypoxia.

Safety and efficacy of oral formulations have not been established in pediatric patients <2 years of age.

Varicella-zoster: Treatment should begin within 24 hours of appearance of rash; oral route not recommended for routine use in otherwise healthy children with varicella, but may be effective in patients at increased risk of moderate-to-severe infection (>12 years of age, chronic cutaneous or pulmonary disorders, long-term salicylate therapy, corticosteroid therapy).

Genital herpes: Physical contact should be avoided when lesions are present; transmission may also occur in the absence of symptoms. Treatment should begin with the first signs or symptoms.

Herpes labialis: For external use only to the lips and face; do not apply to eye or inside the mouth or nose. Treatment should begin with the first signs or symptoms.

Herpes zoster: Acyclovir should be started within 72 hours of appearance of rash to be effective.

Adverse Reactions

Systemic: Oral:
>10%: Central nervous system: Malaise (≤12%)
1% to 10%:
  Central nervous system: Headache (≤2%)
  Gastrointestinal: Nausea (2% to 5%), vomiting (≤3%), diarrhea (2% to 3%)
Systemic: Parenteral:
1% to 10%:
  Dermatologic: Hives (2%), itching (2%), rash (2%)
  Gastrointestinal: Nausea/vomiting (7%)
  Hepatic: Liver function tests increased (1% to 2%)
  Local: Inflammation at injection site or phlebitis (9%)
  Renal: BUN increased (5% to 10%), creatinine increased (5% to 10%), acute renal failure
Topical:
>10%: Dermatologic: Mild pain, burning, or stinging (ointment 30%)
1% to 10%: Dermatologic: Pruritus (ointment 4%), itching
All forms: <1%, postmarketing, and/or case reports: Abdominal pain, aggression, agitation, alopecia, anaphylaxis, anemia, angioedema, anorexia, ataxia, coma, confusion, consciousness decreased, delirium, desquamation, disseminated intravascular coagulopathy (DIC), dizziness, dry lips,

dysarthria, encephalopathy, erythema multiforme, fatigue, fever, gastro-intestinal distress, hallucinations, hematuria, hemolysis, hepatitis, hyper-bilirubinemia, hypotension, insomnia, jaundice, leukocytoclastic vasculitis, leukocytosis, leukopenia, local tissue necrosis (following extravasation), lymphadenopathy, mental depression, myalgia, neutrophilia, pain, paresthe-sia, peripheral edema, photosensitization, pruritus, psychosis, renal failure, renal pain, seizure, somnolence, sore throat, Stevens-Johnson syndrome, thrombocytopenia, thrombocytopenic purpura/hemolytic uremic syndrome (TTP/HUS), thrombocytosis, toxic epidermal necrolysis, tremor, urticaria, visual disturbances

Drug Interactions

Avoid Concomitant Use

Avoid concomitant use of Acyclovir with any of the following: Zoster Vaccine

Increased Effect/Toxicity

Acyclovir may increase the levels/effects of: Mycophenolate; Tenofovir; Zidovudine

The levels/effects of Acyclovir may be increased by: Mycophenolate

Decreased Effect

Acyclovir may decrease the levels/effects of: Zoster Vaccine

Ethanol/Nutrition/Herb Interactions Food: Does not affect absorption of oral acyclovir.

Storage/Stability

Capsule, tablet: Store at controlled room temperature of 15°C to 25°C (59°F to 77°F). Protect from moisture.

Cream, suspension: Store at controlled room temperature of 15°C to 25°C (59°F to 77°F).

Ointment: Store at controlled room temperature of 15°C to 25°C (59°F to 77°F) in a dry place.

Injection: Store powder at controlled room temperature of 15°C to 25°C (59°F to 77°F). Reconstituted solutions remain stable for 12 hours at room temperature. Do not refrigerate reconstituted solutions or solutions diluted for infusion as they may precipitate as they may precipitate. Once diluted for infusion, use within 24 hours.

Reconstitution Powder for injection: Reconstitute acyclovir 500 mg powder with SWFI 10 mL; do not use bacteriostatic water containing benzyl alcohol or parabens. For intravenous infusion, dilute in D_5W, D_5NS, $D_51/4NS$, $D_51/2NS$, LR, or NS to a final concentration ≤7 mg/mL. Concentrations >10 mg/mL increase the risk of phlebitis.

Compatibility Stable in D_5W, D_5NS, $D_51/4NS$, $D_51/2NS$, LR, NS.

Incompatible with blood products and protein-containing solutions.

Y-site administration: Compatible: Allopurinol, amikacin, amphotericin B cholesteryl sulfate complex, ampicillin, anidulafungin, cefazolin, cefotaxime, cefoxitin, ceftazidime, ceftizoxime, ceftriaxone, cefuroxime, chloramphenicol, cimetidine, clindamycin, co-trimoxazole, dexamethasone sodium phosphate, dimenhydrinate, diphenhydramine, docetaxel, doxorubicin liposome, doxycy-cline, erythromycin lactobionate, etoposide phosphate, famotidine, filgrastim, fluconazole, gallium nitrate, gentamicin, granisetron, heparin, hydrocortisone sodium succinate, hydromorphone, imipenem/cilastatin, linezolid, lorazepam, magnesium sulfate, melphalan, methylprednisolone sodium succinate, metoclopramide, metronidazole, milrinone, multivitamins, nafcillin, oxacillin, paclitaxel, pemetrexed, penicillin G potassium, pentobarbital, piperacillin, potassium chloride, propofol, ranitidine, remifentanil, sodium bicarbonate, teniposide, theophylline, thiotepa, tobramycin, vancomycin, zidovudine.

Incompatible: Amifostine, amsacrine, aztreonam, cefepime, dobutamine, dopamine, fludarabine, foscarnet, gemcitabine, idarubicin, levofloxacin, ondansetron, piperacillin/tazobactam, sargramostim, tacrolimus, vinorelbine.
Variable (consult detailed reference): Cisatracurium, diltiazem, meperidine, meropenem, morphine, TPN.

Compatibility in syringe: Incompatible: Caffeine citrate, pantoprazole.

Compatibility when admixed: Compatible: Fluconazole. **Incompatible:** Dobutamine, dopamine. **Variable (consult detailed reference):** Meropenem.

Mechanism of Action Acyclovir is converted to acyclovir monophosphate by virus-specific thymidine kinase then further converted to acyclovir triphosphate by other cellular enzymes. Acyclovir triphosphate inhibits DNA synthesis and viral replication by competing with deoxyguanosine triphosphate for viral DNA polymerase and being incorporated into viral DNA.

Pharmacodynamics/Kinetics

Absorption: Oral: 15% to 30%

Distribution: V_d: 0.8 L/kg (63.6 L): Widely (eg, brain, kidney, lungs, liver, spleen, muscle, uterus, vagina, CSF)

Protein binding: 9% to 33%

Metabolism: Converted by viral enzymes to acyclovir monophosphate, and further converted to diphosphate then triphosphate (active form) by cellular enzymes

Bioavailability: Oral: 10% to 20% with normal renal function (bioavailability decreases with increased dose)

Half-life elimination: Terminal: Neonates: 4 hours; Children 1-12 years: 2-3 hours; Adults: 3 hours

Time to peak, serum: Oral: Within 1.5-2 hours

Excretion: Urine (62% to 90% as unchanged drug and metabolite)

Dosage Note: Obese patients should be dosed using ideal body weight

Genital HSV:

I.V.: Children ≥12 years and Adults (immunocompetent): Initial episode, severe: 5 mg/kg/dose every 8 hours for 5-7 days

Oral:

Children:

Initial episode (unlabeled use): 40-80 mg/kg/day divided into 3-4 doses for 5-10 days (maximum: 1 g/day)

Chronic suppression (unlabeled use; limited data): 80 mg/kg/day in 3 divided doses (maximum: 1 g/day), re-evaluate after 12 months of treatment

Adults:

Initial episode: 200 mg every 4 hours while awake (5 times/day) for 10 days (per manufacturer's labeling); 400 mg 3 times/day for 5-10 days has also been reported

Recurrence: 200 mg every 4 hours while awake (5 times/day) for 5 days (per manufacturer's labeling; begin at earliest signs of disease); 400 mg 3 times/day for 5 days has also been reported

Chronic suppression: 400 mg twice daily or 200 mg 3-5 times/day, for up to 12 months followed by re-evaluation (per manufacturer's labeling); 400-1200 mg/day in 2-3 divided doses has also been reported

Topical: Adults (immunocompromised): Ointment: Initial episode: 1/2" ribbon of ointment for a 4" square surface area every 3 hours (6 times/day) for 7 days

Herpes labialis (cold sores): Topical: Children ≥12 years and Adults: Cream: Apply 5 times/day for 4 days

◄ **Herpes zoster (shingles):**
Oral: Adults (immunocompetent): 800 mg every 4 hours (5 times/day) for 7-10 days
I.V.:
  Children <12 years (immunocompromised): 20 mg/kg/dose every 8 hours for 7 days
  Children ≥12 years and Adults (immunocompromised): 10 mg/kg/dose or 500 mg/m²/dose every 8 hours for 7 days

HSV encephalitis: I.V.:
  Children 3 months to 12 years: 20 mg/kg/dose every 8 hours for 10 days (per manufacturer's labeling); dosing for 14-21 days also reported
  Children ≥12 years and Adults: 10 mg/kg/dose every 8 hours for 10 days (per manufacturer's labeling); 10-15 mg/kg/dose every 8 hours for 14-21 days also reported

Mucocutaneous HSV:
I.V.:
  Children <12 years (immunocompromised): 10 mg/kg/dose every 8 hours for 7 days
  Children ≥12 years and Adults (immunocompromised): 5 mg/kg/dose every 8 hours for 7 days (per manufacturer's labeling); dosing for up to 14 days also reported
Oral: Adults (immunocompromised, unlabeled use): 400 mg 5 times a day for 7-14 days
Topical: Ointment: Adults (nonlife-threatening, immunocompromised): 1/2" ribbon of ointment for a 4" square surface area every 3 hours (6 times/day) for 7 days

Neonatal HSV: I.V.: Neonate: Birth to 3 months: 10 mg/kg/dose every 8 hours for 10 days (manufacturer's labeling); 15 mg/kg/dose or 20 mg/kg/dose every 8 hours for 14-21 days has also been reported

Varicella-zoster (chickenpox): Begin treatment within the first 24 hours of rash onset:
Oral: **Note:** The AIDS*info* guidelines recommended duration of therapy is 7-10 days or until no new lesions for 48 hours (for patients with mild varicella and no or moderate immune suppression).
  Children ≥2 years and ≤40 kg (immunocompetent): 20 mg/kg/dose (up to 800 mg/dose) 4 times/day for 5 days
  Children >40 kg and Adults (immunocompetent): 800 mg/dose 4 times a day for 5 days
I.V.:
  Manufacturer's labeling (immunocompromised):
    Children <12 years: 20 mg/kg/dose every 8 hours for 7 days
    Children ≥12 years and Adults: 10 mg/kg/dose every 8 hours for 7 days
  AIDSinfo guidelines (immunocompromised):
    Children <1 year: 10 mg/kg/dose every 8 hours for 7-10 days or until no new lesions for 48 hours
    Children ≥1 year: 10 mg/kg/dose or 500 mg/m²/dose every 8 hours for 7-10 days or until no new lesions for 48 hours
    Adolescents and Adults: 10-15 mg/kg/dose every 8 hours for 7-10 days

Prevention of HSV reactivation in HIV-positive patients, for use only when recurrences are frequent or severe (unlabeled use): Oral:
  Children: 80 mg/kg/day in 3-4 divided doses
  Adults: 200 mg 3 times/day or 400 mg 2 times/day

Prevention of HSV reactivation in HSCT (unlabeled use): *CDC recommendations:* **Note:** Start at the beginning of conditioning therapy and continue until engraftment or until mucositis resolves (~30 days)
Oral: Adults: 200 mg 3 times/day
I.V.:
Children: 250 mg/m^2/dose every 8 hours or 125 mg/m^2/dose every 6 hours
Adults: 250 mg/m^2/dose every 12 hours

Prevention of VZV reactivation in allogeneic HSCT (unlabeled use): *NCCN guidelines:* Oral: Adults: 800 mg twice a day

Prevention of CMV reactivation in low-risk allogeneic HSCT (unlabeled use): *NCCN guidelines:* **Note:** Requires close monitoring (due to weak activity); not for use in patients at high risk for CMV disease: Oral: Adults: 800 mg 4 times/day

Treatment of disseminated HSV or VZV or empiric treatment of suspected encephalitis in immunocompromised patients with cancer: (unlabeled use): *NCCN guidelines:* I.V.: Adults: 10-12 mg/kg/dose every 8 hours

Dosing adjustment in renal impairment:
Oral:
Cl_{cr} 10-25 mL/minute/1.73 m^2: Normal dosing regimen 800 mg every 4 hours: Administer 800 mg every 8 hours
Cl_{cr} <10 mL/minute/1.73 m^2:
Normal dosing regimen 200 mg every 4 hours or 400 mg every 12 hours: Administer 200 mg every 12 hours
Normal dosing regimen 800 mg every 4 hours: Administer 800 mg every 12 hours
I.V.:
Cl_{cr} 25-50 mL/minute/1.73 m^2: Administer recommended dose every 12 hours
Cl_{cr} 10-25 mL/minute/1.73 m^2: Administer recommended dose every 24 hours
Cl_{cr} <10 mL/minute/1.73 m^2: Administer 50% of recommended dose every 24 hours
Hemodialysis: Administer dose after dialysis
Continuous ambulatory peritoneal dialysis (CAPD): Administer 50% of normal dose once daily; no supplemental dose needed
Continuous renal replacement therapy (CRRT): Drug clearance is highly dependent on the method of renal replacement, filter type, and flow rate. Appropriate dosing requires close monitoring of pharmacologic response, signs of adverse reactions due to drug accumulation, as well as drug levels in relation to target trough (if appropriate). The following are general recommendations only (based on dialysate flow/ultrafiltration rates of 1 L/hour) and should not supersede clinical judgment:
CVVH or CVVHD/CVVHDF: 5-7.5 mg/kg every 24 hours
Note: The higher dose of 7.5 mg/kg is recommended for infections with CNS involvement (Trotman, 2005).

Administration
Oral: May be administered with or without food.
I.V.: Avoid rapid infusion; infuse over 1 hour to prevent renal damage; maintain adequate hydration of patient; check for phlebitis and rotate infusion sites. Avoid I.M. or SubQ administration.
Topical: Not for use in the eye. Apply using a finger cot or rubber glove to avoid transmission to other parts of the body or to other persons.

◀ **Monitoring Parameters** Urinalysis, BUN, serum creatinine, liver enzymes, CBC

Dietary Considerations May be taken with or without food. Acyclovir 500 mg injection contains sodium ~50 mg (~2 mEq).

Vesicant Irritant at concentrations >7 mg/mL

Dosage Forms Excipient information presented when available (limited, particularly for generics); consult specific product labeling.

Capsule: 200 mg
  Zovirax®: 200 mg
Cream, topical:
  Zovirax®: 5% (2 g, 5 g)
Injection, powder for reconstitution, as sodium: 500 mg [base strength], 1000 mg [base strength]
Injection, solution, as sodium [preservative free]: 50 mg/mL (10 mL, 20 mL) [base strength]
Ointment, topical:
  Zovirax®: 5% (15 g)
Suspension, oral: 200 mg/5 mL (480 mL)
  Zovirax®: 200 mg/5 mL (480 mL) [banana flavor]
Tablet: 400 mg, 800 mg
  Zovirax®: 400 mg, 800 mg

References

Aronoff GR, Bennett WM, Berns JS, et al, *Drug Prescribing in Renal Failure: Dosing Guidelines for Adults and Children*, 5th ed. Philadelphia, PA: American College of Physicians; 2007.

Boeckh M, Kim HW, Flowers ME, et al, "Long-Term Acyclovir for Prevention of Varicella Zoster Virus Disease After Allogeneic Hematopoietic Cell Transplantation- A Randomized Double-Blind Placebo-Controlled Study," *Blood*, 2006, 107(5):1800-5.

Centers for Disease Control and Prevention, "Treating Opportunistic Infections Among HIV-Infected Adults and Adolescents: Recommendations From CDC, the National Institutes of Health, and the HIV Medicine Association/Infectious Diseases Society of America," *MMWR Recomm Rep*, 2004, 53(RR-15):1-112. Available at: http://www.cdc.gov/mmwr/preview/mmwrhtml/rr5315a1.htm. Accessed January 9, 2006.

Centers for Disease Control and Prevention, "Treating Opportunistic Infections Among HIV-Exposed and Infected Children: Recommendations from CDC, the National Institutes of Health, and the Infectious Diseases Society of America," *MMWR Recomm Rep*, 2004, 53(RR-14):1-63. Available at: http://www.cdc.gov/mmwr/preview/mmwrhtml/rr5314a1.htm. Accessed January 9, 2006.

Centers for Disease Control and Prevention, "Guidelines for Preventing Opportunistic Infections Among HIV-Infected Persons. 2002 Recommendations of the U.S. Public Health Service and the Infectious Diseases Society of America," *MMWR Recomm Rep*, 2002, 51(RR-8):1-46. Available at: http://www.cdc.gov/mmwr/preview/mmwrhtml/rr5108a1.htm. Accessed January 26, 2004.

Centers for Disease Control and Prevention, "Guidelines for Preventing Opportunistic Infections Among Hematopoietic Stem Cell Transplant Recipients: Recommendations of CDC, the Infectious Disease Society of America, and the American Society of Blood and Marrow Transplantation," *MMWR Recomm Rep*, 2000, 49(RR-10):1-112. Available at: http://www.cdc.gov/mmwr/preview/mmwrhtml/rr4910a1.htm. Accessed January 26, 2004.

Eisen D, Essell J, Broun ER, et al, "Clinical Utility of Oral Valacyclovir Compared With Oral Acyclovir for the Prevention of Herpes Simplex Virus Mucositis Following Autologous Bone Marrow Transplantation or Stem Cell Rescue Therapy," *Bone Marrow Transplant*, 2003, 31 (1):51-5.

"Guidelines for Prevention and Treatment of Opportunistic Infections Among HIV-Exposed and HIV-Infected Children," June 20, 2008. Available at http://aidsinfo.nih.gov

"Guidelines for Prevention and Treatment of Opportunistic Infections in HIV-Infected Adults and Adolescents," June 18, 2008. Available at http://aidsinfo.nih.gov

National Comprehensive Cancer Network (NCCN), "Clinical Practice Guidelines in Oncology™: Prevention and Treatment of Cancer-Related Infections," Version 1.2008. Available at http://www.nccn.org/professionals/physician_gls/PDF/infections.pdf.

Rayani SA, Nimmo CJ, Frighetto L, et al, "Implementation and Evaluation of a Standardized Herpes Simplex Virus Prophylaxis Protocol on a Leukemia/Bone Marrow Transplant Unit," *Ann Pharmacother*, 1994, 28(7-8):852-6.

Wade JC, Newton B, Flournoy N, et al, "Oral Acyclovir for Prevention of Herpes Simplex Virus Reactivation After Marrow Transplantation," *Ann Intern Med*, 1984, 100(6):823-8.

◆ **AD32** *see* Valrubicin *on page* 1160

◆ **ADR (error-prone abbreviation)** *see* DOXOrubicin *on page* 372

◆ **AdreView™** *see* Iobenguane I 123 *on page* 649

◆ **Adria** *see* DOXOrubicin *on page* 372

◆ **Adriamycin®** *see* DOXOrubicin *on page* 372

◆ **Adrucil®** *see* Fluorouracil *on page* 499

◆ **Advagraf™ (Can)** *see* Tacrolimus *on page* 1062

◆ **Advate** *see* Antihemophilic Factor (Recombinant) *on page* 93

◆ **Afinitor®** *see* Everolimus *on page* 440

◆ **Agrylin®** *see* Anagrelide *on page* 83

◆ **AHF (Human)** *see* Antihemophilic Factor (Human) *on page* 91

◆ **AHF (Recombinant)** *see* Antihemophilic Factor (Recombinant) *on page* 93

◆ **A-hydroCort** *see* Hydrocortisone *on page* 575

◆ **AKTob®** *see* Tobramycin *on page* 1110

◆ **ALA** *see* Aminolevulinic Acid *on page* 60

◆ **5-ALA** *see* Aminolevulinic Acid *on page* 60

◆ **Albumin-Bound Paclitaxel** *see* Paclitaxel (Protein Bound) *on page* 904

◆ **Albumin-Stabilized Nanoparticle Paclitaxel** *see* Paclitaxel (Protein Bound) *on page* 904

◆ **Alcomicin® (Can)** *see* Gentamicin *on page* 542

Aldesleukin (al des LOO kin)

Medication Safety Issues

Sound-alike/look-alike issues:

Aldesleukin may be confused with oprelvekin

Proleukin® may be confused with oprelvekin

High alert medication: The Institute for Safe Medication Practices (ISMP) includes this medication among its list of drug classes which have a heightened risk of causing significant patient harm when used in error.

Related Information

Safe Handling of Hazardous Drugs *on page* 1517

U.S. Brand Names Proleukin®

Index Terms Epidermal Thymocyte Activating Factor; IL-2; Interleukin-2; Lymphocyte Mitogenic Factor; T-Cell Growth Factor; TCGF; Thymocyte Stimulating Factor

Generic Available No

Canadian Brand Names Proleukin®

Pharmacologic Category Antineoplastic Agent, Miscellaneous; Biological Response Modulator

Use Treatment of metastatic renal cell cancer, metastatic melanoma

Unlabeled/Investigational Use Treatment of HIV infection, and AIDS; non-Hodgkin's lymphoma, acute myeloid leukemia

Pregnancy Risk Factor C

Lactation Excretion in breast milk unknown/not recommended

Labeled Contraindications Hypersensitivity to aldesleukin or any component of the formulation; patients with abnormal thallium stress or pulmonary function tests; patients who have had an organ allograft; retreatment in patients who have experienced sustained ventricular tachycardia (≥5 beats), refractory cardiac rhythm disturbances, recurrent chest pain with ECG changes consistent with angina or myocardial infarction, intubation ≥72 hours, pericardial tamponade, renal dialysis for ≥72 hours, coma or toxic psychosis lasting ≥48 hours, repetitive or refractory seizures, bowel ischemia/perforation, GI bleeding requiring surgery

Warnings/Precautions Hazardous agent - use appropriate precautions for handling and disposal. **[U.S. Boxed Warning]: High-dose aldesleukin therapy has been associated with capillary leak syndrome (CLS) resulting in hypotension and reduced organ perfusion which may be severe and can result in death. Therapy should be restricted to patients with normal cardiac and pulmonary functions as defined by thallium stress and formal pulmonary function testing.** Extreme caution should be used in patients with a history of prior cardiac or pulmonary disease. Patients must have a serum creatinine ≤1.5 mg/dL prior to treatment.

[U.S. Boxed Warning]: Should be administered under the supervision of an experienced cancer chemotherapy physician in a facility with cardiopulmonary or intensive specialists and intensive care facilities available. Adverse effects are frequent and sometimes fatal. May exacerbate pre-existing or initial presentation of autoimmune diseases and inflammatory disorders. Patients should be evaluated and treated for CNS metastases and have a negative scan prior to treatment. Mental status changes (irritability, confusion, depression) can occur and may indicate bacteremia, hypoperfusion, CNS malignancy, or CNS toxicity.

[U.S. Boxed Warning]: Impaired neutrophil function is associated with treatment; patients are at risk for sepsis, bacterial endocarditis, and central line-related gram-positive infections. Antibiotic prophylaxis which has been associated with a reduced incidence of staphylococcal infections in aldesleukin studies includes the use of oxacillin, nafcillin, ciprofloxacin, or vancomycin.

[U.S. Boxed Warning]: Withhold treatment for patients developing moderate-to-severe lethargy or somnolence; continued treatment may result in coma. Standard prophylactic supportive care during high-dose aldesleukin treatment includes acetaminophen to relieve constitutional symptoms and an H_2 antagonist to reduce the risk of GI ulceration and/or bleeding. Safety and efficacy have not been established in children.

Adverse Reactions

>10%:

Cardiovascular: Hypotension (71%; grade 4: 3%), peripheral edema (28%), tachycardia (23%), edema (15%), vasodilation (13%), cardiovascular disorder (11%; includes blood pressure changes, CHF and ECG changes)

Central nervous system: Chills (52%), confusion (34%), fever (29%; grade 4: 1%), malaise (27%), somnolence (22%), anxiety (12%), pain (12%), dizziness (11%)

Dermatologic: Rash (42%), pruritus (24%), exfoliative dermatitis (18%)

Endocrine & metabolic: Acidosis (12%), hypomagnesemia (12%), hypocalcemia (11%)

Gastrointestinal: Diarrhea (67%), vomiting (19% to 50%), nausea (19% to 35%), stomatitis (22%), anorexia (20%), weight gain (18%), abdominal pain (11%)

Hematologic: Thrombocytopenia (37%; grade 4: 1%), anemia (29%), leukopenia (16%)

Hepatic: Hyperbilirubinemia (40%), AST increased (23%)

Neuromuscular & skeletal: Weakness (23%)

Renal: Oliguria (63%; grade 4: 6%), creatinine increased (33%)

Respiratory: Dyspnea (43%), lung disorder (24%; includes pulmonary congestion, rales, and rhonchi), cough (11%), respiratory disorder (11%; includes acute respiratory distress syndrome, infiltrates and pulmonary changes)

Miscellaneous: Infection (13%; grade 4: 1%)

1% to 10%:

Cardiovascular: Arrhythmia (10%), cardiac arrest (grade 4: 1%), MI (grade 4: 1%), supraventricular tachycardia (grade 4: 1%), ventricular tachycardia (grade 4: 1%)

Gastrointestinal: Abdomen enlarged (10%)

Hematologic: Coagulation disorder (grade 4: 1%)

Hepatic: Alkaline phosphatase increased (10%)

Renal: Anuria (grade 4: 5%), acute renal failure (grade 4: 1%)

Respiratory: Rhinitis (10%), apnea (grade 4: 1%)

Miscellaneous: Sepsis (grade 4: 1%)

<1%, postmarketing, and/or case reports (limited to important or life threatening): Acute tubular necrosis, allergic interstitial nephritis, allergic reactions, anaphylaxis, atrial arrhythmia, AV block, blindness (transient or permanent), bowel necrosis, bradycardia, bullous pemphigoid, BUN increased, cardiomyopathy, cellulitis, cerebral edema, cerebral lesions, cerebral vasculitis, CHF, cholecystitis, colitis, coma, crescentic IgA glomuleronephritis, Crohn's disease exacerbation, depression (severe; leading to suicide), diabetes mellitus, duodenal ulcer, encephalitis, endocarditis, extrapyramidal syndrome, gastrointestinal hemorrhage, hematemesis, hemoptysis, hemorrhage, hepatic failure, hepatitis, hepatosplenomegaly, hypertension, hyperuricemia, hyperventilation, hypothermia, hyperthyroidism, hypoventilation, hypoxia, inflammatory arthritis, injection site necrosis, intestinal obstruction, intestinal perforation, leukocytosis, malignant hyperthermia, meningitis, myocardial ischemia, myocarditis, myopathy, myositis, neuritis, neuropathy, neutropenia, oculobulbar myasthenia gravis, optic neuritis, pancreatitis, pericardial effusion, pericarditis, peripheral gangrene, phlebitis, pneumonia, pneumothorax, pulmonary edema, pulmonary embolus, renal failure, respiratory acidosis, respiratory arrest, respiratory failure, retroperitoneal hemorrhage, rhabdomyolysis, scleroderma, seizure (including grand mal), shock, Stevens-Johnson syndrome, stroke, syncope, thrombosis, thyroiditis, tracheoesophageal fistula, transient ischemic attack, urticaria, ventricular extrasystoles

Drug Interactions

Avoid Concomitant Use There are no known interactions where it is recommended to avoid concomitant use.

Increased Effect/Toxicity

The levels/effects of Aldesleukin may be increased by: Contrast Media (Nonionic); Interferons (Alfa)

Decreased Effect There are no known significant interactions involving a decrease in effect.

Ethanol/Nutrition/Herb Interactions Ethanol: May increase CNS adverse effects.

Storage/Stability Store vials of lyophilized injection in a refrigerator at 2°C to 8°C (36°F to 46°F). Reconstituted vials and solutions diluted for infusion are stable for 48 hours at room temperature or refrigerated, per the manufacturer. Solution diluted with D₅W to a concentration of 220 mg/mL and repackaged into tuberculin syringes was reported to be stable for 14 days refrigerated.

Reconstitution Reconstitute vials with 1.2 mL SWFI to a concentration of 18 million units/1 mL (sterile water should be injected towards the side of the vial). Gently swirl; do not shake. Further dilute with 50 mL of D₅W. Smaller volumes of D₅W should be used for doses <1.5 mg; avoid concentrations <30 mcg/mL and >70 mcg/mL (an increased variability in drug delivery has been seen).

Note: Filtration will result in significant loss of bioactivity.

Final Dilution Concentration (mcg/mL)	Final Dilution Concentration (10⁶ int. units/mL)	Stability
<30	<0.49	Albumin must be added to bag **prior to addition** of aldesleukin at a final concentration of 0.1% (1 mg/mL) albumin; stable at room temperature or at ≥32°C (89°F) for 6 days[1,2]
≥30 to ≤70	≥0.49 to ≤1.1	Stable at room temperature at 6 days without albumin added or at ≥32°C (89°F) for 6 days only if albumin is added (0.1%)[1,2]
70-100	1.2-1.6	Unstable; avoid use
>100-500	1.7-8.2	Stable at room temperature and at ≥32°C (89°F) for 6 days[1,2]

[1]These solutions do not contain a preservative; use for more than 24 hours may not be advisable.

[2]Continuous infusion via ambulatory infusion device raises aldesleukin to this temperature.

Compatibility Stable in D₅W.

Y-site administration: Compatible: Amikacin, amphotericin B, calcium gluconate, co-trimoxazole, diphenhydramine, dopamine, fat emulsion 10%, fluconazole, foscarnet, gentamicin, heparin, magnesium sulfate, metoclopramide, morphine, ondansetron, piperacillin, potassium chloride, ranitidine, thiethylperazine, ticarcillin, tobramycin. **Incompatible:** Ganciclovir, lorazepam, NS, pentamidine, prochlorperazine edisylate, promethazine.

Compatibility when admixed: Incompatible with NS.

Mechanism of Action Aldesleukin promotes proliferation, differentiation, and recruitment of T and B cells, natural killer (NK) cells, and thymocytes; causes cytolytic activity in a subset of lymphocytes and subsequent interactions between the immune system and malignant cells; can stimulate lymphokine-activated killer (LAK) cells and tumor-infiltrating lymphocytes (TIL) cells.

Pharmacodynamics/Kinetics

Distribution: V_d: 4-7 L; primarily in plasma and then in the lymphocytes

Half-life elimination: I.V.: Initial: 6-13 minutes; Terminal: 80-120 minutes

Dosage Refer to individual protocols.

I.V.:

Renal cell carcinoma: 600,000 int. units/kg every 8 hours for a maximum of 14 doses; repeat after 9 days for a total of 28 doses per course. Retreat if needed 7 weeks after previous course.

Melanoma:

Single-agent use: 600,000 int. units/kg every 8 hours for a maximum of 14 doses; repeat after 9 days for a total of 28 doses per course. Retreat if needed 7 weeks after previous course.

In combination with cytotoxic agents (unlabeled use): 24 million int. units/m^2 days 12-16 and 19-23

SubQ (unlabeled route):

Single-agent doses: 3-18 million int. units/day for 5 days each week, up to 6 weeks

In combination with interferon:

5 million int. units/m^2 3 times/week

1.8 million int. units/m^2 twice daily 5 days/week for 6 weeks

Investigational regimen: SubQ: 11 million int. units (flat dose) daily for 4 days per week for 4 consecutive weeks; repeat every 6 weeks

Dosage adjustment in renal impairment: No specific recommendations by manufacturer. Use with caution.

Combination Regimens

Melanoma:

Cisplatin-Dacarbazine-Interferon Alfa-2b-Aldesleukin on page 1266

CVD-Interleukin-Interferon (Melanoma) on page 1282

Dacarbazine-Carboplatin-Aldesleukin-Interferon on page 1286

Renal cell cancer:

Interleukin 2-Interferon Alfa-2 on page 1359

Interleukin 2 (Low Dose)-Interferon Alfa 2b on page 1359

Administration Administer as I.V. infusion over 15 minutes (do not administer with an inline filter). Flush before and after with D_5W, particularly if maintenance I.V. line contains sodium chloride. May also be administered by SubQ injection (unlabeled route)

Management of symptoms related to vascular leak syndrome:

If actual body weight increases >10% above baseline, or rales or rhonchi are audible:

Administer furosemide at dosage determined by patient response

Administer dopamine hydrochloride 1-5 mcg/kg/minute to maintain renal blood flow and urine output

If patient has dyspnea at rest: Administer supplemental oxygen by face mask

If patient has severe respiratory distress: Intubate patient and provide mechanical ventilation; administer ranitidine (as the hydrochloride salt) 50 mg I.V. every 8-12 hours as prophylaxis against stress ulcers

Monitoring Parameters

The following clinical evaluations are recommended for all patients prior to beginning treatment and then frequently during drug administration:

CBC with differential, blood chemistries including electrolytes, renal and hepatic function tests

Chest x-rays

Monitoring during therapy should include vital signs (temperature, pulse, blood pressure, and respiration rate) and weight; in a patient with a decreased blood pressure, especially <90 mm Hg, cardiac monitoring for rhythm should be conducted. If an abnormal complex or rhythm is seen, an ECG should be performed; vital signs in these hypotension patients should be taken hourly and central venous pressure (CVP) checked; monitor for change in mental status.

Pulmonary function (baseline and periodic) basis.

◀ **Additional Information**
1 Cetus unit = 6 int. units
1.1 mg = 18×10^6 int. units (or 3×10^6 Cetus units)
1 Roche unit (Teceleukin) = 3 int. units

Emetic Potential
>12 million units/m^2: Moderate (30% to 90%)
≤12 million units/m^2: Low (10% to 30%)

Dosage Forms Excipient information presented when available (limited, particularly for generics); consult specific product labeling.
Injection, powder for reconstitution:
Proleukin®: 22×10^6 int. units [18 million int. units/mL = 1.1 mg/mL when reconstituted]

References

Atkins MB, Lotze MT, Dutcher JP, et al, "High-Dose Recombinant Interleukin 2 Therapy for Patients With Metastatic Melanoma: Analysis of 270 Patients Treated Between 1985 and 1993," *J Clin Oncol*, 1999, 17(7):2105-16.

Kintzel PE and Calis KA, "Recombinant Interleukin-2: Biological Response Modifier," *Clin Pharm*, 1991, 10(2):110-28.

Sundin DJ and Wolin MJ, "Toxicity Management in Patients Receiving Low-Dose Aldesleukin Therapy," *Ann Pharmacother*,1998, 32(12):1344-52.

Yang JC, Topalian SL, Parkinson D, et al, "Randomized Comparison of High-Dose and Low-Dose Intravenous Interleukin-2 for the Therapy of Metastatic Renal Cell Carcinoma: An Interim Report," *J Clin Oncol*, 1994, 12(8):1572-6.

Alemtuzumab (ay lem TU zoo mab)

Medication Safety Issues
High alert medication: The Institute for Safe Medication Practices (ISMP) includes this medication among its list of drug classes which have a heightened risk of causing significant patient harm when used in error.

Related Information
Safe Handling of Hazardous Drugs *on page 1517*

U.S. Brand Names Campath®

Index Terms Anti-CD52 Monoclonal Antibody ; Campath-1H; Humanized IgG1 Anti-CD52 Monoclonal Antibody; MoAb CD52; Monoclonal Antibody Campath-1H; Monoclonal Antibody CD52

Generic Available No

Canadian Brand Names MabCampath®

Pharmacologic Category Antineoplastic Agent, Monoclonal Antibody

Use Treatment of B-cell chronic lymphocytic leukemia (B-CLL)

Unlabeled/Investigational Use Treatment of cutaneous T-cell lymphoma, peripheral T-cell lymphoma, refractory T-cell prolymphocytic leukemia, refractory or resistant autoimmune cytopenias; preconditioning regimen and prophylaxis of graft-versus-host disease (GVHD) in allogeneic stem cell transplant; immunosuppressant in solid organ transplant (induction and rejection)

Pregnancy Risk Factor C

Lactation Excretion in breast milk unknown/not recommended

Labeled Contraindications There are no contraindications listed in the manufacturer's labeling

Warnings/Precautions Hazardous agent - use appropriate precautions for handling and disposal. **[U.S. Boxed Warning]: Serious infections (bacterial, viral, fungal, and protozoan) have been reported. Prophylactic medications against PCP pneumonia and herpes viral infections are recommended upon initiation of therapy** and for at least 2 months following last dose or until CD4$^+$ counts are ≥200 cells/μL (whichever is later). Severe and prolonged lymphopenia may occur; $CD4^+$ counts usually return to ≥200 cells/μL within 2-6 months; however, $CD4^+$ and $CD8^+$ lymphocyte counts may not return to baseline levels for more than 1 year. Monitor for CMV infection (during and for at least 2 months after completion of therapy). Withhold treatment during serious infections; may be reinitiated upon resolution of infection. Monitor for CMV infection (during and for at least 2 months after completion of therapy); initiate appropriate antiviral treatment and withhold alemtuzumab for CMV infection or confirmed CMV viremia (withhold alemtuzumab during CMV antiviral treatment).

[U.S. Boxed Warning]: Serious and potentially fatal infusion-related reactions may occur; withhold treatment for grade 3 or 4 infusion reactions. Gradual escalation to the recommended maintenance dose is required at initiation and with therapy interruption (for ≥7 days) to minimize infusion-related reactions. Infusion reaction symptoms may include acute respiratory distress syndrome, anaphylactic shock, angioedema, bronchospasm, cardiac arrest, cardiac arrhythmias, chills, dyspnea, fever, hypotension, myocardial infarction, pulmonary infiltrates, rash, rigors, syncope, or urticaria. The incidence of infusion reaction is highest during the first week of treatment. Premedication with acetaminophen and an oral antihistamine is recommended. Medications for the treatment of reactions should be available for immediate use. Use caution and carefully monitor blood pressure in patients with ischemic heart disease and patients on antihypertensive therapy. Reinitiate with gradual dose escalation if treatment is withheld ≥7 days.

[U.S. Boxed Warning]: Serious and fatal cytopenias (including pancytopenia, bone marrow hypoplasia, autoimmune hemolytic anemia, and autoimmune idiopathic thrombocytopenia) have occurred. Single doses >30 mg or cumulative weekly doses >90 mg are associated with an increased incidence of pancytopenia. Severe prolonged myelosuppression, hemolytic anemia, pure red cell aplasia, and bone marrow aplasia have also been reported. Discontinue therapy during serious hematologic or other serious toxicity (except lymphopenia) until the event resolves. Permanently discontinue if autoimmune anemia or autoimmune thrombocytopenia occurs. Patients receiving blood products should only receive irradiated blood products due to the potential for transfusion-associated GVHD during lymphopenia.

Patients should not be immunized with live, viral vaccines during or recently after treatment. The ability to respond to any vaccine following therapy is unknown. Women of childbearing potential and men of reproductive potential should use effective contraceptive methods during treatment and for a minimum of 6 months following therapy. Safety and efficacy have not been established in pediatric patients.

Adverse Reactions

>10%:

Cardiovascular: Hypotension (15% to 32%), peripheral edema (13%), hypertension (11% to 15%), dysrhythmia/tachycardia/SVT (10% to 14%)

Central nervous system: Fever (69% to 85%), chills (53%), fatigue (22% to 34%), headache (13% to 24%), dysthesias (15%), dizziness (12%)

Dermatologic: Rash (13% to 40%), urticaria (16% to 30%), pruritus (14% to 24%)

Gastrointestinal: Nausea (47% to 54%), vomiting (33% to 41%), anorexia (20%), diarrhea (10% to 22%), stomatitis/mucositis (14%), abdominal pain (11%)

Hematologic: Lymphopenia (grades 3/4: 97%), neutropenia (77% to 85%; grade 3/4: 42% to 70% [median onset: 31 days, median duration: 28-37 days]), anemia (76% to 80%; grade 3/4: 12% to 47% [median onset: 31 days, median duration 8 days]), thrombocytopenia (71% to 72%; grade 3/4: 13% to 52% [median onset: 9 days; median duration: 14-21 days])

Local: Injection site reaction (SubQ administration: 90%)

Neuromuscular & skeletal: Rigors (86% to 89%), skeletal pain (24%), weakness (13%), myalgia (11%)

Respiratory: Dyspnea (14% to 26%), cough (25%), bronchitis/pneumonitis (21%), pneumonia (16%), pharyngitis (12%)

Miscellaneous: Infection (43% to 74%; grades 3/4: 21% to 37%; incidence is lower if prophylactic anti-infectives are utilized), CMV viremia (55%), infusion reactions (grades 3/4: 10% to 35%), diaphoresis (19%), CMV infection (6% to 16%), sepsis (15%; grades 3/4: 3% to 10%), herpes viral infections (1% to 11%)

1% to 10%:

Cardiovascular: Chest pain (10%)

Central nervous system: Insomnia (10%), malaise (9%), anxiety (8%), depression (7%), temperature change sensation (5%), somnolence (5%)

Dermatologic: Purpura (8%), erythema (4%)

Gastrointestinal: Dyspepsia (10%), constipation (9%)

Hematologic: Neutropenic fever (10%; grades 3/4: 5% to 10%), pancytopenia/marrow hypoplasia (5% to 6%; grade 3/4: 3%), positive Coombs' test without hemolysis (2%), autoimmune thrombocytopenia (2%), autoimmune hemolytic anemia (1%)

Neuromuscular & skeletal: Back pain (10%), tremor (3% to 7%)

Respiratory: Bronchospasm (9%), epistaxis (7%), rhinitis (7%)

Miscellaneous: Moniliasis (8%)

<1%, postmarketing, and/or case reports (limited to important or life-threatening): Acidosis, acute renal failure, acute respiratory distress syndrome, agranulocytosis, alkaline phosphatase increased, allergic reactions, anaphylactoid reactions, angina pectoris, angioedema, anuria, aphasia, aplastic anemia, arrhythmia, ascites, asthma, atrial fibrillation, bacterial infection, biliary pain, bone marrow aplasia, bullous eruption, capillary fragility, cardiac arrest, cardiac failure, cardiac insufficiency, cardiomyopathy, cellulitis, cerebral hemorrhage, cerebrovascular disorder, chronic inflammatory demyelinating polyradiculoneuropathy (CIDP), coagulation abnormality, colitis, coma, COPD, coronary artery disorder, cyanosis, deep vein thrombosis, dehydration, diabetes mellitus exacerbation, disseminated intravascular coagulation (DIC), duodenal ulcer, ejection fraction decreased, endophthalmitis, Epstein-Barr virus associated lymphoproliferative disorder, esophagitis, fluid overload, flu-like syndrome, gastrointestinal hemorrhage, Goodpasture's syndrome, Graves' disease, Guillain-Barré syndrome, hallucinations, hematemesis, hematoma, hematuria, hemolysis, hemolytic anemia, hemoptysis, hepatic failure, hepatocellular damage, HF, hyperbilirubinemia, hyper-/hypoglycemia, hyper-/hypokalemia, hypersensitivity, hyperthyroidism, hypoalbuminemia, hyponatremia, hypovolemia, hypoxia, idiopathic thrombocytopenic purpura (ITP), interstitial pneumonitis, intestinal obstruction, intestinal perforation, intracranial hemorrhage, *Legionella* pneumonia, *Listeria* meningitis, lymphadenopathy, marrow depression, melena, MI, mouth edema, myositis, optic neuropathy, osteomyelitis, pancreatitis, paralysis, paralytic ileus, paroxysmal nocturnal hemoglobinuria-like monocytes, peptic ulcer, pericarditis, peritonitis, plasma cell dyscrasia, phlebitis, pleural effusion, pleurisy, *Pneumocystis jiroveci* pneumonia, pneumothorax, polymyositis, progressive multifocal leukoencephalopathy,

pseudomembranous colitis, pulmonary edema, pulmonary embolism, pulmonary fibrosis, pulmonary infiltration, pure red cell aplasia, purpuric rash, renal dysfunction, respiratory alkalosis, respiratory arrest, respiratory depression, respiratory insufficiency, seizure (grand mal), serum sickness, sinus bradycardia, splenic infarction, splenomegaly, stridor, subarachnoid hemorrhage, syncope, toxic nephropathy, thrombocythemia, thrombophlebitis, throat tightness, transfusion-associated GVHD, tuberculosis, tumor lysis syndrome, ureteric obstruction, urinary retention, urinary tract infection, ventricular arrhythmia, ventricular tachycardia, viral meningitis, virus reactivation (latent)

Drug Interactions

Avoid Concomitant Use
Avoid concomitant use of Alemtuzumab with any of the following: Natalizumab; Vaccines (Live)

Increased Effect/Toxicity
Alemtuzumab may increase the levels/effects of: Leflunomide; Natalizumab; Vaccines (Live)

The levels/effects of Alemtuzumab may be increased by: Abciximab; Trastuzumab

Decreased Effect
Alemtuzumab may decrease the levels/effects of: Vaccines (Inactivated); Vaccines (Live)

The levels/effects of Alemtuzumab may be decreased by: Echinacea

Ethanol/Nutrition/Herb Interactions Herb/Nutraceutical: Echinacea may diminish the therapeutic effect of alemtuzumab.

Storage/Stability Prior to dilution, store at 2°C to 8°C (36°F to 46°F); do not freeze (if accidentally frozen, thaw in refrigerator prior to administration). Do not shake; protect from light. Following dilution, store at room temperature or refrigerate; protect from light; use within 8 hours.

Reconstitution Dilute with 100 mL NS or D_5W. Gently invert the bag to mix the solution. Do not shake prior to use.

Compatibility Stable in D_5W, NS. Medications should not be added to the solution or simultaneously infused through the same I.V. line.

Mechanism of Action Binds to CD52, a nonmodulating antigen present on the surface of B and T lymphocytes, a majority of monocytes, macrophages, NK cells, and a subpopulation of granulocytes. After binding to $CD52^+$ cells, an antibody-dependent lysis of leukemic cells occurs.

Pharmacodynamics/Kinetics

Distribution: V_d: I.V.: 0.1-0.4 L/kg

Metabolism: Clearance decreases with repeated dosing (due to loss of CD52 receptors in periphery), resulting in a sevenfold increase in AUC.

Half-life elimination: I.V.: 11 hours (following first 30 mg dose; range: 2-32 hours); 6 days (following the last 30 mg dose; range: 1-14 days)

Dosage Note: Dose escalation is required; usually accomplished in 3-7 days. Single doses >30 mg or cumulative doses >90 mg/week increase the incidence of pancytopenia. Pretreatment (with acetaminophen and diphenhydramine) is recommended prior to the first dose, with dose escalations, and as clinically indicated; I.V. hydrocortisone may be used for severe infusion-related reactions. Reinitiate with gradual dose escalation if treatment is withheld ≥7 days.

I.V. infusion: Adults:

B-cell CLL: Initial: 3 mg/day beginning on day 1; if tolerated (infusion reaction ≤grade 2), increase to 10 mg/day; if tolerated (infusion reaction ≤grade 2), increase to maintenance of 30 mg/dose 3 times/week on alternate days for a total duration of therapy of up to 12 weeks

Cutaneous T-cell lymphoma (unlabeled use): 3 mg on day 1; if tolerated increase the next dose to 10 mg; if tolerated increase the next dose to 30 mg; Maintenance dose: 30 mg/dose 3 times/week for up to 12 weeks (Lundin, 2003)

Peripheral T-cell lymphoma (unlabeled use): 3 mg on day 1; 10 mg on day 3, followed by 30 mg/dose 3 times/week for a duration of therapy of up to 12 weeks (Enblad, 2004)

T-cell prolymphocytic leukemia (unlabeled use): Initial test dose 3 mg or 10 mg, followed by dose escalation to 30 mg/dose 3 times/week as tolerated (Dearden, 2001)

or

Week 1: 3 mg on day 1; 10 mg on day 2; 30 mg on day 3, followed in subsequent weeks by 30 mg/dose on alternate days 3 times/week for a total of 4-12 weeks (Ferrajoli, 2003)

or

Initial dose: 3 mg day 1, if tolerated increase to 10 mg day 2, if tolerated increase to 30 mg on day 3 (days 1, 2, and 3 are consecutive days), followed by 30 mg/dose every Monday, Wednesday, Friday for a total of 4-12 weeks (Keating, 2002)

SubQ (unlabeled route): Adults: B-cell CLL: Initial: 3 mg on day 1; if tolerated 10 mg on day 3; if tolerated increase to 30 mg on day 5; maintenance: 30 mg/dose 3 times/week for a maximum of 18 weeks (Lundin, 2002) **or** 3 mg on day 1; if tolerated 10 mg on day 2; if tolerated 30 mg on day 3, followed by 30 mg/dose 3 times/week for 4-12 weeks (Stilgenbauer, 2009)

Dosage adjustment for nonhematologic toxicity:

Grade 3 or 4 infusion reaction: Withhold infusion

Serious infection or other serious adverse reaction: Withhold alemtuzumab until resolution

Autoimmune anemia or autoimmune thrombocytopenia: Discontinue alemtuzumab

Dosage adjustment for hematologic toxicity (severe neutropenia or thrombocytopenia, not autoimmune):

First occurrence: ANC <250/μL and/or platelet count ≤25,000/μL: Hold therapy; resume at 30 mg/dose when ANC ≥500/μL and platelet count ≥50,000/μL

Second occurrence: ANC <250/μL and/or platelet count ≤25,000/μL: Hold therapy; resume at 10 mg/dose when ANC ≥500/μL and platelet count ≥50,000/μL

Third occurrence: ANC <250/μL and/or platelet count ≤25,000/μL: Discontinue alemtuzumab

Patients with a baseline ANC ≤250/μL and/or a baseline platelet count ≤25,000/μL at initiation of therapy: If ANC and/or platelet counts decrease to ≤50% of the baseline value, hold therapy

First occurrence: When ANC and/or platelet count return to baseline, resume therapy at 30 mg/dose

Second occurrence: When ANC and/or platelet count return to baseline, resume therapy at 10 mg/dose

Third occurrence: Discontinue alemtuzumab

Administration Administer by I.V. infusion over 2 hours. Consider premedicating with diphenhydramine 50 mg and acetaminophen 500-1000 mg 30 minutes before initiation of infusion. Hydrocortisone 200 mg has been effective in decreasing severe infusion-related events. Start anti-infective prophylaxis. Other drugs should not be added to or simultaneously infused through the same I.V. line. Do not give I.V. push.

SubQ (unlabeled route): SubQ administration has been studied (Lundin, 2002; Stilgenbauer, 2009); an increased rate of injection site reactions has been observed, with only rare incidences of chills or infusion-like reactions typically observed with I.V. infusion. A longer dose escalation time (1-2 weeks) may be needed due to injection site reactions (Lundin, 2002). Premedication and anti-infective prophylaxis regimens should be given as are recommended with I.V. administration.

Monitoring Parameters Vital signs; carefully monitor BP especially in patient with ischemic heart disease or on antihypertensive medications; CBC with differential and platelets (weekly, more frequent if worsening); signs and symptoms of infection; $CD4^+$ lymphocyte counts (after treatment until recovery); CMV antigen (every 1-2 weeks). Monitor closely for infusion reactions (including hypotension, rigors, fever, shortness of breath, broncho-spasm, chills, and/or rash).

Test Interactions May interfere with diagnostic serum tests that utilize antibodies.

Emetic Potential Very low (<10%)

Dosage Forms Excipient information presented when available (limited, particularly for generics); consult specific product labeling.

Injection, solution [preservative free]:

Campath®: 30 mg/mL (1 mL) [contains polysorbate 80; disodium edetate]

References

Dearden CE, Matutes E, Cazin B, et al, "High Remission Rate in T-Cell Prolymphocytic Leukemia With CAMPATH-1H," *Blood*, 2001, 98(6):1721-6.

Enblad G, Hagberg H, Erlanson M, et al, "A Pilot Study of Alemtuzumab (Anti-CD52 Monoclonal Antibody) Therapy for Patients With Relapsed or Chemotherapy-Refractory Peripheral T-cell Lymphomas," *Blood*, 2003, 103(8):2920-4.

Ferrajoli A, O'Brien SM, Cortes JE, et al, "Phase II Study of Alemtuzumab in Chronic Lymphoproliferative Disorders," *Cancer*, 2003, 98(4):773-8.

Hale G, Rebello P, Brettman LR, et al, "Blood Concentrations of Alemtuzumab and Antiglobulin Responses in Patients With Chronic Lymphocytic Leukemia Following Intravenous or Subcutaneous Routes of Administration, *Blood*, 2004, 104(4):948-55.

Hillmen P, Skotnicki A, Robak T, et al, "Alemtuzumab Compared With Chlorambucil as First-Line Therapy for Chronic Lymphocytic Leukemia," *J Clin Oncol*, 2007, 25(35):5616-23.

Keating MJ, Cazin B, Coutré S, et al, "Campath-1H Treatment of T-Cell Prolymphocytic Leukemia in Patients for Whom at Least One Prior Chemotherapy Regimen Has Failed," *J Clin Oncol*, 2002, 20(1):205-13.

Keating MJ, Flinn I, Jain V, et al, "Therapeutic Role of Alemtuzumab (Campath-1H) in Patients Who Have Failed Fludarabine: Results of a Large International Study," *Blood*, 2002, 99(10):3554-61.

Kennedy B and Hillmen P, "Immunological Effects and Safe Administration of Alemtuzumab (MabCampath) in Advanced B-cLL," *Med Oncol*, 2002, 19(Suppl):49-55.

Lundin J, Hagberg H, Repp R, et al, "Phase 2 Study of Alemtuzumab (Anti-CD52 Monoclonal Antibody) in Patients With Advanced Mycosis Fungoides/Sézary Syndrome," *Blood*, 2003, 101 (11):4267-72.

Lundin J, Kimby E, Bjorkholm M, et al, "Phase II Trial of Subcutaneous Anti-CD52 Monoclonal Antibody Alemtuzumab (Campath-1H) as First-Line Treatment for Patients With B-Cell Chronic Lymphocytic Leukemia (B-CLL)," *Blood*, 2002, 100(3):768-73.

Lundin J, Osterborg A, Brittinger G, et al, "CAMPATH-1H Monoclonal Antibody in Therapy for Previously Treated Low-Grade Non-Hodgkin's Lymphomas: A Phase II Multicenter Study. European Study Group of CAMPATH-1H Treatment in Low-Grade Non-Hodgkin's Lymphoma," *J Clin Oncol*, 1998, 16(10):3257-63.

Magliocca JF and Knechtle SJ, "The Evolving Role of Alemtuzumab (Campath-1H) for Immunosuppressive Therapy in Organ Transplantation," *Transpl Int*, 2006, 19(9):705-14.

National Comprehensive Cancer Network (NCCN)®, "Clinical Practice Guidelines in Oncology™: Non-Hodgkin's Lymphomas," Version 2.2009. Available at http://www.nccn.org/professionals/physician_gls/PDF/nhl.pdf

Osterborg A, Dyer MJ, Bunjes D, et al, "Phase II Multicenter Study of Human CD52 Antibody in Previously Treated Chronic Lymphocytic Leukemia. European Study Group of CAMPATH-1H Treatment in Chronic Lymphocytic Leukemia," *J Clin Oncol*, 1997, 15(4):1567-74.

Rai KR, Freter CE, Mercier RJ, et al, "Alemtuzumab in Previously Treated Chronic Lymphocytic Leukemia Patients Who Also Had Received Fludarabine," *J Clin Oncol*, 2002, 20(18):3891-7.

Stilgenbauer S, Zenz T, Winkler D, et al, "Subcutaneous Alemtuzumab in Fludarabine-Refractory Chronic Lymphocytic Leukemia: Clinical Results and Prognostic Marker Analyses from the CLL2H Study of the German Chronic Lymphocytic Leukemia Study Group," *J Clin Oncol*, 2009, 27(24):3994-4001.

van Besien K, Artz A, Smith S, et al, "Fludarabine, Melphalan, and Alemtuzumab Conditioning in Adults With Standard-Risk Advanced Acute Myeloid Leukemia and Myelodysplastic Syndrome," *J Clin Oncol*, 2005, 23(24):5728-38.

van Besien K, Kunavakkam R, Rondon G, et al, "Fludarabine-Melphalan Conditioning for AML and MDS: Alemtuzumab Reduces Acute and Chronic GVHD Without Affecting Long-term Outcomes," *Biol Blood Marrow Transplant*, 2009, 15(5):610-7.

Vo AA, Wechsler EA, Wang J, et al, "Analysis of Subcutaneous (SQ) Alemtuzumab Induction Therapy in Highly Sensitized Patients Desensitized With IVIG and Rituximab," *Am J Transplant*, 2008, 8(1):144-9.

Willis F, Marsh JC, Bevan DH, et al, "The Effect of Treatment With Campath-1H in Patients With Autoimmune Cytopenias," *Br J Haematol*, 2001, 114(4):891-8.

◆ **Alimta®** *see Pemetrexed on page 939*

Alitretinoin (a li TRET i noyn)

Medication Safety Issues
Sound-alike/look-alike issues:
Panretin® may be confused with pancreatin

High alert medication: The Institute for Safe Medication Practices (ISMP) includes this medication among its list of drugs which have a heightened risk of causing significant patient harm when used in error.

Related Information
Safe Handling of Hazardous Drugs *on page 1517*

U.S. Brand Names Panretin®

Generic Available No

Canadian Brand Names Panretin®

Pharmacologic Category Antineoplastic Agent, Miscellaneous; Retinoic Acid Derivative

Use Orphan drug: Topical treatment of cutaneous lesions in AIDS-related Kaposi's sarcoma

Unlabeled/Investigational Use Cutaneous T-cell lymphomas

Pregnancy Risk Factor D

Lactation Excretion in breast milk unknown/not recommended

Labeled Contraindications Hypersensitivity to alitretinoin, other retinoids, or any component of the formulation; pregnancy

Warnings/Precautions Hazardous agent - use appropriate precautions for handling and disposal. May cause fetal harm if absorbed by a woman who is pregnant. May be photosensitizing (based on experience with other retinoids); minimize sun or other UV exposure of treated areas. Do not use concurrently with topical products containing DEET. Safety in pediatric patients or geriatric patients has not been established.

Adverse Reactions
>10%:
Central nervous system: Pain (0% to 34%)
Dermatologic: Rash (25% to 77%), pruritus (8% to 11%)
Neuromuscular & skeletal: Paresthesia (3% to 22%)

5% to 10%:
  Cardiovascular: Edema (3% to 8%)
  Dermatologic: Exfoliative dermatitis (3% to 9%), skin disorder (0% to 8%)

Drug Interactions

Avoid Concomitant Use There are no known interactions where it is recommended to avoid concomitant use.

Increased Effect/Toxicity There are no known significant interactions involving an increase in effect.

Decreased Effect There are no known significant interactions involving a decrease in effect.

Storage/Stability Store at room temperature.

Mechanism of Action Binds to retinoid receptors to inhibit growth of Kaposi's sarcoma

Pharmacodynamics/Kinetics Absorption: Not extensive

Dosage Topical: Apply gel twice daily to cutaneous lesions

Administration Do not use occlusive dressings.

Dosage Forms Excipient information presented when available (limited, particularly for generics); consult specific product labeling.
  Gel:
    Panretin®: 0.1% (60 g)

◆ **Alkeran®** *see* Melphalan *on page 745*

◆ **Alloprin® (Can)** *see* Allopurinol *on page 37*

Allopurinol (al oh PURE i nole)

Medication Safety Issues
  Sound-alike/look-alike issues:
    Allopurinol may be confused with Apresoline
    Zyloprim® may be confused with Xylo-Pfan®, ZORprin®, Zovirax®

Related Information
  Oral Mucositis / Stomatitis *on page 1460*
  Tumor Lysis Syndrome *on page 1468*

U.S. Brand Names Aloprim®; Zyloprim®

Index Terms Allopurinol Sodium

Generic Available Yes

Canadian Brand Names Alloprin®; Apo-Allopurinol®; Novo-Purol; Zyloprim®

Pharmacologic Category Xanthine Oxidase Inhibitor

Use
Oral: Prevention of attack of gouty arthritis and nephropathy; treatment of secondary hyperuricemia which may occur during treatment of tumors or leukemia; prevention of recurrent calcium oxalate calculi

I.V.: Treatment of elevated serum and urinary uric acid levels when oral therapy is not tolerated in patients with leukemia, lymphoma, and solid tumor malignancies who are receiving cancer chemotherapy

Pregnancy Risk Factor C

Lactation Enters breast milk/use caution (AAP rates "compatible")

Labeled Contraindications Hypersensitivity to allopurinol or any component of the formulation

Warnings/Precautions Do not use to treat asymptomatic hyperuricemia. Has been associated with a number of hypersensitivity reactions, including severe reactions (vasculitis and Stevens-Johnson syndrome); discontinue at first sign of rash. Reversible hepatotoxicity has been reported; use with caution in patients with pre-existing hepatic impairment. Bone marrow suppression has been reported; use caution with other drugs causing myelosuppression. Caution in renal impairment, dosage adjustments needed. Use with caution in patients taking diuretics concurrently. Risk of skin rash may be increased in patients receiving amoxicillin or ampicillin. The risk of hypersensitivity may be increased in patients receiving thiazides, and possibly ACE inhibitors. Use caution with mercaptopurine or azathioprine; dosage adjustment necessary.

Adverse Reactions

Most commonly reported:

Dermatologic: Rash

Endocrine & metabolic: Gout (acute)

Gastrointestinal: Diarrhea, nausea

Hepatic: Alkaline phosphatase increased, liver enzymes increased

<1%: Abdominal pain, agranulocytosis, alopecia, angioedema, aplastic anemia, arthralgia, bronchospasm, cataracts, cholestatic jaundice, dermatitis (eczematoid, exfoliative, vascular bullous), dyspepsia, ecchymosis, eosinophilia, epistaxis, fever, gastritis, granuloma annulare, hepatitis, gynecomastia, headache, hepatic necrosis, hepatomegaly, hyperbilirubinemia, hypersensitivity reactions, leukocytosis, leukopenia, lichen planus, loss of taste perception, macular retinitis, myopathy, necrotizing angiitis, nephritis, neuritis, neuropathy, onycholysis, pancreatitis, paresthesia, purpura, pruritus, renal failure, somnolence, Stevens-Johnson syndrome, taste perversion, thrombocytopenia, toxic epidermal necrolysis, toxic pustuloderma, uremia, vasculitis, vomiting

Drug Interactions

Avoid Concomitant Use

Avoid concomitant use of Allopurinol with any of the following: Didanosine

Increased Effect/Toxicity

Allopurinol may increase the levels/effects of: Amoxicillin; Ampicillin; AzaTHIOprine; CarBAMazepine; ChlorproPAMIDE; Cyclophosphamide; Didanosine; Mercaptopurine; Pivampicillin; Theophylline Derivatives; Vitamin K Antagonists

The levels/effects of Allopurinol may be increased by: ACE Inhibitors; Loop Diuretics; Thiazide Diuretics

Decreased Effect

The levels/effects of Allopurinol may be decreased by: Antacids

Ethanol/Nutrition/Herb Interactions

Ethanol: May decrease effectiveness.

Iron supplements: Hepatic iron uptake may be increased.

Vitamin C: Large amounts of vitamin C may acidify urine and increase kidney stone formation.

Storage/Stability

Powder for injection: Store at controlled room temperature of 15°C to 30°C (59°F to 86°F). Following reconstitution, intravenous solutions should be stored at 20°C to 25°C. Do not refrigerate reconstituted and/or diluted product. Must be administered within 10 hours of solution preparation.

Tablet: Store at controlled room temperature of 15°C to 25°C (59°F to 77°F).

Reconstitution Further dilution with NS or D_5W (50-100 mL) to ≤6 mg/mL is recommended.

Compatibility Stable in D_5W, NS, sterile water for injection.

Y-site administration: Compatible: Acyclovir, aminophylline, aztreonam, bleomycin, bumetanide, buprenorphine, butorphanol, calcium gluconate, carboplatin, cefazolin, cefoperazone, cefotetan, ceftazidime, ceftizoxime, ceftriaxone, cefuroxime, cisplatin, co-trimoxazole, cyclophosphamide,

dactinomycin, dexamethasone sodium phosphate, doxorubicin liposome, enalaprilat, etoposide, famotidine, fluconazole, fludarabine, fluorouracil, furosemide, ganciclovir, heparin, hydrocortisone sodium phosphate, hydrocortisone sodium succinate, hydromorphone, ifosfamide, lorazepam, mannitol, mesna, methotrexate, metronidazole, mitoxantrone, morphine, piperacillin, plicamycin, potassium chloride, ranitidine, thiotepa, ticarcillin, ticarcillin/clavulanate, vancomycin, vinblastine, vincristine, zidovudine.
Incompatible: Amikacin, amphotericin B, carmustine, cefotaxime, chlorpromazine, cimetidine, clindamycin, cytarabine, dacarbazine, daunorubicin, diphenhydramine, doxorubicin, doxycycline, droperidol, floxuridine, gentamicin, haloperidol, hydroxyzine, idarubicin, imipenem/cilastatin, mechlorethamine, meperidine, methylprednisolone sodium succinate, metoclopramide, minocycline, nalbuphine, netilmicin, ondansetron, prochlorperazine edisylate, promethazine, sodium bicarbonate, streptozocin, tobramycin, vinorelbine.

Mechanism of Action Allopurinol inhibits xanthine oxidase, the enzyme responsible for the conversion of hypoxanthine to xanthine to uric acid. Allopurinol is metabolized to oxypurinol which is also an inhibitor of xanthine oxidase; allopurinol acts on purine catabolism, reducing the production of uric acid without disrupting the biosynthesis of vital purines.

Pharmacodynamics/Kinetics

Onset of action: Peak effect: 1-2 weeks

Absorption: Oral: ~80%; Rectal: Poor and erratic

Distribution: V_d: ~1.6 L/kg; V_{ss}: 0.84-0.87 L/kg; enters breast milk

Protein binding: <1%

Metabolism: ~75% to active metabolites, chiefly oxypurinol

Bioavailability: 49% to 53%

Half-life elimination:
  Normal renal function: Parent drug: 1-3 hours; Oxypurinol: 18-30 hours
  End-stage renal disease: Prolonged

Time to peak, plasma: Oral: 30-120 minutes

Excretion: Urine (76% as oxypurinol, 12% as unchanged drug)

Allopurinol and oxypurinol are dialyzable

Dosage

Oral: Doses >300 mg should be given in divided doses.
  Children ≤10 years: Secondary hyperuricemia associated with chemotherapy: 10 mg/kg/day in 2-3 divided doses **or** 200-300 mg/m^2/day in 2-4 divided doses, maximum: 800 mg/24 hours
    Alternative (manufacturer labeling): <6 years: 150 mg/day in 3 divided doses; 6-10 years: 300 mg/day in 2-3 divided doses
  Children >10 years and Adults:
    Secondary hyperuricemia associated with chemotherapy: 600-800 mg/day in 2-3 divided doses for prevention of acute uric acid nephropathy for 2-3 days starting 1-2 days before chemotherapy
    Gout: Mild: 200-300 mg/day; Severe: 400-600 mg/day; to reduce the possibility of acute gouty attacks, initiate dose at 100 mg/day and increase weekly to recommended dosage. Maximum daily dose: 800 mg/day.
    Recurrent calcium oxalate stones: 200-300 mg/day in single or divided doses
  Elderly: Initial: 100 mg/day, increase until desired uric acid level is obtained
I.V.: Hyperuricemia secondary to chemotherapy: Intravenous daily dose can be given as a single infusion or in equally divided doses at 6-, 8-, or 12-hour intervals. A fluid intake sufficient to yield a daily urinary output of at least 2 L in adults and the maintenance of a neutral or, preferably, slightly alkaline urine are desirable.

Children ≤10 years: Starting dose: 200 mg/m^2/day
Children >10 years and Adults: 200-400 mg/m^2/day (maximum: 600 mg/day)

Dosing adjustment in renal impairment: Must be adjusted due to accumulation of allopurinol and metabolites:

Oral: Removed by hemodialysis; adult maintenance doses of allopurinol (mg) based on creatinine clearance (mL/minute): See table.

Adult Maintenance Doses of Allopurinol[1]

Creatinine Clearance (mL/min)	Maintenance Dose of Allopurinol (mg)
140	400 daily
120	350 daily
100	300 daily
80	250 daily
60	200 daily
40	150 daily
20	100 daily
10	100 every 2 days
0	100 every 3 days

[1]This table is based on a standard maintenance dose of 300 mg of allopurinol per day for a patient with a creatinine clearance of 100 mL/min.

I.V.:
Cl$_{cr}$ 10-20 mL/minute: 200 mg/day
Cl$_{cr}$ 3-10 mL/minute: 100 mg/day
Cl$_{cr}$ <3 mL/minute: 100 mg/day at extended intervals

Hemodialysis: Administer dose posthemodialysis or administer 50% supplemental dose

Administration

Oral: Should administer oral forms after meals with plenty of fluid.

I.V.: Infuse over 15-60 minutes. The rate of infusion depends on the volume of the infusion. Whenever possible, therapy should be initiated at 24-48 hours before the start of chemotherapy known to cause tumor lysis (including adrenocorticosteroids). I.V. daily dose can be administered as a single infusion or in equally divided doses at 6-, 8-, or 12-hour interval.

Monitoring Parameters CBC, serum uric acid levels, I & O, hepatic and renal function, especially at start of therapy

Dietary Considerations Should take oral forms after meals with plenty of fluid. Fluid intake should be administered to yield neutral or slightly alkaline urine and an output of ~2 L (in adults).

Dosage Forms Excipient information presented when available (limited, particularly for generics); consult specific product labeling.

Injection, powder for reconstitution, as sodium: 500 mg (base)
  Aloprim®: 500 mg (base)
Tablet: 100 mg, 300 mg
  Zyloprim®: 100 mg, 300 mg

Extemporaneous Preparations Crush tablets to make a 5 mg/mL suspension in simple syrup; stable 14 days under refrigeration

Nahata MC and Hipple TF, *Pediatric Drug Formulations*, 1st ed, Harvey Whitney Books Co, 1990.

References

Bennett WM, Aronoff GR, Golper TA, et al, *Drug Prescribing in Renal Failure*, Philadelphia, PA: American College of Physicians, 1987.

Hande KR and Garrow GC, "Acute Tumor Lysis Syndrome in Patients With High-Grade Non-Hodgkin's Lymphoma," *Am J Med*, 1993, 94(2):133-9.

Krakoff IH and Murphy ML, "Hyperuricemia in Neoplastic Disease in Children: Prevention With Allopurinol, A Xanthine Oxidase Inhibitor," *Pediatrics*, 1968, 41(1):52-6.

McInnes GT, Lawson DH, and Jick H, "Acute Adverse Reactions Attributed to Allopurinol in Hospitalized Patients," *Ann Rheum Dis*, 1981, 40(3):245-9.

Murrell GA and Rapeport WG, "Clinical Pharmacokinetics of Allopurinol," *Clin Pharmacokinet*, 1986, 11(5):343-53.

Parra E, Gota R, Gamen A, et al, "Granulomatous Interstitial Nephritis Secondary to Allopurinol Treatment," *Clin Nephrol*, 1995, 43(5):350.

◆ **Allopurinol Sodium** *see* Allopurinol *on page 37*

◆ **All-*trans* Retinoic Acid** *see* Tretinoin, Systemic *on page 1141*

◆ **All-*trans* Vitamin A Acid** *see* Tretinoin, Systemic *on page 1141*

◆ **Aloprim®** *see* Allopurinol *on page 37*

◆ **Aloxi®** *see* Palonosetron *on page 911*

◆ **AlphaNine® SD** *see* Factor IX *on page 449*

Alteplase (AL te plase)

Medication Safety Issues

Sound-alike/look-alike issues:

Activase® may be confused with Cathflo® Activase®, TNKase®

Alteplase may be confused with Altace®

"tPA" abbreviation should not be used when writing orders for this medication; has been misread as TNKase (tenecteplase)

High alert medication: The Institute for Safe Medication Practices (ISMP) includes this medication (I.V.) among its list of drugs which have a heightened risk of causing significant patient harm when used in error.

U.S. Brand Names Activase®; Cathflo® Activase®

Index Terms Alteplase, Recombinant; Alteplase, Tissue Plasminogen Activator, Recombinant; tPA

Generic Available No

Canadian Brand Names Activase® rt-PA; Cathflo® Activase®

Pharmacologic Category Thrombolytic Agent

Use Management of ST-elevation myocardial infarction (STEMI) for the lysis of thrombi in coronary arteries; management of acute ischemic stroke (AIS); management of acute pulmonary embolism

Recommended criteria for treatment:

STEMI: Chest pain ≥20 minutes duration, onset of chest pain within 12 hours of treatment (or within prior 12-24 hours in patients with continuing ischemic symptoms), and ST-segment elevation >0.1 mV in at least two contiguous precordial leads or two adjacent limb leads on ECG or new or presumably new left bundle branch block (LBBB)

AIS: Onset of stroke symptoms within 3 hours of treatment

Acute pulmonary embolism: Age ≤75 years: Documented massive pulmonary embolism by pulmonary angiography or echocardiography or high probability lung scan with clinical shock

Cathflo® Activase®: Restoration of central venous catheter function

Unlabeled/Investigational Use Acute ischemic stroke presenting 3-4.5 hours after symptom onset; acute peripheral arterial occlusive disease

Pregnancy Risk Factor C

Lactation Excretion in breast milk unknown/use caution

Labeled Contraindications Hypersensitivity to alteplase or any component of the formulation

Treatment of STEMI or PE: Active internal bleeding; history of CVA; recent intracranial or intraspinal surgery or trauma; intracranial neoplasm; arteriovenous malformation or aneurysm; known bleeding diathesis; severe uncontrolled hypertension; suspected aortic dissection

Treatment of acute ischemic stroke: Evidence of intracranial hemorrhage or suspicion of subarachnoid hemorrhage on pretreatment evaluation; intracranial or intraspinal surgery within 3 months; stroke or serious head injury within 3 months; history of intracranial hemorrhage; uncontrolled hypertension at time of treatment (eg, >185 mm Hg systolic or >110 mm Hg diastolic); seizure at the onset of stroke; active internal bleeding; intracranial neoplasm; arteriovenous malformation or aneurysm; multilobar cerebral infarction (hypodensity >1/3 cerebral hemisphere; Adams, 2007); clinical presentation suggesting post-MI pericarditis; known bleeding diathesis including but not limited to current use of oral anticoagulants producing an INR >1.7, an INR >1.7, administration of heparin within 48 hours preceding the onset of stroke with an elevated aPTT at presentation; platelet count <100,000/mm^3.

Additional exclusion criteria within clinical trials:

Presentation <3 hours after initial symptoms (NINDS, 1995): Time of symptom onset unknown, rapidly improving or minor symptoms, major surgery within 2 weeks, GI or urinary tract hemorrhage within 3 weeks, aggressive treatment required to lower blood pressure, glucose level <50 or >400 mg/dL, and arterial puncture at a noncompressible site or lumbar puncture within 1 week.

Presentation 3-4.5 hours after initial symptoms (ECASS-III; Hacke, 2008): Age >80 years, time of symptom onset unknown, rapidly improving or minor symptoms, current use of anticoagulants regardless of INR, glucose level <50 or >400 mg/dL, aggressive intravenous treatment required to lower blood pressure, major surgery or severe trauma within 3 months, baseline National Institutes of Health Stroke Scale (NIHSS) score >25, and history of both stroke and diabetes.

Warnings/Precautions Concurrent heparin anticoagulation may contribute to bleeding. In the treatment of acute ischemic stroke, concurrent use of anticoagulants was not permitted during the initial 24 hours of the <3 hour window trial (NINDS, 1995). Initiation of SubQ heparin (≤10,000 units) or equivalent doses of low molecular weight heparin for prevention of DVT during the first 24 hours of the 3-4.5 hour window trial was permitted and did not increase the incidence of intracerebral hemorrhage (Hacke, 2008). Monitor all potential bleeding sites. Do not use doses >150 mg; associated with increased risk of intracranial hemorrhage. Intramuscular injections and nonessential handling of the patient should be avoided. Venipunctures should be performed carefully and only when necessary. If arterial puncture is necessary, use an upper extremity vessel that can be manually compressed. If serious bleeding occurs, the infusion of alteplase and heparin should be stopped. Avoid aspirin for 24 hours following administration of alteplase; administration within 24 hours increases the risk of hemorrhagic transformation.

For the following conditions, the risk of bleeding is higher with use of thrombolytics and should be weighed against the benefits of therapy: Recent major surgery (eg, CABG, obstetrical delivery, organ biopsy, pregnancy, previous puncture of noncompressible vessels), prolonged CPR with evidence of thoracic trauma, lumbar puncture within 1 week, cerebrovascular disease, recent gastrointestinal or genitourinary bleeding, recent trauma, hypertension (systolic BP >175 mm Hg and/or diastolic BP >110 mm Hg), high likelihood of left heart thrombus (eg, mitral stenosis with atrial fibrillation), acute pericarditis, subacute bacterial endocarditis, hemostatic defects including ones caused by severe renal or hepatic dysfunction, significant hepatic dysfunction, pregnancy, diabetic hemorrhagic retinopathy or other hemorrhagic ophthalmic conditions, septic thrombophlebitis or occluded AV cannula at seriously infected site, advanced age (eg, >75 years), any other condition in which bleeding constitutes a significant hazard or would be particularly difficult to manage because of location. When treating acute MI or pulmonary embolism, use with caution in patients receiving oral anticoagulants. In the treatment of acute ischemic stroke within 3 hours of stroke symptom onset, the current use of oral anticoagulants producing an INR >1.7 is contraindicated.

Coronary thrombolysis may result in reperfusion arrhythmias. Patients who present **within 3 hours** of stroke symptom onset should be treated with alteplase unless contraindications exist. A longer time window (**3-4.5 hours** after symptom onset) has now been formally evaluated and shown to be safe and efficacious for select individuals (del Zoppo, 2009; Hacke, 2008). Treatment of patients with minor neurological deficit or with rapidly improving symptoms is not recommended. Follow standard management for STEMI while infusing alteplase.

Cathflo® Activase®: When used to restore catheter function, use Cathflo® cautiously in those patients with known or suspected catheter infections. Evaluate catheter for other causes of dysfunction before use. Avoid excessive pressure when instilling into catheter.

Adverse Reactions As with all drugs which may affect hemostasis, bleeding is the major adverse effect associated with alteplase. Hemorrhage may occur at virtually any site. Risk is dependent on multiple variables, including the dosage administered, concurrent use of multiple agents which alter hemostasis, and patient predisposition. Rapid lysis of coronary artery thrombi by thrombolytic agents may be associated with reperfusion-related atrial and/or ventricular arrhythmia. **Note:** Lowest rate of bleeding complications expected with dose used to restore catheter function.

1% to 10%:
Cardiovascular: Hypotension
Central nervous system: Fever
Dermatologic: Bruising (1%)
Gastrointestinal: GI hemorrhage (5%), nausea, vomiting
Genitourinary: GU hemorrhage (4%)
Hematologic: Bleeding (0.5% major, 7% minor: GUSTO trial)
Local: Bleeding at catheter puncture site (15.3%, accelerated administration)
<1% (Limited to important or life-threatening): Intracranial hemorrhage (0.4% to 0.87% when dose is ≤100 mg), retroperitoneal hemorrhage, pericardial hemorrhage, gingival hemorrhage, epistaxis, allergic reactions: anaphylaxis, anaphylactoid reactions, laryngeal edema, rash, and urticaria (<0.02%).
Additional cardiovascular events associated **with use in STEMI:** AV block, cardiogenic shock, heart failure, cardiac arrest, recurrent ischemia/infarction, myocardial rupture, electromechanical dissociation, pericardial effusion, pericarditis, mitral regurgitation, cardiac tamponade, thromboembolism, pulmonary edema, asystole, ventricular tachycardia, bradycardia, ruptured

intracranial AV malformation, seizure, hemorrhagic bursitis, cholesterol crystal embolization

Additional events associated **with use in pulmonary embolism:** Pulmonary re-embolization, pulmonary edema, pleural effusion, thromboembolism

Additional events associated **with use in stroke:** Cerebral edema, cerebral herniation, seizure, new ischemic stroke

Drug Interactions

Avoid Concomitant Use There are no known interactions where it is recommended to avoid concomitant use.

Increased Effect/Toxicity

Alteplase may increase the levels/effects of: Anticoagulants; Drotrecogin Alfa

The levels/effects of Alteplase may be increased by: Antiplatelet Agents; Herbs (Anticoagulant/Antiplatelet Properties); Nonsteroidal Anti-Inflammatory Agents; Salicylates

Decreased Effect

The levels/effects of Alteplase may be decreased by: Aprotinin; Nitroglycerin

Ethanol/Nutrition/Herb Interactions Herb/Nutraceutical: Avoid cat's claw, dong quai, evening primrose, feverfew, red clover, horse chestnut, garlic, green tea, ginseng, ginkgo (all have additional antiplatelet activity).

Storage/Stability

Activase®: The lyophilized product may be stored at room temperature (not to exceed 30°C/86°F), or under refrigeration. Once reconstituted it should be used within 8 hours.

Cathflo® Activase®: Store lyophilized product in refrigerator. Once reconstituted, store at 2°C to 30°C (36°F to 86°F) and use within 8 hours.

Reconstitution

Activase®:

50 mg vial: Use accompanying diluent (50 mL sterile water for injection); do not shake. Final concentration: 1 mg/mL.

100 mg vial: Use transfer set with accompanying diluent (100 mL vial of sterile water for injection); no vacuum is present in 100 mg vial. Final concentration: 1 mg/mL.

Cathflo® Activase®: Add 2.2 mL SWFI to vial; do not shake. Final concentration: 1 mg/mL.

Compatibility Stable in NS, sterile water for injection; **incompatible** with bacteriostatic water; **variable stability (consult detailed reference)** in D_5W.

Y-site administration: Compatible: Lidocaine, metoprolol, propranolol. **Incompatible:** Dobutamine, dopamine, heparin, nitroglycerin.

Compatibility when admixed: Compatible: Lidocaine, morphine, nitroglycerin. **Incompatible:** Dobutamine, dopamine, heparin.

Mechanism of Action Initiates local fibrinolysis by binding to fibrin in a thrombus (clot) and converts entrapped plasminogen to plasmin

Pharmacodynamics/Kinetics

Duration: >50% present in plasma cleared ~5 minutes after infusion terminated, ~80% cleared within 10 minutes

Excretion: Clearance: Rapidly from circulating plasma (550-650 mL/minute), primarily hepatic; >50% present in plasma is cleared within 5 minutes after the infusion is terminated, ~80% cleared within 10 minutes

Dosage

I.V. (Activase®):

ST-elevation myocardial infarction (STEMI): Front loading dose (weight-based):

Patients >67 kg: Total dose: 100 mg over 1.5 hours; infuse 15 mg over 1-2 minutes. Infuse 50 mg over 30 minutes. Infuse remaining 35 mg of alteplase over the next hour. See **"Note."**

Patients ≤67 kg: Infuse 15 mg I.V. bolus over 1-2 minutes, then infuse 0.75 mg/kg (not to exceed 50 mg) over next 30 minutes, followed by 0.5 mg/kg over next 60 minutes (not to exceed 35 mg). See **"Note."**

Note: All patients should receive 162-325 mg of chewable nonenteric coated aspirin as soon as possible and then daily. Administer concurrently with heparin 60 units/kg bolus (maximum: 4000 units) followed by continuous infusion of 12 units/kg/hour (maximum: 1000 units/hour) and adjust to aPTT target of 50-70 seconds (or 1.5-2 times the upper limit of control).

Acute pulmonary embolism: 100 mg over 2 hours.

Acute ischemic stroke: Within 3 hours of the onset of symptom onset (labeled use) **or** within 3-4.5 hours of symptom onset (unlabeled use; del Zoppo, 2009; Hacke, 2008): **Note:** Initiation of anticoagulants (eg, heparin) or antiplatelet agents (eg, aspirin) within 24 hours after starting alteplase is not recommended; however, initiation of aspirin between 24-48 hours after stroke onset is recommended (Adams, 2007). Initiation of SubQ heparin (≤10,000 units) or equivalent doses of low molecular weight heparin for prevention of DVT during the first 24 hours of the 3-4.5 hour window trial did not increase incidence of intracerebral hemorrhage (Hacke, 2008).

Recommended total dose: 0.9 mg/kg (maximum total dose: 90 mg)

Patients ≤100 kg: Load with 0.09 mg/kg (10% of 0.9 mg/kg dose) as an I.V. bolus over 1 minute, followed by 0.81 mg/kg (90% of 0.9 mg/kg dose) as a continuous infusion over 60 minutes.

Patients >100 kg: Load with 9 mg (10% of 90 mg) as an I.V. bolus over 1 minute, followed by 81 mg (90% of 90 mg) as a continuous infusion over 60 minutes.

Intracatheter: Central venous catheter clearance (Cathflo® Activase® 1 mg/mL):

Patients <30 kg: 110% of the internal lumen volume of the catheter, not to exceed 2 mg/2 mL; retain in catheter for 0.5-2 hours; may instill a second dose if catheter remains occluded

Patients ≥30 kg: 2 mg (2 mL); retain in catheter for 0.5-2 hours; may instill a second dose if catheter remains occluded

Intra-arterial: Acute peripheral arterial occlusive disease (unlabeled use): 0.02-0.1 mg/kg/hour for up to 36 hours

Advisory Panel to the Society for Cardiovascular and Interventional Radiology on Thrombolytic Therapy recommendation: ≤2 mg/hour and subtherapeutic heparin (aPTT <1.5 times baseline)

Administration

Activase®: ST-elevation MI: Accelerated infusion: Bolus dose may be prepared by one of three methods:

1) Removal of 15 mL reconstituted (1 mg/mL) solution from vial

2) Removal of 15 mL from a port on the infusion line after priming

3) Programming an infusion pump to deliver a 15 mL bolus at the initiation of infusion

Activase®: Acute ischemic stroke: Bolus dose (10% of total dose) may be prepared by one of three methods:

1) Removal of the appropriate volume from reconstituted solution (1 mg/mL)
2) Removal of the appropriate volume from a port on the infusion line after priming
3) Programming an infusion pump to deliver the appropriate volume at the initiation of infusion

Note: Remaining dose for STEMI, AIS, or total dose for acute pulmonary embolism may be administered as follows: Any quantity of drug not to be administered to the patient must be removed from vial(s) prior to administration of remaining dose.

50 mg vial: Either PVC bag or glass vial and infusion set

100 mg vial: Insert spike end of the infusion set through the same puncture site created by transfer device and infuse from vial

If further dilution is desired, may be diluted in equal volume of 0.9% sodium chloride or D_5W to yield a final concentration of 0.5 mg/mL.

Cathflo® Activase®: Intracatheter: Instill dose into occluded catheter. Do not force solution into catheter. After a 30-minute dwell time, assess catheter function by attempting to aspirate blood. If catheter is functional, aspirate 4-5 mL of blood in patients ≥10 kg or 3 mL in patients <10 kg to remove Cathflo® Activase® and residual clots. Gently irrigate the catheter with NS. If catheter remains nonfunctional, let Cathflo® Activase® dwell for another 90 minutes (total dwell time: 120 minutes) and reassess function. If catheter function is not restored, a second dose may be instilled.

Monitoring Parameters

Acute ischemic stroke: In addition to monitoring for bleeding complications, the 2007 AHA/ASA Guidelines for the early management of acute ischemic stroke recommends the following:

Perform neurological assessments every 15 minutes during infusion and every 30 minutes thereafter for the next 6 hours, then hourly until 24 hours after treatment.

If severe headache, acute hypertension, nausea, or vomiting occurs, discontinue the infusion and obtain emergency CT scan.

Measure BP every 15 minutes for the first 2 hours then every 30 minutes for the next 6 hours, then hourly until 24 hours after initiation of alteplase. Increase frequency if a systolic BP is ≥180 mm Hg or if a diastolic BP is ≥105 mm Hg; administer antihypertensive medications to maintain BP at or below these levels.

Obtain a follow-up CT scan at 24 hours before starting anticoagulants or antiplatelet agents.

Central venous catheter clearance: Assess catheter function by attempting to aspirate blood.

ST-elevation MI: Assess for evidence of cardiac reperfusion through resolution of chest pain, resolution of baseline ECG changes, preserved left ventricular function, cardiac enzyme washout phenomenon, and/or the appearance of reperfusion arrhythmias; assess for bleeding potential through clinical evidence of GI bleeding, hematuria, gingival bleeding, fibrinogen levels, fibrinogen degradation products, prothrombin times, and partial thromboplastin times.

Test Interactions Altered results of coagulation and fibrinolytic agents

Dosage Forms Excipient information presented when available (limited, particularly for generics); consult specific product labeling.

Injection, powder for reconstitution, recombinant:

Activase®: 50 mg [29 million int. units; contains polysorbate 80; packaged with diluent]; 100 mg [58 million int. units; contains polysorbate 80; packaged with diluent and transfer device]

Cathflo® Activase®: 2 mg [contains polysorbate 80]

References

Adams HP Jr, del Zoppo G, Alberts MJ, et al, "Guidelines for the Early Management of Adults With Ischemic Stroke: A Guideline From the American Heart Association/American Stroke Association Stroke Council, Clinical Cardiology Council, Cardiovascular Radiology and Intervention Council, and the Atherosclerotic Peripheral Vascular Disease and Quality of Care Outcomes in Research Interdisciplinary Working Groups: The American Academy of Neurology Affirms the Value of This Guideline as an Educational Tool for Neurologists," *Stroke*, 2007, 38(5):1655-711.

Böttiger BW, Bode C, Kern S, et al,"Efficacy and Safety of Thrombolytic Therapy After Initially Unsuccessful Cardiopulmonary Resuscitation: A Prospective Clinical Trial," *Lancet*, 2001, 357 (9268):1583-5.

Broderick J, Connolly S, Feldmann E, et al, "Guidelines for the Management of Spontaneous Intracerebral Hemorrhage in Adults: 2007 Update: A Guideline From the American Heart Association/American Stroke Association Stroke Council, High Blood Pressure Research Council, and the Quality of Care and Outcomes in Research Interdisciplinary Working Group," *Stroke*, 2007, 38(6):2001-23. Available at http://stroke.ahajournals.org/cgi/content/short/STROKEAHA.107.183689.

del Zoppo GJ, Saver JL, Jauch EC, et al, "Expansion of the Time Window for Treatment of Acute Ischemic Stroke With Intravenous Tissue Plasminogen Activator: A Science Advisory From the American Heart Association/American Stroke Association," *Stroke*, 2009, [epub ahead of print]

ECC Committee, Subcommittees and Task Forces of the American Heart Association, "2005 American Heart Association Guidelines for Cardiopulmonary Resuscitation and Emergency Cardiovascular Care," *Circulation*, 2005, 112(24 Suppl):IV1-203.

Goodman SG, Menon V, Cannon CP, et al, "Acute ST-Segment Elevation Myocardial Infarction: American College of Chest Physicians Evidence-Based Clinical Practice," *Chest*, 2008, 133(6 Suppl):708-75.

Hacke W, Kaste M, Bluhmki E, et al, "Thrombolysis With Alteplase 3 to 4.5 Hours After Acute Ischemic Stroke," *N Engl J Med*, 2008, 359(13):1317-29.

Hirsh J, Guyatt G, Albers GW, et al, "Executive Summary: American College of Chest Physicians Evidence-Based Clinical Practice Guidelines (8th Edition)," *Chest*, 2008, 133(6 Suppl):71-109.

Kearon C, Kahn SR, Agnelli G, et al, "Antithrombotic Therapy for Venous Thromboembolic Disease: American College of Chest Physicians Evidence-Based Clinical Practice Guidelines (8th Edition)," *Chest*, 2008, 33(6 Suppl):454-545.

Ponec D, Irwin D, Haire WD, et al, "Recombinant Tissue Plasminogen Activator (Alteplase) for Restoration of Flow in Occluded Central Venous Access Devices: A Double-Blind Placebo-Controlled Trial - The Cardiovascular Thrombolytic to Open Occluded Lines (COOL) Efficacy Trial," *J Vasc Interv Radiol*, 2001, 12(8):951-5.

Semba CP, Murphy TP, Bakal CW, et al, "Thrombolytic Therapy With Use of Alteplase (rtPA) in Peripheral Arterial Occlusive Disease: Review of the Clinical Literature. The Advisory Panel," *J Vasc Interv Radiol*, 2000, 11(2 Pt 1):149-61.

Sugimoto K, Hofmann LV, Razavi MK, et al, "The Safety, Efficacy, and Pharmacoeconomics of Low-Dose Alteplase Compared With Urokinase for Catheter-Directed Thrombolysis of Arterial and Venous Occlusions," *J Vasc Surg*, 2003, 37(3):512-7.

The Gusto Angiographic Investigators, "The Effects of Tissue Plasminogen Activator, Streptokinase, or Both on Coronary-Artery Patency, Ventricular Function, and Survival After Acute Myocardial Infarction," *N Engl J Med*, 1993, 329(22):1615-22.

"Thrombolysis in the Management of Lower Limb Peripheral Arterial Occlusion - A Consensus Document. Working Party on Thrombolysis in the Management of Limb Ischemia," *Am J Cardiol*, 1998, 81(2):207-18.

Zacharias JM, Weatherston CP, Spewak CR, et al, "Alteplase Versus Urokinase for Occluded Hemodialysis Catheters," *Ann Pharmacother*, 2003, 37(1):27-33.

◆ **Alteplase, Recombinant** *see* Alteplase *on page 41*

◆ **Alteplase, Tissue Plasminogen Activator, Recombinant** *see* Alteplase *on page 41*

◆ **Alti-MPA (Can)** *see* MedroxyPROGESTERone *on page 739*

Altretamine (al TRET a meen)

Medication Safety Issues

High alert medication: The Institute for Safe Medication Practices (ISMP) includes this medication among its list of drugs which have a heightened risk of causing significant patient harm when used in error.

International issues:

Hexalen®: Brand name for hexetidine in Greece

Related Information

Safe Handling of Hazardous Drugs on page 1517

U.S. Brand Names Hexalen®

Index Terms Hexamethylmelamine; HEXM; HMM; HXM; NSC-13875

Generic Available No

Canadian Brand Names Hexalen®

Pharmacologic Category Antineoplastic Agent, Miscellaneous

Use Palliative treatment of persistent or recurrent ovarian cancer

Pregnancy Risk Factor D

Lactation Excretion in breast milk unknown/not recommended

Labeled Contraindications Hypersensitivity to altretamine or any component of the formulation; pre-existing severe bone marrow suppression or severe neurologic toxicity; pregnancy

Warnings/Precautions Hazardous agent - use appropriate precautions for handling and disposal. **[U.S. Boxed Warning]: Peripheral blood counts and neurologic examinations should be done routinely before and after drug therapy.** Myelosuppression and neurotoxicity are common; use with caution in patients previously treated with other myelosuppressive drugs or with pre-existing neurotoxicity. Use with caution in patients with renal or hepatic dysfunction. **[U.S. Boxed Warning]: Should be administered under the supervision of an experienced cancer chemotherapy physician.** Safety and efficacy in children have not been established.

Adverse Reactions

>10%:

Central nervous system: Peripheral sensory neuropathy (31%; moderate-to-severe 9%), neurotoxicity (21%; may be progressive and dose limiting)

Gastrointestinal: Nausea/vomiting (33% to 70%; severe 1%), diarrhea (48%)

Hematologic: Anemia (33%), leukopenia (5% to 15%; grade 4: 1%), neutropenia

1% to 10%:

Central nervous system: Fatigue (1%), seizure (1%)

Gastrointestinal: Stomach cramps, anorexia (1%)

Hematologic: Thrombocytopenia (9%)

Hepatic: Alkaline phosphatase increased (9%)

<1%: Alopecia, ataxia, depression, dizziness, hepatotoxicity, mood disorders, pruritus, rash, tremor, vertigo

Drug Interactions

Avoid Concomitant Use

Avoid concomitant use of Altretamine with any of the following: Natalizumab; Vaccines (Live)

Increased Effect/Toxicity

Altretamine may increase the levels/effects of: Leflunomide; MAO Inhibitors; Natalizumab; Tricyclic Antidepressants; Vaccines (Live)

The levels/effects of Altretamine may be increased by: MAO Inhibitors; Trastuzumab

Decreased Effect

Altretamine may decrease the levels/effects of: Vaccines (Inactivated); Vaccines (Live)

The levels/effects of Altretamine may be decreased by: Echinacea; Pyridoxine

Storage/Stability Store at 15°C to 30°C (59°F to 86°F).

Mechanism of Action Although altretamine's clinical antitumor spectrum resembles that of alkylating agents, the drug has demonstrated activity in alkylator-resistant patients. The drug selectively inhibits the incorporation of radioactive thymidine and uridine into DNA and RNA, inhibiting DNA and RNA synthesis; reactive intermediates covalently bind to microsomal proteins and DNA; can spontaneously degrade to demethylated melamines and form-aldehyde which are also cytotoxic.

Pharmacodynamics/Kinetics

Absorption: Well absorbed (75% to 89%)

Distribution: Highly concentrated hepatically and renally; low in other organs

Protein binding: 50% to 94%

Metabolism: Hepatic; rapid and extensive demethylation to active metabolites (pentamethylmelamine and tetramethylmelamine)

Half-life elimination: 13 hours

Time to peak, plasma: 0.5-3 hours

Excretion: Urine (90%, <1% as unchanged drug)

Dosage Refer to individual protocols. Oral: Adults:

Ovarian cancer: 260 mg/m^2/day in 4 divided doses for 14 or 21 days of a 28-day cycle

Alternatively (unlabeled use): 4-12 mg/kg/day in 3-4 divided doses for 21-90 days

Alternatively (unlabeled use): 240-320 mg/m^2/day in 3-4 divided doses for 21 days, repeated every 6 weeks

Alternatively (unlabeled use): 150 mg/m^2/day in 3-4 divided doses for 14 days of a 28-day cycle

Dosage adjustment for toxicity: Temporarily withhold for 14 days or longer, and resume dose at 200 mg/m^2/day for any of the following:

Platelet count <75,000/mm^3

White blood cell count <2000/mm^3 or granulocyte count <1000/mm^3

Progressive neurotoxicity

Gastrointestinal intolerance not responsive to antiemetic regimens

Administration Administer total daily dose as 3-4 divided doses after meals and at bedtime.

Monitoring Parameters CBC with differential, liver function tests; neurologic examination

Dietary Considerations Should be taken after meals at bedtime.

Emetic Potential High (>90%)

Dosage Forms Excipient information presented when available (limited, particularly for generics); consult specific product labeling.

Gelcap:

Hexalen®: 50 mg

References

Damia G and D'Incalci M, "Clinical Pharmacokinetics of Altretamine," *Clin Pharmacokinet*, 1995, 28 (6):439-48.

Lee CR and Faulds D, "Altretamine. A Review of Its Pharmacodynamic and Pharmacokinetic Properties, and Therapeutic Potential in Cancer Chemotherapy," *Drugs*, 1995, 49(6):932-53.

Manetta A, Mac Neill C, Lyter JA, et al, "Hexamethylmelamine as a Single Second-Line Agent in Ovarian Cancer," *Gynecol Oncol*, 1990, 36(1):93-6.

Sutton GP, "Secondary Therapy for Epithelial Ovarian Cancer - 1994," *Semin Oncol*, 1994, 21(4 Suppl 7):32-6.

Thigpen JT, Vance RB, and Khansur T, "Second-Line Chemotherapy for Recurrent Carcinoma of the Ovary," *Cancer*, 1993, 71(4 Suppl):1559-64.

◆ **AmBisome®** see Amphotericin B (Liposomal) on page 74

◆ **AMD3100** see Plerixafor on page 965

◆ **A-Methapred** see MethylPREDNISolone on page 782

◆ **A-Methapred®** see MethylPREDNISolone on page 782

◆ **Amethopterin** see Methotrexate on page 768

◆ **AMG 073** see Cinacalcet on page 225

◆ **AMG 531** see Romiplostim on page 1024

◆ **Amicar®** see Aminocaproic Acid on page 57

Amifostine (am i FOS teen)

Medication Safety Issues
Sound-alike/look-alike issues:
Ethyol® may be confused with ethanol

U.S. Brand Names Ethyol®

Index Terms Ethiofos; Gammaphos; WR-2721; YM-08310

Generic Available Yes

Canadian Brand Names Ethyol®

Pharmacologic Category Adjuvant, Chemoprotective Agent (Cytoprotective); Antidote

Use Reduce the incidence of moderate-to-severe xerostomia in patients undergoing postoperative radiation treatment for head and neck cancer, where the radiation port includes a substantial portion of the parotid glands; reduce the cumulative renal toxicity associated with repeated administration of cisplatin

Unlabeled/Investigational Use Prevention of radiation proctitis in patients with rectal cancer

Pregnancy Risk Factor C

Lactation Excretion in breast milk unknown/not recommended

Labeled Contraindications Hypersensitivity to aminothiol compounds or any component of the formulation

Warnings/Precautions Patients who are hypotensive or dehydrated should not receive amifostine. Interrupt antihypertensive therapy for 24 hours before treatment; patients who cannot safely stop their antihypertensives 24 hours before, should not receive amifostine. Adequately hydrated prior to treatment and keep in a supine position during infusion. Monitor blood pressure every 5 minutes during the infusion. If hypotension requiring interruption of therapy occurs, patients should be placed in the Trendelenburg position and given an infusion of normal saline using a separate I.V. line; subsequent infusions may require a dose reduction. Infusions >15 minutes are associated with a higher incidence of adverse effects. Use caution in patients with cardiovascular and cerebrovascular disease and any other patients in whom the adverse effects of hypotension may have serious adverse events.

Serious cutaneous reactions, including erythema multiforme, Stevens-Johnson syndrome, toxic epidermal necrolysis, toxoderma and exfoliative dermatitis have been reported with amifostine. May be delayed, developing up to weeks after treatment initiation. Cutaneous reactions have been reported more frequently when used as a radioprotectant. Discontinue treatment for severe/serious cutaneous reaction, or with fever. Withhold treatment and obtain dermatologic consultation for rash involving lips or mucosa (of unknown etiology outside of radiation port) and for bullous, edematous or erythematous lesions on hands, feet, or trunk; reinitiate only after careful evaluation.

It is recommended that antiemetic medication, including dexamethasone 20 mg I.V. and a serotonin 5-HT$_3$ receptor antagonist be administered prior to and in conjunction with amifostine. Rare hypersensitivity reactions, including anaphylaxis and allergic reaction, have been reported; discontinue if allergic reaction occurs; do not rechallenge. Medications for the treatment of hypersensitivity reactions should be available.

Reports of clinically-relevant hypocalcemia are rare, but serum calcium levels should be monitored in patients at risk of hypocalcemia, such as those with nephrotic syndrome; may require calcium supplementation. Should not be used (in patients receiving chemotherapy for malignancies other than ovarian cancer) where chemotherapy is expected to provide significant survival benefit or in patients receiving definitive radiotherapy, unless within the context of a clinical trial. Safety and efficacy in children have not been established.

Adverse Reactions

>10%:

Cardiovascular: Hypotension (15% to 61%; grades 3/4: 3% to 8%; dose dependent)

Gastrointestinal: Nausea/vomiting (53% to 96%; grades 3/4: 8% to 30%; dose dependent)

1% to 10%: Endocrine & metabolic: Hypocalcemia (clinically significant: 1%)

<1%, postmarketing, and/or case reports: Apnea, anaphylactoid reactions, anaphylaxis, arrhythmia, atrial fibrillation, atrial flutter, back pain, bradycardia, cardiac arrest, chest pain, chest tightness, chills, cutaneous eruptions, dizziness, erythema multiforme, exfoliative dermatitis, extrasystoles, dyspnea, fever, flushing, hiccups, hypersensitivity reactions (fever, rash, hypoxia, dyspnea, laryngeal edema), hypertension (transient), hypoxia, malaise, MI, myocardial ischemia, pruritus, rash (mild), renal failure, respiratory arrest, rigors, seizure, sneezing, somnolence, Stevens-Johnson syndrome, supraventricular tachycardia, syncope, tachycardia, toxic epidermal necrolysis, toxoderma, urticaria

Drug Interactions

Avoid Concomitant Use There are no known interactions where it is recommended to avoid concomitant use.

Increased Effect/Toxicity

The levels/effects of Amifostine may be increased by: Antihypertensives

Decreased Effect There are no known significant interactions involving a decrease in effect.

Storage/Stability Store intact vials of lyophilized powder at room temperature of 20°C to 25°C (68°F to 77°F). Reconstituted solutions (500 mg/10 mL) and solutions for infusion are chemically stable for up to 5 hours at room temperature (25°C) or up to 24 hours under refrigeration (2°C to 8°C).

Reconstitution For I.V. infusion, reconstitute intact vials with 9.7 mL 0.9% sodium chloride injection and dilute in 0.9% sodium chloride to a final concentration of 5-40 mg/mL. For SubQ administration, reconstitute with 2.5 mL NS or SWFI.

Compatibility Stable in NS.

Y-site administration: Compatible: Amikacin, aminophylline, ampicillin, ampicillin/sulbactam, aztreonam, bleomycin, bumetanide, buprenorphine, butorphanol, calcium gluconate, carboplatin, carmustine, cefazolin, ▶

cefotaxime, cefotetan, cefoxitin, ceftazidime, ceftizoxime, ceftriaxone, cefuroxime, cimetidine, ciprofloxacin, clindamycin, co-trimoxazole, cyclophosphamide, cytarabine, dacarbazine, dactinomycin, daunorubicin HCl, dexamethasone sodium phosphate, diphenhydramine, dobutamine, docetaxel, dopamine, doxorubicin HCl, doxycycline, droperidol, enalaprilat, etoposide, famotidine, floxuridine, fluconazole, fludarabine, fluorouracil, furosemide, gallium nitrate, gemcitabine, gentamicin, granisetron, haloperidol lactate, heparin, hydrocortisone sodium succinate, hydromorphone, idarubicin, ifosfamide, imipenem/cilastatin, leucovorin calcium, lorazepam, magnesium sulfate, mannitol, mechlorethamine, meperidine, mesna, methotrexate, methylprednisolone sodium succinate, metoclopramide, metronidazole, mitomycin, mitoxantrone, morphine, nalbuphine, ondansetron, pemetrexed, piperacillin, potassium chloride, promethazine, ranitidine, sodium bicarbonate, streptozocin, teniposide, thiotepa, ticarcillin/clavulanate, tobramycin, vancomycin, vinblastine, vincristine, zidovudine. **Incompatible:** Acyclovir, amphotericin B, chlorpromazine, cisplatin, ganciclovir, hydroxyzine HCl, prochlorperazine edisylate.

Mechanism of Action Prodrug that is dephosphorylated by alkaline phosphatase in tissues to a pharmacologically-active free thiol metabolite. The free thiol is available to bind to, and detoxify, reactive metabolites of cisplatin; and can also act as a scavenger of free radicals that may be generated (by cisplatin or radiation therapy) in tissues.

Pharmacodynamics/Kinetics

Distribution: V_d: 3.5 L

Metabolism: Hepatic dephosphorylation to two metabolites (active-free thiol and disulfide)

Half-life elimination: ~8-9 minutes

Excretion: Urine

Clearance, plasma: 2.17 L/minute

Dosage Note: Antiemetic medication, including dexamethasone 20 mg I.V. and a serotonin 5-HT$_3$ receptor antagonist, is recommended prior to and in conjunction with amifostine.

Adults:

Cisplatin-induced renal toxicity, reduction: I.V.: 910 mg/m^2 over 15 minutes once daily 30 minutes prior to cisplatin

For 910 mg/m^2 doses, the manufacturer suggests the following blood pressure-based adjustment schedule:

The infusion of amifostine should be interrupted if the systolic blood pressure decreases significantly from baseline, as defined below:

Decrease of 20 mm Hg if baseline systolic blood pressure <100

Decrease of 25 mm Hg if baseline systolic blood pressure 100-119

Decrease of 30 mm Hg if baseline systolic blood pressure 120-139

Decrease of 40 mm Hg if baseline systolic blood pressure 140-179

Decrease of 50 mm Hg if baseline systolic blood pressure ≥180

If blood pressure returns to normal within 5 minutes (assisted by fluid administration and postural management) and the patient is asymptomatic, the infusion may be restarted so that the full dose of amifostine may be administered. If the full dose of amifostine cannot be administered, the dose of amifostine for subsequent cycles should be 740 mg/m^2.

Xerostomia from head and neck cancer, reduction:

I.V.: 200 mg/m^2 over 3 minutes once daily 15-30 minutes prior to radiation therapy **or**

SubQ (unlabeled route): 500 mg once daily prior to radiation therapy

Prevention of radiation proctitis in rectal cancer (unlabeled use): I.V.: 340 mg/m^2 once daily prior to radiation therapy (Keefe, 2007; Peterson, 2008)

Administration I.V.: Administer over 3 minutes (prior to radiation therapy) or 15 minutes (prior to cisplatin); administration as a longer infusion is associated with a higher incidence of side effects. Patients should be kept in supine position during infusion. **Note:** SubQ administration (unlabeled) has been used.

Monitoring Parameters Blood pressure should be monitored every 5 minutes during the infusion and after administration if clinically indicated; serum calcium levels (in patients at risk for hypocalcemia). Evaluate for cutaneous reactions prior to each dose.

Additional Information Oncology Comment: The American Society of Clinical Oncology (ASCO) guidelines for the use of protectants for chemotherapy and radiation (Hensley, 2008) recommend the use of amifostine for prevention of nephrotoxicity due to cisplatin-based chemotherapy and to decrease the incidence of acute and delayed radiation therapy-induced xerostomia. The ASCO guidelines do not recommend the use of amifostine to reduce the incidence of neutropenia or thrombocytopenia associated with chemotherapy or radiation therapy, neurotoxicity or ototoxicity associated with platinum-based chemotherapy, radiation therapy-induced mucositis associated with head and neck cancer, or esophagitis due to chemotherapy in patients with nonsmall cell lung cancer. Additionally, the guidelines do not support the use of amifostine in patients with head and neck cancer receiving concurrent platinum-based chemotherapy.

Emetic Potential
>300 mg/m^2: Moderate (30% to 90%)
≤300 mg/m^2: Low (10% to 30%)

Dosage Forms Excipient information presented when available (limited, particularly for generics); consult specific product labeling.
Injection, powder for reconstitution: 500 mg
Ethyol®: 500 mg

References

Anne PR and Curran WJ Jr, "A Phase II Trial of Subcutaneous Amifostine and Radiation Therapy in Patients With Head and Neck Cancer," *Semin Radiat Oncol*, 2002, 12(1 Suppl 1):18-9.

Bonner HS and Shaw LM, "New Dosing Regimens for Amifostine: A Pilot Study to Compare the Relative Bioavailability of Oral and Subcutaneous Administration With Intravenous Infusion," *J Clin Pharmacol*, 2002, 42(2):166-74.

Brizel DM, Wasserman TH, Henke M, et al, "Phase III Randomized Trial of Amifostine as a Radioprotector in Head and Neck Cancer," *J Clin Oncol*, 2000, 18(19): 3339-45.

Hensley ML, Hagerty KL, Kewalramani T, et al, "American Society of Clinical Oncology 2008 Clinical Practice Guideline Update: Use of Chemotherapy and Radiotherapy Protectants," *J Clin Oncol*, 2009, 27(1): 127-45.

Keefe DM, Schubert MM, Elting LS, et al, "Updated Clinical Practice Guidelines for the Prevention and Treatment of Mucositis," *Cancer*, 2007, 109(5): 820-31.

Koukourakis MI, Kyrias G, and Kakolyris S, "Subcutaneous Administration of Amifostine During Fractionated Radiotherapy: A Randomized Phase II Study," *J Clin Oncol*, 2000, 18(11):2226-33.

Peterson DE, Bensadiun RJ, and Roila F, "Management of Oral and Gastrointestinal Mucositis: ESMO Clinical Recommendations," *Ann Oncol*, 2008, 19(Suppl 2): 122-5.

Samuels MA, Chico IM, Hirsch RL, et al, "Ongoing Prospective Multicenter Safety Study of the Cytoprotectant Amifostine Given Subcutaneously: Overview of Trial Design," *Semin Oncol*, 2003, 30(6 Suppl 18):94-5.

Amikacin (am i KAY sin)

Medication Safety Issues

Sound-alike/look-alike issues:

Amikacin may be confused with Amicar®, anakinra
Amikin® may be confused with Amicar®, Kineret®

◄ **Index Terms** Amikacin Sulfate

Generic Available Yes

Canadian Brand Names Amikacin Sulfate Injection, USP; Amikin®

Pharmacologic Category Antibiotic, Aminoglycoside

Use Treatment of serious infections (bone infections, respiratory tract infections, endocarditis, and septicemia) due to organisms resistant to gentamicin and tobramycin, including *Pseudomonas*, *Proteus*, *Serratia*, and other gram-negative bacilli; documented infection of mycobacterial organisms susceptible to amikacin

Unlabeled/Investigational Use Bacterial endophthalmitis

Pregnancy Risk Factor D

Lactation Enters breast milk/compatible

Labeled Contraindications Hypersensitivity to amikacin sulfate or any component of the formulation; cross-sensitivity may exist with other aminoglycosides

Warnings/Precautions [U.S. Boxed Warning]: Amikacin may cause neurotoxicity, nephrotoxicity, and/or neuromuscular blockade and respiratory paralysis; usual risk factors include pre-existing renal impairment, concomitant neuro-/nephrotoxic medications, advanced age and dehydration. Dose and/or frequency of administration must be monitored and modified in patients with renal impairment. Drug should be discontinued if signs of ototoxicity, nephrotoxicity, or hypersensitivity occur. Ototoxicity is proportional to the amount of drug given and the duration of treatment. Tinnitus or vertigo may be indications of vestibular injury and impending bilateral irreversible damage. Renal damage is usually reversible. Use with caution in patients with neuromuscular disorders, hearing loss and hypocalcemia. Prolonged use may result in fungal or bacterial superinfection, including *C. difficile*-associated diarrhea (CDAD) and pseudomembranous colitis; CDAD has been observed >2 months postantibiotic treatment. Solution contains sodium metabisulfate; use caution in patients with sulfite allergy.

Adverse Reactions

1% to 10%:

Central nervous system: Neurotoxicity

Otic: Ototoxicity (auditory), ototoxicity (vestibular)

Renal: Nephrotoxicity

<1%: Allergic reaction, arthralgia, drowsiness, drug fever, dyspnea, eosinophilia, headache, hypotension, nausea, paresthesia, rash, tremor, vomiting, weakness

Drug Interactions

Avoid Concomitant Use

Avoid concomitant use of Amikacin with any of the following: Gallium Nitrate

Increased Effect/Toxicity

Amikacin may increase the levels/effects of: AbobotulinumtoxinA; Bisphosphonate Derivatives; CARBOplatin; Colistimethate; CycloSPORINE; Gallium Nitrate; Neuromuscular-Blocking Agents; OnabotulinumtoxinA; RimabotulinumtoxinB

The levels/effects of Amikacin may be increased by: Amphotericin B; Capreomycin; CISplatin; Loop Diuretics; Nonsteroidal Anti-Inflammatory Agents; Vancomycin

Decreased Effect

Amikacin may decrease the levels/effects of: Typhoid Vaccine

The levels/effects of Amikacin may be decreased by: Penicillins

Storage/Stability Store at controlled room temperature. Following admixture at concentrations of 0.25-5 mg/mL, amikcain is stable for 24 hours at room temperature and 2 days at refrigeration when mixed in D_5W, NS, and LR.

Compatibility Stable in dextran 75 6% in NS, D_5LR, $D_5$1/4NS, $D_5$1/3NS, $D_5$1/2NS, D_5NS, D_{10}NS, D_5W, $D_{10}W$, $D_{20}W$, mannitol 20%, 1/4NS, 1/2NS, NS; **variable stability (consult detailed reference)** in peritoneal dialysis solutions.

Y-site administration: Compatible: Acyclovir, alatrofloxacin, amifostine, amiodarone, amsacrine, aztreonam, cefpirome, cisatracurium, cyclophosphamide, dexamethasone sodium phosphate, diltiazem, docetaxel, enalaprilat, esmolol, etoposide, filgrastim, fluconazole, fludarabine, foscarnet, furosemide, gatifloxacin, gemcitabine, granisetron, idarubicin, IL-2, labetalol, levofloxacin, linezolid, lorazepam, magnesium sulfate, melphalan, midazolam, morphine, ondansetron, paclitaxel, perphenazine, remifentanil, sargramostim, teniposide, thiotepa, vinorelbine, warfarin, zidovudine. **Incompatible:** Allopurinol, amphotericin B cholesteryl sulfate complex, hetastarch, propofol.

Compatibility in syringe: Compatible: Clindamycin, doxapram. **Incompatible:** Heparin.

Compatibility when admixed: Compatible: Amobarbital, ascorbic acid injection, bleomycin, calcium chloride, calcium gluconate, cefepime, cefoxitin, chloramphenicol, chlorpheniramine, cimetidine, ciprofloxacin, clindamycin, colistimethate, dimenhydrinate, diphenhydramine, epinephrine, ergonovine, fluconazole, furosemide, hyaluronidase, hydrocortisone sodium phosphate, hydrocortisone sodium succinate, lincomycin, metaraminol, metronidazole, metronidazole with sodium bicarbonate, norepinephrine, pentobarbital, phenobarbital, phytonadione, polymyxin B sulfate, prochlorperazine edisylate, promethazine, ranitidine, sodium bicarbonate, succinylcholine, vancomycin, verapamil. **Incompatible:** Amphotericin B, ampicillin, cefazolin, chlorothiazide, heparin, phenytoin, thiopental, vitamin B complex with C. **Variable (consult detailed reference):** Aminophylline, dexamethasone sodium phosphate, oxacillin, penicillin G potassium, potassium chloride.

Mechanism of Action Inhibits protein synthesis in susceptible bacteria by binding to 30S ribosomal subunits

Pharmacodynamics/Kinetics

Absorption:

I.M.: Rapid

Oral: Poorly absorbed

Distribution: Primarily into extracellular fluid (highly hydrophilic); penetrates blood-brain barrier when meninges inflamed

Relative diffusion of antimicrobial agents from blood into CSF: Good only with inflammation (exceeds usual MICs)

CSF:blood level ratio: Normal meninges: 10% to 20%; Inflamed meninges: 15% to 24%

Protein-binding: 0% to 11%

Half-life elimination (renal function and age dependent):

Infants: Low birth weight (1-3 days): 7-9 hours; Full-term >7 days: 4-5 hours

Children: 1.6-2.5 hours

Adults: Normal renal function: 1.4-2.3 hours; Anuria/end-stage renal disease: 28-86 hours

Time to peak, serum: I.M.: 45-120 minutes

Excretion: Urine (94% to 98%)

Dosage Note: Individualization is critical because of the low therapeutic index

Use of ideal body weight (IBW) for determining the mg/kg/dose appears to be more accurate than dosing on the basis of total body weight (TBW)

In morbid obesity, dosage requirement may best be estimated using a dosing weight of IBW + 0.4 (TBW - IBW)

Initial and periodic peak and trough plasma drug levels should be determined, particularly in critically-ill patients with serious infections or in disease states known to significantly alter aminoglycoside pharmacokinetics (eg, cystic fibrosis, burns, or major surgery). Manufacturer recommends a maximum daily dose of 15 mg/kg/day (or 1.5 g/day in heavier patients). Higher doses may be warranted based on therapeutic drug monitoring or susceptibility information.

Usual dosage range:

Infants and Children: I.M., I.V.: 5-7.5 mg/kg/dose every 8 hours

Adults: I.M., I.V.: 5-7.5 mg/kg/dose every 8 hours

Note: Some clinicians suggest a daily dose of 15-20 mg/kg for all patients with normal renal function. This dose is at least as efficacious with similar, if not less, toxicity than conventional dosing.

Indication-specific dosing:

Adults:

Endophthalmitis, bacterial (unlabeled use): Intravitreal: 0.4 mg/0.1 mL NS in combination with vancomycin

Hospital-acquired pneumonia (HAP): I.V.: 20 mg/kg/day with antipseudomonal beta-lactam or carbapenem (American Thoracic Society/ATS guidelines)

Meningitis *(Pseudomonas aeruginosa):* I.V.: 5 mg/kg every 8 hours (administered with another bacteriocidal drug)

Mycobacterium fortuitum, M. chelonae, or M. abscessus: I.V.: 10-15 mg/kg daily for at least 2 weeks with high dose cefoxitin

Dosing interval in renal impairment: Some patients may require larger or more frequent doses if serum levels document the need (ie, cystic fibrosis or febrile granulocytopenic patients).

Cl_{cr} ≥60 mL/minute: Administer every 8 hours

Cl_{cr} 40-60 mL/minute: Administer every 12 hours

Cl_{cr} 20-40 mL/minute: Administer every 24 hours

Cl_{cr} <20 mL/minute: Loading dose, then monitor levels

Hemodialysis: Dialyzable (50% to 100%); administer dose postdialysis or administer 2/3 normal dose as a supplemental dose postdialysis and follow levels

Peritoneal dialysis: Dose as Cl_{cr} <20 mL/minute: Follow levels

Continuous arteriovenous or venovenous hemodiafiltration effects: Dose as for Cl_{cr} 10-40 mL/minute and follow levels

Administration Administer around-the-clock to promote less variation in peak and trough serum levels. Do not mix with other drugs, administer separately.

I.M.: Administer I.M. injection in large muscle mass.

I.V.: Infuse over 30-60 minutes.

Some penicillins (eg, carbenicillin, ticarcillin, and piperacillin) have been shown to inactivate *in vitro*. This has been observed to a greater extent with tobramycin and gentamicin, while amikacin has shown greater stability against inactivation. Concurrent use of these agents may pose a risk of reduced antibacterial efficacy *in vivo*, particularly in the setting of profound renal impairment. However, definitive clinical evidence is lacking. If combination penicillin/aminoglycoside therapy is desired in a patient with renal dysfunction, separation of doses (if feasible), and routine monitoring of aminoglycoside levels, CBC, and clinical response should be considered.

Monitoring Parameters Urinalysis, BUN, serum creatinine, appropriately timed peak and trough concentrations, vital signs, temperature, weight, I & O, hearing parameters

Some penicillin derivatives may accelerate the degradation of aminoglycosides *in vitro*. This may be clinically-significant for certain penicillin (ticarcillin, piperacillin, carbenicillin) and aminoglycoside (gentamicin, tobramycin) combination therapy in patients with significant renal impairment. Close monitoring of aminoglycoside levels is warranted.

Test Interactions Some penicillin derivatives may accelerate the degradation of aminoglycosides *in vitro*, leading to a potential underestimation of aminoglycoside serum concentration.

Dietary Considerations Sodium content of 1 g: 29.9 mg (1.3 mEq)

Additional Information Aminoglycoside levels measured from blood taken from Silastic® central catheters can sometimes give falsely high readings (draw levels from alternate lumen or peripheral stick, if possible).

Dosage Forms Excipient information presented when available (limited, particularly for generics); consult specific product labeling.

Injection, solution, as sulfate: 50 mg/mL (2 mL); 250 mg/mL (2 mL, 4 mL)

References

American Thoracic Society and Infectious Diseases Society of America, "Guidelines for the Management of Adults With Hospital-Acquired, Ventilator-Associated, and Healthcare-Associated Pneumonia," *Am J Respir Crit Care Med*, 2005, 171(4):388-416.

Lortholary O, Tod M, Cohen Y, et al, "Aminoglycosides," *Med Clin North Am*, 1995, 79(4):761-87.

McCormack JP and Jewesson PJ, "A Critical Re-evaluation of the "Therapeutic Range" of Aminoglycosides," *Clin Infect Dis*, 1992, 14(1):320-39

Nicolau DP, Freeman CD, Belliveau PP, et al, "Experience With a Once-Daily Aminoglycoside Program Administered to 2184 Adult Patients," *Antimicrob Agents Chemother*, 1995, 39(3):650-5.

Preston SL and Briceland LL, "Single Daily Dosing of Aminoglycosides," *Pharmacotherapy*, 1995, 15(3):297-316.

Van der Auwera P, "Pharmacokinetic Evaluation of Single Daily Dose Amikacin," *J Antimicrob Chemother*, 1991, 27(Suppl C):63-71.

Vanhaeverbeek M, Siska G, Douchamps J, et al, "Comparison of the Efficacy and Safety of Amikacin Once or Twice-a-Day in the Treatment of Severe Gram-Negative Infections in the Elderly," *Int J Clin Pharmacol Ther Toxicol*, 1993, 31(3):153-6.

♦ **Amikacin Sulfate** *see* Amikacin *on page 53*

♦ **Amikacin Sulfate Injection, USP (Can)** *see* Amikacin *on page 53*

♦ **Amikin® (Can)** *see* Amikacin *on page 53*

♦ **2-Amino-6-Mercaptopurine** *see* Thioguanine *on page 1098*

♦ **2-Amino-6-Methoxypurine Arabinoside** *see* Nelarabine *on page 843*

Aminocaproic Acid (a mee noe ka PROE ik AS id)

Medication Safety Issues

Sound-alike/look-alike issues:

Amicar® may be confused with amikacin, Amikin®, Omacor®

U.S. Brand Names Amicar®

Index Terms EACA; Epsilon Aminocaproic Acid

Generic Available Yes

Pharmacologic Category Antifibrinolytic Agent; Antihemophilic Agent; Hemostatic Agent; Lysine Analog

Use To enhance hemostasis when fibrinolysis contributes to bleeding (causes may include cardiac surgery, hematologic disorders, neoplastic disorders, abruption placentae, hepatic cirrhosis, and urinary fibrinolysis)

Unlabeled/Investigational Use Treatment of traumatic hyphema; control bleeding in thrombocytopenia; control oral bleeding in congenital and acquired coagulation disorders; topical treatment (mouth rinse) of bleeding associated with dental procedures in patients on oral anticoagulant therapy; prevention of perioperative bleeding associated with cardiac surgery

Pregnancy Risk Factor C

Lactation Excretion in breast milk unknown/use caution

Labeled Contraindications Disseminated intravascular coagulation (without heparin); evidence of an active intravascular clotting process

Warnings/Precautions Avoid rapid I.V. administration (may induce hypotension, bradycardia, or arrhythmia); rapid injection of undiluted solution is not recommended. Use with caution in patients with renal disease; aminocaproic acid may accumulate in patients with decreased renal function. Intrarenal obstruction may occur secondary to glomerular capillary thrombosis or clots in the renal pelvis and ureters. Do not use in hematuria of upper urinary tract origin unless possible benefits outweigh risks. Do not administer without a definite diagnosis of laboratory findings indicative of hyperfibrinolysis. Inhibition of fibrinolysis may promote clotting or thrombosis; more likely due to the presence of DIC. Skeletal muscle weakness ranging from mild myalgias and fatigue to severe myopathy with rhabdomyolysis and acute renal failure has been reported with prolonged use. Monitor CPK; discontinue treatment with a rise in CPK. Benzyl alcohol is used as a preservative in the injection; therefore, these products should not be used in the neonate. Do not administer with factor IX complex concentrates or anti-inhibitor coagulant complexes; may increase risk for thrombosis.

Adverse Reactions Frequency not defined.

Cardiovascular: Arrhythmia, bradycardia, edema, hypotension, intracranial hypertension, peripheral ischemia, syncope, thrombosis

Central nervous system: Confusion, delirium, dizziness, fatigue, hallucinations, headache, malaise, seizure, stroke

Dermatologic: Rash, pruritus

Gastrointestinal: Abdominal pain, anorexia, cramps, diarrhea, GI irritation, nausea, vomiting

Genitourinary: Dry ejaculation

Hematologic: Agranulocytosis, bleeding time increased, leukopenia, thrombocytopenia

Local: Injection site necrosis, injection site pain, injectionsite reactions

Neuromuscular & skeletal: CPK increased, myalgia, myositis, myopathy, rhabdomyolysis (rare), weakness

Ophthalmic: Vision decreased, watery eyes

Otic: Tinnitus

Renal: BUN increased, intrarenal obstruction (glomerular capillary thrombosis), myoglobinuria (rare), renal failure (rare)

Respiratory: Dyspnea, nasal congestion, pulmonary embolism

Miscellaneous: Allergic reaction, anaphylactoid reaction, anaphylaxis

Postmarketing and/or case reports: Hepatic lesion, myocardial lesion

Drug Interactions

Avoid Concomitant Use

Avoid concomitant use of Aminocaproic Acid with any of the following: Anti-inhibitor Coagulant Complex; Factor IX; Factor IX Complex (Human)

Increased Effect/Toxicity

Aminocaproic Acid may increase the levels/effects of: Anti-inhibitor Coagulant Complex; Factor IX; Factor IX Complex (Human); Fibrinogen Concentrate (Human)

The levels/effects of Aminocaproic Acid may be increased by: Fibrinogen Concentrate (Human); Tretinoin (Oral)

Decreased Effect There are no known significant interactions involving a decrease in effect.

Storage/Stability Store intact vials, tablets, and syrup at 15°C to 30°C (59°F to 86°F). Do not freeze injection or syrup. Solutions diluted for I.V. use in D_5W or NS to concentrations of 10-100 mg/mL are stable at 4°C (39°F) and 23°C (73°F) for 7 days (Zhang, 1997).

Reconstitution Dilute I.V. solution in D_5W, 0.9% sodium chloride, or Ringer's injection.

Compatibility Stable in D_5W, NS, Ringer's injection

Mechanism of Action Binds competitively to plasminogen; blocking the binding of plasminogen to fibrin and the subsequent conversion to plasmin, resulting in inhibition of fibrin degradation (fibrinolysis).

Pharmacodynamics/Kinetics

Onset of action: ~1-72 hours

Distribution: Widely through intravascular and extravascular compartments
V_d: Oral: 23 L, I.V.: 30 L

Metabolism: Minimally hepatic

Half-life elimination: ~2 hours

Time to peak: Oral: Within 2 hours

Excretion: Urine (65% as unchanged drug, 11% as metabolite)

Dosage

Acute bleeding syndrome:
   Children (unlabeled use): Oral, I.V.: Loading dose: 100-200 mg/kg during the first hour, followed by continuous infusion at 33.3 mg/kg/hour (I.V.) or 100 mg/kg (oral or I.V.) every 6 hours
   Adults: Oral, I.V.: Loading dose: 4-5 g during the first hour, followed by 1 g/hour (or 1.25 g/hour using oral solution) for 8 hours or until bleeding controlled (maximum daily dose: 30 g)

Control of bleeding in thrombocytopenia (unlabeled use): Adults:
   Initial: I.V.: 100 mg/kg over 30-60 minutes
   Maintenance: Oral: 1-3 g every 6 hours

Control of oral bleeding in congenital and acquired coagulation disorder (unlabeled use): Adults: Oral: 50-60 mg/kg every 4 hours

Prevention of dental procedure bleeding in patients on oral anticoagulant therapy (unlabeled use): Oral rinse: Hold 4 g/10 mL in mouth for 2 minutes then spit out. Repeat every 6 hours for 2 days after procedure (Souto, 1996). Concentration and frequency may vary by institution and product availability.

Prevention of perioperative bleeding associated with cardiac surgery (unlabeled use): I.V.:
   Children: 100 mg/kg given over 20-30 minutes after induction and prior to incision, 100 mg/kg during cardiopulmonary bypass, and 100 mg/kg after protamine reversal of heparin
   Adults: 10 g over 20-30 minutes prior to skin incision, followed by 1-2.5 g/hour (usual dose 2 g/hour) until the end of operation (may continue infusion for 4 hours after protamine reversal of heparin). May add 10 g to cardiopulmonary bypass circuit priming solution.
   or
   10 g over 20-30 minutes prior to skin incision, followed by 10 g after heparin administration then 10 g at discontinuation of cardiopulmonary bypass prior to protamine reversal of heparin

Traumatic hyphema (unlabeled use): Children and Adults: Oral: 100 mg/kg/dose every 4 hours (maximum daily dose: 30 g)

◄ **Dosing adjustment in renal impairment:** May accumulate in patients with decreased renal function.

Administration Rapid I.V. injection (IVP) of undiluted solution is not recommended due to possible hypotension, bradycardia, and arrhythmia.

I.V.: Acute bleeding syndrome: Administer loading dose over 1 hour, followed by a continuous infusion

I.V.: Prevention of perioperative bleeding associated with cardiac surgery (unlabeled use): Administer loading dose over 20-30 minutes prior to skin incision, followed by a continuous infusion until the end of operation **or** as 2 additional bolus doses (over 20-30 minutes) given after heparin administration and at discontinuation of cardiopulmonary bypass prior to protamine reversal of heparin.

Monitoring Parameters Fibrinogen, fibrin split products, creatine phosphokinase (with long-term therapy), BUN, creatinine

Dosage Forms Excipient information presented when available (limited, particularly for generics); consult specific product labeling.

Injection, solution: 250 mg/mL (20 mL)

Solution, oral: 1.25 g/5 mL (240 mL, 480 mL)

Syrup:

Amicar®: 1.25 g/5 mL (480 mL) [raspberry flavor]

Tablet [scored]: 500 mg

Amicar®: 500 mg, 1000 mg

References

Bartholomew JR, Salgia R, and Bell WR, "Control of Bleeding in Patients With Immune and Nonimmune Thrombocytopenia With Aminocaproic Acid," *Arch Intern Med*, 1989, 149 (9):1959-61.

Gardner FH and Helmer RE 3rd, "Aminocaproic Acid. Use in Control of Hemorrhage in Patients With Amegakaryocytic Thrombocytopenia," *JAMA*, 1980, 243(1):35-7.

Haut MT, Mauro VF, and Davis HH, "Effect of Renal Failure and Hemodialysis on Aminocaproic Acid Plasma Concentrations," *DICP*, 1989, 23(11):922-3.

Mannucci P, "Hemostatic Drugs," *N Engl J Med*, 1998, 339(4):245-53.

Zhang YP and Trissel LA, "Stability of Aminocaproic Acid Injection Admixtures in 5% Dextrose Injection and 0.9% Sodium Chloride Injection," *Int J Pharm Compound*, 1997, 1(2):132-4.

Aminolevulinic Acid (a MEE noh lev yoo lin ik AS id)

Medication Safety Issues

Sound-alike/look-alike issues:

Aminolevulinic acid may be confused with methyl aminolevulinate

U.S. Brand Names Levulan® Kerastick®

Index Terms 5-ALA; 5-Aminolevulinic Acid; ALA; Amino Levulinic Acid; Aminolevulinic Acid Hydrochloride

Generic Available No

Canadian Brand Names Levulan® Kerastick®

Pharmacologic Category Photosensitizing Agent, Topical; Topical Skin Product

Use Treatment of minimally to moderately thick actinic keratoses (grade 1 or 2) of the face or scalp; to be used in conjunction with blue light illumination

Unlabeled/Investigational Use Photodynamic treatment of low-risk superficial basal cell skin cancer and low-risk squamous cell skin cancer *in situ* (Bowen's disease)

Pregnancy Risk Factor C

Lactation Excretion in breast milk unknown/use caution

Labeled Contraindications Hypersensitivity to aminolevulinic acid or any component of the formulation; individuals with cutaneous photosensitivity at wavelengths of 400-450 nm; porphyria; allergy to porphyrins

Warnings/Precautions Treatment site will become photosensitive following application. Patients should be instructed to avoid exposure to sunlight, bright indoor lights, or tanning beds during the period prior to blue light treatment (exposure may result in lesion burning, edema, erythema and/or stinging). Sunscreen will not protect against visible light; head should be covered with light-opaque material or wide-brimmed hat. If unable to return the next day for blue light treatment, avoid sunlight/bright light exposure to treated lesions for at least 40 hours. Concomitant use of other known photosensitizing agents may increase the degree of photosensitivity reaction.

For external use only. Do not apply to eyes or mucous membranes. Excessive skin irritation may occur if applied under occlusion. Application should involve either scalp or face lesions, although not simultaneously. Should be applied by a qualified health professional to avoid application to perilesional skin. Has not been tested in individuals with coagulation defects (acquired or inherited).

Adverse Reactions Transient stinging, burning, itching, erythema, and edema result from the photosensitizing properties of this agent. Symptoms subside between 1 minute and 24 hours after turning off the blue light illuminator. Severe stinging or burning was reported in at least 50% of patients from at least 1 lesional site during treatment.

>10%: Dermatologic: Stinging or burning (most patients; severe: ≥50%), erythema (99%), scaling/crusted skin (64% to 71%), hyper-/hypopigmentation (22% to 36%), edematous lesions (35%), itching (14% to 25%), erosion (2% to 14%), skin disorder (5% to 12%)

1% to 10%:

Central nervous system: Dysesthesia (≤2%)

Dermatologic: Vesiculation (4% to 5%), skin ulceration (2% to 4%), pustular drug eruption (≤4%)

Hematologic: Bleeding/hemorrhage (2% to 4%)

Local: Wheal/flare (2% to 7%), scabbing (≤2%), tenderness (1% to 2%), edema (≤1%), excoriation (≤1%), local pain (≤1%), oozing (≤1%)

Drug Interactions

Avoid Concomitant Use There are no known interactions where it is recommended to avoid concomitant use.

Increased Effect/Toxicity There are no known significant interactions involving an increase in effect.

Decreased Effect There are no known significant interactions involving a decrease in effect.

Storage/Stability Store at 20°C to 25°C (68°F to 77°F); excursions permitted to 15°C to 30°C (59°F to 86°F). Once prepared, the topical solution should be used immediately and application must be completed within 2 hours of solution preparation.

Reconstitution Follow instructions on Kerastick® Krusher or mix manually: Prepare solution by holding applicator tube with cap pointing up, applying finger pressure to "Position A" on cardboard sleeve to crush ampul containing solution vehicle. Apply finger pressure to "Position B" to crush ampul containing aminolevulinic acid powder. Shake gently for at least 30 seconds to dissolve; point applicator cap away from face while shaking tube. Remove cap; dab dry applicator tip on gauze pad until wet with solution.

Mechanism of Action Aminolevulinic acid is a metabolic precursor of the photosensitizer protoporphyrin IX (PpIX). Photosensitization following local application of aminolevulinic acid occurs through the metabolic conversion to PpIX. When exposed to light of appropriate wavelength and energy, accumulated PpIX produces a photodynamic reaction resulting in local cytotoxicity. Precancerous and cancerous cells exhibit a higher rate of porphyrin induction compared to normal cells.

Pharmacodynamics/Kinetics

Peak fluorescence intensity of protoporphyrin IX (PpIX): Actinic keratosis: 11 hours ± 1 hour; Perilesional skin: 12 hours ± 1 hour

Half-life elimination: Mean fluorescence clearance half-life of PpIX for lesions: 30 ± 10 hours

Dosage Adults: Topical: Apply to actinic keratoses (**not** perilesional skin) followed 14-18 hours later by blue light illumination. Application/treatment may be repeated at a treatment site (once) after 8 weeks.

Administration Dab lesion gently with wet applicator tip (applying enough to uniformly wet lesion without excess running or dripping). Only apply to affected skin. Do not apply to periorbital area, ocular tissue, or mucosal surfaces. Allow to dry, then reapply to same lesion. Apply to either scalp or facial lesions, but not to both simultaneously. Follow application with blue light exposure in 14-18 hours. Do not wash the application area during the time between application and photosensitization; after photosensitization, gently rinse actinic keratosis with water and pat dry. Stinging or burning may occur during blue light treatment. Following blue light treatment, the lesion will temporarily redden, swell and/or scale, which should resolve within 4 weeks after treatment.

Additional Information Use in conjunction with the BLU-U™ Blue Light Photodynamic Therapy Illuminator.

Dosage Forms Excipient information presented when available (limited, particularly for generics); consult specific product labeling.

Powder for topical solution:

Levulan® Kerastick®: 20% (1s, 6s) [2-component system containing aminolevulinic acid hydrochloride 354 mg (powder) and diluent containing ethanol 48% (1.5 mL) packaged together in an applicator tube]

References

Braathen LR, Szeimies RM, Basset-Seguin N, et al, "Guidelines on the Use of Photodynamic Therapy for Nonmelanoma Skin Cancer: An International Consensus. International Society for Photodynamic Therapy in Dermatology, 2005," *J Am Acad Dermatol*, 2007, 56(1):125-43.

Moloney FJ and Collins P, et al, "Randomized, Double-Blind, Prospective Study to Compare Topical 5-Aminolevulinic Acid Methylester With Topical 5-Aminolaevulinic Acid Photodynamic Therapy for Extensive Scalp Actinic Keratosis," *Br J Dermatol*, 2007, 157(1):87-91.

National Comprehensive Cancer Network® (NCCN), "Clinical Practice Guidelines in Oncology™: Basal Cell and Squamous Cell Skin Cancers," Version 1.2009. Available at http://www.nccn.org/professionals/physician_gls/PDF/nmsc.pdf.

Tierney E, Barker A, Ahdout J, et al, "Photodynamic Therapy for the Treatment of Cutaneous Neoplasia, Inflammatory Disorders, and Photoaging," *Dermatol Surg*, 2009, 35(5):725-46.

Amphotericin B Cholesteryl Sulfate Complex
(am foe TER i sin bee kole LES te ril SUL fate KOM plecks)

Medication Safety Issues

Safety issues:

Lipid-based amphotericin formulations (Amphotec®) may be confused with conventional formulations (Amphocin®, Fungizone®)

Large overdoses have occurred when conventional formulations were dispensed inadvertently for lipid-based products. Single daily doses of conventional amphotericin formulation never exceed 1.5 mg/kg.

High alert medication: The Institute for Safe Medication Practices (ISMP) includes this medication among its list of drugs which have a heightened risk of causing significant patient harm when used in error.

U.S. Brand Names Amphotec®

Index Terms ABCD; Amphotericin B Colloidal Dispersion

Generic Available No

Canadian Brand Names Amphotec®

Pharmacologic Category Antifungal Agent, Parenteral

Use Treatment of invasive aspergillosis in patients who have failed amphotericin B deoxycholate treatment, or who have renal impairment or experience unacceptable toxicity which precludes treatment with amphotericin B deoxycholate in effective doses.

Unlabeled/Investigational Use Effective in patients with serious *Candida* species infections

Pregnancy Risk Factor B

Lactation Excretion in breast milk unknown/contraindicated

Labeled Contraindications Hypersensitivity to amphotericin B or any component of the formulation

Warnings/Precautions Anaphylaxis has been reported with amphotericin B-containing drugs. If severe respiratory distress occurs, the infusion should be immediately discontinued. During the initial dosing, the drug should be administered under close clinical observation. Infusion reactions, sometimes severe, usually subside with continued therapy - manage with decreased rate of infusion and pretreatment with antihistamines/corticosteroids.

Adverse Reactions

>10%: Central nervous system: Chills, fever

1% to 10%:

Cardiovascular: Hypotension, tachycardia

Central nervous system: Headache

Dermatologic: Rash

Endocrine & metabolic: Hypokalemia, hypomagnesemia

Gastrointestinal: Nausea, diarrhea, abdominal pain

Hematologic: Thrombocytopenia

Hepatic: LFT change

Neuromuscular & skeletal: Rigors

Renal: Creatinine increased

Respiratory: Dyspnea

Note: Amphotericin B colloidal dispersion has an improved therapeutic index compared to conventional amphotericin B, and has been used safely in patients with amphotericin B-related nephrotoxicity; however, continued decline of renal function has occurred in some patients.

Drug Interactions

Avoid Concomitant Use

Avoid concomitant use of Amphotericin B Cholesteryl Sulfate Complex with any of the following: Gallium Nitrate

Increased Effect/Toxicity

Amphotericin B Cholesteryl Sulfate Complex may increase the levels/effects of: Aminoglycosides; Colistimethate; CycloSPORINE; Flucytosine; Gallium Nitrate

The levels/effects of Amphotericin B Cholesteryl Sulfate Complex may be increased by: Corticosteroids (Orally Inhaled); Corticosteroids (Systemic)

Decreased Effect

Amphotericin B Cholesteryl Sulfate Complex may decrease the levels/effects of: Saccharomyces boulardii

The levels/effects of Amphotericin B Cholesteryl Sulfate Complex may be decreased by: Antifungal Agents (Azole Derivatives, Systemic)

Storage/Stability Store intact vials under refrigeration. After reconstitution, the solution should be refrigerated at 2°C to 8°C (36°F to 46°F) and used within 24 hours. Concentrations of 0.1-2 mg/mL in dextrose 5% in water are stable for 14 days at 4°C and 23°C if protected from light, however, due to the occasional formation of subvisual particles, solutions should be used within 48 hours.

Reconstitution Reconstitute 50 mg and 100 mg vials with 10 mL and 20 mL of SWI, respectively. The reconstituted vials contain 5 mg/mL of amphotericin B. Shake the vial gently by hand until all solid particles have dissolved. Further dilute amphotericin B colloidal dispersion with dextrose 5% in water.

Compatibility Stable in D$_5$W; **incompatible** with NS.

Y-site administration: Compatible: Acyclovir, aminophylline, cefoxitin, ceftizoxime, clindamycin, dexamethasone sodium phosphate, fentanyl, furosemide, ganciclovir, granisetron, hydrocortisone sodium succinate, ifosfamide, lorazepam, mannitol, methotrexate, methylprednisolone sodium succinate, nitroglycerin, sufentanil, trimethoprim/sulfamethoxazole, vinblastine, vincristine, zidovudine. **Incompatible:** Alfentanil, amikacin, ampicillin, ampicillin/sulbactam, atenolol, aztreonam, bretylium, buprenorphine, butorphanol, calcium chloride, calcium gluconate, carboplatin, cefazolin, cefepime, cefoperazone, ceftazidime, ceftriaxone, chlorpromazine, cimetidine, cisatracurium, cisplatin, cyclophosphamide, cyclosporine, cytarabine, diazepam, digoxin, diphenhydramine, dobutamine, dopamine, doxorubicin, doxorubicin liposome, droperidol, enalaprilat, esmolol, famotidine, fluconazole, fluorouracil, gatifloxacin, gentamicin, haloperidol, heparin, hydromorphone, hydroxyzine, imipenem/cilastatin, labetalol, leucovorin, lidocaine, magnesium sulfate, meperidine, mesna, metoclopramide, metoprolol, metronidazole, midazolam, mitoxantrone, morphine, nalbuphine, naloxone, ofloxacin, ondansetron, paclitaxel, pentobarbital, phenobarbital, phenytoin, piperacillin, piperacillin/tazobactam, potassium chloride, prochlorperazine, promethazine, propranolol, ranitidine, remifentanil, sodium bicarbonate, ticarcillin, ticarcillin/clavulanate, tobramycin, vancomycin, vecuronium, verapamil, vinorelbine.

Mechanism of Action Binds to ergosterol altering cell membrane permeability in susceptible fungi and causing leakage of cell components with subsequent cell death. Proposed mechanism suggests that amphotericin causes an oxidation-dependent stimulation of macrophages (Lyman, 1992).

Pharmacodynamics/Kinetics

Distribution: V$_d$: Total volume increases with higher doses, reflects increasing uptake by tissues (with 4 mg/kg/day = 4 L/kg); predominantly distributed in the liver; concentrations in kidneys and other tissues are lower than observed with conventional amphotericin B

Half-life elimination: 28-29 hours; prolonged with higher doses

Dosage Children and Adults: I.V.:

Premedication: For patients who experience chills, fever, hypotension, nausea, or other nonanaphylactic infusion-related immediate reactions, premedicate with the following drugs 30-60 minutes prior to drug administration: A nonsteroidal (eg, ibuprofen, choline magnesium trisalicylate) with or without diphenhydramine **or** acetaminophen with diphenhydramine **or** hydrocortisone 50-100 mg. If the patient experiences rigors during the infusion, meperidine may be administered.

Range: 3-4 mg/kg/day (infusion of 1 mg/kg/hour); maximum: 7.5 mg/kg/day

A regimen of 6 mg/kg/day has been used for treatment of life-threatening invasive mold infections in immunocompromised patients; maximum: 7.5 mg/kg/day

Initially infuse at 1 mg/kg/hour. Rate of infusion may be increased with subsequent doses to 3 mg/kg/hour as patient tolerance allows. Treatment should continue as patient tolerance allows, until complete resolution of microbiologic and clinical evidence of fungal disease.

Administration Avoid injection faster than 1 mg/kg/hour. For a patient who experiences chills, fever, hypotension, nausea, or other nonanaphylactic infusion-related reactions, premedicate with the following drugs 30-60 minutes prior to drug administration: A nonsteroidal (eg, ibuprofen, choline magnesium trisalicylate) with or without diphenhydramine **or** acetaminophen with diphenhydramine **or** hydrocortisone 50-100 mg. If the patient experiences rigors during the infusion, meperidine may be administered. If severe respiratory distress occurs, the infusion should be immediately discontinued.

Monitoring Parameters Liver function tests, electrolytes, BUN, Cr, temperature, CBC, I/O, signs of hypokalemia (muscle weakness, cramping, drowsiness, ECG changes)

Additional Information Controlled trials which compare the original formulation of amphotericin B to the newer liposomal formulations (ie, Amphotec®) are lacking. Thus, comparative data discussing differences among the formulations should be interpreted cautiously. Although the risk of nephrotoxicity and infusion-related adverse effects may be less with Amphotec®, the efficacy profiles of Amphotec® and the original amphotericin formulation are comparable. Consequently, Amphotec® should be restricted to those patients who cannot tolerate or fail a standard amphotericin B formulation.

Dosage Forms Excipient information presented when available (limited, particularly for generics); consult specific product labeling.

Injection, powder for reconstitution:

Amphotec®: 50 mg, 100 mg

References

Edwards JE Jr, Bodey GP, Bowden RA, et al, "International Conference for the Development of a Consensus on the Management and Prevention of Severe Candidal Infections," *Clin Infect Dis*, 1997, 25(1):43-59.

Hiemenz JW and Walsh TJ, "Lipid Formulations of Amphotericin B: Recent Progress and Future Directions," *Clin Infect Dis*, 1996, 22(Suppl 2):133-44.

Lister J, "Amphotericin B Lipid Complex (Abelcet®) in the Treatment of Invasive Mycoses: The North American Experience," *Eur J Haematol Suppl*, 1996, 57:18-23.

Lyman CA and Walsh TJ, "Systemically Administered Antifungal Agents. A Review of Their Clinical Pharmacology and Therapeutic Applications," *Drugs*, 1992, 44(1):9-35.

Mora-Duarte J, Betts R, Rotstein C, et al, "Comparison of Caspofungin and Amphotericin B for Invasive Candidiasis," *N Engl J Med*, 2002, 347(25):2020-9.

Prentice HG, Hann IM, Herbrecht R, et al, "A Randomized Comparison of Liposomal Versus Conventional Amphotericin B for the Treatment of Pyrexia of Unknown Origin in Neutropenic Patients," *Br J Haematol*, 1997, 98(3):711-8.

Rex JH, Bennett JE, and Sugar AM, "A Randomized Trial Comparing Fluconazole With Amphotericin B for the Treatment of Candidemia in Patients Without Neutropenia. Candidemia Study Group and the National Institute," *N Engl J Med*, 1994, 331(20):1325-30.

Rex JH, Pappas PG, Karchmer AW, et al, "A Randomized and Blinded Multicenter Trial of High-Dose Fluconazole Plus Placebo Versus Fluconazole Plus Amphotericin B as Therapy for Candidemia and Its Consequences in Nonneutropenic Subjects," *Clin Infect Dis*, 2003, 36 (10):1221-8.

Rex JH, Walsh TJ, Sobel JD, et al, "Practice Guidelines for the Treatment of Candidiasis. Infectious Diseases Society of America," *Clin Infect Dis*, 2000, 30(4):662-78.

♦ **Amphotericin B Colloidal Dispersion** *see* Amphotericin B Cholesteryl Sulfate Complex *on page 62*

Amphotericin B (Conventional)

(am foe TER i sin bee con VEN sha nal)

Medication Safety Issues

Safety issues:

Conventional amphotericin formulations (Amphocin®, Fungizone®) may be confused with lipid-based formulations (AmBisome®, Abelcet®, Amphotec®).

Large overdoses have occurred when conventional formulations were dispensed inadvertently for lipid-based products. Single daily doses of conventional amphotericin formulation never exceed 1.5 mg/kg.

High alert medication: The Institute for Safe Medication Practices (ISMP) includes this medication (intrathecal administration) among its list of drugs which have a heightened risk of causing significant patient harm when used in error.

Related Information

Oral Mucositis / Stomatitis *on page 1460*

Index Terms Amphotericin B Desoxycholate

Generic Available Yes

Canadian Brand Names Fungizone®

Pharmacologic Category Antifungal Agent, Parenteral

Use Treatment of severe systemic and central nervous system infections caused by susceptible fungi such as *Candida* species, *Histoplasma capsulatum*, *Cryptococcus neoformans*, *Aspergillus* species, *Blastomyces dermatitidis*, *Torulopsis glabrata*, and *Coccidioides immitis*; fungal peritonitis; irrigant for bladder fungal infections; used in fungal infection in patients with bone marrow transplantation, amebic meningoencephalitis, ocular aspergillosis (intraocular injection), candidal cystitis (bladder irrigation), chemoprophylaxis (low-dose I.V.), immunocompromised patients at risk of aspergillosis (intranasal/nebulized), refractory meningitis (intrathecal), coccidioidal arthritis (intra-articular/I.M.).

Low-dose amphotericin B has been administered after bone marrow transplantation to reduce the risk of invasive fungal disease.

Pregnancy Risk Factor B

Lactation Excretion in breast milk unknown/contraindicated

Labeled Contraindications Hypersensitivity to amphotericin or any component of the formulation

Warnings/Precautions Anaphylaxis has been reported with amphotericin B-containing drugs. During the initial dosing, the drug should be administered under close clinical observation. Avoid use with other nephrotoxic drugs; drug-induced renal toxicity usually improves with interrupting therapy, decreasing dosage, or increasing dosing interval. Infusion reactions are most common 1-3 hours after starting the infusion and diminish with continued therapy.

[U.S. Boxed Warning]: Should be used primarily for treatment of progressive, potentially life-threatening fungal infections, not non-invasive forms of infection. **[U.S. Boxed warning]:** Verify the product name and dosage if dose exceeds 1.5 mg/kg.

Adverse Reactions

Systemic:

>10%:

Cardiovascular: Hypotension, tachypnea

Central nervous system: Fever, chills, headache (less frequent with I.T.), malaise

Endocrine & metabolic: Hypokalemia, hypomagnesemia

Gastrointestinal: Anorexia, nausea (less frequent with I.T.), vomiting (less frequent with I.T.), diarrhea, heartburn, cramping epigastric pain

Hematologic: Normochromic-normocytic anemia

Local: Pain at injection site with or without phlebitis or thrombophlebitis (incidence may increase with peripheral infusion of admixtures)

Neuromuscular & skeletal: Generalized pain, including muscle and joint pains (less frequent with I.T.)

Renal: Decreased renal function and renal function abnormalities including azotemia, renal tubular acidosis, nephrocalcinosis (>0.1 mg/mL)

1% to 10%:

Cardiovascular: Hypertension, flushing

Central nervous system: Delirium, arachnoiditis, pain along lumbar nerves (especially I.T. therapy)

Genitourinary: Urinary retention

Hematologic: Leukocytosis

Neuromuscular & skeletal: Paresthesia (especially with I.T. therapy)

<1% (Limited to important or life-threatening): Acute liver failure, agranulocytosis, anuria, bone marrow suppression, cardiac arrest, coagulation defects, convulsions, dyspnea, hearing loss, leukopenia, maculopapular rash, renal failure, renal tubular acidosis, thrombocytopenia, vision changes

Drug Interactions

Avoid Concomitant Use

Avoid concomitant use of Amphotericin B (Conventional) with any of the following: Gallium Nitrate

Increased Effect/Toxicity

Amphotericin B (Conventional) may increase the levels/effects of: Aminoglycosides; Colistimethate; CycloSPORINE; Flucytosine; Gallium Nitrate

The levels/effects of Amphotericin B (Conventional) may be increased by: Corticosteroids (Orally Inhaled); Corticosteroids (Systemic)

Decreased Effect

Amphotericin B (Conventional) may decrease the levels/effects of: Saccharomyces boulardii

The levels/effects of Amphotericin B (Conventional) may be decreased by: Antifungal Agents (Azole Derivatives, Systemic)

Storage/Stability Store intact vials under refrigeration. Protect from light. Reconstituted vials are stable, protected from light, for 24 hours at room temperature and 1 week when refrigerated. Parenteral admixtures are stable, protected from light, for 24 hours at room temperature and 2 days under refrigeration. Short-term exposure (<24 hours) to light during I.V. infusion does **not** appreciably affect potency.

◀ **Reconstitution** Add 10 mL of SWFI (without a bacteriostatic agent) to each vial of amphotericin B. Further dilute with 250-500 mL D_5W; final concentration should not exceed 0.1 mg/mL (peripheral infusion) or 0.25 mg/mL (central infusion).

Compatibility
Solution compatibility:
Compatible: Heparin sodium, hydrocortisone, sodium bicarbonate.

Incompatible: Ampicillin, calcium gluconate, carbenicillin, cimetidine, dopamine, gentamicin, lidocaine, potassium chloride, sodium chloride, tetracycline, verapamil.

Mechanism of Action Binds to ergosterol altering cell membrane permeability in susceptible fungi and causing leakage of cell components with subsequent cell death. Proposed mechanism suggests that amphotericin causes an oxidation-dependent stimulation of macrophages (Lyman, 1992).

Pharmacodynamics/Kinetics
Distribution: Minimal amounts enter the aqueous humor, bile, CSF (inflamed or noninflamed meninges), amniotic fluid, pericardial fluid, pleural fluid, and synovial fluid

Protein binding, plasma: 90%

Half-life elimination: Biphasic: Initial: 15-48 hours; Terminal: 15 days

Time to peak: Within 1 hour following a 4- to 6-hour dose

Excretion: Urine (2% to 5% as biologically active form); ~40% eliminated over a 7-day period and may be detected in urine for at least 7 weeks after discontinued use

Dosage Premedication: For patients who experience infusion-related immediate reactions, premedicate with the following drugs 30-60 minutes prior to drug administration: NSAID (with or without diphenhydramine) **or** acetaminophen with diphenhydramine **or** hydrocortisone 50-100 mg. If the patient experiences rigors during the infusion, meperidine may be administered.

Usual dosage ranges:
Infants and Children:
Test dose: I.V.: 0.1 mg/kg/dose to a maximum of 1 mg; infuse over 30-60 minutes. Many clinicians believe a test dose is unnecessary.

Maintenance: 0.25-1 mg/kg/day given once daily; infuse over 2-6 hours. Once therapy has been established, amphotericin B can be administered on an every-other-day basis at 1-1.5 mg/kg/dose; cumulative dose: 1.5-2 g over 6-10 weeks.

Duration of therapy: Varies with nature of infection, usual duration is 4-12 weeks or cumulative dose of 1-4 g

Adults:
Test dose: 1 mg infused over 20-30 minutes. Many clinicians believe a test dose is unnecessary.

Maintenance dose: Usual: 0.05-1.5 mg/kg/day; 1-1.5 mg/kg over 4-6 hours every other day may be given once therapy is established; aspergillosis, rhinocerebral mucormycosis, often require 1-1.5 mg/kg/day; do not exceed 1.5 mg/kg/day

Indication-specific dosing:
Children: **Meningitis, coccidioidal or cryptococcal:** I.T.: 25-100 mcg every 48-72 hours; increase to 500 mcg as tolerated

Adults:
Aspergillosis, disseminated: I.V.: 0.6-0.7 mg/kg/day for 3-6 months

Bone marrow transplantation (prophylaxis): I.V.: Low-dose amphotericin B 0.1-0.25 mg/kg/day has been administered after bone marrow transplantation to reduce the risk of invasive fungal disease.

Candidemia (neutropenic or non-neutropenic): I.V.: 0.5-1 mg/kg/day until 14 days after last positive blood culture and resolution of signs and symptoms (Pappas, 2009)

Candidiasis, chronic, disseminated: I.V.: 0.5-0.7 mg/kg/day for 3-6 months and resolution of radiologic lesions (Pappas, 2009)

Dematiaceous fungi: I.V.: 0.7 mg/kg/day in combination with an azole

Endocarditis: I.V.: 0.6-1 mg/kg/day (with or without flucytosine) for 6 weeks after valve replacement; **Note:** If isolates susceptible and/or clearance demonstrated, guidelines recommend step-down to fluconazole; also for long-term suppression therapy if valve replacement is not possible (Pappas, 2009)

Endophthalmitis, fungal:

Intravitreal (unlabeled use): 10 mcg in 0.1 mL (in conjunction with systemic therapy)

I.V.: 0.7-1 mg/kg/day (with or without flucytosine) for at least 4-6 weeks (Pappas, 2009)

Esophageal: I.V.: 0.3-0.7 mg/kg/day for 14-21 days after clinical improvement

Histoplasmosis: Chronic, severe pulmonary or disseminated: I.V.: 0.5-1 mg/kg/day for 7 days, then 0.8 mg/kg every other day (or 3 times/week) until total dose of 10-15 mg/kg; may continue itraconazole as suppressive therapy (lifelong for immunocompromised patients)

Meningitis:

Candidal: I.V.: 0.7-1 mg/kg/day (with or without flucytosine) for at least 4 weeks; **Note:** Liposomal amphotericin favored by IDSA guidelines based on decreased risk of nephrotoxicity and potentially better CNS penetration (Pappas, 2009)

Cryptococcal or Coccidioides: I.T.: Initial: 25-300 mcg every 48-72 hours; increase to 500 mcg to 1 mg as tolerated; maximum total dose: 15 mg has been suggested

Histoplasma: I.V.: 0.5-1 mg/kg/day for 7 days, then 0.8 mg/kg every other day (or 3 times/week) for 3 months total duration; follow with fluconazole suppressive therapy for up to 12 months

Meningoencephalitis, cryptococcal: I.V.:

HIV positive: 0.7-1 mg/kg/day (plus flucytosine 100 mg/kg/day) for 2 weeks, then change to oral fluconazole for at least 10 weeks; alternatively, amphotericin and flucytosine may be continued uninterrupted for 6-10 weeks

HIV negative: 0.5-0.7 mg/kg/day (plus flucytosine) for 2 weeks

Oropharyngeal candidiasis: I.V.: 0.3 mg/kg/day for 7-14 days (Pappas, 2009)

Osteoarticular candidiasis: I.V.: 0.5-1 mg/kg/day for several weeks, followed by fluconazole for 6-12 months (osteomyelitis) or 6 weeks (septic arthritis)

Penicillium marneffei: I.V.: 0.6 mg/kg/day for 2 weeks

Pneumonia: Cryptococcal (mild-to-moderate): I.V.:

HIV positive: 0.5-1 mg/kg/day

HIV negative: 0.5-0.7 mg/kg/day (plus flucytosine) for 2 weeks

Sporotrichosis: Pulmonary, meningeal, osteoarticular, or disseminated: I.V.: Total dose of 1-2 g, then change to oral itraconazole or fluconazole for suppressive therapy

Urinary tract candidiasis (Pappas, 2009):

Fungus balls: I.V.: 0.5-0.7 mg/kg/day with or without flucytosine 25 mg/kg 4 times daily

Pyelonephritis: I.V.: 0.5-0.7 mg/kg/day with or without flucytosine 25 mg/kg 4 times daily for 2 weeks

Symptomatic cystitis: I.V.: 0.3-0.6 mg/kg/day for 1-7 days

Bladder irrigation: Irrigate with 50 mcg/mL solution instilled periodically or continuously for 5-10 days or until cultures are clear for fluconazole-resistant *Candida*

Dosing adjustment in renal impairment: If renal dysfunction is due to the drug, the daily total can be decreased by 50% or the dose can be given every other day; I.V. therapy may take several months

Dialysis: Poorly dialyzed; no supplemental dosage necessary when using hemo- or peritoneal dialysis or continuous renal replacement therapy (CRRT)

Administration in dialysate: Children and Adults: 1-2 mg/L of peritoneal dialysis fluid either with or without low-dose I.V. amphotericin B (a total dose of 2-10 mg/kg given over 7-14 days). Precipitate may form in ionic dialysate solutions.

Administration May be infused over 4-6 hours. For a patient who experiences chills, fever, hypotension, nausea, or other nonanaphylactic infusion-related reactions, premedicate with the following drugs 30-60 minutes prior to drug administration: A nonsteroidal (eg, ibuprofen, choline magnesium trisalicylate) with or without diphenhydramine **or** acetaminophen with diphenhydramine **or** hydrocortisone 50-100 mg. If the patient experiences rigors during the infusion, meperidine may be administered. Bolus infusion of normal saline immediately preceding, or immediately preceding and following amphotericin B may reduce drug-induced nephrotoxicity. Risk of nephrotoxicity increases with amphotericin B doses >1 mg/kg/day. Infusion of admixtures more concentrated than 0.25 mg/mL should be limited to patients absolutely requiring volume contraction.

Monitoring Parameters Renal function (monitor frequently during therapy), electrolytes (especially potassium and magnesium), liver function tests, temperature, PT/PTT, CBC; monitor input and output; monitor for signs of hypokalemia (muscle weakness, cramping, drowsiness, ECG changes, etc)

Test Interactions Increased BUN (S), serum creatinine, alkaline phosphate, bilirubin; decreased magnesium, potassium (S)

Additional Information Premedication with diphenhydramine and acetaminophen may reduce the severity of acute infusion-related reactions. Meperidine reduces the duration of amphotericin B-induced rigors and chilling. Hydrocortisone may be used in patients with severe or refractory infusion-related reactions. Bolus infusion of normal saline immediately preceding, or immediately preceding and following amphotericin B may reduce drug-induced nephrotoxicity. Risk of nephrotoxicity increases with amphotericin B doses >1 mg/kg/day. Infusion of admixtures more concentrated than 0.25 mg/mL should be limited to patients absolutely requiring volume restriction. Amphotericin B does not have a bacteriostatic constituent, subsequently admixture expiration is determined by sterility more than chemical stability.

Dosage Forms Excipient information presented when available (limited, particularly for generics); consult specific product labeling.

Injection, powder for reconstitution, as desoxycholate: 50 mg

References

Benson JM and Nahata MC, "Clinical Use of Systemic Antifungal Agents," *Clin Pharm*, 1988, 7 (6):424-38.

Bianco JA, Almgren J, Kern DL, et al, "Evidence That Oral Pentoxifylline Reverses Acute Renal Dysfunction in Bone Marrow Transplant Recipients Receiving Amphotericin B and Cyclosporine," *Transplantation*, 1991, 51(4):925-7.

Branch RA, "Prevention of Amphotericin B-Induced Renal Impairment. A Review on the Use of Sodium Supplementation," *Arch Intern Med*, 1988, 148(11):2389-94.

Cruz JM, Peacock JE Jr, Loomer L, et al, "Rapid Intravenous Infusion of Amphotericin B: A Pilot Study," *Am J Med*, 1992, 93:123-30.

Edwards JE Jr, Bodey GP, Bowden RA, et al, "International Conference for the Development of a Consensus on the Management and Prevention of Severe Candidal Infections," *Clin Infect Dis*, 1997, 25(1):43-59.

Gales MA and Gales BJ, "Rapid Infusion of Amphotericin B in Dextrose," *Ann Pharmacother*, 1995, 29(5):523-9.

Kintzel PE and Smith GH, "Practical Guidelines for Preparing and Administering Amphotericin B," *Am J Hosp Pharm*, 1992, 49(5):1156-64.

Pappas PG, Kauffman CA, Andes D, et al, "Clinical Practice Guidelines for the Management of Candidiasis: 2009 Update by the Infectious Diseases Society of America," *Clin Infect Dis*, 2009, 48(5):503-35.

Rex JH, Bennett JE, Sugar AM, "A Randomized Trial Comparing Fluconazole With Amphotericin B for the Treatment of Candidemia in Patients Without Neutropenia. Candidemia Study Group and the National Institute," *N Engl J Med*, 1994, 331(20):1325-30.

Rex JH, Walsh TJ, Sobel JD, et al, "Practice Guidelines for the Treatment of Candidiasis. Infectious Diseases Society of America," *Clin Infect Dis*, 2000, 30(4):662-78.

◆ **Amphotericin B Desoxycholate** *see* Amphotericin B (Conventional) *on page 66*

Amphotericin B (Lipid Complex)
(am foe TER i sin bee LIP id KOM pleks)

Medication Safety Issues
Safety issues:

Lipid-based amphotericin formulations (Abelcet®) may be confused with conventional formulations (Amphocin®, Fungizone®)

Large overdoses have occurred when conventional formulations were dispensed inadvertently for lipid-based products. Single daily doses of conventional amphotericin formulation never exceed 1.5 mg/kg.

High alert medication: The Institute for Safe Medication Practices (ISMP) includes this medication among its list of drugs which have a heightened risk of causing significant patient harm when used in error.

U.S. Brand Names Abelcet®

Index Terms ABLC

Generic Available No

Canadian Brand Names Abelcet®

Pharmacologic Category Antifungal Agent, Parenteral

Use Treatment of aspergillosis or any type of progressive fungal infection in patients who are refractory to or intolerant of conventional amphotericin B therapy

Unlabeled/Investigational Use Effective in patients with serious *Candida* species infections

Pregnancy Risk Factor B

Lactation Enters breast milk/contraindicated

Labeled Contraindications Hypersensitivity to amphotericin or any component of the formulation

Warnings/Precautions Anaphylaxis has been reported with amphotericin B-containing drugs. If severe respiratory distress occurs, the infusion should be immediately discontinued. During the initial dosing, the drug should be administered under close clinical observation. Acute reactions (including fever and chills) may occur 1-2 hours after starting an intravenous infusion. These reactions are usually more common with the first few doses and generally diminish with subsequent doses.

Adverse Reactions Nephrotoxicity and infusion-related hyperpyrexia, rigor, and chilling are reduced relative to amphotericin deoxycholate.

>10%:
Central nervous system: Chills, fever
Renal: Serum creatinine increased
Miscellaneous: Multiple organ failure
1% to 10%:
Cardiovascular: Hypotension, cardiac arrest
Central nervous system: Headache, pain
Dermatologic: Rash
Endocrine & metabolic: Bilirubinemia, hypokalemia, acidosis
Gastrointestinal: Nausea, vomiting, diarrhea, gastrointestinal hemorrhage, abdominal pain
Renal: Renal failure
Respiratory: Respiratory failure, dyspnea, pneumonia

Drug Interactions

Avoid Concomitant Use
Avoid concomitant use of Amphotericin B (Lipid Complex) with any of the following: Gallium Nitrate

Increased Effect/Toxicity
Amphotericin B (Lipid Complex) may increase the levels/effects of: Aminoglycosides; Colistimethate; CycloSPORINE; Flucytosine; Gallium Nitrate

The levels/effects of Amphotericin B (Lipid Complex) may be increased by: Corticosteroids (Orally Inhaled); Corticosteroids (Systemic)

Decreased Effect
Amphotericin B (Lipid Complex) may decrease the levels/effects of: Saccharomyces boulardii

The levels/effects of Amphotericin B (Lipid Complex) may be decreased by: Antifungal Agents (Azole Derivatives, Systemic)

Storage/Stability Intact vials should be stored at 2°C to 8°C (35°F to 46°F); do not freeze. Protect intact vials from exposure to light. Solutions for infusion are stable for 48 hours under refrigeration and 6 hours at room temperature. Protect from light. Following reconstitution, protect from light.

Reconstitution Shake vial gently to disperse yellow sediment at bottom of container. Dilute with D_5W to 1-2 mg/mL.

Compatibility
Incompatible with any blood products, intravenous drugs, or intravenous fluids other than D_5W when admixed or as Y-site administration.

Mechanism of Action Binds to ergosterol altering cell membrane permeability in susceptible fungi and causing leakage of cell components with subsequent cell death. Proposed mechanism suggests that amphotericin causes an oxidation-dependent stimulation of macrophages.

Pharmacodynamics/Kinetics
Distribution: V_d: Increases with higher doses; reflects increased uptake by tissues (131 L/kg with 5 mg/kg/day)
Half-life elimination: ~24 hours
Excretion: Clearance: Increases with higher doses (5 mg/kg/day): 400 mL/hour/kg

Dosage Children and Adults: I.V.:

Premedication: For patients who experience infusion-related immediate reactions, premedicate with the following drugs 30-60 minutes prior to drug administration: A nonsteroidal anti-inflammatory agent ± diphenhydramine **or** acetaminophen with diphenhydramine **or** hydrocortisone 50-100 mg. If the patient experiences rigors during the infusion, meperidine may be administered.

Range: 2.5-5 mg/kg/day as a single infusion

Dosing adjustment in renal impairment: None necessary; effects of renal impairment are not currently known

Hemodialysis: No supplemental dosage necessary

Peritoneal dialysis: No supplemental dosage necessary

Continuous renal replacement therapy (CRRT): No supplemental dosage necessary

Administration For patients who experience nonanaphylactic infusion-related reactions, premedicate 30-60 minutes prior to drug administration with a nonsteroidal anti-inflammatory agent ± diphenhydramine **or** acetaminophen with diphenhydramine **or** hydrocortisone 50-100 mg. If the patient experiences rigors during the infusion, meperidine may be administered.

Administer at an infusion rate of 2.5 mg/kg/hour (over 2 hours). Invert infusion container several times prior to administration and every 2 hours during infusion if it exceeds 2 hours.

Monitoring Parameters Renal function (monitor frequently during therapy), electrolytes (especially potassium and magnesium), liver function tests, temperature, PT/PTT, CBC; monitor input and output; monitor for signs of hypokalemia (muscle weakness, cramping, drowsiness, ECG changes, etc)

Test Interactions Increased BUN (S), serum creatinine, alkaline phosphate, bilirubin; decreased magnesium, potassium (S)

Additional Information As a modification of dimyristoyl phosphatidylcholine: dimyristoyl phosphatidylglycerol 7:3 (DMPC:DMPG) liposome, amphotericin B lipid-complex has a higher drug to lipid ratio and the concentration of amphotericin B is 33 M. ABLC is a ribbon-like structure, not a liposome.

Controlled trials which compare the original formulation of amphotericin B to the newer liposomal formulations (ie, Abelcet®) are lacking. Thus, comparative data discussing differences among the formulations should be interpreted cautiously. Although the risk of nephrotoxicity and infusion-related adverse effects may be less with Abelcet®, the efficacy profiles of Abelcet® and the original amphotericin formulation are comparable. Consequently, Abelcet® should be restricted to those patients who cannot tolerate or fail a standard amphotericin B formulation.

Dosage Forms Excipient information presented when available (limited, particularly for generics); consult specific product labeling.

Injection, suspension [preservative free]:

Abelcet®: 5 mg/mL (20 mL)

References

De Marie S, "Clinical Use of Liposomal and Lipid-Complexed Amphotericin B," *J Antimicrob Chemother*, 1994, 33(5):907-16.

Edwards JE Jr, Bodey GP, Bowden RA, et al, "International Conference for the Development of a Consensus on the Management and Prevention of Severe Candidal Infections," *Clin Infect Dis*, 1997, 25(1):43-59.

Hiemenz JW and Walsh TJ, "Lipid Formulations of Amphotericin B: Recent Progress and Future Directions," *Clin Infect Dis*, 1996, 22(Suppl 2):133-44.

Kline S, Larsen TA, Fieber L, et al, "Limited Toxicity of Prolonged Therapy With High Doses of Amphotericin B Lipid Complex," *Clin Infect Dis*, 1995, 21(5):1154-8.

◄ Mora-Duarte J, Betts R, Rotstein C, et al, "Comparison of Caspofungin and Amphotericin B for Invasive Candidiasis," *N Engl J Med*, 2002, 347(25):2020-9.

Rapp RP, Gubbins PO, and Evans ME, "Amphotericin B Lipid Complex," *Ann Pharmacother*, 1997, 31(10):1174-86.

Rex JH, Bennett JE, and Sugar AM, "A Randomized Trial Comparing Fluconazole With Amphotericin B for the Treatment of Candidemia in Patients Without Neutropenia. Candidemia Study Group and the National Institute," *N Engl J Med*, 1994, 331(20):1325-30.

Rex JH, Pappas PG, Karchmer AW, et al, "A Randomized and Blinded Multicenter Trial of High-Dose Fluconazole Plus Placebo Versus Fluconazole Plus Amphotericin B as Therapy for Candidemia and Its Consequences in Nonneutropenic Subjects," *Clin Infect Dis*, 2003, 36 (10):1221-8.

Rex JH, Walsh TJ, Sobel JD, et al, "Practice Guidelines for the Treatment of Candidiasis. Infectious Diseases Society of America," *Clin Infect Dis*, 2000, 30(4):662-78.

Slain D, "Lipid-Based Amphotericin B for the Treatment of Fungal Infections," *Pharmacotherapy*, 1999, 19(3):306-23.

Amphotericin B (Liposomal) (am foe TER i sin bee lye po SO mal)

Medication Safety Issues

Safety issues:

Lipid-based amphotericin formulations (AmBisome®) may be confused with conventional formulations (Amphocin®, Fungizone®) or with other lipid-based amphotericin formulations (Abelcet®, Amphotec®)

Large overdoses have occurred when conventional formulations were dispensed inadvertently for lipid-based products. Single daily doses of conventional amphotericin formulation never exceed 1.5 mg/kg.

High alert medication: The Institute for Safe Medication Practices (ISMP) includes this medication among its list of drugs which have a heightened risk of causing significant patient harm when used in error.

U.S. Brand Names AmBisome®

Index Terms L-AmB

Generic Available No

Canadian Brand Names AmBisome®

Pharmacologic Category Antifungal Agent, Parenteral

Use Empirical therapy for presumed fungal infection in febrile, neutropenic patients; treatment of patients with *Aspergillus* species, *Candida* species, and/or *Cryptococcus* species infections refractory to amphotericin B desoxycholate (conventional amphotericin), or in patients where renal impairment or unacceptable toxicity precludes the use of amphotericin B desoxycholate; treatment of cryptococcal meningitis in HIV-infected patients; treatment of visceral leishmaniasis

Unlabeled/Investigational Use Treatment of systemic *Histoplasmosis* infection

Pregnancy Risk Factor B

Lactation Excretion in breast milk unknown/not recommended

Labeled Contraindications Hypersensitivity to amphotericin B desoxycholate or any component of the formulation

Warnings/Precautions Patients should be under close clinical observation during initial dosing. As with other amphotericin B-containing products, anaphylaxis has been reported. Facilities for cardiopulmonary resuscitation should be available during administration. Acute infusion reactions (including fever and chills) may occur 1-2 hours after starting infusions; reactions are more common with the first few doses and generally diminish with subsequent doses. Immediately discontinue infusion if severe respiratory distress occurs; the patient should not receive further infusions. Concurrent use of amphotericin B with other nephrotoxic drugs may enhance the potential for drug-induced renal toxicity. Concurrent use with antineoplastic agents may enhance the potential for renal toxicity, bronchospasm or hypotension. Acute pulmonary toxicity has been reported in patients receiving simultaneous leukocyte transfusions and amphotericin B. Safety and efficacy have not been established in patients <1 month of age.

Adverse Reactions Percentage of adverse reactions is dependent upon population studied and may vary with respect to premedications and underlying illness. Incidence of decreased renal function and infusion-related events are lower than rates observed with amphotericin B deoxycholate.

>10%:
Cardiovascular: Peripheral edema (15%), edema (12% to 14%), tachycardia (9% to 19%), hypotension (7% to 14%), hypertension (8% to 20%), chest pain (8% to 12%), hypervolemia (8% to 12%)

Central nervous system: Chills (29% to 48%), insomnia (17% to 22%), headache (9% to 20%), anxiety (7% to 14%), pain (14%), confusion (9% to 13%)

Dermatologic: Rash (5% to 25%), pruritus (11%)

Endocrine & metabolic: Hypokalemia (31% to 51%), hypomagnesemia (15% to 50%), hyperglycemia (8% to 23%), hypocalcemia (5% to 18%), hyponatremia (9% to 12%)

Gastrointestinal: Nausea (16% to 40%), vomiting (11% to 32%), diarrhea (11% to 30%), abdominal pain (7% to 20%), constipation (15%), anorexia (10% to 14%)

Hematologic: Anemia (27% to 48%), blood transfusion reaction (9% to 18%), leukopenia (15% to 17%), thrombocytopenia (6% to 13%)

Hepatic: Alkaline phosphatase increased (7% to 22%), bilirubinemia (≤18%), ALT increased (15%), AST increased (13%), liver function tests abnormal (not specified) (4% to 13%)

Local: Phlebitis (9% to 11%)

Neuromuscular & skeletal: Weakness (6% to 13%), back pain (12%)

Renal: Nephrotoxicity (14% to 47%), creatinine increased (18% to 40%), BUN increased (7% to 21%), hematuria (14%)

Respiratory: Dyspnea (18% to 23%), lung disorder (14% to 18%), cough (2% to 18%), epistaxis (9% to 15%), pleural effusion (13%), rhinitis (11%)

Miscellaneous: Infusion reactions (4% to 21%), sepsis (7% to 14%), infection (11% to 13%)

2% to 10%:
Cardiovascular: Arrhythmia, atrial fibrillation, bradycardia, cardiac arrest, cardiomegaly, facial swelling, flushing, postural hypotension, valvular heart disease, vascular disorder, vasodilation

Central nervous system: Agitation, abnormal thinking, coma, depression, dysesthesia, dizziness (7% to 9%), hallucinations, malaise, nervousness, seizure, somnolence

Dermatologic: Alopecia, bruising, cellulitis, dry skin, maculopapular rash, petechia, purpura, skin discoloration, skin disorder, skin ulcer, urticaria, vesiculobullous rash

Endocrine & metabolic: Acidosis, fluid overload, hypernatremia (4%), hyperchloremia, hyperkalemia, hypermagnesemia, hyperphosphatemia, hypophosphatemia, hypoproteinemia, lactate dehydrogenase increased, nonprotein nitrogen increased

Gastrointestinal: Abdomen enlarged, amylase increased, dyspepsia, dysphagia, eructation, fecal incontinence, flatulence, gastrointestinal hemorrhage (10%), hematemesis, hemorrhoids, gum/oral hemorrhage, ileus, mucositis, rectal disorder, stomatitis, ulcerative stomatitis, xerostomia

Genitourinary: Vaginal hemorrhage

Hematologic: Coagulation disorder, hemorrhage, prothrombin decreased

Hepatic: Hepatocellular damage, hepatomegaly, veno-occlusive liver disease

Local: Injection site inflammation

Neuromuscular & skeletal: Arthralgia, bone pain, dystonia, myalgia, neck pain, paresthesia, rigors, tremor

Ocular: Conjunctivitis, dry eyes, eye hemorrhage

Renal: Abnormal renal function, acute renal failure, dysuria, renal failure, toxic nephropathy, urinary incontinence

Respiratory: Asthma, atelectasis, dry nose, hemoptysis, hyperventilation, pharyngitis, pneumonia, pulmonary edema, respiratory alkalosis, respiratory insufficiency, respiratory failure, sinusitis, hypoxia (6% to 8%)

Miscellaneous: Allergic reaction, cell-mediated immunological reaction, flu-like syndrome, graft-versus-host disease, herpes simplex, hiccup, procedural complication (8% to 10%), diaphoresis (7%)

Postmarketing and/or case reports: Agranulocytosis, angioedema, bronchospasm, cyanosis/hypoventilation, erythema, hemorrhagic cystitis

Drug Interactions

Avoid Concomitant Use

Avoid concomitant use of Amphotericin B (Liposomal) with any of the following: Gallium Nitrate

Increased Effect/Toxicity

Amphotericin B (Liposomal) may increase the levels/effects of: Aminoglycosides; Colistimethate; CycloSPORINE; Flucytosine; Gallium Nitrate

The levels/effects of Amphotericin B (Liposomal) may be increased by: Corticosteroids (Orally Inhaled); Corticosteroids (Systemic)

Decreased Effect

Amphotericin B (Liposomal) may decrease the levels/effects of: Saccharomyces boulardii

The levels/effects of Amphotericin B (Liposomal) may be decreased by: Antifungal Agents (Azole Derivatives, Systemic)

Storage/Stability Store intact vials at ≤25°C (≤77°F). Reconstituted vials are stable refrigerated at 2°C to 8°C (36°F to 46°F) for 24 hours. Do not freeze. Manufacturer's labeling states infusion should begin within 6 hours of dilution with D_5W; data on file with Astellas Pharma shows extended formulation stability when admixed in D_5W at 0.2-2 mg/mL (in polyolefin or PVC bags) for up to 11 days when stored refrigerated at 2°C to 8°C (36°F to 46°F).

Reconstitution Reconstitute with 12 mL SWFI to a concentration of 4 mg/mL. The use of any solution other than those recommended, or the presence of a bacteriostatic agent in the solution, may cause precipitation. **Shake the vial vigorously** for 30 seconds, until dispersed into a translucent yellow suspension.

Filtration and dilution: The 5-micron filter should be on the syringe used to remove the reconstituted AmBisome®. Dilute to a final concentration of 1-2 mg/mL (0.2-0.5 mg/mL for infants and small children).

Compatibility Stable in D_5W; **incompatible** with NS, 1/2NS, other saline-containing solutions, or preservatives.

Y-site administration: Compatible: Anidulafungin

Mechanism of Action Binds to ergosterol altering cell membrane permeability in susceptible fungi and causing leakage of cell components with subsequent cell death. Proposed mechanism suggests that amphotericin causes an oxidation-dependent stimulation of macrophages (Lyman, 1992).

Pharmacodynamics/Kinetics

Distribution: V_d: 131 L/kg

Half-life elimination: Terminal: 174 hours

Dosage

Usual dosage range:

Children ≥1 month: I.V.: 3-6 mg/kg/day

Adults: I.V.: 3-6 mg/kg/day; **Note:** Higher doses (15 mg/kg/day) have been used clinically (Walsh, 2001)

Note: Premedication: For patients who experience nonanaphylactic infusion-related immediate reactions, premedicate with the following drugs 30-60 minutes prior to drug administration: A nonsteroidal anti-inflammatory agent ± diphenhydramine; **or** acetaminophen with diphenhydramine; **or** hydrocortisone 50-100 mg. If the patient experiences rigors during the infusion, meperidine may be administered.

Indication-specific dosing:

Children ≥1 month: I.V.:

Cryptococcal meningitis (HIV-positive): 6 mg/kg/day (may consider addition of oral flucytosine 25 mg/kg 4 times daily [unlabeled combination; AIDS*info* guidelines, 2008])

Empiric therapy: 3 mg/kg/day

Systemic fungal infections (*Aspergillus, Candida, Cryptococcus, Histoplasmosis*): 3-5 mg/kg/day

General invasive Candidal disease: 3-5 mg/kg/day (may consider addition of oral flucytosine 25-37.5 mg/kg 4 times daily [unlabeled combination; AIDS*info* guidelines, 2008])

Candidal meningitis: 5 mg/kg/day; (may consider addition of oral flucytosine 25-37.5 mg/kg 4 times daily [unlabeled combination; AIDS*info* guidelines, 2008])

Histoplasmosis (unlabeled use): 3-5 mg/kg/day (AIDS*info* guidelines, 2008)

Visceral leishmaniasis:

Immunocompetent: 3 mg/kg/day on days 1-5, and 3 mg/kg/day on days 14 and 21; a repeat course may be given in patients who do not achieve parasitic clearance

Note: Alternate regimen of 10 mg/kg/day for 2 days has been reportedly effective.

Immunocompromised: 4 mg/kg/day on days 1-5, and 4 mg/kg/day on days 10, 17, 24, 31, and 38

Adults: I.V.:

Cryptococcal meningitis (HIV-positive): 6 mg/kg/day or 4-6 mg/kg/day in combination with addition of oral flucytosine 25 mg/kg 4 times daily (unlabeled combination; AIDS*info* guidelines, 2008)

Empiric candidiasis therapy: 3-5 mg/kg/day (Pappas, 2009)

Endocarditis: I.V.: 3-5 mg/kg/day (with or without flucytosine 25 mg/kg 4 times daily) for 6 weeks after valve replacement; **Note:** If isolates susceptible and/or clearance demonstrated, guidelines recommend step-down to fluconazole; also for long-term suppression therapy if valve replacement is not possible (Pappas, 2009)

Fungal sinusitis: Limited data in immunocompromised patients have shown efficacy with 3-10 mg/kg/day (Pagano, 2004; Rokicka, 2006; Barron, 2005). **Note:** An azole antifungal is recommended if causative organism is *Aspergillus* spp or *Pseudallescheria boydii* (*Scedosporium* sp).

Osteoarticular candidiasis: I.V.: 3-5 mg/kg/day for several weeks, followed by fluconazole for 6-12 months (osteomyelitis) or 6 weeks (septic arthritis)

Systemic fungal infections *(Aspergillus, Candida, Cryptococcus, Histoplasmosis)*: 3-5 mg/kg/day

General invasive Candidal disease: 3-5 mg/kg/day with oral flucytosine 25 mg/kg 4 times daily (unlabeled combination; Pappas, 2009)

Candidal meningitis: 3-5 mg/kg/day with or without oral flucytosine 25 mg/kg 4 times daily (unlabeled combination; Pappas, 2009)

Histoplasmosis (unlabeled use): 3-5 mg/kg/day (AIDS*info* guidelines, 2008)

Visceral leishmaniasis:

Immunocompetent: 3 mg/kg/day on days 1-5, and 3 mg/kg/day on days 14 and 21; a repeat course may be given in patients who do not achieve parasitic clearance

Note: Alternate regimen of 2 mg/kg/day for 5 days has been reportedly effective.

Immunocompromised: 4 mg/kg/day on days 1-5, and 4 mg/kg/day on days 10, 17, 24, 31, and 38

Dosing adjustment in renal impairment: None necessary; effects of renal impairment are not currently known

Hemodialysis: No supplemental dosage necessary

Peritoneal dialysis effects: No supplemental dosage necessary

Continuous renal replacement therapy (CRRT): No supplemental dosage necessary

Administration Administer via intravenous infusion, over a period of approximately 2 hours. Infusion time may be reduced to approximately 1 hour in patients in whom the treatment is well-tolerated. If the patient experiences discomfort during infusion, the duration of infusion may be increased. Administer at a rate of 2.5 mg/kg/hour. Existing intravenous line should be flushed with D_5W prior to infusion (if not feasible, administer through a separate line). An in-line membrane filter (not less than 1 micron) may be used.

For a patient who experiences chills, fever, hypotension, nausea, or other nonanaphylactic infusion-related reactions, premedicate with the following drugs, 30-60 minutes prior to drug administration: A nonsteroidal (eg, ibuprofen, choline magnesium trisalicylate) with or without diphenhydramine **or** acetaminophen with diphenhydramine **or** hydrocortisone 50-100 mg. If the patient experiences rigors during the infusion, meperidine may be administered.

Monitoring Parameters Renal function (monitor frequently during therapy), electrolytes (especially potassium and magnesium), liver function tests, temperature, PT/PTT, CBC; monitor input and output; monitor for signs of hypokalemia (muscle weakness, cramping, drowsiness, ECG changes, etc); monitor cardiac function if used concurrently with corticosteroids

Additional Information Amphotericin B (liposomal) is a true single bilayer liposomal drug delivery system. Liposomes are closed, spherical vesicles created by mixing specific proportions of amphophilic substances such as phospholipids and cholesterol so that they arrange themselves into multiple concentric bilayer membranes when hydrated in aqueous solutions. Single bilayer liposomes are then formed by microemulsification of multilamellar vesicles using a homogenizer. Amphotericin B (liposomal) consists of these unilamellar bilayer liposomes with amphotericin B intercalated within the membrane. Due to the nature and quantity of amphophilic substances used, and the lipophilic moiety in the amphotericin B molecule, the drug is an integral part of the overall structure of the amphotericin B liposomal liposomes. Amphotericin B (liposomal) contains true liposomes that are <100 nm in diameter.

Dosage Forms Excipient information presented when available (limited, particularly for generics); consult specific product labeling.
Injection, powder for reconstitution:
AmBisome®: 50 mg [contains soy and sucrose]

References

Barron MA, Lay M, Madinger NE, "Surgery and Treatment with High-Dose Liposomal Amphotericin B for Eradication of Craniofacial Zygomycosis in a Patient with Hodgkin's Disease Who Had Undergone Allogeneic Hematopoietic Stem Cell Transplantation," *J Clin Microbiol*, 2005, 43 (4):2012-14.

Edwards JE Jr, Bodey GP, Bowden RA, et al, "International Conference for the Development of a Consensus on the Management and Prevention of Severe Candidal Infections," *Clin Infect Dis*, 1997, 25(1):43-59.

Emminger W, Graninger W, Emminger-Schmidmeir W, et al, "Tolerance of High Doses of Amphotericin B by Infusion of a Liposomal Formulation in Children With Cancer," *Ann Hematol*, 1994, 68:27-31.

"Guidelines for Prevention and Treatment of Opportunistic Infections Among HIV-Exposed and HIV-Infected Children," June 20, 2008. Available at http://aidsinfo.nih.gov

"Guidelines for Prevention and Treatment of Opportunistic Infections in HIV-Infected Adults and Adolescents," June 18, 2008. Available at http://aidsinfo.nih.gov

Pagano L, Offidani M, Fianchi L, et al, "Mucormycosis in Hematologic Patients," *Haematologica*, 2004, 89(2):207-14.

Pappas PG, Kauffman CA, Andes D, et al, "Clinical Practice Guidelines for the Management of Candidiasis: 2009 Update by the Infectious Diseases Society of America," *Clin Infect Dis*, 2009, 48(5):503-35.

Rex JH, Bennett JE, and Sugar AM, "A Randomized Trial Comparing Fluconazole With Amphotericin B for the Treatment of Candidemia in Patients Without Neutropenia. Candidemia Study Group and the National Institute," *N Engl J Med*, 1994, 331(20):1325-30.

Rex JH, Pappas PG, Karchmer AW, et al, "A Randomized and Blinded Multicenter Trial of High-Dose Fluconazole Plus Placebo Versus Fluconazole Plus Amphotericin B as Therapy for Candidemia and Its Consequences in Nonneutropenic Subjects," *Clin Infect Dis*, 2003, 36 (10):1221-8.

Rex JH, Walsh TJ, Sobel JD, et al, "Practice Guidelines for the Treatment of Candidiasis. Infectious Diseases Society of America," *Clin Infect Dis*, 2000, 30(4):662-78.

Ringden O, Andstrom E, Remberger M, et al, "Safety of Liposomal Amphotericin B (AmBisome®) in 187 Transplant Recipients Treated With Cyclosporin," *Bone Marrow Transplant*, 1994, 14 (Suppl 5):10-4.

Rokicka M, "AmBisome® Treatment of Fungal Sinusitis in Severe Immunocompromised Patient With Acute Lymphoblastic Leukemia Relapsed after Autologous Peripheral Blood Transplantation," *ACTA Biomed*, 2006, 77(Suppl 2):26-7.

Walsh TH, Goodman JL, Pappas P, et al, "Safety, Tolerability, and Pharmacokinetics of High-Dose Liposomal Amphotericin B (AmBisome) in Patients Infected With *Aspergillus* Species and Other Filamentous Fungi: Maximum Tolerated Dose Study," *Antimicrob Agents Chemother*, 2001, 45 (12):3487-96.

Walsh TJ, Finberg RW, Arndt C, et al, "Liposomal Amphotericin B for Empirical Therapy in Patients With Persistent Fever and Neutropenia," *N Engl J Med*, 1999, 340:764-71.

◆ **AMSA** *see Amsacrine on page 79*

Amsacrine (AM sah kreen)

Related Information

Management of Drug Extravasations *on page 1447*
Safe Handling of Hazardous Drugs *on page 1517*

Index Terms 4-(9-Acridinylamino) Methanesulfon-m-Anisidide; Acridinyl Anisidide; AMSA; m-AMSA; NSC-249992

Generic Available No

Canadian Brand Names AMSA PD

Pharmacologic Category Antineoplastic Agent

Use Canada: Refractory acute leukemia

◀ **Unlabeled/Investigational Use** Acute myeloid leukemia (AML)

Restrictions Not available in U.S.

Lactation Excretion in breast milk unknown/not recommended

Labeled Contraindications Hypersensitivity to amsacrine, acridine derivatives, or any component of the formulation; pre-existing bone marrow suppression due to chemotherapy or radiation therapy

Warnings/Precautions Hazardous agent - use appropriate precautions for handling and disposal. Myelosuppression, including transient leukopenia, is a common toxicity; prolonged marrow aplasia may occur; may require dose reduction, therapy interruption or treatment delay. Acute cardiotoxicity, including arrhythmia, ECG changes, and rarely, cardiomyopathy and CHF, have been reported with use, although generally not considered to be a cumulative dose effect; use with caution in patients with underlying cardiovascular disease. Risk factors for cardiotoxicity may include hypokalemia and a history of anthracycline therapy; correct fluid and electrolyte imbalance prior to treatment initiation. Serum potassium should be >4 mEq/L prior to administration (Arlin, 1998). Use with caution in patients who have received high cumulative doses of anthracyclines Tumor lysis syndrome may occur; adequate hydration and prophylactic uric acid reduction should be considered prior to or during treatment; monitor closely. Hepatic metabolism and biliary excretion are major routes of elimination. Use with caution in patients with significant hepatic impairment (bilirubin >2 mg/dL); toxicity may be increased; dosage reductions may be required. Use with caution in patients with significant renal impairment (BUN >20 mg/dL; serum creatinine >1.2 mg/dL); toxicity may be increased; dosage reductions may be recommended. Evaluate renal and hepatic function prior to and during treatment. Avoid vaccination with live virus vaccines during treatment.

Adverse Reactions

>10%:
  Gastrointestinal: Nausea (>10%), vomiting (>10%), stomatitis (>10%), diarrhea (>10%), perirectal abscess (>10%), abdominal pain (>10%)
  Hematologic: Myelosuppression, leukopenia (nadir: 11-13 days; recovery: days 17-25)

Frequency not defined:
Cardiovascular: Atrial tachyarrhythmia, atrial tachycardia, atrial fibrillation, bradycardia, cardiomyopathy (rare), cardiopulmonary arrest, CHF (rare); ECG changes (QT prolongation, nonspecific ST segment or T wave changes); ejection fraction decreased, hypotension, sinus tachycardia, tachycardia, ventricular arrhythmia, ventricular extrasystoles, ventricular fibrillation, ventricular tachyarrhythmia
Central nervous system: Confusion, dizziness, emotional lability, fever, headache, hypoesthesia, lethargy, seizure
Dermatologic: Alopecia, cutaneous inflammatory reaction, dermatologic reaction, purpura, rash (purpuric or maculopapular), urticaria
Gastrointestinal: Anorexia, dysphagia, gingivitis, gum hemorrhage, hematemesis, weight changes
Genitourinary: Orange-red discoloration of the urine
Hematologic: Anemia, granulocytopenia, hemorrhage, pancytopenia, thrombocytopenia
Hepatic: Alkaline phosphatase increased, AST increased, bilirubin increased, hepatic insufficiency, hepatitis, hepatotoxicity, jaundice, progressive liver failure
Local: Injection site inflammation, phlebitis
Neuromuscular & skeletal: Musculoskeletal pain, paresthesia, weakness

Renal: BUN increased, creatinine increased, hematuria, proteinuria, renal failure

Respiratory: Dyspnea

Miscellaneous: Allergic reaction, infection

Drug Interactions

Avoid Concomitant Use

Avoid concomitant use of Amsacrine with any of the following: Natalizumab; Vaccines (Live)

Increased Effect/Toxicity

Amsacrine may increase the levels/effects of: Leflunomide; Natalizumab; Vaccines (Live); Vitamin K Antagonists

The levels/effects of Amsacrine may be increased by: Trastuzumab

Decreased Effect

Amsacrine may decrease the levels/effects of: Cardiac Glycosides; Vaccines (Inactivated); Vaccines (Live); Vitamin K Antagonists

The levels/effects of Amsacrine may be decreased by: Echinacea

Storage/Stability Store intact ampuls and diluent vials at controlled room temperature of 15°C to 25°C (59°F to 77°F). Concentrated amsacrine should not be stored in plastic syringes for >15 minutes. Reconstituted vials may be stored at room temperature for up to 24 hours, under ambient light conditions. Solutions diluted for administration are stable for up to 7 days in glass or plastic containers, however, the manufacturer recommends use with in 24 hours when stored at room temperature and 72 hours if refrigerated.

Reconstitution Use appropriate precautions for handling and disposal. Reconstitute by adding 1.5 mL amsacrine to diluent vial (containing 13.5 mL L-lactic acid), resulting in a 5 mg/mL reconstituted solution. Glass syringes should be used, however if using plastic syringes, do not allow concentrated amsacrine to remain in plastic syringe for >15 minutes. Further dilute appropriate dose in 500 mL D_5W (the solution may be mixed in plastic bags when diluted for infusion).

Compatibility Stable in D_5W; **incompatible** with BNS, D_5NS, $D_5^{1/4}NS$, $D_5^{1/2}NS$, D_5LR, $D_{10}NS$, NSS, LR, chloride ion. Amsacrine forms an immediate precipitate in the presence of chloride ion; do not mix with drugs that are chloride or hydrochloride salts.

Y-site administration: Compatible: Amikacin, chlorpromazine, clindamycin, cytarabine, dexamethasone, diphenhydramine, famotidine, fludarabine, gentamicin, granisetron, haloperidol, hydrocortisone sodium succinate, hydromorphone, lorazepam, morphine, prochlorperazine, promethazine, ranitidine, sodium bicarbonate, tobramycin, vancomycin. **Incompatible:** Acyclovir, amphotericin, aztreonam, calcium chloride, ceftazidime, ceftriaxone, cephalothin, cimetidine, cisplatin, filgrastim, furosemide, ganciclovir, heparin, methylprednisolone, metoclopramide, ondansetron, potassium chloride, sargramostim.

Compatibility when admixed: Compatible: Sodium bicarbonate, bleomycin

Mechanism of Action Amsacrine has been shown to inhibit DNA synthesis by binding to, and intercalating with, DNA; inhibits topoisomerase II activity.

Pharmacodynamics/Kinetics

Distribution: V_d: 1.67 L/kg; minimal CNS penetration

Protein binding: 96% to 98%

Metabolism: Hepatic, to inactive metabolites (major metabolite is 5' glutathione conjugate)

Half-life elimination: 1.4-5 hours; Terminal: 8-9 hours

Excretion: Bile; urine (35%; 20% as unchanged drug)

◀ **Dosage** Details concerning dosing in combination regimens should also be consulted. I.V.: Adults: Acute leukemia:

Induction: 75-125 mg/m^2/day for 5 days every 3-4 weeks (125 mg/m^2/day is preferred; two courses may be necessary to achieve induction; increase dose by 20% in second and subsequent cycles if marrow hypoplasia not achieved and in absence of significant toxicity in previous course.)

Maintenance: Once remission has been achieved, maintenance dose should be ~50% of induction dose, administered every 4-8 weeks, depending on blood counts and marrow recovery

Dosage adjustment for toxicity: Consider decreasing dose by 20% if life-threatening infection or hemorrhage occurred in previous cycle; delay second and subsequent cycles until recovery from myelosuppression or evidence of leukemic infiltrate is evident.

Dosage adjustment in renal impairment: Dosage reduction recommended; specific guidelines from the manufacturer are not available; the following guidelines have been used by some clinicians:

Hall, 1983:
Serum creatinine 1.2-1.8 mg/dL: No adjustment recommended
Serum creatinine 2-3 mg/dL, oliguric patients: Administer 60% to 70% of dose; may increase subsequent dose based on toxicity.
Hornedo, 1985: BUN >20 mg/dL or serum creatinine >1.5 mg/dL: Administer 75% of dose

Dosage adjustment in hepatic impairment: Bilirubin >2 mg/dL: Dosage reduction recommended; specific guidelines from the manufacturer are not available; the following guidelines have been used by some clinicians:

Hall, 1983: Bilirubin >2 mg/dL: Administer 60% to 70% of dose; may increase subsequent dose based on toxicity.
Hornedo, 1985: Bilirubin >2 mg/dL: Administer 75% of dose
Koren, 1992: Severe hepatic dysfunction: Administer ≤50% of dose

Administration I.V.: Infuse over 60-90 minutes; avoid extravasation.

Monitoring Parameters

CBC with differential, bone marrow studies, serum potassium, hepatic function, renal function; ECG (during and after infusion)

Vesicant Yes; see Management of Drug Extravasations on page 1447.

Dosage Forms Excipient information presented when available (limited, particularly for generics); consult specific product labeling. [CAN] = Canadian brand name

Injection, solution [preservative free]:
AMSA PD [CAN]: 50 mg/mL (1.5 mL) [supplied with L-lactic acid 0.0353 M 13.5 mL] [not available in the U.S.]

References

Arlin ZA, "A Special Role for Amsacrine in the Treatment of Acute Leukemia," *Cancer Invest*, 1989, 7(6):607-9.

Arlin ZA, Feldman, E. Kempin S, et al, "Amsacrine With High-Dose Cytarabine is Highly Effective Therapy for Refractory and Relapsed Acute Lymphoblastic Leukemia in Adults," *Blood*, 1988, 72 (2):433-5.

Hall SW, Friedman J, Legha SS, et al, "Human Pharmacokinetics of a New Acridine Derivative, 4'-(9-Acridinylamino)methanesulfon-m-anisidide (NSC 249992)," *Cancer Res*, 1983, 43(7):3422-6.

Hornedo J and Van Echo DA, "Amsacrine (m-AMSA): A New Antineoplastic Agent. Pharmacology, Clinical Activity and Toxicity," *Pharmacotherapy*, 1985, 5(2):78-90.

Koren G, Beatty K, Seto A, et al, "The Effects of Impaired Liver Function on the Elimination of Antineoplastic Agents," *Ann Pharmacother*, 1992, 26(3):363-71.

Louie AC and Issell BF, "Amsacrine (AMSA) - A Clinical Review," *J Clin Oncol*, 1985, 3(4):562-92.

Pai VB and Nahata MC, "Cardiotoxicity of Chemotherapuetic: Incidence, Treatment and Prevention," *Drug Saf*, 2000, 22(4):263-302.

◆ **AMSA PD (Can)** *see* Amsacrine *on page 79*

Anagrelide (an AG gre lide)

Medication Safety Issues
Sound-alike/look-alike issues:
Anagrelide may be confused with anastrozole

U.S. Brand Names Agrylin®

Index Terms Anagrelide Hydrochloride; BL4162A; NSC-724577

Generic Available Yes

Canadian Brand Names Agrylin®; Dom-Anagrelide; Mylan-Anagrelide; PHL-Anagrelide; PMS-Anagrelide; Sandoz-Anagrelide

Pharmacologic Category Phospholipase A_2 Inhibitor

Use Treatment of thrombocythemia associated with myeloproliferative disorders (eg, chronic myelogenous leukemia, essential thrombocythemia, polycythemia vera, myeloid metaplasia with myelofibrosis, or other myeloproliferative disorder)

Pregnancy Risk Factor C

Lactation Excretion in breast milk unknown/not recommended

Labeled Contraindications Severe hepatic impairment

Warnings/Precautions Use caution in patients with known or suspected heart disease; tachycardia, orthostatic hypotension, and CHF; a pretreatment cardiovascular evaluation and careful monitoring during treatment is recommended. Interstitial lung disease (including allergic alveolitis, eosinophilic pneumonia, and interstitial pneumonitis) has been associated with use; onset is from 1 week to several years, usually presenting with progressive dyspnea with lung infiltrations; symptoms usually improve after discontinuation. Use caution in patients with mild-to-moderate hepatic dysfunction; dosage reduction and careful monitoring are required for moderate hepatic impairment; use is contraindicated in severe hepatic impairment. Renal abnormalities (including renal failure) have been observed with anagrelide use; may be associated with pre-existing renal impairment, although dosage adjustment due to renal insufficiency was not required; monitor closely in patients with renal insufficiency.

Adverse Reactions
>10%:
Cardiovascular: Palpitation (26%), edema (21%)
Central nervous system: Headache (44%), dizziness (15%), pain (15%)
Gastrointestinal: Diarrhea (26%), nausea (17%), abdominal pain (16%)
Neuromuscular & skeletal: Weakness (23%)
Respiratory: Dyspnea (12%)
1% to 10%:
Cardiovascular: Peripheral edema (9%), chest pain (8%), tachycardia (8%), angina, arrhythmia, HF, hypertension, postural hypotension, syncope, thrombosis, vasodilatation
Central nervous system: Fever (9%), malaise (6%), amnesia, chills, confusion, depression, insomnia, migraine, nervousness, somnolence
Dermatologic: Rash (8%), pruritus (6%), alopecia, bruising, photosensitivity, urticaria
Endocrine & skeletal: Dehydration
Gastrointestinal: Flatulence (10%), vomiting (10%), anorexia (8%), dyspepsia (5%), aphthous stomatitis, constipation, eructation, gastritis, GI distress, GI hemorrhage, melena
Genitourinary: Dysuria
Hematologic: Thrombocytopenia (9%; grades 3/4: 5%), anemia, hemorrhage ▶

Hepatic: Liver enzymes increased

Neuromuscular & skeletal: Back pain (6%), paresthesia (6%), arthralgia, leg cramps, myalgia

Ocular: Amblyopia, diplopia, visual field abnormality

Otic: Tinnitus

Renal: Renal abnormality (1% to <5%), renal failure (1%), hematuria

Respiratory: Pharyngitis (7%), cough (6%), asthma, bronchitis, epistaxis, pneumonia, rhinitis, sinusitis

Miscellaneous: Flu-like syndrome, lymphadenopathy

Frequency not defined: Atrial fibrillation, cardiomegaly, cardiomyopathy, cerebrovascular accident, complete heart block, deep vein thrombosis, gastric/duodenal ulceration; interstitial lung disease (allergic alveolitis, eosinophilic pneumonia, interstitial pneumonitis); leukocyte count increased, MI, myelofibrosis, pancreatitis, pericarditis, pericardial effusion, pleural effusion, polycythemia, pulmonary fibrosis, pulmonary hypertension, pulmonary infiltrates, seizure, stroke, transient ischemic attack

Drug Interactions

Metabolism/Transport Effects Substrate of CYP1A2 (minor)

Avoid Concomitant Use There are no known interactions where it is recommended to avoid concomitant use.

Increased Effect/Toxicity

Anagrelide may increase the levels/effects of: Anticoagulants; Antiplatelet Agents; Drotrecogin Alfa; Ibritumomab; Salicylates; Thrombolytic Agents; Tositumomab and Iodine I 131 Tositumomab

The levels/effects of Anagrelide may be increased by: Dasatinib; Herbs (Anticoagulant/Antiplatelet Properties); MAO Inhibitors; Nonsteroidal Anti-Inflammatory Agents; Omega-3-Acid Ethyl Esters; Pentosan Polysulfate Sodium; Pentoxifylline; Prostacyclin Analogues

Decreased Effect

The levels/effects of Anagrelide may be decreased by: Nonsteroidal Anti-Inflammatory Agents

Ethanol/Nutrition/Herb Interactions

Ethanol: May increase CNS adverse effects.

Food: No clinically significant effect on absorption.

Herb/Nutraceutical: Avoid herbs with anticoagulant/antiplatelet properties (alfalfa, anise, bilberry, bladderwrack, bromelain, cat's claw, celery, chamomile, coleus, cordyceps, dong quai, evening primrose oil, fenugreek, feverfew, garlic, ginger, ginkgo biloba, ginseng [American], ginseng [Panax], ginseng [Siberian], grape seed, green tea, guggul, horse chestnut seed, horseradish, licorice, prickly ash, red clover, reishi, SAMe [S-adenosylme-thionine], sweet clover, turmeric, white willow); may enhance the adverse effect of antiplatelets agents.

Storage/Stability Store at 27°C (77°F); excursions permitted to 15°C to 30°C (59°F to 86°F). Protect from light.

Mechanism of Action Anagrelide appears to inhibit cyclic nucleotide phosphodiesterase and the release of arachidonic acid from phospholipase, possibly by inhibiting phospholipase A_2. It also causes a dose-related reduction in platelet production, which results from decreased megakaryocyte hypermaturation (disrupts the postmitotic phase of maturation).

Pharmacodynamics/Kinetics

Onset of action: Initial: Within 7-14 days; complete response (platelets ≤600,000/mm^3): 4-12 weeks

Duration: 6-24 hours; upon discontinuation, platelet count begins to rise within 4 days

Metabolism: Hepatic; to RL603 and 3-hydroxy anagrelide

Half-life elimination, plasma: 1.3 hours

Time to peak, serum: 1 hour

Excretion: Urine (<1% as unchanged drug)

Dosage Note: Maintain initial dose for ≥1 week, then adjust to the lowest effective dose to reduce and maintain platelet count <600,000/μL ideally to the normal range; the dose must not be increased by >0.5 mg/day in any 1 week; maximum dose: 10 mg/day or 2.5 mg/dose

Oral: Thrombocythemia:

Children: Initial: 0.5 mg/day (range: 0.5 mg 1-4 times/day)

Adults: Initial: 0.5 mg 4 times/day or 1 mg twice daily (most patients will experience adequate response at dose ranges of 1.5-3 mg/day)

Elderly: There are no special requirements for dosing in the elderly

Dosage adjustment in renal impairment: No adjustment required in renal insufficiency

Dosage adjustment in hepatic impairment:

Moderate impairment: Initial: 0.5 mg once daily; maintain for at least 1 week with careful monitoring of cardiovascular status; the dose must not be increased by >0.5 mg/day in any 1 week.

Severe impairment: Contraindicated

Administration May be administered without regard to food.

Monitoring Parameters Platelet count (every 2 days during the first week of treatment and at least weekly until the maintenance dose is reached); CBC with differential, ALT, AST, BUN, and serum creatinine (monitor closely during first weeks of treatment); blood pressure; cardiovascular exam (pretreatment; monitor during therapy). Monitor for thrombosis or bleeding.

Dietary Considerations May be taken without regard to food.

Dosage Forms Excipient information presented when available (limited, particularly for generics); consult specific product labeling.

Capsule: 0.5 mg, 1 mg

Agrylin®: 0.5 mg

References

Harrison CN, Campbell PJ, Buck G, et al, "Hydroxyurea Compared With Anagrelide in High-Risk Essential Thrombocythemia," *N Engl J Med*, 2005, 353(1):33-45.

Petitt RM, Silverstein MN, and Petrone ME, "Anagrelide for Control of Thrombocythemia in Polycythemia and Other Myeloproliferative Disorders," *Semin Hematol*, 1997, 34(1):51-4.

Steurer M, Gastl G, Jedrzejczak WW, et al, Anagrelide for Thrombocytosis in Myeloproliferative Disorders: A Prospective Study to Assess Efficacy and Adverse Event Profile," *Cancer*, 2004, 101(10):2239-46.

Tefferi A and Vardiman JW, "Classification and Diagnosis of Myeloproliferative Neoplasms: The 2008 World Health Organization Criteria and Point-of-Care Diagnostic Algorithms," *Leukemia*, 2008, 22(1):14-22.

♦ **Anagrelide Hydrochloride** see Anagrelide on page 83

♦ **Anandron® (Can)** see Nilutamide on page 851

Anastrozole (an AS troe zole)

Medication Safety Issues

Sound-alike/look-alike issues:

Anastrozole may be confused with anagrelide, letrozole

Arimidex® may be confused with Aromasin®

◄ **Related Information**
Safe Handling of Hazardous Drugs *on page 1517*
U.S. Brand Names Arimidex®
Index Terms ICI-D1033; ZD1033
Generic Available No
Canadian Brand Names Arimidex®
Pharmacologic Category Antineoplastic Agent, Aromatase Inhibitor
Use Treatment of locally-advanced or metastatic breast cancer (hormone receptor-positive or unknown) in postmenopausal women; treatment of advanced breast cancer in postmenopausal women with disease progression following tamoxifen therapy; adjuvant treatment of early hormone receptor-positive breast cancer in postmenopausal women
Unlabeled/Investigational Use Treatment of recurrent or metastatic endometrial or uterine cancers, treatment of recurrent ovarian cancer
Pregnancy Risk Factor X
Lactation Excretion in breast milk unknown/not recommended
Labeled Contraindications Hypersensitivity to anastrozole or any component of the formulation; pregnancy or women who may become pregnant
Warnings/Precautions Hazardous agent - use appropriate precautions for handling and disposal. Use is contraindicated in women who are or may become pregnant. Anastrozole offers no clinical benefit in premenopausal women with breast cancer. Patients with pre-existing ischemic cardiac disease have an increased risk for ischemic cardiovascular events.

Due to decreased circulating estrogen levels, anastrozole is associated with a reduction in bone mineral density (BMD); decreases (from baseline) in total hip and lumbar spine BMD have been reported. Patients with pre-existing osteopenia are at higher risk for developing osteoporosis (Eastell, 2008). When initiating anastrozole treatment, follow available guidelines for bone mineral density management in postmenopausal women with similar fracture risk; concurrent use of bisphosphonates may be useful in patients at risk for fractures.

Elevated total cholesterol levels (contributed to by LDL cholesterol increases) have been reported in patients receiving anastrozole; use with caution in patients with hyperlipidemias; cholesterol levels should be monitored/managed in accordance with current guidelines for patients with LDL elevations. Plasma concentrations in patients with stable hepatic cirrhosis were within the range of concentrations seen in normal subjects across all clinical trials; use has not been studied in patients with severe hepatic impairment. Safety and efficacy in children have not been established.

Adverse Reactions
>10%:
Cardiovascular: Vasodilatation (25% to 36%), ischemic cardiovascular disease (4%; 17% in patients with pre-existing ischemic heart disease), hypertension (2% to 13%), angina (2%; 12% in patients with pre-existing ischemic heart disease)
Central nervous system: Mood disturbance (19%), fatigue (19%), pain (11% to 17%), headache (9% to 13%), depression (5% to 13%)
Dermatologic: Rash (6% to 11%)
Endocrine & metabolic: Hot flashes (12% to 36%)
Gastrointestinal: Nausea (11% to 19%), vomiting (8% to 13%)
Neuromuscular & skeletal: Weakness (16% to 19%), arthritis (17%), arthralgia (2% to 15%), back pain (10% to 12%), bone pain (6% to 11%), osteoporosis (11%)

Respiratory: Pharyngitis (6% to 14%), cough increased (8% to 11%)

1% to 10%:

Cardiovascular: Peripheral edema (5% to 10%), chest pain (5% to 7%), venous thromboembolic events (2% to 4%), ischemic cerebrovascular events (2%), MI (1%)

Central nervous system: Insomnia (2% to 10%), dizziness (6% to 8%), anxiety (2% to 6%), fever (2% to 5%), malaise (2% to 5%), confusion (2% to 5%), nervousness (2% to 5%), somnolence (2% to 5%), lethargy (1%)

Dermatologic: Alopecia (2% to 5%), pruritus (2% to 5%)

Endocrine & metabolic: Hypercholesterolemia (9%), breast pain (2% to 8%)

Gastrointestinal: Diarrhea (8% to 9%), constipation (7% to 9%), abdominal pain (7% to 9%), weight gain (2% to 9%), anorexia (5% to 7%), xerostomia (6%), dyspepsia (7%), weight loss (2%)

Genitourinary: Urinary tract infection (2% to 8%), vulvovaginitis (6%), pelvic pain (5%), vaginal bleeding (1% to 5%), vaginitis (4%), vaginal discharge (4%), vaginal hemorrhage (2% to 4%), leukorrhea (2% to 3%), vaginal dryness (2%)

Hematologic: Anemia (2% to 5%), leukopenia (2% to 5%)

Hepatic: Liver function tests increased (1% to 10%), alkaline phosphatase increased (1% to 10%), gamma GT increased (≤5%)

Local: Thrombophlebitis (2% to 5%)

Neuromuscular & skeletal: Fracture (1% to 10%), arthrosis (7%), paresthesia (5% to 7%), joint disorder (6%), myalgia (2% to 6%), neck pain (2% to 5%), carpal tunnel syndrome (3%), hypertonia (3%)

Ocular: Cataracts (6%)

Respiratory: Dyspnea (8% to 10%), sinusitis (2% to 6%), bronchitis (2% to 5%), rhinitis (2% to 5%)

Miscellaneous: Lymphedema (10%), infection (2% to 9%), flu-like syndrome (2% to 7%), diaphoresis (2% to 5%), cyst (5%), neoplasm (5%), tumor flare (3%)

<1%, postmarketing, and/or case reports: Anaphylaxis, angioedema, bilirubin increased, CVA, cerebral ischemia, cerebral infarct, endometrial cancer, erythema multiforme, hepatitis, jaundice, joint pain, joint stiffness, liver inflammation, liver pain, liver swelling, myocardial ischemia, pulmonary embolus, retinal vein thrombosis; skin reactions (eg, blisters, lesions, ulcers); Stevens-Johnson syndrome, trigger finger, urticaria

Drug Interactions

Metabolism/Transport Effects Inhibits CYP1A2 (weak), 2C8 (weak), 2C9 (weak), 3A4 (weak)

Avoid Concomitant Use

Avoid concomitant use of Anastrozole with any of the following: Estrogen Derivatives

Increased Effect/Toxicity There are no known significant interactions involving an increase in effect.

Decreased Effect

The levels/effects of Anastrozole may be decreased by: Estrogen Derivatives; Tamoxifen

Storage/Stability Store at 20°C to 25°C (68°F to 77°F).

Mechanism of Action Potent and selective nonsteroidal aromatase inhibitor. By inhibiting aromatase, the conversion of androstenedione to estrone, and testosterone to estradiol, is prevented, thereby decreasing tumor mass or delaying progression in patients with tumors responsive to hormones. Anastrozole causes an 85% decrease in estrone sulfate levels.

Pharmacodynamics/Kinetics
Onset of estradiol reduction: 70% reduction after 24 hours; 80% after 2 weeks therapy

Duration of estradiol reduction: 6 days

Absorption: Well absorbed; extent of absorption not affected by food

Protein binding, plasma: 40%

Metabolism: Extensively hepatic (~85%) via N-dealkylation, hydroxylation, and glucuronidation; primary metabolite (triazole) inactive

Half-life elimination: ~40-50 hours

Time to peak, plasma: ~2 hours without food; 5 hours with food

Excretion: Feces; urine (urinary excretion accounts for ~11% of total elimination, mostly as metabolites)

Dosage Oral: Adults: Breast cancer: 1 mg once daily

Dosage adjustment in renal impairment: Dosage adjustment not necessary

Dosage adjustment in hepatic impairment:

Mild-to-moderate impairment or stable hepatic cirrhosis: Dosage adjustment is not required

Severe hepatic impairment: Has not been studied in this population

Administration May be administered with or without food.

Monitoring Parameters Bone mineral density; total cholesterol and LDL

Dietary Considerations May be taken with or without food.

Dosage Forms Excipient information presented when available (limited, particularly for generics); consult specific product labeling.

Tablet:

Arimidex®: 1 mg

References
Buzdar AU, Robertson JF, Eiermann W, et al, "An Overview of the Pharmacology and Pharmacokinetics of the Newer Generation Aromatase Inhibitors Anastrozole, Letrozole, and Exemestane," *Cancer*, 2002, 95(9):2006-16.

del Carmen MG, Fuller AF, Matulonis U, et al, "Phase II Trial of Anastrozole in Women With Asymptomatic Müllerian Cancer," *Gynecol Oncol*, 2003, 91(3):596-602.

Eastell R, Adams JE, Coleman RE, et al, "Effect of Anastrozole on Bone Mineral Density: 5-Year Results From the Anastrozole, Tamoxifen, Alone or in Combination Trial 18233230," *J Clin Oncol*, 2008, 26(7):1051-7.

Forbes JF, Cuzick J, Buzdar A, et al, "Effect of Anastrozole and Tamoxifen as Adjuvant Treatment for Early-Stage Breast Cancer: 100-month Analysis of the ATAC Trial," *Lancet Oncol*, 2008, 9 (1):45-53.

Kaufmann M, Jonat W, Hilfrich J, et al, "Improved Overall Survival in Postmenopausal Women With Early Breast Cancer After Anastrozole Initiated After Treatment With Tamoxifen Compared With Continued Tamoxifen: The ARNO 95 Study," *J Clin Oncol*, 2007, 25(19):2664-70.

Lonning P, Pfister C, Martoni A, et al, "Pharmacokinetics of Third-Generation Aromatase Inhibitors," *Semin Oncol*, 2003, 30(4 Suppl 14):23-32.

National Comprehensive Cancer Network (NCCN)®, "Clinical Practice Guidelines in Oncology™: Ovarian Cancer," Version 1.2009. Available at http://www.nccn.org/professionals/physician_gls/PDF/ovarian.pdf

National Comprehensive Cancer Network (NCCN)®, "Clinical Practice Guidelines in Oncology™: Uterine Neoplasms," Version 2.2009. Available at http://www.nccn.org/professionals/physician_gls/PDF/uterine.pdf

National Osteoporosis Foundation, *Clinician's Guide to Prevention and Treatment of Osteoporosis*, National Osteoporosis Foundation, Washington, DC, 2008. Available at http://www.nof.org

Rose PG, Brunetto VL, VanLe L, et al, "A Phase II Trial of Anastrozole in Advanced Recurrent or Persistent Endometrial Carcinoma: A Gynecologic Oncology Group Study," *Gynecol Oncol*, 2000, 78(2):212-6.

Winer EP, Hudis C, Burstein HJ, et al, "American Society of Clinical Oncology Technology Assessment on the Use of Aromatase Inhibitors as Adjuvant Therapy for Postmenopausal Women With Hormone Receptor-Positive Breast Cancer: Status Report 2004," *J Clin Oncol*, 2005, 23(3):619-29.

◆ **Ancobon®** *see* Flucytosine *on page 490*

◆ **Androcur® (Can)** *see* Cyproterone *on page 279*

♦ **Androcur® Depot (Can)** *see* Cyproterone *on page* 279

♦ **Androxy™** *see* Fluoxymesterone *on page* 505

Anidulafungin (ay nid yoo la FUN jin)

U.S. Brand Names Eraxis™

Index Terms LY303366

Generic Available No

Canadian Brand Names Eraxis™

Pharmacologic Category Antifungal Agent, Parenteral; Echinocandin

Use Treatment of candidemia and other forms of *Candida* infections (including those of intra-abdominal, peritoneal, and esophageal locus)

Unlabeled/Investigational Use Treatment of infections due to *Aspergillus* spp.

Pregnancy Risk Factor C

Lactation Excretion in breast milk unknown/use caution

Labeled Contraindications Hypersensitivity to anidulafungin, other echinocandins, or any component of the formulation

Warnings/Precautions Histamine-mediated reactions (eg, urticaria, flushing, hypotension) have been observed; these may be related to infusion rate. Elevated liver function tests, hepatitis, and worsening hepatic failure have been reported. Monitor for progressive hepatic impairment if increased transaminase enzymes noted. Safety and efficacy in pediatric patients, neutropenic patients, or other *Candida* infections (eg, endocarditis, osteomyelitis, meningitis) have not been established.

Adverse Reactions

2% to 10%:

Endocrine & metabolic: Hypokalemia (3%)

Gastrointestinal: Diarrhea (3%)

Hepatic: Transaminase increased (<1% to 2%)

<2%: Abdominal pain, alkaline phosphatase increased, amylase increased, angioneurotic edema, atrial fibrillation, back pain, bilirubin increased, bundle branch block (right), candidiasis, cholestasis, clostridial infection, coagulopathy, constipation, cough, CPK increased, creatinine increased, diaphoresis, diarrhea, dizziness, DVT, dyspepsia, ECG abnormality (including QT prolongation), erythema, eye pain, fecal incontinence, flushing, fungemia, GGT increased, headache, hepatic necrosis, hepatitis, hepatic dysfunction, hot flushes, hypercalcemia, hyperglycemia, hyperkalemia, hypernatremia, hyper-/hypotension, hypomagnesemia, infusion-related reaction, leukopenia (0.7%), lipase increased, nausea, neutropenia (1%), peripheral edema, phlebitis, platelet count increased, prothrombin time prolonged, pruritus, pyrexia, rash, rigors, seizure, sinus arrhythmia, thrombocytopenia, thrombophlebitis, urea increased, urticaria, ventricular extrasystoles, vision blurred, visual disturbance, vomiting

Drug Interactions

Avoid Concomitant Use There are no known interactions where it is recommended to avoid concomitant use.

Increased Effect/Toxicity There are no known significant interactions involving an increase in effect.

Decreased Effect

Anidulafungin may decrease the levels/effects of: Saccharomyces boulardii

Storage/Stability Store between 15°C to 30°C (59°F to 86°F). Reconstituted and diluted solutions are stable for 24 hours at room temperature. Do not refrigerate or freeze.

Reconstitution Aseptically add 15 mL (50 mg vial) or 30 mL (100 mg vial) of companion diluent (20% w/w dehydrated alcohol in water for injection) to each vial. Swirl to dissolve; do not shake. Further dilute 50 mg, 100 mg, or 200 mg in 100 mL, 250 mL, or 500 mL, respectively, of D_5W or NS.

Compatibility Stable in D_5W, NS.

Y-site administration: Compatible: Acyclovir, amikacin, aminophylline, ampicillin-sulbactam, carboplatin, cefazolin, cefepime, cefoxitin, ceftazidime, ceftizoxime, ceftriaxone, cefuroxime, cimetidine, ciprofloxacin, cisplatin, clindamycin, cyclophosphamide, cyclosporine, cytarabine, daunorubicin, dexamethasone, digoxin, dobutamine, docetaxel, dopamine, doxorubicin, epinephrine, erythromycin, etoposide, famotidine, fentanyl, fluconazole, fluorouracil, furosemide, ganciclovir, gatifloxacin, gemcitabine, gentamicin, heparin, hydrocortisone, hydromorphone, ifosfamide, imipenem–cilastatin, leucovorin, levofloxacin, linezolid, meperidine, meropenem, methylprednisolone, metronidazole, midazolam, morphine, mycophenolate mofetil, norepinephrine, paclitaxel, pantoprazole, phenylephrine, piperacillin-tazobactam, potassium chloride, quinupristin–dalfopristin, ranitidine, sulfamethoxazole-trimethoprim, tacrolimus, ticarcillin, tobramycin, vancomycin, vincristine, voriconazole, zidovudine. **Incompatible:** Amphotericin B, ertapenem, sodium bicarbonate.

Mechanism of Action Noncompetitive inhibitor of 1,3-beta-D-glucan synthase resulting in reduced formation of 1,3-beta-D-glucan, an essential polysaccharide comprising 30% to 60% of *Candida* cell walls (absent in mammalian cells); decreased glucan content leads to osmotic instability and cellular lysis

Pharmacodynamics/Kinetics

Distribution: 30-50 L

Protein binding: 84%

Metabolism: No hepatic metabolism observed; undergoes slow chemical hydrolysis to open-ring peptide-lacking antifungal activity

Half-life elimination: 27 hours

Excretion: Feces (30%, 10% as unchanged drug); urine (<1%)

Dosage I.V.: Adults:

Candidemia, intra-abdominal or peritoneal candidiasis: 200 mg loading dose on day 1, followed by 100 mg daily for at least 14 days after last positive culture

Esophageal candidiasis: 100 mg loading dose on day 1, followed by 50 mg daily for at least 14 days and for at least 7 days after symptom resolution

Dosage adjustment in renal impairment: No adjustment necessary, including dialysis patients

Dosage adjustment in hepatic impairment: No adjustment necessary

Administration For intravenous use only; infusion rate should not exceed 1.1 mg/minute

Monitoring Parameters Liver function tests

Dosage Forms Excipient information presented when available (limited, particularly for generics); consult specific product labeling.

Injection, powder for reconstitution:

Eraxis™: 50 mg [contains polysorbate 80; packaged with dehydrated alcohol as diluent]; 100 mg [contains polysorbate 80; packaged with dehydrated alcohol as diluent]

References

Trissel LA and Ogundele AB, "Compatibility of Anidulafungin With Other Drugs During Simulated Y-Site Administration," *Am J Health-Sys Pharm*, 2005, 62:834-7.

Vazquez JA, "Anidulafungin: A New Echinocandin With a Novel Profile," *Clin Ther*, 2005, 27 (6):657-73.

Walsh TJ, Anaissie EJ, Denning DW, et al, "Treatment of Aspergillosis: Clinical Practice Guidelines of the Infectious Diseases Society of America," *Clin Infect Dis*, 2008, 46(3):327-60.

Antihemophilic Factor (Human)
(an tee hee moe FIL ik FAK tor HYU man)

U.S. Brand Names Hemofil M; Koāte®-DVI; Monarc-M™; Monoclate-P®

Index Terms AHF (Human); Factor VIII (Human)

Generic Available Yes

Canadian Brand Names Hemofil M

Pharmacologic Category Antihemophilic Agent; Blood Product Derivative

Use Prevention and treatment of hemorrhagic episodes in patients with hemophilia A (classic hemophilia); perioperative management of hemophilia A; can be of significant therapeutic value in patients with acquired factor VIII inhibitors not exceeding 10 Bethesda units/mL

Pregnancy Risk Factor C

Lactation Excretion in breast milk unknown/use caution

Labeled Contraindications Hypersensitivity to any component of the formulation

Warnings/Precautions Risk of viral transmission is not totally eradicated. Because antihemophilic factor is prepared from pooled plasma, it may contain the causative agent of viral hepatitis and other viral diseases. Hepatitis B vaccination is recommended for all patients. Hepatitis A vaccination is also recommended for seronegative patients. Antihemophilic factor contains trace amounts of blood groups A and B isohemagglutinins and when large or frequently repeated doses are given to individuals with blood groups A, B, and AB, the patient should be monitored for signs of progressive anemia and the possibility of intravascular hemolysis should be considered. The dosage requirement will vary in patients with factor VIII inhibitors; optimal treatment should be determined by clinical response. Natural rubber latex is a component of Hemofil M and Monarc-M™ packaging. Hemofil M, Monoclate-P®, and Monarc-M™ contain trace amounts of mouse protein. Products contain naturally-occurring von Willebrand factor for stabilization, however efficacy has not been established for the treatment of von Willebrand disease. Products vary by preparation method; final formulations contain human albumin.

Adverse Reactions <1%: Acute hemolytic anemia, AHF inhibitor development, allergic reactions (rare), anaphylaxis (rare), bleeding tendency increased, blurred vision, chest tightness, chills, fever, headache, hyperfibrinogenemia, jittery feeling, lethargy, nausea, somnolence, stinging at the infusion site, stomach discomfort, tingling, urticaria, vasomotor reactions with rapid infusion, vomiting

Drug Interactions

Avoid Concomitant Use There are no known interactions where it is recommended to avoid concomitant use.

Increased Effect/Toxicity There are no known significant interactions involving an increase in effect.

Decreased Effect There are no known significant interactions involving a decrease in effect.

Storage/Stability Store under refrigeration, 2°C to 8°C (36°F to 46°F); avoid freezing. Use within 3 hours of reconstitution. Do not refrigerate after reconstitution, precipitation may occur.

Hemofil M, Monarc-M™: May also be stored at room temperature not to exceed 30°C (86°F).

Koāte®-DVI; Monoclate-P®: May also be stored at room temperature of 25°C (77°F) for ≤6 months.

Reconstitution If refrigerated, the dried concentrate and diluent should be warmed to room temperature before reconstitution. Gently swirl or rotate vial after adding diluent; do not shake vigorously.

Mechanism of Action Protein (factor VIII) in normal plasma which is necessary for clot formation and maintenance of hemostasis; activates factor X in conjunction with activated factor IX; activated factor X converts prothrombin to thrombin, which converts fibrinogen to fibrin, and with factor XIII forms a stable clot

Pharmacodynamics/Kinetics Half-life elimination: Mean: 8-27 hours

Dosage Children and Adults: I.V.: Individualize dosage based on coagulation studies performed prior to treatment and at regular intervals during treatment. In general, administration of factor VIII 1 int. unit/kg will increase circulating factor VIII levels by ~2 int. units/dL. (General guidelines presented; consult individual product labeling for specific dosing recommendations.)

Dosage based on desired factor VIII increase (%):

To calculate dosage needed based on desired factor VIII increase (%):

Body weight (kg) x 0.5 int. units/kg x desired factor VIII increase (%) = int. units factor VIII required

For example:

50 kg x 0.5 int. units/kg x 30 (% increase) = 750 int. units factor VIII

Dosage based on expected factor VIII increase (%):

It is also possible to calculate the **expected** % factor VIII increase:

(# int. units administered x 2%/int. units/kg) divided by body weight (kg) = expected % factor VIII increase

For example:

(1400 int. units x 2%/int. units/kg) divided by 70 kg = 40%

General guidelines:

Minor hemorrhage: 10-20 int. units/kg as a single dose to achieve FVIII plasma level ~20% to 40% of normal. Mild superficial or early hemorrhages may respond to a single dose; may repeat dose every 12-24 hours for 1-3 days until bleeding is resolved or healing achieved.

Moderate hemorrhage/minor surgery: 15-25 int. units/kg to achieve FVIII plasma level 30% to 50% of normal. If needed, may continue with a maintenance dose of 10-15 int. units/kg every 8-12 hours.

Major to life-threatening hemorrhage: Initial dose 40-50 int. units/kg, followed by a maintenance dose of 20-25 int. units/kg every 8-12 hours until threat is resolved, to achieve FVIII plasma level 80% to 100% of normal.

Major surgery: 50 int. units/kg given preoperatively to raise factor VIII level to 100% before surgery begins. May repeat as necessary after 6-12 hours initially and for a total of 10-14 days until healing is complete. Intensity of therapy may depend on type of surgery and postoperative regimen.

Bleeding prophylaxis: May be administered on a regular basis for bleeding prophylaxis. Doses of 24-40 int. units/kg 3 times/week have been reported in patients with severe hemophilia to prevent joint bleeding.

If bleeding is not controlled with adequate dose, test for presence of inhibitor. It may not be possible or practical to control bleeding if inhibitor titers are >10 Bethesda units/mL.

Elderly: Response in the elderly is not expected to differ from that of younger patients; dosage should be individualized

Administration Administer I.V. over 5-10 minutes (maximum: 10 mL/minute). Infuse Monoclate-P® at 2 mL/minute.

Monitoring Parameters Heart rate and blood pressure (before and during I.V. administration); AHF levels prior to and during treatment; in patients with circulating inhibitors, the inhibitor level should be monitored; hematocrit; monitor for signs and symptoms of intravascular hemolysis; bleeding

Dosage Forms Excipient information presented when available (limited, particularly for generics); consult specific product labeling.

Injection, powder for reconstitution:

Hemofil M: Vial labeled with international units [contains albumin; derived from mouse proteins; packaging may contain natural rubber latex]

Koate®-DVI: ~250 int. units, ~500 int. units, ~1000 int. units [contains albumin]

Monarc-M™: Vial labeled with international units [contains albumin; derived from mouse proteins; packaging may contain natural rubber latex]

Monoclate-P®: ~250 int. units, ~500 int. units, ~1000 int. units, ~1500 int. units [contains albumin; derived from mouse proteins]

References

Nilsson IM, Berntorp E, Lofqvist T, et al, "Twenty-five Years' Experience of Prophylactic Treatment in Severe Haemophilia A and B," *J Intern Med*, 1992, 232(1):25-32.

White GC, Rosendaal F, Aledort LM, et al, "Definitions in Hemophilia. Recommendation of the Scientific Subcommittee on Factor VIII and Factor IX of the Scientific and Standardization Committee of the International Society on Thrombosis and Haemostasis," *Thromb Haemost*, 2001, 85(3):560.

Antihemophilic Factor (Recombinant)

(an tee hee moe FIL ik FAK tor ree KOM be nant)

Medication Safety Issues Confusion may occur due to the omitting of "Factor VIII" from some product labeling. Review product contents carefully prior to dispensing any antihemophilic factor.

U.S. Brand Names Advate; Helixate® FS; Kogenate® FS; Recombinate; ReFacto® [DSC]; Xyntha™

Index Terms AHF (Recombinant); Factor VIII (Recombinant); rAHF

Generic Available No

Canadian Brand Names Helixate® FS; Kogenate®; Kogenate® FS; Recombinate; ReFacto®

Pharmacologic Category Antihemophilic Agent

Use Prevention and treatment of hemorrhagic episodes in patients with hemophilia A (classic hemophilia or congenital factor VIII deficiency); perioperative management of hemophilia A; prophylaxis of joint bleeding and to reduce risk of joint damage in children with hemophilia A with no preexisting joint damage; can be of significant therapeutic value in patients with acquired factor VIII inhibitors ≤10 Bethesda units/mL

Pregnancy Risk Factor C

Lactation Excretion in breast milk unknown/use caution

◀ **Labeled Contraindications** Hypersensitivity to any component of the formulation

Warnings/Precautions Monitor for signs of formation of antibodies to factor VIII; may occur at anytime but more common in young children with severe hemophilia. The dosage requirement will vary in patients with factor VIII inhibitors; optimal treatment should be determined by clinical response. Allergic hypersensitivity reactions (including anaphylaxis) may occur; monitor. Products vary by preparation method. Recombinate is stabilized using human albumin. Helixate® FS and Kogenate® FS are stabilized with sucrose. Advate, Helixate® FS, Kogenate® FS, ReFacto®, and Xyntha™ may contain trace amounts of mouse or hamster protein. Recombinate may contain mouse, hamster or bovine protein. Products may contain von Willebrand factor for stabilization; however, efficacy has not been established for the treatment of von Willebrand's disease.

Adverse Reactions Actual frequency may vary by product.

>1%:

Central nervous system: Chills, dizziness, fever, headache, pain

Dermatologic: Pruritus, rash, urticaria

Gastrointestinal: Diarrhea, nausea, taste perversion, vomiting

Hematologic: Hemorrhage

Local: Injection site pain, injection site inflammation, infusion site reaction

Neuromuscular & skeletal: Arthralgia, weakness

Respiratory: Cough, dyspnea, nasopharyngitis, pharyngolaryngeal pain

Miscellaneous: Catheter thrombosis, factor VIII inhibitor formation

≤1%, postmarketing, and/or case reports: Abdominal pain, adenopathy, allergic reactions, anaphylaxis, anemia, anorexia, arthralgia, AST increased, blood pressure decreased, chest discomfort, chest pain, constipation, depersonalization, diaphoresis, edema, epistaxis, facial edema, facial flushing, factor VIII decreased, fatigue, fever, GI hemorrhage, hives, hot flashes, hypersensitivity reaction, hyper-/hypotension (slight), infection, joint swelling, lethargy, otitis media, pallor, paresthesia, restlessness, rhinitis, rigors, shortness of breath, somnolence, tachycardia, urinary tract infection, vasodilation, venous catheter access complications

Drug Interactions

Avoid Concomitant Use There are no known interactions where it is recommended to avoid concomitant use.

Increased Effect/Toxicity There are no known significant interactions involving an increase in effect.

Decreased Effect There are no known significant interactions involving a decrease in effect.

Storage/Stability Store under refrigeration, 2°C to 8°C (36°F to 46°F); avoid freezing. Use within 3 hours of reconstitution. Do not refrigerate after reconstitution, a precipitation may occur.

Advate: May also be stored at room temperature for up to 6 months.

Helixate® FS, Kogenate® FS, ReFacto®, Xyntha™: May also be stored at room temperature (not to exceed 25°C [36°F]) up to 3 months. Avoid prolonged exposure to light during storage.

Recombinate: May also be stored at room temperature, not to exceed 30°C (86°F).

Reconstitution If refrigerated, the dried concentrate and diluent should be warmed to room temperature before reconstitution. Gently agitate or rotate vial after adding diluent, do not shake vigorously.

Mechanism of Action Factor VIII replacement, necessary for clot formation and maintenance of hemostasis. It activates factor X in conjunction with activated factor IX; activated factor X converts prothrombin to thrombin, which converts fibrinogen to fibrin, and with factor XIII forms a stable clot.

Pharmacodynamics/Kinetics

Distribution: V_{ss}: 0.36-0.57 dL/kg

Half-life elimination: Mean: 8-19 hours

Dosage I.V.:

Hemophilia: Children and Adults: Individualize dosage based on coagulation studies performed prior to treatment and at regular intervals during treatment. In general, administration of factor VIII 1 int. unit/kg will increase circulating factor VIII levels by ~2 int. units/dL. (General guidelines presented; consult individual product labeling for specific dosing recommendations.)

Joint bleeding prophylaxis (Helixate® FS, Kogenate® FS): Children: 25 int. units/kg every other day

Dosage based on desired factor VIII increase (%):

To calculate dosage needed based on desired factor VIII increase (%):

[Body weight (kg) x desired factor VIII increase (%)] divided by 2%/int. units/kg = int. units factor VIII required

For example:

50 kg x 30 (% increase) divided by 2%/int. units/kg = 750 int. units factor VIII

Dosage based on expected factor VIII increase (%):

It is also possible to calculate the **expected** % factor VIII increase:

(# int. units administered x 2%/int. units/kg) divided by body weight (kg) = expected % factor VIII increase

For example:

(1400 int. units x 2%/int. units/kg) divided by 70 kg = 40%

General guidelines:

Minor hemorrhage: 10-20 int. units/kg as a single dose to achieve FVIII plasma level ~20% to 40% of normal. Mild superficial or early hemorrhages may respond to a single dose; may repeat dose every 12-24 hours for 1-3 days until bleeding is resolved or healing achieved.

Moderate hemorrhage/minor surgery: 15-30 int. units/kg to achieve FVIII plasma level 30% to 60% of normal. May repeat 1 dose at 12-24 hours if needed. Some products suggest continuing for ≥3 days until pain and disability are resolved.

Major to life-threatening hemorrhage: Initial dose 40-50 int. units/kg followed by a maintenance dose of 20-25 int. units/kg every 8-24 hours until threat is resolved, to achieve FVIII plasma level 60% to 100% of normal.

Major surgery: 50 int. units/kg given preoperatively to raise factor VIII level to 100% before surgery begins. May repeat as necessary after 6-12 hours initially and for a total of 10-14 days until healing is complete. Intensity of therapy may depend on type of surgery and postoperative regimen.

Bleeding prophylaxis: May be administered on a regular basis for bleeding prophylaxis. Doses of 24-40 int. units/kg 3 times/week have been reported in patients with severe hemophilia to prevent joint bleeding.

If bleeding is not controlled with adequate dose, test for presence of inhibitor. It may not be possible or practical to control bleeding if inhibitor titers >10 Bethesda units/mL.

Elderly: Response in the elderly is not expected to differ from that of younger patients; dosage should be individualized

Administration I.V. infusion over 5-10 minutes (maximum: 10 mL/minute).

Advate: Infuse over ≤5 minutes (maximum: 10 mL/minute)

Helixate® FS, Kogenate® FS: Infuse over 1-15 minutes; based on patient tolerability

Xyntha™: Infuse over several minutes; adjust based on patient comfort. Do not admix or administer in same tubing as other medications.

Monitoring Parameters Heart rate and blood pressure (before and during I.V. administration); plasma factor VIII activity prior to and during treatment; development of factor VIII inhibitors; signs of bleeding

Dietary Considerations Some products may contain sodium and/or sucrose.

Product Availability Xyntha™: FDA approved February 2008; availability anticipated in September 2008

Wyeth is replacing ReFacto® with Xyntha™.

Dosage Forms Excipient information presented when available (limited, particularly for generics); consult specific product labeling. [DSC] = Discontinued product

Injection, powder for reconstitution, recombinant [preservative free]:

Advate: 250 int. units, 500 int. units, 1000 int. units, 1500 int. units, 2000 int. units, 3000 int. units [plasma/albumin free; contains polysorbate 80, sodium 108 mEq/L, mannitol; derived from hamster or mouse proteins]

Helixate® FS: 250 int. units, 500 int. units, 1000 int. units, 2000 int. unit, 3000 int. units [contains sucrose 28-52 mg/vial, sodium 26-36 mEq/L, polysorbate 80; derived from hamster or mouse protein]

Kogenate® FS: 250 int. units, 500 int. units, 1000 int. units, 2000 int. units, 3000 int. units [contains sucrose 28-56 mg/vial, sodium 27-36 mEq/L, polysorbate 80; derived from hamster or mouse protein]

Recombinate: 250 int. units, 500 int. units, 1000 int. units [contains human albumin, sodium 180 mEq/L, polysorbate 80; derived from bovine, hamster or mouse proteins; packaging contains natural rubber latex]

ReFacto®: 250 int. units, 500 int. units, 1000 int. units, 2000 int. units [contains polysorbate 80, sucrose; derived from hamster or mouse proteins] [DSC]

Xyntha™: 250 int. units, 500 int. units, 1000 int. units, 2000 int. units [albumin free; contains sucrose, polysorbate 80; derived from hamster proteins]

References

Manco-Johnson MJ, Abshire TC, Shapiro AD, et al, "Prophylaxis Versus Episodic Treatment to Prevent Joint Disease in Boys With Severe Hemophilia," *N Engl J Med*, 2007, 357(6):535-44.

Manucci PM, "Impact of Recombinant Factor VIII on Hemophilia Care," *Vox Sang*, 1994, 67(Suppl 3):49-52.

Nilsson IM, Berntorp E, Lofqvist T, et al, "Twenty-five Years' Experience of Prophylactic Treatment in Severe Haemophilia A and B," *J Intern Med*, 1992, 232(1):25-32.

White GC, Rosendaal F, Aledort LM, et al, "Definitions in Hemophilia. Recommendation of the Scientific Subcommittee on Factor VIII and Factor IX of the Scientific and Standardization Committee of the International Society on Thrombosis and Haemostasis," *Thromb Haemost*, 2001, 85(3):560.

◆ **Antithrombin III** *see* Antithrombin III *on page 96*

Antithrombin III (an tee THROM bin)

U.S. Brand Names ATryn®; Thrombate III®

Index Terms Antithrombin III; AT; AT-III; Heparin Cofactor I

Generic Available No

Canadian Brand Names Thrombate III®

Pharmacologic Category Anticoagulant; Blood Product Derivative

Use Treatment of hereditary antithrombin (AT or AT-III) deficiency in connection with surgical procedures, obstetrical procedures, or thromboembolism

Pregnancy Risk Factor B

Lactation Excretion in breast milk unknown/use caution

Labeled Contraindications Hypersensitivity to any component of the formulation

Warnings/Precautions Product of human plasma; may potentially contain infectious agents which could transmit disease; screening of donors, as well as testing and/or inactivation or removal of certain viruses, reduces this risk. Infections thought to be transmitted by this product should be reported to Talecris Biotherapeutics at 1-800-520-2807. Safety and efficacy in children have not been established.

Adverse Reactions

1% to 10%: Central nervous system: Dizziness (2%)

<1%: Bowel fullness, chest pain, chest tightness, chills, cramps, dyspnea, fever, film over eye, foul taste, hematoma, hives, lightheadedness, nausea

Drug Interactions

Avoid Concomitant Use There are no known interactions where it is recommended to avoid concomitant use.

Increased Effect/Toxicity

Antithrombin may increase the levels/effects of: Anticoagulants; Drotrecogin Alfa; Ibritumomab; Tositumomab and Iodine I 131 Tositumomab

The levels/effects of Antithrombin may be increased by: Antiplatelet Agents; Dasatinib; Herbs (Anticoagulant/Antiplatelet Properties); Nonsteroidal Anti-Inflammatory Agents; Pentosan Polysulfate Sodium; Prostacyclin Analogues; Salicylates; Thrombolytic Agents

Decreased Effect There are no known significant interactions involving a decrease in effect.

Ethanol/Nutrition/Herb Interactions Herb/Nutraceutical: Recent use/intake of herbs with anticoagulant or antiplatelet activity (including cat's claw, dong quai, evening primrose, garlic, ginkgo and ginseng) may increase the risk of bleeding.

Storage/Stability Thrombate III®: Prior to reconstitution, store vials refrigerated or at room temperature not exceeding 25°C (77°F); avoid freezing. Bring drug and diluent to room temperature prior to reconstitution. Administer within 3 hours after reconstitution. Do not refrigerate reconstituted product.

Reconstitution Thrombate III®: Reconstitute with sterile water for injection. Do not shake; swirl to mix to avoid foaming. Filter through sterile filter needle provided prior to administration.

Mechanism of Action Antithrombin is the primary physiologic inhibitor of *in vivo* coagulation. It is an alpha$_2$-globulin. Its principal actions are the inactivation of thrombin, plasmin, and other active serine proteases of coagulation, including factors IXa, Xa, XIa, and XIIa. The inactivation of proteases is a major step in the normal clotting process. The strong activation of clotting enzymes at the site of every bleeding injury facilitates fibrin formation and maintains normal hemostasis. Thrombosis in the circulation would be caused by active serine proteases if they were not inhibited by antithrombin after the localized clotting process.

Pharmacodynamics/Kinetics Half-life elimination: Biologic: 2.5 days (immunologic assay); 3.8 days (functional AT assay). Half-life may be decreased following surgery, with hemorrhage, acute thrombosis, and/or during heparin administration.

Dosage I.V.: Adults:

Initial loading dose: Dosing is individualized based on pretherapy antithrombin (AT) levels. The initial dose should raise AT levels to 120% and may be calculated based on the following formula:

[(desired AT level % - baseline AT level %) x body weight (kg)] **divided** by 1.4 = int. units of antithrombin required

For example, if a 70 kg adult patient had a baseline AT level of 57%, the initial dose would be

[(120% - 57%) x 70] divided by 1.4 = 3150 int. units

Maintenance dose: In general, subsequent dosing should be targeted to keep levels between 80% to 120% which may be achieved by administering 60% of the initial loading dose every 24 hours. Adjustments may be made by adjusting dose or interval. Maintain level within normal range for 2-8 days depending on type of procedure.

Administration I.V.: Infuse over 10-20 minutes.

Monitoring Parameters Initially, monitor AT at baseline, 20 minutes postinfusion (peak), 12 hours postinfusion, then preceding next infusion (trough level). Measure peak and trough AT levels with each subsequent dose until predictable levels achieved (between 80% and 120%). Some situations (eg, following surgery, hemorrhage or acute thrombosis, concurrent I.V. heparin administration), may require more frequent AT monitoring.

Dietary Considerations Some products may contain sodium.

Additional Information Thromboembolism has been reported in children of women with hereditary antithrombin (AT) deficiency; AT levels in neonates of parents with hereditary AT deficiency should be measured immediately after birth. Plasma AT levels are typically lower in neonates and infants than in adults. Low plasma AT levels in neonates may not be indicative of deficiency; consultation with a coagulation expert is recommended.

Product Availability

ATryn®: FDA approved February 2009; anticipated availability is currently undetermined

ATryn® is the first recombinant antithrombin product approved in the U.S.

Dosage Forms Excipient information presented when available (limited, particularly for generics); consult specific product labeling.

Injection, powder for reconstitution [preservative free]:

ATryn®: ~1750 int. units [exact potency labeled on each vial]

Thrombate III®: 500 int. units, 1000 int. units [contains heparin, sodium chloride 110-210 mEq/L; packaged with diluent]

References

Schwartz RS, Bauer KA, Rosenberg RD, et al, "Clinical Experience With Antithrombin III Concentrate in Treatment of Congenital and Acquired Deficiency of Antithrombin. The Antithrombin III Study Group," *Am J Med*, 1989, 87(3B):53S-60S.

Antithymocyte Globulin (Equine)

(an te THY moe site GLOB yu lin, E kwine)

Medication Safety Issues

Sound-alike/look-alike issues:

Atgam® may be confused with Ativan®

Related Information

Hematopoietic Stem Cell Transplantation *on page 1501*

U.S. Brand Names Atgam®

Index Terms Antithymocyte Immunoglobulin; ATG; Horse Antihuman Thymocyte Gamma Globulin; Lymphocyte Immune Globulin

Generic Available No

Canadian Brand Names Atgam®

Pharmacologic Category Immune Globulin; Immunosuppressant Agent

Use Prevention and treatment of acute renal allograft rejection; treatment of moderate-to-severe aplastic anemia in patients not considered suitable candidates for bone marrow transplantation

Unlabeled/Investigational Use Prevention and treatment of other solid organ allograft rejection; prevention of graft-versus-host disease following bone marrow transplantation; treatment of myelodysplastic syndrome (MDS)

Pregnancy Risk Factor C

Lactation Excretion in breast milk unknown/use caution

Labeled Contraindications History of severe systemic reaction to prior administration of antithymocyte globulin or other equine gamma globulins

Warnings/Precautions For I.V. use only. Must be administered via central line due to chemical phlebitis. **[U.S. Boxed Warning]: Should only be used by physicians experienced in immunosuppressive therapy or management of solid organ or bone marrow transplant patients. Adequate laboratory and supportive medical resources must be readily available in the facility for patient management.** Hypersensitivity and anaphylactic reactions can occur; immediate treatment (including epinephrine 1:1000) should be available. Rash, dyspnea, hypotension, or anaphylaxis precludes further administration of the drug. Discontinue if severe and unremitting thrombocytopenia and/or leukopenia occur. Dose must be administered over at least 4 hours. Patient may need to be pretreated with an antipyretic, antihistamine, and/or corticosteroid. Intradermal skin testing is recommended prior to first-dose administration.

Adverse Reactions

>10%:

Central nervous system: Fever, chills

Dermatologic: Pruritus, rash, urticaria

Hematologic: Leukopenia, thrombocytopenia

1% to 10%:

Cardiovascular: Bradycardia, chest pain, CHF, edema, encephalitis, hyper-/hypotension, myocarditis, tachycardia

Central nervous system: Agitation, headache, lethargy, lightheadedness, listlessness, seizure

Gastrointestinal: Diarrhea, nausea, stomatitis, vomiting

Hepatic: Hepatosplenomegaly, liver function tests abnormal

Local: Pain at injection site, phlebitis, thrombophlebitis, burning soles/palms

Neuromuscular & skeletal: Arthralgia, back pain, myalgia

Ocular: Periorbital edema

Renal: Abnormal renal function tests

Respiratory: Dyspnea, respiratory distress

Miscellaneous: Anaphylaxis, diaphoresis, lymphadenopathy, night sweats, serum sickness, viral infection

<1%: Dizziness, epigastric pain, faintness, herpes simplex reactivation, hiccups, hyperglycemia, iliac vein obstruction, infection, laryngospasm, malaise, paresthesia, pulmonary edema, renal artery thrombosis, serum sickness, toxic epidermal necrosis, weakness, wound dehiscence

Postmarketing and/or case reports: Acute renal failure, anemia, aplasia, confusion, cough, deep vein thrombosis, disorientation, GI bleeding, granulocytopenia, hemolysis, kidney enlarged, neutropenia, nosebleed, pancytopenia, vasculitis

Drug Interactions

Avoid Concomitant Use

Avoid concomitant use of Antithymocyte Globulin (Equine) with any of the following: Natalizumab; Vaccines (Live)

Increased Effect/Toxicity

Antithymocyte Globulin (Equine) may increase the levels/effects of: Leflunomide; Natalizumab; Vaccines (Live)

The levels/effects of Antithymocyte Globulin (Equine) may be increased by: Trastuzumab

Decreased Effect

Antithymocyte Globulin (Equine) may decrease the levels/effects of: Vaccines (Inactivated); Vaccines (Live)

The levels/effects of Antithymocyte Globulin (Equine) may be decreased by: Echinacea

Storage/Stability Ampuls must be refrigerated; do not freeze. Diluted solution is stable for 24 hours (including infusion time) at refrigeration.

Reconstitution Dilute into inverted bottle of sterile vehicle to ensure that undiluted lymphocyte immune globulin does not contact air. Gently rotate or swirl to mix. Final concentration should be 4 mg/mL. May be diluted in NS, $D_5$1/4NS, $D_5$1/2NS.

Mechanism of Action May involve elimination of antigen-reactive T lymphocytes (killer cells) in peripheral blood or alteration of T-cell function

Pharmacodynamics/Kinetics

Distribution: Poorly into lymphoid tissues; binds to circulating lymphocytes, granulocytes, platelets, bone marrow cells

Half-life elimination, plasma: 1.5-12 days

Excretion: Urine (~1%)

Dosage An intradermal skin test is recommended prior to administration of the initial dose of ATG; use 0.1 mL of a 1:1000 dilution of ATG in normal saline. A positive skin reaction consists of a wheal ≥10 mm in diameter. If a positive skin test occurs, the first infusion should be administered in a controlled environment with intensive life support immediately available. A systemic reaction precludes further administration of the drug. The absence of a reaction does **not** preclude the possibility of an immediate sensitivity reaction.

Premedication with diphenhydramine, hydrocortisone, and acetaminophen is recommended prior to first dose.

Children: I.V.:

Aplastic anemia protocol: 10-20 mg/kg/day for 8-14 days; then administer every other day for 7 more doses; additional doses may be given every other day for 21 total doses in 28 days **or**

Unlabeled dosing: Children >10 kg: 40 mg/kg/day for 4 days (Rosenfeld, 1995)

Renal allograft: 5-25 mg/kg/day

Adults: I.V.:

Aplastic anemia protocol: 10-20 mg/kg/day for 8-14 days, then administer every other day for 7 more doses, for a total of 21 doses in 28 days **or**

Unlabeled dosing: 40 mg/kg/day for 4 days (Rosenfeld, 1995)

Renal allograft:

Rejection prophylaxis: 15 mg/kg/day for 14 days, then give every other day for 7 more doses for a total of 21 doses in 28 days; the initial dose should be administered within 24 hours before or after transplantation

Rejection treatment: 10-15 mg/kg/day for 14 days, then administer every other day for 7 more doses for a total of 21 doses in 28 days

Administration Infuse dose over at least 4 hours. Any severe systemic reaction to the skin test, such as generalized rash, tachycardia, dyspnea, hypotension, or anaphylaxis, should preclude further therapy. Epinephrine and resuscitative equipment should be nearby. Patient may need to be pretreated with an antipyretic, antihistamine, and/or corticosteroid. Mild itching and erythema can be treated with antihistamines. Infuse into a vascular shunt, arterial venous fistula, or high-flow central vein through a 0.2-1 micron in-line filter.

First dose: Premedicate with diphenhydramine orally 30 minutes prior to and hydrocortisone I.V. 15 minutes prior to infusion and acetaminophen 2 hours after start of infusion.

Monitoring Parameters Lymphocyte profile, CBC with differential and platelet count, vital signs during administration

Dosage Forms Excipient information presented when available (limited, particularly for generics); consult specific product labeling.

Injection, solution:

Atgam® 50 mg/mL (5 mL)

References

Rosenfeld SJ, Kimball J, Vining D, et al, "Intensive Immunosuppression With Antithymocyte Globulin and Cyclosporine as Treatment for Severe Acquired Aplastic Anemia," *Blood*, 1995, 85 (11):3058-65.

Antithymocyte Globulin (Rabbit)

(an te THY moe site GLOB yu lin RAB bit)

Related Information

Hematopoietic Stem Cell Transplantation *on page 1501*

U.S. Brand Names Thymoglobulin®

Index Terms Antithymocyte Immunoglobulin; rATG

Generic Available No

Pharmacologic Category Immune Globulin; Immunosuppressant Agent

Use Treatment of acute rejection of renal transplant; used in conjunction with concomitant immunosuppression

Unlabeled/Investigational Use Induction therapy in renal transplant; treatment of myelodysplastic syndrome (MDS)

Pregnancy Risk Factor C

Lactation Excretion in breast milk unknown/use caution

Labeled Contraindications Hypersensitivity to antithymocyte globulin, rabbit proteins, or any component of the formulation; acute viral illness

Warnings/Precautions [U.S. Boxed Warning]: Should only be used by physicians experienced in immunosuppressive therapy for the treatment of renal transplant patients. Medical surveillance is required during the infusion. Initial dose must be administered over at least 6 hours into a high flow vein; patient may need pretreatment with an antipyretic, antihistamine, and/or corticosteroid. Hypersensitivity and anaphylactic reactions can occur; immediate treatment (including epinephrine 1:1000) should be available. An increased incidence of lymphoma, post-transplant lymphoproliferative disease (PTLD), other malignancies, or severe infections may develop following concomitant use of immunosuppressants and prolonged use or overdose of antithymocyte globulin. Appropriate antiviral, antibacterial, antiprotozoal, and/ or antifungal prophylaxis is recommended. Reversible neutropenia or thrombocytopenia may result from the development of cross-reactive antibodies.

Adverse Reactions

>10%:

Cardiovascular: Hypertension, peripheral edema, tachycardia

Central nervous system: Chills, fever, headache, pain, malaise

Endocrine & metabolic: Hyperkalemia

Gastrointestinal: Abdominal pain, diarrhea, nausea

Genitourinary: Urinary tract infection

Hematologic: Leukopenia, thrombocytopenia

Neuromuscular & skeletal: Weakness

Respiratory: Dyspnea

Miscellaneous: Antirabbit antibody development, sepsis, systemic infection

1% to 10%:

Central nervous system: Dizziness

Gastrointestinal: Gastritis, gastrointestinal moniliasis

Miscellaneous: Herpes simplex infection, moniliasis

Postmarketing and/or case reports: Anaphylaxis, cytokine release syndrome, PTLD, neutropenia, serum sickness (delayed)

Drug Interactions

Avoid Concomitant Use

Avoid concomitant use of Antithymocyte Globulin (Rabbit) with any of the following: Natalizumab; Vaccines (Live)

Increased Effect/Toxicity

Antithymocyte Globulin (Rabbit) may increase the levels/effects of: Leflunomide; Natalizumab; Vaccines (Live)

The levels/effects of Antithymocyte Globulin (Rabbit) may be increased by: Trastuzumab

Decreased Effect

Antithymocyte Globulin (Rabbit) may decrease the levels/effects of: Vaccines (Inactivated); Vaccines (Live)

The levels/effects of Antithymocyte Globulin (Rabbit) may be decreased by: Echinacea

Storage/Stability Store powder under refrigeration at 2°C to 8°C (36°F to 46°F); do not freeze. Protect from light. Use immediately following reconstitution.

Reconstitution Allow vials to reach room temperature, then reconstitute each vial with SWFI 5 mL. Rotate vial gently until dissolved. Prior to administration, further dilute one vial in 50 mL saline or dextrose (total volume is usually 50-500 mL depending on total number of vials needed per dose). Mix by gently inverting infusion bag once or twice.

Mechanism of Action Polyclonal antibody which appears to cause immunosuppression by acting on T-cell surface antigens and depleting CD4 lymphocytes

Pharmacodynamics/Kinetics

Duration: Lymphopenia may persist ≥1 year

Half-life elimination, plasma: 2-3 days

Dosage I.V.: Children and Adults: Treatment of acute rejection: 1.5 mg/kg/day for 7-14 days

Dosage adjustment for toxicity:
WBC count 2000-3000 cells/mm^3 or platelet count 50,000-75,000 cells/mm^3: Reduce dose by 50%
WBC count <2000 cells/mm^3 or platelet count <50,000 cells/mm^3: Consider discontinuing treatment

Administration The first dose should be infused over at least 6 hours through a high-flow vein. Subsequent doses should be administered over at least 4 hours. Administer through an in-line 0.22 micron filter. Premedication with corticosteroids, acetaminophen, and/or an antihistamine may reduce infusion-related reactions.

Monitoring Parameters Lymphocyte profile, CBC with differential and platelet count; vital signs during administration; signs and symptoms of infection

Dosage Forms Excipient information presented when available (limited, particularly for generics); consult specific product labeling.
Injection, powder for reconstitution:
Thymoglobulin®: 25 mg

References

Broliden PA, Dahl IM, Hast R, et al, "Antithymocyte Globulin and Cyclosporine A as Combination Therapy for Low-Risk Non-Sideroblastic Myelodysplastic Syndromes," *Haematologica*, 2006, 91 (5):667-70.

Hardinger KL, "Rabbit Antithymocyte Globulin Induction Therapy in Adult Renal Transplantation," *Pharmacotherapy*, 2006, 26(12):1771-83.

◆ **Antithymocyte Immunoglobulin** *see* Antithymocyte Globulin (Equine) *on page 98*

◆ **Antithymocyte Immunoglobulin** *see* Antithymocyte Globulin (Rabbit) *on page 101*

◆ **Anti-VEGF Monoclonal Antibody** *see* Bevacizumab *on page 137*

◆ **Anti-VEGF rhuMAb** *see* Bevacizumab *on page 137*

◆ **Anucort-HC®** *see* Hydrocortisone *on page 575*

◆ **Anusol-HC®** *see* Hydrocortisone *on page 575*

◆ **Anusol® HC-1 [OTC]** *see* Hydrocortisone *on page 575*

◆ **Anzemet®** *see* Dolasetron *on page 368*

◆ **Apo-Acyclovir® (Can)** *see* Acyclovir *on page 18*

◆ **Apo-Allopurinol® (Can)** *see* Allopurinol *on page 37*

◆ **Apo-Benzydamine® (Can)** *see* Benzydamine *on page 136*

◆ **Apo-Bicalutamide® (Can)** *see* Bicalutamide *on page 147*

◆ **Apo-Calcitonin® (Can)** *see* Calcitonin *on page 165*

◆ **Apo-Ciproflox® (Can)** *see* Ciprofloxacin *on page 228*

◆ **Apo-Cyclosporine (Can)** *see* CycloSPORINE *on page 268*

◆ **Apo-Cyproterone® (Can)** *see* Cyproterone *on page 279*

◆ **Apo-Desmopressin® (Can)** *see* Desmopressin *on page 344*

◆ **Apo-Dexamethasone® (Can)** *see* Dexamethasone *on page 350*

◆ **Apo-Famciclovir® (Can)** *see* Famciclovir *on page 455*

◆ **Apo-Fluconazole® (Can)** *see* Fluconazole *on page 485*

◆ **Apo-Flutamide® (Can)** *see* Flutamide *on page 506*

◆ **Apo-Granisetron (Can)** *see* Granisetron *on page 552*

◆ **Apo-Haloperidol® (Can)** *see* Haloperidol *on page 556*

◆ **Apo-Haloperidol LA® (Can)** *see* Haloperidol *on page 556*

Aprepitant (ap RE pi tant)

Medication Safety Issues

Sound-alike/look-alike issues:

Aprepitant may be confused with fosaprepitant

Emend® (aprepitant) oral capsule formulation may be confused with Emend® for injection (fosaprepitant).

Related Information

Management of Chemotherapy-Induced Nausea and Vomiting *on page 1434*

U.S. Brand Names Emend®

Index Terms L 754030; MK 869

Generic Available No

Canadian Brand Names Emend®

Pharmacologic Category Antiemetic; Substance P/Neurokinin 1 Receptor Antagonist

Use Prevention of acute and delayed nausea and vomiting associated with moderately- and highly-emetogenic chemotherapy (in combination with other antiemetics); prevention of postoperative nausea and vomiting (PONV)

Pregnancy Risk Factor B

Lactation Excretion in breast milk unknown/not recommended

Labeled Contraindications Hypersensitivity to aprepitant or any component of the formulation; concurrent use with cisapride or pimozide

Warnings/Precautions Use caution with agents primarily metabolized via CYP3A4; aprepitant is a 3A4 inhibitor. Effect on orally administered 3A4 substrates is greater than those administered intravenously. Chronic continuous use is not recommended; however, a single 40 mg aprepitant oral dose is not likely to alter plasma concentrations of CYP3A4 substrates. Use caution with severe hepatic impairment; has not been studied in patients with severe hepatic impairment (Child-Pugh class C). Not intended for treatment of existing nausea and vomiting or for chronic continuous therapy.

Adverse Reactions Note: Adverse reactions reported as part of a combination chemotherapy regimen or with general anesthesia.

>10%:
Central nervous system: Fatigue (18% to 22%)
Gastrointestinal: Nausea (7% to 13%), constipation (9% to 12%)
Neuromuscular & skeletal: Weakness (3% to 18%)
Miscellaneous: Hiccups (≤11%)

1% to 10%:
Cardiovascular: Hypotension (≤6%), bradycardia (≤4%), flushing (≤3%)
Central nervous system: Dizziness (≤7%)
Endocrine & metabolic: Dehydration (≤6%)
Gastrointestinal: Diarrhea (6% to 10%), dyspepsia (≤8%), abdominal pain (≤5%), stomatitis (≤5%), epigastric discomfort (≤4%), gastritis (≤4%), throat pain (≤3%)
Hepatic: ALT increased (1% to 6%), AST increased (3%)
Renal: Proteinuria (7%), BUN increased (5%)

>0.5%: Acid reflux, acne, albumin decreased, alkaline phosphatase increased, anemia, anxiety, appetite decreased, arthralgia, back pain, bilirubin increased, candidiasis, confusion, conjunctivitis, cough, deglutition disorder, depression, diabetes mellitus, diaphoresis, DVT, dysphagia, dyspnea, dysuria, edema, eructation, erythrocytulia, febrile neutropenia, flatulence, herpes simplex, hyperglycemia, hypertension, hypoesthesia, hypokalemia, hyponatremia, hypothermia, hypovolemia, hypoxia, glucosuria, leukocytes increased, leukocyturia, malaise, MI, muscular weakness, musculoskeletal pain, myalgia, nasal secretion, obstipation, pain, palpitation, pelvic pain, peripheral neuropathy, pharyngitis, pneumonitis, pulmonary embolism, rash, renal insufficiency, respiratory infection, respiratory insufficiency, rigors, salivation increased, sensory neuropathy, septic shock, syncope, tachycardia, taste disturbance, thrombocytopenia, tremor, urinary tract infection, urticaria, vocal disturbance, weight loss, xerostomia

<0.5%, postmarketing, and/or case reports: Anaphylactic reaction, angioedema, disorientation, duodenal ulcer (perforating), dysarthria, enterocolitis, hypersensitivity reaction, miosis, neutropenic sepsis, pneumonia, pruritus, sensory disturbance, Stevens-Johnson syndrome, visual acuity decreased, wheezing

Drug Interactions
Metabolism/Transport Effects Substrate of CYP1A2 (minor), 2C19 (minor), 3A4 (major); **Inhibits** CYP2C9 (weak), 2C19 (weak), 3A4 (moderate); **Induces** CYP2C9 (weak), 3A4 (weak)

Avoid Concomitant Use
Avoid concomitant use of Aprepitant with any of the following: Cisapride; Everolimus; Pimozide; Tolvaptan

Increased Effect/Toxicity
Aprepitant may increase the levels/effects of: Benzodiazepines (metabolized by oxidation); Cisapride; Colchicine; Corticosteroids (Systemic); CYP3A4 Substrates; Diltiazem; Eplerenone; Everolimus; FentaNYL; Halofantrine;

Pimecrolimus; Pimozide; Ranolazine; Salmeterol; Saxagliptin; TOLBUTamide; Tolvaptan

The levels/effects of Aprepitant may be increased by: Antifungal Agents (Azole Derivatives, Systemic); CYP3A4 Inhibitors (Moderate); CYP3A4 Inhibitors (Strong); Dasatinib; Diltiazem

Decreased Effect

Aprepitant may decrease the levels/effects of: Contraceptive (Progestins); CYP2C9 Substrates (High risk); Oral Contraceptive (Estrogens); Saxagliptin; Warfarin

The levels/effects of Aprepitant may be decreased by: CYP3A4 Inducers (Strong); Deferasirox; Herbs (CYP3A4 Inducers); Rifamycin Derivatives

Ethanol/Nutrition/Herb Interactions

Food: Aprepitant serum concentration may be increased when taken with grapefruit juice; avoid concurrent use.

Herb/Nutraceutical: Avoid St John's wort (may decrease aprepitant levels).

Storage/Stability Store at room temperature of 20°C to 25°C (68°F to 77°F).

Mechanism of Action Prevents acute and delayed vomiting by inhibiting the substance P/neurokinin 1 (NK_1) receptor; augments the antiemetic activity of $5-HT_3$ receptor antagonists and corticosteroids to inhibit acute and delayed phases of chemotherapy-induced emesis.

Pharmacodynamics/Kinetics

Distribution: V_d: ~70 L; crosses the blood brain barrier

Protein binding: >95%

Metabolism: Extensively hepatic via CYP3A4 (major); CYP1A2 and CYP2C19 (minor); forms 7 metabolites (weakly active)

Bioavailability: ~60% to 65%

Half-life elimination: Terminal: ~9-13 hours

Time to peak, plasma: ~3-4 hours

Dosage Oral: Adults:

Prevention of chemotherapy-induced nausea/vomiting: 125 mg 1 hour prior to chemotherapy on day 1, followed by 80 mg once daily on days 2 and 3 (in combination with a corticosteroid and $5-HT_3$ antagonist antiemetic); **Note:** Fosaprepitant 115 mg 30 minutes prior to chemotherapy may be substituted for aprepitant 125 mg on day 1

Prevention of PONV: 40 mg within 3 hours prior to induction

Dosage adjustment in renal impairment: No dose adjustment necessary in patients with renal disease or end-stage renal disease maintained on hemodialysis.

Dosage adjustment in hepatic impairment:

Mild-to-moderate impairment (Child-Pugh classes A and B): No adjustment necessary

Severe impairment (Child-Pugh class C): Use caution; no data available

Administration

Chemotherapy induced nausea/vomiting: Administer with or without food. First dose should be given 1 hour prior to antineoplastic therapy; subsequent doses should be given in the morning.

PONV: Administer within 3 hours prior to induction; follow healthcare providers instructions about food/drink restrictions prior to surgery.

Dietary Considerations May be taken with or without food.

Additional Information Oncology Comment: Aprepitant is recommended in the American Society of Clinical Oncology (ASCO) oncology antiemetic guidelines for use in combination with a serotonin receptor antagonist and dexamethasone for chemotherapy with high emetic risk and for chemotherapy regimens of moderate emetic risk which contain an anthracycline and cyclophosphamide (Kris, 2006). The National Comprehensive Cancer Network® (NCCN) Clinical Practice Guidelines in Oncology for Antiemesis (version 4.2009) recommend the same use of aprepitant as is in the ASCO recommendation. In addition to the moderately emetogenic chemotherapy listed above, the NCCN guidelines suggest that aprepitant may also be used for select moderately emetogenic regimens containing carboplatin, cisplatin, doxorubicin, epirubicin, ifosfamide, irinotecan and methotrexate. Either fosaprepitant 115 mg or aprepitant (125 mg orally) are administered on day 1; for day 2 and 3, patients should receive aprepitant 80 mg orally.

Dosage Forms Excipient information presented when available (limited, particularly for generics); consult specific product labeling.

Capsule:

Emend®: 40 mg, 80 mg, 125 mg

Combination package [each package contains]:

Emend®:

Capsule: 80 mg (2s)

Capsule: 125 mg (1s)

References

Kris MG, Hesketh PJ, Somerfield MR, et al, "American Society of Clinical Oncology Guideline for Antiemetics in Oncology: Update 2006," *J Clin Oncol*, 2006, 24(18):2932-47.

National Comprehensive Cancer Network® (NCCN), "Clinical Practice Guidelines in Oncology™: Antiemesis," Version 4.2009. Available at http://www.nccn.org/professionals/physician_gls/PDF/antiemesis.pdf.

- ◆ **Aprepitant Injection** *see* Fosaprepitant *on page 513*
- ◆ **Aquacort® (Can)** *see* Hydrocortisone *on page 575*
- ◆ **AquaMEPHYTON® (Can)** *see* Phytonadione *on page 953*
- ◆ **Aquanil™ HC [OTC]** *see* Hydrocortisone *on page 575*
- ◆ **Aquoral™** *see* Saliva Substitute *on page 1027*
- ◆ **Ara-C** *see* Cytarabine *on page 281*
- ◆ **Arabinosylcytosine** *see* Cytarabine *on page 281*
- ◆ **Aranesp®** *see* Darbepoetin Alfa *on page 308*
- ◆ **Aredia®** *see* Pamidronate *on page 914*
- ◆ **Arimidex®** *see* Anastrozole *on page 85*
- ◆ **Arixtra®** *see* Fondaparinux *on page 509*
- ◆ **Aromasin®** *see* Exemestane *on page 444*
- ◆ **Arranon®** *see* Nelarabine *on page 843*

Arsenic Trioxide (AR se nik tri OKS id)

Medication Safety Issues

High alert medication: The Institute for Safe Medication Practices (ISMP) includes this medication among its list of drugs which have a heightened risk of causing significant patient harm when used in error.

Related Information

Management of Drug Extravasations *on page 1447*

Safe Handling of Hazardous Drugs *on page 1517*

U.S. Brand Names Trisenox®

Index Terms As_2O_3; NSC-706363

Generic Available No

Pharmacologic Category Antineoplastic Agent, Miscellaneous

◄ **Use** Induction of remission and consolidation in patients with relapsed or refractory acute promyelocytic leukemia (APL) which is specifically characterized by t(15;17) translocation or PML/RAR-alpha gene expression

Unlabeled/Investigational Use Treatment of myelodysplastic syndrome (MDS), multiple myeloma

Pregnancy Risk Factor D

Lactation Enters breast milk/not recommended

Labeled Contraindications Hypersensitivity to arsenic or any component of the formulation

Warnings/Precautions Hazardous agent - use appropriate precautions for handling and disposal. **[U.S. Boxed Warnings]: May prolong the QT interval. May lead to torsade de pointes or complete AV block.** Risk factors for torsade de pointes include HF, a history of torsade de pointes, pre-existing QT interval prolongation, patients taking potassium-wasting diuretics, and conditions which cause hypokalemia or hypomagnesemia. If possible, discontinue all medications known to prolong the QT interval. **[U.S. Boxed Warning]: A baseline 12-lead ECG, serum electrolytes (potassium, calcium, magnesium), and creatinine should be obtained prior to treatment.** Correct electrolyte abnormalities prior to treatment and monitor potassium and magnesium levels during therapy (potassium should stay >4 mEq/dL and magnesium >1.8 mg/dL). Correct QT_c >500 msec prior to treatment. Discontinue therapy and hospitalize patient if QT_c >500 msec, syncope, or irregular heartbeats develop during therapy; do not reinitiate until QT_c <460 msec.

[U.S. Boxed Warning]: May cause retinoic-acid-acute promyelocytic leukemia (RA-APL) syndrome or APL differentiation syndrome (dyspnea, fever, weight gain, pulmonary infiltrates, and pleural or pericardial effusions) in patients with APL. High-dose steroids have been used for treatment. May lead to the development of hyperleukocytosis (leukocytes ≥10,000/mm^3). Use with caution in renal impairment; arsenic is eliminated renally. **[U.S. Boxed Warning]: Should be administered under the supervision of an experienced cancer chemotherapy physician.** Safety and efficacy in children <5 years of age have not been established (limited experience with children 5-16 years of age).

Adverse Reactions

>10%:

Cardiovascular: Tachycardia (55%), edema (40%), QT interval >500 msec (40%), chest pain (25%; grades 3/4: 5%), hypotension (25%; grades 3/4: 5%)

Central nervous system: Fatigue (63%), fever (63%), headache (60%), insomnia (43%), anxiety (30%), dizziness (23%), depression (20%), pain (15%)

Dermatologic: Dermatitis (43%), pruritus (33%), bruising (20%), dry skin (13%)

Endocrine & metabolic: Hypokalemia (50%; grades 3/4: 13%), hyperglycemia (45%; grades 3/4: 13%), hypomagnesemia (45%; grades 3/4: 13%), hyperkalemia (18%; grades 3/4: 5%)

Gastrointestinal: Nausea (75%), abdominal pain (58%), vomiting (58%), diarrhea (53%), sore throat (35% to 40%), constipation (28%), anorexia (23%), appetite decreased (15%), weight gain (13%)

Genitourinary: Vaginal hemorrhage (13%)

Hematologic: Leukocytosis (50%; grades 3/4: 3%), APL differentiation syndrome (23%), anemia (20%; grades 3/4: 5%), thrombocytopenia (18%; grades 3/4: 13%), febrile neutropenia (13%; grades 3/4: 8%)

Hepatic: ALT increased (20%; grades 3/4: 5%), AST increased (13%; grades 3/4: 3%)

Local: Injection site: Pain (20%), erythema (13%)

Neuromuscular & skeletal: Neuropathy (43%), rigors (38%), arthralgia (33%), paresthesia (33%), myalgia (25%), bone pain (23%), back pain (18%), limb pain (13%), neck pain (13%), tremor (13%)

Respiratory: Cough (65%), dyspnea (38% to 53%; grades 3/4: 10%), epistaxis (25%), hypoxia (23%), pleural effusion (20%), sinusitis (20%), postnasal drip (13%), upper respiratory tract infection (13%), wheezing (13%)

Miscellaneous: Herpes simplex (13%)

1% to 10%:

Cardiovascular: Hypertension (10%), flushing (10%), pallor (10%), palpitation (10%), facial edema (8%), abnormal ECG (not QT prolongation) (7%)

Central nervous system: Convulsion (8%; grades 3/4: 5%), somnolence (8%), agitation (5%), coma (5%), confusion (5%)

Dermatologic: Erythema (10%), hyperpigmentation (8%), petechia (8%), skin lesions (8%), urticaria (8%), local exfoliation (5%)

Endocrine & metabolic: Hypocalcemia (10%), hypoglycemia (8%), acidosis (5%)

Gastrointestinal: Dyspepsia (10%), loose stools (10%), abdominal distension (8%), abdominal tenderness (8%), xerostomia (8%), fecal incontinence (8%), gastrointestinal hemorrhage (8%), hemorrhagic diarrhea (8%), oral blistering (8%), weight loss (8%), oral candidiasis (5%)

Genitourinary: Intermenstrual bleeding (8%), incontinence (5%)

Hematologic: Neutropenia (10%; grades 3/4: 10%), DIC (8%), hemorrhage (8%), lymphadenopathy (8%)

Local: Injection site edema (10%)

Neuromuscular & skeletal: Weakness (10%)

Ocular: Blurred vision (10%), eye irritation (10%), dry eye (8%), eyelid edema (5%), painful eye (5%)

Otic: Earache (8%), tinnitus (5%)

Renal: Renal failure (8%; grades 3/4: 3%), renal impairment (8%), oliguria (5%)

Respiratory: Crepitations (10%), breath sounds decreased (10%), rales (10%), hemoptysis (8%), rhonchi (8%), tachypnea (8%), nasopharyngitis (5%)

Miscellaneous: Diaphoresis increased (10%), APL differentiation syndrome (8%), bacterial infection (8%), herpes zoster (8%), night sweats (8%), hypersensitivity (5%), sepsis (5%; grades 3/4: 5%)

Postmarketing and/or case reports: Atrial dysrhythmia, AV block, torsade de pointes

Drug Interactions

Avoid Concomitant Use

Avoid concomitant use of Arsenic Trioxide with any of the following: Artemether; Dronedarone; Lumefantrine; Nilotinib; Pimozide; QuiNINE; Tetrabenazine; Thioridazine; Ziprasidone

Increased Effect/Toxicity

Arsenic Trioxide may increase the levels/effects of: Dronedarone; Hypoglycemic Agents; Pimozide; QTc-Prolonging Agents; QuiNINE; Tetrabenazine; Thioridazine; Ziprasidone

The levels/effects of Arsenic Trioxide may be increased by: Alfuzosin; Artemether; Chloroquine; Ciprofloxacin; Gadobutrol; Herbs (Hypoglycemic Properties); Lumefantrine; Nilotinib; QuiNINE

Decreased Effect There are no known significant interactions involving a decrease in effect.

Ethanol/Nutrition/Herb Interactions Herb/Nutraceutical: Avoid homeopathic products (arsenic is present in some homeopathic medications). Avoid hypoglycemic herbs, including alfalfa, aloe, bilberry, bitter melon, burdock, celery, damiana, fenugreek, garcinia, garlic, ginger, ginseng, gymnema, marshmallow, and stinging nettle (may enhance the hypoglycemic effect of arsenic trioxide).

Storage/Stability Store at room temperature of 15°C to 30°C (59°F to 86°F); do not freeze. Following dilution, stable for 24 hours at room temperature or 48 hours when refrigerated.

Reconstitution Dilute in 100-250 mL D_5W or 0.9% NaCl. Discard unused portion.

Mechanism of Action Not fully understood; causes *in vitro* morphological changes and DNA fragmentation to NB4 human promyelocytic leukemia cells; also damages or degrades the fusion protein PML-RAR alpha

Pharmacodynamics/Kinetics

Distribution: V_d: ~4 L

Metabolism: Hepatic; pentavalent arsenic is reduced to trivalent arsenic (active) by arsenate reductase; trivalent arsenic is methylated to monomethylarsinic acid, which is then converted to dimethylarsinic acid via methyltransferases

Half-life elimination: Initial: 0.6-1.2 hours; Elimination: 9-15 hours

Excretion: Urine (as methylated metabolite)

Dosage I.V.:

APL: Children ≥5 years and Adults:

Induction: 0.15 mg/kg/day; administer daily until bone marrow remission; maximum induction: 60 doses

Consolidation: 0.15 mg/kg/day starting 3-6 weeks after completion of induction therapy; maximum consolidation: 25 doses over 5 weeks

MDS, multiple myeloma (unlabeled uses): Adults: 0.25 mg/kg/day 5 consecutive days/week for 2 weeks, followed by a 2-week rest period

Elderly: Safety and efficacy have not been established; clinical trials included patients ≤72 years of age; use with caution due to the increased risk of renal impairment in the elderly

Dosage adjustment in renal impairment: Safety and efficacy have not been established; use with caution due to renal elimination

Dosage adjustment in hepatic impairment: Safety and efficacy have not been established

Combination Regimens

Leukemia, acute promyelocytic:

Tretinoin-Arsenic Trioxide (APL) on page 1410

Tretinoin-Arsenic Trioxide-Gemtuzumab (APL) on page 1411

Administration Administer as I.V. infusion over 1-2 hours. If acute vasomotor reactions occur, infuse over a maximum of 4 hours. Does not require administration via a central venous catheter.

Monitoring Parameters Baseline then weekly 12-lead ECG, baseline then twice weekly serum electrolytes, hematologic and coagulation profiles at least twice weekly during induction and at least weekly during consolidation; more frequent monitoring may be necessary in unstable patients

Additional Information Arsenic is stored in liver, kidney, heart, lung, hair, and nails. Arsenic trioxide is a human carcinogen.

Oncology Comment: Arsenic trioxide is listed within National Comprehensive Cancer Network (NCCN) guidelines for the treatment of acute myeloid leukemia as the recommended salvage therapy for relapsed or persistent APL. For patients with APL in their second complete response, who are not candidates for stem cell transplant, in the absence of an appropriate clinical trial, maintenance therapy with arsenic trioxide is an option.

Emetic Potential Moderate (30% to 90%)

Vesicant May be an irritant

Dosage Forms Excipient information presented when available (limited, particularly for generics); consult specific product labeling.

Injection, solution [preservative free]:

Trisenox®: 1 mg/mL (10 mL)

References

Barbey JT, Pezzullo JC, and Soignet SL, "Effect of Arsenic Trioxide on QT Interval in Patients With Advanced Malignancies," *J Clin Oncol*, 2003, 21(19):3609-15.

Chen Z, Chen GQ, Shen ZX, et al, "Expanding the Use of Arsenic Trioxide: Leukemias and Beyond," *Semin Hematol*, 2002, 39(2 Suppl 1):22-6.

Davison K, Mann KK, and Miller WH, "Arsenic Trioxide: Mechanisms of Action," *Semin Hematol*, 2002, 39(2 Suppl 1):3-7.

Hussein MA, Saleh M, Ravandi F, et al, "Phase 2 Study of Arsenic Trioxide in Patients With Relapsed or Refractory Multiple Myeloma," *Br J Haematol*, 2004, 125(4):470-6.

Liu P and Han ZC, "Treatment of Acute Promyelocytic Leukemia and Other Hematologic Malignancies With Arsenic Trioxide: Review of Clinical and Basic Studies," *Int J Hematol*, 2003, 78(1):32-9.

National Comprehensive Cancer Network (NCCN), "Practice Guidelines in Oncology: Acute Myeloid Leukemia, Version 1, 2006." Accessible at http://www.nccn.org/professionals/physician_gls/PDF/aml.pdf

Schiller GJ, Slack J, Hainsworth JD, et al, "Phase II Multicenter Study of Arsenic Trioxide in Patients With Myelodysplastic Syndromes," *J Clin Oncol*, 2006, 24(16):2456-64.

Shen ZX, Chen GQ, Ni JH, et al, "Use of Arsenic Trioxide (As2O3) in the Treatment of Acute Promyelocytic Leukemia (APL): II. Clinical Efficacy and Pharmacokinetics in Relapsed Patients," *Blood*, 1997, 89(9):3354-60.

Soignet SL, Frankel SR, Douer D, et al, "United States Multicenter Study of Arsenic Trioxide in Relapsed Acute Promyelocytic Leukemia," *J Clin Oncol*, 2001, 19(18):3852-60.

◆ **Artificial Saliva** *see* Saliva Substitute *on page 1027*

◆ **As$_2$O$_3$** *see* Arsenic Trioxide *on page 107*

Asparaginase (a SPEAR a ji nase)

Medication Safety Issues

Sound-alike/look-alike issues:

Asparaginase may be confused with pegaspargase

Elspar® may be confused with Elaprase™, Oncaspar®

High alert medication: The Institute for Safe Medication Practices (ISMP) includes this medication among its list of classes of drugs which have a heightened risk of causing significant patient harm when used in error.

Related Information

Safe Handling of Hazardous Drugs *on page 1517*

U.S. Brand Names Elspar®

Index Terms *E. coli* Asparaginase; *Erwinia* Asparaginase; L-asparaginase; NSC-106977 (*Erwinia*); NSC-109229 (*E. coli*)

Generic Available No

Canadian Brand Names Kidrolase®

Pharmacologic Category Antineoplastic Agent, Miscellaneous

Use Treatment of acute lymphocytic leukemia (ALL)

Unlabeled/Investigational Use Treatment of lymphoma

Pregnancy Risk Factor C

◄ **Lactation** Excretion in breast milk unknown/not recommended

Labeled Contraindications History of serious allergic reaction to asparaginase or any *E. coli*-derived asparaginase; history of serious thrombosis with prior asparaginase treatment; history of pancreatitis with prior asparaginase treatment; serious hemorrhagic events with prior asparaginase treatment

Warnings/Precautions Hazardous agent - use appropriate precautions for handling and disposal. Monitor for severe allergic reactions; immediate treatment for hypersensitivity reactions should be available during administration. May alter hepatic function; use caution with pre-existing liver impairment. Serious thrombosis, including sagittal sinus thrombosis may occur; discontinue with serious thrombotic events. Increased prothrombin time, partial thromboplastin time and hypofibrinogenemia may occur; cerebrovascular hemorrhage has been reported; monitor coagulation parameters; use cautiously in patients with an underlying coagulopathy. Monitor blood glucose; may cause hyperglycemia/glucose intolerance (possibly irreversible). May cause serious and possibly fatal pancreatitis; promptly evaluate patients with abdominal pain; discontinue permanently if pancreatitis develops. Appropriate measures must be taken to prevent tumor lysis syndrome and subsequent hyperuricemia and uric acid nephropathy; monitor, consider allopurinol, hydration and urinary alkalization.

Severe allergic reactions may occur; monitor; immediate treatment for hypersensitivity reactions should be available during administration. Risk factors for allergic reactions include: I.V. administration, doses >6000-12,000 units/m^2, patients who have received previous cycles of asparaginase, and intervals of even a few days between doses. Up to 33% of patients who have an allergic reaction to *E. coli* asparaginase will also react to the *Erwinia* form or pegaspargase. A test dose may be administered prior to the first dose of asparaginase, or prior to restarting therapy after a hiatus of several days. **False-negative rates of up to 80% to test doses of 2-50 units are reported.** Desensitization may be performed in patients found to be hypersensitive by the intradermal test dose or who have received previous courses of therapy with the drug.

Adverse Reactions Note: Immediate effects: Fever, chills, nausea, and vomiting occur in 50% to 60% of patients.

>10%:
  Central nervous system: Fatigue, fever, chills, depression, agitation, seizure (10% to 60%), somnolence, stupor, confusion, coma (25%)
  Endocrine & metabolic: Hyperglycemia/glucose intolerance (10%)
  Gastrointestinal: Nausea, vomiting (50% to 60%), anorexia, abdominal cramps (70%), acute pancreatitis (15%, may be severe in some patients)
  Hematologic: Hypofibrinogenemia and depression of clotting factors V and VIII, variable decrease in factors VII and IX, severe protein C deficiency and decrease in antithrombin III (may be dose limiting or fatal)
  Hepatic: Transaminases, bilirubin, and alkaline phosphatase increased (transient)
  Hypersensitivity: Acute allergic reactions (fever, rash, urticaria, arthralgia, hypotension, angioedema, bronchospasm, respiratory distress, anaphylaxis (15% to 35%); may be dose limiting in some patients, may be fatal)
  Renal: Azotemia (66%)
1% to 10%:
  Endocrine & metabolic: Hyperuricemia
  Gastrointestinal: Stomatitis

Miscellaneous: Allergic reaction (including anaphylaxis), antibody formation/immunogenicity (~25%)

<1%, postmarketing case reports, and/or frequency not defined: Acute renal failure, albumin decreased, cerebrovascular hemorrhage, cerebrovascular thrombosis, cough, disorientation, drowsiness, fatty liver, fibrinogen decreased, glucosuria, hallucinations, headache, hemorrhagic pancreatitis, hyper-/hypolipidemia, hyperthermia, hypocholesterolemia, hypotension, insulin-dependent diabetes, intracranial hemorrhage, irritability, ketoacidosis, laryngospasm, malabsorption syndrome, pancreatic pseudocyst, Parkinsonian symptoms (including tremor and increased muscle tone), partial thromboplastin time increased, peripheral edema, polyuria, proteinuria, prothrombin time increased, pruritus, rash, renal insufficiency, serum ammonia increased, serum cholesterol decreased, sagittal sinus thrombosis, thrombosis, urticaria, venous thrombosis, weight loss; mild-to-moderate myelosuppression, leukopenia, anemia, thrombocytopenia (onset: 7 days, nadir: 14 days, recovery: 21 days)

Drug Interactions

Avoid Concomitant Use

Avoid concomitant use of Asparaginase with any of the following: Natalizumab; Vaccines (Live)

Increased Effect/Toxicity

Asparaginase may increase the levels/effects of: Dexamethasone; Leflunomide; Natalizumab; Vaccines (Live)

The levels/effects of Asparaginase may be increased by: Trastuzumab

Decreased Effect

Asparaginase may decrease the levels/effects of: Vaccines (Inactivated); Vaccines (Live)

The levels/effects of Asparaginase may be decreased by: Echinacea

Storage/Stability Intact vials of powder should be refrigerated at 2°C to 8°C (36°F to 48°F). Reconstituted solutions are stable 1 week refrigerated at 8°C (Stecher, 1999), although the manufacturer recommends use within 8 hours. Solutions for I.V. infusion are stable for 8 hours at room temperature or under refrigeration.

Reconstitution Lyophilized powder should be reconstituted with 1-5 mL sterile water for injection or NS for I.V. administration; NS for I.M. use. Shake well, but not too vigorously. A 5 micron filter may be used to remove fiber-like particles in the solution (do not use a 0.2 micron filter; has been associated with loss of potency).

Standard I.M. dilution: 2000, 5000, or 10,000 int. units/mL
Standard I.V. dilution: Dilute in 50-250 mL NS or D_5W

Test dose preparation: Reconstitute a 10,000 unit vial with 5 mL NS or SWFI (concentration = 2000 units/mL); withdraw 0.1 mL and add to 9.9 mL NS (concentration = 20 units/mL); test dose is 0.1 mL (2 units)

Compatibility Stable in D_5W, NS.

Y-site administration: Compatible: Methotrexate, sodium bicarbonate

Mechanism of Action Asparaginase inhibits protein synthesis by hydrolyzing asparagine to aspartic acid and ammonia. Leukemia cells, especially lymphoblasts, require exogenous asparagine; normal cells can synthesize asparagine. Asparaginase is cycle-specific for the G_1 phase.

◀ **Pharmacodynamics/Kinetics**

Absorption: I.M.: Produces peak blood levels 50% lower than those from I.V. administration

Distribution: V_d: 4-5 L/kg; 70% to 80% of plasma volume; <1% CSF penetration

Metabolism: Systemically degraded

Half-life elimination: I.M.: 39-49 hours; I.V.: 8-30 hours

Time to peak, plasma: I.M.: 14-24 hours

Dosage Refer to individual protocols. **Note:** Dose, frequency, number of doses, and start date may vary by protocol and treatment phase.

Children:

I.V.:

6000 units/m^2/dose 3 times/week for ~6-9 doses **or**

1000 units/kg/day for 10 days **or**

High-dose therapy (unlabeled dose): 10,000 units/m^2/dose every ~3 days for ~4-8 doses

I.M.:

6000 units/m^2/dose 3 times/week **or** 6000 units/m^2/dose every ~3 days for ~6-9 doses

High-dose therapy (unlabeled dose): 10,000 units/m^2/dose every ~3 days for ~4-8 doses **or** 25,000 units/m^2/dose weekly for ~9 doses (generally used in high-risk continuation therapy)

Adults:

I.V.:

6000 units/m^2/dose 3 times/week for ~6-9 doses **or**

1000 units/kg/day for 10 days **or**

High-dose therapy (unlabeled dose): 10,000 units/m^2/day for ~3-12 doses

Single agent therapy (rare): 200 units/kg/day for 28 days

I.M.:

6000 units/m^2/dose 3 times/week for ~6-9 doses **or** 6000 units/m^2/dose every ~3 days for ~6-9 doses

High-dose therapy (unlabeled dose): 10,000 units/m^2/day for ~3-12 doses

Test dose: A test dose is often recommended prior to the first dose of asparaginase, or prior to restarting therapy after a hiatus of several days. Most commonly, 0.1 mL of a 20 units/mL (2 units) asparaginase dilution is injected intradermally, and the patient observed for at least 1 hour. False-negative rates of up to 80% to test doses of 2-50 units are reported.

Some practitioners recommend an asparaginase desensitization regimen for patients who react to a test dose, or are being retreated following a break in therapy. Doses are doubled and given every 10 minutes until the total daily dose for that day has been administered. One schedule begins with a total of 1 unit given I.V. and doubles the dose every 10 minutes until the total amount given is the planned dose for that day. For example, if a patient was to receive a total dose of 4000 units, he/she would receive injections 1 through 12 during the desensitization. See table on next page.

Asparaginase Desensitization

Injection No.	Elspar Dose (int. units)	Accumulated Total Dose
1	1	1
2	2	3
3	4	7
4	8	15
5	16	31
6	32	63
7	64	127
8	128	255
9	256	511
10	512	1023
11	1024	2047
12	2048	4095
13	4096	8191
14	8192	16,383
15	16,384	32,767
16	32,768	65,535
17	65,536	131,071
18	131,072	262,143

Combination Regimens

Leukemia, acute lymphocytic:
Leukemia, acute myeloid:

Administration May be administered I.M., I.V., or intradermal (skin test only); has been administered SubQ in specific protocols

I.M.: Doses should be given as a deep intramuscular injection into a large muscle; volumes >2 mL should be divided and administered in 2 separate sites

Note: I.V. administration greatly increases the risk of allergic reactions and should be avoided if possible.

I.V.: I.V. infusion in 50-250 mL of D_5W or NS over at least 30-60 minutes. The manufacturer recommends a test dose (0.1 mL of a dilute 20 unit/mL solution) prior to initial administration and when given after an interval of 7 days or more. Institutional policies vary. The skin test site should be observed for at least 1 hour for a wheal or erythema. Note that a negative skin test does not preclude the possibility of an allergic reaction. Desensitization may be performed in patients who have been found to be hypersensitive by the intradermal skin test or who have received previous courses of therapy with the drug. Have epinephrine, diphenhydramine, and hydrocortisone at the bedside. Have a running I.V. in place. A physician should be readily accessible.

Gelatinous fiber-like particles may develop on standing. Filtration through a 5-micron filter during administration will remove the particles with no loss of potency.

Monitoring Parameters Vital signs during administration; CBC with differential, urinalysis, amylase, liver enzymes, coagulation parameters (baseline and periodic), renal function tests, urine dipstick for glucose, blood glucose, uric acid. Monitor for allergic reaction, be prepared to treat anaphylaxis at each administration; monitor for onset of abdominal pain and mental status changes.

Test Interactions Decreased thyroxine and thyroxine-binding globulin

Additional Information Some institutions recommended the following precautions for asparaginase administration: Parenteral epinephrine, diphenhydramine, and hydrocortisone available at bedside; freely running I.V. in place; physician readily accessible; monitor the patient closely for 30-60 minutes; avoid administering at night.

The *E. coli* and the *Erwinia* strains of asparaginase differ slightly in their gene sequencing, and have slight differences in their enzyme characteristics. Both are highly specific for asparagine and have <10% activity for the D-isomer. The *E. coli* form is more commonly used. The *Erwinia* variety is no longer commercially available in the U.S., although may be obtained through clinical trials or on a compassionate use basis.

Emetic Potential Very low (<10%)

Dosage Forms Excipient information presented when available (limited, particularly for generics); consult specific product labeling.

Injection, powder for reconstitution:

Elspar®: 10,000 int. units

References

Avramis VI, Sencer S, Periclou AP, et al, "A Randomized Comparison of Native Escherichia Coli Asparaginase and Polyethylene Glycol Conjugated Asparaginase for Treatment of Children With Newly Diagnosed Standard-Risk Acute Lymphoblastic Leukemia: A Children's Cancer Group Study," *Blood*, 2002, 99(6):1986-94.

Duval M, Suciu S, Ferster A, et al, "Comparison of *Escherichia Coli* -Asparaginase With *Erwinia*-Asparaginase in the Treatment of Childhood Lymphoid Malignancies: Results of a Randomized European Organisation for Research and Treatment of Cancer – Children's Leukemia Group Phase 3 Trial," *Blood*, 2002, 99(8):2734-9.

Larson RA, Dodge RK, Burns P, et al, "A Five-Drug Remission Induction Regimen With Intensive Consolidation for Adults With Acute Lymphoblastic Leukemia: Cancer and Leukemia Group B Study 8811," *Blood*, 1995, 85(8):2025-37.

Lazarus HM, Richards SM, Chopra R, et al, "Central Nervous System Involvement in Adult Acute Lymphoblastic Leukemia at Diagnosis: Results from the International ALL Trial MRC UKALL XII/ ECOG E2993," *Blood*, 2006, 108(2):465-72.

Pession A, Valsecchi MG, Masera G, et al, "Long-Term Results of a Randomized Trial on Extended Use of High Dose L-Asparaginase for Standard Risk Childhood Acute Lymphoblastic Leukemia," *J Clin Oncol*, 2005, 23(28):7161-7.

Stecher AL, de Deus PM, Polikarpov I, et al, "Stability of L-Asparaginase: An Enzyme Used in Leukemia Treatment," *Pharm Acta Helv*, 1999, 74(1):1-9.

- **ATRA** *see* Tretinoin, Systemic *on page 1141*
- **Atriance™ (Can)** *see* Nelarabine *on page 843*
- **ATryn®** *see* Antithrombin III *on page 96*
- **Avakine** *see* InFLIXimab *on page 635*
- **Avastin®** *see* Bevacizumab *on page 137*
- **Avinza®** *see* Morphine Sulfate *on page 816*
- **Avodart®** *see* Dutasteride *on page 393*
- **AY-25650** *see* Triptorelin *on page 1150*
- **5-Aza-2'-deoxycytidine** *see* Decitabine *on page 327*
- **5-AzaC** *see* Decitabine *on page 327*

AzaCITIDine (ay za SYE ti deen)

Medication Safety Issues
Sound-alike/look-alike issues:
AzaCITIDine may be confused with azaTHIOprine

High alert medication: The Institute for Safe Medication Practices (ISMP) includes this medication among its list of drug classes which have a heightened risk of causing significant patient harm when used in error.

Related Information
Safe Handling of Hazardous Drugs *on page 1517*

U.S. Brand Names Vidaza®

Index Terms 5-Azacytidine; 5-AZC; AZA-CR; Azacytidine; Ladakamycin

Generic Available No

Pharmacologic Category Antineoplastic Agent, DNA Methylation Inhibitor

Use Treatment of myelodysplastic syndrome (MDS)

Unlabeled/Investigational Use Treatment of acute myelogenous leukemia (AML)

Pregnancy Risk Factor D

Lactation Excretion in breast milk unknown/not recommended

Labeled Contraindications Hypersensitivity to azacitidine, mannitol, or any component of the formulation; advanced malignant hepatic tumors

Warnings/Precautions Hazardous agent - use appropriate precautions for handling and disposal. Azacitidine may be hepatotoxic, use caution with hepatic impairment; use is contraindicated in patients with advanced malignant hepatic tumors. Progressive hepatic coma leading to death has been reported (rare) in patients with extensive tumor burden, especially those with a baseline albumin <30 g/L. Use caution with renal impairment; dose adjustment may be required. Serum creatinine elevations, renal tubular acidosis, and renal failure have been reported with combination chemotherapy; decrease or withhold dose for unexplained elevations in BUN or serum creatinine or reductions in serum bicarbonate to <20 mEq/L. Patients with renal and hepatic impairment were excluded from clinical studies. Neutropenia, thrombocytopenia, and anemia are common; may cause therapy delays and/or dosage reductions. Not FDA approved for use in children.

Adverse Reactions
>10%:
Cardiovascular: Peripheral edema (7% to 19%), chest pain (16%), pallor (16%), pitting edema (15%)
Central nervous system: Fever (30% to 52%), fatigue (13% to 36%), headache (22%), dizziness (19%), anxiety (5% to 13%), depression (12%), insomnia (9% to 11%), malaise (11%), pain (11%)

Dermatologic: Bruising (19% to 31%), petechiae (11% to 24%), erythema (7% to 17%), skin lesion (15%), rash (10% to 14%), pruritus (12%)

Endocrine & metabolic: Hypokalemia (6% to 13%)

Gastrointestinal: Nausea (48% to 71%), vomiting (27% to 54%), diarrhea (36%), constipation (34% to 50%), anorexia (13% to 21%), weight loss (16%), abdominal pain (11% to 16%), abdominal tenderness (12%)

Hematologic: Thrombocytopenia (66% to 70%; grades 3/4: 58%), anemia (51% to 70%; grades 3/4: 14%), neutropenia (32% to 66%; grades 3/4: 61%), leukopenia (18% to 48%; grades 3/4: 15%), febrile neutropenia (14% to 16%; grades 3/4: 13%), myelosuppression (nadir: days 10-17; recovery: days 28-31)

Local: Injection site reactions (14% to 29%): Erythema (35% to 43%; more common with I.V. administration), pain (19% to 23%; more common with I.V. administration), bruising (5% to 14%)

Neuromuscular & skeletal: Weakness (29%), rigors (26%), arthralgia (22%), limb pain (20%), back pain (19%), myalgia (16%)

Respiratory: Cough (11% to 30%), dyspnea (5% to 29%), pharyngitis (20%), epistaxis (16%), nasopharyngitis (15%), upper respiratory tract infection (9% to 13%), pneumonia (11%), crackles (11%)

Miscellaneous: Diaphoresis (11%)

5% to 10%:

Cardiovascular: Cardiac murmur (10%), hypertension (≤9%), tachycardia (9%), hypotension (7%), syncope (6%), chest wall pain (5%)

Central nervous system: Lethargy (7% to 8%), hypoesthesia (5%), postprocedural pain (5%)

Dermatologic: Cellulitis (8%), urticaria (6%), dry skin (5%), skin nodule (5%)

Gastrointestinal: Gingival bleeding (10%), oral mucosal petechiae (8%), stomatitis (8%), weight loss (≤8%), dyspepsia (6% to 7%), hemorrhoids (7%), abdominal distension (6%), loose stools (6%), dysphagia (5%), oral hemorrhage (5%), tongue ulceration (5%)

Genitourinary: Dysuria (8%), urinary tract infection (8% to 9%)

Hematologic: Hematoma (9%), postprocedural hemorrhage (6%)

Local: Injection site reactions: Pruritus (7%), hematoma (6%), rash (6%), granuloma (5%), induration (5%), pigmentation change (5%), swelling (5%)

Neuromuscular & skeletal: Muscle cramps (6%)

Renal: Hematuria (≤6%)

Respiratory: Rhinorrhea (10%), rales (9%), wheezing (9%), breath sounds decreased (8%), pharyngolaryngeal pain (6%), pleural effusion (6%), postnasal drip (6%), rhinitis (6%), rhonchi (6%), nasal congestion (6%), atelectasis (5%), sinusitis (5%)

Miscellaneous: Lymphadenopathy (10%), herpes simplex (9%), night sweats (9%), transfusion reaction (7%), mouth hemorrhage (5%)

<5%, postmarketing, and/or case reports (limited to important or life-threatening): Abscess (limb), agranulocytosis, anaphylactic shock, atrial fibrillation, azotemia, blastomycosis, bone marrow depression/failure, bone pain aggravated, cardiac failure, cardiorespiratory arrest, catheter site hemorrhage, cellulitis, cerebral hemorrhage, CHF, cholecystectomy, cholecystitis, congestive cardiomyopathy, dehydration, diverticulitis, eye hemorrhage, fibrosis (interstitial and alveolar), gastrointestinal hemorrhage, glycosuria, hemoptysis, hepatic coma, hypersensitivity reaction, hypophosphatemia, infection (bacterial), injection site infection, intracranial hemorrhage, leukemia cutis, lung infiltration, melena, neutropenic sepsis, orthostatic hypotension, pancytopenia, pneumonitis, polyuria, pyoderma gangrenosum, renal failure, renal tubular acidosis, seizure, respiratory distress, sepsis, septic shock, serum bicarbonate levels decreased, serum

creatinine increased, splenomegaly, systemic inflammatory response syndrome, toxoplasmosis

Drug Interactions

Avoid Concomitant Use

Avoid concomitant use of AzaCITIDine with any of the following: Natalizumab; Vaccines (Live)

Increased Effect/Toxicity

AzaCITIDine may increase the levels/effects of: Leflunomide; Natalizumab; Vaccines (Live)

The levels/effects of AzaCITIDine may be increased by: Trastuzumab

Decreased Effect

AzaCITIDine may decrease the levels/effects of: Vaccines (Inactivated); Vaccines (Live)

The levels/effects of AzaCITIDine may be decreased by: Echinacea

Storage/Stability Prior to reconstitution, store powder at room temperature of 25°C (77°F); excursions permitted to 15°C to 30°C (59°F to 86°F).

SubQ: Following reconstitution, suspension may be stored at room temperature for up to 1 hour, or immediately refrigerated at 2°C to 8°C (36°F to 46°F) and stored for up to 8 hours.

I.V.: **Solutions for I.V. administration have very limited stability and must be prepared immediately prior to each dose.** Administration must be completed within 1 hour of (vial) reconstitution.

Reconstitution Use appropriate precautions for handling and disposal.

SubQ: To prepare a 25 mg/mL suspension, slowly add 4 mL SWFI to each vial. Vigorously shake or roll vial until a suspension is formed (suspension will be cloudy).

I.V.: Reconstitute vial with 10 mL SWFI to form a 10 mg/mL solution; vigorously shake until solution is dissolved and clear. Mix in 50-100 mL of NS or lactated Ringer's injection for infusion.

Compatibility Stable in LR, NS

Compatibility when admixed: Incompatible with D_5W, hetastarch, or solutions containing bicarbonate

Mechanism of Action Antineoplastic effects may be a result of azacitidine's ability to promote hypomethylation of DNA leading to direct toxicity of abnormal hematopoietic cells in the bone marrow.

Pharmacodynamics/Kinetics

Absorption: SubQ: Rapid and complete

Distribution: V_d: I.V.: 76 ± 26 L; does not cross blood-brain barrier

Metabolism: Hepatic; hydrolysis to several metabolites

Bioavailability: SubQ: ~89%

Half-life elimination: I.V., SubQ: ~4 hours

Time to peak, plasma: SubQ: 30 minutes

Excretion: Urine (50% to 85%); feces (minor)

Dosage

Children: I.V.: Refractory AML (unlabeled use): 250 mg/m^2/dose days 4 and 5 every 4 weeks (Steuber, 1996) **or** 300 mg/m^2/dose days 4 and 5 every 4 weeks (Hurwitz, 1995)

Adults:

MDS: I.V., SubQ: 75 mg/m^2/day for 7 days repeated every 4 weeks. Dose may be increased to 100 mg/m^2/day if no benefit is observed after 2 cycles and no toxicity other than nausea and vomiting have occurred. Treatment is recommended for at least 4 cycles; treatment may be continued as long as patient continues to benefit.

Note: Alternate (unlabeled) schedules (which have produced hematologic response) have been used for convenience in community oncology centers (Lyons, 2009):

75 mg/m^2/day for 5 days (Mon-Fri), 2 days rest (Sat, Sun), then 75 mg/m^2/day for 2 days (Mon, Tues); repeat cycle every 28 days **or**

50 mg/m^2/day for 5 days (Mon-Fri), 2 days rest (Sat, Sun), then 50 mg/m^2/day for 5 days (Mon-Fri); repeat cycle every 28 days **or**

75 mg/m^2/day for 5 days (Mon-Fri), repeat cycle every 28 days

AML (unlabeled use): SubQ: 75 mg/m^2/day for 7 days repeated every 4 weeks (Sudan, 2006)

Elderly: Refer to adult dosing; due to the potential for decreased renal function in the elderly, select dose carefully and closely monitor renal function

Dosage adjustment based on hematology: Adults: MDS: I.V., SubQ:

For baseline WBC ≥3.0 x 10^9/L, ANC ≥1.5 x 10^9/L, and platelets ≥75 x 10^9/L:

Nadir count: ANC <0.5 x 10^9/L or platelets <25 x 10^9/L: Administer 50% of dose during next treatment course

Nadir count: ANC 0.5-1.5 x 10^9/L or platelets 25-50 x 10^9/L: Administer 67% of dose during next treatment course

Nadir count: ANC >1.5 x 10^9/L or platelets >50 x 10^9/L: Administer 100% of dose during next treatment course

For baseline WBC <3 x 10^9/L, ANC <1.5 x 10^9/L, or platelets <75 x 10^9/L: Adjust dose as follows based on nadir counts and bone marrow biopsy cellularity at the time of nadir, unless clear improvement in differentiation at the time of the next cycle:

WBC or platelet nadir decreased 50% to 75% from baseline and bone marrow biopsy cellularity at time of nadir 30% to 60%: Administer 100% of dose during next treatment course

WBC or platelet nadir decreased 50% to 75% from baseline and bone marrow biopsy cellularity at time of nadir 15% to 30%: Administer 50% of dose during next treatment course

WBC or platelet nadir decreased 50% to 75% from baseline and bone marrow biopsy cellularity at time of nadir <15%: Administer 33% of dose during next treatment course

WBC or platelet nadir decreased >75% from baseline and bone marrow biopsy cellularity at time of nadir 30% to 60%: Administer 75% of dose during next treatment course

WBC or platelet nadir decreased >75% from baseline and bone marrow biopsy cellularity at time of nadir 15% to 30%: Administer 50% of dose during next treatment course

WBC or platelet nadir decreased >75% from baseline and bone marrow biopsy cellularity at time of nadir <15%: Administer 33% of dose during next treatment course

Note: If a nadir defined above occurs, administer the next treatment course 28 days after the start of the preceding course as long as WBC and platelet counts are >25% above the nadir and rising. If a >25% increase above the nadir is not seen by day 28, reassess counts every 7 days. If a 25% increase is not seen by day 42, administer 50% of the scheduled dose.

Dosage adjustment based on serum electrolytes: The manufacturer recommends that if serum bicarbonate falls to <20 mEq/L (unexplained decrease): Reduce dose by 50% for next treatment course

Dosage adjustment based on renal toxicity: If increases in BUN or serum creatinine (unexplained) occur, delay next cycle until values reach baseline or normal, then reduce dose by 50% for next treatment course.

Dosage adjustment in renal impairment: Not studied in patients with renal impairment; select dose carefully (excretion is primarily renal; consider dose reduction); monitor closely for toxicity

Dosage adjustment in hepatic impairment: Not studied in patients with hepatic impairment; use caution. Contraindicated in patients with advanced malignant hepatic tumors.

Administration

SubQ: Premedication for nausea and vomiting is recommended. The manufacturer recommends equally dividing volumes >4 mL into 2 syringes and injecting into 2 separate sites; however, policies for maximum SubQ administration volume may vary by institution; interpatient variations may also apply. Administer subsequent injections at least 1 inch from previous injection sites. Allow refrigerated suspensions to come to room temperature (up to 30 minutes) prior to administration. Resuspend by inverting the syringe 2-3 times and then rolling the syringe between the palms for 30 seconds. If azacitidine suspension comes in contact with the skin, immediately wash with soap and water.

I.V.: Premedication for nausea and vomiting is recommended. Infuse over 10-40 minutes; infusion must be completed within 1 hour of (vial) reconstitution.

Monitoring Parameters Liver function tests, electrolytes, CBC with differential and platelets, renal function tests (BUN and serum creatinine) should be obtained prior to initiation of therapy. Electrolytes, renal function (BUN and creatinine), CBC should be monitored prior to each cycle and periodically as needed to monitor response and toxicity.

Additional Information Oncology Comment: Azacitidine treatment for MDS is associated with an improvement in quality of life (including a reduction in transfusion requirements), a decrease in transformation to AML, and improved survival, when compared to best supportive care. Treatment should be continued for a minimum of 4-6 cycles (NCCN MDS guidelines v.2.2009).

Emetic Potential Moderate (30% to 90%)

Vesicant No. Subcutaneous injection of undissolved crystals may cause localized reactions.

Dosage Forms Excipient information presented when available (limited, particularly for generics); consult specific product labeling.

Injection, powder for suspension [preservative free]:

Vidaza®: 100 mg [contains mannitol 100 mg]

References

Hurwitz CA, Krance R, Schell MJ, et al, "Current Strategies for Treatment of Acute Myeloid Leukemia at St Jude Children's Research Hospital," *Leukemia*, 1992, (6 Suppl 2):39-43.

Hurwitz CA, Mounce KG, and Grier HE, "Treatment of Patients With Acute Myelogenous Leukemia: Review of Clinical Trials of the Past Decade," *J Pediatr Hematol Oncol*, 1995, 17 (3):185-97.

Jehn U, "Long-Term Outcome of Postremission Chemotherapy for Adults With Acute Myeloid Leukemia Using Different Dose-Intensities," *Leuk Lymphoma*, 1994, 15(1-2):99-112.

Kornblith AB, Herndon JE 2nd, Silverman LR, et al, "Impact of Azacytidine on the Quality of Life of Patients With Myelodysplastic Syndrome Treated in a Randomized Phase III Trial: A Cancer and Leukemia Group B Study," *J Clin Oncol*, 2002, 20(10):2441-52.

Lyons RM, Cosgriff TM, Modi SS, et al, "Hematologic Response to Three Alternative Dosing Schedules of Azacitidine in Patients With Myelodysplastic Syndrome," *J Clin Oncol*, 2009, 27 (11):1850-6.

National Comprehensive Cancer Network® (NCCN), "Practice Guidelines in Oncology™: Acute Myeloid Leukemia," Version 1, 2009. Accessible at http://www.nccn.org/professionals/physician_gls/PDF/aml.pdf

National Comprehensive Cancer Network (NCCN), "Clinical Practice Guidelines in Oncology™: Myelodysplastic Syndromes," Version 2.2009. Available at http://www.nccn.org/professionals/physician_gls/PDF/mds.pdf.

◄ Peterson BA, Collins AJ, Vogelzang NJ, et al, "5-Azacytidine and Renal Tubular Dysfunction," Blood, 1981, 57(1):182-5.

Silverman LR, Demakos EP, Peterson BL, et al, "Randomized Controlled Trial of Azacitidine in Patients With the Myelodysplastic Syndrome: A Study of the Cancer and Leukemia Group B," J Clin Oncol, 2002, 20(10):2429-40.

Silverman LR, McKenzie DR, Peterson BL, et al, "Further Analysis of Trials With Azacitidine in Patients With Myelodysplastic Syndrome: Studies 8421, 8921, and 9221 by the Cancer and Leukemia Group B," J Clin Oncol, 2006, 24(24):3895-903.

Steuber CP, Krischer J, Holbrook T, et al, "Therapy of Refractory or Recurrent Childhood Acute Myeloid Leukemia Using Amsacrine and Etoposide With or Without Azacitidine: A Pediatric Oncology Group Randomized Phase II Study," J Clin Oncol, 1996, 14(5):1521-5.

Sudan N, Rossetti JM, Shadduck RK, et al, "Treatment of Acute Myelogenous Leukemia With Outpatient Azacitidine," Cancer, 2006, 107(8):1839-43.

Volger WR, Weiner RS, Moore JO, et al, "Long-Term Follow-up of a Randomized Postinduction Therapy Trial in Acute Myelogenous Leukemia (A Southeastern Cancer Study Group Trial)," Leukemia, 1995, 9(9):1456-60.

◆ **AZA-CR** see AzaCITIDine on page 117

◆ **Azactam®** see Aztreonam on page 122

◆ **Azacytidine** see AzaCITIDine on page 117

◆ **5-Azacytidine** see AzaCITIDine on page 117

◆ **Azaepothilone B** see Ixabepilone on page 672

◆ **5-AZC** see AzaCITIDine on page 117

◆ **Azthreonam** see Aztreonam on page 122

Aztreonam (AZ tree oh nam)

Medication Safety Issues

Sound-alike/look-alike issues:

Aztreonam may be confused with azidothymidine

U.S. Brand Names Azactam®

Index Terms Azthreonam

Generic Available No

Canadian Brand Names Azactam®

Pharmacologic Category Antibiotic, Miscellaneous

Use Treatment of patients with urinary tract infections, lower respiratory tract infections, septicemia, skin/skin structure infections, intra-abdominal infections, and gynecological infections caused by susceptible gram-negative bacilli

Pregnancy Risk Factor B

Lactation Enters breast milk/not recommended (AAP rates "compatible")

Labeled Contraindications Hypersensitivity to aztreonam or any component of the formulation

Warnings/Precautions Rare cross-allergenicity to penicillins and cephalosporins has been reported. Use caution in renal impairment; dosing adjustment required. Prolonged use may result in fungal or bacterial superinfection, including *C. difficile*-associated diarrhea (CDAD) and pseudomembranous colitis; CDAD has been observed >2 months postantibiotic treatment.

Adverse Reactions As reported in adults:

1% to 10%:

Dermatologic: Rash

Gastrointestinal: Diarrhea, nausea, vomiting

Local: Thrombophlebitis, pain at injection site

<1%: Abdominal cramps, abnormal taste, anaphylaxis, anemia, angioedema, aphthous ulcer, breast tenderness, bronchospasm, *C. difficile*-associated diarrhea, chest pain, confusion, diaphoresis, diplopia, dizziness, dyspnea, eosinophilia, erythema multiforme, exfoliative dermatitis, fever, flushing,

halitosis, headache, hepatitis, hypotension, insomnia, jaundice, leukopenia, liver enzymes increased, muscular aches myalgia, neutropenia, numb tongue, pancytopenia, paresthesia, petechiae, pruritus, pseudomembranous colitis, purpura, seizure, sneezing, thrombocytopenia, tinnitus, toxic epidermal necrolysis, urticaria, vaginitis, vertigo, weakness, wheezing

Drug Interactions

Avoid Concomitant Use There are no known interactions where it is recommended to avoid concomitant use.

Increased Effect/Toxicity There are no known significant interactions involving an increase in effect.

Decreased Effect

Aztreonam may decrease the levels/effects of: Typhoid Vaccine

Storage/Stability Prior to reconstitution, store at room temperature; avoid excessive heat. Reconstituted solutions are colorless to light yellow straw and may turn pink upon standing without affecting potency. Use reconstituted solutions and I.V. solutions (in NS and D_5W) within 48 hours if kept at room temperature (25°C) or 7 days under refrigeration (4°C).

Infusion: Solution for infusion may be frozen at less than -2°C (less than -4°F) for up to 3 months. Thawed solution should be used within 24 hours if thawed at room temperature or within 72 hours if thawed under refrigeration. **Do not refreeze.**

Reconstitution

I.M.: Reconstitute with at least 3 mL SWFI, sterile bacteriostatic water for injection, NS, or bacteriostatic sodium chloride.

I.V.:

Bolus injection: Reconstitute with 6-10 mL SWFI.

Infusion: Reconstitute to a final concentration ≤2%; the final concentration should not exceed 20 mg/mL.

Compatibility Solution for infusion: Stable in D_5LR, $D_5^{1}/_4NS$, $D_5^{1}/_2NS$, D_5NS, D_5W, $D_{10}W$, mannitol 5%, mannitol 10%, LR, NS; **variable stability (consult detailed reference)** in peritoneal dialysis solution.

Y-site administration: Compatible: Allopurinol, amifostine, amikacin, aminophylline, ampicillin, ampicillin/sulbactam, bleomycin, bumetanide, buprenorphine, butorphanol, calcium gluconate, carboplatin, carmustine, cefazolin, cefepime, cefoperazone, cefotaxime, cefotetan, cefoxitin, ceftazidime, ceftizoxime, ceftriaxone, cefuroxime, cimetidine, ciprofloxacin, cisatracurium, cisplatin, clindamycin, co-trimoxazole, cyclophosphamide, cytarabine, dacarbazine, dactinomycin, dexamethasone sodium phosphate, diltiazem, diphenhydramine, dobutamine, docetaxel, dopamine, doxorubicin, doxorubicin liposome, doxycycline, droperidol, enalaprilat, etoposide, etoposide phosphate, famotidine, filgrastim, floxuridine, fluconazole, fludarabine, fluorouracil, foscarnet, furosemide, gatifloxacin, gemcitabine, gentamicin, granisetron, haloperidol, heparin, hydrocortisone sodium phosphate, hydrocortisone sodium succinate, hydromorphone, hydroxyzine, idarubicin, ifosfamide, imipenem/cilastatin, insulin (regular), leucovorin, linezolid, magnesium sulfate, mannitol, mechlorethamine, melphalan, meperidine, mesna, methotrexate, methylprednisolone sodium succinate, metoclopramide, minocycline, morphine, nalbuphine, netilmicin, ondansetron, piperacillin, piperacillin/tazobactam, plicamycin, potassium chloride, promethazine, propofol, ranitidine, remifentanil, sargramostim, sodium bicarbonate, teniposide, theophylline, thiotepa, ticarcillin, ticarcillin/clavulanate, tobramycin, vinblastine, vincristine, vinorelbine, zidovudine. **Incompatible:** Acyclovir, alatrofloxacin, amphotericin B, amphotericin B cholesteryl sulfate complex, amsacrine, chlorpromazine, daunorubicin, ganciclovir, lorazepam,

123

metronidazole, mitomycin, mitoxantrone, prochlorperazine edisylate, strepto-zocin. **Variable (consult detailed reference):** Vancomycin.

Compatibility in syringe: Compatible: Clindamycin.

Compatibility when admixed: Compatible: Ampicillin/sulbactam, cefazolin, ciprofloxacin, clindamycin, gentamicin, linezolid, tobramycin. **Incompatible:** Metronidazole, nafcillin. **Variable (consult detailed reference):** Ampicillin, cefoxitin, vancomycin.

Mechanism of Action Inhibits bacterial cell wall synthesis by binding to one or more of the penicillin binding proteins (PBPs) which in turn inhibits the final transpeptidation step of peptidoglycan synthesis in bacterial cell walls, thus inhibiting cell wall biosynthesis. Bacteria eventually lyse due to ongoing activity of cell wall autolytic enzymes (autolysins and murein hydrolases) while cell wall assembly is arrested. Monobactam structure makes cross-allergenicity with beta-lactams unlikely.

Pharmacodynamics/Kinetics

Absorption: I.M.: Well absorbed; I.M. and I.V. doses produce comparable serum concentrations; Oral: <1%

Distribution: Widely to most body fluids and tissues

V_d: Children: 0.2-0.29 L/kg; Adults: 0.2 L/kg

Relative diffusion of antimicrobial agents from blood into CSF: Good only with inflammation (exceeds usual MICs)

CSF:blood level ratio: Meninges: Inflamed: 8% to 40%; Normal: ~1%

Protein binding: 56%

Metabolism: Hepatic (minor %)

Half-life elimination:

Children 2 months to 12 years: 1.7 hours

Adults: Normal renal function: 1.7-2.9 hours

End-stage renal disease: 6-8 hours

Time to peak: I.M., I.V. push: Within 60 minutes; I.V. infusion: 1.5 hours

Excretion: Urine (60% to 70% as unchanged drug); feces (~13% to 15%)

Dosage

Children >1 month: I.M., I.V.:

Mild-to-moderate infections: I.M., I.V.: 30 mg/kg every 8 hours

Moderate-to-severe infections: I.M., I.V.: 30 mg/kg every 6-8 hours; maximum: 120 mg/kg/day (8 g/day)

Cystic fibrosis: I.V.: 50 mg/kg/dose every 6-8 hours (ie, up to 200 mg/kg/day); maximum: 8 g/day

Adults:

Urinary tract infection: I.M., I.V.: 500 mg to 1 g every 8-12 hours

Moderately-severe systemic infections: 1 g I.V. or I.M. or 2 g I.V. every 8-12 hours

Severe systemic or life-threatening infections (especially caused by *Pseudomonas aeruginosa*): I.V.: 2 g every 6-8 hours; maximum: 8 g/day

Meningitis (gram-negative): I.V.: 2 g every 6-8 hours

Dosing adjustment in renal impairment: Adults: Following initial dose, maintenance doses should be given as follows:

Cl_{cr} 10-30 mL/minute: 50% of usual dose at the usual interval

Cl_{cr} <10 mL/minute: 25% of usual dosage at the usual interval

Hemodialysis: Moderately dialyzable (20% to 50%); Loading dose of 500 mg, 1 g, or 2 g, followed by 25% of initial dose at usual interval; for serious/life-threatening infections, administer 1/8 of initial dose after each hemodialysis session (given in addition to the maintenance doses)

Continuous ambulatory peritoneal dialysis (CAPD): Administer as for Cl_{cr} <10 mL/minute

Continuous renal replacement therapy (CRRT): Drug clearance is highly dependent on the method of renal replacement, filter type, and flow rate. Appropriate dosing requires close monitoring of pharmacologic response, signs of adverse reactions due to drug accumulation, as well as drug levels in relation to target trough (if appropriate). The following are general recommendations only (based on dialysate flow/ultrafiltration rates of 1 L/hour) and should not supersede clinical judgment:

CVVH: 1-2 g every 12 hours

CVVHD/CVVHDF: 2 g every 12 hours

Administration Doses >1 g should be administered I.V.

I.M.: Administer by deep injection into large muscle mass, such as upper outer quadrant of gluteus maximus or the lateral part of the thigh

I.V.: Administer by slow I.V. push over 3-5 minutes or by intermittent infusion over 20-60 minutes.

Monitoring Parameters Periodic liver function test; monitor for signs of anaphylaxis during first dose

Test Interactions May interfere with urine glucose tests containing cupric sulfate (Benedict's solution, Clinitest®); positive Coombs' test

Additional Information Although marketed as an agent similar to aminoglycosides, aztreonam is a monobactam antimicrobial with almost pure gram-negative aerobic activity. It cannot be used for gram-positive infections. Aminoglycosides are often used for synergy in gram-positive infections.

Dosage Forms Excipient information presented when available (limited, particularly for generics); consult specific product labeling. [DSC] = Discontinued product

Infusion premixed iso-osmotic solution:

Azactam®: 1 g (50 mL); 2 g (50 mL)

Injection, powder for reconstitution:

Azactam®: 500 mg [DSC], 1 g, 2 g

References

Brogden RN and Heel RC, "Aztreonam. A Review of Its Antibacterial Activity, Pharmacokinetic Properties and Therapeutic Use," *Drugs*, 1986, 31(2):96-130.

Hellinger WC and Brewer NS, "Carbapenems and Monobactams: Imipenem, Meropenem, and Aztreonam," *Mayo Clin Proc*, 1999, 74(4):420-34.

Settler FR, Schramm M, and Swabb EA, "Safety of Aztreonam and SQ 26,992 in Elderly Patients With Renal Insufficiency," *Rev Infect Dis*, 1985, (Suppl 4):5622.

♦ **Bacillus Calmette-Guérin (BCG) Live** *see* BCG Vaccine *on page 128*

♦ **Bactrim™** *see* Sulfamethoxazole and Trimethoprim *on page 1051*

♦ **Bactrim™ DS** *see* Sulfamethoxazole and Trimethoprim *on page 1051*

Basiliximab (ba si LIK si mab)

U.S. Brand Names Simulect®

Generic Available No

Canadian Brand Names Simulect®

Pharmacologic Category Monoclonal Antibody

Use Prophylaxis of acute organ rejection in renal transplantation

Pregnancy Risk Factor B (manufacturer)

Lactation Excretion in breast milk unknown/not recommended

Labeled Contraindications Hypersensitivity to basiliximab, murine proteins, or any component of the formulation

◀ **Warnings/Precautions** To be used as a component of immunosuppressive regimen which includes cyclosporine and corticosteroids. The incidence of lymphoproliferative disorders and/or opportunistic infections may be increased by immunosuppressive therapy. Severe hypersensitivity reactions, occurring within 24 hours, have been reported. Reactions, including anaphylaxis, have occurred both with the initial exposure and/or following re-exposure after several months. Use caution during re-exposure to a subsequent course of therapy in a patient who has previously received basiliximab. Discontinue the drug permanently if a reaction occurs. Medications for the treatment of hypersensitivity reactions should be available for immediate use. Treatment may result in the development of human antimurine antibodies (HAMA); however, limited evidence suggesting the use of muromonab-CD3 or other murine products is not precluded. **[U.S. Boxed Warning]: Should be administered under the supervision of a physician experienced in immunosuppression therapy.**

Adverse Reactions Administration of basiliximab did not appear to increase the incidence or severity of adverse effects in clinical trials. Adverse events were reported in 96% of both the placebo and basiliximab groups.

>10%:
Cardiovascular: Hypertension, peripheral edema
Central nervous system: Fever, headache, insomnia, pain
Dermatologic: Acne, wound complications
Endocrine & metabolic: Hypercholesterolemia, hyperglycemia, hyper-/hypokalemia, hyperuricemia, hypophosphatemia
Gastrointestinal: Abdominal pain, constipation, diarrhea, dyspepsia, nausea, vomiting
Genitourinary: Urinary tract infection
Hematologic: Anemia
Neuromuscular & skeletal: Tremor
Respiratory: Dyspnea, infection (upper respiratory)
Miscellaneous: Viral infection

3% to 10%:
Cardiovascular: Abnormal heart sounds, angina pectoris, arrhythmia, atrial fibrillation, cardiac failure, chest pain, generalized edema, hypotension, tachycardia
Central nervous system: Agitation, anxiety, depression, dizziness, fatigue, hypoesthesia, malaise, neuropathy, rigors
Dermatologic: Cyst, hypertrichosis, pruritus, rash, skin disorder, skin ulceration
Endocrine & metabolic: Acidosis, dehydration, diabetes mellitus, fluid overload, hyper-/hypocalcemia, hyperlipidemia, hypertriglyceridemia, hypoglycemia, hypomagnesemia, hyponatremia
Gastrointestinal: Abdomen enlarged, esophagitis, flatulence, gastroenteritis, GI hemorrhage, gingival hyperplasia, melena, moniliasis, stomatitis (including ulcerative), weight gain
Genitourinary: Albuminuria, bladder disorder, dysuria, genital edema, hematuria, impotence, oliguria, renal function abnormal, renal tubular necrosis, ureteral disorder, urinary frequency, urinary retention
Hematologic: Hematoma, hemorrhage, leukopenia, polycythemia, purpura, thrombocytopenia, thrombosis
Neuromuscular & skeletal: Arthralgia, arthropathy, back pain, cramps, fracture, hernia, leg pain, myalgia, paresthesia, weakness
Ocular: Abnormal vision, cataract, conjunctivitis

Respiratory: Bronchitis, bronchospasm, cough, pharyngitis, pneumonia, pulmonary edema, sinusitis, rhinitis

Miscellaneous: Accidental trauma, facial edema, glucocorticoids increased, herpes infection, sepsis

Postmarketing and/or case reports: Capillary leak syndrome, cytokine release syndrome; severe hypersensitivity reactions, including anaphylaxis, have been reported (symptoms may include hypotension, tachycardia, cardiac failure, dyspnea, bronchospasm, pulmonary edema, urticaria, rash, pruritus, sneezing, and respiratory failure)

Drug Interactions

Avoid Concomitant Use

Avoid concomitant use of Basiliximab with any of the following: Natalizumab; Vaccines (Live)

Increased Effect/Toxicity

Basiliximab may increase the levels/effects of: Hypoglycemic Agents; Leflunomide; Natalizumab; Vaccines (Live)

The levels/effects of Basiliximab may be increased by: Abciximab; Herbs (Hypoglycemic Properties); Trastuzumab

Decreased Effect

Basiliximab may decrease the levels/effects of: Vaccines (Inactivated); Vaccines (Live)

The levels/effects of Basiliximab may be decreased by: Echinacea

Ethanol/Nutrition/Herb Interactions Herb/Nutraceutical: Echinacea may diminish the therapeutic effect of basiliximab. Avoid hypoglycemic herbs, including alfalfa, bilberry, bitter melon, burdock, celery, damiana, fenugreek, garcinia, garlic, ginger, ginseng, gymnema, marshmallow, and stinging nettle (may enhance the hypoglycemic effect of basiliximab).

Storage/Stability Store intact vials under refrigeration 2°C to 8°C (36°F to 46°F). It is recommended that after reconstitution, the solution should be used immediately. If not used immediately, it can be stored at 2°C to 8°C for up to 24 hours or at room temperature for up to 4 hours. Discard the reconstituted solution within 24 hours.

Reconstitution Reconstitute vials with sterile water for injection, USP. Shake the vial gently to dissolve. Further dilute reconstituted solution with 25-50 mL 0.9% sodium chloride or dextrose 5% in water. When mixing the solution, gently invert the bag to avoid foaming. Do not shake.

Mechanism of Action Chimeric (murine/human) monoclonal antibody which blocks the alpha-chain of the interleukin-2 (IL-2) receptor complex; this receptor is expressed on activated T lymphocytes and is a critical pathway for activating cell-mediated allograft rejection

Pharmacodynamics/Kinetics

Duration: Mean: 36 days (determined by IL-2R alpha saturation)

Distribution: Mean: V_d: Children 1-11 years: 4.8 ± 2.1 L; Adolescents 12-16 years: 7.8 ± 5.1 L; Adults: 8.6 ± 4.1 L

Half-life elimination: Children 1-11 years: 9.5 days; Adolescents 12-16 years: 9.1 days; Adults: Mean: 7.2 days

Excretion: Clearance: Children 1-11 years: 17 mL/hour; Adolescents 12-16 years: 31 mL/hour; Adults: Mean: 41 mL/hour

Dosage Note: Patients previously administered basiliximab should only be re-exposed to a subsequent course of therapy with extreme caution.

I.V.:

Children <35 kg: Renal transplantation: 10 mg within 2 hours prior to transplant surgery, followed by a second 10 mg dose 4 days after transplantation; the second dose should be withheld if complications occur (including severe hypersensitivity reactions or graft loss)

Children ≥35 kg and Adults: Renal transplantation: 20 mg within 2 hours prior to transplant surgery, followed by a second 20 mg dose 4 days after transplantation; the second dose should be withheld if complications occur (including severe hypersensitivity reactions or graft loss)

Dosing adjustment/comments in renal or hepatic impairment: No specific dosing adjustment recommended

Administration For intravenous administration only. Infuse as a bolus or I.V. infusion over 20-30 minutes. (Bolus dosing is associated with nausea, vomiting, and local pain at the injection site.)

Monitoring Parameters Signs and symptoms of acute rejection

Dosage Forms Excipient information presented when available (limited, particularly for generics); consult specific product labeling.

Injection, powder for reconstitution [preservative free]:

Simulect®: 10 mg, 20 mg

◆ **BAY 43-9006** see Sorafenib on page 1042

◆ **Baycadron™** see Dexamethasone on page 350

◆ **BCG, Live** see BCG Vaccine on page 128

BCG Vaccine (bee see jee vak SEEN)

Medication Safety Issues

High alert medication: The Institute for Safe Medication Practices (ISMP) includes this medication among its list of drugs which have a heightened risk of causing significant patient harm when used in error.

Related Information

Safe Handling of Hazardous Drugs on page 1517

U.S. Brand Names TheraCys®; TICE® BCG

Index Terms Bacillus Calmette-Guérin (BCG) Live; BCG Vaccine U.S.P. (percutaneous use product); BCG, Live

Generic Available No

Canadian Brand Names ImmuCyst®; Oncotice™; Pacis™

Pharmacologic Category Biological Response Modulator; Vaccine

Use Immunization against tuberculosis and immunotherapy for cancer; treatment and prophylaxis of carcinoma in situ of the bladder; prophylaxis of primary or recurrent superficial papillary tumors following transurethral resection

Pregnancy Risk Factor C

Lactation Excretion in breast milk unknown/not recommended

Labeled Contraindications Hypersensitivity to BCG vaccine or any component of the formulation; immunocompromised state, HIV-infected, and burn patients; active tuberculosis; intravesicular BCG is contraindicated in febrile illness, urinary tract infection, gross hematuria and recent (<7-14 days) biopsy, transurethral resection (TUR), or traumatic catheterization

Warnings/Precautions [U.S. Boxed Warnings]: Hazardous agent - use appropriate precautions for handling and disposal. BCG is a biohazardous agent; proper technique and disposal of all equipment in contact with BCG vaccine as a biohazardous material is recommended. BCG infections have been reported in healthcare workers due to accidental exposure (needlestick, skin laceration); nosocomial infections have been reported in patients receiving parenteral medications prepared in areas where BCG vaccine was prepared. To avoid cross contamination, do not

prepare parenteral medications in an area where BCG vaccine has been prepared. Systemic reactions have been reported in patients treated as immunotherapy for bladder cancer.

BCG should be administered with caution to persons in groups at high risk for HIV infection or persons known to be severely immunocompromised (including leukemia or lymphoma patients), patients undergoing chemotherapy, or patients on immunosuppressive therapy. Safety and efficacy of intravesicular BCG in children have not been established.

Although limited data suggest that the vaccine may be safe for use in asymptomatic children infected with HIV, BCG vaccination is not recommended for HIV-infected adults or for persons with a positive PPD reaction. Until further research can clearly define the risks and benefits of BCG vaccination for this population, vaccination should be restricted to persons at exceptionally high risk for tuberculosis infection. HIV-infected persons thought to be infected with *Mycobacterium tuberculosis* should be strongly recommended for tuberculosis preventive therapy.

Adverse Reactions All serious adverse reactions must be reported to the U.S. Department of Health and Human Services (DHHS) Vaccine Adverse Event Reporting System (VAERS) 1-800-822-7967.

Adverse reactions associated with **intravesicular administration**:

>10%:

Central nervous system: Malaise (7% to 40%), fever (20% to 38%), chills (34%)

Gastrointestinal: Nausea/vomiting (3% to 16%), anorexia/weight loss (2% to 11%)

Genitourinary: Dysuria (52% to 60%), bladder irritation (50% to 60%), polyuria (40% to 42%), hematuria (26% to 39%), cystitis (6% to 29%), urinary urgency (6% to 18%), urinary tract infection (2% to 18%)

Hematological: Anemia (<1% to 21%)

Miscellaneous: Flu-like syndrome (33%)

1% to 10%:

Central nervous system: Fatigue (7%), headache/dizziness (2%)

Dermatologic: Rash (2%)

Gastrointestinal: Diarrhea (6%), abdominal pain (2% to 3%)

Genitourinary: Genital pain (10%), bladder cramps/pain (6%), urinary incontinence (2% to 6%), bladder spasm (5%), nocturia (5%), urinary debris (2%), genital inflammation/abscess (2%)

Hematological: Leukopenia (5%), coagulopathy (3%)

Neuromuscular & skeletal: Arthralgia/myalgia (3% to 7%), cramps/pain (4% to 6%), rigors (3%)

Renal: Renal toxicity (10%)

Respiratory: Pulmonary infection (3%)

Miscellaneous: Infection (3%), allergy (2%)

<1%: Abscesses, conjunctivitis, constipation, disseminated sepsis, epididymitis, granulomatous chorioretinitis, hepatitis, hepatic granuloma, keratitis, *M. bovis* infection (lung, liver, bone, bone marrow, kidney, lymph nodes, prostate), orchitis, pneumonitis, prostatitis, skin ulceration, thrombocytopenia, urethritis, urinary obstruction, uveitis

Adverse reactions associated with **BCG vaccination**: Axillary lymphadenopathy, cervical lymphadenopathy, disseminated BCG infection (BCG osteomyelitis), local reactions (induration, itching, lesions, lymphadenitis, pustule, tenderness, ulceration). Local reactions may persist for up to 3 months; more severe manifestations may occur up to 5 months after vaccination and persist for several weeks.

Drug Interactions

Avoid Concomitant Use

Avoid concomitant use of BCG Vaccine with any of the following: Immunosuppressants

Increased Effect/Toxicity

The levels/effects of BCG Vaccine may be increased by: Immunosuppressants

Decreased Effect

BCG Vaccine may decrease the levels/effects of: Tuberculin Tests

The levels/effects of BCG Vaccine may be decreased by: Immune Globulins; Immunosuppressants

Storage/Stability Store vials under refrigeration at 2°C to 8°C (36°F to 46°F). Protect from light. Use within 2 hours of mixing.

Reconstitution

TheraCys®: Reconstitute with 3 mL of diluent provided and shake gently. Withdraw contents and add 50 mL of 0.9% NaCl (preservative free).

TICE® BCG: Reconstitute with 1 mL 0.9% NaCl (preservative free) using a 3 mL syringe. Mix by drawing and expelling solution into ampul three times. Add to a catheter tip syringe containing 49 mL of 0.9% NaCl (preservative free).

BCG Vaccine U.S.P.: Reconstitute with 1 mL of SWFI; swirl gently, do not vigorously shake. For children <1 month, reconstitute with 2 mL SWFI.

Mechanism of Action BCG live is an attenuated strain of bacillus Calmette-Guérin (*Mycobacterium bovis*) used as a biological response modifier. BCG live, when used intravesicularly for treatment of bladder carcinoma *in situ*, is thought to cause a local, chronic inflammatory response involving macrophage and leukocyte infiltration of the bladder. By a mechanism not fully understood, this local inflammatory response leads to destruction of superficial tumor cells of the urothelium. BCG is active immunotherapy which stimulates the host's immune mechanism to reject the tumor. Evidence of systemic immune response is also commonly seen, manifested by a positive PPD tuberculin skin test reaction, however, its relationship to clinical efficacy is not well-established.

Dosage

Immunization against tuberculosis: Percutaneous: **Note:** Initial lesion usually appears after 10-14 days consisting of small, red papule at injection site and reaches maximum diameter of 3 mm in 4-6 weeks.

Children <1 month: 0.2-0.3 mL (half-strength dilution). Administer tuberculin test (5 TU) after 2-3 months; repeat vaccination after 1 year of age for negative tuberculin test if indications persist.

Children >1 month and Adults: 0.2-0.3 mL (full strength dilution); conduct postvaccinal tuberculin test (5 TU of PPD) in 2-3 months; if test is negative, repeat vaccination.

Immunotherapy for bladder cancer: Intravesicular: Adults:

TheraCys®: One dose instilled into bladder (for 2 hours) once weekly for 6 weeks followed by one treatment at 3, 6, 12, 18, and 24 months after initial treatment

TICE® BCG: One dose instilled into the bladder (for 2 hours) once weekly for 6 weeks followed by once monthly for 6-12 months

Administration Should only be given intravesicularly (bladder irrigation) or percutaneously; **do not administer I.V., SubQ, or intradermally**.

Intravesicular: Empty or drain bladder. Instill BCG vaccine; retain for up to 2 hours. Patient should lie prone, rotating positions every 15 minutes to maximize bladder surface exposure.

Percutaneous: Apply vaccine with syringe and needle by dropping onto 1-2 inch area of horizontally positioned surface of cleansed, dry site (deltoid region of arm preferred); pulling skin tight, puncture skin with multiple puncture device centered over the vaccine; apply pressure for 5 seconds; spread vaccine evenly over puncture area. Apply loose covering and keep dry for 24 hours.

Test Interactions PPD intradermal test; BCG vaccination results in reactive tuberculin skin test; rule out active tuberculosis prior to initiating intravesicular BCG treatment

Additional Information When used for immunization against tuberculosis, Federal law requires that the date of administration, the vaccine manufacturer, lot number of vaccine, and the administering person's name, title, and address be entered into the patient's permanent medical record. Multiple puncture device for vaccination available from Organon Tenika (1-800-662-6842).

BCG vaccination is not recommended by the CDC for general use in the U.S. for prevention of tuberculosis (TB).

BCG vaccination is recommended for infants and children with negative tuberculin skin tests who:
- are at high risk of intimate and prolonged exposure to persistently untreated or ineffectively treated patients with infectious pulmonary tuberculosis
- cannot be removed from the source of exposure
- cannot be placed on long-term preventive therapy
- are continuously exposed with tuberculosis who have bacilli resistant to isoniazid and rifampin

BCG vaccination is recommended for healthcare workers (HCW) in high-risk settings where:
- a high percentage of TB patients are infected with *M. tuberculosis* strains resistant to both isoniazid and rifampin
- transmission of drug-resistant *M. tuberculosis* strains and subsequent infection are likely
- comprehensive TB infection control precautions have been implemented yet have not been successful

BCG vaccination in not recommended for HCWs in low-risk settings.

Dosage Forms Excipient information presented when available (limited, particularly for generics); consult specific product labeling.

Injection, powder for reconstitution, intravesical [preservative free]:
TheraCys®: 81 mg [contains natural rubber/natural latex in packaging, polysorbate 80 (in diluent)]
TICE® BCG: 50 mg

Injection, powder for reconstitution, percutaneous [preservative free]:
BCG Vaccine: 50 mg

References

Alexandroff AB, Jackson AM, O'Donnell MA, et al, "BCG Immunotherapy of Bladder Cancer: 20 Years On," *Lancet*, 1999, 353(9165):1689-94.

Badalament RA and Farah RN, "Treatment of Superficial Bladder Cancer With Intravesicle Chemotherapy," *Semin Surg Oncol*, 1997, 13(5):335-41.

Bassi P, "BCG (Bacillus of Calmette Guerin) Therapy of High-Risk Superficial Bladder Cancer," *Surg Oncol*, 2002, 11(1-2):77-83.

Centers for Disease Control, "Recommendations of the Advisory Committee on Immunization Practices (ACIP): General Recommendations on Immunization," *MMWR Recomm Rep*, 2002, 51 (RR-2):1-36.

Centers for Disease Control and Prevention,"TB Elimination: BCG Vaccine," Document 250120, January, 2005; available at http://www.cdc.gov/nchstp/tb/pubs/tbfactsheets/250120.pdf

Meyer JP, Persad R, and Gillatt DA, "Use of Bacille Calmette-Guerin in Superficial Bladder Cancer," *Postgrad Med J*, 2002, 78(922):449-54.

Rischmann P, Desgrandchamps F, Malavaud B, et al, "BCG Intravesical Instillations: Recommendations for Side-Effects Management," *Eur Urol*, 2000, 37(Suppl 1):33-6.

◆ **BCG Vaccine U.S.P.** *(percutaneous use product)* see BCG Vaccine on page 128

◆ **BCNU** see Carmustine on page 183

◆ **Bebulin® VH** see Factor IX Complex (Human) on page 452

Bendamustine (ben da MUS teen)

Medication Safety Issues

Sound-alike/look-alike issues:

Bendamustine may be confused with carmustine, lomustine

High alert medication: The Institute for Safe Medication Practices (ISMP) includes this medication among its list of drug classes which have a heightened risk of causing significant patient harm when used in error.

Related Information

Safe Handling of Hazardous Drugs on page 1517

U.S. Brand Names Treanda®

Index Terms Bendamustine Hydrochloride; Cytostasan; SDX-105

Generic Available No

Pharmacologic Category Antineoplastic Agent; Antineoplastic Agent, Alkylating Agent; Antineoplastic Agent, Alkylating Agent (Nitrogen Mustard)

Use Treatment of chronic lymphocytic leukemia (CLL); treatment of progressed indolent B-cell non-Hodgkin's lymphoma (NHL)

Unlabeled/Investigational Use Treatment of mantle cell lymphoma; salvage therapy for relapsed multiple myeloma

Pregnancy Risk Factor D

Lactation Excretion in breast milk unknown/not recommended

Labeled Contraindications Hypersensitivity to bendamustine, mannitol, or any component of the formulation

Warnings/Precautions Hazardous agent - use appropriate precautions for handling and disposal. Myelosuppression (neutropenia, thrombocytopenia, and anemia) is a common toxicity; may require therapy delay and/or dose reduction; monitor. Complications due to febrile neutropenia and severe thrombocytopenia have been reported. ANC should recover to ≥1000/mm^3 and platelets to ≥75,000/mm^3 prior to therapy/cycle initiation. Infections, including pneumonia and sepsis have been reported with use; may require hospitalization; septic shock and fatalities have occurred. Patients with myelosuppression are more susceptible to infection; monitor closely.

Infusion reactions, including chills, fever, pruritus, and rash are common; rarely, anaphylactic and anaphylactoid reactions have occurred, particularly with the second or subsequent cycle(s). In general, patients who experienced grade 3 or 4 allergic reactions were not rechallenged in CLL clinical trials. Consider premedication with antihistamines, antipyretics and/or corticosteroids for patients with a history of grade 1 or 2 infusion reaction. Discontinue for severe allergic reaction; consider discontinuation with grade 3 or 4 infusion reaction. Rash, toxic skin reactions and bullous exanthema have been reported with monotherapy and in combination with other antineoplastics; may be progressive or worsen with continued treatment; discontinue bendamustine treatment for severe or progressive skin reaction; monitor closely; discontinue bendamustine treatment for severe or progressive skin reaction. The risk for severe skin toxicity is increased with concurrent use of allopurinol and other medications known to cause skin toxicity; Stevens-Johnson syndrome and toxic epidermal necrolysis (TEN) have been reported. TEN has also been reported when used in combination with rituximab.

Tumor lysis syndrome may occur as a consequence of leukemia treatment, including treatment with bendamustine, usually occurring in the first treatment cycle. May lead to life threatening acute renal failure; adequate hydration and prophylactic allopurinol should be instituted prior to treatment in high risk patients; monitor closely.

Use is not recommended in patients with moderate (AST or ALT 2.5-10 times ULN and total bilirubin 1.5-3 times ULN) or severe (total bilirubin >3 times ULN) hepatic impairment; use with caution in patients with mild hepatic impairment. Use is not recommended in patient with Cl_{cr} <40 mL/minute; use with caution in patients with mild-to-moderate renal impairment. Malignancies (including myelodysplastic syndrome, myeloproliferative disorders, acute myeloid leukemia and bronchial cancer) and premalignant diseases have been reported in patients who have received bendamustine. Safety and efficacy have not been established in children.

Adverse Reactions

>10%:

Cardiovascular: Peripheral edema (≤13%)

Central nervous system: Fatigue (9% to 57%), fever (24% to 34%), headache (≤21%), chills (6% to 14%), dizziness (≤14%), insomnia (≤13%)

Dermatologic: Rash (8% to 16%; grades 3/4: ≤3%)

Endocrine & metabolic: Dehydration (≤14%)

Gastrointestinal: Nausea (20% to 75%), vomiting (16% to 40%), diarrhea (9% to 37%), constipation (≤29%), anorexia (≤23%), weight loss (7% to 18%), stomatitis (≤15%), abdominal pain (5% to 13%), appetite loss (≤13%), dyspepsia (≤11%)

Hematologic: Myelosuppression (nadir: in week 3), lymphopenia (68% to 99%; grades 3/4: 47% to 94%), leukopenia (61% to 94%; grades 3/4: 28% to 56%), anemia (88% to 89%; grades 3/4: 11% to 13%), thrombocytopenia (77% to 86%; grades 3/4: 11% to 25%), neutropenia (75% to 86%; grades 3/4: 43% to 60%)

Hepatic: Bilirubin increased (≤34%; grades 3/4: 3%)

Neuromuscular & skeletal: Back pain (≤14%), weakness (8% to 11%)

Respiratory: Cough (4% to 22%), dyspnea (≤16%)

1% to 10%:

Cardiovascular: Tachycardia (≤7%), hypotension (≤6%), chest pain (≤6%), hypertension aggravated (≤3%)

Central nervous system: Anxiety (≤8%), depression (≤6%), pain (≤6%)

Dermatologic: Pruritus (5% to 6%), dry skin (≤5%)

Endocrine & metabolic: Hypokalemia (≤9%), hyperuricemia (≤7%; grades 3/4: 2%), hyperglycemia (grades 3/4: ≤3%), hypocalcemia (grades 3/4: ≤2%), hyponatremia (grades 3/4: ≤2%)

Gastrointestinal: Gastroesophageal reflux disease (≤10%), xerostomia (9%), taste alteration (≤7%), oral candidiasis (≤6%), abdominal distention (≤5%)

Genitourinary: Urinary tract infection (≤10%)

Hematologic: Febrile neutropenia (3% to 6%)

Hepatic: ALT increased (grades 3/4: ≤3%), AST increased (grades 3/4: ≤1%)

Local: Infusion site pain (≤6%), catheter site pain (≤5%)

Neuromuscular & skeletal: Arthralgia (≤6%), bone pain (≤5%), limb pain (≤5%)

Renal: Creatinine increased (grades 3/4: ≤2%)

Respiratory: Upper respiratory infection (10%), sinusitis (≤9%), pharyngolaryngeal pain (≤8%), pneumonia (≤8%), nasopharyngitis (6% to 7%), wheezing (≤5%), nasal congestion (≤5%)

Miscellaneous: Herpes infection (3% to 10%), infection (≤6%; grades 3/4: 2%), hypersensitivity (≤5%; grades 3/4: 1%), diaphoresis (≤5%), night sweats (≤5%)

<1%, postmarketing, and/or case reports: Acute myeloid leukemia, acute renal failure, alopecia, anaphylaxis, bronchial carcinoma, bullous exanthema, cardiac failure, dermatitis, erythema, hemolysis, infusion reaction, injection/infusion site reaction (irritation, pruritus, swelling), malaise, mucosal inflammation, myelodysplastic syndrome, myeloproliferative disorders, pulmonary fibrosis, sepsis, septic shock, skin necrosis, somnolence, Stevens-Johnson syndrome, toxic epidermal necrolysis, toxic skin reactions, tumor lysis syndrome

Drug Interactions

Metabolism/Transport Effects Substrate of CYP1A2; P-glycoprotein (ABCB1); BCRP (ABCG2)

Avoid Concomitant Use There are no known interactions where it is recommended to avoid concomitant use.

Increased Effect/Toxicity
The levels/effects of Bendamustine may be increased by: CYP1A2 Inhibitors (Strong)

Decreased Effect
The levels/effects of Bendamustine may be decreased by: CYP1A2 Inducers (Strong)

Storage/Stability Prior to reconstitution, store intact vials at 25°C (77°F); excursions permitted up to 30°C (86°F). Protect from light. The solution in the vial (reconstituted with SWFI) is stable for 30 minutes (transfer to 500 mL infusion bag within that 30 minutes). The solution diluted in 500 mL for infusion is stable for 24 hours refrigerated or 3 hours at room temperature and room light. Infusion must be completed within these time frames.

Reconstitution Use appropriate precautions for handling and disposal. Reconstitute 100 mg vial with 20 mL of sterile water for injection to a concentration of 5 mg/mL; powder usually dissolves within 5 minutes. Prior to administration, dilute appropriate dose in 500 mL NS (or $D_{2.5}^{1/2}NS$) to a final concentration of 0.2-0.6 mg/mL; mix thoroughly.

Compatibility Stable in NS, $D_{2.5}^{1/2}NS$

Mechanism of Action Bendamustine is an alkylating agent (nitrogen mustard derivative) with a benzimidazole ring (purine analog) which demonstrates only partial cross-resistance (in vitro) with other alkylating agents. It leads to cell death via single and double strand DNA cross-linking. Bendamustine is active against quiescent and dividing cells. The primary cytotoxic activity is due to bendamustine (as compared to metabolites).

Pharmacodynamics/Kinetics

Distribution: V_{ss}: ~25 L

Protein binding: 94% to 96%

Metabolism: Hepatic, via CYP1A2 to active (minor) metabolites gamma-hydroxy bendamustine (M3) and N-desmethyl-bendamustine (M4)

Half-life elimination: Bendamustine: ~40 minutes; M3: ~3 hours; M4: ~30 minutes

Time to peak, serum: At end of infusion

Excretion: Feces (~90%); urine (1% to 10%)

Dosage I.V.: Adults:

CLL: 100 mg/m^2 on days 1 and 2 of a 28-day treatment cycle (for up to 6 cycles)

NHL: 120 mg/m^2 on days 1 and 2 of a 21-day treatment cycle for up to 8 cycles

Mantle cell lymphoma (unlabeled use): 90 mg/m^2 days 2 and 3 of a 28-day treatment cycle for up to 4 cycles (Rummel, 2005)

Multiple myeloma (unlabeled use): 90-100 mg/m^2 on days 1 and 2 of a 28-day treatment cycle for at least 2 cycles (Knop, 2005)

Dosage adjustment for toxicity:

Infusion reactions:

Grade 1 or 2: Consider premedication with antihistamines, antipyretics, and corticosteroids in subsequent cycles

Grade 3 or 4: Consider discontinuing treatment

Treatment delay:

Hematologic toxicity ≥grade 4: Delay treatment until resolves (ANC ≥1000/mm^3, platelets ≥75,000/mm^3)

Nonhematologic toxicity ≥grade 2 (clinically significant): Delay treatment until resolves to ≤grade 1

Dose modification in CLL:

Hematologic toxicity ≥grade 3: Reduce dose to 50 mg/m^2 on days 1 and 2 of each treatment cycle. For recurrent hematologic toxicity (≥grade 3), further reduce dose to 25 mg/m^2 on days 1 and 2 of the treatment cycle. May cautiously re-escalate dose in subsequent cycles.

Nonhematologic toxicity ≥grade 3 (clinically significant): Reduce dose to 50 mg/m^2 on days 1 and 2 of the treatment cycle with discretion. May cautiously re-escalate dose in subsequent cycles.

Dose modification in NHL:

Hematologic toxicity grade 4: Reduce dose to 90 mg/m^2 on days 1 and 2 of each treatment cycle. For recurrent hematologic toxicity (grade 4), further reduce dose to 60 mg/m^2 on days 1 and 2 of each treatment cycle.

Nonhematologic toxicity ≥grade 3: Reduce dose to 90 mg/m^2 on days 1 and 2 of the treatment cycle with discretion. For recurrent toxicity ≥grade 3, further reduce dose to 60 mg/m^2 on days 1 and 2 of each treatment cycle.

Dosage adjustment in renal impairment:

Mild-to-moderate renal impairment: Use with caution

Cl$_{cr}$ <40 mL/minute: Use is not recommended

Dosage adjustment in hepatic impairment:

Mild hepatic impairment: Use with caution

Moderate hepatic impairment (AST or ALT 2.5-10 times ULN and total bilirubin 1.5-3 times ULN): Use is not recommended

Severe hepatic impairment (total bilirubin >3 times ULN): Use is not recommended

Combination Regimens

Lymphoma, non-Hodgkin's: Bendamustine-Rituximab on page 1229

Lymphoma, non-Hodgkin's: (Mantle Cell): Bendamustine-Rituximab on page 1229

Administration Infuse over 30 minutes for the treatment of CLL and over 60 minutes for NHL. Prophylactic treatment with allopurinol may be needed in patients at risk for tumor lysis syndrome. Consider premedication with antihistamines, antipyretics, and/or corticosteroids for patients with a previous grade 1 or 2 infusion reaction to bendamustine.

Monitoring Parameters CBC with differential (monitored weekly [initially] in clinical trials); serum creatinine (pretreatment); ALT, AST, and total bilirubin (pretreatment); monitor potassium and uric acid levels in patients at risk for tumor lysis syndrome; monitor for infusion reactions anaphylaxis, infection and dermatologic toxicity

Emetic Potential Moderate (30% to 90%)

Dosage Forms Excipient information presented when available (limited, particularly for generics); consult specific product labeling.

Injection, powder for reconstitution:

Treanda®: 100 mg [contains mannitol 170 mg]

References

Aivado M, Schulte K, Henze L, et al, "Bendamustine in the Treatment of Chronic Lymphocytic Leukemia: Results and Future Perspectives," *Semin Oncol*, 2002, 29(4 Suppl 13):19-22.

Friedberg JW, Cohen P, Chen L, et al, "Bendamustine in Patients With Rituximab-Refractory Indolent and Transformed Non-Hodgkin's Lymphoma: Results From a Phase II Multicenter, Single-Agent Study," *J Clin Oncol*, 2008, 26(2):204-10.

Kahl B, Bartlett NL, Leonard JP, et al, "Bendamustine Is Safe and Effective in Patients with Rituximab-Refractory, Indolent B-Cell Non-Hodgkin Lymphoma," *Blood*, 2007, 110(11) [ASH Abstract 1351].

Knauf WU, Lissichkov T, Aldaoud A, et al, "Bendamustine Versus Chlorambucil in Treatment - Naïve Patients With B-Cell Chronic Lymphocytic Leukemia (B-CLL): Results of an International Phase III Study," *Blood*, 2007, 110(11) [ASH Abstract 2043].

Knop S, Straka C, Haen M, et al, "The Efficacy and Toxicity of Bendamustine in Recurrent Multiple Myeloma After High-Dose Chemotherapy," *Haematologica*, 2005, 90(9):1287-8.

National Comprehensive Cancer Network (NCCN), "Clinical Practice Guidelines in Oncology™: Multiple Myeloma," Version 2.2009. Available at http://www.nccn.org/professionals/physician_gls/PDF/myeloma.pdf.

National Comprehensive Cancer Network® (NCCN), "Clinical Practice Guidelines in Oncology™: Non-Hodgkin's Lymphomas," Version 2.2009. Available at http://www.nccn.org/professionals/physician_gls/PDF/nhl.pdf

Ponisch W and Niederwieser D, "Bendamustine in the Treatment of Multiple Myeloma: Results and Future Perspectives," *Semin Oncol*, 2002, 29(4 Suppl 13):23-6.

Robinson KS, Williams ME, van der Jagt RH, et al, "Phase II Multicenter Study of Bendamustine Plus Rituximab in Patients With Relapsed Indolent B-Cell and Mantle Cell Non-Hodgkin's Lymphoma," *J Clin Oncol*, 2008, 26(27):4473-9.

Rummel MJ, Al-Batran SE, Kim SZ, et al, "Bendamustine Plus Rituximab is Effective and has a Favorable Toxicity Profile in the Treatment of Mantle Cell and Low-Grade Non-Hodgkin's Lymphoma," *J Clin Oncol*, 2005, 23(15):3383-9.

◆ **Bendamustine Hydrochloride** see Bendamustine on page 132

◆ **BeneFix®** see Factor IX on page 449

◆ **Benzmethyzin** see Procarbazine on page 989

Benzydamine (ben ZID a meen)

Index Terms Benzydamine Hydrochloride

Generic Available Yes

Canadian Brand Names Apo-Benzydamine®; Dom-Benzydamine; Novo-Benzydamine; PMS-Benzydamine; ratio-Benzydamine; Sun-Benz®; Tantum®

Pharmacologic Category Local Anesthetic, Oral

Use Symptomatic treatment of pain associated with acute pharyngitis; treatment of pain associated with radiation-induced oropharyngeal mucositis

Restrictions Not available in U.S.

Lactation Excretion in breast milk unknown/use caution

Labeled Contraindications Hypersensitivity to benzydamine or any component of the formulation

Warnings/Precautions May cause local irritation and/or burning sensation in patients with altered mucosal integrity. Dilution (1:1 in warm water) may attenuate this effect. Use caution in renal impairment. Safety and efficacy have not been established in children ≤5 years of age.

Adverse Reactions
Central nervous system: Drowsiness, headache
Gastrointestinal: Nausea and/or vomiting (2%), dry mouth
Local: Numbness (10%), burning/stinging sensation (8%)
Respiratory: Pharyngeal irritation, cough

Drug Interactions
Metabolism/Transport Effects Substrate (minor) of CYP1A2, 2C19, 2D6, 3A4

Avoid Concomitant Use There are no known interactions where it is recommended to avoid concomitant use.

Increased Effect/Toxicity There are no known significant interactions involving an increase in effect.

Decreased Effect There are no known significant interactions involving a decrease in effect.

Storage/Stability Store at 15°C to 30°C; protect from freezing.

Mechanism of Action Local anesthetic and anti-inflammatory, reduces local pain and inflammation. Does not interfere with arachidonic acid metabolism.

Pharmacodynamics/Kinetics
Absorption: Oral rinse may be absorbed, at least in part, through the oral mucosa
Excretion: Urine (primarily as unchanged drug)

Dosage Oral rinse: Adults:
Acute pharyngitis: Gargle with 15 mL of undiluted solution every 1½-3 hours until symptoms resolve. Patient should expel solution from mouth following use; solution should not be swallowed.
Mucositis: 15 mL of undiluted solution as a gargle or rinse 3-4 times/day; contact should be maintained for at least 30 seconds, followed by expulsion from the mouth. Clinical studies maintained contact for ~2 minutes, up to 8 times/day. Patient should not swallow the liquid. Begin treatment 1 day prior to initiation of radiation therapy and continue daily during treatment. Continue oral rinse treatments after the completion of radiation therapy until desired result/healing is achieved.

Dosage adjustment in renal impairment: No adjustment required.

Dosage Forms Excipient information presented when available (limited, particularly for generics); consult specific product labeling.
Oral rinse: 0.15% (100 mL, 250 mL) [not available in the U.S.]

References
Epstein JB, Silverman S Jr, Paggiarino DA, et al, "Benzydamine HCl for Prophylaxis of Radiation-Induced Oral Mucositis: Results From a Multicenter, Randomized, Double-Blind, Placebo-Controlled Clinical Trial," Cancer, 2001, 92(4):875-85.
Ribldi E, Frascaroli G, Transidico P, "Benzydamine Inhibits Monocyte Migration and MAPK Activation Induced by Chemotactic Agonists," Br J Pharmacol, 2003, 140(2):377-83.

♦ **Benzydamine Hydrochloride** see Benzydamine on page 136

♦ **Beta-HC®** see Hydrocortisone on page 575

Bevacizumab (be vuh SIZ uh mab)
Medication Safety Issues
Sound-alike/look-alike issues:
Bevacizumab may be confused with cetuximab, riTUXimab

High alert medication: The Institute for Safe Medication Practices (ISMP) includes this medication among its list of drug classes which have a heightened risk of causing significant patient harm when used in error.

U.S. Brand Names Avastin®

◀ **Index Terms** Anti-VEGF Monoclonal Antibody; Anti-VEGF rhuMAb; rhuMAb-VEGF

Generic Available No

Canadian Brand Names Avastin®

Pharmacologic Category Antineoplastic Agent, Monoclonal Antibody; Vascular Endothelial Growth Factor (VEGF) Inhibitor

Use Treatment of metastatic colorectal cancer; treatment of advanced nonsquamous, nonsmall cell lung cancer; treatment of metastatic HER-2 negative breast cancer (who have not received chemotherapy for metastatic disease); treatment of progressive glioblastoma (not an approved use in Canada); treatment of metastatic renal cell cancer (not an approved use in Canada)

Unlabeled/Investigational Use Treatment of recurrent ovarian cancer, age-related macular degeneration (AMD)

Pregnancy Risk Factor C

Lactation Excretion in breast milk unknown/not recommended

Labeled Contraindications There are no contraindications listed in the FDA-approved manufacturer's labeling.

Canadian labeling: Hypersensitivity to bevacizumab, any component of the formulation, Chinese hamster ovary cell products or other recombinant human or humanized antibodies; untreated CNS metastases

Warnings/Precautions [U.S. Boxed Warning]: Gastrointestinal perforation, fistula (including gastrointestinal, enterocutaneous, esophageal, duodenal, and rectal fistulas), intra-abdominal abscess, and wound dehiscence/wound healing complications have been reported in patients receiving bevacizumab for colorectal cancer and other cancers (not related to treatment duration). Most cases occur within 50 days of treatment initiation; may be fatal in some cases; monitor patients for signs/symptoms (eg, fever, abdominal pain with constipation and/or nausea/vomiting). Permanently discontinue in patients who develop these complications. Nongastrointestinal fistula formation (including tracheoesophageal, bronchopleural, biliary, vaginal, renal, and bladder fistulas) has been observed, most commonly within the first 6 months of treatment; permanently discontinue in patients who develop internal organ fistulas. The appropriate intervals between administration of bevacizumab and surgical procedures to avoid impairment in wound healing has not been established. Therapy should not be initiated within 28 days of major surgery and only following complete healing of the incision. Bevacizumab should be discontinued at least 28 days prior to elective surgery.

Use with caution in patients with cardiovascular disease; patients with significant recent cardiovascular disease were excluded from clinical trials. Bevacizumab is associated with an increased risk for arterial thromboembolic events (ATE), including cerebral infarction, stroke, MI, TIA, angina, and other ATEs, when used in combination with chemotherapy. History of ATE or ≥65 years of age may present an even greater risk; permanently discontinue with serious ATE; the safety of treatment reinitiation after ATE has not been studied. Although patients with cancer are at risk for venous thromboembolism (VTE), a meta-analysis of 15 controlled trials has demonstrated an increased risk for VTE in patients who received bevacizumab (Nalluri, 2008).

The incidence of heart failure (HF) and/or left ventricular dysfunction, is higher in patients receiving bevacizumab plus chemotherapy when compared to chemotherapy alone. May potentiate the cardiotoxic effects of anthracyclines. HF is more common with prior anthracycline exposure and/or left chest wall irradiation. The safety of therapy resumption or continuation in patients with cardiac dysfunction has not been studied. Bevacizumab may cause and/or worsen hypertension significantly; use caution in patients with pre-existing hypertension and monitor BP closely in all patients. Permanent discontinuation is recommended in patients who experience a hypertensive crisis or encephalopathy. Temporarily discontinue in patients who develop uncontrolled hypertension. Cases of reversible posterior leukoencephalopathy syndrome (RPLS) have been reported. Symptoms (which include headache, seizure, confusion, lethargy, blindness and/or other vision, or neurologic disturbances) may occur from 16 hours to 1 year after treatment initiation. Resolution of symptoms usually occurs within days after discontinuation; however, neurologic sequelae may remain. RPLS may be associated with hypertension; discontinue bevacizumab and begin management of hypertension, if present.

[U.S. Boxed Warning]: Severe or fatal hemorrhage, including hemoptysis, gastrointestinal bleeding, central nervous system hemorrhage, epistaxis, and vaginal bleeding have been observed. Avoid use in patients with serious hemorrhage or recent hemoptysis (≥2.5 mL blood). Serious pulmonary hemorrhage has been reported in patients receiving bevacizumab (primarily in patients with nonsmall cell lung cancer with squamous cell histology [not an FDA-approved indication]). Intracranial hemorrhage, including cases of grade 3 or 4 hemorrhage, has occurred in patients with previously treated glioblastoma. Treatment discontinuation is recommended in all patients with intracranial or other serious hemorrhage. Use with caution in patients with CNS metastases; once case of CNS hemorrhage was observed in an ongoing study of NSCLC patients with CNS metastases. Use in patients with CNS metastases is contraindicated in the Canadian labeling. Use with caution in patients at risk for thrombocytopenia.

Infusion reactions (eg, hypertension, hypertensive crisis, wheezing, oxygen desaturation, hypersensitivity, chest pain, rigors, headache, diaphoresis) may occur with the first infusion (uncommon); interrupt therapy in patients experiencing severe infusion reactions; there are no data to address reinstitution of therapy in patients who experience severe infusion reactions. Proteinuria and/or nephrotic syndrome have been associated with bevacizumab; risk may be increased in patients with a history of hypertension; thrombotic microangiopathy has been associated with bevacizumab-induced proteinuria. Withhold treatment for ≥2 g proteinuria/24 hours and resume when proteinuria is <2 g/24 hours; discontinue in patients with nephrotic syndrome. Elderly patients (≥65 years of age) are at higher risk for adverse events, including thromboembolic events and proteinuria; serious adverse events occurring more frequently in the elderly also include deep thrombophlebitis, sepsis, hyper-/hypotension, MI, CHF, leukopenia, anemia, dehydration, hypokalemia, and hyponatremia. Microangiopathic hemolytic anemia (MAHA) has been reported when bevacizumab has been used in combination with sunitinib. Concurrent therapy with sunitinib and bevacizumab is also associated with dose-limiting hypertension in patients with metastatic renal cell cancer. The incidence of hand-foot syndrome is increased in patients treated with bevacizumab plus sorafenib in comparison to those treated with sorafenib monotherapy. When used in combination with myelosuppressive chemotherapy, increased rates of severe or febrile neutropenia and neutropenic infection were reported. Safety and efficacy in children have not been established.

Adverse Reactions Percentages reported as monotherapy and as part of combination chemotherapy regimens. Some studies only reported hematologic toxicities grades ≥4 and nonhematologic toxicities grades ≥3.

>10%:
Cardiovascular: Hypertension (23% to 67%; grades 3/4: 5% to 18%), thromboembolic event (≤21%; grades 3/4: 15%; venous thrombus/embolus: 8%; grades 3/4: 5% to 7%), arterial thrombosis 6%; grades 3/4: 3%), hypotension (7% to 15%)
Central nervous system: Pain (31% to 62%), headache (24% to 37%; grades 3/4: 2% to 4%), dizziness (19% to 26%), fatigue (≤45%; grades 3/4: 4% to 19%), sensory neuropathy (grades 3/4: 1% to 17%; in combination with paclitaxel: 24%)
Dermatologic: Alopecia (6% to 32%), dry skin (7% to 20%), exfoliative dermatitis (3% to 19%), skin discoloration (2% to 16%)
Endocrine & metabolic: Hypokalemia (12% to 16%)
Gastrointestinal: Abdominal pain (50% to 61%; grades 3/4: 8%), vomiting (47% to 52%; grades 3/4: 6% to 11%), anorexia (35% to 43%), constipation (29% to 40%), diarrhea (grades 3/4: 1% to 34%), stomatitis (25% to 32%), gastrointestinal hemorrhage (19% to 24%), dyspepsia (17% to 24%), taste disorder (14% to 21%), flatulence (11% to 19%), weight loss (9% to 20%), nausea (grades 3/4: 4% to 12%)
Hematologic: Hemorrhage (≤40%; grades 3/4: 1% to 5%), leukopenia (grades 3/4: 37%), neutropenia (grade 4: 6% to 27%)
Neuromuscular & skeletal: Weakness (57% to 74%), myalgia (8% to 19%), back pain (≤12%)
Ocular: Tearing increased (6% to 18%)
Renal: Proteinuria (4% to 36%; grades 3/4: ≤7%; median onset: 5.6 months; median time to resolution: 6.1 months)
Respiratory: Upper respiratory infection (40% to 47%), epistaxis (16% to 35%), dyspnea (25% to 26%), rhinitis
Miscellaneous: Infection (≤55%; serious: 9% to 14%; pneumonia, catheter, or wound infections)
1% to 10%:
Cardiovascular: DVT (6% to 9%; grades 3/4: 9%), syncope (grades 3/4: 3%), intra-abdominal venous thrombosis (grades 3/4: 3%), cardio-/cerebrovascular arterial thrombotic event (2% to 4%), CHF (with prior anthracycline therapy: 4%; grades 3/4: 2%), left ventricular dysfunction (grades 3/4: 1%)
Central nervous system: Confusion (1% to 6%), abnormal gait (1% to 5%); CNS hemorrhage (1% to 5%; grades 3/4: 1%), reversible posterior leukoencephalopathy syndrome ([RPLS] ≤1%)
Dermatologic: Nail disorder (2% to 8%), skin ulcer (≤6%), rash desquamation (grades 3/4: 3%), wound dehiscence (1% to 6%), acne (≤1%)
Endocrine & metabolic: Dehydration (grades 3/4: 3% to 10%), hyponatremia (grades 3/4: 4%)
Gastrointestinal: Xerostomia (4% to 7%), colitis (1% to 6%), ileus (grades 3/4: 4% to 5%), gingival bleeding (2% to 4%), fistula (1%), gastrointestinal perforation (≤4%), gastroesophageal reflux (≤2%), gingivitis (≤2%), mouth ulceration (≤2%), tooth abscess (≤2%), intra-abdominal abscess (1%), gastritis (≤1%), gingival pain (≤1%)
Genitourinary: Polyuria/urgency (3% to 6%), vaginal hemorrhage (4%)
Hematologic: Neutropenic fever/infection (5%; grades 3 and/or 4: 4% to 5%), thrombocytopenia (5%)
Hepatic: Bilirubinemia (1% to 6%)

Neuromuscular & skeletal: Bone pain (grades 3/4: 4%), neuropathy (other than sensory: grades 3/4: 1% to 5%)

Ocular: Blurred vision (≤2%)

Otic: Tinnitus (≤2%), deafness (≤1%)

Respiratory: Voice alteration (5% to 9%), pneumonitis/pulmonary infiltrates (grades 3/4: 5%), hemoptysis (nonsquamous histology 2%), pulmonary embolism (≤1%)

Miscellaneous: Infusion reactions (<3%)

<1%, postmarketing, and/or case reports (limited to important or life-threatening): Anaphylaxis, anastomotic ulceration, angina, cerebral infarction; fistula (biliary, bladder, bronchopleural, duodenal, endophthalmitis, enterocutaneous, esophageal, eye inflammation, gastrointestinal, rectal, renal, tracheoesophageal [TE] and vaginal); hemorrhagic stroke, hypersensitivity, hypertensive crises, hypertensive encephalopathy, intestinal necrosis, intestinal obstruction, mesenteric venous occlusion, microangiopathic hemolytic anemia (when used in combination with sunitinib), MI, nasal septum perforation, nephrotic syndrome, pancytopenia, polyserositis, pulmonary hemorrhage, pulmonary hypertension, renal failure, renal thrombotic microangiopathy, sepsis, subarachnoid hemorrhage, toxic anterior segment syndrome (TASS), transient ischemic attack, ureteral stricture wound healing complications

Drug Interactions

Avoid Concomitant Use

Avoid concomitant use of Bevacizumab with any of the following: Sunitinib

Increased Effect/Toxicity

Bevacizumab may increase the levels/effects of: Antineoplastic Agents (Anthracycline); Irinotecan; Sorafenib; Sunitinib

The levels/effects of Bevacizumab may be increased by: Sunitinib

Decreased Effect There are no known significant interactions involving a decrease in effect.

Storage/Stability Store vials at 2°C to 8°C (36°F to 46°F); do not freeze. Protect from light; do not shake. Diluted solutions are stable for up to 8 hours under refrigeration.

Reconstitution Prior to infusion, dilute prescribed dose of bevacizumab in 100 mL NS. Do not mix with dextrose-containing solutions.

Mechanism of Action Bevacizumab is a recombinant, humanized monoclonal antibody which binds to, and neutralizes, vascular endothelial growth factor (VEGF), preventing its association with endothelial receptors, Flt-1 and KDR. VEGF binding initiates angiogenesis (endothelial proliferation and the formation of new blood vessels). The inhibition of microvascular growth is believed to retard the growth of all tissues (including metastatic tissue).

Pharmacodynamics/Kinetics

Distribution: V_d: 46 mL/kg

Half-life elimination: ~20 days (range: 11-50 days)

Excretion: Clearance: 2.75-5 mL/kg/day

Dosage Adults: Details concerning dosing in combination regimens should also be consulted.

I.V.:

Breast cancer: 10 mg/kg every 2 weeks (in combination with paclitaxel)

Colorectal cancer: 5 or 10 mg/kg every 2 weeks (in combination with fluorouracil-based chemotherapy)

Canadian labeling: 5 mg/kg every 2 weeks (in combination with fluorouracil-based chemotherapy)

Glioblastoma: 10 mg/kg every 2 weeks as monotherapy **or** in combination (unlabeled) with irinotecan (Vredenburgh, 2007)

Lung cancer, nonsquamous cell nonsmall cell: 15 mg/kg every 3 weeks (in combination with carboplatin and paclitaxel)

Renal cell cancer: 10 mg/kg every 2 weeks in combination with interferon alfa or as monotherapy (unlabeled; Yang, 2003)

Ovarian cancer (unlabeled use): 15 mg/kg every 3 weeks (Burger, 2007; Cannistra, 2007)

Intravitreal: AMD (unlabeled use): 1.25 mg (0.05 mL) monthly until improvement/resolution, usually ~1-3 injections (Avery, 2006) or 2.5 mg (0.1 mL) every 4 weeks for 3 doses (Bashshur, 2006)

Dosage adjustment for toxicity: I.V. administration (systemic): Temporary suspension is recommended for severe infusion reactions, at least 4 weeks prior to elective surgery, in moderate-to-severe proteinuria (in most studies, treatment was withheld for ≥2 g proteinuria/24 hours), or in patients with severe hypertension which is not controlled with medical management. Permanent discontinuation is recommended (by the manufacturer) in patients who develop wound dehiscence requiring intervention, fistula (gastrointestinal and nongastrointestinal), gastrointestinal perforation, intra-abdominal abscess, hypertensive crisis, hypertensive encephalopathy, serious bleeding/hemorrhage, severe arterial thromboembolic event, nephrotic syndrome, or RPLS.

Combination Regimens

Brain tumors: Bevacizumab-Irinotecan (Glioblastoma) on page 1233
Breast cancer:
  Bevacizumab-Capecitabine on page 1231
  Docetaxel-Bevacizumab on page 1289
  Paclitaxel-Bevacizumab on page 1385
Colorectal cancer:
  Bevacizumab-Fluorouracil-Leucovorin on page 1232
  Bevacizumab-Irinotecan-Fluorouracil-Leucovorin on page 1233
  Bevacizumab-Oxaliplatin-Fluorouracil-Leucovorin on page 1233
Lung cancer (nonsmall cell):
  Bevacizumab-Cisplatin-Gemcitabine (NSCLC) on page 1232
  Paclitaxel-Carboplatin-Bevacizumab on page 1385
Renal cell cancer: Bevacizumab-Interferon Alfa (RCC) on page 1232

Administration

I.V. infusion, usually after the other antineoplastic agents. Infuse the initial dose over 90 minutes. Infusion may be shortened to 60 minutes if the initial infusion is well tolerated. The third and subsequent infusions may be shortened to 30 minutes if the 60-minute infusion is well tolerated. Monitor closely during the infusion for signs/symptoms of an infusion reaction. Some institutions use a 10-minute infusion (0.5 mg/kg/minute) for bevacizumab dosed at 5 mg/kg (Reidy, 2007).

Intravitreal injection (unlabeled use): Adequate anesthesia and a broad-spectrum antimicrobial agent should be administered prior to the procedure; administer topical antibiotics for 3 days after procedure.

Monitoring Parameters Monitor closely during the infusion for signs/symptoms of an infusion reaction. Monitor CBC with differential; signs/symptoms of gastrointestinal perforation, fistula, or abscess (including abdominal pain, constipation, vomiting, and fever); signs/symptoms of bleeding, including hemoptysis, gastrointestinal, and/or CNS bleeding, and/or epistaxis. Monitor blood pressure every 2-3 weeks; more frequently if hypertension develops during therapy. Continue to monitor blood pressure after discontinuing due to bevacizumab-induced hypertension. Monitor for proteinuria/nephrotic syndrome with urine dipstick; collect 24 hour urine in patients with ≥2+ reading.

AMD: Monitor intraocular pressure and retinal artery perfusion

Emetic Potential Very low <10%

Dosage Forms Excipient information presented when available (limited, particularly for generics); consult specific product labeling.

Injection, solution [preservative free]:

Avastin®: 25 mg/mL (4 mL, 16 mL)

References

Avery RL, Pieramici DJ, Rabena MD, et al, "Intravitreal Bevacizumab (Avastin) for Neovascular Age-Related Macular Degeneration," *Ophthalmology*, 2006, 113(3):363-72.

Azad NS, Aragon-Ching JB, Dahut WL, et al, "Hand-Foot Skin Reaction Increases With Cumulative Sorafenib Dose and With Combination Anti-Vascular Endothelial Growth Factor Therapy," *Clin Cancer Res*, 2009, 15(4):1411-16.

Bashshur AF, Bazarbachi A, Schakal A, et al, "Intravitreal Bevacizumab for the Management of Choroidal Neovascularization in Age-Related Macular Degeneration," *Am J Ophthalmol*, 2006, 142(1):1-9.

Burger RA, Sill MW, Monk BJ, et al, "Phase II Trial of Bevacizumab in Persistent or Recurrent Epithelial Ovarian Cancer or Primary Peritoneal Cancer: A Gynecologic Oncology Group Study," *J Clin Oncol*, 2007, 25(33):5165-71.

Cannistra SA, Matulonis UA, Penson RT, et al, "Phase II Study of Bevacizumab in Patients With Platinum-Resistant Ovarian Cancer or Peritoneal Serous Cancer," *J Clin Oncol*, 2007, 25 (33):5180-6.

Cloughesy TF, Prados MD, Wen PY, et al, "A Phase II, Randomized, Non-Comparative Clinical Trial of the Effect of Bevacizumab (BV) Alone or in Combination With Irinotecan (CPT) on 6-Month Progression Free Survival (PFS6) in Recurrent, Treatment-Refractory Glioblastoma (GBM)," *J Clin Oncol*, 2008, 26(Supp) [abstract 2010b from 2008 ASCO Annual Meeting]

Escudier B, Pluzanska A, Koralewski P, et al, "Bevacizumab Plus Interferon Alfa-2a for Treatment of Metastatic Renal Cell Carcinoma: A Randomised, Double-Blind Phase III Trial," *Lancet*, 2007, 370(9605):2103-11.

Feldman DR, Baum MS, Ginsberg MS, et al, "Phase I Trial of Bevacizumab Plus Escalated Doses of Sunitinib in Patients With Metastatic Renal Cell Carcinoma," *J Clin Oncol*, 2009, 27(9):1432-9.

Johnson DH, Fehrenbacher L, Novotny WF, et al, "Randomized Phase II Trial Comparing Bevacizumab Plus Carboplatin and Paclitaxel With Carboplatin and Paclitaxel Alone in Previously Untreated Locally Advanced or Metastatic Non-Small-Cell Lung Cancer," *J Clin Oncol*, 2004, 22(11):2184-91.

Kreisl TN, Kim L, Moore K, et al, "Phase II Trial of Single-Agent Bevacizumab Followed by Bevacizumab Plus Irinotecan at Tumor Progression in Recurrent Glioblastoma," *J Clin Oncol*, 2009, 27(5):740-5.

Miller KD, "E2100: A Phase III Trial of Paclitaxel Versus Paclitaxel/Bevacizumab for Metastatic Breast Cancer," *Clin Breast Cancer*, 2003, 3(6):421-2.

Miller K, Wang M, Gralow J, et al, "Paclitaxel Plus Bevacizumab Versus Paclitaxel Alone for Metastatic Breast Cancer," *N Engl J Med*, 2007, 357(26):2666-76.

Nalluri SR, Chu D, Keresztes R, et al, "Risk of Venous Thromboembolism With the Angiogenesis Inhibitor Bevacizumab in Cancer Patients: A Meta-Analysis," *JAMA*, 2008, 300(19): 2277-85.

National Comprehensive Cancer Network (NCCN)®, "Clinical Practice Guidelines in Oncology™: Breast Cancer," Version 1.2009. Available at http://www.nccn.org/professionals/physician_gls/PDF/breast.pdf.

National Comprehensive Cancer Network (NCCN)®, "Clinical Practice Guidelines in Oncology™: Central Nervous System Cancers," Version 2.2009. Available at http://www.nccn.org/professionals/physician_gls/PDF/cns.pdf

National Comprehensive Cancer Network (NCCN)®, "Clinical Practice Guidelines in Oncology™: Colon Cancer," Version 2.2009. Accessible at http://www.nccn.org/professionals/physician_gls/PDF/colon.pdf

National Comprehensive Cancer Network (NCCN)®, "Clinical Practice Guidelines in Oncology™: Kidney Cancer," Version 2.2009. Available at http://www.nccn.org/professionals/physician_gls/PDF/kidney.pdf

National Comprehensive Cancer Network (NCCN)®, "Clinical Practice Guidelines in Oncology™: Non-Small Cell Lung Cancer," Version 2.2009. Accessible at http://www.nccn.org/professionals/physician_gls/PDF/nscl.pdf.

National Comprehensive Cancer Network (NCCN)®, "Clinical Practice Guidelines in Oncology™: Ovarian Cancer," Version 2.2009. Available at http://www.nccn.org/professionals/physician_gls/PDF/ovarian.pdf

Reidy DL, Chung KY, Timoney JP, et al, "Bevacizumab 5 mg/kg Can be Infused Safely over 10 minutes," *J Clin Oncol*, 2007, 25(19):2691-5.

Rini BI, Halabi S, Rosenberg JE, et al, "Bevacizumab Plus Interferon Alfa Compared With Interferon Alfa Monotherapy in Patients With Metastatic Renal Cell Carcinoma: CALGB 90206," *J Clin Oncol*, 2008, 26(33):5422-8.

Sandler A, Gray R, Perry MC, et al, "Paclitaxel-Carboplatin Alone or With Bevacizumab for Non-Small-Cell Lung Cancer," *N Engl J Med*, 2006, 355(24):2542-50.

Scappaticci FA, Skillings JR, Holden SN, et al, "Arterial Thromboembolic Events in Patients with Metastatic Carcinoma Treated With Chemotherapy and Bevacizumab," *J Natl Cancer Inst*, 2007, 99(16):1232-9.

Vredenburgh JJ, Desjardins A, Herndon JE 2nd, et al, "Bevacizumab Plus Irinotecan in Recurrent Glioblastoma Multiforme," *J Clin Oncol*, 2007, 25(30):4722-9.

Yang JC, Haworth L, Sherry RM, et al, "A Randomized Trial of Bevacizumab, An Antivascular Endothelial Growth Factor Antibody, for Metastatic Renal Cancer," *N Engl J Med*, 2003, 349 (5):427-34.

Bexarotene (beks AIR oh teen)

Medication Safety Issues

High alert medication: The Institute for Safe Medication Practices (ISMP) includes this medication among its list of drugs which have a heightened risk of causing significant patient harm when used in error.

Related Information

Safe Handling of Hazardous Drugs *on page 1517*

U.S. Brand Names Targretin®

Generic Available No

Canadian Brand Names Targretin®

Pharmacologic Category Antineoplastic Agent, Miscellaneous

Use

Oral: Treatment of cutaneous manifestations of cutaneous T-cell lymphoma in patients who are refractory to at least one prior systemic therapy

Topical: Treatment of cutaneous lesions in patients with refractory cutaneous T-cell lymphoma (stage 1A and 1B) or who have not tolerated other therapies

Pregnancy Risk Factor X

Lactation Excretion in breast milk unknown/contraindicated

Labeled Contraindications Hypersensitivity to bexarotene or any component of the formulation; pregnancy

Warnings/Precautions Hazardous agent - use appropriate precautions for handling and disposal. **[U.S. Boxed Warning]: Bexarotene is a retinoid, a drug class associated with birth defects in humans; do not administer during pregnancy.** Pregnancy test needed 1 week before initiation and every month thereafter. Effective contraception must be in place 1 month before initiation, during therapy, and for at least 1 month after discontinuation. Male patients with sexual partners who are pregnant, possibly pregnant, or who could become pregnant, must use condoms during sexual intercourse during treatment and for 1 month after last dose. Induces significant lipid abnormalities in a majority of patients (triglyceride, total cholesterol, and HDL); reversible on discontinuation. Use extreme caution in patients with underlying hypertriglyceridemia. Pancreatitis secondary to hypertriglyceridemia has been reported. Patients with risk factors for pancreatitis (eg, prior pancreatitis, uncontrolled hyperlipidemia, excess ethanol consumption, uncontrolled diabetes, biliary tract disease) should generally not receive bexarotene (oral). Monitor for liver function test abnormalities and discontinue drug if tests are three times the upper limit of normal values for AST, ALT, or bilirubin. Hypothyroidism occurs in about a third of patients. Monitor for signs

and symptoms of infection about 4-8 weeks after initiation (leukopenia may occur). Any new visual abnormalities experienced by the patient should be evaluated by an ophthalmologist (cataracts can form, or worsen, especially in the geriatric population). May cause photosensitization. Safety and efficacy are not established in the pediatric population. Use only with extreme caution in patients with hepatic impairment. Limit additional vitamin A intake to <15,000 int. units/day. Use caution with diabetic patients.

Adverse Reactions

Oral: First percentage is at a dose of 300 mg/m^2/day; the second percentage is at a dose >300 mg/m^2/day.

>10%:

Cardiovascular: Peripheral edema (13% to 11%)

Central nervous system: Headache (30% to 42%), chills (10% to 13%)

Dermatologic: Rash (17% to 23%), exfoliative dermatitis (10% to 28%)

Endocrine & metabolic: Hyperlipidemia (about 79% in both dosing ranges), hypercholesteremia (32% to 62%), hypothyroidism (29% to 53%)

Hematologic: Leukopenia (17% to 47%)

Neuromuscular & skeletal: Weakness (20% to 45%)

Miscellaneous: Infection (13% to 23%)

<10%:

Cardiovascular: Hemorrhage, hypertension, angina pectoris, right heart failure, tachycardia, cerebrovascular accident, syncope

Central nervous system: Fever (5% to 17%), insomnia (5% to 11%), subdural hematoma, depression, agitation, ataxia, confusion, dizziness, hyperesthesia

Dermatologic: Dry skin (about 10% for both dosing ranges), alopecia (4% to 11%), skin ulceration, acne, skin nodule, maculopapular rash, serous drainage, vesicular bullous rash, cheilitis

Endocrine & metabolic: Hypoproteinemia, hyperglycemia, weight loss/gain, breast pain

Gastrointestinal: Abdominal pain (11% to 4%), nausea (16% to 8%), diarrhea (7% to 42%), vomiting (4% to 13%), anorexia (2% to 23%), constipation, xerostomia, flatulence, colitis, dyspepsia, gastroenteritis, gingivitis, melena, pancreatitis, serum amylase increased

Genitourinary: Albuminuria, hematuria, urinary incontinence, urinary tract infection, urinary urgency, dysuria, kidney function abnormality

Hematologic: Hypochromic anemia (4% to 13%), anemia (6% to 25%), eosinophilia, thrombocythemia, coagulation time increased, lymphocytosis, thrombocytopenia

Hepatic: LDH increased (7% to 13%), hepatic failure

Neuromuscular & skeletal: Back pain (2% to 11%), arthralgia, myalgia, bone pain, myasthenia, arthrosis, neuropathy

Ocular: Dry eyes, conjunctivitis, blepharitis, corneal lesion, visual field defects, keratitis

Otic: Ear pain, otitis externa

Renal: Creatinine increased

Respiratory: Pharyngitis, rhinitis, dyspnea, pleural effusion, bronchitis, cough increased, lung edema, hemoptysis, hypoxia

Miscellaneous: Flu-like syndrome (4% to 13%), bacterial infection (1% to 13%)

Topical:

Cardiovascular: Edema (10%)

Central nervous system: Headache (14%), weakness (6%), pain (30%)

Dermatologic: Rash (14% to 72%), pruritus (6% to 40%), contact dermatitis (14%), exfoliative dermatitis (6%)

Hematologic: Leukopenia (6%), lymphadenopathy (6%)
Neuromuscular & skeletal: Paresthesia (6%)
Respiratory: Cough (6%), pharyngitis (6%)
Miscellaneous: Diaphoresis (6%), infection (18%)

Drug Interactions

Metabolism/Transport Effects Substrate of CYP3A4 (minor); **Induces** CYP3A4 (weak)

Avoid Concomitant Use

Avoid concomitant use of Bexarotene with any of the following: Tetracycline Derivatives; Vitamin A

Increased Effect/Toxicity

Bexarotene may increase the levels/effects of: Vitamin A

The levels/effects of Bexarotene may be increased by: Tetracycline Derivatives

Decreased Effect

Bexarotene may decrease the levels/effects of: Oral Contraceptive (Estrogens); Oral Contraceptive (Progestins); Saxagliptin

Ethanol/Nutrition/Herb Interactions

Food: Bioavailability is increased when administered with a fat-containing meal. Bexarotene serum levels may be increased by grapefruit juice; avoid concurrent use.

Herb/Nutraceutical: Avoid dong quai, St John's wort (may also cause photosensitization). St John's wort may decrease bexarotene levels. Additional vitamin A supplements may lead to vitamin A toxicity (dry skin, irritation, arthralgias, myalgias, abdominal pain, hepatic changes).

Storage/Stability Store at 2°C to 25°C (36°F to 77°F). Protect from light.

Mechanism of Action The exact mechanism is unknown. Binds and activates retinoid X receptor subtypes. Once activated, these receptors function as transcription factors that regulate the expression of genes which control cellular differentiation and proliferation. Bexarotene inhibits the growth *in vitro* of some tumor cell lines of hematopoietic and squamous cell origin.

Pharmacodynamics/Kinetics

Absorption: Significantly improved by a fat-containing meal

Protein binding: >99%

Metabolism: Hepatic via CYP3A4 isoenzyme; four metabolites identified; further metabolized by glucuronidation

Half-life elimination: 7 hours

Time to peak: 2 hours

Excretion: Primarily feces; urine (<1% as unchanged drug and metabolites)

Dosage Adults:

Oral: 300-400 mg/m^2/day taken as a single daily dose.

Topical: Apply once every other day for first week, then increase on a weekly basis to once daily, 2 times/day, 3 times/day, and finally 4 times/day, according to tolerance

Dosing adjustment in renal impairment: No studies have been conducted; however, renal insufficiency may result in significant protein binding changes and alter pharmacokinetics of bexarotene

Dosing adjustment in hepatic impairment: No studies have been conducted; however, hepatic impairment would be expected to result in decreased clearance of bexarotene due to the extensive hepatic contribution to elimination

Administration

Oral: Administer capsule following a fat-containing meal.

Topical: Allow gel to dry before covering with clothing. Avoid application to normal skin. Use of occlusive dressings is not recommended.

Monitoring Parameters If female, pregnancy test 1 week before initiation then monthly while on bexarotene; lipid panel before initiation, then weekly until lipid response established and then at 8-week intervals thereafter; baseline LFTs, repeat at 1, 2, and 4 weeks after initiation then at 8-week intervals thereafter if stable; baseline and periodic thyroid function tests; baseline CBC with periodic monitoring

Dietary Considerations It is preferable to take the oral capsule following a fat-containing meal. Avoid grapefruit juice.

Emetic Potential Low (10% to 30%)

Dosage Forms Excipient information presented when available (limited, particularly for generics); consult specific product labeling.

Capsule:

Targretin®: 75 mg

Gel: 1% (60 g)

Targretin®: 1% (60 g) [contains dehydrated alcohol]

References

Duvic M, "Bexarotene and DAB(389)IL-2 (Denileukin Diftitox, ONTAK) in Treatment of Cutaneous T-Cell Lymphomas: Algorithms," *Clin Lymphoma*, 2000, 1(Suppl 1):51-5.

Farol LT and Hymes KB, "Bexarotene: A Clinical Review," *Expert Rev Anticancer Ther*, 2004, 4 (2):180-8.

Martin AG, "Bexarotene Gel: A New Skin-Directed Treatment Option for Cutaneous T-Cell Lymphomas," *J Drugs Dermatol*, 2003, 2(2):155-67.

♦ **Bexxar®** *see* Tositumomab and Iodine I 131 Tositumomab *on page 1123*

Bicalutamide (bye ka LOO ta mide)

Medication Safety Issues

Sound-alike/look-alike issues:

Casodex® may be confused with Kapidex™

Related Information

Safe Handling of Hazardous Drugs *on page 1517*

U.S. Brand Names Casodex®

Index Terms CDX; ICI-176334

Generic Available Yes

Canadian Brand Names Apo-Bicalutamide®; Casodex®; CO Bicalutamide; Dom-Bicalutamide; Gen-Bicalutamide; Mylan-Bicalutamide; Novo-Bicaluta-mide; PHL-Bicalutamide; PMS-Bicalutamide; Pro-Bicalutamide; ratio-Bicaluta-mide; Sandoz-Bicalutamide; ZYM-Bicalutamide

Pharmacologic Category Antineoplastic Agent, Antiandrogen

Use Treatment of metastatic prostate cancer (in combination with an LHRH agonist)

Unlabeled/Investigational Use Monotherapy for locally-advanced prostate cancer

Pregnancy Risk Factor X

Lactation Excretion in breast milk unknown/contraindicated

Labeled Contraindications Hypersensitivity to bicalutamide or any component of the formulation; use in women, especially women who are or may become pregnant

Warnings/Precautions Hazardous agent - use appropriate precautions for handling and disposal. Rare cases of death or hospitalization due to hepatitis have been reported postmarketing. Use with caution in moderate-to-severe ▶

hepatic dysfunction. Hepatotoxicity generally occurs within the first 3-4 months of use; patients should be monitored for signs and symptoms of liver dysfunction. Bicalutamide should be discontinued if patients have jaundice or ALT is >2 times the upper limit of normal. May cause gynecomastia, breast pain, or lead to spermatogenesis inhibition. When used in combination with LHRH agonists, a loss of glycemic control and decrease in glucose tolerance has been reported in patients with diabetes; monitor. May cause gynecomastia, breast pain, or lead to spermatogenesis inhibition. Safety and efficacy have not been established in children. Not indicated for use in women.

Adverse Reactions Adverse reaction percentages reported as part of combination regimen with an LHRH analogue unless otherwise noted.

>10%:
  Cardiovascular: Peripheral edema (13%)
  Central nervous system: Pain (35%)
  Endocrine & metabolic: Hot flashes (53%), breast pain (6%; monotherapy: 39% to 85%), gynecomastia (9%; monotherapy: 38% to 73%)
  Gastrointestinal: Constipation (22%), nausea (15%), diarrhea (12%), abdominal pain (11%)
  Genitourinary: Pelvic pain (21%), hematuria (12%), nocturia (12%)
  Hematologic: Anemia (11%)
  Neuromuscular & skeletal: Back pain (25%), weakness (22%)
  Respiratory: Dyspnea (13%)
  Miscellaneous: Infection (18%)
≥2% to 10%:
  Cardiovascular: Chest pain (8%), hypertension (8%), angina pectoris (2% to <5%), cardiac arrest (2% to <5%), CHF (2% to <5%), edema (2% to <5%), MI (2% to <5%), coronary artery disorder (2% to <5%), syncope (2% to <5%)
  Central nervous system: Dizziness (10%), headache (7%), insomnia (7%), anxiety (5%), depression (4%), chills (2% to <5%), confusion (2% to <5%), fever (2% to <5%), nervousness (2% to <5%), somnolence (2% to <5%)
  Dermatologic: Rash (9%), alopecia (2% to <5%), dry skin (2% to <5%), pruritus (2% to <5%), skin carcinoma (2% to <5%)
  Endocrine & metabolic: Hyperglycemia (6%), dehydration (2% to <5%), gout (2% to <5%), hypercholesterolemia (2% to <5%), libido decreased (2% to <5%)
  Gastrointestinal: Dyspepsia (7%), weight loss (7%), anorexia (6%), flatulence (6%), vomiting (6%), weight gain (5%), dysphagia (2% to <5%), gastrointestinal carcinoma (2% to <5%), melena (2% to <5%), periodontal abscess (2% to <5%), rectal hemorrhage (2% to <5%), xerostomia (2% to <5%)
  Genitourinary: Urinary tract infection (9%), impotence (7%), polyuria (6%), urinary retention (5%), urinary impairment (5%), urinary incontinence (4%), dysuria (2% to <5%), urinary urgency (2% to <5%)
  Hepatic: LFTs increased (7%), alkaline phosphatase increased (5%)
  Neuromuscular & skeletal: Bone pain (9%), paresthesia (8%), myasthenia (7%), arthritis (5%), pathological fracture (4%), hypertonia (2% to <5%), leg cramps (2% to <5%), myalgia (2% to <5%), neck pain (2% to <5%), neuropathy (2% to <5%)
  Ocular: Cataract (2% to <5%)
  Renal: BUN increased (2% to <5%), creatinine increased (2% to <5%), hydronephrosis (2% to <5%)

Respiratory: Cough (8%), pharyngitis (8%), bronchitis (6%), pneumonia (4%), rhinitis (4%), asthma (2% to <5%), epistaxis (2% to <5%), sinusitis (2% to <5%)

Miscellaneous: Flu-like syndrome (7%), diaphoresis (6%), cyst (2% to <5%), hernia (2% to <5%), herpes zoster (2% to <5%), sepsis (2% to <5%)

Postmarketing and/or case reports: Bilirubin increased, glucose tolerance decreased, hemoglobin decreased, hepatitis, hepatotoxicity, hypersensitivity reactions (including angioneurotic edema and urticaria), interstitial pneumonitis, pulmonary fibrosis, WBC decreased

Drug Interactions

Avoid Concomitant Use

Avoid concomitant use of Bicalutamide with any of the following: Everolimus; Tolvaptan

Increased Effect/Toxicity

Bicalutamide may increase the levels/effects of: Colchicine; CYP3A4 Substrates; Eplerenone; Everolimus; FentaNYL; Halofantrine; Pimecrolimus; Ranolazine; Salmeterol; Saxagliptin; Tolvaptan; Vitamin K Antagonists

Decreased Effect There are no known significant interactions involving a decrease in effect.

Storage/Stability Store at room temperature of 20°C to 25°C (68°F to 77°F).

Mechanism of Action Androgen receptor inhibitor; pure nonsteroidal antiandrogen that binds to androgen receptors; specifically a competitive inhibitor for the binding of dihydrotestosterone and testosterone; prevents testosterone stimulation of cell growth in prostate cancer

Pharmacodynamics/Kinetics

Absorption: Rapid and complete; unaffected by food

Protein binding: 96%

Metabolism: Extensively hepatic; glucuronidation and oxidation of the R (active) enantiomer to inactive metabolites; the S enantiomer is inactive

Half-life elimination: Active enantiomer: ~6 days, ~10 days in severe liver disease

Time to peak, plasma: Active enantiomer: ~31 hours

Excretion: Urine (36%, as inactive metabolites); feces (42%, as unchanged drug and inactive metabolites)

Dosage Adults: Oral:

Metastatic prostate cancer: 50 mg once daily (in combination with an LHRH analogue)

Locally-advanced prostate cancer, monotherapy (unlabeled use): 150 mg once daily (McLeod, 2006)

Dosage adjustment in renal impairment: No adjustment required

Dosage adjustment in hepatic impairment: No adjustment required for mild, moderate, or severe hepatic impairment; use caution with moderate-to-severe impairment. Discontinue if ALT >2 times ULN or patient develops jaundice.

Combination Regimens

Prostate cancer:

Bicalutamide-Goserelin on page 1234

Bicalutamide-Leuprolide on page 1234

Administration Dose should be taken at the same time each day with or without food. Treatment should be started concomitantly with an LHRH analogue.

◄ **Monitoring Parameters** Periodically monitor CBC, ECG, echocardiograms, serum testosterone, luteinizing hormone, and prostate specific antigen (PSA). Liver function tests should be obtained at baseline and repeated regularly during the first 4 months of treatment, and periodically thereafter; monitor for signs and symptoms of liver dysfunction (discontinue if jaundice is noted or ALT is >2 times the upper limit of normal). Monitor blood glucose in patients with diabetes. If initiating bicalutamide in patients who are on warfarin, closely monitor prothrombin time.

Dietary Considerations May be taken with or without food.

Additional Information Oncology Comment: According to the 2007 update of the American Society of Clinical Oncology (ASCO) guidelines for initial hormonal management of androgen-sensitive advanced prostate cancer, the standard of care is initial treatment with a luteinizing hormone-releasing hormone (LHRH) agonist, however, bicalutamide should be considered in combination with an LHRH agonist for combined androgen blockade (CAB) treatment. Although the incidence of adverse effects is increased, the addition of a nonsteroidal antiandrogen (NSAA) such a s bicalutamide, increases overall survival (OS) (Loblaw, 2007).

The National Comprehensive Cancer Network® (NCCN) Guidelines for Prostate Cancer (v.2.2009) also recommend an LHRH agonist as medical castration, which may be given alone or in combination with an NSAA. Certain patients (with evidence of metastases) receiving LHRH agonists are at risk for tumor flare, a condition in which an initial transient increase in testosterone levels induced by an LHRH agonist, results in worsening symptoms. These patients, according to the NCCN guidelines, should receive an antiandrogen with the LHRH agonist for at least 7 days, which may begin with or just prior to the LHRH agonist. The NCCN guidelines also address monotherapy with bicalutamide (150 mg orally daily) and while, to date, no OS advantage has been demonstrated in early, localized, or locally advanced prostate cancer, an improvement in progression-free survival has been demonstrated in locally advanced prostate cancer.

Dosage Forms Excipient information presented when available (limited, particularly for generics); consult specific product labeling.

Tablet: 50 mg

Casodex®: 50 mg

References

Iversen, P, Johansson JE, Lodding P, et al, "Bicalutamide (150 mg) Versus Placebo as Immediate Therapy Alone or as Adjuvant to Therapy With Curative Intent for Early Nonmetastatic Prostate Cancer: 5.3 Year Median Followup from the Scandinavian Prostate Cancer Group Study Number 6," J Urol 2004, 172(5 Pt 1):1871-6.

Loblaw DA, Virgo KS, Nam R, et al, "Initial Hormonal Management of Androgen-Sensitive Metastatic, Recurrent, or Progressive Prostate Cancer: 2007 Update of an American Society of Clinical Oncology Practice Guideline," J Clin Oncol, 2007, 25(12):1596-605.

McLeod DG, Iversen P, See WA, et al, "Bicalutamide 150 mg Plus Standard Care vs Standard Care Alone for Early Prostate Cancer," BJU Int, 2005, 97(2):247-54.

McLeod DG, See WA, Klimberg I, et al, "The Bicalutamide 150 mg Early Prostate Cancer Program: Findings of the North American Trial at 7.7-Year Median Followup," J Urol, 2006, 176(1):75-80.

National Comprehensive Cancer Network® (NCCN), "Clinical Practice Guidelines in Oncology™: Prostate Carcinoma," Version 2.2009. Available at http://www.nccn.org/professionals/physician_gls/PDF/prostate.pdf

Schellhammer P, Sharifi R, Block N, et al, "A Controlled Trial of Bicalutamide Versus Flutamide, Each in Combination With Luteinizing Hormone-Releasing Hormone Analogue Therapy, in Patients With Advanced Prostate Cancer. Casodex Combination Study Group." Urology, 1995, 45(5):745-52.

Schellhammer PF, Sharifi R, Block NL, et al, "Clinical Benefits of Bicalutamide Compared With Flutamide in Combined Androgen Blockade for Patients With Advanced Prostatic Carcinoma: Final Report of a Double-Blind, Randomized, Multicenter Trial. Casodex Combination Study Group," Urology, 1997, 50(3):330-6.

Tyrell CJ, Denis L, Newling D, et al, "Casodex 10-200 mg Daily, Used as Monotherapy for the Treatment of Patients With Advanced Prostate Cancer. An Overview of the Efficacy, Tolerability and Pharmacokinetics from Three Phase II Dose-Ranging Studies. Casodex Study Group," *Eur Urol*, 1998, 33(1):39-53.

◆ **BiCNU®** *see* Carmustine *on page 183*

◆ **Bioniche Promethazine (Can)** *see* Promethazine *on page 997*

◆ **Bio-Statin®** *see* Nystatin *on page 855*

◆ **bis-chloronitrosourea** *see* Carmustine *on page 183*

◆ **BL4162A** *see* Anagrelide *on page 83*

◆ **Blenoxane® [DSC]** *see* Bleomycin *on page 151*

◆ **Blenoxane® (Can)** *see* Bleomycin *on page 151*

◆ **Bleo** *see* Bleomycin *on page 151*

Bleomycin (blee oh MYE sin)

Medication Safety Issues
Sound-alike/look-alike issues:
Bleomycin may be confused with Cleocin®

High alert medication: The Institute for Safe Medication Practices (ISMP) includes this medication among its list of drugs which have a heightened risk of causing significant patient harm when used in error.

Related Information
Management of Drug Extravasations *on page 1447*
Safe Handling of Hazardous Drugs *on page 1517*

U.S. Brand Names Blenoxane® [DSC]

Index Terms Bleo; Bleomycin Sulfate; BLM; NSC-125066

Generic Available Yes

Canadian Brand Names Blenoxane®; Bleomycin Injection, USP

Pharmacologic Category Antineoplastic Agent, Antibiotic

Use Treatment of squamous cell carcinomas, melanomas, sarcomas, testicular carcinoma, Hodgkin's lymphoma, and non-Hodgkin's lymphoma; sclerosing agent for malignant pleural effusion

Pregnancy Risk Factor D

Lactation Excretion in breast milk unknown/not recommended

Labeled Contraindications Hypersensitivity to bleomycin or any component of the formulation; severe pulmonary disease; pregnancy

Warnings/Precautions Hazardous agent - use appropriate precautions for handling and disposal. **[U.S. Boxed Warnings]: Occurrence of pulmonary fibrosis (commonly presenting as pneumonitis) is higher in elderly patients, patients receiving >400 units total lifetime dose or single doses >30 units, smokers, and patients with prior radiation therapy or receiving concurrent oxygen. A severe idiosyncratic reaction consisting of hypotension, mental confusion, fever, chills, and wheezing (similar to anaphylaxis) has been reported in 1% of lymphoma patients treated with bleomycin.** Since these reactions usually occur after the first or second dose, careful monitoring is essential after these doses. Use caution when administering O_2 during surgery to patients who have received bleomycin. Use caution with renal impairment, may require dose adjustment. May cause renal or hepatic toxicity. **[U.S. Boxed Warning]: Should be administered under the supervision of an experienced cancer chemotherapy physician.**

Adverse Reactions

>10%:

Dermatologic: Pain at the tumor site, phlebitis. About 50% of patients develop erythema, rash, striae, induration, hyperkeratosis, vesiculation, and peeling of the skin, particularly on the palmar and plantar surfaces of the hands and feet. Hyperpigmentation (50%), alopecia, nailbed changes may also occur. These effects appear dose related and reversible with discontinuation.

Gastrointestinal: Stomatitis and mucositis (30%), anorexia, weight loss

Respiratory: Tachypnea, rales, acute or chronic interstitial pneumonitis, and pulmonary fibrosis (5% to 10%); hypoxia and death (1%). Symptoms include cough, dyspnea, and bilateral pulmonary infiltrates. The pathogenesis is not certain, but may be due to damage of pulmonary, vascular, or connective tissue. Response to steroid therapy is variable and somewhat controversial.

Miscellaneous: Acute febrile reactions (25% to 50%)

1% to 10%:

Dermatologic: Skin thickening, diffuse scleroderma, onycholysis, pruritus

Miscellaneous: Anaphylactoid-like reactions (characterized by hypotension, confusion, fever, chills, and wheezing; onset may be immediate or delayed for several hours); idiosyncratic reactions (1% in lymphoma patients)

<1%: Angioedema, cerebrovascular accident, cerebral arteritis, hepatotoxicity, malaise, MI, nausea, Raynaud's phenomenon, renal toxicity, scleroderma-like skin changes, thrombotic microangiopathy, vomiting; Myelosuppression (rare); Onset: 7 days, Nadir: 14 days, Recovery: 21 days

Drug Interactions

Avoid Concomitant Use

Avoid concomitant use of Bleomycin with any of the following: Natalizumab; Vaccines (Live)

Increased Effect/Toxicity

Bleomycin may increase the levels/effects of: Leflunomide; Natalizumab; Vaccines (Live)

The levels/effects of Bleomycin may be increased by: Gemcitabine; Trastuzumab

Decreased Effect

Bleomycin may decrease the levels/effects of: Cardiac Glycosides; Vaccines (Inactivated); Vaccines (Live)

The levels/effects of Bleomycin may be decreased by: Echinacea

Storage/Stability Refrigerate intact vials of powder. Intact vials are stable for up to 1 month at 45°C. Solutions for infusion are stable for 96 hours at room temperature and 14 days under refrigeration.

Reconstitution Reconstitute powder with 1-5 mL BWFI or BNS which is stable at room temperature or under refrigeration for 28 days.

Standard I.V. dilution: Dose/50-1000 mL NS.

Compatibility Stable in NS; **variable stability (consult detailed reference)** in D_5W.

Y-site administration: Compatible: Allopurinol, amifostine, aztreonam, cefepime, cisplatin, cyclophosphamide, doxorubicin, doxorubicin liposome, droperidol, etoposide phosphate, filgrastim, fludarabine, fluorouracil, gemcitabine, granisetron, heparin, leucovorin, melphalan, methotrexate, metoclopramide, mitomycin, ondansetron, paclitaxel, piperacillin/tazobactam, sargramostim, teniposide, thiotepa, vinblastine, vincristine, vinorelbine.

Compatibility in syringe: Compatible: Cisplatin, cyclophosphamide, doxorubicin, droperidol, fluorouracil, furosemide, heparin, leucovorin, methotrexate, metoclopramide, mitomycin, vinblastine, vincristine.

Compatibility when admixed: Compatible: Amikacin, dexamethasone sodium phosphate, diphenhydramine, fluorouracil, gentamicin, heparin, hydrocortisone sodium phosphate, phenytoin, streptomycin, tobramycin, vinblastine, vincristine. **Incompatible:** Aminophylline, ascorbic acid injection, cefazolin, diazepam, hydrocortisone sodium succinate, methotrexate, mitomycin, nafcillin, penicillin G sodium, terbutaline.

Mechanism of Action Inhibits synthesis of DNA; binds to DNA leading to single- and double-strand breaks

Pharmacodynamics/Kinetics

Absorption: I.M. and intrapleural administration: 30% to 50% of I.V. serum concentrations; intraperitoneal and SubQ routes produce serum concentrations equal to those of I.V.

Distribution: V_d: 22 L/m^2; highest concentrations in skin, kidney, lung, heart tissues; lowest in testes and GI tract; does not cross blood-brain barrier

Protein binding: 1%

Metabolism: Via several tissues including hepatic, GI tract, skin, pulmonary, renal, and serum

Half-life elimination: Biphasic (renal function dependent):

Normal renal function: Initial: 1.3 hours; Terminal: 9 hours

End-stage renal disease: Initial: 2 hours; Terminal: 30 hours

Time to peak, serum: I.M.: Within 30 minutes

Excretion: Urine (50% to 70% as active drug)

Dosage Maximum cumulative lifetime dose: 400 units; refer to individual protocols; 1 unit = 1 mg

May be administered I.M., I.V., SubQ, or intracavitary

Children and Adults:

Test dose for lymphoma patients: I.M., I.V., SubQ: Because of the possibility of an anaphylactoid reaction, administer 1-2 units of bleomycin before the first 1-2 doses; monitor vital signs every 15 minutes; wait a minimum of 1 hour before administering remainder of dose; if no acute reaction occurs, then the regular dosage schedule may be followed. **Note:** Test doses may produce false-negative results.

Single-agent therapy:

I.M./I.V./SubQ: Squamous cell carcinoma, lymphoma, testicular carcinoma: 0.25-0.5 units/kg (10-20 units/m^2) 1-2 times/week

CIV: 15 units/m^2 over 24 hours daily for 4 days

Pleural sclerosing: Intrapleural: 60 units as a single instillation (some recommend limiting the dose in the elderly to 40 units/m^2; usual maximum: 60 units). Dose may be repeated at intervals of several days if fluid continues to accumulate (mix in 50-100 mL of NS); may add lidocaine 100-200 mg to reduce local discomfort.

Dosing adjustment in renal impairment:

The FDA-approved labeling recommends the following adjustments:

Cl_{cr} 40-50 mL/minute: Administer 70% of normal dose

Cl_{cr} 30-40 mL/minute: Administer 60% of normal dose

Cl_{cr} 20-30 mL/minute: Administer 55% of normal dose

Cl_{cr} 10-20 mL/minute: Administer 45% of normal dose

Cl_{cr} 5-10 mL/minute: Administer 40% of normal dose

The following guidelines have been used by some clinicians:

Aronoff, 2007: Adults: Continuous renal replacement therapy (CRRT): Administer 75% of dose

◀ Kintzel, 1995:

Cl$_{cr}$ 46-60 mL/minute: Administer 70% of dose

Cl$_{cr}$ 31-45 mL/minute: Administer 60% of dose

Cl$_{cr}$ <30 mL/minute: Consider use of alternative drug

Dosing adjustment in hepatic impairment: Not studied in patients with hepatic impairment; adjustment for hepatic impairment may be needed.

Combination Regimens

Cervical cancer: BIP on page 1235

Head and neck cancer: CABO on page 1241

Lymphoma, Hodgkin's:

ABVD on page 1222

BEACOPP on page 1229

CAD/MOPP/ABV on page 1242

MOPP/ABV Hybrid on page 1372

MOPP/ABVD on page 1369

Stanford V Regimen on page 1403

Lymphoma, non-Hodgkin's:

CEPP(B) on page 1254

COP-BLAM on page 1280

MACOP-B on page 1364

m-BACOD on page 1365

Pro-MACE-CytaBOM on page 1397

Melanoma:

BOLD on page 1235

BOLD + Interferon on page 1235

BOLD (Melanoma) on page 1237

Osteosarcoma: POG-8651 on page 1396

Ovarian cancer:

BEP (Ovarian Cancer) on page 1230

BEP (Ovarian Cancer, Testicular Cancer) on page 1230

Testicular cancer:

BEP (Ovarian Cancer, Testicular Cancer) on page 1230

BEP (Testicular Cancer) on page 1230

PVB on page 1400

VBP on page 1419

Administration

I.V. doses should be administered slowly (over 10-60 minutes).

I.M. or SubQ: May cause pain at injection site

Intrapleural: 60 units in 50-100 mL NS; use of topical anesthetics or narcotic analgesia is usually not necessary

Monitoring Parameters Pulmonary function tests (total lung volume, forced vital capacity, carbon monoxide diffusion), renal function, liver function, chest x-ray, temperature initially; check body weight at regular intervals

Emetic Potential Very low (<10%)

Vesicant May be an irritant

Dosage Forms Excipient information presented when available (limited, particularly for generics); consult specific product labeling. [DSC] = Discontinued product

Injection, powder for reconstitution, as sulfate: 15 units, 30 units

Blenoxane®: 30 units [DSC]

References

Aronoff GR, Bennett WM, Berns JS, et al, *Drug Prescribing in Renal Failure: Dosing Guidelines for Adults and Children*, 5th ed. Philadelphia, PA: American College of Physicians; 2007, p 97.

Kintzel PE and Dorr RT, "Anticancer Drug Renal Toxicity and Elimination: Dosing Guidelines for Altered Renal Function," *Cancer Treat Rev*, 1995, 21(1):33-64.

- ◆ **Bleomycin Injection, USP (Can)** *see Bleomycin on page 151*
- ◆ **Bleomycin Sulfate** *see Bleomycin on page 151*
- ◆ **BLM** *see Bleomycin on page 151*
- ◆ **BMS-247550** *see Ixabepilone on page 672*
- ◆ **BMS-354825** *see Dasatinib on page 314*
- ◆ **Bondronat® (Can)** *see Ibandronate on page 597*
- ◆ **Bonefos® (Can)** *see Clodronate on page 247*
- ◆ **Boniva®** *see Ibandronate on page 597*

Bortezomib (bore TEZ oh mib)

Medication Safety Issues
High alert medication: The Institute for Safe Medication Practices (ISMP) includes this medication among its list of drug classes which have a heightened risk of causing significant patient harm when used in error.

Related Information
Management of Drug Extravasations *on page 1447*
Safe Handling of Hazardous Drugs *on page 1517*

U.S. Brand Names Velcade®

Index Terms LDP-341; MLN341; NSC-681239; PS-341

Generic Available No

Canadian Brand Names Velcade®

Pharmacologic Category Antineoplastic Agent; Proteasome Inhibitor

Use Treatment of multiple myeloma; treatment of relapsed or refractory mantle cell lymphoma

Unlabeled/Investigational Use Treatment of non-Hodgkin's lymphomas (other than mantle cell lymphoma); treatment of Waldenstrom's macroglobulinemia

Pregnancy Risk Factor D

Lactation Excretion in breast milk unknown/not recommended

Labeled Contraindications Hypersensitivity to bortezomib, boron, mannitol, or any component of the formulation

Warnings/Precautions Hazardous agent - use appropriate precautions for handling and disposal. May cause peripheral neuropathy (usually sensory but may be mixed sensorimotor); risk may be increased with previous use of neurotoxic agents or pre-existing peripheral neuropathy; adjustment of dose and schedule may be required. May cause hypotension (including postural and orthostatic); use caution with dehydration, history of syncope, or medications associated with hypotension. Has been associated with the development or exacerbation of congestive heart failure and decreased left ventricular ejection fraction; use caution in patients with risk factors or existing heart disease. Has also been associated with QT_c prolongation.

Pulmonary disorders including pneumonitis, interstitial pneumonia, lung infiltrates, and acute respiratory distress syndrome (ARDS) have been reported. Pulmonary hypertension (without left heart failure or significant pulmonary disease has been reported rarely). May cause tumor lysis syndrome; risk is increased in patients with high tumor burden prior to treatment. Reversible posterior leukoencephalopathy syndrome (RPLS) has been reported (rarely). Symptoms of RPLS include confusion, headache, hypertension, lethargy, seizure, blindness and/or other vision, or neurologic disturbances; discontinue if RPLS occurs. The safety of reinitiating bortezomib in patients previously experiencing RPLS is unknown. Herpes (zoster and simplex) reactivation has been reported with bortezomib; consider antiviral prophylaxis during therapy. Hematologic toxicity, including neutropenia and severe thrombocytopenia, may occur; risk is increased in patients with pretreatment platelet counts <75,000/μL; frequent monitoring is required throughout treatment; may require dosage adjustments; withhold treatment for platelets <25,000/μL. Hemorrhage (gastrointestinal and intracerebral) due to low platelet count has been observed. Acute liver failure has been reported (rarely) in patients receiving multiple concomitant medications; hepatitis, transaminase increases, and hyperbilirubinemia have also been reported. Use caution in patients with hepatic dysfunction; toxicities may be increased. Hyper- and hypoglycemia may occur in diabetic patients receiving oral hypoglycemics; may require adjustment of diabetes medications. Safety and efficacy have not been established in pediatric patients.

Adverse Reactions

>10%:

Cardiovascular: Edema (11% to 28%), hypotension (12% to 15%; grades 3/4: 3%)

Central nervous system: Fever (19% to 37%), psychiatric disturbance (35%), headache (17% to 26%), dysesthesia (9% to 27%), insomnia (18% to 21%), dizziness (14% to 23%; excludes vertigo), anxiety (5% to 11%)

Dermatologic: Rash (17% to 28%), pruritus (11%)

Endocrine & metabolic: Dehydration (7% to 11%)

Gastrointestinal: Diarrhea (47% to 57%), nausea (44% to 57%), constipation (40% to 50%), anorexia (34% to 39%), vomiting (27% to 35%), abdominal pain (14% to 16%), abnormal taste (13%), dyspepsia (13%)

Hematologic: Thrombocytopenia (21% to 38%; grade 4: 4% to 5%; nadir: day 11; recovery: by day 21), anemia (17% to 30%; grade 4: <1%), neutropenia (6% to 19%; grade 4: 2% to 3%; nadir: day 11; recovery: by day 21)

Neuromuscular & skeletal: Weakness (61% to 72%; grades 3/4: 12% to 19%), peripheral neuropathy (36% to 55%; grade 3: 7% to 11%; grade 4: <1%), paresthesia (9% to 27%), arthralgia (13% to 18%), limb pain (5% to 17%), bone pain (2% to 16%), back pain (<1 % to 15%), myalgia (10% to 12%), muscle cramps (5% to 12%), rigors (11%)

Ocular: Blurred vision (11%)

Respiratory: Dyspnea (20% to 23%), cough (19% to 21%), lower respiratory infection (15%), upper respiratory tract infection (11% to 15%), nasopharyngitis (8% to 14%), pneumonia (9% to 12%)

Miscellaneous: Herpesvirus infections (7% to 13%)

1% to 10%:

Cardiovascular: Syncope (2%)

Endocrine & metabolic: Hypercalcemia (grade 4: 2%)

Frequency not defined (including postmarketing and/or case reports; limited to important or life-threatening): Acute diffuse infiltrative pulmonary disease, acute respiratory distress syndrome, alkaline phosphatase increased, allergic reaction, amyloidosis, anaphylaxis, angina, angioedema, ascites, aspergillosis, atelectasis, atrial fibrillation, atrial flutter, AV block, bacteremia, bradycardia, cardiac amyloidosis, cardiac arrest, cardiac tamponade, cardiogenic shock, cardiopulmonary arrest, cerebral hemorrhage, cerebrovascular accident, CHF, cholestasis, coma, complete heart block, confusion, cranial palsy, deafness, deep venous thrombosis, diplopia, disseminated intravascular coagulation (DIC), duodenitis (hemorrhagic), dysautonomia, dysphagia, edema (facial), encephalopathy, embolism, epistaxis, fecal impaction, fracture, gastritis (hemorrhagic), gastroenteritis, GGT increased, glomerular nephritis, hematemesis, hematuria, hemoptysis, hemorrhagic cystitis, hepatic failure, hepatic hemorrhage, hepatitis, hepatocellular

damage, herpes meningoencephalitis, hyperbilirubinemia, hyper-/hypoglyce-
mia, hyper-/hypokalemia, hyper-/hyponatremia, hypersensitivity, hyperuricemia, hypocalcemia, hypoxia, immune complex hypersensitivity, injection site
reaction, intestinal obstruction, intestinal perforation, intracerebral hemorrhage, ischemic colitis, ischemic stroke, laryngeal edema, leukocytoclastic
vasculitis, leukopenia, listeriosis, lymphopenia, melena, mental status
change, MI, myocardial ischemia, neuralgia, neutropenic fever, ophthalmic
herpes, oral candidiasis, pancreatitis, paralytic ileus, paraplegia, pericardial
effusion, pericarditis, peritonitis, pleural effusion, pneumonia, pneumonitis,
portal vein thrombosis, proliferative glomerular nephritis, psychosis, pulmonary alveolar hemorrhage, pulmonary edema, pulmonary embolism,
pulmonary hypertension, psychosis, QT_c prolongation, renal calculus, renal
failure, respiratory failure, respiratory insufficiency, reversible posterior
leukoencephalopathy syndrome (RPLS), seizure, septic shock, sepsis, sinus
arrest, spinal cord compression, stomatitis, stroke (hemorrhagic), stroke,
subarachnoid hemorrhage, subdural hematoma, suicidal ideation, tachycardia, torsade de pointes, toxic epidermal necrolysis, toxoplasmosis, transaminases increased, transient ischemic attack, tumor lysis syndrome, urinary
incontinence, urinary retention, urinary tract infection, urticaria, ventricular
tachycardia

Drug Interactions

Metabolism/Transport Effects Substrate of CYP1A2 (minor), 2C9
(minor), 2C19 (major), 2D6 (minor), 3A4 (major); **Inhibits** CYP1A2 (weak),
2C9 (weak), 2C19 (moderate), 2D6 (weak), 3A4 (weak)

Avoid Concomitant Use

Avoid concomitant use of Bortezomib with any of the following: Clopidogrel;
Green Tea

Increased Effect/Toxicity

Bortezomib may increase the levels/effects of: CYP2C19 Substrates

The levels/effects of Bortezomib may be increased by: CYP2C19 Inhibitors
(Moderate); CYP2C19 Inhibitors (Strong); CYP3A4 Inhibitors (Moderate);
CYP3A4 Inhibitors (Strong); Dasatinib

Decreased Effect

Bortezomib may decrease the levels/effects of: Clopidogrel

The levels/effects of Bortezomib may be decreased by: CYP2C19 Inducers
(Strong); CYP3A4 Inducers (Strong); Deferasirox; Green Tea; Herbs
(CYP3A4 Inducers); Peginterferon Alfa-2b

Ethanol/Nutrition/Herb Interactions

Food: Avoid grapefruit juice (may increase bortezomib levels).

Herb/Nutraceutical: Avoid St John's wort (may decrease bortezomib levels).
Avoid green tea and green tea extracts (may diminish the therapeutic effect of
bortezomib) (Golden, 2009).

Storage/Stability Prior to reconstitution, store at room temperature of 25°C
(77°F); excursions permitted between 15°C to 30°C (59°F to 86°F). Protect
from light. Once reconstituted, although the manufacturer recommends use
within 8 hours, solution may be stored at room temperature for up to 3 days, or
under refrigeration for up to 5 days, in vial or syringe (Andre, 2005). Protect
from light.

Reconstitution Dilute each 3.5 mg vial with 3.5 mL NS to a final concentration
of 1 mg/mL. Use appropriate precautions for handling and disposal.

◄ **Mechanism of Action** Bortezomib inhibits proteasomes, enzyme complexes which regulate protein homeostasis within the cell. Specifically, it reversibly inhibits chymotrypsin-like activity at the 26S proteasome, leading to activation of signaling cascades, cell-cycle arrest, and apoptosis.

Pharmacodynamics/Kinetics

Distribution: 498-1884 L/m^2

Protein binding: ~83%

Metabolism: Hepatic primarily via CYP2C19 and 3A4 and to a lesser extent CYP1A2; forms metabolites (inactive) via deboronization followed by hydroxylation

Half-life elimination: Single dose: 9-15 hours; multiple dosing: 1 mg/m^2: 40-193 hours; 1.3 mg/m^2: 76-108 hours

Dosage Details concerning dosing in combination regimens should also be consulted. I.V.: Adults:

Multiple myeloma (first-line therapy; in combination with melphalan and prednisone): 1.3 mg/m^2 days 1, 4, 8, 11, 22, 25, 29, and 32 of a 42-day treatment cycle for 4 cycles, followed by 1.3 mg/m^2 days 1, 8, 22, and 29 of a 42-day treatment cycle for 5 cycles.

Relapsed multiple myeloma and mantle cell lymphoma: 1.3 mg/m^2 twice weekly for 2 weeks on days 1, 4, 8, and 11 of a 21-day treatment cycle. Consecutive doses should be separated by at least 72 hours. Therapy extending beyond 8 cycles may be given once weekly for 4 weeks (days 1, 8, 15, and 22), followed by a 13-day rest (days 23 through 35).

Non-Hodgkin's lymphoma, other than mantle cell (unlabeled use): 1.3-1.5 mg/m^2 twice weekly for 2 weeks on days 1, 4, 8, and 11 of a 21-day treatment cycle.

Waldenstrom's macroglobinemia (unlabeled use): 1.3 mg/m^2 days 1, 4, 8, and 11 of a 21-day treatment cycle (Chen, 2007)

Dosage adjustment in renal impairment: Dosage adjustment not necessary. **Note:** Dialysis may reduce bortezomib concentrations; administer postdialysis.

Dosage adjustment in hepatic impairment: Specific guidelines are not available; clearance may be decreased; monitor closely for toxicity

Dosage adjustment for toxicity:

Myeloma (first-line therapy):

Platelets should be ≥70,000/mm^3, ANC should be ≥1000/mm^3, and nonhematologic toxicities should resolve to grade 1 or baseline prior to therapy initiation.

Platelets ≤30,000/mm^3 or ANC <750/mm^3 on bortezomib day(s): Withhold bortezomib; if several consecutive bortezomib doses are withheld, reduce dose 1 level (1.3 mg/m^2/dose reduced to 1 mg/m^2/dose; 1 mg/m^2/dose reduced to 0.7 mg/m^2/dose).

Grade ≥3 nonhematological toxicity (other than neuropathy): Withhold bortezomib until toxicity resolves to grade 1 or baseline. May reinitiate bortezomib at 1 dose level reduction (1.3 mg/m^2/dose reduced to 1 mg/m^2/dose; 1 mg/m^2/dose reduced to 0.7 mg/m^2/dose).

Neuropathic pain and/or peripheral sensory neuropathy: See "Neuropathic pain and/or peripheral sensory neuropathy" toxicity adjustment guidelines.

Relapsed multiple myeloma and mantle cell lymphoma:

Grade 3 nonhematological (excluding neuropathy) or Grade 4 hematological toxicity: Withhold until toxicity resolved; may reinitiate with a 25% dose reduction (1.3 mg/m^2/dose reduced to 1 mg/m^2/dose; 1 mg/m^2/dose reduced to 0.7 mg/m^2/dose)

Neuropathic pain and/or peripheral sensory neuropathy:

Grade 1 without pain or loss of function: No action needed

Grade 1 with pain or Grade 2 interfering with function but not activities of daily living: Reduce dose to 1 mg/m^2

Grade 2 with pain or Grade 3 interfering with activities of daily living: Withhold until toxicity resolved, may reinitiate at 0.7 mg/m^2 once weekly

Grade 4: Discontinue therapy

Combination Regimens

Multiple myeloma:

Administration Administer via rapid I.V. push (3-5 seconds)

Monitoring Parameters Signs/symptoms of peripheral neuropathy, dehydration, or hypotension; CBC with differential and platelets (monitor frequently throughout therapy); renal function, pulmonary function (with new or worsening pulmonary symptoms), liver function tests (in patients with existing hepatic impairment)

Dietary Considerations Green tea and green tea extracts may diminish the therapeutic effect of bortezomib and should be avoided (Golden, 2009). Avoid grapefruit juice.

Emetic Potential Low (10% to 30%)

Vesicant May be an irritant

Dosage Forms Excipient information presented when available (limited, particularly for generics); consult specific product labeling.

Injection, powder for reconstitution [preservative free]:

Velcade®: 3.5 mg [contains mannitol 35 mg]

References

Andre P, Cisternino S, Chiadmi F, et al, "Stability of Bortezomib 1-mg/mL Solution in Plastic Syringe and Glass Vial," *Ann Pharmacother*, 2005, 39(9):1462-6.

Chanan-Khan AA, Kaufman JL, Mehta J, et al, "Activity and Safety of Bortezomib in Multiple Myeloma Patients With Advanced Renal Failure: A Multicenter Retrospective Study," *Blood*, 2006, 109(9):2604-6.

Chen CI, Kouroukis CT, White D, et al, "Bortezomib is Active in Patients With Untreated or Relapsed Waldenstrom's Macroglobulinemia: A Phase II Study of the National Cancer Institute of Canada Clinical Trials Group," *J Clin Oncol*, 2007, 25(12):1570-5.

Fisher RI, Bernstein SH, Kahl BS, et al, "Multicenter Phase II Study of Bortezomib in Patients With Relapsed or Refractory Mantle Cell Lymphoma," *J Clin Oncol*, 2006, 24(30):4867-74.

Golden EB, Lam PY, Kardosh A, et al, "Green Tea Polyphenols Block the Anticancer Effects of Bortezomib and Other Boronic Acid-Based Proteasome Inhibitors," *Blood*, 2009.

Goy A, Younes A, McLaughlin P, et al, "Phase II Study of Proteasome Inhibitor Bortezomib in Relapsed or Refractory B-cell Non-Hodgkin's Lymphoma," *J Clin Oncol*, 2005, 23(4):667-75.

Jagannath S, Barlogie B, Berenson JR, et al, "Bortezomib in Recurrent and/or Refractory Multiple Myeloma; Initial Clinical Experience in Patients With Impaired Renal Function," *Cancer*, 2005, 103(6):1195-200.

Kastritis E, Anagnostopoulos A, Bamias A, et al, "Reversibility of Renal Failure in Newly Diagnosed Patients With Multiple Myeloma Treated With High-Dose Dexamethasone Containing Regimens and the Impact of Novel Agents," *Blood*, 2006, 108(11):3586. Abstract from ASH Annual Meeting.

Mulkerin D, Remick S, Ramanathan R, et al, "A Dose-Escalating and Pharmacologic Study of Bortezomib in Adult Cancer Patients With Impaired Renal Function," *J Clin Oncol*, ASCO Annual Meeting Proceedings, 2006, Part I, 24(18S):2032.

O'Connor OA, Wright J, Moskowitz C, et al "Phase II Clinical Experience With the Novel Proteasome Inhibitor Bortezomib in Patients With Indolent Non-Hodgkin's Lymphoma and Mantle Cell Lymphoma," *J Clin Oncol*, 2005, 23(4):676-84.

Richardson PG, Sonneveld P, Schuster MW, et al, "Bortezomib or High-Dose Dexamethasone for Relapsed Multiple Myeloma," *N Engl J Med*, 2005, 352(24):2487-98.

San-Miguel JF, Richardson PG, Sonneveld P, et al, "Efficacy and Safety of Bortezomib in Patients With Renal Impairment: Results from the APEX Phase 3 Study," *Leukemia*, 2008, 22(4):842-9.
San-Miguel JF, Schlag R, Khuageva N, et al, "Bortezomib Plus Melphalan and Prednisone for Initial Treatment of Multiple Myeloma," *N Engl J Med*2008, 359(9):906-17.

◆ **BRL 43694** *see* Granisetron *on page 552*

Busulfan (byoo SUL fan)

Medication Safety Issues

Sound-alike/look-alike issues:

Busulfan may be confused with Butalan®

Myleran® may be confused with Alkeran®, Leukeran®, melphalan, Mylicon®

High alert medication: The Institute for Safe Medication Practices (ISMP) includes this medication among its list of drugs which have a heightened risk of causing significant patient harm when used in error.

Related Information

Fertility and Cancer Therapy *on page 1430*

Hematopoietic Stem Cell Transplantation *on page 1501*

Management of Drug Extravasations *on page 1447*

Safe Handling of Hazardous Drugs *on page 1517*

U.S. Brand Names Busulfex®; Myleran®

Index Terms NSC-750

Generic Available No

Canadian Brand Names Busulfex®; Myleran®

Pharmacologic Category Antineoplastic Agent, Alkylating Agent

Use

Oral: Chronic myelogenous leukemia (CML); conditioning regimens for bone marrow transplantation

I.V.: Combination therapy with cyclophosphamide as a conditioning regimen prior to allogeneic hematopoietic progenitor cell transplantation for chronic myelogenous leukemia

Unlabeled/Investigational Use Oral: Bone marrow disorders, such as polycythemia vera and myeloid metaplasia; thrombocytosis

Pregnancy Risk Factor D

Lactation Excretion in breast milk unknown/not recommended

Labeled Contraindications Hypersensitivity to busulfan or any component of the formulation; oral busulfan is contraindicated in patients without a definitive diagnosis of CML

Warnings/Precautions Hazardous agent - use appropriate precautions for handling and disposal. **[U.S. Boxed Warning]: May induce severe bone marrow suppression.** May result in severe neutropenia, thrombocytopenia and/or anemia. Seizures have been reported with use; use caution in patients predisposed to seizures; initiate prophylactic anticonvulsant therapy (eg, phenytoin) prior to treatment; use caution with history of seizures or head trauma. May cause delayed pulmonary toxicity (known as "busulfan lung" - bronchopulmonary dysplasia with pulmonary fibrosis); the average onset is 4 years (range: 4 months to 10 years). Cardiac tamponade as been reported in children with thalassemia treated with high-dose oral busulfan in combination with cyclophosphamide. Busulfan has been causally related to the development of secondary malignancies (tumors and acute leukemias). Busulfan has been associated with ovarian failure (including failure to achieve puberty).

High busulfan area under the concentration versus time curve (AUC) values (>1500 μM/minute) are associated with increased risk of hepatic veno-occlusive disease during conditioning for allogenic BMT; patients with of history of radiation therapy, prior chemotherapy (≥3 cycles) and prior stem cell transplantation are at increased risk. Oral busulfan doses above 16 mg/kg (based on IBW) and concurrent use with alkylating agents may also increase the risk for hepatic VOD. The solvent in I.V. busulfan, DMA, may impair fertility. DMA may also be associated with hepatotoxicity, hallucinations, somnolence, lethargy, and confusion. **[U.S. Boxed Warning]: Should be administered under the supervision of an experienced cancer chemotherapy physician.**

Adverse Reactions

I.V.:

>10%:

Cardiovascular: Tachycardia (44%), hypertension (36%; grades 3/4: 7%), edema (28% to 79%), thrombosis (33%), chest pain (26%), vasodilation (25%), hypotension (11%; grades 3/4: 3%)

Central nervous system: Insomnia (84%), fever (80%), anxiety (72% to 75%), headache (69%), chills (46%), pain (44%), dizziness (30%), depression (23%), confusion (11%)

Dermatologic: Rash (57%), pruritus (28%), alopecia (2% to 15%)

Endocrine & metabolic: Hypomagnesemia (77%), hyperglycemia (66%; grades 3/4: 15%), hypokalemia (64%), hypocalcemia (49%), hypophosphatemia (17%)

Gastrointestinal: Nausea (98%), mucositis/stomatitis (97%; grades 3/4: 26%), vomiting (43% to 95%), anorexia (85%), diarrhea (84%; grades 3/4: 5%), abdominal pain (72%), dyspepsia (44%), constipation (38%), xerostomia (26%), rectal disorder (25%), abdominal fullness (23%)

Hematologic: Myelosuppression (≤100%), neutropenia (100%; median recovery: 13 days), thrombocytopenia (98%; median onset: 5-6 days), lymphopenia (children: 79%), anemia (69%)

Hepatic: Hyperbilirubinemia (49%; grades 3/4: 30%), ALT increased (31%; grades 3/4: 7%), veno-occlusive disease (adults: 8% to 12%; children: 21%), jaundice (12%)

Local: Injection site inflammation (25%), injection site pain (15%)

Neuromuscular & skeletal: Weakness (51%), back pain (23%), myalgia (16%), arthralgia (13%)

Renal: Creatinine increased (21%), oliguria (15%)

Respiratory: Rhinitis (44%), lung disorder (34%), cough (28%), epistaxis (25%), dyspnea (25%), pneumonia (children: 21%), hiccup (18%), pharyngitis (18%)

Miscellaneous: Infection (51%), allergic reaction (26%)

1% to 10%:

Cardiovascular: Arrhythmia (5%), cardiomegaly (5%), atrial fibrillation (2%), ECG abnormal (2%), heart block (2%), heart failure (grade 3/4: 2%), pericardial effusion (2%), tamponade (children with thalassemia: 2%), ventricular extrasystoles (2%), hypervolemia

Central nervous system: Lethargy (7%), hallucination (5%), agitation (2%), delirium (2%), encephalopathy (2%), seizure (2%), somnolence (2%), cerebral hemorrhage (1%)

Dermatologic: Vesicular rash (10%), vesiculobullous rash (10%), skin discoloration (8%), maculopapular rash (8%), acne (7%), exfoliative dermatitis (5%), erythema nodosum (2%)

Endocrine & metabolic: Hyponatremia (2%)

Gastrointestinal: Ileus (8%), weight gain (8%), hematemesis (2%), pancreatitis (2%)

Hematologic: Prothrombin time increased (2%)

Hepatic: Hepatomegaly (6%)

◄ Renal: Hematuria (8%), dysuria (7%), hemorrhagic cystitis (grade 3/4: 7%), BUN increased (3%)

Respiratory: Asthma (8%), alveolar hemorrhage (5%), hyperventilation (5%), hemoptysis (3%), pleural effusion (3%), sinusitis (3%), atelectasis (2%), hypoxia (2%)

Oral: Frequency not defined:

Central nervous system: Seizure

Dermatologic: Hyperpigmentation of skin (busulfan tan 5% to 10%), alopecia, rash, urticaria

Endocrine & metabolic: Amenorrhea, ovarian suppression

Hematologic: Myelosuppression (anemia, leukopenia, thrombocytopenia), pancytopenia

I.V. and/or Oral: Infrequent, postmarketing, and/or case reports: Acute leukemias, adrenal suppression, alopecia (permanent), aplastic anemia (may be irreversible), azoospermia, blurred vision, cataracts, cheilosis, cholestatic jaundice, corneal thinning, dry skin, endocardial fibrosis, erythema multiforme, erythema nodosum, esophageal varices, gynecomastia, hemorrhagic cystitis, hepatic dysfunction, hepatocellular atrophy, hyperuricemia, hyperuricosuria, interstitial pulmonary fibrosis (busulfan lung; manifested by a diffuse interstitial pulmonary fibrosis and persistent cough, fever, rales, and dyspnea; may be relieved by corticosteroids); malignant tumors, myasthenia gravis, ocular (lens) changes, ovarian failure, porphyria cutanea tarda, radiation myelopathy, radiation recall (skin rash), sepsis, sterility, testicular atrophy

Drug Interactions

Metabolism/Transport Effects Substrate of CYP3A4 (major)

Avoid Concomitant Use

Avoid concomitant use of Busulfan with any of the following: Natalizumab; Vaccines (Live)

Increased Effect/Toxicity

Busulfan may increase the levels/effects of: Leflunomide; Natalizumab; Vaccines (Live); Vitamin K Antagonists

The levels/effects of Busulfan may be increased by: Antifungal Agents (Azole Derivatives, Systemic); CYP3A4 Inhibitors (Moderate); CYP3A4 Inhibitors (Strong); Dasatinib; MetroNIDAZOLE; Trastuzumab

Decreased Effect

Busulfan may decrease the levels/effects of: Vaccines (Inactivated); Vaccines (Live); Vitamin K Antagonists

The levels/effects of Busulfan may be decreased by: CYP3A4 Inducers (Strong); Deferasirox; Echinacea; Herbs (CYP3A4 Inducers)

Ethanol/Nutrition/Herb Interactions

Ethanol: Avoid ethanol due to GI irritation.

Food: No clear or firm data on the effect of food on busulfan bioavailability.

Herb/Nutraceutical: Avoid St John's wort (may decrease busulfan levels).

Storage/Stability

Injection: Store unopened ampuls and vials under refrigeration (2°C to 8°C). Final solution is stable for up to 8 hours at room temperature (25°C); the infusion must be completed within that 8-hour timeframe. Dilution of busulfan injection in 0.9% sodium chloride is stable for up to 12 hours at refrigeration (2°C to 8°C); the infusion must be completed within that 12-hour timeframe.

Tablet: Store at room temperature at 15°C to 30°C (59°F to 86°F).

Reconstitution Injection: Dilute (using manufacturer provided 5-micron filters for ampuls) in 0.9% sodium chloride injection or dextrose 5% in water. The dilution volume of busulfan injection, ensuring that the final concentration of busulfan is 0.5 mg/mL.

Compatibility Variable stability (consult detailed reference) in D_5W, NS.

Mechanism of Action Busulfan is an alkylating agent which reacts with the N-7 position of guanosine and interferes with DNA replication and transcription of RNA. Busulfan has a more marked effect on myeloid cells than on lymphoid cells and is also very toxic to hematopoietic stem cells. Busulfan exhibits little immunosuppressive activity. Interferes with the normal function of DNA by alkylation and cross-linking the strands of DNA.

Pharmacodynamics/Kinetics

Duration: 28 days

Absorption: Rapid and complete

Distribution: V_d: ~1 L/kg; into CSF and saliva with levels similar to plasma

Protein binding: 32% to plasma proteins and 47% to red blood cells

Metabolism: Extensively hepatic (may increase with multiple doses); glutathione conjugation followed by oxidation

Half-life elimination: After first dose: 3.4 hours; After last dose: 2.3 hours

Time to peak, serum: Oral: Within 4 hours; I.V.: Within 5 minutes

Excretion: Urine (10% to 50% as metabolites) within 24 hours (<2% as unchanged drug)

Dosage Note: Premedicate with prophylactic anticonvulsant therapy (eg, phenytoin) prior to high-dose busulfan treatment.

Children:

CML, remission induction: Oral: 0.06-0.12 mg/kg/day **or** 1.8-4.6 mg/m²/day; titrate dosage to maintain leukocyte count above 40,000/mm³; reduce dosage by 50% if the leukocyte count reaches 30,000-40,000/mm³; discontinue drug if counts fall to ≤20,000/mm³

BMT marrow-ablative conditioning regimen:

Oral: 1 mg/kg/dose (ideal body weight) every 6 hours for 16 doses

I.V.:

≤12 kg: 1.1 mg/kg/dose (ideal body weight) every 6 hours for 16 doses

>12 kg: 0.8 mg/kg/dose (ideal body weight) every 6 hours for 16 doses

Adjust dose to desired AUC [1125 µmol(min)] using the following formula:

Adjusted dose (mg) = Actual dose (mg) x [target AUC µmol(min) / actual AUC µmol(min)]

Adults:

CML, remission induction: Oral: 60 mcg/kg/day or 1.8 mg/m²/day; usual range: 4-8 mg/day (may be as high as 12 mg/day); Maintenance doses: 1-4 mg/day to 2 mg/week to maintain WBC 10,000-20,000 cells/mm³

BMT marrow-ablative conditioning regimen:

Oral: 1 mg/kg/dose (ideal body weight) every 6 hours for 16 doses

I.V.: 0.8 mg/kg (ideal body weight or actual body weight, whichever is lower); for obese or severely-obese patients adjusted ideal body weight is recommended) every 6 hours for 4 days (a total of 16 doses)

Polycythemia vera (unlabeled use): Oral: 2-6 mg/day

Thrombocytosis (unlabeled use): Oral: 4-6 mg/day

Dosing adjustment in renal impairment: I.V.: Has not been studied in patients with renal impairment per the FDA-approved labeling. Some clinicians suggest adjustment is not necessary (Aronoff, 2007).

◄

Dosing adjustment in hepatic impairment: I.V.: Has not been administered in clinical studies in patients with hepatic impairment per the FDA-approved labeling. Busulfan has extensive hepatic metabolism and risk of hepatic veno-occlusive disease with high doses; dosage adjustment may be needed.

Administration Intravenous busulfan should be administered as a 2-hour via central line.

BMT only: To facilitate ingestion of high oral doses, insert multiple tablets into gelatin capsules.

Monitoring Parameters CBC with differential and platelet count, liver function tests (evaluate transaminases, alkaline phosphatase, and bilirubin daily for at least 28 days post transplant)

Additional Information Oncology Comment: Low-dose monotherapy with oral busulfan for the palliative treatment of CML is no longer common. Treatment with imatinib or hematopoietic stem cell transplant (HSCT) are considered the primary treatments for CML (NCCN v1.2008).

Emetic Potential

≥4 mg/day: Moderate (30% to 90%)

<4 mg/day: Very low (<10%)

Vesicant May be an irritant

High Dose Considerations

Comments Phenytoin or clonazepam should be administered prophylacti-cally during and for at least 48 hours following completion of busulfan. Risk of seizures is increased in patients with sickle cell disease. Increased risk of VOD when busulfan AUC >3000 µmol(min)/L (mean AUC, 2012 µmol (min)/L). Increased risk of failure to engraft for allogeneic BMT patients when AUC is <900 µmol (min)/L. To facilitate ingestion of high doses, multiple tablets may be inserted into gelatin capsules. Ursodiol 9-12 mg/kg/day may reduce the level of regimen-related hyperbilirubinemia.

High Dose Note: Generally combined with other high-dose chemo-therapeutic drugs or total body irradiation.

Oral:

0.875-1 mg/kg/dose every 6 hours for 16 doses; total dose: 12-16 mg/kg

37.5 mg/m^2 every 6 hours for 16 doses; total dose: 600 mg/m^2 (studied primarily in pediatric patients)

150 mg/m^2 daily for 4 days; total dose: 600 mg/m^2 (studied primarily in pediatric patients)

I.V.: 0.8 mg/kg every 6 hours for 16 doses (4 days)

Unique Toxicities

Central nervous system: Generalized or myoclonic seizures and loss of consciousness, abnormal electroencephalographic findings

Gastrointestinal: Mucositis, anorexia, moderately emetogenic

Hepatic: Veno-occlusive disease (VOD), hyperbilirubinemia

Respiratory: Idiopathic pneumonia syndrome

Miscellaneous: Transient pain at tumor sites, transient autoimmune disorders

Dosage Forms Excipient information presented when available (limited, particularly for generics); consult specific product labeling.

Injection, solution:

Busulfex®: 6 mg/mL (10 mL) [contains N,N-dimethylacetamide (DMA)]

Tablet:

Myleran®: 2 mg

References

Aronoff GR, Bennett WM, Berns JS, et al, *Drug Prescribing in Renal Failure: Dosing Guidelines for Adults and Children*, 5th ed. Philadelphia, PA: American College of Physicians; 2007, p 97.

Booth BP, Rahman A, Dagher R, et al, "Population Pharmacokinetic-Based Dosing of Intravenous Busulfan in Pediatric Patients," *J Clin Pharmacol*, 2007, 47(1):101-11.

National Comprehensive Cancer Network (NCCN) "Practice Guidelines in Oncology: Antiemesis Version 3.2008." Available at http://www.nccn.org/professionals/physician_gls/PDF/antiemesis.pdf

National Comprehensive Cancer Network (NCCN) "Practice Guidelines in Oncology: Chronic Myelogenous Leukemia Version 1.2008." Available at http://www.nccn.org/professionals/physician_gls/PDF/cml.pdf

Seddon BM, Cassoni AM, Galloway MJ, et al, "Fatal Radiation Myelopathy After High-Dose Busulfan and Melphalan Chemotherapy and Radiotherapy for Ewing's Sarcoma: A Review of the Literature and Implications for Practice," *Clin Oncol (R Coll Radiol)*, 2005, 17(5):385-90.

Shaw PJ, Nath C, Berry A, et al, "Busulphan Given as Four Single Daily Doses of 150 mg/m² Is Safe and Effective in Children of All Ages," *Bone Marrow Transplant*, 2004, 34(3):197-205.

Vassal G, Gouyette A, Hartmann O, et al, "Pharmacokinetics of High-Dose Busulfan in Children," *Cancer Chemother Pharmacol*, 1989, 24(6):386-90.

- ◆ **Busulfex®** *see Busulfan on page 160*
- ◆ **C2B8 Monoclonal Antibody** *see RiTUXimab on page 1017*
- ◆ **C225** *see Cetuximab on page 211*
- ◆ **Caelyx® (Can)** *see DOXOrubicin (Liposomal) on page 379*
- ◆ **CAFdA** *see Clofarabine on page 250*
- ◆ **Calcijex®** *see Calcitriol on page 168*
- ◆ **Calcimar® (Can)** *see Calcitonin on page 165*

Calcitonin (kal si TOE nin)

Medication Safety Issues

Sound-alike/look-alike issues:
Calcitonin may be confused with calcitriol
Miacalcin® may be confused with Micatin®

Calcitonin nasal spray is administered as a single spray into **one** nostril daily, using alternate nostrils each day.

U.S. Brand Names Fortical®; Miacalcin®

Index Terms Calcitonin (Salmon)

Generic Available Yes: Intranasal solution

Canadian Brand Names Apo-Calcitonin®; Calcimar®; Caltine®; Miacalcin® NS; Pro-Calcitonin

Pharmacologic Category Antidote; Hormone

Use Calcitonin (salmon): Treatment of Paget's disease of bone (osteitis deformans); adjunctive therapy for hypercalcemia; treatment of osteoporosis in women >5 years postmenopause

Pregnancy Risk Factor C

Lactation Excretion in breast milk unknown/not recommended

Labeled Contraindications Hypersensitivity to calcitonin salmon or any component of the formulation

Warnings/Precautions A skin test should be performed prior to initiating therapy of calcitonin salmon in patients with suspected sensitivity; have epinephrine immediately available for a possible hypersensitivity reaction. A detailed skin testing protocol is available from the manufacturers. Temporarily withdraw use of nasal spray if ulceration of nasal mucosa occurs. Patients >65 years of age may experience a higher incidence of nasal adverse events with calcitonin nasal spray. Safety and efficacy have not been established in pediatric patients.

Adverse Reactions Unless otherwise noted, frequencies reported are with nasal spray.

>10%: Respiratory: Rhinitis (12%)

1% to 10%:

Cardiovascular: Flushing (nasal spray: <1%; injection: 2% to 5%), angina (1% to 3%), hypertension (1% to 3%)

Central nervous system: Depression (1% to 3%), dizziness (1% to 3%), fatigue (1% to 3%)

Dermatologic: Erythematous rash (1% to 3%)

Gastrointestinal: Abdominal pain (1% to 3%), constipation (1% to 3%), diarrhea (1% to 3%), dyspepsia (1% to 3%), nausea (injection: 10%; nasal spray: 1% to 3%)

Genitourinary: Cystitis (1% to 3%)

Local: Injection site reactions (injection: 10%)

Neuromuscular & skeletal: Back pain (5%), arthrosis (1% to 3%), myalgia (1% to 3%), paresthesia (1% to 3%)

Ocular: Conjunctivitis (1% to 3%), lacrimation abnormality (1% to 3%)

Respiratory: Bronchospasm (1% to 3%), sinusitis (1% to 3%), upper respiratory tract infection (1% to 3%)

Miscellaneous: Flu-like syndrome (1% to 3%), infection (1% to 3%), lymphadenopathy (1% to 3%)

<1%: Agitation, allergic reactions, alopecia, anaphylaxis, anemia, anorexia, anxiety, appetite increased, arthritis, blurred vision, bronchitis, bundle branch block, cerebrovascular accident, cholelithiasis, cough, diaphoresis, dyspnea, earache, eczema, fever, flatulence, gastritis, goiter, hearing loss, hematuria, hepatitis, hyperthyroidism, insomnia, migraine, myocardial infarction, neuralgia, nocturia, palpitation, parosmia, periorbital edema, pharyngitis, pneumonia, polymyalgia rheumatica, pruritus, pyelonephritis, rash, renal calculus, skin ulceration, stiffness, tachycardia, taste perversion, thirst, thrombophlebitis, tinnitus, vertigo, vitreous floater, vomiting, weight gain, xerostomia

Drug Interactions

Avoid Concomitant Use There are no known interactions where it is recommended to avoid concomitant use.

Increased Effect/Toxicity There are no known significant interactions involving an increase in effect.

Decreased Effect There are no known significant interactions involving a decrease in effect.

Ethanol/Nutrition/Herb Interactions Ethanol: Avoid ethanol (may increase risk of osteoporosis).

Storage/Stability

Injection: Store under refrigeration at 2°C to 8°C (36°F to 46°F); protect from freezing.

Nasal: Store unopened bottle under refrigeration at 2°C to 8°C (36°F to 46°F); do not freeze.

Fortical®: After opening, store for up to 30 days at 20°C to 25°C (68°F to 77°F); excursions permitted to 15°C to 30°C (59°F to 86°F). Store in upright position.

Miacalcin®: After opening, store for up to 35 days at room temperature of 15°C to 30°C (59°F to 86°F). Store in upright position.

Reconstitution Injection: NS has been recommended for the dilution to prepare a skin test in patients with suspected sensitivity.

Mechanism of Action Peptide sequence similar to human calcitonin; functionally antagonizes the effects of parathyroid hormone. Directly inhibits osteoclastic bone resorption; promotes the renal excretion of calcium, phosphate, sodium, magnesium, and potassium by decreasing tubular reabsorption; increases the jejunal secretion of water, sodium, potassium, and chloride

Pharmacodynamics/Kinetics

Hypercalcemia: I.M. or SubQ:
  Onset of action: ~2 hours
  Duration: 6-8 hours
Absorption: Nasal: ~3% of I.M. level (range: 0.3% to 31%)
Distribution: Does not cross placenta
Half-life elimination: SubQ: 1.2 hours; Nasal: 43 minutes
Time to peak: Nasal: ~30-40 minutes
Excretion: Urine (as inactive metabolites)

Dosage

Children: Dosage not established
Adults:
  Paget's disease (Miacalcin®): I.M., SubQ: Initial: 100 units/day; maintenance: 50 units/day or 50-100 units every 1-3 days
  Hypercalcemia (Miacalcin®): Initial: I.M., SubQ: 4 units/kg every 12 hours; may increase up to 8 units/kg every 12 hours to a maximum of every 6 hours
  Postmenopausal osteoporosis:
    I.M., SubQ: Miacalcin®: 100 units/every other day
    Intranasal: Fortical®, Miacalcin®: 200 units (1 spray) in one nostril daily

Administration

Injection solution: Administer I.M. or SubQ; intramuscular route is recommended over the subcutaneous route when the volume of calcitonin to be injected exceeds 2 mL.

Nasal spray: Before first use, allow bottle to reach room temperature, then prime pump by releasing at least 5 sprays until full spray is produced. To administer, place nozzle into nostril with head in upright position. Alternate nostrils daily. Do not prime pump before each daily use. Discard after 30 doses.

Monitoring Parameters Serum electrolytes and calcium; alkaline phosphatase and 24-hour urine collection for hydroxyproline excretion (Paget's disease), urinalysis (urine sediment); bone mineral density
Nasal formulation: Visualization of nasal mucosa, turbinate, septum, and mucosal blood vessels)

Dietary Considerations Adequate vitamin D and calcium intake is essential for preventing/treating osteoporosis. Patients with Paget's disease and hypercalcemia should follow a low calcium diet as prescribed.

Dosage Forms Excipient information presented when available (limited, particularly for generics); consult specific product labeling.
Injection, solution [calcitonin-salmon]:
  Miacalcin®: 200 int. units/mL (2 mL)
Solution, intranasal [spray, calcitonin-salmon]: 2200 int. units/mL (3.7 mL)
  Fortical®: 200 int. units/0.09 mL (3.7 mL) [rDNA origin; contains benzyl alcohol; delivers 30 doses, 200 units/actuation]
  Miacalcin®: 200 int. units/0.09 mL (3.7 mL) [contains benzalkonium chloride; delivers 30 doses, 200 units/actuation]

References

Bergqvist E, Sjoberg HE, Hjern B, et al, "Calcitonin in the Treatment of Hypercalcaemic Crisis," *Acta Med Scand*, 1972, 192(5):385-9.
Stevenson JC, "Current Management of Malignant Hypercalcemia," *Drugs*, 1988, 36(2):229-30.

◆ **Calcitonin (Salmon)** *see* Calcitonin *on page 165*

Calcitriol (kal si TRYE ole)

Medication Safety Issues

Sound-alike/look-alike issues:

Calcitriol may be confused with calcifediol, Calciferol®, calcitonin, calcium carbonate, captopril, colestipol, paricalcitol, ropinirole

Dosage is expressed in mcg (micrograms), **not** mg (milligrams); rare cases of acute overdose have been reported

U.S. Brand Names Calcijex®; Rocaltrol®; Vectical™

Index Terms 1,25 Dihydroxycholecalciferol

Generic Available Yes: Excludes ointment

Canadian Brand Names Calcijex®; Rocaltrol®

Pharmacologic Category Vitamin D Analog

Use

Oral, injection: Management of hypocalcemia in patients on chronic renal dialysis; management of secondary hyperparathyroidism in patients with chronic kidney disease (CKD); management of hypocalcemia in hypoparathyroidism and pseudohypoparathyroidism

Topical: Management of mild-to-moderate plaque psoriasis

Unlabeled/Investigational Use Decrease severity of psoriatic lesions in psoriatic vulgaris; vitamin D-dependent rickets

Pregnancy Risk Factor C (manufacturer); A/D (dose exceeding RDA recommendation) (expert analysis)

Lactation Enters breast milk/not recommended

Labeled Contraindications Hypersensitivity to calcitriol or any component of the formulation; hypercalcemia, vitamin D toxicity

Topical: There are no contraindications listed in the manufacturer's labeling.

Warnings/Precautions

Oral, injection: Adequate dietary (supplemental) calcium is necessary for clinical response to vitamin D. Excessive vitamin D may cause severe hypercalcemia, hypercalciuria, and hyperphosphatemia; calcium-phosphate product (serum calcium times phosphorus) must not exceed 70 mg^2/dL^2. Other forms of vitamin D should be withheld during therapy. Immobilization may increase risk of hypercalcemia and/or hypercalciuria. Maintain adequate hydration. Use caution in patients with malabsorption syndromes (efficacy may be limited and/or response may be unpredictable). Use of calcitriol for the treatment of secondary hyperparathyroidism associated with CKD is not recommended in patients with rapidly worsening kidney function or in noncompliant patients. Increased serum phosphate levels in patients with renal failure may lead to calcification; the use of an aluminum-containing phosphate binder is recommended along with a low phosphate diet in these patients. Use with caution in patients taking cardiac glycosides; digitalis toxicity is potentiated by hypocalcemia. Products may contain coconut (capsule) or palm seed oil (oral solution). Some products may contain tartrazine.

Topical: May cause hypercalcemia; if alterations in calcium occur, discontinue treatment until levels return to normal. For external use only; not for ophthalmic, oral, or intravaginal use. Do not apply to facial skin, eyes, or lips. Absorption may be increased with occlusive dressings. Avoid or limit excessive exposure to natural or artificial sunlight, or phototherapy. The safety and effectiveness has not been evaluated in patients with erythrodermic, exfoliative, or pustular psoriasis.

Adverse Reactions

Oral, I.V.: Frequency not defined.

Cardiovascular: Cardiac arrhythmia, hypertension

Central nervous system: Apathy, headache, hypothermia, psychosis, sensory disturbances, somnolence

Dermatologic: Erythema multiforme, pruritus

Endocrine & metabolic: Dehydration, growth suppression, hypercalcemia, hypercholesterolemia, hypermagnesemia, hyperphosphatemia, libido decreased, polydipsia

Gastrointestinal: Abdominal pain, anorexia, constipation, metallic taste, nausea, pancreatitis, stomach ache, vomiting, weight loss, xerostomia

Genitourinary: Nocturia, urinary tract infection

Hepatic: ALT increased, AST increased

Local: Injection site pain (mild)

Neuromuscular & skeletal: Bone pain, myalgia, dystrophy, soft tissue calcification, weakness

Ocular: Conjunctivitis, photophobia

Renal: Albuminuria, BUN increased, creatinine increased, hypercalciuria, nephrocalcinosis, polyuria

Respiratory: Rhinorrhea

Miscellaneous: Allergic reaction

Topical:

>10%: Endocrine: Hypercalcemia (≤24%)

1% to 10%:

Dermatologic: Skin discomfort (3%), pruritus (1% to 3%)

Genitourinary: Urine abnormality (4%)

Renal: Hypercalciuria (3%)

Postmarketing and/or case reports: Dermatitis (acute; blistering), erythema, hypercalcemia, kidney stones, skin burning

Drug Interactions

Metabolism/Transport Effects Induces CYP3A4 (weak)

Avoid Concomitant Use There are no known interactions where it is recommended to avoid concomitant use.

Increased Effect/Toxicity

Calcitriol may increase the levels/effects of: Cardiac Glycosides; Magnesium Salts

The levels/effects of Calcitriol may be increased by: CYP3A4 Inhibitors (Moderate); CYP3A4 Inhibitors (Strong); Dasatinib; Thiazide Diuretics

Decreased Effect

Calcitriol may decrease the levels/effects of: Saxagliptin

The levels/effects of Calcitriol may be decreased by: Bile Acid Sequestrants; Corticosteroids (Systemic); CYP3A4 Inducers (Strong); Deferasirox; Herbs (CYP3A4 Inducers)

Storage/Stability

Injection: Store at room temperature of 15°C to 30°C (59°F to 86°F). Protect from light.

Oral capsule, solution: Store at room temperature of 20°C to 25°C (68°F to 77°F). Protect from light.

Topical: Store at room temperature of 25°C (77°F); excursions permitted to 15°C to 30°C (59°F to 86°F); do not refrigerate; do not freeze.

Compatibility Stable in D_5W, NS, sterile water for injection.

◀ **Mechanism of Action** Calcitriol is a potent active metabolite of vitamin D. Vitamin D promotes absorption of calcium in the intestines and retention at the kidneys thereby increasing calcium levels in the serum; decreases excessive serum phosphatase levels, parathyroid hormone levels, and decreases bone resorption; increases renal tubule phosphate resorption

The mechanism by which calcitriol is beneficial in the treatment of psoriasis has not been established.

Pharmacodynamics/Kinetics

Onset of action: Oral: ~2-6 hours

Duration: Oral, I.V.: 3-5 days

Absorption: Oral: Rapid

Protein binding: 99.9%

Metabolism: Primarily to 1,24,25-trihydroxycholecalciferol and 1,24,25-trihydroxy ergocalciferol

Half-life elimination: Children ~27 hours; Normal adults: 5-8 hours; Hemodialysis: 16-22 hours

Time to peak, serum: Oral: 3-6 hours; Hemodialysis: 8-12 hours

Excretion: Primarily feces; urine

Dosage

Hypocalcemia in patients on chronic renal dialysis (manufacturer labeling): *Adults:*

Oral: 0.25 mcg/day or every other day (may require 0.5-1 mcg/day); increases should be made at 4- to 8-week intervals

I.V.: Initial: 1-2 mcg 3 times/week (0.02 mcg/kg) approximately every other day. Adjust dose at 2-4 week intervals; dosing range: 0.5-4 mcg 3 times/week

Hypocalcemia in hypoparathyroidism/pseudohypoparathyroidism (manufacturers labeling): Oral (evaluate dosage at 2- to 4-week intervals):

Children <1 year (unlabeled use): 0.04-0.08 mcg/kg once daily

Children 1-5 years: 0.25-0.75 mcg once daily

Children ≥6 years and Adults: Initial: 0.25 mcg/day, range: 0.5-2 mcg once daily

Secondary hyperparathyroidism associated with moderate-to-severe CKD in patients not on dialysis (manufacturer labeling): Oral:

Children <3 years: Initial dose: 0.01-0.015 mcg/kg/day

Children ≥3 years and Adults: 0.25 mcg/day; may increase to 0.5 mcg/day

K/DOQI guidelines for vitamin D therapy in CKD:

Children:

CKD stage 2, 3: Oral:

<10 kg: 0.05 mcg every other day

10-20 kg: 0.1-0.15 mcg/day

>20 kg: 0.25 mcg/day

Note: Treatment should only be started with serum 25(OH) D >30 ng/mL, serum iPTH >70 pg/mL, serum calcium <10 mg/dL and serum phosphorus less than or equal to the age appropriate level.

CKD stage 4: Oral:

<10 kg: 0.05 mcg every other day

10-20 kg: 0.1-0.15 mcg/day

>20 kg: 0.25 mcg/day

Note: Treatment should only be started with serum 25(OH) D >30 ng/mL, serum iPTH >110 pg/mL, serum calcium <10 mg/dL and serum phosphorus less than or equal to the age appropriate level.

CKD stage 5: Oral, I.V.: **Note:** The following initial doses are based on plasma PTH and serum calcium levels for patients with serum phosphorus <5.5 mg/dL in adolescents or <6.5 in infants and children, and Ca-P product <55 in adolescents or <65 in infants and children <12 years. Adjust dose based on serum phosphate, calcium and PTH levels. Administer dose with each dialysis session (3 times/week). Intermittent I.V./oral administration is more effective than daily oral dosing.

Plasma PTH 300-500 pg/mL and serum Ca <10 mg/dL: 0.0075 mcg/kg (maximum: 0.25 mcg/day)

Plasma PTH >500-1000 pg/mL and serum Ca <10 mg/dL: 0.015 mcg/kg (maximum: 0.5 mcg/day)

Plasma PTH >1000 pg/mL and serum Ca <10.5 mg/dL: 0.025 mcg/kg (maximum: 1 mcg/day)

Adults:

CKD stage 3: Oral: 0.25 mcg/day. Treatment should only be started with serum 25(OH) D >30 ng/mL, serum iPTH >70 pg/mL, serum calcium <9.5 mg/dL and serum phosphorus <4.6 mg/dL

CKD stage 4: Oral: 0.25 mcg/day. Treatment should only be started with serum 25(OH) D >30 ng/mL, serum iPTH >110 pg/mL, serum calcium <9.5 mg/dL and serum phosphorus <4.6 mg/dL

CKD stage 5:

Peritoneal dialysis: Oral: Initial: 0.5-1 mcg 2-3 times/week or 0.25 mcg/day

Hemodialysis: **Note:** The following initial doses are based on plasma PTH and serum calcium levels for patients with serum phosphorus <5.5 mg/dL and Ca-P product <55. Adjust dose based on serum phosphate, calcium, and PTH levels. Intermittent I.V. administration may be more effective than daily oral dosing.

Plasma PTH 300-600 pg/mL and serum Ca <9.5 mg/dL: Oral, I.V.: 0.5-1.5 mcg

Plasma PTH 600-1000 pg/mL and serum Ca <9.5 mg/dL:

Oral: 1-4 mcg

I.V.: 1-3 mcg

Plasma PTH >1000 pg/mL and serum Ca <10 mg/dL:

Oral: 3-7 mcg

I.V.: 3-5 mcg

Psoriasis: Adults: Topical: Apply twice daily to affected areas (maximum: 200 g/week)

Vitamin D-dependent rickets (unlabeled use): Children and Adults: Oral: 1 mcg once daily

Elderly: No dosage recommendations, but start at the lower end of the dosage range

Dosage adjustment for toxicity: K/DOQI guidelines: Children and Adults: CKD stage 3 and 4:

iPTH below target: Hold calcitriol until levels rise then resume treatment at half the previous dose. If the lowest dose was being used, switch to alternate day therapy.

Corrected total calcium >9.5 mg/dL (adults) or 10.2 mg/dL (children): Hold calcitriol until serum calcium returns to <9.5 mg/dL (adults) or <9.8 mg/dL (children) then resume treatment at half the previous dose. If the lowest dose was being used, switch to alternate day therapy.

Serum phosphorus >4.6 mg/dL (adults) or greater than the age appropriate limits in children: Hold calcitriol (or add/increase dose of phosphate binder) until levels of phosphorous decrease, then resume at half the prior dose.

◄ **Combination Regimens**
  Prostate cancer: Estramustine + Docetaxel + Calcitriol on page 1313
Administration
  I.V.: May be administered as a bolus dose I.V. through the catheter at the end of hemodialysis.
  Oral: May be administered without regard to food. Administer with meals to reduce GI problems.
  Topical: Apply externally; not for ophthalmic, oral, or intravaginal use. Do not apply to eyes, lips, or facial skins. Rub in gently so that no medication remains visible. Limit application to only the areas of skin affected by psoriasis.
Monitoring Parameters Signs and symptoms of vitamin D intoxication; alkaline phosphatase, serum creatinine
  Serum calcium and phosphorus:
    CKD stage 2-4: Every month for the first 3 months, then every 3 months
    CKD stage 5: Every 2 weeks for 1 month, then monthly
  Serum or plasma intact PTH (iPTH):
    CKD stage 3 and 4: Every 3 months for 6 months, then every 3 months
    CKD stage 5: Monthly for 3 months, then every 3 months
Dietary Considerations May be taken without regard to food. Give with meals to reduce GI problems. Adequate calcium intake should be maintained during therapy; dietary phosphorous may need to be restricted.
Dosage Forms Excipient information presented when available (limited, particularly for generics); consult specific product labeling.
  Capsule, softgel: 0.25 mcg, 0.5 mcg
    Rocaltrol®: 0.25 mcg [contains coconut oil]; 0.5 mcg [contains coconut oil]
  Injection, solution: 1 mcg/mL (1 mL)
    Calcijex®: 1 mcg/mL (1 mL) [contains aluminum]
  Ointment, topical:
    Vectical™: 3 mcg/g (100 g)
  Solution, oral: 1 mcg/mL (15 mL)
    Rocaltrol®: 1 mcg/mL (15 mL) [contains palm seed oil]
References
  "K/DOQI Clinical Practice Guidelines for Bone Metabolism and Disease in Children With Chronic Kidney Disease," *Am J Kidney Dis*, 2005, 46(4 Suppl 1):1-121.
  "K/DOQI Clinical Practice Guidelines for Bone Metabolism and Disease in Chronic Kidney Disease. Guideline 1. Evaluation of Calcium and Phosphorus Metabolism," *Am J Kidney Dis*, 2003, 42(4 Suppl 3):52-7.
  "K/DOQI Clinical Practice Guidelines for Chronic Kidney Disease: Evaluation, Classification, and Stratification, Part 4. Definition and Classification of Stages of Chronic Kidney Disease," *Am J Kidney Dis*, 2002, 39(2 Suppl 1):46-75.
  "K/DOQI Clinical Practice Guidelines for Bone Metabolism and Disease in Chronic Kidney Disease. Guideline 3. Evaluation of Serum Phosphorus Levels," *Am J Kidney Dis*, 2003, 42(4 Suppl 3):62-3.
  "K/DOQI Clinical Practice Guidelines for Chronic Kidney Disease: Evaluation, Classification, and Stratification, Part 6. Serum Calcium and Calcium-Phosphorus Product," *Am J Kidney Dis*, 2003, 42(4 Suppl 3):77-84.
  "K/DOQI Clinical Practice Guidelines for Bone Metabolism and Disease in Chronic Kidney Disease. Guideline 8A. Active Vitamin D Therapy in Patients With Stages 3 and 4 CKD," *Am J Kidney Dis*, 2003, 42(4 Suppl 3):89-92.
  "K/DOQI Clinical Practice Guidelines for Bone Metabolism and Disease in Chronic Kidney Disease. Guideline 8B. Vitamin D Therapy in Patients on Dialysis (CKD Stage 5)," *Am J Kidney Dis*, 2003, 42(4 Suppl 3):92-98.

◆ **Calcium Leucovorin** *see* Leucovorin Calcium *on page* 697

◆ **Calcium Levoleucovorin** *see* LEVOleucovorin *on page* 714

◆ **Caldecort® [OTC]** *see* Hydrocortisone *on page* 575

- **Caltine® (Can)** *see* Calcitonin *on page* 165
- **Campath®** *see* Alemtuzumab *on page* 30
- **Campath-1H** *see* Alemtuzumab *on page* 30
- **Camptosar®** *see* Irinotecan *on page* 651
- **Camptothecin-11** *see* Irinotecan *on page* 651
- **Cancidas®** *see* Caspofungin *on page* 188
- **Candistatin® (Can)** *see* Nystatin *on page* 855
- **Canesten® Topical (Can)** *see* Clotrimazole *on page* 253
- **Canesten® Vaginal (Can)** *see* Clotrimazole *on page* 253
- **Cannabidiol and Tetrahydrocannabinol** *see* Tetrahydrocannabinol and Cannabidiol *on page* 1090

Capecitabine (ka pe SITE a been)

Medication Safety Issues

Sound-alike/look-alike issues:
Xeloda® may be confused with Xenical®

High alert medication: The Institute for Safe Medication Practices (ISMP) includes this medication among its list of drug classes which have a heightened risk of causing significant patient harm when used in error.

Related Information

Safe Handling of Hazardous Drugs *on page* 1517

U.S. Brand Names Xeloda®

Index Terms NSC-712807

Generic Available No

Canadian Brand Names Xeloda®

Pharmacologic Category Antineoplastic Agent, Antimetabolite; Antineoplastic Agent, Antimetabolite (Pyrimidine Analog)

Use Treatment of metastatic colorectal cancer; adjuvant therapy of Dukes' C colon cancer; treatment of metastatic breast cancer

Unlabeled/Investigational Use Treatment of gastric cancer, pancreatic cancer, esophageal cancer, ovarian cancer, metastatic renal cell cancer, neuroendocrine tumors, metastatic CNS lesions

Pregnancy Risk Factor D

Lactation Excretion in breast milk unknown/not recommended

Labeled Contraindications Hypersensitivity to capecitabine, fluorouracil, or any component of the formulation; known deficiency of dihydropyrimidine dehydrogenase (DPD); severe renal impairment (Cl_{cr} <30 mL/minute)

Warnings/Precautions Hazardous agent - use appropriate precautions for handling and disposal. Use with caution in patients with bone marrow suppression, ≥80 years of age, or renal or hepatic dysfunction. Patients with baseline moderate renal impairment require dose reduction. Patients with mild-to-moderate renal impairment require careful monitoring and subsequent dose reduction with any grade 2 or higher adverse event. Use with caution in patients who have received extensive pelvic radiation or alkylating therapy. Use cautiously with warfarin. Rare and unexpected severe toxicity may be attributed to dihydropyrimidine dehydrogenase (DPD) deficiency. Necrotizing enterocolitis (typhlitis) has been reported.

Capecitabine can cause severe diarrhea; median time to first occurrence is 34 days. Subsequent doses should be reduced after grade 3 or 4 diarrhea or recurrence of grade 2 diarrhea.

Hand-and-foot syndrome is characterized by numbness, dysesthesia/paresthesia, tingling, painless or painful swelling, erythema, desquamation, blistering, and severe pain. If grade 2 or 3 hand-and-foot syndrome occurs, interrupt administration of capecitabine until decreases to grade 1. Following grade 3 hand-and-foot syndrome, decrease subsequent doses of capecitabine. In patients with colorectal cancer, treatment with capecitabine immediately following 6 weeks of fluorouracil/leucovorin (FU/LV) therapy has been associated with an increased incidence of grade ≥3 toxicity, when compared to patients receiving the reverse sequence, capecitabine (two 3-week courses) followed by FU/LV (Hennig, 2008).

There has been cardiotoxicity associated with fluorinated pyrimidine therapy. May be more common in patients with a history of coronary artery disease. **[U.S. Boxed Warning]: Capecitabine may increase the anticoagulant effects of warfarin; monitor closely.**

Safety and efficacy in children <18 years of age have not been established.

Adverse Reactions Frequency listed derived from monotherapy trials.

>10%:

Cardiovascular: Edema (9% to 15%)

Central nervous system: Fatigue (16% to 42%), fever (7% to 18%), pain (12%)

Dermatologic: Palmar-plantar erythrodysesthesia (hand-and-foot syndrome) (54% to 60%; grade 3: 11% to 17%; may be dose limiting), dermatitis (27% to 37%)

Gastrointestinal: Diarrhea (47% to 57%; may be dose limiting; grade 3: 12% to 13%; grade 4: 2% to 3%), nausea (34% to 53%), vomiting (15% to 37%), abdominal pain (7% to 35%), stomatitis (22% to 25%), appetite decreased (26%), anorexia (9% to 23%), constipation (9% to 15%)

Hematologic: Lymphopenia (94%; grade 4: 14%), anemia (72% to 80%; grade 4: <1% to 1%), neutropenia (2% to 26%; grade 4: 2%), thrombocytopenia (24%; grade 4: 1%)

Hepatic: Bilirubin increased (22% to 48%; grades 3/4: 11% to 23%)

Neuromuscular & skeletal: Paresthesia (21%)

Ocular: Eye irritation (13% to 15%)

Respiratory: Dyspnea (14%)

5% to 10%:

Cardiovascular: Venous thrombosis (8%), chest pain (6%)

Central nervous system: Headache (5% to 10%), lethargy (10%), dizziness (6% to 8%), insomnia (7% to 8%), mood alteration (5%), depression (5%)

Dermatologic: Nail disorder (7%), rash (7%), skin discoloration (7%), alopecia (6%), erythema (6%)

Endocrine & metabolic: Dehydration (7%)

Gastrointestinal: Motility disorder (10%), oral discomfort (10%), dyspepsia (6% to 8%), upper GI inflammatory disorders (colorectal cancer: 8%), hemorrhage (6%), ileus (6%), taste perversion (colorectal cancer: 6%)

Neuromuscular & skeletal: Back pain (10%), weakness (10%), neuropathy (10%), myalgia (9%), arthralgia (8%), limb pain (6%)

Ocular: Abnormal vision (colorectal cancer: 5%), conjunctivitis (5%)

Respiratory: Cough (7%)

Miscellaneous: Viral infection (colorectal cancer: 5%)

<5%: Abdominal distension, angina, appetite increased, arthritis, ascites, asthma, ataxia, atrial fibrillation, bone pain, bradycardia, bronchitis, bronchopneumonia, bronchospasm, cachexia, cardiac arrest, cardiac failure, cardiomyopathy, cerebral vascular accident, cholestasis, coagulation

disorder, colitis, confusion, deep vein thrombosis, diaphoresis, duodenitis, dysarthria, dysphagia, dysrhythmia, ecchymoses, ECG changes, encephalopathy, epistaxis, esophagitis, fibrosis, fungal infection, gastric ulcer, gastritis, gastroenteritis, hematemesis, hemoptysis, hepatic fibrosis, hepatitis, hoarseness, hot flushes, hypokalemia, hypomagnesemia, hyper-/hypotension, hypersensitivity, hypertriglyceridemia, idiopathic thrombocytopenia purpura, ileus, impaired balance, infection, influenza-like illness, intestinal obstruction (~1%), irritability, joint stiffness, keratoconjunctivitis, laryngitis, leukopenia, loss of consciousness, lymphedema, MI, myocardial ischemia, myocarditis, necrotizing enterocolitis (typhlitis), nocturia, oral candidiasis, pericardial effusion, thrombocytopenic purpura, pancytopenia, photosensitivity reaction, pneumonia, proctalgia, pruritus, pulmonary embolism, radiation recall syndrome, renal impairment, respiratory distress, sedation, sepsis, skin ulceration, sore throat, tachycardia, thirst, thrombophlebitis, toxic megacolon, tremor, ventricular extrasystoles, vertigo, weight gain

Postmarketing and/or case reports: Fingerprint distortion (secondary to hand-and-foot syndrome), hepatic failure, lacrimal duct stenosis, multifocal leukoencephalopathy

Drug Interactions

Avoid Concomitant Use

Avoid concomitant use of Capecitabine with any of the following: Natalizumab; Vaccines (Live)

Increased Effect/Toxicity

Capecitabine may increase the levels/effects of: Carvedilol; CYP2C9 Substrates (High risk); Leflunomide; Natalizumab; Phenytoin; Vaccines (Live); Vitamin K Antagonists

The levels/effects of Capecitabine may be increased by: Leucovorin-Levoleucovorin; Trastuzumab

Decreased Effect

Capecitabine may decrease the levels/effects of: Vaccines (Inactivated); Vaccines (Live)

The levels/effects of Capecitabine may be decreased by: Echinacea

Ethanol/Nutrition/Herb Interactions Food: Food reduced the rate and extent of absorption of capecitabine.

Storage/Stability Store at room temperature of 25°C (77°F); excursions permitted between 15°C and 30°C (59°F and 86°F).

Mechanism of Action Capecitabine is a prodrug of fluorouracil. It undergoes hydrolysis in the liver and tissues to form fluorouracil which is the active moiety. Fluorouracil is a fluorinated pyrimidine antimetabolite that inhibits thymidylate synthetase, blocking the methylation of deoxyuridylic acid to thymidylic acid, interfering with DNA, and to a lesser degree, RNA synthesis. Fluorouracil appears to be phase specific for the G_1 and S phases of the cell cycle.

Pharmacodynamics/Kinetics

Absorption: Rapid and extensive

Protein binding: <60%; ~35% to albumin

Metabolism:

Hepatic: Inactive metabolites: 5'-deoxy-5-fluorocytidine, 5'-deoxy-5-fluorouridine

Tissue: Active metabolite: Fluorouracil

Half-life elimination: 0.5-1 hour

Time to peak: 1.5 hours; Fluorouracil: 2 hours

Excretion: Urine (96%, 57% as α-fluoro-β-alanine); feces (<3%)

Dosage Oral:

Adults: **Note:** Details concerning dosing in combination regimens should also be consulted. Capecitabine toxicities, particularly hand-foot syndrome, may be higher in North American populations (for the treatment of colorectal cancer); therapy initiation at doses of 1000 mg/m^2 twice daily (for 2 weeks every 21 days) may be considered (Haller, 2006; NCCN Colon Cancer Guidelines)

Metastatic breast cancer, metastatic colorectal cancer: 1250 mg/m^2 twice daily (morning and evening) for 2 weeks, every 21 days

Adjuvant therapy of Dukes' C colon cancer: Recommended for a total of 24 weeks (8 cycles of 2 weeks of drug administration and 1 week rest period.

Pancreatic cancer (unlabeled use): 1000-1250 mg/m^2 twice daily (morning and evening) for 2 weeks, every 21 days

Elderly: The elderly may be more sensitive to the toxic effects of fluorouracil. Insufficient data are available to provide dosage modifications.

Dosing adjustment in renal impairment:

Cl$_{cr}$ 51-80 mL/minute: No adjustment of initial dose

Cl$_{cr}$ 30-50 mL/minute: Administer 75% of normal dose

Cl$_{cr}$ <30 mL/minute: Use is contraindicated

Dosing adjustment in hepatic impairment:

Mild-to-moderate impairment: No starting dose adjustment is necessary; however, carefully monitor patients

Severe hepatic impairment: Patients have not been studied

Dosage modification guidelines: See table.

Refer to package labeling for modifications when administered in combination with docetaxel.

Recommended Dose Modifications

Toxicity NCI Grades	During a Course of Therapy (Monotherapy)	Dose Adjustment for Next Cycle (% of starting dose)
Grade 1	Maintain dose level	Maintain dose level
Grade 2 1st appearance	Interrupt until resolved to grade 0-1	100%
2nd appearance	Interrupt until resolved to grade 0-1	75%
3rd appearance	Interrupt until resolved to grade 0-1	50%
4th appearance	Discontinue treatment permanently	
Grade 3 1st appearance	Interrupt until resolved to grade 0-1	75%
2nd appearance	Interrupt until resolved to grade 0-1	50%
3rd appearance	Discontinue treatment permanently	
Grade 4 1st appearance	Discontinue permanently or If physician deems it to be in the patient's best interest to continue, interrupt until resolved to grade 0-1	50%

Dosage adjustments for hematologic toxicity in combination therapy with ixabepilone:
Neutrophils <500/mm^3 for ≥7 days or neutropenic fever: Hold for concurrent diarrhea or stomatitis until neutrophils recover to >1000/mm^3, then continue at same dose
Platelets <25,000/mm^3 (or <50,000/mm^3 with bleeding): Hold for concurrent diarrhea or stomatitis until platelets recover to >50,000/mm^3, then continue at same dose

Combination Regimens
Biliary adenocarcinoma:
CAPOX (Biliary Cancer) on page 1246
Gemcitabine-Capecitabine on page 1340
Breast cancer:
Bevacizumab-Capecitabine on page 1231
Capecitabine + Docetaxel (Breast Cancer) on page 1243
Capecitabine + Lapatinib on page 1245
Capecitabine-Trastuzumab on page 1245
Ixabepilone-Capecitabine on page 1361
TEX (Capecitabine + Docetaxel + Epirubicin) on page 1405
Colorectal cancer: CAPOX (Colorectal Cancer) on page 1246
Esophageal cancer:
Epirubicin-Cisplatin-Capecitabine (Esophageal Cancer) on page 1305
Epirubicin-Oxaliplatin-Capecitabine on page 1306
Gastric cancer:
Capecitabine + Docetaxel (Gastric Cancer) on page 1244
Epirubicin-Oxaliplatin-Capecitabine on page 1306
Lung cancer (nonsmall cell): Capecitabine-Docetaxel (NSCLC) on page 1244
Pancreatic cancer:
CAPOX (Pancreatic Cancer) on page 1247
Gemcitabine-Capecitabine on page 1340

Administration Usually administered in 2 divided doses taken 12 hours apart. Doses should be taken with water within 30 minutes after a meal.

Monitoring Parameters Renal function should be estimated at baseline to determine initial dose. During therapy, CBC with differential, hepatic function, and renal function should be monitored.

Dietary Considerations Because current safety and efficacy data are based upon administration with food, it is recommended that capecitabine be administered with food. In all clinical trials, patients were instructed to take with water within 30 minutes after a meal.

Additional Information Oncology Comment: An investigational uridine prodrug, vistonuridine, has been studied in a limited number of cases of fluorouracil overdose. Of 17 patients receiving vistonuridine beginning within 8-96 hours after fluorouracil overdose, all patients fully recovered (von Borstel, 2009); refer to Vistonuridine monograph.

Emetic Potential Low (10% to 30%)

Dosage Forms Excipient information presented when available (limited, particularly for generics); consult specific product labeling.
Tablet:
Xeloda®: 150 mg, 500 mg

Extemporaneous Preparations Capecitabine oral solution: A solution of capecitabine in water may be prepared by adding 2000 mg capecitabine (powder) to 200 mL water. Capecitabine tablets are water soluble (data on file from Roche). Administer immediately after preparation, 30 minutes after a meal. Use appropriate precautions for handling and disposal.

Judson IR, Beale PJ, Trigo JM, et al, "A Human Capecitabine Excretion Balance and Pharmacokinetic Study After Administration of a Single Oral Dose of ^{14}C-Labelled Drug," *Invest New Drugs*, 1999, 17(1):49-56.

References

Cartwright TH, Cohn A, Varkey JA, et al, "Phase II Study of Oral Capecitabine in Patients With Advanced or Metastatic Pancreatic Cancer," J Clin Oncol, 2002, 20(1):160-4.

Cassidy J, Tabernero J, Twelves C, et al, "XELOX (Capecitabine Plus Oxaliplatin): Active First-Line Therapy for Patients With Metastatic Colorectal Cancer," J Clin Oncol, 2004, 22(11):2084-91.

Haller DG, Cassidy J, Clarke S, et al, "Tolerability of Fluoropyrimidines Appears to Differ by Region," J Clin Oncol, 2006, 24(18S):3514 [abstract from 2006 ASCO Annual Meeting Proceedings]

Hennig IM, Naik JD, Brrown S, et al, "Severe Sequence-Specific Toxicity When Capecitabine Is Given After Fluorouracil and Leucovorin," J Clin Oncol, 2008, 26(20):3411-7.

Hoff PM, Ansari R, Batist G, et al, "Comparison of Oral Capecitabine Versus Intravenous Fluorouracil Plus Leucovorin as First-Line Treatment in 605 Patients With Metastatic Colorectal Cancer: Results of a Randomized Phase III Study," J Clin Oncol, 2001, 19(8):2282-92.

National Comprehensive Cancer Network (NCCN), "Clinical Practice Guidelines in Oncology™: Prevention and Treatment of Colon Cancer," Version 1.2008. Available at http://www.nccn.org/professionals/physician_gls/PDF/colon.pdf.

National Comprehensive Cancer Network (NCCN), "Clinical Practice Guidelines in Oncology™: Prevention and Treatment of Pancreatic Adenocarcinoma," Version 1.2008. Available at http://www.nccn.org/professionals/physician_gls/PDF/pancreatic.pdf.

Twelves C, Wong A, Nowacki MP, et al, "Capecitabine as Adjuvant Treatment for Stage III Colon Cancer," N Engl J Med, 2005, 352(26):2696-704.

Van Cutsem E, Twelves C, Cassidy J, et al, "Oral Capecitabine Compared With Intravenous Fluorouracil Plus Leucovorin in Patients With Metastatic Colorectal Cancer: Results of a Large Phase III Study," J Clin Oncol, 2001, 19(21):4097-106.

von Borstel R, O'Neil J, and Bamat M, "Vistonuridine: An Orally Administered, Life-Saving Antidote for 5-Fluorouracil (5FU) Overdose," J Clin Oncol, 2009, 27(15S):9616 [abstract from 2009 ASCO Annual Meeting].

Wong M, Choo SP, and Tan EH, "Travel Warning With Capecitabine," Ann Oncol, 2009, 20 (7):2081.

◆ **Caphosol®** *see* Saliva Substitute *on page 1027*

◆ **Carac®** *see* Fluorouracil *on page 499*

CARBOplatin (KAR boe pla tin)

Medication Safety Issues

Sound-alike/look-alike issues:

CARBOplatin may be confused with CISplatin, oxaliplatin

Paraplatin® may be confused with Platinol®

High alert medication: The Institute for Safe Medication Practices (ISMP) includes this medication among its list of drugs which have a heightened risk of causing significant patient harm when used in error.

Related Information

Hematopoietic Stem Cell Transplantation *on page 1501*

Management of Chemotherapy-Induced Nausea and Vomiting *on page 1434*

Management of Drug Extravasations *on page 1447*

Safe Handling of Hazardous Drugs *on page 1517*

Index Terms CBDCA; NSC-241240

Generic Available Yes

Canadian Brand Names Paraplatin-AQ

Pharmacologic Category Antineoplastic Agent, Alkylating Agent; Antineoplastic Agent, Platinum Analog

Use Treatment of ovarian cancer

Unlabeled/Investigational Use Lung cancer, head and neck cancer, endometrial cancer, esophageal cancer, bladder cancer, breast cancer, cervical cancer, CNS tumors, germ cell tumors, osteogenic sarcoma, and high-dose therapy with stem cell/bone marrow support

Pregnancy Risk Factor D

Lactation Excretion in breast milk unknown/contraindicated

Labeled Contraindications History of severe allergic reaction to cisplatin, carboplatin, other platinum-containing formulations, or any component of the formulation; pregnancy; breast-feeding

Warnings/Precautions Hazardous agent - use appropriate precautions for handling and disposal. High doses have resulted in severe abnormalities of liver function tests. **[U.S. Boxed Warning]: Bone marrow suppression, which may be severe, and vomiting are dose related;** reduce dosage in patients with bone marrow suppression and impaired renal function. Anemia is cumulative. Clinically significant hearing loss has been reported to occur in pediatric patients when carboplatin was administered at higher than recommended doses in combination with other ototoxic agents.

[U.S. Boxed Warning]: Increased risk of allergic reactions in patients previously exposed to platinum therapy. When administered as sequential infusions, taxane derivatives (docetaxel, paclitaxel) should be administered before the platinum derivatives (carboplatin, cisplatin) to limit myelosuppression and to enhance efficacy. Loss of vision (reversible) has been reported with higher than recommended doses. The elderly (≥65 years) and patients who have previously received cisplatin have an increased incidence of peripheral neuropathy. **[U.S. Boxed Warning]: Should be administered under the supervision of an experienced cancer chemotherapy physician.**

Adverse Reactions Percentages reported with single-agent therapy.

>10%:

Central nervous system: Pain (23%)

Endocrine & metabolic: Hyponatremia (29% to 47%), hypomagnesemia (29% to 43%), hypocalcemia (22% to 31%), hypokalemia (20% to 28%)

Gastrointestinal: Vomiting (65% to 81%), abdominal pain (17%), nausea (10% to 15%)

Hematologic: Myelosuppression (dose related and dose limiting; nadir at ~21 days; recovery by ~28 days), leukopenia (85%; grades 3/4: 15% to 26%), anemia (71% to 90%; grades 3/4: 21%), neutropenia (67%; grades 3/4: 16% to 21%), thrombocytopenia (62%; grades 3/4: 25% to 35%)

Hepatic: Alkaline phosphatase increased (24% to 37%), AST increased (15% to 19%)

Neuromuscular & skeletal: Weakness (11%)

Renal: Creatinine clearance decreased (27%), BUN increased (14% to 22%)

1% to 10%:

Central nervous system: Neurotoxicity (5%)

Dermatologic: Alopecia (2% to 3%)

Gastrointestinal: Constipation (5%), diarrhea (6%), stomatitis/mucositis (1%), taste dysgeusia (1%)

Hematologic: Hemorrhagic complications (5%)

Hepatic: Bilirubin increased (5%)

Local: Pain at injection site

Neuromuscular & skeletal: Peripheral neuropathy (4% to 6%; up to 10% in older and/or previously-treated patients)

Ocular: Visual disturbance (1%)

Otic: Ototoxicity (1%)

Renal: Creatinine increased (6% to 10%)

Miscellaneous: Infection (5%), hypersensitivity (2%)

<1%, postmarketing, and/or case reports (limited to important or life-threatening): Anaphylaxis, anorexia, bronchospasm, cardiac failure, cerebrovascular accident, embolism, erythema, fever, hemolytic uremic syndrome (HUS), hyper-/hypotension, malaise, necrosis (associated with extravasation), nephrotoxicity, neurotoxicity, pruritus, rash, secondary malignancies, urticaria, vision loss

Drug Interactions

Avoid Concomitant Use

Avoid concomitant use of CARBOplatin with any of the following: Natalizumab; Vaccines (Live)

Increased Effect/Toxicity

CARBOplatin may increase the levels/effects of: Leflunomide; Natalizumab; Taxane Derivatives; Topotecan; Vaccines (Live)

The levels/effects of CARBOplatin may be increased by: Aminoglycosides; Trastuzumab

Decreased Effect

CARBOplatin may decrease the levels/effects of: Vaccines (Inactivated); Vaccines (Live)

The levels/effects of CARBOplatin may be decreased by: Echinacea

Ethanol/Nutrition/Herb Interactions Herb/Nutraceutical: Avoid black cohosh, dong quai in estrogen-dependent tumors.

Storage/Stability Store intact vials at room temperature of 15°C to 30°C (59°F to 86°F). Protect from light. Further dilution to a concentration as low as 0.5 mg/mL is stable at room temperature (25°C) for 8 hours in NS; stable at room temperature or under refrigeration for at least 9 days in D_5W, although the manufacturer states to use within 8 hours due to lack of preservative.

Powder for reconstitution: Reconstituted to a final concentration of 10 mg/mL is stable for 5 days at room temperature (25°C).

Solution for injection: Multidose vials are stable for up to 14 days after opening when stored at room temperature.

Reconstitution Reconstitute powder to yield a final concentration of 10 mg/mL. Reconstituted carboplatin 10 mg/mL should be further diluted to a final concentration of 0.5-2 mg/mL with D_5W or NS for administration.

Compatibility Stable in $D_5$1/4NS, $D_5$1/2NS, D_5NS, D_5W, NS.

Y-site administration: **Compatible:** Allopurinol, amifostine, aztreonam, cefepime, cladribine, doxorubicin liposome, etoposide phosphate, filgrastim, fludarabine, gatifloxacin, gemcitabine, granisetron, linezolid, melphalan, ondansetron, paclitaxel, piperacillin/tazobactam, propofol, sargramostim, teniposide, thiotepa, topotecan, vinorelbine. **Incompatible:** Amphotericin B cholesteryl sulfate complex.

Compatibility when admixed: **Compatible:** Cisplatin, etoposide, floxuridine, ifosfamide, ifosfamide with etoposide, paclitaxel. **Incompatible:** Fluorouracil, mesna.

Mechanism of Action Carboplatin is an alkylating agent which covalently binds to DNA; possible cross-linking and interference with the function of DNA

Pharmacodynamics/Kinetics

Distribution: V_d: 16 L/kg; into liver, kidney, skin, and tumor tissue

Protein binding: 0%; platinum is 30% irreversibly bound

Metabolism: Minimally hepatic to aquated and hydroxylated compounds

Half-life elimination: Terminal: 22-40 hours; Cl_{cr} >60 mL/minute: 2.5-5.9 hours

Excretion: Urine (~60% to 90%) within 24 hours

Dosage Details concerning dosing in combination regimens should also be consulted. **Note:** Doses for adults are usually determined by the AUC using the Calvert formula.

IVPB, I.V. infusion:
Children:
Solid tumor (unlabeled use): 300-600 mg/m² once every 4 weeks
Brain tumor (unlabeled use): 175 mg/m² weekly for 4 weeks every 6 weeks, with a 2-week recovery period between courses
Adults:
Ovarian cancer: 300-360 mg/m² every 4 weeks **or** target AUC 5-7.5 every 3 weeks (unlabeled dose; Ozols, 2003; Parmar, 2003)
Autologous BMT (unlabeled use): 1600 mg/m² (total dose) divided over 4 days
In adults, dosing is commonly calculated using the Calvert formula:
Total dose (mg) = Target AUC x (GFR+ 25)
Usual target AUCs:
Previously untreated patients: 6-8
Previously treated patients: 4-6
Elderly: The Calvert formula should be used to calculate dosing for elderly patients.
Intraperitoneal: Ovarian cancer (unlabeled use): Adults: 200-650 mg/m² in 2 L of dialysis fluid have been administered into the peritoneum **or** target AUC: 5-7
Dosage adjustment for toxicity: Platelets <50,000 cells/mm³ or ANC <500 cells/mm³: Administer 75% of dose

Dosing adjustment in renal impairment: Note: Dose determination with Calvert formula uses GFR and, therefore, inherently adjusts for renal dysfunction.
The FDA-approved labeling recommends the following dosage adjustment guidelines:
Baseline Cl_{cr} 41-59 mL/minute: Initiate at 250 mg/m² and adjust subsequent doses based on bone marrow toxicity
Baseline Cl_{cr} 16-40 mL/minute: Initiate at 200 mg/m² and adjust subsequent doses based on bone marrow toxicity
Baseline Cl_{cr} ≤15 mL/minute: No guidelines are available.
The following dosage adjustments have been used by some clinicians (Aronoff, 2007): Adults (for dosing based on mg/m²):
Hemodialysis: Administer 50% of dose
Continuous ambulatory peritoneal dialysis (CAPD): Administer 25% of dose
Continuous renal replacement therapy (CRRT): 200 mg/m²
Dosing adjustment in hepatic impairment: Minimal hepatic metabolism; dosage adjustment may not be needed. No specific dosage adjustment guidelines are available.

Combination Regimens
Adenocarcinoma, unknown primary:
Carbo-Tax (Adenocarcinoma) on page 1250
Paclitaxel-Carboplatin-Etoposide on page 1386
PCE on page 1390
Bladder cancer:
Gemcitabine-Carboplatin (Bladder Cancer) on page 1340
Paclitaxel-Carboplatin (Bladder Cancer) on page 1386
Paclitaxel-Carboplatin-Gemcitabine on page 1387

Breast cancer:

Administration Infuse over 15 minutes to 24 hours. May also be administered intraperitoneally. When administered as sequential infusions, taxane derivatives (docetaxel, paclitaxel) should be administered before platinum derivatives to limit myelosuppression and to enhance efficacy.

Monitoring Parameters CBC (with differential and platelet count), serum electrolytes, creatinine clearance, liver function tests, BUN, creatinine

Emetic Potential Moderate (30% to 90%)

Vesicant May be an irritant

High Dose Considerations

  Comments Observe serum creatinine. Carboplatin is nephrotoxic and drug accumulation occurs with decreased creatinine clearance.

High Dose I.V.: 1.2-2.4 g/m^2 administered as 3-4 divided doses every 24-48 hours; generally infused over at least 60 minutes; 400 mg/m^2 has been infused over 15-30 minutes; generally combined with other high-dose chemotherapeutic drugs.

Unique Toxicities

Dermatologic: Alopecia

Endocrine & metabolic: Hypokalemia, hypomagnesemia

Gastrointestinal: Nausea, vomiting, mucositis

Hepatic: Liver function tests elevated

Otic: Ototoxicity

Renal: Nephrotoxicity

Dosage Forms Excipient information presented when available (limited, particularly for generics); consult specific product labeling.

Injection, powder for reconstitution: 50 mg, 150 mg, 450 mg

Injection, solution: 10 mg/mL (5 mL, 15 mL, 45 mL, 60 mL)

Injection, solution [preservative free]: 10 mg/mL (5 mL, 15 mL, 45 mL)

References

Aronoff GR, Bennett WM, Berns JS, et al, *Drug Prescribing in Renal Failure: Dosing Guidelines for Adults and Children*, 5th ed. Philadelphia, PA: American College of Physicians; 2007, p 97, 169.

Benaji B, Dine T, Luyckx M, et al, "Stability and Compatibility of Cisplatin and Carboplatin With PVC Infusion Bags," *J Clin Pharm Ther*, 1994, 19(2):95-100.

Calvert AH, Newell DR, Grumbell LA, et al, "Carboplatin Dosage: Prospective Evaluation of a Simple Formula Based on Renal Function," *J Clin Oncol*, 1989, 7(11):1748-56.

Cheung Y-W, Cradock JC, Vishnuvajjala BR, et al, "Stability of Cisplatin, Iproplatin, Carboplatin, and Tetraplatin in Commonly Used Intravenous Solutions," *Am J Hosp Pharm*, 1987, 44:124-30.

Fujiwara K, Markman M, Morgan M, et al, "Intraperitoneal Carboplatin-Based Chemotherapy for Epithelial Ovarian Cancer," *Gynecol Oncol*, 2005, 97(1):10-5.

Lovett D, Kelsen D, Eisenberger M, et al, "A Phase II Trial of Carboplatin and Vinblastine in the Treatment of Advanced Squamous Cell Carcinoma of the Esophagus," *Cancer*, 1991, 67 (2):354-6.

Markman M and Walker JL, "Intraperitoneal Chemotherapy of Ovarian Cancer: a Review, With a Focus on Practical Aspects of Treatment," *J Clin Oncol*, 2006, 24(6):988-94.

National Comprehensive Cancer Network® (NCCN), "Clinical Practice Guidelines in Oncology™: Ovarian Cancer," Version 1.2009. Available at http://www.nccn.org/professionals/physician_gls/PDF/ovarian.pdf

Ozols RF, Bundy BN, Greer BE, et al, "Phase III Trial of Carboplatin and Paclitaxel Compared with Cisplatin and Paclitaxel in Patients With Optimally Resected Stage III Ovarian Cancer: A Gynecologic Oncology Group Study," *J Clin Oncol*, 2003, 21(17):3194-200.

Parmar MK, Ledermann JA, Colombo N, et al, "Paclitaxel Plus Platinum-Based Chemotherapy Versus Conventional Platinum-Based Chemotherapy in Women With Relapsed Ovarian Cancer: The ICON4/AGO-OVAR-2.2 Trial," *Lancet*, 2003, 361(9375):2099-106.

Polyzos A, Tsavaris N, Kosmas C, et al, "A Comparative Study of Intraperitoneal Carboplatin versus Intravenous Carboplatin With Intravenous Cyclophosphamide in Both Arms as Initial Chemotherapy for Stage III Ovarian Cancer," *Oncology*, 1999, 56(4):291-6.

Wandt H, Birkmann J, Denzel T, et al, "Sequential Cycles of High-Dose Chemotherapy With Dose Escalation of Carboplatin With or Without Paclitaxel Supported by G-CSF Mobilized Peripheral Blood Progenitor Cells: A Phase I/II Study in Advanced Ovarian Cancer," *Bone Marrow Transplant*, 1999, 23(8):763-70.

◆ **Carboxypeptidase-G2** *see* Glucarpidase *on page 547*

◆ **Carimune® NF** *see* Immune Globulin (Intravenous) *on page 627*

Carmustine (kar MUS teen)

Medication Safety Issues

Sound-alike/look-alike issues:

Carmustine may be confused with bendamustine, lomustine

High alert medication: The Institute for Safe Medication Practices (ISMP) includes this medication among its list of drugs which have a heightened risk of causing significant patient harm when used in error.

◀ **Related Information**
Hematopoietic Stem Cell Transplantation *on page 1501*
Management of Drug Extravasations *on page 1447*
Safe Handling of Hazardous Drugs *on page 1517*
U.S. Brand Names BiCNU®; Gliadel®
Index Terms BCNU; bis-chloronitrosourea; Carmustinum; WR-139021
Generic Available No
Canadian Brand Names BiCNU®; Gliadel Wafer®
Pharmacologic Category Antineoplastic Agent; Antineoplastic Agent, Alkylating Agent; Antineoplastic Agent, Alkylating Agent (Nitrosourea)
Use
Injection: Treatment of brain tumors (glioblastoma, brainstem glioma, medulloblastoma, astrocytoma, ependymoma, and metastatic brain tumors), multiple myeloma, Hodgkin's disease (relapsed or refractory), non-Hodgkin's lymphomas (relapsed or refractory)

Wafer (implant): Adjunct to surgery in patients with recurrent glioblastoma multiforme; adjunct to surgery and radiation in patients with high-grade malignant glioma

Unlabeled/Investigational Use Treatment of metastatic melanoma
Pregnancy Risk Factor D
Lactation Excretion in breast milk unknown/not recommended
Labeled Contraindications Hypersensitivity to carmustine or any component of the formulation
Warnings/Precautions Hazardous agent - use appropriate precautions for handling and disposal. **[U.S. Boxed Warning]: Bone marrow suppression (thrombocytopenia, leukopenia) is the major toxicity and may be delayed; monitor blood counts weekly for at least 6 weeks after administration. Myelosuppression is cumulative; consider nadir blood counts from prior dose for dosage adjustment. May cause bleeding (due to thrombocytopenia) or infections (due to neutropenia); monitor closely.** Administer with caution to patients with depressed platelet, leukocyte, or erythrocyte counts; renal or hepatic impairment. Diluent contains significant amounts of ethanol; use caution with aldehyde dehydrogenase-2 deficiency or history of "alcohol-flushing syndrome."

[U.S. Boxed Warning]: Dose-related pulmonary toxicity may occur; patients receiving cumulative doses >1400 mg/m^2 are at higher risk. Baseline pulmonary function tests are recommended. **[U.S. Boxed Warning]: Delayed onset of pulmonary fibrosis has occurred up to 17 years after treatment** in children (1-16 years) who received carmustine in cumulative doses ranging from 770-1800 mg/m^2 combined with cranial radiotherapy for intracranial tumors. **[U.S. Boxed Warning]: Should be administered under the supervision of an experienced cancer chemotherapy physician.** Long-term use may be associated with the development of secondary malignancies. Safety and efficacy in children have not been established.

Adverse Reactions
>10%:
Cardiovascular: Hypotension (with high-dose I.V. therapy, due to the alcohol content of the diluent)

Central nervous system: Ataxia, dizziness
Postoperatively: Seizure (wafer 5% to 54%), brain edema (wafer 4% to 23%)

Dermatologic: Burning (with skin contact), hyperpigmentation of skin (with skin contact)

Gastrointestinal: Severe nausea and vomiting, usually begins within 2-4 hours of drug administration and lasts for 4-6 hours; dose related. Patients should receive a prophylactic antiemetic regimen.

Hematologic: Myelosuppression (cumulative, dose related, delayed, and dose limiting), thrombocytopenia (onset: 28 days; recovery: 35-42 days), leukopenia (onset: 35-42 days; recovery: 42-56 days)

Hepatic: Reversible increases in bilirubin, alkaline phosphatase, and AST occur in 20% to 25% of patients

Local: Pain and burning at injection site, phlebitis

Neuromuscular & skeletal: Weakness (wafer 22%)

Ocular: Ocular toxicities (transient conjunctival flushing and blurred vision), retinal hemorrhages

Respiratory: Interstitial fibrosis occurs in up to 50% of patients receiving a cumulative dose >1400 mg/m^2, or bone marrow transplantation doses; may be delayed up to 3 years; rare in patients receiving lower doses. A history of lung disease or concomitant bleomycin therapy may increase the risk of this reaction. Patients with forced vital capacity (FVC) or carbon monoxide diffusing capacity of the lungs (DLCO) <70% of predicted are at higher risk.

Miscellaneous: Disease progression/performance deterioration (wafer 82%)

1% to 10%:

Cardiovascular: Chest pain, deep thrombophlebitis (wafer), facial edema (wafer), peripheral edema (wafer)

Central nervous system: Wafer: Amnesia, anxiety, aphasia, ataxia, brain abscess, confusion, convulsion, CSF leaks, depression, diplopia, dizziness, facial paralysis, headache, hemiplegia, hydrocephalus, hypoesthesia, insomnia, intracranial hypertension, meningitis, somnolence, speech disorder, stupor

Dermatologic: Facial flushing, probably due to the alcohol diluent; alopecia, rash (wafer), wound healing abnormal (wafer)

Gastrointestinal: Abdominal pain, anorexia, constipation, diarrhea, stomatitis

Hematologic: Anemia, hemorrhage (wafer)

Local: Abscess (wafer)

Neuromuscular & skeletal: Back pain

<1%: Allergic reaction, azotemia (progressive), cerebral hemorrhage infarction (wafer), cyst formation (wafer), dermatitis, hepatic coma, hyperpigmentation, hypotension, kidney size decreased, neuroretinitis, painless jaundice, renal failure, subacute hepatitis, tachycardia, thrombosis

Drug Interactions

Avoid Concomitant Use

Avoid concomitant use of Carmustine with any of the following: Natalizumab; Vaccines (Live)

Increased Effect/Toxicity

Carmustine may increase the levels/effects of: Leflunomide; Natalizumab; Vaccines (Live)

The levels/effects of Carmustine may be increased by: Cimetidine; Trastuzumab

Decreased Effect

Carmustine may decrease the levels/effects of: Cardiac Glycosides; Vaccines (Inactivated); Vaccines (Live)

The levels/effects of Carmustine may be decreased by: Echinacea

Ethanol/Nutrition/Herb Interactions Ethanol: Diluent for infusion contains ethanol; avoid concurrent use of medications that inhibit aldehyde dehydrogenase-2 or cause disulfiram-like reactions.

◀ **Storage/Stability**

Injection: Store intact vials under refrigeration at 2°C to 8°C (36°F to 46°F); vials are stable for 36 days at room temperature. Reconstituted solutions are stable for 8 hours at room temperature (25°C) and 24 hours under refrigeration (2°C to 8°C) and protected from light. Further dilution in D_5W or NS is stable for 8 hours at room temperature (25°C) and 48 hours under refrigeration (4°C) in glass or polyolefin containers and protected from light.

Wafer: Store at or below -20°C (-4°F). Unopened foil pouches may be kept at room temperature for up to 6 hours.

Reconstitution Injection: Initially, dilute with 3 mL of absolute alcohol. Further dilute with SWFI (27 mL) to a concentration of 3.3 mg/mL; protect from light; may further dilute with D_5W or NS, using a non-PVC container.

Compatibility Compatible with D_5W, NS, SWFI, dacarbazine.

Y-site administration: Compatible: Amifostine, aztreonam, cefepime, filgrastim, fludarabine, gemcitabine, granisetron, ondansetron, piperacillin/tazobactam, sargramostim, teniposide, thiotepa, vinorelbine. **Incompatible:** Allopurinol, sodium bicarbonate.

Compatibility when admixed: Incompatible with sodium bicarbonate.

Mechanism of Action Interferes with the normal function of DNA and RNA by alkylation and cross-linking the strands of DNA and RNA, and by possible protein modification; may also inhibit enzyme processes by carbamylation of amino acids in protein

Pharmacodynamics/Kinetics

Distribution: 3.3 L/kg; readily crosses blood-brain barrier producing CSF levels equal to >50% of blood plasma levels; highly lipid soluble

Metabolism: Rapidly hepatic; forms active metabolites

Half-life elimination: Biphasic: Initial: 1.4 minutes; Secondary: 20 minutes (active metabolites: plasma half-life of 67 hours)

Excretion: Urine (~60% to 70%) within 96 hours; lungs (6% to 10% as CO_2)

Dosage

I.V. (refer to individual protocols):

Children (unlabeled use): 200-250 mg/m^2 every 4-6 weeks as a single dose

Adults: Usual dosage (per manufacturer labeling): 150-200 mg/m^2 every 6 weeks **or** 75-100 mg/m^2/day for 2 days every 6 weeks

Alternative regimens (unlabeled):

75-120 mg/m^2 days 1 and 2 every 6-8 weeks **or**

50-80 mg/m^2 days 1,2,3 every 6-8 weeks

Primary brain cancer:

150-200 mg/m^2 every 6-8 weeks as a single dose **or**

75-120 mg/m^2 days 1 and 2 every 6-8 weeks **or**

20-65 mg/m^2 every 4-6 weeks **or**

0.5-1 mg/kg every 4-6 weeks **or**

40-80 mg/m^2/day for 3 days every 6-8 weeks

Autologous BMT:

Combination therapy: Up to 300-900 mg/m^2

Single-agent therapy: Up to 1200 mg/m^2 (fatal necrosis is associated with doses >2 g/m^2)

Implantation (wafer): Adults: Recurrent glioblastoma multiforme, malignant glioma: Up to 8 wafers may be placed in the resection cavity (total dose 62.6 mg); should the size and shape not accommodate 8 wafers, the maximum number of wafers allowed should be placed

Dosing adjustment in renal impairment: I.V.: The FDA-approved labeling does not contain renal dosing adjustment guidelines. The following dosage adjustments have been used by some clinicians (Kintzel, 1995):

Cl_{cr} 46-60 mL/minute: Administer 80% of dose

Cl_{cr} 31-45 mL/minute: Administer 75% of dose

Cl_{cr} ≤30 mL/minute: Consider use of alternative drug

Dosing adjustment in hepatic impairment: Dosage adjustment may be necessary; however, no specific guidelines are available.

Combination Regimens

Lymphoma, Hodgkin's disease: mini-BEAM on page 1367

Melanoma:

CCDT (Melanoma) on page 1253

Cisplatin-Dacarbazine-Carmustine (Melanoma) on page 1265

Dartmouth Regimen on page 1286

Multiple myeloma:

M-2 on page 1364

VBAP on page 1418

VBMCP on page 1419

Administration

Injection: Significant absorption to PVC containers - should be administered in either glass or polyolefin containers. I.V. infusion over 1-2 hours is recommended; infusion through a free-flowing saline or dextrose infusion, or administration through a central catheter can alleviate venous pain/irritation.

High-dose carmustine: Maximum rate of infusion of ≤3 mg/m^2/minute to avoid excessive flushing, agitation, and hypotension; infusions should run over at least 2 hours; some investigational protocols dictate shorter infusions. **(High-dose carmustine is fatal if not followed by bone marrow or peripheral stem cell infusions.)**

Extravasation management: Elevate extremity. Inject long-acting dexamethasone (Decadron® LA) or by hyaluronidase throughout tissue with a 25- to 37-gauge needle. Apply warm, moist compresses.

Implant: Use appropriate precautions for handling and disposal; double glove before handling; outer gloves should be discarded as chemotherapy waste after handling wafers. Any wafer or remnant that is removed upon repeat surgery should be discarded as chemotherapy waste. The outer surface of the external foil pouch is not sterile. Open pouch gently; avoid pressure on the wafers to prevent breakage. Wafer that are broken in half may be used, however, wafers broken into more than 2 pieces should be discarded. Oxidized regenerated cellulose (Surgicel®) may be placed over the wafer to secure; irrigate cavity prior to closure.

Monitoring Parameters CBC with differential and platelet count, pulmonary function, liver function, and renal function tests; monitor blood pressure during administration

Wafer: Complications of craniotomy (seizures, intracranial infection, brain edema)

Additional Information Accidental skin contact may cause transient burning and brown discoloration of the skin. Delayed onset pulmonary fibrosis occurring up to 17 years after treatment has been reported in patients who received cumulative doses >1400 mg/m^2.

Emetic Potential

>250 mg/m^2: Very high (>90%)

≤250 mg/m^2: Moderate (30% to 90%)

◀ **Vesicant** Irritant; the alcohol-based diluent may be an irritant, especially with high doses.

High Dose Considerations

Comments Due to risk of hypotension, patients receiving high-dose carmustine must be supine and may require the Trendelenburg position, fluid support, and vasopressor support. Vital signs must be monitored frequently during the infusion of high-dose carmustine.

Infusion-related cardiovascular effects are primarily due to concomitant ethanol and acetaldehyde. Use with great caution in patients with aldehyde dehydrogenase-2 deficiency or history of "alcohol flushing syndrome". Avoid concurrent use of medications that inhibit aldehyde dehydrogenase-2 or cause disulfiram-like reactions. Acute lung injury tends to occur 1-3 months following carmustine infusion. Patients must be counseled to contact their BMT physician for dyspnea, cough, or fever following carmustine. Acute lung injury is managed with a course of corticosteroids.

High Dose I.V.: 300-800 mg/m² infused over at least 2 hours; may be divided into two doses administered every 12 hours; generally combined with other high-dose chemotherapeutic drugs. **(High-dose carmustine is fatal if not followed by bone marrow or peripheral stem cell infusions.)**

Unique Toxicities

Cardiovascular: Hypotension (infusion related), arrhythmias (infusion related)

Central nervous system: Encephalopathy, ethanol intoxication, seizures, fever

Endocrine & metabolic: Hyperprolactinemia and hypothyroidism in patients with brain tumors treated with radiation

Gastrointestinal: Severe nausea and vomiting

Hepatic Hepatitis, hepatic veno-occlusive disease

Pulmonary: Dyspnea

Dosage Forms Excipient information presented when available (limited, particularly for generics); consult specific product labeling.

Implant:
Gliadel®: 7.7 mg (8s)

Injection, powder for reconstitution:
BiCNU®: 100 mg [packaged with 3 mL of absolute alcohol as diluent]

References

Durando X, Lemaire JJ, Tortochaux J, et al, "High-Dose BCNU Followed by Autologous Hematopoietic Stem Cell Transplantation in Supratentorial High-Grade Malignant Gliomas: A Retrospective Analysis of 114 Patients," *Bone Marrow Transplant*, 2003, 31(7):559-64.

Fleming AB and Saltzman WM, "Pharmacokinetics of the Carmustine Implant," *Clin Pharmacokinet*, 2002, 41(6):403-19.

Kintzel PE and Dorr RT, "Anticancer Drug Renal Toxicity and Elimination: Dosing Guidelines for Altered Renal Function," *Cancer Treat Rev*, 1995, 21(1):33-64.

Lesser GJ and Grossman SA, "The Chemotherapy of Adult Primary Brain Tumors," *Cancer Treat Rev*, 1993, 19(3):261-81.

Mahendra P, Johnson D, Scott MA, et al, "Peripheral Blood Progenitor Cell Transplantation: A Single Centre Experience Comparing Two Mobilisation Regimens in 67 Patients," *Bone Marrow Transplant*, 1996, 17(4):503-7.

Weingart JD and Brem H, "Carmustine Implants: Potential in the Treatment of Brain Tumors," *CNS Drugs*, 1996, 4:263-9.

◆ **Carmustinum** *see* Carmustine *on page 183*

◆ **Casodex®** *see* Bicalutamide *on page 147*

Caspofungin (kas poe FUN jin)

U.S. Brand Names Cancidas®

Index Terms Caspofungin Acetate

Generic Available No

Canadian Brand Names Cancidas®

Pharmacologic Category Antifungal Agent, Parenteral; Echinocandin

Use Treatment of invasive *Aspergillus* infections in patients who are refractory or intolerant of other therapy; treatment of candidemia and other *Candida* infections (intra-abdominal abscesses, esophageal, peritonitis, pleural space); empirical treatment for presumed fungal infections in febrile neutropenic patient

Pregnancy Risk Factor C

Lactation Excretion in breast milk unknown/use caution

Labeled Contraindications Hypersensitivity to caspofungin or any component of the formulation

Warnings/Precautions Concurrent use of cyclosporine should be limited to patients for whom benefit outweighs risk, due to a high frequency of hepatic transaminase elevations observed during concurrent use. Limited data are available concerning treatment durations longer than 4 weeks, however, treatment appears to be well tolerated. Use caution in hepatic impairment; dosage reduction required with moderate impairment. Safety and efficacy have not been established in children <3 months of age.

Adverse Reactions

>10%:

Cardiovascular: Hypotension (6% to 20%), peripheral edema (6% to 11%), tachycardia (4% to 11%)

Central nervous system: Fever (13% to 30%), chills (8% to 23%), headache (5% to 15%)

Dermatologic: Rash (4% to 23%)

Endocrine & metabolic: Hypokalemia (5% to 23%)

Gastrointestinal: Diarrhea (7% to 27%), vomiting (7% to 17%), nausea (4% to 15%)

Hematologic: Hemoglobin decreased (5% to 21%), hematocrit decreased (13% to 18%), WBC decreased (12%), anemia (2% to 11%)

Hepatic: Serum alkaline phosphatase increased (13% to 22%), transaminases increased (2% to 18%), bilirubin increased (5% to 13%)

Local: Phlebitis/thrombophlebitis (18%)

Renal: Serum creatinine increased (3% to 11%), urinary RBCs increased (10%)

Respiratory: Respiratory failure (11% to 20%), cough (6% to 11%), pneumonia (4% to 11%)

Miscellaneous: Infusion reactions (20% to 35%), septic shock (11%)

1% to 10%:

Cardiovascular: Hypertension (children 9% to 10%), edema (3% to 4%)

Dermatologic: Erythema (4% to 9%), pruritus (5% to 7%)

Endocrine & metabolic: Hypomagnesemia (7%), hyperglycemia (6%), hyperkalemia (3%)

Gastrointestinal: Mucosal inflammation (4% to 10%), abdominal pain (4% to 9%)

Hepatic: Albumin decreased (7%)

Local: Infection (1% to 9%, central line)

Neuromuscular & skeletal: Back pain (children up to 4%)

Renal: Nephrotoxicity (13%), blood urea nitrogen increased (4% to 9%)

Note: Nephrotoxicity defined as serum creatinine ≥2x baseline value or ≥1 mg/dL in patients with serum creatinine above ULN range (patients with Cl_{cr} <30 mL/minute were excluded)

Respiratory: Dyspnea (9%), pleural effusion (9%), **respiratory** distress (children up to 8%), rales (7%), tachypnea (1%)

<1%, postmarketing. and/or case reports: Abdominal distention, anaphylaxis, anorexia, anxiety, appetite decrease, arrhythmia, arthralgia, atrial fibrillation, bradycardia, coagulopathy, confusion, constipation, depression, dizziness, dyspepsia, dystonia, epistaxis, erythema multiforme, fatigue, febrile neutropenia, fluid overload, flushing, hematuria, hepatic necrosis, hepatomegaly, hepatotoxicity, hypercalcemia, hypoxia, infusion site reactions (pain/pruritus/swelling), insomnia, jaundice, liver failure, MI, pain (extremities), pancreatitis, petechiae, pulmonary edema, renal failure/insufficiency, seizure, skin exfoliation, skin lesion, somnolence, stridor, Stevens-Johnson syndrome, tachypnea, thrombocytopenia, tremor, urinary tract infection, urticaria, weakness; histamine-mediated reactions (including facial swelling, bronchospasm, sensation of warmth) have been reported

Drug Interactions

Avoid Concomitant Use There are no known interactions where it is recommended to avoid concomitant use.

Increased Effect/Toxicity

The levels/effects of Caspofungin may be increased by: CycloSPORINE

Decreased Effect

Caspofungin may decrease the levels/effects of: Saccharomyces boulardii; Tacrolimus

The levels/effects of Caspofungin may be decreased by: Inducers of Drug Clearance; Rifampin

Storage/Stability Store vials at 2°C to 8°C (36°F to 46°F). Reconstituted solution may be stored at ≤25°C (≤77°F) for 1 hour prior to preparation of infusion solution. Infusion solutions may be stored at ≤25°C (≤77°F) and should be used within 24 hours; up to 48 hours if stored at 2°C to 8°C (36°F to 46°F).

Reconstitution Bring refrigerated vial to room temperature. Reconstitute vials using 0.9% sodium chloride for injection, SWFI, or bacteriostatic water for injection. Mix gently until clear solution is formed; do not use if cloudy or contains particles. Solution should be further diluted with 0.9%, 0.45%, or 0.225% sodium chloride or LR (do not exceed final concentration of 0.5 mg/mL).

Compatibility Stable in NS, ½NS, ¼NS, LR. Do not mix with dextrose-containing solutions. Do not coadminister with other medications.

Mechanism of Action Inhibits synthesis of β(1,3)-D-glucan, an essential component of the cell wall of susceptible fungi. Highest activity in regions of active cell growth. Mammalian cells do not require β(1,3)-D-glucan, limiting potential toxicity.

Pharmacodynamics/Kinetics

Protein binding: ~97% to albumin

Metabolism: Slowly, via hydrolysis and *N*-acetylation as well as by spontaneous degradation, with subsequent metabolism to component amino acids. Overall metabolism is extensive.

Half-life elimination: Beta (distribution): 9-11 hours; Terminal: 40-50 hours

Excretion: Urine (41% as metabolites, 1% to 9% unchanged) and feces (35% as metabolites)

Dosage I.V.:

Children: 3 months to 17 years: Initial dose: 70 mg/m^2 on day 1, subsequent dosing: 50 mg/m^2 once daily, if clinical response inadequate, may increase to 70 mg/m^2 once daily if tolerated, but increased efficacy not demonstrated (maximum dose: 70 mg/day)

Adults: **Note:** Duration of caspofungin treatment should be determined by patient status and clinical response. Empiric therapy should be given until neutropenia resolves. In patients with positive cultures, treatment should continue until 14 days after last positive culture. In neutropenic patients, treatment should be given at least 7 days after both signs and symptoms of infection **and** neutropenia resolve.

Aspergillosis, invasive: Initial dose: 70 mg on day 1; subsequent dosing: 50 mg/day. If clinical response inadequate, may increase up to 70 mg/day if tolerated, but increased efficacy not demonstrated. **Note:** Duration of therapy should be a minimum of 6-12 weeks or throughout period of immunosuppression.

Candidiasis: Initial dose: 70 mg on day 1; subsequent dosing: 50 mg/day
Esophageal: 50 mg/day; **Note:** The majority of patients studied for this indication also had oropharyngeal involvement.

Empiric therapy: Initial dose: 70 mg on day 1; subsequent dosing: 50 mg/day; if clinical response inadequate, may increase up to 70 mg/day if tolerated, but increased efficacy not demonstrated

Concomitant use of an enzyme inducer:

Children: Patients receiving carbamazepine, dexamethasone, efavirenz, nevirapine, phenytoin, or rifampin (and possibly other enzyme inducers): Consider 70 mg/m^2 once daily (maximum: 70 mg/day)

Adults:

Patients receiving rifampin: 70 mg caspofungin daily

Patients receiving carbamazepine, dexamethasone, efavirenz, nevirapine, **or** phenytoin (and possibly other enzyme inducers) may require an increased daily dose of caspofungin (70 mg/day).

Elderly: The number of patients >65 years of age in clinical studies was not sufficient to establish whether a difference in response may be anticipated.

Dosage adjustment in renal impairment: No specific dosage adjustment is required; supplemental dose is not required following dialysis

Dosage adjustment in hepatic impairment:

Children: Mild-to-severe hepatic insufficiency: No clinical experience

Adults:

Mild hepatic insufficiency (Child-Pugh score 5-6): No adjustment necessary

Moderate hepatic insufficiency (Child-Pugh score 7-9): 35 mg/day; initial 70 mg loading dose should still be administered in treatment of invasive infections

Severe hepatic insufficiency (Child-Pugh score >9): No clinical experience

Administration Infuse slowly, over 1 hour; monitor during infusion. Isolated cases of possible histamine-related reactions have occurred during clinical trials (rash, flushing, pruritus, facial edema).

Monitoring Parameters Liver function

Dosage Forms Excipient information presented when available (limited, particularly for generics); consult specific product labeling.

Injection, powder for reconstitution, as acetate:

Cancidas®: 50 mg [contains sucrose 39 mg], 70 mg [contains sucrose 54 mg]

References

Mora-Duarte J, Betts R, Rotstein C, et al, "Comparison of Caspofungin and Amphotericin B for Invasive Candidiasis," *N Engl J Med*, 2002, 347(25):2020-9.

Pappas PG, Rex JH, Sobel JD, et al, "Guidelines for Treatment of Candidiasis," *Clin Infect Dis*, 2004, 38:161-89.

Walsh TJ, Anaissie EJ, Denning DW, et al, "Treatment of Aspergillosis: Clinical Practice Guidelines of the Infectious Diseases Society of America," *Clin Infect Dis*, 2008, 46(3):327-60.

- ◆ **Caspofungin Acetate** *see* Caspofungin *on page 188*
- ◆ **Cathflo® Activase®** *see* Alteplase *on page 41*
- ◆ **CB-1348** *see* Chlorambucil *on page 216*
- ◆ **CBDCA** *see* CARBOplatin *on page 178*
- ◆ **CC-5013** *see* Lenalidomide *on page 688*
- ◆ **CCI-779** *see* Temsirolimus *on page 1083*
- ◆ **CCNU** *see* Lomustine *on page 727*
- ◆ **2-CdA** *see* Cladribine *on page 244*
- ◆ **CDDP** *see* CISplatin *on page 237*
- ◆ **CDX** *see* Bicalutamide *on page 147*
- ◆ **CeeNU®** *see* Lomustine *on page 727*

Cefepime (SEF e pim)

U.S. Brand Names Maxipime®

Index Terms Cefepime Hydrochloride

Generic Available Yes

Canadian Brand Names Maxipime®

Pharmacologic Category Antibiotic, Cephalosporin (Fourth Generation)

Use Treatment of uncomplicated and complicated urinary tract infections, including pyelonephritis caused by typical urinary tract pathogens; monotherapy for febrile neutropenia; uncomplicated skin and skin structure infections caused by *Streptococcus pyogenes*; moderate-to-severe pneumonia caused by pneumococcus, *Pseudomonas aeruginosa*, and other gram-negative organisms; complicated intra-abdominal infections (in combination with metronidazole). Also active against methicillin-susceptible staphylococci, *Enterobacter* sp, and many other gram-negative bacilli.

Children 2 months to 16 years: Empiric therapy of febrile neutropenia patients, uncomplicated skin/soft tissue infections, pneumonia, and uncomplicated/complicated urinary tract infections.

Pregnancy Risk Factor B

Lactation Enters breast milk/use caution

Labeled Contraindications Hypersensitivity to cefepime, any component of the formulation, or other cephalosporins

Warnings/Precautions Modify dosage in patients with severe renal impairment; use with caution in patients with a history of penicillin or cephalosporin allergy, especially IgE-mediated reactions (eg, anaphylaxis, urticaria). Prolonged use may result in fungal or bacterial superinfection, including *C. difficile*-associated diarrhea (CDAD) and pseudomembranous colitis; CDAD has been observed >2 months postantibiotic treatment. May be associated with increased INR, especially in nutritionally-deficient patients, prolonged treatment, hepatic or renal disease. Use with caution in patients with a history of seizure disorder; high levels, particularly in the presence of renal impairment, may increase risk of seizures.

Adverse Reactions
>10%: Hematologic: Positive Coombs' test without hemolysis
1% to 10%:
Central nervous system: Fever (1%), headache (1%)
Dermatologic: Rash, pruritus
Gastrointestinal: Diarrhea, nausea, vomiting
Local: Pain, erythema at injection site
<1%, postmarketing, and/or case reports: Agranulocytosis, anaphylactic shock, anaphylaxis, coma, encephalopathy, hallucinations, leukopenia, myoclonus, neuromuscular excitability, neutropenia, seizure, status epilepticus (nonconvulsive), thrombocytopenia
Reactions reported with other cephalosporins: Aplastic anemia, erythema multiforme, hemolytic anemia, hemorrhage, pancytopenia, PT prolonged, renal dysfunction, Stevens-Johnson syndrome, superinfection, toxic epidermal necrolysis, toxic nephropathy, vaginitis

Drug Interactions
Avoid Concomitant Use There are no known interactions where it is recommended to avoid concomitant use.

Increased Effect/Toxicity
The levels/effects of Cefepime may be increased by: Uricosuric Agents

Decreased Effect
Cefepime may decrease the levels/effects of: Typhoid Vaccine

Storage/Stability
Vials: Store at 20°C to 25°C (68°F to 77°F). Protect from light. After reconstitution, stable in normal saline, D₅W, and a variety of other solutions for 24 hours at room temperature and 7 days refrigerated.
Premixed solution: Store frozen at -20°C (-4°F). Thawed solution is stable for 24 hours at room temperature or 7 days under refrigeration; do not refreeze.

Compatibility Stable in D₅LR, D₅NS, D₅W, D₁₀W, NS, bacteriostatic water, sterile water for injection; **variable stability (consult detailed reference)** in peritoneal dialysis solutions.

Y-site administration: Compatible: Ampicillin/sulbactam, aztreonam, bleomycin, bumetanide, buprenorphine, butorphanol, calcium gluconate, carboplatin, carmustine, co-trimoxazole, cyclophosphamide, cytarabine, dactinomycin, dexamethasone sodium phosphate, docetaxel, doxorubicin liposome, fluconazole, fludarabine, fluorouracil, furosemide, granisetron, hydrocortisone sodium phosphate, hydrocortisone sodium succinate, hydromorphone, imipenem/cilastatin, leucovorin, lorazepam, melphalan, mesna, methotrexate, methylprednisolone sodium succinate, metronidazole, paclitaxel, piperacillin/tazobactam, ranitidine, sargramostim, sodium bicarbonate, thiotepa, ticarcillin/clavulanate, zidovudine. **Incompatible:** Acyclovir, amphotericin B, amphotericin B cholesteryl sulfate complex, chlordiazepoxide, chlorpromazine, cimetidine, ciprofloxacin, cisplatin, dacarbazine, daunorubicin, diazepam, diphenhydramine, dobutamine, dopamine, doxorubicin, droperidol, enalaprilat, etoposide, etoposide phosphate, famotidine, filgrastim, floxuridine, ganciclovir, haloperidol, hydroxyzine, idarubicin, ifosfamide, magnesium sulfate, mannitol, mechlorethamine, meperidine, metoclopramide, mitomycin, mitoxantrone, morphine, nalbuphine, ofloxacin, ondansetron, plicamycin, prochlorperazine edisylate, promethazine, streptozocin, vancomycin, vinblastine, vincristine.

Compatibility when admixed: Compatible: Amikacin, clindamycin, heparin, potassium chloride, theophylline, vancomycin. **Incompatible:** Aminophylline, gentamicin, netilmicin, tobramycin. **Variable (consult detailed reference):** Ampicillin, metronidazole.

◀ **Mechanism of Action** Inhibits bacterial cell wall synthesis by binding to one or more of the penicillin-binding proteins (PBPs) which in turn inhibits the final transpeptidation step of peptidoglycan synthesis in bacterial cell walls, thus inhibiting cell wall biosynthesis. Bacteria eventually lyse due to ongoing activity of cell wall autolytic enzymes (autolysis and murein hydrolases) while cell wall assembly is arrested.

Pharmacodynamics/Kinetics

Absorption: I.M.: Rapid and complete

Distribution: V_d: Adults: 14-20 L; penetrates into inflammatory fluid at concentrations ~80% of serum levels and into bronchial mucosa at levels ~60% of those reached in the plasma; crosses blood-brain barrier

Protein binding, plasma: 16% to 19%

Metabolism: Minimally hepatic

Half-life elimination: 2 hours

Time to peak: 0.5-1.5 hours

Excretion: Urine (85% as unchanged drug)

Dosage

Usual dosage range:

Children: I.M., I.V.: 50 mg/kg every 8-12 hours (maximum not to exceed adult dosing)

Adults: I.V.: 1-2 g every 8-12 hours; I.M.: 500-1000 mg every 12 hours

Indication-specific dosing:

Children ≥2 months to 16 years (<40 kg):

Febrile neutropenia: I.V.: 50 mg/kg every 8 hours for 7 days or until neutropenia resolves

Skin and skin structure infections (uncomplicated) and pneumonia: I.V.: 50 mg/kg every 12 hours for 10 days

Urinary tract infections, complicated and uncomplicated: I.M., I.V.: 50 mg/kg every 12 hours for 7-10 days; **Note:** I.M. may be considered for mild-to-moderate infection only

Adults:

Brain abscess, postneurosurgical prevention (unlabeled use): I.V.: 2 g every 8 hours with vancomycin

Febrile neutropenia, monotherapy: I.V: 2 g every 8 hours for 7 days or until the neutropenia resolves

Intra-abdominal infections, complicated: I.V.: 2 g every 12 hours for 7-10 days with metronidazole

Otitis externa, malignant (unlabeled use): I.V.: 2 g every 12 hours

Pneumonia: I.V.:

Nosocomial (HAP/VAP): 1-2 g every 8-12 hours; **Note:** Duration of therapy may vary considerably (7-21 days); usually longer courses are required if *Pseudomonas*. In absence of *Pseudomonas*, and if appropriate empiric treatment used and patient responsive, it may be clinically appropriate to reduce duration of therapy to 7-10 days (American Thoracic Society Guidelines, 2005).

Community-acquired (including pseudomonal): 1-2 g every 12 hours for 10 days

Septic lateral/cavernous sinus thrombosis (unlabeled use): I.V.: 2 g every 8-12 hours; with metronidazole for lateral

Skin and skin structure, uncomplicated: I.V.: 2 g every 12 hours for 10 days

Urinary tract infections, complicated and uncomplicated:

Mild-to-moderate: I.M., I.V.: 500-1000 mg every 12 hours for 7-10 days

Severe: I.V.: 2 g every 12 hours for 10 days

Dosing adjustment in renal impairment: Adults: Recommended maintenance schedule based on creatinine clearance (mL/minute), compared to normal dosing schedule: See table.

Cefepime Hydrochloride

Creatinine Clearance (mL/minute)	Recommended Maintenance Schedule			
>60 (normal recommended dosing schedule)	500 mg every 12 hours	1 g every 12 hours	2 g every 12 hours	2 g every 8 hours
30-60	500 mg every 24 hours	1 g every 24 hours	2 g every 24 hours	2 g every 12 hours
11-29	500 mg every 24 hours	500 mg every 24 hours	1 g every 24 hours	2 g every 24 hours
<11	250 mg every 24 hours	250 mg every 24 hours	500 mg every 24 hours	1 g every 24 hours

Hemodialysis: Initial: 1 g (single dose) on day 1. Maintenance: 500 mg once daily (1 g once daily in febrile neutropenic patients). Dosage should be administered after dialysis on dialysis days.

Continuous ambulatory peritoneal dialysis (CAPD): Removed to a lesser extent than hemodialysis; administer normal recommended dose every 48 hours

Continuous renal replacement therapy (CRRT) (Trotman, 2005): Drug clearance is highly dependent on the method of renal replacement, filter type, and flow rate. Appropriate dosing requires close monitoring of pharmacologic response, signs of adverse reactions due to drug accumulation, as well as drug levels in relation to target trough (if appropriate). The following are general recommendations only (based on dialysate flow/ultrafiltration rates of 1 L/hour) and should not supersede clinical judgment:
CVVH: 1-2 g every 12 hours
CVVHDF: 2 g every 12 hours

Note: Consider higher dosage of 4 g/day if treating *Pseudomonas* or life-threatening infections in order to maximize time above MIC.

Administration May be administered either I.M. or I.V.

Inject deep I.M. into large muscle mass. Inject direct I.V. over 5 minutes. Infuse intermittent infusion over 30 minutes.

Monitoring Parameters Obtain specimen for culture and sensitivity prior to the first dose. Monitor for signs of anaphylaxis during first dose.

Test Interactions Positive direct Coombs', false-positive urinary glucose test using cupric sulfate (Benedict's solution, Clinitest®, Fehling's solution), false-positive serum or urine creatinine with Jaffé reaction, false-positive urinary proteins and steroids

Dosage Forms Excipient information presented when available (limited, particularly for generics); consult specific product labeling.

Infusion, premixed iso-osmotic dextrose solution: 1 g (50 mL); 2 g (100 mL)
Injection, powder for reconstitution, as hydrochloride: 500 mg, 1 g, 2 g
Maxipime®: 500 mg, 1 g, 2 g

References

Barbhaiya RH, Knupp CA, and Pittman KA, "Effects of Age and Gender on Pharmacokinetics of Cefepime," *J Antimicrob Chemother*, 1992, 36(6):1181-5.

Barradell LB and Bryson HM, "Cefepime. A Review of Its Antibacterial Activity, Pharmacokinetic Properties, and Therapeutic Use," *Drugs*, 1994, 47(3):471-505.

Blumer JL, Reed MD, Lemon E, et al, "Pharmacokinetics (PK) of Cefepime in Pediatric Patients Administered Single and Multiple 50 mg/kg Doses Every 8 Hours by the Intravenous (I.V.) or Intramuscular (I.M.) Route," 34th Interscience Conference on Antimicrobial Agents and Chemotherapy, 1994, Orlando, Fl. Abs. A69.

Okamoto MP, Nakahiro RK, Chin A, et al, "Cefepime: A New Fourth-Generation Cephalosporin," *Am J Hosp Pharm*, 1994, 51(4):463-77.

Wynd MA and Paladino JA, "Cefepime: A Fourth-Generation Parenteral Cephalosporin," *Ann Pharmacother*, 1996, 30(12):1414-24.

Yahav D, Paul M, Fraser A, et al, "Efficacy and Safety of Cefepime: A Systematic Review and Meta-Analysis," *Lancet Infect Dis*, 2007, 7(5):338-48.

◆ **Cefepime Hydrochloride** see Cefepime on page 192

Ceftazidime (SEF tay zi deem)

Medication Safety Issues

Sound-alike/look-alike issues:

Ceftazidime may be confused with ceftizoxime

Ceptaz® may be confused with Septra®

Tazicef® may be confused with Tazidime®

Tazidime® may be confused with Tazicef®

International issues:

Ceftim® [Italy] may be confused with Ceftin® which is a brand name for cefuroxime in the U.S.

Ceftim® [Italy] may be confused with Cefiton® which is a brand name for cefixime in Portugal

Ceftim® [Italy] may be confused with Ceftina® which is a brand name for cefalotin in Mexico

U.S. Brand Names Fortaz®; Tazicef®

Generic Available Yes: Injection

Canadian Brand Names Fortaz®

Pharmacologic Category Antibiotic, Cephalosporin (Third Generation)

Use Treatment of documented susceptible *Pseudomonas aeruginosa* infection and infections due to other susceptible aerobic gram-negative organisms; empiric therapy of a febrile, granulocytopenic patient

Unlabeled/Investigational Use Bacterial endophthalmitis

Pregnancy Risk Factor B

Lactation Enters breast milk (small amounts)/use caution (AAP rates "compatible")

Labeled Contraindications Hypersensitivity to ceftazidime, any component of the formulation, or other cephalosporins

Warnings/Precautions Modify dosage in patients with severe renal impairment. Use with caution in patients with a history of penicillin allergy, especially IgE-mediated reactions (eg, anaphylaxis, urticaria). Prolonged use may result in fungal or bacterial superinfection, including *C. difficile*-associated diarrhea (CDAD) and pseudomembranous colitis; CDAD has been observed >2 months postantibiotic treatment. May be associated with increased INR, especially in nutritionally-deficient patients, prolonged treatment, hepatic or renal disease. Use with caution in patients with a history of seizure disorder; high levels, particularly in the presence of renal impairment, may increase risk of seizures.

Adverse Reactions

1% to 10%:

Gastrointestinal: Diarrhea (1%)

Local: Pain at injection site (1%)

Miscellaneous: Hypersensitivity reactions (2%)

<1%: Anaphylaxis, angioedema, asterixis, BUN increased, candidiasis, creatinine increased, dizziness, encephalopathy, eosinophilia, erythema multiforme, fever, headache, hemolytic anemia, hyperbilirubinemia, jaundice, leukopenia, myoclonus, nausea, neuromuscular excitability, paresthesia, phlebitis, pruritus, pseudomembranous colitis, rash, Stevens-Johnson syndrome, thrombocytosis, toxic epidermal necrolysis, transaminases increased, vaginitis, vomiting

Reactions reported with other cephalosporins: Seizure, urticaria, serum-sickness reactions, renal dysfunction, interstitial nephritis, toxic nephropathy, elevated BUN, elevated creatinine, cholestasis, aplastic anemia, hemolytic anemia, pancytopenia, agranulocytosis, colitis, prolonged PT, hemorrhage, superinfection

Drug Interactions

Avoid Concomitant Use There are no known interactions where it is recommended to avoid concomitant use.

Increased Effect/Toxicity

The levels/effects of Ceftazidime may be increased by: Uricosuric Agents

Decreased Effect

Ceftazidime may decrease the levels/effects of: Typhoid Vaccine

Storage/Stability

Vials: Reconstituted solution and solution further diluted for I.V. infusion are stable for 12 hours at room temperature, for 3 days when refrigerated, or for 12 weeks when frozen at -20°C (-4°F). After freezing, thawed solution in SWFI for I.M. administration is stable for 3 hours at room temperature or for 3 days when refrigerated, thawed solution in NS in a Viaflex® small volume container for I.V. administration is stable for 12 hours at room temperature or for 3 days when refrigerated, and thawed solution in SWFI in the original container is stable for 8 hours at room temperature or for 3 days when refrigerated.

Premixed frozen solution: Store frozen at -20°C (-4°F). Thawed solution is stable for 8 hours at room temperature or for 3 days under refrigeration; do not refreeze.

Compatibility Stable in D_5NS, D_5W, NS, sterile water for injection; **variable stability (consult detailed reference)** in peritoneal dialysis solutions.

Y-site administration: Compatible: Acyclovir, allopurinol, amifostine, aminophylline, aztreonam, ciprofloxacin, diltiazem, docetaxel, enalaprilat, esmolol, etoposide phosphate, famotidine, filgrastim, fludarabine, foscarnet, gatifloxacin, gemcitabine, granisetron, heparin, hydromorphone, labetalol, linezolid, melphalan, meperidine, morphine, ondansetron, paclitaxel, propofol, ranitidine, remifentanil, tacrolimus, teniposide, theophylline, thiotepa, vinorelbine, zidovudine. **Incompatible:** Alatrofloxacin, amphotericin B cholesteryl sulfate complex, amsacrine, doxorubicin liposome, fluconazole, idarubicin, midazolam, pentamidine, warfarin. **Variable (consult detailed reference):** Cisatracurium, sargramostim, vancomycin.

Compatibility in syringe: Compatible: Hydromorphone.

Compatibility when admixed: Compatible: Ciprofloxacin, clindamycin, fluconazole, linezolid, metronidazole, ofloxacin. **Incompatible:** Aminoglycosides (in same bottle/bag), aminophylline, ranitidine. **Variable (consult detailed reference):** Vancomycin.

Mechanism of Action Inhibits bacterial cell wall synthesis by binding to one or more of the penicillin-binding proteins (PBPs) which in turn inhibits the final transpeptidation step of peptidoglycan synthesis in bacterial cell walls, thus inhibiting cell wall biosynthesis. Bacteria eventually lyse due to ongoing activity of cell wall autolytic enzymes (autolysins and murein hydrolases) while cell wall assembly is arrested.

◀ **Pharmacodynamics/Kinetics**

Distribution: Widely throughout the body including bone, bile, skin, CSF (higher concentrations achieved when meninges are inflamed), endometrium, heart, pleural and lymphatic fluids

Protein binding: 17%

Half-life elimination: 1-2 hours, prolonged with renal impairment; Neonates <23 days: 2.2-4.7 hours

Time to peak, serum: I.M.: ~1 hour

Excretion: Urine (80% to 90% as unchanged drug)

Dosage

Usual dosage range:

Infants and Children 1 month to 12 years: I.V.: 30-50 mg/kg/dose every 8 hours (maximum dose: 6 g/day)

Adults: I.M., I.V.: 500 mg to 2 g every 8-12 hours

Indication-specific dosing:

Bacterial arthritis (gram-negative bacilli): I.V.: 1-2 g every 8 hours

Cystic fibrosis: I.V.: 30-50 mg/kg every 8 hours (maximum: 6 g/day)

Endophthalmitis, bacterial (unlabeled use): Intravitreal: 2.25 mg/0.1 mL NS in combination with vancomycin

Melioidosis: I.V.: 40 mg/kg every 8 hours for 10 days, followed by oral therapy with doxycycline or TMP/SMX

Otitis externa: I.V.: 2 g every 8 hours

Peritonitis (CAPD):

Anuric, intermittent: 1000-1500 mg/day

Anuric, continuous (per liter exchange): Loading dose: 250 mg; maintenance dose: 125 mg

Severe infections, including meningitis, complicated pneumonia, endophthalmitis, CNS infection, osteomyelitis, intra-abdominal and gynecological, skin and soft tissue: I.V.: 2 g every 8 hours

Dosing interval in renal impairment:

Cl_{cr} 30-50 mL/minute: Administer every 12 hours

Cl_{cr} 10-30 mL/minute: Administer every 24 hours

Cl_{cr} <10 mL/minute: Administer every 48-72 hours

Hemodialysis: Dialyzable (50% to 100%)

Continuous renal replacement therapy (CRRT): Drug clearance is highly dependent on the method of renal replacement, filter type, and flow rate. Appropriate dosing requires close monitoring of pharmacologic response, signs of adverse reactions due to drug accumulation, as well as drug levels in relation to target trough (if appropriate). The following are general recommendations only (based on dialysate flow/ultrafiltration rates of 1 L/hour) and should not supersede clinical judgment:

CVVH: 1-2 g every 12 hours

CVVHD/CVVHDF: 2 g every 12 hours

Administration Any carbon dioxide bubbles that may be present in the withdrawn solution should be expelled prior to injection. Administer around-the-clock to promote less variation in peak and trough serum levels. Ceftazidime can be administered deep I.M. into large mass muscle, IVP over 3-5 minutes, or I.V. intermittent infusion over 15-30 minutes. Do not admix with aminoglycosides in same bottle/bag. Final concentration for I.V. administration should not exceed 100 mg/mL.

Monitoring Parameters Observe for signs and symptoms of anaphylaxis during first dose

Test Interactions Positive direct Coombs', false-positive urinary glucose test using cupric sulfate (Benedict's solution, Clinitest®, Fehling's solution), false-positive serum or urine creatinine with Jaffé reaction

Dietary Considerations Sodium content of 1 g: 2.3 mEq

Additional Information With some organisms, resistance may develop during treatment (including *Enterobacter* spp and *Serratia* spp). Consider combination therapy or periodic susceptibility testing for organisms with inducible resistance.

Dosage Forms Excipient information presented when available (limited, particularly for generics); consult specific product labeling.

Infusion [premixed iso-osmotic solution, frozen]:

Fortaz®: 1 g (50 mL) [contains sodium carbonate, sodium ~54 mg (2.3 mEq)/g]; 2 g (50 mL) [contains sodium ~54 mg (2.3 mEq)/g]

Injection, powder for reconstitution: 1 g, 2 g, 6 g

Fortaz®: 500 mg, 1 g, 2 g, 6 g [contains sodium ~54 mg (2.3 mEq)/g]

Tazicef®: 1 g, 2 g, 6 g [contains sodium ~54 mg (2.3 mEq)/g]

References

Donowitz GR and Mandell GL, "Beta-Lactam Antibiotics," *N Engl J Med*, 1988, 318(7):419-26 and 318(8):490-500.

Klein NC and Cunha BA, "Third-Generation Cephalosporins," *Med Clin North Am*, 1995, 79 (4):705-19.

Marshall WF and Blair JE, "The Cephalosporins," *Mayo Clin Proc*, 1999, 74(2):187-95.

Rains CP, Bryson HM, and Peters DH, "Ceftazidime. An Update of Its Antibacterial Activity, Pharmacokinetic Properties and Therapeutic Efficacy," *Drugs*, 1995, 49(4):577-617.

Robinson DG, Cookson TL, and Frisafe JA, "Concentration Guidelines for Parenteral Antibiotics in Fluid-Restricted Patients," *Drug Intell Clin Pharm*, 1987, 21(12):985-9.

Sirgo MA and Norris S, "Ceftazidime in the Elderly: Appropriateness of Twice-Daily Dosing," *DICP Ann Pharmacother*, 1991, 25(3):284-8.

Slaker RA and Danielson B, "Neurotoxicity Associated With Ceftazidime Therapy in Geriatric Patients With Renal Dysfunction," *Pharmacotherapy*, 1991, 11(4):351-2.

CefTRIAXone (sef trye AKS one)

Medication Safety Issues

Sound-alike/look-alike issues:

CefTRIAXone may be confused with CeFAZolin, Cetraxal®

Rocephin® may be confused with Roferon®

U.S. Brand Names Rocephin®

Index Terms Ceftriaxone Sodium

Generic Available Yes

Canadian Brand Names Rocephin®

Pharmacologic Category Antibiotic, Cephalosporin (Third Generation)

Use Treatment of lower respiratory tract infections, acute bacterial otitis media, skin and skin structure infections, bone and joint infections, intra-abdominal and urinary tract infections, pelvic inflammatory disease (PID), uncomplicated gonorrhea, bacterial septicemia, and meningitis; used in surgical prophylaxis

Unlabeled/Investigational Use Treatment of chancroid, epididymitis, complicated gonococcal infections; sexually-transmitted diseases (STD); periorbital or buccal cellulitis; salmonellosis or shigellosis; atypical community-acquired pneumonia; epiglottitis, Lyme disease; used in chemoprophylaxis for high-risk contacts and persons with invasive meningococcal disease; sexual assault; typhoid fever, Whipple's disease

Pregnancy Risk Factor B

Lactation Enters breast milk/use caution (AAP rates "compatible")

Labeled Contraindications Hypersensitivity to ceftriaxone sodium, any component of the formulation, or other cephalosporins; **do not use in hyperbilirubinemic neonates**, particularly those who are premature since ceftriaxone is reported to displace bilirubin from albumin binding sites; concomitant use with intravenous calcium-containing solutions/products in neonates (≤28 days)

Warnings/Precautions Use with caution in patients with a history of penicillin allergy, especially IgE-mediated reactions (eg, anaphylaxis, urticaria). Abnormal gallbladder sonograms have been reported, possibly due to cetriaxone-calcium precipitates; discontinue in patients with signs and symptoms of gallbladder disease. Secondary to biliary obstruction, pancreatitis has been reported rarely. Use with caution in patients with a history of GI disease, especially colitis. Severe cases (including some fatalities) of immune-related hemolytic anemia have been reported in patients receiving cephalosporins, including ceftriaxone. Prolonged use may result in fungal or bacterial superinfection, including *C. difficile*-associated diarrhea (CDAD) and pseudomembranous colitis; CDAD has been observed >2 months postanti-biotic treatment.

May be associated with increased INR (rarely), especially in nutritionally-deficient patients, prolonged treatment, hepatic or renal disease. No adjustment is generally necessary in patients with renal impairment; use with caution in patients with concurrent hepatic dysfunction and significant renal disease, dosage should not exceed 2 g/day. Ceftriaxone may complex with calcium causing precipitation. Fatal lung and kidney damage associated with calcium-ceftriaxone precipitates has been observed in premature and term neonates. Do not reconstitute, admix, or coadminister with calcium-containing solutions, even via separate infusion lines/sites or at different times in any neonatal patient. Ceftriaxone should not be diluted or administered simultaneously with any calcium-containing solution via a Y-site in any patient. However, ceftriaxone and calcium-containing solution may be administered sequentially of one another for use in patients **other than neonates** if infusion lines are thoroughly flushed, with a compatible fluid, between infusions

Adverse Reactions

>10%: Local: Induration (I.M. 5% to 17%), warmth (I.M.), tightness (I.M.)

1% to 10%:

  Dermatologic: Rash (2%)

  Gastrointestinal: Diarrhea (3%)

  Hematologic: Eosinophilia (6%), thrombocytosis (5%), leukopenia (2%)

  Hepatic: Transaminases increased (3%)

  Local: Tenderness at injection site (I.V. 1%), pain

  Renal: BUN increased (1%)

<1%: Abdominal pain, agranulocytosis, alkaline phosphatase increased, allergic pneumonitis, anaphylaxis, anemia, basophilia, biliary lithiasis, bilirubin increased, bronchospasm, chills, colitis, creatinine increased, diaphoresis, dizziness, dysgeusia, dyspepsia, epistaxis, fever, flatulence, flushing, gallbladder sludge, gallstones, glycosuria, headache, hematuria, hemolytic anemia, jaundice, leukocytosis, lymphocytosis, lymphopenia, monocytosis, moniliasis, nausea, nephrolithiasis, neutropenia, palpitation, pancreatitis, phlebitis, prolonged or decreased PT, pruritus, pseudomem-branous colitis, seizure, serum sickness, thrombocytopenia, urinary casts, vaginitis, vomiting

Postmarketing and/or case reports: Allergic dermatitis, edema, erythema multiforme, exanthema, glossitis, Lyell's syndrome, oliguria, renal and pulmonary ceftriaxone-calcium precipitations (neonates; including some fatalities), Stevens-Johnson syndrome, stomatitis, toxic epidermal necrolysis, urticaria

Reactions reported with other cephalosporins: Angioedema, allergic reaction, aplastic anemia, asterixis, cholestasis, encephalopathy, hemorrhage, hepatic dysfunction, hyperactivity (reversible), hypertonia, interstitial nephritis, LDH increased, neuromuscular excitability, pancytopenia, paresthesia, renal dysfunction, superinfection, toxic nephropathy

Drug Interactions

Avoid Concomitant Use There are no known interactions where it is recommended to avoid concomitant use.

Increased Effect/Toxicity

CefTRIAXone may increase the levels/effects of: Vitamin K Antagonists

The levels/effects of CefTRIAXone may be increased by: Calcium Salts (Intravenous); Ringer's Injection (Lactated); Uricosuric Agents

Decreased Effect

CefTRIAXone may decrease the levels/effects of: Typhoid Vaccine

Storage/Stability

Powder for injection: Prior to reconstitution, store at room temperature ≤25°C (≤77°F). Protect from light.

Premixed solution (manufacturer premixed): Store at -20°C; once thawed, solutions are stable for 3 days at room temperature of 25°C (77°F) or for 21 days refrigerated at 5°C (41°F). Do not refreeze.

Stability of reconstituted solutions:

10-40 mg/mL: Reconstituted in D_5W, $D_{10}W$, NS, or SWFI: Stable for 2 days at room temperature of 25°C (77°F) or for 10 days when refrigerated at 4°C (39°F). Stable for 26 weeks when frozen at -20°C when reconstituted with D_5W or NS. Once thawed (at room temperature), solutions are stable for 2 days at room temperature of 25°C (77°F) or for 10 days when refrigerated at 4°C (39°F); does not apply to manufacturer's premixed bags. Do not refreeze.

100 mg/mL:

Reconstituted in D_5W, SWFI, or NS: Stable for 2 days at room temperature of 25°C (77°F) or for 10 days when refrigerated at 4°C (39°F).

Reconstituted in lidocaine 1% solution or bacteriostatic water: Stable for 24 hours at room temperature of 25°C (77°F) or for 10 days when refrigerated at 4°C (39°F).

250-350 mg/mL: Reconstituted in D_5W, NS, lidocaine 1% solution, bacteriostatic water, or SWFI: Stable for 24 hours at room temperature of 25°C (77°F) or for 3 days when refrigerated at 4°C (39°F).

Reconstitution

I.M. injection: Vials should be reconstituted with appropriate volume of diluent (including D_5W, NS, SWFI, bacteriostatic water, or 1% lidocaine) to make a final concentration of 250 mg/mL or 350 mg/mL.

Volume to add to create a **250 mg/mL** solution:

250 mg vial: 0.9 mL

500 mg vial: 1.8 mL

1 g vial: 3.6 mL

2 g vial: 7.2 mL

Volume to add to create a **350 mg/mL** solution:

500 mg vial: 1.0 mL

1 g vial: 2.1 mL

2 g vial: 4.2 mL

I.V. infusion: Infusion is prepared in two stages: Initial reconstitution of powder, followed by dilution to final infusion solution.

Vials: Reconstitute powder with appropriate I.V. diluent (including SWFI, D_5W, $D_{10}W$, NS) to create an initial solution of ~100 mg/mL. Recommended volume to add:

250 mg vial: 2.4 mL

500 mg vial: 4.8 mL

1 g vial: 9.6 mL

2 g vial: 19.2 mL

Note: After reconstitution of powder, further dilution into a volume of compatible solution (eg, 50-100 mL of D_5W or NS) is recommended.

Piggyback bottle: Reconstitute powder with appropriate I.V. diluent (D_5W or NS) to create a resulting solution of ~100 mg/mL. Recommended initial volume to add:

1 g bottle: 10 mL

2 g bottle: 20 mL

Note: After reconstitution, to prepare the final infusion solution, further dilution to 50 mL or 100 mL volumes with the appropriate I.V. diluent (including D_5W or NS) is recommended.

Compatibility Stable in D_5W with KCl 10 mEq, $D_5^1/4NS$ with KCl 20 mEq, $D_5^1/2NS$, D_5W, $D_{10}W$, NS, mannitol 5%, mannitol 10%, sodium bicarbonate 5%, bacteriostatic water, sterile water for injection. **Incompatible** with calcium-containing solutions (eg, LR, Hartmann's solution, parenteral nutrition solutions). **Variable stability (consult detailed reference)** in peritoneal dialysis solutions.

Y-site administration: Compatible: Acyclovir, allopurinol, amifostine, amiodarone, anidulafungin, aztreonam, bivalirudin, cisatracurium, daptomycin, dexmedetomidine, diltiazem, docetaxel, doxorubicin liposome, drotrecogin alfa, etoposide phosphate, famotidine, fenoldopam, fludarabine, foscarnet, gallium nitrate, gatifloxacin, gemcitabine, granisetron, heparin, lansoprazole, linezolid, melphalan, meperidine, methotrexate, morphine, paclitaxel, pantoprazole, pemetrexed, propofol, remifentanil, sargramostim, sodium bicarbonate, tacrolimus, teniposide, theophylline, thiotepa, warfarin, zidovudine. **Incompatible:** Alatrofloxacin, amphotericin B cholesteryl sulfate complex, amsacrine, azithromycin, calcium, filgrastim, fluconazole, Hartmann's solution, labetalol, LR, pentamidine, parenteral nutrition solutions (containing calcium), vinorelbine. **Variable (consult detailed reference):** Anakinra, vancomycin.

Compatibility in syringe: Variable (consult detailed reference): Lidocaine.

Compatibility when admixed: Compatible: Amikacin, metronidazole. **Incompatible:** Aminophylline, amsacrine, calcium, clindamycin, fluconazole, linezolid, theophylline. **Variable (consult detailed reference):** Gentamicin, metronidazole hydrochloride, vancomycin.

Mechanism of Action Inhibits bacterial cell wall synthesis by binding to one or more of the penicillin-binding proteins (PBPs) which in turn inhibits the final transpeptidation step of peptidoglycan synthesis in bacterial cell walls, thus inhibiting cell wall biosynthesis. Bacteria eventually lyse due to ongoing activity of cell wall autolytic enzymes (autolysins and murein hydrolases) while cell wall assembly is arrested.

Pharmacodynamics/Kinetics

Absorption: I.M.: Well absorbed

Distribution: V_d: 6-14 L; widely throughout the body including gallbladder, lungs, bone, bile, CSF (higher concentrations achieved when meninges are inflamed)

Protein binding: 85% to 95%

Half-life elimination: Normal renal and hepatic function: 5-9 hours; Renal impairment (mild-to-severe): 12-16 hours

Time to peak, serum: I.M.: 2-3 hours

Excretion: Urine (33% to 67% as unchanged drug); feces (as inactive drug)

Dosage

Usual dosage range:

Infants and Children: I.M., I.V.: 50-100 mg/kg/day in 1-2 divided doses (maximum: 4 g/day [meningitis]; 2 g/day [nonmeningeal infections])

Adults: I.M., I.V.: 1-2 g every 12-24 hours

Indication-specific dosing:

Infants and Children:

Epiglottitis (unlabeled use): I.M., I.V.: 50-100 mg/kg once daily; reported duration of treatment ranged from 2-14 days

Gonococcal infections:

Conjunctivitis, complicated (unlabeled use): I.M.:

<45 kg: 50 mg/kg in a single dose (maximum: 1 g)

≥45 kg: 1 g in a single dose

Disseminated (unlabeled use): I.M., I.V.:

<45 kg: 25-50 mg/kg once daily (maximum: 1 g)

≥45 kg: 1 g once daily for 7 days

Endocarditis (unlabeled use):

<45 kg: I.M., I.V.: 50 mg/kg/day every 12 hours (maximum: 2 g/day) for at least 28 days

≥45 kg: I.V.: 1-2 g every 12 hours, for at least 28 days

Prophylaxis (due to maternal gonococcal infection): I.M., I.V.: 25-50 mg/kg as a single dose (maximum: 125 mg)

Uncomplicated: I.M.: 125 mg in a single dose

Infective endocarditis: I.M., I.V.:

Native valve: 100 mg/kg once daily for 2-4 weeks; **Note:** If using 2-week regimen, concurrent gentamicin is recommended

Prosthetic valve: 100 mg/kg once daily for 6 weeks (with or without 2 weeks of gentamicin [dependent on penicillin MIC]); **Note:** For HACEK organisms, duration of therapy is 4 weeks

Enterococcus faecalis (resistant to penicillin, aminoglycoside, and vancomycin), native or prosthetic valve: 100 mg/kg once daily for ≥8 weeks administered concurrently with ampicillin

Prophylaxis: 50 mg/kg 30-60 minutes before procedure; maximum dose: 1 g. Intramuscular injections should be avoided in patients who are receiving anticoagulant therapy. In these circumstances, orally administered regimens should be given whenever possible. Intravenously administered antibiotics should be used for patients who are unable to tolerate or absorb oral medications.

Note: American Heart Association (AHA) guidelines now recommend prophylaxis only in patients undergoing invasive procedures and in whom underlying cardiac conditions may predispose to a higher risk of adverse outcomes should infection occur. As of April 2007, routine prophylaxis for GI/GU procedures is no longer recommended by the AHA.

Lyme disease, persistent arthritis (unlabeled use): I.M., I.V.: 75-100 mg/kg (maximum: 2 g) for 2-4 weeks

Mild-to-moderate infections: I.M., I.V.: 50-75 mg/kg/day in 1-2 divided doses every 12-24 hours (maximum: 2 g/day); continue until at least 2 days after signs and symptoms of infection have resolved

Meningitis:
Gonococcal, complicated:
<45 kg: I.V.: 50 mg/kg/day given every 12 hours (maximum: 2 g/day); usual duration of treatment is 10-14 days
>45 kg: I.V.: 1-2 g every 12 hours; usual duration of treatment is 10-14 days
Uncomplicated: I.M., I.V.: Loading dose of 100 mg/kg (maximum: 4 g), followed by 100 mg/kg/day divided every 12-24 hours (maximum: 4 g/day); usual duration of treatment is 7-14 days

Otitis media:
Acute: I.M.: 50 mg/kg in a single dose (maximum: 1 g)
Persistent or relapsing (unlabeled use): I.M., I.V.: 50 mg/kg once daily for 3 days

Pneumonia: I.V.: 50-75 mg/kg once daily
Serious infections: I.V.: 80-100 mg/kg/day in 1-2 divided doses (maximum: 4 g/day)
Skin/skin structure infections: I.M., I.V.: 50-75 mg/kg/day in 1-2 divided doses (maximum: 2 g/day)
STD, sexual assault (unlabeled use): I.M.: 125 mg in a single dose
Typhoid fever (unlabeled use): I.V.: 75-80 mg/kg once daily for 5-14 days

Children >8 years (≥45 kg) and Adolescents:
Epididymitis, acute (unlabeled use): I.M.: 125 mg in a single dose

Children ≤15 years:
Chemoprophylaxis for high-risk contacts and persons with invasive meningococcal disease (unlabeled use): I.M.: 125 mg in a single dose. Children >15 years: Refer to adult dosing.

Adults:
Arthritis, septic (unlabeled use): I.V.: 1-2 g once daily
Brain abscess (unlabeled use): I.V.: 2 g every 12 hours with metronidazole
Cavernous sinus thrombosis (unlabeled use): I.V.: 2 g once daily with vancomycin or linezolid
Chancroid (unlabeled use): I.M.: 250 mg as single dose
Chemoprophylaxis for high-risk contacts and persons with invasive meningococcal disease (unlabeled use): I.M.: 250 mg in a single dose
Gonococcal infections:
Conjunctivitis, complicated (unlabeled use): I.M.: 1 g in a single dose
Disseminated (unlabeled use): I.M., I.V.: 1 g once daily for 7 days
Endocarditis (unlabeled use): I.M., I.V.: 1-2 g every 12 hours for at least 28 days
Epididymitis, acute (unlabeled use): I.M.: 250 mg in a single dose with doxycycline
Prostatitis (unlabeled use): I.M.: 125-250 mg in a single dose with doxycycline
Uncomplicated: I.M.: 125-250 mg in a single dose
Infective endocarditis: I.M., I.V.:
Native valve: 2 g once daily for 2-4 weeks; **Note:** If using 2-week regimen, concurrent gentamicin is recommended
Prosthetic valve: I.M., I.V.: 2 g once daily for 6 weeks (with or without 2 weeks of gentamicin [dependent on penicillin MIC]); **Note:** For HACEK organisms, duration of therapy is 4 weeks
Enterococcus faecalis (resistant to penicillin, aminoglycoside, and vancomycin), native or prosthetic valve: 2 g twice daily for ≥8 weeks administered concurrently with ampicillin

Prophylaxis: I.M., I.V.: 1 g 30-60 minutes before procedure. Intramuscular injections should be avoided in patients who are receiving anticoagulant therapy. In these circumstances, orally administered regimens should be given whenever possible. Intravenously administered antibiotics should be used for patients who are unable to tolerate or absorb oral medications.

Note: American Heart Association (AHA) guidelines now recommend prophylaxis only in patients undergoing invasive procedures and in whom underlying cardiac conditions may predispose to a higher risk of adverse outcomes should infection occur. As of April 2007, routine prophylaxis for GI/GU procedures is no longer recommended by the AHA.

Lyme disease (unlabeled use): I.V.: 2 g once daily for 14-28 days

Mastoiditis (hospitalized; unlabeled use): I.V.: 2 g once daily; >60 years old: 1 g once daily

Meningitis: I.V.: 2 g every 12 hours for 7-14 days (longer courses may be necessary for selected organisms)

Orbital cellulitis (unlabeled use) and endophthalmitis: I.V.: 2 g once daily

Pelvic inflammatory disease: I.M.: 250 mg in a single dose

Pneumonia, community-acquired: I.V.: 1 g once daily, usually in combination with a macrolide; consider 2 g/day for patients at risk for more severe infection and/or resistant organisms (ICU status, age >65 years, disseminated infection)

Pyelonephritis (acute, uncomplicated): Females: I.V.: 1-2 g once daily (Stamm, 1993). Many physicians administer a single parenteral dose before initiating oral therapy (Warren, 1999).

Septic/toxic shock/necrotizing fasciitis (unlabeled use): I.V.: 2 g once daily; with clindamycin for toxic shock

STD prophylaxis in sexual assault victims: I.M.: 125 mg as a single dose

Surgical prophylaxis: I.V.: 1 g 30 minutes to 2 hours before surgery

Syphilis (unlabeled use): I.M., I.V.: 1 g once daily for 8-10 days

Typhoid fever (unlabeled use): I.V.: 2 g once daily for 14 days

Whipple's disease (unlabeled use): Initial: 2 g once daily for 10-14 days, then oral therapy for ~1 year.

Dosage adjustment in renal impairment: No adjustment is generally necessary; **Note:** Concurrent renal and hepatic dysfunction: Maximum dose ≤2 g/day

Hemodialysis: Not dialyzable (0% to 5%); administer dose postdialysis

Continuous ambulatory peritoneal dialysis (CAPD): Administer 1 g every 12 hours

Continuous renal replacement therapy (CRRT): Drug clearance is highly dependent on the method of renal replacement, filter type, and flow rate. Appropriate dosing requires close monitoring of pharmacologic response, signs of adverse reactions due to drug accumulation, as well as drug levels in relation to target trough (if appropriate). The following are general recommendations only (based on dialysate flow/ultrafiltration rates of 1 L/hour) and should not supersede clinical judgment:

CVVH or CVVHD/CVVHDF: 2 g every 12-24 hours

Dosage adjustment in hepatic impairment: No adjustment necessary unless there is concurrent renal dysfunction (see dosage adjustment in renal impairment).

◄ **Administration** Do not admix with aminoglycosides in same bottle/bag. Do not reconstitute, admix, or coadminister with calcium-containing solutions. Infuse intermittent infusion over 30 minutes.

I.M.: Inject deep I.M. into large muscle mass; a concentration of 250 mg/mL or 350 mg/mL is recommended for all vial sizes except the 250 mg size (250 mg/mL is suggested); can be diluted with 1:1 water and 1% lidocaine for I.M. administration.

I.V.: Infuse intermittent infusion over 30 minutes.

Monitoring Parameters Observe for signs and symptoms of anaphylaxis

Test Interactions Positive direct Coombs', false-positive urinary glucose test using cupric sulfate (Benedict's solution, Clinitest®, Fehling's solution), false-positive serum or urine creatinine with Jaffé reaction

Dietary Considerations Some products may contain sodium.

Dosage Forms Excipient information presented when available (limited, particularly for generics); consult specific product labeling. [DSC] = Discontinued product

Infusion [premixed in dextrose]: 1 g (50 mL); 2 g (50 mL)

Injection, powder for reconstitution: 250 mg, 500 mg, 1 g, 2 g, 10 g

Rocephin®: 250 mg [DSC], 500 mg, 1 g, 2 g [DSC], 10 g [contains sodium ~83 mg (3.6 mEq) per ceftriaxone 1 g] [DSC]

References

Hayton WL and Stoeckel K, "Age-Associated Changes in Ceftriaxone Pharmacokinetics," *Clin Pharmacokinet*, 1986, 11(1):76-82.

Marshall WF and Blair JE, "The Cephalosporins," *Mayo Clin Proc*, 1999, 74(2):187-95.

Schaad UB, Suter S, Gianella-Borradori A, et al, "A Comparison of Ceftriaxone and Cefuroxime for the Treatment of Bacterial Meningitis in Children," *N Engl J Med*, 1990, 322(3):141-7.

Stamm WE, Hooton TM, "Management of Urinary Tract Infections in Adults," *N Engl J Med*, 1993, 329(18):1328-34.

Warren JW, Abrutyn E, Hebel JR, et al, "Guidelines for Antimicrobial Treatment of Uncomplicated Acute Bacterial Cystitis and Acute Pyelonephritis in Women," *Clin Infect Dis*, 1999, 29(4):745-58.

♦ **Ceftriaxone Sodium** *see* CefTRIAXone *on page* 199

♦ **Celebrex®** *see* Celecoxib *on page* 206

Celecoxib (se le KOKS ib)

Medication Safety Issues

Sound-alike/look-alike issues:

Celebrex® may be confused with Celexa®, cerebra, Cerebyx®, Clarinex®

Related Information

Oral Mucositis / Stomatitis *on page* 1460

U.S. Brand Names Celebrex®

Generic Available No

Canadian Brand Names Celebrex®; GD-Celecoxib

Pharmacologic Category Nonsteroidal Anti-inflammatory Drug (NSAID), COX-2 Selective

Use Relief of the signs and symptoms of osteoarthritis, ankylosing spondylitis, juvenile rheumatoid arthritis (JRA), and rheumatoid arthritis; management of acute pain; treatment of primary dysmenorrhea; to reduce the number of intestinal polyps in familial adenomatous polyposis (FAP)

Canadian note: Celecoxib is only indicated for relief of symptoms of rheumatoid arthritis, osteoarthritis, and relief of acute pain in adults

Pregnancy Risk Factor C (prior to 30 weeks gestation)/D (≥30 weeks gestation)

Lactation Enters breast milk/use caution

Labeled Contraindications Hypersensitivity to celecoxib, sulfonamides, aspirin, other NSAIDs, or any component of the formulation; perioperative pain in the setting of coronary artery bypass graft (CABG) surgery

Canadian labeling: Additional contraindications (not in U.S. labeling): Pregnancy (3rd trimester); women who are breast-feeding; severe, uncontrolled heart failure; active gastrointestinal ulcer (gastric, duodenal, peptic) or bleeding; inflammatory bowel disease; cerebrovascular bleeding; severe liver impairment or active hepatic disease; severe renal impairment (Cl_{cr} <30 mL/minute) or deteriorating renal disease; known hyperkalemia; use in children

Warnings/Precautions [U.S. Boxed Warning]: NSAIDs are associated with an increased risk of adverse cardiovascular thrombotic events, including MI and stroke. Risk may be increased with duration of use or pre-existing cardiovascular risk factors or disease. Carefully evaluate individual cardiovascular risk profiles prior to prescribing. New-onset or worsening of pre-existing hypertension may occur. May cause sodium and fluid retention; use with caution in patients with edema, cerebrovascular disease, or ischemic heart disease. Avoid use in heart failure. Long-term cardiovascular risk in children has not been evaluated.

[U.S. Boxed Warning]: Celecoxib is contraindicated for treatment of perioperative pain in the setting of coronary artery bypass graft (CABG) surgery. Risk of MI and stroke may be increased with use following CABG surgery.

[U.S. Boxed Warning]: NSAIDs may increase risk of gastrointestinal irritation, ulceration, bleeding, and perforation. These events may occur at any time during therapy and without warning. Use caution with a history of GI disease (bleeding or ulcers), concurrent therapy with aspirin, anticoagulants and/or corticosteroids, smoking, use of alcohol, the elderly or debilitated patients. When used concomitantly with ≤325 mg of aspirin, a substantial increase in the risk of gastrointestinal complications (eg, ulcer) occurs; concomitant gastroprotective therapy (eg, proton pump inhibitors) is recommended (Bhatt, 2008).

Use the lowest effective dose for the shortest duration of time, consistent with individual patient goals, to reduce risk of cardiovascular or GI adverse events. Alternate therapies should be considered for patients at high risk.

NSAIDs may cause serious skin adverse events including exfoliative dermatitis, Stevens-Johnson syndrome (SJS), and toxic epidermal necrolysis (TEN). Anaphylactoid reactions may occur, even without prior exposure; patients with "aspirin triad" (bronchial asthma, aspirin intolerance, rhinitis) may be at increased risk. Do not use in patients who experience bronchospasm, asthma, rhinitis, or urticaria with NSAID or aspirin therapy. Use caution in other forms of asthma.

Use with caution in patients with decreased hepatic (dosage adjustments are recommended for moderate hepatic impairment; not recommended for patients with severe hepatic impairment) or renal function. Transaminase elevations have been reported with use; closely monitor patients with any abnormal LFT. Severe hepatic reactions (eg, fulminant hepatitis, liver failure) have occurred with NSAID use, rarely; discontinue if signs or symptoms of liver disease develop, if systemic manifestations occur, or with persistent or worsening abnormal hepatic function tests. NSAID use may compromise existing renal function; dose-dependent decreases in prostaglandin synthesis may result from NSAID use, causing a reduction in renal blood flow which may cause renal decompensation. Patients with impaired renal function, dehydration, heart failure, liver dysfunction, those taking diuretics and ACEI, and the elderly are at greater risk for renal toxicity. Rehydrate patient before starting therapy; monitor renal function closely. Not recommended for use in patients with advanced renal disease or severe renal insufficiency; discontinue use with persistent or worsening abnormal renal function tests. Long-term NSAID use may result in renal papillary necrosis.

Anaphylactoid reactions may occur, even with no prior exposure to celecoxib. Use with caution in patients with known or suspected deficiency of cytochrome P450 isoenzyme 2C9; poor metabolizers may have higher plasma levels due to reduced metabolism; consider reduced initial doses. Alternate therapies should be considered in patients with JRA who are poor metabolizers of CYP2C9.

Anemia may occur with use; monitor hemoglobin or hematocrit in patients on long-term treatment. Celecoxib does not affect PT, PTT or platelet counts; does not inhibit platelet aggregation at approved doses.

When used for the treatment of FAP, routine monitoring and care should be continued. When used for JRA, celecoxib is not FDA-approved in children <2 years of age or in children <10 kg. Use caution with systemic onset JRA (may be at risk for disseminated intravascular coagulation). Safety and efficacy have not been established for use in children for indications other than JRA.

Adverse Reactions

>10%:
  Cardiovascular: Hypertension (≤13%)
  Central nervous system: Headache (10% to 16%)
  Gastrointestinal: Diarrhea (4% to 11%)
2% to 10%:
  Cardiovascular: Peripheral edema (2%)
  Central nervous system: Fever (≤9%), insomnia (2%), dizziness (1% to 2%)
  Dermatologic: Skin rash (2%)
  Gastrointestinal: Dyspepsia (9%), nausea (4% to 7%), gastroesophageal reflux (≤5%), abdominal pain (4% to 8%), vomiting (≤6%), flatulence (2%)
  Neuromuscular & skeletal: Arthralgia (≤7%), back pain (3%)
  Respiratory: Upper respiratory tract infection (8%), cough (≤7%), nasopharyngitis (≤6%), sinusitis (5%), dyspnea (≤3%), pharyngitis (2%), rhinitis (2%)
  Miscellaneous: Accidental injury (3%)
0.1% to 2%:
  Cardiovascular: Angina, aortic valve incompetence, chest pain, coronary artery disorder, DVT, edema, facial edema, hypertension (aggravated), MI, palpitation, sinus bradycardia, tachycardia, ventricular hypertrophy
  Central nervous system: Anxiety, cerebral infarction, depression, fatigue, hypoesthesia, migraine, nervousness, pain, somnolence, vertigo
  Dermatologic: Alopecia, bruising, cellulitis, dermatitis, dry skin, nail disorder, photosensitivity, pruritus, rash (erythematous), rash (maculopapular), urticaria
  Endocrine & metabolic: Breast fibroadenosis, breast neoplasm, breast pain, diabetes mellitus, dysmenorrhea, hot flashes, hypercholesterolemia, hyperglycemia, hyper-/hypokalemia, hypernatremia, menstrual disturbances, ovarian cyst, testosterone decreased
  Gastrointestinal: Anorexia, appetite increased, constipation, diverticulitis, dysphagia, eructation, esophagitis, gastritis, gastroenteritis, gastrointestinal ulcer, hemorrhoids, hiatal hernia, melena, stomatitis, taste disturbance, tenesmus, tooth disorder, weight gain, xerostomia

Genitourinary: Cystitis, dysuria, incontinence, monilial vaginitis, prostate disorder, urinary frequency, urinary tract infection, vaginal bleeding, vaginitis

Hematologic: Anemia, thrombocytopenia

Hepatic: Alkaline phosphatase increased, transaminases increased

Neuromuscular & skeletal: Arthrosis, bone disorder, CPK increased, fracture, hypertonia, leg cramps, myalgia, neck stiffness, neuralgia, neuropathy, paresthesia, synovitis, tendon rupture, tendonitis, weakness

Ocular: Blurred vision, cataract, conjunctival hemorrhage, conjunctivitis, eye pain, glaucoma, vitreous floaters

Otic: Deafness, earache, labyrinthitis, otitis media, tinnitus

Renal: Albuminuria, BUN increased, creatinine increased, hematuria, nonprotein nitrogen increased, renal calculi

Respiratory: Bronchitis, bronchospasm, epistaxis, laryngitis, pneumonia

Miscellaneous: Allergic reactions, allergy aggravated, diaphoresis, flu-like syndrome, herpes infection, infection (bacterial, fungal, viral), moniliasis

<0.1%, postmarketing, and/or case reports (limited to important or life-threatening): Acute renal failure, agranulocytosis, anaphylactoid reactions, angioedema, aplastic anemia, aseptic meningitis, ataxia, cerebrovascular accident, CHF, cholelithiasis, colitis, erythema multiforme, esophageal perforation, exfoliative dermatitis, gangrene, gastrointestinal bleeding, hepatic failure, hepatic necrosis, hepatitis (including fulminant), hypoglycemia, hyponatremia, ileus, interstitial nephritis, intestinal obstruction, intestinal perforation, intracranial hemorrhage, jaundice, leukopenia, pancreatitis, pancytopenia, pulmonary embolism, renal papillary necrosis, sepsis, Stevens-Johnson syndrome, sudden death, suicide, syncope, thrombophlebitis, toxic epidermal necrolysis, vasculitis, ventricular fibrillation

Drug Interactions

Metabolism/Transport Effects Substrate of CYP2C9 (major), 3A4 (minor); **Inhibits** CYP2C8 (moderate), 2D6 (weak)

Avoid Concomitant Use

Avoid concomitant use of Celecoxib with any of the following: Ketorolac; Thioridazine

Increased Effect/Toxicity

Celecoxib may increase the levels/effects of: Aminoglycosides; Anticoagulants; Antiplatelet Agents; Bisphosphonate Derivatives; CycloSPORINE; CYP2C8 Substrates (High risk); CYP2D6 Substrates; Desmopressin; Eplerenone; Fesoterodine; Lithium; Methotrexate; Nebivolol; Nonsteroidal Anti-Inflammatory Agents; Potassium-Sparing Diuretics; Quinolone Antibiotics; Tamoxifen; Thioridazine; Thrombolytic Agents; Vancomycin; Vitamin K Antagonists

The levels/effects of Celecoxib may be increased by: Antidepressants (Tricyclic, Tertiary Amine); Corticosteroids (Systemic); CYP2C9 Inhibitors (Moderate); CYP2C9 Inhibitors (Strong); Herbs (Anticoagulant/Antiplatelet Properties); Ketorolac; Probenecid; Selective Serotonin Reuptake Inhibitors; Treprostinil

Decreased Effect

Celecoxib may decrease the levels/effects of: ACE Inhibitors; Angiotensin II Receptor Blockers; Antiplatelet Agents; Beta-Blockers; Codeine; Eplerenone; HydrALAZINE; Loop Diuretics; Potassium-Sparing Diuretics; Thiazide Diuretics; TraMADol

The levels/effects of Celecoxib may be decreased by: Bile Acid Sequestrants; CYP2C9 Inducers (Highly Effective); Peginterferon Alfa-2b

Ethanol/Nutrition/Herb Interactions

Ethanol: Avoid ethanol (increased GI irritation).

Food: Peak concentrations are delayed and AUC is increased by 10% to 20% when taken with a high-fat meal.

Herb/Nutraceutical: Avoid concomitant use with herbs possessing anti-coagulation/antiplatelet properties, including alfalfa, anise, bilberry, bladder-wrack, bromelain, cat's claw, celery, chamomile, coleus, cordyceps, dong quai, evening primrose, fenugreek, feverfew, garlic, ginger, ginkgo biloba, ginseng (American, Panax, Siberian), grapeseed, green tea, guggul, horse chestnuts, horseradish, licorice, prickly ash, red clover, reishi, SAMe (S-adenosylmethionine), sweet clover, turmeric, white willow.

Storage/Stability Store at controlled room temperature of 25°C (77°F); excursions permitted to 15°C to 30°C (59°F to 86°F).

Mechanism of Action Inhibits prostaglandin synthesis by decreasing the activity of the enzyme, cyclooxygenase-2 (COX-2), which results in decreased formation of prostaglandin precursors; has antipyretic, analgesic, and anti-inflammatory properties. Celecoxib does not inhibit cyclooxygenase-1 (COX-1) at therapeutic concentrations.

Pharmacodynamics/Kinetics

Distribution: V_d (apparent): ~400 L

Protein binding: ~97% primarily to albumin

Metabolism: Hepatic via CYP2C9; forms inactive metabolites

Bioavailability: Absolute: Unknown

Half-life elimination: ~11 hours (fasted)

Time to peak: ~3 hours

Excretion: Feces (~57% as metabolites, <3% as unchanged drug); urine (27% as metabolites, <3% as unchanged drug)

Dosage Note: Use the lowest effective dose for the shortest duration of time, consistent with individual patient goals. Oral:

Children ≥2 years: JRA

≥10 kg to ≤25 kg: 50 mg twice daily

>25 kg: 100 mg twice daily

Adults:

Acute pain or primary dysmenorrhea: Initial dose: 400 mg, followed by an additional 200 mg if needed on day 1; maintenance dose: 200 mg twice daily as needed

Ankylosing spondylitis: 200 mg/day as a single dose or in divided doses twice daily; if no effect after 6 weeks, may increase to 400 mg/day. If no response following 6 weeks of treatment with 400 mg/day, consider discontinuation and alternative treatment.

Familial adenomatous polyposis: 400 mg twice daily (with food)

Osteoarthritis: 200 mg/day as a single dose or in divided dose twice daily

Rheumatoid arthritis: 100-200 mg twice daily

Elderly: No specific adjustment based on age is recommended. However, the AUC in elderly patients may be increased by 50% as compared to younger subjects. Initiate at the lowest recommended dose in patients weighing <50 kg.

Dosing adjustment in poor CYP2C9 metabolizers: Consider reducing initial dose by 50%; consider alternative treatment in patients with JRA who are poor CYP2C9 metabolizers

Dosing adjustment in renal impairment:

Advanced renal disease: Use is not recommended, however, if celecoxib treatment cannot be avoided, monitor renal function closely

Severe renal insufficiency: Use is not recommended

Abnormal renal function tests (persistent or worsening): Discontinue use

Dosing adjustment in hepatic impairment:

Moderate hepatic impairment (Child-Pugh class B): Reduce dose by 50%

Severe hepatic impairment: Use is not recommended

Abnormal liver function tests (persistent or worsening): Discontinue use

Administration Lower doses (200 mg twice daily) may be taken without regard to meals. Larger doses (400 mg twice daily) should be taken with food to improve absorption. Capsules may be swallowed whole or the entire contents emptied onto a teaspoon of cool or room temperature applesauce. The contents of the capsules sprinkled onto applesauce may be stored under refrigeration for up to 6 hours.

Monitoring Parameters CBC; blood chemistry profile; occult blood loss and periodic liver function tests; monitor renal function (urine output, serum BUN and creatinine); monitor response (pain, range of motion, grip strength, mobility, ADL function), inflammation; observe for weight gain, edema; observe for bleeding, bruising; evaluate gastrointestinal effects (abdominal pain, bleeding, dyspepsia); blood pressure

FAP: Continue routine endoscopic exams

JRA: Monitor for development of abnormal coagulation tests with systemic onset JRA

Dietary Considerations Lower doses (200 mg twice daily) may be taken without regard to meals. Larger doses (400 mg twice daily) should be taken with food to improve absorption.

Dosage Forms Excipient information presented when available (limited, particularly for generics); consult specific product labeling.

Capsule:

Celebrex®: 50 mg, 100 mg, 200 mg, 400 mg

References

Arbor N, Eagle CJ, Spicak J, et al, "Celecoxib for the Prevention of Colorectal Adenomatous Polyps," *N Engl J Med*, 2006, 355(9):885-95.

Bertagnolli MM, Eagle CJ, Zauber AG, et al, "Celecoxib for the Prevention of Sporadic Colorectal Adenomas," *N Engl J Med*, 2006, 355(9):873-84.

Bhatt DL, Scheiman J, Abraham NS, et al, "ACCF/ACG/AHA 2008 Expert Consensus Document on Reducing the Gastrointestinal Risk of Antiplatelet Therapy and NSAID Use. A Report of the American College of Cardiology Foundation Task Force on Clinical Expert Consensus Documents," *J Am Coll Cardiol*, 2008, 52(18):1502-17.

Solomon SD, McMurray JJ, Pfeffer MA, et al, "Cardiovascular Risk Associated With Celecoxib in a Clinical Trial for Colorectal Adenoma Prevention," *N Engl J Med*, 2005, 352(11):1071-80.

Steinbach G, Lynch PM, Phillips RK, et al, "The Effect of Celecoxib, a Cyclooxygenase-2 Inhibitor, in Familial Adenomatous Polyposis," *N Engl J Med*, 2000, 342(26):1946-52.

◆ **CellCept®** *see* Mycophenolate *on page 831*

◆ **Cerubidine®** *see* DAUNOrubicin Hydrochloride *on page 323*

◆ **Cesamet™** *see* Nabilone *on page 838*

◆ **Cetacort® [DSC]** *see* Hydrocortisone *on page 575*

◆ **Cetraxal®** *see* Ciprofloxacin *on page 228*

Cetuximab (se TUK see mab)

Medication Safety Issues

Sound-alike/look-alike issues:

Cetuximab may be confused with bevacizumab

U.S. Brand Names Erbitux®

Index Terms C225; IMC-C225; MOAB C225

Generic Available No

Canadian Brand Names Erbitux®

Pharmacologic Category Antineoplastic Agent, Monoclonal Antibody; Epidermal Growth Factor Receptor (EGFR) Inhibitor

Use Treatment of metastatic colorectal cancer; treatment of squamous cell cancer of the head and neck

Note: Subset analyses (retrospective) in metastatic colorectal cancer trials have not shown a benefit with EGFR inhibitor treatment in patients whose tumors have codon 12 or 13 *KRAS* mutations; use is not recommended in these patients.

Unlabeled/Investigational Use Treatment of EGFR-expressing advanced nonsmall cell lung cancer (NSCLC)

Pregnancy Risk Factor C

Lactation Excretion in breast milk is unknown/not recommended

Labeled Contraindications There are no contraindications listed in the manufacturer's labeling

Warnings/Precautions [U.S. Boxed Warning]: Severe infusion reactions (bronchospasm, stridor, hoarseness, urticaria, hypotension, loss of consciousness, shock, MI, cardiac arrest) have been reported in ~3% of patients; fatal outcome has been reported rarely. Approximately 90% of reactions occur with the first infusion despite the use of prophylactic antihistamines. **Note:** Although a 20 mg test dose was used in some studies, it did not reliably predict the risk of an infusion reaction, and is not recommended. In case of severe reaction, treatment should be stopped and permanently discontinued. Immediate treatment for anaphylactic/anaphylactoid reactions should be available during administration. The manufacturer recommends monitoring patients for at least 1 hour following completion of infusion, or longer if a reaction occurs. Mild-to-moderate infusion reactions are managed by slowing the infusion rate (by 50%) and administering antihistamines. Patients with pre-existing IgE antibody against cetuximab (specific for galactose-α-1,3-galactose) are reported to have a higher incidence of severe hypersensitivity reaction. Severe hypersensitivity reaction has been reported more frequently in patients living in the middle south area of the United States, including North Carolina and Tennessee (O'Neil, 2007; Chung, 2008).

[U.S. Boxed Warning]: Cardiopulmonary arrest has occurred in 2% of patients receiving radiation therapy in combination with cetuximab; closely monitor serum electrolytes during and after (for at least 8 weeks) cetuximab therapy; use caution with history of coronary artery disease, HF, and arrhythmias. Interstitial lung disease (ILD) has been reported; use caution with pre-existing lung disease; permanently discontinue with confirmed ILD. Acneiform rash has been reported in 76% to 88% of patients (severe in 1% to 17%), usually developing within the first 2 weeks of therapy; may require dose modification. Acneiform rash should be treated with topical and/or oral antibiotics; topical corticosteroids are not recommended. Other dermatologic toxicities, including dry skin, fissures, hypertrichosis, paronychial inflammation, and skin infections have been reported; related ocular toxicities (blepharitis, conjunctivitis, keratitis) may also occur. Sunlight may exacerbate skin reactions (limit sun exposure). Hypomagnesemia is common; the onset of electrolyte disturbance may occur within days to months after initiation of treatment; monitor during treatment and for at least 8 weeks after completion. Nonneutralizing anticetuximab antibodies were detected in 5% of evaluable patients. Safety and efficacy have not been established when used in combination with radiation therapy and cisplatin. Patients with colorectal cancer with tumors with a codon 12 or 13 *KRAS* mutation are unlikely to benefit from EGFR inhibitor therapy and should not receive cetuximab treatment. Safety and efficacy in children have not been established.

Adverse Reactions Except where noted, percentages reported for cetuximab monotherapy.

>10%:

Central nervous system: Fatigue (89%), pain (17% to 51%), headache (26% to 33%), insomnia (10% to 30%), fever (27% to 30%), confusion (15%), anxiety (14%), chills/rigors (13%), depression (7% to 13%)

Dermatologic: Acneiform rash (76% to 90%; grades 3/4: 1% to 17%; onset: ≤14 days), rash (89%), dry skin (49%), pruritus (11% to 40%), nail changes/disorder (16% to 21%)

Endocrine & metabolic: Hypomagnesemia (55%; grades 3/4: 6% to 17%)

Gastrointestinal: Abdominal pain (26% to 59%), constipation (26% to 46%), diarrhea (25% to 39%), vomiting (25% to 37%), nausea (mild-to-moderate 29%), weight loss (7% to 27%), anorexia (23%), stomatitis (10% to 25%), xerostomia (11%)

Neuromuscular & skeletal: Weakness (45% to 48%), bone pain (15%)

Respiratory: Dyspnea (17% to 48%), cough (11% to 29%)

Miscellaneous: Infection (13% to 35%), infusion reaction (15% to 21%; grades 3/4: 2% to 5%; 90% of severe reactions occurred with first infusion)

1% to 10%:

Cardiovascular: Peripheral edema (10%), cardiopulmonary arrest (2%; with radiation therapy)

Dermatologic: Alopecia (4%), skin disorder (4%)

Endocrine & metabolic: Dehydration (2% to 10%)

Gastrointestinal: Dyspepsia (6%)

Hematologic: Anemia (9%)

Hepatic: Alkaline phosphatase increased (5% to 10%), transaminases increased (5% to 10%)

Neuromuscular & skeletal: Back pain (10%)

Ocular: Conjunctivitis (7%)

Renal: Renal failure (1%)

Respiratory: Pulmonary embolus (1%)

Miscellaneous: Sepsis (1% to 4%)

<1%, postmarketing, and/or case reports: Abscess formation, arrhythmia, blepharitis, bronchospasm, cardiac arrest, cellulitis, cheilitis, hoarseness, hypertrichosis, hypotension, interstitial lung disease (occurred between the fourth and eleventh doses), keratitis, leukopenia, loss of consciousness, MI, paronychial inflammation, sepsis, shock, skin fissure, skin infection, stridor

Drug Interactions

Avoid Concomitant Use There are no known interactions where it is recommended to avoid concomitant use.

Increased Effect/Toxicity There are no known significant interactions involving an increase in effect.

Decreased Effect There are no known significant interactions involving a decrease in effect.

Storage/Stability Store unopened vials under refrigeration at 2°C to 8°C (36°F to 46°F); do not freeze. Preparations in infusion containers are stable for up to 12 hours under refrigeration at 2°C to 8°C (36°F to 46°F) and up to 8 hours at room temperature of 20°C to 25°C (68°F to 77°F).

Reconstitution Reconstitution is not required. Appropriate dose should be added to empty sterile container; do not shake or dilute.

Mechanism of Action Recombinant human/mouse chimeric monoclonal antibody which binds specifically to the epidermal growth factor receptor (EGFR, HER1, c-ErbB-1) and competitively inhibits the binding of epidermal growth factor (EGF) and other ligands. Binding to the EGFR blocks phosphorylation and activation of receptor-associated kinases, resulting in inhibition of cell growth, induction of apoptosis, and decreased matrix metalloproteinase and vascular endothelial growth factor production. EGFR signal transduction results in *KRAS* wild-type activation; cells with *KRAS* mutations appear to be unaffected by EGFR inhibition.

Pharmacodynamics/Kinetics

Distribution: V_d: ~2-3 L/m^2

Half-life elimination: ~112 hours (range: 63-230 hours)

Dosage I.V.: Adults: **Note:** Premedicate with an H$_1$ antagonist (eg, diphenhydramine) I.V. 30-60 minutes prior to the first dose; premedication for subsequent doses is based on clinical judgement.

Colorectal cancer:

Initial loading dose: 400 mg/m^2 infused over 120 minutes

Maintenance dose: 250 mg/m^2 infused over 60 minutes weekly

Biweekly administration (unlabeled dosing): 500 mg/m^2 every 2 weeks (initial dose infused over 120 minutes, subsequent doses infused over 60 minutes) (Pfeiffer, 2007)

Head and neck cancer:

Initial loading dose: 400 mg/m^2 infused over 120 minutes

Maintenance dose: 250 mg/m^2 infused over 60 minutes weekly

Note: If given in combination with radiation therapy, administer loading dose 1 week prior to initiation of radiation course. Weekly maintenance dose should be completed 1 hour prior to radiation for the duration of radiation therapy (6-7 weeks).

NSCLC (unlabeled use): Initial loading dose: 400 mg/m^2, followed by maintenance dose: 250 mg/m^2 weekly (Pirker, 2008)

Dosage adjustment for toxicity:

Infusion reactions, grade 1 or 2 and nonserious grades 3 or 4: Reduce the infusion rate by 50% and continue to use prophylactic antihistamines

Infusion reactions, severe: Immediately and permanently discontinue treatment

Pulmonary toxicity:

Acute onset or worsening pulmonary symptoms: Hold treatment

Interstitial lung disease: Permanently discontinue

Skin toxicity, mild-to-moderate: No dosage modification required

Acneiform rash, severe (grade 3 or 4):

First occurrence: Delay cetuximab infusion 1-2 weeks

If improvement, continue at 250 mg/m^2

If no improvement, discontinue therapy

Second occurrence: Delay cetuximab infusion 1-2 weeks

If improvement, continue at reduced dose of 200 mg/m^2

If no improvement, discontinue therapy

Third occurrence: Delay cetuximab infusion 1-2 weeks

If improvement, continue at reduced dose of 150 mg/m^2

If no improvement, discontinue therapy

Fourth occurrence: Discontinue therapy

Note: Dose adjustments are not recommended for severe **radiation** dermatitis.

Combination Regimens

Colorectal cancer:

Cetuximab (Biweekly)-Irinotecan on page 1255
Cetuximab-FOLFOX4 on page 1257
Cetuximab-Irinotecan on page 1258

Head and neck cancer:

Carboplatin-Cetuximab on page 1248
Cetuximab-Carboplatin-Fluorouracil on page 1255
Cetuximab-Cisplatin-Fluorouracil on page 1256
Cisplatin-Cetuximab on page 1264
Paclitaxel-Cetuximab on page 1387

Lung cancer (nonsmall cell): Cetuximab-Cisplatin-Vinorelbine on page 1256

Administration Administer via I.V. infusion; loading dose over 2 hours, weekly maintenance dose over 1 hour. Do not administer as I.V. push or bolus. Do not shake or dilute. Administer via infusion pump or syringe pump. Following the infusion, an observation period (1 hour) is recommended; longer observation time (following an infusion reaction) may be required. Premedication with an H_1 antagonist prior to the initial dose is recommended. The maximum infusion rate is 10 mg/minute. Administer through a low protein-binding 0.22 micrometer in-line filter. Use 0.9% NaCl to flush line at the end of infusion.

For biweekly administration (unlabeled frequency and dose), the initial dose was infused over 120 minutes and subsequent doses infused over 60 minutes (Pfeiffer, 2007).

Monitoring Parameters Vital signs during infusion and observe for at least 1 hour postinfusion. Patients developing dermatologic toxicities should be monitored for the development of complications. Periodic monitoring of serum magnesium, calcium, and potassium are recommended to continue over an interval consistent with the half-life (8 weeks); monitor closely (during and after treatment) for cetuximab plus radiation therapy. KRAS genotyping of tumor tissue in patients with colorectal cancer.

Additional Information Oncology Comment: EGFR expression is detected in nearly all patients with head and neck cancer; laboratory evidence of EGFR expression is not necessary for head and neck cancers.

The National Comprehensive Cancer Network® (NCCN) guidelines for colon cancer (v.2.2009) and the American Society of Clinical Oncology (ASCO) provisional clinical opinion (Allegra, 2009) recommend genotyping tumor tissue for KRAS mutation in all patients with metastatic colorectal cancer (genotyping may be done on archived specimens). Patients with known codon 12 or 13 KRAS gene mutations are unlikely to respond to EGFR inhibitors and should not receive cetuximab. Favorable progression-free survival and overall survival has been demonstrated with cetuximab in patients with KRAS wild-type (Karapetis, 2008; Van Cutsem, 2008). Because EGFR testing in colorectal tumors does not correlate with response, the NCCN guidelines do not recommend routine EGFR testing in colorectal cancer. Dermatologic toxicity with cetuximab is predictive for response; the presence of acneiform rash correlates with treatment response and prolonged survival (Cunningham, 2004).

The NCCN Non-Small Cell Lung cancer guidelines (v.2.2009) recommend cetuximab in combination with cisplatin and vinorelbine as a first-line therapy option in patients with advanced (stage IIIB or IV disease), with EGFR expression and a performance status of 0-2.

Emetic Potential Low (10% to 30%)

◀ **Dosage Forms** Excipient information presented when available (limited, particularly for generics); consult specific product labeling.

Injection, solution [preservative free]:

Erbitux®: 2 mg/mL (50 mL, 100 mL)

References

Allegra CJ, Jessup JM, Somerfield MR, et al, "American Society of Clinical Oncology Provisional Clinical Opinion: Testing for *KRAS* Gene Mutations in Patients With Metastatic Colorectal Carcinoma to Predict Response to Anti-Epidermal Growth Factor Receptor Monoclonal Antibody Therapy, " *J Clin Oncol*, 2009, 27(12):2091-6.

Bonner JA, Harari PM, Giralt J, et al, "Radiotherapy Plus Cetuximab for Squamous-Cell Carcinoma of the Head and Neck," *N Engl J Med*, 2006, 354(6):567-78.

Chung CH, Mirakhur B, Chan E, et al, "Cetuximab-Induced Anaphylaxis and IgE Specific for Galactose-alpha-1,3-galactose," *N Engl J Med*, 2008, 358(11):1109-17

Cunningham D, Humblet Y, Siena S, et al, "Cetuximab Monotherapy and Cetuximab Plus Irinotecan in Irinotecan-Refractory Metastatic Colorectal Cancer," *N Engl J Med*, 2004, 351 (4):337-45.

Jonker DJ, O'Callaghan CJ, Karapetis CS, et al, "Cetuximab for the Treatment of Colorectal Cancer," *N Engl J Med*, 2007, 357(20):2040-8.

Karapetis CS, Khambata-Ford S, Jonker DJ, et al, "K-ras Mutations and Benefit From Cetuximab in Advanced Colorectal Cancer," *N Engl J Med*, 2008, 359(17):1757-65.

National Comprehensive Cancer Network (NCCN), "Clinical Practice Guidelines in Oncology™: Colon Cancer," Version 2.2009. Accessible at http://www.nccn.org/professionals/physician_gls/PDF/colon.pdf

National Comprehensive Cancer Network (NCCN), "Clinical Practice Guidelines in Oncology™: Non-Small Cell Lung Cancer," Version 2.2009. Accessible at http://www.nccn.org/professionals/physician_gls/PDF/nscl.pdf.

O'Neil BH, Allen R, Spigel DR, et al, "High Incidence of Cetuximab-Related Infusion Reactions in Tennessee and North Carolina and the Association With Atopic History," *J Clin Oncol*, 2007, 25 (24):3644-8.

Pfeiffer P, Bjerregarrd JK, Qvortrup C, et al, "Simplification of Cetuximab (Cet) Administration: Double Dose Every Second Week as a 60 Minute Infusion," *J Clin Oncol*, 2007, 25(18S):4133 [abstract from 2007 ASCO Annual Meeting Proceedings, Part I]

Pfeiffer P, Nielsen D, Bjerregaard J, et al, "Biweekly Cetuximab and Irinotecan as Third-Line Therapy in Patients With Advanced Colorectal Cancer After Failure to Irinotecan, Oxaliplatin and 5-Fluorouracil," *Ann Oncol*, 2008, 19(6):1141-5.

Pirker R, Szczesna A, von Pawel J, et al, "FLEX: A Randomized, Multicenter, Phase III Study of Cetuximab in Combination With Cisplatin/Vinorelbine (CV) Versus CV Alone in the First-Line Treatment of Patients With Advanced Non-Small Cell Lung Cancer (NSCLC),"*J Clin Oncol*, 2008, 26(Supp) [abstract 3 from 2008 ASCO Annual Meeting].

Van Cutsem E, Lang, I, D'haens G, et al, "*KRAS* Status and Efficacy in the First-Line Treatment of Patients With Metastatic Colorectal Cancer (mCRC) Treated With FOLFIRI With or Without Cetuximab: The CRYSTAL Experience," *J Clin Oncol*, 2008, 26(Supp) [abstract 2 from 2008 ASCO Annual Meeting].

◆ **CGP-42446** *see* Zoledronic Acid *on page 1199*

◆ **CGP-57148B** *see* Imatinib *on page 613*

◆ **CGS-20267** *see* Letrozole *on page 694*

◆ **Chloditan** *see* Mitotane *on page 807*

◆ **Chlodithane** *see* Mitotane *on page 807*

Chlorambucil (klor AM byoo sil)

Medication Safety Issues

Sound-alike/look-alike issues:

Chlorambucil may be confused with Chloromycetin®

Leukeran® may be confused with Alkeran®, leucovorin, Leukine®, Myleran®

High alert medication: The Institute for Safe Medication Practices (ISMP) includes this medication among its list of drugs which have a heightened risk of causing significant patient harm when used in error.

Related Information
Fertility and Cancer Therapy *on page 1430*
Safe Handling of Hazardous Drugs *on page 1517*

U.S. Brand Names Leukeran®

Index Terms CB-1348; Chlorambucilum; Chloraminophene; Chlorbutinum; WR-139013

Generic Available No

Canadian Brand Names Leukeran®

Pharmacologic Category Antineoplastic Agent, Alkylating Agent

Use Management of chronic lymphocytic leukemia (CLL), Hodgkin's lymphoma, non-Hodgkin's lymphoma (NHL)

Unlabeled/Investigational Use Treatment of nephrotic syndrome, Waldenström's macroglobulinemia

Pregnancy Risk Factor D

Lactation Excretion in breast milk unknown/not recommended

Labeled Contraindications Hypersensitivity to chlorambucil or any component of the formulation; hypersensitivity to other alkylating agents (may have cross-hypersensitivity); pregnancy

Warnings/Precautions Hazardous agent - use appropriate precautions for handling and disposal. Seizures have been observed; use with caution in patients with seizure disorder or head trauma; history of nephrotic syndrome and high pulse doses are at higher risk of seizures. **[U.S. Boxed Warning]: May cause bone marrow suppression;** reduce initial dosage if patient has received myelosuppressive or radiation therapy, or has a depressed baseline leukocyte or platelet count within the previous 4 weeks. Lymphopenia may occur. Avoid administration of live vaccines to immunocompromised patients. Rare instances of severe skin reactions (eg, erythema multiforme, Stevens-Johnson syndrome) have been reported; discontinue if a reaction occurs.

[U.S. Boxed Warning]: Affects human fertility; carcinogenic in humans and probably mutagenic and teratogenic as well; chromosomal damage has been documented. Fertility effects (reversible and irreversible sterility) include azoospermia (when administered to prepubertal and pubertal males) and amenorrhea. Secondary malignancies and acute myelocytic leukemia may be associated with chronic therapy. Safety and efficacy in pediatric patients have not been established.

Adverse Reactions Frequency not always defined.
Central nervous system: Agitation (rare), ataxia (rare), confusion (rare), drug fever, focal/generalized seizure (rare), hallucinations (rare)
Dermatologic: Angioneurotic edema, erythema multiforme (rare), rash, skin hypersensitivity, Stevens-Johnson syndrome (rare), toxic epidermal necrolysis (rare), urticaria
Endocrine & metabolic: Amenorrhea, infertility, SIADH (rare)
Gastrointestinal: Diarrhea (infrequent), nausea (infrequent), oral ulceration (infrequent), vomiting (infrequent)
Genitourinary: Azoospermia, cystitis (sterile)
Hematologic: Neutropenia (25%; dose- and duration-related; onset: 3 weeks; recovery: 10 days after last dose), bone marrow failure (irreversible), bone marrow suppression, anemia, leukemia (secondary), leukopenia, lymphopenia, pancytopenia, thrombocytopenia
Hepatic: Hepatotoxicity, jaundice
Neuromuscular & skeletal: Flaccid paresis (rare), muscular twitching (rare), myoclonia (rare), peripheral neuropathy, tremor (rare)
Respiratory: Interstitial pneumonia, pulmonary fibrosis

Miscellaneous: Allergic reactions, malignancies (secondary)

Drug Interactions

Avoid Concomitant Use

Avoid concomitant use of Chlorambucil with any of the following: Natalizumab; Vaccines (Live)

Increased Effect/Toxicity

Chlorambucil may increase the levels/effects of: Leflunomide; Natalizumab; Vaccines (Live)

The levels/effects of Chlorambucil may be increased by: Trastuzumab

Decreased Effect

Chlorambucil may decrease the levels/effects of: Vaccines (Inactivated); Vaccines (Live)

The levels/effects of Chlorambucil may be decreased by: Echinacea

Storage/Stability Store in refrigerator at 2°C to 8°C (36°F to 46°F). Protect from light.

Mechanism of Action Interferes with DNA replication and RNA transcription by alkylation and cross-linking the strands of DNA

Pharmacodynamics/Kinetics

Absorption: Rapid and complete

Distribution: V_d: 0.14-0.24 L/kg

Protein binding: ~99%

Metabolism: Hepatic; forms a major active metabolite (phenylacetic acid mustard) and inactive metabolites

Bioavailability: Reduced 10% to 20% with food

Half-life elimination: ~1.5 hours; Phenylacetic acid mustard: ~1.8 hours

Time to peak, plasma: Within 1 hour; Phenylacetic acid mustard: 1.2-2.6 hours

Excretion: Urine (15% to 60% primarily as inactive metabolites, <1% unchanged drug or phenylacetic acid mustard)

Dosage Oral (refer to individual protocols):

Children (unlabeled uses):

General short courses: 0.1-0.2 mg/kg/day for 3-6 weeks **or** maintenance therapy: 0.03-0.1 mg/kg/day

Nephrotic syndrome: 0.1-0.2 mg/kg/day every day for ~8-12 weeks with low-dose prednisone

Chronic lymphocytic leukemia (CLL):

Biweekly regimen: Initial: 0.4 mg/kg/dose every 2 weeks; increase dose by 0.1 mg/kg every 2 weeks until a response occurs and/or myelosuppression occurs

Monthly regimen: Initial: 0.4 mg/kg, increase dose by 0.1 mg/kg every 4 weeks until a response occurs and/or myelosuppression occurs

Malignant lymphomas:

Non-Hodgkin's lymphoma: 0.1 mg/kg/day

Hodgkin's lymphoma: 0.2 mg/kg/day

Adults:

CLL, NHL: 0.1 mg/kg/day for 3-6 weeks **or** 0.4 mg/kg (increased by 0.1mg/kg/dose until response/toxicity observed) biweekly **or** 0.4 mg/kg (increased by 0.1mg/kg/dose until response/toxicity observed) monthly **or** 0.03-0.1 mg/kg/day continuously

Hodgkin's lymphoma: 0.2 mg/kg/day for 3-6 weeks **or** 0.4 mg/kg (increased by 0.1mg/kg/dose until response/toxicity observed) biweekly **or** 0.4 mg/kg (increased by 0.1mg/kg/dose until response/toxicity observed) monthly **or** 0.03-0.1 mg/kg/day continuously

Waldenström's macroglobulinemia (unlabeled use): 0.1 mg/kg/day (continuously) for at least 6 months **or** 0.3 mg/kg/day for 7 days every 6 weeks for at least 6 months

Elderly: Refer to adult dosing; begin at the lower end of dosing range(s)

Dosage adjustment for toxicity:

Skin reactions: Discontinue treatment

Hematologic: Persistent neutropenia, thrombocytopenia, and/or lymphocytosis: Do not exceed 0.1 mg/kg/day

Concurrent or within 4 weeks of chemotherapy/radiotherapy: Initiate treatment cautiously; reduce dose; monitor closely. (May use the usual dose if radiation therapy is small doses of palliative radiation over isolated foci remote from bone marrow.)

Dosing adjustment in renal impairment: The FDA-apppproved labeling does not contain renal dosing adjustment guidelines. The following guidelines have been used by some clinicians (Aronoff, 2007): Adults:

Cl_{cr} 10-50 mL/minute: Administer 75% of dose

Cl_{cr} <10 mL/minute: Administer 50% of dose

Continuous ambulatory peritoneal dialysis (CAPD): Administer 50% of dose

Dosing adjustment in hepatic impairment: The FDA-approved labeling does not contain hepatic dosing adjustment guidelines. Chlorambucil is hepatically metabolized into active and inactive metabolites; dosage adjustment may be needed in patients with hepatic impairment.

Combination Regimens

Leukemia, chronic lymphocytic:

CHL + PRED on page 1262

CP (Leukemia) on page 1281

Lymphoma, Hodgkin's disease:

Chlorambucil-VPP (Hodgkin's Lymphoma) on page 1262

LOPP on page 1363

Administration Usually administered as a single dose; preferably on an empty stomach.

Monitoring Parameters Liver function tests, CBC with differential and platelets (weekly, with WBC monitored twice weekly during the first 3-6 weeks of treatment), serum uric acid

Emetic Potential Very low (<10%)

Dosage Forms Excipient information presented when available (limited, particularly for generics); consult specific product labeling.

Tablet:

Leukeran®: 2 mg

Extemporaneous Preparations A 2 mg/mL oral suspension can be prepared by crushing sixty 2 mg tablets in a mortar and then mixing in small amounts of methylcellulose (mix in a total of 30 mL of methylcellulose). Next, add a sufficient quantity of syrup to make 60 mL of final product. Transfer to amber container. Label "shake well," "refrigerate," and "protect from light." Refrigerated stability is 7 days.

Nahata MC and Hipple TF, *Pediatric Drug Formulations*, 4th ed, Cincinnati, OH: Harvey Whitney Books Co, 2000.

Dressman JB and Poust RI, "Stability of Allopurinol and of Five Antineoplastics in Suspension," *Am J Hosp Pharm*, 1983, 40(4):616-8.

References

Aronoff GR, Bennett WM, Berns JS, et al, *Drug Prescribing in Renal Failure: Dosing Guidelines for Adults and Children*, 5th ed. Philadelphia, PA: American College of Physicians; 2007, p 98.

Begleiter A, Mowat M, Israels LG, et al, "Chlorambucil in Chronic Lymphocytic Leukemia: Mechanism of Action," *Leuk Lymphoma*, 1996, 23(3-4):187-201.

Brittinger G, Hellriegel KP, and Hiddemann W, "Chronic Lymphocytic Leukemia and Hairy-Cell Leukemia-Diagnosis and Treatment: Results of a Consensus Meeting of the German CLL Cooperative Group," *Ann Hematol*, 1997, 74(6):291-4.

Hogg RH, Portman RJ, Milliner D, et al, "Evaluation and Management of Proteinuria and Nephrotic Syndrome in Children: Recommendations From a Pediatric Nephrology Panel Established at the National Kidney Foundation Conference on Proteinuria, Albuminuria, Risk, Assessment, Detection, and Elimination (PARADE)," *Pediatrics*, 2000, 105(6):1242-9.

Kyle RA, Greipp PR, Gertz MA, et al, "Waldenström's Macroglobulinemia: A Prospective Study Comparing Daily With Intermittent Oral Chlorambucil," *Br J Haematol*, 2000, 108(4):737-42.

Robinson RF, Nahata MC, Mahan JD, "Management of Nephrotic Syndrome in Children," *Pharmacotherapy*, 2003, 23(8):1021-36.

ChlorproMAZINE (klor PROE ma zeen)

Medication Safety Issues

Sound-alike/look-alike issues:

ChlorproMAZINE may be confused with chlordiazePOXIDE, chlorproPA-MIDE, clomiPRAMINE, prochlorperazine, promethazine

Thorazine® may be confused with thiamine, thioridazine

Index Terms Chlorpromazine Hydrochloride; CPZ; Thorazine

Generic Available Yes

Canadian Brand Names Largactil®; Novo-Chlorpromazine

Pharmacologic Category Antimanic Agent; Antipsychotic Agent, Typical, Phenothiazine

Use Control of mania; treatment of schizophrenia; control of nausea and vomiting; relief of restlessness and apprehension before surgery; acute intermittent porphyria; adjunct in the treatment of tetanus; intractable hiccups; combativeness and/or explosive hyperexcitable behavior in children 1-12 years of age and in short-term treatment of hyperactive children

Unlabeled/Investigational Use Management of psychotic disorders; behavioral symptoms associated with dementia (elderly); psychosis/agitation related to Alzheimer's dementia

Pregnancy Risk Factor C

Lactation Enters breast milk/not recommended (AAP rates "of concern")

Labeled Contraindications Hypersensitivity to chlorpromazine or any component of the formulation (cross-reactivity between phenothiazines may occur); severe CNS depression; coma

Warnings/Precautions [U.S. Boxed Warning]: Elderly patients with dementia-related psychosis treated with antipsychotics are at an increased risk of death compared to placebo. Most deaths appeared to be either cardiovascular (eg, heart failure, sudden death) or infectious (eg, pneumonia) in nature. Chlorpromazine is not approved for the treatment of dementia-related psychosis. Highly sedating, use with caution in disorders where CNS depression is a feature and in patients with Parkinson's disease. Use with caution in patients with hemodynamic instability, predisposition to seizures, subcortical brain damage, severe cardiac, hepatic, or renal disease. Use caution in respiratory disease (eg, severe asthma, emphysema) due to potential for CNS effects.

Esophageal dysmotility and aspiration have been associated with antipsychotic use; use with caution in patients at risk of aspiration pneumonia (ie, Alzheimer's disease). Use associated with increased prolactin levels; clinical significance of hyperprolactinemia in patients with breast cancer or other prolactin-dependent tumors is unknown. May alter temperature regulation or mask toxicity of other drugs due to antiemetic effects. May alter cardiac conduction; life-threatening arrhythmias have occurred with therapeutic doses of neuroleptics. May cause blood dyscrasias; check blood counts periodically. May cause pigmentary retinopathy, and lenticular and corneal deposits, particularly with prolonged therapy.

Use with caution in patients at risk of hypotension (orthostasis is common) or those who would tolerate transient hypotensive episodes (cerebrovascular disease, cardiovascular disease, or other medications which may predispose). Significant hypotension may occur, particularly with parenteral administration. Injection contains sulfites.

Use with caution in patients with decreased gastrointestinal motility, urinary retention, BPH, xerostomia, or visual problems (ie, narrow-angle glaucoma), and myasthenia gravis. Relative to other neuroleptics, chlorpromazine has a moderate potency of cholinergic blockade.

May cause extrapyramidal symptoms (EPS), including pseudoparkinsonism, acute dystonic reactions, akathisia, and tardive dyskinesia (risk of these reactions is low-moderate relative to other neuroleptics). Risk of dystonia (and possibly other EPS) may be greater with increased doses, use of conventional antipsychotics, males, and younger patients. May cause neuroleptic malignant syndrome (NMS). Use with caution in the elderly.

Adverse Reactions Frequency not defined.

Cardiovascular: Postural hypotension, tachycardia, dizziness, nonspecific QT changes

Central nervous system: Drowsiness, dystonias, akathisia, pseudoparkinsonism, tardive dyskinesia, neuroleptic malignant syndrome, seizure

Dermatologic: Photosensitivity, dermatitis, skin pigmentation (slate gray)

Endocrine & metabolic: Lactation, breast engorgement, false-positive pregnancy test, amenorrhea, gynecomastia, hyper- or hypoglycemia

Gastrointestinal: Xerostomia, constipation, nausea

Genitourinary: Urinary retention, ejaculatory disorder, impotence

Hematologic: Agranulocytosis, eosinophilia, leukopenia, hemolytic anemia, aplastic anemia, thrombocytopenic purpura

Hepatic: Jaundice

Ocular: Blurred vision, corneal and lenticular changes, epithelial keratopathy, pigmentary retinopathy

Drug Interactions

Metabolism/Transport Effects Substrate of CYP1A2 (minor), 2D6 (major), 3A4 (minor); **Inhibits** CYP2D6 (strong), 2E1 (weak)

Avoid Concomitant Use

Avoid concomitant use of ChlorproMAZINE with any of the following: Artemether; Dronedarone; Lumefantrine; Nilotinib; Pimozide; QuiNINE; Tamoxifen; Tetrabenazine; Thioridazine; Ziprasidone

Increased Effect/Toxicity

ChlorproMAZINE may increase the levels/effects of: Alcohol (Ethyl); Analgesics (Opioid); Anticholinergics; Atomoxetine; Beta-Blockers; CNS Depressants; CYP2D6 Substrates; Desmopressin; Dronedarone; Fesoterodine; Haloperidol; Pimozide; QTc-Prolonging Agents; QuiNINE; Tamoxifen; Tetrabenazine; Thioridazine; Valproic Acid; Ziprasidone

◄ *The levels/effects of ChlorproMAZINE may be increased by:* Acetylcholinesterase Inhibitors (Central); Alfuzosin; Antimalarial Agents; Artemether; Beta-Blockers; Chloroquine; Ciprofloxacin; CYP2D6 Inhibitors (Moderate); CYP2D6 Inhibitors (Strong); Darunavir; Gadobutrol; Haloperidol; Lithium formulations; Lumefantrine; Nilotinib; Pramlintide; QuiNINE; Tetrabenazine

Decreased Effect

ChlorproMAZINE may decrease the levels/effects of: Amphetamines; Anti-Parkinson's Agents (Dopamine Agonist); TraMADol

The levels/effects of ChlorproMAZINE may be decreased by: Antacids; Lithium formulations; Peginterferon Alfa-2b

Ethanol/Nutrition/Herb Interactions

Ethanol: Avoid ethanol (may increase CNS depression).

Herb/Nutraceutical: Avoid St John's wort (may decrease chlorpromazine levels, increase photosensitization, or enhance sedative effect). Avoid dong quai (may enhance photosensitization). Avoid kava kava, gotu kola, valerian (may increase CNS depression).

Storage/Stability Injection: Protect from light. A slightly yellowed solution does not indicate potency loss, but a markedly discolored solution should be discarded. Diluted injection (1 mg/mL) with NS and stored in 5 mL vials remains stable for 30 days.

Reconstitution Dilute injection (1 mg/mL) with NS for I.V. administration.

Compatibility Stable in dextran 6% in dextrose, dextran 6% in NS, D_5LR, $D_5^{1/4}NS$, $D_5^{1/2}NS$, D_5NS, D_5W, $D_{10}W$, LR, $^{1/2}NS$, NS.

Y-site administration: **Compatible:** Amsacrine, cisatracurium, cisplatin, cladribine, cyclophosphamide, cytarabine, docetaxel, doxorubicin, doxorubicin liposome, famotidine, filgrastim, fluconazole, gatifloxacin, gemcitabine, granisetron, heparin, hydrocortisone sodium succinate, ondansetron, potassium chloride, propofol, teniposide, thiotepa, vinorelbine, vitamin B complex with C. **Incompatible:** Allopurinol, amifostine, amphotericin B cholesteryl sulfate complex, aztreonam, cefepime, etoposide phosphate, fludarabine, furosemide, linezolid, melphalan, methotrexate, paclitaxel, piperacillin/tazobactam, sargramostim. **Variable (consult detailed reference):** Remifentanil, TPN.

Compatibility in syringe: **Compatible:** Atropine, benztropine, butorphanol, diphenhydramine, doxapram, droperidol, fentanyl, glycopyrrolate, hydromorphone, hydroxyzine, meperidine, metoclopramide, midazolam, morphine, pentazocine, perphenazine, prochlorperazine edisylate, promazine, promethazine, scopolamine. **Incompatible:** Cimetidine, dimenhydrinate, heparin, pentobarbital, thiopental. **Variable (consult detailed reference):** Ranitidine.

Compatibility when admixed: **Compatible:** Ascorbic acid injection, ethacrynate, netilmicin, theophylline, vitamin B complex with C. **Incompatible:** Aminophylline, amphotericin B, ampicillin, chloramphenicol, chlorothiazide, floxacillin, furosemide, methohexital, penicillin G potassium, penicillin G sodium, phenobarbital. **Variable (consult detailed reference):** Pentobarbital.

Mechanism of Action Chlorpromazine is an aliphatic phenothiazine antipsychotic which blocks postsynaptic mesolimbic dopaminergic receptors in the brain; exhibits a strong alpha-adrenergic blocking effect and depresses the release of hypothalamic and hypophyseal hormones; believed to depress the reticular activating system, thus affecting basal metabolism, body temperature, wakefulness, vasomotor tone, and emesis

Pharmacodynamics/Kinetics

Onset of action: I.M.: 15 minutes; Oral: 30-60 minutes

Absorption: Rapid

Distribution: V_d: 20 L/kg; crosses the placenta; enters breast milk
Protein binding: 92% to 97%
Metabolism: Extensively hepatic to active and inactive metabolites
Bioavailability: 20%
Half-life, biphasic: Initial: 2 hours; Terminal: 30 hours
Excretion: Urine (<1% as unchanged drug) within 24 hours

Dosage

Children ≥6 months:

Schizophrenia/psychoses:

Oral: 0.5-1 mg/kg/dose every 4-6 hours; older children may require 200 mg/day or higher

I.M., I.V.: 0.5-1 mg/kg/dose every 6-8 hours

<5 years (22.7 kg): Maximum: 40 mg/day

5-12 years (22.7-45.5 kg): Maximum: 75 mg/day

Nausea and vomiting:

Oral: 0.5-1 mg/kg/dose every 4-6 hours as needed

I.M., I.V.: 0.5-1 mg/kg/dose every 6-8 hours

<5 years (22.7 kg): Maximum: 40 mg/day

5-12 years (22.7-45.5 kg): Maximum: 75 mg/day

Adults:

Schizophrenia/psychoses:

Oral: Range: 30-800 mg/day in 1-4 divided doses, initiate at lower doses and titrate as needed; usual dose: 200-600 mg/day; some patients may require 1-2 g/day

I.M., I.V.: Initial: 25 mg, may repeat (25-50 mg) in 1-4 hours, gradually increase to a maximum of 400 mg/dose every 4-6 hours until patient is controlled; usual dose: 300-800 mg/day

Intractable hiccups: Oral, I.M.: 25-50 mg 3-4 times/day

Nausea and vomiting:

Oral: 10-25 mg every 4-6 hours

I.M., I.V.: 25-50 mg every 4-6 hours

Elderly: Behavioral symptoms associated with dementia (unlabeled use): Initial: 10-25 mg 1-2 times/day; increase at 4- to 7-day intervals by 10-25 mg/day. Increase dose intervals (bid, tid, etc) as necessary to control behavior response or side effects; maximum daily dose: 800 mg; gradual increases (titration) may prevent some side effects or decrease their severity.

Dosing comments in renal impairment: Hemodialysis: Not dialyzable (0% to 5%)

Dosing adjustment/comments in hepatic impairment: Avoid use in severe hepatic dysfunction

Administration Do not administer SubQ (tissue damage and irritation may occur); for direct I.V. injection: Dilute with NS to a maximum concentration of 1 mg/mL, administer slow I.V. at a rate not to exceed 0.5 mg/minute in children and 1 mg/minute in adults. **Note:** Avoid skin contact with solution; may cause contact dermatitis.

Monitoring Parameters Vital signs; lipid profile, fasting blood glucose/Hgb A_{1c}; BMI; mental status; abnormal involuntary movement scale (AIMS); extrapyramidal symptoms (EPS)

Test Interactions False-positives for phenylketonuria, amylase, uroporphyrins, urobilinogen. May cause false-positive pregnancy test.

Dosage Forms Excipient information presented when available (limited, particularly for generics); consult specific product labeling.

Injection, solution, as hydrochloride: 25 mg/mL (1 mL, 2 mL)

Tablet, as hydrochloride: 10 mg, 25 mg, 50 mg, 100 mg, 200 mg

References

American Academy of Pediatrics Committee on Drugs, "Reappraisal of Lytic Cocktail/Demerol®, Phenergan®, and Thorazine® (DPT) for the Sedation of Children," *Pediatrics*, 1995, 95 (4):598-602.

Gez E, Ben-Yosef R, Catane R, et al, "Chlorpromazine and Dexamethasone Versus High-Dose Metoclopramide and Dexamethasone in Patients Receiving Cancer Chemotherapy, Particularly Cis-Platinum: A Prospective Randomized Crossover Study," *Oncology*, 1989, 46(3):150-4.

Gez E, Brufman G, Kaufman B, et al, "Methylprednisolone and Chlorpromazine in Patients Receiving Cancer Chemotherapy: A Prospective Nonrandomized Study," *J Chemother*, 1989, 1 (2):140-3.

Hutcheon AW, Palmer JB, Soukop M, et al, "A Randomized Multicentre Single Blind Comparison of a Cannabinoid Antiemetic (Levonantradol) With Chlorpromazine in Patients Receiving Their First Cytotoxic Chemotherapy," *Eur J Cancer Clin Oncol*, 1983, 19(8):1087-90.

Peabody CA, Warner MD, Whiteford HA, et al, "Neuroleptics and the Elderly," *J Am Geriatr Soc*, 1987, 35(3):233-8.

Relling MV, Mulhern RK, Fairclough D, et al, "Chlorpromazine With and Without Lorazepam as Antiemetic Therapy in Children Receiving Uniform Chemotherapy," *J Pediatr*, 1993, 123(5):811-6.

Saab GA, Shamseddine A, and Habbal Z, "Prolonged Chlorpromazine Infusion as Antiemetic in Patients on Daily Cisplating Infusion. A Pilot Study," *Am J Clin Oncol*, 1988, 11(4):470-3.

Schneeweiss S, Setoguchi S, Brookhart A, et al, "Risk of Death Associated With the Use of Conventional Versus Atypical Antipsychotic Drugs Among Elderly Patients," *CMAJ*, 2007, 176(5): 627-32.

♦ **Chlorpromazine Hydrochloride** see ChlorproMAZINE *on page 220*

Chromic Phosphate P 32 (KROME ik FOS fate pe THUR tee too)

U.S. Brand Names Phosphocol® P 32

Index Terms P32; Phosphorus p32

Generic Available No

Pharmacologic Category Radiopharmaceutical

Use Treatment of peritoneal or pleural effusions caused by metastatic disease by intracavitary instillation; may be injected interstitially for the treatment of cancer

Lactation Excretion in breast milk unknown/not recommended

Labeled Contraindications Should not be used in patients with ulcerative tumors or in exposed cavities or where there is evidence of loculation, unless the extent of loculation has been determined

Warnings/Precautions Radiopharmaceutical: use appropriate precautions for handling, disposal, and minimizing exposure to patients and healthcare personnel. Use under supervision of experienced personnel. Use of this medication may increase risk of developing acute lymphocytic leukemia. Cases have been reported in children following intra-articular injection of this medication for hemarthroses (**not** an approved use). Intestinal fibrosis/necrosis and chronic fibrosis of the body wall may result from misplacement of the medication. Avoid placing into intrapleural or intraperitoneal loculations, bowel lumen, or body wall. May be less effective in bloody effusions. This product is not for intravascular use. Patients must be instructed in measures to minimize exposure of others. Should only be used by nuclear medicine physicians and/or radiopharmacists qualified and experienced in use and handling of radionuclides. Safety and efficacy have not been established in children.

Adverse Reactions Frequency not defined.

Gastrointestinal: Abdominal cramps, nausea

Hematologic: Bone marrow suppression

Respiratory: Pleuritis

Miscellaneous: Peritonitis, radiation sickness

Postmarketing and/or case reports: Radiation damage (interstitial or loculation injection), leukemia (children)

Drug Interactions

Avoid Concomitant Use There are no known interactions where it is recommended to avoid concomitant use.

Increased Effect/Toxicity There are no known significant interactions involving an increase in effect.

Decreased Effect There are no known significant interactions involving a decrease in effect.

Storage/Stability Store at controlled room temperature of 20°C to 25°C (68°F to 77°F).

Dosage Adults: **Note:** Consult manufacturer potency tables when applicable. All doses should be individualized.

General dosing ranges (based on 70 kg patient):

Intraperitoneal instillation: 370-740 megabecquerels (10-20 millicuries)

Intrapleural instillation: 222-444 megabecquerels (6-12 millicuries)

Interstitial use: ~3.7-18.5 megabecquerels/g of tumor weight (0.1-0.5 millicuries/g)

Administration This product is for intraperitoneal or intrapleural instillation; **not** for intravascular use.

Dosage Forms Excipient information presented when available (limited, particularly for generics); consult specific product labeling.

Injection, suspension:

Phosphocol® P 32: 185 MBq (5mCi) per mL

♦ **Ciloxan®** see Ciprofloxacin on page 228

Cinacalcet (sin a KAL cet)

U.S. Brand Names Sensipar®

Index Terms AMG 073; Cinacalcet Hydrochloride

Generic Available No

Canadian Brand Names Sensipar®

Pharmacologic Category Calcimimetic

Use Treatment of secondary hyperparathyroidism in patients with chronic kidney disease (CKD) on dialysis; treatment of hypercalcemia in patients with parathyroid carcinoma

Note: In Canada, cinacalcet is approved only for the treatment of secondary hyperparathyroidism in patients with chronic kidney disease (CKD) on dialysis

Unlabeled/Investigational Use Primary hyperparathyroidism

Pregnancy Risk Factor C

Lactation Excretion in breast milk unknown/not recommended

Labeled Contraindications Hypersensitivity to cinacalcet or any component of the formulation

Warnings/Precautions If hypocalcemia develops or symptoms of hypocalcemia (eg, cramps, myalgia, paresthesia, seizure, tetany) occur during treatment, consider initiating supplemental calcium, calcium-based phosphate binder, or vitamin D or temporarily withholding cinacalcet (dosage reductions may be necessary upon reinitiation of cinacalcet). Serum calcium levels should be ≥8.4 mg/dL prior to initiating treatment. Use caution in patients with a seizure disorder; monitor calcium levels closely. Adynamic bone disease may develop if iPTH levels are suppressed (<100 pg/mL). Use caution in patients with moderate-to-severe hepatic impairment (Child-Pugh classes B & C). In the U.S., the long-term safety and efficacy of cinacalcet has not been evaluated in chronic kidney disease (CKD) patients with hyperparathyroidism not requiring dialysis. Not indicated for CKD patients not receiving dialysis. Although possibly related to lower baseline calcium levels, clinical studies have shown an increased incidence of hypocalcemia (<8.4 mg/dL) in patients not requiring dialysis. May cause a decrease in testosterone levels (free and total); although below normal testosterone levels may occur in patients with end-stage renal disease, the clinical significance has not been determined. Use with caution in patients with cardiovascular disease; idiosyncratic hypotension, worsening of heart failure, and/or arrhythmia have been reported in patients with impaired cardiovascular function. Safety and efficacy have not been established in pediatric patients.

Adverse Reactions

>10%:
  Endocrine & metabolic: Hypocalcemia
  Gastrointestinal: Nausea (31%), vomiting (27%), diarrhea (21%)
  Neuromuscular & skeletal: Myalgia (15%)

1% to 10%:
  Cardiovascular: Hypertension (7%)
  Central nervous system: Dizziness (10%), seizure (1%)
  Endocrine & metabolic: Testosterone decreased
  Gastrointestinal: Anorexia (6%)
  Neuromuscular & skeletal: Weakness (7%), chest pain (noncardiac; 6%)

Postmarketing and/or case reports: Adynamic bone disease, arrhythmia (in patients with cardiac dysfunction), heart failure (worsening; in patients with cardiac dysfunction), hypersensitivity reactions, hypotension (idiosyncratic; in patients with cardiac dysfunction), rash

Drug Interactions

Metabolism/Transport Effects Substrate of CYP1A2, 2D6, 3A4; **Inhibits** CYP2D6 (major)

Avoid Concomitant Use
  Avoid concomitant use of Cinacalcet with any of the following: Tamoxifen; Thioridazine

Increased Effect/Toxicity
  Cinacalcet may increase the levels/effects of: Atomoxetine; CYP2D6 Substrates; Fesoterodine; Nebivolol; Tamoxifen; Tetrabenazine; Thioridazine; Tricyclic Antidepressants

  The levels/effects of Cinacalcet may be increased by: Antifungal Agents (Azole Derivatives, Systemic); CYP3A4 Inhibitors (Moderate); CYP3A4 Inhibitors (Strong); Dasatinib

Decreased Effect
  Cinacalcet may decrease the levels/effects of: Codeine; Tacrolimus; TraMADol

  The levels/effects of Cinacalcet may be decreased by: Peginterferon Alfa-2b

Ethanol/Nutrition/Herb Interactions Food: Food increases bioavailability.

Storage/Stability Store at 25°C (77°F); excursions permitted to 15°C to 30°C (59°F to 86°F).

Mechanism of Action Increases the sensitivity of the calcium-sensing receptor on the parathyroid gland thereby, concomitantly lowering PTH and serum calcium levels.

Pharmacodynamics/Kinetics

Distribution: V_d: ~1000 L
Protein binding: ~93% to 97%
Metabolism: Hepatic (extensive) via CYP3A4, 2D6, 1A2; forms inactive metabolites

Half-life elimination: Terminal: 30-40 hours; moderate hepatic impairment: prolonged 33%; severe hepatic impairment: prolonged 70%

Time to peak, plasma: Nadir in iPTH levels: ~2-6 hours postdose

Excretion: Urine ~80% (as metabolites); feces ~15%

Dosage Oral: Adults: **Do not titrate dose more frequently than every 2-4 weeks.**

Secondary hyperparathyroidism: Initial: 30 mg once daily (maximum daily dose: 180 mg); increase dose incrementally (60 mg, 90 mg, 120 mg, 180 mg once daily) as necessary to maintain iPTH level between 150-300 pg/mL.

Parathyroid carcinoma: Initial: 30 mg twice daily (maximum daily dose: 360 mg daily as 90 mg 4 times/day); increase dose incrementally (60 mg twice daily, 90 mg twice daily, 90 mg 3-4 times/day) as necessary to normalize serum calcium levels.

Elderly: No adjustment required; refer to adult dosing

Dosage adjustment for hypocalcemia:

If serum calcium >7.5 mg/dL but <8.4 mg/dL **or** if hypocalcemia symptoms occur: Use calcium-containing phosphate binders and/or vitamin D to raise calcium levels.

If serum calcium <7.5 mg/dL **or** if hypocalcemia symptoms persist and the dose of vitamin D cannot be increased: Withhold cinacalcet until serum calcium ≥8 mg/dL and/or symptoms of hypocalcemia resolve. Reinitiate cinacalcet at the next lowest dose.

If iPTH <150-300 pg/mL: Reduce dose or discontinue cinacalcet and/or vitamin D.

Dosage adjustment in renal impairment: No adjustment required.

Dosage adjustment in hepatic impairment: Patients with moderate-to-severe dysfunction (Child-Pugh classes B and C) have an increased exposure to cinacalcet and increased half-life.

Administration Administer with food or shortly after a meal. Do not break tablet; should be taken whole.

Monitoring Parameters

Hyperparathyroidism: Serum calcium and phosphorus levels prior to initiation and within a week of initiation or dosage adjustment; iPTH should be measured 1-4 weeks after initiation or dosage adjustment. After the maintenance dose is established, monthly calcium and phosphorus levels and iPTH every 1-3 months are required. Wait at least 12 hours after dose before drawing PTH levels.

Parathyroid carcinoma: Serum calcium levels prior to initiation and within a week of initiation or dosage adjustment; once maintenance dose is established, obtain serum calcium level every 2 months.

Dietary Considerations Take with food or shortly after a meal. May be taken with vitamin D and/or phosphate binders.

Dosage Forms Excipient information presented when available (limited, particularly for generics); consult specific product labeling.

Tablet:

Sensipar®: 30 mg, 60 mg, 90 mg

References

Eknoyan G, Levin A, and Levin NW, "Bone Metabolism and Disease in Chronic Kidney Disease," Am J Kidney Dis, 2003, 42(4 Suppl 3):1-201.

National Kidney Foundation. K/DOQI Clinical Practice Guidelines for Bone Metabolism and Disease in Chronic Kidney Disease. Guideline 13: Treatment of Bone Disease in Chronic Kidney Disease. Available at: www.kidney.org/professionals/kdoqi/guidelines_bone/index.htm. Accessed March 18, 2004.

◆ **Cinacalcet Hydrochloride** see Cinacalcet on page 225

♦ **Cipro®** *see* Ciprofloxacin *on page 228*

♦ **Cipro® XL (Can)** *see* Ciprofloxacin *on page 228*

Ciprofloxacin (sip roe FLOKS a sin)

Medication Safety Issues

Sound-alike/look-alike issues:

Cetraxal® may be confused with cefTRIAXone

Ciprofloxacin may be confused with cephalexin

Ciloxan® may be confused with cinoxacin, Cytoxan®

Cipro® may be confused with Ceftin®

U.S. Brand Names Cetraxal®; Ciloxan®; Cipro®; Cipro® I.V.; Cipro® XR; Proquin® XR

Index Terms Ciprofloxacin Hydrochloride

Generic Available Yes: Excludes ointment, otic solution, suspension

Canadian Brand Names Apo-Ciprofloxan®; Ciloxan®; Cipro®; Cipro® XL; CO Ciprofloxacin; Dom-Ciprofloxacin; Mint-Ciprofloxacin; Mylan-Ciprofloxacin; Novo-Ciprofloxacin; PHL-Ciprofloxacin; PMS-Ciprofloxacin; PRO-Ciprofloxacin; RAN-Ciprofloxacin; ratio-Ciprofloxacin; Riva-Ciprofloxacin; Sandoz-Ciprofloxacin; Taro-Ciprofloxacin

Pharmacologic Category Antibiotic, Ophthalmic; Antibiotic, Otic; Antibiotic, Quinolone

Use

Children: Complicated urinary tract infections and pyelonephritis due to *E. coli*.
Note: Although effective, ciprofloxacin is not the drug of first choice in children.

Children and Adults: To reduce incidence or progression of disease following exposure to aerolized *Bacillus anthracis*. Ophthalmologically, for superficial ocular infections (corneal ulcers, conjunctivitis) due to susceptible strains. Auricularly, for acute otitis externa due to susceptible strains of *Pseudomonas aeruginosa* or *Staphylococcus aureus*

Adults: Treatment of the following infections when caused by susceptible bacteria: Urinary tract infections; acute uncomplicated cystitis in females; chronic bacterial prostatitis; lower respiratory tract infections (including acute exacerbations of chronic bronchitis); acute sinusitis; skin and skin structure infections; bone and joint infections; complicated intra-abdominal infections (in combination with metronidazole); infectious diarrhea; typhoid fever due to *Salmonella typhi* (eradication of chronic typhoid carrier state has not been proven); uncomplicated cervical and urethra gonorrhea (due to *N. gonorrhoeae*); nosocomial pneumonia; empirical therapy for febrile neutropenic patients (in combination with piperacillin)
Note: As of April 2007, the CDC no longer recommends the use of fluoroquinolones for the treatment of gonococcal disease.

Unlabeled/Investigational Use Acute pulmonary exacerbations in cystic fibrosis (children); cutaneous/gastrointestinal/oropharyngeal anthrax (treatment, children and adults); disseminated gonococcal infection (adults); chancroid (adults); prophylaxis to *Neisseria meningitidis* following close contact with an infected person; empirical therapy (oral) for febrile neutropenia in low-risk cancer patients; HACEK group endocarditis; infectious diarrhea (children)

Pregnancy Risk Factor C

Lactation Enters breast milk/not recommended (AAP rates "compatible")

Labeled Contraindications Hypersensitivity to ciprofloxacin, any component of the formulation, or other quinolones; concurrent administration of tizanidine

Warnings/Precautions [U.S. Boxed Warning]: There have been reports of tendon inflammation and/or rupture with quinolone antibiotics; risk may be increased with concurrent corticosteroids, organ transplant recipients, and in patients >60 years of age. Rupture of the Achilles tendon sometimes requiring surgical repair has been reported most frequently; but other tendon sites (eg, rotator cuff, biceps) have also been reported. Strenuous physical activity, rheumatoid arthritis, and renal impairment may be an independent risk factor for tendonitis. Discontinue at first sign of tendon inflammation or pain. May occur even after discontinuation of therapy. Use with caution in patients with rheumatoid arthritis; may increase risk of tendon rupture. CNS stimulation may occur (tremor, restlessness, confusion, and very rarely hallucinations or seizures). Use with caution in patients with known or suspected CNS disorder. Potential for seizures, although very rare, may be increased with concomitant NSAID therapy. Use with caution in individuals at risk of seizures. Fluoroquinolones may prolong QT_c interval; avoid use in patients with a history of QT_c prolongation, uncorrected hypokalemia, hypomagnesemia, or concurrent administration of other medications known to prolong the QT interval (including Class Ia and Class III antiarrhythmics, cisapride, erythromycin, antipsychotics, and tricyclic antidepressants). Prolonged use may result in fungal or bacterial superinfection, including *C. difficile*-associated diarrhea (CDAD) and pseudomembranous colitis; CDAD has been observed >2 months postantibiotic treatment. Rarely crystalluria has occurred; urine alkalinity may increase the risk. Ensure adequate hydration during therapy. Adverse effects, including those related to joints and/or surrounding tissues, are increased in pediatric patients and therefore, ciprofloxacin should not be considered as drug of choice in children (exception is anthrax treatment). Rare cases of peripheral neuropathy may occur.

Fluoroquinolones have been associated with the development of serious, and sometimes fatal, hypoglycemia, most often in elderly diabetics but also in patients without diabetes. This occurred most frequently with gatifloxacin (no longer available systemically), but may occur at a lower frequency with other quinolones.

Severe hypersensitivity reactions, including anaphylaxis, have occurred with quinolone therapy. Reactions may present as typical allergic symptoms after a single dose, or may manifest as severe idiosyncratic dermatologic, vascular, pulmonary, renal, hepatic, and/or hematologic events, usually after multiple doses. Prompt discontinuation of drug should occur if skin rash or other symptoms arise. Quinolones may exacerbate myasthenia gravis, use with caution (rare, potentially life-threatening weakness of respiratory muscles may occur). Use caution in renal impairment. Avoid excessive sunlight and take precautions to limit exposure (eg, loose fitting clothing, sunscreen); may cause moderate-to-severe phototoxicity reactions. Discontinue use if photosensitivity occurs. Since ciprofloxacin is ineffective in the treatment of syphilis and may mask symptoms, all patients should be tested for syphilis at the time of gonorrheal diagnosis and 3 months later. Hemolytic reactions may (rarely) occur with quinolone use in patients with latent or actual G6PD deficiency.

Ciprofloxacin is a potent inhibitor of CYP1A2. Coadministration of drugs which depend on this pathway may lead to substantial increases in serum concentrations and adverse effects.

◀ **Adverse Reactions**
Systemic:
1% to 10%:
Central nervous system: Neurologic events (children 2%, includes dizziness, insomnia, nervousness, somnolence); fever (children 2%); headache (I.V. administration); restlessness (I.V. administration)
Dermatologic: Rash (children 2%, adults 1%)
Gastrointestinal: Nausea (children/adults 3%); diarrhea (children 5%, adults 2%); vomiting (children 5%, adults 1%); abdominal pain (children 3%, adults <1%); dyspepsia (children 3%)
Hepatic: ALT increased, AST increased (adults 1%)
Local: Injection site reactions (I.V. administration)
Respiratory: Rhinitis (children 3%)
<1%: Abnormal gait, acute renal failure, agitation, allergic reactions, anaphylaxis, anemia, angina pectoris, angioedema, anorexia, arthralgia, ataxia, atrial flutter, breast pain, bronchospasm, candidiasis, cardiopulmonary arrest, cerebral thrombosis, chills, cholestatic jaundice, confusion, chromatopsia, crystalluria (particularly in alkaline urine), cylindruria, depersonalization, depression, dizziness, drowsiness, dyspnea, edema, eosinophilia, erythema nodosum, fever (adults), gastrointestinal bleeding, hallucinations, headache (oral), hematuria, hyperpigmentation, hyper-/hypotension, insomnia, interstitial nephritis, intestinal perforation, irritability, joint pain, laryngeal edema, lightheadedness, lymphadenopathy, malaise, manic reaction, migraine, MI, nephritis, nightmares, palpitation, paranoia, paresthesia, peripheral neuropathy, petechia, photosensitivity, pulmonary edema, seizure, syncope, tachycardia, thrombophlebitis, tinnitus, tremor, urethral bleeding, vaginitis, ventricular ectopy, visual disturbance, weakness
Postmarketing and/or case reports: Agranulocytosis, albuminuria, anaphylactic shock, anosmia, bone marrow depression (life-threatening), candiduria, constipation, delirium, dyspepsia (adults), dysphagia, erythema multiforme, exfoliative dermatitis, fixed eruption, flatulence, hemolytic anemia, hepatic failure (some fatal), hepatic necrosis, hyperesthesia, hyperglycemia, hypertonia, jaundice, methemoglobinemia, moniliasis, myalgia, myasthenia gravis, myoclonus, nystagmus, orthostatic hypotension, pancreatitis, pancytopenia (life-threatening or fatal), pneumonitis, prolongation of PT/INR, pseudomembranous colitis, psychosis, renal calculi, serum cholesterol increased, serum glucose increased, serum sickness-like reactions, serum triglycerides increased, Stevens-Johnson syndrome, taste loss, tendon rupture, tendonitis, toxic epidermal necrolysis (Lyell's syndrome), torsade de pointes, twitching, vaginal candidiasis, vasculitis

Otic:
1% to 10%:
Central nervous system: Headache (2% to 3%)
Local: Application site pain (2% to 3%), fungal superinfection (2% to 3%), pruritus (2% to 3%)
Drug Interactions
Metabolism/Transport Effects Inhibits CYP1A2 (strong), 3A4 (weak)
Avoid Concomitant Use
Avoid concomitant use of Ciprofloxacin with any of the following: TiZANidine
Increased Effect/Toxicity
Ciprofloxacin may increase the levels/effects of: Bendamustine; Caffeine; Corticosteroids (Systemic); CYP1A2 Substrates; Erlotinib; Methotrexate; Pentoxifylline; QTc-Prolonging Agents; Ropinirole; Ropivacaine; Sulfonylureas; Theophylline Derivatives; TiZANidine; Vitamin K Antagonists

The levels/effects of Ciprofloxacin may be increased by: Insulin; Nonsteroidal Anti-Inflammatory Agents; P-Glycoprotein Inhibitors; Probenecid

Decreased Effect

Ciprofloxacin may decrease the levels/effects of: Mycophenolate; Phenytoin; Sulfonylureas; Typhoid Vaccine

The levels/effects of Ciprofloxacin may be decreased by: Antacids; Calcium Salts; Didanosine; Iron Salts; Magnesium Salts; P-Glycoprotein Inducers; Quinapril; Sevelamer; Sucralfate; Zinc Salts

Ethanol/Nutrition/Herb Interactions

Food: Food decreases rate, but not extent, of absorption. Ciprofloxacin serum levels may be decreased if taken with dairy products or calcium-fortified juices. Ciprofloxacin may increase serum caffeine levels if taken with caffeine.

Enteral feedings may decrease plasma concentrations of ciprofloxacin probably by >30% inhibition of absorption. Ciprofloxacin should not be administered with enteral feedings. The feeding would need to be discontinued for 1-2 hours prior to and after ciprofloxacin administration. Nasogastric administration produces a greater loss of ciprofloxacin bioavailability than does nasoduodenal administration.

Herb/Nutraceutical: Avoid dong quai, St John's wort (may also cause photosensitization).

Storage/Stability

Injection:

Premixed infusion: Store between 5°C to 25°C (41°F to 77°F); avoid freezing. Protect from light.

Vial: Store between 5°C to 30°C (41°F to 86°F); avoid freezing. Protect from light. Diluted solutions of 0.5-2 mg/mL are stable for up to 14 days refrigerated or at room temperature.

Ophthalmic solution/ointment: Store at 2°C to 25°C (36°F to 77°F). Protect from light.

Otic solution: Store at 15°C to 25°C (59°F to 77°F). Protect from light. Store unused single-dose containers in foil overwrap pouch until immediately prior to use.

Microcapsules for oral suspension: Prior to reconstitution, store below 25°C (77°F). Protect from freezing. Following reconstitution, store below 30°C (86°F) for up to 14 days. Protect from freezing.

Tablet:

Immediate release: Store below 30°C (86°F).

Extended release: Store at room temperature of 15°C to 30°C (59°F to 86°F).

Reconstitution Injection, vial: May be diluted with NS, D_5W, SWFI, $D_{10}W$, $D_5^{1/4}NS$, $D_5^{1/2}NS$, LR.

Compatibility Stable in $D_5^{1/4}NS$, $D_5^{1/2}NS$, D_5W, $D_{10}W$, LR, NS; **variable stability (consult detailed reference)** in peritoneal dialysis solution.

Y-site administration: Compatible: Amifostine, amino acids (dextrose), aztreonam, calcium gluconate, ceftazidime, cisatracurium, clarithromycin, digoxin, diltiazem, diphenhydramine, dobutamine, docetaxel, dopamine, doxorubicin liposome, etoposide phosphate, gemcitabine, gentamicin, granisetron, hydroxyzine, lidocaine, linezolid, lorazepam, metoclopramide, midazolam, midodrine, piperacillin, potassium acetate, potassium chloride, potassium phosphates, promethazine, ranitidine, remifentanil, Ringer's injection (lactated), sodium chloride, tacrolimus, teniposide, thiotepa, tobramycin, verapamil. **Incompatible:** Aminophylline, ampicillin/sulbactam, cefepime, dexamethasone sodium phosphate, furosemide, heparin, hydrocortisone sodium succinate, methylprednisolone sodium succinate, phenytoin, propofol, sodium phosphates, warfarin. **Variable (consult detailed reference):** Magnesium sulfate, sodium bicarbonate, teicoplanin, TPN.

Compatibility when admixed: Compatible: Amikacin, aztreonam, ceftazidime, cyclosporine, gentamicin, metronidazole, netilmicin, piperacillin, potassium chloride, ranitidine, tobramycin, vitamin B complex. **Incompatible:** Aminophylline, clindamycin, floxacillin, heparin.

Mechanism of Action Inhibits DNA-gyrase in susceptible organisms; inhibits relaxation of supercoiled DNA and promotes breakage of double-stranded DNA

Pharmacodynamics/Kinetics

Absorption: Oral: Immediate release tablet: Rapid (~50% to 85%)

Distribution: V_d: 2.1-2.7 L/kg; tissue concentrations often exceed serum concentrations especially in kidneys, gallbladder, liver, lungs, gynecological tissue, and prostatic tissue; CSF concentrations: 10% of serum concentrations (noninflamed meninges), 14% to 37% (inflamed meninges)

Protein binding: 20% to 40%

Metabolism: Partially hepatic; forms 4 metabolites (limited activity)

Half-life elimination: Children: 2.5 hours; Adults: Normal renal function: 3-5 hours

Time to peak: Oral:

Immediate release tablet: 0.5-2 hours

Extended release tablet: Cipro® XR: 1-2.5 hours, Proquin® XR: 3.5-8.7 hours

Excretion: Urine (30% to 50% as unchanged drug); feces (15% to 43%)

Dosage Note: Extended release tablets and immediate release formulations are not interchangeable. Unless otherwise specified, oral dosing reflects the use of immediate release formulations.

Usual dosage ranges:

Children (see Warnings/Precautions):

Oral: 20-30 mg/kg/day in 2 divided doses; maximum dose: 1.5 g/day

I.V.: 20-30 mg/kg/day divided every 12 hours; maximum dose: 800 mg/day

Adults:

Oral: 250-750 mg every 12 hours

I.V.: 200-400 mg every 12 hours

Indication-specific dosing:

Children:

Acute otitis externa: Children ≥1 year: Refer to adult dosing

Anthrax:

Inhalational (postexposure prophylaxis):

Oral: 15 mg/kg/dose every 12 hours for 60 days; maximum: 500 mg/dose

I.V.: 10 mg/kg/dose every 12 hours for 60 days; do **not** exceed 400 mg/dose (800 mg/day)

Cutaneous (treatment, CDC guidelines): Oral: 10-15 mg/kg every 12 hours for 60 days (maximum: 1 g/day); amoxicillin 80 mg/kg/day divided every 8 hours is an option for completion of treatment after clinical improvement. **Note:** In the presence of systemic involvement, extensive edema, lesions on head/neck, refer to I.V. dosing for treatment of inhalational/gastrointestinal/oropharyngeal anthrax.

Inhalational/gastrointestinal/oropharyngeal (treatment, CDC guidelines): I.V.: Initial: 10-15 mg/kg every 12 hours for 60 days (maximum: 500 mg/dose); switch to oral therapy when clinically appropriate; refer to adult dosing for notes on combined therapy and duration

Bacterial conjunctivitis: See adult dosing

Corneal ulcer: See adult dosing

Cystic fibrosis (unlabeled use):

Oral: 40 mg/kg/day divided every 12 hours administered following 1 week of I.V. therapy has been reported in a clinical trial; total duration of therapy: 10-21 days

I.V.: 30 mg/kg/day divided every 8 hours for 1 week, followed by oral therapy, has been reported in a clinical trial

Urinary tract infection (complicated) or pyelonephritis:

Oral: 20-30 mg/kg/day in 2 divided doses (every 12 hours) for 10-21 days; maximum: 1.5 g/day

I.V.: 6-10 mg/kg every 8 hours for 10-21 days (maximum: 400 mg/dose)

Adults:

Acute otitis externa: Otic solution: Instill 0.25 mL (contents of 1 single-dose container) into affected ear twice daily for 7 days

Anthrax:

Inhalational (postexposure prophylaxis):

Oral: 500 mg every 12 hours for 60 days

I.V.: 400 mg every 12 hours for 60 days

Cutaneous (treatment, CDC guidelines): Oral: Immediate release formulation: 500 mg every 12 hours for 60 days. **Note:** In the presence of systemic involvement, extensive edema, lesions on head/neck, refer to I.V. dosing for treatment of inhalational/gastrointestinal/oropharyngeal anthrax

Inhalational/gastrointestinal/oropharyngeal (treatment, CDC guidelines): I.V.: 400 mg every 12 hours. **Note:** Initial treatment should include two or more agents predicted to be effective (per CDC recommendations). Continue combined therapy for 60 days.

Bacterial conjunctivitis:

Ophthalmic solution: Instill 1-2 drops in eye(s) every 2 hours while awake for 2 days and 1-2 drops every 4 hours while awake for the next 5 days

Ophthalmic ointment: Apply a 1/2" ribbon into the conjunctival sac 3 times/day for the first 2 days, followed by a 1/2" ribbon applied twice daily for the next 5 days

Bone/joint infections:

Oral: 500-750 mg twice daily for 4-6 weeks

I.V.: Mild-to-moderate: 400 mg every 12 hours for 4-6 weeks; Severe/complicated: 400 mg every 8 hours for 4-6 weeks

Chancroid (CDC guidelines): Oral: 500 mg twice daily for 3 days

Corneal ulcer: Ophthalmic solution: Instill 2 drops into affected eye every 15 minutes for the first 6 hours, then 2 drops into the affected eye every 30 minutes for the remainder of the first day. On day 2, instill 2 drops into the affected eye hourly. On days 3-14, instill 2 drops into affected eye every 4 hours. Treatment may continue after day 14 if re-epithelialization has not occurred.

Endocarditis due to HACEK organisms (AHA guidelines, unlabeled use): Note: Not first-line option; use only if intolerant of beta-lactam therapy:

Oral: 500 mg every 12 hours for 4 weeks

I.V.: 400 mg every 12 hours for 4 weeks

Febrile neutropenia*: I.V.: 400 mg every 8 hours for 7-14 days

Gonococcal infections:

Urethral/cervical gonococcal infections: Oral: 250-500 mg as a single dose (CDC recommends concomitant doxycycline or azithromycin due to possible coinfection with *Chlamydia*; **Note:** As of April 2007, the CDC no longer recommends the use of fluoroquinolones for the treatment of uncomplicated gonococcal disease.

Disseminated gonococcal infection (CDC guidelines): Oral: 500 mg twice daily to complete 7 days of therapy (initial treatment with ceftriaxone 1 g I.M./I.V. daily for 24-48 hours after improvement begins); **Note:** As of April 2007, the CDC no longer recommends the use of fluoroquinolones for the treatment of more serious gonococcal disease, unless no other options exist and susceptibility can be confirmed via culture.

Infectious diarrhea: Oral:
Salmonella: 500 mg twice daily for 5-7 days
Shigella: 500 mg twice daily for 3 days
Traveler's diarrhea: Mild: 750 mg for one dose; Severe: 500 mg twice daily for 3 days
Vibrio cholerae: 1 g for one dose

Intra-abdominal*:
Oral: 500 mg every 12 hours for 7-14 days
I.V.: 400 mg every 12 hours for 7-14 days

Lower respiratory tract, skin/skin structure infections:
Oral: 500-750 mg twice daily for 7-14 days
I.V.: Mild-to-moderate: 400 mg every 12 hours for 7-14 days; Severe/complicated: 400 mg every 8 hours for 7-14 days

Nosocomial pneumonia: I.V.: 400 mg every 8 hours for 10-14 days

Prostatitis (chronic, bacterial): Oral: 500 mg every 12 hours for 28 days

Sinusitis (acute): Oral: 500 mg every 12 hours for 10 days

Typhoid fever: Oral: 500 mg every 12 hours for 10 days

Urinary tract infection:
Acute uncomplicated, cystitis:
Oral:
Immediate release formulation: 250 mg every 12 hours for 3 days
Extended release formulation (Cipro® XR, Proquin® XR): 500 mg every 24 hours for 3 days
I.V.: 200 mg every 12 hours for 7-14 days
Complicated (including pyelonephritis):
Oral:
Immediate release formulation: 500 mg every 12 hours for 7-14 days
Extended release formulation (Cipro® XR): 1000 mg every 24 hours for 7-14 days
I.V.: 400 mg every 12 hours for 7-14 days

*Combination therapy generally recommended.

Elderly: No adjustment needed in patients with normal renal function

Dosing adjustment in renal impairment: Adults:
Cl_{cr} 30-50 mL/minute: Oral: 250-500 mg every 12 hours
Cl_{cr} <30 mL/minute: Acute uncomplicated pyelonephritis or complicated UTI: Oral: Extended release formulation: 500 mg every 24 hours
Cl_{cr} 5-29 mL/minute:
Oral: 250-500 mg every 18 hours
I.V.: 200-400 mg every 18-24 hours
Dialysis: Only small amounts of ciprofloxacin are removed by hemo- or peritoneal dialysis (<10%); usual dose: Oral: 250-500 mg every 24 hours following dialysis
Continuous renal replacement therapy (CRRT): I.V.:
CVVH: 200 mg every 12 hours
CVVHD or CVVHDF: 200-400 mg every 12 hours

Administration

Ophthalmic ointment/solution: For topical ophthalmic use only; avoid touching tip of applicator to eye or other surfaces.

Oral: May administer with food to minimize GI upset; avoid antacid use; maintain proper hydration and urine output. Administer immediate release ciprofloxacin and Cipro® XR at least 2 hours before or 6 hours after, and Proquin® XR at least 4 hours before or 6 hours after antacids or other products containing calcium, iron, or zinc (including dairy products or calcium-fortified juices). Separate oral administration from drugs which may impair absorption (see Drug Interactions).

Oral suspension: Should not be administered through feeding tubes (suspension is oil-based and adheres to the feeding tube). Patients should avoid chewing on the microcapsules.

Nasogastric/orogastric tube: Crush immediate-release tablet and mix with water. Flush feeding tube before and after administration. Hold tube feedings at least 1 hour before and 2 hours after administration.

Tablet, extended release: Do not crush, split, or chew. May be administered with meals containing dairy products (calcium content <800 mg), but not with dairy products alone. Proquin® XR should be administered with a main meal of the day; evening meal is preferred.

Otic solution: For otic use only. Prior to use, warm solution by holding container in hands for at least 1 minute. Patient should lie down with affected ear upward and medication instilled. Patients should remain in the position for at least 1 minute to allow penetration of solution.

Parenteral: Administer by slow I.V. infusion over 60 minutes to reduce the risk of venous irritation (burning, pain, erythema, and swelling); final concentration for administration should not exceed 2 mg/mL.

Monitoring Parameters CBC, renal and hepatic function during prolonged therapy

Test Interactions Some quinolones may produce a false-positive urine screening result for opiates using commercially-available immunoassay kits. This has been demonstrated most consistently for levofloxacin and ofloxacin, but other quinolones have shown cross-reactivity in certain assay kits. Confirmation of positive opiate screens by more specific methods should be considered.

Dietary Considerations

Food: Drug may cause GI upset; take without regard to meals (manufacturer prefers that immediate release tablet is taken 2 hours after meals). Extended release tablet may be taken with meals that contain dairy products (calcium content <800 mg), but not with dairy products alone.

Dairy products, calcium-fortified juices, oral multivitamins, and mineral supplements: Absorption of ciprofloxacin is decreased by divalent and trivalent cations. The manufacturer states that the usual dietary intake of calcium (including meals which include dairy products) has not been shown to interfere with ciprofloxacin absorption. Immediate release ciprofloxacin and Cipro® XR may be taken 2 hours before or 6 hours after, and Proquin® XR may be taken 4 hours before or 6 hours after, any of these products.

Caffeine: Patients consuming regular large quantities of caffeinated beverages may need to restrict caffeine intake if excessive cardiac or CNS stimulation occurs.

Additional Information Although the systemic use of ciprofloxacin is only FDA approved in children for the treatment of complicated UTI and postexposure treatment of inhalation anthrax, use of the fluoroquinolones in pediatric patients is increasing. Current recommendations by the American

Academy of Pediatrics note that the systemic use of these agents in children should be restricted to infections caused by multidrug resistant pathogens with no safe or effective alternative, and when parenteral therapy is not feasible or other oral agents are not available.

Dosage Forms Excipient information presented when available (limited, particularly for generics); consult specific product labeling.

Infusion [premixed in D_5W]: 200 mg (100 mL); 400 mg (200 mL)

    Cipro® I.V.: 200 mg (100 mL); 400 mg (200 mL)

Injection, solution [concentrate]: 10 mg/mL (20 mL, 40 mL, 120 mL)

    Cipro® I.V.: 10 mg/mL (20 mL, 40 mL [DSC])

Microcapsules for suspension, oral:

    Cipro®: 250 mg/5 mL (100 mL); 500 mg/5 mL (100 mL) [strawberry flavor]

Ointment, ophthalmic, as hydrochloride:

    Ciloxan®: 3.33 mg/g (3.5 g) [equivalent to ciprofloxacin base 0.3%]

Solution, ophthalmic, as hydrochloride: 3.5 mg/mL (2.5 mL, 5mL, 10 mL) [equivalent to ciprofloxacin base 0.3%]

    Ciloxan®: 3.5 mg/mL (5 mL) [0.3% base; contains benzalkonium chloride]

Solution, otic, as hydrochloride [preservative free]:

    Cetraxal®: 0.5 mg/0.25 mL (14s) [equivalent to ciprofloxacin base 0.2%]

Tablet, as hydrochloride: 100 mg [strength expressed as base], 250 mg [strength expressed as base], 500 mg [strength expressed as base], 750 mg [strength expressed as base]

    Cipro®: 250 mg [strength expressed as base], 500 mg [strength expressed as base], 750 mg [strength expressed as base]

Tablet, extended release, as base and hydrochloride: 500 mg [strength expressed as base], 1000 mg [strength expressed as base]

    Cipro® XR: 500 mg [strength expressed as base], 1000 mg [strength expressed as base]

Tablet, extended release, as hydrochloride:

    Proquin® XR: 500 mg [strength expressed as base]

Tablet, extended release, as hydrochloride [dose pack]:

    Proquin® XR: 500 mg (3s) [strength expressed as base]

References

American Thoracic Society and Infectious Diseases Society of America, "Guidelines for the Management of Adults With Hospital-Acquired, Ventilator-Associated, and Healthcare-Associated Pneumonia," *Am J Respir Crit Care Med*, 2005, 171(4):388-416.

Bayer A, Gajewska A, Stephens M, et al, "Pharmacokinetics of Ciprofloxacin in the Elderly," *Respiration*, 1987, 51(4):292-5.

Centers for Disease Control and Prevention, "Prevention and Control of Meningococcal Disease. Recommendations of the Advisory Committee on Immunization Practices (ACIP)," *MMWR Recomm Rep*, 2000, 49(RR-7):1-10. Available at: http://www.cdc.gov/mmwr/preview/mmwrhtml/rr4907a1.htm. Accessed May 5, 2004.

Committee on Infectious Diseases, "The Use of Systemic Fluoroquinolones," *Pediatrics*, 2006, 118 (3):1287-92.

Gamboa F, Rivera JM, Gomez Mateos JM, et al, "Ciprofloxacin-Induced Henoch-Schönlein Purpura," *Ann Pharmacother*, 1995, 29(1):84.

Guay DRP, Awni WM, Peterson PK, et al, "Single and Multiple Dose Pharmacokinetics of Oral Ciprofloxacin in Elderly Patients," *Int J Clin Pharmacol Ther Toxicol*, 1988, 26(6):279-84.

Guharoy SR, "Serum Sickness Secondary to Ciprofloxacin Use," *Vet Hum Toxicol*, 1994, 36 (6):540-1.

Hughes WT, Armstrong D, Bodey GP, et al, "2002 Guidelines for the Use of Antimicrobial Agents in Neutropenic Patients With Cancer," *Clin Infect Dis*, 2002, 15;34(6):730-51.

Khaliq Y and Zhanel GG, "Fluoroquinolone-Associated Tendinopathy: A Critical Review of the Literature," *Clin Infect Dis*, 2003, 36(11):1404-10.

Mackay AD and Mehta A, "Autoimmune Haemolytic Anemia Associated With Ciprofloxacin," *Clin Lab Haematol*, 1995, 17(1):97-8.

Mullen CA, "Ciprofloxacin in Treatment of Fever and Neutropenia in Pediatric Cancer Patients," *Pediatr Infect Dis J*, 2003, 22(12):1138-42.

Schaad UB, abdus Salam M, Aujard Y, et al, "Use of Fluoroquinolones in Pediatrics: Consensus Report of an International Society of Chemotherapy Commission," *Pediatr Infect Dis J*, 1995, 14 (1):1-9.

Szarfman A, Chen M, and Blum MD, "More on Fluoroquinolone Antibiotics and Tendon Rupture," *N Engl J Med*, 1995, 332(3):193.

Villenueve JP, Davies C, and Cote J, "Suspected Ciprofloxacin-Induced Hepatotoxicity," *Ann Pharmacother*, 1995, 29(3):257-9.

Zacher JL and Givone DM, "False-Positive Urine Opiate Screening Associated With Fluoroquinolone Use," *Ann Pharmacother*, 2004, 38:1525-28.

♦ **Ciprofloxacin Hydrochloride** *see* Ciprofloxacin *on page 228*

♦ **Cipro® I.V.** *see* Ciprofloxacin *on page 228*

♦ **Cipro® XR** *see* Ciprofloxacin *on page 228*

CISplatin (SIS pla tin)

Medication Safety Issues

Sound-alike/look-alike issues:

CISplatin may be confused with CARBOplatin, oxaliplatin

High alert medication: The Institute for Safe Medication Practices (ISMP) includes this medication among its list of drugs which have a heightened risk of causing significant patient harm when used in error.

Doses >100 mg/m^2 once every 3-4 weeks are rarely used and should be verified with the prescriber.

Related Information

Fertility and Cancer Therapy *on page 1430*
Hematopoietic Stem Cell Transplantation *on page 1501*
Management of Drug Extravasations *on page 1447*
Safe Handling of Hazardous Drugs *on page 1517*

Index Terms CDDP

Generic Available Yes

Pharmacologic Category Antineoplastic Agent, Alkylating Agent; Antineoplastic Agent, Platinum Analog

Use Treatment of bladder, testicular, and ovarian cancer

Unlabeled/Investigational Use Treatment of head and neck cancer, breast cancer, gastric cancer, esophageal cancer, cervical cancer, prostate cancer, nonsmall cell lung cancer, small cell lung cancer; Hodgkin's and non-Hodgkin's lymphoma; neuroblastoma; sarcomas, myeloma, melanoma, mesothelioma, and osteosarcoma

Pregnancy Risk Factor D

Lactation Enters breast milk/contraindicated

Labeled Contraindications Hypersensitivity to cisplatin, other platinum-containing compounds, or any component of the formulation (anaphylactic-like reactions have been reported); pre-existing renal insufficiency; myelosuppression; hearing impairment; pregnancy

Warnings/Precautions Hazardous agent - use appropriate precautions for handling and disposal. **[U.S. Boxed Warning]: Doses >100 mg/m^2 once every 3-4 weeks are rarely used and should be verified with the prescriber.** Patients should receive adequate hydration, with or without diuretics, prior to and for 24 hours after cisplatin administration. Reduce dosage in renal impairment. **[U.S. Boxed Warning]: Cumulative renal toxicity may be severe.** Elderly patients may be more susceptible to nephrotoxicity and peripheral neuropathy; select dose cautiously and monitor closely. **[U.S. Boxed Warnings]: Dose-related toxicities include myelosuppression, nausea, and vomiting. Ototoxicity, especially pronounced** ▶

◀ in children, is manifested by tinnitus or loss of high frequency hearing and occasionally, deafness. Severe and possibly irreversible neuropathies may occur with higher than recommended doses or more frequent regimen. Serum electrolytes, particularly magnesium and potassium, should be monitored and replaced as needed during and after cisplatin therapy. When administered as sequential infusions, taxane derivatives (docetaxel, paclitaxel) should be administered before platinum derivatives (carboplatin, cisplatin). **[U.S. Boxed Warnings]: Anaphylactic-like reactions have been reported; may be managed with epinephrine, corticosteroids, and/or antihistamines. Should be administered under the supervision of an experienced cancer chemotherapy physician.**

Adverse Reactions

>10%:

Central nervous system: Neurotoxicity: Peripheral neuropathy is dose- and duration-dependent.

Dermatologic: Mild alopecia

Gastrointestinal: Nausea and vomiting (76% to 100%)

Hematologic: Myelosuppression (25% to 30%; mild with moderate doses, mild-to-moderate with high-dose therapy)

WBC: Mild

Platelets: Mild

Onset: 10 days

Nadir: 14-23 days

Recovery: 21-39 days

Hepatic: Liver enzymes increased

Renal: Nephrotoxicity (acute renal failure and chronic renal insufficiency)

Otic: Ototoxicity (10% to 30%; manifested as high frequency hearing loss; ototoxicity is especially pronounced in children)

1% to 10%:

Gastrointestinal: Diarrhea

Local: Tissue irritation

<1%: Anaphylactic reaction, arrhythmias, blurred vision, bradycardia, hemolytic uremic syndrome, mild alopecia, mouth sores, optic neuritis, orthostatic hypotension, papilledema, phlebitis, SIADH, thrombophlebitis

Drug Interactions

Avoid Concomitant Use

Avoid concomitant use of CISplatin with any of the following: Natalizumab; Vaccines (Live)

Increased Effect/Toxicity

CISplatin may increase the levels/effects of: Aminoglycosides; Leflunomide; Natalizumab; Taxane Derivatives; Topotecan; Vaccines (Live); Vinorelbine

The levels/effects of CISplatin may be increased by: Trastuzumab

Decreased Effect

CISplatin may decrease the levels/effects of: Vaccines (Inactivated); Vaccines (Live)

The levels/effects of CISplatin may be decreased by: Echinacea

Ethanol/Nutrition/Herb Interactions Herb/Nutraceutical: Avoid black cohosh, dong quai in estrogen-dependent tumors.

Storage/Stability Store intact vials at room temperature 15°C to 25°C (59°F to 77°F). Protect from light. Do not refrigerate solution as a precipitate may form. Further dilution **stability is dependent on the chloride ion concentration** and should be mixed in solutions of NS (at least 0.3% NaCl). After initial entry into the vial, solution is stable for 28 days protected from light or for at least 7 days under fluorescent room light at room temperature.

Further dilutions in NS, D_5/0.45% NaCl or D_5/NS to a concentration of 0.05-2 mg/mL are stable for 72 hours at 4°C to 25°C. The infusion solution should have a final sodium chloride concentration ≥0.2%.

Reconstitution The infusion solution should have a final sodium chloride concentration ≥0.2%.

Compatibility Stable in D_5¼NS, D_5½NS, D_5NS, ¼NS, ⅓NS, ½NS, NS; **incompatible** with sodium bicarbonate; **variable stability (consult detailed reference)** in D_5W.

Y-site administration: Compatible: Allopurinol, aztreonam, bleomycin, chlorpromazine, cimetidine, cladribine, cyclophosphamide, dexamethasone sodium phosphate, diphenhydramine, doxorubicin, doxorubicin liposome, droperidol, etoposide phosphate, famotidine, filgrastim, fludarabine, fluorouracil, furosemide, ganciclovir, gatifloxacin, gemcitabine, granisetron, heparin, hydromorphone, leucovorin, linezolid, lorazepam, melphalan, methotrexate, methylprednisolone sodium succinate, metoclopramide, mitomycin, morphine, ondansetron, paclitaxel, prochlorperazine edisylate, promethazine, propofol, ranitidine, sargramostim, teniposide, topotecan, vinblastine, vincristine, vinorelbine. **Incompatible:** Amifostine, amphotericin B cholesteryl sulfate complex, cefepime, piperacillin/tazobactam, thiotepa.

Compatibility in syringe: Compatible: Bleomycin, cyclophosphamide, doxapram, doxorubicin, droperidol, fluorouracil, furosemide, heparin, leucovorin, methotrexate, metoclopramide, mitomycin, vinblastine, vincristine.

Compatibility when admixed: Compatible: Carboplatin, cyclophosphamide with etoposide, etoposide, etoposide with floxuridine, floxuridine, floxuridine with leucovorin, hydroxyzine, ifosfamide, ifosfamide with etoposide, leucovorin, magnesium sulfate, mannitol, ondansetron. **Incompatible:** Fluorouracil, mesna, thiotepa. **Variable (consult detailed reference):** Etoposide with mannitol and potassium chloride, paclitaxel.

Mechanism of Action Inhibits DNA synthesis by the formation of DNA cross-links; denatures the double helix; covalently binds to DNA bases and disrupts DNA function; may also bind to proteins; the *cis*-isomer is 14 times more cytotoxic than the *trans*-isomer; both forms cross-link DNA but cis-platinum is less easily recognized by cell enzymes and, therefore, not repaired. Cisplatin can also bind two adjacent guanines on the same strand of DNA producing intrastrand cross-linking and breakage.

Pharmacodynamics/Kinetics

Distribution: I.V.: Rapidly into tissue; high concentrations in kidneys, liver, ovaries, uterus, and lungs

Protein binding: >90%

Metabolism: Nonenzymatic; inactivated (in both cell and bloodstream) by sulfhydryl groups; covalently binds to glutathione and thiosulfate

Half-life elimination: Initial: 20-30 minutes; Beta: 60 minutes; Terminal: ~24 hours; Secondary half-life: 44-73 hours

Excretion: Urine (>90%); feces (10%)

Dosage Refer to individual protocols. **VERIFY ANY CISPLATIN DOSE EXCEEDING 100 mg/m² PER COURSE.**

Children (unlabeled uses):

Intermittent dosing schedule: 37-75 mg/m² once every 2-3 weeks or 50-100 mg/m² over 4-6 hours, once every 21-28 days

Daily dosing schedule: 15-20 mg/m²/day for 5 days every 3-4 weeks

Osteogenic sarcoma or neuroblastoma: 60-100 mg/m² on day 1 every 3-4 weeks

Recurrent brain tumors: 60 mg/m^2 once daily for 2 consecutive days every 3-4 weeks

Bone marrow/blood cell transfusion: Continuous Infusion: High dose: 55 mg/m^2/day for 72 hours; total dose = 165 mg/m^2

Adults:

Advanced bladder cancer: 50-70 mg/m^2 every 3-4 weeks

Head and neck cancer (unlabeled use): 100-120 mg/m^2 every 3-4 weeks

Malignant pleural mesothelioma in combination with pemetrexed: 75 mg/m^2 on day 1 of each 21-day cycle; see Pemetrexed monograph for additional details

Metastatic ovarian cancer: 75-100 mg/m^2 every 3-4 weeks

Intraperitoneal: Cisplatin has been administered intraperitoneal with systemic sodium thiosulfate for ovarian cancer; doses up to 90-270 mg/m^2 have been administered and retained for 4 hours before draining

Testicular cancer: 10-20 mg/m^2/day for 5 days repeated every 3-4 weeks

Dosing adjustment in renal impairment: Note: The manufacturer(s) recommend that repeat courses of cisplatin should not be given until serum creatinine is <1.5 mg/dL and/or BUN is <25 mg/dL. The FDA-approved labeling does not contain renal dosing adjustment guidelines. The following guidelines have been used by some clinicians:

Aronoff, 2007:

Cl$_{cr}$ 10-50 mL/minute: Administer 75% of dose

Cl$_{cr}$ <10 mL/minute: Administer 50% of dose

Hemodialysis: Partially cleared by hemodialysis

Administer 50% of dose posthemodialysis

Continuous ambulatory peritoneal dialysis (CAPD): Administer 50% of dose

Continuous renal replacement therapy (CRRT): Administer 75% of dose

Kintzel, 1995:

Cl$_{cr}$ 46-60 mL/minute: Administer 75% of dose

Cl$_{cr}$ 31-45 mL/minute: Administer 50% of dose

Cl$_{cr}$ <30 mL/minute: Consider use of alternative drug

Combination Regimens

Adenocarcinoma, unknown primary: EP (Adenocarcinoma) on page 1304

Biliary adenocarcinoma: Gemcitabine-Cisplatin (Biliary Cancer) on page 1341

Bladder cancer:

CAP on page 1243

CISCA on page 1264

Cisplatin-Docetaxel on page 1266

Cisplatin-Fluorouracil (Bladder Cancer) on page 1267

CMV on page 1277

Gemcitabine-Cisplatin (Bladder Cancer) on page 1342

M-VAC (Bladder Cancer) on page 1375

Brain tumors:

8 in 1 (Brain Tumors) on page 1221

CDDP/VP-16 on page 1253

COPE on page 1280

Breast Cancer:

Docetaxel-Trastuzumab-Cisplatin on page 1294

M-VAC (Breast Cancer) on page 1378

Cervical cancer:

BIP on page 1235

Cisplatin-Fluorouracil (Cervical Cancer) on page 1267

Lymphoma, non-Hodgkin's:
Malignant pleural mesothelioma:
Melanoma:
Multiple myeloma:
Neuroblastoma:
Osteosarcoma:
Ovarian cancer:
Retinoblastoma:
Testicular cancer:
Administration Pretreatment hydration with 1-2 L of fluid is recommended prior to cisplatin administration; adequate hydration and urinary output (>100 mL/hour) should be maintained for 24 hours after administration.
I.V.: Rate of administration has varied from a 15- to 120-minute infusion, 1 mg/minute infusion, 6- to 8-hour infusion, 24-hour infusion, or per protocol; maximum rate of infusion of 1 mg/minute in patients with CHF.

Monitoring Parameters Renal function (serum creatinine, BUN, Cl$_{cr}$); electrolytes (particularly magnesium, calcium, potassium) before and within 48 hours after cisplatin therapy; audiography (baseline and prior to each subsequent dose), neurologic exam (with high dose); liver function tests periodically, CBC with differential and platelet count; urine output, urinalysis

Dietary Considerations Some products may contain sodium.

Emetic Potential

≥50 mg/m^2: Very high (>90%)

<50 mg/m^2: Moderate (30% to 90%)

Vesicant >0.5 mg/mL: Yes; <0.5 mg/mL: Irritant; see Management of Drug Extravasations on page 1447

High Dose Considerations

High Dose Continuous I.V.: 55 mg/m^2/24 hours for 72 hours; total dose: 165 mg/m^2; generally combined with other high-dose chemotherapy

Unique Toxicities

Central nervous system: Autonomic neuropathy, ototoxicity

Gastrointestinal: Highly emetogenic

Hematologic: Myelosuppression

Endocrine & metabolic: Hypokalemia, hypomagnesemia

Neuromuscular & skeletal: Peripheral neuropathy

Ocular: Optic neuropathy, retinal vascular occlusion and myelopathy (concurrent administration of high-dose carmustine)

Renal: Acute renal failure, serum creatinine increased, azotemia

Miscellaneous: Transient pain at tumor, transient autoimmune disorders

Dosage Forms Excipient information presented when available (limited, particularly for generics); consult specific product labeling.

Injection, solution [preservative free]: 1 mg/mL (50 mL, 100 mL, 200 mL)

References

Aronoff GR, Bennett WM, Berns JS, et al, *Drug Prescribing in Renal Failure: Dosing Guidelines for Adults and Children*, 5th ed. Philadelphia, PA: American College of Physicians; 2007, p 97, 170.

Costello MA, Dominick C, and Clerico A, "A Pilot Study of 5-Day Continuous Infusion of High-Dose Cisplatin and Pulsed Etoposide in Childhood Solid Tumors," *Am J Pediatr Hematol Oncol*, 1988, 10:103-8.

Go RS and Adjei AA, "Review of the Comparative Pharmacology and Clinical Activity of Cisplatin and Carboplatin," *J Clin Oncol*, 1999, 17(1):409-22.

Howell SB, Pfeifle CL, Wung WE, et al, "Intraperitoneal Cisplatin With Systemic Thiosulfate Protection," *Ann Intern Med*, 1982, 97(6):845-51.

Kintzel PE and Dorr RT, "Anticancer Drug Renal Toxicity and Elimination: Dosing Guidelines for Altered Renal Function," *Cancer Treat Rev*, 1995, 21(1):33-64.

Reece PA, Stafford I, Abbott RL, et al, "Two- Versus 24-Hour Infusion of Cisplatin: Pharmacokinetic Considerations," *J Clin Oncol*, 1989, 7(2):270-5.

Rothmann SA and Weick JK, "Cisplatin Toxicity for Erythroid Precursors," *N Engl J Med*, 1981, 304 (6):360.

Schilsky RL and Anderson T, "Hypomagnesemia and Renal Magnesium Wasting in Patients Receiving Cisplatin," *Ann Intern Med*, 1979, 90(6):929-31.

Schuchter LM, Hensley ML, Meropol NJ, et al, "2002 Update of Recommendations for the Use of Chemotherapy and Radiotherapy Protectants: Clinical Practice Guidelines of the American Society of Clinical Oncology," *J Clin Oncol*, 2002, 20(12):2895-903.

Shlebak AA, Clark PI, and Green JA, "Hypersensitivity and Cross-Reactivity to Cisplatin and Analogues," *Cancer Chemother Pharmacol*, 1995, 35(4):349-51.

Siddik ZH, "Cisplatin: Mode of Cytotoxic Action and Molecular Basis of Resistance," *Oncogene*, 2003, 22(47):7265-79.

◆ **Citrovorum Factor** see Leucovorin Calcium on page 697

◆ **CL-118,532** see Triptorelin on page 1150

◆ **CL-184116** see Porfimer on page 967

◆ **CL-232315** see Mitoxantrone on page 810

Cladribine (KLA dri been)

Medication Safety Issues

Sound-alike/look-alike issues:

Cladribine may be confused with clevidipine, clofarabine, fludarabine

Leustatin® may be confused with lovastatin

High alert medication: The Institute for Safe Medication Practices (ISMP) includes this medication among its list of drugs which have a heightened risk of causing significant patient harm when used in error.

Related Information

Management of Drug Extravasations *on page 1447*

Safe Handling of Hazardous Drugs *on page 1517*

U.S. Brand Names Leustatin®

Index Terms 2-CdA; 2-Chlorodeoxyadenosine; NSC-105014

Generic Available Yes

Canadian Brand Names Leustatin®

Pharmacologic Category Antineoplastic Agent, Antimetabolite; Antineoplastic Agent, Antimetabolite (Purine Antagonist)

Use Treatment of hairy cell leukemia

Unlabeled/Investigational Use Treatment of chronic lymphocytic leukemia (CLL), chronic myelogenous leukemia (CML), non-Hodgkin's lymphomas, progressive multiple sclerosis

Pregnancy Risk Factor D

Lactation Excretion in breast milk unknown/not recommended

Labeled Contraindications Hypersensitivity to cladribine or any component of the formulation

Warnings/Precautions Hazardous agent - use appropriate precautions for handling and disposal. **[U.S. Boxed Warnings]: Dose-dependent, reversible myelosuppression will occur; use with caution in patients with pre-existing hematologic or immunologic abnormalities. Neurologic toxicity has been reported, usually with higher doses, but may occur at normal doses. Acute renal toxicity has been reported with high doses; use caution when administering with other nephrotoxic agents.** Use caution with renal or hepatic impairment. Fever may occur, with or without neutropenia. Use caution in patients with high tumor burden; tumor lysis syndrome may occur. **[U.S. Boxed Warning]: Should be administered under the supervision of an experienced cancer chemotherapy physician.** Safety and efficacy in children have not been established.

Adverse Reactions

>10%:

Central nervous system: Fever (69%; ≥104°F: 11%), fatigue (11% to 45%), headache (7% to 22%)

Dermatologic: Rash (10% to 27%)

Gastrointestinal: Nausea (28%), appetite decreased (17%), vomiting (13%)

Hematologic: Myelosuppression, common, dose limiting (nadir: 5-10 days, recovery: 4-8 weeks); neutropenia (70%); anemia (37%); thrombocytopenia (12%)

Local: Injection site reactions (9% to 19%)

Respiratory: Abnormal breath sounds (11%)

Miscellaneous: Infection (28%)

1% to 10%:

Cardiovascular: Edema (6%), tachycardia (6%), thrombosis (2%)

Central nervous system: Dizziness (9%), chills (9%), insomnia (7%), malaise (5% to 7%), pain (6%)

Dermatologic: Purpura (10%), petechiae (8%), pruritus (6%), erythema (6%)

Gastrointestinal: Diarrhea (10%), constipation (9%), abdominal pain (6%)

Local: Phlebitis (2%)

Neuromuscular & skeletal: Weakness (9%), myalgia (7%), arthralgia (5%)

Respiratory: Cough (7% to 10%), abnormal chest sounds (9%), dyspnea (7%), epistaxis (5%)

Miscellaneous: Diaphoresis (9%)

<1%, postmarketing and/or case reports: Aplastic anemia, bilirubin increased, hemolytic anemia, hypereosinophilia, myelodysplastic syndrome, neurologic toxicity, opportunistic infections, pancytopenia, paraparesis, pneumonia, polyneuropathy (with high doses), pulmonary interstitial infiltrates, quadriplegia (reported at high doses); renal dysfunction (with high doses), Stevens-Johnson syndrome, toxic epidermal necrolysis, transaminases increased, tumor lysis syndrome, urticaria

Drug Interactions

Avoid Concomitant Use

Avoid concomitant use of Cladribine with any of the following: Natalizumab; Vaccines (Live)

Increased Effect/Toxicity

Cladribine may increase the levels/effects of: Leflunomide; Natalizumab; Vaccines (Live)

The levels/effects of Cladribine may be increased by: Trastuzumab

Decreased Effect

Cladribine may decrease the levels/effects of: Vaccines (Inactivated); Vaccines (Live)

The levels/effects of Cladribine may be decreased by: Echinacea

Ethanol/Nutrition/Herb Interactions Ethanol: Avoid ethanol (due to GI irritation).

Storage/Stability Store intact vials under refrigeration 2°C to 8°C (36°F to 46°F). Protect from light. Dilutions in 500 mL NS are stable for 72 hours. Stable in PVC containers for 24 hours at room temperature of 15°C to 30°C (59°F to 86°F) and 7 days in Pharmacia Deltec® cassettes.

Reconstitution Dilute in 500 mL; dilute to a total volume of 100 mL for 7-day infusion. Solutions for 7-day infusion should be prepared in bacteriostatic NS; the manufacturer recommends filtering with a 0.22 micron filter when preparing 7-day infusions.

Compatibility Stable in NS; **incompatible** with D_5W.

Y-site administration: Compatible: Aminophylline, bumetanide, buprenorphine, butorphanol, calcium gluconate, carboplatin, chlorpromazine, cimetidine, cisplatin, cyclophosphamide, cytarabine, dexamethasone sodium phosphate, diphenhydramine, dobutamine, dopamine, doxorubicin, droperidol, enalaprilat, etoposide, famotidine, furosemide, granisetron, haloperidol, heparin, hydrocortisone sodium phosphate, hydrocortisone sodium succinate, hydromorphone, hydroxyzine, idarubicin, leucovorin, lorazepam, mannitol, meperidine, mesna, methylprednisolone sodium succinate, metoclopramide, mitoxantrone, morphine, nalbuphine, ondansetron, paclitaxel, potassium chloride, prochlorperazine edisylate, promethazine, ranitidine, sodium bicarbonate, teniposide, vincristine.

Mechanism of Action A purine nucleoside analogue; prodrug which is activated via phosphorylation by deoxycytidine kinase to a 5'-triphosphate derivative. This active form incorporates into DNA to result in the breakage of DNA strand and shutdown of DNA synthesis. This also results in a depletion of nicotinamide adenine dinucleotide and adenosine triphosphate (ATP). Cladribine is cell-cycle nonspecific.

◄ **Pharmacodynamics/Kinetics**
  Absorption: Oral: 55%; SubQ: 100%; Rectal: 20%
  Distribution: V_d: 4.52 ± 2.82 L/kg
  Protein binding: 20%
  Metabolism: Hepatic; 5'-triphosphate moiety-active
  Half-life elimination: Biphasic: Alpha: 25 minutes; Beta: 6.7 hours; Terminal, mean: Normal renal function: 5.4 hours
  Excretion: Urine (18% to 44%)
  Clearance: Estimated systemic: 640 mL/hour/kg

Dosage I.V.: Refer to individual protocols.
  Children (unlabeled use): Acute leukemias: 6.2-7.5 mg/m²/day continuous infusion for days 1-5; maximum tolerated dose was 8.9 mg/m²/day.
  Adults:
    Hairy cell leukemia: Continuous infusion:
      0.09 mg/kg/day days 1-7; may be repeated every 28-35 days **or**
      3.4 mg/m²/day SubQ days 1-7 (unlabeled dose)
    Chronic lymphocytic leukemia (unlabeled use): Continuous infusion:
      0.1 mg/kg/day days 1-7 **or**
      0.028-0.14 mg/kg/day as a 2-hour infusion days 1-5
    Chronic myelogenous leukemia (unlabeled use): 15 mg/m²/day as a 1-hour infusion days 1-5; if no response, increase dose to 20 mg/m²/day in the second course.

  Dosing adjustment in renal impairment: The FDA-approved labeling recommends that caution should be used in patients with renal impairment; however, no specific dosage adjustment guidelines are available due to lack of data. The following guidelines have been used by some clinicians (Aronoff, 2007):
    Children:
      Cl_{cr} 10-50 mL/minute: Administer 50% of dose
      Cl_{cr} <10 mL/minute: Administer 30% of dose
      Hemodialysis: Administer 30% of dose
      Continuous renal replacement therapy (CRRT): Administer 50% of dose
    Adults:
      Cl_{cr} 10-50 mL/minute: Administer 75% of dose
      Cl_{cr} <10 mL/minute: Administer 50% of dose
      Continuous ambulatory peritoneal dialysis (CAPD): Administer 50% of dose
  Dosing adjustment in hepatic impairment: The FDA-approved labeling recommends that caution should be used in patients with hepatic impairment; however, no specific dosage adjustment guidelines are available due to lack of data.

Administration I.V.: Administer as a 1- to 2-hour infusion or by continuous infusion

Monitoring Parameters CBC with differential, renal and hepatic function; monitor for fever
  Periodic assessment of peripheral blood counts, particularly during the first 4-8 weeks post-treatment, is recommended to detect the development of anemia, neutropenia, and thrombocytopenia and for early detection of any potential sequelae (eg, infection or bleeding)

Emetic Potential Very low (<10%)

Dosage Forms Excipient information presented when available (limited, particularly for generics); consult specific product labeling.
  Injection, solution [preservative free]: 1 mg/mL (10 mL)

References

Aronoff GR, Bennett WM, Berns JS, et al, *Drug Prescribing in Renal Failure: Dosing Guidelines for Adults and Children*, 5th ed. Philadelphia, PA: American College of Physicians; 2007, p 98, 170.

Baltz JK and Montello MJ, "Cladribine for the Treatment of Hematologic Malignancies," *Clin Pharm*, 1993, 12(11):805-13.

Kearns CM, Biakley RL, Santane VM, et al, "Pharmacokinetics of Cladribine (2-Chlorodioxyadenosine) in Children With Acute Leukemia," *Cancer Res*, 1994, 54:1235-39.

Larson RA, Mick R, Spielberger RT, et al, "Dose Escalation Trial of Cladribine Using 5 Daily I.V. Infusions in Patients With Advanced Hematologic Malignancies," *J Clin Oncol*, 1996, 14 (1):188-95.

Liliemark J, "The Clinical Pharmacokinetics of Cladribine," *Clin Pharmacokinet*, 1997, 32 (2):120-31.

Piro LD, "2-Chlorodeoxyadenosine Treatment of Lymphoid Malignancies," *Blood*, 1992, 79 (4):843-5.

Robak T, "Cladribine in the Treatment of Chronic Lymphocytic Leukemia," *Leuk Lymphoma*, 2001, 40(5-6):551-64.

Stine KC, Saylors RL, Williams LL, et al, "2-Chlorodeoxyadenosine (2-CDA) for the Treatment of Refractory or Recurrent Langerhans Cell Histiocytosis (LCH) in Pediatric Patients," *Med Pediatr Oncol*, 1997, 29:288-92.

Tallman MS and Hakimian D, "Current Results and Prospective Trials of Cladribine in Chronic Lymphocytic Leukemia," *Semin Hematol*, 1996, 33(Suppl 1):23-7.

◆ **Clasteon® (Can)** *see* Clodronate *on page* 247

Clodronate (KLOE droh nate)

Index Terms Clodronate Disodium

Canadian Brand Names Bonefos®; Clasteon®

Pharmacologic Category Bisphosphonate Derivative

Use Management of hypercalcemia of malignancy; management of osteolysis due to bone metastases of malignancy

Restrictions Not available in U.S.

Lactation Excretion in breast milk unknown/contraindicated

Labeled Contraindications Hypersensitivity to clodronate, bisphosphonates, or any component of the formulation; severe GI inflammation; renal impairment (serum creatinine >5 mg/dL, SI 440 µmol/L); concomitant use with other bisphosphonates; pregnancy or breast-feeding

Warnings/Precautions Use caution in patients with renal impairment; dose reductions, as well as close monitoring of serum creatinine and BUN, are necessary. Use is contraindicated when serum creatinine >5 mg/dL, SI 440 µmol/L. May cause irritation to upper gastrointestinal mucosa. Esophagitis, dysphagia, esophageal ulcers, esophageal erosions, and esophageal stricture (rare) have been reported with bisphosphonates (oral). Use with caution in patients with dysphagia, esophageal disease, gastritis, duodenitis, or ulcers (may worsen underlying condition). Discontinue use if new or worsening symptoms develop.

Bisphosphonate therapy has been associated with osteonecrosis, primarily of the jaw; this has been observed mostly in cancer patients, but also in patients with postmenopausal osteoporosis and other diagnoses. Most reported cases occurred after I.V. bisphosphonate therapy; however, cases have been reported following oral therapy. Dental exams and preventative dentistry should be performed prior to placing patients with risk factors on chronic bisphosphonate therapy. Invasive dental procedures should be avoided during treatment.

Infrequently, severe (and occasionally debilitating) bone, joint, and/or muscle pain have been reported during bisphosphonate treatment. The onset of pain ranged from a single day to several months. Consider discontinuing therapy in patients who experience severe symptoms; symptoms usually resolve upon ▶

discontinuation. Some patients experienced recurrence when rechallenged with same drug or another bisphosphonate; avoid use in patients with a history of these symptoms in association with bisphosphonate therapy. May cause hypocalcemia (increased risk with intravenous administration) or transient hypophosphatemia.

For I.V. preparation: Dilute prior to use; adequate hydration should be ensured prior to infusion; avoid infiltration/extravasation. Do not administer as bolus injection (may precipitate acute renal failure, severe local reactions, and thrombophlebitis). Monitor renal function during and after intravenous administration. Interrupt infusion in patients experiencing deteriorating renal function during therapy.

Adverse Reactions

>10%: Hepatic: Transaminases increased (≤18%; >2 x ULN: 2%)

1% to 10%:

Endocrine & metabolic: Hypocalcemia (≤3%)

Gastrointestinal: Vomiting (4%), nausea (≤3%), diarrhea (≤2%), anorexia (1%)

Renal: Serum creatinine increased (1%), BUN increased

<1%, postmarketing, and/or case reports: Alkaline phosphatase increased, bronchospasm, erythematous rash; hypersensitivity reactions (angioedema, pruritus, rash, urticaria); macropapular rash, mouth irritation, oliguria, osteonecrosis (primarily of jaw), parathyroid hormone increased, proteinuria, renal failure, ulcerative pharyngitis

Drug Interactions

Avoid Concomitant Use There are no known interactions where it is recommended to avoid concomitant use.

Increased Effect/Toxicity

Clodronate may increase the levels/effects of: Estramustine; Phosphate Supplements

The levels/effects of Clodronate may be increased by: Aminoglycosides; Nonsteroidal Anti-Inflammatory Agents

Decreased Effect

The levels/effects of Clodronate may be decreased by: Antacids; Calcium Salts; Iron Salts; Magnesium Salts

Ethanol/Nutrition/Herb Interactions Food: All food and beverages may interfere with absorption. Coadministration with dairy products may decrease absorption. Beverages (especially orange juice and coffee), food, and medications (eg, antacids, calcium, iron, and multivalent cations) may reduce the absorption of bisphosphonates as much as 60%.

Storage/Stability Store capsules and undiluted ampuls at room temperature (15°C to 30°C).

Clasteon®: Diluted solution should be infused within 12 hours of preparation.

Bonefos®: Diluted solution should be infused within 24 hours of preparation. Once diluted, Bonefos® may be stored up to 24 hours at room temperature.

Reconstitution Injection must be diluted (in 500 mL of NS or D_5W).

Compatibility Stable in D_5W or 0.9% NS. **Incompatible** with calcium-containing solutions (eg, Ringer's solution).

Mechanism of Action A bisphosphonate which lowers serum calcium by inhibition of bone resorption via actions on osteoclasts or on osteoclast precursors.

Pharmacodynamics/Kinetics

Onset of effect: Within 48 hours
  Peak effect: 5-7 days
Duration: 2-3 weeks
Absorption: Oral: Rapid but low absorption (~1% to 3%)
Distribution: V_d: ~20 L; 20% of absorbed clodronate is bound to bone
Protein binding: Variable (2% to 36%)
Bioavailability: Oral: 1% to 3%
Half-life elimination: Terminal: Oral: ~6 hours; I.V.: 13 hours (serum); prolonged in bone tissue
Time to peak, plasma: Oral: 30 minutes
Excretion: Urine (60% to 80% as unchanged drug); feces (as unabsorbed drug)

Dosage Adults:

Clasteon®: Hypercalcemia of malignancy/osteolytic bone metastases:
  I.V.:
    Single infusion: 1500 mg as a single dose
    Multiple infusions: 300 mg/day; should not be prolonged beyond 10 days
  Oral: Recommended daily maintenance dose following I.V. therapy: Range: 1600 mg (4 capsules) to 2400 mg (6 capsules) given in a single or 2 divided doses; maximum recommended daily dose: 3200 mg (8 capsules). Should be taken at least 1 hour before or after food since food may decrease clodronate absorption.

Bonefos®:
  Hypercalcemia of malignancy:
    I.V.: Multiple infusions: 300 mg/day; should not be prolonged beyond 7 days
    Oral: Recommended daily maintenance dose following I.V. therapy: Range: 1600 mg (4 capsules) to 2400 mg (6 capsules) given in single or 2 divided doses; maximum recommended daily dose: 3200 mg (8 capsules). Should be taken at least 2 hours before or after food since food may decrease clodronate absorption.
  Osteolytic bone metastases:
    I.V.: Multiple infusions: 300 mg/day; should not be prolonged beyond 7 days
    Oral: Initial: 1600 mg/day; may be increased to a maximum of 3200 mg/day

Dosage adjustment in renal impairment:

Clasteon®:
  Serum creatinine (S_{cr}) >5 mg/dL: Use is contraindicated
  S_{cr} ≥2.5-5 mg/dL: Dosage reduction is recommended; no specific guidelines available
Bonefos®:
  S_{cr} >5 mg/dL: Use is contraindicated
  Cl_{cr}: 50-80 mL/minute: Administer 75% to 100% of normal dose
  Cl_{cr}: 12-49 mL/minute: Administer 50% to 75% of normal dose
  Cl_{cr}: <12 mL/minute: Administer 50% of normal dose

Administration

Capsules: Administer with a glass of plain water at least 2 hours (Bonefos®) or 1 hour (Clasteon®) before or after food.
Injection: Do not administer as bolus injection; for single infusion therapy administer over at least 4 hours; for multiple-infusion therapy administered once daily, infuse over 2-6 hours. Patients should be adequately hydrated with oral or I.V. fluids prior to infusion.

Monitoring Parameters Serum electrolytes including calcium, phosphorous, magnesium, and potassium; monitor for hypocalcemia for at least 2 weeks after therapy; serum creatinine, BUN, CBC with differential, hepatic function

◀ **Test Interactions** Bisphosphonates may interfere with diagnostic imaging agents such as technetium-99m-diphosphonate in bone scans.

Dosage Forms Excipient information presented when available (limited, particularly for generics); consult specific product labeling. [CAN] = Canadian brand name

Injection:
Bonefos® [CAN]: 60 mg/mL (5 mL) [not available in the U.S.]
Clasteon® [CAN]: 30 mg/mL (10 mL) [not available in the U.S.]

Capsule:
Bonefos® [CAN], Clasteon® [CAN]: 400 mg [not available in the U.S.]

References

American Dental Association Council on Scientific Affairs, "Dental Management of Patients Receiving Oral Bisphosphonate Therapy," *JADA*, 2006, 137(8):1144-50. Available at http://www.ada.org/prof/resources/pubs/jada/reports/report bisphosphonate.pdf

McMahon RE, Bouquot JE, Glueck CJ, et al, "Osteonecrosis: A Multifactorial Etiology," *J Oral Maxillofac Surg*, 2004, 62(7):904-5.

Tarassoff P and Csermak K, "Avascular Necrosis of the Jaws: Risk Factors in Metastatic Cancer Patients," *J Oral Maxillofac Surg*, 2003, 61(10):1238-9.

◆ **Clodronate Disodium** see Clodronate *on page 247*

Clofarabine (klo FARE a been)

Medication Safety Issues

Sound-alike/look-alike issues:
Clofarabine may be confused with cladribine, clevidipine

High alert medication: The Institute for Safe Medication Practices (ISMP) includes this medication among its list of drug classes which have a heightened risk of causing significant patient harm when used in error.

Related Information

Safe Handling of Hazardous Drugs *on page 1517*

U.S. Brand Names Clolar®

Index Terms CAFdA; Clofarex; NSC606869

Generic Available No

Pharmacologic Category Antineoplastic Agent, Antimetabolite (Purine Antagonist)

Use Treatment of relapsed or refractory acute lymphoblastic leukemia (ALL)

Unlabeled/Investigational Use Relapsed and refractory acute myeloid leukemia (AML) and myelodysplastic syndrome (MDS)

Pregnancy Risk Factor D

Lactation Excretion in breast milk unknown/not recommended

Labeled Contraindications There are no contraindications listed within the manufacturer's labeling.

Warnings/Precautions Hazardous agent - use appropriate precautions for handling and disposal. Tumor lysis syndrome and cytokine release may develop into systemic inflammatory response syndrome (SIRS)/capillary leak syndrome, and organ dysfunction; discontinuation of clofarabine should be considered with the presentation of SIRS or capillary leak syndrome (see Tumor Lysis Syndrome on page 1468). Safety and efficacy have not been established with renal or hepatic dysfunction; use with caution. Safety and efficacy in pediatric patients <1 year of age or adults >21 years have not been established.

Adverse Reactions

>10%:
Cardiovascular: Tachycardia (35%), hypotension (29%), flushing (19%), hypertension (13%), edema (12%)

Central nervous system: Headache (43%), fever (39%), chills (34%), fatigue (34%), anxiety (21%), pain (15%)

Dermatologic: Pruritus (43%), rash (38%), petechiae (26%), palmar-plantar erythrodysesthesia syndrome (16%), erythema (11%)

Gastrointestinal: Vomiting (78%; grades 3/4: 9%), nausea (73%; grades 3/4: 15%), diarrhea (56%), abdominal pain (8% to 35%), anorexia (30%), mucosal inflammation (16%), gingival bleeding (14%), oral candidiasis (11%)

Genitourinary: Hematuria (13%)

Hematologic: Leukopenia (grades 3/4: 88%), anemia (83%; grades 3/4: 75%), lymphopenia (grades 3/4: 82%), thrombocytopenia (81%; grades 3/4: 80%), neutropenia (grades 3/4: 10% to 64%), febrile neutropenia (55%; grade 4: 3%)

Hepatic: ALT increased (81%; grades 3/4: 43% to 44%), AST increased (74%; grades 3/4: 36%), bilirubin increased (45%; grades 3/4: 13%)

Neuromuscular & skeletal: Limb pain (30%), myalgia (14%)

Renal: Creatinine increased (50%; grades 3/4: 8%)

Respiratory: Epistaxis (27%), dyspnea (13%), pleural effusion (12%)

Miscellaneous: Infection (83%; includes bacterial, fungal, and viral), catheter-related infection (12%)

1% to 10%:

Cardiovascular: Pericardial effusion (8%)

Central nervous system: Irritability (10%), lethargy (10%), somnolence (10%), agitation (5%), mental status change

Dermatologic: Cellulitis (8%), pruritic rash (8%)

Gastrointestinal: Proctalgia (8%), clostridium colitis (7%), stomatitis (7%), mouth hemorrhage (5%), oral mucosal petechiae (5%), cecitis (1% to 4%), pancreatitis (1% to 4%)

Hepatic: Jaundice (8%)

Neuromuscular & skeletal: Back pain (10%), bone pain (10%), weakness (10%), arthralgia (9%)

Respiratory: Pneumonia (10%), respiratory distress (10%), tachypnea (9%), upper respiratory tract infection (5%), pulmonary edema (1% to 4%)

Miscellaneous: Herpes simplex (10%), sepsis (10%), bacteremia (9%), candidiasis (7%), herpes zoster (7%), septic shock (7%), staphylococcus bacteremia (6%), tumor lysis syndrome (grade 3: 6%), capillary leak syndrome (4%), hypersensitivity (1% to 4%), SIRS (2%)

<1%, postmarketing, and/or case reports: Bone marrow failure, dermatitis, hallucination, hepatic veno-occlusive disease, hepatomegaly, hypokalemia, hypophosphatemia, left ventricular systolic function decreased, right ventricular pressure increased, Stevens-Johnson syndrome, toxic epidermal necrolysis

Drug Interactions

Avoid Concomitant Use

Avoid concomitant use of Clofarabine with any of the following: Natalizumab; Vaccines (Live)

Increased Effect/Toxicity

Clofarabine may increase the levels/effects of: Leflunomide; Natalizumab; Vaccines (Live); Vitamin K Antagonists

The levels/effects of Clofarabine may be increased by: Trastuzumab

◀ **Decreased Effect**

Clofarabine may decrease the levels/effects of: Cardiac Glycosides; Vaccines (Inactivated); Vaccines (Live); Vitamin K Antagonists

The levels/effects of Clofarabine may be decreased by: Echinacea

Storage/Stability Store undiluted and diluted solutions at room temperature of 25°C (77°F); excursions permitted to 15°C to 30°C (59°F to 86°F). Solutions diluted in 100-500 mL of D_5W or NS are stable for 24 hours at room temperature.

Reconstitution Clofarabine should be diluted with 100-500 mL NS or D_5W to a final concentration of 0.15-0.4 mg/mL. Manufacturer recommends the product be filtered through a 0.2 micrometer filter before dilution. Use appropriate precautions for handling and disposal.

Compatibility Stable in D_5W or NS.

Mechanism of Action Clofarabine, a purine (deoxyadenosine) nucleoside analog, is metabolized to clofarabine 5'-triphosphate. Clofarabine 5'-triphosphate decreases cell replication and repair as well as causing cell death. To decrease cell replication and repair, clofarabine 5'-triphosphate competes with deoxyadenosine triphosphate for the enzymes ribonucleotide reductase and DNA polymerase. Cell replication is decreased when clofarabine 5'-triphosphate inhibits ribonucleotide reductase from reacting with deoxyadenosine triphosphate to produce deoxynucleotide triphosphate which is needed for DNA synthesis. Cell replication is also decreased when clofarabine 5'-triphosphate competes with DNA polymerase for incorporation into the DNA chain; when done during the repair process, cell repair is affected. To cause cell death, clofarabine 5'-triphosphate alters the mitochondrial membrane by releasing proteins, an inducing factor and cytochrome C.

Pharmacodynamics/Kinetics

Distribution: V_d: 172 L/m^2

Protein binding: 47%, primarily to albumin

Metabolism: Intracellular by deoxycytidine kinase and mono- and diphosphokinases to active metabolite clofarabine 5'-triphosphate; limited hepatic metabolism (0.2%)

Half-life elimination: ~5.2 hours

Excretion: Urine (49% to 60%, as unchanged drug)

Dosage Consider prophylactic corticosteroids (hydrocortisone 100 mg/m^2 on days 1-3; to prevent signs/symptoms of capillary leak syndrome or SIRS), hydration and allopurinol (to reduce the risk of tumor lysis syndrome/hyperuricemia), and prophylactic antiemetics.

I.V.: Children ≥1 year and Adults ≤21 years: ALL: 52 mg/m^2/day days 1 through 5; repeat every 2-6 weeks; subsequent cycles should begin no sooner than 14 days from day 1 of the previous cycle (subsequent cycles may be administered when ANC ≥750/mm^3)

Dosage adjustment for toxicity:

Hematologic toxicity: ANC <500/mm^3 lasting ≥4 weeks: Reduce clofarabine dose by 25% for next cycle

Nonhematologic toxicity:

Clinically significant infection: Withhold treatment until infection is under control, then restart clofarabine at full dose

Grade 3 toxicity excluding infection, nausea and vomiting, and transient elevations in transaminases and bilirubin: Withhold treatment; may reinitiate clofarabine with a 25% dose-reduction with resolution or return to baseline

Grade ≥3 increase in creatinine or bilirubin: Discontinue clofarabine; may reinitiate with 25% dosage reduction when creatinine or bilirubin return to baseline and patient is stable; administer allopurinol for hyperuricemia

Grade 4 toxicity (noninfectious): Discontinue clofarabine treatment

Capillary leak or systemic inflammatory response syndrome (SIRS) signs/ symptoms (eg, hypotension, tachycardia, tachypnea, pulmonary edema): Discontinue clofarabine; institute supportive measures

Dosage adjustment in renal/hepatic impairment: Safety not established; use with caution

Administration I.V. infusion: Over 2 hours. Continuous I.V. fluids are encouraged to decrease adverse events and tumor lysis effects. Hypotension may be a sign of capillary leak syndrome or systemic inflammatory response syndrome (SIRS). Discontinue if the patient becomes hypotensive during administration. Retreatment should only be considered if the hypotension is not related to capillary leak syndrome or SIRS.

Monitoring Parameters Blood pressure, cardiac function, and respiratory status during infusion; periodic CBC with platelet count (increase frequency in patients who develop cytopenias); liver and kidney function during 5 days of clofarabine administration; signs and symptoms of tumor lysis syndrome and cytokine release syndrome (tachypnea, tachycardia, hypotension, pulmonary edema); hydration status

Emetic Potential Moderate (30% to 90%)

Dosage Forms Excipient information presented when available (limited, particularly for generics); consult specific product labeling.

Injection, solution [preservative free]:

Clolar®: 1 mg/mL (20 mL)

References

Faderl S, Ravandi F, Huang X, et al, "A Randomized Study of Clofarabine versus Clofarabine Plus Low-Dose Cytarabine as Front-Line Therapy for Patients Aged 60 Years and Older With Acute Myeloid Leukemia and High-Risk Myelodysplastic Syndrome," *Blood*, 2008, 112(5):1638-45.

Jeha S, Gandhi V, Chan KW, et al, "Clofarabine, a Novel Nucleoside Analog, is Active in Pediatric Patients With Advanced Leukemia," *Blood*, 2004, 103(3):784-9.

Jeha S, Gaynon PS, Razzouk BI, et al, "Phase II Study of Clofarabine in Pediatric Patients With Refractory or Relapsed Acute Lymphoblastic Leukemia," *J Clin Oncol*, 2008, 24(12):1917-23.

Kantarjian H, Gandhi V, Cortes J, et al, "Phase 2 Clinical and Pharmacologic Study of Clofarabine in Patients With Refractory or Relapsed Acute Leukemia," *Blood*, 2003, 102(7):2379-86.

◆ **Clofarex** *see* Clofarabine *on page 250*

◆ **Clolar®** *see* Clofarabine *on page 250*

◆ **Clotrimaderm (Can)** *see* Clotrimazole *on page 253*

Clotrimazole (kloe TRIM a zole)

Medication Safety Issues

Sound-alike/look-alike issues:

Clotrimazole may be confused with co-trimoxazole

Lotrimin® may be confused with Lotrisone®, Otrivin®

Mycelex® may be confused with Myoflex®

International issues:

Cloderm®: Brand name for clocortolone in the United States

Canesten® [multiple international markets] may be confused with Cenestin® which is a brand name for estrogens (conjugated a/synthetic) in the U.S.

Canesten® [multiple international markets]: Brand name for fluconazole in Great Britain

Mycelex® may be confused with Mucolex® which is a brand name for carbocysteine in Ireland, Portugal, and Thailand; a brand name for guaifenesin in Hong Kong

Related Information

Oral Mucositis / Stomatitis *on page 1460*

U.S. Brand Names Cruex® Cream [OTC]; Gyne-Lotrimin® 3 [OTC]; Gyne-Lotrimin® 7 [OTC]; Lotrimin® AF Athlete's Foot Cream [OTC]; Lotrimin® AF for Her [OTC]; Lotrimin® AF Jock Itch Cream [OTC]; Mycelex®

Generic Available Yes: Cream, solution, troche

Canadian Brand Names Canesten® Topical; Canesten® Vaginal; Clotrima-derm; Trivagizole-3®

Pharmacologic Category Antifungal Agent, Oral Nonabsorbed; Antifungal Agent, Topical; Antifungal Agent, Vaginal

Use Treatment of susceptible fungal infections, including oropharyngeal candidiasis, dermatophytoses, superficial mycoses, and cutaneous candidiasis, as well as vulvovaginal candidiasis; limited data suggest that clotrimazole troches may be effective for prophylaxis against oropharyngeal candidiasis in neutropenic patients

Pregnancy Risk Factor B (topical); C (troches)

Lactation Excretion in breast milk unknown

Labeled Contraindications Hypersensitivity to clotrimazole or any component of the formulation

Warnings/Precautions Clotrimazole should not be used for treatment of systemic fungal infection. Safety and effectiveness of clotrimazole lozenges (troches) in children <3 years of age have not been established. When using topical formulation, avoid contact with eyes.

Adverse Reactions

Oral:

>10%: Hepatic: Abnormal liver function tests

1% to 10%:

Gastrointestinal: Nausea and vomiting may occur in patients on clotrimazole troches

Local: Mild burning, irritation, stinging to skin or vaginal area

Vaginal:

1% to 10%: Genitourinary: Vulvar/vaginal burning

<1% (Limited to important or life-threatening): Vulvar itching, soreness, edema, or discharge; polyuria; burning or itching of penis of sexual partner

Drug Interactions

Metabolism/Transport Effects Inhibits CYP1A2 (weak), 2A6 (weak), 2B6 (weak), 2C8 (weak), 2C9 (weak), 2C19 (weak), 2D6 (weak), 2E1 (weak), 3A4 (moderate)

Avoid Concomitant Use

Avoid concomitant use of Clotrimazole with any of the following: Everolimus; Tolvaptan

Increased Effect/Toxicity

Clotrimazole may increase the levels/effects of: Colchicine; CYP3A4 Substrates; Eplerenone; Everolimus; FentaNYL; Halofantrine; Pimecrolimus; Ranolazine; Salmeterol; Saxagliptin; Tolvaptan

Decreased Effect

Clotrimazole may decrease the levels/effects of: Saccharomyces boulardii

Mechanism of Action Binds to phospholipids in the fungal cell membrane altering cell wall permeability resulting in loss of essential intracellular elements

Pharmacodynamics/Kinetics

Absorption: Topical: Negligible through intact skin

Time to peak, serum:

Oral topical (troche): Salivary levels occur within 3 hours following 30 minutes of dissolution time

Vaginal cream: High vaginal levels: 8-24 hours

Vaginal tablet: High vaginal levels: 1-2 days

Excretion: Feces (as metabolites)

Dosage

Children >3 years and Adults:

Oral:

Prophylaxis: 10 mg troche dissolved 3 times/day for the duration of chemotherapy or until steroids are reduced to maintenance levels

Treatment: 10 mg troche dissolved slowly 5 times/day for 14 consecutive days

Topical (cream, solution): Apply twice daily; if no improvement occurs after 4 weeks of therapy, re-evaluate diagnosis

Children >12 years and Adults:

Vaginal:

Cream:

1%: Insert 1 applicatorful vaginal cream daily (preferably at bedtime) for 7 consecutive days

2%: Insert 1 applicatorful vaginal cream daily (preferably at bedtime) for 3 consecutive days

Tablet: Insert 100 mg/day for 7 days or 500 mg single dose

Topical (cream, solution): Apply to affected area twice daily (morning and evening) for 7 consecutive days

Administration

Oral (troche): Allow to dissolve slowly over 15-30 minutes.

Topical: Avoid contact with eyes. For external use only. Apply sparingly. Protect hands with latex gloves. Do not use occlusive dressings.

Monitoring Parameters Periodic liver function tests during oral therapy with clotrimazole troche

Dosage Forms Excipient information presented when available (limited, particularly for generics); consult specific product labeling. [DSC] = Discontinued product

Cream, topical: 1% (15 g, 30 g, 45 g)

Cruex®: 1% (15 g) [contains benzyl alcohol]

Lotrimin® AF Athlete's Foot: 1% (12 g) [contains benzyl alcohol]

Lotrimin® AF Jock Itch: 1% (12 g) [contains benzyl alcohol]

Lotrimin® AF for Her: 1% (24 g) [contains benzyl alcohol]

Cream, topical/vaginal: 1% (45 g)

Gyne-Lotrimin® 7: 1% (45 g) [contains benzyl alcohol; packaged with refillable applicator]

Cream, vaginal: 2% (21 g)

Gyne-Lotrimin® 3: 2% (21 g) [contains benzyl alcohol; packaged with 3 disposable applicators]

Solution, topical: 1% (10 mL, 30 mL)

Tablet, vaginal:

Gyne-Lotrimin® 3: 200 mg (3s) [DSC]

Troche, oral: 10 mg

Mycelex®: 10 mg

References

Duhm B, Medenwald H, Puetter J, et al, "The Pharmacokinetics of Clotrimazole 14C," *Postgrad Med J*, 1974, 50(Suppl 1):13-6.

◆ **CMA-676** *see* Gemtuzumab Ozogamicin *on page 537*

◆ **CMV-IGIV** *see* Cytomegalovirus Immune Globulin (Intravenous-Human) *on page 290*

◆ **Coagulation Factor I** *see* Fibrinogen Concentrate (Human) *on page 474*

◆ **Coagulation Factor VIIa** *see* Factor VIIa (Recombinant) *on page 446*

◆ **CO Bicalutamide (Can)** *see* Bicalutamide *on page 147*

◆ **CO Ciprofloxacin (Can)** *see* Ciprofloxacin *on page 228*

Codeine (KOE deen)

Medication Safety Issues

Sound-alike/look-alike issues: *

Codeine may be confused with Cardene®, Cophene®, Cordran®, iodine, Lodine®

High alert medication: The Institute for Safe Medication Practices (ISMP) includes this medication among its list of drug classes which have a heightened risk of causing significant patient harm when used in error.

Index Terms Codeine Phosphate; Codeine Sulfate; Methylmorphine

Generic Available Yes

Canadian Brand Names Codeine Contin®

Pharmacologic Category Analgesic, Opioid; Antitussive

Use Treatment of mild-to-moderate pain; antitussive in lower doses

Restrictions C-II

Pregnancy Risk Factor C/D (prolonged use or high doses at term)

Lactation Enters breast milk/use caution (AAP rates "compatible")

Labeled Contraindications Hypersensitivity to codeine or any component of the formulation; pregnancy (prolonged use or high doses at term)

Warnings/Precautions Use with caution in patients with hypersensitivity reactions to other phenanthrene-derivative opioid agonists (morphine, hydrocodone, hydromorphone, levorphanol, oxycodone, oxymorphone); respiratory diseases including asthma, emphysema, COPD, adrenal insufficiency, biliary tract impairment, CNS depression/coma, head trauma, morbid obesity, prostatic hyperplasia, urinary stricture, thyroid dysfunction, or severe liver or renal insufficiency; some preparations contain sulfites which may cause allergic reactions; tolerance or drug dependence may result from extended use. May obscure diagnosis or clinical course of patients with acute abdominal conditions. May cause CNS depression, which may impair physical or mental abilities; patients must be cautioned about performing tasks which require mental alertness (eg, operating machinery or driving). May cause hypotension; use with caution in patients with hypovolemia, cardiovascular disease (including acute MI), or drugs which may exaggerate hypotensive effects (including phenothiazines or general anesthetics). Use caution in patients with two or more copies of the variant CYP2D6*2 allele; may have extensive conversion to morphine and thus increased opioid-mediated effects.

Not recommended for use for cough control in patients with a productive cough; not recommended as an antitussive for children <2 years of age; the elderly and debilitated patients may be particularly susceptible to adverse effects of narcotics

Not approved for I.V. administration (although this route has been used clinically). If given intravenously, must be given slowly and the patient should be lying down. Rapid intravenous administration of narcotics may increase the incidence of serious adverse effects, in part due to limited opportunity to assess response prior to administration of the full dose. Access to respiratory support should be immediately available.

Concurrent use of agonist/antagonist analgesics may precipitate withdrawal symptoms and/or reduced analgesic efficacy in patients following prolonged therapy with mu opioid agonists. Abrupt discontinuation following prolonged use may also lead to withdrawal symptoms.

Adverse Reactions

Frequency not defined: ALT increased, AST increased

>10%:

Central nervous system: Drowsiness

Gastrointestinal: Constipation

1% to 10%:

Cardiovascular: Hypotension, tachycardia or bradycardia

Central nervous system: Confusion, dizziness, false feeling of well being, headache, lightheadedness, malaise, paradoxical CNS stimulation, restlessness

Dermatologic: Rash, urticaria

Gastrointestinal: Anorexia, nausea, vomiting, xerostomia

Genitourinary: Ureteral spasm, urination decreased

Hepatic: LFTs increased

Local: Burning at injection site

Neuromuscular & skeletal: Weakness

Ocular: Blurred vision

Respiratory: Dyspnea

Miscellaneous: Histamine release

<1%: Biliary spasm, convulsions, hallucinations, insomnia, mental depression, muscle rigidity, nightmares, paralytic ileus, stomach cramps

Drug Interactions

Metabolism/Transport Effects Substrate of CYP2D6 (major), 3A4 (minor); **Inhibits** CYP2D6 (weak)

Avoid Concomitant Use There are no known interactions where it is recommended to avoid concomitant use.

Increased Effect/Toxicity

Codeine may increase the levels/effects of: Alcohol (Ethyl); Alvimopan; CNS Depressants; Desmopressin; Selective Serotonin Reuptake Inhibitors; Thiazide Diuretics

The levels/effects of Codeine may be increased by: Amphetamines; Antipsychotic Agents (Phenothiazines); Somatostatin Analogs; Succinylcholine

Decreased Effect

Codeine may decrease the levels/effects of: Pegvisomant

The levels/effects of Codeine may be decreased by: Ammonium Chloride; CYP2D6 Inhibitors (Moderate); CYP2D6 Inhibitors (Strong)

Ethanol/Nutrition/Herb Interactions

Ethanol: Avoid or limit ethanol (may increase CNS depression).

Herb/Nutraceutical: St John's wort may decrease codeine levels. Avoid valerian, St John's wort, kava kava, gotu kola (may increase CNS depression).

◄ **Storage/Stability** Store injection between 15°C to 30°C; avoid freezing. Do not use if injection is discolored or contains a precipitate. Protect injection from light.

Compatibility Compatibility in syringe: **Compatible:** Glycopyrrolate, hydroxyzine.

Mechanism of Action Binds to opiate receptors in the CNS, causing inhibition of ascending pain pathways, altering the perception of and response to pain; causes cough supression by direct central action in the medulla; produces generalized CNS depression

Pharmacodynamics/Kinetics

Onset of action: Oral: 0.5-1 hour; I.M.: 10-30 minutes

Peak effect: Oral: 1-1.5 hours; I.M.: 0.5-1 hour

Duration: 4-6 hours

Absorption: Oral: Adequate

Distribution: Crosses placenta; enters breast milk

Protein binding: 7%

Metabolism: Hepatic to morphine (active)

Half-life elimination: 2.5-3.5 hours

Excretion: Urine (3% to 16% as unchanged drug, norcodeine, and free and conjugated morphine)

Dosage Note: These are guidelines and do not represent the maximum doses that may be required in all patients. Doses should be titrated to pain relief/prevention. Doses >1.5 mg/kg body weight are not recommended.

Analgesic:

Children: Oral, I.M., SubQ: 0.5-1 mg/kg/dose every 4-6 hours as needed; maximum: 60 mg/dose

Adults:

Oral: 30 mg every 4-6 hours as needed; patients with prior opiate exposure may require higher initial doses. Usual range: 15-120 mg every 4-6 hours as needed. **Note:** The American Pain Society recommends an initial dose of 30-60 mg for adults with moderate pain.

Oral, controlled release formulation (Codeine Contin®, not available in U.S.): 50-300 mg every 12 hours. **Note:** A patient's codeine requirement should be established using prompt release formulations; conversion to long acting products may be considered when chronic, continuous treatment is required. Higher dosages should be reserved for use only in opioid-tolerant patients.

I.M., SubQ: 30 mg every 4-6 hours as needed; patients with prior opiate exposure may require higher initial doses. Usual range: 15-120 mg every 4-6 hours as needed; more frequent dosing may be needed

Antitussive: Oral (for nonproductive cough):

Children: 1-1.5 mg/kg/day in divided doses every 4-6 hours as needed: Alternative dose according to age:

2-6 years: 2.5-5 mg every 4-6 hours as needed; maximum: 30 mg/day

6-12 years: 5-10 mg every 4-6 hours as needed; maximum: 60 mg/day

Adults: 10-20 mg/dose every 4-6 hours as needed; maximum: 120 mg/day

Dosing adjustment in renal impairment:

Cl_{cr} 10-50 mL/minute: Administer 75% of dose

Cl_{cr} <10 mL/minute: Administer 50% of dose

Dosing adjustment in hepatic impairment: Probably necessary in hepatic insufficiency

Administration Not approved for I.V. administration (although this route has been used clinically). If given intravenously, must be given slowly and the patient should be lying down. Rapid intravenous administration of narcotics may increase the incidence of serious adverse effects, in part due to limited opportunity to assess response prior to administration of the full dose. Access to respiratory support should be immediately available.

Monitoring Parameters Pain relief, respiratory and mental status, blood pressure, heart rate

Test Interactions Some quinolones may produce a false-positive urine screening result for opiates using commercially-available immunoassay kits. This has been demonstrated most consistently for levofloxacin and ofloxacin, but other quinolones have shown cross-reactivity in certain assay kits. Confirmation of positive opiate screens by more specific methods should be considered.

Dosage Forms Excipient information presented when available (limited, particularly for generics); consult specific product labeling. [CAN] = Canadian brand name

Injection, as phosphate: 15 mg/mL (2 mL); 30 mg/mL (2 mL) [contains sodium metabisulfite]

Powder, for prescription compounding: 10 g, 25 g

Tablet, as phosphate: 30 mg, 60 mg

Tablet, as sulfate: 15 mg, 30 mg, 60 mg

Tablet, controlled release (Codeine Contin®) [CAN]: 50 mg, 100 mg, 150 mg, 200 mg [not available in U.S.]

References

Desjardins PJ, Cooper SA, Gallegos TL, et al, "The Relative Analgesic Efficacy of Propiram Fumarate, Codeine, Aspirin, and Placebo in Postimpaction Dental Pain," *J Clin Pharmacol*, 1984, 24(1):35-42.

"Drugs for Pain," *Med Lett Drugs Ther*, 2000, 42(1085):73-8.

Ferrell BA, "Pain Management in Elderly People," *J Am Geriatr Soc*, 1991, 39(1):64-73.

Jacobi J, Fraser GL, Coursin DB, et al, "Clinical Practice Guidelines for the Sustained Use of Sedatives and Analgesics in the Critically Ill Adult," *Crit Care Med*, 2002, 30(1):119-41. Available at: http://www.sccm.org/pdf/sedatives.pdf. Accessed August 2, 2003.

Kaiko RF, Wallenstein SL, Rogers AG, et al, "Narcotics in the Elderly," *Med Clin North Am*, 1982, 66 (5):1079-89.

"Principles of Analgesic Use in the Treatment of Acute Pain and Chronic Cancer Pain," 5th ed, Glenview, IL: American Pain Society, 2003.

- ◆ **Cortifoam®** *see* Hydrocortisone *on page 575*
- ◆ **Cortifoam™ (Can)** *see* Hydrocortisone *on page 575*
- ◆ **Cortisol** *see* Hydrocortisone *on page 575*
- ◆ **Cortizone-10® Maximum Strength [OTC]** *see* Hydrocortisone *on page 575*
- ◆ **Cortizone-10® Maximum Strength Cooling Relief [OTC]** *see* Hydrocortisone *on page 575*
- ◆ **Cortizone-10® Maximum Strength Easy Relief [OTC]** *see* Hydrocortisone *on page 575*
- ◆ **Cortizone-10® Maximum Strength Intensive Healing Formula [OTC]** *see* Hydrocortisone *on page 575*
- ◆ **Cortizone-10® Plus Maximum Strength [OTC]** *see* Hydrocortisone *on page 575*
- ◆ **Cortizone-10® Quick Shot [OTC] [DSC]** *see* Hydrocortisone *on page 575*
- ◆ **Cosmegen®** *see* DACTINomycin *on page 299*
- ◆ **Co-Trimoxazole** *see* Sulfamethoxazole and Trimethoprim *on page 1051*
- ◆ **Co-Vidarabine** *see* Pentostatin *on page 949*
- ◆ **CP358774** *see* Erlotinib *on page 420*
- ◆ **CPDG2** *see* Glucarpidase *on page 547*
- ◆ **CPG2** *see* Glucarpidase *on page 547*
- ◆ **CPM** *see* Cyclophosphamide *on page 260*
- ◆ **CPT-11** *see* Irinotecan *on page 651*
- ◆ **CPZ** *see* ChlorproMAZINE *on page 220*
- ◆ **Cruex® Cream [OTC]** *see* Clotrimazole *on page 253*
- ◆ **CsA** *see* CycloSPORINE *on page 268*
- ◆ **CTX** *see* Cyclophosphamide *on page 260*
- ◆ **CyA** *see* CycloSPORINE *on page 268*

Cyclophosphamide (sye kloe FOS fa mide)

Medication Safety Issues

Sound-alike/look-alike issues:

Cyclophosphamide may be confused with cycloSPORINE, ifosfamide

Cytoxan® may be confused with cefoxitin, Centoxin®, Ciloxan®, cytarabine, CytoGam®, Cytosar®, Cytosar-U®, Cytotec®

High alert medication: The Institute for Safe Medication Practices (ISMP) includes this medication among its list of drugs which have a heightened risk of causing significant patient harm when used in error.

Related Information

Fertility and Cancer Therapy *on page 1430*
Hematopoietic Stem Cell Transplantation *on page 1501*
Management of Drug Extravasations *on page 1447*
Safe Handling of Hazardous Drugs *on page 1517*

U.S. Brand Names Cytoxan® [DSC]

Index Terms CPM; CTX; CYT; Neosar

Generic Available Yes

Canadian Brand Names Cytoxan®; Procytox®

Pharmacologic Category Antineoplastic Agent, Alkylating Agent

Use

Oncology-related uses: Treatment of Hodgkin's lymphoma, non-Hodgkin's lymphoma (including Burkitt's lymphoma), chronic lymphocytic leukemia (CLL), chronic myelocytic leukemia (CML), acute myelocytic leukemia (AML), acute lymphocytic leukemia (ALL), mycosis fungoides, multiple myeloma, neuroblastoma, retinoblastoma; breast cancer; ovarian adenocarcinoma

Nononcology uses: Treatment of nephrotic syndrome in children

Unlabeled/Investigational Use

Oncology-related uses: Ewing's sarcoma, rhabdomyosarcoma, Wilms tumor, ovarian germ cell tumors, small cell lung cancer, testicular cancer, pheochromocytoma, bone marrow transplantation conditioning regimen

Nononcology uses: Severe rheumatoid disorders, Wegener's granulomatosis, myasthenia gravis, multiple sclerosis, systemic lupus erythematosus, lupus nephritis, autoimmune hemolytic anemia, idiopathic thrombocytic purpura (ITP), and antibody-induced pure red cell aplasia

Pregnancy Risk Factor D

Lactation Enters breast milk/contraindicated

Labeled Contraindications Hypersensitivity to cyclophosphamide or any component of the formulation; pregnancy

Warnings/Precautions Hazardous agent - use appropriate precautions for handling and disposal. Dosage adjustment may be needed for renal or hepatic failure. Hemorrhagic cystitis may occur; increased hydration and frequent voiding is recommended. Immunosuppression may occur; monitor for infections. May cause cardiotoxicity (HF, usually with higher doses); may potentiate the cardiotoxicity of anthracyclines. May impair fertility; interferes with oogenesis and spermatogenesis. Secondary malignancies (usually delayed) have been reported

Adverse Reactions

>10%:

Dermatologic: Alopecia (40% to 60%) but hair will usually regrow although it may be a different color and/or texture. Hair loss usually begins 3-6 weeks after the start of therapy.

Endocrine & metabolic: Fertility: May cause sterility; interferes with oogenesis and spermatogenesis; may be irreversible in some patients; gonadal suppression (amenorrhea)

Gastrointestinal: Nausea and vomiting (usually beginning 6-10 hours after administration); anorexia, diarrhea, mucositis, and stomatitis are also seen

Genitourinary: Severe, potentially fatal, acute hemorrhagic cystitis or urinary fibrosis (7% to 40%)

Hematologic: Thrombocytopenia and anemia are less common than leukopenia

Onset: 7 days

Nadir: 10-14 days

Recovery: 21 days

1% to 10%:

Cardiovascular: Facial flushing

Central nervous system: Headache

Dermatologic: Skin rash

Renal: SIADH may occur, usually with doses >50 mg/kg (or 1 g/m^2); renal tubular necrosis, which usually resolves with discontinuation of the drug, is also reported

Respiratory: Nasal congestion occurs when I.V. doses are administered too rapidly; patients experience runny eyes, rhinorrhea, sinus congestion, and sneezing during or immediately after the infusion.

<1%, postmarketing, and/or case reports: High-dose therapy may cause cardiac dysfunction manifested as CHF; cardiac necrosis or hemorrhagic myocarditis has occurred rarely, but may be fatal. Interstitial pneumonitis and pulmonary fibrosis are occasionally seen with high doses. Cyclophosphamide may also potentiate the cardiac toxicity of anthracyclines. Other adverse reactions include anaphylactic reactions, darkening of skin/fingernails, dizziness, hemorrhagic colitis, hemorrhagic ureteritis, hepatotoxicity, hyperuricemia, hypokalemia, jaundice, malaise, neutrophilic eccrine hidradenitis, radiation recall, renal tubular necrosis, secondary malignancy (eg, bladder carcinoma), SAIDH, Stevens-Johnson syndrome, toxic epidermal necrolysis, weakness.

Drug Interactions

Metabolism/Transport Effects Substrate of CYP2A6 (minor), 2B6 (major); 2C9 (minor), 2C19 (minor), 3A4 (major); **Inhibits** CYP3A4 (weak); **Induces** CYP2B6 (weak), 2C8 (weak), 2C9 (weak)

Avoid Concomitant Use

Avoid concomitant use of Cyclophosphamide with any of the following: Natalizumab; Vaccines (Live)

Increased Effect/Toxicity

Cyclophosphamide may increase the levels/effects of: Leflunomide; Mivacurium [Off Market]; Natalizumab; Succinylcholine; Vaccines (Live); Vitamin K Antagonists

The levels/effects of Cyclophosphamide may be increased by: Allopurinol; CYP2B6 Inhibitors (Moderate); CYP2B6 Inhibitors (Strong); Etanercept; Pentostatin; Trastuzumab

Decreased Effect

Cyclophosphamide may decrease the levels/effects of: Cardiac Glycosides; Vaccines (Inactivated); Vaccines (Live); Vitamin K Antagonists

The levels/effects of Cyclophosphamide may be decreased by: CYP2B6 Inducers (Strong); Echinacea

Ethanol/Nutrition/Herb Interactions Herb/Nutraceutical: Avoid black cohosh, dong quai in estrogen-dependent tumors.

Storage/Stability Store intact vials of powder at room temperature of 15°C to 30°C (59°F to 86°F). Reconstituted solutions are stable for 24 hours at room temperature and 6 days under refrigeration 2°C to 8°C (36°F to 46°F). Further dilutions in D_5W or NS are stable for 24 hours at room temperature (25°C) and 6 days at refrigeration.

Reconstitution Reconstitute vials with SWI, NS, or D_5W to a concentration of 20 mg/mL.

Compatibility Stable in D_5LR, D_5NS, D_5W, LR, ½NS, NS.

Y-site administration: Compatible: Allopurinol, amifostine, amikacin, ampicillin, azlocillin, aztreonam, bleomycin, cefamandole, cefazolin, cefepime, cefoperazone, cefotaxime, cefoxitin, cefuroxime, chloramphenicol, chlorpromazine, cimetidine, cisplatin, cladribine, clindamycin, co-trimoxazole, dexamethasone sodium phosphate, diphenhydramine, doxorubicin, doxorubicin liposome, doxycycline, droperidol, erythromycin lactobionate, etoposide phosphate, famotidine, filgrastim, fludarabine, fluorouracil, furosemide, ganciclovir, gatifloxacin, gemcitabine, gentamicin, granisetron, heparin, hydromorphone, idarubicin, kanamycin, leucovorin, linezolid, lorazepam, melphalan, methotrexate, methylprednisolone sodium succinate, metoclopramide, metronidazole, minocycline, mitomycin, morphine, nafcillin, ondansetron, oxacillin, paclitaxel, penicillin G potassium, piperacillin, piperacillin/tazobactam, prochlorperazine edisylate, promethazine, propofol, ranitidine, sargramostim, sodium bicarbonate, teniposide, thiotepa, ticarcillin, ticarcillin/ clavulanate, tobramycin, topotecan, vancomycin, vinblastine, vincristine, vinorelbine. **Incompatible:** Amphotericin B cholesteryl sulfate complex.

Compatibility in syringe: Compatible: Bleomycin, cisplatin, doxapram, doxorubicin, droperidol, fluorouracil, furosemide, heparin, leucovorin, methotrexate, metoclopramide, mitomycin, vinblastine, vincristine.

Compatibility when admixed: Compatible: Cisplatin with etoposide, dacarbazine, fluorouracil, hydroxyzine, mesna, methotrexate, methotrexate with fluorouracil, mitoxantrone, ondansetron.

Mechanism of Action Cyclophosphamide is an alkylating agent that prevents cell division by cross-linking DNA strands and decreasing DNA synthesis. It is a cell cycle phase nonspecific agent. Cyclophosphamide also possesses potent immunosuppressive activity. Cyclophosphamide is a prodrug that must be metabolized to active metabolites in the liver.

Pharmacodynamics/Kinetics

Absorption: Oral: Well absorbed

Distribution: V_d: 0.48-0.71 L/kg; crosses placenta; crosses into CSF (not in high enough concentrations to treat meningeal leukemia)

Protein binding: 10% to 60%

Metabolism: Hepatic to active metabolites acrolein, 4-aldophosphamide, 4-hydroperoxycyclophosphamide, and nor-nitrogen mustard

Bioavailability: >75%

Half-life elimination: 3-12 hours

Time to peak, serum: Oral: ~1 hour

Excretion: Urine (<30% as unchanged drug, 85% to 90% as metabolites)

Dosage Details concerns dosing in combination regimens should also be consulted.

Children:

Nephrotic syndrome: Oral: 2-3 mg/kg/day every day for up to 12 weeks when corticosteroids are unsuccessful

SLE (unlabeled use): I.V.: 500-750 mg/m^2 every month; maximum dose: 1 g/m^2

Children and Adults:

Oral: 50-100 mg/m^2/day as continuous therapy or 400-1000 mg/m^2 in divided doses over 4-5 days as intermittent therapy

I.V.:

Single doses: 400-1800 mg/m^2 (30-50 mg/kg) per treatment course (1-5 days) which can be repeated at 2-4 week intervals

Continuous daily doses: 60-120 mg/m^2 (1-2.5 mg/kg) per day

Autologous BMT (unlabeled use): IVPB: 50 mg/kg/dose x 4 days or 60 mg/ kg/dose for 2 days; total dose is usually divided over 2-4 days

JRA/vasculitis (unlabeled use): 10 mg/kg every 2 weeks

Adults: Nephrotic syndrome (unlabeled use): Oral: 2-3 mg/kg/day every day for up to 12 weeks when corticosteroids are unsuccessful

Dosing adjustment in renal impairment: The FDA-approved labeling states there is insufficient evidence to recommend dosage adjustment and therefore, does not contain renal dosing adjustment guidelines. The following guidelines have been used by some clinicians (Aronoff, 2007): Children and Adults:

Cl_{cr} <10 mL/minute: Administer 75% of normal dose

Hemodialysis effects: Moderately dialyzable (20% to 50%)

Administer 50% of dose posthemodialysis

Continuous ambulatory peritoneal dialysis (CAPD): Administer 75% of normal dose

Continuous renal replacement therapy (CRRT): Administer 100% of normal dose

Dosing adjustment in hepatic impairment: The pharmacokinetics of cyclophosphamide are not significantly altered in the presence of hepatic insufficiency. The FDA-approved labeling does not contain hepatic dosing adjustment guidelines. The following guidelines have been used by some clinicians (Floyd, 2006):

Serum bilirubin 3.1-5 mg/dL or transaminases >3 times ULN: Administer 75% of dose

Serum bilirubin >5 mg/mL: Avoid use

Combination Regimens

Retinoblastoma:
  CCCDE (Retinoblastoma) on page 1252
  CO on page 1278
  CV on page 1282
Rhabdomyosarcoma:
  VAC Pulse on page 1417
  VAC (Rhabdomyosarcoma) on page 1417
Sarcoma:
  CYVADIC on page 1285
  VAC Alternating With IE (Ewing's Sarcoma) on page 1416
Wilms' tumor: VDA-C (Wilms' Tumor) on page 1420

Administration
  Injection: Administer I.P., intrapleurally, IVPB, or continuous I.V. infusion; may also be administered slow IVP in doses ≤1 g.
  I.V. infusions may be administered over 1-24 hours
  Doses >500 mg to approximately 2 g may be administered over 20-30 minutes
  To minimize bladder toxicity, increase normal fluid intake during and for 1-2 days after cyclophosphamide dose. Most adult patients will require a fluid intake of at least 2 L/day. High-dose regimens should be accompanied by vigorous hydration with or without mesna therapy.
  Oral: Tablets are not scored and should not be cut or crushed. To minimize the risk of bladder irritation, do not administer tablets at bedtime.

Monitoring Parameters CBC with differential and platelet count, BUN, UA, serum electrolytes, serum creatinine

Dietary Considerations Tablets should be administered during or after meals.

Additional Information In patients with CYP2B6 G516T variant allele, cyclophosphamide metabolism is markedly increased; metabolism is not influenced by CYP2C9 and CYP2C19 isotypes.

Emetic Potential
  >1500 mg/m^2: Very high (>90%)
  ≤1500 mg/m^2: Moderate (30% to 90%)
  Oral: Moderate (30% to 90%)

Vesicant
  May be an irritant

High Dose Considerations
  Comments Approaches to reduction of hemorrhagic cystitis include infusion of 0.9% NaCl 3 L/m^2/24 hours, infusion of 0.9% NaCl 3 L/m^2/24 hours with continuous 0.9% NaCl bladder irrigation 300-1000 mL/hour, and infusion of 0.9% NaCl 1.5-3 L/m^2/24 hours with intravenous mesna. Hydration should begin at least 4 hours before cyclophosphamide and continue at least 24 hours after completion of cyclophosphamide. The dose of daily mesna used should equal the daily dose of cyclophosphamide. Mesna can be administered as a continuous 24-hour intravenous infusion or be given in divided doses every 4 hours. Mesna should begin at the start of treatment, and continue at least 24 hours following the last dose of cyclophosphamide.

  Enhanced bioactivation of cyclophosphamide may increase the risk of cardiotoxicity. A 30-minute infusion of thiotepa administered 1 hour before a 60-minute infusion of cyclophosphamide reduced bioactivation of cyclophosphamide to 4-hydroxycyclophosphamide in 20 patients. This effect did not occur with administration of thiotepa 1 hour following infusion of cyclophosphamide. Intravascular red blood cell hemolysis requiring transfusion support occurred during continuous flow plasmapheresis performed 12 hours following infusion of cyclophosphamide 60 mg/kg.

High Dose

I.V.:

60 mg/kg/day for 2 days (total dose: 120 mg/kg)

50 mg/kg/day for 4 days (total dose: 200 mg/kg)

1.8 g/m^2/day for 4 days (total dose: 7.2 g/m^2)

Continuous I.V.:

1875 mg/m^2/24 hours for 72 hours (total dose: 5625 mg/m^2)

1.5 g/m^2/24 hours for 96 hours (total dose: 6 g/m^2)

Duration of infusion is 1-24 hours; generally combined with other high-dose chemotherapeutic drugs, lymphocyte immune globulin, or total body irradiation (TBI).

Unique Toxicities

Cardiovascular: Heart failure, cardiac necrosis, pericardial tamponade, heart block

Endocrine & metabolic: Hyponatremia, acquired pseudocholinesterase deficiency, transient diabetes insipidus

Hematologic: Methemoglobinemia

Neuromuscular & skeletal: Rhabdomyolysis

Respiratory: Pleural effusion, interstitial pneumonitis

Dosage Forms Excipient information presented when available (limited, particularly for generics); consult specific product labeling. [DSC] = Discontinued product

Injection, powder for reconstitution: 500 mg, 1 g, 2 g

Cytoxan®: 500 mg, 1 g, 2 g [DSC]

Tablet: 25 mg, 50 mg

Cytoxan®: 25 mg, 50 mg [DSC]

Extemporaneous Preparations A 2 mg/mL oral elixir was stable for 14 days when refrigerated when made as follows: Reconstitute a 200 mg vial with aromatic elixir, withdraw the solution, and add sufficient aromatic elixir to make a final volume of 100 mL (store in amber glass container).

Brook D, Davis RE, and Bequette RJ, "Chemical Stability of Cyclophosphamide in Aromatic Elixir U.S.P.," *Am J Health Syst Pharm*, 1973, 30:618-20.

References

Aronoff GR, Bennett WM, Berns JS, et al, *Drug Prescribing in Renal Failure: Dosing Guidelines for Adults and Children*, 5th ed. Philadelphia, PA: American College of Physicians; 2007, p 97, 170.

Brade W, Seeber S, and Herdrich K, "Comparative Activity of Ifosfamide and Cyclophosphamide," *Cancer Chemother Pharmacol*, 1986, 18(Suppl 2):1-9.

deJonge ME, Huitema AD, vanDam SM, et al, "Significant Induction of Cyclophosphamide and Thiotepa Metabolism by Phenytoin," *Cancer Chemother Pharmacol*, 2005, 55(5):507-10.

Eder JP, Elias A, Shea TC, et al, "A Phase I-II Study of Cyclophosphamide, Thiotepa, and Carboplatin With Autologous Bone Marrow Transplantation in Solid Tumor Patients," *J Clin Oncol*, 1990, 8(7):1239-45.

Floyd J, Mirza I, Sachs B, et al, "Hepatotoxicity of Chemotherapy," *Semin Oncol*, 2006, 33 (1):50-67.

Giralt SA, LeMaistre CF, Vriesendorp HM, et al, "Etoposide, Cyclophosphamide, Total-Body Irradiation and Allogeneic Bone Marrow Transplantation for Hematologic Malignancies," *J Clin Oncol*, 1994, 12(9):1923-30.

Xie H, Griskevicius L, Stahle L, et al, "Pharmacogenetics of Cyclophosphamide in Patients With Hematologic Malignancies," *Eur J Pharm Sci*, 2006, 27(1):54-61.

◆ **Cyclosporin A** see CycloSPORINE on page 268

CycloSPORINE (SYE kloe spor een)

Medication Safety Issues

Sound-alike/look-alike issues:

CycloSPORINE may be confused with cyclophosphamide, Cyklokapron®, cycloSERINE

CycloSPORINE modified (Neoral®, Gengraf®) may be confused with cycloSPORINE non-modified (Sandimmne®)

Gengraf® may be confused with Prograf®

Neoral® may be confused with Neurontin®, Nizoral®

Sandimmune® may be confused with Sandostatin®

Related Information

Hematopoietic Stem Cell Transplantation *on page 1501*

Safe Handling of Hazardous Drugs *on page 1517*

U.S. Brand Names Gengraf®; Neoral®; Restasis®; Sandimmune®

Index Terms CsA; CyA; Cyclosporin A

Generic Available Yes: Excludes ophthalmic emulsion

Canadian Brand Names Apo-Cyclosporine; Neoral®; Rhoxal-cyclosporine; Sandimmune® I.V.; Sandoz-Cyclosporine

Pharmacologic Category Immunosuppressant Agent

Use Prophylaxis of organ rejection in kidney, liver, and heart transplants, has been used with azathioprine and/or corticosteroids; severe, active rheumatoid arthritis (RA) not responsive to methotrexate alone; severe, recalcitrant plaque psoriasis in nonimmunocompromised adults unresponsive to or unable to tolerate other systemic therapy

Ophthalmic emulsion (Restasis®): Increase tear production when suppressed tear production is presumed to be due to keratoconjunctivitis sicca-associated ocular inflammation (in patients not already using topical anti-inflammatory drugs or punctal plugs)

Unlabeled/Investigational Use Short-term, high-dose cyclosporine as a modulator of multidrug resistance in cancer treatment; allogenic bone marrow transplants for prevention and treatment of graft-versus-host disease; also used in some cases of severe autoimmune disease (eg, SLE, myasthenia gravis, inflammatory bowel disease) that are resistant to corticosteroids and other therapy; focal segmental glomerulosclerosis

Pregnancy Risk Factor C

Lactation Enters breast milk/not recommended

Labeled Contraindications Hypersensitivity to cyclosporine or any component of the formulation. Rheumatoid arthritis and psoriasis: Abnormal renal function, uncontrolled hypertension, malignancies. Concomitant treatment with PUVA or UVB therapy, methotrexate, other immunosuppressive agents, coal tar, or radiation therapy are also contraindications for use in patients with psoriasis. Ophthalmic emulsion is contraindicated in patients with active ocular infections.

Warnings/Precautions [U.S. Boxed Warning]: Renal impairment, including structural kidney damage has occurred (when used at high doses); monitor renal function closely. Use caution with other potentially nephrotoxic drugs (eg, acyclovir, aminoglycoside antibiotics, amphotericin B, ciprofloxacin). **[U.S. Boxed Warning]: Increased risk of lymphomas and other malignancies, particularly those of the skin;** risk is related to intensity/duration of therapy and the use of >1 immunosuppressive agent; all patients should avoid excessive sun/UV light exposure. **[U.S. Boxed Warning]: Increased risk of infection; fatal infections have been reported. [U.S. Boxed Warning]: May cause hypertension.** Use caution when changing dosage forms. **[U.S. Boxed Warning]: Cyclosporine (modified) has increased bioavailability as compared to cyclosporine (non-modified) and cannot be used interchangeably without close monitoring.** Monitor cyclosporine concentrations closely following the addition, modification, or deletion of other medications; live, attenuated vaccines may be less effective; use should be avoided. Increased hepatic enzymes and bilirubin have occurred (when used at high doses); improvement usually seen with dosage reduction.

Transplant patients: To be used initially with corticosteroids. May cause significant hyperkalemia and hyperuricemia, seizures (particularly if used with high dose corticosteroids), and encephalopathy. Make dose adjustments based on cyclosporine blood concentrations. **[U.S. Boxed Warning]: Adjustment of dose should only be made under the direct supervision of an experienced physician.** Anaphylaxis has been reported with I.V. use; reserve for patients who cannot take oral form. **[U.S. Boxed Warning]: Risk of skin cancer may be increased in transplant patients.**

Psoriasis: Patients should avoid excessive sun exposure; safety and efficacy in children <18 years of age have not been established. **[U.S. Boxed Warning]: Risk of skin cancer may be increased with a history of PUVA and possibly methotrexate or other immunosuppressants, UVB, coal tar, or radiation.**

Rheumatoid arthritis: Safety and efficacy for use in juvenile rheumatoid arthritis have not been established. If receiving other immunosuppressive agents, radiation or UV therapy, concurrent use of cyclosporine is not recommended.

Ophthalmic emulsion: Safety and efficacy have not been established in patients <16 years of age.

Products may contain corn oil, ethanol, or propylene glycol; injection also contains Cremophor® EL (polyoxyethylated castor oil), which has been associated with rare anaphylactic reactions.

Adverse Reactions Adverse reactions reported with systemic use, including rheumatoid arthritis, psoriasis, and transplantation (kidney, liver, and heart). Percentages noted include the highest frequency regardless of indication/dosage. Frequencies may vary for specific conditions or formulation.

>10%:
Cardiovascular: Hypertension (8% to 53%), edema (5% to 14%)
Central nervous system: Headache (2% to 25%)
Dermatologic: Hirsutism (21% to 45%), hypertrichosis (5% to 19%)
Endocrine & metabolic: Triglycerides increased (15%), female reproductive disorder (9% to 11%)
Gastrointestinal: Nausea (23%), diarrhea (3% to 13%), gum hyperplasia (2% to 16%), abdominal discomfort (<1% to 15%), dyspepsia (2% to 12%)
Neuromuscular & skeletal: Tremor (7% to 55%), paresthesia (1% to 11%), leg cramps/muscle contractions (2% to 12%)
Renal: Renal dysfunction/nephropathy (10% to 38%), creatinine increased (16% to ≥50%)
Respiratory: Upper respiratory infection (1% to 14%)
Miscellaneous: Infection (3% to 25%)
Kidney, liver, and heart transplant only (≤2% unless otherwise noted):
Cardiovascular: Flushes (<1% to 4%), MI
Central nervous system: Convulsions (1% to 5%), anxiety, confusion, fever, lethargy

Dermatologic: Acne (1% to 6%), brittle fingernails, hair breaking, pruritus

Endocrine & metabolic: Gynecomastia (<1% to 4%), hyperglycemia

Gastrointestinal: Nausea (2% to 10%), vomiting (2% to 10%), diarrhea (3% to 8%), abdominal discomfort (<1% to 7%), cramps (0% to 4%), anorexia, constipation, gastritis, mouth sores, pancreatitis, swallowing difficulty, upper GI bleed, weight loss

Hematologic: Leukopenia (<1% to 6%), anemia, thrombocytopenia

Hepatic: Hepatotoxicity (<1% to 7%)

Neuromuscular & skeletal: Paresthesia (1% to 3%), joint pain, muscle pain, tingling, weakness

Ocular: Conjunctivitis, visual disturbance

Otic: Hearing loss, tinnitus

Renal: Hematuria

Respiratory: Sinusitis (<1% to 7%)

Miscellaneous: Lymphoma (<1% to 6%), allergic reactions, hiccups, night sweats

Rheumatoid arthritis only (1% to <3% unless otherwise noted):

Cardiovascular: Hypertension (8%), edema (5%), chest pain (4%), arrhythmia (2%), abnormal heart sounds, cardiac failure, MI, peripheral ischemia

Central nervous system: Dizziness (8%), pain (6%), insomnia (4%), depression (3%), migraine (2%), anxiety, hypoesthesia, emotional lability, impaired concentration, malaise, nervousness, paranoia, somnolence, vertigo

Dermatologic: Purpura (3%), abnormal pigmentation, angioedema, cellulitis, dermatitis, dry skin, eczema, folliculitis, nail disorder, pruritus, skin disorder, urticaria

Endocrine & metabolic: Menstrual disorder (3%), breast fibroadenosis, breast pain, diabetes mellitus, goiter, hot flashes, hyperkalemia, hyperuricemia, hypoglycemia, libido increased/decreased

Gastrointestinal: Vomiting (9%), flatulence (5%), gingivitis (4%), gum hyperplasia (2%), constipation, dry mouth, dysphagia, enanthema, eructation, esophagitis, gastric ulcer, gastritis, gastroenteritis, gingival bleeding, glossitis, peptic ulcer, salivary gland enlargement, taste perversion, tongue disorder, tooth disorder, weight loss/gain

Genitourinary: Leukorrhea (1%), abnormal urine, micturition urgency, nocturia, polyuria, pyelonephritis, urinary incontinence, uterine hemorrhage

Hematologic: Anemia, leukopenia

Hepatic: Bilirubinemia

Neuromuscular & skeletal: Paresthesia (8%), tremor (8%), leg cramps/muscle contractions (2%), arthralgia, bone fracture, joint dislocation, myalgia, neuropathy, stiffness, synovial cyst, tendon disorder, weakness

Ocular: Abnormal vision, cataract, conjunctivitis, eye pain

Otic: Tinnitus, deafness, vestibular disorder

Renal: BUN increased, hematuria, renal abscess

Respiratory: Cough (5%), dyspnea (5%), sinusitis (4%), abnormal chest sounds, bronchospasm, epistaxis

Miscellaneous: Infection (9%), abscess, allergy, bacterial infection, carcinoma, fungal infection, herpes simplex, herpes zoster, lymphadenopathy, moniliasis, diaphoresis increased, tonsillitis, viral infection

Psoriasis only (1% to <3% unless otherwise noted):

Cardiovascular: Chest pain, flushes

Central nervous system: Psychiatric events (4% to 5%), pain (3% to 4%), dizziness, fever, insomnia, nervousness, vertigo

Dermatologic: Hypertrichosis (5% to 7%), acne, dry skin, folliculitis, keratosis, pruritus, rash, skin malignancies

Endocrine & metabolic: Hot flashes

Gastrointestinal: Nausea (5% to 6%), diarrhea (5% to 6%), gum hyperplasia (4% to 6%), abdominal discomfort (3% to 6%), dyspepsia (2% to 3%), abdominal distention, appetite increased, constipation, gingival bleeding

Genitourinary: Micturition increased

Hematologic: Bleeding disorder, clotting disorder, platelet disorder, red blood cell disorder

Hepatic: Hyperbilirubinemia

Neuromuscular & skeletal: Paresthesia (5% to 7%), arthralgia (1% to 6%)

Ocular: Abnormal vision

Respiratory: Bronchospasm (5%), cough (5%), dyspnea (5%), rhinitis (5%), respiratory infection

Miscellaneous: Flu-like syndrome (8% to 10%)

Postmarketing and/or case reports (any indication): Anaphylaxis/anaphylactoid reaction (possibly associated with Cremophor® EL vehicle in injection formulation), benign intracranial hypertension, cholesterol increased, death (due to renal deterioration), encephalopathy, gout, hyperbilirubinemia, hyperkalemia, hypomagnesemia (mild), impaired consciousness, neurotoxicity, papilloedema, pulmonary edema (noncardiogenic), uric acid increased

Ophthalmic emulsion (Restasis®):

>10%: Ocular: Burning (17%)

1% to 10%: Ocular: Hyperemia (conjunctival 5%), eye pain, pruritus, stinging

Drug Interactions

Metabolism/Transport Effects Substrate of CYP3A4 (major); **Inhibits** CYP2C9 (weak), 3A4 (moderate)

Avoid Concomitant Use

Avoid concomitant use of CycloSPORINE with any of the following: Aliskiren; Bosentan; Dabigatran Etexilate; Dronedarone; Everolimus; Natalizumab; Pitavastatin; Silodosin; Sitaxsentan; Tacrolimus; Tolvaptan; Topotecan; Vaccines (Live)

Increased Effect/Toxicity

CycloSPORINE may increase the levels/effects of: Aliskiren; Ambrisentan; Bosentan; Calcium Channel Blockers (Dihydropyridine); Calcium Channel Blockers (Nondihydropyridine); Cardiac Glycosides; Caspofungin; Colchicine; Corticosteroids (Systemic); CYP3A4 Substrates; Dabigatran Etexilate; DOXOrubicin; Dronedarone; Eplerenone; Etoposide; Etoposide Phosphate; Everolimus; Ezetimibe; FentaNYL; Fibric Acid Derivatives; Halofantrine; HMG-CoA Reductase Inhibitors; Leflunomide; Methotrexate; Minoxidil; Natalizumab; P-Glycoprotein Substrates; Pimecrolimus; Pitavastatin; Protease Inhibitors; Ranolazine; Repaglinide; Rivaroxaban; Salmeterol; Saxagliptin; Silodosin; Sirolimus; Sitaxsentan; Tacrolimus; Tolvaptan; Topotecan; Vaccines (Live)

The levels/effects of CycloSPORINE may be increased by: ACE Inhibitors; Aminoglycosides; Amiodarone; Amphotericin B; Androgens; Antifungal Agents (Azole Derivatives, Systemic); Bromocriptine; Calcium Channel Blockers (Nondihydropyridine); Carvedilol; Corticosteroids (Systemic); CYP3A4 Inhibitors (Moderate); CYP3A4 Inhibitors (Strong); Dasatinib; Ezetimibe; Fluconazole; Grapefruit Juice; Imatinib; Macrolide Antibiotics; Melphalan; Methotrexate; Metoclopramide; MetroNIDAZOLE; Nonsteroidal Anti-Inflammatory Agents; Norfloxacin; Omeprazole; P-Glycoprotein Inhibitors; Protease Inhibitors; Quinupristin; Sirolimus; Sulfonamide Derivatives; Sulfonylureas; Tacrolimus; Temsirolimus; Trastuzumab

Decreased Effect

CycloSPORINE may decrease the levels/effects of: Mycophenolate; Vaccines (Inactivated); Vaccines (Live)

The levels/effects of CycloSPORINE may be decreased by: Antacids; Barbiturates; Bosentan; CarBAMazepine; CYP3A4 Inducers (Strong); Deferasirox; Echinacea; Fibric Acid Derivatives; Griseofulvin; Nafcillin; P-Glycoprotein Inducers; Phenytoin; Probucol; Pyrazinamide; Rifamycin Derivatives; Somatostatin Analogs; St Johns Wort; Sulfinpyrazone [Off Market]; Sulfonamide Derivatives; Terbinafine

Ethanol/Nutrition/Herb Interactions

Food: Grapefruit juice increases cyclosporine serum concentrations.

Herb/Nutraceutical: Avoid St John's wort; as an enzyme inducer, it may increase the metabolism of and decrease plasma levels of cyclosporine; organ rejection and graft loss have been reported. Avoid cat's claw, echinacea (have immunostimulant properties).

Storage/Stability

Capsule: Store at controlled room temperature.

Injection: Store at controlled room temperature; do not refrigerate. Ampuls should be protected from light. Stability of injection of parenteral admixture at room temperature (25°C) is 6 hours in PVC; 24 hours in Excel®, PAB® containers, or glass.

Ophthalmic emulsion: Store at 15°C to 25°C (59°F to 77°F). Vials are single-use; discard immediately following administration.

Oral solution: Store at controlled room temperature; do not refrigerate. Use within 2 months after opening; should be mixed in glass containers.

Reconstitution Sandimmune® injection: Injection should be further diluted [1 mL (50 mg) of concentrate in 20-100 mL of D_5W or NS] for administration by intravenous infusion.

Compatibility Stable in D_5W, fat emulsion 10%, fat emulsion 20%, NS.

Y-site administration: Compatible: Alatrofloxacin, gatifloxacin, linezolid, propofol, sargramostim. Incompatible: Amphotericin B cholesteryl sulfate complex.

Compatibility when admixed: Compatible: Ciprofloxacin. Incompatible: Magnesium sulfate.

Mechanism of Action Inhibition of production and release of interleukin II and inhibits interleukin II-induced activation of resting T-lymphocytes.

Pharmacodynamics/Kinetics

Absorption:

Ophthalmic emulsion: Serum concentrations not detectable.

Oral:

Cyclosporine (non-modified): Erratic and incomplete; dependent on presence of food, bile acids, and GI motility; larger oral doses are needed in pediatrics due to shorter bowel length and limited intestinal absorption

Cyclosporine (modified): Erratic and incomplete; increased absorption, up to 30% when compared to cyclosporine (non-modified); less dependent on food, bile acids, or GI motility when compared to cyclosporine (non-modified)

Distribution: Widely in tissues and body fluids including the liver, pancreas, and lungs; crosses placenta; enters breast milk

V_{dss}: 4-6 L/kg in renal, liver, and marrow transplant recipients (slightly lower values in cardiac transplant patients; children <10 years have higher values)

Protein binding: 90% to 98% to lipoproteins

Metabolism: Extensively hepatic via CYP3A4; forms at least 25 metabolites; extensive first-pass effect following oral administration

Bioavailability: Oral:

Cyclosporine (non-modified): Dependent on patient population and transplant type (<10% in adult liver transplant patients and as high as 89% in renal transplant patients); bioavailability of Sandimmune® capsules and oral solution are equivalent; bioavailability of oral solution is ~30% of the I.V. solution

Children: 28% (range: 17% to 42%); gut dysfunction common in BMT patients and oral bioavailability is further reduced

Cyclosporine (modified): Bioavailability of Neoral® capsules and oral solution are equivalent:

Children: 43% (range: 30% to 68%)

Adults: 23% greater than with cyclosporine (non-modified) in renal transplant patients; 50% greater in liver transplant patients

Half-life elimination: Oral: May be prolonged in patients with hepatic impairment and shorter in pediatric patients due to the higher metabolism rate

Cyclosporine (non-modified): Biphasic: Alpha: 1.4 hours; Terminal: 19 hours (range: 10-27 hours)

Cyclosporine (modified): Biphasic: Terminal: 8.4 hours (range: 5-18 hours)

Time to peak, serum: Oral:

Cyclosporine (non-modified): 2-6 hours; some patients have a second peak at 5-6 hours

Cyclosporine (modified): Renal transplant: 1.5-2 hours

Excretion: Primarily feces; urine (6%, 0.1% as unchanged drug and metabolites)

Dosage Neoral®/Genraf® and Sandimmune® are not bioequivalent and cannot be used interchangeably.

Children: Refer to adult dosing; children may require, and are able to tolerate, larger doses than adults.

Adults:

Newly-transplanted patients: Adjunct therapy with corticosteroids is recommended. Initial dose should be given 4-12 hours prior to transplant or may be given postoperatively; adjust initial dose to achieve desired plasma concentration

Oral: Dose is dependent upon type of transplant and formulation:

Cyclosporine (modified):

Renal: 9 ± 3 mg/kg/day, divided twice daily

Liver: 8 ± 4 mg/kg/day, divided twice daily

Heart: 7 ± 3 mg/kg/day, divided twice daily

Cyclosporine (non-modified): Initial dose: 15 mg/kg/day as a single dose (range 14-18 mg/kg); lower doses of 10-14 mg/kg/day have been used for renal transplants. Continue initial dose daily for 1-2 weeks; taper by 5% per week to a maintenance dose of 5-10 mg/kg/day; some renal transplant patients may be dosed as low as 3 mg/kg/day

Note: When using the non-modified formulation, cyclosporine levels may increase in liver transplant patients when the T-tube is closed; dose may need decreased

I.V.: Cyclosporine (non-modified): Manufacturer's labeling: Initial dose: 5-6 mg/kg/day as a single dose ($1/3$ the oral dose), infused over 2-6 hours; use should be limited to patients unable to take capsules or oral solution; patients should be switched to an oral dosage form as soon as possible

Note: Many transplant centers administer cyclosporine as "divided dose" infusions (2-3 doses/day) or as a continuous (24-hour) infusion; dosages range from 3-7.5 mg/kg/day. Specific institutional protocols should be consulted.

Conversion to cyclosporine (modified) from cyclosporine (non-modified): Start with daily dose previously used and adjust to obtain preconversion cyclosporine trough concentration. Plasma concentrations should be monitored every 4-7 days and dose adjusted as necessary, until desired trough level is obtained. When transferring patients with previously poor absorption of cyclosporine (non-modified), monitor trough levels at least twice weekly (especially if initial dose exceeds 10 mg/kg/day); high plasma levels are likely to occur.

Rheumatoid arthritis: Oral: Cyclosporine (modified): Initial dose: 2.5 mg/kg/day, divided twice daily; salicylates, NSAIDs, and oral glucocorticoids may be continued (refer to Drug Interactions); dose may be increased by 0.5-0.75 mg/kg/day if insufficient response is seen after 8 weeks of treatment; additional dosage increases may be made again at 12 weeks (maximum dose: 4 mg/kg/day). Discontinue if no benefit is seen by 16 weeks of therapy.

Note: Increase the frequency of blood pressure monitoring after each alteration in dosage of cyclosporine. Cyclosporine dosage should be decreased by 25% to 50% in patients with no history of hypertension who develop sustained hypertension during therapy and, if hypertension persists, treatment with cyclosporine should be discontinued.

Psoriasis: Oral: Cyclosporine (modified): Initial dose: 2.5 mg/kg/day, divided twice daily; dose may be increased by 0.5 mg/kg/day if insufficient response is seen after 4 weeks of treatment. Additional dosage increases may be made every 2 weeks if needed (maximum dose: 4 mg/kg/day). Discontinue if no benefit is seen by 6 weeks of therapy. Once patients are adequately controlled, the dose should be decreased to the lowest effective dose. Doses lower than 2.5 mg/kg/day may be effective. Treatment longer than 1 year is not recommended.

Note: Increase the frequency of blood pressure monitoring after each alteration in dosage of cyclosporine. Cyclosporine dosage should be decreased by 25% to 50% in patients with no history of hypertension who develop sustained hypertension during therapy and, if hypertension persists, treatment with cyclosporine should be discontinued.

Focal segmental glomerulosclerosis (unlabeled use): Initial: 3 mg/kg/day divided every 12 hours

Autoimmune diseases (unlabeled use): 1-3 mg/kg/day

Keratoconjunctivitis sicca: Ophthalmic (Restasis®): Children ≥16 years and Adults: Instill 1 drop in each eye every 12 hours

Dosage adjustment in renal impairment: For severe psoriasis:

Serum creatinine levels ≥25% above pretreatment levels: Take another sample within 2 weeks; if the level remains ≥25% above pretreatment levels, decrease dosage of cyclosporine (modified) by 25% to 50%. If two dosage adjustments do not reverse the increase in serum creatinine levels, treatment should be discontinued.

Serum creatinine levels ≥50% above pretreatment levels: Decrease cyclosporine dosage by 25% to 50%. If two dosage adjustments do not reverse the increase in serum creatinine levels, treatment should be discontinued.

Hemodialysis: Supplemental dose is not necessary.

Peritoneal dialysis: Supplemental dose is not necessary.

Dosage adjustment in hepatic impairment: Probably necessary; monitor levels closely

Administration

Oral solution: Do not administer liquid from plastic or styrofoam cup. May dilute Neoral® oral solution with orange juice or apple juice. May dilute

Sandimmune® oral solution with milk, chocolate milk, or orange juice. Avoid changing diluents frequently. Mix thoroughly and drink at once. Use syringe provided to measure dose. Mix in a glass container and rinse container with more diluent to ensure total dose is taken. Do not rinse syringe before or after use (may cause dose variation).

I.V.: The manufacturer recommends that following dilution, intravenous admixture be administered over 2-6 hours. However, many transplant centers administer as divided doses (2-3 doses/day) or as a 24-hour continuous infusion. Discard solution after 24 hours. Anaphylaxis has been reported with I.V. use; reserve for patients who cannot take oral form. Patients should be under continuous observation for at least the first 30 minutes of the infusion, and should be monitored frequently thereafter. Maintain patent airway; other supportive measures and agents for treating anaphylaxis should be present when I.V. drug is given.

Ophthalmic emulsion: Prior to use, invert vial several times to obtain a uniform emulsion. Remove contact lenses prior to instillation of drops; may be reinserted 15 minutes after administration. May be used with artificial tears; allow 15 minute interval between products.

Monitoring Parameters Monitor blood pressure and serum creatinine after any cyclosporine dosage changes or addition, modification, or deletion of other medications. Monitor plasma concentrations periodically.

Transplant patients: Cyclosporine trough levels, serum electrolytes, renal function, hepatic function, blood pressure, lipid profile

Psoriasis therapy: Baseline blood pressure, serum creatinine (2 levels each), BUN, CBC, serum magnesium, potassium, uric acid, lipid profile. Biweekly monitoring of blood pressure, complete blood count, and levels of BUN, uric acid, potassium, lipids, and magnesium during the first 3 months of treatment for psoriasis. Monthly monitoring is recommended after this initial period. Also evaluate any atypical skin lesions prior to therapy. Increase the frequency of blood pressure monitoring after each alteration in dosage of cyclosporine. Cyclosporine dosage should be decreased by 25% to 50% in patients with no history of hypertension who develop sustained hypertension during therapy and, if hypertension persists, treatment with cyclosporine should be discontinued.

Rheumatoid arthritis: Baseline blood pressure, and serum creatinine (2 levels each); serum creatinine every 2 weeks for first 3 months, then monthly if patient is stable. Increase the frequency of blood pressure monitoring after each alteration in dosage of cyclosporine. Cyclosporine dosage should be decreased by 25% to 50% in patients with no history of hypertension who develop sustained hypertension during therapy and, if hypertension persists, treatment with cyclosporine should be discontinued.

Test Interactions Specific whole blood, HPLC assay for cyclosporine may be falsely elevated if sample is drawn from the same line through which dose was administered (even if flush has been administered and/or dose was given hours before).

Dietary Considerations Administer this medication consistently with relation to time of day and meals. Avoid grapefruit juice with oral cyclosporine use.

Additional Information Cyclosporine (modified): Refers to the capsule dosage formulation of cyclosporine in an aqueous dispersion (previously referred to as "microemulsion"). Cyclosporine (modified) has increased bioavailability as compared to cyclosporine (non-modified) and cannot be used interchangeably without close monitoring.

◀ **Dosage Forms** Excipient information presented when available (limited, particularly for generics); consult specific product labeling.

Capsule [modified]:
Gengraf®: 25 mg [contains alcohol 12.8%]; 100 mg [contains alcohol 12.8%]

Capsule [non-modified]: 25 mg, 100 mg

Capsule, soft gel [modified]: 25 mg, 50 mg, 100 mg
Neoral®: 25 mg [contains alcohol 11.9% and corn oil]; 100 mg [contains alcohol 11.9% and corn oil]

Capsule, soft gel [non-modified]:
Sandimmune®: 25 mg [contains alcohol 12.7% and corn oil]; 100 mg [contains alcohol 12.7% and corn oil]

Emulsion, ophthalmic [preservative free]:
Restasis®: 0.05% (0.4 mL) [contains 30 single-use vials/box]

Injection, solution [non-modified]: 50 mg/mL (5 mL)
Sandimmune®: 50 mg/mL (5 mL) [contains Cremophor® EL (polyoxyethylated castor oil) and alcohol 32.9%]

Solution, oral [modified]: 100 mg/mL (50 mL)
Gengraf®: 100 mg/mL (50 mL) [contains propylene glycol]
Neoral®: 100 mg/mL (50 mL) [contains alcohol 11.9%, corn oil, and propylene glycol]

Solution, oral [non-modified]: 100 mg/mL (50 mL)
Sandimmune®: 100 mg/mL (50 mL) [contains alcohol 12.5%]

References

Andrews DJ and Cramb R, "Cyclosporin: Revisions in Monitoring Guidelines and Review of Current Analytical Methods," *Ann Clin Biochem*, 2002, 39(Pt 5):424-35.

Back DJ and Tjia JF, "Comparative Effects of the Antimycotic Drugs Ketoconazole, Fluconazole, Itraconazole and Terbinafine on the Metabolism of Cyclosporin by Human Liver Microsomes," *Br J Clin Pharmacol*, 1991, 32(5):624-6.

Bulengo-Ransby SM, Sahn EE, Metcalf JS, et al, "Bowenoid Change in Association With Graft-Versus-Host Disease: A Cyclosporine Toxicity?" *J Am Acad Dermatol*, 1994, 31(6):1052-4.

Davies MG and Bowers PW, "Alopecia Areata Arising in Patients Receiving Cyclosporin Immunosuppression," *Br J Dermatol*, 1995, 132(5):835-6.

Ducharme MP, Warbasse LH, and Edwards DJ, "Disposition of Intravenous and Oral Cyclosporine After Administration With Grapefruit Juice," *Clin Pharmacol Ther*, 1995, 57(5):485-91.

Dunn CJ, Wagstaff AJ, Perry CM, et al, "Cyclosporin: An Updated Review of the Pharmacokinetic Properties, Clinical Efficacy and Tolerability of a Microemulsion-Based Formulation (Neoral)1 in Organ Transplantation," *Drugs*, 2001, 61(13):2075-2016.

Hollander AA, van Rooij J, Lentjes GW, et al, "The Effect of Grapefruit Juice on Cyclosporine and Prednisone Metabolism in Transplant Patients," *Clin Pharmacol Ther*, 1995, 57(3):318-24.

Kahan BD, "Cyclosporine," *N Engl J Med*, 1989, 321(25):1725-38.

Kino KJ and Wittkowsky AK, "Influence of Bile Acid Replacement on Cyclosporine Absorption in a Patient With Jejunoileal Bypass," *Pharmacotherapy*, 1995, 15(3):350-2.

Lin CY and Lee SF, "Comparison of Pharmacokinetics Between CsA Capsules and Sandimmune® Neoral® in Pediatric Patients," *Transplant Proc*, 1994, 26(5):2973-4.

Memon M, de Magalhace-Silverman M, Bloom EJ, et al, "Reversible Cyclosporine-Induced Cortical Blindness in Allogeneic Bone Marrow Transplant Recipients," *Bone Marrow Transplant*, 1995, 15 (2):283-6.

Pollard S, Nashan B, Johnston A, et al, "A Pharmacokinetic and Clinical Review of the Potential Clinical Impact of Using Different Formulations of Cyclosporin A. Berlin, Germany, November 19, 2001," *Clin Ther*, 2003, 25(6): 1654-69.

Ratanatharathorn V, Nash RA, Przepiorka D, et al, "Phase III Study Comparing Methotrexate and Tacrolimus (Prograf, FK506) With Methotrexate and Cyclosporine for Graft-Versus-Host Disease Prophylaxis After HLA-Identical Sibling Bone Marrow Transplantation," *Blood*, 1998, 92 (7):2303-14.

Taesch S, Niese D, and Mueller EA, "Sandimmune® Neoral®, A New Oral Formulation of Cyclosporine With Improved Pharmacokinetic Characteristics: Safety and Tolerability in Renal Transplant Patients," *Transplant Proc*, 1994, 26(6):3147-9.

Yee GC and McGuire TR, "Pharmacokinetic Drug Interactions With Cyclosporine," *Clin Pharmacokinet*, 1990, 19(4):319-32 and 19(5):400-15.

Yee GC, "Recent Advances in Cyclosporine Pharmacokinetics," *Pharmacotherapy*, 1991, 11 (5):130S-134S.

♦ **Cyklokapron®** *see* Tranexamic Acid *on page 1134*

Cyproheptadine (si proe HEP ta deen)

Medication Safety Issues
Sound-alike/look-alike issues:
Cyproheptadine may be confused with cyclobenzaprine
Periactin may be confused with Perative®, Percodan®, Persantine®

Index Terms Cyproheptadine Hydrochloride; Periactin

Generic Available Yes

Pharmacologic Category Histamine H₁ Antagonist; Histamine H₁ Antagonist, First Generation

Use Perennial and seasonal allergic rhinitis and other allergic symptoms including urticaria

Unlabeled/Investigational Use Appetite stimulation, blepharospasm, cluster headaches, migraine headaches, Nelson's syndrome, pruritus, schizophrenia, spinal cord damage associated spasticity, and tardive dyskinesia

Pregnancy Risk Factor B

Lactation Excretion in breast milk unknown/contraindicated

Labeled Contraindications Hypersensitivity to cyproheptadine or any component of the formulation; narrow-angle glaucoma; bladder neck obstruction; symptomatic prostatic hyperplasia; acute asthmatic attack; stenosing peptic ulcer; GI tract obstruction; concurrent use of MAO inhibitors; avoid use in premature and term newborns due to potential association with SIDS

Warnings/Precautions May cause CNS depression, which may impair physical or mental abilities; patients must be cautioned about performing tasks which require mental alertness (eg, operating machinery or driving). Effects may be potentiated when used with other sedative drugs or ethanol. Use with caution in patients with cardiovascular disease; increased intraocular pressure; respiratory disease; or thyroid dysfunction. Use with caution in the elderly; may be more sensitive to adverse effects. In case reports, cyproheptadine has promoted weight gain in anorexic adults, though it has not been specifically studied in the elderly. All cases of weight loss or decreased appetite should be adequately assessed. Antihistamines may cause excitation in young children. Safety and efficacy have not been established in children <2 years of age.

Adverse Reactions
>10%:
Central nervous system: Slight-to-moderate drowsiness
Respiratory: Thickening of bronchial secretions
1% to 10%:
Central nervous system: Dizziness, fatigue, headache, nervousness
Gastrointestinal: Abdominal pain, appetitie stimulation, diarrhea, nausea, xerostomia
Neuromuscular & skeletal: Arthralgia
Respiratory: Pharyngitis
<1%: Allergic reaction, angioedema, bronchospasm, CNS stimulation, depression, edema, epistaxis, hemolytic anemia, hepatitis, leukopenia, myalgia, palpitation, paresthesia, photosensitivity, rash, sedation, seizure, tachycardia, thrombocytopenia

Drug Interactions
Avoid Concomitant Use There are no known interactions where it is recommended to avoid concomitant use.

Increased Effect/Toxicity
Cyproheptadine may increase the levels/effects of: Alcohol (Ethyl); Anticholinergics; CNS Depressants

The levels/effects of Cyproheptadine may be increased by: Pramlintide

Decreased Effect
Cyproheptadine may decrease the levels/effects of: Acetylcholinesterase Inhibitors (Central); Betahistine; Selective Serotonin Reuptake Inhibitors

The levels/effects of Cyproheptadine may be decreased by: Acetylcholinesterase Inhibitors (Central); Amphetamines

Ethanol/Nutrition/Herb Interactions Ethanol: Avoid ethanol (may increase CNS sedation).

Mechanism of Action A potent antihistamine and serotonin antagonist, competes with histamine for H_1-receptor sites on effector cells in the gastrointestinal tract, blood vessels, and respiratory tract

Pharmacodynamics/Kinetics
Absorption: Completely
Metabolism: Almost completely hepatic
Excretion: Urine (>50% primarily as metabolites); feces (~25%)

Dosage Oral:
Children:
  Allergic conditions: 0.25 mg/kg/day or 8 mg/m^2/day in 2-3 divided doses **or**
    2-6 years: 2 mg every 8-12 hours (not to exceed 12 mg/day)
    7-14 years: 4 mg every 8-12 hours (not to exceed 16 mg/day)
  Migraine headaches: 4 mg 2-3 times/day
Children ≥12 years and Adults: Spasticity associated with spinal cord damage: 4 mg at bedtime; increase by a 4 mg dose every 3-4 days; average daily dose: 16 mg in divided doses; not to exceed 36 mg/day
Children >13 years and Adults: Appetite stimulation (anorexia nervosa): 2 mg 4 times/day; may be increased gradually over a 3-week period to 8 mg 4 times/day
Adults:
  Allergic conditions: 4-20 mg/day divided every 8 hours (not to exceed 0.5 mg/kg/day)
  Cluster headaches: 4 mg 4 times/day
  Migraine headaches: 4-8 mg 3 times/day

Dosage adjustment in hepatic impairment: Reduce dosage in patients with significant hepatic dysfunction

Test Interactions Diagnostic antigen skin test results may be suppressed; false positive serum TCA screen

Additional Information May stimulate appetite. In case reports, cyproheptadine has promoted weight gain in anorexic adults.

Dosage Forms Excipient information presented when available (limited, particularly for generics); consult specific product labeling.
Syrup, as hydrochloride: 2 mg/5 mL (473 mL) [contains alcohol 5%; mint flavor]
Tablet, as hydrochloride: 4 mg

References
Carlton MC, Kunkel DB, and Curry SC, "Ergotism Treated With Cyproheptadine," *Clin Toxicol*, 1995, 33(5):552.
Lappin RI and Auchincloss EL, "Treatment of the Serotonin Syndrome With Cyproheptadine," *N Engl J Med*, 1994, 331(15):1021-2.

◆ **Cyproheptadine Hydrochloride** *see* Cyproheptadine *on page* 277

Cyproterone (sye PROE ter one)

Index Terms Cyproterone Acetate

Generic Available Yes

Canadian Brand Names Androcur®; Androcur® Depot; Apo-Cyproterone®; Gen-Cyproterone; Mylan-Cyproterone; Novo-Cyproterone

Pharmacologic Category Antiandrogen

Use Palliative treatment of advanced prostate carcinoma

Restrictions Not available in U.S.

Pregnancy Risk Factor Not indicated for use in women

Labeled Contraindications Hypersensitivity to cyproterone or any component of the formulation; active liver disease or hepatic dysfunction; renal impairment

Warnings/Precautions Cyproterone has been associated with hepatic toxicity (jaundice, hepatitis, hepatic failure); typically this toxicity develops after several months of therapy. Monitor hepatic function and consider discontinuation of therapy in patients with evidence of hepatic injury.

Use caution in patients with a history of depression. Cyproterone has been associated with an increased incidence of depression, particularly early in the course of therapy (initial 6-8 weeks). Use with caution in patients with diabetes or impaired glucose tolerance, may cause alterations in glucose metabolism. Use with caution in conditions that may be aggravated by fluid retention, or cardiovascular disease. May increase the risk of thromboembolism and/or alter lipid profiles.

Adverse Reactions Frequency not defined.

Cardiovascular: Heart failure, hemorrhage, hypotension, MI, stroke, shock, stroke, syncope, tachycardia, thrombosis (DVT, pulmonary embolism, retinal vein thrombosis)

Central nervous system: Depression, dizziness, encephalopathy, fatigue, headache, lassitude

Dermatologic: Dry skin (sebum reduction), eczema, erythema, exfoliative dermatitis, hirsutism, nodosum, patchy loss of body hair, photosensitivity, pruritus, rash, scleroderma, skin discoloration, urticaria

Endocrine & metabolic: Adrenal suppression (dose related), benign nodular breast hyperplasia, diabetes mellitus, galactorrhea, gynecomastia, hot flashes, hypercalcemia, hyperglycemia, impotence, inhibition of spermatogenesis, libido increased, negative nitrogen balance, weight gain/loss

Gastrointestinal: Anorexia, constipation, diarrhea, dyspepsia, glossitis, nausea, pancreatitis, vomiting

Genitourinary: Bladder carcinoma, hematuria, urinary frequency

Hematologic: Anemia, fibrinogen increased, hemolytic anemia, leukopenia, leukocytosis, PT decreased, thrombocytopenia

Hepatic: Ascites, cholestatic jaundice, cirrhosis, hepatic dysfunction (dose related), hepatic carcinoma, hepatic coma, hepatic failure, hepatic necrosis, hepatitis, hepatoma, hepatomegaly, transaminases increased

Local: Injection site reaction

Neuromuscular and skeletal: Myasthenia, osteoporosis, weakness

Ocular: Abnormal accommodation, abnormal vision, blindness, optic neuritis, optic atrophy, retinal disorder

Renal: Renal failure, serum creatinine increased

Respiratory: Asthma, bronchospasm, cough, dyspnea, pulmonary embolism, pulmonary fibrosis

Miscellaneous: Allergic reaction

Drug Interactions
Avoid Concomitant Use There are no known interactions where it is recommended to avoid concomitant use.
Increased Effect/Toxicity
The levels/effects of Cyproterone may be increased by: Herbs (Progestogenic Properties)
Decreased Effect
The levels/effects of Cyproterone may be decreased by: Aminoglutethimide
Ethanol/Nutrition/Herb Interactions
Ethanol: May reduce the effect of cyproterone (not established in the treatment of prostatic carcinoma); avoid concurrent use.

Storage/Stability Store at controlled room temperature of 25°C (77°F).

Mechanism of Action Cyproterone is a steroidal compound with antiandrogenic, antigonadotropic, and progestin-like activity.

Pharmacodynamics/Kinetics
Absorption: Oral: Rapid and complete
Metabolism: Hepatic, some metabolites have activity
Half-life elimination: Oral: 38 hours; Depot injection: 4 days
Time to peak, plasma: Oral: 3-4 hours; Depot injection: 3 days
Excretion: Urine (35%, as metabolites); feces (60%)

Dosage Adults: Males: Prostatic carcinoma (palliative treatment):
Oral: 200-300 mg/day in 2-3 divided doses; following orchiectomy, reduce dose to 100-200 mg/day; should be taken with meals
I.M. (depot): 300 mg (3 mL) once weekly; reduce dose in orchiectomized patients to 300 mg every 2 weeks

Dosage adjustment in renal impairment: Use is contraindicated
Dosage adjustment in hepatic impairment: Use is contraindicated with hepatic impairment or active liver disease

Administration Administer at the same time each day, with meals.

Monitoring Parameters Liver function tests should be performed at baseline and periodically thereafter, or whenever signs or symptoms suggestive of hepatotoxicity are noted. Adrenal function should be monitored periodically.

Dietary Considerations Take with meals.

Dosage Forms Excipient information presented when available (limited, particularly for generics); consult specific product labeling.
Injection, solution, as acetate (Androcur® Depot): 100 mg/mL (3 mL) [contains benzyl benzoate and castor oil]
Tablet, as acetate (Androcur®): 50 mg

References
Barradell LB and Faulds D, "Cyproterone. A Review of its Pharmacology and Therapeutic Efficacy in Prostate Cancer," *Drugs Aging*, 1994, 5(1):59-80.
Goldenberg SL and Bruchovsky N, "Use of Cyproterone Acetate in Prostate Cancer," *Urol Clin North Am*, 1991, 18(1):111-22.
Neumann F, "Pharmacology and Potential Use of Cyproterone Acetate," *Horm Metab Res*, 1977, 9 (1):1-13.
Neumann F, "The Antiandrogen Cyproterone Acetate: Discovery, Chemistry, Basic Pharmacology, Clinical Use and Tool in Basic Research," *Exp Clin Endocrinol*, 1994, 102(1):1-32.
Schroder FH, "Cyproterone Acetate–Mechanism of Action and Clinical Effectiveness in Prostate Cancer Treatment," *Cancer*, 1993, 72(12 Suppl):3810-5.

◆ **Cyproterone Acetate** *see* Cyproterone *on page 279*
◆ **CYT** *see* Cyclophosphamide *on page 260*

Cytarabine (sye TARE a been)

Medication Safety Issues

Sound-alike/look-alike issues:

Cytarabine may be confused with Cytadren®, Cytosar®, Cytoxan®, vidarabine

Cytarabine (conventional) may be confused with cytarabine liposomal

Cytosar-U may be confused with cytarabine, Cytovene®, Cytoxan®, Neosar®

High alert medication: The Institute for Safe Medication Practices (ISMP) includes this medication among its list of drugs which have a heightened risk of causing significant patient harm when used in error.

Related Information

Hematopoietic Stem Cell Transplantation *on page 1501*

Safe Handling of Hazardous Drugs *on page 1517*

Index Terms Ara-C; Arabinosylcytosine; Cytarabine (Conventional); Cytarabine Hydrochloride; Cytosar-U; Cytosine Arabinosine Hydrochloride; NSC-63878

Generic Available Yes

Canadian Brand Names Cytosar®

Pharmacologic Category Antineoplastic Agent, Antimetabolite; Antineoplastic Agent, Antimetabolite (Pyrimidine Analog)

Use Treatment of acute myeloid leukemia (AML), acute lymphocytic leukemia (ALL), chronic myelocytic leukemia (CML; blast phase), and lymphomas; prophylaxis and treatment of meningeal leukemia

Pregnancy Risk Factor D

Lactation Excretion in breast milk unknown/not recommended

Labeled Contraindications Hypersensitivity to cytarabine or any component of the formulation

Warnings/Precautions Hazardous agent - use appropriate precautions for handling and disposal. **[U.S. Boxed Warning]: Potent myelosuppressive agent;** use with caution in patients with prior bone marrow suppression; monitor for signs of febrile neutropenia.

High-dose regimens are associated with CNS, gastrointestinal, ocular (prophylaxis with ophthalmic corticosteroid drops is recommended), pulmonary toxicities and cardiomyopathy. Neurotoxicity associated with high dose treatment may present as acute cerebellar toxicity, or may be severe with seizure and/or coma; may be delayed, occurring up to 3 to 8 days after treatment has begun. Risk factors for neurotoxicity include cumulative cytarabine dose, prior CNS disease and renal impairment. Tumor lysis syndrome and subsequent hyperuricemia may occur with high dose cytarabine; monitor, consider allopurinol and hydrate accordingly. There have been case reports of fatal cardiomyopathy when high dose cytarabine was used in combination with cyclophosphamide as a preparation regimen for transplantation.

Use with caution in patients with impaired renal and hepatic function; may be at higher risk for CNS toxicities; dosage adjustments may be necessary. Cytarabine syndrome is characterized by fever, myalgia, bone pain, chest pain, maculopapular rash, conjunctivitis, and malaise, and may occur 6-12 hours following administration; may be managed with corticosteroids. There have been reports of acute pancreatitis in patients receiving continuous infusion and in patients previously treated with L-asparaginase. **[U.S. Boxed Warning]: Should be administered under the supervision of an** ▶

◄ **experienced cancer chemotherapy physician.** Some products may contain benzyl alcohol; do not use products containing benzyl alcohol or products reconstituted with bacteriostatic diluent intrathecally or for high-dose cytarabine regimens.

Adverse Reactions Note: Frequency not defined.

Frequent:

Central nervous system: Fever

Dermatologic: Rash

Gastrointestinal: Anal inflammation, anal ulceration, anorexia, diarrhea, mucositis, nausea, vomiting

Hematologic: Myelosuppression, neutropenia (onset: 1-7 days; nadir [biphasic]: 7-9 days and at 15-24 days; recovery [biphasic]: 9-12 and at 24-34 days), thrombocytopenia (onset: 5 days; nadir: 12-15 days; recovery 15-25 days), anemia, bleeding, leukopenia, megaloblastosis, reticulocytes decreased

Hepatic: Hepatic dysfunction, transaminases increased (acute)

Local: Thrombophlebitis

Less frequent:

Cardiovascular: Chest pain, pericarditis

Central nervous system: Dizziness, headache, neural toxicity, neuritis

Dermatologic: Alopecia, pruritus, skin freckling, skin ulceration, urticaria

Gastrointestinal: Abdominal pain, bowel necrosis, esophageal ulceration, esophagitis, pancreatitis, sore throat

Genitourinary: Urinary retention

Hepatic: Jaundice

Local: Injection site cellulitis

Ocular: Conjunctivitis

Renal: Renal dysfunction

Respiratory: Dyspnea

Miscellaneous: Allergic edema, anaphylaxis, sepsis

Infrequent and/or case reports: Amylase increased, aseptic meningitis, cardiopulmonary arrest (acute), cerebral dysfunction, cytarabine syndrome (bone pain, chest pain, conjunctivitis, fever, maculopapular rash, malaise, myalgia); exanthematous pustulosis, hyperuricemia, injection site inflammation (SubQ injection), injection site pain (SubQ injection), interstitial pneumonitis, lipase increased, paralysis (intrathecal and I.V. combination therapy), rhabdomyolysis, veno-occlusive liver disease

Adverse events associated with high-dose cytarabine (CNS, gastrointestinal, ocular, and pulmonary toxicities are more common with high-dose regimens):

Cardiovascular: Cardiomegaly, cardiomyopathy (in combination with cyclophosphamide)

Central nervous system: Coma, neurotoxicity (dose-related, cerebellar toxicity may occur in patients receiving high-dose cytarabine [>36-48 $g/m^2/cycle$]; incidence may up to 55% in patients with renal impairment), personality change, somnolence

Dermatologic: Alopecia (complete), desquamation, rash (severe)

Gastrointestinal: Gastrointestinal ulcer, peritonitis, pneumatosis cystoides intestinalis

Hepatic: Hyperbilirubinemia, liver abscess, liver damage, necrotizing colitis

Neuromuscular & skeletal: Peripheral neuropathy (motor and sensory)

Ocular: Corneal toxicity, hemorrhagic conjunctivitis

Respiratory: Pulmonary edema, syndrome of sudden respiratory distress

Miscellaneous: Sepsis

Adverse events associated with intrathecal cytarabine administration:

Central nervous system: Accessory nerve paralysis, fever, necrotizing leukoencephalopathy (with concurrent cranial irradiation, I.T. methotrexate, and I.T. hydrocortisone), neurotoxicity, paraplegia

Gastrointestinal: Dysphagia, nausea, vomiting

Ocular: Blindness (with concurrent systemic chemotherapy and cranial irradiation), diplopia

Respiratory: Cough, hoarseness

Miscellaneous: Aphonia

Drug Interactions

Avoid Concomitant Use

Avoid concomitant use of Cytarabine with any of the following: Natalizumab; Vaccines (Live)

Increased Effect/Toxicity

Cytarabine may increase the levels/effects of: Leflunomide; Natalizumab; Vaccines (Live)

The levels/effects of Cytarabine may be increased by: Trastuzumab

Decreased Effect

Cytarabine may decrease the levels/effects of: Cardiac Glycosides; Flucytosine; Vaccines (Inactivated); Vaccines (Live)

The levels/effects of Cytarabine may be decreased by: Echinacea

Storage/Stability

Powder for reconstitution: Store intact vials of powder at room temperature 15°C to 30°C (59°F to 86°F). Reconstituted solutions are stable for up to 8 days at room temperature, although the manufacturer recommends use within 48 hours.

Solution: Prior to dilution, store at room temperature, 15°C to 30°C (59°F to 86°F). Protect from light. Do not refrigerate solution; precipitate may form.

Reconstitution Reconstitute powder with bacteriostatic water for injection, bacteriostatic 0.9% NaCl.

For I.T. use: Reconstitute with preservative free diluent.

For I.V. infusion: Dilute in 250-1000 mL 0.9% NaCl or D$_5$W.

Note: Solutions containing bacteriostatic agents should not be used for the preparation of either high doses or intrathecal doses of cytarabine; may be used for I.M., SubQ, and low-dose (100-200 mg/m^2) I.V. solution.

Compatibility Stable in D$_5$LR, D$_5$¼NS, D$_5$NS, D$_{10}$W, LR, NS.

Y-site administration: **Compatible:** Amifostine, amsacrine, aztreonam, cefepime, chlorpromazine, cimetidine, cladribine, dexamethasone sodium phosphate, diphenhydramine, doxorubicin liposome, droperidol, etoposide phosphate, famotidine, filgrastim, fludarabine, furosemide, gatifloxacin, gemcitabine, gentamicin, granisetron, heparin, hydrocortisone sodium succinate, hydromorphone, idarubicin, linezolid, lorazepam, melphalan, methotrexate, methylprednisolone sodium succinate, metoclopramide, morphine, ondansetron, paclitaxel, piperacillin/tazobactam, prochlorperazine edisylate, promethazine, propofol, ranitidine, sargramostim, sodium bicarbonate, teniposide, thiotepa, vinorelbine. **Incompatible:** Allopurinol, amphotericin B cholesteryl sulfate complex, ganciclovir.

Compatibility in syringe: **Compatible:** Metoclopramide.

Compatibility when admixed: **Compatible:** Corticotropin, dacarbazine, daunorubicin with etoposide, etoposide, hydroxyzine, lincomycin, methotrexate, mitoxantrone, ondansetron, potassium chloride, sodium bicarbonate, vincristine. **Incompatible:** Fluorouracil, heparin, insulin (regular), nafcillin, oxacillin, penicillin G sodium. **Variable (consult detailed reference):** Gentamicin, hydrocortisone sodium succinate, methylprednisolone sodium succinate.

◀ **Mechanism of Action** Inhibits DNA synthesis. Cytosine gains entry into cells by a carrier process, and then must be converted to its active compound, aracytidine triphosphate. Cytosine is a pyrimidine analog and is incorporated into DNA; however, the primary action is inhibition of DNA polymerase resulting in decreased DNA synthesis and repair. The degree of cytotoxicity correlates linearly with incorporation into DNA; therefore, incorporation into the DNA is responsible for drug activity and toxicity. Cytarabine is specific for the S phase of the cell cycle (blocks progression from the G_1 to the S phase).

Pharmacodynamics/Kinetics

Distribution: V_d: Total body water; widely and rapidly since it enters the cells readily; crosses blood-brain barrier with CSF levels of 40% to 50% of plasma level

Metabolism: Primarily hepatic; metabolized by deoxycytidine kinase and other nucleotide kinases to aracytidine triphosphate (active); about 86% to 96% of dose is metabolized to inactive uracil arabinoside (ARA-U); intrathecal administration results in little conversion to ARA-U due to the low levels of deaminase in the cerebral spinal fluid

Half-life elimination: I.V.: Initial: 7-20 minutes; Terminal: 1-3 hours

Time to peak, plasma: I.M., SubQ: 20-60 minutes

Excretion: Urine (~80%; 90% as metabolite ARA-U) within 24 hours

Dosage Refer to individual protocols. Children and Adults:

Remission induction:

I.V.: 75-200 mg/m^2/day for 5-10 days; a second course, beginning 2-4 weeks after the initial therapy, may be required in some patients.

or 100 mg/m^2 for 7 days

or 100 mg/m^2/dose every 12 hours for 7 days

I.T.: Usual dose 30 mg/m^2 every 4 days; range: 5-75 mg/m^2 every 2-7 days until CNS findings normalize; or age-based dosing (frequency of administration usually defined by protocol):

<1 year of age: 15-20 mg per dose

1-2 years of age: 16-30 mg per dose

2-3 years of age: 20-50 mg per dose

>3 years of age: 24-75 mg per dose

Remission maintenance:

I.V.: 70-200 mg/m^2/day for 2-5 days at monthly intervals

I.M., SubQ: 1-1.5 mg/kg single dose for maintenance at 1- to 4-week intervals

High-dose therapies (unlabeled use):

Doses of 1-3 g/m^2 have been used for refractory or secondary leukemias or refractory non-Hodgkin's lymphoma.

Doses of 1-3 g/m^2 every 12 hours for up to 12 doses have been used for leukemia

Bone marrow transplant (unlabeled use): 1.5 g/m^2 continuous infusion over 48 hours

Dosage adjustment in renal impairment: The FDA-approved labeling does not contain renal dosing adjustment guidelines; the following guidelines have been used by some clinicians:

Aronoff, 2007 (Cytarabine 100-200 mg/m^2): Children and Adults: No adjustment necessary

Kintzel, 1995 (High-dose cytarabine 1-3 g/m^2):

Cl_{cr} 46-60 mL/minute: Administer 60% of dose

Cl_{cr} 31-45 mL/minute: Administer 50% of dose

Cl_{cr} <30 mL/minute: Consider use of alternative drug

Smith, 1997 (High-dose cytarabine ≥2 g/m^2/dose):

Serum creatinine 1.5-1.9 mg/dL or increase (from baseline) of 0.5-1.2 mg/dL: Reduce dose to 1 g/m^2/dose

Serum creatinine ≥2 mg/dL or increase (from baseline) of >1.2 mg/dL: Reduce dose to 0.1 g/m^2/day as a continuous infusion

Dosage adjustment in hepatic impairment: Dose may need to be adjusted in patients with liver failure since cytarabine is partially detoxified in the liver. The FDA-approved labeling does not contain hepatic dosing adjustment guidelines; the following guideline has been used by some clinicians:

Floyd, 2006: Transaminases (any elevation): Administer 50% of dose; may increase subsequent doses in the absence of toxicities

Koren, 1992 (dose level not specified): Bilirubin >2 mg/dL: Administer 50% of dose; may increase subsequent doses in the absence of toxicities

Combination Regimens

Brain tumors: 8 in 1 (Brain Tumors) on page 1221

Leukemia, acute lymphocytic:
FIS-HAM on page 1322
Hyper-CVAD + Imatinib on page 1348
Hyper-CVAD (Leukemia, Acute Lymphocytic) on page 1349
Linker Protocol on page 1362
PVA (POG 8602) on page 1398

Leukemia, acute myeloid:
5 + 2 on page 1220
7 + 3 (Daunorubicin) on page 1220
7 + 3 (Idarubicin) on page 1221
7 + 3 (Mitoxantrone) on page 1221
7 + 3 + 7 on page 1220
CA on page 1241
DA on page 1285
DAT on page 1288
DAV on page 1288
EMA 86 on page 1300
FIS-HAM on page 1322
FLAG (AML) on page 1323
FLAG-IDA on page 1324
Idarubicin, Cytarabine, Etoposide (ICE Protocol) on page 1357
Idarubicin-Cytarabine (High Dose)-Etoposide (AML) on page 1358
TAD on page 1405
V-TAD on page 1427

Leukemia, acute promyelocytic: Tretinoin-Daunorubicin-Cytarabine (APL) on page 1412

Leukemia, chronic lymphocytic: OFAR (CLL) on page 1381

Lymphoma, Hodgkin's disease: mini-BEAM on page 1367

Lymphoma, non-Hodgkin's:
Cisplatin-Cytarabine-Dexamethasone (NHL Regimen) on page 1265
CODOX-M on page 1278
COMLA on page 1279
ESHAP on page 1312
Hyper-CVAD (Lymphoma, non-Hodgkin's) on page 1355
IVAC on page 1361
Oxaliplatin-Cytarabine-Dexamethasone (NHL Regimen) on page 1383
Pro-MACE-CytaBOM on page 1397

Lymphoma, non-Hodgkin's (Burkitt's): CODOX-M/IVAC on page 1278

Lymphoma, non-Hodgkin's (Mantle cell): Hyper-CVAD + Rituximab on page 1356

Neuroblastoma: N4SE Protocol on page 1380
Retinoblastoma: 8 in 1 (Retinoblastoma) on page 1222

Administration May be administered I.M., I.T., or SubQ at a concentration not to exceed 100 mg/mL. When administered via I.V. infusion, infuse over 1-3 hours or as a continuous infusion. GI effects may be more pronounced with divided I.V. bolus doses than with continuous infusion.

Monitoring Parameters Liver function tests, CBC with differential and platelet count, serum creatinine, BUN, serum uric acid

Additional Information I.V. doses ≥1.5 g/m^2 may produce conjunctivitis which can be ameliorated with prophylactic use of corticosteroid (0.1% dexamethasone) eye drops. Dexamethasone eye drops should be administered at 1-2 drops every 6 hours during and for 2-7 days after cytarabine is done.

Emetic Potential
>1000 mg/m^2: Moderate (30% to 90%)
100-200 mg/m^2: Low (10% to 30%)

High Dose Considerations

Comments Risk of cerebellar toxicity increases with creatinine clearance <60 mL/minute, age older than 50 years, pre-existing CNS lesion, and alkaline phosphatase levels exceeding 3 times the upper limit of normal. Conjunctivitis is prevented and treated with saline or corticosteroid eye drops. As prophylaxis, eye drops should be started 6-12 hours before initiation of cytarabine and continued 24 hours following the last dose.

High Dose I.V.: 2-3 g/m^2/dose every 12-24 hours for 4-12 doses; duration of infusion is 1-3 hours; maximum single-agent dose: 36 g/m^2; generally combined with other high-dose chemotherapeutic drugs or total body irradiation (TBI).

Unique Toxicities

Central nervous system: Cerebellar toxicity which includes nystagmus, dysarthria, disdiadochokinesis, slurred speech; cerebral toxicity which includes somnolence, confusion

Dermatologic: Rash, desquamation may occur

Gastrointestinal: Severe nausea and vomiting, mucositis, diarrhea, ageusia

Ocular: Photophobia, excessive tearing, blurred vision, local discomfort, chemical conjunctivitis, optic neuropathy, visual loss

Respiratory: Noncardiogenic pulmonary edema (onset 22-27 days following completion of therapy)

Miscellaneous: Anosmia

Dosage Forms Excipient information presented when available (limited, particularly for generics); consult specific product labeling.

Injection, powder for reconstitution: 100 mg, 500 mg, 1 g, 2 g [contains benzyl alcohol (in diluent)]

Injection, solution: 100 mg/mL (20 mL)

Injection, solution: 20 mg/mL (25 mL) [contains benzyl alcohol]

Injection, solution [preservative free]: 20 mg/mL (5 mL, 50 mL); 100 mg/mL (20 mL)

References

Aronoff GR, Bennett WM, Berns JS, et al, *Drug Prescribing in Renal Failure: Dosing Guidelines for Adults and Children*, 5th ed. Philadelphia, PA: American College of Physicians; 2007, p 98, 170.

Capizzi RL, White JC, Powell BL, et al, "Effect of Dose on the Pharmacokinetic and Pharmacodynamic Effects of Cytarabine," *Semin Hematol*, 1991, 28(3 Suppl 4):54-69.

Cassileth PA, Harrington DP, Appelbaum FR, et al, "Chemotherapy Compared With Autologous or Allogeneic Bone Marrow Transplantation in the Management of Acute Myeloid Leukemia in First Remission," *N Engl J Med*, 1998, 339(23):1649-56.

Floyd J, Mirza I, Sachs B, et al, "Hepatotoxicity of Chemotherapy," *Semin Oncol*, 2006, 33 (1):50-67.

Gaynor PS, Steinherz PG, Bleyer WA, et al, "Improved Therapy for Children With Acute Lymphoblastic Leukemia and Unfavorable Presenting Features: A Follow-Up Report of the Childrens Cancer Group Study CCG-106," *J Clin Oncol*, 1993, 11(11):2234-42.

Hamada A, Kawaguchi T, and Nakano M, "Clinical Pharmacokinetics of Cytarabine Formulations," *Clin Pharmacokinet*, 2002, 41(10):705-18.

Hiddemann W, "Cytosine Arabinoside in the Treatment of Acute Myeloid Leukemia: The Role and Place of High-Dose Regimens," *Ann Hematol*, 1991, 62(4):119-28.

Kintzel PE and Dorr RT, "Anticancer Drug Renal Toxicity and Elimination: Dosing Guidelines for Altered Renal Function," *Cancer Treat Rev*, 1995, 21(1):33-64.

Koren G, Beatty K, Seto A, et al, "The Effects of Impaired Liver Function on the Elimination of Antineoplastic Agents," *Ann Pharmacother*, 1992, 26(3):363-71.

Matloub Y, Lindemulder S, Gaynon PS, et al, "Intrathecal Triple Therapy Decreases Central Nervous System Relapse but Fails to Improve Event-Free Survival When Compared With Intrathecal Methotrexate: Results of the Children's Cancer Group (CCG) 1952 Study for Standard-Risk Acute Lymphoblastic Leukemia, Reported by the Children's Oncology Group," *Blood*, 2006, 108(4):1165-73.

National Comprehensive Cancer Network (NCCN), "Clinical Practice Guidelines in Oncology™: Antiemesis," Version 1.2008. Available at http://www.nccn.org/professionals/physician_gls/PDF/antiemesis.pdf.

Pease CL, Horton TM, McClain KL, et al, "Aseptic Meningitis in a Child After Systemic Treatment With High Dose Cytarabine," *Pediatr Infect Dis J*, 2001, 20(1):87-9.

Pegram AA and Kennedy LD, "Prevention and Treatment of Veno-Occlusive Disease," *Ann Pharmacother*, 2001, 35(7-8):935-42.

Pieters R, Schrappe M, De Lorenzo P, et al, "A Treatment Protocol for Infants Younger Than 1 Year With Acute Lymphoblastic Leukaemia (Interfant-99): An Observational Study and a Multicentre Randomised Trial," *Lancet*, 2007, 370(9583):240-50.

Smith G, Damon LE, Rugo HS, et al. "High-Dose Cytarabine Dose Modification Reduces the Incidence of Neurotoxicity in Patients With Renal Insufficiency," *J Clin Oncol*, 1997, 15(2): 833-9.

Stasi R, Venditti A, Del Poeta G, et al, "High-Dose Chemotherapy in Adult Acute Myeloid Leukemia: Rationale and Results," *Leuk Res*, 1996, 20(7):535-49.

Truica CI and Frankel SR, "Acute Rhabdomyolysis as a Complication of Cytarabine Chemotherapy for Acute Myeloid Leukemia: Case Report and Review of Literature," *Am J Hematol*, 2002, 70 (4):320-3.

◆ **Cytarabine (Conventional)** *see Cytarabine on page 281*

◆ **Cytarabine Hydrochloride** *see Cytarabine on page 281*

Cytarabine (Liposomal) (sye TARE a been lip po SOE mal)

Medication Safety Issues

Sound-alike/look-alike issues:

Cytarabine may be confused with Cytadren®, Cytosar®, Cytoxan®, vidarabine

Cytarabine liposomal may be confused with conventional cytarabine

DepoCyt® may be confused with Depoject®

High alert medication: The Institute for Safe Medication Practices (ISMP) includes this medication among its list of drugs which have a heightened risk of causing significant patient harm when used in error.

Related Information

Management of Drug Extravasations *on page 1447*
Safe Handling of Hazardous Drugs *on page 1517*

U.S. Brand Names DepoCyt®

Generic Available No

Canadian Brand Names DepoCyt®

Pharmacologic Category Antineoplastic Agent, Antimetabolite (Pyrimidine Antagonist)

Use Treatment of lymphomatous meningitis

Pregnancy Risk Factor D

Lactation Excretion in breast milk unknown/not recommended

◀ **Labeled Contraindications** Hypersensitivity to cytarabine or any component of the formulation; active meningeal infection

Warnings/Precautions Hazardous agent - use appropriate precautions for handling and disposal. **[U.S. Boxed Warning]: Chemical arachnoiditis (nausea, vomiting, headache, fever) occurs commonly; may be fatal if untreated. The incidence and severity of chemical arachnoiditis is reduced by coadministration with dexamethasone.** Hydrocephalus has been reported and may be precipitated by chemical arachnoiditis. May cause neurotoxicity (including myelopathy), which may lead to permanent neurologic deficit. Blockage to CSF flow may increase the risk of neurotoxicity. Peripheral neurotoxicity has also been reported. Monitor for neurotoxicity; reduce subsequent doses; discontinue with persistent neurotoxicity. The risk of adverse events, including neurotoxicity, is increased with concurrent radiation therapy or systemic chemotherapy. Infectious meningitis may be associated with intrathecal administration. **[U.S. Boxed Warning]: Should be administered under the supervision of an experienced cancer chemotherapy physician.** For intrathecal use only. Safety and efficacy in pediatric patients have not been established.

Adverse Reactions

>10%:

Cardiovascular: Peripheral edema (11%)

Central nervous system: Chemical arachnoiditis (without dexamethasone premedication: 100%; with dexamethasone premedication: 33% to 42%; grade 4: 19% to 30%; onset: ≤5 days); headache (56%), confusion (33%), fever (32%), fatigue (25%), seizure (20% to 22%), dizziness (18%), lethargy (16%), insomnia (14%), memory impairment (14%), pain (14%)

Endocrine & metabolic: Dehydration (13%)

Gastrointestinal: Nausea (46%), vomiting (44%), constipation (25%), diarrhea (12%), appetite decreased (11%)

Genitourinary: Urinary tract infection (14%)

Hematologic: Anemia (12%), thrombocytopenia (3% to 11%)

Neuromuscular & skeletal: Weakness (40%), back pain (24%), abnormal gait (23%), limb pain (15%), neck pain (14%), arthralgia (11%), neck stiffness (11%)

Ocular: Blurred vision (11%)

1% to 10%:

Cardiovascular: Tachycardia (9%), hypotension (8%), hypertension (6%), syncope (3%), edema (2%)

Central nervous system: Agitation (10%), hypoesthesia (10%), depression (8%), anxiety (7%), sensory neuropathy (3%)

Dermatologic: Pruritus (2%)

Endocrine & metabolic: Hypokalemia (7%), hyponatremia (7%), hyperglycemia (6%)

Gastrointestinal: Abdominal pain (9%), dysphagia (8%), anorexia (5%), hemorrhoids (3%), mucosal inflammation (3%)

Genitourinary: Incontinence (7%), urinary retention (5%)

Hematologic: Neutropenia (10%), contusion (2%)

Neuromuscular & skeletal: Muscle weakness (10%), tremor (9%), peripheral neuropathy (4%), abnormal reflexes (3%)

Otic: Hypoacusis (6%)

Respiratory: Dyspnea (10%), cough (7%), pneumonia (6%)

Miscellaneous: Diaphoresis (2%)

<1%, postmarketing, and/or case reports: Anaphylaxis, bladder control impaired, blindness, bowel control impaired, cauda equine syndrome, cranial

nerve palsies, CSF protein increased, CSF WBC increased, deafness, encephalopathy, hemiplegia, hydrocephalus, infectious meningitis, intracranial pressure increased, myelopathy, neurologic deficit, numbness, papilledema, somnolence, visual disturbance

Drug Interactions

Avoid Concomitant Use

Avoid concomitant use of Cytarabine (Liposomal) with any of the following: Natalizumab; Vaccines (Live)

Increased Effect/Toxicity

Cytarabine (Liposomal) may increase the levels/effects of: Leflunomide; Natalizumab; Vaccines (Live)

The levels/effects of Cytarabine (Liposomal) may be increased by: Trastuzumab

Decreased Effect

Cytarabine (Liposomal) may decrease the levels/effects of: Vaccines (Inactivated); Vaccines (Live)

The levels/effects of Cytarabine (Liposomal) may be decreased by: Echinacea

Storage/Stability Store under refrigeration at 2°C to 8°C (36°F to 46°F); protect from freezing. Avoid aggressive agitation. Solutions should be used within 4 hours of withdrawal from the vial.

Reconstitution Allow vial to warm to room temperature prior to withdrawal from vial. Particles may settle in diluent over time, and may be resuspended by gentle agitation or inversion of the vial. Further reconstitution or dilution is not required.

Mechanism of Action Cytarabine liposomal is a sustained-release formulation of the active ingredient cytarabine, an antimetabolite which acts through inhibition of DNA synthesis and is cell cycle-specific for the S phase of cell division. Cytarabine is converted intracellularly to its active metabolite cytarabine-5'-triphosphate (ara-CTP). Ara-CTP also appears to be incorporated into DNA and RNA; however, the primary action is inhibition of DNA polymerase, resulting in decreased DNA synthesis and repair. The liposomal formulation allows for gradual release, resulting in prolonged exposure.

Pharmacodynamics/Kinetics

Absorption: Systemic exposure following intrathecal administration is negligible since transfer rate from CSF to plasma is slow

Half-life elimination, CSF: 6-82 hours

Time to peak, CSF: Intrathecal: <1 hour

Dosage Note: Patients should be started on dexamethasone 4 mg twice daily (oral or I.V.) for 5 days, beginning on the day of cytarabine liposomal injection.

Intrathecal: Adults:

Induction: 50 mg every 14 days for a total of 2 doses (weeks 1 and 3)

Consolidation: 50 mg every 14 days for 3 doses (weeks 5, 7, and 9), followed by an additional dose at week 13

Maintenance: 50 mg every 28 days for 4 doses (weeks 17, 21, 25, and 29)

Dosage reduction for toxicity: If drug-related neurotoxicity develops, reduce dose to 25 mg. If toxicity persists, discontinue treatment.

Administration For intrathecal use only. Dose should be removed from vial immediately before administration (must be administered within 4 hours of removal). An in-line filter should **not** be used. Administer directly into the CSF via an intraventricular reservoir or by direct injection into the lumbar sac. ▶

Injection should be made slowly (over 1-5 minutes). Patients should lie flat for 1 hour after lumbar puncture.

Monitoring Parameters Monitor closely for signs of an immediate reaction; neurotoxicity

Test Interactions Since cytarabine liposomes are similar in appearance to WBCs, care must be taken in interpreting CSF examinations in patients receiving cytarabine liposomal.

Vesicant May be an irritant

Dosage Forms Excipient information presented when available (limited, particularly for generics); consult specific product labeling.

Injection, suspension, intrathecal [preservative free]:

DepoCyt®: 10 mg/mL (5 mL)

References

Cole BF, Glantz MJ, Jaeckle KA, et al, "Quality-of-Life-Adjusted Survival Comparison of Sustained-Release Cytosine Arabinoside Versus Intrathecal Methotrexate for Treatment of Solid Tumor Neoplastic Meningitis," *Cancer*, 2003, 97(12):3053-60.

Glantz MJ, LaFollette S, Jaeckle KA, et al, "Randomized Trial of a Slow-Release Versus a Standard Formulation of Cytarabine for the Intrathecal Treatment of Lymphomatous Meningitis," *J Clin Oncol*, 1999, 17(10):3110-6.

Jabbour E, O'Brien S, Kantarjian H, et al, "Neurologic Complications Associated With Intrathecal Liposomal Cytarabine in Combination With High-Dose Methotrexate and Cytarabine to Patients With Acute Lymphocytic Leukemia," *Blood*, 2007, 109(8):3214-8.

◆ **CytoGam®** see Cytomegalovirus Immune Globulin (Intravenous-Human) on page 290

Cytomegalovirus Immune Globulin (Intravenous-Human) (sye toe meg a low VYE rus i MYUN GLOB yoo lin in tra VEE nus HYU man)

Medication Safety Issues

Sound-alike/look-alike issues:

CytoGam® may be confused with Cytoxan®, Gamimune® N

U.S. Brand Names CytoGam®

Index Terms CMV-IGIV

Generic Available No

Canadian Brand Names CytoGam®

Pharmacologic Category Blood Product Derivative; Immune Globulin

Use Prophylaxis of cytomegalovirus (CMV) disease associated with kidney, lung, liver, pancreas, and heart transplants; concomitant use with ganciclovir should be considered in organ transplants (other than kidney) from CMV seropositive donors to CMV seronegative recipients

Unlabeled/Investigational Use Adjunct therapy in the treatment of CMV disease in immunocompromised patients

Pregnancy Risk Factor C

Lactation Excretion in breast milk unknown

Labeled Contraindications Hypersensitivity to CMV-IGIV, other immunoglobulins, or any component of the formulation; immunoglobulin A deficiency

Warnings/Precautions Hypersensitivity and anaphylactic reactions can occur; immediate treatment (including epinephrine 1:1000) should be available. Aseptic meningitis syndrome (AMS) has been reported with intravenous immune globulin administration (rare); may occur with high doses (≥2 g/kg). Intravenous immune globulin has been associated with antiglobulin hemolysis; monitor for signs of hemolytic anemia. Monitor for transfusion-related acute lung injury (TRALI); noncardiogenic pulmonary edema has been reported with intravenous immune globulin use. Acute renal dysfunction (increased serum creatinine, oliguria, acute renal failure) can rarely occur;

usually within 7 days of use (more likely with products stabilized with sucrose). Use with caution in the elderly, patients with renal disease, diabetes mellitus, volume depletion, sepsis, paraproteinemia, and nephrotoxic medications due to risk of renal dysfunction. In patients at risk of renal dysfunction, the rate of infusion and concentration of solution should be minimized. discontinue if renal function deteriorates. Patients should not be volume depleted prior to therapy. Thrombotic events have been reported with administration of intravenous immune globulin; use with caution in patients with cardiovascular risk factors. Use with caution in patients >65 years of age. Product is stabilized with albumin. Product of human plasma; may potentially contain infectious agents which could transmit disease. Screening of donors, as well as testing and/or inactivation or removal of certain viruses, reduces the risk. Infections thought to be transmitted by this product should be reported to the manufacturer. Product is stabilized with sucrose.

Adverse Reactions

<6%:

Cardiovascular: Flushing

Central nervous system: Chills, fever

Gastrointestinal: Nausea, vomiting

Neuromuscular & skeletal: Arthralgia, back pain, muscle cramps

Respiratory: Wheezing

<1%: Blood pressure decreased

Postmarketing and/or case reports: Acute renal failure, acute tubular necrosis, anaphylactic shock, angioneurotic edema, anuria, aseptic meningitis syndrome (AMS), BUN increased, oliguria, osmotic nephrosis, proximal tubular nephropathy, serum creatinine increased

Drug Interactions

Avoid Concomitant Use There are no known interactions where it is recommended to avoid concomitant use.

Increased Effect/Toxicity There are no known significant interactions involving an increase in effect.

Decreased Effect

Cytomegalovirus Immune Globulin (Intravenous-Human) may decrease the levels/effects of: Vaccines (Live)

Storage/Stability Store between 2°C and 8°C (35.6°F and 46.4°F). Use reconstituted product within 6 hours.

Reconstitution Do not admix with other medications; do not use if turbid. Do not shake vials. Dilution is not recommended.

Compatibility Infusion with other products is not recommended. If unavoidable, may be piggybacked into an I.V. line of sodium chloride, 2.5% dextrose in water, 5% dextrose in water, 10% dextrose in water, or 20% dextrose in water. Do not dilute more than 1:2. Do not admix with other medications.

Mechanism of Action CMV-IGIV is a preparation of immunoglobulin G derived from pooled healthy blood donors with a high titer of CMV antibodies; administration provides a passive source of antibodies against cytomegalovirus

Dosage I.V.: Adults:

Kidney transplant:

Initial dose (within 72 hours of transplant): 150 mg/kg/dose

2-, 4-, 6-, and 8 weeks after transplant: 100 mg/kg/dose

12 and 16 weeks after transplant: 50 mg/kg/dose

Liver, lung, pancreas, or heart transplant:
  Initial dose (within 72 hours of transplant): 150 mg/kg/dose
  2-, 4-, 6-, and 8 weeks after transplant: 150 mg/kg/dose
  12 and 16 weeks after transplant: 100 mg/kg/dose
Severe CMV pneumonia (unlabeled): Various regimens have been used, including 400 mg/kg CMV-IGIV in combination with ganciclovir on days 1, 2, 7, or 8, followed by 200 mg/kg CMV-IGIV on days 14 and 21
Elderly: Use with caution in patients >65 years of age, may be at increased risk of renal insufficiency
Dosage adjustment in renal impairment: Use with caution; specific dosing adjustments are not available. Infusion rate should be the minimum practical; do not exceed 180 mg/kg/hour

Administration Administer through an I.V. line containing an in-line filter (pore size 15 micron) using an infusion pump. Do not mix with other infusions; do not use if turbid. Begin infusion within 6 hours of entering vial, complete infusion within 12 hours.

Infuse at 15 mg/kg/hour. If no adverse reactions occur within 30 minutes, may increase rate to 30 mg/kg/hour. If no adverse reactions occur within the second 30 minutes, may increase rate to 60 mg/kg/hour; maximum rate of infusion: 75 mL/hour. When infusing subsequent doses, may decrease titration interval from 30 minutes to 15 minutes. If patient develops nausea, back pain, or flushing during infusion, slow the rate or temporarily stop the infusion. Discontinue if blood pressure drops or in case of anaphylactic reaction.

Monitoring Parameters Vital signs (throughout infusion), flushing, chills, muscle cramps, back pain, fever, nausea, vomiting, wheezing, decreased blood pressure, or anaphylaxis; renal function and urine output

Dietary Considerations CytoGam® solution for injection 50 mg (± 10 mg/mL) contains sodium 20-30 mEq/L

Dosage Forms Excipient information presented when available (limited, particularly for generics); consult specific product labeling.
Injection, solution [preservative free]:
  CytoGam®: 50 mg ± 10 mg/mL (50 mL) [contains sodium 20-30 mEq/L, human albumin, and sucrose]

References
Levinson ML and Jacobson PA, "Treatment and Prophylaxis of Cytomegalovirus Disease," *Pharmacotherapy*, 1992, 12(4):300-18.
Reed EC, Bowden RA, Dandliker PS, et al, "Efficacy of Cytomegalovirus Immunoglobulin in Marrow Transplant Recipients With Cytomegalovirus Pneumonia," *J Infect Dis*, 1987, 156:641-5.
Reed EC, Bowden RA, Dandliker PS, et al, "Treatment of Cytomegalovirus Pneumonia With Ganciclovir and Intravenous Cytomegalovirus Immunoglobulin in Patients With Bone Marrow Transplants," *Ann Intern Med*, 1988, 109:783-8.
"Renal Insufficiency and Failure Associated With Immune Globulin Intravenous Therapy - United States, 1985-1998." *MMWR*, 1999, 48(24):518-21.

♦ **DABIL2** *see* Denileukin Diftitox *on page 340*

Dacarbazine (da KAR ba zeen)
Medication Safety Issues
Sound-alike/look-alike issues:
Dacarbazine may be confused with Dicarbosil®, procarbazine

High alert medication: The Institute for Safe Medication Practices (ISMP) includes this medication among its list of drugs which have a heightened risk of causing significant patient harm when used in error.

Related Information
Management of Drug Extravasations *on page 1447*
Safe Handling of Hazardous Drugs *on page 1517*

Index Terms DIC; Dimethyl Triazeno Imidazole Carboxamide; DTIC; Imidazole Carboxamide; Imidazole Carboxamide Dimethyltriazene; WR-139007

Generic Available Yes

Canadian Brand Names DTIC®

Pharmacologic Category Antineoplastic Agent, Alkylating Agent (Triazene)

Use Treatment of malignant melanoma, Hodgkin's disease

Unlabeled/Investigational Use Treatment of soft-tissue sarcomas, islet cell tumors, pheochromocytoma, medullary carcinoma of the thyroid

Pregnancy Risk Factor C

Lactation Excretion in breast milk unknown/not recommended

Labeled Contraindications Hypersensitivity to dacarbazine or any component of the formulation

Warnings/Precautions Hazardous agent - use appropriate precautions for handling and disposal. **[U.S. Boxed Warnings]: Bone marrow suppression is a common toxicity; monitor closely. Hepatotoxicity with hepatocellular necrosis and hepatic vein thrombosis has been reported,** usually with combination chemotherapy, but may occur with dacarbazine alone. The half-life is increased in patients with renal and/or hepatic impairment; use caution, monitor for toxicity and consider dosage reduction. Anaphylaxis may occur. Extravasation may result in tissue damage and pain. **[U.S. Boxed Warnings]: May be carcinogenic and/or teratogenic. Should be administered under the supervision of an experienced cancer chemotherapy physician.**

Adverse Reactions
>10%:
Gastrointestinal: Nausea and vomiting (>90%), can be severe and dose limiting; nausea and vomiting decrease on successive days when dacarbazine is given daily for 5 days; diarrhea

Hematologic: Myelosuppression, leukopenia, thrombocytopenia - dose limiting
Onset: 5-7 days
Nadir: 7-10 days
Recovery: 21-28 days

Local: Pain on infusion, may be minimized by administration through a central line, or by administration as a short infusion (eg, 1-2 hours as opposed to bolus injection)

1% to 10%:
Dermatologic: Alopecia, rash, photosensitivity
Gastrointestinal: Anorexia, metallic taste
Miscellaneous: Flu-like syndrome (fever, myalgia, malaise)

◄ <1%: Anaphylactic reactions, diarrhea (following high-dose bolus injection), eosinophilia, headache, hepatic necrosis, hepatic vein occlusion, liver enzymes increased (transient), paresthesia

Drug Interactions

Metabolism/Transport Effects Substrate (major) of CYP1A2, 2E1

Avoid Concomitant Use

Avoid concomitant use of Dacarbazine with any of the following: Natalizumab; Vaccines (Live)

Increased Effect/Toxicity

Dacarbazine may increase the levels/effects of: Leflunomide; Natalizumab; Vaccines (Live)

The levels/effects of Dacarbazine may be increased by: CYP1A2 Inhibitors (Moderate); CYP1A2 Inhibitors (Strong); CYP2E1 Inhibitors (Moderate); CYP2E1 Inhibitors (Strong); MAO Inhibitors; Trastuzumab

Decreased Effect

Dacarbazine may decrease the levels/effects of: Vaccines (Inactivated); Vaccines (Live)

The levels/effects of Dacarbazine may be decreased by: CYP1A2 Inducers (Strong); Echinacea; Sorafenib

Ethanol/Nutrition/Herb Interactions

Ethanol: Avoid ethanol (due to GI irritation).

Herb/Nutraceutical: Avoid dong quai, St John's wort (may also cause photosensitization).

Storage/Stability Store intact vials under refrigeration (2°C to 8°C) and protect from light. Vials are stable for 4 weeks at room temperature. Reconstituted solution is stable for 24 hours at room temperature (20°C) and 96 hours under refrigeration (4°C). Solutions for infusion (in D_5W or NS) are stable for 24 hours at room temperature and protected from light. Decomposed drug turns pink.

Reconstitution The manufacturer recommends reconstituting 100 mg and 200 mg vials with 9.9 mL and 19.7 mL SWFI, respectively, to a concentration of 10 mg/mL; some institutions use different standard dilutions (eg, 20 mg/mL).

Standard I.V. dilution: Dilute in 250-1000 mL D_5W or NS.

Compatibility Stable in NS, sterile water for injection; **variable stability (consult detailed reference)** in D_5W.

Y-site administration: Compatible: Amifostine, aztreonam, etoposide phosphate, filgrastim, fludarabine, granisetron, melphalan, ondansetron, paclitaxel, sargramostim, teniposide, thiotepa, vinorelbine. **Incompatible:** Allopurinol, cefepime, piperacillin/tazobactam. **Variable (consult detailed reference):** Heparin.

Compatibility when admixed: Compatible: Bleomycin, carmustine, cyclophosphamide, cytarabine, dactinomycin, doxorubicin, fluorouracil, hydrocortisone sodium phosphate, lidocaine, mercaptopurine, methotrexate, ondansetron, vinblastine. **Incompatible:** Hydrocortisone sodium succinate. **Variable (consult detailed reference):** Ondansetron with doxorubicin.

Mechanism of Action Alkylating agent which appears to form methylcarbonium ions that attack nucleophilic groups in DNA; cross-links strands of DNA resulting in the inhibition of DNA, RNA, and protein synthesis, the exact mechanism of action is still unclear.

Pharmacodynamics/Kinetics

Onset of action: I.V.: 18-24 days

Distribution: V_d: 0.6 L/kg, exceeding total body water; suggesting binding to some tissue (probably liver)

Protein binding: 5%

Metabolism: Extensively hepatic; hepatobiliary excretion is probably of some importance; metabolites may also have an antineoplastic effect

Half-life elimination: Biphasic: Initial: 20-40 minutes; Terminal: 5 hours

Excretion: Urine (~30% to 50% as unchanged drug)

Dosage Details concerning dosing in combination regimens should also be consulted. Some dosage regimens include:

Intra-arterial (unlabeled route): 50-400 mg/m^2 for 5-10 days

I.V.:

Hodgkin's disease, ABVD: 375 mg/m^2 days 1 and 15 every 4 weeks **or** 100 mg/m^2/day for 5 days

Metastatic melanoma (alone or in combination with other agents): 150-250 mg/m^2 days 1-5 every 3-4 weeks

Metastatic melanoma (unlabeled dosing): 850 mg/m^2 every 3 weeks

Dosage adjustment in renal impairment: The FDA-approved labeling does not contain dosage adjustment guidelines. The following guidelines have been used by some clinicians (Kintzel, 1995):

Cl_{cr} 46-60 mL/minute: Administer 80% of dose

Cl_{cr} 31-45 mL/minute: Administer 75% of dose

Cl_{cr} <30 mL/minute: Administer 70% of dose

Dosage adjustment in hepatic impairment: The FDA-approved labeling does not contain adjustment guidelines. May cause hepatotoxicity; monitor closely for signs of toxicity.

Combination Regimens

Brain tumors: 8 in 1 (Brain Tumors) on page 1221

Lymphoma, Hodgkin's:

ABVD on page 1222

MOPP/ABVD on page 1369

Melanoma:

BOLD on page 1235

BOLD (Melanoma) on page 1237

BOLD + Interferon on page 1235

CCDT (Melanoma) on page 1253

Cisplatin-Dacarbazine-Carmustine (Melanoma) on page 1265

Cisplatin-Dacarbazine-Interferon Alfa-2b-Aldesleukin on page 1266

Cisplatin-Vinblastine-Dacarbazine (Melanoma) on page 1274

CVD-Interleukin-Interferon (Melanoma) on page 1282

Dacarbazine-Carboplatin-Aldesleukin-Interferon on page 1286

Dartmouth Regimen on page 1286

Neuroblastoma: CCDDT (Neuroblastoma) on page 1252

Sarcoma: CYVADIC on page 1285

Soft tissue sarcoma:

AD on page 1225

MAID on page 1365

Administration Infuse over 30-60 minutes; rapid infusion may cause severe venous irritation.

Extravasation management: Local pain, burning sensation, and irritation at the injection site may be relieved by local application of hot packs. If extravasation occurs, apply cold packs. Protect exposed tissue from light following extravasation.

Monitoring Parameters CBC with differential, liver function

Emetic Potential High (>90%)

Vesicant May be an irritant

High Dose Considerations

Comments Doses of 6591 mg/m^2 have been administered, although hypotension is considered the nonhematologic dose-limiting side effect for doses >3380 mg/m^2. Infusion-related hypotension may be secondary to calcium chelation by citric acid in formulation.

High Dose I.V.: 1-3 g/m^2; maximum dose as a single agent: 3.38 g/m^2; generally combined with other high-dose chemotherapeutic drugs.

Unique Toxicities

Cardiovascular: Hypotension (infusion-related)

Gastrointestinal: Severe nausea and vomiting

Dosage Forms Excipient information presented when available (limited, particularly for generics); consult specific product labeling.

Injection, powder for reconstitution: 100 mg, 200 mg

References

Berg SL, Grisell DL, DeLaney TF, et al, "Principles of Treatment of Pediatric Solid Tumors," *Pediatr Clin North Am*, 1991, 38(2):249-67.

Bonfante V, Santoro A, Viviani S, et al, "ABVD in the Treatment of Hodgkin's Disease," *Semin Oncol*, 1992, 19(2 Suppl 5):38-44.

Buesa JM and Urrechaga E, "Clinical Pharmacokinetics of High-Dose DTIC," *Cancer Chemother Pharmacol*, 1991, 28(6):475-9.

Eggermont AM and Kirkwood JM, "Re-Evaluating the Role of Dacarbazine in Metastatic Melanoma: What Have We Learned in 30 years?" *Eur J Cancer*, 2004, 40(12):1825-36.

Finklestein JZ, Albo V, Ertel I, et al, "5-(3,3-Dimethyl-l-triazeno) imidazole-4-carboxamide (NSC-45388) in the Treatment of Solid Tumors in Children," *Cancer Chemother Rep*, 1975, 59(2 Pt 1):351-7.

Keohan ML and Taub RN, "Chemotherapy for Advanced Sarcoma: Therapeutic Decisions and Modalities," *Semin Oncol*, 1997, 24(5):572-9.

Kintzel PE and Dorr RT, "Anticancer Drug Renal Toxicity and Elimination: Dosing Guidelines for Altered Renal Function," *Cancer Treat Rev*, 1995, 21(1):33-64.

Rusthoven JJ, Quirt IC, Iscoe NA, et al, "Randomized, Double-Blind, Placebo-Controlled Trial Comparing the Response Rates of Carmustine, Dacarbazine, and Cisplatin With and Without Tamoxifen in Patients With Metastatic Melanoma. National Cancer Institute of Canada Clinical Trials Group" *J Clin Oncol*, 1996, 14(7):2083-90.

Yuen AR and Horning SJ, "Hodgkin's Disease: Management of First Relapse," *Oncology*, 1996, 10 (2):233-40, 245.

Daclizumab (dac KLYE zue mab)

U.S. Brand Names Zenapax®

Generic Available No

Canadian Brand Names Zenapax®

Pharmacologic Category Immunosuppressant Agent

Use Part of an immunosuppressive regimen (including cyclosporine and corticosteroids) for the prophylaxis of acute organ rejection in patients receiving renal transplant

Unlabeled/Investigational Use Graft-versus-host disease; prevention of organ rejection after heart transplant

Pregnancy Risk Factor C

Lactation Excretion in breast milk unknown/use caution

Labeled Contraindications Hypersensitivity to daclizumab or any component of the formulation

Warnings/Precautions Patients on immunosuppressive therapy are at increased risk for infectious complications and secondary malignancies. Long-term effects of daclizumab on immune function are unknown. Severe hypersensitivity reactions have been rarely reported; anaphylaxis has been observed on initial exposure and following re-exposure; medications for the management of severe allergic reaction should be available for immediate use. Anti-idiotype antibodies have been measured in patients who have received daclizumab (adults 14%; children 34%); detection of antibodies may be influenced by multiple factors and may therefore be misleading.

In cardiac transplant patients, the combined use of daclizumab, cyclosporine, mycophenolate mofetil, and corticosteroids has been associated with an increased mortality. Higher mortality may be associated with the use of antilymphocyte globulin and a higher incidence of severe infections. **[U.S. Boxed Warning]: Should be administered under the supervision of a physician experienced in immunosuppressive therapy.**

Adverse Reactions Although reported adverse events are frequent, when daclizumab is compared with placebo the incidence of adverse effects is similar between the two groups. Many of the adverse effects reported during clinical trial use of daclizumab may be related to the patient population, transplant procedure, and concurrent transplant medications. Diarrhea, fever, postoperative pain, pruritus, respiratory tract infection, urinary tract infection, and vomiting occurred more often in children than adults.

≥5%:
Cardiovascular: Chest pain, edema, hyper-/hypotension, tachycardia, thrombosis
Central nervous system: Dizziness, fatigue, fever, headache, insomnia, pain, post-traumatic pain, tremor
Dermatologic: Acne, cellulitis, wound healing impaired
Gastrointestinal: Abdominal distention, abdominal pain, constipation, diarrhea, dyspepsia, epigastric pain, nausea, pyrosis, vomiting
Genitourinary: Dysuria
Hematologic: Bleeding
Neuromuscular & skeletal: Back pain, musculoskeletal pain
Renal: Oliguria, renal tubular necrosis
Respiratory: Cough, dyspnea, pulmonary edema
Miscellaneous: Lymphocele, wound infection
≥2% to <5%:
Central nervous system: Anxiety, depression, shivering
Dermatologic: Hirsutism, pruritus, rash
Endocrine & metabolic: Dehydration, diabetes mellitus, fluid overload
Gastrointestinal: Flatulence, gastritis, hemorrhoids
Genitourinary: Urinary retention, urinary tract bleeding
Local: Application site reaction
Neuromuscular & skeletal: Arthralgia, leg cramps, myalgia, weakness
Ocular: Vision blurred
Renal: Hydronephrosis, renal damage, renal insufficiency
Respiratory: Atelectasis, congestion, hypoxia, pharyngitis, pleural effusion, rales, rhinitis
Miscellaneous: Night sweats, prickly sensation, diaphoresis
<1%, postmarketing, and/or case reports: Severe hypersensitivity reactions (rare): Anaphylaxis, bronchospasm, cardiac arrest, cytokine release syndrome, hypotension, laryngeal edema, pulmonary edema, pruritus, urticaria

Drug Interactions
Avoid Concomitant Use
Avoid concomitant use of Daclizumab with any of the following: Natalizumab; Vaccines (Live)
Increased Effect/Toxicity
Daclizumab may increase the levels/effects of: Leflunomide; Natalizumab; Vaccines (Live)

The levels/effects of Daclizumab may be increased by: Trastuzumab

Decreased Effect

Daclizumab may decrease the levels/effects of: Vaccines (Inactivated); Vaccines (Live)

The levels/effects of Daclizumab may be decreased by: Echinacea

Storage/Stability Refrigerate vials at 2°C to 8°C (36°F to 46°F). Do not shake or freeze; protect undiluted solution against direct sunlight. Diluted solution is stable for 24 hours at 4°C or for 4 hours at room temperature.

Reconstitution Dose should be further diluted in 50 mL 0.9% sodium chloride solution. When mixing, gently invert bag to avoid foaming; do not shake. Do not use if solution is discolored.

Compatibility Do not mix with other medications or infuse other medications through same I.V. line.

Mechanism of Action Daclizumab is a chimeric (90% human, 10% murine) monoclonal IgG antibody produced by recombinant DNA technology. Daclizumab inhibits immune reactions by binding and blocking the alpha-chain of the interleukin-2 receptor (CD25) located on the surface of activated lymphocytes.

Pharmacodynamics/Kinetics

Distribution: V_d:

Adults: Central compartment: 0.031 L/kg; Peripheral compartment: 0.043 L/kg

Children: Central compartment: 0.067 L/kg; Peripheral compartment: 0.047 L/kg

Half-life elimination (estimated): Adults: Terminal: 20 days; Children: 13 days

Dosage Daclizumab is used adjunctively with other immunosuppressants (eg, cyclosporine, corticosteroids, mycophenolate mofetil, and azathioprine): I.V.:

Children: Use same weight-based dose as adults

Adults:

Immunoprophylaxis against acute renal allograft rejection: 1 mg/kg infused over 15 minutes within 24 hours before transplantation (day 0), then every 14 days for 4 additional doses

Treatment of graft-versus-host disease (unlabeled use, limited data): 0.5-1.5 mg/kg, repeat same dosage for transient response. Repeat doses have been administered 11-48 days following the initial dose.

Prevention of organ rejection after heart transplant (unlabeled use): 1 mg/kg up to a maximum of 100 mg; administer within 12 hours after heart transplant and on days 8, 22, 36, and 50 post-transplant

Dosage adjustment in renal impairment: No adjustment needed.

Dosage adjustment in hepatic impairment: No data available for patients with severe impairment.

Administration For I.V. administration following dilution. Daclizumab solution should be administered within 4 hours of preparation if stored at room temperature; infuse over a 15-minute period via a peripheral or central vein.

Dosage Forms Excipient information presented when available (limited, particularly for generics); consult specific product labeling.

Injection, solution [concentrate; preservative free]:

Zenapax® : 5 mg/mL (5 mL) [contains polysorbate 80]

References

Carswell CI, Plosker GL, and Wagstaff AJ, "Daclizumab: A Review of its Use in the Management of Organ Transplantation," *BioDrugs*, 2001, 15(11):745-73.

Hershberger RE, Starling RC, Eisen HJ, et al, "Daclizumab to Prevent Rejection After Cardiac Transplantation," *N Engl J Med*, 2005, 352(26):2705-13.

Vincenti F, Kirkman R, Light S, et al, "Interleukin-2-Receptor Blockade With Daclizumab to Prevent Acute Rejection in Renal Transplantation. Daclizumab Triple Therapy Study Group," *N Engl J Med*, 1998, 338(3):161-5.

◆ **Dacogen™** *see* Decitabine *on page 327*

◆ **DACT** *see* DACTINomycin *on page 299*

DACTINomycin (dak ti noe MYE sin)

Medication Safety Issues
Sound-alike/look-alike issues:
DACTINomycin may be confused with DAPTOmycin, DAUNOrubicin
Actinomycin may be confused with achromycin

High alert medication: The Institute for Safe Medication Practices (ISMP) includes this medication among its list of drug classes which have a heightened risk of causing significant patient harm when used in error.

Related Information
Management of Drug Extravasations *on page 1447*
Safe Handling of Hazardous Drugs *on page 1517*

U.S. Brand Names Cosmegen®

Index Terms ACT-D; Actinomycin; Actinomycin CI; Actinomycin D; DACT

Generic Available No

Canadian Brand Names Cosmegen®

Pharmacologic Category Antineoplastic Agent, Antibiotic

Use Treatment of Wilms' tumor, childhood rhabdomyosarcoma, Ewing's sarcoma, metastatic testicular tumors (nonseminomatous), gestational trophoblastic neoplasm; regional perfusion (palliative or adjunctive) of locally recurrent or locoregional solid tumors (sarcomas, carcinomas and adenocarcinomas)

Unlabeled/Investigational Use Treatment of ovarian cancer (germ cell or stromal tumors), osteosarcoma, soft tissue sarcoma (other than rhabdomyosarcoma)

Pregnancy Risk Factor D

Lactation Excretion in breast milk unknown/not recommended

Labeled Contraindications Hypersensitivity to dactinomycin or any component of the formulation; patients with concurrent or recent chickenpox or herpes zoster

Warnings/Precautions [U.S. Boxed Warnings]: Hazardous agent - use appropriate precautions for handling and disposal. Dactinomycin is extremely irritating to tissues; if extravasation occurs during I.V. use, severe damage to soft tissues will occur; has led to contracture of the arm (rare). Avoid inhalation of vapors or contact with skin, mucous membrane, or eyes; avoid exposure during pregnancy. Recommended for I.V. administration only. The manufacturer recommends intermittent ice (15 minutes 4 times/day) for suspected extravasation.

May cause veno-occlusive liver disease (VOD); use with caution in hepatobiliary dysfunction. Monitor for signs or symptoms of hepatic VOD, including bilirubin >1.4 mg/dL, unexplained weight gain, ascites, hepatomegaly, or unexplained right upper quadrant pain (Arndt, 2004). The risk of fatal VOD is increased in children <4 years of age.

Dactinomycin potentiates the effects of radiation therapy; use with caution in patients who have received radiation therapy; reduce dosages in patients who are receiving dactinomycin and radiation therapy simultaneously; combination with radiation therapy may result in increased GI toxicity and myelosuppression. Avoid dactinomycin use within 2 months of radiation treatment for right-sided Wilms' tumor, may increase the risk of hepatotoxicity.

Toxic effects may be delayed in onset (2-4 days following a course of treatment) and may require 1-2 weeks to reach maximum severity. Long-term observation of cancer survivors is recommended due to the increased risk of second primary tumors following treatment with radiation and antineoplastic agents. Regional perfusion therapy may result in local limb edema, soft tissue damage, and possible venous thrombosis; leakage of dactinomycin into systemic circulation may result in hematologic toxicity, infection, impaired wound healing, and mucositis. Dosage is usually expressed in **MICRO**grams and should be calculated on the basis of body surface area (BSA) in obese or edematous adult patients (to relate dose to lean body mass). Avoid administration of live vaccines during dactinomycin treatment. Avoid use in infants <6 months of age (toxic effects may occur more frequently). May be associated with an increased risk of myelosuppression in the elderly; use with caution. **[U.S. Boxed Warning]: Should be administered under the supervision of an experienced cancer chemotherapy physician.**

Adverse Reactions Frequency not defined.

Central nervous system: Fatigue, fever, lethargy, malaise

Dermatologic: Acne, alopecia (reversible), cheilitis; increased pigmentation, sloughing, or erythema of previously irradiated skin; skin eruptions

Endocrine & metabolic: Growth retardation, hyperuricemia, hypocalcemia

Gastrointestinal: Abdominal pain, anorexia, diarrhea, dysphagia, esophagitis, GI ulceration, mucositis, nausea, pharyngitis, proctitis, stomatitis, vomiting

Hematologic: Agranulocytosis, anemia, aplastic anemia, febrile neutropenia, leukopenia, neutropenia, pancytopenia, reticulocytopenia, thrombocytopenia, myelosuppression (onset: 7 days, nadir: 14-21 days, recovery: 21-28 days)

Hepatic: Ascites, bilirubin increased, hepatic failure, hepatitis, hepatomegaly, hepatopathy thrombocytopenia syndrome, hepatotoxicity, liver function test abnormality, veno-occlusive disease

Local: Erythema, edema, epidermolysis, pain, tissue necrosis, and ulceration (following extravasation)

Neuromuscular & skeletal: Myalgia

Renal: Renal function abnormality

Respiratory: Pneumonitis

Miscellaneous: Anaphylactoid reaction, infection

Drug Interactions

Avoid Concomitant Use

Avoid concomitant use of DACTINomycin with any of the following: Natalizumab; Vaccines (Live)

Increased Effect/Toxicity

DACTINomycin may increase the levels/effects of: Leflunomide; Natalizumab; Vaccines (Live)

The levels/effects of DACTINomycin may be increased by: Trastuzumab

Decreased Effect

DACTINomycin may decrease the levels/effects of: Vaccines (Inactivated); Vaccines (Live)

The levels/effects of DACTINomycin may be decreased by: Echinacea

Storage/Stability Store at controlled room temperature of 15°C to 30°C (59°F to 86°F). Protect from light and humidity. Reconstituted solutions retain potency for 24 hours at room temperature or refrigerated. Solutions in 50 mL D_5W are stable for 24 hours at room temperature.

Reconstitution Use appropriate precautions for handling and disposal. Dilute with 1.1 mL of preservative-free SWFI to yield a final concentration of 500 mcg/mL (diluent containing preservatives will cause precipitation). May further dilute in D_5W or NS. Cellulose ester membrane filters may partially remove dactinomycin from solution and should not be used during preparation or administration.

Compatibility Stable in D_5W, NS, SWFI.

Y-site administration: Compatible: Allopurinol, amifostine, aztreonam, cefepime, etoposide phosphate, fludarabine, gemcitabine, granisetron, melphalan, ondansetron, sargramostim, teniposide, thiotepa, vinorelbine. **Incompatible:** Filgrastim.

Compatibility when admixed: Compatible: Dacarbazine.

Mechanism of Action Binds to the guanine portion of DNA intercalating between guanine and cytosine base pairs inhibiting DNA and RNA synthesis and protein synthesis

Pharmacodynamics/Kinetics

Distribution: Children: Extensive extravascular distribution (59-714 L); does not penetrate blood brain barrier

Metabolism: Minimal

Half-life elimination: ~36 hours; Children: Range: 14-43 hours

Excretion: Urine and feces

Dosage Details concerning dosing in combination regimens should also be consulted.

Note: Medication orders for dactinomycin are commonly written in MICROgrams (eg, 150 mcg) although many regimens list the dose in MILLIgrams (eg, mg/kg or mg/m^2). One-time doses for >1000 mcg, or multiple-day doses for >500 mcg/day are not common. The dose intensity per 2-week cycle for adults and children should not exceed 15 mcg/kg/day for 5 days or 400-600 mcg/m^2/day for 5 days. Some practitioners recommend calculation of the dosage for obese or edematous adult patients on the basis of body surface area in an effort to relate dosage to lean body mass.

I.V.:

Children >6 months:

Usual dose: 15 mcg/kg/day for 5 days every 3-6 weeks **or** 400-600 mcg/m^2/day for 5 days every 3-6 weeks

Wilms' tumor, rhabdomyosarcoma, Ewing's sarcoma: 15 mcg/kg/day for 5 days (in various combination regimens and schedules)

Osteosarcoma (unlabeled use): 600 mcg/m^2/dose days 1, 2, and 3 as part of a combination chemotherapy regimen (Goorin, 2003)

Adults:

Usual doses: 15 mcg/kg/day for 5 days every 3-6 weeks **or** 400-600 mcg/m^2/day for 5 days every 3-6 weeks **or** 1000 mcg/m^2 on day 1 **or** 12 mcg/kg/day for 5 days (monotherapy) **or** 500 mcg/dose days 1 and 2 (as part of a combination chemotherapy regimen)

Testicular cancer: 1000 mcg/m^2 on day 1 (as part of a combination chemotherapy regimen)

Gestational trophoblastic neoplasm: 12 mcg/kg/day for 5 days (monotherapy) **or** 500 mcg/dose days 1 and 2 (as part of a combination chemotherapy regimen)

Wilms' tumor, Ewing's sarcoma, rhabdomyosarcoma: 15 mcg/kg/day for 5 days (in various combination regimens and schedules)

Osteosarcoma (unlabeled use): 600 mcg/m^2/dose days 1, 2, and 3 as part of a combination chemotherapy regimen (Goorin, 2003)

Ovarian (germ cell) tumor (unlabeled use): 500 mcg/day for 5 days every 4 weeks (Gershenson, 1985) **or** 300 mcg/m^2/day for 5 days every 4 weeks (Slayton,1985)

Regional perfusion: Adults (dosages and techniques may vary by institution; obese patients and patients with prior chemotherapy or radiation therapy may require lower doses): Lower extremity or pelvis: 50 mcg/kg; Upper extremity: 35 mcg/kg

Elderly: Elderly patients are at increased risk of myelosuppression; dosing should begin at the low end of the dosing range.

Dosage adjustment in renal impairment: No adjustment required

Combination Regimens

Gestational trophoblastic tumor:

CHAMOCA (Modified Bagshawe Regimen) on page 1259

CHAMOMA (Bagshawe Regimen) on page 1261

EMA/CO on page 1301

EP/EMA on page 1304

Osteosarcoma: POG-8651 on page 1396

Ovarian cancer: Vincristine-Dactinomycin-Cyclophosphamide (Ovarian Cancer) on page 1421

Rhabdomyosarcoma:

VAC Pulse on page 1417

VAC (Rhabdomyosarcoma) on page 1417

Sarcoma: VAC Alternating With IE (Ewing's Sarcoma) on page 1416

Wilms' tumor:

AAV (DD) on page 1222

AV (EE) on page 1228

AV (K) on page 1228

AV (L) on page 1228

AV (Wilms' Tumor) on page 1228

AVD on page 1227

EE on page 1299

EE-4A on page 1299

VDA-C (Wilms' Tumor) on page 1420

Administration I.V.: Administer by slow I.V. push or infuse over 10-15 minutes. Avoid extravasation. Do not filter with cellulose ester membrane filters. Do not administer I.M. or SubQ.

Monitoring Parameters CBC with differential and platelet count, liver function tests, and renal function tests; monitor for signs/symptoms of hepatic VOD, including unexplained weight gain, ascites, hepatomegaly, or unexplained right upper quadrant pain (Arndt, 2004)

Test Interactions May interfere with bioassays of antibacterial drug levels

Emetic Potential Moderate (30% to 90%)

Vesicant Yes; see Management of Drug Extravasations on page 1447.

Dosage Forms Excipient information presented when available (limited, particularly of generics); consult specific product labeling.

Injection, powder for reconstitution:

Cosmegen®: 0.5 mg [contains mannitol 20 mg]

References

Arndt C, Hawkins, D, Anderson JR, et a;, "Age is a Risk Factor for Chemotherapy-Induced Hepatopathy With Vincristine, Dactinomycin and Cyclophosphamide," *J Clin Oncol*, 2004, 22 (10):1894-901.

Bagshawe KD, "High-Risk Metastatic Trophoblastic Disease," *Obstet Gynecol Clin North Am*, 1988, 15(3):531-43.

Berkowitz RS and Goldstein DP, "Gestational Trophoblastic Disease," *Cancer*, 1995, 76(10 Suppl):2079-85.

Carli M, Pastore G, Perilongo G, et al, "Tumor Response and Toxicity After Single High-Dose Versus Standard Five-Day Divided Dose Dactinomycin in Childhood Rhabdomyosarcoma," *J Clin Oncol*, 1988, 6(4):654-8.

Czauderna P, Katski K, Kowalczyk J, et al, "Venoocclusive Liver Disease (VOD) as a Complication of Wilms' Tumour Management in the Series of Consecutive 206 Patients," *Eur J Pediatr Surg*, 2000, 10(5):300-3.

D'Antiga L, Baker A, Pritchard J. et al, "Veno-Occlusive Disease With Multi-Organ Involvement Following Actinomycin-D," *Eur J Cancer*, 2001, 37(9):1141-8.

Gershenson DM, Copeland LJ, Kavanagh JJ, et al, "Treatment of Malignant Nondysgerminomatous Germ Cell Tumors of the Ovary With Vincristine, Dactinomycin, and Cyclophosphamide," *Cancer*, 1985, 56(12):2756-61.

Goorin AM, Schwartzentruber DJ, Devidas M, et al, "Presurgical Chemotherapy Compared With Immediate Surgery and Adjuvant Chemotherapy for Nonmetastatic Osteosarcoma: Pediatric Oncology Group Study POG-8651," *J Clin Oncol*, 2003, 21(8):1574-80.

Slayton RE, Park RC, Silverberg SG, et al, "Vincristine, Dactinomycin, and Cyclophosphamide in the Treatment of Malignant Germ Cell Tumors of the Ovary. A Gynecologic Oncology Group Study (A Final Report)," *Cancer*, 1985, 56(2):243-8.

Sulis ML, Bessmertny O, Granowetter L, et al, "Veno-Occlusive Disease in Pediatric Patients Receiving Actinomycin D and Vincristine Only for the Treatment of Rhabdomyosarcoma, *J Pediatr Hematol Oncol*, 2004, 26(12):843-6.

Veal GJ, Cole M, Errington J, et al, "Pharmacokinetics of Dactinomycin in a Pediatric Patient Population: A United Kingdom Children's Cancer Study Group Study," *Clin Cancer Res*, 2005, 11 (16):5893-9.

Dalteparin (dal TE pa rin)

Medication Safety Issues

High alert medication: The Institute for Safe Medication Practices (ISMP) includes this medication among its list of drugs which have a heightened risk of causing significant patient harm when used in error.

2009 National Patient Safety Goals: The Joint Commission on Accreditation of Healthcare Organizations requires healthcare organizations that provide anticoagulant therapy to have a process in place to reduce the risk of anticoagulant-associated patient harm. Patients receiving anticoagulants should receive individualized care through a defined process that includes standardized ordering, dispensing, administration, monitoring and education. This does not apply to routine short-term use of anticoagulants for prevention of venous thromboembolism when the expectation is that the patient's laboratory values will remain within or close to normal values (NPSG.03.05.01).

U.S. Brand Names Fragmin®

Index Terms Dalteparin Sodium; NSC-714371

Generic Available No

Canadian Brand Names Fragmin®

Pharmacologic Category Low Molecular Weight Heparin

Use Prevention of deep vein thrombosis which may lead to pulmonary embolism, in patients requiring abdominal surgery who are at risk for thromboembolism complications (eg, patients >40 years of age, obesity, patients with malignancy, history of deep vein thrombosis or pulmonary embolism, and surgical procedures requiring general anesthesia and lasting >30 minutes); prevention of DVT in patients undergoing hip-replacement surgery; patients immobile during an acute illness; acute treatment of unstable angina or non-Q-wave myocardial infarction; prevention of ischemic complications in patients on concurrent aspirin therapy; in patients with cancer, extended treatment (6 months) of acute symptomatic venous thromboembolism (DVT and/or PE) to reduce the recurrence of venous thromboembolism

Unlabeled/Investigational Use Active treatment of deep vein thrombosis (noncancer patients)

Pregnancy Risk Factor B

Lactation Enters breast milk/use caution

Labeled Contraindications Hypersensitivity to dalteparin or any component of the formulation; thrombocytopenia associated with a positive *in vitro* test for antiplatelet antibodies in the presence of dalteparin; hypersensitivity to heparin or pork products; patients with active major bleeding; patients with unstable angina, non-Q-wave MI, or acute venous thromboembolism undergoing regional anesthesia; not for I.M. or I.V. use

Warnings/Precautions [U.S. Boxed Warning]: Patients with recent or anticipated neuraxial anesthesia (epidural or spinal anesthesia) are at risk of spinal or epidural hematoma and subsequent paralysis. Consider risk versus benefit prior to neuraxial anesthesia. Risk is increased by concomitant agents which may alter hemostasis, as well as traumatic or repeated epidural or spinal puncture. Patient should be observed closely for bleeding if dalteparin is administered during or immediately following diagnostic lumbar puncture, epidural anesthesia, or spinal anesthesia.

Use with caution in patients with pre-existing thrombocytopenia, recent childbirth, subacute bacterial endocarditis, peptic ulcer disease, pericarditis or pericardial effusion, liver or renal function impairment, recent lumbar puncture, vasculitis, concurrent use of aspirin (increased bleeding risk), previous hypersensitivity to heparin, heparin-associated thrombocytopenia. Monitor platelet count closely. Rare thrombocytopenia may occur. Consider discontinuation of dalteparin in any patient developing significant thrombocytopenia related to initiation of dalteparin. Rare cases of thrombocytopenia with thrombosis have occurred. Use caution in patients with congenital or drug-induced thrombocytopenia or platelet defects. Cancer patients with thrombocytopenia may require dose adjustments for treatment of acute venous thromboembolism.

Use with caution in patients with known hypersensitivity to methylparaben and propylparaben. Monitor patient closely for signs or symptoms of bleeding. Certain patients are at increased risk of bleeding. Risk factors include bacterial endocarditis; congenital or acquired bleeding disorders; active ulcerative or angiodysplastic GI diseases; severe uncontrolled hypertension; hemorrhagic stroke; or use shortly after brain, spinal, or ophthalmology surgery; in patient treated concomitantly with platelet inhibitors; recent GI bleeding; thrombocytopenia or platelet defects; severe liver disease; hypertensive or diabetic retinopathy; or in patients undergoing invasive procedures.

Use with caution in patients with severe renal failure (has not been studied). Safety and efficacy in pediatric patients have not been established. Rare cases of thrombocytopenia with thrombosis have occurred. Multidose vials contain benzyl alcohol and should not be used in pregnant women. In neonates, large amounts of benzyl alcohol (>100 mg/kg/day) have been associated with fatal toxicity (gasping syndrome). Heparin can cause hyperkalemia by affecting aldosterone. Similar reactions could occur with dalteparin. Monitor for hyperkalemia. Do **not** administer intramuscularly. Not to be used interchangeably (unit for unit) with heparin or any other low molecular weight heparins.

There is no consensus for adjusting/correcting the weight-based dosage of LMWH for patients who are morbidly obese (BMI ≥40 kg/m^2). For patients undergoing inpatient bariatric surgery, the American College of Chest Physicians Practice Guidelines suggest using a higher thromboprophylaxis dose of LMWH for obese patients (Geerts, 2008).

Adverse Reactions

Note: As with all anticoagulants, bleeding is the major adverse effect of dalteparin. Hemorrhage may occur at virtually any site. Risk is dependent on multiple variables.

>10%:

Hematologic: Bleeding (3% to 14%)

1% to 10%:

Hematologic: Wound hematoma (up to 3%)

Hepatic: AST >3 times upper limit of normal (5% to 9%), ALT >3 times upper limit of normal (4% to 10%)

Local: Pain at injection site (up to 12%), injection site hematoma (up to 7%)

<1% (Limited to important or life-threatening): Thrombocytopenia (including heparin-induced thrombocytopenia), allergic reaction (fever, pruritus, rash, injections site reaction, bullous eruption), alopecia, anaphylactoid reaction, operative site bleeding, gastrointestinal bleeding, hemoptysis, skin necrosis, subdural hematoma, thrombosis (associated with heparin-induced thrombocytopenia). Spinal or epidural hematomas can occur following neuraxial anesthesia or spinal puncture, resulting in paralysis.

Drug Interactions

Avoid Concomitant Use There are no known interactions where it is recommended to avoid concomitant use.

Increased Effect/Toxicity

Dalteparin may increase the levels/effects of: Anticoagulants; Drotrecogin Alfa; Ibritumomab; Tositumomab and Iodine I 131 Tositumomab

The levels/effects of Dalteparin may be increased by: Antiplatelet Agents; Dasatinib; Herbs (Anticoagulant/Antiplatelet Properties); Nonsteroidal Anti-Inflammatory Agents; Pentosan Polysulfate Sodium; Pentoxifylline; Prostacyclin Analogues; Salicylates; Thrombolytic Agents

Decreased Effect There are no known significant interactions involving a decrease in effect.

Ethanol/Nutrition/Herb Interactions Herb/Nutraceutical: Alfalfa, anise, bilberry, bladderwrack, bromelain, cat's claw, celery, chamomile, coleus, cordyceps, dong quai, evening primrose oil, fenugreek, feverfew, garlic, ginger, ginkgo biloba, Ginseng (american), Ginseng (panax), Ginseng (siberian), grapeseed, green tea, guggul, horse chestnut seed, horseradish, licorice, prickly ash, red clover, reishi, SAMe (s-adenosylmethionine), sweet clover, turmeric, white willow (all have additional antiplatelet/anticoagulant activity)

Storage/Stability Store at temperatures of 20°C to 25°C (68°F to 77°F). Multidose vials may be stored for up to 2 weeks at room temperature after entering.

Mechanism of Action Low molecular weight heparin analog with a molecular weight of 4000-6000 daltons; the commercial product contains 3% to 15% heparin with a molecular weight <3000 daltons, 65% to 78% with a molecular weight of 3000-8000 daltons and 14% to 26% with a molecular weight >8000 daltons; while dalteparin has been shown to inhibit both factor Xa and factor IIa (thrombin), the antithrombotic effect of dalteparin is characterized by a higher ratio of antifactor Xa to antifactor IIa activity (ratio = 4)

◄ **Pharmacodynamics/Kinetics**
Onset of action: 1-2 hours
Duration: >12 hours
Distribution: V_d: 40-60 mL/kg
Bioavailability: SubQ: 81% to 93%
Half-life elimination (route dependent): 2-5 hours
Time to peak, serum: 4 hours

Dosage Adults: SubQ:
Abdominal surgery:
Low-to-moderate DVT risk: 2500 int. units 1-2 hours prior to surgery, then once daily for 5-10 days postoperatively
High DVT risk: 5000 int. units the evening prior to surgery and then once daily for 5-10 days postoperatively. Alternatively in patients with malignancy: 2500 int. units 1-2 hours prior to surgery, 2500 int. units 12 hours later, then 5000 int. units once daily for 5-10 days postoperatively.

Patients undergoing total hip surgery: **Note:** Three treatment options are currently available. Dose is given for 5-10 days, although up to 14 days of treatment have been tolerated in clinical trials:
Postoperative start:
Initial: 2500 int. units 4-8 hours* after surgery
Maintenance: 5000 int. units once daily; start at least 6 hours after postsurgical dose
Preoperative (starting day of surgery):
Initial: 2500 int. units within 2 hours before surgery
Adjustment: 2500 int. units 4-8 hours* after surgery
Maintenance: 5000 int. units once daily; start at least 6 hours after postsurgical dose
Preoperative (starting evening prior to surgery):
Initial: 5000 int. units 10-14 hours before surgery
Adjustment: 5000 int. units 4-8 hours* after surgery
Maintenance: 5000 int. units once daily, allowing 24 hours between doses.
*Dose may be delayed if hemostasis is not yet achieved.

Unstable angina or non-Q-wave myocardial infarction: 120 int. units/kg body weight (maximum dose: 10,000 int. units) every 12 hours for 5-8 days with concurrent aspirin therapy. Discontinue dalteparin once patient is clinically stable.

Venous thromboembolism: Cancer patients:
Initial (month 1): 200 int. units/kg (maximum dose: 18,000 int. units) once daily for 30 days
Maintenance (months 2-6): ~150 int. units/kg (maximum dose: 18,000 int. units) once daily. If platelet count between 50,000-100,000/mm^3, reduce dose by 2,500 int. units until platelet count recovers to ≥100,000/mm^3. If platelet count <50,000/mm^3, discontinue dalteparin until platelet count recover to >50,000/mm^3.

Immobility during acute illness: 5000 int. units once daily

Dosing adjustment in renal impairment: Half-life is increased in patients with chronic renal failure, use with caution, accumulation can be expected; specific dosage adjustments have not been recommended. In cancer patients, receiving treatment for venous thromboembolism, if Cl_{cr} <30 mL/minute, manufacturer recommends monitoring anti-Xa levels to determine appropriate dose.

Dosing adjustment in hepatic impairment: Use with caution in patients with hepatic insufficiency; specific dosage adjustments have not been recommended

Administration Do **not** administer I.M.; for deep SubQ injection only. May be injected in a U-shape to the area surrounding the navel, the upper outer side of the thigh, or the upper outer quadrangle of the buttock. Use thumb and forefinger to lift a fold of skin when injecting dalteparin to the navel area or thigh. Insert needle at a 45- to 90-degree angle. The entire length of needle should be inserted. Do not expel air bubble from fixed-dose syringe prior to injection. Air bubble (and extra solution, if applicable) may be expelled from graduated syringes. In order to minimize bruising, do not rub injection site.

To convert from I.V. unfractionated heparin (UFH) infusion to SubQ dalteparin (Nutescu, 2007): Calculate specific dose for dalteparin based on indication, discontinue UFH and begin dalteparin within 1 hour

To convert from SubQ dalteparin to I.V. UFH infusion (Nutescu, 2007): Discontinue dalteparin; calculate specific dose for I.V. UFH infusion based on indication; omit heparin bolus/loading dose
Converting from SubQ dalteparin dosed every 12 hours: Start I.V. UFH infusion 10-11 hours after last dose of dalteparin
Converting from SubQ dalteparin dosed every 24 hours: Start I.V. UFH infusion 22-23 hours after last dose of dalteparin

Monitoring Parameters Periodic CBC including platelet count; stool occult blood tests; monitoring of PT and PTT is not necessary. Once patient has received 3-4 doses, anti-Xa levels, drawn 4-6 hours after dalteparin administration, may be used to monitor effect in patients with severe renal dysfunction or if abnormal coagulation parameters or bleeding should occur.

Additional Information Multidose vial contains 14 mg/mL benzyl alcohol.

Dosage Forms Excipient information presented when available (limited, particularly for generics); consult specific product labeling.
Injection, solution:
Fragmin®: Antifactor Xa 10,000 int. units per 1 mL (9.5 mL) [contains benzyl alcohol]; antifactor Xa 25,000 units per 1 mL (3.8 mL) [contains benzyl alcohol]
Injection, solution [preservative free]:
Fragmin®: Antifactor Xa 2500 int. units per 0.2 mL (0.2 mL); antifactor Xa 5000 int. units per 0.2 mL (0.2 mL); antifactor Xa 7500 int. units per 0.3 mL (0.3 mL); antifactor Xa 10,000 int. units per 1 mL (1 mL); antifactor Xa 12,500 int. units per 0.5 mL (0.5 mL); antifactor Xa 15,000 int. units per 0.6 mL (0.6 mL); antifactor Xa 18,000 int. units per 0.72 mL (0.72 mL)

References
Geerts WH, Bergqvist D, Pineo GF, et al, "Prevention of Venous Thromboembolism: American College of Chest Physicians Evidence-Based Clinical Practice Guidelines (8th Edition)," *Chest*, 2008, 133(6 Suppl):381S-453S.

Lee AY, Levine MN, Baker RI, et al, "Low-Molecular-Weight Heparin Versus a Coumarin for the Prevention of Recurrent Venous Thromboembolism in Patients with Cancer," *N Engl J Med*, 2003, 349(2):146-53.

Lee AY, Rickels FR, Julian JA, et al, "Randomized Comparison of Low Molecular Weight Heparin and Coumarin Derivatives on the Survival of Patients With Cancer and Venous Thromboembolism," *J Clin Oncol*, 2005, 23(10):2123-9.

Mechanick JI, Kushner RF, Sugerman HJ, et al, "American Association of Clinical Endocrinologists, The Obesity Society, and American Society for Metabolic & Bariatric Surgery Medical Guidelines for Clinical Practice for the Perioperative Nutritional, Metabolic, and Nonsurgical Support of the Bariatric Surgery Patient," *Obesity*, 2009, 17(Suppl 1):1-70.

Nagge J, Crowther M, and Hirsh J, "Is Impaired Renal Function a Contraindication to the Use of Low-Molecular Weight Heparin?" *Arch Intern Med*, 2002, 162(22):2605-9.

Nutescu EA, Spinler SA, Wittkowsky A, et al, "Low-Molecular-Weight Heparins in Renal Impairment and Obesity: Available Evidence and Clinical Practice Recommendations Across Medical and Surgical Settings," *Ann Pharmacother*, 2009, 43(6):1064-83.

◆ **Dalteparin Sodium** *see* Dalteparin *on page 303*

Darbepoetin Alfa (dar be POE e tin AL fa)

Medication Safety Issues

Sound-alike/look-alike issues:

Aranesp® may be confused with Aralast, Aricept®

Darbepoetin alfa may be confused with dalteparin, epoetin alfa, epoetin beta

U.S. Brand Names Aranesp®

Index Terms Erythropoiesis-Stimulating Agent (ESA); Erythropoiesis-Stimulating Protein; NSC-729969

Generic Available No

Canadian Brand Names Aranesp®

Pharmacologic Category Colony Stimulating Factor; Growth Factor; Recombinant Human Erythropoietin

Use Treatment of anemia (elevate/maintain red blood cell level and decrease the need for transfusions) associated with chronic renal failure (including patients on dialysis and not on dialysis); treatment of anemia due to concurrent chemotherapy in patients with metastatic cancer (nonmyeloid malignancies)

Note: Darbepoetin is **not** indicated for use in cancer patients under the following conditions:
- receiving hormonal therapy, therapeutic biologic products, or radiation therapy unless also receiving concurrent myelosuppressive chemotherapy
- receiving myelosuppressive therapy when the expected outcome is curative

Unlabeled/Investigational Use Treatment of symptomatic anemia in myelodysplastic syndrome (MDS)

Pregnancy Risk Factor C

Lactation Excretion in breast milk unknown/use caution

Labeled Contraindications Hypersensitivity to darbepoetin or any component of the formulation; uncontrolled hypertension

Warnings/Precautions [U.S. Boxed Warning]: ESAs increased the risk of serious cardiovascular events, thromboembolic events, mortality, and/or tumor progression in clinical studies; a rapid rise in hemoglobin (>1 g/dL over 2 weeks) or maintaining higher hemoglobin levels may contribute to these risks. **[U.S. Boxed Warning]: A shortened overall survival and/or increased risk of tumor progression or recurrence has been reported in studies with breast,cervical, head and neck, lymphoid, and non small cell lung cancer patients.** It is of note that in these studies, patients received ESAs to a target hemoglobin of ≥12 g/dL; although risk has not been excluded when dosed to achieve a target hemoglobin of <12 g/dL. **[U.S. Boxed Warnings]: To decrease these risks, and risk of cardio- and thrombovascular events, use ESAs in cancer patients only for the treatment of anemia related to concurrent chemotherapy and use the lowest dose needed to avoid red blood cell transfusions. Discontinue ESA following completion of the chemotherapy course. ESAs are <u>not</u> indicated for patients receiving myelosuppressive therapy when the anticipated outcome is curative. [U.S. Boxed Warning]: An increased risk of death and serious cardiovascular events was reported in chronic renal failure patients administered ESAs to target higher versus lower hemoglobin levels (13.5 vs 11.3 g/dL; 14 vs 10 g/dL) in two clinical studies; dosing should be individualized to achieve and maintain hemoglobin levels within 10-12 g/dL range.** Hemoglobin rising >1 g/dL in a 2-week period may contribute to the risk. Chronic renal failure patients who exhibit an inadequate hemoglobin response to ESA therapy may be at a higher risk for cardiovascular events and mortality compared to other patients. ESA therapy may reduce dialysis efficacy (due to increase in red blood cells and decrease in plasma volume); adjustments in dialysis parameters may be needed. An increased risk of DVT has been observed in patients treated with epoetin undergoing surgical orthopedic procedures. Darbepoetin is **not** approved for reduction in red blood cell transfusions in patients scheduled for surgical procedures. During therapy in any patient, hemoglobin levels should not exceed a target range of 10-12 g/dL and should not rise >1 g/dL per 2-week time period.

Use with caution in patients with hypertension or with a history of seizures; hypertensive encephalopathy and seizures have been reported. If hypertension is difficult to control, reduce or hold darbepoetin alfa. **Not** recommended for acute correction of severe anemia or as a substitute for transfusion. Consider discontinuing in patients who receive a renal transplant.

Prior to treatment, correct or exclude deficiencies of iron, vitamin B_{12}, and/or folate, as well as other factors which may impair erythropoiesis (aluminum toxicity, inflammatory conditions, infections). Prior to and during therapy, iron stores must be evaluated. Supplemental iron is recommended if serum ferritin <100 mcg/L or serum transferrin saturation <20%. Poor response should prompt evaluation of these potential factors, as well as possible malignant processes, occult blood loss, hemolysis, and/or bone marrow fibrosis. Severe anemia and pure red cell aplasia (PRCA) with associated neutralizing antibodies to erythropoietin has been reported, predominantly in patients with CRF receiving SubQ darbepoetin (the I.V. route is preferred for hemodialysis patients). Patients with loss of response to darbepoetin should be evaluated; discontinue treatment in patients with PRCA secondary to neutralizing antibodies to erythropoietin. Antibodies may cross-react; do not switch to another ESA in patients who develop antibody-mediated anemia.

Due to the delayed onset of erythropoiesis, darbepoetin is of no value in the acute treatment of anemia. Safety and efficacy in patients with underlying hematologic diseases have not been established, including porphyria, thalassemia, hemolytic anemia, and sickle cell disease. Potentially serious allergic reactions have been reported. Some products may contain albumin and the packaging of some formulations may contain latex. Safety and efficacy in children with cancer have not been established; children >1 year of age with CRF have been converted from epoetin alfa to darbepoetin.

Adverse Reactions

>10%:
  Cardiovascular: Edema (21%), hypertension (4% to 20%), hypotension (20%)
  Central nervous system: Fatigue (9% to 33%), fever (4% to 19%), headache (12% to 16%), dizziness (7% to 14%)
  Gastrointestinal: Diarrhea (14% to 22%), constipation (5% to 18%), vomiting (2% to 14%), nausea (11%)
  Neuromuscular & skeletal: Muscle spasm (17%), arthralgia (9% to 13%)
  Respiratory: Upper respiratory infection (15%)
  Miscellaneous: Infection (24%)
1% to 10%:
  Cardiovascular: Peripheral edema (10%), arrhythmia/arrest (8%), angina/chest pain (7% to 8%), fluid overload (6%), thrombosis (6%), CHF (5%), MI (2%)
  Central nervous system: Stroke (2%), seizure (≤1%), TIA (≤1%)
  Dermatologic: Rash (7%), pruritus (6%)
  Endocrine & metabolic: Dehydration (3% to 5%)
  Gastrointestinal: Abdominal pain (10%)

Local: Vascular access hemorrhage (7%), injection site pain (6%), vascular access infection (6%), vascular access thrombosis (6%)

Neuromuscular & skeletal: Limb pain (8%), myalgia (8%), back pain (7%), weakness (5%)

Respiratory: Dyspnea (2% to 10%), cough (9%), bronchitis (5%), pneumonia (3%), pulmonary embolism (1%)

Miscellaneous: Death (7% to 10 %; similar to placebo), flu-like syndrome (6%)

<1%, postmarketing, and/or case reports: Abscess, allergic reaction, bacteremia, deep vein thrombosis, GI hemorrhage, hypertensive encephalopathy, peritonitis, pure red cell aplasia (PRCA), sepsis, severe anemia (with or without other cytopenias), thromboembolism, thrombophlebitis, thrombosis, tumor progression (cancer patients)

Drug Interactions

Avoid Concomitant Use There are no known interactions where it is recommended to avoid concomitant use.

Increased Effect/Toxicity There are no known significant interactions involving an increase in effect.

Decreased Effect There are no known significant interactions involving a decrease in effect.

Ethanol/Nutrition/Herb Interactions Ethanol: Should be avoided due to adverse effects on erythropoiesis.

Storage/Stability Store at 2°C to 8°C (36°F to 46°F); do not freeze. Do not shake. Protect from light.

Compatibility Do not dilute or administer with other solutions.

Mechanism of Action Induces erythropoiesis by stimulating the division and differentiation of committed erythroid progenitor cells; induces the release of reticulocytes from the bone marrow into the bloodstream, where they mature to erythrocytes. There is a dose response relationship with this effect. This results in an increase in reticulocyte counts followed by a rise in hematocrit and hemoglobin levels. When administered SubQ or I.V., darbepoetin's half-life is ~3 times that of epoetin alfa concentrations.

Pharmacodynamics/Kinetics

Onset of action: Increased hemoglobin levels not generally observed until 2-6 weeks after initiating treatment

Absorption: SubQ: Slow

Distribution: V_d: 0.06 L/kg

Bioavailability: CRF: SubQ: Adults: ~37% (range: 30% to 50%); Children: 54% (range: 32% to 70%)

Half-life elimination:

CRF: Adults:

I.V.: 21 hours

SubQ: Nondialysis patients: 70 hours (range: 35-139 hours); Dialysis patients: 46 hours (range: 12-89 hours)

Cancer: Adults: SubQ: 74 hours (range: 24-144 hours); Children: 49 hours

Note: Darbepoetin half-life is approximately threefold longer than epoetin alfa following I.V. administration

Time to peak: SubQ:

CRF: Adults: 48 hours (range: 12-72 hours; independent of dialysis); Children: 36 hours (range: 10-58 hours)

Cancer: Adults: 71-90 hours (range: 28-123 hours); Children: 71 hours (range: 21-143 hours)

Dosage Note: Hemoglobin levels should not exceed 12 g/dL and should not rise >1 g/dL per 2-week time period during therapy in any patient.

Anemia associated with CRF: Individualize dosing to achieve and maintain hemoglobin levels at a target range of 10-12 g/dL. Hemoglobin levels should not exceed 12 g/dL. **Note:** I.V. route is preferred in hemodialysis patients.

Children ≥1 year: Conversion from epoetin alfa: I.V., SubQ: Initial dose: Epoetin alfa doses of 1500 to ≥90,000 units per week may be converted to doses ranging from 6.25-200 mcg darbepoetin alfa per week (see pediatric column in conversion table on next page).

Children 11-18 years: Initial treatment (unlabeled use): I.V., SubQ: Initial dose: 0.45 mcg/kg once weekly; titrate to hemoglobin response

Adults: I.V., SubQ: Initial: 0.45 mcg/kg once weekly; alternative dose for nondialysis patients: 0.75 mcg/kg once every 2 weeks; Maintenance: titrate to maintain hemoglobin levels between 10-12 g/dL as described below (may be administered once weekly or every 2 weeks; nondialysis patients may require lower maintenance doses)

Dosage adjustment:

Decrease dose by ~25%: If hemoglobin approaches 12 g/dL **or** hemoglobin increases >1 g/dL in any 2-week period. If hemoglobin continues to increase, temporarily discontinue therapy until hemoglobin begins to decrease, then resume therapy with a ~25% reduction from previous dose.

Increase dose by ~25%: If hemoglobin does not increase by 1 g/dL after 4 weeks of therapy (with adequate iron stores). Do not increase dose more frequently than at 4-week intervals.

Inadequate or lack of response: If patient does not attain target hemoglobin range of 10-12 g/dL after appropriate dose titrations over 12 weeks:

Do not continue to increase dose and use the minimum effective dose that will maintain a hemoglobin level sufficient to avoid red blood cell transfusions **and** evaluate patient for other causes of anemia.

Monitor hemoglobin closely thereafter, and if responsiveness improves, may resume making dosage adjustments as recommended above. If responsiveness does not improve and recurrent red blood cell transfusions continue to be needed, discontinue therapy.

Maintenance dose: Individualize to target hemoglobin range of 10-12 g/dL; limit additional dosage increase to every 4 weeks or longer. Patients generally require lower maintenance doses than initial doses to maintain target range.

Conversion from epoetin alfa: I.V., SubQ: Initial dose: Epoetin alfa doses may be converted to doses ranging from 6.25-200 mcg darbepoetin alfa per week (see conversion table on next page).

Anemia associated with chemotherapy: Titrate dosage to use the minimum effective dose that will maintain a hemoglobin level sufficient to avoid red blood cell transfusions. Do not initiate therapy if hemoglobin ≥10 g/dL. Discontinue darbepoetin following completion of chemotherapy.

Children (unlabeled use): SubQ: 2.25 mcg/kg once weekly

Adults: SubQ: Initial: 2.25 mcg/kg once weekly **or** 500 mcg once every 3 weeks

Dosage adjustment:

Increase dose: If hemoglobin does not increase by 1 g/dL after 6 weeks of therapy (for patients receiving weekly therapy), the dose should be increased up to 4.5 mcg/kg once weekly.

Decrease dose by 40%: If hemoglobin increases >1 g/dL in any 2-week period **or** hemoglobin reaches a level sufficient to avoid red blood cell transfusion.

Withhold dose: If hemoglobin exceeds a level needed to avoid red blood cell transfusion. Resume treatment with a dose 40% below the previous dose when hemoglobin approaches a level where transfusions may be required.

Discontinue: On completion of chemotherapy or if after 8 weeks of therapy there is no hemoglobin response or transfusions still required

Anemia associated with MDS (unlabeled use): Adults: SubQ: 150-300 mcg once weekly

Conversion from epoetin alfa to darbepoetin alfa: See table.

Conversion From Epoetin Alfa to Darbepoetin Alfa (Initial Dose)

Previous Dosage of Epoetin Alfa (units/week)	Children Darbepoetin Alfa Dosage (mcg/week)	Adults Darbepoetin Alfa Dosage (mcg/week)
<1500	Not established	6.25
1500-2499	6.25	6.25
2500-4999	10	12.5
5000-10,999	20	25
11,000-17,999	40	40
18,000-33,999	60	60
34,000-89,999	100	100
≥90,000	200	200

Note: In patients receiving epoetin alfa 2-3 times per week, darbepoetin alfa is administered once weekly. In patients receiving epoetin alfa once weekly, darbepoetin alfa is administered once every 2 weeks. The darbepoetin dose to be administered every 2 weeks is derived by adding together 2 weekly epoetin alfa doses and then converting to the appropriate darbepoetin dose. Titrate dose to hemoglobin response thereafter (see dosage adjustment in renal impairment).

Dosage adjustment in renal impairment: Dosage requirements for patients with chronic renal failure who do not require dialysis may be lower than in dialysis patients. Monitor patients closely during the time period in which a dialysis regimen is initiated, dosage requirement may increase. The National Kidney Foundation Clinical Practice Guidelines for Anemia in Chronic Kidney Disease: 2007 Update of Hemoglobin Target (September, 2007) recommend hemoglobin levels in the range of 11-12 g/dL for dialysis and nondialysis patients receiving ESAs; hemoglobin levels should not be maintained >13 g/dL.

Hemodialysis: I.V. route is preferred in hemodialysis patients.

Administration May be administered by SubQ or I.V. injection. The I.V. route is recommended in hemodialysis patients. Do not shake; vigorous shaking may denature darbepoetin alfa, rendering it biologically inactive. Do not dilute or administer in conjunction with other drug solutions. Discard any unused portion of the vial; do not pool unused portions.

Monitoring Parameters Hemoglobin (at least once per week until maintenance dose established and after dosage changes; monitor at regular intervals at least once per month once hemoglobin is stabilized); iron stores (transferrin saturation and ferritin) prior to and during therapy; serum chemistry (CRF patients); blood pressure

Dietary Considerations Supplemental iron intake may be required in patients with low iron stores.

Additional Information Oncology Comment: The American Society of Hematology (ASH) and American Society of Clinical Oncology (ASCO) 2007 updates to the clinical practice guidelines for the use of erythropoiesis-stimulating agents (ESAs) indicate that ESAs are most appropriate when used according to the dosage parameters within the Food and Drug Administration (FDA) approved labeling for epoetin and darbepoetin (Rizzo, 2008). While the previous guidelines addressed only the use of epoetin, the 2007 guidelines also address the use of darbepoetin, which is assessed as being equivalent to epoetin with respect to safety and efficacy. When used as an option for the treatment of chemotherapy-associated anemia (to increase hemoglobin and decrease red blood cell transfusions), therapy with ESAs should begin as the hemoglobin level approaches or falls below 10 g/dL. The ASH/ASCO guidelines recommend following the FDA approved dosing (and dosing adjustment) guidelines and target hemoglobin ranges as alternate dosing and schedules have not demonstrated consistent differences in effectiveness with regard to hemoglobin response. In patients who do not have a response within 6-8 weeks (hemoglobin rise <1-2 g/dL or no reduction in transfusions) ESA therapy should be discontinued.

The guidelines note that patients with an increased risk of thromboembolism (generally includes previous history of thrombosis, surgery, and/or prolonged periods of immobilization) and patients receiving concomitant medications that may increase thromboembolic risk, should begin ESA therapy only after careful consideration. With the exception of low-risk myelodysplasia-associated anemia (which has evidence supporting the use of ESAs without concurrent chemotherapy), the guidelines do not support the use of ESAs in the absence of concurrent chemotherapy.

Dosage Forms Excipient information presented when available (limited, particularly for generics); consult specific product labeling.

Injection, solution [preservative free]:

Aranesp®: 25 mcg/0.42 mL (0.42 mL); 40 mcg/ 0.4 mL (0.4 mL); 60 mcg/0.3 mL (0.3 mL); 100 mcg/0.5 mL (0.5 mL); 150 mcg/0.3 mL (0.3 mL); 200 mcg/0.4 mL (0.4 mL); 300 mcg/0.6 mL (0.6 mL); 500 mcg/mL (1 mL) [contains polysorbate 80; prefilled syringe; needle cover contains latex]

Aranesp®: 25 mcg/mL (1 mL); 40 mcg/mL (1 mL); 60 mcg/mL (1 mL); 100 mcg/mL (1 mL); 150 mcg/0.75 mL (0.75 mL); 200 mcg/mL (1 mL); 300 mcg/mL (1 mL) [contains polysorbate 80; single-dose vial]

References

Andre JL, Deschenes G, Boudaillies B, et al, "Darbepoetin, Effective Treatment of Anaemia in Paediatric Patients With Chronic Renal Failure," *Pediatr Nephrol*, 2007, 22(5):708-14.

Bennett CL, Silver SM, Djulbegovic B, et al, "Venous Thromboembolism and Mortality Associated With Recombinant Erythropoietin and Darbepoetin Administration for the Treatment of Cancer-Associated Anemia," *JAMA*, 2008, 299(8):914-24.

Blumer J, Berg S, Adamson PC, et al, "Pharmacokinetic Evaluation of Darbepoetin Alfa for the Treatment of Pediatric Patients With Chemotherapy-Induced Anemia," *Pediatr Blood Cancer*, 2007, 49(5):687-93.

Bristoyiannis G, Germanos N, Grekas D, et al, "Unit Dosing of Darbepoetin Alfa for the Treatment of Anemia in Patients With End-Stage Renal Disease Being Switched From Recombinant Human Erythropoietin: Results of a Phase IIIb, 27-Week, Multicenter, Open-Label Study in Greek Patients," *Curr Ther Res*, 2005, 66(3):195-211.

Canon JL, Vansteenkiste J, Bodoky G, et al, "Randomized, Double-Blind, Active-Controlled Trial of Every-3-Week Darbepoetin Alfa for the Treatment of Chemotherapy-Induced Anemia," *J Natl Cancer Inst*, 2006, 98(4):273-84.

Corwin HL, Gettinger A, Pearl RG, et al, "Efficacy of Recombinant Human Erythropoietin in Critically Ill Patients: A Randomized Controlled Trial," *JAMA*, 2002, 288(22):2827-35.

Dellinger RP, Levy MM, Carlet JM, et al, "Surviving Sepsis Campaign: International Guidelines for Management of Severe Sepsis and Septic Shock: 2008," *Intensive Care Med*, 2008, 34(1):17-60. Available at http://www.survivingsepsis.org/system/files/images/2008_20International_20SSC_20Guidelines_1_.pdf

Drueke TB, Locatelli F, Clyne N, et al, "Normalization of Hemoglobin Level in Patients With Chronic Kidney Disease and Anemia," *N Engl J Med*, 2006, 355(20): 2071-84.

Giraldo P, Nomdedeu B, Loscertales J, et al, "Darbepoetin Alpha for the Treatment of Anemia in Patients With Myelodysplastic Syndromes," *Cancer*, 2006, 107(12):2807-16.

Hesketh PJ, Arena F, Patel D, et al, "A Randomized Controlled Trial of Darbepoetin Alfa Administered as a Fixed or Weight-Based Dose Using a Front-Loading Schedule in Patients With Anemia Who Have Nonmyeloid Malignancies," *Cancer*, 2004, 100(4):859-68.

Jadoul M, Vanrenterghem Y, Foret M, et al, "Darbepoetin Alfa Administered Once Monthly Maintains Haemoglobin Levels in Stable Dialysis Patients," *Nephrol Dial Transplant*, 2004, 19 (4):898-903.

Lerner G, Kale AS, Warady BA, et al, "Pharmacokinetics of Darbepoetin Alfa in Pediatric Patients With Chronic Kidney Disease," *Pediatr Nephrol*, 2002, 17(11):933-7.

National Comprehensive Cancer Network® (NCCN), "Practice Guidelines in Oncology™: Cancer- and Chemotherapy-Induced Anemia Version 2.2009." Available at http://www.nccn.org/professionals/physician_gls/PDF/anemia.pdf

National Comprehensive Cancer Network® (NCCN), "Practice Guidelines in Oncology™: Myelodysplastic Syndromes Version 1.2009." Available at http://www.nccn.org/professionals/physician_gls/PDF/mds.pdf

National Kidney Foundation, "KDOQI Clinical Practice Guidelines and Clinical Practice Recommentaions for Anemia in Chronic Kidney Disease," *Am J Kidney Dis*, 2007, 50 (3):529-30. Available at http://www.kidney.org/professionals/kdoqi/pdf/KDOQI_finalPDF.pdf or http://www.kidney.org/professionals/KDOQI.

Phronmmintikul A, Haas SJ, Elsik M, et al, "Mortality and Target Haemoglobin Concentrations in Anaemic Patients with Chronic Kidney Disease Treated With Erythropoietin: A Meta-Analysis," *Lancet*, 2007, 369(9559):381-88.

Rizzo JD, Somerfield MR, Hagerty LK, et al, "American Society of Hematology/American Society of Clinical Oncology 2007 Clinical Practice Guideline Update on the Use of Epoetin and Darbepoetin," *Blood*, 2008, 111(1):25-41.

Singh AJ, Szczech L, Tang KI, et al, "Correction of Anemia with Epoetin Alfa in Chronic Kidney Disease," *N Engl J Med*, 2006, 355(20):2085-98.

Thames W, Yao B, Scheifele A, et al, "Drug Use Evaluation (DUE) of Darbepoetin Alfa in Anemic Patients Undergoing Chemotherapy Supports a Fixed Dose of 200 mcg Q2W Given Every 2 Weeks (Q2W)," Asco Annual Meeting, 2003.

Toto RD, Pichette V, Brenner R, et al, "Darbepoetin Alfa Effectively Treats Anemia in Patients With Chronic Kidney Disease With de novo Every-Other-Week Administration," *Am J Nephrol*, 2004, 24(4):453-60.

Vadhan-Raj S, Mirtsching B, Charu V, et al, "Assessment of Hematologic Effects and Fatigue in Cancer Patients With Chemotherapy-Induced Anemia Given Darbepoetin Alfa Every Two Weeks," *J Support Oncol*, 2003, 1(2):131-8.

Warady BA, Arar MY, Lerner G, et al, "Darbepoetin Alfa for the Treatment of Anemia in Pediatric Patients With Chronic Kidney Disease," *Pediatr Nephrol*, 2006, 21(8):1144-52.

Dasatinib (da SA ti nib)

Medication Safety Issues

Sound-alike/look-alike issues:

Dasatinib may be confused with imatinib

High alert medication: The Institute for Safe Medication Practices (ISMP) includes this medication among its list of drug classes which have a heightened risk of causing significant patient harm when used in error.

Related Information

Safe Handling of Hazardous Drugs *on page 1517*

U.S. Brand Names Sprycel®

Index Terms BMS-354825

Generic Available No

Canadian Brand Names Sprycel®

Pharmacologic Category Antineoplastic Agent, Tyrosine Kinase Inhibitor

Use Treatment of chronic myelogenous leukemia (CML) in chronic, accelerated or blast (myeloid or lymphoid) phase resistant or intolerant to prior therapy (including imatinib); treatment of Philadelphia chromosome-positive (Ph+) acute lymphoblastic leukemia (ALL) resistant or intolerant to prior therapy

Unlabeled/Investigational Use Post-stem cell transplant (allogeneic) follow-up treatment of CML

Pregnancy Risk Factor D

Lactation Excretion in breast milk unknown/not recommended

Labeled Contraindications There are no contraindications listed within the FDA-approved manufacturer's labeling.

Canadian labeling: Hypersensitivity to dasatinib or any other component of the formulation

Warnings/Precautions Hazardous agent - use appropriate precautions for handling and disposal. Severe dose-related bone marrow suppression (thrombocytopenia, neutropenia, anemia) is associated with treatment; dosage adjustment or temporary interruption may be required for severe myelosuppression; the incidence of myelosuppression is higher in patients with advanced CML and Ph+ ALL. Fatal intracranial hemorrhage has been reported in association with dasatinib use. Severe hemorrhage (including CNS, GI) may occur due to thrombocytopenia; in addition to thrombocytopenia, dasatinib may also cause platelet dysfunction. Use caution with patients taking anticoagulants or medications interfering with platelet function; not studied in clinical trials. Use with caution in patients receiving concurrent therapy which alters CYP3A4 activity; avoid concomitant use or consider dasatinib dosage adjustments. Fluid retention, including pleural and pericardial effusions, severe ascites, severe pulmonary edema, and generalized edema were reported; may be dose-related. A chest x-ray is recommended for symptoms suggestive of effusion (dyspnea or dry cough). Utilizing once-daily dosing is associated with a decreased frequency of fluid retention. The risk for pleural effusion is increased in patients with hypertension, prior cardiac history and a twice a day administration schedule; interrupt treatment for grade ≥2 effusion; may consider reinitiating at a reduced dose after resolution (Quintás-Cardama, 2007). Use caution in patients where fluid accumulation may be poorly tolerated, such as in cardiovascular disease (HF or hypertension) and pulmonary disease. Elderly may be more likely to experience dyspnea and fluid retention.

May prolong QT interval; use caution in patients at risk for QT prolongation, including patients with long QT syndrome; patients taking antiarrhythmic medications or other medications that lead to QT prolongation or potassium-wasting diuretics; patients with cumulative high-dose anthracycline therapy; and conditions which cause hypokalemia or hypomagnesemia. Correct hypokalemia and hypomagnesemia prior to initiation of therapy. Use caution with hepatic impairment due to extensive hepatic metabolism; patients with ALT or AST >2.5 times the upper limit of normal (ULN) or total bilirubin >2 times the ULN were excluded from clinical trials. Safety and efficacy in children <18 years of age have not been established.

Adverse Reactions

≥10%:

Cardiovascular: Fluid retention (21% to 35%; grades 3/4: 4% to 8%), superficial edema (3% to 19%; grades 3/4: ≤1%)

Central nervous system: Headache (15% to 33%), fatigue (9% to 24%), fever (5% to 18%)

Dermatologic: Rash (15% to 21%; includes drug eruption, erythema, erythema multiforme, erythematous rash, erythrosis, exfoliative rash, follicular rash, heat rash, macular rash, maculopapular rash, milia, papular rash, pruritic rash, pustular rash, skin exfoliation, skin irritation, systemic lupus erythematosus rash, urticaria vesiculosa, vesicular rash)

Endocrine & metabolic: Hypophosphatemia (grades 3/4: 10% to 18%), hypokalemia (grades 3/4: 2% to 15%), hypocalcemia (grades 3/4: <1% to 12%)

Gastrointestinal: Diarrhea (18% to 31%; grades 3/4: ≤5%), nausea (18% to 24%), vomiting (7% to 16%), abdominal pain (3% to 12%)

Hematologic: Thrombocytopenia (grades 3/4: 23% to 85%), neutropenia (grades 3/4: 36% to 79%), anemia (grades 3/4: 13% to 74%), hemorrhage (11% to 26%; grades 3/4: 1% to 9%), neutropenic fever (grades 3/4: 1% to 12%)

Neuromuscular & skeletal: Musculoskeletal pain (≤19%), myalgia (3% to 13%), arthralgia (≤12%)

Respiratory: Pleural effusion (18% to 24%; grades 3/4: 2% to 11%), dyspnea (3% to 20%; grades 3/4: 2% to 3%), cough

Miscellaneous: Infection (9% to 12%, includes bacterial, fungal, viral)

1% to <10%:

Cardiovascular: Generalized edema (≤3%), pericardial effusion (≤3%; grades 3/4: ≤3%), CHF/cardiac dysfunction (≤4%; includes cardiac failure, cardiomyopathy, diastolic dysfunction, ejection fraction decreased, ventricular dysfunction, ventricular failure); arrhythmia, chest pain, flushing, hypertension, palpitation

Central nervous system: CNS bleeding (≤3%; grades 3/4: ≤1%), chills, depression, dizziness, insomnia, pain, somnolence

Dermatologic: Acne, alopecia, dermatitis, dry skin, eczema, hyperhydrosis, pruritus, urticaria

Endocrine & metabolic: Hyperuricemia

Gastrointestinal: Gastrointestinal bleeding (2% to 9%; grades 3/4: 1% to 7%), abdominal distention, anorexia, colitis (including neutropenic colitis), constipation, dyspepsia, enterocolitis, gastritis, mucositis/stomatitis, oral soft tissue disorder, taste alteration, weight loss/gain

Hematologic: Contusion, pancytopenia

Hepatic: Bilirubin increased (grades 3/4: ≤6%), ALT increased (grades 3/4: ≤5%), AST increased (grades 3/4: ≤4%)

Neuromuscular & skeletal: Arthralgia, muscle inflammation, muscle stiffness, muscle weakness, myalgia, neuropathy, peripheral neuropathy, weakness

Ocular: Visual disorder (blurred vision, acuity reduced, visual disturbance), xerophthalmia

Otic: Tinnitus

Renal: Serum creatinine increased (grades 3/4: ≤8%)

Respiratory: Pulmonary edema (≤4%; grades 3/4: ≤3%), lung infiltration, pneumonia (bacterial, viral or fungal), pneumonitis, pulmonary hypertension, upper respiratory tract infection/inflammation

Miscellaneous: Herpes virus infection, sepsis

<1%, postmarketing, and/or case reports (limited to important or life-threatening): Acute coronary syndrome, acute febrile neutrophilic dermatosis, acute respiratory distress syndrome, affect lability, amnesia, anal fissure, angina, anxiety, ascites, asthma, bronchospasm, bullous conditions, cardiomegaly, cerebrovascular accident, cholecystitis, cholestasis, coagulopathy, confusion, conjunctivitis, cor pulmonale, creatine phosphokinase increased, dysphagia, erythema nodosum, esophagitis, gynecomastia, hand-foot syndrome (palmar-plantar erythrodysesthesia syndrome), hepatitis, hypersensitivity, hypoalbuminemia, hypotension, ileus, libido decreased, livedo reticularis, malaise, menstrual irregularities, MI, myocarditis, nail disorder, neutropenic colitis, pancreatitis, panniculitis, pericarditis, periorbital

edema, photosensitivity, pigmentation disorder, platelet aggregation abnormal, polyuria, proteinuria, pure red cell aplasia, QT_c prolongation, renal failure, reversible posterior leukoencephalopathy syndrome, rhabdomyolysis, seizure, skin ulcer, syncope, temperature intolerance, tendonitis, thrombophlebitis, TIA, tremor, troponin increased, tumor lysis syndrome, upper gastrointestinal ulcer, ventricular arrhythmia, ventricular tachycardia, vertigo

Drug Interactions

Metabolism/Transport Effects Substrate of CYP3A4 (major); **Inhibits** CYP3A4 (weak)

Avoid Concomitant Use

Avoid concomitant use of Dasatinib with any of the following: Artemether; Dronedarone; Lumefantrine; Nilotinib; Pimozide; QuiNINE; Tetrabenazine; Thioridazine; Ziprasidone

Increased Effect/Toxicity

Dasatinib may increase the levels/effects of: Anticoagulants; Antiplatelet Agents; CYP3A4 Substrates; Dronedarone; Pimozide; QTc-Prolonging Agents; QuiNINE; Tetrabenazine; Thioridazine; Ziprasidone

The levels/effects of Dasatinib may be increased by: Alfuzosin; Artemether; Chloroquine; Ciprofloxacin; CYP3A4 Inhibitors (Moderate); CYP3A4 Inhibitors (Strong); Gadobutrol; Lumefantrine; Nilotinib; QuiNINE

Decreased Effect

The levels/effects of Dasatinib may be decreased by: Antacids; CYP3A4 Inducers (Strong); Deferasirox; H2-Antagonists; Herbs (CYP3A4 Inducers); Proton Pump Inhibitors

Ethanol/Nutrition/Herb Interactions Herb/Nutraceutical: Avoid St John's wort (may increase metabolism and decrease dasatinib plasma concentration).

Storage/Stability Store at 25°C (77°F); excursions permitted to 15°C to 30°C (59°F to 86°F).

Mechanism of Action BCR-ABL tyrosine kinase inhibitor; targets most imatinib-resistant BCR-ABL mutations (except the T315I and F317V mutants) by distinctly binding to active and inactive ABL-kinase. Kinase inhibition halts proliferation of leukemia cells. Also inhibits SRC family (including SRC, LKC, YES, FYN); c-KIT, EPHA2 and platelet derived growth factor receptor (PDGFRβ)

Pharmacodynamics/Kinetics

Distribution: 2505 L

Protein binding: Dasatinib: 96%; metabolite (active): 93%

Metabolism: Hepatic (extensive); metabolized by CYP3A4 (primarily), flavin-containing mono-oxygenase-3 (FOM-3) and uridine diphosphate-glucurono-syltransferase (UGT) to an active metabolite and other inactive metabolites (the active metabolite plays only a minor role in the pharmacology of dasatinib)

Half-life elimination: Terminal: 3-5 hours

Time to peak, plasma: 0.5-6 hours

Excretion: Feces (85%, 19% as unchanged drug); urine (4%, 0.1% as unchanged drug)

Dosage Oral: Adults:

CML:

Chronic phase: 100 mg once daily. In clinical studies, a dose escalation to 140 mg once daily was allowed in patients not achieving cytogenetic response at recommended initial dosage.

Accelerated or blast phase: 140 mg once daily. In clinical studies, a dose escalation to 180 mg once daily was allowed in patients not achieving cytogenetic response at recommended initial dosage.

Ph+ ALL: 140 mg once daily. In clinical studies, a dose escalation to 180 mg once daily was allowed in patients not achieving cytogenetic response at recommended initial dosage.

Dosage adjustment for concomitant CYP3A4 inhibitors/inducers: Dose reductions are likely to be needed when dasatinib is administered concomitantly with a strong CYP3A4 inhibitor (eg, itraconazole, ketoconazole, voriconazole, clarithromycin, telithromycin, nefazodone, atazanavir, indinavir, nelfinavir, ritonavir, saquinavir, grapefruit juice; an alternate medication for CYP3A4 enzyme inhibitors should be investigated first). In the event that dasatinib must be administered concomitantly with a potent enzyme inhibitor, consider reducing dasatinib from 100 mg/day to 20 mg daily **or** from 140 mg/day to 40 mg daily, with careful monitoring. If reduced dose is not tolerated, the strong CYP3A4 inhibitor must be discontinued or dasatinib therapy temporarily held until concomitant inhibitor use has ceased. When a strong CYP3A4 inhibitor is discontinued, allow a washout period (~1 week) prior to adjusting dasatinib dose upward.

Concomitant administration with strong CYP3A4 inducers (eg, dexamethasone, phenytoin, carbamazepine, rifamycins, phenobarbital, St John's wort) may require increased dasatinib doses, with careful monitoring; alternatives to the enzyme-inducing agent should be utilized first.

Dosage adjustment for toxicity:
Hematologic toxicity:
Chronic phase CML (100 mg daily starting dose): For ANC <0.5 x 10^9/L or platelets <50 x 10^9/L, withhold treatment until ANC ≥1 x 10^9/L and platelets ≥50 x 10^9/L; then resume treatment at the original starting dose if recovery occurs in ≤7 days. If platelets <25 x 10^9/L or recurrence of ANC <0.5 x 10^9/L for >7 days, withhold treatment until ANC ≥1 x 10^9/L and platelets ≥50 x 10^9/L; then resume treatment at 80 mg once daily (2nd episode) or discontinue (3rd episode)

Accelerated or blast phase CML and Ph+ ALL (140 mg once daily starting dose): For ANC <0.5 x 10^9/L or platelets <10 x 10^9/L, if cytopenia unrelated to leukemia, withhold treatment until ANC ≥1 x 10^9/L and platelets ≥20 x 10^9/L; then resume treatment at the original starting dose. If cytopenia recurs, withhold treatment until ANC ≥1 x 10^9/L and platelets ≥20 x 10^9/L; then resume treatment at 100 mg once daily (2nd episode) or 80 mg once daily (3rd episode). For cytopenias related to leukemia (confirm with marrow aspirate or biopsy), consider dose escalation to 180 mg once daily (*Canadian labeling:* 100 mg twice daily) with careful monitoring.

Nonhematologic toxicity: Withhold treatment until toxicity improvement or resolution; if appropriate, resume treatment at a reduced dose based on the event severity.

Dosage adjustment for hepatic impairment: No adjustment required; use with caution

Administration Administer once daily (morning or evening). May be taken without regard to food. Do not break, crush, or chew tablets.

Monitoring Parameters CBC with differential (weekly for 2 months, then monthly or as clinically necessary); bone marrow biopsy; liver function tests, electrolytes including calcium, phosphorus, magnesium; monitor for fluid retention; ECG monitoring if at risk for QT_c prolongation; chest x-ray is recommended for symptoms suggestive of pleural effusion (eg, cough, dyspnea)

Dietary Considerations May be taken without regard to food. Avoid grapefruit juice.

Additional Information Oncology Comment: In a dose finding study in chronic-phase CML, dasatinib 100 mg once daily provided comparable efficacy to the original FDA-approved dose of 70 mg twice daily. The 100 mg once daily dose was better tolerated (lower rates of pleural effusion and grades 3/4 thrombocytopenia), required fewer dose reductions, and fewer dosing interruptions or discontinuations (Shah, 2008).

Emetic Potential Very low (<10%)

Dosage Forms Excipient information presented when available (limited, particularly for generics); consult specific product labeling.

Tablet, oral:

Sprycel®: 20 mg, 50 mg, 70 mg, 100 mg

References

Apperley JF, Cortes JE, Kim DW, et al, "Dasatinib in the Treatment of Chronic Myeloid Leukemia in Accelerated Phase After Imatinib Failure: The START A Trial," *J Clin Oncol*, 2009 [epub ahead of print]

Assouline S, Laneuville P and Gambacorti-Passerini C, "Panniculitis During Dasatinib Therapy for Imatinib-Resistant Chronic Myelogenous Leukemia," *N Engl J Med*, 2006, 354(24):2623-4.

Bradeen HA, Eide CA, O'Hare T, et al, "Comparison of Imatinib, Dasatinib (BMS-354825), and Nilotinib (AMN107) in an N-Ethyl-N-Nitrosourea (ENU)-Based Mutagenesis Screen: High Efficacy of Drug Combinations," *Blood*, 2006, 108(7):2332-8.

Copland M, Hamilton A, Elrick LJ, et al, "Dasatinib (BMS-354825) Targets an Earlier Progenitor Population Than Imatinib in Primary CML But Does Not Eliminate the Quiescent Fraction," *Blood*, 2006, 107(11):4532-9.

Cortes J, Rousselot P, Kim DW, et al, "Dasatinib Induces Complete Hematologic and Cytogenetic Responses in Patients With Imatinib-Resistant or Intolerant Chronic Myeloid Leukemia in Blast Crisis," *Blood*, 2007, 109(8):3207-13.

Guilhot F, Apperley J, Kim DW, et al, "Dasatinib Induces Significant Hematologic and Cytogenetic Responses in Patients with Imatinib-Resistant or Intolerant Chronic Myeloid Leukemia in Accelerated Phase," *Blood*, 2007, 109(10):4143-50.

Hochhaus A, Kantarjian HM, Baccarani M, et al, "Dasatinib Induces Notable Hematologic and Cytogenetic Responses in Chronic-Phase Chronic Myeloid Leukemia After Failure of Imatinib Therapy," *Blood*, 2007, 109(6):2303-09.

National Comprehensive Cancer Network® (NCCN) "Practice Guidelines in Oncology™: Chronic Myelogenous Leukemia Version 1.2010." Available at http://www.nccn.org/professionals/physician_gls/PDF/cml.pdf

Ottmann O, Dombret H, Martinelli G, et al, "Dasatinib Induces Rapid Hematologic and Cytogenetic Responses in Adult Patients with Philadelphia Chromosome-Positive Acute Lymphoblastic Leukemia with Intolerance to Imatinib: Interim Results of a Phase 2 Study," *Blood*, 2007, 110 (7):2309-15.

Quintas-Cardama A, Han X, Kantarjian H, et al, "Dasatinib-Induced Platelet Dysfunction," *Blood* (ASH Annual Meeting Abstracts), 2007, 110: Abstract 2941.

Quintás-Cardama A, Kantarjian H, O'brien S, et al, "Pleural Effusion in Patients With Chronic Myelogenous Leukemia Treated With Dasatinib After Imatinib Failure," *J Clin Oncol*, 2007, 25 (25):3908-14.

Shah NP, Kantarjian HM, Kim DW, et al, "Intermittent Target Inhibition With Dasatinib 100 mg Once Daily Preserves Efficacy and Improves Tolerability in Imatinib-Resistant and -Intolerant Chronic-Phase Chronic Myeloid Leukemia," *J Clin Oncol*, 2008, 26(19):3204-12.

Talpaz M, Shah NP, Kantarjian H, et al, "Dasatinib in Imatinib-Resistant Philadelphia Chromosome-Positive Leukemias," *N Engl J Med*, 2006, 354(24):2531-41.

◆ **Daunomycin** see DAUNORubicin Hydrochloride *on page 323*

DAUNOrubicin Citrate (Liposomal)
(daw noe ROO bi sin SI trate lip po SOE mal)

Medication Safety Issues

Sound-alike/look-alike issues:

DAUNOrubicin liposomal may be confused with DACTINomycin, DOXOrubicin, DOXOrubicin liposomal, epirubicin, IDArubicin, valrubicin

Liposomal formulation (DaunoXome®) may be confused with the conventional formulation (Cerubidine®, Rubex®)

High alert medication: The Institute for Safe Medication Practices (ISMP) includes this medication among its list of drug classes which have a heightened risk of causing significant patient harm when used in error.

Related Information
Management of Drug Extravasations *on page 1447*
Safe Handling of Hazardous Drugs *on page 1517*

U.S. Brand Names DaunoXome®

Index Terms DAUNOrubicin Liposomal; Liposomal DAUNOrubicin; NSC-697732

Generic Available No

Pharmacologic Category Antineoplastic Agent, Anthracycline

Use First-line treatment of advanced HIV-associated Kaposi's sarcoma (KS)

Pregnancy Risk Factor D

Lactation Excretion in breast milk unknown/not recommended

Labeled Contraindications Hypersensitivity to daunorubicin citrate (liposomal), daunorubicin, or any component of the formulation

Warnings/Precautions Hazardous agent - use appropriate precautions for handling and disposal. **[U.S. Boxed Warning]: Monitor cardiac function regularly; especially in patients with previous therapy with high cumulative doses of anthracyclines, cyclophosphamide, or thoracic radiation, or who have pre-existing cardiac disease.** Although the risk increases with cumulative dose, irreversible cardiotoxicity may occur with anthracycline treatment at any dose level. Patients with pre-existing heart disease, hypertension, concurrent administration of other antineoplastic agents, prior or concurrent chest irradiation, and advanced age are at increased risk. Evaluate left ventricular ejection fraction (LVEF) prior to treatment and periodically during treatment.

[U.S. Boxed Warning]: May cause bone marrow suppression, particularly neutropenia; monitor closely for infections. **[U.S. Boxed Warning]: Use caution with hepatic impairment;** dosage reduction is recommended. Use caution with renal impairment; may require dose adjustment. **[U.S. Boxed Warning]: The lipid component is associated with infusion-related reactions (back pain, flushing, chest tightness) usually within the first 5 minutes of infusion;** monitor, interrupt infusion, and resume at reduced infusion rate. Safety and efficacy in children and the elderly have not been established. **[U.S. Boxed Warning]: Should be administered under the supervision of an experienced cancer chemotherapy physician.**

Adverse Reactions
>10%:
Cardiovascular: Edema (11%)
Central nervous system: Fatigue (49%), fever (47%), headache (25%), neutropenic fever (17%)
Gastrointestinal: Nausea (54%), diarrhea (38%), abdominal pain (23%), anorexia (23%), vomiting (23%)
Hematologic: Myelosuppression (onset: 7 days; nadir: 14 days; recovery 21 days), neutropenia (up to 55%; grade 4: 15%), anemia (up to 55%; grade 4: 2%), thrombocytopenia (up to 12%; grade 4: 1%)
Neuromuscular & skeletal: Rigors (19%), back pain (16%), neuropathy (13%)
Respiratory: Cough (28%), dyspnea (26%), rhinitis (12%)

Miscellaneous: Opportunistic infections (40%), allergic reactions (24%), diaphoresis (14%), infusion-related reactions (14%; includes back pain, flushing, chest tightness)

1% to 10%:

Cardiovascular: Chest pain (10%), hypertension (≤5%), palpitation (≤5%), syncope (≤5%), tachycardia (≤5%), LVEF decreased (3%), CHF/cardiomyopathy

Central nervous system: Depression (10%), malaise (10%), dizziness (8%), insomnia (6%), abnormal thinking (≤5%), amnesia (≤5%), anxiety (≤5%), ataxia (≤5%), confusion (≤5%), emotional lability (≤5%), hallucination (≤5%), meningitis (≤5%), seizure (≤5%), somnolence (≤5%)

Dermatologic: Alopecia (8%), pruritus (7%), dry skin (≤5%), folliculitis (≤5%), seborrhea (≤5%)

Endocrine & metabolic: Dehydration (≤5%), hot flashes (≤5%)

Gastrointestinal: Stomatitis (10%), constipation (7%), tenesmus (5%), appetite increased (≤5%), dental caries (≤5%), dysphagia (≤5%), gastro-intestinal hemorrhage (≤5%), gastritis (≤5%), gingival bleeding (≤5%), hemorrhoids (≤5%), melena (≤5%), splenomegaly (≤5%), taste perversion (≤5%), xerostomia (≤5%)

Genitourinary: Dysuria (≤5%), nocturia (≤5%), polyuria (≤5%)

Hepatic: Hepatomegaly (≤5%)

Local: Injection site inflammation (≤5%)

Neuromuscular & skeletal: Arthralgia (7%), myalgia (7%), gait abnormal (≤5%), hyperkinesia (≤5%), hypertonia (≤5%), tremor (≤5%)

Ocular: Abnormal vision (5%) conjunctivitis (≤5%), eye pain (≤5%)

Otic: Deafness (≤5%), earache (≤5%), tinnitus (≤5%)

Respiratory: Sinusitis (8%), hemoptysis (≤5%), pulmonary infiltrate (≤5%), sputum increased (≤5%)

Miscellaneous: Flu-like syndrome (5%), hiccups (≤5%), lymphadenopathy (≤5%), thirst (≤5%)

Postmarketing and/or case reports: Angina, atrial fibrillation, cardiac arrest, MI, pericardial effusion, pericardial tamponade, pulmonary hypertension, supra-ventricular tachycardia, ventricular extrasystoles

Drug Interactions

Avoid Concomitant Use

Avoid concomitant use of DAUNOrubicin Citrate (Liposomal) with any of the following: Natalizumab; Vaccines (Live)

Increased Effect/Toxicity

DAUNOrubicin Citrate (Liposomal) may increase the levels/effects of: Leflunomide; Natalizumab; Vaccines (Live)

The levels/effects of DAUNOrubicin Citrate (Liposomal) may be increased by: Bevacizumab; P-Glycoprotein Inhibitors; Taxane Derivatives; Trastuzumab

Decreased Effect

DAUNOrubicin Citrate (Liposomal) may decrease the levels/effects of: Cardiac Glycosides; Vaccines (Inactivated); Vaccines (Live)

The levels/effects of DAUNOrubicin Citrate (Liposomal) may be decreased by: Cardiac Glycosides; Echinacea; P-Glycoprotein Inducers

Storage/Stability Store intact vials of solution under refrigeration at 2°C to 8°C (36°F to 46°F); do not freeze. Protect from light. Diluted daunorubicin liposomal for infusion may be refrigerated at 2°C to 8°C (36°F to 46°F) for a maximum of 6 hours. Do not use with in-line filters.

Reconstitution Only fluid which may be mixed with DaunoXome® is D_5W. Dilute to a 1:1 solution (1 mg daunorubicin liposomal/mL D_5W). Must **not** be mixed with saline, bacteriostatic agents (such as benzyl alcohol), or any other solution.

Compatibility Stable in D_5W. **Incompatible** with normal saline, sodium bicarbonate and fluorouracil, heparin, dexamethasone.

Mechanism of Action Liposomes have been shown to penetrate solid tumors more effectively, possibly because of their small size and longer circulation time. Once in tissues, daunorubicin is released. Daunorubicin inhibits DNA and RNA synthesis by intercalation between DNA base pairs and by steric obstruction; and intercalates at points of local uncoiling of the double helix. Although the exact mechanism is unclear, it appears that direct binding to DNA (intercalation) and inhibition of DNA repair (topoisomerase II inhibition) result in blockade of DNA and RNA synthesis and fragmentation of DNA.

Pharmacodynamics/Kinetics

Distribution: V_d: 5-8 L

Metabolism: Similar to daunorubicin, but metabolite plasma levels are low

Half-life elimination: Distribution: 4.4 hours; Terminal: 3-5 hours

Excretion: Primarily feces; some urine

Clearance, plasma: 17.3 mL/minute

Dosage Refer to individual protocols. I.V.:

Adults: HIV-associated KS: 40 mg/m² every 2 weeks

Elderly: Use with caution.

Dosage adjustment for toxicity: Withhold treatment for ANC <750/mm³

Elderly: Use with caution.

Dosing adjustment in renal impairment: Serum creatinine >3 mg/dL: Administer 50% of normal dose

Dosing adjustment in hepatic impairment:

Bilirubin 1.2-3 mg/dL: Administer 75% of normal dose

Bilirubin >3 mg/dL: Administer 50% of normal dose

Combination Regimens

Leukemia, acute lymphocytic: Hyper-CVAD (Leukemia, Acute Lymphocytic) on page 1349

Administration Infuse over 1 hour; do not mix with other drugs. Avoid extravasation.

Monitoring Parameters CBC with differential and platelets (prior to each dose), liver function tests, renal function tests; evaluate cardiac function (baseline left ventricular ejection fraction [LVEF] prior to treatment initiation; repeat LVEF at total cumulative doses of 320 mg/m², and every 160 mg/m² thereafter; patients with pre-existing cardiac disease, history of prior chest irradiation, or history of prior anthracycline treatment should have baseline LVEF and every 160 mg/m² thereafter); signs and symptoms of infection or disease progression; monitor closely for infusion reactions

Vesicant May be an irritant

Dosage Forms Excipient information presented when available (limited, particularly for generics); consult specific product labeling.

Injection, solution [preservative free]:

DaunoXome®: 2 mg/mL (25 mL) [contains sucrose 2125 mg/25 mL]

References

Eckardt JR, Campbell E, Burris HA, et al, "A Phase II Trial of DaunoXome®, Liposome-Encapsulated Daunorubicin, in Patients With Metastatic Adenocarcinoma of the Colon," *Am J Clin Oncol*, 1994, 17(5):498-501.

Gill PS, Espina BM, Muggia F, et al, "Phase I/II Clinical and Pharmacokinetic Evaluation of Liposomal Daunorubicin," *J Clin Oncol*, 1995, 13(4):996-1003.

Gill PS, Wernz J, Scadden DT, et al, "Randomized Phase III Trial of Liposomal Daunorubicin Versus Doxorubicin, Bleomycin, and Vincristine in AIDS-Related Kaposi's Sarcoma," *J Clin Oncol*, 1996, 14(8):2353-64.

DAUNOrubicin Hydrochloride (daw noe ROO bi sin hye droe KLOR ide)

Medication Safety Issues

Sound-alike/look-alike issues:

DAUNOrubicin may be confused with DACTINomycin, DOXOrubicin, DOXOrubicin liposomal, epirubicin, IDArubicin, valrubicin

Conventional formulation (Cerubidine®, DAUNOrubicin hydrochloride) may be confused with the liposomal formulation (DaunoXome®)

High alert medication: The Institute for Safe Medication Practices (ISMP) includes this medication among its list of drug classes which have a heightened risk of causing significant patient harm when used in error.

Related Information

Management of Drug Extravasations *on page 1447*
Safe Handling of Hazardous Drugs *on page 1517*

U.S. Brand Names Cerubidine®

Index Terms Daunomycin; Rubidomycin Hydrochloride

Generic Available Yes

Canadian Brand Names Cerubidine®

Pharmacologic Category Antineoplastic Agent, Anthracycline

Use Treatment of acute lymphocytic leukemia (ALL) and acute myeloid leukemia (AML)

Pregnancy Risk Factor D

Lactation Excretion in breast milk unknown/not recommended

Labeled Contraindications Hypersensitivity to daunorubicin or any component of the formulation

Warnings/Precautions Hazardous agent - use appropriate precautions for handling and disposal. Use with caution in patients who have received radiation therapy; reduce dosage in patients who are receiving radiation therapy simultaneously. **[U.S. Boxed Warnings]: Use caution with renal impairment or in the presence of hepatic dysfunction; dosage reduction is recommended. Potent vesicant; if extravasation occurs, severe local tissue damage leading to ulceration and necrosis, and pain may occur. For I.V. administration only. Severe bone marrow suppression may occur.**

[U.S. Boxed Warning]: May cause cumulative, dose-related myocardial toxicity (concurrent or delayed). Total cumulative dose should take into account previous or concomitant treatment with cardiotoxic agents or irradiation of chest. The incidence of irreversible myocardial toxicity increases as the total cumulative (lifetime) dosages approach:

550 mg/m^2 in adults
400 mg/m^2 in adults receiving chest radiation
300 mg/m^2 in children >2 years of age
10 mg/kg in children <2 years of age

Although the risk increases with cumulative dose, irreversible cardiotoxicity may occur at any dose level. Patients with pre-existing heart disease, hypertension, concurrent administration of other antineoplastic agents, prior or concurrent chest irradiation, advanced age; and infants and children are at increased risk. Monitor left ventricular (LV) function (baseline and periodic) with ECHO or MUGA scan; monitor ECG.

◄ Secondary leukemias may occur when used with combination chemotherapy or radiation therapy. **[U.S. Boxed Warning]: Should be administered under the supervision of an experienced cancer chemotherapy physician].**

Adverse Reactions

>10%:

Cardiovascular: Transient ECG abnormalities (supraventricular tachycardia, S-T wave changes, atrial or ventricular extrasystoles); generally asymptomatic and self-limiting. CHF, dose related, may be delayed for 7-8 years after treatment.

Dermatologic: Alopecia (reversible), radiation recall

Gastrointestinal: Mild nausea or vomiting, stomatitis

Genitourinary: Discoloration of urine (red)

Hematologic: Myelosuppression (onset: 7 days; nadir: 10-14 days; recovery: 21-28 days), primarily leukopenia; thrombocytopenia and anemia

1% to 10%:

Dermatologic: Skin "flare" at injection site; discoloration of saliva, sweat, or tears

Endocrine & metabolic: Hyperuricemia

Gastrointestinal: Abdominal pain, GI ulceration, diarrhea

<1%: Anaphylactoid reaction, bilirubin increased, hepatitis, infertility; local (cellulitis, pain, thrombophlebitis at injection site); MI, myocarditis, nail banding, onycholysis, pericarditis, pigmentation of nailbeds, secondary leukemia, skin rash, sterility, systemic hypersensitivity (including urticaria, pruritus, angioedema, dysphagia, dyspnea); transaminases increased

Drug Interactions

Avoid Concomitant Use

Avoid concomitant use of DAUNOrubicin Hydrochloride with any of the following: Natalizumab; Vaccines (Live)

Increased Effect/Toxicity

DAUNOrubicin Hydrochloride may increase the levels/effects of: Leflunomide; Natalizumab; Vaccines (Live)

The levels/effects of DAUNOrubicin Hydrochloride may be increased by: Bevacizumab; P-Glycoprotein Inhibitors; Taxane Derivatives; Trastuzumab

Decreased Effect

DAUNOrubicin Hydrochloride may decrease the levels/effects of: Cardiac Glycosides; Vaccines (Inactivated); Vaccines (Live)

The levels/effects of DAUNOrubicin Hydrochloride may be decreased by: Cardiac Glycosides; Echinacea; P-Glycoprotein Inducers

Ethanol/Nutrition/Herb Interactions Ethanol: Avoid ethanol (due to GI irritation).

Storage/Stability Store intact vials of powder for injection at room temperature of 15°C to 30°C (59°F to 86°F); intact vials of solution for injection should be refrigerated at 2°C to 8°C (36°F to 46°F). Protect from light. Reconstituted solution is stable for 4 days at 15°C to 25°C. Further dilution in D$_5$W, LR, or NS is stable at room temperature (25°C) for up to 4 weeks if protected from light.

Reconstitution Dilute vials of powder for injection with 4 mL SWFI for a final concentration of 5 mg/mL. May further dilute in 100 mL D$_5$W or NS.

Compatibility Stable in D$_5$W, LR, NS, sterile water for injection. **Incompatible** with heparin, sodium bicarbonate, fluorouracil, and dexamethasone.

Y-site administration: Compatible: Amifostine, etoposide phosphate, filgrastim, gemcitabine, granisetron, melphalan, methotrexate, ondansetron, sodium bicarbonate, teniposide, thiotepa, vinorelbine. **Incompatible:** Allopurinol, aztreonam, cefepime, fludarabine, piperacillin/tazobactam.

Compatibility when admixed: Compatible: Cytarabine with etoposide, hydrocortisone sodium succinate. **Incompatible:** Dexamethasone sodium phosphate, heparin.

Mechanism of Action Inhibition of DNA and RNA synthesis by intercalation between DNA base pairs and by steric obstruction. Daunomycin intercalates at points of local uncoiling of the double helix. Although the exact mechanism is unclear, it appears that direct binding to DNA (intercalation) and inhibition of DNA repair (topoisomerase II inhibition) result in blockade of DNA and RNA synthesis and fragmentation of DNA.

Pharmacodynamics/Kinetics

Distribution: Many body tissues, particularly the liver, kidneys, lung, spleen, and heart; not into CNS; crosses placenta; V_d: 40 L/kg

Metabolism: Primarily hepatic to daunorubicinol (active), then to inactive aglycones, conjugated sulfates, and glucuronides

Half-life elimination: Distribution: 2 minutes; Elimination: 14-20 hours; Terminal: 18.5 hours; Daunorubicinol plasma half-life: 24-48 hours

Excretion: Feces (40%); urine (~25% as unchanged drug and metabolites)

Dosage I.V. (refer to individual protocols):

Children: **Note:** Cumulative dose should not exceed 300 mg/m^2 in children >2 years or 10 mg/kg in children <2 years of age; maximum cumulative doses for younger children are unknown.

Children <2 years or BSA <0.5 m^2: ALL combination therapy: 1 mg/kg/dose per protocol, with frequency dependent on regimen employed

Children ≥2 years and BSA ≥0.5 m^2:

ALL combination therapy: Remission induction: 25 mg/m^2 on day 1 every week for up to 4-6 cycles

AML combination therapy: Induction: I.V. continuous infusion: 30-60 mg/m^2/day on days 1-3 of cycle

Adults: **Note:** Cumulative dose should not exceed 550 mg/m^2 in adults without risk factors for cardiotoxicity and should not exceed 400 mg/m^2 in adults receiving chest irradiation.

Range: 30-60 mg/m^2/day for 3 days, repeat dose in 3-4 weeks

ALL combination therapy: 45 mg/m^2/day for 3 days

AML combination therapy:

Adults <60 years: Induction: 45 mg/m^2/day for 3 days of the first course of induction therapy; subsequent courses: 45 mg/m^2/day for 2 days

Adults ≥60 years: Induction: 30 mg/m^2/day for 3 days of the first course of induction therapy; subsequent courses: 30 mg/m^2/day for 2 days

Dosing adjustment in renal impairment:

The FDA-approved labeling recommends the following adjustment: S_{cr} >3 mg/dL: Administer 50% of normal dose

The following guidelines have been used by some clinicians (Aronoff, 2007): Children:

Cl_{cr} <30 mL/minute: Administer 50% of dose

Hemodialysis/continuous ambulatory peritoneal dialysis (CAPD): Administer 50% of dose

Adults: No adjustment recommended

Dosing adjustment in hepatic impairment:

The FDA-approved labeling recommends the following adjustments:

Serum bilirubin 1.2-3 mg/dL: Administer 75% of dose

Serum bilirubin >3 mg/dL: Administer 50% of dose

The following guidelines have been used by some clinicians (Floyd, 2006):

Serum bilirubin 1.2-3 mg/dL: Administer 75% of dose

Serum bilirubin 3.1-5 mg/dL: Administer 50% of dose

Serum bilirubin >5 mg/dL: Avoid use

◀ **Combination Regimens**

Leukemia, acute lymphocytic:

Leukemia, acute myeloid:

Leukemia, acute promyelocytic:

Administration Not for I.M. or SubQ administration. Administer as slow I.V. push over 1-5 minutes into the tubing of a rapidly infusing I.V. solution of D_5W or NS or dilute in 100 mL of D_5W or NS and infuse over 15-30 minutes.

Monitoring Parameters CBC with differential and platelet count, liver function test, ECG, left ventricular ejection function (echocardiography [ECHO] or multigated radionuclide angiography [MUGA] scan), renal function test

Emetic Potential Moderate (30% to 90%)

Vesicant Yes; see Management of Drug Extravasations on page 1447.

Dosage Forms Excipient information presented when available (limited, particularly for generics); consult specific product labeling. **Note: Strength expressed as base**

Injection, powder for reconstitution: 20 mg

Cerubidine®: 20 mg [contains mannitol 100 mg]

Injection, solution: 5 mg/mL (4 mL, 10 mL)

References

Aronoff GR, Bennett WM, Berns JS, et al, *Drug Prescribing in Renal Failure: Dosing Guidelines for Adults and Children*, 5th Ed. Philadelphia, PA: American College of Physicians, 2007, 98.

Crom WR, Glynn-Barnhart AM, Rodman JH, et al, "Pharmacokinetics of Anticancer Drugs in Children," *Clin Pharmacokinet*, 1987, 12(3):168-213.

Cuttner J, Mick R, Budman DR, et al, "Phase III Trial of Brief Intensive Treatment of Adult Acute Lymphocytic Leukemia Comparing Daunorubicin and Mitoxantrone: A CALGB Study," *Leukemia*, 1991, 5(5):425-31.

Davis HL and Davis TE, "Daunorubicin and Adriamycin in Cancer Treatment: An Analysis of Their Roles and Limitations," *Cancer Treat Rep*, 1979, 63(5):809-15.

Floyd J, Mirza I, Sachs B, et al, "Hepatotoxicity of Chemotherapy," *Semin Oncol*, 2006, 33 (1):50-67.

Floyd JD, Nguyen DT, Lobins RL, et al, "Cardiotoxicity of Cancer Therapy," *J Clin Oncol*, 2005, 23 (30):7685-96.

Keefe DL, "Anthracycline-Induced Cardiomyopathy," *Semin Oncol*, 2001, 28(4 Suppl 12):2-7.

Masaoka T, Ogawa M, Yamada K, et al, "A Phase II Comparative Study of Idarubicin Plus Cytarabine Versus Daunorubicin Plus Cytarabine in Adult Acute Myeloid Leukemia," *Semin Hematol*, 1996, 33(4 Suppl 3):12-7.

Riggs CE Jr., "Clinical Pharmacology of Daunorubicin in Patients With Acute Leukemia," *Semin Oncol*, 1984, 11(4 Suppl 3):2-11.

Speth PA, Minderman H, and Haanen C, "Idarubicin v Daunorubicin: Preclinical and Clinical Pharmacokinetic Studies," *Semin Oncol*, 1989, 16(1 Suppl 2):2-9.

Weick JK, Kopecky KJ, Appelbaum FR, et al, "A Randomized Investigation of High-Dose Versus Standard-Dose Cytosine Arabinoside With Daunorubicin in Patients With Previously Untreated Acute Myeloid Leukemia: A Southwest Oncology Group Study," *Blood*, 1996, 88(8):2841-51.

◆ **DAUNOrubicin Liposomal** *see* DAUNOrubicin Citrate (Liposomal) *on page 319*

◆ **DaunoXome®** *see* DAUNOrubicin Citrate (Liposomal) *on page 319*

◆ **DAVA** *see* Vindesine *on page 1180*

◆ **dCF** *see* Pentostatin *on page 949*

◆ **DDAVP®** *see* Desmopressin *on page 344*

◆ **DDAVP® Melt (Can)** *see* Desmopressin *on page 344*

◆ **Deacetyl Vinblastine Carboxamide** *see* Vindesine *on page 1180*

◆ **1-Deamino-8-D-Arginine Vasopressin** *see* Desmopressin *on page 344*

Decitabine (de SYE ta been)

Medication Safety Issues
High alert medication: The Institute for Safe Medication Practices (ISMP) includes this medication among its list of drug classes which have a heightened risk of causing significant patient harm when used in error.

Related Information
Safe Handling of Hazardous Drugs *on page 1517*

U.S. Brand Names Dacogen™

Index Terms 5-Aza-2'-deoxycytidine; 5-AzaC; NSC-127716

Generic Available No

Pharmacologic Category Antineoplastic Agent, DNA Methylation Inhibitor

Use Treatment of myelodysplastic syndrome (MDS)

Unlabeled/Investigational Use Treatment of acute myelogenous leukemia (AML), chronic myelogenous leukemia (CML), sickle cell anemia

Pregnancy Risk Factor D

Lactation Excretion in breast milk unknown/not recommended

Labeled Contraindications Hypersensitivity to decitabine or any component of the formulation

Warnings/Precautions Hazardous agent - use appropriate precautions for handling and disposal. The dose-limiting toxicity is bone marrow suppression; worsening neutropenia is common in first two treatment cycles and may not correlate with progression of underlying MDS; may require growth factor support. Not studied in hepatic and renal disease; use caution. Safety and efficacy in children have not been established.

Adverse Reactions
>10%:
Cardiovascular: Peripheral edema (25%), pallor (23%), edema (18%), cardiac murmur (16%)

Central nervous system: Pyrexia (6% to 53%), headache (28%), insomnia (28%), dizziness (18%), pain (13%), confusion (12%), lethargy (12%), anxiety (11%), hypoesthesia (11%)

Dermatologic: Petechiae (39%), bruising (22%), rash (19%), erythema (14%), cellulitis (12%), lesions (11%), pruritus (11%)

Endocrine & metabolic: Hyperglycemia (33%), hypoalbuminemia (7% to 24%), hypomagnesemia (24%), hypokalemia (22%), hyperkalemia (13%), hyponatremia (13%)

Gastrointestinal: Nausea (42%), constipation (35%), diarrhea (34%), vomiting (25%), anorexia (16%), appetite decreased (16%), abdominal pain (5% to 14%), oral mucosal petechiae (13%), stomatitis (12%), dyspepsia (12%)

Hematologic: Neutropenia (90%; recovery 28-50 days), thrombocytopenia (89%), anemia (82%), febrile neutropenia (29%), leukopenia (28%), lymphadenopathy (12%)

Hepatic: Hyperbilirubinemia (14%), alkaline phosphatase increased (11%)

Local: Tenderness (11%)

Neuromuscular & skeletal: Rigors (22%), arthralgia (20%), limb pain (19%), back pain (17%)

Respiratory: Cough (40%), pneumonia (22%), pharyngitis (16%), lung crackles (14%)

5% to 10%:

Cardiovascular: Chest discomfort (7%), facial swelling (6%), hypotension (6%)

Central nervous system: Malaise (5%)

Dermatologic: Alopecia (8%), urticaria (6%)

Endocrine & metabolic: Hyperuricemia (10%), LDH increased (8%), bicarbonate increased (6%), dehydration (6%), hypochloremia (6%), bicarbonate decreased (5%), hypoproteinemia (5%)

Gastrointestinal: Gingival bleeding (8%), hemorrhoids (8%), loose stools (7%), tongue ulceration (7%), dysphagia (6%), oral candidiasis (6%), lip ulceration (5%), abdominal distension (5%), gastroesophageal reflux (5%), glossodynia (5%)

Genitourinary: Urinary tract infection (7%), dysuria (6%), polyuria (5%)

Hematologic: Hematoma (5%), thrombocythemia (5%), bacteremia (5%)

Hepatic: Ascites (10%), AST increased (10%), hypobilirubinemia (5%)

Local: Catheter infection (8%), catheter site erythema (5%), catheter site pain (5%), injection site swelling (5%)

Neuromuscular & skeletal: Falling (8%), chest wall pain (7%), musculoskeletal discomfort (6%), crepitation (5%), myalgia (5%)

Ocular: Blurred vision (6%)

Respiratory: Breath sounds diminished (10%), hypoxia (10%), rales (8%), pulmonary edema (6%), postnasal drip (5%), sinusitis (5%)

Miscellaneous: Candidal infection (10%), staphylococcal infection (7%), transfusion reaction (7%)

<5%, postmarketing, and/or case reports: Anaphylactic reaction, atrial fibrillation, bronchopulmonary aspergillosis, cardiomyopathy, cardiorespiratory failure, catheter site hemorrhage, chest pain, CHF, cholecystitis, dyspnea, fungal infection, gastrointestinal hemorrhage, gingival pain, hemoptysis, hypersensitivity, intracranial hemorrhage, mental status change, MI, mucosal inflammation, mycobacterium avium complex infection, peridiverticular abscess, pseudomonal lung infection, pulmonary embolism, pulmonary infiltrates, pulmonary mass, renal failure, respiratory arrest, respiratory tract infection, sepsis, splenomegaly, supraventricular tachycardia, urethral hemorrhage, weakness

Drug Interactions

Avoid Concomitant Use There are no known interactions where it is recommended to avoid concomitant use.

Increased Effect/Toxicity There are no known significant interactions involving an increase in effect.

Decreased Effect There are no known significant interactions involving a decrease in effect.

Storage/Stability Store vials at 15°C to 30°C (59°F to 86°F). Solutions diluted for infusion may be stored for up to 7 hours under refrigeration at 2°C to 8°C (36°F to 46°F) if prepared with cold infusion fluids.

Reconstitution Vials should be reconstituted with 10 mL SWFI to a concentration of 5 mg/mL. Further dilute with 50-250 mL NS, D$_5$W, or lactated Ringer's to a final concentration of 0.1-1 mg/mL. Solutions not administered within 15 minutes of preparation should be prepared with cold (2°C to 8°C [36°F to 46°F]) infusion solutions.

Compatibility Stable in NS, D$_5$W, and lactated Ringer's.

Mechanism of Action After phosphorylation, decitabine is incorporated into DNA and inhibits DNA methyltransferase causing hypomethylation and subsequent cell death.

Pharmacodynamics/Kinetics

Distribution: 63-89 L/m^2

Protein binding: <1%

Metabolism: Extrahepatic; possibly via deamination by cytidine deaminase

Half-life elimination: ~30-35 minutes

Time to peak: At end of infusion

Dosage Adults:

MDS: I.V.: 15 mg/m^2 over 3 hours every 8 hours (45 mg/m^2/day) for 3 days (135 mg/m^2/cycle) every 6 weeks (treatment is recommended for at least 4 cycles and may continue until the patient no longer continues to benefit) **or** Low-dose schedule (unlabeled): 20 mg/m^2 over 1 hour daily for 5 days every 28 days

AML (investigational use): I.V.:

5-15 mg/m^2 over 1 hour daily, 5 days/week for 2 weeks (5 days on, 2 days off, 5 days on; 10 doses total) every 6 weeks

or

15 mg/m^2 over 1 hour daily for 10 days every 6 weeks

CML (investigational use): I.V.:

20 mg/m^2 over 1 hour daily for 5 days every 28 days

or

10-15 mg/m^2 over 1 hour daily, 5 days/week for 2 weeks (5 days on, 2 days off, 5 days on; 10 doses total) every 6 weeks

or

50-75 mg/m^2 over 6 hours every 12 hours for 5 days every 4-8 weeks

Sickle cell anemia (investigational use): I.V., SubQ: 0.15-0.3 mg/kg/day over 2 minutes 5 days/week for 2 weeks (5 days on, 2 days off, 5 days on; 10 doses total) every 6 weeks

Dosage adjustment for toxicity:

For delayed hematologic recovery (ANC ≥1000/mm^3 and platelets ≥50,000/mm^3):

Greater than 6 weeks but less than 8 weeks: Delay dose for up to 2 weeks and temporarily reduce dose to 11 mg/m^2 every 8 hours (33 mg/m^2/day) for 3 days

Greater than 8 weeks but less than 10 weeks: Assess for disease progression; if no disease progression, delay dose for up to 2 weeks and reduce dose to 11 mg/m^2 every 8 hours (33 mg/m^2/day) for 3 days; maintain or increase dose with subsequent cycles if clinically indicated

Temporarily hold treatment until resolution for any of the following non-hematologic toxicities:

Serum creatinine ≥2 mg/dL

ALT, bilirubin ≥2 times ULN

Active or uncontrolled infection

Combination Regimens

Leukemia, chronic myelogenous: Decitabine (Low Dose Regimen) on page 1288

Myelodysplastic syndrome: Decitabine (Low Dose Regimen) on page 1288

Administration Infuse over 1-6 hours. Premedication with antiemetics is recommended.

Monitoring Parameters CBC and platelets with each cycle, more frequently if needed; liver enzymes; serum creatinine

◄ **Emetic Potential** Very low (<10%)

Dosage Forms Excipient information presented when available (limited, particularly for generics); consult specific product labeling.

Injection, powder for reconstitution:

Dacogen™: 50 mg

References

Cashen AF, Shah AK, Todt L, et al, "Pharmacokinetics of Decitabine Administered as a 3-h Infusion to Patients With Acute Myeloid Leukemia (AML) or Myelodysplastic Syndrome (MDS)," *Cancer Chemother Pharmacol*, 2008, 61(5):759-66

DeSimone J, Koshy M, Dorn L, et al, "Maintenance of Elevated Fetal Hemoglobin Levels by Decitabine During Dose Interval Treatment of Sickle Cell Anemia," *Blood*, 2002, 99(11):3905-8.

Issa JP, Garcia-Manero G, and Giles FJ, "Phase 1 Study of Low-Dose Prolonged Exposure Schedules of the Hypomethylating Agent 5-Aza-2'Deoxycytidine (Decitabine) in Hematopoietic Malignancies," *Blood*, 2004, 103(5):1635-40.

Issa JP, Gharibyan V, Cortes J, et al, "Phase II Study of Low-Dose Decitabine in Patients With Chronic Myelogenous Leukemia Resistant to Imatinib Mesylate," *J Clin Oncol*, 2005, 23 (17):3948-56.

Kantarjian H, Issa JP, Rosenfeld CS, et al, "Decitabine Improves Patient Outcomes in Myelodysplastic Syndromes," *Cancer*, 2006, 106(8):1794-803.

Kantarjian HM, O'Brien S, Cortes J, et al, "Results of Decitabine (5-Aza-2'Dexoxycytidine) Therapy in 130 Patients With Chronic Myelogenous Leukemia," *Cancer*, 2003, 98(3):522-8.

Kantarjian H, Oki Y, Garcia-Manero G, et al, "Results of a Randomized Study of 3 Schedules of Low-Dose Decitabine in Higher-Risk Myelodysplastic Syndrome and Chronic Myelomonocytic Leukemia," *Blood*, 2007, 109(1):52-7.

Momparler RL, "Pharmacology of 5-Aza-2'-Deoxycytidine (Decitabine)," *Semin Hematol*, 2005, 42 (3 Suppl 2):9-16.

Deferasirox (de FER a sir ox)

Medication Safety Issues

Sound-alike/look-alike issues:

Deferasirox may be confused with deferoxamine

U.S. Brand Names Exjade®

Index Terms ICL670

Generic Available No

Canadian Brand Names Exjade®

Pharmacologic Category Antidote; Chelating Agent

Use Treatment of chronic iron overload due to blood transfusions (transfusional hemosiderosis)

Pregnancy Risk Factor B

Lactation Excretion in breast milk unknown/use caution

Labeled Contraindications Hypersensitivity to deferasirox or any component of the formulation

Canadian labeling: Additional contraindications (not in U.S. labeling): Cl$_{cr}$ <60 mL/minute

Warnings/Precautions Cases of acute renal failure (some fatal) and dose-related elevations in serum creatinine have been reported. Monitor serum creatinine in all patients; monitor patients at risk for renal complications (eg, pre-existing renal conditions, elderly, comorbid conditions, and/or with concurrent medications that may affect renal function) more closely; consider dose reduction, interruption, or discontinuation for serum creatinine elevations. Has not been studied in patients with renal impairment; patients with baseline serum creatinine above the upper limit of normal (ULN) were excluded from clinical trials. May cause proteinuria; closely monitor.

Severe hepatic dysfunction or failure (including fatalities) have occurred (postmarketing reports), mostly in patients >55 years of age with underlying comorbidities (including hepatic cirrhosis and multiorgan failure). Hepatitis and elevated transaminases have also been reported; monitor transaminases and consider dose modification or interruption of therapy with severe or persistent hepatic function test abnormalities. Has not been studied in patients with hepatic impairment, although has been used in patients with baseline transaminases ≤5 times ULN (deferasirox pharmacokinetics were not altered with these transaminase levels); use with caution. Gastrointestinal (GI) irritation, as well as upper GI ulceration and hemorrhage have been reported. Use caution with concurrent medications that may increase risk of adverse GI effects (eg, NSAIDs, corticosteroids, anticoagulants, oral bisphosphonates). Monitor patients closely for signs/symptoms of GI ulceration/bleeding.

May cause skin rash (dose-related); mild-to-moderate rashes may resolve without treatment interruption; for severe rash, interrupt and consider restarting at a lower dose with dose escalation and oral steroids. Hypersensitivity reactions, including severe reactions (anaphylaxis and angioedema) have been reported, usually within the first month of treatment. Discontinuation of therapy may be necessary. Auditory (decreased hearing and high frequency hearing loss) or ocular disturbances (lens opacities, cataracts, intraocular pressure elevation, and retinal disorders) have been reported; monitor and consider dose reduction or treatment interruption. Cytopenias (including agranulocytosis, neutropenia, and thrombocytopenia) have been reported, predominately in patients with preexisting hematologic disorders; monitor closely; interrupt treatment for unexplained cytopenias. Potent UGT inducers (eg, rifampin) may decrease the efficacy of deferasirox; dosage modifications may be needed; monitor serum ferritin and clinical response. Do not combine with other iron chelation therapies; safety of combinations has not been established. Treatment should be initiated with evidence of chronic iron overload (eg, transfusion of ~100 mL/kg of packed RBCs [~20 units for a 40 kg individual] and serum ferritin consistently >1000 mcg/L). Use with caution in the elderly due to the higher incidence of hepatic, renal and cardiac dysfunction in the elderly. Safety and efficacy in children <2 years of age have not been established.

Adverse Reactions

>10%:

Central nervous system: Fever (19%), headache (16%)

Dermatologic: Rash (dose related; 8% to 11%)

Gastrointestinal: Abdominal pain (dose related; 21% to 28%), diarrhea (dose related; 12% to 20%), nausea (dose related; 11% to 23%), vomiting (dose related; 10% to 21%)

Renal: Serum creatinine increased (dose related; 7% to 38%), proteinuria (19%)

Respiratory: Cough (14%), nasopharyngitis (13%), pharyngolaryngeal pain (11%)

Miscellaneous: Influenza (11%)

1% to 10%:

Central nervous system: Fatigue (6%)

Dermatologic: Urticaria (4%)

Hepatic: ALT increased (2% to 8%), transaminitis (4%)

Neuromuscular & skeletal: Arthralgia (7%), back pain (6%)

Otic: Ear infection (5%)

Respiratory: Respiratory tract infection (10%), bronchitis (9%), pharyngitis (8%), acute tonsillitis (6%), rhinitis (6%)

<1%, postmarketing, and/or case reports: Acute renal failure, agranulocytosis, anaphylaxis, angioedema, anxiety, ascites, bilirubin increased, cataract, cholecystitis, cholelithiasis, constipation, cytopenias, dizziness, drug fever, duodenal ulcer, edema, erythema multiforme, esophagitis, gastric ulcer,

gastritis, gastrointestinal bleeding, glomerulonephritis, glucosuria, hearing loss (including high frequency), hematuria, Henoch-Schönlein purpura, hepatic dysfunction, hepatic encephalopathy, hepatic failure (including fatalities), hepatic transaminases increased, hepatitis, hyperactivity, hypersensitivity reaction, hypocalcemia, insomnia, interstitial nephritis, intraocular pressure increased, jaundice, lens opacities, leukocytoclastic vasculitis, maculopathy, neutropenia, optic neuritis, pigment disorder, purpura, renal tubular necrosis, renal tubulopathy, retinal disorder, sleep disorder, thrombocytopenia, visual disturbance

Drug Interactions

Avoid Concomitant Use There are no known interactions where it is recommended to avoid concomitant use.

Increased Effect/Toxicity

Deferasirox may increase the levels/effects of: CYP2C8 Substrates (High risk)

Decreased Effect

Deferasirox may decrease the levels/effects of: CYP3A4 Substrates

The levels/effects of Deferasirox may be decreased by: Aluminum Hydroxide; PHENobarbital; Phenytoin; Rifampin; Ritonavir

Storage/Stability Store at room temperature of 25°C (77°F); excursions permitted to 15°C and 30°C (59°F and 86°F). Protect from moisture.

Mechanism of Action Selectively binds iron, forming a complex which is excreted primarily through the feces.

Pharmacodynamics/Kinetics

Distribution: Adults: 11.7-17.1 L

Protein binding: ~99% to serum albumin

Metabolism: Hepatic via glucuronidation by UGT1A1(primarily) and UGT1A3; minor oxidation by CYP450; undergoes enterohepatic recirculation

Bioavailability: 70%

Half-life elimination: 8-16 hours

Time to peak, plasma: ~1.5-4 hours

Excretion: Feces (84%), urine (8%)

Dosage Oral: Children ≥2 years and Adults:

Initial: 20 mg/kg daily (calculate dose to nearest whole tablet)

Maintenance: Adjust dose every 3-6 months based on serum ferritin levels; adjust by 5-10 mg/kg/day (calculate dose to nearest whole tablet); titrate. Usual range: 20-30 mg/kg/day; doses up to 40 mg/kg/day may be considered for serum ferritin levels persistently >2500 mcg/L (doses above 40 mg/kg/day are not recommended). In clinical trials, doses were individualized based on iron burden determined by liver iron concentrations (LIC); transfusional iron intake should be considered when individualizing maintenance dose. **Note:** Consider interrupting therapy for serum ferritin <500 mcg/L and dose reduction or interruption for hearing loss or visual disturbances.

Dosage adjustment with concomitant potent UGT inducers: Increased deferasirox doses may be required with concomitant potent UGT inducers (eg, rifampin); monitor serum ferritin and clinical response. Doses above 40 mg/kg are not recommended.

Dosage adjustment in renal impairment: Interrupt treatment for progressive increase in serum creatinine above the age-appropriate ULN; once serum creatinine recovers to within the normal range, reinitiate treatment at a reduced dose; gradually escalate the dose if the clinical benefit outweighs potential risk.

Children: For increase in serum creatinine above the age-appropriate ULN for 2 consecutive levels, reduce daily dose by 10 mg/kg

Adults: For increase in serum creatinine >33% above the average pretreatment level at 2 consecutive levels (and cannot be attributed to other causes), reduce daily dose by 10 mg/kg

Dosage adjustment in hepatic impairment: Consider dose adjustment or discontinuation for severe or persistent elevations in liver function tests.

Administration Oral: **Do not chew or swallow whole tablets.** Take at same time each day on an empty stomach, 30 minutes before food. Disperse tablets in water, orange juice, or apple juice (use 3.5 ounces for total doses <1 g; 7 ounces for doses ≥1 g); stir to form suspension and drink entire contents. Rinse remaining residue with more fluid; drink. Do not take simultaneously with aluminum-containing antacids.

Monitoring Parameters Serum ferritin (monthly), CBC with differential, serum creatinine (2 baseline assessments then monthly; in patients who are at increased risk of complications [eg, pre-existing renal conditions, elderly, comorbid conditions, or receiving other potentially nephrotoxic medications]: weekly for the first month then monthly thereafter); urine protein (monthly); liver function tests (baseline, every 2 weeks for 1 month, then monthly); baseline and annual auditory and ophthalmic function (including slit lamp examinations and dilated fundoscopy); number of RBC units received

Dietary Considerations Bioavailability increased variably when taken with food; take on empty stomach 30 minutes before a meal.

Additional Information Deferasirox has a low affinity for binding with zinc and copper, may cause variable decreases in the serum concentration of these trace minerals.

Oncology Comment: The National Comprehensive Cancer Network (NCCN) guidelines for myelodysplastic syndromes (MDS) recommend considering iron chelation therapy in low- or intermediate-risk MDS patients to decrease iron overload due to multiple transfusions (v.1.2009). Treatment is generally recommended in MDS patients who have received ≥20 units of RBC transfusions and for those with serum ferritin levels >2500 mcg/L, with a goal to decrease ferritin levels to <1000 mcg/L. Although clinical trials in MDS are ongoing, deferasirox may be useful in the management of iron overload of these patients.

Dosage Forms Excipient information presented when available (limited, particularly for generics); consult specific product labeling.

Tablet, for oral suspension:

Exjade®: 125 mg, 250 mg, 500 mg

References

Cappellini MD, "Long-Term Efficacy and Safety of Deferasirox," *Blood Rev*, 2008, 22(Suppl 2):35-41.

Cappellini MD, Cohen A, Piga A, et al, "A Phase 3 Study of Deferasirox (ICL670), a Once-Daily Oral Iron Chelator, in Patients With Beta-Thalassemia," *Blood*, 2006, 107(9):3455-62.

Cohen AR, Glimm E, and Porter JB, "Effect of Transfusional Iron Intake on Response to Chelation Therapy in β-Thalassemia," *Blood*, 2008, 111(2):583-7.

Galanello R, Piga A, Alberti D, et al, "Safety, Tolerability, and Pharmacokinetics of ICL670, a New Orally Active Iron-Chelating Agent in Patients With Transfusion-Dependent Iron Overload Due to Beta-Thalassemia," *J Clin Pharmacol*, 2003, 43(6):565-72.

National Comprehensive Cancer Network (NCCN), "Clinical Practice Guidelines in Oncology™: Myelodysplastic Syndromes," Version 1.2009. Available at http://www.nccn.org/professionals/physician_gls/PDF/mds.pdf.

Nisbet-Brown E, Oliveri NF, Giardina PJ, et al, "Effectiveness and Safety of ICL670 in Iron-Loaded Patients With Thalassaemia: A Randomised, Double-Blind, Placebo-Controlled, Dose-Escalation Trial," *Lancet*, 2003, 361(9369):1597-602.

Porter J, Galanello R, Saglio G, et al, "Relative Response of Patients With Myelodysplastic Syndromes and Other Transfusion-Dependent Anaemias to Deferasirox (ICL670): A 1-Yr Prospective Study," *Eur J Haematol*, 2008, 80(2):168-76.

Raphael JL, Bernhardt MB, Mahoney DH, et al, "Oral Iron Chelation and the Treatment of Iron Overload in a Pediatric Hematology Center," *Pediatr Blood Cancer*, 2009, 52(5):616-20.

Vichinsky E, Onyekwere O, Porter J, et al, "A Randomised Comparison of Deferasirox Versus Deferoxamine for the Treatment of Transfusional Iron Overload in Sickle Cell Disease," *Br J Haematol*, 2007, 136(3):501-8.

Deferoxamine (de fer OKS a meen)

Medication Safety Issues

Sound-alike/look-alike issues:

Deferoxamine may be confused with cefuroxime, deferasirox

Desferal® may be confused with desflurane, Dexferrum®, Disophrol®

International issues:

Desferal® may be confused with Deseril® which is a brand name for methysergide in multiple international markets

U.S. Brand Names Desferal®

Index Terms Deferoxamine Mesylate; Desferrioxamine; NSC-644468

Generic Available Yes

Canadian Brand Names Desferal®; PMS-Deferoxamine

Pharmacologic Category Antidote; Chelating Agent

Use Acute iron intoxication or when clinical signs of significant iron toxicity exist; chronic iron overload secondary to multiple transfusions

Unlabeled/Investigational Use Removal of corneal rust rings following surgical removal of foreign bodies; diagnosis or treatment of aluminum induced toxicity associated with chronic kidney disease (CKD)

Pregnancy Risk Factor C

Lactation Excretion in breast milk unknown/use caution

Labeled Contraindications Hypersensitivity to deferoxamine or any component of the formulation; patients with severe renal disease or anuria, primary hemochromatosis

Warnings/Precautions Patients with iron overload are at increased susceptibility to infection with *Yersinia enterocolitica* and *Yersinia pseudotuberculosis;* treatment with deferoxamine may enhance this risk; if infection develops, discontinue deferoxamine until resolved. Rare and serious cases of mucormycosis have been reported with use; withhold treatment with signs and symptoms of mucormycosis. Combination treatment with ascorbic acid may impair cardiac function (rare). If combination treatment is warranted, therapy may need adjusted; monitor cardiac function. Do not administer deferoxamine in combination with ascorbic acid in patients with pre-existing cardiac failure.

High doses may exacerbate neurological symptoms, including seizure in patients with aluminum-related encephalopathy. Deferoxamine treatment in patients with aluminum toxicity may cause hypocalcemia and aggravate hyperparathyroidism. Deferoxamine is associated with dialysis dementia onset. Ocular and auditory disturbances have been reported following prolonged administration at high doses, or in patients with low ferritin levels; elderly patients are at increased risk for ocular and auditory disorders. Has been associated with adult respiratory distress syndrome (ARDS) following excessively high-dose treatment of acute intoxication or thalassemia; has also been reported in children. Flushing, hypotension, urticaria and shock are associated with rapid infusions. Patients should be informed that urine may have a reddish color. High deferoxamine doses and low ferritin levels are also associated with growth retardation. Safety and efficacy have not been established in children <3 years of age.

Adverse Reactions Frequency not defined.

Cardiovascular: Flushing, hypotension, tachycardia, shock, edema

Central nervous system: Fever, dizziness, neuropathy, seizure, exacerbation of aluminum-related encephalopathy (dialysis), headache

Dermatologic: Angioedema, rash, urticaria

Endocrine & metabolic: Growth retardation (children), hypocalcemia

Gastrointestinal: Abdominal discomfort, abdominal pain, diarrhea, nausea, vomiting

Genitourinary: Dysuria

Hematologic: Thrombocytopenia, leukopenia

Local: Injection site: Burning, crust, edema, erythema, eschar, induration, infiltration, irritation, pain, pruritus, swelling, vesicles, wheal formation

Neuromuscular & skeletal: Arthralgia, leg cramps, metaphyseal dysplasia (dose related), myalgia, paresthesia

Ocular: Acuity decreased, blurred vision, dichromatopsia, maculopathy, night vision impaired, peripheral vision impaired, visual loss, scotoma, visual field defects, optic neuritis, cataracts, retinal pigmentary abnormalities, night blindness

Otic: Hearing loss, tinnitus

Renal: Renal impairment, urine discoloration (vin-rose color)

Respiratory: Acute/adult respiratory distress syndrome, asthma

Miscellaneous: Anaphylaxis, hypersensitivity reaction, infections (*Yersinia*, mucormycosis)

Drug Interactions

Avoid Concomitant Use There are no known interactions where it is recommended to avoid concomitant use.

Increased Effect/Toxicity

The levels/effects of Deferoxamine may be increased by: Ascorbic Acid

Decreased Effect There are no known significant interactions involving a decrease in effect.

Storage/Stability Prior to reconstitution, do not store above 25°C (77°F). Following reconstitution, may be stored at room temperature for 7 days; protect from light. Do not refrigerate reconstituted solution.

Reconstitution

I.M.: Reconstitute with sterile water for injection (500 mg vial with 2 mL to a final concentration of 210 mg/mL; 2000 mg vial with 8 mL to a final concentration of 213 mg/mL)

I.V.: Reconstitute with sterile water for injection to a final solution of 100 mg/mL

SubQ: Reconstitute with sterile water for injection (500 mg vial with 5 mL; 2000 mg vial with 20 mL) to a final concentration of 95 mg/mL

Compatibility Stable in D_5W, LR, NS, sterile water for injection.

Mechanism of Action Complexes with trivalent ions (ferric ions) to form ferrioxamine, which are removed by the kidneys

Pharmacodynamics/Kinetics

Absorption: I.M.: Erratic

Metabolism: Plasma enzymes; binds with iron to form ferrioxamine

Half-life elimination: Parent drug: 6.1 hours; Ferrioxamine: 5.8 hours

Excretion: Primarily urine (as unchanged drug and ferrioxamine); feces (via bile)

Dosage

Acute iron toxicity: **Note:** I.V. route is used when severe toxicity is evidenced by systemic symptoms (coma, shock, metabolic acidosis, or severe gastrointestinal bleeding) or potentially severe intoxications (serum iron level >500 mcg/dL). When severe symptoms are not present, the I.M. route may be preferred (per manufacturer); however, the use of deferoxamine in situations where the serum iron concentration is <500 mcg/dL or when severe toxicity is not evident is a subject of some clinical debate.

Children ≥3 years:

    I.M.: 90 mg/kg/dose every 8 hours (maximum: 6 g/24 hours)

    I.V.: 15 mg/kg/hour (maximum: 6 g/24 hours)

    Adults: I.M., I.V.: Initial: 1000 mg, may be followed by 500 mg every 4 hours for up to 2 doses; subsequent doses of 500 mg have been administered every 4-12 hours

    Maximum recommended dose: 6 g/day (per manufacturer, however, higher doses have been administered)

Chronic iron overload:

    Children ≥3 years:

        I.V.: 15 mg/kg/hour (maximum: 12 g/24 hours)

        SubQ: 20-40 mg/kg/day over 8-12 hours (maximum: 1000-2000 mg/day)

    Adults:

        I.M., I.V.: 500-1000 mg/day I.M.; in addition, 2000 mg should be given I.V. with each unit of blood transfused (administer separately from blood); maximum: 1 g/day in absence of transfusions; 6 g/day if patient received transfusions

        SubQ: 1-2 g every day or 20-40 mg/kg/day over 8-24 hours

Diagnosis of aluminum induced toxicity with CKD (unlabeled use): Children and Adults: I.V.: Test dose: 5 mg/kg during the last hour of dialysis if serum aluminum levels are 60-200 mcg/L and there are clinical signs/symptoms of toxicity. Do not use if aluminum serum levels are >200 mcg/L

Treatment of aluminum toxicity with CKD (unlabeled use): Children and Adults: I.V.: 5-10 mg/kg 4-6 hours before dialysis. Administer every 7-10 days with 3-4 dialysis procedures between doses. Do not use if aluminum serum levels are >200 mcg/L.

Dosing adjustment in renal impairment: Cl$_{cr}$ <10 mL/minute: Administer 50% of dose

Administration

I.V.: Urticaria, hypotension, and shock have occurred following rapid I.V. administration; limiting infusion rate to 15mg/kg/hour may help avoid infusion-related adverse effects.

    Acute iron toxicity: The manufacturer states that the I.M. route is preferred; however, the I.V. route is generally preferred in patients with severe toxicity (ie, patients in shock). For the first 1000 mg, infuse at 15 mg/kg/hour (although rates up to 40-50 mg/kg/hour have been given in patients with massive iron intoxication). Subsequent doses may be given over 4-12 hours at a rate not to exceed 125 mg/hour.

    Diagnosis or treatment of aluminum induced toxicity with CKD: Administer dose over 1 hour

SubQ: When administered for chronic iron overload, daily dose should be given over 8-24 hours using portable pump.

Monitoring Parameters Serum iron; ophthalmologic exam (fundoscopy, slit-lamp exam) and audiometry with chronic therapy; growth and body weight in children (every 3 months)

Dialysis patients: Serum aluminum (yearly; every 3 months in patients on aluminum-containing medications)

Aluminum-induced bone disease: Serum aluminum 2 days following test dose; test is considered positive if serum aluminum increases ≥50 mcg/L

Test Interactions TIBC may be falsely elevated with high serum iron concentrations or deferoxamine therapy. Imaging results may be distorted due to rapid urinary excretion of deferoxamine-bound gallium-67; discontinue deferoxamine 48 hours prior to scintigraphy.

Dietary Considerations Vitamin C supplements may need to be limited. The manufacturer recommends a maximum of 200 mg/day in adults (given in divided doses) and avoiding use in patients with heart failure.

Dosage Forms Excipient information presented when available (limited, particularly for generics); consult specific product labeling.

Injection, powder for reconstitution, as mesylate: 500 mg, 2 g

Desferal®: 500 mg, 2 g

References

Allain P, Mauras Y, Chaleil D, et al, "Pharmacokinetics and Renal Elimination of Desferrioxamine and Ferrioxamine in Healthy Subjects and Patients With Haemochromatosis," *Br J Clin Pharmacol*, 1987, 24(2):207-12.

Cohen AR, Mizanin J, and Schwartz E, "Rapid Removal of Excessive Iron With Daily, High-Dose Intravenous Chelation Therapy," *J Pediatr*, 1989, 115(1):151-5.

Freedman MH, Olivieri N, Benson L, et al, "Clinical Studies on Iron Chelation in Patients With Thalassemia Major," *Haematologica*, 1990, 75(Suppl 5):74-83.

Hershko C, Konijn AM, and Link G, "Iron Chelators for Thalassaemia," *Br J Haematol*, 1998, 101 (3):399-406.

Kirking MH, "Treatment of Chronic Iron Overload," *Clin Pharm*, 1991, 10(10):775-83.

National Kidney Foundation, K/DOQI Clinical Practice Guidelines for Bone Metabolism and Disease in Chronic Kidney Failure," *Am J Kidney Dis*, 2003, 42(4 Supple3):1-201.

◆ **Deferoxamine Mesylate** *see* Deferoxamine on page 334

Degarelix (deg a REL ix)

Medication Safety Issues

Sound-alike/look-alike issues:

Degarelix may be confused with cetrorelix, ganirelix

Related Information

Safe Handling of Hazardous Drugs on page 1517

U.S. Brand Names Firmagon®

Index Terms Degarelix Acetate; FE200486

Generic Available No

Pharmacologic Category Antineoplastic Agent, Gonadotropin-Releasing Hormone Antagonist; Gonadotropin Releasing Hormone Antagonist

Use Treatment of advanced prostate cancer

Pregnancy Risk Factor X

Lactation Excretion in breast milk unknown/not recommended

Labeled Contraindications Hypersensitivity to degarelix or any component of the formulation; pregnancy (or potential to become pregnant)

Warnings/Precautions Hazardous agent - use appropriate precautions for handling and disposal. Long-term androgen deprivation therapy may prolong the QT interval; use with caution in patients with a known history of QT prolongation or other risk factors for QT prolongation (eg, concomitant use of medications known to prolong QT interval, heart failure, and/or electrolyte abnormalities). Androgen deprivation therapy may increase the risk for cardiovascular disease and decreased bone mineral density. Androgen deprivation therapy may cause obesity and insulin resistance; the risk for diabetes is increased.

◄ Degarelix exposure is decreased in patients with hepatic impairment, dosage adjustment is not recommended in patients with mild-to-moderate hepatic impairment, although testosterone levels should be monitored. Has not been studied in patients with severe hepatic impairment; use with caution. Data for use in patients with moderate-to-severe renal impairment (Cl_{cr} <50 mL/minute) is limited; use with caution. Safety and efficacy have not been established in children.

Adverse Reactions

>10%:
  Endocrine & metabolic: Hot flashes (26%)
  Local: Injections site reactions (35%, grade 3: ≤2%; pain 28%, erythema 17%, swelling 6%, induration 4%, nodule 3%)

1% to 10%:
  Cardiovascular: Hypertension (6%)
  Central nervous system: Chills (5%), dizziness (1% to 5%), fever (1% to 5%), headache (1% to 5%), insomnia (1% to 5%), fatigue (3%)
  Dermatologic: Hyperhydrosis
  Endocrine & metabolic: Hypercholesterolemia (3%), gynecomastia, testicular atrophy
  Gastrointestinal: Weight gain (9%), constipation (5%), nausea (1% to 5%), diarrhea
  Genitourinary: Urinary tract infection (5%), erectile dysfunction
  Hepatic: ALT increased (10%; grade 3: <1%), AST increased (5%; grade 3: <1%), GGT increased
  Neuromuscular & skeletal: Back pain (6%), arthralgia (5%), weakness (1% to 5%)
  Miscellaneous: Antidegarelix antibody formation (10%), night sweats (1% to 5%)

<1%, postmarketing, and/or case reports: Bone metastases worsening, cerebral stroke, depression, injection site pruritus, injection site soreness, lymphoma (malignant), mental status changes, MI, osteoarthritis, QT interval prolongation, squamous cell cancer, unstable angina

Drug Interactions

Avoid Concomitant Use
Avoid concomitant use of Degarelix with any of the following: Artemether; Dronedarone; Lumefantrine; Nilotinib; Pimozide; QuiNINE; Tetrabenazine; Thioridazine; Ziprasidone

Increased Effect/Toxicity
Degarelix may increase the levels/effects of: Dronedarone; Pimozide; QTc-Prolonging Agents; QuiNINE; Tetrabenazine; Thioridazine; Ziprasidone

The levels/effects of Degarelix may be increased by: Alfuzosin; Artemether; Chloroquine; Ciprofloxacin; Gadobutrol; Lumefantrine; Nilotinib; QuiNINE

Decreased Effect There are no known significant interactions involving a decrease in effect.

Storage/Stability Store at 25°C (77°F); excursions permitted to 15°C to 30°C (59°F to 86°F).

Reconstitution Use appropriate precautions (wear gloves for preparation and administration) for handling and disposal. Reconstitute with preservative free sterile water for injection (reconstitute each 120 mg vial with 3 mL; reconstitute the 80 mg vial with 4.2 mL). Swirl gently; do not shake (to prevent foaming). Dissolution may take up to 15 minutes. Keep vial upright at all times. Tilt vial slightly, keeping needle in lowest section of vial to withdraw for administration. Administer within 1 hour of reconstitution.

Mechanism of Action Gonadotropin-releasing hormone (GnRH) antagonist which reversibly binds to GnRH receptors in the anterior pituitary gland, blocking the receptor and decreasing secretion of luteinizing hormone (LH) and follicle stimulation hormone (FSH), resulting in rapid androgen deprivation by decreasing testosterone production, thereby decreasing testosterone levels. Testosterone levels do not exhibit an initial surge, or flare, as is typical with GnRH agonists.

Pharmacodynamics/Kinetics

Onset of action: Rapid; ~96% of patients had testosterone levels ≤50 ng/dL within 3 days (Klotz, 2008)

Distribution: V_d: >1000 L

Protein binding: ~90%

Metabolism: Hepatobiliary, via peptide hydrolysis

Bioavailability: Biphasic release: Rapid release initially, then slow release from depot formed after subcutaneous injection administration (Tornoe, 2007)

Half-life elimination: Loading dose: SubQ: ~53 days

Time to peak, plasma: Loading dose: SubQ: Within 2 days

Excretion: Feces (~70% to 80%, primarily as peptide fragments); urine (~20% to 30%)

Dosage SubQ: Adults: Prostate cancer:

Loading dose: 240 mg administered as two 120 mg (3 mL) injections

Maintenance dose: 80 mg every 28 days (beginning 28 days after initial loading dose)

Dosage adjustment in renal impairment: Cl_{cr} <50 mL/minute: Use with caution

Dosage adjustment in hepatic impairment:

Mild-to-moderate hepatic impairment: No adjustment required; monitor serum testosterone levels

Severe hepatic impairment: Has not been studied; use with caution

Administration Not for I.V. use. Administer SubQ in the abdominal area by grasping skin and elevating SubQ tissue; inject at an angle ≤45 degrees. Avoid pressure exposed areas (eg, waistband, belt, or near ribs); rotate injection site. Inject loading dose as two 3 mL injections (40 mg/mL); maintenance dose should be administered as a single 4 mL injection (20 mg/mL); begin maintenance dose 28 days after initial loading dose.

Monitoring Parameters Prostate-specific antigen (PSA) periodically, serum testosterone levels (if PSA increases; in patients with hepatic impairment: monitor testosterone levels monthly until achieve castration levels, then consider monitoring every other month), liver function tests (at baseline), serum electrolytes (calcium, magnesium, potassium, sodium); bone mineral density

Screen for diabetes and cardiovascular risk prior to initiating treatment.

Test Interactions Suppression of pituitary-gonadal function may affect diagnostic tests of pituitary gonadotropic and gonadal functions.

Dietary Considerations Supplementation with 500 mg calcium and 400 int. units of vitamin D is recommended (due to the increased risk for osteoporosis with androgen deprivation therapy).

Dosage Forms Excipient information presented when available (limited, particularly for generics); consult specific product labeling.

Injection, powder for reconstitution, as acetate:

Firmagon®: 80 mg, 120 mg

References

Gittelman M, Pommerville PJ, Persson BE, et al, "A 1-Year, Open Label, Randomized Phase II Dose Finding Study of Degarelix for the Treatment of Prostate Cancer in North America," *J Urol*, 2008, 180(5):1986-92.

Klotz L, Boccon-Gibod L, Shore ND, et al, "The Efficacy and Safety of Degarelix: A 12-month, Comparative, Randomized, Open-Label, Parallel-Group Phase III Study in Patients With Prostate Cancer," *BJU Int*, 2008, 102(11):1531-8.

National Comprehensive Cancer Network® (NCCN), "Clinical Practice Guidelines in Oncology™: Prostate Cancer," Version 2.2009. Available at http://www.nccn.org/professionals/physician_gls/PDF/prostate.pdf

Tornoe CW, Agerso H, Senderovitz T, et al, "Population Pharmacokinetic/Pharmacodynamic (PK/PD) Modelling of the Hypothalamic-Pituitary-Gonadal Axis Following Treatment With GnRH Analogues," *Br J Clin Pharmacol*, 2007, 63(6):648-64.

◆ **Degarelix Acetate** *see* Degarelix *on page 337*

◆ **Dehydrobenzperidol** *see* Droperidol *on page 389*

◆ **Delta-9-tetrahydro-cannabinol** *see* Dronabinol *on page 387*

◆ **Delta-9-Tetrahydrocannabinol and Cannabinol** *see* Tetrahydrocannabinol and Cannabidiol *on page 1090*

◆ **Delta-9 THC** *see* Dronabinol *on page 387*

◆ **Deltacortisone** *see* PredniSONE *on page 982*

◆ **Deltadehydrocortisone** *see* PredniSONE *on page 982*

◆ **Deltahydrocortisone** *see* PrednisoLONE *on page 977*

◆ **Demerol®** *see* Meperidine *on page 750*

◆ **4-Demethoxydaunorubicin** *see* IDArubicin *on page 605*

Denileukin Diftitox (de ni LOO kin DIF ti toks)

Medication Safety Issues

High alert medication: The Institute for Safe Medication Practices (ISMP) includes this medication among its list of drug classes which have a heightened risk of causing significant patient harm when used in error.

Related Information

Safe Handling of Hazardous Drugs *on page 1517*

U.S. Brand Names ONTAK®

Index Terms DAB389 Interleukin-2; DAB$_{389}$IL-2; DABIL2

Generic Available No

Pharmacologic Category Antineoplastic Agent, Miscellaneous

Use Treatment of persistent or recurrent cutaneous T-cell lymphoma (CTCL) whose malignant cells express the CD25 component of the IL-2 receptor

Unlabeled/Investigational Use Treatment of CTCL types mycosis fungoides (MF) and Sézary syndrome (SS); peripheral T-cell lymphoma (second-line treatment)

Lactation Excretion in breast milk unknown/not recommended

Labeled Contraindications There are no contraindications listed within the manufacturer's labeling.

Warnings/Precautions Hazardous agent - use appropriate precautions for handling and disposal. **[U.S. Boxed Warning]: Has been associated with a potentially severe, including life-threatening, capillary leak syndrome; monitor weight, edema, blood pressure, and serum albumin prior to and during treatment.** Symptoms of capillary leak syndrome (hypotension, edema, hypoalbuminemia) may be delayed, occurring up to 2 weeks post infusion; symptoms may persist or worsen after cessation of denileukin diftitox. Withhold treatment if serum albumin <3 g/dL; pre-existing low serum albumin levels may correlate with capillary leak syndrome. **[U.S. Boxed Warning]: Serious and fatal infusion reactions have occurred. Administer in a facility appropriate for cardiopulmonary resuscitation. Discontinue immediately and permanently with serious infusion reaction.** Infusion reaction symptoms usually occur within 24 hours of infusion and resolve within 48 hours of last infusion of cycle. Incidence of infusion reaction has been reported to be lower in cycles 3 and 4 (compared to cycles 1 and 2). The manufacturer recommends premedicating with an antihistamine and acetaminophen; corticosteroid (eg, dexamethasone) premedication may help to reduce the incidence of hypersensitivity and edema (Foss, 2001). **[U.S. Boxed Warning]: Loss of visual acuity, usually associated with loss of color vision (with or without retinal pigment mottling) has been reported;** most patients have persistent visual impairment.

Confirm CD25 expression on malignant cells prior to treatment. May develop immunogenicity; patients with antibodies have a two- to threefold increase in clearance; the presence of antibodies does not correlate with risk for hypersensitivity/infusion related reactions. Monitor closely for infection; may impair immune function. Use with caution in patients >65 years of age; adverse events (anemia, anorexia, confusion, hypotension, rash, nausea/vomiting) may occur more frequently. Safety and efficacy in children have not been established. Should be administered under the supervision of an experienced cancer chemotherapy physician.

Adverse Reactions

>10%:

Cardiovascular: Capillary leak syndrome (33%; serious: 11%), peripheral edema (20% to 26%), vasodilation (22%), hypotension (7% to 16%), chest pain (4% to 13%), tachycardia (12%), thrombosis-related events (7% to 11%)

Central nervous system: Fever (49% to 64%), fatigue (44% to 47%), headache (26% to 29%), dizziness (11% to 13%), pain (11% to 13%)

Dermatologic: Rash (20% to 24%), pruritus (16% to 18%)

Endocrine & metabolic: Hypoalbuminemia (14% to 17%)

Gastrointestinal: Nausea (47% to 60%), vomiting (13% to 35%), diarrhea (22%), anorexia (9% to 20%), taste disturbance (11% to 13%)

Hematologic: Lymphopenia (70%; 24% had lymphopenia at baseline)

Hepatic: ALT increased (84%), AST increased (84%)

Neuromuscular & skeletal: Rigors (42% to 47%), myalgia (18% to 20%), weakness (18%), back pain (16% to 18%), arthralgia (13% to 16%)

Respiratory: Cough (18% to 20%), upper respiratory infection (13%), dyspnea (11% to 13%)

Miscellaneous: Antibody formation (76% to 100%) neutralizing antibodies (45% to 97%), flu-like syndrome (≤85%), infusion reaction (71%; serious: 8%), infection (48%)

1% to 10%:

Cardiovascular: Arrhythmia (6%), hypertension (6%)

Hematologic: Leukopenia (grades 3/4: 3% to 6%), neutropenia (grades 3/4: 3%), thrombocytopenia (grades 3/4: 3%)

Local: Injection site reaction (8%)

Ocular: Visual changes (serious: 4%; includes loss of visual acuity)

Renal: Serum creatinine increased (3% to 10%), proteinuria/casts/hematuria (6%)

Postmarketing and/or case reports: Acute renal insufficiency, hyper-/hypo-thyroidism, oral ulcer, pancreatitis, thyroiditis, thyrotoxicosis, toxic epidermal necrolysis

Drug Interactions

Avoid Concomitant Use

Avoid concomitant use of Denileukin Diftitox with any of the following: Natalizumab; Vaccines (Live)

Increased Effect/Toxicity

Denileukin Diftitox may increase the levels/effects of: Leflunomide; Natalizumab; Vaccines (Live)

The levels/effects of Denileukin Diftitox may be increased by: Trastuzumab

Decreased Effect

Denileukin Diftitox may decrease the levels/effects of: Vaccines (Inactivated); Vaccines (Live)

The levels/effects of Denileukin Diftitox may be decreased by: Echinacea

Storage/Stability Store intact vials frozen at or below -10°C (14°F); do not refreeze after thawing. Solutions ≥15 mcg/mL in NS should be used within 6 hours.

Reconstitution Must be brought to room temperature (25°C or 77°F) before preparing the dose. Do **not** heat vials. Thaw in refrigerator for not more than 24 hours or at room temperature for 1-2 hours. Solution may be mixed by gentle swirling; avoid vigorous agitation. Dilute with NS to a concentration of ≥15 mcg/mL; the concentration must be ≥15 mcg/mL during all steps of preparation. Add drug to the empty sterile I.V. bag first, then add NS. Do not prepare with glass syringes or in glass containers.

Mechanism of Action Denileukin diftitox is a fusion protein (a combination of amino acid sequences from diphtheria toxin and interleukin-2) which selectively delivers the cytotoxic activity of diphtheria toxin to targeted cells. It interacts with the high-affinity IL-2 receptor on the surface of malignant cells to inhibit intracellular protein synthesis, rapidly leading to cell death.

Pharmacodynamics/Kinetics

Distribution: V_d: 0.06-0.09 L/kg

Metabolism: Hepatic via proteolytic degradation (animal studies)

Half-life elimination: Distribution: 2-5 minutes; Terminal: 70-80 minutes

Dosage Note: Premedicate with an antihistamine and acetaminophen prior to each infusion; corticosteroid premedication (eg, dexamethasone) may reduce the incidence of hypersensitivity and edema (Foss, 2001). Withhold treatment if serum albumin <3 g/dL.

I.V.: Adults: CTCL: 9 or 18 mcg/kg/day days 1 through 5 every 21 days for 8 cycles

Dosage adjustment for toxicity:

Serum albumin <3 g/dL: Withhold treatment

Severe infusion reaction: Permanently discontinue treatment

Administration For I.V. use only. Infuse over 30-60 minutes. Should **not** be given as a rapid I.V. bolus. Discontinue or reduce infusion rate for infusion related reactions; discontinue for severe infusion reaction. Do not administer through an in-line filter. Premedicate with an antihistamine and acetaminophen; consider corticosteroid premedication.

Monitoring Parameters Baseline CD25 expression (on malignant cells); serum albumin level (prior to each treatment), CBC, blood chemistry panel, renal and hepatic function tests (prior to initiation of therapy and weekly during therapy). During the infusion, the patient should be monitored for symptoms of an infusion reaction. After infusion, the patient should be monitored for the development of a delayed capillary leak syndrome (usually in the first 2 weeks), including careful monitoring of weight, blood pressure, and serum albumin.

Information on assay for malignant cell CD25 expression is available at 1-877-873-4724.

Additional Information Oncology Comment: The National Comprehensive Cancer Network® (NCCN) Non-Hodgkin's Lymphoma Guidelines (v.2.2009) list denileukin diftitox as a second-line treatment option for systemic therapy of peripheral (cutaneous) T-cell lymphoma in patients who are not candidates for high dose therapy or autologous stem cell rescue. In mycosis fungoides (MF) and Sézary syndrome (SS), denileukin diftitox is a therapy option, either as monotherapy or in combination with bexarotene (Foss, 2005). Participation in a clinical trial is encouraged for this patient population.

Corticosteroids may be considered for prevention of hypersensitivity reaction. In a small study (Foss, 2001) reviewing denileukin diftitox and premedication with either prednisone 20 mg orally or dexamethasone 8 mg I.V. on day 1 followed by dexamethasone 8 mg I.V. on days 2-5, a reduction in adverse events was observed when compared to a previous (Olsen, 2001) phase III study. A statistically significant reduction in the incidence of edema was demonstrated. Improved response rates (compared to the phase III study) were noted, likely due to in increase in tolerability due to corticosteroid premedication. While some studies did not allow premedication with cortico-steroids (Kuzel, 2007; Olsen, 2001) as part of the trial design, dexamethasone premedication has been utilized in other studies and case reports (Foss, 2005; Frankel, 2006; Gerena-Lewis, 2009; Talpur, 2002) with denileukin diftitox use for cutaneous T-cell lymphoma as well as other (unlabeled) uses.

Emetic Potential Very low (<10%)

Dosage Forms Excipient information presented when available (limited, particularly for generics); consult specific product labeling.

Injection, solution [frozen]:

ONTAK®: 150 mcg/mL (2 mL) [contains EDTA]

References

Foss FM, Bacha P, Osann KE, et al, "Biological Correlates of Acute Hypersensitivity Events With DAB389IL-2 (Denileukin Diftitox, Ontak®) in Cutaneous T-Cell Lymphoma: Decreased Frequency and Severity With Steroid Premedication," *Clin Lymphoma*, 2001, 1(4):298-302.

Foss F, Demierre MF, and DiVenuti F, "A Phase-1 Trial of Bexarotene and Denileukin Diftitox in Patients With Relapsed or Refractory Cutaneous T-Cell Lymphoma," *Blood*, 2005, 106(2):454-7.

Frankel AE, Surendranathan A, Black JH, et al, "Phase II Clinical Studies of Denileukin Diftitox Diphtheria Toxin Fusion Protein in Patients With Previously Treated Chronic Lymphocytic Leukemia," *Cancer*, 2006, 106(10):2158-64.

Gerena-Lewis M, Crawford J, Bonomi P, et al, "A Phase II Trial of Denileukin Diftitox in Patients With Previously Treated Advanced Non-Small Cell Lung Cancer," *Am J Clin Oncol*, 2009, 32 (3):269-73.

National Comprehensive Cancer Network (NCCN)®, "Clinical Practice Guidelines in Oncology™: Non-Hodgkin's Lymphomas," Version 2.2009. Available at http://www.nccn.org/professionals/physician_gls/PDF/nhl.pdf

Olsen E, Duvic M, Frankel A, et al, "Pivotal Phase III Trial of Two Dose Levels of Denileukin Diftitox for the Treatment of Cutaneous T-Cell Lymphoma," *J Clin Oncol*, 2001, 19(2):376-88.

Polder K, Wang C, Duvic M, et al, "Toxic Epidermal Necrolysis Associated With Denileukin Diftitox (DAB389IL-2) Administration in a Patient With Follicular Large Cell Lymphoma," *Leuk Lymphoma*, 2005, 46(12):1807-11.

Talpur R, Apisarnthanarax N, Ward S, et al, "Treatment of Refractory Peripheral T-Cell Lymphoma With Denileukin Diftitox (Ontak®)," *Leuk Lymphoma*, 2002, 43(1):121-6.

Desmopressin (des moe PRES in)

U.S. Brand Names DDAVP®; Stimate®
Index Terms 1-Deamino-8-D-Arginine Vasopressin; Desmopressin Acetate
Generic Available Yes
Canadian Brand Names Apo-Desmopressin®; DDAVP®; DDAVP® Melt; Minirin®; Novo-Desmopressin; Octostim®; PMS-Desmopressin
Pharmacologic Category Antihemophilic Agent; Hemostatic Agent; Vasopressin Analog, Synthetic

Use

Injection: Treatment of diabetes insipidus; maintenance of hemostasis and control of bleeding in hemophilia A with factor VIII coagulant activity levels >5% and mild-to-moderate classic von Willebrand's disease (type 1) with factor VIII coagulant activity levels >5%

Nasal solutions (DDAVP® Nasal Spray and DDAVP® Rhinal Tube): Treatment of central diabetes insipidus

Nasal spray (Stimate®): Maintenance of hemostasis and control of bleeding in hemophilia A with factor VIII coagulant activity levels >5% and mild-to-moderate classic von Willebrand's disease (type 1) with factor VIII coagulant activity levels >5%

Tablet: Treatment of central diabetes insipidus, temporary polyuria and polydipsia following pituitary surgery or head trauma, primary nocturnal enuresis

Unlabeled/Investigational Use Uremic bleeding associated with acute or chronic renal failure; prevention of surgical bleeding in patients with uremia

Pregnancy Risk Factor B

Lactation Excretion in breast milk unknown/use caution

Labeled Contraindications Hypersensitivity to desmopressin or any component of the formulation; hyponatremia or a history of hyponatremia; moderate-to-severe renal impairment (Cl$_{cr}$<50 mL/minute)

Canadian labeling: Additional contraindications (not in U.S. labeling): Type 2B or platelet-type (pseudo) von Willebrand's disease (injection, intranasal, oral, sublingual); known hyponatremia, habitual or psychogenic polydipsia, cardiac insufficiency or other conditions requiring diuretic therapy (intranasal, sublingual); nephrosis, severe hepatic dysfunction (sublingual); primary nocturnal enuresis (intranasal)

Warnings/Precautions Allergic reactions and anaphylaxis have been reported rarely with both the I.V. and intranasal formulations. Fluid intake should be adjusted downward in the elderly and very young patients to decrease the possibility of water intoxication and hyponatremia. Use may rarely lead to extreme decreases in plasma osmolality, resulting in seizures, coma, and death. Use caution with cystic fibrosis, heart failure, renal dysfunction, polydipsia (habitual or psychogenic [contraindicated in Canadian labeling]), or other conditions associated with fluid and electrolyte imbalance due to potential hyponatremia. Use caution with coronary artery insufficiency or hypertensive cardiovascular disease; may increase or decrease blood pressure leading to changes in heart rate. Consider switching from nasal to intravenous solution if changes in the nasal mucosa (scarring, edema) occur leading to unreliable absorption. Use caution in patients predisposed to thrombus formation; thrombotic events (acute cerebrovascular thrombosis, acute myocardial infarction) have occurred (rare).

Desmopressin (intranasal and I.V.), when used for hemostasis in hemophilia, is not for use in hemophilia B, type 2B von Willebrand disease, severe classic von Willebrand disease (type 1), or in patients with factor VIII antibodies. In general, desmopressin is also not recommended for use in patients with ≤5% factor VIII activity level, although it may be considered in selected patients with activity levels between 2% and 5%.

Consider switching from nasal to intravenous administration if changes in the nasal mucosa (scarring, edema) occur leading to unreliable absorption. Consider alternative rout of administration (I.V. or intranasal) with inadequate therapeutic response at maximum recommended oral doses. Therapy should be interrupted if patient experiences an acute illness (eg, fever, recurrent vomiting or diarrhea), vigorous exercise, or any condition associated with an increase in water consumption. Some patients may demonstrate a change in response after long-term therapy (>6 months) characterized as decreased response or a shorter duration of response.

Adverse Reactions Frequency may not be defined (may be dose or route related).

Cardiovascular: Blood pressure increased/decreased (I.V.), facial flushing

Central nervous system: Headache (2% to 5%), dizziness (intranasal; ≤3%), chills (intranasal; 2%)

Dermatologic: Rash

Endocrine & metabolic: Hyponatremia, water intoxication

Gastrointestinal: Abdominal pain (intranasal; 2%), gastrointestinal disorder (intranasal; ≤2%), nausea (intranasal; ≤2%), abdominal cramps, sore throat

Hepatic: Transient increases in liver transaminases (associated primarily with tablets)

Local: Injection: Burning pain, erythema, and swelling at the injection site

Neuromuscular & Skeletal: Weakness (intranasal; ≤2%)

Ocular: Conjunctivitis (intranasal; ≤2%), eye edema (intranasal; ≤2%), lacrimation disorder (intranasal; ≤2%)

Respiratory: Rhinitis (intranasal; 3% to 8%), epistaxis (intranasal; ≤3%), nostril pain (intranasal; ≤2%), cough, nasal congestion, upper respiratory infection

<1%, postmarketing, and/or case reports: Acute cerebrovascular thrombosis (I.V.), acute MI (I.V.), agitation, allergic reactions (rare), anaphylaxis (rare), balanitis, chest pain, coma, diarrhea, dyspepsia, edema, insomnia, itching eyes, light-sensitive eyes, pain, palpitation, seizure, somnolence, tachycardia, thinking abnormal, vomiting, vulval pain, warmth

Drug Interactions

Avoid Concomitant Use There are no known interactions where it is recommended to avoid concomitant use.

Increased Effect/Toxicity

Desmopressin may increase the levels/effects of: Lithium

The levels/effects of Desmopressin may be increased by: Analgesics (Opioid); CarBAMazepine; ChlorproMAZINE; LamoTRIgine; Nonsteroidal Anti-Inflammatory Agents; Selective Serotonin Reuptake Inhibitors; Tricyclic Antidepressants

Decreased Effect

The levels/effects of Desmopressin may be decreased by: Demeclocycline; Lithium

Ethanol/Nutrition/Herb Interactions Ethanol: Avoid ethanol (may decrease antidiuretic effect).

Storage/Stability

DDAVP®:

Nasal spray: Store at controlled room temperature of 20°C to 25°C (68°F to 77°F). Keep nasal spray in upright position.

Rhinal Tube solution: Store refrigerated at 2°C to 8°C (36°F to 46°F). May store at controlled room temperature of 20°C to 25°C (68°F to 77°F) for up to 3 weeks.

Solution for injection: Store refrigerated at 2°C to 8°C (36°F to 46°F).

Tablet: Store at controlled room temperature of 20°C to 25°C (68°F to 77°F).

DDAVP® Melt (CAN; not available in U.S.): Store at 15°C to 25°C (59°F to 77°F) in original container. Protect from moisture.

Stimate® nasal spray: Store at controlled room temperature of 20°C to 25°C (68°F to 77°F). Keep nasal spray in upright position. Discard 6 months after opening.

Reconstitution DDAVP®: Dilute solution for injection in 10-50 mL NS for I.V. infusion (10 mL for children ≤10 kg: 50 mL for adults and children >10 kg).

Compatibility Stable in NS.

Mechanism of Action In a dose dependent manner, desmopressin increases cyclic adenosine monophosphate (cAMP) in renal tubular cells which increases water permeability resulting in decreased urine volume and increased urine osmolality; increases plasma levels of von Willebrand factor, factor VIII, and t-PA contributing to a shortened activated partial thromboplastin time (aPTT) and bleeding time.

Pharmacodynamics/Kinetics

Onset of action:

Intranasal: Antidiuretic: 15-30 minutes; Increased factor VIII and von Willebrand factor (vWF) activity (dose related): 30 minutes

Peak effect: Antidiuretic: 1 hour; Increased factor VIII and vWF activity: 1.5 hours

I.V. infusion: Increased factor VIII and vWF activity: 30 minutes (dose related)

Peak effect: 1.5-2 hours

Oral tablet: Antidiuretic: ~1 hour

Peak effect: 4-7 hours

Duration: Intranasal, I.V. infusion, Oral tablet: ~6-14 hours

Absorption: Sublingual: Rapid

Bioavailability: Intranasal: ~3.5%; Oral tablet: 5% compared to intranasal, 0.16% compared to I.V.

Half-life elimination: Intranasal: ~3.5 hours; I.V. infusion: 3 hours; Oral tablet: 2-3 hours

Renal impairment: ≤9 hours

Excretion: Urine

Dosage

Children:

Diabetes insipidus:

I.M., I.V., SubQ: Canadian labeling (not in U.S. labeling): ≥3 months: 0.4 mcg (0.1 mL) once daily or 1/10 of the maintenance intranasal dose. Fluid restriction should be observed.

I.V., SubQ: Children <12 years: No definitive dosing available. Adult dosing should **not** be used in this age group; adverse events such as hyponatremia-induced seizures may occur. Dose should be reduced. Some have suggested an initial dosage range of 0.1-1 mcg in 1 or 2 divided doses (Cheetham, 2002). Initiate at low dose and increase as necessary. Closely monitor serum sodium levels and urine output; fluid restriction is recommended.

Intranasal (using 100 mcg/mL nasal solution): 3 months to 12 years: Initial: 5 mcg/day (0.05 mL/day) divided 1-2 times/day; range: 5-30 mcg/day (0.05-0.3 mL/day) divided 1-2 times/day; adjust morning and evening doses separately for an adequate diurnal rhythm of water turnover. **Note:** The nasal spray pump can only deliver doses of 10 mcg (0.1 mL) or multiples of 10 mcg (0.1 mL); if doses other than this are needed, the rhinal tube delivery system is preferred. Fluid restriction should be observed.

Oral:

U.S. labeling: ≥4 years: Initial: 0.05 mg twice daily; total daily dose should be increased or decreased as needed to obtain adequate antidiuresis (range: 0.1-1.2 mg divided 2-3 times/day). Fluid restriction should be observed.

Canadian labeling (not in U.S. labeling): ≥5 years: Initial: 0.1 mg 3 times/day; total daily dose should be increased or decreased as needed to obtain adequate antidiuresis (range: 0.3-1.2 mg divided 3 times/day). Divide daily doses so that the evening dose is 2 times higher than the morning or afternoon dose to ensure adequate antidiuresis during the night. Fluid restriction should be observed.

Sublingual formulation: Canadian labeling (not in U.S. labeling): ≥3 months: Initial: 60 mcg 3 times/day; total daily dose should be increased or decreased as needed to obtain adequate antidiuresis. Usual maintenance: 60-120 mcg 3 times/day (range: 120-720 mcg divided 2-3 times/day); divide daily doses so that the evening dose is 2 times higher than the morning or afternoon dose to ensure adequate antidiuresis during the night. Fluid restriction should be observed.

Hemophilia A and von Willebrand disease (type 1):

I.V.: ≥3 months: 0.3 mcg/kg by slow infusion; may repeat dose if needed; if used preoperatively, administer 30 minutes before procedure

Canadian labeling (not in U.S. labeling): Maximum I.V. dose: 20 mcg

Note: Adverse events such as hyponatremia-induced seizures have been reported especially in young children using this dosing regimen (Das, 2005; Molnar, 2005; Smith, 1989; Thumfart, 2005; Weinstein, 1989). Fluid restriction and careful monitoring of serum sodium levels and urine output are necessary.

Intranasal (using high concentration spray [1.5 mg/mL]): ≥11 months: Refer to adult dosing.

Nocturnal enuresis:

Oral: ≥6 years: 0.2 mg at bedtime; dose may be titrated up to 0.6 mg to achieve desired response. Fluid intake should be limited 1 hour prior to dose until the next morning, or at least 8 hours after administration. **Note:** In the Canadian labeling, use is approved for patients ≥5 years.

Sublingual formulation: Canadian labeling (not in U.S. labeling): ≥5 years: Initial: 120 mcg at bedtime; dose may be titrated up to 360 mcg to achieve desired response. Fluid intake should be limited 1 hour prior to dose until the next morning, or at least 8 hours after administration.

Children ≥12 years and Adults:

Diabetes insipidus:

I.V., SubQ: 2-4 mcg/day (0.5-1 mL) in 2 divided doses or $^{1}/_{10}$ of the maintenance intranasal dose. Fluid restriction should be observed.

Intranasal (using 100 mcg/mL nasal solution): 10-40 mcg/day (0.1-0.4 mL) divided 1-3 times/day; adjust morning and evening doses separately for an adequate diurnal rhythm of water turnover. **Note:** The nasal spray pump can only deliver doses of 10 mcg (0.1 mL) or multiples of 10 mcg (0.1 mL); if doses other than this are needed, the rhinal tube delivery system is preferred. Fluid restriction should be observed.

Oral:

U.S. labeling: Initial: 0.05 mg twice daily; total daily dose should be increased or decreased as needed to obtain adequate antidiuresis (range: 0.1-1.2 mg divided 2-3 times/day). Fluid restriction should be observed.

Canadian labeling (not in U.S. labeling): Initial: 0.1 mg 3 times/day; total daily dose should be increased or decreased as needed to obtain adequate antidiuresis (range: 0.3-1.2 mg divided 3 times/day). Fluid restriction should be observed.

Sublingual formulation: Canadian labeling (not in U.S. labeling): Initial: 60 mcg 3 times/day; total daily dose should be increased or decreased as needed to obtain adequate antidiuresis. Usual maintenance: 60-120 mcg 3 times/day (range: 120-720 mcg divided 2-3 times/day). Fluid restriction should be observed.

Hemophilia A and mild-to-moderate von Willebrand disease (type 1):

I.V.: 0.3 mcg/kg by slow infusion; if used preoperatively, administer 30 minutes before procedure

Canadian labeling (not in U.S. labeling): Maximum I.V. dose: 20 mcg

Intranasal (using high concentration spray [1.5 mg/mL]): <50 kg: 150 mcg (1 spray); >50 kg: 300 mcg (1 spray each nostril); repeat use is determined by the patient's clinical condition and laboratory work; if using preoperatively, administer 2 hours before surgery

Adults:

Diabetes insipidus: I.M., I.V., SubQ: Canadian label (not in U.S. labeling): 1-4 mcg (0.25-1 mL) once daily or $^1/_{10}$ of the maintenance intranasal dose. Fluid restriction should be observed.

Uremic bleeding associated with acute or chronic renal failure (unlabeled use; Watson, 1984): I.V.: 0.4 mcg/kg over 10 minutes

Prevention of surgical bleeding in patients with uremia (unlabeled use; Mannucci, 1983): I.V.: 0.3 mcg/kg over 30 minutes

Dosage adjustment in renal impairment: Cl_{cr} <50 mL/minute: Use is contraindicated according to the manufacturer; however, has been used in acute and chronic renal failure patients experiencing uremic bleeding or for prevention of surgical bleeding (unlabeled uses; Mannuccio, 1983; Watson, 1984)

Administration

I.M., I.V. push, SubQ injection: Central diabetes insipidus: Withdraw dose from ampul into appropriate syringe size (eg, insulin syringe). Further dilution is not required. Administer as direct injection.

I.V. infusion:

Hemophilia A, von Willebrand disease (type 1), and prevention of surgical bleeding in patients with uremia (unlabeled; Mannucci, 1983): Infuse over 15-30 minutes

Acute uremic bleeding (unlabeled; Watson, 1984): May infuse over 10 minutes

Intranasal:

DDAVP®: Nasal pump spray: Delivers 0.1 mL (10 mcg); for doses <10 mcg or for other doses which are not multiples, use rhinal tube. DDAVP® Nasal spray delivers fifty 10 mcg doses. For 10 mcg dose, administer in one nostril. Any solution remaining after 50 doses should be discarded. Pump must be primed prior to first use.

DDAVP® Rhinal tube: Insert top of dropper into tube (arrow marked end) in downward position. Squeeze dropper until solution reaches desired calibration mark. Disconnect dropper. Grasp the tube ¾ inch from the end and insert tube into nostril until the fingertips reach the nostril. Place opposite end of tube into the mouth (holding breath). Tilt head back and blow with a strong, short puff into the nostril (for very young patients, an adult should blow solution into the child's nose). Reseal dropper after use.

Monitoring Parameters Blood pressure and pulse should be monitored during I.V. infusion

Note: For all indications, fluid intake, urine volume, and signs and symptoms of hyponatremia should be closely monitored especially in high-risk patient subgroups (eg, young children, elderly, patients with heart failure).

Diabetes insipidus: Urine specific gravity, plasma and urine osmolality, serum electrolytes

Hemophilia A: Factor VIII coagulant activity, factor VIII ristocetin cofactor activity, and factor VIII antigen levels, aPTT

von Willebrand disease: Factor VIII coagulant activity, factor VIII ristocetin cofactor activity, and factor VIII von Willebrand antigen levels, bleeding time

Nocturnal enuresis: Serum electrolytes if used for >7 days

Additional Information 10 mcg of desmopressin acetate is equivalent to 40 int. units

Dosage Forms Excipient information presented when available (limited, particularly for generics); consult specific product labeling. [CAN] = Canadian product

Injection, solution, as acetate: 4 mcg/mL (1 mL, 10 mL)
DDAVP®: 5 mcg/mL (1 mL, 10 mL)

Solution, intranasal, as acetate: 100 mcg/mL (2.5 mL)
DDAVP®: 100 mcg/mL (2.5 mL) [contains benzalkonium chloride; with rhinal tube]

Solution, as acetate, intranasal [spray]: 100 mcg/mL (5 mL)
DDAVP®: 100 mcg/mL (5 mL) [contains benzalkonium chloride; delivers 10 mcg/spray]

Stimate®: 1.5 mg/mL (2.5 mL) [delivers 150 mcg/spray]

Tablet, as acetate, oral: 0.1 mg, 0.2 mg
DDAVP®: 0.1 mg, 0.2 mg [scored]

Tablet, as acetate, sublingual:
DDAVP® Melt (CAN) [not available in U.S.]: 60 mcg, 120 mcg, 240 mcg

References

Byrnes JJ, Larcada A, and Moake JL, "Thrombosis Following Desmopressin for Uremic Bleeding," *Am J Hematol*, 1988, 28(1):63-5.

Cattaneo M, "Review of Clinical Experience of Desmopressin in Patients With Congenital and Acquired Bleeding Disorder," *Eur J Anesthesiol Suppl*, 1997, 14:10-4.

Chistolini A, Dragoni F, Ferrari A, et al, "Intranasal DDAVP®: Biological and Clinical Evaluation in Mild Factor VIII Deficiency," *Haemostasis*, 1991, 21(5):273-7.

Couch P and Stumpf JL, "Management of Uremic Bleeding," *Clin Pharm*, 1990, 9(9):673-81.

Das P, Carcao M, and Hitzler J, "DDAVP-Induced Hyponatremia in Young Children," *J Pediatr Hematol Oncol*, 2005, 27(6):330-2.

Das P, Carcao M, and Hitzler J, "Use of Recombinant Factor VIIa Prior to Lumbar Puncture in Pediatric Patients With Acute Leukemia," *Pediatr Blood Cancer*, 2006, 47(2):206-9.

Dave SP, Greenstein AJ, Sachar DB, et al, "Bleeding Diathesis in Amyloidosis With Renal Insufficiency Associated With Crohn's Disease: Response to Desmopressin," *Am J Gastroenterol*, 2002, 97(1):187-9.

Lusher JM, "Response to 1-Deamino-8-D-Arginine Vasopressin in von Willebrand Disease," *Haemostasis*, 1994, 24(5):276-84.

Mannucci PM and Cattaneo M, "Desmopressin: A Nontransfusional Treatment of Hemophilia and von Willebrand Disease," *Haemostasis*, 1992, 22(5)276-80.

Mannucci PM, Remuzzi G, Pusineri F, et al, "Deamino-8-D-Arginine Vasopressin Shortens the Bleeding Time in Uremia," *N Engl J Med*, 1983, 308(1):8-12.

♦ **Desmopressin Acetate** *see* Desmopressin *on page 344*

Dexamethasone (deks a METH a sone)

Medication Safety Issues

Sound-alike/look-alike issues:

Dexamethasone may be confused with desoximetasone, dextro-amphetamine

Decadron® may be confused with Percodan®

Maxidex® may be confused with Maxzide®

Related Information

Management of Chemotherapy-Induced Nausea and Vomiting *on page 1434*

U.S. Brand Names Baycadron™; Dexamethasone Intensol™; DexPak® 10 Day TaperPak®; DexPak® 13 Day TaperPak®; DexPak® 6 Day TaperPak®; DexPak® TaperPak® [DSC]; Maxidex®

Index Terms Dexamethasone Sodium Phosphate

Generic Available Yes: Excludes ophthalmic suspension

Canadian Brand Names Apo-Dexamethasone®; Dexasone®; Diodex®; Maxidex®; PMS-Dexamethasone

Pharmacologic Category Anti-inflammatory Agent; Anti-inflammatory Agent, Ophthalmic; Antiemetic; Corticosteroid, Ophthalmic; Corticosteroid, Systemic

Use

Systemic: Primarily as an anti-inflammatory or immunosuppressant agent in the treatment of a variety of diseases including those of allergic, dermatologic, endocrine, hematologic, inflammatory, neoplastic, nervous system, renal, respiratory, rheumatic, and autoimmune origin; may be used in management of cerebral edema, chronic swelling, as a diagnostic agent, diagnosis of Cushing's syndrome, antiemetic

Ophthalmic: Management of steroid responsive inflammatory conditions such as allergic conjunctivitis, iritis, or cyclitis; symptomatic treatment of corneal injury from chemical, radiation, or thermal burns, or penetration of foreign bodies.

Unlabeled/Investigational Use

Dexamethasone suppression test: General indicator consistent with depression and/or suicide

Accelerate fetal lung maturation in patients with preterm labor

Pregnancy Risk Factor C

Lactation Excretion in breast milk unknown/use caution

Labeled Contraindications Hypersensitivity to dexamethasone or any component of the formulation; systemic fungal infections, cerebral malaria; ophthalmic use in viral (active ocular herpes simplex), fungal, or tuberculosis diseases of the eye

Warnings/Precautions Use with caution in patients with thyroid disease, hepatic impairment, renal impairment, cardiovascular disease, diabetes, glaucoma, cataracts, myasthenia gravis, patients at risk for osteoporosis, patients at risk for seizures, or GI diseases (diverticulitis, peptic ulcer, ulcerative colitis) due to perforation risk. Use caution following acute MI (corticosteroids have been associated with myocardial rupture). Because of the risk of adverse effects, systemic corticosteroids should be used cautiously in the elderly in the smallest possible effective dose for the shortest duration. May affect growth velocity; growth should be routinely monitored in pediatric patients. Withdraw therapy with gradual tapering of dose.

May cause hypercorticism or suppression of hypothalamic-pituitary-adrenal (HPA) axis, particularly in younger children or in patients receiving high doses for prolonged periods. HPA axis suppression may lead to adrenal crisis. Withdrawal and discontinuation of a corticosteroid should be done slowly and carefully. Particular care is required when patients are transferred from systemic corticosteroids to inhaled products due to possible adrenal insufficiency or withdrawal from steroids, including an increase in allergic symptoms. Patients receiving >20 mg per day of prednisone (or equivalent) may be most susceptible. Fatalities have occurred due to adrenal insufficiency in asthmatic patients during and after transfer from systemic corticosteroids to aerosol steroids; aerosol steroids do not provide the systemic steroid needed to treat patients having trauma, surgery, or infections. Dexamethasone does not provide adequate mineralocorticoid activity in adrenal insufficiency (may be employed as a single dose while cortisol assays are performed). The lowest possible dose should be used during treatment; discontinuation and/or dose reductions should be gradual.

Acute myopathy has been reported with high dose corticosteroids, usually in patients with neuromuscular transmission disorders; may involve ocular and/or respiratory muscles; monitor creatine kinase; recovery may be delayed. Corticosteroid use may cause psychiatric disturbances, including depression, euphoria, insomnia, mood swings, and personality changes. Pre-existing psychiatric conditions may be exacerbated by corticosteroid use. Prolonged use of corticosteroids may also increase the incidence of secondary infection, mask acute infection (including fungal infections), prolong or exacerbate viral infections, or limit response to vaccines. Exposure to chickenpox should be avoided; corticosteroids should not be used to treat ocular herpes simplex. Corticosteroids should not be used for cerebral malaria or viral hepatitis. Close observation is required in patients with latent tuberculosis and/or TB reactivity; restrict use in active TB (only in conjunction with antituberculosis treatment). Prolonged treatment with corticosteroids has been associated with the development of Kaposi's sarcoma (case reports); if noted, discontinuation of therapy should be considered. High-dose corticosteroids should not be used to manage acute head injury.

Adverse Reactions Frequency not defined.

Cardiovascular: Arrhythmia, bradycardia, cardiac arrest, cardiomyopathy, CHF, circulatory collapse, edema, hypertension, myocardial rupture (post-MI), syncope, thromboembolism, vasculitis

Central nervous system: Depression, emotional instability, euphoria, headache, intracranial pressure increased, insomnia, malaise, mood swings, neuritis, personality changes, pseudotumor cerebri (usually following discontinuation), psychic disorders, seizure, vertigo

Dermatologic: Acne, allergic dermatitis, alopecia, angioedema, bruising, dry skin, erythema, fragile skin, hirsutism, hyper-/hypopigmentation, hypertrichosis, perianal pruritus (following I.V. injection), petechiae, rash, skin atrophy, skin test reaction impaired, striae, urticaria, wound healing impaired

Endocrine & metabolic: Adrenal suppression, carbohydrate tolerance decreased, Cushing's syndrome, diabetes mellitus, glucose intolerance decreased, growth suppression (children), hyperglycemia, hypokalemic alkalosis, menstrual irregularities, negative nitrogen balance, pituitary-adrenal axis suppression, protein catabolism, sodium retention

Gastrointestinal: Abdominal distention, appetite increased, gastrointestinal hemorrhage, gastrointestinal perforation, nausea, pancreatitis, peptic ulcer, ulcerative esophagitis, weight gain

Genitourinary: Altered (increased or decreased) spermatogenesis

Hepatic: Hepatomegaly, transaminases increased

Local: Postinjection flare (intra-articular use), thrombophlebitis

Neuromuscular & skeletal: Arthropathy, aseptic necrosis (femoral and humoral heads), fractures, muscle mass loss, myopathy (particularly in conjunction with neuromuscular disease or neuromuscular-blocking agents), neuropathy, osteoporosis, parasthesia, tendon rupture, vertebral compression fractures, weakness

Ocular: Cataracts, exophthalmos, glaucoma, intraocular pressure increased

Renal: Glucosuria

Respiratory: Pulmonary edema

Miscellaneous: Abnormal fat deposition, anaphylactoid reaction, anaphylaxis, avascular necrosis, diaphoresis, hiccups, hypersensitivity, impaired wound healing, infections, Kaposi's sarcoma, moon face, secondary malignancy

Drug Interactions

Metabolism/Transport Effects Substrate of CYP3A4 (major); **Induces** CYP2A6 (weak), 2B6 (weak), 2C8 (weak), 2C9 (weak), 3A4 (strong)

Avoid Concomitant Use

Avoid concomitant use of Dexamethasone with any of the following: Dronedarone; Everolimus; Natalizumab; Nilotinib; Nisoldipine; Ranolazine; Tolvaptan; Vaccines (Live)

Increased Effect/Toxicity

Dexamethasone may increase the levels/effects of: Acetylcholinesterase Inhibitors; Amphotericin B; CycloSPORINE; Leflunomide; Lenalidomide; Loop Diuretics; Natalizumab; NSAID (COX-2 Inhibitor); NSAID (Non-selective); Thalidomide; Thiazide Diuretics; Vaccines (Live); Warfarin

The levels/effects of Dexamethasone may be increased by: Antifungal Agents (Azole Derivatives, Systemic); Aprepitant; Asparaginase; Calcium Channel Blockers (Nondihydropyridine); CycloSPORINE; CYP3A4 Inhibitors (Moderate); CYP3A4 Inhibitors (Strong); Dasatinib; Estrogen Derivatives; Fluconazole; Fosaprepitant; Macrolide Antibiotics; Neuromuscular-Blocking Agents (Nondepolarizing); P-Glycoprotein Inhibitors; Quinolone Antibiotics; Salicylates; Trastuzumab

Decreased Effect

Dexamethasone may decrease the levels/effects of: Antidiabetic Agents; Calcitriol; Caspofungin; Corticorelin; CYP3A4 Substrates; Dabigatran Etexilate; Dronedarone; Everolimus; Isoniazid; Maraviroc; Nilotinib; Nisoldipine; P-Glycoprotein Substrates; Ranolazine; Salicylates; Sorafenib; Tadalafil; Tolvaptan; Vaccines (Inactivated); Vaccines (Live)

The levels/effects of Dexamethasone may be decreased by: Aminoglutethimide; Antacids; Barbiturates; Bile Acid Sequestrants; CYP3A4 Inducers (Strong); Deferasirox; Echinacea; Herbs (CYP3A4 Inducers); Mitotane; P-Glycoprotein Inducers; Primidone; Rifamycin Derivatives

Ethanol/Nutrition/Herb Interactions

Ethanol: Avoid ethanol (may enhance gastric mucosal irritation).

Food: Dexamethasone interferes with calcium absorption. Limit caffeine.

Herb/Nutraceutical: Avoid cat's claw, echinacea (have immunostimulant properties).

Storage/Stability

Injection solution: Store at room temperature; protect from light and freezing.

Stability of injection of parenteral admixture at room temperature (25°C): 24 hours.

Stability of injection of parenteral admixture at refrigeration temperature (4°C): 2 days; protect from light and freezing.

Reconstitution Injection should be diluted in 50-100 mL NS or D_5W.

Compatibility Stable in D_5W, NS.

Y-site administration: Compatible: Acyclovir, allopurinol, amifostine, amikacin, amphotericin B cholesteryl sulfate complex, amsacrine, aztreonam, cefepime, cefpirome, cisatracurium, cisplatin, cladribine, cyclophosphamide, cytarabine, docetaxel, doxorubicin, doxorubicin liposome, etoposide phosphate, famotidine, filgrastim, fluconazole, fludarabine, foscarnet, gatifloxacin, gemcitabine, granisetron, heparin, heparin with hydrocortisone sodium succinate, levofloxacin, linezolid, lorazepam, melphalan, meperidine, meropenem, morphine, ondansetron, paclitaxel, piperacillin/tazobactam, potassium chloride, propofol, remifentanil, sargramostim, sodium bicarbonate, sufentanil, tacrolimus, teniposide, theophylline, thiotepa, vinorelbine, vitamin B complex with C, zidovudine. **Incompatible:** Ciprofloxacin, idarubicin, midazolam, topotecan. **Variable (consult detailed reference):** Methotrexate.

Compatibility in syringe: Compatible: Granisetron, metoclopramide, palonosetron, ranitidine, sufentanil. **Incompatible:** Doxapram, glycopyrrolate. **Variable (consult detailed reference):** Diphenhydramine, hydromorphone, ondansetron.

Compatibility when admixed: Compatible: Aminophylline, bleomycin, cimetidine, floxacillin, furosemide, granisetron, lidocaine, meropenem, mitomycin, nafcillin, netilmicin, ondansetron, palonosetron, prochlorperazine edisylate, ranitidine, verapamil. **Incompatible:** Daunorubicin, diphenhydramine with lorazepam and metoclopramide, metaraminol, vancomycin. **Variable (consult detailed reference):** Amikacin.

Mechanism of Action Decreases inflammation by suppression of neutrophil migration, decreased production of inflammatory mediators, and reversal of increased capillary permeability; suppresses normal immune response. Dexamethasone's mechanism of antiemetic activity is unknown.

Pharmacodynamics/Kinetics

Onset of action: Acetate: Prompt

Duration of metabolic effect: 72 hours; acetate is a long-acting repository preparation

Metabolism: Hepatic

Half-life elimination: Normal renal function: 1.8-3.5 hours; Biological half-life: 36-54 hours

Time to peak, serum: Oral: 1-2 hours; I.M.: ~8 hours

Excretion: Urine and feces

Dosage Refer to individual protocols.

Children:

Antiemetic (prior to chemotherapy): I.V.: 10 mg/m^2 (initial dose) followed by 5 mg/m^2 every 6 hours as needed **or** 5-20 mg given 15-30 minutes before treatment

Anti-inflammatory immunosuppressant: Oral, I.M., I.V.: 0.08-0.3 mg/kg/day **or** 2.5-10 mg/m^2/day in divided doses every 6-12 hours

Extubation or airway edema: Oral, I.M., I.V.: 0.5-2 mg/kg/day in divided doses every 6 hours beginning 24 hours prior to extubation and continuing for 4-6 doses afterwards

Cerebral edema: I.V.: Loading dose: 1-2 mg/kg/dose as a single dose; maintenance: 1-1.5 mg/kg/day (maximum: 16 mg/day) in divided doses every 4-6 hours, taper off over 1-6 weeks

Bacterial meningitis in infants and children >2 months: I.V.: 0.6 mg/kg/day in 4 divided doses every 6 hours for the first 4 days of antibiotic treatment; start dexamethasone at the time of the first dose of antibiotic

Physiologic replacement: Oral, I.M., I.V.: 0.03-0.15 mg/kg/day **or** 0.6-0.75 mg/m^2/day in divided doses every 6-12 hours

Adults:

Antiemetic:

Prophylaxis: Oral, I.V.: 10-20 mg 15-30 minutes before treatment on each treatment day

Continuous infusion regimen: Oral or I.V.: 10 mg every 12 hours on each treatment day

Mildly emetogenic therapy: Oral, I.M., I.V.: 4 mg every 4-6 hours

Delayed nausea/vomiting: Oral: 4-10 mg 1-2 times/day for 2-4 days **or**

8 mg every 12 hours for 2 days; then

4 mg every 12 hours for 2 days **or**

20 mg 1 hour before chemotherapy; then

10 mg 12 hours after chemotherapy; then

8 mg every 12 hours for 4 doses; then

4 mg every 12 hours for 4 doses

Anti-inflammatory:

Oral, I.M., I.V. (injections should be given as sodium phosphate): 0.75-9 mg/day in divided doses every 6-12 hours

Intra-articular, intralesional, or soft tissue (as sodium phosphate): 0.4-6 mg/day

Ophthalmic:

Solution: Instill 1-2 drops into conjunctival sac every hour during the day and every other hour during the night; gradually reduce dose to every 3-4 hours, then to 3-4 times/day

Suspension: Instill 1-2 drops into conjunctival sac up to 4-6 times per day; may use hourly in severe disease; taper prior to discontinuation

Multiple myeloma: Oral, I.V.: 40 mg/day, days 1 to 4, 9 to 12, and 17 to 20, repeated every 4 weeks (alone or as part of a regimen)

Cerebral edema: I.V. 10 mg stat, 4 mg I.M./I.V. every 6 hours until response is maximized, then switch to oral regimen, then taper off if appropriate; dosage may be reduced after 24 days and gradually discontinued over 5-7 days

Extubation or airway edema: Oral, I.M., I.V. (injections should be given as sodium phosphate): 0.5-2 mg/kg/day in divided doses every 6 hours beginning 24 hours prior to extubation and continuing for 4-6 doses afterwards

Dexamethasone suppression test (depression/suicide indicator) (unlabeled use): Oral: 1 mg at 11 PM, draw blood at 8 AM the following day for plasma cortisol determination

Cushing's syndrome, diagnostic: Oral: 1 mg at 11 PM, draw blood at 8 AM; greater accuracy for Cushing's syndrome may be achieved by the following:

Dexamethasone 0.5 mg by mouth every 6 hours for 48 hours (with 24-hour urine collection for 17-hydroxycorticosteroid excretion)

Differentiation of Cushing's syndrome due to ACTH excess from Cushing's due to other causes: Oral: Dexamethasone 2 mg every 6 hours for 48 hours (with 24-hour urine collection for 17-hydroxycorticosteroid excretion)

Multiple sclerosis (acute exacerbation): 30 mg/day for 1 week, followed by 4-12 mg/day for 1 month

Physiological replacement: Oral, I.M., I.V. (should be given as sodium phosphate): 0.03-0.15 mg/kg/day **or** 0.6-0.75 mg/m^2/day in divided doses every 6-12 hours

Treatment of shock:

Addisonian crisis/shock (ie, adrenal insufficiency/responsive to steroid therapy): I.V. (given as sodium phosphate): 4-10 mg as a single dose, which may be repeated if necessary

Unresponsive shock (ie, unresponsive to steroid therapy): I.V. (given as sodium phosphate): 1-6 mg/kg as a single I.V. dose or up to 40 mg initially followed by repeat doses every 2-6 hours while shock persists

Hemodialysis: Supplemental dose is not necessary

Peritoneal dialysis: Supplemental dose is not necessary

Combination Regimens

Leukemia, acute lymphocytic:
Hyper-CVAD + Imatinib on page 1348
Hyper-CVAD (Leukemia, Acute Lymphocytic) on page 1349
TVTG on page 1416
VAD/CVAD on page 1418
Leukemia, acute myeloid: TVTG on page 1416
Lymphoma, Hodgkin's: VIM-D (Hodgkin's Lymphoma) on page 1420
Lymphoma, non-Hodgkin's:
Cisplatin-Cytarabine-Dexamethasone (NHL Regimen) on page 1265
Fludarabine-Mitoxantrone-Dexamethasone (NHL) on page 1328
Fludarabine-Mitoxantrone-Dexamethasone-Rituximab on page 1329
Hyper-CVAD (Lymphoma, non-Hodgkin's) on page 1355
m-BACOD on page 1365
Oxaliplatin-Cytarabine-Dexamethasone (NHL Regimen) on page 1383
Lymphoma, non-Hodgkin's (Mantle cell): Hyper-CVAD + Rituximab on page 1356
Multiple myeloma:
Bortezomib-Dexamethasone on page 1237
Bortezomib-Doxorubicin (Liposomal)-Dexamethasone on page 1240
Bortezomib-Doxorubicin-Dexamethasone on page 1238
DTPACE on page 1297
Doxorubicin (Liposomal)-Vincristine-Dexamethasone on page 1297
Hyper-CVAD (Multiple Myeloma) on page 1355
Lenalidomide-Dexamethasone on page 1362
Lenalidomide-Dexamethasone (Low Dose) on page 1362
Thalidomide-Dexamethasone on page 1405
VAD on page 1417

Administration

Oral: Administer with meals to decrease GI upset.

I.V.: Administer as a 5-10 minute bolus; rapid injection is associated with a high incidence of perineal discomfort.

Ophthalmic: Remove soft contact lenses prior to using solutions containing benzalkonium chloride. Do not touch tip of container to eye.

Monitoring Parameters Hemoglobin, occult blood loss, serum potassium, and glucose; intraocular pressure (with use >6 weeks)

Dietary Considerations May be taken with meals to decrease GI upset. May need diet with increased potassium, pyridoxine, vitamin C, vitamin D, folate, calcium, and phosphorus.

Additional Information Effects of inhaled/intranasal steroids on growth have been observed in the absence of laboratory evidence of HPA axis suppression, suggesting that growth velocity is a more sensitive indicator of systemic corticosteroid exposure in pediatric patients than some commonly used tests of HPA axis function. The long-term effects of this reduction in growth velocity associated with orally-inhaled and intranasal corticosteroids, including the ▶

◄ impact on final adult height, are unknown. The potential for "catch up" growth following discontinuation of treatment with inhaled corticosteroids has not been adequately studied.

Withdrawal/tapering of therapy: Corticosteroid tapering following short-term use is limited primarily by the need to control the underlying disease state; tapering may be accomplished over a period of days. Following longer-term use, tapering over weeks to months may be necessary to avoid signs and symptoms of adrenal insufficiency and to allow recovery of the HPA axis. Testing of HPA axis responsiveness may be of value in selected patients. Subtle deficits in HPA response may persist for months after discontinuation of therapy, and may require supplemental dosing during periods of acute illness or surgical stress.

Dosage Forms Excipient information presented when available (limited, particularly for generics); consult specific product labeling. [DSC] = Discontinued product

Elixir: 0.5 mg/5 mL (240 mL)

Baycadron™: 0.5 mg/5 mL (237 mL) [contains benzoic acid; ethanol 5.1%; propylene glycol; raspberry flavor]

Injection, solution, as sodium phosphate: 4 mg/mL (1 mL, 5 mL, 30 mL); 10 mg/mL (10 mL)

Injection, solution, as sodium phosphate [preservative free]: 10 mg/mL (1 mL)

Solution, ophthalmic, as sodium phosphate [drops]: 0.1% (5 mL)

Solution, oral: 0.5 mg/5 mL (500 mL)

Solution, oral [concentrate]:

Dexamethasone Intensol™: 1 mg/mL (30 mL) [dye free; sugar free; contains alcohol 30% and propylene glycol]

Suspension, ophthalmic [drops]:

Maxidex®: 0.1% (5 mL) [contains benzalkonium chloride]

Tablet [scored]: 0.5 mg, 0.75 mg, 1 mg, 1.5 mg, 2 mg, 4 mg, 6 mg

DexPak® 10 Day TaperPak®: 1.5 mg [35 tablets on taper dose card]

DexPak® 13 Day TaperPak®: 1.5 mg [51 tablets on taper dose card]

DexPak® 6 Day TaperPak®: 1.5 mg [21 tablets on taper dose card]

DexPak® TaperPak®: 1.5 mg [51 tablets on taper dose card] [DSC]

References

Abraham E and Evans T, "Corticosteroids and Septic Shock [editorial]," *JAMA*, 2002, 288(7):886-7.

Annane D, Sebille V, Charpentier C, et al, "Effect of Treatment With Low Doses of Hydrocortisone and Fludrocortisone on Mortality in Patients With Septic Shock," *JAMA*, 2002, 288(7):862-71.

Cooper MS and Stewart PM, "Corticosteroid Insufficiency in Acutely Ill Patients," *N Engl J Med*, 2003, 348(8):727-34.

Coursin DB and Wood KE, "Corticosteroid Supplementation for Adrenal Insufficiency," *JAMA*, 2002, 287(2):236-40.

Dellinger RP, Levy MM, Carlet JM, et al, "Surviving Sepsis Campaign: International Guidelines for Management of Severe Sepsis and Septic Shock: 2008," *Intensive Care Med*, 2008, 34(1):17-60. Available at http://www.survivingsepsis.org/system/files/images/2008_20International_20SSC_20Guidelines_1_.pdf

"Dexamethasone, Granisetron, or Both for the Prevention of Nausea and Vomiting During Chemotherapy for Cancer. The Italian Group for Antiemetic Research," *N Engl J Med*, 1995, 332 (1):1-5.

Goedert JJ, Vitale F, Lauria C, et al, "Risk Factors for Classical Kaposi's Sarcoma," *J Natl Cancer Inst*, 2002, 94(22):1712-8.

Kyle RA and Rajkumar SV, "Multiple Myeloma," *N Engl J Med*, 2004, 351(18): 1860-73.

Kris MG, Baltzer L, Pisters KM, et al, "Enhancing the Effectiveness of the Specific Serotonin Antagonists. Combination Antiemetic Therapy With Dexamethasone," *Cancer*, 1993, 72(11 Suppl):3436-42.

Latreille J, Stewart D, Laberge F, et al, "Dexamethasone Improves the Efficacy of Granisetron in the First 24 h Following High-Dose Cisplatin Chemotherapy," *Support Care Cancer*, 1995, 3 (5):307-12.

Marik PE, Pastores SM, Annane D, et al, "Recommendations for the Diagnosis and Management of Corticosteroid Insufficiency in Critically III Adult Patients: Consensus Statements From an International Task Force by the American College of Critical Care Medicine," *Crit Care Med*, 2008, 36(6):1937-49.

McDonnell M and Evans N, "Upper and Lower Gastrointestinal Complications With Dexamethasone Despite H2 Antagonists," *J Paediatr Child Health*, 1995, 31(2):152-4.

Peterson C, Hursti TJ, Borjeson S, et al, "Single High-Dose Dexamethasone Improves the Effect of Ondansetron on Acute Chemotherapy-Induced Nausea and Vomiting But Impairs the Control of Delayed Symptoms," *Support Care Cancer*, 1996, 4(6):440-6.

Trissel LA and Zhang Y, "Compatibility and Stability of Aloxi (Palonosetron Hydrochloride) Admixed With Dexamethasone Sodium Phosphate," *Intl J Pharm Compounding*, 2004, 8(5):398-403.

◆ **Dexamethasone Intensol™** *see* Dexamethasone *on page 350*

◆ **Dexamethasone Sodium Phosphate** *see* Dexamethasone *on page 350*

◆ **Dexasone® (Can)** *see* Dexamethasone *on page 350*

◆ **Dexferrum®** *see* Iron Dextran Complex *on page 658*

◆ **Dexiron™ (Can)** *see* Iron Dextran Complex *on page 658*

◆ **DexPak® 6 Day TaperPak®** *see* Dexamethasone *on page 350*

◆ **DexPak® 10 Day TaperPak®** *see* Dexamethasone *on page 350*

◆ **DexPak® 13 Day TaperPak®** *see* Dexamethasone *on page 350*

◆ **DexPak® TaperPak® [DSC]** *see* Dexamethasone *on page 350*

Dexrazoxane (deks ray ZOKS ane)

Medication Safety Issues
Sound-alike/look-alike issues:
Zinecard® may be confused with Gemzar®

Related Information
Management of Drug Extravasations *on page 1447*
Safe Handling of Hazardous Drugs *on page 1517*

U.S. Brand Names Totect™; Zinecard®

Index Terms ICRF-187; NSC-169780

Generic Available Yes

Canadian Brand Names Zinecard®

Pharmacologic Category Antidote; Cardioprotectant

Use
Zinecard®: Reduction of the incidence and severity of cardiomyopathy associated with doxorubicin administration in women with metastatic breast cancer who have received a cumulative doxorubicin dose of 300 mg/m^2 and who would benefit from continuing therapy with doxorubicin. (Not recommended for use with initial doxorubicin therapy.)

Totect™: Treatment of anthracycline-induced extravasation.

Unlabeled/Investigational Use Reduction of the incidence and severity of cardiomyopathy associated with doxorubicin administration (cumulative doses >300 mg/m^2) in patients with malignancies other than metastatic breast cancer who would benefit from continuing therapy with doxorubicin; reduction of the incidence and severity of cardiomyopathy associated with continued epirubicin administration for advanced breast cancer

Pregnancy Risk Factor C (Zinecard®) / D (Totect™)

Lactation Excretion in breast milk unknown/not recommended

Labeled Contraindications
Zinecard®: Use with chemotherapy regimens that do not contain an anthracycline

Totect™: There are no contraindications listed within the manufacturer's labeling.

Warnings/Precautions Hazardous agent - use appropriate precautions for handling and disposal. Dexrazoxane may cause mild myelosuppression activity; myelosuppression may be additive with concurrently administered chemotherapeutic agents. Does not eliminate the potential for anthracycline-induced cardiac toxicity; carefully monitor cardiac function. May interfere with the antitumor effect of chemotherapy when given concurrently with fluorouracil, doxorubicin and cyclophosphamide (FAC). When used for the prevention of cardiomyopathy, doxorubicin should be administered 30 minutes after the beginning of the dexrazoxane infusion. Dosage adjustment required for moderate or severe renal insufficiency (clearance is reduced). Due to dosage adjustments for doxorubicin in hepatic impairment, a proportional dose reduction in dexrazoxane is recommended to maintain the dosage ratio of 10:1. Do not use DMSO in patients receiving dexrazoxane for anthracycline-induced extravasation; may diminish dexrazoxane efficacy. For I.V. administration; **not** for local infiltration into extravasation site. Safety and efficacy in children have not been established.

Adverse Reactions Adverse reactions listed are those which were greater in the dexrazoxane arm in a trial comparison of dexrazoxane plus fluorouracil, doxorubicin, and cyclophosphamide (FAC) to FAC alone for the prevention of cardiomyopathy. Most adverse reactions are thought to be attributed to chemotherapy, except for increased myelosuppression, pain at injection site, and phlebitis.

Central nervous system: Fatigue/malaise, fever
Dermatologic: Alopecia, streaking/erythema
Endocrine & metabolic: Serum calcium decreased, serum triglycerides increased
Gastrointestinal: Serum amylase increased
Hematologic: Anemia, granulocytopenia, hemorrhage, leukopenia, myelosuppression, neutropenia, thrombocytopenia
Hepatic: ALT increased, AST increased, bilirubin increased
Local: Injection site pain (12% to 16%), phlebitis (6% to 8%), extravasation
Neuromuscular & skeletal: Neurotoxicity
Miscellaneous: Infection, sepsis
Postmarketing and/or case reports (Zinecard® or Totect™): Abdominal pain, alkaline phosphatase increased, anorexia, calcium increased, constipation, cough, creatinine increased, depression, diarrhea, dizziness, dyspnea, headache, insomnia, LDH increased, nausea, peripheral edema, pneumonia, stomatitis, vomiting

Drug Interactions

Avoid Concomitant Use
Avoid concomitant use of Dexrazoxane with any of the following: Dimethyl Sulfoxide

Increased Effect/Toxicity There are no known significant interactions involving an increase in effect.

Decreased Effect
The levels/effects of Dexrazoxane may be decreased by: Dimethyl Sulfoxide

Storage/Stability Store intact vials at room temperature of 25°C (77°F); excursions permitted to 15°C to 30°C (59°F to 86°F). Protect from light. According to the manufacturers, infusion solutions diluted in 1000 mL NS (Totect™) are stable for 4 hours when stored at temperatures <25°C (<77°F); solutions diluted in D_5W or NS (Zinecard®) are stable for 6 hours at room temperature of 15°C to 30°C (59°F to 86°F) or under refrigeration at 2°C to 8°C (36°F to 46°F). When studied as a 24-hour continuous infusion for the prevention of cardiomyopathy, solutions diluted to a final concentration of

0.1 or 0.5 mg/mL in D_5W were found to retain ≥90% of their initial concentration when stored at room temperature (ambient light conditions) for ≤24 hours (Tetef, 2007).

Reconstitution Must be reconstituted with 0.167 Molar (M/6) sodium lactate injection to a concentration of 10 mg dexrazoxane/mL sodium lactate. Reconstituted dexrazoxane solution may be diluted with either 0.9% sodium chloride injection or 5% dextrose injection to a final concentration of 1.3-5 mg/mL in intravenous infusion bags for prevention of cardiomyopathy. For anthracycline-induced extravasation, add the reconstituted solution to 1000 mL NS. Use appropriate precautions for handling and disposal.

Compatibility Stable in NS, D_5W.

Y-site administration: Compatible: Gemcitabine, pemetrexed.

Mechanism of Action Derivative of ethylenediaminetetraacetic acid (EDTA); potent intracellular chelating agent. The mechanism of cardioprotectant activity is not fully understood. Appears to be converted intracellularly to a ring-opened chelating agent that interferes with iron-mediated oxygen free radical generation thought to be responsible, in part, for anthracycline-induced cardiomyopathy. In the management of anthracycline-induced extravasation, dexrazoxane may act by reversibly inhibiting topoisomerase II, protecting tissue from anthracycline cytotoxicity, thereby decreasing tissue damage.

Pharmacodynamics/Kinetics
Distribution: V_d: 22 L/m^2
Protein binding: None
Half-life elimination: 2-2.5 hours
Excretion: Urine (42%)

Dosage Adults: I.V.:

Prevention of doxorubicin cardiomyopathy: A 10:1 ratio of dexrazoxane: doxorubicin (500 mg/m² dexrazoxane: 50 mg/m² doxorubicin). **Note:** Cardiac monitoring should continue during dexrazoxane therapy; doxorubicin/ dexrazoxane should be discontinued in patients who develop a decline in LVEF or clinical CHF.

Treatment of anthracycline extravasation: 1000 mg/m² on days 1 and 2 (maximum dose: 2000 mg), followed by 500 mg/m² on day 3 (maximum dose: 1000 mg); begin treatment as soon as possible, within 6 hours of extravasation

Dosage adjustment in renal impairment: Moderate-to-severe (Cl_{cr}<40 mL/ minute):

Prevention of cardiomyopathy: Reduce dose by 50%, using a 5:1 dexrazoxane:doxorubicin ratio (250 mg/m² dexrazoxane: 50 mg/m² doxorubicin)

Anthracycline-induced extravasation: Reduce dose by 50%

Dosage adjustment in hepatic impairment:

Prevention of cardiomyopathy: Since doxorubicin dosage is reduced in hyperbilirubinemia, a proportional reduction in dexrazoxane dosage is recommended (maintain a 10:1 ratio of dexrazoxane:doxorubicin)

Anthracycline-induced extravasation: Use has not been evaluated in patients with hepatic dysfunction

Administration

Prevention of doxorubicin cardiomyopathy: Administer by slow I.V. push or rapid (5-15 minutes) I.V. infusion. Administer doxorubicin within 30 minutes after beginning the infusion with dexrazoxane.

Treatment of anthracycline extravasation: Administer over 1-2 hours; begin infusion as soon as possible, within 6 hours of extravasation. Infuse in a large vein in an area remote from the extravasation. If extravasation is also being managed with cooling, withhold cooling beginning 15 minutes before dexrazoxane infusion; continue withholding cooling until 15 minutes after infusion is completed. Day 2 and 3 doses should be administered at approximately the same time (±3 hours) as the dose on day 1. For I.V. administration; **not** for local infiltration into extravasation

Monitoring Parameters Since dexrazoxane will always be used with cytotoxic drugs, and may add to the myelosuppressive effects of cytotoxic drugs, frequent complete blood counts are recommended; liver function; serum creatinine; cardiac function (repeat monitoring at 400 mg/m^2, 500 mg/m^2 and with every 50 mg/m^2 of doxorubicin thereafter); monitor site of extravasation

Additional Information Oncology Comment: Guidelines from the American Society of Clinical Oncology (ASCO) for the use of chemotherapy and radiotherapy protectants (Schuchter, 2002; Hensley, 2008 [update]) recommend the use of dexrazoxane as a cardioprotectant in patients with metastatic breast cancer who may benefit from further doxorubicin-based chemotherapy after a cumulative doxorubicin dose >300 mg/m^2 has been reached. In patients with metastatic breast cancer who had previously received >300 mg/m^2 doxorubicin in the adjuvant setting, the decision to use dexrazoxane should be individualized, weighing the benefits of cardioprotection against the possibility of decreased response rates (due to dexrazoxane). Dexrazoxane use is not recommended in patients with metastatic breast cancer receiving doxorubicin as initial therapy. In the adjuvant setting, dexrazoxane use is not recommended outside of a clinical trial. Dexrazoxane may be considered for reduction of the incidence and severity of cardiomyopathy associated with continued epirubicin administration in patients with advanced breast cancer. In adults with malignancies other than breast cancer, dexrazoxane may be considered in patients who have received >300 mg/m^2 of doxorubicin-based therapy. Cardiac monitoring should continue during dexrazoxane therapy; discontinue doxorubicin/dexrazoxane in patients who develop a decline in LVEF or clinical CHF.

Emetic Potential Very low (<10%)

Dosage Forms Excipient information presented when available (limited, particularly for generics); consult specific product labeling.

Injection, powder for reconstitution: 250 mg, 500 mg

Totect™: 500 mg [provided with 0.167 Molar sodium lactate injection, USP]

Zinecard®: 250 mg, 500 mg [provided with 0.167 Molar sodium lactate injection, USP]

References

Hensley ML, Hagerty KL, Kewalramani T, et al, "American Society of Clinical Oncology 2008 Clinical Practice Guideline Update: Use of Chemotherapy and Radiotherapy Protectants," *J Clin Oncol*, 2009, 27(1): 127-45.

Hochster HS, "Clinical Pharmacology of Dexrazoxane," *Semin Oncol*, 1998, 25(4 Suppl 10):37-42.

Kwok JC and Richardson DR, "The Cardioprotective Effect of the Iron Chelator Dexrazoxane (ICRF-187) on Anthracycline-Mediated Cardiotoxicity," *Redox Rep*, 2000, 5(6):317-24.

Langer SW, Sehested M, and Jensen PB, "Treatment of Anthracycline Extravasation With Dexrazoxane," *Clin Cancer Res*, 2000, 6(9):3680-6.

Langer SW, Thougaard AV, Sehested M, et al, "Treatment of Anthracycline Extravasation in Mice With Dexrazoxane With or Without DMSO and Hydrocortisone," *Cancer Chemother Pharmacol*, 2006, 57(1):125-8.

Lopez M and Vici P, "European Trials With Dexrazoxane in Amelioration of Doxorubicin and Epirubicin-Induced Cardiotoxicity," *Semin Oncol*, 1998, 25(4 Suppl 10):55-60.

Mouridsen HT, Langer SW, Buter J, et al, "Treatment of Anthracycline Extravasation With Savene (Dexrazoxane): Results From Two Prospective Clinical Multicentre Studies," *Ann Oncol*, 2007, 18 (3):546-50.

Schuchter LM, Hensley ML, Meropol NJ, et al, "2002 Update of Recommendations for the Use of Chemotherapy and Radiotherapy Protectants: Clinical Practice Guidelines of the American Society of Clinical Oncology," *J Clin Oncol*, 2002, 20(12):2895-903.

Sehested M, et al, "Dexrazoxane for Protection Against Cardiotoxic Effects of Anthracyclines," *J Clin Oncol*, 1996, 14:2884.

Tetef ML, Synold TW, Chow W, et al, "Phase I Trial of 96-Hour Continuous Infusion of Dexrazoxane I Patients With Advanced Malignancies," *Clin Cancer Res*, 2001, 7(6):1569-76.

Wiseman LR and Spencer CM, "Dexrazoxane. A Review of Its Use as a Cardioprotective Agent in Patients Receiving Anthracycline-Based Chemotherapy," *Drugs*, 1998. 56(3):385-403.

- ◆ **DHAD** *see* Mitoxantrone *on page 810*
- ◆ **DHAQ** *see* Mitoxantrone *on page 810*
- ◆ **DHPG Sodium** *see* Ganciclovir *on page 525*
- ◆ **Diaminocyclohexane Oxalatoplatinum** *see* Oxaliplatin *on page 882*
- ◆ **DIC** *see* Dacarbazine *on page 293*
- ◆ **Diflucan®** *see* Fluconazole *on page 485*
- ◆ **Dihematoporphyrin Ether** *see* Porfimer *on page 967*
- ◆ **Dihydrohydroxycodeinone** *see* OxyCODONE *on page 889*
- ◆ **Dihydromorphinone** *see* HYDROmorphone *on page 584*
- ◆ **Dihydroxyanthracenedione** *see* Mitoxantrone *on page 810*
- ◆ **Dihydroxyanthracenedione Dihydrochloride** *see* Mitoxantrone *on page 810*
- ◆ **1,25 Dihydroxycholecalciferol** *see* Calcitriol *on page 168*
- ◆ **Dihydroxydeoxynorvinkaleukoblastine** *see* Vinorelbine *on page 1181*
- ◆ **Dilaudid®** *see* HYDROmorphone *on page 584*
- ◆ **Dilaudid-HP®** *see* HYDROmorphone *on page 584*
- ◆ **Dilaudid-HP-Plus® (Can)** *see* HYDROmorphone *on page 584*
- ◆ **Dilaudid® Sterile Powder (Can)** *see* HYDROmorphone *on page 584*
- ◆ **Dilaudid-XP® (Can)** *see* HYDROmorphone *on page 584*
- ◆ **Dimethyl Triazeno Imidazole Carboxamide** *see* Dacarbazine *on page 293*
- ◆ **Diocarpine (Can)** *see* Pilocarpine *on page 956*
- ◆ **Diodex® (Can)** *see* Dexamethasone *on page 350*
- ◆ **Diogent® (Can)** *see* Gentamicin *on page 542*
- ◆ **Diopred® (Can)** *see* PrednisoLONE *on page 977*
- ◆ **Disodium Thiosulfate Pentahydrate** *see* Sodium Thiosulfate *on page 1040*
- ◆ **5071-1DL(6)** *see* Megestrol *on page 743*
- ◆ **4-DMDR** *see* IDArubicin *on page 605*

Docetaxel (doe se TAKS el)

Medication Safety Issues

Sound-alike/look-alike issues:

Taxotere® may be confused with Taxol®

High alert medication: The Institute for Safe Medication Practices (ISMP) includes this medication among its list of drug classes which have a heightened risk of causing significant patient harm when used in error.

Related Information

Management of Drug Extravasations *on page 1447*

Safe Handling of Hazardous Drugs *on page 1517*

U.S. Brand Names Taxotere®

Index Terms NSC-628503; RP-6976

Generic Available No

Canadian Brand Names Taxotere®

◀ **Pharmacologic Category** Antineoplastic Agent, Antimicrotubular; Antineoplastic Agent, Natural Source (Plant) Derivative; Antineoplastic Agent, Taxane Derivative

Use Treatment of breast cancer; locally-advanced or metastatic nonsmall cell lung cancer (NSCLC); hormone refractory, metastatic prostate cancer; advanced gastric adenocarcinoma; locally-advanced squamous cell head and neck cancer

Unlabeled/Investigational Use Treatment of bladder cancer, ovarian cancer, small cell lung cancer, and soft tissue sarcoma

Pregnancy Risk Factor D

Lactation Excretion in breast milk unknown/not recommended

Labeled Contraindications Hypersensitivity to docetaxel or any component of the formulation; prior hypersensitivity to medications containing polysorbate 80; pre-existing bone marrow suppression (neutrophils <1500 cells/mm^3)

Warnings/Precautions Hazardous agent - use appropriate precautions for handling and disposal. **[U.S. Boxed Warnings]: Use caution in hepatic disease; avoid use in patients with bilirubin exceeding upper limit of normal (ULN) or AST and/or ALT >1.5 times ULN in conjunction with alkaline phosphatase >2.5 times ULN; patients with abnormal liver function are at increased risk of treatment-related adverse events. Severe hypersensitivity reactions characterized by rash/erythema, hypotension, bronchospasms, or anaphylaxis may occur; minor reactions including flushing or localized skin reactions may also occur. Fluid retention syndrome characterized by pleural effusions, ascites, edema, and weight gain (2-15 kg) has also been reported.** The incidence and severity of the syndrome increase sharply at cumulative doses ≥400 mg/m^2. Patients should be premedicated with a corticosteroid to prevent hypersensitivity reactions and fluid retention; severity is reduced with dexamethasone premedication starting one day prior to docetaxel administration.

[U.S. Boxed Warning]: Patients with abnormal liver function, those receiving higher doses, and patients with nonsmall cell lung cancer and a history of prior treatment with platinum derivatives who receive docetaxel doses higher than 100 mg/m^2 are at higher risk for treatment-related mortality.

Neutropenia is the dose-limiting toxicity; however, this rarely results in treatment delays and prophylactic colony stimulating factors have not been routinely used. Patients with increased liver function tests experienced more episodes of neutropenia with a greater number of severe infections. **[U.S. Boxed Warning]: Patients with an absolute neutrophil count <1500 cells/mm^3 should not receive docetaxel.** When administered as sequential infusions, taxane derivatives (docetaxel, paclitaxel) should be administered before platinum derivatives (carboplatin, cisplatin) to limit myelosuppression and to enhance efficacy.

Cutaneous reactions including erythema and desquamation have been reported; may require dose reduction. Dosage adjustment is recommended with severe neurosensory symptoms (paresthesia, dysesthesia, pain). Safety and efficacy in children have not been established.

Adverse Reactions Percentages reported for docetaxel monotherapy; frequency may vary depending on diagnosis, dose, liver function, prior treatment, and premedication. The incidence of adverse events was usually higher in patients with elevated liver function tests.

>10%:

Cardiovascular: Fluid retention (13% to 60%; dose dependent)

Central nervous system: Neurosensory events (20% to 58%; including neuropathy), fever (31% to 35%), neuromotor events (16%)

Dermatologic: Alopecia (56% to 76%), cutaneous events (20% to 48%), nail disorder (11% to 41%)

Gastrointestinal: Stomatitis (19% to 53%; severe 1% to 8%), diarrhea (23% to 43%; severe: 5% to 6%), nausea (34% to 42%), vomiting (22% to 23%)

Hematologic: Neutropenia (84% to 99%; grade 4: 75% to 86%; onset: 4-7 days, nadir: 5-9 days, recovery: 21 days; dose dependent), leukopenia (84% to 99%; grade 4: 32% to 44%), anemia (65% to 94%; dose dependent; grades 3/4: 8% to 9%), thrombocytopenia (8% to 14%; grade 4: 1%; dose dependent), febrile neutropenia (6% to 12%; dose dependent)

Hepatic: Transaminases increased (4% to 19%)

Neuromuscular & skeletal: Weakness (53% to 66%; severe 13% to 18%), myalgia (3% to 23%)

Respiratory: Pulmonary events (41%)

Miscellaneous: Infection (1% to 34%; dose dependent), hypersensitivity (1% to 21%; with premedication 15%)

1% to 10%:

Cardiovascular: Left ventricular ejection fraction decreased (prostate cancer: 10%; metastatic breast cancer: 8%), hypotension (3%)

Dermatologic: Rash/erythema (2%)

Gastrointestinal: Taste perversion (6%)

Hepatic: Bilirubin increased (9%), alkaline phosphatase increased (4% to 7%)

Local: Infusion-site reactions (4%, including hyperpigmentation, inflammation, redness, dryness, phlebitis, extravasation, swelling of the vein)

Neuromuscular and skeletal: Arthralgia (3% to 9%)

Ocular: Epiphora associated with canalicular stenosis (≤77% with weekly administration; ≤1% with every 3-week administration)

<1%, postmarketing and/or case reports (limited to important or life-threatening): Acute myeloid leukemia (AML), acute respiratory distress syndrome (ARDS), anaphylactic shock, angina, ascites, atrial fibrillation, atrial flutter, bleeding episodes, bronchospasm, cardiac tamponade, chest pain, chest tightness, colitis, conjunctivitis, constipation, cutaneous lupus erythematosus, deep vein thrombosis, dehydration, disseminated intravascular coagulation (DIC), drug fever, duodenal ulcer, dyspnea, dysrhythmia, ECG abnormalities, erythema multiforme, esophagitis, gastrointestinal hemorrhage, gastrointestinal obstruction, gastrointestinal perforation, hand and foot syndrome, hearing loss, heart failure, hepatitis, hypertension, ileus, interstitial pneumonia, ischemic colitis, lacrimal duct obstruction, loss of consciousness (transient), MI, multiorgan failure, myelodysplastic syndrome, neutropenic enterocolitis, ototoxicity, pleural effusion, pruritus, pulmonary edema, pulmonary embolism, pulmonary fibrosis, radiation recall, radiation pneumonitis, renal insufficiency, seizure, sepsis, sinus tachycardia, Stevens-Johnson syndrome, syncope, toxic epidermal necrolysis, tachycardia, thrombophlebitis, unstable angina, visual disturbances (transient)

Drug Interactions

Metabolism/Transport Effects Substrate of CYP3A4 (major); **Inhibits** CYP3A4 (weak)

Avoid Concomitant Use

Avoid concomitant use of Docetaxel with any of the following: Natalizumab; Vaccines (Live)

◀ **Increased Effect/Toxicity**

Docetaxel may increase the levels/effects of: Antineoplastic Agents (Anthracycline); Leflunomide; Natalizumab; Vaccines (Live)

The levels/effects of Docetaxel may be increased by: Antifungal Agents (Azole Derivatives, Systemic); CYP3A4 Inhibitors (Moderate); CYP3A4 Inhibitors (Strong); Dasatinib; P-Glycoprotein Inhibitors; Platinum Derivatives; Trastuzumab

Decreased Effect

Docetaxel may decrease the levels/effects of: Vaccines (Inactivated); Vaccines (Live)

The levels/effects of Docetaxel may be decreased by: CYP3A4 Inducers (Strong); Deferasirox; Echinacea; Herbs (CYP3A4 Inducers); P-Glycoprotein Inducers

Ethanol/Nutrition/Herb Interactions

Ethanol: Avoid ethanol (due to GI irritation).

Herb/Nutraceutical: Avoid St John's wort (may decrease docetaxel levels).

Storage/Stability Intact vials should be stored at 2°C to 25°C (36°F to 77°F) and protected from light. Freezing does not adversely affect the product. If refrigerated, vials should be stored at room temperature for approximately 5 minutes before using. Diluted solutions in the vial are stable for 8 hours at room temperature or under refrigeration. Solutions diluted for infusion in D_5W or NS are stable for up to 4 weeks at room temperature of 15°C to 25°C (59°F to 77°F) in polyolefin containers; however, the manufacturer recommends use within 4 hours.

Reconstitution Vials should be diluted with 13% (w/w) ethanol/water (provided with the drug) to a final concentration of 10 mg/mL. Do not shake. The solution should be further diluted in 250-1000 mL of NS or D_5W to a final concentration of 0.3-0.9 mg/mL (although the manufacturer recommends a final concentration of 0.3-0.74) and dispensed in a non-DEHP container (eg, glass, polypropylene, polyolefin).

Compatibility Stable in D_5W, NS.

Y-site administration: Compatible: Acyclovir, amifostine, amikacin, aminophylline, ampicillin, ampicillin/sulbactam, anidulafungin, aztreonam, bumetanide, buprenorphine, butorphanol, calcium gluconate, cefazolin, cefepime, cefotaxime, cefotetan, cefoxitin, ceftazidime, ceftizoxime, ceftriaxone, cefuroxime, chlorpromazine, cimetidine, ciprofloxacin, clindamycin, cotrimoxazole, dexamethasone sodium phosphate, diphenhydramine, dobutamine, dopamine, doxycycline, droperidol, enalaprilat, famotidine, fluconazole, furosemide, ganciclovir, gemcitabine, gentamicin, granisetron, haloperidol, heparin, hydrocortisone sodium succinate, hydromorphone, hydroxyzine, imipenem/cilastatin, leucovorin calcium, lorazepam, magnesium sulfate, mannitol, meperidine, meropenem, mesna, metoclopramide, metronidazole, morphine, ofloxacin, ondansetron, oxaliplatin, palonosetron, pemetrexed, piperacillin, piperacillin/tazobactam, potassium chloride, prochlorperazine edisylate, promethazine, ranitidine, Ringer's injection (lactated), sodium bicarbonate, ticarcillin/clavulanate, tobramycin, vancomycin, zidovudine. **Incompatible:** Amphotericin B, doxorubicin liposome, methylprednisolone sodium succinate, nalbuphine.

Mechanism of Action Docetaxel promotes the assembly of microtubules from tubulin dimers, and inhibits the depolymerization of tubulin which stabilizes microtubules in the cell. This results in inhibition of DNA, RNA, and protein synthesis. Most activity occurs during the M phase of the cell cycle.

Pharmacodynamics/Kinetics Exhibits linear pharmacokinetics at the recommended dosage range

Distribution: Extensive extravascular distribution and/or tissue binding; V_d: 80-90 L/m^2, V_{dss}: 113 L (mean steady state)

Protein binding: ~94% to 97%, primarily to alpha$_1$-acid glycoprotein, albumin, and lipoproteins

Metabolism: Hepatic; oxidation via CYP3A4 to metabolites

Half-life elimination: Terminal: 11 hours

Excretion: Feces (75%, <8% as unchanged drug); urine (6%); ~80% within 48 hours

Clearance: Total body: Mean: 21 L/hour/m^2

Dosage Adults: I.V. infusion: Refer to individual protocols: **Note:** Premedicate with corticosteroids, beginning the day before docetaxel administration, (administer for 1-5 days) to reduce the severity of hypersensitivity reactions and pulmonary/peripheral edema

Breast cancer:

Locally-advanced or metastatic: 60-100 mg/m^2 every 3 weeks; patients initially started at 60 mg/m^2 who do not develop toxicity may tolerate higher doses

Operable, node-positive (adjuvant treatment): 75 mg/m^2 every 3 weeks for 6 courses (in combination with doxorubicin and cyclophosphamide)

Nonsmall cell lung cancer: 75 mg/m^2 every 3 weeks (as monotherapy or in combination with cisplatin)

Prostate cancer: 75 mg/m^2 every 3 weeks (in combination with prednisone)

Gastric adenocarcinoma: 75 mg/m^2 every 3 weeks (in combination with cisplatin and fluorouracil)

Head and neck cancer: 75 mg/m^2 every 3 weeks (in combination with cisplatin and fluorouracil) for 3 or 4 cycles, followed by radiation therapy

Dosing adjustment for toxicity:

Note: Toxicity includes febrile neutropenia, neutrophils ≤500/mm^3 for >1 week, severe or cumulative cutaneous reactions; in nonsmall cell lung cancer, this may also include platelets <25,000/mm^3 and other grade 3/4 nonhematologic toxicities.

Breast cancer: Patients dosed initially at 100 mg/m^2; reduce dose to 75 mg/m^2; **Note:** If the patient continues to experience these adverse reactions, the dosage should be reduced to 55 mg/m^2 or therapy should be discontinued; discontinue for peripheral neuropathy ≥ grade 3

Breast cancer, adjuvant treatment: TAC regimen should be administered when neutrophils are ≥1500 cells/mm^3. Patients experiencing febrile neutropenia should receive G-CSF in all subsequent cycles. Patients with persistent febrile neutropenia (while on G-CSF) or patients experiencing severe/cumulative cutaneous reactions or moderate neurosensory effects (signs/symptoms) should receive a reduced dose (60 mg/m^2) of docetaxel. Patients who experience grade 3 or 4 stomatitis should also receive a reduced dose (60 mg/m^2) of docetaxel. Discontinue therapy with persistent toxicities after dosage reduction.

Nonsmall cell lung cancer:

Monotherapy: Patients dosed initially at 75 mg/m^2 should have dose held until toxicity is resolved, then resume at 55 mg/m^2; discontinue for peripheral neuropathy ≥ grade 3.

Combination therapy (with cisplatin): Patients dosed initially at 75 mg/m^2 should have the docetaxel dosage reduced to 65 mg/m^2 in subsequent cycles; if further adjustment is required, dosage may be reduced to 50 mg/m^2

◀ Prostate cancer: Reduce dose to 60 mg/m^2; discontinue therapy if toxicities persist at lower dose.

Gastric cancer, head and neck cancer: **Note:** Cisplatin may require dose reductions/therapy delays for peripheral neuropathy, ototoxicity, and/or nephrotoxicity. Patients experiencing febrile neutropenia, documented infection with neutropenia or neutropenia >7 days should receive G-CSF in all subsequent cycles. For neutropenic complications despite G-CSF use, further reduce dose to 60 mg/m^2. Neutropenic complications in subsequent cycles should be further dose reduced to 45 mg/m^2. Patients who experience grade 4 thrombocytopenia should receive a dose reduction from 75 mg/m^2 to 60 mg/m^2. Discontinue therapy for persistent toxicities.

Gastrointestinal toxicity for docetaxel in combination with cisplatin and fluorouracil for treatment of gastric cancer or head and neck cancer:

Diarrhea, grade 3:
First episode: Reduce fluorouracil dose by 20%
Second episode: Reduce docetaxel dose by 20%

Diarrhea, grade 4:
First episode: Reduce fluorouracil and docetaxel doses by 20%
Second episode: Discontinue treatment

Stomatitis, grade 3:
First episode: Reduce fluorouracil dose by 20%
Second episode: Discontinue fluorouracil for all subsequent cycles
Third episode: Reduce docetaxel dose by 20%

Stomatitis, grade 4:
First episode: Discontinue fluorouracil for all subsequent cycles
Second episode: Reduce docetaxel dose by 20%

Dosing adjustment in renal impairment: Docetaxel has minimal renal excretion; dosage adjustments for renal dysfunction may not be needed.

Dosing adjustment in hepatic impairment:

The FDA-approved labeling recommends the following adjustments:

Total bilirubin greater than the ULN, or AST and/or ALT >1.5 times ULN concomitant with alkaline phosphatase >2.5 times ULN: Docetaxel **generally should not be administered**.

Hepatic impairment dosing adjustment specific for gastric adenocarcinoma:

AST/ALT >2.5 to ≤5 times ULN and alkaline phosphatase ≤2.5 times ULN: Administer 80% of dose

AST/ALT >1.5 to ≤5 times ULN and alkaline phosphatase >2.5 to ≤5 times ULN: Administer 80% of dose

AST/ALT >5 times ULN and /or alkaline phosphatase >5 times ULN: Discontinue docetaxel

The following guidelines have been used by some clinicians (Floyd, 2006):

Transaminases 1.6-6 times ULN: Administer 75% of dose
Transaminases >6 times ULN: Use clinical judgment

Combination Regimens

Bladder cancer:
Cisplatin-Docetaxel on page 1266
Gemcitabine-Docetaxel (Bladder Cancer) on page 1344
Breast cancer:
AT on page 1226
Capecitabine + Docetaxel (Breast Cancer) on page 1243
Docetaxel-Bevacizumab on page 1289
Docetaxel-Cyclophosphamide (TC) on page 1291
Docetaxel-FEC on page 1292
Docetaxel-Trastuzumab on page 1293

Docetaxel-Trastuzumab-Carboplatin on page 1293
Docetaxel-Trastuzumab-Cisplatin on page 1294
Docetaxel-Trastuzumab-FEC on page 1294
Docetaxel (Weekly)-Trastuzumab on page 1295
Doxorubicin (Liposomal)-Docetaxel (Breast Cancer) on page 1296
TAC on page 1404
TEX (Capecitabine + Docetaxel + Epirubicin) on page 1405
Esophageal cancer: Docetaxel-Cisplatin-Fluorouracil (Gastric/Esophageal Cancer) on page 1290
Gastric cancer:
Capecitabine + Docetaxel (Gastric Cancer) on page 1244
Docetaxel-Cisplatin-Fluorouracil (Gastric/Esophageal Cancer) on page 1290
Head and neck cancer: Docetaxel-Cisplatin-Fluorouracil (Head and Neck Cancer) on page 1291
Lung cancer (nonsmall cell):
Capecitabine-Docetaxel (NSCLC) on page 1244
Docetaxel-Cisplatin on page 1290
Prostate cancer:
Docetaxel-Prednisone on page 1292
Docetaxel-Thalidomide on page 1292
Docetaxel (Weekly Regimen) on page 1295
Estramustine + Docetaxel on page 1313
Estramustine + Docetaxel + Calcitriol on page 1313
Estramustine + Docetaxel + Carboplatin on page 1314
Estramustine + Docetaxel + Hydrocortisone on page 1314
Estramustine + Docetaxel + Prednisone on page 1314
Osteosarcoma: Gemcitabine-Docetaxel (Sarcoma) on page 1344
Ovarian cancer:
Docetaxel-Carboplatin (Ovarian Cancer) on page 1289
Docetaxel-Oxaliplatin (Ovarian Cancer) on page 1292
Soft tissue sarcoma: Gemcitabine-Docetaxel (Sarcoma) on page 1344

Administration Administer I.V. infusion over 1-hour through nonsorbing polyethylene lined (non-DEHP) tubing; in-line filter is not necessary (the use of a filter during administration is not recommended by the manufacturer). **Note:** Premedication with corticosteroids for 1-5 days, beginning the day before docetaxel administration, is recommended to prevent hypersensitivity reactions and pulmonary/peripheral edema (see Additional Information).

Monitoring Parameters CBC with differential, liver function tests, bilirubin, alkaline phosphatase, renal function; monitor for hypersensitivity reactions, fluid retention, epiphora, and canalicular stenosis

Additional Information Premedication with oral corticosteroids is recommended to decrease the incidence and severity of fluid retention and severity of hypersensitivity reactions. Dexamethasone 8-10 mg orally twice daily for 3-5 days, starting the day before docetaxel administration, is usually recommended. When prednisone is part of the antineoplastic regimen (eg, prostate cancer), the prednisone is sometimes withheld on the days dexamethasone is administered.

Emetic Potential Low (10% to 30%)

Vesicant May be an irritant

Dosage Forms Excipient information presented when available (limited, particularly for generics); consult specific product labeling.
Injection, solution [concentrate]:
Taxotere®: 20 mg/0.5 mL (0.5 mL, 2 mL) [contains Polysorbate 80®; diluent contains ethanol 13%]

References

Ajani JA, Fodor MD, Tjulandin SA, et al, "Phase II Multi-Institutional Randomized Trial of Docetaxel Plus Cisplatin With or Without Fluorouracil in Patients With Untreated, Advanced Gastric, or Gastroesophageal Adenocarcinoma," *J Clin Oncol*, 2005, 23(24):5660-7.

Floyd J, Mirza I, Sachs B, et al, "Hepatotoxicity of Chemotherapy," *Semin Oncol*, 2006, 33 (1):50-67.

Posner MR, Glisson B, Frenette G, et al, "Multicenter Phase I-II Trial of Docetaxel, Cisplatin, and Fluorouracil Induction Chemotherapy for Patients With Locally Advanced Squamous Cell Cancer of the Head and Neck," *J Clin Oncol*, 2001, 19(4):1096-104.

Posner MR, Hershock DM, Blajman CR, et al, "Cisplatin and Fluorouracil Alone or With Docetaxel in Head and Neck Cancer," *N Engl J Med*, 2007, 357(17):1705-15.

Schrijvers D, Van Herpen C, Kerger J, et al, "Docetaxel, Cisplatin and 5-Fluorouracil in Patients With Locally Advanced Unresectable Head and Neck Cancer: A Phase I-II Feasibility Study," *Ann Oncol*, 2004, 15(4):638-45.

Thiesen J and Kramer I, "Physico-Chemical Stability of Docetaxel Premix Solution and Docetaxel Infusion Solutions in PVC Bags and Polyolefine Containers," *Pharm World Sci*, 1999, 21 (3):137-41.

Vermorken JB, Remenar E, van Herpen C, et al, "Cisplatin, Fluorouracil, and Docetaxel in Unresectable Head and Neck Cancer," *N Engl J Med*, 2007, 357(17):1695-704.

Dolasetron (dol A se tron)

Medication Safety Issues

Sound-alike/look-alike issues:

Anzemet® may be confused with Aldomet®, Avandamet®

Dolasetron may be confused with granisetron, ondansetron, palonosetron

Related Information

Management of Chemotherapy-Induced Nausea and Vomiting *on page 1434*

U.S. Brand Names Anzemet®

Index Terms Dolasetron Mesylate; MDL 73,147EF

Generic Available No

Canadian Brand Names Anzemet®

Pharmacologic Category Antiemetic; Selective 5-HT₃ Receptor Antagonist

Use Prevention of nausea and vomiting associated with emetogenic cancer chemotherapy; prevention of postoperative nausea and vomiting; treatment of postoperative nausea and vomiting (injectable form only).

Note: In Canada, the use of dolasetron is contraindicated in children <18 years of age and for the prevention and treatment of postoperative nausea and vomiting in adults. These are not labeled contraindications in the U.S.

Unlabeled/Investigational Use Breakthrough treatment of nausea and vomiting associated with chemotherapy

Pregnancy Risk Factor B

Lactation Excretion in breast milk unknown/use caution

Labeled Contraindications Hypersensitivity to dolasetron or any component of the formulation

Note: In Canada, the use of dolasetron is contraindicated for all uses in children <18 years of age or in the treatment of postoperative nausea and vomiting in adults. These are not labeled contraindications in the U.S.

Warnings/Precautions Dolasetron should be administered with caution in patients with congenital long QT syndrome or other risk factors for QT prolongation (eg, medications known to prolong QT interval, electrolyte abnormalities, and cumulative high-dose anthracycline therapy). Dolasetron has been associated with a number of dose-dependent increases in ECG intervals (eg, PR, QRS duration, QT/QT_c, JT), usually occurring 1-2 hours after I.V. administration and usually lasting 6-8 hours; however, may last ≥24 hours and rarely lead to heart block or arrhythmia. Clinically relevant QT interval prolongation may occur resulting in torsade de pointes, when used in conjunction with other agents that prolong the QT interval (eg, Class I and III antiarrhythmics). Use with caution in patients at risk of QT prolongation and/or ventricular arrhythmia. Reduction in heart rate may also occur with the 5-HT$_3$ antagonists. I.V. formulations of 5-HT$_3$ antagonists have more association with ECG interval changes, compared to oral formulations. Use with caution in children and adolescents who have or may develop QT$_c$ prolongation; rare cases of supraventricular and ventricular arrhythmias, cardiac arrest, and MI have been reported in this population.

Use with caution in patients allergic to other 5-HT$_3$ receptor antagonists; cross-reactivity has been reported. **For chemotherapy, should be used on a scheduled basis, not on an "as needed" (PRN) basis,** since data support the use of this drug only in the prevention of nausea and vomiting (due to antineoplastic therapy) and not in the rescue of nausea and vomiting. Not intended for treatment of nausea and vomiting or for chronic continuous therapy. Safety and efficacy in children <2 years of age have not been established.

Adverse Reactions Adverse events may vary according to indication

>10%:
  Central nervous system: Headache (7% to 24%)
  Gastrointestinal: Diarrhea (2% to 12%)

1% to 10%:
  Cardiovascular: Bradycardia (4% to 5%), hypotension (5%), hypertension (2% to 3%), tachycardia (2% to 3%)
  Central nervous system: Dizziness (1% to 6%), fatigue (3% to 6%), fever (4% to 5%), pain (≤3%), chills/shivering (1% to 2%), sedation (2%)
  Dermatological: Pruritus (3% to 4%)
  Gastrointestinal: Dyspepsia (2% to 3%), abdominal pain (≤3%)
  Hepatic: Abnormal hepatic function (4%)
  Neuromuscular & skeletal: Pain (3%)
  Renal: Oliguria (1% to 3%)

<1% (Limited to important or life-threatening): Abnormal vision, abnormal dreaming, acute renal failure, alkaline phosphatase increased, ALT increased, anaphylactic reaction, anemia, anorexia, anxiety, arrhythmia (supraventricular and ventricular), AST increased, ataxia, AV block, bronchospasm, cardiac arrest, cardiac conduction abnormalities, chest pain, confusion, constipation, diaphoresis, dyspnea, dysuria, edema, epistaxis, facial edema, flushing, GGT increased, heart block, hematuria, hyper-bilirubinemia, ischemia (peripheral), local injection site reaction, MI, myocardial ischemia, orthostatic hypotension, palpitation, pancreatitis, paresthesia, peripheral edema, photophobia, polyuria; prolonged PR, QRS, JT, and QT$_c$ intervals; prothrombin time increased, PTT increased, purpura/hematoma, rash, sleep disorder, syncope, taste perversion, thrombocytopenia, thrombophlebitis/phlebitis, tinnitus, tremor, twitching, urticaria, vertigo

Drug Interactions

Metabolism/Transport Effects Substrate (minor) of CYP2C9, 3A4; **Inhibits** CYP2D6 (weak)

Avoid Concomitant Use
  Avoid concomitant use of Dolasetron with any of the following: Apomorphine; Artemether; Dronedarone; Lumefantrine; Nilotinib; Pimozide; QuiNINE; Tetrabenazine; Thioridazine; Ziprasidone

Increased Effect/Toxicity
  Dolasetron may increase the levels/effects of: Apomorphine; Dronedarone; Pimozide; QTc-Prolonging Agents; QuiNINE; Tetrabenazine; Thioridazine; Ziprasidone

◀ *The levels/effects of Dolasetron may be increased by:* Alfuzosin; Artemether; Chloroquine; Ciprofloxacin; Gadobutrol; Lumefantrine; Nilotinib; QuiNINE

Decreased Effect There are no known significant interactions involving a decrease in effect.

Storage/Stability Store intact vials and tablets at room temperature. Protect from light. A 20 mg/mL solution in syringes is stable for 8 months at room temperature. Solutions diluted for infusion are stable at room temperature for 24 hours or under refrigeration for 48 hours.

Reconstitution Dilute in 50-100 mL of a compatible solution (ie, 0.9% NS, D_5W, $D_5\frac{1}{2}NS$, D_5LR, LR, and 10% mannitol injection).

Compatibility Stable in 0.9% NS, D_5W, $D_5\frac{1}{2}NS$, D_5LR, LR, and 10% mannitol injection.

Mechanism of Action Selective serotonin receptor (5-HT_3) antagonist, blocking serotonin both peripherally (primary site of action) and centrally at the chemoreceptor trigger zone

Pharmacodynamics/Kinetics

Absorption: Rapid and complete

Distribution: Hydrodolasetron: 5.8 L/kg

Protein binding: Hydrodolasetron: 69% to 77% (50% bound to alpha$_1$-acid glycoprotein)

Metabolism: Hepatic; reduction by carbonyl reductase to hydrodolasetron (active metabolite); further metabolized by CYP2D6, CYP3A, and flavin monooxygenase

Bioavailability: 75%

Half-life elimination: Dolasetron: 10 minutes; hydrodolasetron: Adults: 6-8 hours; Children: 4-6 hours

Time to peak, plasma: Hydrodolasetron: I.V.: 0.6 hours; Oral: 1 hour

Excretion: Urine ~67% (53% to 61% as active metabolite hydrodolasetron); feces ~33%

Dosage

Prevention of chemotherapy-associated nausea and vomiting (including initial and repeat courses):

Children 2-16 years:

Oral: 1.8 mg/kg within 1 hour before chemotherapy; maximum: 100 mg/dose

I.V.: 1.8 mg/kg ~30 minutes before chemotherapy; maximum: 100 mg/dose

Adults:

Oral:100 mg single dose 1 hour prior to chemotherapy

I.V.: 1.8 mg/kg or 100 mg 30 minutes prior to chemotherapy

Prevention of postoperative nausea and vomiting:

Children 2-16 years:

Oral: 1.2 mg/kg within 2 hours before surgery; maximum: 100 mg/dose

I.V.: 0.35 mg/kg (maximum: 12.5 mg) ~15 minutes before stopping anesthesia

Adults:

Oral: 100 mg within 2 hours before surgery

I.V.: 12.5 mg ~15 minutes before stopping anesthesia

Treatment of postoperative nausea and vomiting: I.V. (only):

Children: 0.35 mg/kg (maximum: 12.5 mg) as soon as needed

Adults: 12.5 mg as soon as needed

Dosing adjustment for elderly, renal/hepatic impairment: No dosage adjustment is recommended

Administration I.V. injection may be given either undiluted IVP over 30 seconds or diluted in 50 mL of compatible fluid and infused over 15 minutes.

Line should be flushed, prior to and after, dolasetron administration. Dolasetron injection may be diluted in apple or apple-grape juice and taken orally; this dilution is stable for 2 hours at room temperature.

Monitoring Parameters Liver function tests, blood pressure and pulse, and ECG in patients with cardiovascular disease

Additional Information Efficacy of dolasetron, for chemotherapy treatment, is enhanced with concomitant administration of dexamethasone 20 mg (increases complete response by 10% to 20%). Oral administration of the intravenous solution is equivalent to tablets. A single I.V. dose of dolasetron mesylate (1.8 or 2.4 mg/kg) has comparable safety and efficacy to a single 32 mg I.V. dose of ondansetron in patients receiving cisplatin chemotherapy.

Dosage Forms Excipient information presented when available (limited, particularly for generics); consult specific product labeling.

Injection, solution, as mesylate:

Anzemet®: 20 mg/mL (0.625 mL) [single-use Carpuject® or vial; contains mannitol 38.2 mg/mL]; 20 mg/mL (5 mL) [single-use vial; contains mannitol 38.2 mg/mL]; 20 mg/mL (25 mL) [multidose vial; contains mannitol 29 mg/mL]

Tablet, as mesylate:

Anzemet®: 50 mg, 100 mg

Extemporaneous Preparations Dolasetron injection may be diluted in apple or apple-grape juice and taken orally; this dilution is stable for 2 hours at room temperature.

References

Fauser AA, Russ W, and Bischoff M, "Oral Dolasetron Mesilate (MDL 73, 147EF) for the Control of Emesis During Fractionated Total-Body Irradiation and High-Dose Cyclophosphamide in Patients Undergoing Allogeneic Bone Marrow Transplantation," *Support Care Cancer*, 1997, 5(3):219-22.

Gan TJ, Meyer TA, Apfel CC, et al, "Society for Ambulatory Anesthesia Guidelines for the Management of Postoperative Nausea and Vomiting," *Anesth Analg*, 2007, 105(6):1615-28.

Hesketh P, Navari R, Grote T, et al, "Double-Blind, Randomized Comparison of the Antiemetic Efficacy of Intravenous Dolasetron Mesylate and Intravenous Ondansetron in the Prevention of Acute Cisplatin-Induced Emesis in Patients With Cancer: Dolasetron Comparative Chemotherapy-induced Emesis Prevention Group," *J Clin Oncol*, 1996, 14(8):2242-9.

Kris MG, Hesketh PJ, Somerfield MR, et al, "American Society of Clinical Oncology Guideline for Antiemetics in Oncology: Update 2006," *J Clin Oncol*, 2006, 24(18):2932-47.

Kris MG, Pendergrass KB, Navari RM, et al, "Prevention of Acute Emesis in Cancer Patients Following High-Dose Cisplatin With the Combination of Oral Dolasetron and Dexamethasone," *J Clin Oncol*, 1997, 15(5):2135-8.

Navari RM and Koeller JM, "Electrocardiographic and Cardiovascular Effects of the 5-Hydroxytryptamine₃ Receptor Antagonists," *Ann Pharmacother*, 2003, 37(9):1276-86.

Steiner ME, Lensmeyer G, and Vermeulen LC, "Stability and Sterility of Dolasetron Mesylate in Syringes Stored at Room Temperature," *Am J Health Syst Pharm*, 2005, 62(9):896-9.

DOXOrubicin (doks oh ROO bi sin)

Medication Safety Issues

Sound-alike/look-alike issues:

DOXOrubicin may be confused with DACTINomycin, DAUNOrubicin, DAUNOrubicin liposomal, doxacurium, doxapram, doxazosin, DOXOrubicin liposomal, epirubicin, IDArubicin, valrubicin

Adriamycin PFS® may be confused with achromycin, Aredia®, Idamycin®

Conventional formulation (Adriamycin PFS®, Adriamycin RDF®) may be confused with the liposomal formulation (Doxil®)

Use caution when selecting product for preparation and dispensing; indications, dosages and adverse event profiles differ between conventional DOXOrubicin hydrochloride solution and DOXOrubicin liposomal. Both formulations are the same concentration. As a result, serious errors have occurred.

High alert medication: The Institute for Safe Medication Practices (ISMP) includes this medication among its list of drug classes which have a heightened risk of causing significant patient harm when used in error.

ADR is an error-prone abbreviation

International issues:

Doxil® may be confused with Doxal® which is a brand name for doxepin in Finland, a brand name for doxycycline in Austria, and a brand name for pyridoxine/thiamine combination in Brazil

Rubex, a discontinued brand name for DOXOrubicin in the U.S, is a brand name for ascorbic acid in Ireland

Related Information

Fertility and Cancer Therapy *on page 1430*
Management of Drug Extravasations *on page 1447*
Safe Handling of Hazardous Drugs *on page 1517*

U.S. Brand Names Adriamycin®

Index Terms ADR (error-prone abbreviation); Adria; Doxorubicin Hydrochloride; Hydroxydaunomycin Hydrochloride; Hydroxyldaunorubicin Hydrochloride

Generic Available Yes

Canadian Brand Names Adriamycin®

Pharmacologic Category Antineoplastic Agent, Anthracycline

Use Treatment of acute lymphocytic leukemia (ALL), acute myeloid leukemia (AML), Hodgkin's disease, malignant lymphoma, soft tissue and bone sarcomas, thyroid cancer, small cell lung cancer, breast cancer, gastric cancer, ovarian cancer, bladder cancer, neuroblastoma, and Wilms' tumor

Unlabeled/Investigational Use Treatment of multiple myeloma, endometrial carcinoma, uterine sarcoma, head and neck cancer, liver cancer, kidney cancer

Pregnancy Risk Factor D

Lactation Enters breast milk/not recommended

Labeled Contraindications Hypersensitivity to doxorubicin, any component of the formulation, or to other anthracyclines or anthracenediones; recent MI, severe myocardial insufficiency, severe arrhythmia; previous therapy with high cumulative doses of doxorubicin, daunorubicin, idarubicin, or other anthracycline and anthracenediones; baseline neutrophil count <1500/mm^3; severe hepatic impairment

Warnings/Precautions Hazardous agent - use appropriate precautions for handling and disposal. **[U.S. Boxed Warning]: May cause cumulative, dose-related, myocardial toxicity (early or delayed).** Cardiotoxicity is dose-limiting. Total cumulative dose should take into account previous or concomitant treatment with cardiotoxic agents or irradiation of chest. The incidence of irreversible myocardial toxicity increases as the total cumulative (lifetime) dosages approach 450-500 mg/m². Although the risk increases with cumulative dose, irreversible cardiotoxicity may occur at any dose level. Patients with pre-existing heart disease,, hypertension, concurrent administration of other antineoplastic agents, prior or concurrent chest irradiation, advanced age; and infants and children are at increased risk. Alternative administration schedules (weekly or continuous infusions) have are associated with less cardiotoxicity Baseline and periodic monitoring of ECG and LVEF (with either ECHO or MUGA scan) is recommended. **[U.S. Boxed Warnings]: Reduce dose in patients with impaired hepatic function; dose-limiting severe myelosuppression (primarily leukopenia and neutropenia) may occur. Secondary acute myelogenous leukemia and myelodysplastic syndrome have been reported following treatment.** May cause tumor lysis syndrome and hyperuricemia (in patients with rapidly growing tumors).

Children are at increased risk for developing delayed cardiotoxicity; follow-up cardiac function monitoring is recommended. Doxorubicin may contribute to prepubertal growth failure in children; may also contribute to gonadal impairment (usually temporary). Radiation recall pneumonitis has been reported in children receiving concomitant dactinomycin and doxorubicin. **[U.S. Boxed Warnings]: For I.V. administration only. Potent vesicant; if extravasation occurs, severe local tissue damage leading to ulceration, necrosis, and pain may occur. Should be administered under the supervision of an experienced cancer chemotherapy physician.**

Adverse Reactions Frequency not defined.

Cardiovascular:

Acute cardiotoxicity: Atrioventricular block, bradycardia, bundle branch block, ECG abnormalities, extrasystoles (atrial or ventricular), sinus tachycardia, ST-T wave changes, supraventricular tachycardia, tachyarrhythmia, ventricular tachycardia

Delayed cardiotoxicity: LVEF decreased, CHF (manifestations include ascites, cardiomegaly, dyspnea, edema, gallop rhythm, hepatomegaly, oliguria, pleural effusion, pulmonary edema, tachycardia); myocarditis, pericarditis

Central nervous system: Malaise

Dermatologic: Alopecia, itching, photosensitivity, radiation recall, rash; discoloration of saliva, sweat, or tears

Endocrine & metabolic: Amenorrhea, dehydration, infertility (may be temporary), hyperuricemia

Gastrointestinal: Abdominal pain, anorexia, colon necrosis, diarrhea, GI ulceration, mucositis, nausea, vomiting

Genitourinary: Discoloration of urine

Hematologic: Leukopenia/neutropenia (75%; nadir: 10-14 days; recovery: by day 21); thrombocytopenia and anemia

Local: Skin "flare" at injection site, urticaria

Neuromuscular & skeletal: Weakness

Postmarketing and/or case reports: Anaphylaxis, azoospermia, bilirubin increased, chills, coma (when in combination with cisplatin or vincristine), conjunctivitis, fever, gonadal impairment (children), growth failure (prepubertal), hepatitis, hyperpigmentation (nail, skin & oral mucosa), infection, keratitis, lacrimation, myelodysplastic syndrome, neutropenic fever, oligo-spermia, onycholysis, peripheral neurotoxicity (with intra-arterial doxorubicin), phlebosclerosis, radiation recall pneumonitis (children), secondary acute myelogenous leukemia, seizure (when in combination with cisplatin or vincristine), sepsis, shock, systemic hypersensitivity (including urticaria, pruritus, angioedema, dysphagia, and dyspnea), transaminases increased, urticaria

Drug Interactions

Metabolism/Transport Effects Substrate (major) of CYP2D6, 3A4; **Inhibits** CYP2B6 (moderate), 2D6 (weak), 3A4 (weak)

Avoid Concomitant Use

Avoid concomitant use of DOXOrubicin with any of the following: Natalizumab; Vaccines (Live)

Increased Effect/Toxicity

DOXOrubicin may increase the levels/effects of: CYP2B6 Substrates; Leflunomide; Natalizumab; Vaccines (Live); Vitamin K Antagonists; Zidovudine

The levels/effects of DOXOrubicin may be increased by: Bevacizumab; CycloSPORINE; CYP2D6 Inhibitors (Moderate); CYP2D6 Inhibitors (Strong); CYP3A4 Inhibitors (Moderate); CYP3A4 Inhibitors (Strong); Darunavir; Dasatinib; P-Glycoprotein Inhibitors; Sorafenib; Taxane Derivatives; Trastuzumab

Decreased Effect

DOXOrubicin may decrease the levels/effects of: Cardiac Glycosides; Dabigatran Etexilate; P-Glycoprotein Substrates; Stavudine; Vaccines (Inactivated); Vaccines (Live); Vitamin K Antagonists; Zidovudine

The levels/effects of DOXOrubicin may be decreased by: Cardiac Glyco-sides; CYP3A4 Inducers (Strong); Deferasirox; Echinacea; Herbs (CYP3A4 Inducers); Peginterferon Alfa-2b; P-Glycoprotein Inducers

Ethanol/Nutrition/Herb Interactions Herb/Nutraceutical: Avoid St John's wort (may decrease doxorubicin levels). Avoid black cohosh, dong quai in estrogen-dependent tumors.

Storage/Stability Store intact vials of solution under refrigeration at 2°C to 8°C. Protected from light. Store intact vials of lyophilized powder at room temperature (15°C to 30°C). Reconstituted vials are stable for 7 days at room temperature (25°C) and 15 days under refrigeration (5°C) when protected from light. Infusions are stable for 48 hours at room temperature (25°C) when protected from light. Solutions diluted in 50-1000 mL D_5W or NS are stable for 48 hours at room temperature (25°C) when protected from light.

Reconstitution Reconstitute lyophilized powder with NS to a final concen-tration of 2 mg/mL (may further dilute in 50-1000 mL D_5W or NS for infusion). Unstable in solutions with a pH <3 or >7.

Compatibility Stable in D_5W, LR, NS.

Y-site administration: Compatible: Amifostine, aztreonam, bleomycin, chlorpromazine, cimetidine, cisplatin, cladribine, cyclophosphamide, dexa-methasone sodium phosphate, diphenhydramine, droperidol, etoposide phosphate, famotidine, filgrastim, fludarabine, fluorouracil, gatifloxacin, gemcitabine, granisetron, hydromorphone, leucovorin, linezolid, lorazepam, melphalan, methotrexate, methylprednisolone sodium succinate, metoclo-pramide, mitomycin, morphine, ondansetron, paclitaxel, prochlorperazine edisylate, promethazine, ranitidine, sargramostim, sodium bicarbonate, teniposide, thiotepa, topotecan, vinblastine, vincristine, vinorelbine. **Incom-patible:** Allopurinol, amphotericin B cholesteryl sulfate complex, cefepime, ganciclovir, piperacillin/tazobactam, propofol. **Variable (consult detailed reference):** Furosemide, heparin.

Compatibility in syringe: Compatible: Bleomycin, cisplatin, cyclophosphamide, droperidol, leucovorin, methotrexate, metoclopramide, mitomycin, vinblastine, vincristine. **Incompatible:** Furosemide, heparin. **Variable (consult detailed reference):** Fluorouracil.

Compatibility when admixed: Compatible: Dacarbazine, ondansetron, ondansetron with vincristine, paclitaxel, vinblastine. **Incompatible:** Aminophylline, diazepam, fluorouracil. **Variable (consult detailed reference):** Dacarbazine with ondansetron, etoposide with vincristine.

Mechanism of Action Inhibition of DNA and RNA synthesis by intercalation between DNA base pairs by inhibition of topoisomerase II and by steric obstruction. Doxorubicin intercalates at points of local uncoiling of the double helix. Although the exact mechanism is unclear, it appears that direct binding to DNA (intercalation) and inhibition of DNA repair (topoisomerase II inhibition) result in blockade of DNA and RNA synthesis and fragmentation of DNA. Doxorubicin is also a powerful iron chelator; the iron-doxorubicin complex can bind DNA and cell membranes and produce free radicals that immediately cleave the DNA and cell membranes.

Pharmacodynamics/Kinetics

Absorption: Oral: Poor (<50%)

Distribution: V_d: 809-1214 L/m^2; to many body tissues, particularly liver, spleen, kidney, lung, heart; does not distribute into the CNS; crosses placenta

Protein binding, plasma: 70% to 76%

Metabolism: Primarily hepatic to doxorubicinol (active), then to inactive aglycones, conjugated sulfates, and glucuronides

Half-life elimination:

Distribution: 5-10 minutes

Elimination: Doxorubicin: 1-3 hours; Metabolites: 3-3.5 hours

Terminal: 17-48 hours

Male: 54 hours; Female: 35 hours

Excretion: Feces (~40% to 50% as unchanged drug); urine (~5% to 12% as unchanged drug and metabolites)

Clearance: Male: 113 L/hour; Female: 44 L/hour

Dosage I.V.: Refer to individual protocols. **Note:** Lower dosage should be considered for patients with inadequate marrow reserve (due to old age, prior treatment or neoplastic marrow infiltration)

Children:

35-75 mg/m^2/dose every 21 days **or**

20-30 mg/m^2/dose once weekly **or**

60-90 mg/m^2/dose given as a continuous infusion over 96 hours every 3-4 weeks

Adults: Usual or typical dose: 60-75 mg/m^2/dose every 21 days **or**

60 mg/m^2/dose every 2 weeks (dose dense) **or**

40-60 mg/m^2/dose every 3-4 weeks **or**

20-30 mg/m^2/day for 2-3 days every 4 weeks **or**

20 mg/m^2/dose once weekly

Dosing adjustment in toxicity: The following delays and/or dose reductions have been used:

Neutropenic fever/infection: Consider reducing to 75% of dose in subsequent cycles

ANC <1000/mm^3: Delay treatment until ANC recovers to ≥1000/mm^3

Platelets <100,000/mm^3: Delay treatment until platelets recover to ≥100,000/mm^3

◄ **Dosing adjustment in renal impairment:**
  Adjustments are not required.
  Hemodialysis: Supplemental dose is not necessary.
Dosing adjustment in hepatic impairment:
  The FDA-approved labeling recommends the following adjustments:
  Serum bilirubin 1.2-3 mg/dL: Administer 50% of dose
  Serum bilirubin 3.1-5 mg/dL: Administer 25% of dose
  Severe hepatic impairment: Use is contraindicated
  The following guidelines have been used by some clinicians: Floyd, 2006:
  Transaminases 2-3 times ULN: Administer 75% of dose
  Transaminases >3 times ULN or serum bilirubin 1.2-3 mg/dL: Administer
    50% of dose
  Serum bilirubin 3.1-5 mg/dL: Administer 25% of dose
  Serum bilirubin >5 mg/dL: Do not administer

Combination Regimens

Soft tissue sarcoma:
Wilms' tumor:

Administration Vesicant. Administer I.V. push over at least 3-5 minutes, IVPB over 15-60 minutes, or continuous infusion. May be further diluted in either NS of D₅W for I.V. administration. Avoid extravasation associated with severe ulceration and soft tissue necrosis. Flush with 5-10 mL of I.V. solution before and after drug administration. Incompatible with heparin. Monitor for local erythematous streaking along vein and/or facial flushing (may indicate rapid infusion rate).

Monitoring Parameters CBC with differential and platelet count; liver function tests (bilirubin, ALT/AST, alkaline phosphatase); serum uric acid, calcium, potassium, phosphate and creatinine; cardiac function (baseline, periodic, and followup): ECG, left ventricular ejection fraction (echocardiography [ECHO] or multigated radionuclide angiography [MUGA])

Emetic Potential Moderate (30% to 90%)

Vesicant Yes; see Management of Drug Extravasations on page 1447.

Dosage Forms Excipient information presented when available (limited, particularly for generics); consult specific product labeling.

Injection, powder for reconstitution, as hydrochloride: 10 mg, 50 mg
    Adriamycin®: 10 mg, 20 mg, 50 mg, [contains lactose]
Injection, solution, as hydrochloride: 2 mg/mL (5 mL, 10 mL, 25 mL, 100 mL)
    Adriamycin®: 2 mg/mL (5 mL, 10 mL, 25 mL, 100 mL)

References

Davis HL and Davis TE, "Daunorubicin and Adriamycin in Cancer Treatment: An Analysis of Their Roles and Limitations," *Cancer Treat Rep*, 1979, 63(5):809-15.

Floyd J, Mirza I, Sachs B, et al, "Hepatotoxicity of Chemotherapy," *Semin Oncol*, 2006, 33 (1):50-67.

Floyd JD, Nguyen DT, Lobins RL, et al, "Cardiotoxicity of Cancer Therapy," *J Clin Oncol*, 2005, 23 (30):7685-96.

Ishii E, Hara T, Ohkubo K, et al, "Treatment of Childhood Acute Lymphoblastic Leukemia With Intermediate Dose Cytosine Arabinoside and Adriamycin," *Med Pediatr Oncol*, 1986, 14(2):73-7.

King PD and Perry MC, "Hepatotoxicity of Chemotherapy," *Oncologist*, 2001, 6(2):162-76.

Lauvin R, Miglianico L, and Hellegouarc'h R, "Skin Cancer Occurring 10 Years After the Extravasation of Doxorubicin," *N Engl J Med*, 1995, 332(11):754.

Legha SS, Benjamin RS, Mackay B, et al, "Reduction of Doxorubicin Cardiotoxicity by Prolonged Continuous Intravenous Infusion," *Ann Intern Med*, 1982, 96(2):133-9.

National Comprehensive Cancer Network (NCCN), "Clinical Practice Guidelines in Oncology™: Breast Cancer," Version 1.2008. Available at http://www.nccn.org/professionals/physician_gls/PDF/breast.pdf.

Seifert CF, Nesser ME, and Thompson DF, "Dexrazoxane in the Prevention of Doxorubicin-Induced Cardiotoxicity," *Ann Pharmacother*, 1994, 28(9):1063-72.

Speth PA, van Hoesel QG, and Haanen C, "Clinical Pharmacokinetics of Doxorubicin," *Clin Pharmacokinet*, 1988, 15(1):15-31.

Speyer JL, Green MD, Kramer E, et al, "Protective Effect of the Bispiperazinedione ICRF-187 Against Doxorubicin-Induced Cardiac Toxicity in Women With Advanced Breast Cancer," *N Engl J Med*, 1988, 319(12):745-52.

Zimmerman S, Adkins D, Graham M, et al, "Irreversible, Severe, Congestive Cardiomyopathy Occurring in Association With Interferon Alpha Therapy," *Cancer Biother*, 1994, 9(4):291-9.

◆ **Doxorubicin Hydrochloride** *see* DOXOrubicin *on page 372*

◆ **DOXOrubicin Hydrochloride (Liposomal)** *see* DOXOrubicin (Liposomal) *on page 379*

◆ **DOXOrubicin Hydrochloride Liposome** *see* DOXOrubicin (Liposomal) *on page 379*

DOXOrubicin (Liposomal) (doks oh ROO bi sin lip pah SOW mal)

Medication Safety Issues

Sound-alike/look-alike issues:

DOXOrubicin liposomal may be confused with DACTINomycin, DAUNOrubicin, DAUNOrubicin liposomal, doxacurium, doxapram, doxazosin, DOXOrubicin, epirubicin, IDArubicin, valrucibin

DOXOrubicin liposomal may be confused with DAUNOrubicin liposomal

Doxil® may be confused with Doxy®, Paxil®

Liposomal formulation (Doxil®) may be confused with the conventional formulation (Adriamycin PFS®, Adriamycin RDF®)

High alert medication: The Institute for Safe Medication Practices (ISMP) includes this medication among its list of drug classes which have a heightened risk of causing significant patient harm when used in error.

Use caution when selecting product for preparation and dispensing; indications, dosages and adverse event profiles differ between conventional DOXOrubicin hydrochloride solution and DOXOrubicin liposomal. Both formulations are the same concentration. As a result, serious errors have occurred. Liposomal formulation of doxorubicin should NOT be substituted for doxorubicin hydrochloride on a mg-per-mg basis.

Related Information

Management of Drug Extravasations *on page 1447*
Safe Handling of Hazardous Drugs *on page 1517*

U.S. Brand Names Doxil®

Index Terms DOXOrubicin Hydrochloride (Liposomal); DOXOrubicin Hydrochloride Liposome; Liposomal DOXOrubicin; Pegylated DOXOrubicin Liposomal; Pegylated Liposomal DOXOrubicin

Generic Available No

Canadian Brand Names Caelyx®

Pharmacologic Category Antineoplastic Agent, Anthracycline

Use Treatment of ovarian cancer, multiple myeloma, and AIDS-related Kaposi's sarcoma

Unlabeled/Investigational Use Treatment of metastatic breast cancer, Hodgkin's lymphoma, cutaneous T-cell lymphomas (mycosis fungoides and Sézary syndrome); advanced soft tissue sarcomas; recurrent or metastatic cervical cancer, advanced or metastatic uterine sarcoma

Pregnancy Risk Factor D

Lactation Excretion in breast milk unknown/contraindicated

Labeled Contraindications Hypersensitivity to doxorubicin liposomal, conventional doxorubicin, or any component of the formulation; breast-feeding

Warnings/Precautions Hazardous agent - use appropriate precautions for handling and disposal.

[U.S. Boxed Warning]: Doxorubicin may cause cumulative, dose-related myocardial toxicity (concurrent or delayed). Doxorubicin liposomal should be used with caution in patients with high cumulative doses of any anthracycline. Total cumulative dose should also account for previous or concomitant treatment with other cardiotoxic agents or irradiation of chest. The incidence of irreversible myocardial toxicity increases as the total cumulative (lifetime) dosages approach 450-550 mg/m^2; or 400 mg/m^2 in patients who have received prior mediastinal radiation therapy or concurrent therapy with other cardiotoxic agents (eg, cyclophosphamide). Although the risk increases with cumulative dose, irreversible cardiotoxicity may occur with anthracycline treatment at any dose level. Patients with pre-existing heart disease, hypertension, concurrent administration of other antineoplastic agents, prior or concurrent chest irradiation, and advanced age are at increased risk. Evaluate left ventricular ejection fraction (LVEF) prior to treatment and periodically during treatment. The onset of symptoms of anthracycline-induced HF and/or cardiomyopathy may be delayed.

[U.S. Boxed Warning]: Acute infusion reactions may occur, some may be serious/life-threatening, including fatal allergic/anaphylactoid-like reactions. Infusion reactions typically occur with the first infusion and may include flushing, dyspnea, facial swelling, headache, chills, back pain, hypotension, and/or tightness of chest/throat. Reactions usually resolve with termination of infusion, or in some cases, slowing the infusion rate. Medication for the treatment of reactions should be readily available in the event of severe reactions. Infuse doxorubicin liposomal at 1 mg/minute initially to minimize risk of infusion reaction.

[U.S. Boxed Warning]: Use with caution in patients with hepatic impairment; dosage reduction is recommended. Use in patients with hepatic impairment has not been adequately studied; dosing adjustment recommendations in multiple myeloma patients with hepatic impairment is not available. **[U.S. Boxed Warning]: Severe myelosuppression may occur.** Palmar-plantar erythrodysesthesia (hand-foot syndrome) has been reported in up to 51% of patients with ovarian cancer, 19% of patients with multiple myeloma, and ~3% in patients with Kaposi's sarcoma. May occur early in treatment, but is usually seen after 2-3 treatment cycles. Dosage modification may be required. In severe cases, treatment discontinuation may be required. **[U.S. Boxed Warning]: Liposomal formulations of doxorubicin should NOT be substituted for conventional doxorubicin hydrochloride on a mg-per-mg basis.**

Doxorubicin may potentiate the toxicity of cyclophosphamide (hemorrhagic cystitis) and mercaptopurine (hepatotoxicity). Radiation recall reaction has been reported with doxorubicin liposomal treatment after radiation therapy. Radiation-induced toxicity (to the myocardium, mucosa, skin, and liver) may be increased by doxorubicin. Safety and efficacy in children have not been established.

Adverse Reactions

>10%:

Cardiovascular: Peripheral edema (≤11%)

Central nervous system: Fever (8% to 21%), headache (≤11%), pain (≤21%)

Dermatologic: Palmar-plantar erythrodysesthesia/hand-foot syndrome (≤51% in ovarian cancer [grades 3/4: 24%]; 3% in Kaposi's sarcoma), rash (≤29% in ovarian cancer, ≤5% in Kaposi's sarcoma), alopecia (9% to 19%)

Gastrointestinal: Nausea (17% to 46%), stomatitis (5% to 41%), vomiting (8% to 33%), constipation (≤30%), diarrhea (5% to 21%), anorexia (≤20%), mucositis (≤14%), dyspepsia (≤12%), intestinal obstruction (≤11%)

Hematologic: Myelosuppression (onset: 7 days; nadir: 10-14 days; recovery: 21-28 days), thrombocytopenia (13% to 65%; grades 3/4: 1%), neutropenia (12% to 62%; grade 4: 4%), leukopenia (36%), anemia (6% to 74%; grade 4: <1%)

Neuromuscular & skeletal: Weakness (7% to 40%), back pain (≤12%)

Respiratory: Pharyngitis (≤16%), dyspnea (≤15%)

Miscellaneous: Infection (≤12%)

1% to 10%:

Cardiovascular: Cardiac arrest, chest pain, deep thrombophlebitis, edema, hypotension, pallor, tachycardia, vasodilation

Central nervous system: Agitation, anxiety, chills, confusion, depression, dizziness, emotional lability, insomnia, somnolence, vertigo

Dermatologic: Acne, bruising, dry skin (6%), exfoliative dermatitis, fungal dermatitis, furunculosis, maculopapular rash, pruritus, skin discoloration, vesiculobullous rash

Endocrine & metabolic: Dehydration, hypercalcemia, hyperglycemia, hypokalemia, hyponatremia

Gastrointestinal: Abdomen enlarged, anorexia, ascites, cachexia, dyspepsia, dysphagia, esophagitis, flatulence, gingivitis, glossitis, ileus, mouth ulceration, oral moniliasis, rectal bleeding, taste perversion, weight loss, xerostomia

Genitourinary: Cystitis, dysuria, leukorrhea, pelvic pain, polyuria, urinary incontinence, urinary tract infection, urinary urgency, vaginal bleeding, vaginal moniliasis

Hematologic: Hemolysis, prothrombin time increased

Hepatic: ALT increased, alkaline phosphatase increased, hyperbilirubinemia

Local: Thrombophlebitis

Neuromuscular & skeletal: Arthralgia, hypertonia, myalgia, neuralgia, neuritis (peripheral), neuropathy, paresthesia (≤10%), pathological fracture

Ocular: Conjunctivitis, dry eyes, retinitis

Otic: Ear pain

Renal: Albuminuria, hematuria

Respiratory: Apnea, cough (≤10%), epistaxis, pleural effusion, pneumonia, rhinitis, sinusitis

Miscellaneous: Allergic reaction; infusion-related reactions (7%; includes bronchospasm, chest tightness, chills, dyspnea, facial edema, flushing, headache, herpes simplex/zoster, hypotension, pruritus); moniliasis, diaphoresis

<1%, postmarketing, and/or case reports (limited to important or life-threatening): Abscess, acute brain syndrome, abnormal vision, acute myeloid leukemia (secondary), alkaline phosphatase increased, anaphylactic or anaphylactoid reaction, asthma, balanitis, blindness, bone pain, bronchitis, BUN increased, bundle branch block, cardiomegaly, cardiomyopathy, cellulitis, CHF, colitis, creatinine increased, cryptococcosis, diabetes mellitus, erythema multiforme, erythema nodosum, eosinophilia, fecal impaction, flu-like syndrome, gastritis, glucosuria, hemiplegia, hemorrhage, hepatic failure, hepatitis, hepatosplenomegaly, hyperkalemia, hypernatremia, hyperuricemia, hyperventilation, hypoglycemia, hypolipidemia, hypomagnesemia, hypophosphatemia, hypoproteinemia, hypothermia, injection site hemorrhage, injection site pain, jaundice, ketosis, lactic dehydrogenase increased, kidney failure, lymphadenopathy, lymphangitis, migraine, myositis, optic neuritis, palpitation, pancreatitis, pericardial effusion, petechia, pneumothorax, pulmonary embolism, radiation injury, sclerosing cholangitis, seizure, sepsis, skin necrosis, skin ulcer, syncope, Stevens-Johnson syndrome, tenesmus, thromboplastin decreased, thrombosis, tinnitus, toxic epidermal necrolysis, urticaria, visual field defect, ventricular arrhythmia

◄ **Drug Interactions**

Metabolism/Transport Effects Substrate (major) of CYP2D6, 3A4; Inhibits CYP2B6 (moderate), 2D6 (weak), 3A4 (weak)

Avoid Concomitant Use

Avoid concomitant use of DOXOrubicin (Liposomal) with any of the following: Natalizumab; Vaccines (Live)

Increased Effect/Toxicity

DOXOrubicin (Liposomal) may increase the levels/effects of: CYP2B6 Substrates; Leflunomide; Natalizumab; Vaccines (Live); Zidovudine

The levels/effects of DOXOrubicin (Liposomal) may be increased by: Bevacizumab; CYP2D6 Inhibitors (Moderate); CYP2D6 Inhibitors (Strong); CYP3A4 Inhibitors (Moderate); CYP3A4 Inhibitors (Strong); Darunavir; Dasatinib; Taxane Derivatives; Trastuzumab

Decreased Effect

DOXOrubicin (Liposomal) may decrease the levels/effects of: Cardiac Glycosides; Stavudine; Vaccines (Inactivated); Vaccines (Live); Zidovudine

The levels/effects of DOXOrubicin (Liposomal) may be decreased by: Cardiac Glycosides; CYP3A4 Inducers (Strong); Deferasirox; Echinacea; Herbs (CYP3A4 Inducers); Peginterferon Alfa-2b

Ethanol/Nutrition/Herb Interactions

Ethanol: Avoid ethanol (due to GI irritation).

Herb/Nutraceutical: St John's wort may decrease doxorubicin levels.

Storage/Stability Store intact vials of solution under refrigeration at 2°C to 8°C (36°F to 46°F); avoid freezing. Prolonged freezing may adversely affect liposomal drug products, however, short-term freezing (<1 month) does not appear to have a deleterious effect. Diluted doxorubicin hydrochloride liposome injection may be refrigerated at 2°C to 8°C (36°F to 46°F); administer within 24 hours. **Do not infuse with in-line filters.**

Reconstitution Doses of doxorubicin liposomal ≤90 mg must be diluted in 250 mL of D_5W prior to administration. Doses >90 mg should be diluted in 500 mL D_5W. Solution is not a clear, but has a red, translucent appearance due to the liposomal dispersion. Use appropriate precautions for handling and disposal.

Compatibility Stable in D_5W.

Y-site administration: Compatible: Acyclovir, allopurinol, aminophylline, ampicillin, aztreonam, bleomycin, butorphanol, calcium gluconate, carboplatin, cefazolin, cefepime, cefoxitin, ceftizoxime, ceftriaxone, chlorpromazine, cimetidine, ciprofloxacin, cisplatin, clindamycin, co-trimoxazole, cyclophosphamide, cytarabine, dacarbazine, dexamethasone sodium phosphate, diphenhydramine, dobutamine, dopamine, droperidol, enalaprilat, etoposide, famotidine, fluconazole, fluorouracil, furosemide, ganciclovir, gentamicin, granisetron, haloperidol lactate, heparin, hydrocortisone sodium succinate, hydromorphone, ifosfamide, leucovorin calcium, lorazepam, magnesium sulfate, mesna, methotrexate, methylprednisolone sodium succinate, metronidazole, ondansetron, piperacillin, potassium chloride, prochlorperazine edisylate, ranitidine, ticarcillin/clavulanate, tobramycin, vancomycin, vinblastine, vincristine, vinorelbine, zidovudine. **Incompatible:** Amphotericin B, amphotericin B cholesteryl sulfate complex, buprenorphine, ceftazidime, docetaxel, hydroxyzine HCl, mannitol, meperidine, metoclopramide, mitoxantrone, morphine, ofloxacin, paclitaxel, piperacillin/tazobactam, promethazine, sodium bicarbonate.

Mechanism of Action Doxorubicin inhibits DNA and RNA synthesis by intercalating between DNA base pairs causing steric obstruction and inhibits topoisomerase-II at the point of DNA cleavage. Doxorubicin is also a powerful iron chelator. The iron-doxorubicin complex can bind DNA and cell membranes, producing free hydroxyl (OH) radicals that cleave DNA and cell membranes. Active throughout entire cell cycle. Doxorubicin liposomal is a pegylated formulation which protects the liposomes, and thereby increases blood circulation time.

Pharmacodynamics/Kinetics

Distribution: V_{dss}: 2.7-2.8 L/m^2

Protein binding, plasma: Unknown; nonliposomal (conventional) doxorubicin: 70%

Half-life elimination: Terminal: Distribution: 4.7-5.2 hours, Elimination: 44-55 hours

Metabolism: Hepatic and in plasma to doxorubicinol and the sulfate and glucuronide conjugates of 4-demethyl,7-deoxyaglycones

Excretion: Urine (5% as doxorubicin or doxorubicinol)

Dosage Details concerning dosing in combination regimens should also be consulted. **Liposomal formulations of doxorubicin should NOT be substituted for conventional doxorubicin hydrochloride on a mg-per-mg basis.**

AIDS-related Kaposi's sarcoma: I.V.: 20 mg/m^2/dose once every 3 weeks

Multiple myeloma: I.V.: 30 mg/m^2/dose every 3 weeks (in combination with bortezomib) **or**

Unlabeled dosing: I.V.: 40 mg/m^2/dose every 4 weeks (in combination with vincristine and dexamethasone) (Rifkin, 2006)

Ovarian cancer: I.V.: 50 mg/m^2/dose every 4 weeks (minimum of 4 cycles is recommended)

Breast cancer (unlabeled use): I.V.: 50 mg/m^2/dose every 4 weeks (Keller, 2004)

Uterine sarcoma (unlabeled use): I.V.: 50 mg/m^2/dose every 4 weeks (Sutton, 2005)

Dosing adjustment in hepatic impairment: Note: Dosage adjustment information is not available in patients with multiple myeloma.

Bilirubin 1.2-3 mg/dL: Administer 50% of dose

Bilirubin >3 mg/dL: Administer 25% of dose

Dosing adjustment for toxicity:

Recommended Dose Modification Guidelines

Toxicity Grade	Dose Adjustment
HAND FOOT SYNDROME (HFS)	
1 (Mild erythema, swelling, or desquamation not interfering with daily activities)	Redose unless patient has experienced previous Grade 3 or 4 HFS toxicity. If so, delay up to 2 weeks and decrease dose by 25%; return to original dosing interval.
2 (Erythema, desquamation, or swelling interfering with, but not precluding, normal physical activities; small blisters or ulcerations <2 cm in diameter)	Delay dosing up to 2 weeks or until resolved to Grade 0-1. If after 2 weeks there is no resolution, discontinue liposomal doxorubicin. Otherwise, if no prior Grade 3-4 HFS, continue treatment at previous dose and dosage interval. If a prior Grade 3-4 HFS has occurred, continue prior dosage interval, but decrease dose by 25%.
3 (Blistering, ulceration, or swelling interfering with walking or normal daily activities; cannot wear regular clothing)	Delay dosing up to 2 weeks or until resolved to Grade 0-1. Decrease dose by 25% and return to original dosing interval; if after 2 weeks there is no resolution, discontinue liposomal doxorubicin.
4 (Diffuse or local process causing infectious complications, or a bedridden state or hospitalization)	Delay dosing up to 2 weeks or until resolved to Grade 0-1. Decrease dose by 25% and return to original dosing interval. If after 2 weeks there is no resolution, discontinue liposomal doxorubicin.
STOMATITIS	
1 (Painless ulcers, erythema, or mild soreness)	Redose unless patient has experienced previous Grade 3 or 4 toxicity. If so, delay up to 2 weeks and decrease by 25%. Return to original dosing interval.
2 (Painful erythema, edema, or ulcers, but can eat)	Delay dosing up to 2 weeks or until resolved to Grade 0-1. If after 2 weeks there is no resolution, discontinue liposomal doxorubicin. Otherwise, if not prior Grade 3-4 stomatitis, continue treatment at previous dose and dosage interval. If prior Grade 3-4 toxicity, continue treatment with previous dosage interval, but decrease dose by 25%.
3 (Painful erythema, edema, or ulcers, and cannot eat)	Delay dosing up to 2 weeks or until resolved to Grade 0-1. Decrease dose by 25% and return to original dosing interval. If after 2 weeks there is no resolution, discontinue liposomal doxorubicin.
4 (Requires parenteral or enteral support)	Delay dosing up to 2 weeks or until resolved to Grade 0-1. Decrease dose by 25% and return to original dosing interval. If after 2 weeks there is no resolution, discontinue liposomal doxorubicin.

See table: "Hematological Toxicity"

Hematological Toxicity (see below for multiple myeloma)

Grade	ANC	Platelets	Modification
1	1500-1900	75,000-150,000	Resume treatment with no dose reduction.
2	1000-<1500	50,000-<75,000	Wait until ANC ≥1500 and platelets ≥75,000; redose with no dose reduction.
3	500-999	25,000-<50,000	Wait until ANC ≥1500 and platelets ≥75,000; redose with no dose reduction.
4	<500	<25,000	Wait until ANC ≥1500 and platelets ≥75,000; redose at 25% dose reduction or continue full dose with cytokine support.

Dosing Adjustment for Toxicity in Treatment with Bortezomib (for Multiple Myeloma) (see Bortezomib monograph for bortezomib dosage reduction with toxicity guidelines):

Fever ≥38°C and ANC <1000/mm³: If prior to doxorubicin liposomal treatment (day 4), do not administer; if after doxorubicin liposomal administered, reduce dose by 25% in next cycle.

ANC <500/mm³, platelets <25,000/mm³, hemoglobin <8 g/dL: If prior to doxorubicin liposomal treatment (day 4); do not administer; if after doxorubicin liposomal administered, reduce dose by 25% in next cycle if bortezomib dose reduction occurred for hematologic toxicity.

Grade 3 or 4 nonhematologic toxicity: Delay dose until resolved to grade <2; reduce dose by 25% for all subsequent doses.

Neuropathic pain or peripheral neuropathy: No dose reductions needed for doxorubicin liposomal, refer to Bortezomib monograph for bortezomib dosing adjustment.

Combination Regimens

Breast cancer: Doxorubicin (Liposomal)-Docetaxel (Breast Cancer) on page 1296

Lymphoma, Hodgkin's disease: Gemcitabine-Vinorelbine-Doxorubicin (Liposomal) on page 1346

Multiple myeloma:

Bortezomib-Doxorubicin (Liposomal) on page 1239

Bortezomib-Doxorubicin (Liposomal)-Dexamethasone on page 1240

Doxorubicin (Liposomal)-Vincristine-Dexamethasone on page 1297

Administration Administer IVPB over 60 minutes; manufacturer recommends administering at initial rate of 1 mg/minute to minimize risk of infusion reactions until the absence of a reaction has been established, then increase the infusion rate for completion over 1 hour. **Do not administer I.M. or SubQ. Do not infuse with in-line filters.** Avoid extravasation (irritant), monitor site; extravasation may occur without stinging or burning. Flush with 5-10 mL of D₅W solution before and after drug administration (do not rapidly flush through the I.V. line), incompatible with heparin flushes. Monitor for local erythematous streaking along vein and/or facial flushing (may indicate rapid infusion rate).

Monitoring Parameters CBC with differential and platelet count, liver function tests (ALT/AST, bilirubin, alkaline phosphatase); monitor for infusion reactions

Cardiac function (left ventricular ejection fraction [LVEF]), should be carefully monitored; echocardiography, or MUGA scan may be used. Endomyocardial biopsy is the most definitive test for anthracycline myocardial injury.

◄ **Additional Information Oncology Comment:** Doxorubicin liposomal is listed within National Comprehensive Cancer Network® (NCCN) guidelines for the treatment of the following types of malignancies:

Breast cancer: As a preferred single-agent therapy for recurrent or metastatic breast cancer

Cervical cancer: As second-line treatment for recurrent or metastatic cervical cancer

Hodgkin's lymphoma: As second-line chemotherapy (in combination with gemcitabine and vinorelbine)

Non-Hodgkin's lymphomas: As a first-line systemic treatment for cutaneous T-cell lymphomas, mycosis fungoides, and Sezary syndrome, in patients with generalized tumor disease or tumor disease with blood involvement

Ovarian cancer: As a preferred agent for recurrent ovarian cancer

Multiple myeloma: As primary induction therapy for both transplant candidates and nontransplant candidates (in combination with vincristine and dexamethasone), and as salvage therapy (in combination with bortezomib)

Soft tissue sarcoma: As a systemic single-agent treatment for metastatic disease for extremity, retroperitoneal, or intra-abdominal (other than GIST) soft tissue sarcomas

Uterine cancer: As a single-agent treatment for advanced or metastatic uterine sarcoma

Emetic Potential Low (10% to 30%)

Vesicant No; may be an irritant

Dosage Forms Excipient information presented when available (limited, particularly for generics); consult specific product labeling.

Injection, solution, as hydrochloride:

Doxil®: 2 mg/mL (10 mL, 25 mL)

References

Bartlett NL, Niedzwiecki D, Johnson JL, et al, "Gemcitabine, Vinorelbine, and Pegylated Liposomal Doxorubicin (GVD), A Salvage Regimen in Relapsed Hodgkin's Lymphoma: CALGB 59804," *Ann Oncol*, 2007, 18(6):1071-9.

Biehn SE, Moore DT, Voorhees PM, et al, "Extended Follow-Up of Outcome Measures in Multiple Myeloma Patients Treated on a Phase I Study With Bortezomib and Pegylated Liposomal Doxorubicin," *Ann Hematol*, 2007, 86(3):211-6.

Gordon AN, Fleagle JT, Guthrie D, et al, "Recurrent Epithelial Ovarian Carcinoma: A Randomized Phase III Study of Pegylated Liposomal Doxorubicin Versus Topotecan," *J Clin Oncol*, 2001, 19 (14):3312-22.

Hussein MA, Wood L, Hsi E, et al, "A Phase II Trial of Pegylated Liposomal Doxorubicin, Vincristine, and Reduced-Dose Dexamethasone Combination Therapy in Newly Diagnosed Multiple Myeloma Patients," *Cancer*, 2002, 95(10):2160-8.

Keller AM, Mennel RG, Georgoulias VA, et al, "Randomized Phase III Trial of Pegylated Liposomal Doxorubicin Versus Vinorelbine or Mitomycin C Plus Vinblastine in Women With Taxane-Refractory Advanced Breast Cancer," *J Clin Oncol*, 2004, 22(19):3893-901.

King PD and Perry MC, "Hepatotoxicity of Chemotherapy," *Oncologist*, 2001, 6(2):162-76.

National Comprehensive Cancer Network® (NCCN), "Clinical Practice Guidelines in Oncology™: Breast Cancer," Version 1.2009. Available at http://www.nccn.org/professionals/physician_gls/PDF/breast.pdf.

National Comprehensive Cancer Network® (NCCN), "Clinical Practice Guidelines in Oncology™: Cervical Cancer." Version 1.2009. Available at http://www.nccn.org/professionals/physician_gls/PDF/cervical.pdf

National Comprehensive Cancer Network® (NCCN), "Clinical Practice Guidelines in Oncology™: Hodgkin Disease/Lymphoma," Version 2.2009. Available at http://www.nccn.org/professionals/physician_gls/PDF/hodgkins.pdf

National Comprehensive Cancer Network® (NCCN), "Clinical Practice Guidelines in Oncology™: Multiple Myeloma," Version 2.2010. Available at http://www.nccn.org/professionals/physician_gls/PDF/myeloma.pdf.

National Comprehensive Cancer Network® (NCCN), "Clinical Practice Guidelines in Oncology™: Non-Hodgkin's Lymphomas," Version 2.2009. Available at http://www.nccn.org/professionals/physician_gls/PDF/nhl.pdf

National Comprehensive Cancer Network® (NCCN), "Clinical Practice Guidelines in Oncology™: Ovarian Cancer," Version 2.2009. Available at http://www.nccn.org/professionals/physician_gls/PDF/ovarian.pdf.

National Comprehensive Cancer Network® (NCCN), "Clinical Practice Guidelines in Oncology™: Soft Tissue Sarcoma," Version 2.2009. Available at http://www.nccn.org/professionals/physician_gls/PDF/sarcoma.pdf

National Comprehensive Cancer Network® (NCCN), "Clinical Practice Guidelines in Oncology™: Uterine Neoplasms," Version 2.2009. Available at http://www.nccn.org/professionals/physician_gls/PDF/uterine.pdf

Northfelt DW, Dezebe BJ, Thommes JA, et al, "Pegylated-Liposomal Doxorubicin Versus Doxorubicin, Bleomycin, and Vincristine in the Treatment of AIDS-Related Kaposi's Sarcoma: Results of a Randomized Phase III Clinical Trial," J Clin Oncol, 1998, 16(7):2445-51.

O'Brien ME, Wigler N, Inbar M, et al, "Reduced Cardiotoxicity and Comparable Efficacy in a Phase III Trial of Pegylated Liposomal Doxorubicin HCl (CAELYX™/Doxil®) Versus Conventional Doxorubicin for First-Line Treatment of Metastatic Breast Cancer," Ann Oncol, 2004, 15(3):440-9.

Orditura M, Quaglia F, Morgillo F, et al, "Pegylated Liposomal Doxorubicin: Pharmacologic and Clinical Evidence of Potent Antitumor Activity With Reduced Anthracycline-induced Cardiotoxicity (Review)," Oncol Rep, 2004, 12(3):549-56.

Orlowski RZ, Voorhees PM, Garcia RA, et al, "Phase I Trial of the Proteasome Inhibitor Bortezomib and Pegylated Liposomal Doxorubicin in Patients With Advanced Hematologic Malignancies," Blood, 2005, 105(8):3058-65.

O'Shaughnessy JA, "Pegylated Liposomal Doxorubicin in the Treatment of Breast Cancer," Clin Breast Cancer, 2003, 4(5):318-28.

Rifkin RM, Gregory SA, Mohrbacher A, et al, "Pegylated Liposomal Doxorubicin, Vincristine, and Dexamethasone Provide Significant Reduction in Toxicity Compared With Doxorubicin, Vincristine, and Dexamethasone in Patients With Newly Diagnosed Multiple Myeloma," Cancer, 2006, 106(4):848-58.

Theodoulou M and Hudis C, "Cardiac Profiles of Liposomal Anthracyclines: Greater Cardiac Safety Versus Conventional Doxorubicin?" Cancer, 2004, 100(10):2052-63.

Vorbiof DA, Rapoport BL, Chasen C, et al, "First Line Therapy With Paclitaxel (Taxol) and Pegylated Liposomal Doxorubicin (Caelyx) in Patients With Metastatic Breast Cancer: A Multicentre Phase II Study," Breast, 2004, 13(3):219-26.

Wollina U, Dummer R, Brockmeyer NH, "Multicenter Study of Pegylated Liposomal Doxorubicin in Patients With Cutaneous T-Cell Lymphoma," Cancer, 2003, 98(5):993-1001.

Dronabinol (droe NAB i nol)

Medication Safety Issues
Sound-alike/look-alike issues:

Dronabinol may be confused with droperidol

Related Information
Management of Chemotherapy-Induced Nausea and Vomiting on page 1434

U.S. Brand Names Marinol®

Index Terms Delta-9 THC; Delta-9-tetrahydro-cannabinol; Tetrahydrocannabinol; THC

Generic Available Yes

Canadian Brand Names Marinol®

Pharmacologic Category Antiemetic; Appetite Stimulant

Use Chemotherapy-associated nausea and vomiting refractory to other antiemetic(s); AIDS-related anorexia

Unlabeled/Investigational Use Cancer-related anorexia

Restrictions C-III

Pregnancy Risk Factor C

Lactation Enters breast milk/contraindicated

Labeled Contraindications Hypersensitivity to dronabinol, cannabinoids, sesame oil, or any component of the formulation, or marijuana; should be avoided in patients with a history of schizophrenia

Warnings/Precautions Use with caution in patients with hepatic disease or seizure disorders. Reduce dosage in patients with severe hepatic impairment. May cause additive CNS effects with sedatives, hypnotics or other psychoactive agents; patients must be cautioned about performing tasks which require mental alertness (eg, operating machinery or driving).

May have potential for abuse; drug is psychoactive substance in marijuana; use caution in patients with a history of substance abuse or potential. May cause withdrawal symptoms upon abrupt discontinuation. Use with caution in patients with mania, depression, or schizophrenia; careful psychiatric monitoring is recommended. Use caution in elderly; they are more sensitive to adverse effects. Safety and efficacy have not been established in children.

Adverse Reactions Frequency not always specified.

>1%:

Cardiovascular: Palpitations, tachycardia, vasodilation/facial flushing

Central nervous system: Euphoria (8% to 24%, dose related), abnormal thinking (3% to 10%), dizziness (3% to 10%), paranoia (3% to 10%), somnolence (3% to 10%), amnesia, anxiety, ataxia, confusion, depersonalization, hallucination

Gastrointestinal: Abdominal pain (3% to 10%), nausea (3% to 10%), vomiting (3% to 10%)

Neuromuscular & skeletal: Weakness

<1%, postmarketing, and/or case reports: Conjunctivitis, depression, diarrhea, fatigue, fecal incontinence, flushing, hypotension, myalgia, nightmares, seizure, speech difficulties, tinnitus, vision difficulties

Drug Interactions

Avoid Concomitant Use There are no known interactions where it is recommended to avoid concomitant use.

Increased Effect/Toxicity

Dronabinol may increase the levels/effects of: Alcohol (Ethyl); CNS Depressants; Methotrimeprazine; Sympathomimetics

The levels/effects of Dronabinol may be increased by: Anticholinergic Agents; Cocaine; MAO Inhibitors; Methotrimeprazine; Ritonavir

Decreased Effect There are no known significant interactions involving a decrease in effect.

Ethanol/Nutrition/Herb Interactions

Ethanol: Avoid ethanol (may increase CNS depression).

Food: Administration with high-lipid meals may increase absorption.

Herb/Nutraceutical: St John's wort may decrease dronabinol levels.

Storage/Stability Store under refrigeration (or in a cool environment) between 8°C and 15°C (46°F and 59°F); protect from freezing.

Mechanism of Action Unknown, may inhibit endorphins in the brain's emetic center, suppress prostaglandin synthesis, and/or inhibit medullary activity through an unspecified cortical action. Some pharmacologic effects appear to involve sympathimometic activity; tachyphylaxis to some effect (eg, tachycardia) may occur, but appetite-stimulating effects do not appear to wane over time. Antiemetic activity may be due to effect on cannabinoid receptors (CB1) within the central nervous system.

Pharmacodynamics/Kinetics

Onset of action: Within 1 hour

Peak effect: 2-4 hours

Duration: 24 hours (appetite stimulation)

Absorption: Oral: 90% to 95%; 10% to 20% of dose gets into systemic circulation

Distribution: V_d: 10 L/kg; dronabinol is highly lipophilic and distributes to adipose tissue

Protein binding: 97% to 99%

Metabolism: Hepatic to at least 50 metabolites, some of which are active; 11-hydroxy-delta-9-tetrahydrocannabinol (11-OH-THC) is the major metabolite; extensive first-pass effect

Half-life elimination: Dronabinol: 25-36 hours (terminal); Dronabinol metabolites: 44-59 hours

Time to peak, serum: 0.5-4 hours

Excretion: Feces (50% as unconjugated metabolites, 5% as unchanged drug); urine (10% to 15% as acid metabolites and conjugates)

Dosage Refer to individual protocols. Oral:

Antiemetic: Children and Adults: 5 mg/m^2 1-3 hours before chemotherapy, then 5 mg/m^2/dose every 2-4 hours after chemotherapy for a total of 4-6 doses/day; increase doses in increments of 2.5 mg/m^2 to a maximum of 15 mg/m^2/dose.

Appetite stimulant: Adults: Initial: 2.5 mg twice daily (before lunch and dinner); titrate up to a maximum of 20 mg/day.

Monitoring Parameters CNS effects, heart rate, blood pressure, behavioral profile

Test Interactions Decreased FSH, LH, growth hormone, and testosterone

Dietary Considerations Capsules contain sesame oil.

Dosage Forms Excipient information presented when available (limited, particularly for generics); consult specific product labeling.

Capsule, soft gelatin: 2.5 mg, 5 mg, 10 mg

Marinol®: 2.5 mg, 5 mg, 10 mg [contains sesame oil]

References

Anderson PO and Muire GG, "Delta-9-Tetrahydrocannabinol as an Antiemetic," *Am J Hosp Pharm,* 1981, 38:639-46.

Tramer MR, Carroll D, Campbell FA, et al, "Cannabinoids for Control of Chemotherapy Induced Nausea and Vomiting: Quantitative Systematic Review," *BMJ,* 2001, 323(7303):16-21.

Droperidol (droe PER i dole)

Medication Safety Issues

Sound-alike/look-alike issues:

Droperidol may be confused with dronabinol

Inapsine® may be confused with asenapine, Nebcin®

Related Information

Management of Chemotherapy-Induced Nausea and Vomiting on page 1434

U.S. Brand Names Inapsine® [DSC]

Index Terms Dehydrobenzperidol

Generic Available Yes

Canadian Brand Names Droperidol Injection, USP

Pharmacologic Category Antiemetic; Antipsychotic Agent, Typical

Use Prevention and/or treatment of nausea and vomiting from surgical and diagnostic procedures

Pregnancy Risk Factor C

Lactation Excretion in breast milk unknown

Labeled Contraindications Hypersensitivity to droperidol or any component of the formulation; known or suspected QT prolongation, including congenital long QT syndrome (prolonged QT$_c$ is defined as >440 msec in males or >450 msec in females)

Warnings/Precautions May alter cardiac conduction. **[U.S. Boxed Warning]: Cases of QT prolongation and torsade de pointes, including some fatal cases, have been reported.** Use extreme caution in patients with bradycardia (<50 bpm), cardiac disease, concurrent MAO inhibitor therapy, Class I and Class III antiarrhythmics or other drugs known to prolong QT interval, and electrolyte disturbances (hypokalemia or hypomagnesemia), including concomitant drugs which may alter electrolytes (diuretics).

Use with caution in patients with seizures or severe liver disease. May be sedating, use with caution in disorders where CNS depression is a feature. Caution in patients with hemodynamic instability, predisposition to seizures, subcortical brain damage, pheochromocytoma or renal disease. Esophageal dysmotility and aspiration have been associated with antipsychotic use - use with caution in patients at risk of pneumonia (ie, Alzheimer's disease). Caution in breast cancer or other prolactin-dependent tumors (may elevate prolactin levels). May alter temperature regulation or mask toxicity of other drugs due to antiemetic effects. May cause orthostatic hypotension - use with caution in patients at risk of this effect or those who would tolerate transient hypotensive episodes (cerebrovascular disease, cardiovascular disease, or other medications which may predispose). Significant hypotension may occur.

May cause anticholinergic effects (confusion, agitation, constipation, xerostomia, blurred vision, urinary retention). Therefore, they should be used with caution in patients with decreased gastrointestinal motility, urinary retention, BPH, xerostomia, or visual problems. Conditions which also may be exacerbated by cholinergic blockade include narrow-angle glaucoma (screening is recommended) and worsening of myasthenia gravis. Relative to other neuroleptics, droperidol has a low potency of cholinergic blockade.

May cause extrapyramidal symptoms (EPS), including pseudoparkinsonism, acute dystonic reactions, akathisia, and tardive dyskinesia (risk of these reactions is high relative to other neuroleptics). Risk of dystonia (and possibly other EPS) may be greater with increased doses, use of conventional antipsychotics, males, and younger patients. May be associated with neuroleptic malignant syndrome (NMS) or pigmentary retinopathy. May mask toxicity of other drugs or conditions (eg, intestinal obstruction, Reye's syndrome, brain tumor) due to antiemetic effects. Use with caution in the elderly; reduce initial dose. Safety in children <2 years of age has not been established.

Adverse Reactions

>10%:
Cardiovascular: QT_c prolongation (dose dependent)
Central nervous system: Restlessness, anxiety, extrapyramidal symptoms, dystonic reactions, pseudoparkinsonian signs and symptoms, tardive dyskinesia, seizure, altered central temperature regulation, sedation, drowsiness
Endocrine & metabolic: Swelling of breasts
Gastrointestinal: Weight gain, constipation

1% to 10%:
Cardiovascular: Hypotension (especially orthostatic), tachycardia, abnormal T waves with prolonged ventricular repolarization, hypertension
Central nervous system: Hallucinations, persistent tardive dyskinesia, akathisia
Gastrointestinal: Nausea, vomiting
Genitourinary: Dysuria

<1%: Adynamic ileus, agranulocytosis, alopecia, amenorrhea, arrhythmia, blurred vision, cholestatic jaundice, contact dermatitis, galactorrhea, gynecomastia, heat stroke, hyperpigmentation, laryngospasm, leukopenia (usually with large doses for prolonged periods), neuroleptic malignant syndrome (NMS), obstructive jaundice, overflow incontinence, photosensitivity (rare), priapism, pruritus, rash, respiratory depression, retinal

pigmentation, sexual dysfunction, tardive dystonia, torsade de pointes, urinary retention, ventricular tachycardia, visual acuity decreased (may be irreversible), xerostomia

Drug Interactions

Avoid Concomitant Use

Avoid concomitant use of Droperidol with any of the following: Artemether; Dronedarone; Lumefantrine; Nilotinib; Pimozide; QuiNINE; Tetrabenazine; Thioridazine; Ziprasidone

Increased Effect/Toxicity

Droperidol may increase the levels/effects of: Alcohol (Ethyl); Anticholinergics; CNS Depressants; Dronedarone; Pimozide; QTc-Prolonging Agents; QuiNINE; Tetrabenazine; Thioridazine; Ziprasidone

The levels/effects of Droperidol may be increased by: Acetylcholinesterase Inhibitors (Central); Alfuzosin; Artemether; Chloroquine; Ciprofloxacin; Gadobutrol; Lithium formulations; Lumefantrine; MAO Inhibitors; Nilotinib; Pramlintide; QuiNINE; Tetrabenazine

Decreased Effect

Droperidol may decrease the levels/effects of: Amphetamines; Anti-Parkinson's Agents (Dopamine Agonist)

The levels/effects of Droperidol may be decreased by: Lithium formulations

Storage/Stability Droperidol ampuls/vials should be stored at room temperature and protected from light. Solutions diluted in NS or D_5W are stable at room temperature for up to 7 days.

Compatibility Stable in D_5W, LR, NS.

Y-site administration: Compatible: Alatrofloxacin, amifostine, aztreonam, bleomycin, cisatracurium, cisplatin, cladribine, cyclophosphamide, cytarabine, docetaxel, doxorubicin, doxorubicin liposome, etoposide phosphate, famotidine, filgrastim, fluconazole, fludarabine, gatifloxacin, gemcitabine, granisetron, hydrocortisone sodium succinate, idarubicin, linezolid, melphalan, meperidine, metoclopramide, mitomycin, ondansetron, paclitaxel, potassium chloride, propofol, remifentanil, sargramostim, teniposide, thiotepa, vinblastine, vincristine, vinorelbine, vitamin B complex with C. **Incompatible:** Allopurinol, amphotericin B cholesteryl sulfate complex, cefepime, fluorouracil, foscarnet, furosemide, leucovorin, nafcillin, piperacillin/tazobactam. **Variable (consult detailed reference):** Heparin, methotrexate.

Compatibility in syringe: Compatible: Atropine, bleomycin, butorphanol, chlorpromazine, cimetidine, cisplatin, cyclophosphamide, dimenhydrinate, diphenhydramine, doxorubicin, fentanyl, glycopyrrolate, hydroxyzine, meperidine, metoclopramide, midazolam, mitomycin, morphine, nalbuphine, pentazocine, perphenazine, prochlorperazine edisylate, promazine, promethazine, scopolamine, vinblastine, vincristine. **Incompatible:** Fluorouracil, furosemide, heparin, leucovorin, methotrexate, ondansetron, pentobarbital.

Mechanism of Action Droperidol is a butyrophenone antipsychotic; antiemetic effect is a result of blockade of dopamine stimulation of the chemoreceptor trigger zone. Other effects include alpha-adrenergic blockade, peripheral vascular dilation, and reduction of the pressor effect of epinephrine resulting in hypotension and decreased peripheral vascular resistance; may also reduce pulmonary artery pressure

Pharmacodynamics/Kinetics

Onset of action: Peak effect: Parenteral:~30 minutes
Duration: Parenteral: 2-4 hours, may extend to 12 hours
Absorption: I.M.: Rapid

Distribution: Crosses blood-brain barrier and placenta

V_d: Children: ~0.25-0.9 L/kg; Adults: ~2 L/kg

Protein binding: Extensive

Metabolism: Hepatic, to p-fluorophenylacetic acid, benzimidazolone, p-hydroxypiperidine

Half-life elimination: Adults: 2.3 hours

Excretion: Urine (75%, <1% as unchanged drug); feces (22%, 11% to 50% as unchanged drug)

Dosage Titrate carefully to desired effect

Children 2-12 years: Nausea and vomiting: I.M., I.V.: 0.05-0.06 mg/kg (maximum initial dose: 0.1 mg/kg); additional doses may be repeated to achieve effect; administer additional doses with caution

Adults: Prevention of postoperative nausea and vomiting (PONV): I.M., I.V.: Initial: 0.625-2.5 mg; additional doses of 1.25 mg may be administered to achieve desired effect; administer additional doses with caution. Consensus guidelines recommend 0.625-1.25 mg I.V. administered after surgery (Gan, 2003).

Administration Administer I.M. or I.V.; according to the manufacturer, I.V. push administration should be slow (generally regarded as 2-5 minutes); however, many clinicians administer I.V. doses rapidly (over 30-60 seconds) in an effort to reduce the incidence of EPS. The effect, if any, of rapid administration on QT prolongation is unclear. For I.V. infusion, dilute in 50-100 mL NS or D_5W; ECG monitoring for 2-3 hours after administration is recommended regardless of rate of infusion.

Monitoring Parameters To identify QT prolongation, a 12-lead ECG prior to use is recommended; continued ECG monitoring for 2-3 hours following administration is recommended. Vital signs; lipid profile, fasting blood glucose/Hgb A_{1c}, serum magnesium and potassium; BMI; mental status, abnormal involuntary movement scale (AIMS); observe for dystonias, extrapyramidal side effects, and temperature changes

Additional Information Does not possess analgesic effects; has little or no amnesic properties.

Dosage Forms Excipient information presented when available (limited, particularly for generics); consult specific product labeling. [DSC] = Discontinued product

Injection, solution [preservative free]: 2.5 mg/mL (1 mL, 2 mL)

Inapsine®: 2.5 mg/mL (1 mL, 2 mL) [DSC]

References

Cersosimo RJ, Bromer R, Hoffer S, et al, "The Antiemetic Activity of Droperidol Administered by Intramuscular Injection During Cisplatin Chemotherapy: A Pilot Study," Drug Intell Clin Pharm, 1985, 19(2):118-21.

Grunberg SM and Hesketh PJ, "Control of Chemotherapy-Induced Emesis," N Engl J Med, 1993, 329(24):1790-6.

Jackson CW, Sheehan AH, and Reddan JG, "Evidence-Based Review of the Black-Box Warning for Droperidol", AJHP, 2007, 64(11):1174-86.

Kao LW, Kirk MA, Evers SJ, et al, "Droperidol, QT Prolongation, and Sudden Death: What Is the Evidence," Ann Emerg Med, 2003, 41(4):546-58.

Leslie JB and Gan TJ, "Meta-Analysis of the Safety Of 5-HT3 Antagonists With Dexamethasone or Droperidol for Prevention of PONV," Ann Pharacother, 2006, 40(5):856-72.

Sridhar KS and Donnelly E, "Combination Antiemetics for Cisplatin Chemotherapy," Cancer, 1988, 61(8):1508-17.

Tortorice PV and O'Connell MB, "Management of Chemotherapy-Induced Nausea and Vomiting," Pharmacotherapy, 1990, 10(2):129-45.

Wilson J, Weltz M, Solimando D, et al, "Continuous Infusion Droperidol: Antiemetic Therapy for Cis-Platinum (DDP) Toxicity," Proc Am Soc Clin Oncol, 1981, C-351.

◆ **Droperidol Injection, USP (Can)** see Droperidol on page 389

- **Droxia®** *see* Hydroxyurea *on page 589*
- **D-Ser(Bu^t)^6,Azgly^{10}-LHRH** *see* Goserelin *on page 549*
- **DTIC** *see* Dacarbazine *on page 293*
- **DTIC® (Can)** *see* Dacarbazine *on page 293*
- **D-Trp(6)-LHRH** *see* Triptorelin *on page 1150*
- **Duragesic®** *see* FentaNYL *on page 458*
- **Duragesic MAT (Can)** *see* FentaNYL *on page 458*
- **Duramorph®** *see* Morphine Sulfate *on page 816*

Dutasteride (doo TAS teer ide)

Related Information
Safe Handling of Hazardous Drugs *on page 1517*

U.S. Brand Names Avodart®

Generic Available No

Canadian Brand Names Avodart®

Pharmacologic Category 5 Alpha-Reductase Inhibitor

Use Treatment of symptomatic benign prostatic hyperplasia (BPH) as monotherapy or combination therapy with tamsulosin

Unlabeled/Investigational Use Treatment of male patterned baldness; prostate cancer prevention (to reduce the incidence)

Pregnancy Risk Factor X

Lactation Excretion in breast milk unknown/contraindicated

Labeled Contraindications Hypersensitivity to dutasteride, other 5α-reductase inhibitors (eg, finasteride), or any component of the formulation; not indicated for use in women or children; pregnant women or women trying to conceive should not handle the product

Warnings/Precautions Hazardous agent - use appropriate precautions for handling and disposal. Pregnant women or women trying to conceive should not handle the product. Urological diseases including cancer and/or obstructive uropathy should be ruled out before initiating. Avoid donating blood during or for 6 months following treatment due to risk of administration to a pregnant female transfusion recipient. Use caution in hepatic impairment and with concurrent use of potent, chronic CYP3A4 inhibitors. Reduces prostate specific antigen (PSA); re-establish a new baseline after 3-6 months of use. When compared to placebo, 5-alpha-reductase inhibitors (5-ARI) have been shown to reduce the incidence of prostate cancer, although an increase in the incidence of high-grade prostate cancers has been observed with another 5-ARI, finasteride (Thompson, 2003; Kramer, 2009).

Adverse Reactions

>10%: Endocrine & metabolic: Serum testosterone increased, thyroid-stimulating hormone increased

1% to 10%: Endocrine & metabolic: Impotence (1% to 5%), libido decreased (≤3%), ejaculation disorders (≤1%), gynecomastia (including breast tenderness, breast enlargement; ≤1%)

<1%, postmarketing, and/or case reports: Allergic reaction, angioedema, dizziness, edema (localized), hypersensitivity, pruritus, rash, skin reactions (serious), urticaria

Note: Frequency of adverse events (except gynecomastia) tends to decrease with continued use (>6 months).

Drug Interactions

Metabolism/Transport Effects Substrate of CYP3A4 (minor)

◄ **Avoid Concomitant Use** There are no known interactions where it is recommended to avoid concomitant use.

Increased Effect/Toxicity

The levels/effects of Dutasteride may be increased by: CYP3A4 Inhibitors (Strong)

Decreased Effect There are no known significant interactions involving a decrease in effect.

Ethanol/Nutrition/Herb Interactions

Ethanol: No effect or interaction noted.

Food: Maximum serum concentrations reduced by 10% to 15% when taken with food; not clinically significant.

Herb/Nutraceutical: St John's wort may decrease dutasteride levels. Avoid saw palmetto (concurrent use has not been adequately studied).

Storage/Stability Store at controlled room temperature of 25°C (77°F).

Mechanism of Action Dutasteride is a 4-azo analog of testosterone and is a competitive, selective inhibitor of both reproductive tissues (type 2) and skin and hepatic (type 1) 5α-reductase. This results in inhibition of the conversion of testosterone to dihydrotestosterone and markedly suppresses serum dihydrotestosterone levels.

Pharmacodynamics/Kinetics

Absorption: Via skin when handling capsules

Distribution: V_d: 300-500 L, ~12% of serum concentrations partitioned into semen

Protein binding: 99% to albumin; ~97% to α_1-acid glycoprotein; >96% to semen protein

Metabolism: Hepatic via CYP3A4 isoenzyme; forms metabolites: 6-hydroxydutasteride has activity similar to parent compound, 4'-hydroxydutasteride and 1,2-dihydrodutasteride are much less potent than parent *in vitro*

Bioavailability: ~60% (range: 40% to 94%)

Half-life elimination: Terminal: ~5 weeks

Time to peak: 2-3 hours

Excretion: Feces (40% as metabolites, 5% as unchanged drug); urine (<1% as unchanged drug); 55% of dose unaccounted for

Dosage Oral: Adults: Males:

BPH: 0.5 mg once daily alone or in combination with tamsulosin

Prostate cancer prevention (unlabeled use): 0.5 mg once daily; planned duration of treatment was 4 years (Andriole, 2004; Kramer, 2009)

Dosage adjustment in renal impairment: No adjustment required

Dosage adjustment in hepatic impairment: Use caution; no specific adjustments recommended

Administration May be administered with or without food. Capsule should be swallowed whole; do not chew or open; contact with opened capsule can cause oropharyngeal irritation. Should not be touched or handled by women who are pregnant or are of childbearing age.

Monitoring Parameters Objective and subjective signs of relief of benign prostatic hyperplasia, including improvement in urinary flow, reduction in symptoms of urgency, and relief of difficulty in micturition; new baseline PSA level after 3-6 months of therapy

Test Interactions PSA levels decrease in treated patients. After 6 months of therapy, PSA levels stabilize to a new baseline that is ~50% of pretreatment values. If following serial PSAs in a patient, re-establish a new baseline after 3-6 months of use. If interpreting an isolated PSA value in a patient treated for 6 months, then double the PSA value for comparison.

Dietary Considerations May be taken with or without food.

Dosage Forms Excipient information presented when available (limited, particularly for generics); consult specific product labeling.

Capsule, softgel:

Avodart®: 0.5 mg

References

Andriole G, Bostwick D, Brawley O, et al, "Chemoprevention of Prostate Cancer in Men at High Risk: Rationale and Design of the Reduction by Dutasteride of Prostate Cancer Events (REDUCE) Trial," *J Urol*, 2004, 172(4 Pt 1):1314-7.

Andriole G, Roehrborn C, Schulman C, et al, "Effect of Dutasteride on the Detection of Prostate Cancer in Men With Benign Prostatic Hyperplasia," *Urology*, 2004, 64(3):537-41.

Kramer BS, Hagerty KL, Justman S, et al. "Use of 5-α-Reductase Inhibitors for Prostate Cancer Chemoprevention: American Society of Clinical Oncology/American Urological Association 2008 Clinical Practice Guideline," *J Clin Oncol*, 2009, 27(9):1502-16.

Thompson IM, Goodman PJ, Tangen CM, et al, "The Influence of Finasteride on the Development of Prostate Cancer," *N Engl J Med*, 2003, 349(3):215-24.

- ◆ **DVA** see Vindesine *on page 1180*

- ◆ **EACA** see Aminocaproic Acid *on page 57*

- ◆ *E. coli* **Asparaginase** see Asparaginase *on page 111*

- ◆ **Econopred® Plus [DSC]** see PrednisoLONE *on page 977*

- ◆ **Ecteinascidin** see Trabectedin *on page 1127*

- ◆ **Ecteinascidin 743** see Trabectedin *on page 1127*

Eculizumab (e kue LIZ oo mab)

Medication Safety Issues

Sound-alike/look-alike issues:

Eculizumab may be confused with efalizumab

U.S. Brand Names Soliris™

Generic Available No

Pharmacologic Category Monoclonal Antibody; Monoclonal Antibody, Complement Inhibitor

Use Treatment of paroxysmal nocturnal hemoglobinuria (PNH) to reduce hemolysis

Restrictions Patients and providers must enroll with Soliris™ OneSource™ (1-888-765-4747) prior to treatment initiation.

Pregnancy Risk Factor C

Lactation Excretion in breast milk unknown/use caution

Labeled Contraindications Hypersensitivity to eculizumab or any component of the formulation; unresolved serious *Neisseria meningitidis* infection; use in patients who have not received *Neisseria meningitidis* vaccination at least 2 weeks prior to first treatment

Warnings/Precautions [U.S. Boxed Warning]: The risk for meningococcal *(Neisseria meningitides)* **infections (septicemia and/or meningitis) is increased with PNH and may be further increased in patients receiving eculizumab; vaccinate with meningococcal vaccine at least 2 weeks prior to initiation of treatment;** revaccinate according to current guidelines. Quadravalent, conjugated meningococcal vaccines are recommended. Meningococcal infections developed in some patients despite vaccination. Monitor for early signs of meningococcal infections; evaluate and treat promptly. Consider withholding eculizumab during the treatment of serious meningococcal infections. In addition to meningitis, the risk of other infections, especially with encapsulated bacteria (eg, *Streptococcus pneumoniae, H. influenzae*) is increased with eculizumab treatment. Use caution in patients ▶

◄ with concurrent systemic infection. Patients should be brought up to date with all immunizations before initiating therapy.

Infusion reactions, including anaphylaxis or hypersensitivity, may occur; interrupt infusion for severe reaction. Continue monitoring for 1 hour after completion of infusion. Patients with PNH who discontinue treatment may be at increased risk for serious hemolysis; monitor closely for at least 8 weeks after treatment discontinuation. In clinical trials, anticoagulant therapy was continued in patients who were receiving these agents prior to initiation of eculizumab. The effect of anticoagulant therapy withdrawal is unknown. Safety and efficacy have not been established in children.

Adverse Reactions
>10%:
  Central nervous system: Headache (2% to 44%), fatigue (12%)
  Gastrointestinal: Nausea (16%)
  Neuromuscular & skeletal: Back pain (19%)
  Respiratory: Nasopharyngitis (23%), cough (12%)
1% to 10%:
  Central nervous system: Fever (2%)
  Gastrointestinal: Constipation (7%)
  Hematologic: Anemia (2%)
  Neuromuscular & skeletal: Limb pain (7%), myalgia (7%)
  Respiratory: Respiratory tract infection (7%), sinusitis (7%)
  Miscellaneous: Herpes infections (7%), flu-like syndrome (5%), viral infection (2%), meningococcal infection (1%)
<1%, postmarketing, and/or case reports: Chills, dizziness, infusion reaction, vomiting

Drug Interactions
Avoid Concomitant Use
Avoid concomitant use of Eculizumab with any of the following: Natalizumab; Vaccines (Live)

Increased Effect/Toxicity
Eculizumab may increase the levels/effects of: Leflunomide; Natalizumab; Vaccines (Live)

The levels/effects of Eculizumab may be increased by: Trastuzumab

Decreased Effect
Eculizumab may decrease the levels/effects of: Vaccines (Inactivated); Vaccines (Live)

The levels/effects of Eculizumab may be decreased by: Echinacea

Storage/Stability Prior to dilution, store vials at 2°C to 8°C (36°F to 46°F); do not freeze. Protect from light; do not shake. Following dilution, store at room temperature or refrigerate; protect from light; use within 24 hours.

Reconstitution Dilute with an equal volume of D_5W, sodium chloride 0.9%, sodium chloride 0.45%, or Ringer's injection to a final concentration of 5 mg/mL (eg, 600 mg in a total volume of 120 mL or 900 mg in a total volume of 180 mL). Gently invert bag to mix.

Compatibility Compatible with D_5W, sodium chloride 0.9%, sodium chloride 0.45%, Ringer's injection

Mechanism of Action Eculizumab is a humanized monoclonal IgG antibody that binds to complement protein C5, preventing cleavage into C5a and C5b. Blocking the formation of C5b inhibits the subsequent formation of terminal complex C5b-9 or membrane attack complex (MAC). Terminal complement-mediated intravascular hemolysis is a key clinical feature of paroxysmal nocturnal hemoglobinuria. Blocking the formation of MAC results in stabilization of hemoglobin and a reduction in the need for RBC transfusions.

Pharmacodynamics/Kinetics

Onset of action: PNH: Reduced hemolysis: ≤1 week

Distribution: 7.7 L

Half-life elimination: ~11 days (range: ~8-15 days)

Dosage Note: Patients must receive meningococcal vaccine at least 2 weeks prior to treatment initiation; revaccinate according to current guidelines.

I.V.: Adults: PNH: 600 mg once weekly (±2 days) for 4 weeks, followed by 900 mg 1 week (±2 days) later; then maintenance: 900 mg every 2 weeks (±2 days) thereafter

Treatment should be administered at the recommended time interval, however, the administration day may be varied by ±2 days if serum LDH levels suggest increased hemolysis before the end of the dosing interval.

Dosage adjustment in renal impairment: Not studied in renal dysfunction

Dosage adjustment in hepatic impairment: Not studied in hepatic dysfunction

Administration I.V.: Allow to warm to room temperature prior to administration. Infuse over 35 minutes. Decrease infusion rate or discontinue for infusion reactions; do not exceed a maximum 2-hour duration of infusion. Monitor for at least 1 hour following completion of infusion.

Monitoring Parameters Signs and symptoms of infusion reaction (during infusion and for 1 hour after infusion complete); CBC with differential, lactic dehydrogenase (LDH), AST, urinalysis

After discontinuation: Signs and symptoms of intravascular hemolysis, serum LDH (monitor for at least 8 weeks after discontinuation)

Dosage Forms Excipient information presented when available (limited, particularly for generics); consult specific product labeling.

Injection, solution [preservative free]:

Soliris™: 10 mg/mL (30 mL) [contains polysorbate 80]

References

Centers for Disease Control and Prevention, "Prevention and Control of Meningococcal Disease Recommendations of the Advisory Committee on Immunization Practices (ACIP)," *MMWR Recomm Rep*, 2005, 54(RR-7):1-21. Available at http://www.cdc.gov/mmwr/pdf/rr/rr5407.pdf (last accessed March 19, 2007).

Hill A, Hillmen P, Richards SJ, et al, "Sustained Response and Long-Term Safety of Eculizumab in Paroxysmal Nocturnal Hemoglobinuria," *Blood*, 2005, 106(7):2559-65.

Hillmen P, Hall C, Marsh JC, et al, "Effect of Eculizumab on Hemolysis and Transfusion Requirements in Patients With Paroxysmal Nocturnal Hemoglobinuria," *N Engl J Med*, 2004, 350 (6):552-9.

Hillmen P, Young NS, Schubert J, et al, "The Complement Inhibitor Eculizumab in Paroxysmal Nocturnal Hemoglobinuria," *N Engl J Med*, 2006, 355(12):1233-43.

Eltrombopag (el TROM boe pag)

U.S. Brand Names Promacta®

Index Terms Eltrombopag Olamine; Revolade®; SB-497115; SB-497115-GR

Generic Available No

Pharmacologic Category Colony Stimulating Factor; Thrombopoietic Agent

Use Treatment of thrombocytopenia in patients with chronic immune (idiopathic) thrombocytopenic purpura (ITP) at risk for bleeding who have had insufficient response to corticosteroids, immune globulin, or splenectomy

Restrictions Eltrombopag is approved for marketing under a Food and Drug Administration (FDA) approved, risk management, and restricted distribution program called Promacta® Cares™ (1-877-977-6622). Patients, prescribers, and pharmacies must be enrolled in the program.

Pregnancy Risk Factor C

Lactation Excretion in breast milk unknown/ not recommended

Labeled Contraindications There are no contraindications listed within the manufacturer's labeling.

Warnings/Precautions [U.S. Boxed Warning]: May cause hepatotoxicity; obtain ALT/AST and bilirubin prior to treatment initiation, every 2 weeks during adjustment phase, then monthly; obtain fractionation for elevated bilirubin levels. Repeat abnormal liver function tests within 3-5 days; if confirmed abnormal, monitor weekly until resolves, stabilizes, or returns to baseline. Discontinue treatment for ALT levels ≥3 times the upper limit of normal (ULN) and which are progressive, or persistent (≥4 weeks), or accompanied by increased direct bilirubin, or accompanied by clinical signs of liver injury or evidence of hepatic decompensation. Reinitiation is not recommended; hepatotoxicity usually recurred with retreatment after therapy interruption. Use with caution in patients with pre-existing hepatic impairment (clearance may be reduced); dosage reductions are recommended in patients moderate-to-severe hepatic dysfunction; monitor closely.

[U.S. Boxed Warning]: Eltrombopag is available through a restricted access program called Promacta Cares™; prescribers, pharmacies, and patients must be registered with the program. The program maintains a patient registry and requires prescribers to monitor and report baseline and periodic safety information related to hepatotoxicity, thromboembolic events, bone marrow reticulin events, rebound thrombocytopenia (after cessation), and malignancies. May increase the risk for bone marrow reticulin formation or progression; collagen fibrosis (not associated with cytopenias) was observed in clinical trials. Monitor peripheral blood smear for cellular morphologic abnormalities; discontinue treatment with onset of new or worsening abnormalities or cytopenias and consider bone marrow biopsy. Upon discontinuation of therapy, thrombocytopenia may worsen; severity may be greater than pretreatment level. Risk of bleeding is increased during rebound thrombocytopenia, particularly in patients receiving anticoagulants or anti-platelet agents; monitor closely; monitor for at least 4 weeks after treatment discontinuation.

Thromboembolism may occur with excess increases in platelet levels. Use with caution in patients with known risk factors for thromboembolism (eg, Factor V Leiden, AT deficiency, antiphospholipid syndrome). Stimulation of cell surface thrombopoietin (TPO) receptors may increase the risk for hematologic malignancies.

Cataract formation or worsening was observed in clinical trials. Monitor regularly for signs and symptoms of cataracts; obtain ophthalmic exam at baseline and during therapy. Use with caution in patients at risk for cataracts (eg, advanced age, long-term glucocorticoid use). Allow at least 4 hours between dosing of eltrombopag and antacids, minerals (eg, iron, calcium, aluminum, magnesium, selenium, zinc), or foods high in calcium; may reduce eltrombopag levels. Patients of East-Asian ethnicity (eg, Chinese, Japanese, Korean, Taiwanese) may have greater drug exposure (compared to non-east Asians); therapy should be initiated with lower starting doses. Safety and efficacy have not been established in renal impairment or in children.

Indicated only when the degree of thrombocytopenia and clinical conditions increase the risk for bleeding; use the lowest dose necessary to achieve and maintain platelet count ≥50,000/mm³. Do not use to normalize platelet counts. Discontinue if platelet count does not respond to a level to avoid clinically important bleeding after 4 weeks at the maximum recommended dose.

Adverse Reactions

1% to 10%:

Dermatologic: Rash (≤7%), bruising (2%)

Endocrine & metabolic: Menorrhagia (4%)

Gastrointestinal: Nausea (6%), vomiting (4%), dyspepsia (2%)

Hematologic: Rebound thrombocytopenia (10%), thrombocytopenia (2%)

Hepatic: Liver function tests abnormal (10%), ALT increased (2%), AST increased (2%)

Neuromuscular & skeletal: Limb pain (≤7%), myalgia (3%), paresthesia (3%)

Ocular: Cataract (3%), conjunctival hemorrhage (2%)

<1%, postmarketing, and/or case reports: Bone marrow collagen fiber deposits, bone marrow reticulin fiber deposits, cataract worsening, epistaxis, headache, hemorrhage (due to thrombocytopenia or rebound thrombocytopenia), non-Hodgkin's lymphoma, thrombotic/thromboembolic complications

Drug Interactions

Metabolism/Transport Effects

Substrate of CYP1A2, CYP2C8, UGT 1A1, UGT1A3; **Inhibits** OATP1B1, UGT1A1, UGT1A3, UGT1A4, UGT1A6, UGT1A9, UGT2B7, and UGT2B15

Avoid Concomitant Use There are no known interactions where it is recommended to avoid concomitant use.

Increased Effect/Toxicity

Eltrombopag may increase the levels/effects of: CYP2C8 Substrates (High risk); OATP1B1/SLCO1B1 Substrates; Rosuvastatin

Decreased Effect

The levels/effects of Eltrombopag may be decreased by: Aluminum Hydroxide; Calcium Salts; Iron Salts; Magnesium Salts; Sucralfate

Ethanol/Nutrition/Herb Interactions Food: Food, especially dairy products, may decrease the absorption of eltrombopag; allow at least 4 hours between dosing of eltrombopag and polyvalent cation intake (eg, dairy products, calcium-rich foods, multivitamins with minerals).

Storage/Stability Store at room temperature of 25°C (77°F); excursions permitted to 15°C to 30°C (59°F to 86°F).

Mechanism of Action Thrombopoietin (TPO) nonpeptide agonist which increases platelet counts by binding to and activating the human TPO receptor. Activates intracellular signal transduction pathways to increase proliferation and differentiation of marrow progenitor cells. Does not induce platelet aggregation or activation.

Pharmacodynamics/Kinetics
Onset of action: Platelet count increase: Within 1-2 weeks
  Peak platelet count increase: 14-16 days
Duration: Platelets return to baseline: 1-2 weeks after last dose
Protein binding: >99%
Metabolism: Extensive hepatic metabolism; via CYP 1A2, 2C8 oxidation and UGT 1A1, 1A3 glucuronidation
Bioavailability: ~52%
Half-life elimination: ~21-32 hours in healthy individuals; ~26-35 hours in patients with ITP
Time to peak, plasma: 2-6 hours
Excretion: Feces (~59%, 20% as unchanged drug, 21% glutathione-related conjugates); urine (31%, 20% glucuronide of the phenypyrazole moiety)

Dosage Note: Discontinue if platelet count does not respond to a level that avoids clinically important bleeding after 4 weeks at the maximum daily dose of 75 mg.

Oral: Adults: ITP: Initial: 50 mg once daily; adjust dose to achieve and maintain platelet count ≥50,000/mm^3 to reduce the risk of bleeding; Maximum dose: 75 mg once daily

Dosage adjustment recommendations:
Platelet count <50,000/mm^3 (after at least 2 weeks): Increase daily dose by 25 mg; maximum dose: 75 mg/day
Platelet count >200,000/mm^3 (at any time): Reduce daily dose by 25 mg; reassess in 2 weeks
Platelet count >400,000/mm^3: Withhold dose; assess platelet count twice weekly; when platelet count <150,000/mm^3, resume with the daily dose reduced by 25 mg
Platelet count >400,000/mm^3 after 2 weeks at the lowest dose: Permanently discontinue

Dosage adjustment for patients of East-Asian ethnicity (eg, Chinese, Japanese, Korean, Taiwanese): Initial dose: 25 mg once daily

Dosage adjustment for toxicity:
ALT levels ≥3 times the upper limit of normal (ULN) **and** which are progressive, or persistent (≥4 weeks), or accompanied by increased direct bilirubin, or accompanied by clinical signs of liver injury or evidence of hepatic decompensation: Discontinue treatment
New or worsening cellular abnormalities or cytopenias: Discontinue treatment

Dosage adjustment in renal impairment: Has not been evaluated in patients with renal impairment; monitor closely

Dosage adjustment in hepatic impairment:
Mild impairment: No adjustment required
Moderate-to-severe impairment: Initial dose: 25 mg once daily

Administration Administer on an empty stomach, 1 hour before or 2 hours after a meal. Do not administer concurrently with antacids, foods high in calcium, or minerals (eg, iron, calcium, aluminum, magnesium, selenium, zinc); separate by at least 4 hours.

Monitoring Parameters Liver tests, including ALT, AST, and bilirubin (baseline, every 2 weeks during dosage titration, then monthly; monitor weekly if retreating [not recommended] after therapy interruption for hepatotoxicity); bilirubin fractionation (for elevated bilirubin); CBC with differential and platelet count (weekly at initiation and during dosage titration, then monthly when stable; continue monitoring for ≥4 weeks after cessation); peripheral blood smear (baseline and monthly when stable); bone marrow biopsy (if peripheral blood smear reveals abnormality); ophthalmic exam (baseline and during treatment)

Dietary Considerations Take on an empty stomach (1 hour before or 2 hours after a meal). Food, especially dairy products, may decrease the absorption of eltrombopag; allow at least 4 hours between dosing of eltrombopag and polyvalent cation intake (eg, dairy products, calcium-rich foods, multivitamins with minerals).

Dosage Forms Excipient information presented when available (limited, particularly for generics); consult specific product labeling.

Tablet:

Promacta®: 25 mg, 50 mg

References

Bussel JB, Cheng G, Saleh MN, et al, "Eltrombopag for the Treatment of Chronic Idiopathic Thrombocytopenic Purpura," *N Engl J Med*, 2007, 357(22):2237-47.

Jenkins JM, Williams D, Deng Y, et al, "Phase 1 Clinical Study of Eltrombopag, An Oral, Nonpeptide Thrombopoietin Receptor Agonist," *Blood*, 2007, 109(11):4739-41.

Kuter DJ, "New Thrombopoietic Growth Factors," *Blood*, 2007, 109(11):4607-16.

◆ **Eltrombopag Olamine** *see* Eltrombopag *on page 398*

◆ **Emcyt®** *see* Estramustine *on page 426*

◆ **Emend®** *see* Aprepitant *on page 104*

◆ **Emend® for Injection** *see* Fosaprepitant *on page 513*

◆ **EMLA®** *see* Lidocaine and Prilocaine *on page 719*

◆ **Emo-Cort® (Can)** *see* Hydrocortisone *on page 575*

◆ **Encort™** *see* Hydrocortisone *on page 575*

Enoxaparin (ee noks a PA rin)

Medication Safety Issues

Sound-alike/look-alike issues:

Lovenox® may be confused with Lasix®, Levaquin®, Lotronex®, Protonix®

High alert medication: The Institute for Safe Medication Practices (ISMP) includes this medication among its list of drugs which have a heightened risk of causing significant patient harm when used in error.

International issues:

Lovenox® may be confused with Lotanax® which is a brand name for terfenadine in the Czech Republic

2009 National Patient Safety Goals: The Joint Commission on Accreditation of Healthcare Organizations requires healthcare organizations that provide anticoagulant therapy to have a process in place to reduce the risk of anticoagulant-associated patient harm. Patients receiving anticoagulants should receive individualized care through a defined process that includes standardized ordering, dispensing, administration, monitoring and education. This does not apply to routine short-term use of anticoagulants for prevention of venous thromboembolism when the expectation is that the patient's laboratory values will remain within or close to normal values (NPSG.03.05.01).

U.S. Brand Names Lovenox®

Index Terms Enoxaparin Sodium

Generic Available No

Canadian Brand Names Enoxaparin Injection; Lovenox®; Lovenox® HP

Pharmacologic Category Low Molecular Weight Heparin

◀ **Use**
Acute coronary syndromes: Unstable angina (UA), non-ST-elevation (NSTEMI), and ST-elevation myocardial infarction (STEMI)

DVT prophylaxis: Following hip or knee replacement surgery, abdominal surgery, or in medical patients with severely-restricted mobility during acute illness who are at risk for thromboembolic complications

DVT treatment (acute): Inpatient treatment (patients with and without pulmonary embolism) and outpatient treatment (patients without pulmonary embolism)

Note: High-risk patients include those with one or more of the following risk factors: >40 years of age, obesity, general anesthesia lasting >30 minutes, malignancy, history of deep vein thrombosis or pulmonary embolism

Unlabeled/Investigational Use Prophylaxis and treatment of thromboembolism in children; anticoagulant bridge therapy during temporary interruption of vitamin K antagonist therapy in patients at high risk for thromboembolism; DVT prophylaxis following moderate-risk general surgery, major gynecologic surgery and following higher-risk general surgery for cancer; management of venous thromboembolism (VTE) during pregnancy (Hirsh, 2008)

Pregnancy Risk Factor B

Lactation Excretion in breast milk unknown/use caution

Labeled Contraindications Hypersensitivity to enoxaparin, heparin, or any component of the formulation; thrombocytopenia associated with a positive *in vitro* test for antiplatelet antibodies in the presence of enoxaparin; hypersensitivity to pork products; active major bleeding; not for I.M. use

Warnings/Precautions [U.S. Boxed Warning]: Patients with recent or anticipated neuraxial anesthesia (epidural or spinal anesthesia) are at risk of spinal or epidural hematoma and subsequent paralysis. Consider risk versus benefit prior to neuraxial anesthesia; risk is increased by concomitant agents which may alter hemostasis or by the use of indwelling epidural catheters for analgesia, as well as traumatic or repeated epidural or spinal puncture. Patient should be observed closely for bleeding if enoxaparin is administered during or immediately following diagnostic lumbar puncture, epidural anesthesia, or spinal anesthesia.

Do not administer intramuscularly. Not recommended for thromboprophylaxis in patients with prosthetic heart valves (especially pregnant women). Not to be used interchangeably (unit for unit) with heparin or any other low molecular weight heparins. Use caution in patients with history of heparin-induced thrombocytopenia. Monitor patient closely for signs or symptoms of bleeding. Certain patients are at increased risk of bleeding. Risk factors include bacterial endocarditis; congenital or acquired bleeding disorders; active ulcerative or angiodysplastic GI diseases; severe uncontrolled hypertension; history of hemorrhagic stroke; use shortly after brain, spinal, or ophthalmic surgery; patients treated concomitantly with platelet inhibitors; recent GI bleeding; thrombocytopenia or platelet defects; severe liver disease; hypertensive or diabetic retinopathy; or in patients undergoing invasive procedures. Monitor platelet count closely. Rare cases of thrombocytopenia have occurred. Discontinue therapy and consider alternative treatment if platelets are <100,000/mm^3 and/or thrombosis develops. Rare cases of thrombocytopenia with thrombosis have occurred. Use caution in patients with congenital or drug-induced thrombocytopenia or platelet defects. Risk of bleeding may be increased in women <45 kg and in men <57 kg. Use caution in patients with renal failure; dosage adjustment needed if Cl_{cr} <30 mL/minute. Use with caution in the elderly (delayed elimination may occur); dosage alteration/adjustment may be required (eg, omission of I.V. bolus in acute STEMI in patients ≥75 years of age). Monitor for hyperkalemia; can cause hyperkalemia possibly by suppressing aldosterone production. Multiple-dose vials contain benzyl alcohol (use caution in pregnant women). In neonates, large amounts of benzyl alcohol (>100 mg/kg/day) have been associated with fatal toxicity (gasping syndrome).

There is no consensus for adjusting/correcting the weight-based dosage of LMWH for patients who are morbidly obese (BMI ≥40 kg/m^2). For patients undergoing inpatient bariatric surgery, the American College of Chest Physicians Practice Guidelines suggest using a higher thromboprophylaxis dose of LMWH for obese patients (Geerts, 2008).

Adverse Reactions As with all anticoagulants, bleeding is the major adverse effect of enoxaparin. Hemorrhage may occur at virtually any site. Risk is dependent on multiple variables. At the recommended doses, single injections of enoxaparin do not significantly influence platelet aggregation or affect global clotting time (ie, PT or aPTT).

1% to 10%:

Central nervous system: Fever (5% to 8%), confusion, pain

Dermatologic: Erythema, bruising

Gastrointestinal: Nausea (3%), diarrhea

Hematologic: Hemorrhage (major, <1% to 4%; includes cases of intracranial, retroperitoneal, or intraocular hemorrhage; incidence varies with indication/population), thrombocytopenia (moderate 1%; severe 0.1% - see note below), anemia (<2%)

Hepatic: ALT, increased, AST increased

Local: Injection site hematoma (9%), local reactions (irritation, pain, ecchymosis, erythema)

Renal: Hematuria (<2%)

<1% and/or postmarketing case reports (limited to important or life-threatening): Allergic reaction, anaphylactoid reaction, cutaneous vasculitis (hypersensitive), eczematous plaques, hematoma (see note on "Spinal or epidural hematomas" below), hyperkalemia, hyperlipidemia, hypertriglyceridemia, intracranial hemorrhage (up to 0.8%), erythematous pruritic patches, pruritus, purpura, retroperitoneal bleeding, skin necrosis, thrombocytopenia with thrombosis, thrombocytosis, urticaria, vesicobullous rash

Notes:

Spinal or epidural hematomas: Can occur following neuraxial anesthesia or spinal puncture, resulting in paralysis. Risk is increased in patients with indwelling epidural catheters or concomitant use of other drugs affecting hemostasis. Prosthetic valve thrombosis, including fatal cases, has been reported in pregnant women receiving enoxaparin as thromboprophylaxis.

Thrombocytopenia with thrombosis: Cases of heparin-induced thrombocytopenia (some complicated by organ infarction, limb ischemia, or death) have been reported.

Drug Interactions

Avoid Concomitant Use There are no known interactions where it is recommended to avoid concomitant use.

Increased Effect/Toxicity

Enoxaparin may increase the levels/effects of: Anticoagulants; Drotrecogin Alfa; Ibritumomab; Tositumomab and Iodine I 131 Tositumomab

The levels/effects of Enoxaparin may be increased by: Antiplatelet Agents; Dasatinib; Herbs (Anticoagulant/Antiplatelet Properties); Nonsteroidal Anti-Inflammatory Agents; Pentosan Polysulfate Sodium; Pentoxifylline; Prostacyclin Analogues; Salicylates; Thrombolytic Agents

Decreased Effect There are no known significant interactions involving a decrease in effect.

Ethanol/Nutrition/Herb Interactions Herb/Nutraceutical: Avoid cat's claw, dong quai, evening primrose, feverfew, garlic, ginger, ginkgo, red clover, horse chestnut, green tea, ginseng (all have additional antiplatelet activity).

Storage/Stability Store at 25°C (77°F); excursions permitted to 15°C to 30°C (59°F to 86°F); do not freeze.

Compatibility Stable in D_5W, NS; do not mix with other injections or infusions.

Mechanism of Action Standard heparin consists of components with molecular weights ranging from 4000-30,000 daltons with a mean of 16,000 daltons. Heparin acts as an anticoagulant by enhancing the inhibition rate of clotting proteases by antithrombin III impairing normal hemostasis and inhibition of factor Xa. Low molecular weight heparins have a small effect on the activated partial thromboplastin time and strongly inhibit factor Xa. Enoxaparin is derived from porcine heparin that undergoes benzylation followed by alkaline depolymerization. The average molecular weight of enoxaparin is 4500 daltons which is distributed as (≤20%) 2000 daltons (≥68%) 2000-8000 daltons, and (≤15%) >8000 daltons. Enoxaparin has a higher ratio of antifactor Xa to antifactor IIa activity than unfractionated heparin.

Pharmacodynamics/Kinetics

Onset of action: Peak effect: SubQ: Antifactor Xa and antithrombin (antifactor IIa): 3-5 hours

Duration: 40 mg dose: Antifactor Xa activity: ~12 hours

Distribution: 4.3 L (based on antifactor Xa activity)

Metabolism: Hepatic, to lower molecular weight fragments (little activity)

Protein binding: Does not bind to heparin binding proteins

Half-life elimination, plasma: 2-4 times longer than standard heparin, independent of dose; based on anti-Xa activity: 4.5-7 hours

Excretion: Urine (40% of dose; 10% as active fragments)

Dosage SubQ:

Infants and Children (unlabeled use; Monagle, 2008):

Infants <2 months: Initial:

Prophylaxis: 0.75 mg/kg every 12 hours

Treatment: 1.5 mg/kg every 12 hours

Infants >2 months and Children ≤18 years: Initial:

Prophylaxis: 0.5 mg/kg every 12 hours

Treatment: 1 mg/kg every 12 hours

Maintenance: See **Dosage Titration** table on next page.

Enoxaparin Pediatric Dosage Titration

Antifactor Xa	Dose Titration	Time to Repeat Antifactor Xa Level
<0.35 units/mL	Increase dose by 25%	4 h after next dose
0.35-0.49 units/mL	Increase dose by 10%	4 h after next dose
0.5-1 unit/mL	Keep same dosage	Next day, then 1 wk later, then monthly (4 h after dose)
1.1-1.5 units/mL	Decrease dose by 20%	Before next dose
1.6-2 units/mL	Hold dose for 3 h and decrease dose by 30%	Before next dose, then 4 h after next dose
>2 units/mL	Hold all doses until antifactor Xa is 0.5 units/mL, then decrease dose by 40%	Before next dose and every 12 h until antifactor Xa <0.5 units/mL

Modified from Monagle P, Michelson AD, Bovill E, et al, "Antithrombotic Therapy in Children," *Chest,* 2001, 119:344S-70S.

Adults:

DVT prophylaxis:

Hip replacement surgery:

Twice-daily dosing: 30 mg every 12 hours, with initial dose within 12-24 hours after surgery, and every 12 hours for at least 10 days or until risk of DVT has diminished or the patient is adequately anticoagulated on warfarin.

Once-daily dosing: 40 mg once daily, with initial dose within 9-15 hours before surgery, and daily for at least 10 days (or up to 35 days postoperatively) or until risk of DVT has diminished or the patient is adequately anticoagulated on warfarin.

Knee replacement surgery: 30 mg every 12 hours, with initial dose within 12-24 hours after surgery, and every 12 hours for at least 10 days or until risk of DVT has diminished or the patient is adequately anticoagulated on warfarin.

Abdominal surgery: 40 mg once daily, with initial dose given 2 hours prior to surgery; continue until risk of DVT has diminished (usually 7-10 days).

Bariatric surgery: Roux-en-Y gastric bypass: Appropriate dosing strategies have not been clearly defined (Borkgren-Okonek, 2008; Scholten, 2002):

BMI ≤50 kg/m^2: 40 mg every 12 hours

BMI >50 kg/m^2: 60 mg every 12 hours

Note: Bariatric surgery guidelines suggest initiation 30-120 minutes before surgery and postoperatively until patient is fully mobile (Mechanick, 2009). Alternatively, limiting administration to the postoperative period may reduce perioperative bleeding.

Medical patients with severely-restricted mobility during acute illness: 40 mg once daily; continue until risk of DVT has diminished (usually 6-11 days).

DVT treatment (acute): **Note:** Start warfarin on the first treatment day and continue enoxaparin until INR is between 2 and 3 (usually 5-7 days).

Inpatient treatment (with or without pulmonary embolism): 1 mg/kg/dose every 12 hours or 1.5 mg/kg once daily.

Outpatient treatment (without pulmonary embolism): 1 mg/kg/dose every 12 hours.

◀ Percutaneous coronary intervention (PCI), adjunctive therapy: In enoxaparin-treated patients undergoing PCI, if balloon inflation occurs ≤8 hours after the last SubQ enoxaparin dose, no additional dosing is needed. If balloon inflation occurs 8-12 hours after the last SubQ enoxaparin dose, a single I.V. dose of 0.3 mg/kg should be administered (Hirsh, 2008; King, 2007)

ST-elevation myocardial infarction (STEMI):

Patients <75 years of age: Initial: 30 mg I.V. single bolus plus 1 mg/kg (maximum 100 mg for the first 2 doses only) SubQ every 12 hours. The first SubQ dose should be administered with the I.V. bolus. Maintenance: After first 2 doses, administer 1 mg/kg SubQ every 12 hours.

Patients ≥75 years of age: Initial: SubQ: 0.75 mg/kg every 12 hours (**Note:** No I.V. bolus is administered in this population); a maximum dose of 75 mg is recommended for the first 2 doses. Maintenance: After first 2 doses, administer 0.75 mg/kg SubQ every 12 hours

Obesity: Use weight-based dosing; a maximum dose of 100 mg is recommended for the first 2 doses (Nutescu, 2009)

Additional notes on STEMI treatment: Therapy was continued for 8 days or until hospital discharge; optimal duration not defined. Unless contra-indicated, all patients received aspirin (75-325 mg daily) in clinical trials. In patients with STEMI receiving thrombolytics, initiate enoxaparin dosing between 15 minutes before and 30 minutes after fibrinolytic therapy. In patients undergoing PCI, if balloon inflation occurs ≤8 hours after the last SubQ enoxaparin dose, no additional dosing is needed. If balloon inflation occurs 8-12 hours after last SubQ enoxaparin dose, a single I.V. dose of 0.3 mg/kg should be administered (Hirsh, 2008; King, 2007).

Unstable angina or non-ST-elevation myocardial infarction (NSTEMI): 1 mg/kg every 12 hours in conjunction with oral aspirin therapy (100-325 mg once daily); continue until clinical stabilization (a minimum of at least 2 days)

Elderly: Refer to adult dosing. Increased incidence of bleeding with doses of 1.5 mg/kg/day or 1 mg/kg every 12 hours; injection-associated bleeding and serious adverse reactions are also increased in the elderly. Careful attention should be paid to elderly patients, particularly those <45 kg. **Note:** Dosage alteration/adjustment may be required.

Dosing adjustment in renal impairment: SubQ:

Cl_{cr} ≥30 mL/minute: No specific adjustment recommended (per manufacturer); monitor closely for bleeding

Cl_{cr} <30 mL/minute:

DVT prophylaxis in abdominal surgery, hip replacement, knee replacement, or in medical patients during acute illness: 30 mg once daily

DVT treatment (inpatient or outpatient treatment in conjunction with warfarin): 1 mg/kg once daily

STEMI:

<75 years: Initial: I.V.: 30 mg as a single dose with the first dose of the SubQ maintenance regimen administered at the same time as the I.V. bolus

≥75 years of age: Omit I.V. bolus; Maintenance: SubQ: 1 mg/kg every 24 hours in all patients

Unstable angina, NSTEMI: SubQ: 1 mg/kg once daily

Dialysis: Enoxaparin has not been FDA approved for use in dialysis patients. It's elimination is primarily via the renal route. Serious bleeding complications have been reported with use in patients who are dialysis dependent or have severe renal failure. LMWH administration at fixed doses without monitoring has greater unpredictable anticoagulant effects in patients with chronic kidney disease. If used, dosages should be reduced and anti-Xa levels frequently monitored, as accumulation may occur with repeated doses. Many clinicians would not use enoxaparin in this population especially without timely anti-Xa levels.

Hemodialysis: Supplemental dose is not necessary.

Peritoneal dialysis: Significant drug removal is unlikely based on physiochemical characteristics.

Administration Do **not** administer I.M.; should be administered by deep SubQ injection to the left or right anterolateral and left or right posterolateral abdominal wall. A single dose may be administered I.V. as part of treatment for ST-elevation myocardial infarction (STEMI) to patients <75 years of age; no I.V. bolus is given to patients ≥75 years of age. To avoid loss of drug from the 30 mg and 40 mg syringes, do not expel the air bubble from the syringe prior to injection. In order to minimize bruising, do not rub injection site. An automatic injector (Lovenox EasyInjector™) is available with the 30 mg and 40 mg syringes to aid the patient with self-injections. **Note:** Enoxaparin is available in 100 mg/mL and 150 mg/mL concentrations.

To convert from I.V. unfractionated heparin (UFH) infusion to SubQ enoxaparin (Nutescu, 2007): Calculate specific dose for enoxaparin based on indication, discontinue UFH and begin enoxaparin within 1 hour.

To convert from SubQ enoxaparin to I.V. UFH infusion (Nutescu, 2007): Discontinue enoxaparin, calculate specific dose for I.V. UFH infusion based on indication, omit heparin bolus/loading dose:

Converting from SubQ enoxaparin dosed every 12 hours: Start I.V. UFH infusion 10-11 hours after last dose of enoxaparin

Converting from SubQ enoxaparin dosed every 24 hours: Start I.V. UFH infusion 22-23 hours after last dose of enoxaparin

Monitoring Parameters Platelets, occult blood, anti-Xa levels, serum creatinine; monitoring of PT and/or aPTT is not necessary. Routine monitoring of anti-Xa levels is not required, but has been utilized in patients with obesity and/or renal insufficiency. Monitoring anti-Xa levels is recommended in pregnant women receiving therapeutic doses of enoxaparin (Hirsh, 2008).

Dosage Forms Excipient information presented when available (limited, particularly for generics); consult specific product labeling.

Injection, solution, as sodium [graduated prefilled syringe; preservative free]:
Lovenox®: 60 mg/0.6 mL (0.6 mL); 80 mg/0.8 mL (0.8 mL); 100 mg/mL (1 mL); 120 mg/0.8 mL (0.8 mL); 150 mg/mL (1 mL)

Injection, solution, as sodium [multidose vial]:
Lovenox®: 100 mg/mL (3 mL) [contains benzyl alcohol]

Injection, solution, as sodium [prefilled syringe; preservative free]:
Lovenox®: 30 mg/0.3 mL (0.3 mL); 40 mg/0.4 mL (0.4 mL)

References

Borkgren-Okonek MJ, Hart RW, Pantano JE, et al, "Enoxaparin Thromboprophylaxis in Gastric Bypass Patients: Extended Duration, Dose Stratification, and Antifactor Xa Activity," *Surg Obes Relat Dis*, 2008, 4(5):625-31.

Farooq V, Hegarty J, Chandrasekar T, et al, "Serious Adverse Incidents With the Usage of Low Molecular Weight Heparins in Patients With Chronic Kidney Disease," *Am J Kidney Dis*, 2004, 43 (3):531-7.

Geerts WH, Bergqvist D, Pineo GF, et al, "Prevention of Venous Thromboembolism: American College of Chest Physicians Evidence-Based Clinical Practice Guidelines (8th Edition)," *Chest*, 2008, 133(6 Suppl):381-453.

Gerlach AT, Pickworth KK, Seth SK, et al, "Enoxaparin and Bleeding Complications: A Review in Patients With and Without Renal Insufficiency," *Pharmacotherapy*, 2000, 20(7):771-5.

Hirsh J, Dalen J, and Guyatt G, et al, "The Sixth (2000) ACCP Guidelines for Antithrombotic Therapy for Prevention and Treatment of Thrombosis. American College of Chest Physicians," *Chest*, 2001, 119(1 Suppl):346-7.

Hirsh J, Guyatt G, Albers GW, et al, "Executive Summary: American College of Chest Physicians Evidence-Based Clinical Practice Guidelines (8th Edition)," *Chest*, 2008, 133(6 Suppl):71-109.

Kearon C, Kahn SR, Agnelli G, et al, "Antithrombotic Therapy for Venous Thromboembolic Disease: American College of Chest Physicians Evidence-Based Clinical Practice Guidelines (8th Edition)," *Chest*, 2008, 33(6 Suppl):454-545.

Mechanick JI, Kushner RF, Sugerman HJ, et al, "American Association of Clinical Endocrinologists, The Obesity Society, and American Society for Metabolic & Bariatric Surgery Medical Guidelines for Clinical Practice for the Perioperative Nutritional, Metabolic, and Nonsurgical Support of the Bariatric Surgery Patient," *Obesity*, 2009, 17(Suppl 1):1-70.

Monagle P, Michelson AD, Bovill E, et al, "Antithrombotic Therapy in Children," *Chest*, 2001, 119:344S-70S.

Montalescot G, Philippe F, Ankri A, et al, "Early Increase of von Willebrand Factor Predicts Adverse Outcome in Unstable Coronary Artery Disease: Beneficial Effects of Enoxaparin. French Investigators of the ESSENCE Trial," *Circulation*, 1998, 98(4):294-9.

Nagge J, Crowther M, and Hirsh J, "Is Impaired Renal Function a Contraindication to the Use of Low-Molecular Weight Heparin?" *Arch Intern Med*, 2002, 162(22):2605-9.

Nutescu EA, Spinler SA, Wittkowsky A, et al, "Low-Molecular-Weight Heparins in Renal Impairment and Obesity: Available Evidence and Clinical Practice Recommendations Across Medical and Surgical Settings," *Ann Pharmacother*, 2009, 43(6):1064-83.

Polkinghorne KR, McMahon LP, and Becker GJ, "Pharmacokinetic Studies of Dalteparin (Fragmin), Enoxaparin (Clexane), and Danaparoid Sodium (Orgaran) in Stable Chronic Hemodialysis Patients," *Am J Kidney Dis*, 2002, 40(5):990-5.

Reach L, Debure A, de Groc F, et al, "Anticoagulation With Enoxaparin 0.5 mg/kg in 630 Dialysis Sessions," *Haemostasis*, 1994, 24(Suppl 1):280 [Abstract 281]

Sanderink GJ, Le Liboux A, Jariwala N, et al, "The Pharmacokinetic and Pharmacodynamics of Enoxaparin in Obese Volunteers," *Clin Pharmacol Ther*, 2002, 72(3):308-18.

Scholten DJ, Hoedema RM, and Scholten SE, "A Comparison of Two Different Prophylactic Dose Regimens of Low-Molecular Weight Heparin in Bariatric Surgery," *Obes Surg*, 2002, 12(1):19-24.

Simonneau G, Charbonnier B, Decousus H, et al, "Subcutaneous Low-Molecular-Weight Heparin Compared With Continuous Intravenous Unfractionated Heparin in the Treatment of Proximal Deep Vein Thrombosis," *Arch Intern Med*, 1993, 153(13):1541-6.

Von Visger J and Magee C, "Low Molecular Weight Heparins in Renal Failure," *J Nephrol*, 2003, 16 (6):914-6.

◆ **Enoxaparin Injection (Can)** *see* Enoxaparin *on page 401*

◆ **Enoxaparin Sodium** *see* Enoxaparin *on page 401*

◆ **Entertainer's Secret® [OTC]** *see* Saliva Substitute *on page 1027*

◆ **Epidermal Thymocyte Activating Factor** *see* Aldesleukin *on page 25*

◆ **Epipodophyllotoxin** *see* Etoposide *on page 429*

Epirubicin (ep i ROO bi sin)

Medication Safety Issues

Sound-alike/look-alike issues:

Epirubicin may be confused with DOXOrubicin, DAUNOrubicin, idarubicin

Ellence® may be confused with Elase®

High alert medication: The Institute for Safe Medication Practices (ISMP) includes this medication among its list of drugs which have a heightened risk of causing significant patient harm when used in error.

Related Information

Management of Drug Extravasations *on page 1447*
Safe Handling of Hazardous Drugs *on page 1517*

U.S. Brand Names Ellence®

Index Terms Epirubicin Hydrochloride; Pidorubicin; Pidorubicin Hydrochloride

Generic Available Yes

Canadian Brand Names Ellence®; Pharmorubicin®

Pharmacologic Category Antineoplastic Agent, Anthracycline

Use Adjuvant therapy for primary breast cancer

Unlabeled/Investigational Use Treatment of cervical cancer, esophageal cancer, gastric cancer, soft tissue sarcoma, uterine sarcoma

Pregnancy Risk Factor D

Lactation Excretion in breast milk unknown/contraindicated

Labeled Contraindications Hypersensitivity to epirubicin or any component of the formulation, other anthracyclines, or anthracenediones; previous anthracycline treatment up to maximum cumulative dose; severe myocardial insufficiency; severe arrhythmias; recent myocardial infarction; severe hepatic dysfunction; baseline neutrophil count 1500 cells/mm^3; pregnancy

Warnings/Precautions Hazardous agent - use appropriate precautions for handling and disposal.

[U.S. Boxed Warning]: Potential cardiotoxicity, particularly in patients who have received prior anthracyclines, prior or concomitant radiotherapy to the mediastinal/pericardial area, or who have pre-existing cardiac disease, may occur. Acute toxicity (primarily arrhythmias) and delayed toxicity (HF) have been described. Delayed toxicity usually develops late in the course of therapy or within 2-3 months after completion, however, events with an onset of several months to years after termination of treatment have been described. The risk of delayed cardiotoxicity increases more steeply with cumulative doses >900 mg/m^2, and this dose should be exceeded only with extreme caution. (The risk of HF is ~0.9% at a cumulative dose of 550 mg/m^2, ~1.6% at a cumulative dose of 700 mg/m^2, and ~3.3% at a cumulative dose of 900 mg/m^2.) Toxicity may be additive with other anthracyclines or anthracenediones, and may be increased in pediatric patients. Regular monitoring of LVEF and discontinuation at the first sign of impairment is recommended especially in patients with cardiac risk factors or impaired cardiac function.

[U.S. Boxed Warning]: May cause severe myelosuppression; neutropenia is the dose-limiting toxicity; severe thrombocytopenia or anemia may occur. Thrombophlebitis and thromboembolic phenomena (including pulmonary embolism) have occurred.

[U.S. Boxed Warning]: Reduce dosage and use with caution in mild-to-moderate hepatic impairment or in severe renal dysfunction (serum creatinine >5 mg/dL). May cause tumor lysis syndrome. Radiation recall has been reported; epirubicin may have radiosensitizing activity. **[U.S. Boxed Warnings]: Treatment with anthracyclines may increase the risk of secondary leukemias. For I.V. administration only, severe local tissue damage and necrosis will result if extravasation occurs.** Women ≥70 years of age should be especially monitored for toxicity; women of childbearing age should be advised to avoid becoming pregnant. **[U.S. Boxed Warning]: Should be administered under the supervision of an experienced cancer chemotherapy physician.** Safety and efficacy in children have not been established.

Adverse Reactions Percentages reported as part of combination chemotherapy regimens.

>10%:

Central nervous system: Lethargy (1% to 46%)

Dermatologic: Alopecia (69% to 96%)

Endocrine & metabolic: Amenorrhea (69% to 72%), hot flashes (5% to 39%)

Gastrointestinal: Nausea/vomiting (83% to 92%), mucositis (9% to 59%), diarrhea (7% to 25%)

Hematologic: Leukopenia (50% to 80%; grades 3/4: 2% to 59%), neutropenia (54% to 80%; grades 3/4: 11% to 67%; nadir: 10-14 days; recovery: 21 days), anemia (13% to 72%; grades 3/4: 6%), thrombocytopenia (5% to 49%; grades 3/4: 5%)

Local: Injection site reactions (3% to 20%)

Ocular: Conjunctivitis (1% to 15%)

Miscellaneous: Infection (15% to 21%)

1% to 10%:

Cardiovascular: CHF (0.4% to 1.5%), decreased LVEF (asymptomatic) (1% to 2%); recommended maximum cumulative dose: 900 mg/m^2

Central nervous system: Fever (1% to 5%)

Dermatologic: Rash (1% to 9%), skin changes (1% to 5%)

Gastrointestinal: Anorexia (2% to 3%)

Hematologic: Neutropenic fever (grades 3/4: 6%)

<1%, postmarketing, case reports, and/or frequency not defined: Acute lymphoid leukemia; acute myelogenous leukemia (0.3% at 3 years, 0.5% at 5 years, 0.6% at 8 years); anaphylaxis, atrioventricular block, bradycardia, bundle-branch block, cardiomyopathy, ECG abnormalities, hypersensitivity, myelodysplastic syndrome, photosensitivity, premature menopause, premature ventricular contractions, pulmonary embolism, radiation recall, sinus tachycardia, skin and nail hyperpigmentation, ST-T wave changes (nonspecific), tachyarrhythmias, thromboembolism, thrombophlebitis, transaminases increased, urticaria, ventricular tachycardia

Drug Interactions

Avoid Concomitant Use

Avoid concomitant use of Epirubicin with any of the following: Natalizumab; Vaccines (Live)

Increased Effect/Toxicity

Epirubicin may increase the levels/effects of: Leflunomide; Natalizumab; Vaccines (Live)

The levels/effects of Epirubicin may be increased by: Bevacizumab; Taxane Derivatives; Trastuzumab

Decreased Effect

Epirubicin may decrease the levels/effects of: Cardiac Glycosides; Vaccines (Inactivated); Vaccines (Live)

The levels/effects of Epirubicin may be decreased by: Cardiac Glycosides; Echinacea

Ethanol/Nutrition/Herb Interactions

Ethanol: Avoid ethanol (due to GI irritation).

Herb/Nutraceutical: Avoid black cohosh, dong quai in estrogen-dependent tumors.

Storage/Stability Store intact vials of solution under refrigeration at 2°C to 8°C (36°F to 46°F). Store intact vials of lyophilized powder at room temperature 15°C to 30°C (59°F to 86°F). Protect from light. Reconstituted solutions and solutions for infusion are stable for 24 hours when stored at 2°C to 8°C (36°F to 46°F).

Reconstitution Reconstitute lyophilized powder with SWFI to a final concentration of 2 mg/mL. May administer undiluted for IVP or dilute in 50-250 mL NS or D$_5$W for infusion.

Compatibility Stable in D$_5$W, LR, NS; **incompatible** with heparin, fluorouracil, or any solution of alkaline pH.

Compatibility in syringe: Compatible: Ifosfamide. **Incompatible:** Fluorouracil, heparin, ifosfamide with mesna, any solution of alkaline pH.

Mechanism of Action Epirubicin is an anthracycline antibiotic; known to inhibit DNA and RNA synthesis by steric obstruction after intercalating between DNA base pairs; active throughout entire cell cycle. Intercalation triggers DNA cleavage by topoisomerase II, resulting in cytocidal activity. Also inhibits DNA helicase, and generates cytotoxic free radicals.

Pharmacodynamics/Kinetics

Distribution: V_{ss}: 21-27 L/kg

Protein binding: 77% to albumin

Metabolism: Extensively via hepatic and extrahepatic (including RBCs) routes

Half-life elimination: Triphasic; Mean terminal: 33 hours

Excretion: Feces (34% to 35%); urine (20% to 27%)

Dosage Adults: I.V.: 100-120 mg/m^2 once every 3-4 weeks **or** 50-60 mg/m^2 days 1 and 8 every 3-4 weeks

Breast cancer:

CEF-120: 60 mg/m^2 on days 1 and 8 every 28 days for 6 cycles

FEC-100: 100 mg/m^2 on day 1 every 21 days for 6 cycles

Note: Patients receiving 120 mg/m^2/cycle as part of combination therapy should also receive prophylactic therapy with sulfamethoxazole/trimethoprim or a fluoroquinolone.

Dosage modifications:

Delay day 1 dose until platelets are ≥100,000/mm^3, ANC ≥1500/mm^3, and nonhematologic toxicities have recovered to ≤grade 1

Reduce day 1 dose in subsequent cycles to 75% of previous day 1 dose if patient experiences nadir platelet counts <50,000/mm^3, ANC <250/mm^3, neutropenic fever, or grade 3/4 nonhematologic toxicity during the previous cycle

For divided doses (day 1 and day 8), reduce day 8 dose to 75% of day 1 dose if platelet counts are 75,000-100,000/mm^3 and ANC is 1000-1499/mm^3; omit day 8 dose if platelets are <75,000/mm^3, ANC <1000/mm^3, or grade 3/4 nonhematologic toxicity

Dosage adjustment in bone marrow dysfunction: Heavily-treated patients, patients with pre-existing bone marrow depression or neoplastic bone marrow infiltration: Lower starting doses (75-90 mg/mm^2) should be considered.

Elderly: Plasma clearance of epirubicin in elderly female patients was noted to be reduced by 35%. Although no initial dosage reduction is specifically recommended, particular care should be exercised in monitoring toxicity and adjusting subsequent dosage in elderly patients (particularly females >70 years of age).

Dosage adjustment in renal impairment: The FDA-approved labeling recommends that in patients with severe renal impairment (serum creatinine >5 mg/dL), lower doses should be considered. Aronoff (2007) recommends no dosage adjustment needed for Cl_{cr} <50 mL/minute.

Dosage adjustment in hepatic impairment: The FDA-approved labeling recommends the following guidelines (based on clinical trial information):

Bilirubin 1.2-3 mg/dL or AST 2-4 times the upper limit of normal: Administer 50% of recommended starting dose

Bilirubin >3 mg/dL or AST >4 times the upper limit of normal: Administer 25% of recommended starting dose

Severe hepatic impairment: Use is contraindicated

Combination Regimens

Breast cancer:

CEF on page 1254

Docetaxel-FEC on page 1292

Docetaxel-Trastuzumab-FEC on page 1294

FEC on page 1322

Tamoxifen-Epirubicin on page 1405

TEX (Capecitabine + Docetaxel + Epirubicin) on page 1405

Vinorelbine-FEC on page 1423

◀ Vinorelbine-Trastuzumab-FEC on page 1424

Esophageal cancer:
  Epirubicin-Cisplatin-Capecitabine (Esophageal Cancer) on page 1305
  Epirubicin-Cisplatin-Fluorouracil (Gastric/Esophageal Cancer) on page 1305
  Epirubicin-Oxaliplatin-Capecitabine on page 1306
  Epirubicin-Oxaliplatin-Fluorouracil (Esophageal Cancer) on page 1306

Gastric cancer:
  Epirubicin-Cisplatin-Fluorouracil (Gastric/Esophageal Cancer) on page 1305
  Epirubicin-Oxaliplatin-Capecitabine on page 1306

Rhabdomyosarcoma: CEV on page 1259

Administration I.V.: Infuse over 15-20 minutes or slow I.V. push (for lower doses [due to dose modification or organ dysfunction]) over 3-10 minutes

Monitoring Parameters Monitor injection site during infusion for possible extravasation or local reactions; CBC with differential and platelet count, liver function tests, renal function, ECG, and left ventricular ejection fraction. Monitor during therapy for potential cardiotoxicity with ECHO or with MUGA scans (patients with higher cumulative doses).

Emetic Potential Moderate (30% to 90%)

Vesicant Yes; see Management of Drug Extravasations on page 1447.

Dosage Forms Excipient information presented when available (limited, particularly for generics); consult specific product labeling.

Injection, powder for reconstitution, as hydrochloride, [preservative free]:
  50 mg, 200 mg [contains lactose]

Injection, solution, as hydrochloride [preservative free]: 2 mg/mL (5 mL, 25 mL, 75 mL, 100 mL)
  Ellence®: 2 mg/mL (25 mL, 100 mL)

References

Aronoff GR, Bennett WM, Berns JS, et al, *Drug Prescribing in Renal Failure: Dosing Guidelines for Adults and Children*, 5th ed. Philadelphia, PA: American College of Physicians; 2007, p 99.

Coukell AJ and Faulds D, "Epirubicin. An Updated Review of Its Pharmacodynamic and Pharmacokinetic Properties and Therapeutic Efficacy in the Management of Breast Cancer," *Drugs*, 1997, 53(3):453-82.

Murray LS, Jodrell DI, Morrison JG, et al, "The Effect of Cimetidine on the Pharmacokinetics of Epirubicin in Patients With Advanced Breast Cancer: Preliminary Evidence of a Potentially Common Drug Interaction," *Clin Oncol (R Coll Radiol)*, 1998, 10(1):35-8.

Onrust SV, Wiseman LR, and Goa KL, "Epirubicin: A Review of Its Intravesical Use in Superficial Bladder Cancer," *Drugs Aging*, 1999, 15(4):307-33.

Trudeau M and Pagani O, "Epirubicin in Combination With the Taxanes," *Semin Oncol*, 2001, 28(4 Suppl 12):41-50.

◆ **Epirubicin Hydrochloride** see Epirubicin on page 408

◆ **EPO** see Epoetin Alfa on page 412

Epoetin Alfa (e POE e tin AL fa)

Medication Safety Issues

Sound-alike/look-alike issues:
  Epoetin alfa may be confused with darbepoetin alfa, epoetin beta
  Epogen® may be confused with Neupogen®

International issues:
  Epopen® [Spain] may be confused with EpiPen® which is a brand name for epinephrine in the U.S.

U.S. Brand Names Epogen®; Procrit®

Index Terms rHuEPO-α; EPO; Erythropoiesis-Stimulating Agent (ESA); Erythropoietin; NSC-724223

Generic Available No

Canadian Brand Names Eprex®

Pharmacologic Category Colony Stimulating Factor

Use Treatment of anemia (elevate/maintain red blood cell level and decrease the need for transfusions) associated with HIV (zidovudine) therapy, chronic renal failure (including patients on dialysis and not on dialysis); reduction of allogeneic blood transfusion for elective, noncardiac, nonvascular surgery; treatment of anemia due to concurrent chemotherapy in patients with metastatic cancer (nonmyeloid malignancies)

Note: Erythropoietin is **not** indicated for use in cancer patients under the following conditions:
- receiving hormonal therapy, therapeutic biologic products, or radiation therapy unless also receiving concurrent myelosuppressive chemotherapy
- receiving myelosuppressive therapy when the expected outcome is curative
- anemia due to other factors (eg, iron deficiency, folate deficiency, or gastrointestinal bleed)

Unlabeled/Investigational Use Treatment of anemia associated with critical illness; anemia of prematurity; symptomatic anemia in myelodysplastic syndrome (MDS)

Pregnancy Risk Factor C

Lactation Excretion in breast milk unknown/use caution

Labeled Contraindications Hypersensitivity to albumin (human) or mammalian cell-derived products; uncontrolled hypertension

Warnings/Precautions [U.S. Boxed Warning]: ESAs increased the risk of serious cardiovascular events, thromboembolic events, mortality, and/or tumor progression in clinical studies; a rapid rise in hemoglobin (>1 g/dL over 2 weeks) or maintaining higher hemoglobin levels may contribute to these risks. **[U.S. Boxed Warning]: A shortened overall survival and/or increased risk of tumor progression or recurrence has been reported in studies with breast, cervical, head and neck, lymphoid, and non small cell lung cancer patients.** It is of note that in these studies, patients received ESAs to a target hemoglobin of ≥12 g/dL; although risk has not been excluded when dosed to achieve a target hemoglobin of <12 g/dL. **[U.S. Boxed Warnings]: To decrease these risks, and risk of cardio- and thrombovascular events, use the lowest dose needed to avoid red blood cell transfusions. Use ESAs in cancer patients only for the treatment of anemia related to concurrent chemotherapy; discontinue ESA following completion of the chemotherapy course. ESAs are not indicated for patients receiving myelosuppressive therapy when the anticipated outcome is curative.** **[U.S. Boxed Warning]: An increased risk of death and serious cardiovascular events was reported in chronic renal failure patients administered ESAs to target higher versus lower hemoglobin levels (13.5 vs 11.3 g/dL; 14 vs 10 g/dL) in two clinical studies; dosing should be individualized to achieve and maintain hemoglobin levels within 10-12 g/dL range.** Hemoglobin rising >1 g/dL in a 2-week period may contribute to the risk. Chronic renal failure patients who exhibit an inadequate hemoglobin response to ESA therapy may be at a higher risk for cardiovascular events and mortality compared to other patients. ESA therapy may reduce dialysis efficacy (due to increase in red blood cells and decrease in plasma volume); adjustments in dialysis parameters may be needed. Patients treated with epoetin may require increased heparinization during dialysis to prevent clotting of the artificial kidney. **[U.S. Boxed Warning]: Epoetin alfa increased the rate of DVT in perisurgery patients not receiving anticoagulant prophylaxis; consider DVT prophylaxis.** Increased mortality was also observed in patients undergoing coronary artery bypass surgery who received epoetin alfa; these deaths were associated with thrombotic events. Epoetin is not approved for reduction of red blood cell transfusion in patients undergoing cardiac or vascular surgery. During therapy in any patient, hemoglobin levels should not exceed a target range of 10-12 g/dL and should not rise >1 g/dL per 2-week time period.

Use with caution in patients with hypertension or with a history of seizures; hypertensive encephalopathy and seizures have been reported. If hypertension is difficult to control, reduce or hold epoetin alfa. An excessive rate of rise of hemoglobin is associated with hypertension or exacerbation of hypertension; decrease the epoetin dose if the hemoglobin increase exceeds 1 g/dL in any 2-week period. Blood pressure should be controlled prior to start of therapy and monitored closely throughout treatment. **Not** recommended for acute correction of severe anemia or as a substitute for transfusion.

Prior to treatment, correct or exclude deficiencies of iron, vitamin B_{12}, and/or folate, as well as other factors which may impair erythropoiesis (aluminum toxicity, inflammatory conditions, infections). Prior to and periodically during therapy, iron stores must be evaluated. Supplemental iron is recommended if serum ferritin <100 mcg/L or serum transferrin saturation <20%. Poor response should prompt evaluation of these potential factors, as well as possible malignant processes, occult blood loss, hemolysis, and/or bone marrow fibrosis. Severe anemia and pure red cell aplasia (PRCA) with associated neutralizing antibodies to erythropoietin has been reported, predominantly in patients with CRF receiving SubQ epoetin (the I.V. route is preferred for hemodialysis patients). Patients with loss of response to epoetin alfa should be evaluated; discontinue treatment in patients with PRCA secondary to neutralizing antibodies to epoetin. Antibodies may cross-react; do not switch to another ESA in patients who develop antibody-mediated anemia.

Due to the delayed onset of erythropoiesis, epoetin is of no value in the acute treatment of anemia. Safety and efficacy in patients with underlying hematologic diseases have not been established, including hypercoagulation disorders and sickle cell disease. Potentially serious allergic reactions have been reported. Use caution with porphyria, exacerbation of porphyria has been reported (rarely) in patients with chronic renal failure. Some products may contain albumin. Multidose vials contain benzyl alcohol; do not use in premature infants. Safety and efficacy in children <1 month of age have not been established.

Adverse Reactions

>10%:
Cardiovascular: Hypertension (5% to 24%), thrombotic/vascular events (coronary artery bypass graft surgery: 23%), edema (6% to 17%), deep vein thrombosis (3% to 11%)
Central nervous system: Fever (29% to 51%), dizziness (<7% to 21%), insomnia (13% to 21%), headache (10% to 19%)
Dermatologic: Pruritus (14% to 22%), skin pain (4% to 18%), rash (≤16%)
Gastrointestinal: Nausea (11% to 58%), constipation (42% to 53%), vomiting (8% to 29%), diarrhea (9% to 21%), dyspepsia (7% to 11%)
Genitourinary: Urinary tract infection (3% to 12%)
Local: Injection site reaction (<10% to 29%)
Neuromuscular & skeletal: Arthralgia (11%), paresthesia (11%)
Respiratory: Cough (18%), congestion (15%), dyspnea (13% to 14%), upper respiratory infection (11%)
1% to 10%:
Central nervous system: Seizure (1% to 3%)
Local: Clotted vascular access (7%)

<1%, postmarketing, and/or case reports: Allergic reaction, anemia (severe; with or without other cytopenias), CVA, flu-like syndrome, hyperkalemia, hypersensitivity reactions, hypertensive encephalopathy, microvascular thrombosis, MI, myalgia, neutralizing antibodies, pulmonary embolism, pure red cell aplasia (PRCA), renal vein thrombosis, retinal artery thrombosis, tachycardia, temporal vein thrombosis, thrombophlebitis, thrombosis, TIA, urticaria

Drug Interactions

Avoid Concomitant Use There are no known interactions where it is recommended to avoid concomitant use.

Increased Effect/Toxicity There are no known significant interactions involving an increase in effect.

Decreased Effect There are no known significant interactions involving a decrease in effect.

Storage/Stability Vials should be stored at 2°C to 8°C (36°F to 46°F); **do not freeze or shake**. Protect from light.

Single-dose 1 mL vial contains no preservative: Use one dose per vial. Do not re-enter vial; discard unused portions.

Single-dose vials (except 40,000 units/mL vial) are stable for 2 weeks at room temperature. Single-dose 40,000 units/mL vial is stable for 1 week at room temperature.

Multidose 1 mL or 2 mL vial contains preservative. Store at 2°C to 8°C after initial entry and between doses. Discard 21 days after initial entry.

Multidose vials (with preservative) are stable for 1 week at room temperature.

Prefilled syringes containing the 20,000 units/mL formulation with preservative are stable for 6 weeks refrigerated (2°C to 8°C).

Dilutions of 1:10 in $D_{10}W$ with human albumin 0.05% or 0.1% are stable for 24 hours.

Reconstitution Prior to SubQ administration, preservative free solutions may be mixed with bacteriostatic NS containing benzyl alcohol 0.9% in a 1:1 ratio.

Compatibility Stable in $D_{10}W$ with albumin 0.05%, $D_{10}W$ with albumin 0.1%; **incompatible** with $D_{10}W$ with albumin 0.01%, $D_{10}W$, NS; **variable stability (consult detailed reference)** in TPN.

Mechanism of Action Induces erythropoiesis by stimulating the division and differentiation of committed erythroid progenitor cells; induces the release of reticulocytes from the bone marrow into the bloodstream, where they mature to erythrocytes. There is a dose response relationship with this effect. This results in an increase in reticulocyte counts followed by a rise in hematocrit and hemoglobin levels.

Pharmacodynamics/Kinetics

Onset of action: Several days

Peak effect: 2-3 weeks

Distribution: V_d: 9 L; rapid in the plasma compartment; concentrated in liver, kidneys, and bone marrow

Metabolism: Some degradation does occur

Bioavailability: SubQ: ~21% to 31%; intraperitoneal epoetin: 3% (a few patients)

Half-life elimination: Cancer: SubQ: 16-67 hours; Chronic renal failure: I.V.: 4-13 hours

Time to peak, serum: Chronic renal failure: SubQ: 5-24 hours

Excretion: Feces (majority); urine (small amounts, 10% unchanged in normal volunteers)

Dosage Note: Hemoglobin levels should not exceed 12 g/dL and should not rise >1 g/dL per 2-week time period during therapy in any patient.

Chronic renal failure patients: Individualize dosing to achieve and maintain hemoglobin levels between 10-12 g/dL. Hemoglobin levels should not exceed 12 g/dL. **Note:** I.V. route is preferred for hemodialysis patients.

Children: I.V., SubQ: Initial dose: 50 units/kg 3 times/week

Adults: I.V., SubQ: Initial dose: 50-100 units/kg 3 times/week

Dosage adjustment in Children and Adults: SubQ, I.V.:

Decrease dose by 25%: If hemoglobin approaches 12 g/dL **or** hemoglobin increases >1 g/dL in any 2-week period. If hemoglobin continues to increase, temporarily discontinue therapy until hemoglobin begins to decrease, then resume therapy with a ~25% reduction from previous dose.

Increase dose by 25%: If hemoglobin <10 g/dL and does not increase by 1 g/dL after 4 weeks of therapy (with adequate iron stores) **or** hemoglobin decreases below 10 g/dL. If transferrin saturation >20%, may increase epoetin dose. Do not increase dose more frequently than at 4-week intervals, unless clinically indicated (hemoglobin response time for dose increases may be 2-6 weeks).

Inadequate or lack of response: If patient does not attain target hemoglobin range of 10-12 g/dL after appropriate dose titrations over 12 weeks:

Do not continue to increase dose and use the minimum effective dose that will maintain a hemoglobin level sufficient to avoid red blood cell transfusions **and** evaluate patient for other causes of anemia.

Monitor hemoglobin closely thereafter, and if responsiveness improves, may resume making dosage adjustments as recommended above. If responsiveness does not improve and recurrent red blood cell transfusions continue to be needed, discontinue therapy.

Maintenance dose: Individualize to target hemoglobin range of 10-12 g/dL; limit additional dosage increases to every 4 weeks (or longer)

Dialysis patients: Median dose:

Children: 167 units/kg/week (hemodialysis) **or** 76 units/kg/week (peritoneal dialysis), in 2-3 divided doses per week

Adults: 75 units/kg 3 times/week

Nondialysis patients:

Children: Dosing range: 50-250 units/kg 1-3 times/week

Adults: Dosing range: 75-150 units/kg/week

Zidovudine-treated, HIV-infected patients (patients with erythropoietin levels >500 mU/mL are **unlikely** to respond): Titrate dosage to use the minimum effective dose that will maintain a hemoglobin level sufficient to avoid red blood cell transfusions. Hemoglobin levels should not exceed 12 g/dL.

Children: SubQ, I.V.: Limited data available; reported dosing range: 50-400 units/kg 2-3 times/week

Adults (with serum erythropoietin levels ≤500 and zidovudine doses ≤4200 mg/week): SubQ, I.V.: 100 units/kg 3 times/week for 8 weeks

Dosage adjustment:

Increase dose by 50-100 units/kg 3 times/week: If response is not satisfactory in terms of reducing transfusion requirements **or** increasing hemoglobin after 8 weeks of therapy. Evaluate response every 4-8 weeks thereafter, and adjust the dose accordingly by 50-100 units/kg increments 3 times/week. If patients has not responded satisfactorily to 300 units/kg/dose 3 times/week, a response to higher doses is unlikely.

Withhold dose: If hemoglobin exceeds 12 g/dL. Resume treatment with a 25% dose reduction when hemoglobin drops below 11 g/dL

Cancer patient on chemotherapy: Treatment of patients with erythropoietin levels >200 mU/mL is **not recommended by the manufacturer.** Titrate dosage to use the minimum effective dose that will maintain a hemoglobin level sufficient to avoid red blood cell transfusions. Do not initiate therapy if hemoglobin ≥10 g/dL. Discontinue erythropoietin following completion of chemotherapy.

Children: I.V.: 600 units/kg once weekly (maximum: 40,000 units)

Dosage adjustment:

Increase dose: If response is not satisfactory after a sufficient period of evaluation (no increase in hemoglobin by ≥1 g/dL after 4 weeks of once-weekly therapy), the dose may be increased every 4 weeks (or longer) to 900 units/kg/week; maximum 60,000 units. If patient does not respond, a response to higher doses is unlikely.

Withhold dose: If hemoglobin exceeds a level needed to avoid red blood cell transfusion. Resume treatment with a 25% dose reduction when hemoglobin approaches a level where transfusions may be required.

Reduce dose by 25%: If hemoglobin increases >1 g/dL in any 2-week period **or** hemoglobin reaches a level sufficient to avoid red blood cell transfusion.

Discontinue: If after 8 weeks of therapy there is no response (ie, increased hemoglobin levels) or transfusions still required.

Adults: SubQ: Initial dose: 150 units/kg 3 times/week or 40,000 units once weekly; commonly used doses range from 10,000 units 3 times/week to 40,000-60,000 units once weekly.

Dosage adjustment:

Increase dose: If response is not satisfactory after a sufficient period of evaluation (no reduction in transfusion requirements or increase in hemoglobin after 8 weeks of 3 times/week therapy) **or** (no increase in hemoglobin by ≥1 g/dL after 4 weeks of once-weekly therapy), the dose may be increased every 4 weeks (or longer) to 300 units/kg 3 times/week, **or** when dosed weekly, increased all at once to 60,000 units weekly. If patient does not respond, a response to higher doses is unlikely.

Withhold dose: If hemoglobin exceeds a level needed to avoid red blood cell transfusion. Resume treatment with a 25% dose reduction when hemoglobin approaches a level where transfusions may be required.

Reduce dose by 25%: If hemoglobin increases >1 g/dL in any 2-week period **or** hemoglobin reaches a level sufficient to avoid red blood cell transfusion.

Discontinue: If after 8 weeks of therapy there is no response (ie, increased hemoglobin levels) or transfusions still required.

Surgery patients: Prior to initiating treatment, obtain a hemoglobin to establish that it is >10 g/dL and ≤13 g/dL: Adults: SubQ: Initial dose: 300 units/kg/day for 10 days before surgery, on the day of surgery, and for 4 days after surgery

Alternative dose: 600 units/kg in once weekly doses (21, 14, and 7 days before surgery) plus a fourth dose on the day of surgery

Anemia of critical illness (unlabeled use): Adults: SubQ: 40,000 units once weekly

Symptomatic anemia associated with MDS (unlabeled use): Adults: SubQ: 40,000-60,000 units 1-3 times/week

Anemia of prematurity (unlabeled use): Infants: I.V., SubQ: Dosing range: 500-1250 units/kg/week; commonly used dose: 250 units/kg 3 times/week; supplement with oral iron therapy 3-8 mg/kg/day

Dosage adjustment in renal impairment: The National Kidney Foundation Clinical Practice Guideline for Anemia in Chronic Kidney Disease: 2007 Update of Hemoglobin Target (September, 2007) recommend hemoglobin levels in the range of 11-12 g/dL for dialysis and nondialysis patients receiving ESAs; hemoglobin levels should not be >13 g/dL.

Hemodialysis: Supplemental dose is not necessary. I.V. route is preferred for hemodialysis patients.

Peritoneal dialysis: Supplemental dose is not necessary.

Administration SubQ, I.V.:

Patients with CRF on dialysis: I.V. route preferred; may be administered I.V. bolus into the venous line after dialysis.

Patients with CRF not on dialysis: May be administered I.V. or SubQ

Monitoring Parameters Blood pressure; hemoglobin, CBC with differential and platelets, transferrin saturation and ferritin, serum chemistry (CRF patients)

Suggested tests to be monitored and their frequency: See table.

Test	Initial Phase Frequency	Maintenance Phase Frequency
Hemoglobin	1-2 x/week	2-4 x/month
Blood pressure	3 x/week	3 x/week
Serum ferritin	Monthly	Quarterly
Transferrin saturation	Monthly	Quarterly
Serum chemistries including CBC with differential, creatinine, blood urea nitrogen, potassium, phosphorous	Regularly per routine	Regularly per routine

Additional Information Factors limiting response to epoetin alfa: Delayed onset of erythropoiesis (2-6 weeks to increase hemoglobin), iron deficiency (most patients require iron supplementation); underlying infection, inflammatory or malignant process; blood loss (occult), underlying hematologic disease (thalassemia, refractory anemia, MDS); vitamin deficiency (folic acid or cyanocobalamin), hemolysis, aluminum overload, osteitis fibrosa cystica, and PRCA

Oncology Comment: The American Society of Hematology (ASH) and American Society of Clinical Oncology (ASCO) 2007 updates to the clinical practice guidelines for the use of erythropoiesis-stimulating agents (ESAs) indicate that ESAs are most appropriate when used according to the dosage parameters within the Food and Drug Administration (FDA) approved labeling for epoetin and darbepoetin (Rizzo, 2008). While the previous guidelines addressed only the use of epoetin, the 2007 guidelines also address the use of darbepoetin, which is assessed as being equivalent to epoetin with respect to safety and efficacy. When used as an option for the treatment of chemotherapy-associated anemia (to increase hemoglobin and decrease red blood cell transfusions), therapy with ESAs should begin as the hemoglobin level approaches or falls below 10 g/dL. The ASH/ASCO guidelines recommend following the FDA approved dosing (and dosing adjustment) guidelines and target hemoglobin ranges as alternate dosing and schedules have not demonstrated consistent differences in effectiveness with regard to hemoglobin response. In patients who do not have a response within 6-8 weeks (hemoglobin rise <1-2 g/dL or no reduction in transfusions) ESA therapy should be discontinued.

The guidelines note that patients with an increased risk of thromboembolism (generally includes previous history of thrombosis, surgery, and/or prolonged periods of immobilization) and patients receiving concomitant medications that may increase thromboembolic risk, should begin ESA therapy only after careful consideration. With the exception of low-risk myelodysplasia-associated anemia (which has evidence supporting the use of ESAs without concurrent chemotherapy), the guidelines do not support the use of ESAs in the absence of concurrent chemotherapy.

Dosage Forms Excipient information presented when available (limited, particularly for generics); consult specific product labeling.

Injection, solution [preservative free]:

Epogen®, Procrit®: 2000 units/mL (1 mL); 3000 units/mL (1 mL); 4000 units/mL (1 mL); 10,000 units/mL (1 mL); 40,000 units/mL (1 mL) [contains human albumin]

Injection, solution [with preservative]:

Epogen®, Procrit®: 10,000 units/mL (2 mL); 20,000 units/mL (1 mL) [contains human albumin and benzyl alcohol]

References

Bennett CL, Cournoyer D, Carson KR, et al, "Long-Term Outcome of Individuals With Pure Red Cell Aplasia and Antierythropoietin Antibodies in Patients Treated With Recombinant Epoetin: A Follow-up Report From the Research on Adverse Drug Events and Reports (RADAR) Project,"*Blood*, 2005, 106(10):3343-7.

Bennett CL, Silver SM, Djulbegovic B, et al, "Venous Thromboembolism and Mortality Associated With Recombinant Erythropoietin and Darbepoetin Administration for the Treatment of Cancer-Associated Anemia," *JAMA*, 2008, 299(8):914-24.

Cournoyer D, Toffelmire EB, Wells GA, et al, "Anti-Erythropoietin Antibody-Mediated Pure Red Cell Aplasia After Treatment With Recombinant Erythropoietin Products: Recommendations for Minimization of Risk," *J Am Soc Nephrol*, 2004, 15(10):2728-34.

Dellinger RP, Levy MM, Carlet JM, et al, "Surviving Sepsis Campaign: International Guidelines for Management of Severe Sepsis and Septic Shock: 2008," *Intensive Care Med*, 2008, 34(1): 17-60. Available at http://www.survivingsepsis.org/system/files/images/2008_20International_20SSC_20Guidelines_1_.pdf

Drueke TB, Locatelli F, Clyne N, et al, "Normalization of Hemoglobin Level in Patients With Chronic Kidney Disease and Anemia," *N Engl J Med*, 2006, 355(20): 2071-84.

Feusner J and Hastings C, "Recombinant Human Erythropoietin in Pediatric Oncology: A Review," *Med Pediatr Oncol*, 2002, 39(4):463-8.

Henry DH and Thatcher N, "Patient Selection and Predicting Response to Recombinant Human Erythropoietin in Anemic Cancer Patients," *Semin Hematol*, 1996, 33(1 Suppl 1):2-5.

Joosten E, Van Hove L, Lesaffre E, et al, "Serum Erythropoietin Levels in Elderly Inpatients With Anemia of Chronic Disorders and Iron Deficiency Anemia," *J Am Geriatr Soc*, 1993, 41 (12):1301-4.

Kharagjitsingh AV, Korevaar JC, Vandenbroucke JP, et al, "Incidence of Recombinant Erythropoietin (EPO) Hyporesponse, EPO-Associated Antibodies, and Pure Red Cell Aplasia in Dialysis Patients," *Kidney Int*, 2005, 68(3):1215-22.

Nafziger J, Pailla K, Luciani L, et al, "Decreased Erythropoietin Responsiveness to Iron Deficiency Anemia in the Elderly," *Am J Hematol*, 1993, 43(3):172-6.

National Comprehensive Cancer Network® (NCCN), "Practice Guidelines in Oncology™: Cancer- and Chemotherapy-Induced Anemia Version 2.2009." Available at http://www.nccn.org/professionals/physician_gls/PDF/anemia.pdf

National Comprehensive Cancer Network® (NCCN), "Practice Guidelines in Oncology™: Myelodysplastic Syndromes Version 1.2009." Available at http://www.nccn.org/professionals/physician_gls/PDF/mds.pdf

National Kidney Foundation, "KDOQI Clinical Practice Guidelines and Clinical Practice Recommentaions for Anemia in Chronic Kidney Disease," *Am J Kidney Dis*, 2007, 50 (3):529-30. Available at http://www.kidney.org/professionals/KDOQI/guidelines_anemiaUP/index.htm or http://www.kidney.org/professionals/KDOQI.

Naughton CA, Duppong LM, Forbes KD, et al, "Stability of Multidose, Preserved Formulation Epoetin Alfa in Syringes for Three and Six Weeks," *Am J Health Syst Pharm*, 2003, 60(5):464-8.

Phronmmintikul A, Haas SJ, Elsik M, et al, "Mortality and Target Haemoglobin Concentrations in Anaemic Patients with Chronic Kidney Disease Treated With Erythropoietin: A Meta-Analysis, *Lancet*, 2007, 369(9559):381-88.

Rizzo JD, Somerfield MR, Hagerty LK, et al, "American Society of Hematology/American Society of Clinical Oncology 2007 Clinical Practice Guideline Update on the Use of Epoetin and Darbepoetin," *Blood*, 2008, 111(1):25-41.

Sinai-Trieman L, Salusky IB, and Fine RN, "Use of Subcutaneous Recombinant Human Erythropoietin in Children Undergoing Continuous Cycling Peritoneal Dialysis," *J Pediatr*, 1989, 114(4 Pt 1):550-4.

Singh AJ, Szczech L, Tang KI, et al, "Correction of Anemia With Epoetin Alfa in Chronic Kidney Disease," *N Engl J Med*, 2006, 355(20):2085-98.

Weinthal JA, "The Role of Cytokines Following Bone Marrow Transplantation: Indications and Controversies," *Bone Marrow Transplant*, 1996, 18(Suppl 3):10-4.

◆ **Epogen®** *see* Epoetin Alfa *on page 412*

◆ **Epothilone B Lactam** *see* Ixabepilone *on page 672*

◆ **Eprex® (Can)** *see* Epoetin Alfa *on page 412*

◆ **Epsilon Aminocaproic Acid** *see* Aminocaproic Acid *on page 57*

◆ **EPT** *see* Teniposide *on page 1087*

◆ **Eptacog Alfa (Activated)** *see* Factor VIIa (Recombinant) *on page 446*

◆ **Eraxis™** *see* Anidulafungin *on page 89*

◆ **Erbitux®** *see* Cetuximab *on page 211*

Erlotinib (er LOE tye nib)

Medication Safety Issues

Sound-alike/look-alike issues:

Erlotinib may be confused with gefitinib, imatinib

High alert medication: The Institute for Safe Medication Practices (ISMP) includes this medication among its list of drug classes which have a heightened risk of causing significant patient harm when used in error.

Related Information

Safe Handling of Hazardous Drugs *on page 1517*

U.S. Brand Names Tarceva®

Index Terms CP358774; Erlotinib Hydrochloride; OSI-774

Generic Available No

Canadian Brand Names Tarceva®

Pharmacologic Category Antineoplastic Agent, Tyrosine Kinase Inhibitor; Epidermal Growth Factor Receptor (EGFR) Inhibitor

Use Treatment of locally advanced or metastatic nonsmall cell lung cancer (NSCLC) refractory to at least 1 prior chemotherapy regimen (as mono-therapy); locally advanced, unresectable or metastatic pancreatic cancer (first-line therapy in combination with gemcitabine)

Unlabeled/Investigational Use First-line treatment of NSCLC with known activated EGFR mutation or gene amplification (as single agent or in combination with platinum-based chemotherapy) in patients who have never smoked; treatment of head and neck cancer

Pregnancy Risk Factor D

Lactation Excretion in breast milk unknown/not recommended

Labeled Contraindications There are no contraindications listed within the FDA-approved manufacturer's labeling.

Canadian labeling: Hypersensitivity to erlotinib or any component of the formulation

Warnings/Precautions Hazardous agent - use appropriate precautions for handling and disposal. Rare, sometimes fatal, pulmonary toxicity (interstitial pneumonia, interstitial lung disease [ILD], obliterative bronchiolitis, pulmonary fibrosis) has occurred; symptoms may begin within 5 days to more than 9 months after treatment initiation. Interrupt therapy for unexplained pulmonary symptoms (dyspnea, cough, and fever); discontinue for confirmed ILD.

Liver enzyme elevations have been reported. Hepatic failure and hepatorenal syndrome have also been reported, particularly in patients with baseline hepatic impairment. Monitor liver function; patients with any hepatic impairment (total bilirubin >ULN; Child-Pugh class A, B, or C) should be closely monitored, including those with hepatic disease due to tumor burden; use with extreme caution in patients with total bilirubin >3 times ULN. Dosage reduction, interruption or discontinuation may be recommended for changes in hepatic function. Acute renal failure and renal insufficiency (with/without hypokalemia) have been reported; use with caution in patients with or at risk for renal impairment. Monitor closely for dehydration; monitor renal function and electrolytes in patients at risk for dehydration. Gastrointestinal perforation has been reported with use; risk for perforation is increased with concurrent anti-angiogenic agents, corticosteroids, NSAIDs, and/or taxane based-therapy, and patients with history of peptic ulcers or diverticular disease; permanently discontinue in patients who develop perforation.

Bullous, blistering, or exfoliating skin conditions, some suggestive of Stevens-Johnson or toxic epidermal necrolysis (TEN) have been reported with use. Generalized or severe acneiform, erythematous or maculopapular rash may occur. Skin rash may correlate with treatment response and prolonged survival (Saif, 2008); management of skin rashes that are not serious should include alcohol-free lotions, topical antibiotics or topical corticosteroids, or if necessary, oral antibiotics and systemic corticosteroids; avoid sunlight. Reduce dose or temporarily interrupt treatment for severe skin reactions; interrupt or discontinue treatment for bullous, blistering or exfoliative skin toxicity. Corneal perforation and ulceration have been reported with use; abnormal eyelash growth, keratoconjunctivitis sicca, or keratitis have also been reported and are known risk factors for corneal ulceration/perforation. Interrupt or discontinue treatment in patients presenting with eye pain or other acute or worsening ocular symptoms.

Use caution with cardiovascular disease; MI, CVA, and microangiopathic hemolytic anemia with thrombocytopenia have been noted in patients receiving concomitant erlotinib and gemcitabine. Elevated INR and bleeding events have been reported; use caution with concomitant anticoagulant therapy. Erlotinib levels may be lower in patients who smoke; advise patients to stop smoking. Smokers treated with 300 mg/day exhibited steady-state erlotinib levels comparable to former- and never-smokers receiving 150 mg/day (Hughes, 2009). Concurrent use with CYP3A4 inhibitors and moderate or strong CYP3A4 inducers may affect erlotinib levels; consider alternative agents to CYP3A4 inducers to avoid the potential for CYP-mediated interactions; use with caution in patients taking strong CYP3A4 inhibitors. Consider erlotinib dosage modification if concurrent use with CYP3A4 inhibitors/inducers cannot be avoided. Erlotinib treatment is not recommended in patients with a KRAS mutation; they are not likely to benefit from erlotinib treatment (Miller, 2008; Eberhard, 2005). Product may contain lactose; avoid use in patients with Lapp lactase deficiency, glucose-galactose malabsorption, or glucose intolerance. Safety and efficacy have not been established in children.

Adverse Reactions

Adverse reactions reported with monotherapy:

>10%:

Central nervous system: Fatigue (52% to 79%)

Dermatologic: Rash (75% to 76%; grade 3: 8%; grade 4: <1%; median onset: 8 days), pruritus (13%), dry skin (12%)

Gastrointestinal: Diarrhea (54% to 55%; grade 3: 6%; grade 4: <1%; median onset: 12 days), anorexia (52% to 69%), nausea (33% to 40%), vomiting (23% to 25%), stomatitis (17% to 19%), abdominal pain (11%)

Ocular: Conjunctivitis (12%), keratoconjunctivitis sicca (12%)

Respiratory: Dyspnea (41%), cough (33%)

Miscellaneous: Infection (24% to 34%)

1% to 10%:

Hepatic: ALT increased (grade 2: 4%)

Respiratory: Pneumonitis/pulmonary infiltrate (3%), pulmonary fibrosis (3%)

Significant adverse reactions reported with combination (erlotinib plus gemcitabine) therapy:

Cardiovascular: Deep venous thrombosis (4%), cerebrovascular accident (2%; including cerebral hemorrhage), MI/myocardial ischemia (2%), arrhythmia, syncope

Central nervous system: Fever (36%), depression (19%), headache (15%)

Dermatologic: Rash (69%)

Gastrointestinal: Diarrhea (48%), weight loss (39%), stomatitis (22%), ileus, pancreatitis

Hematologic: Hemolytic anemia, microangiopathic hemolytic anemia with thrombocytopenia (1%)

Hepatic: ALT increased (grade 2: 31%, grade 3: 13%, grade 4: <1%), AST increased (grade 2: 24%, grade 3: 10%, grade 4 <1%), hyperbilirubinemia (grade 2: 17%, grade 3: 10%, grade 4: <1%)

Renal: Renal insufficiency

Respiratory: Dyspnea (24%), cough (16%), ILD-like events (3%)

Miscellaneous: Infection (39%)

Mono- or combination therapy: <1%, postmarketing, and/or case reports (limited to important or life-threatening): Acute renal failure, bronchiolitis, blistering/bullous/exfoliative skin conditions (suggesting Stevens-Johnson syndrome or TEN), corneal perforation, corneal ulcerations, episcleritis, epistaxis, eye lash disorders (ingrown lashes, excessive growth, thickening), gastritis, gastroduodenal ulcers, GI bleeding, GI hemorrhage, GI perforation, hair/nail disorders (alopecia, brittle/loose nails, hirsutism, paronychia), hearing loss, hematemesis, hematochezia, hepatic failure, hepatorenal syndrome, hepatotoxicity, hyperpigmentation, interstitial lung disease, keratitis, melena, peptic ulcer bleeding, pulmonary fibrosis, pulmonary infiltrates, rash (acneiform; sparing prior radiation field), skin fissures, tympanic membrane perforation

Drug Interactions

Metabolism/Transport Effects Substrate of CYP1A2 (minor), 3A4 (major)

Avoid Concomitant Use

Avoid concomitant use of Erlotinib with any of the following: H2-Antagonists; Natalizumab; Proton Pump Inhibitors; Vaccines (Live)

Increased Effect/Toxicity

Erlotinib may increase the levels/effects of: Leflunomide; Natalizumab; Vaccines (Live); Vitamin K Antagonists

The levels/effects of Erlotinib may be increased by: Antifungal Agents (Azole Derivatives, Systemic); Ciprofloxacin; CYP3A4 Inhibitors (Moderate); CYP3A4 Inhibitors (Strong); Dasatinib; Fluvoxamine; Trastuzumab

Decreased Effect

Erlotinib may decrease the levels/effects of: Cardiac Glycosides; Vaccines (Inactivated); Vaccines (Live); Vitamin K Antagonists

The levels/effects of Erlotinib may be decreased by: Antacids; CYP3A4 Inducers (Strong); Deferasirox; Echinacea; H2-Antagonists; Herbs (CYP3A4 Inducers); Proton Pump Inhibitors; Rifampin

Ethanol/Nutrition/Herb Interactions

Food: Erlotinib bioavailability is increased with food. Avoid grapefruit or grapefruit juice (may decrease the metabolism and increase erlotinib levels).

Herb/Nutraceutical: Avoid St John's wort (may increase metabolism and decrease erlotinib concentrations).

Storage/Stability Store at room temperature of 25°C (77°F); excursions permitted to 15°C and 30°C (59°F and 86°F).

Mechanism of Action The mechanism of erlotinib's antitumor action is not fully characterized. The drug is known to inhibit overall epidermal growth factor receptor (HER1/EGFR) - tyrosine kinase. Active competitive inhibition of adenosine triphosphate inhibits downstream signal transduction of ligand dependent HER1/EGFR activation.

Pharmacodynamics/Kinetics

Absorption: Oral: 60% on an empty stomach; almost 100% on a full stomach

Distribution: 94-232 L

Protein binding: 92% to 95% to albumin and α_1-acid glycoprotein

Metabolism: Hepatic, via CYP3A4 (major), CYP1A1 (minor), CYP1A2 (minor), and CYP1C (minor)

Bioavailability: Almost 100% when given with food; 60% without food

Half-life elimination: 24-36 hours

Time to peak, plasma: 1-7 hours

Excretion: Primarily as metabolites: Feces (83%; 1% as unchanged drug); urine (8%)

Dosage Oral: Adults: **Note:** Details concerning dosing in combination regimens should also be consulted. Dose adjustments are likely to be needed when erlotinib is administered concomitantly with strong CYP3A4 inducers or inhibitors. A dose increase to a maximum dose of 300 mg may be required in patients who continue to smoke.

NSCLC (refractory): 150 mg once daily

Pancreatic cancer: 100 mg once daily in combination with gemcitabine

NSCLC, first-line therapy in never-smokers (unlabeled use): 150 mg once daily as monotherapy or in combination with carboplatin and paclitaxel (Herbst, 2005)

Dosage adjustment for concomitant CYP3A4 inhibitors/inducers:

CYP3A4 inhibitors: Consider dose reductions for severe adverse reactions when erlotinib is administered concomitantly with strong CYP3A4 inhibitors (eg, azole antifungals, clarithromycin, erythromycin, nefazodone, protease inhibitors, telithromycin). Dose reduction (if required) should be done in decrements of 50 mg.

Concomitant CYP3A4 and CYP1A2 inhibitor (eg, ciprofloxacin): Consider dose reductions if severe adverse reactions occur.

CYP3A4 inducers: Concomitant administration with CYP3A4 inducers (eg, carbamazepine, phenobarbital, phenytoin, rifamycins, and St John's wort) may require increased doses (increase as tolerated at 2-week intervals);

doses >150 mg/day should be considered with rifampin (the maximum erlotinib dose studied in combination with rifampin was 450 mg); alternatives to the enzyme-inducing agent should be utilized first. Immediately reduce dose to recommended starting dose when CYP3A4 inducer is discontinued.

Dosage adjustment for toxicity: Dose reductions should be made in 50 mg decrements

Diarrhea: Manage with loperamide; Severe diarrhea: Reduce dose or temporarily interrupt treatment

Pulmonary symptoms: Acute onset (or worsening) of pulmonary symptoms (eg, dyspnea, cough, fever): Interrupt treatment and evaluate for drug-induced interstitial lung disease; discontinue permanently with development of interstitial lung disease

Severe skin reaction: Reduce dose or temporarily interrupt treatment

Bullous, blistering or exfoliative skin toxicity, acute or worsening ocular toxicities, or dehydration with risk for renal failure: Interrupt or discontinue treatment

Gastrointestinal perforation, hepatic failure: Discontinue treatment

Dosage adjustment in renal impairment: Interrupt treatment for renal disease due to dehydration; may resume after euvolemia re-established.

Dosage adjustment in hepatic impairment:

The manufacturer recommends the following guidelines:

Patients with normal hepatic function at baseline: Total bilirubin >3 times ULN and/or transaminases >5 times ULN: Interrupt or discontinue treatment

Patients with baseline hepatic impairment:

Total bilirubin >3 times ULN: Use extreme caution

Worsening liver function (not yet severe): Interrupt treatment and/or reduce dose

Severe changes in liver function (eg, doubling of total bilirubin and/or tripling of transaminases): Interrupt or discontinue treatment

A reduced starting dose (75 mg once daily) has been recommended in patients with hepatic dysfunction (AST ≥3 times ULN or direct bilirubin 1-7 mg/dL), with individualized dosage escalation if tolerated (Miller, 2007).

Combination Regimens

Lung cancer, nonsmall cell: Erlotinib-Paclitaxel-Carboplatin (NSCLC) on page 1312

Pancreatic cancer: Gemcitabine-Erlotinib on page 1344

Administration The manufacturer recommends administration on an empty stomach (at least 1 hour before or 2 hours after the ingestion of food) even though this reduces drug absorption by approximately 40%. Administration after a meal results in nearly 100% absorption.

For patients unable to swallow whole, tablets may be dissolved in 100 mL water and administered orally or via feeding tube (silicone-based); to ensure full dose is received, rinse container with 40 mL water, administer residue and repeat rinse (data on file, Genentech; Siu, 2007; Soulieres, 2004).

Monitoring Parameters Periodic liver function tests (transaminases, bilirubin, and alkaline phosphatase); monitor more frequently with worsening liver function; periodic renal function tests and serum electrolytes (in patients at risk for dehydration); hydration status

Dietary Considerations Take this medicine an empty stomach, 1 hour before or 2 hours after a meal. Avoid grapefruit juice.

Additional Information Oncology Comment: According to the National Comprehensive Cancer Network® (NCCN) pancreatic adenocarcinoma guidelines, gemcitabine combination therapy (including gemcitabine plus erlotinib) is an option for patients with good performance status in the treatment of locally-advanced or metastatic pancreatic cancer.

The NCCN guidelines for NSCLC recommend erlotinib as single agent treatment for disease progression after failure of first- or second-line treatment in patients with a performance status of 0-2. Erlotinib may be considered for patients with a performance status of 3. Erlotinib is considered a first-line therapy (alone or in combination with chemotherapy) in patients with advanced or metastatic NSCLC who have never smoked and have known active EGFR mutation or gene amplification.

Factors (in patients with NSCLC) which correlate positively with response to EGFR-tyrosine kinase inhibitor (TKI) therapy include skin rash (due to EGFR-TKI therapy), patients who have never smoked, EGFR mutation, and patients of Asian origin. KRAS mutation correlated with poorer outcome with EGFR-TKI therapy in patients with NSCLC. (Cooley, 2008; Jackman, 2008; Masarelli, 2007; Shepherd 2005)

Emetic Potential Very low (<10%)

Dosage Forms Excipient information presented when available (limited, particularly for generics); consult specific product labeling.
Tablet:
  Tarceva®: 25 mg, 100 mg, 150 mg

Extemporaneous Preparations Erlotinib suspension: A suspension of erlotinib in water may be prepared by dissolving tablets in 100 mL water for oral or feeding tube (silicone-based) administration. To ensure full dose is received, rinse container with 40 mL water, administer residue and repeat rinse.

> Siu LL, Soulieres D, Chen EX, et al, "Phase I/II Trial of Erlotinib and Cisplatin in Patients With Recurrent or Metastatic Squamous Cell Carcinoma of the Head and Neck: A Princess Margaret Hospital Phase II Consortium and National Cancer Institute of Canada Clinical Trials Group Study," *J Clin Oncol*, 2007, 25(16):2178-83.

> Soulieres D, Senzer NN, Vokes EE, et al, "Multicenter Phase II Study of Erlotinib, an Oral Epidermal Growth Factor Receptor Tyrosine Kinase Inhibitor, in Patients With Recurrent or Metastatic Squamous Cell Cancer of the Head and Neck," *J Clin Oncol*, 2004, 22(1):77-85.

> Tarceva® data on file, Genentech

References

Bonomi P, "Erlotinib: A New Therapeutic Approach for Non-Small Cell Lung Cancer," Expert Opin Investig Drugs, 2003, 12(8):1395-1401.

Cooley ME, Emmons KM, Li, H, et al, "Smoking History, Drug Toxicity, and Survival in Non-Small Cell Lung Cancer (NSCLC) Patients Receiving Epidermal Growth Factor Receptor Tyrosine Kinase Inhibitor (EGFI-TKI) Drugs," J Clin Oncol, 2008, 26(15 Supp) [abstract 9570 from 2008 ASCO Annual Meeting].

Eberhard DA, Johnson BE, Amler LC, et al, "Mutations in the Epidermal Growth Factor Receptor and in KRAS are Predictive and Prognostic Indicators in Patients With Non-Small-Cell Lung Cancer Treated With Chemotherapy Alone and in Combination With Erlotinib," J Clin Oncol, 2005, 23(25):5900-9.

Herbst RS, Prager D, Hermann R, et al, "TRIBUTE: A Phase III Trial of Erlotinib Hydrochloride (OSI-774) Combined With Carboplatin and Paclitaxel Chemotherapy in Advanced Non-Small-Cell Lung Cancer," J Clin Oncol, 2005, 23(25):5892-9.

Hidalgo M and Bloedow D, "Pharmacokinetics and Pharmacodynamics: Maximizing the Clinical Potential of Erlotinib (Tarceva)," Semin Oncol, 2003, 30(3 Suppl 7):25-33.

Hughes AN, O'Brien ME, Petty WJ, et al, "Overcoming CYP1A1/1A2 Mediated Induction of Metabolism by Escalating Erlotinib Dose in Current Smokers," J Clin Oncol, 2009, 27(8):1220-6.

Jackman DM, Sequist LV, Cioffrei L, et al, "Impact of EGFR and KRAS Genotype on Outcome in a Clinical Trial Registry of NSCLC Patients Initially Treated With Erlotinib or Gefitinib," *J Clin Oncol*, 2008, 26(15 Supp) [abstract 8035 from 2008 ASCO Annual Meeting].

Massarelli E, Varella-Garcia M, Tang X, et al, "KRAS Mutation is an Important Predictor of Resistance to Therapy With Epidermal Growth Factor Receptor Tyrosine Kinase Inhibitors in Non-Small-Cell Lung Cancer," *Clin Cancer Res*, 2007, 13(10):2890-6.

Miller AA, Murry DJ, Owzar K, et al, "Phase I and Pharmacokinetic Study of Erlotinib for Solid Tumors in Patients With Hepatic or Renal Dysfunction: CALGB 60101," *J Clin Oncol*, 2007, 25 (21):3055-60.

Miller VA, Riely GJ, Zakowski MF, et al, "Molecular Characteristics of Bronchioloalveolar Carcinoma and Adenocarcinoma, Bronchioloalveolar Carcinoma Subtype, Predict Response to Erlotinib," *J Clin Oncol*, 2008, 26(9):1472-8.

Moore MJ, Goldstein D, Hamm J, et al, "Erlotinib Plus Gemcitabine Compared With Gemcitabine Alone in Patients With Advanced Pancreatic Cancer: A Phase III Trial of the National Cancer Institute of Canada Clinical Trials Group," *J Clin Oncol*, 2007, 25(15):1960-6.

National Comprehensive Cancer Network® (NCCN), "Clinical Practice Guidelines in Oncology™: Head and Neck Cancers," Version 2.2008. Accessible at http://www.nccn.org/professionals/physician_gls/PDF/head-and-neck.pdf

National Comprehensive Cancer Network® (NCCN), "Clinical Practice Guidelines in Oncology™: Non-Small Cell Lung Cancer," Version 2.2009. Accessible at http://www.nccn.org/professionals/physician_gls/PDF/nscl.pdf.

National Comprehensive Cancer Network® (NCCN), "Clinical Practice Guidelines in Oncology™: Pancreatic Adenocarcinoma," Version 1.2009. Accessible at http://www.nccn.org/professionals/physician_gls/PDF/pancreatic.pdf.

Pérez-Soler R, Chachoua A, Hammond LA, et al, "Determinants of Tumor Response and Survival With Erlotinib in Patients With Non-Small-Cell Lung Cancer," *J Clin Oncol*, 2004, 22(16):3238-47.

Saif MS, Merikas I, Tsimboukis S, et al, "Erlotinib-Induced Skin Rash. Pathogenesis, Clinical Significance and Management in Pancreatic Cancer Patients," *JOP*, 2008, 9(3):267-74.

Shepherd FA, Rodrigues Pereira J, Ciuleanu T, et al, "Erlotinib in Previously Treated Non-Small-Cell Lung Cancer," *N Engl J Med*, 2005, 353(2):123-32.

Willett CG, Czito BG, Bendell JC, et al, "Locally Advanced Pancreatic Cancer," *J Clin Oncol*, 2005, 23(20):4538-44.

◆ **Erlotinib Hydrochloride** *see* Erlotinib *on page 420*

◆ *Erwinia* **Asparaginase** *see* Asparaginase *on page 111*

◆ **Erythropoiesis-Stimulating Agent (ESA)** *see* Darbepoetin Alfa *on page 308*

◆ **Erythropoiesis-Stimulating Agent (ESA)** *see* Epoetin Alfa *on page 412*

◆ **Erythropoiesis-Stimulating Protein** *see* Darbepoetin Alfa *on page 308*

◆ **Erythropoietin** *see* Epoetin Alfa *on page 412*

Estramustine (es tra MUS teen)

Medication Safety Issues

Sound-alike/look-alike issues:

Emcyt® may be confused with Eryc®

Estramustine may be confused with exemestane.

High alert medication: The Institute for Safe Medication Practices (ISMP) includes this medication among its list of drug classes which have a heightened risk of causing significant patient harm when used in error.

Related Information

Safe Handling of Hazardous Drugs *on page 1517*

U.S. Brand Names Emcyt®

Index Terms Estramustine Phosphate; Estramustine Phosphate Sodium; NSC-89199

Generic Available No

Canadian Brand Names Emcyt®

Pharmacologic Category Antineoplastic Agent, Alkylating Agent; Antineoplastic Agent, Hormone; Antineoplastic Agent, Hormone (Estrogen/Nitrogen Mustard)

Use Palliative treatment of progressive or metastatic prostate cancer

Labeled Contraindications Hypersensitivity to estramustine, estradiol, nitrogen mustard, or any component of the formulation; active thrombophlebitis or thromboembolic disorders (except where tumor mass is the cause of thromboembolic disorder and the benefit may outweigh the risk)

Canadian labeling: Additional contraindications (not in the U.S. labeling): Severe hepatic or cardiac disease

Warnings/Precautions Hazardous agent - use appropriate precautions for handling and disposal. Glucose tolerance may be decreased; use with caution in patients with diabetes. Elevated blood pressure, peripheral edema (new-onset or exacerbation), or congestive heart disease may occur; use with caution in patients where fluid accumulation may be poorly tolerated, including cardiovascular disease (HF or hypertension), migraine, seizure disorder or renal dysfunction. Estrogen treatment for prostate cancer is associated with an increased risk of thrombosis and MI; use caution with history of cardiovascular disease (eg, thrombophlebitis, thrombosis, or thromboembolic disease) and cerebrovascular or coronary artery disease. Use with caution in patients with hepatic impairment (may be metabolized poorly) or with metabolic bone diseases. Allergic reactions and angioedema, including airway involvement, have been reported with use. Patients with prostate cancer and osteoblastic metastases should have their calcium monitored regularly. Estrogen use may cause gynecomastia and/or impotence. Avoid vaccination with live vaccines during treatment (risk of infection may be increased due to immunosuppression). Although the response to vaccines may be diminished, inactivated vaccines may be administered during treatment.

Adverse Reactions

>10%:

Cardiovascular: Edema (20%)

Endocrine & metabolic: Gynecomastia (75%), breast tenderness (71%), libido decreased

Gastrointestinal: Nausea (16%), diarrhea (13%), gastrointestinal upset (12%)

Hepatic: LDH increased (2% to 33%), AST increased (2% to 33%)

Respiratory: Dyspnea (12%)

1% to 10%:

Cardiovascular: CHF (3%), MI (3%), cerebrovascular accident (2%), chest pain (1%), flushing (1%)

Central nervous system: Lethargy (4%), insomnia (3%), emotional lability (2%), anxiety (1%), headache (1%)

Dermatologic: Bruising (3%), dry skin (2%), pruritus (2%), hair thinning (1%), rash (1%), skin peeling (1%)

Gastrointestinal: Anorexia (4%), flatulence (2%), burning throat (1%), gastrointestinal bleeding (1%), thirst (1%), vomiting (1%)

Hematologic: Leukopenia (4%), thrombocytopenia (1%)

Hepatic: Bilirubin increased (1% to 2%)

Local: Thrombophlebitis (3%)

Neuromuscular & skeletal: Leg cramps (9%)

Ocular: Tearing (1%)

Respiratory: Pulmonary embolism (2%), upper respiratory discharge (1%), hoarseness (1%)

<1%, postmarketing, and/or case reports: Allergic reactions, anemia, angina, angioedema, cerebrovascular ischemia, confusion, coronary ischemia, depression, glucose tolerance decreased, hyper-/hypocalcemia, hypertension, impotence, muscle weakness, venous thrombosis

◀ **Drug Interactions**

Avoid Concomitant Use

Avoid concomitant use of Estramustine with any of the following: Natalizumab; Vaccines (Live)

Increased Effect/Toxicity

Estramustine may increase the levels/effects of: Leflunomide; Natalizumab; Vaccines (Live)

The levels/effects of Estramustine may be increased by: Clodronate; Trastuzumab

Decreased Effect

Estramustine may decrease the levels/effects of: Vaccines (Inactivated); Vaccines (Live)

The levels/effects of Estramustine may be decreased by: Calcium Salts; Echinacea

Ethanol/Nutrition/Herb Interactions Food: Estramustine serum levels may be decreased if taken with milk and other dairy products, calcium supplements, and vitamins containing calcium.

Storage/Stability Refrigerate at 2°C to 8°C (36°F to 46°F).

Mechanism of Action Combines the effects of estradiol and nitrogen mustard. It appears to bind to microtubule proteins, preventing normal tubulin function. The antitumor effect may be due solely to an estrogenic effect. Estramustine causes a marked decrease in plasma testosterone and an increase in estrogen levels.

Pharmacodynamics/Kinetics

Absorption: Oral: 75%

Metabolism:

GI tract: Initial dephosphorylation

Hepatic: Oxidation and hydrolysis; metabolites include estramustine, estrone analog, estrone, and estradiol

Half-life elimination: Terminal: 15-24 hours

Time to peak, serum: 2-3 hours

Excretion: Feces (2.9% to 4.8% as unchanged drug)

Dosage Details concerning dosing in combination regimens should also be consulted.

Oral: Adults: Males: Prostate cancer: 14 mg/kg/day (range: 10-16 mg/kg/day) in 3 or 4 divided doses

Combination therapy with docetaxel (unlabeled dose): 280 mg 3 times/day for 5 days (days 1 through 5) of a 21-day treatment cycle for up to 12 cycles (Petrylak, 2004)

Combination Regimens

Prostate cancer:

Doxorubicin + Ketoconazole/Estramustine + Vinblastine on page 1296

Estramustine + Docetaxel on page 1313

Estramustine + Docetaxel + Calcitriol on page 1313

Estramustine + Docetaxel + Carboplatin on page 1314

Estramustine + Docetaxel + Hydrocortisone on page 1314

Estramustine + Docetaxel + Prednisone on page 1314

Estramustine + Etoposide on page 1315

Estramustine-Paclitaxel on page 1315

Estramustine-Vinblastine on page 1316

Estramustine + Vinorelbine on page 1317

Paclitaxel + Estramustine + Carboplatin on page 1388

Paclitaxel + Estramustine + Etoposide on page 1388

Administration Administer on an empty stomach, at least 1 hour before or 2 hours after eating.

Monitoring Parameters Serum calcium, liver function tests; blood pressure

Dietary Considerations Should be taken at least 1 hour before or 2 hours after eating. Milk products and calcium-rich foods or supplements may impair the oral absorption of estramustine phosphate sodium.

Dosage Forms Excipient information presented when available (limited, particularly for generics); consult specific product labeling.

Capsule, as phosphate sodium:

Emcyt®: 140 mg

References

Bergenheim AT and Henriksson R, "Pharmacokinetics and Pharmacodynamics of Estramustine Phosphate," *Clin Pharmacokinet*, 1998, 34(2):163-72.

Floyd JD, Nguyen DT, Lobins RL, et al, "Cardiotoxicity of Cancer Therapy," *J Clin Oncol*, 2005, 23 (30):7685-96.

Hudes GR, "Estramustine-Based Chemotherapy," *Semin Urol Oncol*, 1997, 15(1):13-9.

Lubiniecki GM, Berlin JA, Weinstein RB, et al, "Thromboembolic Events With Estramustine Phosphate-Based Chemotherapy in Patients With Hormone-Refractory Prostate Carcinoma: Results of a Meta-Analysis," *Cancer*, 2004, 101(12):2755-9.

Petrylak DP, Tangen CM, Hussain MH, et al, "Docetaxel and Estramustine Compared With Mitoxantrone and Prednisone for Advanced Refractory Prostate Cancer," *N Engl J Med*, 2004, 351(15):1513-20.

Etoposide (e toe POE side)

Medication Safety Issues

Sound-alike/look-alike issues:

Etoposide may be confused with teniposide

VePesid® may be confused with Versed

High alert medication: The Institute for Safe Medication Practices (ISMP) includes this medication among its list of drugs which have a heightened risk of causing significant patient harm when used in error.

Related Information

Hematopoietic Stem Cell Transplantation on page 1501
Management of Drug Extravasations on page 1447
Safe Handling of Hazardous Drugs on page 1517

U.S. Brand Names Toposar™

Index Terms Epipodophyllotoxin; VP-16; VP-16-213

Generic Available Yes

Pharmacologic Category Antineoplastic Agent, Podophyllotoxin Derivative

Use Treatment of refractory testicular tumors; treatment of small cell lung cancer

Unlabeled/Investigational Use Treatment of lymphomas, acute non-lymphocytic leukemia (ANLL); lung, bladder, and prostate carcinoma; hepatoma, rhabdomyosarcoma, uterine carcinoma, neuroblastoma, mycosis fungoides, Kaposi's sarcoma, histiocytosis, gestational trophoblastic disease, Ewing's sarcoma, Wilms' tumor, brain tumors

Pregnancy Risk Factor D

Lactation Enters breast milk/contraindicated

Labeled Contraindications Hypersensitivity to etoposide or any component of the formulation; pregnancy

Warnings/Precautions Hazardous agent - use appropriate precautions for handling and disposal. **[U.S. Boxed Warning]: Severe myelosuppression with resulting infection or bleeding may occur.** Treatment should be withheld for platelets <50,000/mm^3 or absolute neutrophil count (ANC) <500/mm^3. May cause anaphylactic reaction manifested by chills, fever, tachycardia, bronchospasm, dyspnea, and hypotension. In children, the use of concentrations higher than recommended were associated with higher rates of anaphylactic-like reactions. Infusion should be interrupted and medications for the treatment of anaphylaxis should be available for immediate use. Must be diluted; do not give I.V. push, infuse over at least 30-60 minutes; hypotension is associated with rapid infusion. Dosage should be adjusted in patients with hepatic or renal impairment. **[U.S. Boxed Warning]: Should be administered under the supervision of an experienced cancer chemotherapy physician.** Injectable formula contains polysorbate 80; do not use in premature infants. May contain benzyl alcohol; do not use in newborn infants.

Adverse Reactions

>10%:

Dermatologic: Alopecia (8% to 66%)

Endocrine & metabolic: Ovarian failure (38%), amenorrhea

Gastrointestinal: Nausea/vomiting (31% to 43%), anorexia (10% to 13%), diarrhea (1% to 13%), mucositis/esophagitis (with high doses)

Hematologic: Leukopenia (60% to 91%; grade 4: 3% to 17%; onset: 5-7 days; nadir: 7-14 days; recovery: 21-28 days), thrombocytopenia (22% to 41%; grades 3/4: 1% to 20%; nadir 9-16 days), anemia (up to 33%)

1% to 10%:

Cardiovascular: Hypotension (1% to 2%; due to rapid infusion)

Gastrointestinal: Stomatitis (1% to 6%), abdominal pain (up to 2%)

Hepatic: Hepatic toxicity (up to 3%)

Neuromuscular & skeletal: Peripheral neuropathy (1% to 2%)

Miscellaneous: Anaphylactic-like reaction (I.V. infusion: 1% to 2%; including chills, fever, tachycardia, bronchospasm, dyspnea)

<1%: Anovulatory cycles, back pain; blindness (transient, cortical); CHF, constipation, cough, cyanosis, diaphoresis, dysphagia, erythema; extravasation (induration, necrosis, swelling); facial swelling, fatigue, fever, headache, hepatic toxicity, hepatitis, hyperpigmentation, hypersensitivity, hypersensitivity-associated apnea, hypomenorrhea, interstitial pneumonitis, laryngospasm, maculopapular rash, malaise, metabolic acidosis, MI, optic neuritis, perivasculitis, pruritus, pulmonary fibrosis, radiation-recall dermatitis, rash, seizure, somnolence, Stevens-Johnson syndrome, tachycardia, taste perversion, thrombophlebitis, tongue swelling, toxic epidermal necrolysis, urticaria, weakness

Drug Interactions

Metabolism/Transport Effects Substrate of CYP1A2 (minor), 2E1 (minor), 3A4 (major); **Inhibits** CYP2C9 (weak), 3A4 (weak)

Avoid Concomitant Use

Avoid concomitant use of Etoposide with any of the following: Natalizumab; Vaccines (Live)

Increased Effect/Toxicity

Etoposide may increase the levels/effects of: Leflunomide; Natalizumab; Vaccines (Live); Vitamin K Antagonists

The levels/effects of Etoposide may be increased by: CycloSPORINE; CYP3A4 Inhibitors (Moderate); CYP3A4 Inhibitors (Strong); Dasatinib; P-Glycoprotein Inhibitors; Trastuzumab

Decreased Effect

Etoposide may decrease the levels/effects of: Vaccines (Inactivated); Vaccines (Live); Vitamin K Antagonists

The levels/effects of Etoposide may be decreased by: Barbiturates; CYP3A4 Inducers (Strong); Deferasirox; Echinacea; Herbs (CYP3A4 Inducers); P-Glycoprotein Inducers; Phenytoin

Ethanol/Nutrition/Herb Interactions

Ethanol: Avoid ethanol (may increase GI irritation).

Herb/Nutraceutical: Avoid concurrent St John's wort; may decrease etoposide levels.

Storage/Stability Store intact vials of injection at 15°C to 30°C (59°F to 86°F). Protect from light. Store oral capsules at 2°C to 8°C (36°F to 46°F). Solutions for infusion, at room temperature, in D_5W or NS in polyvinyl chloride, the concentration is stable as follows:

0.2 mg/mL: 96 hours

0.4 mg/mL: 24 hours

Etoposide injection contains polysorbate 80 which may cause leaching of diethylhexyl phthalate (DEHP), a plasticizer contained in polyvinyl chloride (PVC) bags and tubing. Higher concentrations and longer storage time after preparation in PVC bags may increase DEHP leaching. Preparation in glass or polyolefin containers will minimize patient exposure to DEHP.

Etoposide injection diluted for oral use to 10 mg/mL in NS may be stored for 22 days in plastic oral syringes at room temperature. Mix with orange juice, apple juice, or lemonade to a concentration of ≤0.4 mg/mL, and use within a 3-hour period.

Reconstitution Etoposide should be diluted to a concentration of 0.2-0.4 mg/mL in D_5W or NS for administration. Diluted solutions have concentration-dependent stability: More concentrated solutions have shorter stability times. Precipitation may occur with concentrations >0.4 mg/mL.

Compatibility Variable stability (consult detailed reference) in D_5W, LR, NS.

Y-site administration: Compatible: Allopurinol, amifostine, aztreonam, cladribine, doxorubicin liposome, fludarabine, gemcitabine, granisetron, melphalan, ondansetron, paclitaxel, piperacillin/tazobactam, sargramostim, sodium bicarbonate, teniposide, thiotepa, topotecan, vinorelbine. **Incompatible:** Cefepime, filgrastim, idarubicin.

Compatibility when admixed: Compatible: Carboplatin, cisplatin, cisplatin with cyclophosphamide, cisplatin with floxuridine, cytarabine, cytarabine with daunorubicin, floxuridine, fluorouracil, hydroxyzine, ifosfamide, ifosfamide with carboplatin, ifosfamide with cisplatin, ondansetron. **Variable (consult detailed reference):** Cisplatin with mannitol and potassium chloride, doxorubicin with vincristine.

Mechanism of Action Etoposide has been shown to delay transit of cells through the S phase and arrest cells in late S or early G_2 phase. The drug may inhibit mitochondrial transport at the NADH dehydrogenase level or inhibit uptake of nucleosides into HeLa cells. It is a topoisomerase II inhibitor and appears to cause DNA strand breaks. Etoposide does not inhibit microtubular assembly.

Pharmacodynamics/Kinetics

Absorption: Oral: 25% to 75%; significant inter- and intrapatient variation

Distribution: Average V_d: 7-17 L/m^2; poor penetration across the blood-brain barrier; CSF concentrations <10% of plasma concentrations

Protein binding: 94% to 97%

Metabolism: Hepatic to hydroxy acid and cislactone metabolites

Bioavailability: Oral: ~50% (range: 25% to 75%)

Half-life elimination: Terminal: 4-11 hours; Children: Normal renal/hepatic function: 6-8 hours

Time to peak, serum: Oral: 1-1.5 hours

Excretion:

Children: Urine (≤55% as unchanged drug)

Adults: Urine (42% to 67%; 8% to 35% as unchanged drug) within 24 hours; feces (up to 44%)

Dosage Refer to individual protocols:

Children (unlabeled uses): I.V.: 60-120 mg/m^2/day for 3-5 days every 3-6 weeks

AML:

Remission induction: 150 mg/m^2/day for 2-3 days for 2-3 cycles

Intensification or consolidation: 250 mg/m^2/day for 3 days, courses 2-5

Brain tumor: 150 mg/m^2/day on days 2 and 3 of treatment course

Neuroblastoma: 100 mg/m^2/day over 1 hour on days 1-5 of cycle; repeat cycle every 4 weeks

BMT conditioning regimen used in patients with rhabdomyosarcoma or neuroblastoma: I.V. continuous infusion: 160 mg/m^2/day for 4 days

Conditioning regimen for allogenic BMT: 60 mg/kg/dose as a single dose

Adults:

Small cell lung cancer (in combination with other approved chemotherapeutic drugs):

Oral: Due to poor bioavailability, oral doses should be twice the I.V. dose, rounded to the nearest 50 mg given once daily

I.V.: 35 mg/m^2/day for 4 days or 50 mg/m^2/day for 5 days every 3-4 weeks

IVPB: 60-100 mg/m^2/day for 3 days (with cisplatin)

CIV: 500 mg/m^2 over 24 hours every 3 weeks

Testicular cancer (in combination with other approved chemotherapeutic drugs):

IVPB: 50-100 mg/m^2/day for 5 days repeated every 3-4 weeks

I.V.: 100 mg/m^2 every other day for 3 doses repeated every 3-4 weeks

BMT/relapsed leukemia (unlabeled uses): I.V.: 2.4-3.5 g/m^2 or 25-70 mg/kg administered over 4-36 hours

Dosing adjustment in renal impairment:

The FDA-approved labeling recommends the following adjustments:

Cl$_{cr}$ 15-50 mL/minute: Administer 75% of dose

Cl$_{cr}$ <15 mL minute: Data not available; consider further dose reductions

The following guidelines have been used by some clinicians:

Aronoff, 2007:

Cl_{cr} 10-50 mL/minute: Children and Adults: Administer 75% of dose

Cl_{cr} <10 mL minute: Children and Adults: Administer 50% of dose

Hemodialysis:

Children: Administer 50% of dose

Adults: Supplemental dose is not necessary

Continuous ambulatory peritoneal dialysis (CAPD):

Children: Administer 50% of dose

Adults: Supplemental dose is not necessary

Continuous renal replacement therapy (CRRT): Children and Adults: Administer 75% of dose

Kintzel, 1995:

Cl_{cr} 46-60 mL/minute: Administer 85% of dose

Cl_{cr} 31-45 mL/minute: Administer 80% of dose

Cl_{cr} <30 mL/minute: Administer 75% of dose

Dosing adjustment in hepatic impairment: The FDA-approved labeling does not contain dosing adjustment guidelines. The following adjustments have been used by some clinicians:

Donelli, 1998: Liver dysfunction may reduce the metabolism and increase the toxicity of etoposide. Normal doses of I.V. etoposide should be given to patients with liver dysfunction (dose reductions may result in subtherapeutic concentrations); however, use caution with concomitant liver dysfunction (severe) and renal dysfunction as the decreased metabolic clearance cannot be compensated by increased renal clearance.

Floyd, 2006: Bilirubin 1.5-3 mg/dL or AST >3 times ULN: Administer 50% of dose

King, 2001: Bilirubin 1.5-3 mg/dL or ALT or AST >180 units/L: Administer 50% of dose

Koren, 1992: Bilirubin 1.5-3 mg/dL or AST >180 units/L: Administer 50% of dose

Perry, 1982:

Bilirubin 1.5-3 mg/dL or AST 60-180 units/L: Administer 50% of dose

Bilirubin >3 mg/dL or AST >180 units/L: Avoid use

Combination Regimens

Adenocarcinoma, unknown primary:

Brain tumors:

Breast cancer:

Gastric cancer:

Gestational trophoblastic tumor:

Leukemia, acute lymphocytic:

Prostate cancer:
Estramustine + Etoposide on page 1315
Paclitaxel + Estramustine + Etoposide on page 1388
Retinoblastoma:
CCCDE (Retinoblastoma) on page 1252
CE (Retinoblastoma) on page 1255
Sarcoma: VAC Alternating With IE (Ewing's Sarcoma) on page 1416
Soft tissue sarcoma
ICE (Sarcoma) on page 1357
ICE-T on page 1357
IE on page 1358
Testicular cancer:
BEP (Ovarian Cancer, Testicular Cancer) on page 1230
BEP (Testicular Cancer) on page 1230
EP (Testicular Cancer) on page 1311
VIP (Etoposide) (Testicular Cancer) on page 1424

Administration

Oral: Doses ≤400 mg/day as a single once daily dose; doses >400 mg should be given in 2-4 divided doses. If necessary, the injection may be used for oral administration.

I.V.: As a bolus or 24-hour continuous infusion; bolus infusions are usually administered over at least 45-60 minutes. Infusion of doses in ≤30 minutes greatly increases the risk of hypotension. Etoposide injection contains polysorbate 80 which may cause leaching of diethylhexyl phthalate (DEHP), a plasticizer contained in polyvinyl chloride (PVC) tubing. Administration through non-PVC (low sorbing) tubing will minimize patient exposure to DEHP. Concentrations >0.4 mg/mL are very unstable and may precipitate within a few minutes. For large doses, where dilution to ≤0.4 mg/mL is not feasible, consideration should be given to slow infusion of the undiluted drug through a running normal saline, dextrose or saline/dextrose infusion; or use of etoposide phosphate. Etoposide solutions of 0.1-0.4 mg/mL may be filtered through a 0.22 micron filter without damage to the filter or significant loss of drug.

Monitoring Parameters CBC with differential, platelet count, and hemoglobin, vital signs (blood pressure), bilirubin, and renal function tests

Emetic Potential

Oral: Moderate (30% to 90%)

I.V.: Low (10% to 30%)

Vesicant May be an irritant

High Dose Considerations

Comments The etoposide formulation contains ethanol 30.3% (v/v). Etoposide 2.4 mg/m^2 delivers ethanol 45 g/m^2 I.V. Adverse effects may be increased with administration of etoposide to patients with decreased creatinine clearance. Etoposide 400-1600 mg/m^2 has been drawn into plastic syringes undiluted (20 mg/mL) for administration over 3-4 hours. Etoposide 800 mg/m^2 was pharmacokinetically equivalent to etoposide phosphate 910 mg/m^2 in patients with refractory hematologic malignancies.

High Dose I.V.: 750-2400 mg/m^2; 10-60 mg/kg; duration of infusion is 1-4 hours to 24 hours; generally combined with other high-dose chemotherapeutic drugs or total body irradiation (TBI).

Unique Toxicities

Cardiovascular: Hypotension (infusion-related)

Central nervous system: Confusion, somnolence, seizure activity increased

Dermatologic: Skin lesions resembling Stevens-Johnson syndrome, alopecia ▶

◀ Endocrine & metabolic: Metabolic acidosis, parotitis
Gastrointestinal: Severe nausea and vomiting, mucositis
Hepatic: Hepatitis
Neuromuscular & skeletal: Peripheral neuropathy, motor deficits exacerbated
Miscellaneous: Secondary malignancy, ethanol intoxication (infusion-related)

Dosage Forms Excipient information presented when available (limited, particularly for generics); consult specific product labeling.

Capsule, softgel: 50 mg

Injection, solution: 20 mg/mL (5 mL, 25 mL, 50 mL) [contains benzyl alcohol, ethanol 30.5%, polyethylene glycol 300, and polysorbate 80]

Toposar™: 20 mg/mL (5 mL, 25 mL, 50 mL) [contains dehydrated ethanol 33.2%, polyethylene glycol 300, and polysorbate 80]

References

Aronoff GR, Bennett WM, Berns JS, et al, *Drug Prescribing in Renal Failure: Dosing Guidelines for Adults and Children*, 5th ed. Philadelphia, PA: American College of Physicians; 2007, p 99, 171.

Clark PL and Slevin ML, "The Clinical Pharmacology of Etoposide and Teniposide," *Clin Pharmacokinet*, 1987, 12(4):223-52.

de Lemos ML, Hamata L, and Vu T, "Leaching of Diethylhexyl Phthalate from Polyvinyl Chloride Materials into Etoposide Intravenous Solutions," *J Oncol Pharm Pract*, 2005, 11(4):155-7.

Demoré B, Vigneron J, Perrin A, et al, "Leaching of Diethylhexyl Phthalate from Polyvinyl Chloride Bags into Intravenous Etoposide Solution," *J Clin Pharm Ther*, 2002, 27(2):139-42.

Donelli MG, Zucchetti M, Munzone E, et al, "Pharmacokinetics of Anticancer Agents in Patients With Impaired Liver Function," *Eur J Cancer*, 1998, 34(1):33-46.

Floyd J, Mirza I, Sachs B, et al, "Hepatotoxicity of Chemotherapy," *Semin Oncol*, 2006, 33 (1):50-67.

Hainsworth JD and Greco FA, "Etoposide: Twenty Years Later," *Ann Oncol*, 1995, 6(4):325-41.

Joel SP, Shah R, and Slevin ML, "Etoposide Dosage and Pharmacodynamics," *Cancer Chemother Pharmacol*, 1994, 34(Suppl):69-75.

King PD and Perry MC, "Hepatotoxicity of Chemotherapy," *Oncologist*, 2001, 6(2):162-76.

Kintzel PE and Dorr RT, "Anticancer Drug Renal Toxicity and Elimination: Dosing Guidelines for Altered Renal Function," *Cancer Treat Rev*, 1995, 21(1):33-64.

Koren G, Beatty K, Seto A, et al, "The Effects of Impaired Liver Function on the Elimination of Antineoplastic Agents," *Ann Pharmacother*, 1992, 26(3):363-71.

McLeod HL and Relling MV, "Stability of Etoposide Solution for Oral Use," *Am J Hosp Pharm*, 1992, 49(11):2784-5.

Meresse P, Dechaux E, Monneret C, et al, "Etoposide: Discovery and Medicinal Chemistry," *Curr Med Chem*, 2004, 11(18):2443-66.

Perry MC, "Hepatotoxicity of Chemotherapeutic Agents," *Semin Oncol*, 1982, 9(1):65-73.

Toffoli G, Corona G, Basso B, et al "Pharmacokinetic Optimisation of Treatment with Oral Etoposide," *Clin Pharmacokinet*, 2004, 43(7):441-66.

Trissel L, *Handbook of Injectable Drugs*, 13th ed, Bethesda, MD: American Society of Health-System Pharmacists; 2005, p 590-6.

Etoposide Phosphate (e toe POE side FOS fate)

Medication Safety Issues

Sound-alike/look-alike issues:

Etoposide may be confused with teniposide

Etoposide phosphate is a prodrug of etoposide and is rapidly converted in the plasma to etoposide. To avoid confusion or dosing errors, **dosage should be expressed as the desired etoposide dose,** not as the etoposide phosphate dose (eg, etoposide phosphate equivalent to _____ mg etoposide).

High alert medication: The Institute for Safe Medication Practices (ISMP) includes this medication among its list of drugs which have a heightened risk of causing significant patient harm when used in error.

Related Information

Safe Handling of Hazardous Drugs *on page 1517*

U.S. Brand Names Etopophos®

Generic Available No

Pharmacologic Category Antineoplastic Agent, Podophyllotoxin Derivative

Use Treatment of refractory testicular tumors; treatment of small cell lung cancer

Pregnancy Risk Factor D

Lactation Enters breast milk/contraindicated

Labeled Contraindications Hypersensitivity to etoposide, etoposide phosphate, or any component of the formulation; pregnancy

Warnings/Precautions Hazardous agent - use appropriate precautions for handling and disposal. **[U.S. Boxed Warning]: Severe myelosuppression with resulting infection or bleeding may occur.** Treatment should be withheld for platelets <50,000/mm^3 or absolute neutrophil count (ANC) <500/mm^3. May cause anaphylactic reaction manifested by chills, fever, tachycardia, bronchospasm, dyspnea, and hypotension (higher concentrations were associated with higher rates of reactions in children). Infusion should be interrupted and medications for the treatment of anaphylaxis should be available for immediate use. Dosage should be adjusted in patients with hepatic or renal impairment. Use with caution in patients with low serum albumin; may increase risk for toxicities. Doses of etoposide phosphate >175 mg/m^2 have not been evaluated. Use caution in elderly patients (may be more likely to develop severe myelosuppression and/or GI effects. **[U.S. Boxed Warning]: Should be administered under the supervision of an experienced cancer chemotherapy physician.** Safety and efficacy in children have not been established.

Adverse Reactions Note: Also see adverse reactions for **etoposide**. Since etoposide phosphate is converted to etoposide, adverse reactions experienced with etoposide would also be expected with etoposide phosphate.

>10%:
  Central nervous system: Chills/fever (24%)
  Dermatologic: Alopecia (33% to 44%)
  Gastrointestinal: Nausea/vomiting (37%), anorexia (16%), mucositis (11%)
  Hematologic: Leukopenia (91%; grade 4: 17%), neutropenia (88%; grade 4: 37%), anemia (72%; grades 3/4: 19%), thrombocytopenia (23%; grade 4: 9%)
  Neuromuscular & skeletal: Weakness/malaise (39%)
1% to 10%:
  Cardiovascular: Hypotension (5%), hypertension (3%), facial flushing (2%)
  Central nervous system: Dizziness (5%)
  Dermatologic: Skin rash (3%)
  Gastrointestinal: Constipation (8%), abdominal pain (7%), diarrhea (6%), taste perversion (6%)
  Local: Extravasation/phlebitis (5%)
  Miscellaneous: Anaphylactic-type reactions (3%; including chills, diaphoresis, fever, rigor, tachycardia, bronchospasm, dyspnea, pruritus)
<1%, postmarketing, and/or case reports: Acute leukemia (with/without preleukemia phase), anaphylactic-like reactions, back pain, blindness (transient, cortical), cough, cyanosis, diaphoresis, dysphagia, erythema, facial swelling, hepatic toxicity, hyperpigmentation, hypersensitivity-associated apnea, infection, interstitial pneumonitis, laryngospasm, maculopapular rash, neutropenic fever, optic neuritis, perivasculitis, pruritus, pulmonary fibrosis, radiation recall dermatitis, seizure, Stevens-Johnson syndrome, taste perversion, tongue swelling, toxic epidermal necrolysis, urticaria

Drug Interactions

Metabolism/Transport Effects Substrate of CYP1A2 (minor), 2E1 (minor), 3A4 (major); **Inhibits** CYP2C9 (weak), 3A4 (weak)

Avoid Concomitant Use
Avoid concomitant use of Etoposide Phosphate with any of the following:
Natalizumab; Vaccines (Live)

Increased Effect/Toxicity
Etoposide Phosphate may increase the levels/effects of: Leflunomide; Natalizumab; Vaccines (Live)

The levels/effects of Etoposide Phosphate may be increased by: Cyclo-SPORINE; CYP3A4 Inhibitors (Moderate); CYP3A4 Inhibitors (Strong); Dasatinib; P-Glycoprotein Inhibitors; Trastuzumab

Decreased Effect
Etoposide Phosphate may decrease the levels/effects of: Vaccines (Inactivated); Vaccines (Live)

The levels/effects of Etoposide Phosphate may be decreased by: Barbiturates; CYP3A4 Inducers (Strong); Deferasirox; Echinacea; Herbs (CYP3A4 Inducers); P-Glycoprotein Inducers; Phenytoin

Ethanol/Nutrition/Herb Interactions
Ethanol: Avoid ethanol (may increase GI irritation).
Herb/Nutraceutical: Avoid St John's wort (may decrease etoposide levels).

Storage/Stability Store intact vials of injection under refrigeration 2°C to 8°C (36°F to 46°F). Protect from light. Reconstituted etoposide phosphate is stable refrigerated at 2°C to 8°C (36°F to 47°F) for 7 days. Undiluted solutions are stable for 24 hours at room temperature of 20°C to 25°C (68°F to 77°F) when reconstituted with SWI, D_5W or NS; and stable for 48 hours at room temperature when reconstituted with bacteriostatic SWI or NS. Further diluted solutions are stable at room temperature 20°C to 25°C (68°F to 77°F) or under refrigeration 2°C to 8°C (36°F to 47°F) for up to 24 hours.

Reconstitution Reconstitute vials with 5 mL or 10 mL SWI, D_5W, NS, bacteriostatic SWI, or bacteriostatic NS to a concentration of 20 mg/mL or 10 mg/mL etoposide equivalent. These solutions may be administered without further dilution or may be diluted in 50-500 mL of D_5W or NS to a concentration as low as 0.1 mg/mL.

Compatibility Stable in D_5W, NS, sterile water for injection.
Y-site administration: Compatible: Acyclovir, amikacin, aminophylline, ampicillin, ampicillin/sulbactam, aztreonam, bleomycin, bumetanide, buprenorphine, butorphanol, calcium gluconate, carboplatin, carmustine, cefazolin, cefoperazone, cefotaxime, cefotetan, cefoxitin, ceftazidime, ceftizoxime, ceftriaxone, cefuroxime, cimetidine, ciprofloxacin, cisplatin, clindamycin, cotrimoxazole, cyclophosphamide, cytarabine, dacarbazine, dactinomycin, daunorubicin, dexamethasone sodium phosphate, diphenhydramine, dobutamine, dopamine, doxorubicin, doxycycline, droperidol, enalaprilat, famotidine, floxuridine, fluconazole, fludarabine, fluorouracil, furosemide, ganciclovir, gatifloxacin, gemcitabine, gentamicin, granisetron, haloperidol, heparin, hydrocortisone sodium phosphate, hydrocortisone sodium succinate, hydromorphone, hydroxyzine, idarubicin, ifosfamide, leucovorin, linezolid, lorazepam, magnesium sulfate, mannitol, meperidine, mesna, methotrexate, metoclopramide, metronidazole, minocycline, mitoxantrone, morphine, nalbuphine, netilmicin, ofloxacin, ondansetron, paclitaxel, piperacillin, piperacillin/tazobactam, plicamycin, potassium chloride, promethazine, ranitidine, sodium bicarbonate, streptozocin, teniposide, thiotepa, ticarcillin, ticarcillin/clavulanate, tobramycin, vancomycin, vinblastine, vincristine, zidovudine. **Incompatible:** Amphotericin B, cefepime, chlorpromazine, imipenem/cilastatin, methylprednisolone sodium succinate, mitomycin, prochlorperazine edisylate.

Mechanism of Action Etoposide phosphate is converted *in vivo* to the active moiety, etoposide, by dephosphorylation. Etoposide inhibits mitotic activity; inhibits cells from entering prophase; inhibits DNA synthesis. Initially thought to be mitotic inhibitors similar to podophyllotoxin, but actually have no effect on microtubule assembly. However, later shown to induce DNA strand breakage and inhibition of topoisomerase II (an enzyme which breaks and repairs DNA); etoposide acts in late S or early G2 phases.

Pharmacodynamics/Kinetics
Distribution: Average V_d: 7-17 L/m^2; poor penetration across blood-brain barrier; concentrations in CSF being <10% that of plasma

Protein binding: 94% to 97%

Metabolism:
Etoposide phosphate: Rapidly and completely converted to etoposide in plasma

Etoposide: Hepatic, via CYP3A4, to hydroxy acid and cislactone metabolites

Half-life elimination: Terminal: 4-11 hours; Children: Normal renal/hepatic function: 6-8 hours

Excretion: Urine (56%; 45% as etoposide); feces (44% as etoposide and metabolites)

Children: I.V.: Urine (≤55% as etoposide)

Dosage Refer to individual protocols. Adults: **Note:** Etoposide phosphate is a prodrug of etoposide, doses should be expressed as the desired **ETOPOSIDE** dose; **not** as the etoposide phosphate dose. (eg, etoposide phosphate equivalent to _____ mg etoposide).

Small cell lung cancer (in combination with other approved chemotherapeutic drugs): I.V.: Etoposide 35 $mg/m^2/day$ for 4 days to 50 $mg/m^2/day$ for 5 days. Courses are repeated at 3- to 4-week intervals after adequate recovery from any toxicity.

Testicular cancer (in combination with other approved chemotherapeutic agents): I.V.: Etoposide 50-100 $mg/m^2/day$ on days 1-5 to 100 $mg/m^2/day$ on days 1, 3, and 5. Courses are repeated at 3- to 4-week intervals after adequate recovery from any toxicity.

Dosage adjustment in renal impairment:
Manufacturer recommended guidelines:
Cl_{cr} 15-50 mL/minute: Administer 75% of normal dose
Cl_{cr} <15 mL minute: Data are available; consider further dose reductions
Aronoff, 1999:
Cl_{cr} 10-50 mL/minute: Administer 75% of normal dose
Cl_{cr} <10 mL minute: Administer 50% of normal dose
Hemodialysis: Supplemental dose is not necessary
Peritoneal dialysis: Supplemental dose is not necessary
CAPD effects: Unknown
CAVH effects: Dose for Cl_{cr} 10-50 mL/minute (Aronoff, 1999)

Dosage adjustment in hepatic impairment:
Bilirubin 1.5-3 mg/dL or AST 60-180 units: Reduce dose by 50%
Bilirubin 3-5 mg/dL or AST >180 units: Reduce by 75%
Bilirubin >5 mg/dL: Do not administer

Administration Infuse over 5-210 minutes.

Monitoring Parameters CBC with differential, platelet count, bilirubin, renal function

Additional Information Etoposide phosphate 113.5 mg is equivalent to etoposide 100 mg. Dosages should always be expressed, and calculated, as the desired **etoposide** dose.

Emetic Potential Low (10% to 30%)

◀ **Vesicant** May be an irritant

High Dose Considerations

Comments In contrast to etoposide, metabolic acidosis is not a frequent adverse effect of high-dose etoposide phosphate. Etoposide 800 mg/m^2 was pharmacokinetically equivalent to etoposide phosphate 910 mg/m^2 in patients with refractory hematologic malignancies.

High Dose I.V.: 0.5-2 g/m^2 divided into 2 daily doses; maximum single-dose agent: 3.2 g/m^2; generally combined with other high-dose chemotherapeutic drugs.

Unique Toxicities Gastrointestinal: Nausea, vomiting, mucositis

Dosage Forms Excipient information presented when available (limited, particularly for generics); consult specific product labeling.

Injection, powder for reconstitution:
Etopophos®: 100 mg

References

Aronoff GR, Berns JS, Brier ME, et al, "Drug Prescribing in Renal Failure: Dosing Guidelines for Adults," 4th ed. Philadelphia, PA: American College of Physicians; 1999, p 73.

Budman DR, "Early Studies of Etoposide Phosphate, a Water-Soluble Prodrug," *Semin Oncol*, 1996, 23(6 Suppl 13):8-14.

Dorr RT, Briggs A, Kintzel P, et al, "Comparative Pharmacokinetic Study of High-Dose Etoposide and Etoposide Phosphate in Patients With Lymphoid Malignancy Receiving Autologous Stem Cell Transplantation," *Bone Marrow Transplant*, 2003, 31(8):643-9.

Greco FA and Hainsworth JD, "Clinical Studies With Etoposide Phosphate," *Semin Oncol*, 1996, 23(6 Suppl 13):45-50.

Mummaneni V, Kaul S, Igwemezie LN, et al, "Bioequivalence Assessment of Etoposide Phosphate and Etoposide Using Pharmacodynamic and Traditional Pharmacokinetic Parameters," *J Pharmacokinet Biopharm*, 1996, 24(4):313-25.

Schacter LP, Igwemezie LN, Seyedsadr M, et al, "Clinical and Pharmacokinetic Overview of Parenteral Etoposide Phosphate," *Cancer Chemother Pharmacol*, 1994, 34(Suppl):58-63.

Witterland AH, Koks CH, and Beijnen JH, "Etoposide Phosphate, the Water Soluble Prodrug of Etoposide," *Pharm World Sci*, 1996, 18(5):163-70.

◆ **Euflex® (Can)** *see* Flutamide *on page 506*

◆ **Eulexin® (Can)** *see* Flutamide *on page 506*

Everolimus (e ver OH li mus)

Medication Safety Issues

Sound-alike/look-alike issues:

Everolimus may be confused with sirolimus, tacrolimus, temsirolimus

High alert medication: The Institute for Safe Medication Practices (ISMP) includes this medication among its list of drug classes which have a heightened risk of causing significant patient harm when used in error.

U.S. Brand Names Afinitor®

Index Terms RAD001

Generic Available No

Pharmacologic Category Antineoplastic Agent, mTOR Kinase Inhibitor; mTOR Kinase Inhibitor

Use Treatment of advanced renal cell cancer (RCC), after sunitinib or sorafenib failure

Unlabeled/Investigational Use Immunosuppressant following solid organ transplant

Pregnancy Risk Factor D

Lactation Excretion in breast milk unknown/not recommended

Labeled Contraindications Hypersensitivity to everolimus, other rapamycin derivatives, or any component of the formulation.

Warnings/Precautions Hazardous agent - use appropriate precautions for handling and disposal. Noninfectious pneumonitis (sometimes fatal) has been observed with mTOR inhibitors including everolimus; symptoms include dyspnea, cough, hypoxia and/or pleural effusion; promptly evaluate worsening respiratory symptoms; may require dosage modification or corticosteroid therapy; severe symptoms may require discontinuation. Everolimus has immunosuppressant properties; the risk for local, opportunistic, systemic infections, and/or sepsis is increased. Resolve pre-existing invasive fungal infections prior to treatment initiation. Discontinue if invasive systemic fungal infection is diagnosed (and manage with appropriate antifungal therapy). Avoid concomitant use with strong CYP3A4 inducers (eg, dexamethasone, phenytoin, carbamazepine, rifampin, rifabutin, phenobarbital) and strong or moderate CYP3A4 inhibitors (eg, aprepitant, ketoconazole, itraconazole, voriconazole, clarithromycin, erythromycin, telithromycin, atazanavir, nefazodone, saquinavir, ritonavir, amprenavir, indinavir, delavirdine, fosamprenavir, fluconazole, grapefruit juice, verapamil, diltiazem); dosage modification may be needed if concomitant use with CYP3A4 inducers cannot be avoided; avoid concomitant use with P-glycoprotein (P-gp) inhibitors. Use is associated with mouth ulcers, mucositis and stomatitis; avoid the use of alcohol or peroxide based mouthwashes (due to the high potential for drug interactions, avoid the use of systemic antifungals unless fungal infection has been diagnosed).

Everolimus exposure is increased in patients with moderate hepatic impairment; dosage reductions are recommended. Use is not recommended in patients with severe impairment (has not been studied). Elevations in serum creatinine (generally mild) have been observed; monitor renal function. Use with caution in patients with hyperlipidemia; may increase serum lipids (cholesterol and triglycerides). Decreases in hemoglobin, neutrophils, platelets and lymphocytes have been reported with use. Increases in serum glucose are common; may alter insulin and/or oral hypoglycemic therapy requirements in patients with diabetes. Patients should not be immunized with live viral vaccines during or shortly after treatment and should avoid close contact with recently vaccinated (live vaccine) individuals. Continue treatment as long as clinical benefit is demonstrated or until occurrence of unacceptable toxicity.

Adverse Reactions

>10%:

Cardiovascular: Peripheral edema (25%)

Central nervous system: Fever (20%), headache (19%), fatigue (20%)

Dermatologic: Rash (29%), pruritus (14%), dry skin (13%)

Endocrine & metabolic: Hypercholesterolemia (77%; grade 3: 4%), hypertriglyceridemia (73%; grade 3: <1%), hyperglycemia (57%; grade 3: 15%; grade 4: <1%), hypophosphatemia (37%; grade 3: 6%), hypocalcemia (17%)

Gastrointestinal: Stomatitis (44%; grade 3: 4%; grade 4: <1%), diarrhea (30%; grade 3: 1%), nausea (26%; grade 3: 1%), anorexia (25%), vomiting (20%; grade 3: 2%), mucosal inflammation (19%; grade 3: 1%)

Hematologic: Anemia (92%; grade 3: 12%; grade 4: 1%), lymphocytopenia (51%; grade 3: 16%; grade 4: 2%), leukopenia (26%), thrombocytopenia (23%; grade 3: 1%), neutropenia (14%; grade 4: <1%)

Hepatic: Alkaline phosphatase increased (37%), AST increased (25%; grade 3: <1%; grade 4: <1%), ALT increased (21%; grade 3: 1%)

Neuromuscular & skeletal: Weakness (33%)

Renal: Creatinine increased (50%; grade 3: 1%)

Respiratory: Cough (30%), dyspnea (24%; grade 3: 6%; grade 4: 1%), epistaxis (18%), pneumonitis (includes alveolitis, interstitial lung disease, lung infiltrate, pulmonary alveolar hemorrhage, pulmonary toxicity: 14%; grade 3: 4%)

Miscellaneous: Infection (all infections: 37%; grade 3: 7%; grade 4: 3%)

1% to 10%:

Cardiovascular: Chest pain (5%), hypertension (4%), tachycardia (3%), heart failure (1%)

Central nervous system: Insomnia (9%), dizziness (7%), chills (4%)

Dermatologic: Nail disorder (5%), palmar-plantar erythrodysesthesia syndrome ([hand-foot syndrome] 5%), erythema 4%, onychoclasis (4%), skin lesions (4%), acneiform dermatitis (3%)

Endocrine & metabolic: Diabetes mellitus (exacerbation: 2%; new onset: <1%)

Gastrointestinal: Taste alteration (10%), abdominal pain (9%), weight loss (9%), xerostomia (8%), hemorrhoids (5%), dysphagia (4%)

Genitourinary: Urinary tract infection (5%)

Hematologic: Hemorrhage (3%)

Hepatic: Bilirubin increased (3%; grade 3: <1%; grade 4: <1%)

Neuromuscular & skeletal: Limb pain (10%), paresthesia (5%), jaw pain (3%)

Ocular: Eyelid edema (4%), conjunctivitis (2%)

Renal: Renal failure (3%)

Respiratory: Pleural effusion (7%), nasopharyngitis (6%), pneumonia (6%), bronchitis (4%), pharyngolaryngeal pain (4%), rhinorrhea (3%), sinusitis (3%)

<1%, postmarketing, and/or case reports: Aspergillosis, candidiasis; hypersensitivity (anaphylaxis, dyspnea, flushing, chest pain, angioedema); pancytopenia, sepsis

Drug Interactions

Avoid Concomitant Use

Avoid concomitant use of Everolimus with any of the following: CycloSPORINE; CYP3A4 Inducers (Strong); CYP3A4 Inhibitors (Moderate); CYP3A4 Inhibitors (Strong); Natalizumab; Vaccines (Live); Verapamil

Increased Effect/Toxicity

Everolimus may increase the levels/effects of: Leflunomide; Natalizumab; Vaccines (Live); Verapamil

The levels/effects of Everolimus may be increased by: CycloSPORINE; CYP3A4 Inhibitors (Moderate); CYP3A4 Inhibitors (Strong); Dasatinib; P-Glycoprotein Inhibitors; Trastuzumab; Verapamil

Decreased Effect

Everolimus may decrease the levels/effects of: Vaccines (Inactivated); Vaccines (Live)

The levels/effects of Everolimus may be decreased by: CYP3A4 Inducers (Strong); Deferasirox; Echinacea; Herbs (CYP3A4 Inducers); P-Glycoprotein Inducers

Ethanol/Nutrition/Herb Interactions

Food: Avoid grapefruit juice (may increase levels of everolimus).

Herb/Nutraceutical: Avoid St John's wort.

Storage/Stability Store at room temperature of 25°C (77°F); excursions permitted to 15°C to 30°C (59°F to 86°F). Protect from light; protect from moisture.

Mechanism of Action Everolimus has antiproliferative and antiangiogenic properties. Reduces protein synthesis and cell proliferation by binding to the FK binding protein-12 (FKBP-12), an intracellular protein, to form a complex that inhibits activation of mTOR (mammalian target of rapamycin) serine-threonine kinase activity. Also reduces angiogenesis by inhibiting vascular endothelial growth factor (VEGF) and hypoxia-inducible factor (HIF-1) expression.

Pharmacodynamics/Kinetics

Absorption: Rapid, but moderate

Protein binding: ~74%

Metabolism: Extensively metabolized via CYP3A4; forms 6 weak metabolites

Bioavailability: ~30%

Half-life elimination: ~30 hours

Time to peak, plasma: 1-2 hours

Excretion: Feces (80%, based on solid organ transplant studies); Urine (~5%, based on solid organ transplant studies)

Dosage Oral: Adults: RCC: 10 mg once daily

Dosage adjustment for toxicity:

Severe/intolerable adverse reactions: Temporarily reduce dose to 5 mg once daily and/or temporarily interrupt treatment

Noninfectious pneumonitis:

Mild or asymptomatic (radiological changes suggestive of pneumonitis): Continue treatment

Moderate symptoms: Consider interrupting treatment until symptoms improve (may require corticosteroids); may reinitiate at a reduced dose of 5 mg once daily

Severe symptoms: Discontinue treatment and consider corticosteroids until clinical symptoms improve; if appropriate (depending on individual circumstances) may reinitiate at a reduced dose of 5 mg once daily

Dosage adjustment for concomitant CYP3A4 inhibitors/inducers:

CYP3A4 inducers: Avoid concomitant administration with strong CYP3A4 inducers (eg, dexamethasone, phenytoin, carbamazepine, rifampin, rifabutin, phenobarbital) if possible; if coadministration cannot be avoided, consider adjusting everolimus dose upward in 5 mg increments up to 20 mg daily, with careful monitoring. (If the strong CYP3A4 enzyme inducer is discontinued, reduce the everolimus to the dose used prior to initiation of the CYP3A4 inducer.)

CYP3A4 inhibitors: Avoid concomitant administration with P-gp inhibitors or moderate or strong CYP3A4 inhibitors (eg, aprepitant, ketoconazole, itraconazole, voriconazole, clarithromycin, erythromycin, telithromycin, atazanavir, nefazodone, nelfinavir, saquinavir, ritonavir, amprenavir, indinavir, delavirdine, fosamprenavir, fluconazole, grapefruit juice, verapamil, diltiazem).

Dosage adjustment in renal impairment: No adjustment necessary

Dosage adjustment in hepatic impairment:

Moderate hepatic impairment (Child-Pugh class B): Reduce dose to 5 mg once daily

Severe hepatic impairment (Child-Pugh class C): Use is not recommended (not studied in severe hepatic impairment)

Administration Oral: Administer at the same time each day. May be taken with or without food. Swallow whole with a glass of water. Do not chew or crush. Avoid contact with or exposure to crushed or broken tablets.

◀ **Monitoring Parameters** CBC with differential (baseline and periodic), liver function, serum creatinine and BUN (baseline and periodic), fasting serum glucose and lipid profile (baseline and periodic)

Dietary Considerations Avoid grapefruit juice. May be taken with or without food.

Emetic Potential Very low (<10%)

Dosage Forms Excipient information presented when available (limited, particularly for generics); consult specific product labeling.

Tablet:

Afinitor®: 5 mg, 10 mg

References

Amato RJ, Jac J, Geissinger S, et al, "A Phase 2 Study With a Daily Regimen of the Oral mTOR Inhibitor RAD001 (Everolimus) in Patients With Metastatic Clear Cell Renal Cell Cancer," *Cancer*, 2009, 115(11):2438-46.

Kirchner GI, Meier-Wiedenbach I, and Manns MP, "Clinical Pharmacokinetics of Everolimus," *Clin Pharmacokinet*, 2004, 43(2):83-95.

Kovarik JM, Sabia HD, Figuerierdo J, et al, "Influence of Hepatic Impairment on Everolimus Pharmacokinetics: Implications for Dose Adjustment," *Clin Pharmacol Ther*, 2001, 70(5):425-30.

Motzer RJ, Escudier B, Oudard S, et al, "Efficacy of Everolimus in Advanced Renal Cell Carcinoma: A Double-Blind, Randomised, Placebo-Controlled Phase III Trial," *Lancet*, 2008, 372 (9637):449-56.

O'Donnell A, Faivre S, Burris HA 3rd, et al, "Phase I Pharmacokinetic and Pharmacodynamic Study of the Oral Mammalian Target of Rapamycin Inhibitor Everolimus in Patients With Advanced Solid Tumors," *J Clin Oncol*, 2008, 26(10):1588-95.

Tabernero J, Rojo F, Calvo E, et al, "Dose- and Schedule-Dependent Inhibition of the Mammalian Target of Rapamycin Pathway With Everolimus: A Phase I Tumor Pharmacodynamic Study in Patients With Advanced Solid Tumors," *J Clin Oncol*, 2008, 26(10):1603-10.

◆ **Evista®** *see* Raloxifene *on page 1002*

Exemestane (ex e MES tane)

Medication Safety Issues

Sound-alike/look-alike issues:

Aromasin® may be confused with Arimidex®

Exemestane may be confused with estramustine.

Related Information

Safe Handling of Hazardous Drugs *on page 1517*

U.S. Brand Names Aromasin®

Generic Available No

Canadian Brand Names Aromasin®

Pharmacologic Category Antineoplastic Agent, Aromatase Inactivator

Use Treatment of advanced breast cancer in postmenopausal women whose disease has progressed following tamoxifen therapy; adjuvant treatment of postmenopausal estrogen receptor-positive early breast cancer following 2-3 years of tamoxifen (for a total of 5 years of adjuvant therapy)

Pregnancy Risk Factor D

Lactation Excretion in breast milk unknown/use caution

Labeled Contraindications Hypersensitivity to exemestane or any component of the formulation; pregnancy

Warnings/Precautions Hazardous agent - use appropriate precautions for handling and disposal. Not indicated for premenopausal women; not to be given with estrogen-containing agents.

Adverse Reactions

>10%:

Cardiovascular: Hypertension (5% to 15%)

Central nervous system: Fatigue (8% to 22%), insomnia (11% to 14%), pain (13%), headache (7% to 13%), depression (6% to 13%)

Dermatological: Hyperhidrosis (4% to 18%), alopecia (15%)

Endocrine & metabolic: Hot flashes (13% to 21%)

Gastrointestinal: Nausea (9% to 18%), abdominal pain (6% to 11%)

Hepatic: Alkaline phosphatase increased (14% to 15%)

Neuromuscular & skeletal: Arthralgia (15% to 29%)

1% to 10%:

Cardiovascular: Edema (6% to 7%); cardiac ischemic events (2%: MI, angina, myocardial ischemia); chest pain

Central nervous system: Dizziness (8% to 10%), anxiety (4% to 10%), fever (5%), confusion, hypoesthesia

Dermatologic: Dermatitis (8%), itching, rash

Endocrine & metabolic: Weight gain (8%)

Gastrointestinal: Diarrhea (4% to 10%), vomiting (7%), anorexia (6%), constipation (5%), appetite increased (3%), dyspepsia

Genitourinary: Urinary tract infection

Hepatic: Bilirubin increased (5% to 7%)

Neuromuscular & skeletal: Back pain (9%), limb pain (9%), osteoarthritis (6%), weakness (6%), osteoporosis (5%), pathological fracture (4%), paresthesia (3%), carpal tunnel syndrome (2%), cramps (2%)

Ocular: Visual disturbances (5%)

Renal: Creatinine increased (6%)

Respiratory: Dyspnea (10%), cough (6%), bronchitis, pharyngitis, rhinitis, sinusitis, upper respiratory infection

Miscellaneous: Influenza-like symptoms (6%), diaphoresis (6%), lymphedema, infection

<1%: Cardiac failure, endometrial hyperplasia, GGT increased, neuropathy, osteochondrosis, thromboembolism, transaminases increased, trigger finger, uterine polyps

A dose-dependent decrease in sex hormone-binding globulin has been observed with daily doses of 25 mg or more. Serum luteinizing hormone and follicle-stimulating hormone levels have increased with this medicine.

Drug Interactions

Metabolism/Transport Effects Substrate of CYP3A4 (major)

Avoid Concomitant Use There are no known interactions where it is recommended to avoid concomitant use.

Increased Effect/Toxicity There are no known significant interactions involving an increase in effect.

Decreased Effect

Exemestane may decrease the levels/effects of: Saxagliptin

The levels/effects of Exemestane may be decreased by: CYP3A4 Inducers (Strong); Deferasirox; Herbs (CYP3A4 Inducers); Rifampin

Ethanol/Nutrition/Herb Interactions

Food: Plasma levels increased by 40% when exemestane was taken with a fatty meal.

Herb/Nutraceutical: St John's wort may decrease exemestane levels. Avoid black cohosh, dong quai in estrogen-dependent tumors.

Storage/Stability Store at 25°C (77°F)

Mechanism of Action Exemestane is an irreversible, steroidal aromatase inactivator. It prevents conversion of androgens to estrogens by tying up the enzyme aromatase. In breast cancers where growth is estrogen-dependent, this medicine will lower circulating estrogens.

◀ **Pharmacodynamics/Kinetics**
Absorption: Rapid and moderate (~42%) following oral administration; absorption increases ~40% following high-fat meal

Distribution: Extensive

Protein binding: 90%, primarily to albumin and α_1-acid glycoprotein

Metabolism: Extensively hepatic; oxidation (CYP3A4) of methylene group, reduction of 17-keto group with formation of many secondary metabolites; metabolites are inactive

Half-life elimination: 24 hours

Time to peak: Women with breast cancer: 1.2 hours

Excretion: Urine (<1% as unchanged drug, 39% to 45% as metabolites); feces (36% to 48%)

Dosage Adults: Oral: 25 mg once daily

Dosage adjustment with CYP3A4 inducers: 50 mg once daily when used with potent inducers (eg, rifampin, phenytoin)

Dosing adjustment in renal/hepatic impairment: Safety of chronic doses has not been studied

Administration Administer after a meal.

Dietary Considerations Take after a meal; patients on aromatase inhibitor therapy should receive vitamin D and calcium supplements.

Dosage Forms Excipient information presented when available (limited, particularly for generics); consult specific product labeling.

Tablet: 25 mg

References

Buzdar AU, Robertson JF, Eiermann W, et al, "An Overview of the Pharmacology and Pharmacokinetics of the Newer Generation Aromatase Inhibitors Anastrozole, Letrozole, and Exemestane," *Cancer*, 2002, 95(9):2006-16.

Morandi P, Rouzier R, Altundag K, et al, "The Role of Aromatase Inhibitors in the Adjuvant Treatment of Breast Carcinoma: The M. D. Anderson Cancer Center Evidence-Based Approach," *Cancer*, 2004, 101(7):1482-9.

Winer EP, Hudis C, Burstein HJ, et al, "American Society of Clinical Oncology Technology Assessment on the Use of Aromatase Inhibitors as Adjuvant Therapy for Postmenopausal Women With Hormone Receptor-Positive Breast Cancer: Status Report 2004," *J Clin Oncol*, 2005, 23(3):619-29.

◆ **Exjade®** see Deferasirox on page 330

◆ **Extina®** see Ketoconazole on page 677

Factor VIIa (Recombinant) (FAK ter SEV en aye ree KOM be nant)

Medication Safety Issues

Sound-alike/look-alike issues:

NovoSeven® may be confused with Novacet®

U.S. Brand Names NovoSeven [DSC]; NovoSeven® RT

Index Terms Coagulation Factor VIIa; Eptacog Alfa (Activated); rFVIIa

Generic Available No

Canadian Brand Names Niastase®

Pharmacologic Category Antihemophilic Agent; Blood Product

Use Treatment of bleeding episodes and prevention of bleeding in surgical interventions in patients with hemophilia A or B with inhibitors to factor VIII or factor IX, acquired hemophilia, and in patients with congenital factor VII deficiency

Unlabeled/Investigational Use Reduction of hematoma growth in patients with acute intracerebral hemorrhage, warfarin-related intracerebral hemorrhage

Pregnancy Risk Factor C

Lactation Excretion in breast milk unknown/not recommended

Labeled Contraindications There are no contraindications listed within the FDA-approved labeling.

Warnings/Precautions Use with caution in patients with known hypersensitivity to mouse, hamster, or bovine proteins, or factor VIIa, or any components of the product. Patients should be monitored for signs and symptoms of activation of the coagulation system or thrombosis. Thrombotic events may be increased in patients with disseminated intravascular coagulation (DIC), advanced atherosclerotic disease, sepsis, crush injury, or concomitant treatment with prothrombin complex concentrates. Decreased dosage or discontinuation is warranted in confirmed DIC. Efficacy with prolonged infusions and data evaluating this agent's long-term adverse effects are limited.

Adverse Reactions

1% to 10%:

Cardiovascular: Hypertension

Central nervous system: Fever

Hematologic: Hemorrhage, plasma fibrinogen decreased

Neuromuscular & skeletal: Hemarthrosis

<1%: Abnormal renal function, allergic reactions, arthrosis, bradycardia, coagulation disorder, disseminated intravascular coagulation (DIC), edema, fibrinolysis increased, gastrointestinal bleeding, headache, hypotension, injection site reactions, intracranial hemorrhage, localized phlebitis, pain, pneumonia, prothrombin decreased, pruritus, purpura, rash, splenic hematoma, therapeutic response decreased, thrombosis, vomiting

Postmarketing and/or case reports: Anaphylactic reaction, arterial thrombosis, cerebral infarction and/or ischemia, consumptive coagulopathy, deep vein thrombosis, hypersensitivity, MI, myocardial ischemia, pulmonary embolism, thrombophlebitis

Drug Interactions

Avoid Concomitant Use There are no known interactions where it is recommended to avoid concomitant use.

Increased Effect/Toxicity There are no known significant interactions involving an increase in effect.

Decreased Effect There are no known significant interactions involving a decrease in effect.

Storage/Stability

NovoSeven®: Store under refrigeration at 2°C to 8°C (36°F to 46°F). Protect from light. Reconstituted solutions may be stored at room temperature or under refrigeration, but must be infused within 3 hours of reconstitution. Do not freeze reconstituted solutions. Do not store reconstituted solutions in syringes.

NovoSeven® RT: Prior to reconstitution, store under refrigeration or between 2°C to 25°C (36°F to 77°F). Protect from light. Reconstituted solutions may be stored at room temperature or under refrigeration, but must be infused within 3 hours of reconstitution. Do not freeze reconstituted solutions. Do not store reconstituted solutions in syringes.

Reconstitution Prior to reconstitution, bring vials to room temperature. Add recommended diluent along wall of vial; do not inject directly onto powder. Gently swirl until dissolved.

NovoSeven®: Reconstitute each vial to a final concentration of 0.6 mg/mL as follows:

1.2 mg vial: 2.2 mL sterile water
2.4 mg vial: 4.3 mL sterile water
4.8 mg vial: 8.5 mL sterile water

NovoSeven® RT: Reconstitute each vial to a final concentration of 1 mg/mL using the provided histidine diluent as follows:

1 mg vial: 1.1 mL histidine diluent
2 mg vial: 2.1 mL histidine diluent
5 mg vial: 5.2 mL histidine diluent

Mechanism of Action Recombinant factor VIIa, a vitamin K-dependent glycoprotein, promotes hemostasis by activating the extrinsic pathway of the coagulation cascade. It replaces deficient activated coagulation factor VII, which complexes with tissue factor and may activate coagulation factor X to Xa and factor IX to IXa. When complexed with other factors, coagulation factor Xa converts prothrombin to thrombin, a key step in the formation of a fibrin-platelet hemostatic plug.

Pharmacodynamics/Kinetics

Distribution: V_d: 103 mL/kg (78-139)

Half-life elimination: 2.3 hours (1.7-2.7)

Excretion: Clearance: 33 mL/kg/hour (27-49)

Dosage Children and Adults: I.V. administration only:

Hemophilia A or B with inhibitors:

Bleeding episodes: 90 mcg/kg every 2 hours until hemostasis is achieved or until the treatment is judged ineffective. The dose and interval may be adjusted based upon the severity of bleeding and the degree of hemostasis achieved. For patients experiencing severe bleeds, dosing should be continued at 3- to 6-hour intervals after hemostasis has been achieved and the duration of dosing should be minimized.

Surgical interventions: 90 mcg/kg immediately before surgery; repeat at 2-hour intervals for the duration of surgery. Continue every 2 hours for 48 hours, then every 2-6 hours until healed for minor surgery; continue every 2 hours for 5 days, then every 4 hours until healed for major surgery.

Congenital factor VII deficiency: Bleeding episodes and surgical interventions: 15-30 mcg/kg every 4-6 hours until hemostasis. Doses as low as 10 mcg/kg have been effective.

Acquired hemophilia: 70-90 mcg/kg every 2-3 hours until hemostasis is achieved

Intracerebral hemorrhage (warfarin-related) (unlabeled use; Freeman, 2004; Ilyas, 2008): 10-100 mcg/kg (see **"Note"** below) administered concurrently with I.V. vitamin K (to correct the non-factor VII coagulation factors).

Note: Lower doses (10-20 mcg/kg) are generally preferred given the higher risk of thromboembolic complications with higher doses; response is highly variable; monitor INR frequently after administration since rebound increases in INR occur quickly given the short half-life of rFVIIa; duration of INR correction is dose dependent.

Administration I.V. administration only; bolus over 2-5 minutes. Administer within 3 hours after reconstitution.

Monitoring Parameters Monitor for evidence of hemostasis; although the prothrombin time, aPTT, and factor VII clotting activity have no correlation with achieving hemostasis, these parameters may be useful as adjunct tests to evaluate efficacy and guide dose or interval adjustments

Dietary Considerations Contains sodium 0.44 mEq/mg rFVIIa

Product Availability

Novoseven® RT: FDA approved May 2008; formulation is currently available. Novo Nordisk® is replacing Novoseven® with Novoseven® RT, a room temperature formulation that allows the product to be stored either refrigerated or at room temperature (2°C to 25°C/36°F to 77°F) prior to reconstitution. The previously available Novoseven® required refrigeration prior to reconstitution.

Dosage Forms Excipient information presented when available (limited, particularly for generics); consult specific product labeling. [DSC] = Discontinued product

Injection, powder for reconstitution [preservative free]:

NovoSeven®: 1.2 mg, 2.4 mg, 4.8 mg [contains sodium 0.44 mEq/mg rFVIIa, polysorbate 80] [DSC]

NovoSeven® RT:

1 mg [contains polysorbate 80, sodium 0.4 mEq/mg rFVIIa, sucrose 10 mg/vial]

2 mg [contains polysorbate 80, sodium 0.4 mEq/mg rFVIIa, sucrose 20 mg/vial]

5 mg [contains polysorbate 80, sodium 0.4 mEq/mg rFVIIa, sucrose 50 mg/vial]

References

Broderick J, Connolly S, Feldmann E, et al, "Guidelines for the Management of Spontaneous Intracerebral Hemorrhage in Adults: 2007 Update: A Guideline From the American Heart Association/American Stroke Association Stroke Council, High Blood Pressure Research Council, and the Quality of Care and Outcomes in Research Interdisciplinary Working Group," *Stroke*, 2007, 38(6):2001-23. Available at http://stroke.ahajournals.org/cgi/content/short/STROKEAHA.107.183689.

Freeman WD, Brott TG, Barrett KM, et al, "Recombinant Factor VIIa for Rapid Reversal of Warfarin Anticoagulation in Acute Intracranial Hemorrhage," *Mayo Clin Proc*, 2004, 79(12):1495-500.

Ilyas C, Beyer GM, Dutton RP, et al, "Recombinant Factor VIIa for Warfarin-Associated Intracranial Bleeding," *J Clin Anesth*, 2008, 20(4):276-9.

Mayer SA, Brun NC, Begtrup K, et al, "Efficacy and Safety of Recombinant Activated Factor VII for Acute Intracerebral Hemorrhage," *N Engl J Med*, 2008, 358(20):2127-37.

Mayer SA, Brun NC, Begtrup K, et al, "Recombinant Activated Factor VII for Acute Intracerebral Hemorrhage," *N Engl J Med*, 2005, 352(8):777-85.

Mohr AM, Holcomb JB, Dutton RP, et al, "Recombinant Activated Factor VIIa and Hemostasis in Critical Care: A Focus on Trauma," *Crit Care*, 2005, 9 (Suppl 5):37-42.

◆ **Factor VIII (Human)** see Antihemophilic Factor (Human) on page 91

◆ **Factor VIII (Recombinant)** see Antihemophilic Factor (Recombinant) on page 93

Factor IX (FAK ter nyne)

U.S. Brand Names AlphaNine® SD; BeneFix®; Mononine®

Index Terms Factor IX Concentrate

Generic Available No

Canadian Brand Names BeneFix®; Immunine® VH; Mononine®

Pharmacologic Category Antihemophilic Agent; Blood Product Derivative

Use Control bleeding in patients with factor IX deficiency (hemophilia B or Christmas disease)

Pregnancy Risk Factor C

Labeled Contraindications Hypersensitivity to mouse protein (Mononine®) or hamster protein (BeneFix®)

Warnings/Precautions Hypersensitivity and anaphylactic reactions have been reported with use. Delayed reactions (up to 20 days after infusion) in previously untreated patients may also occur. Due to potential for allergic reactions, the initial ~10-20 administrations should be performed under appropriate medical supervision. The development of factor IX antibodies (or inhibitors) has been reported with factor IX therapy; the risk of severe hypersensitivity reactions occurring may be greater in these patients. Patients experiencing allergic reactions should be evaluated for factor IX inhibitors.

Observe closely for signs or symptoms of intravascular coagulation or thrombosis; risk is generally associated with the use of factor IX complex concentrates (containing therapeutic amounts of additional factors); however, potential risk exists with use of factor IX products (containing only factor IX). Use with caution when administering to patients with liver disease, post-operatively, neonates, or patients at risk of thromboembolic phenomena, disseminated intravascular coagulation or patients with signs of fibrinolysis due to the potential risk of thromboembolic complications.

Factor IX is **NOT INDICATED** for the treatment or reversal of coumarin-induced anticoagulation, hemophilia A patients with factor VIII inhibitors, or patients in a hemorrhagic state caused by reduced production of liver-dependent coagulation factors (eg, hepatitis, cirrhosis). AlphaNine® SD and Mononine® contain **nondetectable levels of factors II, VII, and X** and are, therefore, **NOT INDICATED** for replacement therapy of any of these clotting factors. AlphaNine® SD and Mononine® are products of human plasma and may potentially contain infectious agents which could transmit disease. Screening of donors, as well as testing and/or inactivation or removal of certain viruses, reduces the risk. Infections thought to be transmitted by this product should be reported to the manufacturer. Safety and efficacy have not been established with factor IX products in immune tolerance induction. Nephrotic syndrome has occurred following immune tolerance induction in patients with factor IX inhibitors and a history of allergic reactions to therapy.

Adverse Reactions Frequency not defined.

Cardiovascular: Cyanosis, flushing, hypotension, chest tightness, thrombosis

Central nervous system: Chills, dizziness, drowsiness, fever (including transient fever following rapid administration), headache, lethargy, light-headedness, somnolence

Dermatologic: Angioedema, photosensitivity reaction, rash, urticaria

Gastrointestinal: Abnormal taste, diarrhea, nausea, vomiting

Hematologic: Disseminated intravascular coagulation (DIC)

Hepatic: Alkaline phosphatase increased, ALT increased, AST increased

Local: Injection site reactions: Cellulitis, discomfort, pain, phlebitis, stinging

Neuromuscular & skeletal: Neck tightness, paresthesia, rigors

Ocular: Visual disturbance

Respiratory: Allergic rhinitis, asthma, cough, dyspnea, hypoxia, laryngeal edema, lung disorder

Miscellaneous: Allergic reaction, anaphylaxis, burning sensation in jaw/skull, factor IX inhibitor development, hypersensitivity reaction

Postmarketing and/or case reports: HAV seroconversion, inadequate response/recovery, nephrotic syndrome (associated with immune tolerance induction), parvovirus B19 seroconversion, renal infarction

Drug Interactions

Avoid Concomitant Use

Avoid concomitant use of Factor IX with any of the following: Aminocaproic Acid

Increased Effect/Toxicity

The levels/effects of Factor IX may be increased by: Aminocaproic Acid

Decreased Effect There are no known significant interactions involving a decrease in effect.

Storage/Stability When stored at refrigerator temperature, 2°C to 8°C (36°F to 46°F), coagulation factor IX is stable for the period indicated by the expiration date on its label. Avoid freezing which may damage container for the diluent.

AlphaNine® SD: May also be stored at room temperature not to exceed 30°C (86°F) for up to 1 month,

BeneFix®: May also be stored at room temperature not to exceed 25°C (77°F) for up to 6 months. Reconstituted solution at room temperature should be used within 3 hours.

Mononine®: May also be stored at room temperature not to exceed 25°C (77°F) for up to 1 month.

Reconstitution Refer to instructions for individual products. Diluent and factor IX complex should come to room temperature before combining.

Mechanism of Action Replaces deficient clotting factor IX. Hemophilia B, or Christmas disease, is an X-linked inherited disorder of blood coagulation characterized by insufficient or abnormal synthesis of the clotting protein factor IX. Factor IX is a vitamin K-dependent coagulation factor which is synthesized in the liver. Factor IX is activated by factor XIa in the intrinsic coagulation pathway. Activated factor IX (IXa), in combination with factor VII:C activates factor X to Xa, resulting ultimately in the conversion of prothrombin to thrombin and the formation of a fibrin clot. The infusion of exogenous factor IX to replace the deficiency present in hemophilia B temporarily restores hemostasis.

Pharmacodynamics/Kinetics Half-life elimination: IX component: Adults: 21-31 hours; children: 14-28 hours

Dosage Dosage is expressed in int. units of factor IX activity; dosing must be individualized based on severity of factor IX deficiency, extent and location of bleeding, and clinical status of patient. I.V.:

Formula for int. units required to raise blood level %:

AlphaNine® SD, Mononine®: Children and Adults:

Number of factor IX int. units required = body weight (in kg) x desired factor IX level increase (int. units/dL or % of normal) x 1 int. unit/kg

For example, for a 100% level a 70 kg patient who has an actual level of 20%: Number of factor IX int. units needed = 70 kg x 80% x 1 int. unit/kg = 5600 int. units

BeneFix®:

Children <15 years:

Number of factor IX int. units required = body weight (in kg) x desired factor IX level increase (int. units/dL or % of normal) x 1.4 int. units/kg

Children ≥15 years and Adults:

Number of factor IX int. units required = body weight (in kg) x desired factor IX level increase (int. units/dL or % of normal) x 1.3 int. units/kg

Guidelines: As a general rule, the level of factor IX required for treatment of different conditions is listed below:

Minor spontaneous hemorrhage, prophylaxis:

Desired levels of factor IX for hemostasis: 15% to 25%

Initial loading dose to achieve desired level: 20-30 int. units/kg

Frequency of dosing: Every 12-24 hours if necessary

Duration of treatment: 1-2 days

Moderate hemorrhage:

Desired levels of factor IX for hemostasis: 25% to 50%

Initial loading dose to achieve desired level: 25-50 int. units/kg

Frequency of dosing: Every 12-24 hours

Duration of treatment: 2-7 days

◀ Major hemorrhage:
Desired levels of factor IX for hemostasis: >50%
Initial loading dose to achieve desired level: 30-50 int. units/kg
Frequency of dosing: Every 12-24 hours, depending on half-life and measured factor IX levels (after 3-5 days, maintain at least 20% activity)
Duration of treatment: 7-10 days, depending upon nature of insult
Surgery or major trauma:
Desired levels of factor IX for hemostasis: 50% to 100%
Initial loading dose to achieve desired level: 50-100 int. units/kg
Frequency of dosing: Every 12-24 hours or every 18-30 hours, depending on half-life and measured factor IX levels
Duration of treatment: 7-10 days, depending upon nature of insult

Administration Solution should be infused at room temperature
I.V. administration only: Should be infused **slowly**: The rate of administration should be determined by the response and comfort of the patient.
AlphaNine® SD: Administer I.V. at a rate not exceeding 10 mL/minute
BeneFix®: Administer I.V. over several minutes
Mononine®: Administer I.V. at a rate of ~2 mL/minute. Administration rates of up to 225 int. units/minute have been regularly tolerated without incident (when reconstituted as directed to ~100 int. units/mL).

Monitoring Parameters Levels of factors IX, PTT, BP, HR, signs of hypersensitivity reactions

Dosage Forms Excipient information presented when available (limited, particularly for generics); consult specific product labeling.
Injection, powder for reconstitution (**Note:** Exact potency labeled on each vial):
BeneFix® [contains polysorbate 80; sucrose 0.8%; recombinant formulation; supplied with diluent]
Injection, powder for reconstitution [human derived] (**Note:** Exact potency labeled on each vial):
AlphaNine® SD [contains polysorbate 80; solvent detergent treated; virus filtered; contains nondetectable levels of factors II, VII, X; supplied with diluent]
Mononine® [contains polysorbate 80; monoclonal antibody purified; contains nondetectable levels of factors II, VII, X; supplied with diluent]

References
Shord SS and Lindley CM, "Coagulation Products and Their Uses," Am J Health-Syst Pharm, 2000, 57(15):1403-17.
Srivastava A, "Dose and Response in Haemophilia-Optimization of Factor Replacement Therapy," Br J Haematol, 2004, 127(1):12-25.
White GC, Beebe A, and Nielsen B, "Recombinant Factor IX," Thromb Haemost, 1997, 78 (1):261-5.

Factor IX Complex (Human) (FAK ter nyne KOM pleks HYU man)

U.S. Brand Names Bebulin® VH; Profilnine® SD
Index Terms Prothrombin Complex Concentrate
Generic Available No
Pharmacologic Category Antihemophilic Agent; Blood Product Derivative; Prothrombin Complex Concentrate (PCC)
Use Prevention and control of bleeding in patients with factor IX deficiency (hemophilia B or Christmas disease)
Unlabeled/Investigational Use Emergency correction of the coagulopathy of warfarin excess in critical situations. **Note:** Products contain low or nontherapeutic levels of factor VII component.
Pregnancy Risk Factor C

Labeled Contraindications There are no contraindications listed in the manufacturer's labeling.

Warnings/Precautions Thrombosis or disseminated intravascular coagulation (DIC) may occur with use, particularly following surgery. Use with caution in patients with liver dysfunction; may be at increased risk of developing thrombosis or DIC. Products do not contain therapeutic levels of factor VII and should not be used for the treatment of factor VII deficiency. Product of human plasma; may potentially contain infectious agents which could transmit disease. Screening of donors, as well as testing and/or inactivation or removal of certain viruses, reduces the risk. Infections thought to be transmitted by this product should be reported to the manufacturer. Some products may contain heparin. Use with caution in patients with a history of heparin-induced thrombocytopenia type II. Some product packaging may contain natural rubber latex.

Adverse Reactions Frequency not defined.

Cardiovascular: Fatal intracardiac thrombosis (INR reversal [Warren, 2009]), flushing, thrombosis

Central nervous system: Chills, fever, headache, lethargy, somnolence

Dermatologic: Rash, urticaria

Gastrointestinal: Nausea, vomiting

Hematologic: DIC

Neuromuscular & skeletal: Paresthesia

Respiratory: Dyspnea

Miscellaneous: Anaphylactic shock, clotting factor antibodies (development of), heparin-induced thrombocytopenia type II (with products containing heparin)

Drug Interactions

Avoid Concomitant Use

Avoid concomitant use of Factor IX Complex (Human) with any of the following: Aminocaproic Acid

Increased Effect/Toxicity

The levels/effects of Factor IX Complex (Human) may be increased by: Aminocaproic Acid

Decreased Effect There are no known significant interactions involving a decrease in effect.

Storage/Stability

Bebulin® VH: Prior to use, store under refrigeration at 2°C to 8°C (36°F to 46°F); avoid freezing. Following reconstitution, do not refrigerate and use within 3 hours.

Profilnine® SD: Prior to use, store under refrigeration at 2°C to 8°C (36°F to 46°F); avoid freezing; may also stored at room temperature (not to exceed 30°C) for up to 3 months. Following reconstitution, do not refrigerate and use within 3 hours.

Reconstitution Bring diluent and concentrate to room temperature; gently rotate or agitate to dissolve.

Mechanism of Action Replaces deficient clotting factor including factor X; hemophilia B, or Christmas disease, is an X-linked recessively inherited disorder of blood coagulation characterized by insufficient or abnormal synthesis of the clotting protein factor IX. Factor IX is a vitamin K-dependent coagulation factor which is synthesized in the liver. Factor IX is activated by factor XIa in the intrinsic coagulation pathway. Activated factor IX (IXa), in combination with factor VII:C, activates factor X to Xa, resulting ultimately in the conversion of prothrombin to thrombin and the formation of a fibrin clot. The infusion of exogenous factor IX to replace the deficiency present in hemophilia B temporarily restores hemostasis.

◀ **Pharmacodynamics/Kinetics** Half-life elimination: IX component: ~24 hours

Dosage Children and Adults: Dosage is expressed in units of factor IX activity and must be individualized. When multiple doses are required, administer at 24-hour intervals unless otherwise specified. Administer I.V. only:

Formula for units required to raise blood level %:

Bebulin® VH: In general, Factor IX 1 int. unit/kg will increase the plasma factor IX level by 0.8%

Number of Factor IX int. units required = body weight (kg) x desired factor IX increase (% of normal) x 1.2 int. units/kg

Profilnine® SD: In general, Factor IX 1 int. unit/kg will increase the plasma factor IX level by 1%:

Number of Factor IX int. units required = bodyweight (kg) x desired factor IX increase (% of normal) x 1 int. unit/kg

As a general rule, the level of factor IX required for treatment of different conditions is listed below:

Minor bleeding (early hemarthrosis, minor epistaxis, gingival bleeding, mild hematuria: Raise Factor IX level to 20% of normal; generally a single dose required.

Moderate bleeding (severe joint bleeding, early hematoma, major open bleeding, minor trauma, minor hemoptysis, hematemesis, melena, major hematuria: Raise Factor IX level to 40% of normal; average duration of treatment is 2 days or until adequate wound healing.

Major bleeding (severe hematoma, major trauma, severe hemoptysis, hematemesis, melena): Raise Factor IX level to 50 to ≥60% of normal; average duration of treatment is 2-3 days or until adequate wound healing. Do not raise ≥50% in patients who may be predisposed to thrombosis.

Minor surgery: Raise Factor IX level to 40% to 60% of normal on day of surgery then decrease from 40% of normal to 20% of normal during initial postoperative period (1-2 weeks or until adequate wound healing). The preoperative dose should be given 1 hour prior to surgery. The average dosing interval may be every 12 hours initially, then every 24 hours later in the postoperative period.

Dental surgery: Raise Factor IX level to 40% to 60% of normal on day of surgery. One infusion is generally sufficient for the extraction of one tooth; for the extraction of multiple teeth replacement therapy may be required for up to 1 week (See dosing guidelines for Minor Surgery)

Major surgery: Raise Factor IX level to ≥60% of normal on day of surgery; do not raise ≥50% in patients who may be predisposed to thrombosis. Decrease from 60% of normal to 20% of normal during initial post operative period (1-2 weeks), and late postoperative period (≥3 weeks) continuing until adequate wound healing is achieved. The preoperative dose should be given 1 hour prior to surgery. The average dosing interval may be every 12 hours initially, then every 24 hours later in the postoperative period.

Long-term prophylactic treatment: 20-30 int. units/kg once or twice a week may reduce frequency of spontaneous hemorrhage; dosing should be individualized.

Warfarin associated hemorrhage (unlabeled use): I.V.: **Note:** Administer vitamin K (phytonadione) 10 mg by slow I.V. infusion; vitamin K may be repeated every 12 hours if INR is persistently elevated (Ansell, 2008)

Fixed-dose regimen (Yasaka, 2005): INR ≤5: 500 int. units

Adjusted-dose regimen, weight based (Makris, 2001):

INR 2-3.9: 25 int. units/kg

INR 4-5.9: 35 int. units/kg

INR ≥6: 50 int. units/kg

Administration I.V. administration only; should be infused **slowly**. Rate should not exceed 2 mL/minute for Bebulin® VH or 10 mL/minute for Profilnine® SD. Slowing the rate of infusion, changing the lot of medication, or administering antihistamines may relieve some adverse reactions

Monitoring Parameters Levels of factor IX; PT, PTT; signs and symptoms of hypersensitivity reactions, DIC, thrombosis

Additional Information Vaccination with hepatitis A and hepatitis B vaccines are recommended at diagnosis for patients with hemophilia.

Factor IX concentrate containing only factor IX is also available and preferable for this indication. Prothrombin complex concentrates also contain factor II, factor VII, and factor X and are of intermediate purity. Heparin may present in some products to decrease thrombotic effects.

Dosage Forms Excipient information presented when available (limited, particularly for generics); consult specific product labeling. [DSC] = Discontinued product

Injection, powder for reconstitution (**Note:** Exact potency labeled on each vial):
Bebulin® VH [single-dose vial; vapor heated; supplied with sterile water for injection; contains heparin; packaging contains latex]
Profilnine® SD [single-dose vial; solvent detergent treated]

References

Ansell J, Hirsh J, Hylek E, et al, "Pharmacology and Management of the Vitamin K Antagonists: American College of Chest Physicians Evidence-Based Clinical Practice Guidelines (8th Edition)," *Chest*, 2008, 133(6 Suppl):160-98.

Broderick J, Connolly S, Feldmann E, et al, "Guidelines for the Management of Spontaneous Intracerebral Hemorrhage in Adults: 2007 Update: A Guideline From the American Heart Association/American Stroke Association Stroke Council, High Blood Pressure Research Council, and the Quality of Care and Outcomes in Research Interdisciplinary Working Group," *Stroke*, 2007, 38(6):2001-23. Available at http://stroke.ahajournals.org/cgi/content/short/STROKEAHA.107.183689.

Hellstern P, Halbmayer WM, Köhler M, et al, "Prothrombin Complex Concentrates: Indications, Contraindications, and Risks: A Task Force Summary," *Thromb Res*, 1999, 95(4 Suppl 1):3-6.

Lee JW, "Von Willebrand Disease, Hemophilia A and B, and Other Factor Deficiencies," *Int Anesthesiol Clin*, 2004, 42(3):59-76.

Lusher JM, "Thrombogenicity Associated With Factor IX Complex Concentrates," *Semin Hematol*, 1991, 28(3 Suppl 6):3-5.

Makris M and Watson HG, "The Management of Coumarin-Induced Over-Anticoagulation Annotation," *Br J Haematol*, 2001, 114(2):271-80.

Preston FE, Laidlaw ST, Sampson B, et al, "Rapid Reversal of Oral Anticoagulation With Warfarin by a Prothrombin Complex Concentrate (Beriplex): Efficacy and Safety in 42 Patients," *Br J Haematol*, 2002, 116(3):619-24.

Warren O and Simon B. "Massive, Fatal, Intracardiac Thrombosis Associated with Prothrombin Complex Concentrate," *Ann Emerg Med*, 2009, 53(6):758-61.

Yasaka M, Sakata T, Naritomi H, et al, "Optimal Dose of Prothrombin Complex Concentrate for Acute Reversal of Oral Anticoagulation," *Thromb Res*, 2005, 115(6):455-9.

◆ **Factor IX Concentrate** *see* Factor IX *on page 449*

Famciclovir (fam SYE kloe veer)

Medication Safety Issues

Sound-alike/look-alike issues:
Famvir® may be confused with Femara®

U.S. Brand Names Famvir®

Generic Available Yes

Canadian Brand Names Apo-Famciclovir®; CO Famciclovir; Famvir®; PMS-Famciclovir; Sandoz-Famciclovir

Pharmacologic Category Antiviral Agent

Use Treatment of acute herpes zoster (shingles); treatment and suppression of recurrent episodes of genital herpes in immunocompetent patients; treatment of herpes labialis (cold sores) in immunocompetent patients; treatment of recurrent mucocutaneous/genital herpes simplex in HIV-infected patients

Pregnancy Risk Factor B

Lactation Excretion in breast milk unknown/not recommended

Labeled Contraindications Hypersensitivity to famciclovir, penciclovir, or any component of the formulation

Warnings/Precautions Has not been studied in immunocompromised patients or patients with ophthalmic, disseminated zoster, or with initial episode of genital herpes. Dosage adjustment is required in patients with renal insufficiency. Tablets contain lactose; do not use with galactose intolerance, severe lactase deficiency, or glucose-galactose malabsorption syndromes. Safety and efficacy have not been established in children <18 years of age.

Adverse Reactions

Note: Frequencies vary with dose and duration. Single-dose treatment (herpes labialis) was associated only with headache (10%), diarrhea (2%), fatigue (1%), and dysmenorrhea (1%).

>10%:
Central nervous system: Headache (14% to 39%)
Gastrointestinal: Nausea (3% to 13%)
1% to 10%:
Central nervous system: Fatigue (1% to 5%), migraine (1% to 3%)
Dermatologic: Pruritus (≤4%), rash (≤3%)
Endocrine & metabolic: Dysmenorrhea (≤8%)
Gastrointestinal: Diarrhea (5% to 9%), abdominal pain (≤8%), flatulence (1% to 5%), vomiting (1% to 5%)
Hematologic: Neutropenia (3%)
Hepatic: Transaminases increased (2% to 3%), bilirubin increased (2%)
Neuromuscular & skeletal: Paresthesia (≤3%)
<1%, postmarketing, and/or case reports: Anemia, cholestatic jaundice, confusion, delirium, disorientation, dizziness, erythema multiforme, hallucinations, somnolence, Stevens-Johnson syndrome, thrombocytopenia, toxic epidermal necrolysis, urticaria

Drug Interactions

Avoid Concomitant Use

Avoid concomitant use of Famciclovir with any of the following: Zoster Vaccine

Increased Effect/Toxicity There are no known significant interactions involving an increase in effect.

Decreased Effect

Famciclovir may decrease the levels/effects of: Zoster Vaccine

Ethanol/Nutrition/Herb Interactions Food: Rate of absorption and/or conversion to penciclovir and peak concentration are reduced with food, but bioavailability is not affected.

Storage/Stability Store at 25°C (77°F); excursions permitted to 15°C to 30°C (59°F to 86°F).

Mechanism of Action Famciclovir undergoes rapid biotransformation to the active compound, penciclovir (prodrug), which is phosphorylated by viral thymidine kinase in HSV-1, HSV-2, and VZV-infected cells to a monophosphate form; this is then converted to penciclovir triphosphate and competes with deoxyguanosine triphosphate to inhibit HSV-2 polymerase, therefore, herpes viral DNA synthesis/replication is selectively inhibited.

Pharmacodynamics/Kinetics

Absorption: Food decreases maximum peak penciclovir concentration and delays time to penciclovir peak; AUC remains the same

Distribution: V_d: Penciclovir: 0.91-1.25 L/kg

Protein binding: Penciclovir: ≤20%

Metabolism: Famciclovir is rapidly deacetylated and oxidized to penciclovir (active prodrug); not via CYP

Bioavailability: Penciclovir: 69% to 85%

Half-life elimination: Penciclovir: 2-4 hours; Prolonged in renal impairment: Cl_{cr} 20-39 mL/minute: 5-8 hours, Cl_{cr} <20 mL/minute: 3-24 hours

Time to peak: Penciclovir: 0.9 hours; C_{max} and T_{max} are decreased and prolonged with noncompensated hepatic impairment

Excretion: Urine (73% primarily as penciclovir); feces (27%)

Dosage Adults: Oral:

Acute herpes zoster: 500 mg every 8 hours for 7 days (**Note:** Initiate therapy within 72 hours of rash onset.)

Recurrent genital herpes simplex in immunocompetent patients:
Initial: 1000 mg twice daily for 1 day (**Note:** Initiate therapy within 6 hours of symptoms/lesions.)
Suppressive therapy: 250 mg twice daily for up to 1 year

Recurrent herpes labialis (cold sores): 1500 mg as a single dose; initiate therapy at first sign or symptom such as tingling, burning, or itching (initiated within 1 hour in clinical studies)

Recurrent mucocutaneous/genital herpes simplex in HIV patients: 500 mg twice daily for 7 days

Dosing interval in renal impairment:

Herpes zoster:
Cl_{cr} 40-59 mL/minute: Administer 500 mg every 12 hours
Cl_{cr} 20-39 mL/minute: Administer 500 mg every 24 hours
Cl_{cr} <20 mL/minute: Administer 250 mg every 24 hours
Hemodialysis: Administer 250 mg after each dialysis session.

Recurrent genital herpes: Treatment (single day regimen):
Cl_{cr} 40-59 mL/minute: Administer 500 mg every 12 hours for 1 day
Cl_{cr} 20-39 mL/minute: Administer 500 mg as a single dose
Cl_{cr} <20 mL/minute: Administer 250 mg as a single dose
Hemodialysis: Administer 250 mg as a single dose after dialysis session.

Recurrent genital herpes: Suppression:
Cl_{cr} 20-39 mL/minute: Administer 125 mg every 12 hours
Cl_{cr} <20 mL/minute: Administer 125 mg every 24 hours
Hemodialysis: Administer 125 mg after each dialysis session.

Recurrent herpes labialis: Treatment (single day regimen):
Cl_{cr} 40-59 mL/minute: Administer 750 mg as a single dose
Cl_{cr} 20-39 mL/minute: Administer 500 mg as a single dose
Cl_{cr} <20 mL/minute: Administer 250 mg as a single dose
Hemodialysis: Administer 250 mg as a single dose after dialysis session.

Recurrent orolabial or genital herpes in HIV-infected patients:
Cl_{cr} 20-39 mL/minute: Administer 500 mg every 24 hours
Cl_{cr} <20 mL/minute: Administer 250 mg every 24 hours
Hemodialysis: Administer 250 mg after each dialysis session.

Monitoring Parameters Periodic CBC during long-term therapy

Dietary Considerations May be taken with food or on an empty stomach.

Additional Information Most effective for herpes zoster if therapy is initiated within 48 hours of initial lesion. Resistance may occur by alteration of thymidine kinase, resulting in loss of or reduced penciclovir phosphorylation ▶

(cross-resistance occurs between acyclovir and famciclovir). When treatment for herpes labialis is initiated within 1 hour of symptom onset, healing time is reduced by ~2 days.

Dosage Forms Excipient information presented when available (limited, particularly for generics); consult specific product labeling.

Tablet: 125 mg, 250 mg, 500 mg

Famvir®: 125 mg, 250 mg, 500 mg

References

Boike SC, Pue MA, and Freed MI, "Pharmacokinetics of Famciclovir in Subjects With Varying Degrees of Renal Impairment," *Clin Pharmacol Ther*, 1994, 55(4):418-26.

Gill KS and Wood MJ, "The Clinical Pharmacokinetics of Famciclovir," *Clin Pharmacokinet*, 1996, 31(1):1-8.

Hodge RA, "Famciclovir and Penciclovir: The Mode of Action of Famciclovir Including Its Conversion to Penciclovir," *Antivir Chem Chemother*, 1993, 4:67-84.

Luber AD and Flaherty JF Jr, "Famciclovir for Treatment of Herpesvirus Infections," *Ann Pharmacother*, 1996, 30(9):978-85.

Tyring SK, Barbarash RA, Nahlik JE, et al, "Famciclovir for the Treatment of Acute Herpes Zoster: Effects on Acute Disease and Postherpetic Neuralgia," *Ann Intern Med*, 1995, 123(2):89-96.

Tyring SK, "Efficacy of Famciclovir in the Treatment of Herpes Zoster," *Semin Dermatol*, 1996, 15(2 Suppl 1):27-31.

FentaNYL (FEN ta nil)

Medication Safety Issues

Sound-alike/look-alike issues:

FentaNYL may be confused with alfentanil, SUFentanil

Dosing of transdermal fentanyl patches may be confusing. Transdermal fentanyl patches should always be prescribed in mcg/hour, not size. Patch dosage form of Duragesic®-12 actually delivers 12.5 mcg/hour of fentanyl. Use caution, as orders may be written as "Duragesic 12.5" which can be erroneously interpreted as a 125 mcg dose.

Fentora® and Actiq® are not interchangeable; do not substitute doses on a mcg-per-mcg basis.

High alert medication: The Institute for Safe Medication Practices (ISMP) includes this medication among its list of drug classes which have a heightened risk of causing significant patient harm when used in error.

Fentanyl transdermal system patches: Leakage of fentanyl gel from the patch has been reported; patch may be less effective; do not use. Thoroughly wash any skin surfaces coming into direct contact with gel with water (do not use soap).

U.S. Brand Names Actiq®; Duragesic®; Fentora®; Onsolis™; Sublimaze®

Index Terms Fentanyl Citrate; Fentanyl Hydrochloride; OTFC (Oral Trans-mucosal Fentanyl Citrate)

Generic Available Yes: Excludes buccal tablet

Canadian Brand Names Actiq®; Duragesic MAT; Duragesic®; Fentanyl Citrate Injection, USP; Novo-Fentanyl; RAN™-Fentanyl Transdermal System; ratio-Fentanyl

Pharmacologic Category Analgesic, Opioid; Anilidopiperidine Opioid; General Anesthetic

Use

Injection: Relief of pain, preoperative medication, adjunct to general or regional anesthesia

Iontophoretic transdermal system (Ionsys™): Short-term, in-hospital management of acute postoperative pain

Transdermal patch (eg, Duragesic®): Management of persistent moderate-to-severe chronic pain

Transmucosal lozenge (eg, Actiq®), buccal tablet (Fentora®): Management of breakthrough cancer pain in opioid-tolerant patients

Restrictions C-II

Pregnancy Risk Factor C/D (prolonged use or high doses at term)

Lactation Enters breast milk/not recommended (AAP rates "compatible")

Labeled Contraindications Hypersensitivity to fentanyl or any component of the formulation

Transdermal system: Severe respiratory disease or depression including acute asthma (unless patient is mechanically ventilated); paralytic ileus; patients requiring short-term therapy, management of intermittent pain

Transmucosal buccal tablets (Fentora®), lozenges (eg, Actiq®), and/or transdermal patches (eg, Duragesic®): Contraindicated in the management of acute or postoperative pain and in patients who are not opioid tolerant

Warnings/Precautions An opioid-containing analgesic regimen should be tailored to each patient's needs and based upon the type of pain being treated (acute versus chronic), the route of administration, degree of tolerance for opioids (naive versus chronic user), age, weight, and medical condition. The optimal analgesic dose varies widely among patients. Doses should be titrated to pain relief/prevention. When using with other CNS depressants, reduce dose of one or both agents. Fentanyl shares the toxic potentials of opiate agonists, and precautions of opiate agonist therapy should be observed; use with caution in patients with bradycardia or bradyarrhythmias; rapid I.V. infusion may result in skeletal muscle and chest wall rigidity leading to respiratory distress and/or apnea, bronchoconstriction, laryngospasm; inject slowly over 3-5 minutes. **[U.S. Boxed Warning]: Healthcare provider should be alert to problems of abuse, misuse, and diversion.** Tolerance or drug dependence may result from extended use. The elderly may be particularly susceptible to the CNS depressant and constipating effects of narcotics. Use extreme caution in patients with COPD or other chronic respiratory conditions. Use caution with head injuries, morbid obesity, renal impairment, or hepatic dysfunction. **[U.S. Boxed Warning]: Use with strong or moderate CYP3A4 inhibitors may result in increased effects and potential respiratory depression.** Concurrent use of agonist/antagonist analgesics may precipitate withdrawal symptoms and/or reduced analgesic efficacy in patients following prolonged therapy with mu opioid agonists. Abrupt discontinuation following prolonged use may also lead to withdrawal symptoms. Safety and efficacy have not been established in children <16 years of age for the lozenge and <18 years of age for the buccal tablet. **[U.S. Boxed Warning]: Safety and efficacy of the transdermal patch have been limited to children ≥2 years of age who are opioid-tolerant.**

◄

[U.S. Boxed Warning] Actiq®, Duragesic®, Fentora®: May cause potentially life-threatening hypoventilation, respiratory depression, and/or death; Actiq®, Duragesic®, Fentora® should only be prescribed for opioid-tolerant patients. Risk of respiratory depression increased in elderly patients, debilitated patients, and patients with conditions associated with hypoxia or hypercapnia; usually occurs after administration of initial dose in nontolerant patients or when given with other drugs that depress respiratory function.

Transmucosal: Lozenge (eg, Actiq®), buccal tablet (Fentora®): **[U.S. Boxed Warning]: Should be used only for the care of opioid-tolerant cancer patients with breakthrough pain and is intended for use by specialists who are knowledgeable in treating cancer pain.** Not approved for use in management of acute or postoperative pain. **[U.S. Boxed Warning]: Buccal tablet and lozenge preparations contain an amount of medication that can be fatal to children. Keep all units out of the reach of children and discard any open units properly.** Patients and caregivers should be counseled on the dangers to children including the risk of exposure to partially-consumed units.

Transmucosal: Buccal tablet (Fentora®): **[U.S. Boxed Warning]: Due to the higher bioavailability of fentanyl in Fentora®, when converting patients from oral transmucosal fentanyl citrate (OTFC, Actiq®) to Fentora®, do not substitute Fentora®): on a mcg-per-mcg basis for any other fentanyl product. [U.S. Boxed Warning]: Fentora® is contraindicated in the management of acute or postoperative pain, including headache/migraine. Serious adverse events, including death, have been reported when used inappropriately (improper dose or patient selection). [U.S. Boxed Warning]: Patients using Fentora® who experience breakthrough pain may only take one additional dose using the same strength and must wait four hours before taking another dose.**

Transdermal patches (eg, Duragesic®): **[U.S. Boxed Warning]: Indicated for the management of persistent moderate-to-severe pain when around the clock pain control is needed for an extended time period. Should only be used in patients who are already receiving opioid therapy, are opioid tolerant, and who require a total daily dose equivalent to 25 mcg/hour transdermal patch. Contraindicated in patients who are not opioid tolerant, in the management of short-term analgesia, or in the management of postoperative pain. Should be applied only to intact skin. Use of a patch that has been cut, damaged, or altered in any way may result in overdosage.** Serum fentanyl concentrations may increase approximately one-third for patients with a body temperature of 40°C secondary to a temperature-dependent increase in fentanyl release from the patch and increased skin permeability. **[U.S. Boxed Warning]: Avoid exposure of application site and surrounding area to direct external heat sources.** Patients who experience fever or increase in core temperature should be monitored closely. Patients who experience adverse reactions should be monitored for at least 24 hours after removal of the patch.

Adverse Reactions

>10%:

Cardiovascular: Bradycardia, edema

Central nervous system: CNS depression, confusion, dizziness, drowsiness, headache, sedation

Gastrointestinal: Nausea, vomiting, constipation, xerostomia

Local: Application-site reaction erythema

Neuromuscular & skeletal: Chest wall rigidity (high dose I.V.), muscle rigidity, weakness

Ocular: Miosis

Respiratory: Dyspnea, respiratory depression

Miscellaneous: Diaphoresis

1% to 10%:

Cardiovascular: Cardiac arrhythmia, chest pain, flushing, hyper-/hypotension, orthostatic hypotension, pallor, palpitation, peripheral edema, syncope, tachycardia, vasodilation

Central nervous system: Abnormal dreams, abnormal thinking, agitation, amnesia, anxiety, chills, depression, euphoria, fatigue, fever, hallucinations, hypoesthesia, insomnia, lethargy, migraine, nervousness, paranoid reaction, stupor, vertigo

Dermatologic: Alopecia, bruising, cellulitis, erythema, hyperhidrosis, papules, pruritus, rash

Endocrine & metabolic: Breast pain, dehydration, hyper-/hypocalcemia, hyper-/hypoglycemia, hypoalbuminemia, hypokalemia, hypomagnesemia

Gastrointestinal: Abdominal pain, abnormal taste, anorexia, biliary tract spasm, diarrhea, dyspepsia, dysphagia (buccal tablet), flatulence, GI hemorrhage, gingival pain (buccal tablet), gingivitis (lozenge), glossitis (lozenge), ileus, periodontal abscess (lozenge/buccal tablet), stomatitis (lozenge/buccal tablet), weight loss

Genitourinary: Dysuria, urinary incontinence, urinary retention, vaginitis, vaginal hemorrhage

Hematologic: Anemia, leukopenia, neutropenia, thrombocytopenia

Hepatic: Ascites, jaundice

Local: Application site pain, application site irritation

Neuromuscular & skeletal: Abnormal coordination, abnormal gait, arthralgia, back pain, myalgia, neuropathy, paresthesia, rigors, tremor

Renal: Renal failure

Respiratory: Apnea, asthma, bronchitis, cough, epistaxis, hemoptysis, hypoventilation, hypoxia, nasopharyngitis, pharyngolaryngeal pain, pharyngitis, pneumonia, rhinitis, sinusitis, upper respiratory infection, wheezing

Miscellaneous: Hiccups, flu-like syndrome, lymphadenopathy, speech disorder

<1%, postmarketing, and/or case reports: Abdominal distention, amblyopia, allergic reaction, anaphylaxis, angina, anorgasmia, aphasia, bladder pain, blurred vision, bronchospasm, CNS excitation or delirium, cold/clammy skin, dental caries (lozenge), depersonalization, DVT, dysesthesia, ejaculatory difficulty, emotional lability, eructation, esophageal stenosis, exfoliative dermatitis, fecal impaction, flank pain, gum line erosion (lozenge), gum hemorrhage (lozenge), hematuria, hostility, hyper-/hypotonia, laryngospasm, libido decreased, moniliasis (lozenge/buccal tablet), mouth ulceration (lozenge/buccal tablet), myasthenia, nocturia, oliguria, pancytopenia, paradoxical dizziness, physical and psychological dependence with prolonged use, pleural effusion, polyuria, pustules, speech disorder, stertorous breathing, seizure, sputum increased, tooth loss (lozenge), urinary tract spasm, urticaria, vertigo

Drug Interactions

Metabolism/Transport Effects Substrate of CYP3A4 (major); **Inhibits** CYP3A4 (weak)

Avoid Concomitant Use

Avoid concomitant use of FentaNYL with any of the following: MAO Inhibitors ▶

◀ **Increased Effect/Toxicity**

FentaNYL may increase the levels/effects of: Alcohol (Ethyl); Alvimopan; Beta-Blockers; Calcium Channel Blockers (Nondihydropyridine); CNS Depressants; Desmopressin; MAO Inhibitors; Selective Serotonin Reuptake Inhibitors; Thiazide Diuretics

The levels/effects of FentaNYL may be increased by: Amphetamines; Antipsychotic Agents (Phenothiazines); CYP3A4 Inhibitors (Moderate); CYP3A4 Inhibitors (Strong); Dasatinib; MAO Inhibitors; Protease Inhibitors; Succinylcholine

Decreased Effect

FentaNYL may decrease the levels/effects of: Pegvisomant

The levels/effects of FentaNYL may be decreased by: Ammonium Chloride; Rifamycin Derivatives

Ethanol/Nutrition/Herb Interactions

Ethanol: Avoid ethanol (may increase CNS depression).

Herb/Nutraceutical: St John's wort may decrease fentanyl levels. Avoid valerian, St John's wort, kava kava, gotu kola (may increase CNS depression).

Storage/Stability

Injection formulation: Store at controlled room temperature of 20°C to 25°C (68°F to 77°F). Protect from light.

Transdermal patch: Do not store above 25°C (77°F).

Transmucosal (buccal tablets, lozenge): Store at controlled room temperature of 20°C to 25°C (68°F to 77°F). Protect from freezing and moisture.

Compatibility Stable in D_5W, NS.

Y-site administration: **Compatible:** Alatrofloxacin, amphotericin B cholesteryl sulfate complex, atracurium, cisatracurium, diltiazem, dobutamine, dopamine, enalaprilat, epinephrine, esmolol, etomidate, furosemide, gatifloxacin, heparin, hydrocortisone sodium succinate, hydromorphone, labetalol, levofloxacin, linezolid, lorazepam, midazolam, milrinone, morphine, nafcillin, nicardipine, nitroglycerin, norepinephrine, pancuronium, potassium chloride, propofol, ranitidine, remifentanil, sargramostim, thiopental, vecuronium, vitamin B complex with C.

Compatibility in syringe: **Compatible:** Atracurium, atropine, bupivacaine with ketamine, butorphanol, chlorpromazine, cimetidine, clonidine with lidocaine, dimenhydrinate, diphenhydramine, droperidol, heparin, hydromorphone, hydroxyzine, meperidine, metoclopramide, midazolam, morphine, ondansetron, pentazocine, perphenazine, prochlorperazine edisylate, promazine, promethazine, ranitidine, scopolamine. **Incompatible:** Pentobarbital.

Compatibility when admixed: **Compatible:** Bupivacaine. **Incompatible:** Fluorouracil, methohexital, pentobarbital, thiopental.

Mechanism of Action Binds with stereospecific receptors at many sites within the CNS, increases pain threshold, alters pain reception, inhibits ascending pain pathways

Pharmacodynamics/Kinetics

Onset of action: Analgesic: I.M.: 7-8 minutes; I.V.: Almost immediate; Transmucosal: 5-15 minutes

Peak effect: Transmucosal: Analgesic: 15-30 minutes

Duration: I.M.: 1-2 hours; I.V.: 0.5-1 hour; Transmucosal: Related to blood level; respiratory depressant effect may last longer than analgesic effect

Absorption:

Transdermal: Initial application: Gradually absorbed for the first 12-24 hours, followed by a constant absorption for the remainder of the dosing interval

Transmucosal, buccal tablet: Rapid, ~50% from the buccal mucosa; remaining 50% swallowed with saliva and slowly absorbed from GI tract.

Transmucosal, lozenge: Rapid, ~25% from the buccal mucosa; 75% swallowed with saliva and slowly absorbed from GI tract

Distribution: 4-6 L/kg; Highly lipophilic, redistributes into muscle and fat

Protein binding: 80% to 85%

Metabolism: Hepatic, primarily via CYP3A4

Bioavailability: Total (transmucosal and GI absorption): Buccal: 65% (range: 45% to 85%); Lozenge: 47% (range: 37% to 57%)

Half-life elimination:

I.V.: 2-4 hours

Transdermal patch: 17 hours (13-22 hours, half-life is influenced by absorption rate)

Transmucosal: Lozenge: 7 hours; Buccal tablet: 100-200 mcg: 3-4 hours, 400-800 mcg: 11-12 hours

Time to peak: Buccal tablet: 20-240 minutes (median: 47 minutes); Lozenge: 20-480 minutes (median: 20-40 minutes); Transdermal patch: 24-72 hours, after several sequential 72-hour applications, steady state serum concentrations are reached

Excretion: Urine 75% (primarily as metabolites, <7% to 10% as unchanged drug); feces ~9%

Dosage Note: These are guidelines and do not represent the maximum doses that may be required in all patients. Doses and dosage intervals should be titrated to pain relief/prevention. Monitor vital signs routinely. Single I.M. doses have a duration of 1-2 hours, single I.V. doses last 0.5-1 hour.

Minor procedures/analgesia (unlabeled use): I.V.:

Children 1-12 years: 0.5-2 mcg/kg/dose given 3 minutes prior to procedure; may repeat every 1-2 hours

Children >12 years: 0.5-2 mcg/kg/dose (maximum 50 mcg/dose) given 3 minutes prior to procedure; may repeat in 5 minutes if necessary; if more than 2 doses are needed, repeat with a maximum of 25 mcg/dose up to 5 times

Surgery:

Children ≥2 years: Adjunct to anesthesia (induction and maintenance): Slow I.V.: 2-3 mcg/kg/dose every 1-2 hours as needed

Adults:

Premedication: I.M., slow I.V.: 50-100 mcg/dose 30-60 minutes prior to surgery

Adjunct to regional anesthesia: Slow I.V.: 25-100 mcg/dose over 1-2 minutes. **Note:** An I.V. should be in place with regional anesthesia so the I.M. route is rarely used but still maintained as an option in the package labeling.

Adjunct to general anesthesia: Slow I.V.:

Low dose: 0.5-2 mcg/kg/dose depending on the indication

Moderate dose: Initial: 2-20 mcg/kg/dose; Maintenance (bolus or infusion): 1-2 mcg/kg/hour. Discontinuing fentanyl infusion 30-60 minutes prior to the end of surgery will usually allow adequate ventilation upon emergence from anesthesia. For "fast-tracking" and early extubation following major surgery, total fentanyl doses are limited to 10-15 mcg/kg.

High dose: 20-50 mcg/kg/dose; **Note:** Fentanyl is rarely used, but is still maintained in the package labeling.

◀ **Pain management:**
Children (unlabeled use): I.V.: 0.5-2 mcg/kg/dose given every 1-2 hours as needed; continuous infusion: 0.5-2 mcg/kg/hour; titrate to desired effects

Patient-controlled analgesia (PCA) (unlabeled use; American Pain Society, 2008): Children <50 kg: **Note:** Opiate-naive: Consider lower end of dosing range:

Usual concentration: 10 mcg/mL
Demand dose: 0.5-1 mcg/kg/dose
Lockout interval: 6-8 minutes
Usual basal rate: 0-0.5 mcg/kg/hour

Adults:

I.V. (unlabeled use): Bolus at start of infusion: 1-2 mcg/kg **or** 25-100 mcg/dose; continuous infusion rate: 1-2 mcg/kg/hour **or** 25-200 mcg/hour

Severe pain: I.M, I.V. (unlabeled): 50-100 mcg/dose every 1-2 hours as needed; patients with prior opiate exposure may tolerate higher initial doses

Patient-controlled analgesia (PCA) (unlabeled use): I.V.:

Usual concentration: 10 mcg/mL
Demand dose: Usual: 20 mcg; range: 10-50 mcg
Lockout interval: 5-8 minutes
Usual basal rate: ≤50 mcg/hour

Critically-ill patients (unlabeled dose): Slow I.V.: 25-100 mcg (based on ~70 kg patient) **or** 0.35-1.5 mcg/kg every 30-60 minutes as needed. **Note:** More frequent dosing may be needed (eg, mechanically-ventilated patients).

Continuous infusion: 50-700 mcg/hour (based on ~70 kg patient) **or** 0.7-10 mcg/kg/hour

Intrathecal (I.T.) (unlabeled use; American Pain Society, 2008): **Must be preservative-free.** Doses must be adjusted for age, injection site, and patient's medical condition and degree of opioid tolerance.

Single dose: 5-25 mcg/dose; may provide adequate relief for up to 6 hours

Continuous infusion: Not recommended in acute pain management due to risk of excessive accumulation. For chronic cancer pain, infusion of very small doses may be practical (American Pain Society, 2008).

Epidural (unlabeled use; American Pain Society, 2008): **Must be preservative-free.** Doses must be adjusted for age, injection site, and patient's medical condition and degree of opioid tolerance

Single dose: 25-100 mcg/dose; may provide adequate relief for up to 8 hours

Continuous infusion: 25-100 mcg/hour

Breakthrough cancer pain: For patients who are tolerant to and currently receiving opioid therapy for persistent cancer pain; dosing should be individually titrated to provide adequate analgesia with minimal side effects. Dose titration should be done if patient requires more than 1 dose/breakthrough pain episode for several consecutive episodes. Patients experiencing >4 breakthrough pain episodes/day should have the dose of their long-term opioid re-evaluated.

Children ≥16 years and Adults: Lozenge: Initial dose: 200 mcg; the second dose may be started 15 minutes after completion of the first dose. Consumption should be limited to ≤4 units/day. Additional requirements suggest need for improved baseline therapy.

Adults: Buccal tablet (Fentora®): Initial dose: 100 mcg; a second 100 mcg dose, if needed, may be started 30 minutes after the start of the first dose.

Note: For patients previously using the transmucosal lozenge (Actiq®), the initial dose should be selected using the conversions listed below (maximum: 2 doses per breakthrough pain episode every 4 hours).

Dose titration, if required, should be done using multiples of the 100 mcg tablets. Patient can take two 100 mcg tablets (one on each side of mouth). If that dose is not successful, can use four 100 mcg tablets (two on each side of mouth). If titration requires >400 mcg/dose, then use 200 mcg tablets.

Conversion from lozenge to buccal tablet (Fentora®):

Lozenge dose 200-400 mcg, then buccal tablet 100 mcg

Lozenge dose 600-800 mcg, then buccal tablet 200 mcg

Lozenge dose 1200-1600 mcg, then buccal tablet 400 mcg

Note: Four 100 mcg buccal tablets deliver approximately 12% and 13% higher values of C_{max} and AUC, respectively, compared to one 400 mcg buccal tablet. To prevent confusion, patient should only have one strength available at a time. Using more than four buccal tablets at a time has not been studied.

Elderly >65 years: Transmucosal lozenge (eg, Actiq®): In clinical trials, patients who were >65 years of age were titrated to a mean dose that was 200 mcg less than that of younger patients.

Chronic pain management: Children ≥2 years and Adults (opioid-tolerant patients): Transdermal patch (eg, Duragesic®):

Initial: To convert patients from oral or parenteral opioids to transdermal patch, a 24-hour analgesic requirement should be calculated (based on prior opiate use). Using the tables, the appropriate initial dose can be determined. The initial fentanyl dosage may be approximated from the 24-hour morphine dosage equivalent and titrated to minimize adverse effects and provide analgesia. With the initial application, the absorption of transdermal fentanyl requires several hours to reach plateau; therefore transdermal fentanyl is inappropriate for management of acute pain. Change patch every 72 hours.

Conversion from continuous infusion of fentanyl: In patients who have adequate pain relief with a fentanyl infusion, fentanyl may be converted to transdermal dosing at a rate equivalent to the intravenous rate. A two-step taper of the infusion to be completed over 12 hours has been recommended (Kornick, 2001) after the patch is applied. The infusion is decreased to 50% of the original rate six hours after the application of the first patch, and subsequently discontinued twelve hours after application.

Titration: Short-acting agents may be required until analgesic efficacy is established and/or as supplements for "breakthrough" pain. The amount of supplemental doses should be closely monitored. Appropriate dosage increases may be based on daily supplemental dosage using the ratio of 45 mg/24 hours of oral morphine to a 12.5 mcg/hour increase in fentanyl dosage.

Frequency of adjustment: The dosage should not be titrated more frequently than every 3 days after the initial dose or every 6 days thereafter. Patients should wear a consistent fentanyl dosage through two applications (6 days) before dosage increase based on supplemental opiate dosages can be estimated. **Note:** Upon discontinuation, ~17 hours are required for a 50% decrease in fentanyl levels.

Frequency of application: The majority of patients may be controlled on every 72-hour administration; however, a small number of patients require every 48-hour administration.

Dose conversion guidelines for transdermal fentanyl[1]
(see tables below and on next page).

Recommended Initial Duragesic® Dose Based Upon Daily Oral Morphine Dose[1]

Oral 24-Hour Morphine (mg/d)	Duragesic® Dose (mcg/h)
60-134[2]	25
135-224	50
225-314	75
315-404	100
405-494	125
495-584	150
585-674	175
675-764	200
765-854	225
855-944	250
945-1034	275
1035-1124	300

[1]The table should NOT be used to convert from transdermal fentanyl (eg, Duragesic®) to other opioid analgesics. Rather, following removal of the patch, titrate the dose of the new opioid until adequate analgesia is achieved.

[2]Pediatric patients initiating therapy on a 25 mcg/hour Duragesic® system should be opioid-tolerant and receiving at least 60 mg oral morphine equivalents per day.

Dosing Conversion Guidelines[1,2]

Current Analgesic	Daily Dosage (mg/day)			
Morphine (I.M./I.V.)	10-22	23-37	38-52	53-67
Oxycodone (oral)	30-67	67.5-112	112.5-157	157.5-202
Oxycodone (I.M./I.V.)	15-33	33.1-56	56.1-78	78.1-101
Codeine (oral)	150-447	448-747	748-1047	1048-1347
Hydromorphone (oral)	8-17	17.1-28	28.1-39	39.1-51
Hydromorphone (I.V.)	1.5-3.4	3.5-5.6	5.7-7.9	8-10
Meperidine (I.M.)	75-165	166-278	279-390	391-503
Methadone (oral)	20-44	45-74	75-104	105-134
Methadone (I.M.)	10-22	23-37	38-52	53-67
Fentanyl transdermal recommended dose (mcg/h)	25 mcg/h	50 mcg/h	75 mcg/h	100 mcg/h

[1]The table should NOT be used to convert from transdermal fentanyl (eg, Duragesic®) to other opioid analgesics. Rather, following removal of the patch, titrate the dose of the new opioid until adequate analgesia is achieved.

[2]Duragesic® product insert, Janssen Pharmaceutica, Feb 2008.

Opioid Analgesics Initial Oral Dosing Commonly Used for Severe Pain

Drug	Equianalgesic Dose (mg)		Initial Oral Dose	
	Oral[1]	Parenteral[2]	Children (mg/kg)	Adults (mg)
Buprenorphine	—	0.4	—	—
Butorphanol	—	2	—	—
Hydromorphone	7.5	1.5	0.06	4-8
Levorphanol	Acute: 4 Chronic: 1	Acute: 2 Chronic: 1	0.04	2-4
Meperidine	300	75	Not recommended	
Methadone	Acute: 10 Chronic: Varies depending upon opioid dose[3]	Acute: 5	0.2	5-10
Morphine	30	10	0.3	15-30
Nalbuphine	—	10	—	—
Pentazocine	50	30	—	—
Oxycodone	20	—	0.2	10-20
Oxymorphone	10	1	—	5-10

From "Principles of Analgesic Use in the Treatment of Acute Pain and Cancer Pain," *Am Pain Soc*, Sixth Ed.

[1]Elderly: Starting dose should be lower for this population group

[2]Standard parenteral doses for acute pain in adults; can be used to convert doses for I.V. infusions and repeated small I.V. boluses. For single I.V. boluses, use half the I.M. dose. Children >6 months: I.V. dose = parenteral equianalgesic dose x weight (kg)/100

[3]Conversion of higher doses may be guided by the following (consult a pain or palliative care specialist if unfamiliar with methadone prescribing): As the total daily dose of morphine increases, the equianalgesic dose ratio (methadone:morphine) increases in adults with ongoing cancer pain. (American Pain Society, 2008; National Comprehensive Cancer Network®, 2009). Applicability to pediatric patients is unknown.

Dosing adjustment in hepatic impairment: Actiq®: Although fentanyl kinetics may be altered in hepatic disease, Actiq® can be used successfully in the management of breakthrough cancer pain. Doses should be titrated to reach clinical effect with careful monitoring of patients with severe hepatic disease.

Administration

I.V.: Administer as slow I.V. infusion over 1-2 minutes. May also be administered as continuous infusion or PCA (unlabeled use) routes. Muscular rigidity may occur with rapid I.V. administration.

Transdermal patch (eg, Duragesic®): Apply to nonirritated and nonirradiated skin, such as chest, back, flank, or upper arm. Do not shave skin; hair at application site should be clipped. Prior to application, clean site with clear water and allow to dry completely. Do not use damaged, cut or leaking patches; patch may be less effective. Skin exposure from fentanyl gel leaking from patch may lead to serious adverse effects; thoroughly wash affected skin surfaces with water (do not use soap). Firmly press in place and hold for 30 seconds. Change patch every 72 hours. Do **not** use soap, alcohol, or other solvents to remove transdermal gel if it accidentally touches skin; use copious amounts of water. Avoid exposing application site to external heat sources (eg, heating pad, electric blanket, heat lamp, hot tub).

Lozenge: Foil overwrap should be removed just prior to administration. Place the unit in mouth and allow it to dissolve. Do not chew. Lozenge may be moved from one side of the mouth to the other. The unit should be consumed over a period of 15 minutes. Handle should be removed after it is consumed or if patient has achieved an adequate response and/or shows signs of respiratory depression.

Buccal tablet: Patient should not open blister until ready to administer. The blister backing should be peeled back to expose the tablet; tablet should not be pushed out through the blister. Immediately use tablet once removed from blister. Place entire tablet in the buccal cavity (above a rear molar, between the upper cheek and gum). Tablet should not be broken, sucked, chewed, or swallowed. Should dissolve in about 14-25 minutes when left between the cheek and the gum. If remnants remain they may be swallowed with water.

Monitoring Parameters Respiratory and cardiovascular status, blood pressure, heart rate; signs of misuse, abuse, or addiction

Transdermal patch: Monitor for 24 hours after application of first dose

Dietary Considerations Transmucosal lozenge contains 2 g sugar per unit.

Additional Information Fentanyl is 50-100 times as potent as morphine; morphine 10 mg I.M. is equivalent to fentanyl 0.1-0.2 mg I.M.; fentanyl has less hypotensive effects than morphine due to lack of histamine release. However, fentanyl may cause rigidity with high doses. If the patient has required high-dose analgesia or has used for a prolonged period (~7 days), taper dose to prevent withdrawal; monitor for signs and symptoms of withdrawal.

Transmucosal (oral lozenge): Disposal of lozenge units: After consumption of a complete unit, the handle may be disposed of in a trash container that is out of the reach of children. For a partially-consumed unit, or a unit that still has any drug matrix remaining on the handle, the handle should be placed under hot running tap water until the drug matrix has dissolved. Special child-resistant containers are available to temporarily store partially consumed units that cannot be disposed of immediately.

Transdermal patch (Duragesic®): Upon removal of the patch, ~17 hours are required before serum concentrations fall to 50% of their original values. Opioid withdrawal symptoms are possible. Gradual downward titration (potentially by the sequential use of lower-dose patches) is recommended. Keep transdermal patch (both used and unused) out of the reach of children. Do **not** use soap, alcohol, or other solvents to remove transdermal gel if it accidentally touches skin as they may increase transdermal absorption, use copious amounts of water. Avoid exposure of direct external heat sources (eg, heating pads, electric blankets, heat lamps, saunas, hot tubs, heated water beds) to application site.

Product Availability

Onsolis™: FDA approved July 2009; availability expected in the fourth quarter of 2009

Onsolis™ (fentanyl buccal soluble film) is approved for the management of breakthrough pain in adult patients with cancer. It will only be available through a restricted distribution program called the FOCUS program.

Dosage Forms Excipient information presented when available (limited, particularly for generics); consult specific product labeling.

Note: Strengths expressed as base.

Injection, solution, as citrate [preservative free]: 0.05 mg/mL (2 mL, 5 mL, 10 mL, 20 mL; 30 mL [DSC]; 50 mL)

Sublimaze®: 0.05 mg/mL (2 mL, 5 mL, 10 mL [DSC], 20 mL)

Lozenge, oral, as citrate [transmucosal]: 200 mcg, 400 mcg, 600 mcg, 800 mcg, 1200 mcg, 1600 mcg

Actiq®: 200 mcg, 400 mcg, 600 mcg, 800 mcg, 1200 mcg, 1600 mcg [contains sugar 2 g/lozenge; berry flavor]

Powder, for prescription compounding, as citrate: USP (1 g)

Tablet, for buccal application, as citrate:

Fentora®: 100 mcg, 200 mcg, 300 mcg, 400 mcg, 600 mcg, 800 mcg

Transdermal system, topical, as base: 12 (5s) [delivers 12.5 mcg/hour; 3.13 cm^2]; 12 (5s) [delivers 12.5 mcg/hour; 5 cm^2]; 25 (5s) [delivers 25 mcg/hour; 10 cm^2]; 25 (5s) [delivers 25 mcg/hour; 6.25 cm^2]; 50 (5s) [delivers 50 mcg/hour; 12.5 cm^2]; 50 (5s) [delivers 50 mcg/hour; 20 cm^2]; 75 (5s) [delivers 75 mcg/hour; 18.75 cm^2]; 75 (5s) [delivers 75 mcg/hour; 30 cm^2]; 75 (5s) [delivers 75 mcg/hour; 32.1 cm^2]; 100 (5s) [delivers 100 mcg/hour; 25 cm^2]; 100 (5s) [delivers 100 mcg/hour; 40 cm^2]; 100 (5s) [delivers 100 mcg/hour; 42.8 cm^2]

Duragesic®: 12 (5s) [delivers 12.5 mcg/hour; 5 cm^2; contains ethanol 0.1 mL/ 10 cm^2]; 25 (5s) [delivers 25 mcg/hour; 10 cm^2; contains ethanol 0.1 mL/10 cm^2]; 50 (5s) [delivers 50 mcg/hour; 20 cm^2; contains ethanol 0.1 mL/10 cm^2]; 75 (5s) [delivers 75 mcg/hour; 30 cm^2; contains ethanol 0.1 mL/10 cm^2]; 100 (5s) [delivers 100 mcg/hour; 40 cm^2; contains ethanol 0.1 mL/ 10 cm^2]

References

Bailey PL, Pace NL, Ashburn MA, et al, "Frequent Hypoxemia and Apnea After Sedation With Midazolam and Fentanyl," *Anesthesiology*, 1990, 73(5):826-30.

Berde C, Ablin A, Glazer J, et al, "Report of the Subcommittee on Disease-Related Pain in Childhood Cancer," *Pediatrics*, 1990, 86(5 Pt 2):818-25.

"Drugs for Pain," *Med Lett Drugs Ther*, 2000, 42(1085):73-8.

Fine PG, "Fentanyl in the Treatment of Cancer Pain," *Semin Oncol*, 1997, 24(5 Suppl 16):16-20.7.

Friedrichsdorf SJ amd Kand TI, "The Management of Pain in Children With Life-limiting Illnesses," *Pediatr Clin North Am*, 2007, 54(5):645-72.

Greco C and Berde C, "Pain Management for the Hospitalized Pediatric Patient," *Pediat Clin North Am*, 2005, 52(4):995-1027.

Hegenbarth MA and the American Academy of Pediatrics Committee on Drugs, "Preparing for Pediatric Emergencies: Drugs to Consider," *Pediatrics*, 2008, 121(2):433-443.

Jacobi J, Fraser GL, Coursin DB, et al, "Clinical Practice Guidelines for the Sustained Use of Sedatives and Analgesics in the Critically Ill Adult," *Crit Care Med*, 2002, 30(1):119-41. Available at: http://www.sccm.org/pdf/sedatives.pdf. Accessed August 2, 2003.

Jeal W and Benfield P, "Transdermal Fentanyl. A Review of Its Pharmacological Properties and Therapeutic Efficacy in Pain Control," *Drugs*, 1997, 53(1):109-38.

Kornick CA, Santiago-Palma J, Khojainova N, et al, "A Safe and Effective Method for Converting Cancer Patients from Intravenous to Transdermal Fentanyl," *Cancer*, 2001, 92(12):3056-61.

Liu LL and Gropper MA, "Postoperative Analgesia and Sedation in the Adult Intensive Care Unit," *Drugs*, 2003, 63(8):755-67.

"Principles of Analgesic Use in the Treatment of Acute Pain and Chronic Cancer Pain," 5th ed, Glenview, IL: American Pain Society, 2003.

Zeltzer LK, Altman A, Cohen D, et al, "Report of the Subcommittee on the Management of Pain Associated With Procedures in Children With Cancer," *Pediatrics*, 1990, 86(5 Pt 2):826-31.

Ferric Gluconate (FER ik GLOO koe nate)

Medication Safety Issues

Sound-alike/look-alike issues:

Ferric gluconate may be confused with ferumoxytol

Ferrlecit® may be confused with Ferralet®

◀ **U.S. Brand Names** Ferrlecit®
Index Terms Sodium Ferric Gluconate
Generic Available No
Canadian Brand Names Ferrlecit®
Pharmacologic Category Iron Salt
Use Repletion of total body iron content in patients with iron-deficiency anemia who are undergoing hemodialysis in conjunction with erythropoietin therapy
Unlabeled/Investigational Use Cancer-/chemotherapy-associated anemia
Pregnancy Risk Factor B
Lactation Excretion in breast milk unknown/use caution
Labeled Contraindications Hypersensitivity to ferric gluconate or any component of the formulation; use in any anemia not caused by iron deficiency; iron overload
Warnings/Precautions Potentially serious hypersensitivity reactions may occur. Fatal immediate hypersensitivity reactions have occurred with other iron carbohydrate complexes. Avoid rapid administration. Flushing and transient hypotension may occur. May augment hemodialysis-induced hypotension. Use with caution in elderly patients. Use only in patients with documented iron deficiency; caution with hemoglobinopathies or other refractory anemias. Contains benzyl alcohol; do not use in neonates.
Adverse Reactions Frequency not defined.
   Cardiovascular: Angina, bradycardia, chest pain, edema, hyper-/hypotension, hypervolemia, MI, pulmonary edema, syncope, tachycardia, thrombosis, vasodilation
   Central nervous system: Agitation, chills, dizziness, fatigue, fever, headache, insomnia, malaise, pain, somnolence
   Dermatologic: Pruritus, rash
   Endocrine & metabolic: Hyper-/hypokalemia, hypoglycemia
   Gastrointestinal: Abdominal pain, anorexia, diarrhea, dyspepsia, epigastric pain, eructation, flatulence, melena, nausea, vomiting
   Genitourinary: Urinary tract infection
   Hematologic: Abnormal erythrocytes, leukocytosis, lymphadenopathy
   Local: Injection site reactions, injection site pain
   Neuromuscular & skeletal: Arthralgia, back pain, cramps, groin pain, leg cramps, myalgia, paresthesia, rigors, weakness
   Ocular: Blurred vision, conjunctivitis
   Respiratory: Cough, dyspnea, pneumonia, rhinitis, upper respiratory infection
   Miscellaneous: Carcinoma, diaphoresis increased, flu-like syndrome, hypersensitivity reactions, infection, sepsis
   Postmarketing and/or case reports: Dry mouth, dysgeusia, hemorrhage, hypertension, hypoesthesia, loss of consciousness, nervousness, pallor, phlebitis, seizure, shock, skin discoloration
Drug Interactions
   Avoid Concomitant Use
      Avoid concomitant use of Ferric Gluconate with any of the following: Dimercaprol
   Increased Effect/Toxicity
      The levels/effects of Ferric Gluconate may be increased by: ACE Inhibitors; Dimercaprol
   Decreased Effect
      Ferric Gluconate may decrease the levels/effects of: Cefdinir; Eltrombopag; Levothyroxine; Phosphate Supplements; Trientine

The levels/effects of Ferric Gluconate may be decreased by: Pancrelipase; Trientine

Storage/Stability Store at 20°C to 25°C (68°F to 77°F); do not freeze.

Reconstitution For I.V. infusion, dilute 10 mL ferric gluconate in 0.9% sodium chloride (children: 25 mL NS, adults: 100 mL NS); use immediately after dilution.

Compatibility Stable with 0.9% sodium chloride; do not mix with parenteral nutrition solutions or other medications.

Mechanism of Action Supplies a source to elemental iron necessary to the function of hemoglobin, myoglobin and specific enzyme systems; allows transport of oxygen via hemoglobin

Pharmacodynamics/Kinetics Half-life elimination: Bound: 1 hour

Dosage

Children ≥6 years: Repletion of iron in hemodialysis patients: 1.5 mg/kg of elemental iron (maximum: 125 mg/dose) diluted in NS 25 mL, administered over 60 minutes at 8 sequential dialysis sessions

Adults:

Repletion of iron in hemodialysis patients: I.V.: 125 mg elemental iron per 10 mL (either by I.V. infusion or slow I.V. injection). Most patients will require a cumulative dose of 1 g elemental iron over approximately 8 sequential dialysis treatments to achieve a favorable response.

Note: A test dose of 2 mL diluted in NS 50 mL administered over 60 minutes was previously recommended (not in current manufacturer labeling). Doses >125 mg are associated with increased adverse events.

Cancer-/chemotherapy-associated anemia (unlabeled use): I.V. infusion: 125 mg over 1 hour; maximum 250 mg/infusion. Repeat dose every week for 8 doses. Test doses (25 mg slow I.V. push or infusion) are recommended in patients with iron dextran hypersensitivity or those with other drug allergies (NCCN guidelines, v.2.2010)

Administration I.V.: Adults: May be diluted prior to administration; avoid rapid administration. Solutions diluted for infusion should be infused over 1 hour. If administered undiluted, infuse slowly at a rate of up to 12.5 mg/minute.

Monitoring Parameters Hemoglobin and hematocrit, serum ferritin, iron saturation; vital signs

NKF K/DOQI guidelines recommend that iron status should be monitored monthly during initiation through the percent transferrin saturation (TSAT) and serum ferritin.

Test Interactions Serum or transferrin bound iron levels may be falsely elevated if assessed within 24 hours of ferric gluconate administration. Serum ferritin levels may be falsely elevated for 5 days after ferric gluconate administration.

Dosage Forms Excipient information presented when available (limited, particularly for generics); consult specific product labeling.

Injection, solution:

Ferrlecit®: Elemental iron 12.5 mg/mL (5 mL) [contains benzyl alcohol and sucrose 20%]

References

"Dietary Reference Intakes for Vitamin A, Vitamin K, Arsenic, Boron, Chromium, Copper, Iodine, Iron, Manganese, Molybdenum, Nickel, Silicon, Vanadium, and Zinc." Standing Committee on the Scientific Evaluation of Dietary Reference Intakes, Food and Nutrition Board, Institute of Medicine, National Academy of Sciences, Washington, DC: National Academy Press, 2000. Available at http://www.nap.edu.

National Kidney Foundation, "KDOQI Clinical Practice Guidelines and Clinical Practice Recommentations for Anemia in Chronic Kidney Disease," Available at www.kidney.org/professionals/KDOQI/guidelines_anemia/cpr32.htm. Last accessed November 20, 2006.

"Recommendations to Prevent and Control Iron Deficiency in the United States. Centers for Disease Control and Prevention," *MMWR Recomm Rep*, 1998, 47(RR-3):1-29.

◆ **Ferrlecit®** *see* Ferric Gluconate *on page 469*

Ferumoxytol (fer ue MOX i tol)

Medication Safety Issues

Sound-alike/look-alike issues:

Ferumoxytol may be confused with ferric gluconate, iron dextran complex, iron sucrose

U.S. Brand Names Feraheme™

Generic Available No

Pharmacologic Category Iron Salt

Use Treatment of iron-deficiency anemia in chronic kidney disease

Pregnancy Risk Factor C

Lactation Excretion in breast milk unknown/not recommended

Labeled Contraindications Hypersensitivity to ferumoxytol or any component of the formulation; evidence of iron overload; anemia not caused by iron deficiency

Warnings/Precautions Hypersensitivity reactions, including rare anaphylactic and anaphylactoid reactions, may occur; equipment for resuscitation and trained personnel experienced in handling emergencies should be immediately available during use. Monitor patients for signs/symptoms of hypersensitivity reactions for ≥30 minutes after administration. Hypotension, including serious hypotensive reactions, may occur; monitor patients for hypotension following administration.

Withhold iron in the presence of tissue iron overload; periodic monitoring of hemoglobin, serum ferritin, serum iron, and transferrin saturation is recommended. Serum iron and transferrin-bound iron may be overestimated in laboratory assays if level is drawn during the first 24 hours following administration. Administration may alter magnetic resonance (MR) imaging; conduct anticipated MRI studies prior to use. MR imaging alterations may persist for ≤3 months following use, with peak alterations anticipated in the first 2 days following administration. If MR imaging is required within 3 months after administration, use T1- or proton density-weighted MR pulse sequences to decrease effect on imagining. Do not use T2-weighted sequence MR imaging prior to 4 weeks following ferumoxytol administration. Ferumoxytol does not interfere with X-ray, computed tomography (CT), positron emission tomography (PET), single photon emission computed tomography (SPECT), ultrasound or nuclear medicine imaging.

Not FDA-approved for use in children.

Adverse Reactions

1% to 10%:

Cardiovascular: Hypotension (≤3%), edema (2%), peripheral edema (2%), chest pain (1%), hypertension (1%)

Central nervous system: Dizziness (3%), headache (2%), fever (1%)

Dermatologic: Pruritus (1%), rash (1%)

Gastrointestinal: Diarrhea (4%), nausea (3%), constipation (2%), vomiting (2%), abdominal pain (1%)

Neuromuscular & skeletal: Back pain (1%), muscle spasms (1%)

Respiratory: Cough (1%), dyspnea (1%)

Miscellaneous: Hypersensitivity reactions (≤4%; serious reactions: <1%)

<1%, postmarketing, and/or case reports: Fatigue; infusion site reactions (including bruising, burning, erythema, irritation, pain, swelling, warmth); urticaria, wheezing

Drug Interactions

Avoid Concomitant Use

Avoid concomitant use of Ferumoxytol with any of the following: Dimercaprol

Increased Effect/Toxicity

The levels/effects of Ferumoxytol may be increased by: Dimercaprol

Decreased Effect There are no known significant interactions involving a decrease in effect.

Storage/Stability Store vials at controlled room temperature of 20°C to 25°C (68°F to 77°F); do not freeze.

Mechanism of Action Superparamagnetic iron oxide coated with a low molecular weight semisynthetic carbohydrate; iron-carbohydrate complex enters the reticuloendothelial system macrophages of the liver, spleen, and bone marrow where the iron is released from the complex. The released iron is either transported into storage pools or is transported via plasma transferrin for incorporation into hemoglobin.

Pharmacodynamics/Kinetics

Distribution: V_d: 3.16 L

Metabolism: Iron released from iron-carbohydrate complex after uptake in the reticuloendothelial system macrophages of the liver, spleen, and bone marrow

Half-life elimination: ~15 hours

Dialysis: Ferumoxytol is not removed by hemodialysis

Dosage Doses expressed in mg of **elemental** iron. **Note:** Test dose: Product labeling does not indicate need for a test dose.

I.V.: Adults: Iron-deficiency anemia in chronic kidney disease: 510 mg (17 mL) as a single dose, followed by a second 510 mg dose 3-8 days after initial dose. Recommended dose may be readministered in patients with persistent or recurrent iron deficiency anemia.

Dosage adjustment in renal impairment: Hemodialysis patients should receive injection after at least 1 hour of hemodialysis has been completed and once blood pressure has stabilized.

Administration Administer intravenously as an undiluted injection at a rate ≤1 mL/second (30 mg of elemental iron/second). Do not administer if solution has particulate matter or is discolored (solution is black to reddish-brown).

Hemodialysis patients should receive injection after at least 1 hour of hemodialysis has been completed and once blood pressure has stabilized.

Monitoring Parameters Hemoglobin, serum ferritin, serum iron, transferrin saturation (for at least 1 month following second injection and periodically); signs/symptoms of hypotension following administration; signs/symptoms of hypersensitivity reactions (≥30 minutes following administration)

Test Interactions May interfere with MR imaging; alterations may persist for ≤3 months following use, with peak alterations anticipated in the first 2 days following administration. If MR imaging is required within 3 months after administration, use T1- or proton density-weighted MR pulse sequences to decrease effect on imaging. Do not use T2-weighted sequence MR imaging prior to 4 weeks following administration.

Serum iron and transferrin-bound iron may be overestimated in laboratory assays if level is drawn during the first 24 hours following administration (due to contribution of iron in feruxomytol).

◀ **Dosage Forms** Excipient information presented when available (limited, particularly for generics); consult specific product labeling.

Injection, solution:

Feraheme™: Elemental iron 30 mg/mL (17 mL)

References

American College of Obstetricians and Gynecologists, "ACOG Practice Bulletin No. 95: Anemia in Pregnancy," *Obstet Gynecol*, 2008, 112(1):201-7.

Auerbach M, "Ferumoxytol as a New, Safer, Easier-to-Administer Intravenous Iron: Yes or No", *Am J of Kidney Dis*, 2008, 52(5):826-9 [editorial].

Baker WF Jr, "Iron Deficiency in Pregnancy, Obstetrics, and Gynecology," *Hematol Oncol Clin North Am*, 2000, 14(5):1061-77.

"Nutrition During Lactation." Subcommittee on Nutrition During Lactation, Committee on Nutritional Status During Pregnancy and Lactation, Food and Nutrition Board Institute of Medicine, National Academy of Sciences Washington, DC: National Academy Press, 1991. Available at http://www.nap.edu.

"Recommendations to Prevent and Control Iron Deficiency in the United States. Centers for Disease Control and Prevention," *MMWR Recomm Rep*, 1998, 47(RR-3):1-29.

"Routine Iron Supplementation During Pregnancy. Review Article. US Preventive Services Task Force," *JAMA*, 1993, 270(23):2848-54.

Singh A, Patel T, Hertel J, et al, "Safety of Ferumoxytol in Patients With Anemia and CKD", *Am J of Kidney Dis*, 2008, 52(5):907-15.

Fibrinogen Concentrate (Human)

(fi BRIN o gin KON suhn trate HYU man)

U.S. Brand Names RiaSTAP™

Index Terms Coagulation Factor I

Generic Available No

Pharmacologic Category Blood Product Derivative

Use Treatment of acute bleeding episodes in patients with congenital fibrinogen deficiency (afibrinogenemia and hypofibrinogenemia)

Pregnancy Risk Factor C

Labeled Contraindications Severe hypersensitivity reactions to fibrinogen concentrate or any component of the formulation

Warnings/Precautions

Hypersensitivity reactions (eg, urticaria, hives, wheezing, hypotension, anaphylaxis) may occur. In the event of hypersensitivity reactions, treatment should be discontinued immediately. Thrombosis may occur in patients with congenital fibrinogen deficiency with or without fibrinogen replacement therapy. Consider potential risk of thrombosis with use. Product of human plasma; may potentially contain infectious agents which could transmit disease. Screening of donors, as well as testing and/or inactivation or removal of certain viruses, reduces the risk. Infections thought to be transmitted by this product should be reported to the manufacturer. Not for the treatment of dysfibrinogenemia.

Adverse Reactions

>1%: Central nervous system: Fever, headache

Postmarketing and/or case reports: Allergic reactions, anaphylaxis, arterial thrombosis, chills, DVT, dyspnea, MI, nausea, pulmonary embolism, rash, thromboembolism, vomiting

Drug Interactions

Avoid Concomitant Use There are no known interactions where it is recommended to avoid concomitant use.

Increased Effect/Toxicity

Fibrinogen Concentrate (Human) may increase the levels/effects of: Antifibrinolytic Agents

The levels/effects of Fibrinogen Concentrate (Human) may be increased by: Antifibrinolytic Agents

Decreased Effect There are no known significant interactions involving a decrease in effect.

Storage/Stability Store at 2°C to 25°C (36°F to 77°F) in original carton; do not freeze. Protect from light. Stable for 24 hours after reconstitution when stored at 20°C to 25°C (68°F to 77°F). Discard partially used vials.

Reconstitution Transfer sterile water for injection 50 mL into vial. Gently swirl until dissolved; do not shake.

Mechanism of Action Fibrinogen (coagulation factor I), a protein found in normal plasma, is required to clot blood. Fibrinogen concentrate made from pooled human plasma replaces this protein which is missing or reduced in patients with a congenital fibrinogen deficiency.

Pharmacodynamics/Kinetics

Distribution: V_d: 45-60 mL/kg (range: 36-68 mL/kg)

Half-life elimination: 61-97 hours (range: 56-117 hours); may be decreased in children <16 years of age

Dosage I.V.: Children and Adults: Congenital fibrinogen deficiency: **Note:** Adjust dose based on laboratory values and condition of patient. Maintain a target fibrinogen level of 100 mg/dL until hemostasis is achieved.

When baseline fibrinogen level is known:

Dose (mg/kg) = [Target level (mg/dL) - measured level (mg/dL)] **divided by** 1.7 (mg/dL per mg/kg body weight)

When baseline fibrinogen level is not known: 70 mg/kg

Administration For I.V. administration only; infuse at ≤5 mL/minute

Monitoring Parameters Signs and symptoms of hypersensitivity, thrombosis; fibrinogen level

Dosage Forms Excipient information presented when available (limited, particularly for generics); consult specific product labeling. [DSC] = Discontinued product

Injection, powder for reconstitution:

RiaSTAP™: 900-1300 mg [contains albumin (human); exact potency labeled on vial]

References

Acharya SS and Dimichele DM, "Rare Inherited Disorders of Fibrinogen," *Haemophilia*, 2008, 14 (6):1151-8.

Kreuz W, Meili E, Peter-Salonen K, et al. "Efficacy and Tolerability of a Pasteurised Human Fibrinogen Concentrate in Patients With Congenital Fibrinogen Deficiency," *Transfus Apher Sci*, 2005, 32(3):247-53.

Filgrastim (fil GRA stim)

Medication Safety Issues

Sound-alike/look-alike issues:

Neupogen® may be confused with Epogen®, Neulasta®, Neumega®, Neupro®, Nutramigen®

Related Information

Hematopoietic Stem Cell Transplantation on page 1501

U.S. Brand Names Neupogen®

Index Terms G-CSF; Granulocyte Colony Stimulating Factor; NSC-614629

Generic Available No

Canadian Brand Names Neupogen®

Pharmacologic Category Colony Stimulating Factor

Use Stimulation of granulocyte production in chemotherapy-induced neutropenia (nonmyeloid malignancies, acute myeloid leukemia, and bone marrow transplantation); severe chronic neutropenia (SCN); mobilization of hematopoietic progenitor cells in patients undergoing peripheral blood progenitor cell (PBPC) collection

Unlabeled/Investigational Use Treatment of anemia in myelodysplastic syndrome; treatment of drug-induced (nonchemotherapy) agranulocytosis in the elderly

Pregnancy Risk Factor C

Lactation Excretion in breast milk unknown/use caution

Labeled Contraindications Hypersensitivity to filgrastim, *E. coli*-derived proteins, or any component of the formulation

Warnings/Precautions Do not use filgrastim in the period 24 hours before to 24 hours after administration of cytotoxic chemotherapy because of the potential sensitivity of rapidly dividing myeloid cells to cytotoxic chemotherapy. May potentially act as a growth factor for any tumor type, particularly myeloid malignancies; precaution should be exercised in the usage of filgrastim in any malignancy with myeloid characteristics. Increases circulating leukocytes when used in conjunction with plerixafor for stem cell mobilization; monitor WBC; use with caution in patients with neutrophil count >50,000/mm³; tumor cells released from marrow could be collected in leukapheresis product; potential effect of tumor cell re-infusion is unknown. Reports of alveolar hemorrhage, manifested as pulmonary infiltrates and hemoptysis, have occurred in healthy donors undergoing PBPC collection (not FDA approved for use in healthy donors); hemoptysis resolved upon discontinuation. Safety and efficacy have not been established with patients receiving radiation therapy, or with chemotherapy associated with delayed myelosuppression (eg, nitrosoureas, mitomycin C).

Allergic-type reactions (rash, urticaria, wheezing, dyspnea, tachycardia and/or hypotension) have occurred with first or later doses. Reactions tended to occur more frequently with intravenous administration and within 30 minutes of administration. Rare cases of splenic rupture or acute respiratory distress syndrome have been reported in association with filgrastim; patients must be instructed to report left upper quadrant pain or shoulder tip pain or respiratory distress. Cutaneous vasculitis has been reported, generally occurring in SCN patients on long-term therapy; dose reductions may improve symptoms to allow for continued therapy. Use caution in patients with sickle cell diseases; sickle cell crises have been reported following filgrastim therapy. Cytogenetic abnormalities, transformation to AML and MDS have been observed in patients treated with filgrastim for congenital neutropenia; a longer duration of treatment and poorer ANC response appear to increase the risk. The packaging of some forms may contain latex.

Adverse Reactions
>10%:
Central nervous system: Fever (12%)
Dermatologic: Petechiae (17%), rash (12%)
Gastrointestinal: Splenomegaly (severe chronic neutropenia: 30%; rare in other patients)
Hepatic: Alkaline phosphatase increased (21%)
Neuromuscular & skeletal: Bone pain (22% to 33%), commonly in the lower back, posterior iliac crest, and sternum
Respiratory: Epistaxis (9% to 15%)
1% to 10%:
Cardiovascular: Hyper-/hypotension (4%), S-T segment depression (3%), myocardial infarction/arrhythmias (3%)
Central nervous system: Headache (7%)
Gastrointestinal: Nausea (10%), vomiting (7%), peritonitis (2%)
Hematologic: Leukocytosis (2%)

Miscellaneous: Transfusion reaction (10%)

<1%, postmarketing, and/or case reports: Acute respiratory distress syndrome, allergic reactions, alopecia, alveolar hemorrhage, arthralgia, capillary leak syndrome, cerebral hemorrhage, cutaneous vasculitis, dyspnea, edema (facial), erythema nodosum, hematuria, hemoptysis, hepatomegaly, hypersensitivity reaction, injection site reaction, osteoporosis, pericarditis, proteinuria, psoriasis exacerbation, pulmonary infiltrates, renal insufficiency, sickle cell crisis, splenic rupture, Sweet's syndrome (acute febrile dermatosis), tachycardia, thrombocytopenia (in PBPC mobilization), thrombophlebitis, transient supraventricular arrhythmia, urticaria, wheezing

Drug Interactions

Avoid Concomitant Use There are no known interactions where it is recommended to avoid concomitant use.

Increased Effect/Toxicity

Filgrastim may increase the levels/effects of: Topotecan

Decreased Effect There are no known significant interactions involving a decrease in effect.

Storage/Stability Intact vials and prefilled syringes should be stored under refrigeration at 2°C to 8°C (36°F to 46°F) and protected from direct sunlight. Filgrastim should be protected from freezing and temperatures >30°C to avoid aggregation. If inadvertently frozen, thaw in a refrigerator and use within 24 hours; do not use if frozen >24 hours or frozen more than once. Do not shake.

Filgrastim vials and prefilled syringes are stable for 24 hours at 9°C to 30°C (47°F to 86°F).

Undiluted filgrastim is stable for 24 hours at 15°C to 30°C (59°F to 86°F) and for up to 14 days at 2°C to 8°C (36°F to 46°F) (data on file, Amgen Medical Information) in BD tuberculin syringes; however, sterility has only been assessed and maintained for up to 7 days when prepared under strict aseptic conditions (Singh, 1994; Jacobson, 1996). The manufacturer recommends using syringes within 24 hours due to the potential for bacterial contamination.

Filgrastim diluted with D_5W or D_5W with albumin for I.V. infusion (5-15 mcg/mL) is stable for 7 days at 2°C to 8°C (36°F to 46°F), however, should be used within 24 hours due to the possibility for bacterial contamination.

Reconstitution Do not dilute with saline at any time; product may precipitate. Filgrastim may be diluted with D_5W or with D_5W with albumin to a concentration of 5-15 mcg/mL for I.V. infusion administration (minimum concentration: 5 mcg/mL). Dilution to <5 mcg/mL is not recommended. Concentrations 5-15 mcg/mL require addition of albumin (final concentration of 2 mg/mL) to prevent adsorption to plastics.

Compatibility Stable in D_5W; **incompatible** with NS.

Y-site administration: Compatible: Acyclovir, allopurinol, amikacin, aminophylline, ampicillin, ampicillin/sulbactam, aztreonam, bleomycin, bumetanide, buprenorphine, butorphanol, calcium gluconate, carboplatin, carmustine, cefazolin, cefotetan, ceftazidime, chlorpromazine, cimetidine, cisplatin, co-trimoxazole, cyclophosphamide, cytarabine, dacarbazine, daunorubicin HCl, dexamethasone sodium phosphate, diphenhydramine, doxorubicin HCl, doxycycline, droperidol, enalaprilat, famotidine, floxuridine, fluconazole, fludarabine, gallium nitrate, ganciclovir, granisetron, haloperidol lactate, hydrocortisone sodium succinate, hydromorphone, hydroxyzine HCl, idarubicin, ifosfamide, leucovorin calcium, lorazepam, mechlorethamine, melphalan, meperidine, mesna, methotrexate, metoclopramide, mitoxantrone, morphine, nalbuphine, ondansetron, potassium chloride, promethazine, ranitidine, sodium bicarbonate, streptozocin, ticarcillin/clavulanate,

◄ tobramycin, vancomycin, vinblastine, vincristine, vinorelbine, zidovudine.
Incompatible: Amphotericin B, cefepime, cefotaxime, cefoxitin, ceftizoxime, ceftriaxone, cefuroxime, clindamycin, dactinomycin, etoposide, fluorouracil, furosemide, heparin, mannitol, methylprednisolone sodium succinate, metronidazole, mitomycin, piperacillin, prochlorperazine edisylate, thiotepa.
Variable (consult detailed reference): Gentamicin, imipenem/cilastatin.

Mechanism of Action Stimulates the production, maturation, and activation of neutrophils; filgrastim activates neutrophils to increase both their migration and cytotoxicity.

Pharmacodynamics/Kinetics

Onset of action: ~24 hours; plateaus in 3-5 days

Duration: ANC decreases by 50% within 2 days after discontinuing filgrastim; white counts return to the normal range in 4-7 days; peak plasma levels can be maintained for up to 12 hours

Absorption: SubQ: 100%

Distribution: V_d: 150 mL/kg; no evidence of drug accumulation over a 11- to 20-day period

Metabolism: Systemically degraded

Half-life elimination: 1.8-3.5 hours

Time to peak, serum: SubQ: 2-8 hours

Dosage Details concerning dosing in combination regimens and institution protocols should also be consulted.

Dosing, even in morbidly obese patients, should be based on actual body weight. Rounding doses to the nearest vial size often enhances patient convenience and reduces costs without compromising clinical response.

Children and Adults:

Chemotherapy-induced neutropenia: SubQ, I.V.: 5 mcg/kg/day; doses may be increased by 5 mcg/kg according to the duration and severity of the neutropenia; continue for up to 14 days or until the ANC reaches 10,000/mm^3

Bone marrow transplantation: SubQ, I.V.: 10 mcg/kg/day; adjust the dose according to the duration and severity of neutropenia; recommended steps based on neutrophil response:

When ANC >1000/mm^3 for 3 consecutive days: Reduce filgrastim dose to 5 mcg/kg/day

If ANC remains >1000/mm^3 for 3 more consecutive days: Discontinue filgrastim

If ANC decreases to <1000/mm^3: Resume at 5 mcg/kg/day

If ANC decreases <1000/mm^3 during the 5 mcg/kg/day dose, increase filgrastim to 10 mcg/kg/day and follow the above steps

Peripheral blood progenitor cell (PBPC) collection: SubQ: 10 mcg/kg daily in donors, usually for 6-7 days. Begin at least 4 days before the first leukopheresis and continue until the last leukopheresis; consider dose adjustment for WBC >100,000/mm^3

Hematopoietic stem cell mobilization (in combination with plerixafor, for autologous transplantation in patients with non-Hodgkin's lymphoma and multiple myeloma): SubQ: 10 mcg/kg once daily; begin 4 days before initiation of plerixafor; continue G-CSF on each day prior to apheresis

Severe chronic neutropenia: SubQ:

Congenital: 6 mcg/kg twice daily; adjust the dose based on ANC and clinical response

Idiopathic/cyclic: 5 mcg/kg/day; adjust the dose based on ANC and clinical response

Anemia in myelodysplastic syndrome (unlabeled use - in combination with epoetin): SubQ: 0.3-3 mcg/kg daily **or** 30-150 mcg daily **or** 1-2 mcg/kg 2-3 times weekly

Elderly: Refer to adult dosing.

Drug-induced agranulocytosis (nonchemotherapy) in the elderly (unlabeled use): SubQ: 300 mcg daily until ANC >1500/mm^3

Combination Regimens

Breast cancer: AC/Paclitaxel (Sequential) on page 1223

Leukemia, acute myeloid:
FLAG (AML) on page 1323
FLAG-IDA on page 1324

Lymphoma, non-Hodgkin's:
EPOCH Dose-Adjusted (AIDS-Related Lymphoma) on page 1307
EPOCH Dose-Adjusted (NHL) on page 1307
EPOCH (Dose-Adjusted)-Rituximab (NHL) on page 1308
ICE (Lymphoma, non-Hodgkin's) on page 1356
RICE on page 1402

Lymphoma, non-Hodgkin's (Burkitt's): CODOX-M/IVAC on page 1278

Soft tissue sarcoma: AI on page 1225

Administration May be administered undiluted by SubQ injection. May also be administered by I.V. bolus over 15-30 minutes in D$_5$W, or by continuous SubQ or I.V. infusion. Do not administer earlier than 24 hours after or in the 24 hours prior to cytotoxic chemotherapy.

Monitoring Parameters CBC with differential prior to treatment and twice weekly during filgrastim treatment for chemotherapy-induced neutropenia (3 times a week following marrow transplantation). For severe chronic neutropenia, monitor CBC with differential twice weekly during the first month of therapy and for 2 weeks following dose adjustments; monthly thereafter. In PBPC mobilization, monitor platelets.

Test Interactions May interfere with bone imaging studies; increased hematopoietic activity of the bone marrow may appear as transient positive bone imaging changes

Dietary Considerations Solution for injection contains sodium 0.035 mg/mL and sorbitol.

Additional Information

Reimbursement Hotline: 1-800-272-9376
Professional Services [Amgen]: 1-800-77-AMGEN

High Dose Considerations

High Dose 5-10 mcg/kg/day

Dosage Forms Excipient information presented when available (limited, particularly for generics); consult specific product labeling.

Injection, solution [preservative free]:
Neupogen®: 300 mcg/mL (1 mL, 1.6 mL) [vial; contains sodium 0.035 mg/mL and sorbitol]

Injection, solution [preservative free]:
Neupogen®: 600 mcg/mL (0.5 mL, 0.8 mL) [prefilled Singleject® syringe; contains sodium 0.035 mg/mL and sorbitol; needle cover contains latex]

References

Andres E, Kurtz JE, Martin-Hunyadi C, et al, "Nonchemotherapy Drug-Induced Agranulocytosis in Elderly Patients: The Effects of Granulocyte Colony-Stimulating Factor," *Am J Med*, 2002, 112 (6):460-4.

Calandra G, McCarty J, McGuirk J, et al, "AMD3100 Plus G-CSF Can Successfully Mobilize CD34 + Cells From Non-Hodgkin's Lymphoma, Hodgkin's Disease and Multiple Myeloma Patients Previously Failing Mobilization With Chemotherapy and/or Cytokine Treatment: Compassionate Use Data," *Bone Marrow Transplant*, 2008, 41(4):331-8.

Flomenberg N, Devine SM, DiPersio JF, et al, "The Use of AMD3100 Plus G-CSF for Autologous Hematopoietic Progenitor Cell Mobilization is Superior to G-CSF Alone," *Blood*, 2005, 106(5): 1867-74.

Jacobson PA, West NJ, Spadoni V, et al, "Sterility of Filgrastim (G-CSF) in Syringes," *Ann Pharmacother*, 1996, 30(11):1238-42.

Jädersten M, Montgomery SM, Dybedal I, et al, "Long-Term Outcome of Treatment of Anemia in MDS with Erythropoietin and G-CSF," *Blood*, 2005, 106(3):803-11.

National Comprehensive Cancer Network (NCCN), "Clinical Practice Guidelines in Oncology™: Myelodysplastic Syndromes," Version 2.2008. Available at http://www.nccn.org/professionals/physician_gls/PDF/mds.pdf

National Comprehensive Cancer Network (NCCN), "Clinical Practice Guidelines in Oncology™: Myeloid Growth Factors," Version 1.2008. Available at http://www.nccn.org/professionals/physician_gls/PDF/myeloid_growth.pdf

Rosenberg PS, Alter BP, Bolyard AA, et al, "The Incidence of Leukemia and Mortality From Sepsis in Patients With Severe Congenital Neutropenia Receiving Long-Term G-CSF Therapy," *Blood*, 2006, 107(12): 4628-35.

Singh RF, Corelli RL, and Gugliemo BJ, "Sterility of Unit Dose Syringes of Filgrastim and Sargramostim," *Am J Hosp Pharm*, 1994, 51(15):2811-2.

Smith TJ, Khatcheressian J, Lyman GH, et al, "2006 Update of Recommendations for the Use of White Blood Cell Growth Factors: An Evidence-Based Clinical Practice Guideline," *J Clin Oncol*, 2006, 24(19):3187-205.

Finasteride (fi NAS teer ide)

Medication Safety Issues

Sound-alike/look-alike issues:

Finasteride may be confused with furosemide

Proscar® may be confused with ProSom®, Provera®, Prozac®, Psorcon®

Related Information

Safe Handling of Hazardous Drugs *on page 1517*

U.S. Brand Names Propecia®; Proscar®

Generic Available Yes

Canadian Brand Names Propecia®; Proscar®

Pharmacologic Category 5 Alpha-Reductase Inhibitor

Use

Propecia®: Treatment of male pattern hair loss in **men only**. Safety and efficacy were demonstrated in men between 18-41 years of age.

Proscar®: Treatment of symptomatic benign prostatic hyperplasia (BPH); can be used in combination with an alpha-blocker, doxazosin

Unlabeled/Investigational Use Prostate cancer prevention (to reduce the incidence); treatment of female hirsutism

Pregnancy Risk Factor X

Lactation Excretion in breast milk unknown/contraindicated

Labeled Contraindications Hypersensitivity to finasteride or any component of the formulation; pregnancy; not for use in children

Warnings/Precautions Hazardous agent - use appropriate precautions for handling and disposal. Other urological diseases including cancer should be ruled out before initiating. A minimum of 6 months of treatment may be necessary to determine whether an individual will respond to finasteride. Reduces prostate specific antigen (PSA) by 50%; in patients treated for ≥6 months the PSA should be doubled when comparing to normal ranges in untreated patients. Use with caution in those patients with hepatic dysfunction. When compared to placebo, 5-alpha-reductase inhibitors have been shown to reduce the incidence of prostate cancer, although an increase in the incidence of high-grade prostate cancers has been observed (Thompson, 2003; Kramer, 2009). Carefully monitor patients with a large residual urinary volume or severely diminished urinary flow for obstructive uropathy. These patients may not be candidates for finasteride therapy. Safety and efficacy have not been established in children.

Adverse Reactions Note: "Combination therapy" refers to finasteride and doxazosin.

>10%:

Endocrine & metabolic: Impotence (19%; combination therapy 23%), libido decreased (10%; combination therapy 12%)

Neuromuscular & skeletal: Weakness (5%; combination therapy 17%)

1% to 10%:

Cardiovascular: Postural hypotension (9%; combination therapy 18%), edema (1%; combination therapy 3%)

Central nervous system: Dizziness (7%; combination therapy 23%), somnolence (2%; combination therapy 3%)

Genitourinary: Ejaculation disturbances (7%; combination therapy 14%), decreased volume of ejaculate

Endocrine & metabolic: Gynecomastia (2%)

Respiratory: Dyspnea (1%; combination therapy 2%), rhinitis (1%; combination therapy 2%)

<1%, postmarketing, and/or case reports: Hypersensitivity (pruritus, rash, urticaria, swelling of face/lips); breast tenderness, breast enlargement, breast cancer (males), prostate cancer (high grade), testicular pain

Drug Interactions

Metabolism/Transport Effects Substrate of CYP3A4 (minor)

Avoid Concomitant Use There are no known interactions where it is recommended to avoid concomitant use.

Increased Effect/Toxicity There are no known significant interactions involving an increase in effect.

Decreased Effect There are no known significant interactions involving a decrease in effect.

Ethanol/Nutrition/Herb Interactions

Herb/Nutraceutical: St John's wort may decrease finasteride levels. Avoid saw palmetto (concurrent use has not been adequately studied).

Storage/Stability Store below 30°C (86°F). Protect from light.

Mechanism of Action Finasteride is a competitive inhibitor of both tissue and hepatic 5-alpha reductase. This results in inhibition of the conversion of testosterone to dihydrotestosterone and markedly suppresses serum dihydrotestosterone levels

Pharmacodynamics/Kinetics

Onset of action: 3-6 months of ongoing therapy

Duration:

After a single oral dose as small as 0.5 mg: 65% depression of plasma dihydrotestosterone levels persists 5-7 days

After 6 months of treatment with 5 mg/day: Circulating dihydrotestosterone levels are reduced to castrate levels without significant effects on circulating testosterone; levels return to normal within 14 days of discontinuation of treatment

Distribution: V_{dss}: 76 L

Protein binding: 90%

Metabolism: Hepatic via CYP3A4; two active metabolites (<20% activity of finasteride)

Bioavailability: Mean: 63%

Half-life elimination, serum: Elderly: 8 hours; Adults: 6 hours (3-16)

Time to peak, serum: 2-6 hours

Excretion: Feces (57%) and urine (39%) as metabolites

Dosage Oral: Adults:

Male:

Benign prostatic hyperplasia (Proscar®): 5 mg once daily as a single dose; clinical responses occur within 12 weeks to 6 months of initiation of therapy; long-term administration is recommended for maximal response

Male pattern baldness (Propecia®): 1 mg daily

Prostate cancer prevention (unlabeled use): 5 mg once daily; planned duration of treatment was 7 years (Kramer, 2009; Thompson, 2003)

Female hirsutism (unlabeled use): 5 mg/day

Dosing adjustment in renal impairment: No dosage adjustment is necessary

Dosing adjustment in hepatic impairment: Use with caution in patients with liver function abnormalities because finasteride is metabolized extensively in the liver

Administration Administration with food may delay the rate and reduce the extent of oral absorption. Women of childbearing age should not touch or handle broken tablets.

Monitoring Parameters Objective and subjective signs of relief of benign prostatic hyperplasia, including improvement in urinary flow, reduction in symptoms of urgency, and relief of difficulty in micturition

Dosage Forms Excipient information presented when available (limited, particularly for generics); consult specific product labeling.

Tablet: 5 mg

Propecia®: 1 mg

Proscar®: 5 mg

References

Kramer BS, Hagerty KL, Justman S, et al, "Use of 5-α-Reductase Inhibitors for Prostate Cancer Chemoprevention: American Society of Clinical Oncology/American Urological Association 2008 Clinical Practice Guideline," *J Clin Oncol*, 2009, 27(9):1502-16.

McConnell JD, Roehrborn CG, Bautista OM, et al, "The Long-Term Effect of Doxazosin, Finasteride, and Combination Therapy on the Clinical Progression of Benign Prostatic Hyperplasia. Medical Therapy of Prostatic Symptoms (MTOPS) Research Group," *N Engl J Med*, 2003, 349(25):2387-98.

Thompson IM, Goodman PJ, Tangen CM, et al, "The Influence of Finasteride on the Development of Prostate Cancer," *N Engl J Med*, 2003, Jul 349(3):215-24.

◆ **Firmagon®** *see* Degarelix *on page* 337

◆ **FK506** *see* Tacrolimus *on page* 1062

◆ **Flagyl®** *see* MetroNIDAZOLE *on page* 793

◆ **Flagyl® 375** *see* MetroNIDAZOLE *on page* 793

◆ **Flagyl® ER** *see* MetroNIDAZOLE *on page* 793

◆ **Flebogamma®** *see* Immune Globulin (Intravenous) *on page* 627

◆ **Florazole® ER (Can)** *see* MetroNIDAZOLE *on page* 793

◆ **Floxin®** *see* Ofloxacin *on page* 863

◆ **Floxin Otic Singles** *see* Ofloxacin *on page* 863

Floxuridine (floks YOOR i deen)

Medication Safety Issues

Sound-alike/look-alike issues:

Floxuridine may be confused with Fludara®, fludarabine

FUDR® may be confused with Fludara®

High alert medication: The Institute for Safe Medication Practices (ISMP) includes this medication among its list of drugs which have a heightened risk of causing significant patient harm when used in error.

Related Information

Management of Drug Extravasations *on page 1447*
Safe Handling of Hazardous Drugs *on page 1517*

U.S. Brand Names FUDR®

Index Terms Fluorodeoxyuridine; FUDR

Generic Available Yes

Canadian Brand Names FUDR®

Pharmacologic Category Antineoplastic Agent, Antimetabolite (Pyrimidine Analog)

Use Management of hepatic metastases of colorectal and gastric cancers

Pregnancy Risk Factor D

Lactation Excretion in breast milk unknown/contraindicated

Labeled Contraindications Hypersensitivity to floxuridine, fluorouracil, or any component of the formulation; pregnancy

Warnings/Precautions Hazardous agent - use appropriate precautions for handling and disposal. Use caution with impaired kidney or liver function. Discontinue if intractable vomiting, diarrhea, precipitous fall in leukocyte or platelet counts, myocardial ischemia, hemorrhage, gastrointestinal ulcer, or stomatitis occur. Use with caution in patients with poor nutritional status; depressed (leukocyte count <5000/mm^3 or platelet count <100,000/mm^3) bone marrow function; potentially serious infections. Use with caution in patients who have had high-dose pelvic radiation or previous use of alkylating agents. **[U.S. Boxed Warnings]: Should be administered under the supervision of an experienced cancer chemotherapy physician. Patients should be hospitalized for initiation of the first course of therapy due to the risk for severe toxic reactions.**

Adverse Reactions

>10%:

Gastrointestinal: Stomatitis, diarrhea; may be dose limiting

Hematologic: Myelosuppression, may be dose limiting; leukopenia, thrombocytopenia, anemia

Onset: 4-7 days

Nadir: 5-9 days

Recovery: 21 days

1% to 10%:

Dermatologic: Alopecia, photosensitivity, hyperpigmentation of the skin, localized erythema, dermatitis

Gastrointestinal: Anorexia

Hepatic: Biliary sclerosis, cholecystitis, jaundice

<1%: Nausea, vomiting, intrahepatic abscess

Drug Interactions

Avoid Concomitant Use

Avoid concomitant use of Floxuridine with any of the following: Natalizumab; Vaccines (Live)

Increased Effect/Toxicity

Floxuridine may increase the levels/effects of: Carvedilol; CYP2C9 Substrates (High risk); Leflunomide; Natalizumab; Phenytoin; Vaccines (Live); Vitamin K Antagonists

The levels/effects of Floxuridine may be increased by: Trastuzumab

◀ **Decreased Effect**

Floxuridine may decrease the levels/effects of: Cardiac Glycosides; Vaccines (Inactivated); Vaccines (Live); Vitamin K Antagonists

The levels/effects of Floxuridine may be decreased by: Echinacea

Ethanol/Nutrition/Herb Interactions Ethanol: Avoid ethanol (due to GI irritation).

Storage/Stability Store intact vials at room temperature of 15°C to 30°C (59°F to 86°F). Reconstituted vials are stable for up to 2 weeks under refrigeration at 2°C to 8°C (36°C to 46°C). Further dilution in 500-1000 mL D_5W or NS is stable for 2 weeks at room temperature. Solutions in 0.9% sodium chloride are stable in some ambulatory infusion pumps for up to 21 days.

Reconstitution Reconstitute with 5 mL SWI for a final concentration of 100 mg/mL. Further dilute in 500-1000 mL D_5W or NS for I.V. infusion.

Compatibility Stable in D_5W, NS, sterile water for injection.

Y-site administration: Compatible: Amifostine, aztreonam, etoposide phosphate, filgrastim, fludarabine, gemcitabine, granisetron, melphalan, ondansetron, paclitaxel, piperacillin/tazobactam, sargramostim, teniposide, thiotepa, vinorelbine. **Incompatible:** Allopurinol, cefepime.

Compatibility when admixed: Compatible: Carboplatin, cisplatin, cisplatin with etoposide, cisplatin with leucovorin, etoposide, fluorouracil, leucovorin.

Mechanism of Action Mechanism of action and pharmacokinetics are very similar to fluorouracil; floxuridine is the deoxyribonucleotide of fluorouracil. Floxuridine is a fluorinated pyrimidine antagonist which inhibits DNA and RNA synthesis and methylation of deoxyuridylic acid to thymidylic acid.

Pharmacodynamics/Kinetics

Metabolism: Hepatic; Active metabolites: Floxuridine monophosphate (FUDR-MP) and fluorouracil; Inactive metabolites: Urea, CO_2, α-fluoro-β-alanine, α-fluoro-β-guanidopropionic acid, α-fluoro-β-ureidopropionic acid, and dihydrofluorouracil

Excretion: Urine: Fluorouracil, urea, α-fluoro-β-alanine, α-fluoro-β-guanidopropionic acid, α-fluoro-β-ureidopropionic acid, and dihydrofluorouracil; exhaled gases (CO_2)

Dosage Refer to individual protocols.

Intra-arterial:

0.1-0.6 mg/kg/day

4-20 mg/day

I.V. (unlabeled use):

0.15 mg/kg/day for 7-14 days

0.5-1 mg/kg/day for 6-15 days

30 mg/kg/day for 5 days, then 15 mg/kg/day every other day, up to 11 days

Dosage adjustment in renal impairment: The FDA-approved labeling does not contain dosing adjustment guidelines; use with extreme caution.

Dosage adjustment in hepatic impairment: The FDA-approved labeling does not contain dosing adjustment guidelines; use with extreme caution. The following guidelines have been used by some clinicians (Floyd, 2006):

Serum bilirubin 1.2 times ULN or alkaline phosphatase 1.2 times ULN: Administer 80% of dose

Serum bilirubin 1.5 times ULN; transaminases 3 times baseline or alkaline phosphatase 1.5 times ULN: Administer 50% of dose

Serum bilirubin 2 times ULN; transaminases >3 times baseline or alkaline phosphatase 2 times ULN: No recommendation is available

Administration Continuous intra-arterial or I.V. infusion (unlabeled use)

Vesicant May be an irritant

Dosage Forms Excipient information presented when available (limited, particularly for generics); consult specific product labeling.

Injection, powder for reconstitution: 500 mg

References

Davidson BS, Izzo F, Chase JL, et al, "Alternating Floxuridine and 5-Fluorouracil Hepatic Arterial Chemotherapy for Colorectal Liver Metastases Minimizes Biliary Toxicity," *Am J Surg*, 1996, 172 (3):244-7.

DeConti RC, Kaplan SR, Papac RJ, et al, "Continuous Infusions of 5-Fluoro-2-Deoxyuridine in the Treatment of Solid Tumors," *Cancer*, 1973, 31(4):894-8.

de Takats PG, Kerr DJ, Poole CJ, et al, "Hepatic Arterial Chemotherapy for Metastatic Colorectal Carcinoma," *Br J Cancer*, 1994, 69(2):372-8.

Floyd J, Mirza I, Sachs B, et al, "Hepatotoxicity of Chemotherapy," *Semin Oncol*, 2006, 33 (1):50-67.

Hrushesky WJ, von Roemeling R, Lanning RM, et al, "Circadian-Shaped Infusions of Floxuridine for Progressive Metastatic Renal Cell Carcinoma," *J Clin Oncol*, 1990, 8(9):1504-13.

Kemeny N, Seiter K, Conti JA, et al, Hepatic Arterial Floxuridine and Leucovorin for Unresectable Liver Metastases From Colorectal Carcinoma. New Dose Schedules and Survival Update," *Cancer*, 1994, 73(4):1134-42.

Fluconazole (floo KOE na zole)

Medication Safety Issues

Sound-alike/look-alike issues:

Fluconazole may be confused with flecainide, FLUoxetine, furosemide, itraconazole

Diflucan® may be confused with diclofenac, Diprivan®, disulfiram

International issues:

Canesten® [Great Britain]: Brand name for clotrimazole in multiple international markets

U.S. Brand Names Diflucan®

Generic Available Yes

Canadian Brand Names Apo-Fluconazole®; CO Fluconazole; Diflucan®; Dom-Fluconazole; Fluconazole Injection; Fluconazole Omega; Gen-Fluconazole; GMD-Fluconazole; Mylan-Fluconazole; Novo-Fluconazole; PHL-Fluconazole; PMS-Fluconazole; Pro-Fluconazole; Riva-Fluconazole; Taro-Fluconazole; Zym-Fluconazole

Pharmacologic Category Antifungal Agent, Oral; Antifungal Agent, Parenteral

Use Treatment of candidiasis (vaginal, oropharyngeal, esophageal, urinary tract infections, peritonitis, pneumonia, and systemic infections); cryptococcal meningitis; antifungal prophylaxis in allogeneic bone marrow transplant recipients

Pregnancy Risk Factor C

Lactation Enters breast/not recommended (AAP rates "compatible")

Labeled Contraindications Hypersensitivity to fluconazole, other azoles, or any component of the formulation; concomitant administration with cisapride

Warnings/Precautions Should be used with caution in patients with renal and hepatic dysfunction or previous hepatotoxicity from other azole derivatives. Patients who develop abnormal liver function tests during fluconazole therapy should be monitored closely and discontinued if symptoms consistent with liver disease develop. Rare exfoliative skin disorders have been observed; monitor closely if rash develops. The manufacturer reports rare cases of QT_c prolongation and TdP associated with fluconazole use and advises caution in patients with concomitant medications or conditions which are arrhythmogenic. However, given the limited number of cases and the

presence of multiple confounding variables, the likelihood that fluconazole causes conduction abnormalities appears remote.

Adverse Reactions Frequency not always defined.

Cardiovascular: Angioedema, pallor, QT prolongation (rare, case reports), torsade de pointes (rare, case reports)

Central nervous system: Headache (2% to 13%), seizure, dizziness

Dermatologic: Rash (2%), alopecia, toxic epidermal necrolysis, Stevens-Johnson syndrome

Endocrine & metabolic: Hypercholesterolemia, hypertriglyceridemia, hypokalemia

Gastrointestinal: Nausea (4% to 7%), abdominal pain (2% to 6%), diarrhea (2% to 3%), vomiting (2%), dyspepsia, taste perversion

Hematologic: Agranulocytosis, leukopenia, neutropenia, thrombocytopenia

Hepatic: Alkaline phosphatase increased, ALT increased, AST increased, cholestasis, hepatic failure (rare), hepatitis, jaundice

Respiratory: Dyspnea

Miscellaneous: Anaphylactic reactions (rare)

Drug Interactions

Metabolism/Transport Effects Inhibits CYP1A2 (weak), 2C9 (strong), 2C19 (strong), 3A4 (moderate)

Avoid Concomitant Use

Avoid concomitant use of Fluconazole with any of the following: Artemether; Cisapride; Clopidogrel; Conivaptan; Dofetilide; Dronedarone; Everolimus; Lumefantrine; Nilotinib; Pimozide; QuiNIDine; QuiNINE; Ranolazine; Tetrabenazine; Thioridazine; Tolvaptan; Ziprasidone

Increased Effect/Toxicity

Fluconazole may increase the levels/effects of: Alfentanil; Aprepitant; Benzodiazepines (metabolized by oxidation); Bosentan; BusPIRone; Busulfan; Calcium Channel Blockers; CarBAMazepine; Cardiac Glycosides; Carvedilol; Cilostazol; Cinacalcet; Cisapride; Citalopram; Colchicine; Conivaptan; Corticosteroids (Orally Inhaled); Corticosteroids (Systemic); CycloSPORINE; CYP2C19 Substrates; CYP2C9 Substrates (High risk); CYP3A4 Substrates; Docetaxel; Dofetilide; Dronedarone; Eletriptan; Eplerenone; Erlotinib; Eszopiclone; Everolimus; FentaNYL; Fosaprepitant; Gefitinib; HMG-CoA Reductase Inhibitors; Imatinib; Irbesartan; Irinotecan; Losartan; Macrolide Antibiotics; Methadone; Phenytoin; Phosphodiesterase 5 Inhibitors; Pimecrolimus; Pimozide; Protease Inhibitors; Proton Pump Inhibitors; QTc-Prolonging Agents; QuiNIDine; QuiNINE; Ramelteon; Ranolazine; Repaglinide; Rifamycin Derivatives; Salmeterol; Saxagliptin; Sirolimus; Solifenacin; Sulfonylureas; Sunitinib; Tacrolimus; Temsirolimus; Tetrabenazine; Thioridazine; Tolterodine; Tolvaptan; Trimetrexate; Vitamin K Antagonists; Zidovudine; Ziprasidone; Zolpidem

The levels/effects of Fluconazole may be increased by: Alfuzosin; Artemether; Chloroquine; Ciprofloxacin; Gadobutrol; Grapefruit Juice; Lumefantrine; Macrolide Antibiotics; Nilotinib; Protease Inhibitors; QuiNINE

Decreased Effect

Fluconazole may decrease the levels/effects of: Amphotericin B; Clopidogrel; Saccharomyces boulardii

The levels/effects of Fluconazole may be decreased by: Didanosine; Phenytoin; Rifamycin Derivatives; Sucralfate

Storage/Stability

Powder for oral suspension: Store dry powder at ≤30°C (86°F). Following reconstitution, store at 5°C to 30°C (41°F to 86°F). Discard unused portion after 2 weeks. Do not freeze.

Injection: Store injection in glass at 5°C to 30°C (41°F to 86°F). Store injection in Viaflex® at 5°C to 25°C (41°F to 77°F). Do not freeze. Do not unwrap unit until ready for use.

Compatibility Stable in D$_5$W, LR, NS.

Y-site administration: Compatible: Acyclovir, aldesleukin, allopurinol, amifostine, amikacin, aminophylline, ampicillin/sulbactam, aztreonam, benztropine, cefazolin, cefepime, cefotetan, cefoxitin, cefpirome, chlorpromazine, cimetidine, cisatracurium, dexamethasone sodium phosphate, diltiazem, diphenhydramine, dobutamine, docetaxel, dopamine, doxorubicin liposome, droperidol, etoposide phosphate, famotidine, filgrastim, fludarabine, foscarnet, ganciclovir, gatifloxacin, gemcitabine, gentamicin, granisetron, heparin, hydrocortisone sodium phosphate, immune globulin intravenous, leucovorin, linezolid, lorazepam, melphalan, meperidine, meropenem, metoclopramide, metronidazole, midazolam, morphine, nafcillin, nitroglycerin, ondansetron, oxacillin, paclitaxel, pancuronium, penicillin G potassium, phenytoin, piperacillin/tazobactam, prochlorperazine edisylate, promethazine, propofol, ranitidine, remifentanil, sargramostim, tacrolimus, teniposide, theophylline, thiotepa, ticarcillin/clavulanate, tobramycin, vancomycin, vecuronium, vinorelbine, zidovudine. **Incompatible:** Amphotericin B, amphotericin B cholesteryl sulfate complex, ampicillin, calcium gluconate, cefotaxime, ceftazidime, ceftriaxone, cefuroxime, chloramphenicol, clindamycin, co-trimoxazole, diazepam, digoxin, erythromycin lactobionate, furosemide, haloperidol, hydroxyzine, imipenem/cilastatin, pentamidine, piperacillin, ticarcillin.

Compatibility when admixed: Compatible: Acyclovir, amikacin, amphotericin B, cefazolin, ceftazidime, clindamycin, gentamicin, heparin, meropenem, metronidazole, morphine, piperacillin, potassium chloride, ranitidine with ondansetron, theophylline. **Incompatible:** Co-trimoxazole.

Mechanism of Action Interferes with fungal cytochrome P450 activity (lanosterol 14-α-demethylase), decreasing ergosterol synthesis (principal sterol in fungal cell membrane) and inhibiting cell membrane formation

Pharmacodynamics/Kinetics

Distribution: Widely throughout body with good penetration into CSF, eye, peritoneal fluid, sputum, skin, and urine

Relative diffusion blood into CSF: Adequate with or without inflammation (exceeds usual MICs)

CSF:blood level ratio: Normal meninges: 70% to 80%; Inflamed meninges: >70% to 80%

Protein binding, plasma: 11% to 12%

Bioavailability: Oral: >90%

Half-life elimination: Normal renal function: ~30 hours

Time to peak, serum: Oral: 1-2 hours

Excretion: Urine (80% as unchanged drug)

Dosage The daily dose of fluconazole is the same for oral and I.V. administration

Usual dosage ranges:

Neonates: First 2 weeks of life, especially premature neonates: Same dose as older children every 72 hours

Children: Loading dose: 6-12 mg/kg; maintenance: 3-12 mg/kg/day; duration and dosage depends on severity of infection

Adults: 200-800 mg/day; duration and dosage depends on severity of infection

◀ **Indication-specific dosing:**

Children:

Candidiasis:

Oropharyngeal: Loading dose: 6 mg/kg; maintenance: 3 mg/kg/day for 2 weeks

Esophageal: Loading dose: 6 mg/kg; maintenance: 3-12 mg/kg/day for 21 days and at least 2 weeks following resolution of symptoms

Systemic infection: 6 mg/kg every 12 hours for 28 days

Meningitis, cryptococcal: Loading dose: 12 mg/kg; maintenance: 6-12 mg/kg/day for 10-12 weeks following negative CSF culture; relapse suppression (HIV-positive): 6 mg/kg/day

Adults:

Candidiasis (Pappas, 2009):

Candidemia (neutropenic and non-neutropenic): Loading dose: 800 mg on first day, then 400 mg/day for 14 days after last positive blood culture and resolution of signs/symptoms; **Note:** Not recommended for neutropenic patients with recent azole exposure and critical illness

Chronic, disseminated: 400 mg/day until calcification or lesion resolution

CNS candidemia: 400-800 mg/day until CSF/radiological abnormalities resolved; **Note:** Recommended as alternative therapy in patients intolerant of amphotericin B

Oropharyngeal (long-term suppression): 100-200 mg/day for 7-14 days; chronic therapy of 100 mg 3 times weekly is recommended in immunocompromised patients with history of oropharyngeal candidiasis (OPC)

Osteoarticular: 400 mg/day for 6-12 months (osteomyelitis) or 6 weeks (septic arthritis)

Esophageal: 200-400 mg/day for 14-21 days

Prophylaxis:

Solid organ: 200-400 mg/day for 7-14 days

Neutropenic patients: 400 mg/day for duration of neutropenia

Urinary tract:

Fungus balls: 200-400 mg/day

Pyelonephritis: 200-400 mg/day for 2 weeks

Symptomatic cystitis: 200 mg/day for 2 weeks

Vaginal: 150 mg as a single dose

Coccidiomycosis (unlabeled use, IDSA guideline): 400 mg/day; doses of 800-1000 mg/day have been used for meningeal disease; usual duration of therapy ranges from 3-6 months for primary uncomplicated infections and up to 1 year for pulmonary (chronic and diffuse) infection

Endocarditis, prosthetic valve, early (unlabeled use, IDSA guideline): 400-800 mg/day for 6 weeks after valve replacement (as step-down in stable, culture-negative patients); long-term suppression in absence of valve replacement: 400-800 mg/day

Endophthalmitis: 400-800 mg/day for 4-6 weeks until examination indicates resolution

Meningitis, cryptococcal: Amphotericin 0.7-1 mg/kg +/- 5-FC for 2 weeks then fluconazole 400 mg/day for at least 10 weeks (consider life-long in HIV-positive); maintenance (HIV-positive): 200-400 mg/day life-long

Pericarditis or myocarditis: 400-800 mg/day

Pneumonia, cryptococcal (mild-to-moderate) (unlabeled use, IDSA guideline): 200-400 mg/day for 6-12 months (consider life-long in HIV-positive patients)

Dosing adjustment/interval in renal impairment:
No adjustment for vaginal candidiasis single-dose therapy

For multiple dosing, administer usual load then adjust daily doses as follows:
Cl_{cr} ≤50 mL/minute (no dialysis): Administer 50% of recommended dose or administer every 48 hours.

Hemodialysis: 50% is removed by hemodialysis; administer 100% of daily dose (according to indication) after each dialysis treatment.

Continuous renal replacement therapy (CRRT): Drug clearance is highly dependent on the method of renal replacement, filter type, and flow rate. Appropriate dosing requires close monitoring of pharmacologic response, signs of adverse reactions due to drug accumulation, as well as drug levels in relation to target trough (if appropriate). The following are general recommendations only (based on dialysate flow/ultrafiltration rates of 1 L/ hour) and should not supersede clinical judgment:

CVVH: 200-400 mg every 24 hours

CVVHD/CVVHDF: 400-800 mg every 24 hours

Note: Higher daily doses of 400 mg (CVVH) and 800 mg (CVVHD/ CVVHDF) should be considered when treating resistant organisms and/ or when employing combined ultrafiltration and dialysis flow rates of ≥2 L/ hour for CVVHD/CVVHDF (Trotman, 2005).

Administration
I.V.: Infuse over approximately 1-2 hours; do not exceed 200 mg/hour

Oral: May be administered with or without food

Monitoring Parameters Periodic liver function tests (AST, ALT, alkaline phosphatase) and renal function tests, potassium

Dietary Considerations Take with or without regard to food.

Dosage Forms Excipient information presented when available (limited, particularly for generics); consult specific product labeling.

Infusion [premixed in sodium chloride or dextrose]: 200 mg (100 mL); 400 mg (200 mL)

Diflucan® [premixed in sodium chloride or dextrose]: 200 mg (100 mL); 400 mg (200 mL)

Powder for oral suspension: 10 mg/mL (35 mL); 40 mg/mL (35 mL)

Diflucan®: 10 mg/mL (35 mL); 40 mg/mL (35 mL) [contains sodium benzoate; orange flavor]

Tablet: 50 mg, 100 mg, 150 mg, 200 mg

Diflucan®: 50 mg, 100 mg, 150 mg, 200 mg

References
Amichai B and Grunwald MH, "Adverse Drug Reactions of the New Oral Antifungal Agents - Terbinafine, Fluconazole, and Itraconazole," *Int J Dermatol*, 1998, 37(6):410-5.

Berl T, Wilner KD, Gardner M, et al, "Pharmacokinetics of Fluconazole in Renal Failure," *J Am Soc Nephrol*, 1995, 6(2):242-7.

Como JA and Dismukes WE, "Oral Azole Drugs as Systemic Antifungal Therapy," *N Engl J Med*, 1993, 330(4):263-72.

Edwards JE Jr, Bodey GP, Bowden RA, et al, "International Conference for the Development of a Consensus on the Management and Prevention of Severe Candidal Infections," *Clin Infect Dis*, 1997, 25(1):43-59.

Goa KL and Barradell LB, "Fluconazole. An Update of Its Pharmacodynamic and Pharmacokinetic Properties and Therapeutic Use in Major Superficial and Systemic Mycoses in Immunocompromised Patients," *Drugs*, 1995, 50(4):658-90.

Goodman JL, Winston DJ, Greenfield RA, et al, "A Controlled Trial of Fluconazole to Prevent Fungal Infections in Patients Undergoing Bone Marrow Transplantation," *N Engl J Med*, 1992, 326(13):845-51.

Lee JW, Seibel NL, Amantea M, et al, "Safety and Pharmacokinetics of Fluconazole in Children With Neoplastic Diseases," *J Pediatr*, 1992, 120(6):987-93.

Pappas PG, Kauffman CA, Andes D, et al, "Clinical Practice Guidelines for the Management of Candidiasis: 2009 Update by the Infectious Diseases Society of America," *Clin Infect Dis*, 2009, 48(5):503-35.

◀

Rex JH, Bennett JE, Sugar AM, "A Randomized Trial Comparing Fluconazole With Amphotericin B for the Treatment of Candidemia in Patients Without Neutropenia. Candidemia Study Group and the National Institute," *N Engl J Med*, 1994, 331(20):1325-30.

Rex JH, Walsh TJ, Sobel JD, et al, "Practice Guidelines for the Treatment of Candidiasis, Infectious Diseases Society of America," *Clin Infect Dis*, 2000, 30(4):662-78.

Saag MS, Graybill RJ, Larsen RA, et al, "Practice Guidelines for the Management of Cryptococcal Disease. Infectious Diseases Society of America," *Clin Infect Dis*, 2000, 30(4):710-8.

Viscoli C, Castagnola E, Fioredda F, et al, "Fluconazole in the Treatment of Candidiasis in Immunocompromised Children," *Antimicrob Agents Chemother*, 1991, 35(2):365-7.

◆ **Fluconazole Injection (Can)** *see* Fluconazole *on page* 485

◆ **Fluconazole Omega (Can)** *see* Fluconazole *on page* 485

Flucytosine (floo SYE toe seen)

Medication Safety Issues

Sound-alike/look-alike issues:

Flucytosine may be confused with fluorouracil

Ancobon® may be confused with Oncovin®

High alert medication: The Institute for Safe Medication Practices (ISMP) includes this medication among its list of drugs which have a heightened risk of causing significant patient harm when used in error.

U.S. Brand Names Ancobon®

Index Terms 5-FC; 5-Fluorocytosine; 5-Flurocytosine

Generic Available No

Canadian Brand Names Ancobon®

Pharmacologic Category Antifungal Agent, Oral

Use Adjunctive treatment of systemic fungal infections (eg, septicemia, endocarditis, UTI, meningitis, or pulmonary) caused by susceptible strains of *Candida* or *Cryptococcus*

Pregnancy Risk Factor C

Lactation Excretion in breast milk unknown/not recommended

Labeled Contraindications Hypersensitivity to flucytosine or any component of the formulation

Warnings/Precautions [U.S. Boxed Warning]: Use with extreme caution in patients with renal dysfunction; dosage adjustment required. Avoid use as monotherapy; resistance rapidly develops. Use with caution in patients with bone marrow depression; patients with hematologic disease or who have been treated with radiation or drugs that suppress the bone marrow may be at greatest risk. Bone marrow toxicity can be irreversible. **[U.S. Boxed Warning]: Closely monitor hematologic, renal, and hepatic status.** Hepatotoxicity and bone marrow toxicity appear to be dose related; monitor levels closely and adjust dose accordingly. Safety and efficacy in children have not been established.

Adverse Reactions Frequency not defined.

Cardiovascular: Cardiac arrest, myocardial toxicity, ventricular dysfunction, chest pain

Central nervous system: Ataxia, confusion, dizziness, drowsiness, fatigue, hallucinations, headache, parkinsonism, psychosis, pyrexia, sedation, seizure, vertigo

Dermatologic: Rash, photosensitivity, pruritus, toxic epidermal necrolysis, urticaria

Endocrine & metabolic: Hypoglycemia, hypokalemia

Gastrointestinal: Abdominal pain, diarrhea, dry mouth, duodenal ulcer, hemorrhage, loss of appetite, nausea, ulcerative colitis, vomiting

Hematologic: Agranulocytosis, anemia, aplastic anemia, eosinophilia, leukopenia, pancytopenia, thrombocytopenia

Hepatic: Acute hepatic injury, bilirubin increased, hepatic dysfunction, jaundice, liver enzymes increased

Neuromuscular & skeletal: Paresthesia, peripheral neuropathy, weakness

Otic: Hearing loss

Renal: Azotemia, BUN increased, crystalluria, renal failure, serum creatinine increased

Respiratory: Dyspnea, respiratory arrest

Miscellaneous: Allergic reaction

Drug Interactions

Avoid Concomitant Use There are no known interactions where it is recommended to avoid concomitant use.

Increased Effect/Toxicity

The levels/effects of Flucytosine may be increased by: Amphotericin B

Decreased Effect

Flucytosine may decrease the levels/effects of: Saccharomyces boulardii

The levels/effects of Flucytosine may be decreased by: Cytarabine

Ethanol/Nutrition/Herb Interactions Food: Food decreases the rate, but not the extent of absorption.

Storage/Stability Store at room temperature of 15°C to 30°C (59°F to 86°F). Protect from light.

Mechanism of Action Penetrates fungal cells and is converted to fluorouracil which competes with uracil interfering with fungal RNA and protein synthesis

Pharmacodynamics/Kinetics

Absorption: 76% to 89%

Distribution: Into CSF, aqueous humor, joints, peritoneal fluid, and bronchial secretions; V_d: 0.6 L/kg

Protein binding: 3% to 4%

Metabolism: Minimally hepatic; deaminated, possibly via gut bacteria, to 5-fluorouracil

Half-life elimination:

Normal renal function: 2-5 hours

Anuria: 85 hours (range: 30-250)

End stage renal disease: 75-200 hours

Time to peak, serum: ~1-2 hours

Excretion: Urine (>90% as unchanged drug)

Dosage

Usual dosage ranges: Children (unlabeled use) and Adults: Oral: 50-150 mg/kg/day in divided doses every 6 hours

Indication-specific dosing:

Children (unlabeled use) and Adults: Oral:

Endocarditis: 25-37.5 mg/kg every 6 hours (with amphotericin B) for at least 6 weeks after valve replacement

Meningoencephalitis, cryptococcal: Induction: 25 mg/kg/dose (with amphotericin B) every 6 hours for 2 weeks; if clinical improvement, may discontinue both amphotericin and flucytosine and follow with an extended course of fluconazole (400 mg/day); alternatively, may continue flucytosine for 6-10 weeks (with amphotericin B) without conversion to fluconazole treatment

Dosing interval in renal impairment: Use lower initial dose:

Cl_{cr} 20-40 mL/minute: Administer 37.5 mg/kg every 12 hours

Cl_{cr} 10-20 mL/minute: Administer 37.5 mg/kg every 24 hours

Cl_{cr} <10 mL/minute: Administer 37.5 mg/kg every 24-48 hours, but monitor drug concentrations frequently

Hemodialysis: Dialyzable (50% to 100%); administer dose posthemodialysis

Peritoneal dialysis: Adults: Administer 0.5-1 g every 24 hours

Continuous arteriovenous or venovenous hemodiafiltration effects: Change dosing frequency to every 12-24 hours (monitor serum concentrations and adjust)

Administration Administer around-the-clock to promote less variation in peak and trough serum levels. To avoid nausea and vomiting, administer a few capsules at a time over 15 minutes until full dose is taken.

Monitoring Parameters

Pretreatment: Electrolytes (especially potassium), CBC with differential, BUN, renal function, blood culture

During treatment: CBC with differential, and LFTs (eg, alkaline phosphatase, AST/ALT) frequently, serum flucytosine concentration, renal function

Test Interactions Flucytosine causes markedly false elevations in serum creatinine values when the Ektachem® analyzer is used. The Jaffé reaction is recommended for determining serum creatinine.

Dosage Forms Excipient information presented when available (limited, particularly for generics); consult specific product labeling.

Capsule: 250 mg, 500 mg

Extemporaneous Preparations Flucytosine oral liquid has been prepared by using the contents of ten 500 mg capsules triturated in a mortar and pestle with a small amount of distilled water; the mixture was transferred to a 500 mL volumetric flask; the mortar was rinsed several times with a small amount of distilled water and the fluid added to the flask; sufficient distilled water was added to make a total volume of 500 mL of a 10 mg/mL liquid; oral liquid was stable for 70 days when stored in glass or plastic prescription bottles at 4°C or for up to 14 days at room temperature.

Wintermeyer SM and Nahata MC, "Stability of Flucytosine in an Extemporaneously Compounded Oral Liquid," *Am J Health Syst Pharm*, 1996, 53:407-9.

References

Aronoff GR, Berns JS, Brier ME, et al, "Drug Prescribing in Renal Failure: Dosing Guidelines for Adults," 4th ed. Philadelphia, PA: American College of Physicians; 1999.

Mofenson LM, Oleske J, Serchuck L, et al, "Treating Opportunistic Infections Among HIV-Exposed and Infected Children: Recommendations from CDC, the National Institutes of Health, and the Infectious Diseases Society of America," *MMWR Recomm Rep*, 2004, 53(RR-14):1-92. Available at http://www.cdc.gov/MMWR/preview/MMWRhtml/rr5314a1.htm

Saag MS, Graybill RJ, Larsen RA, et al, "Practice Guidelines for the Management of Cryptococcal Disease. Infectious Diseases Society of America," *Clin Infect Dis*, 2000, 30(4):710-8.

Vermes A, Guchelaar H, and Dankert J, "Flucytosine: A Review of its Pharmacology, Clinical Indications, Pharmacokinetics, Toxicity and Drug Interactions," *J Antimicrob Chemother*, 2000, 46 (2):171-9.

◆ **Fludara®** *see* Fludarabine *on page 492*

Fludarabine (floo DARE a been)

Medication Safety Issues

Sound-alike/look-alike issues:

Fludarabine may be confused with cladribine, floxuridine, Flumadine® Fludara® may be confused with FUDR®

High alert medication: The Institute for Safe Medication Practices (ISMP) includes this medication among its list of drug classes which have a heightened risk of causing significant patient harm when used in error.

Related Information

Hematopoietic Stem Cell Transplantation *on page 1501*

Safe Handling of Hazardous Drugs *on page 1517*

U.S. Brand Names Fludara®

Index Terms 2F-ara-AMP; Fludarabine Phosphate; NSC-312887

Generic Available Yes

Canadian Brand Names Fludara®

Pharmacologic Category Antineoplastic Agent, Antimetabolite (Purine Antagonist)

Use

U.S. labeling: Treatment of progressive or refractory B-cell chronic lymphocytic leukemia (CLL)

Canadian labeling: Second-line treatment of chronic lymphocytic leukemia (CLL); second-line treatment of low-grade, refractory non-Hodgkin's lymphoma (NHL)

Unlabeled/Investigational Use Treatment of non-Hodgkin's lymphoma (NHL); refractory acute leukemias and solid tumors (in pediatric patients); Waldenström's macroglobulinemia (WM); reduced-intensity conditioning regimens prior to allogeneic hematopoietic stem cell transplantation (generally administered in combination with busulfan and antithymocyte globulin or lymphocyte immune globulin, or in combination with melphalan and alemtuzumab)

Pregnancy Risk Factor D

Lactation Excretion in breast milk unknown/not recommended

Labeled Contraindications Hypersensitivity of fludarabine or any component of the formulation

Canadian labeling: Additional contraindications (not in U.S. labeling): Severe renal impairment (Cl_{cr} <30 mL/minute); decompensated hemolytic anemia; concurrent use with pentostatin

Warnings/Precautions Hazardous agent - use appropriate precautions for handling and disposal. Use with caution in patients with renal insufficiency (clearance of the primary metabolite 2-fluoro-ara-A is reduced); dosage modifications may be recommended; monitor closely. Use with caution in patients with pre-existing hematological disorders (particularly granulocytopenia) or pre-existing central nervous system disorder (epilepsy), spasticity, or peripheral neuropathy. **[U.S. Boxed Warning]: Higher than recommended doses are associated with severe neurologic toxicity (delayed blindness, coma, death); similar neurotoxicity (agitation, coma, confusion and seizure) has been reported with standard CLL doses.** Neurotoxicity symptoms due to high doses appear from 21-60 days following the last fludarabine dose. Possible neurotoxic effects of chronic administration are unknown. Caution patients about performing tasks which require mental alertness (eg, operating machinery or driving. **[U.S. Boxed Warning]: Life-threatening (and sometimes fatal) autoimmune effects, including hemolytic anemia, autoimmune thrombocytopenia/thrombocytopenic purpura (ITP), Evans syndrome, and acquired hemophilia have occurred;** monitor closely for hemolysis; discontinue fludarabine if hemolysis occurs; the hemolytic effects usually recur with fludarabine rechallenge. **[U.S. Boxed Warning]: Severe bone marrow suppression (anemia, thrombocytopenia, and neutropenia) may occur;** may be cumulative. Severe myelosuppression (trilineage bone marrow hypoplasia/aplasia) has been reported (rare); the ▶

duration of significant cytopenias in these cases may be prolonged (up to 1 year).

Use with caution in patients with documented infection, fever, immunodeficiency, or with a history of opportunistic infection; prophylactic anti-infectives should be considered for patients with an increased risk for developing opportunistic infections. Progressive multifocal leukoencephalopathy (PML) due to JC virus (usually fatal) has been reported with use; usually in patients who had received prior and/or other concurrent chemotherapy; onset ranges from a few weeks to 1 year; evaluate any neurological change promptly. Avoid vaccination with live vaccines during and after fludarabine treatment. May cause tumor lysis syndrome; risk is increased in patients with large tumor burden prior to treatment. Patients receiving blood products should only receive irradiated blood products due to the potential for transfusion related GVHD. **[U.S. Boxed Warnings]: Do not use in combination with pentostatin; may lead to severe, even fatal pulmonary toxicity. Should be administered under the supervision of an experienced cancer chemotherapy physician.**

Adverse Reactions

>10%:

Cardiovascular: Edema (8% to 19%)

Central nervous system: Fever (11% to 69%), fatigue (10% to 38%), pain (5% to 22%), chills (11% to 19%)

Dermatologic: Rash (4% to 15%)

Gastrointestinal: Nausea/vomiting (1% to 38%), anorexia (≤34%), diarrhea (5% to 15%), gastrointestinal bleeding (3% to 13%)

Genitourinary: Urinary tract infection (2% to 15%)

Hematologic: Myelosuppression (nadir: 10-14 days; recovery: 5-7 weeks; dose-limiting toxicity), anemia (14% to 60%), neutropenia (grade 4: 37% to 59%; nadir: ~13 days), thrombocytopenia (17% to 55%; nadir: ~16 days)

Neuromuscular & skeletal: Weakness (9% to 65%), myalgia (4% to 16%), paresthesia (4% to 12%)

Ocular: Visual disturbance (3% to 15%)

Respiratory: Cough (≤44%), pneumonia (3% to 22%), dyspnea (1% to 22%), upper respiratory infection (2% to 16%), rhinitis (≤11%)

Miscellaneous: Infection (12% to 44%), diaphoresis (≤14%)

1% to 10%:

Cardiovascular: Peripheral edema (≤7%), angina (≤6%), chest pain (≤5%), CHF (≤3%), arrhythmia (≤3%), cerebrovascular accident (≤3%), MI (≤3%), supraventricular tachycardia (≤3%), deep vein thrombosis (1% to 3%), phlebitis (1% to 3%), aneurysm (≤1%), transient ischemic attack (≤1%)

Central nervous system: Headache (≤9%), malaise (6% to 8%), sleep disorder (1% to 3%), cerebellar syndrome (≤1%), depression (≤1%), mentation impaired (≤1%)

Dermatologic: Alopecia (≤3%), pruritus (1% to 3%), seborrhea (≤1%)

Endocrine & metabolic: Hyperglycemia (1% to 6%), LDH increased (≤6%), dehydration (≤1%)

Gastrointestinal: Abdominal pain (≤10%), stomatitis (≤9%), weight loss (≤6%), esophagitis (≤3%), constipation (1% to 3%), mucositis (≤2%), dysphagia (≤1%)

Genitourinary: Dysuria (3% to 4%), hesitancy (≤3%)

Hematologic: Hemorrhage (≤1%), myelodysplastic syndrome/acute myeloid leukemia (usually associated with prior or concurrent treatment with other anticancer agents)

Hepatic: Cholelithiasis (≤3%), liver function tests abnormal (1% to 3%), liver failure (≤1%)

Neuromuscular & skeletal: Back pain (≤9%), osteoporosis (≤2%), arthralgia (≤1%)

Otic: Hearing loss (2% to 6%)

Renal: Hematuria (2% to 3%), renal failure (≤1%), renal function test abnormal (≤1%), proteinuria (≤1%)

Respiratory: Bronchitis (≤9%), pharyngitis (≤9%), allergic pneumonitis (≤6%), hemoptysis (1% to 6%), sinusitis (≤5%), epistaxis (≤1%), hypoxia (≤1%)

Miscellaneous: Flu-like syndrome (5% to 8%), herpes simplex infection (≤8%), anaphylaxis (≤1%), tumor lysis syndrome (1%)

<1%, postmarketing, and/or case reports: Acute respiratory distress syndrome, agitation, blindness, blurred vision, bone marrow fibrosis, coma, confusion, diplopia, eosinophilia, Epstein-Barr virus (EBV) associated lymphoproliferation, EBV reactivation, erythema multiforme, Evans syndrome, flank pain, hemolytic anemia (autoimmune), hemophilia (acquired), hemorrhagic cystitis, herpes zoster reactivation, hyperkalemia, hyperphosphatemia, hyperuricemia, hypocalcemia, interstitial pneumonitis, metabolic acidosis, opportunistic infection, optic neuritis, optic neuropathy, pancreatic enzymes abnormal, pancytopenia, pemphigus, pericardial effusion, peripheral neuropathy, photophobia (primarily with high doses), progressive multifocal leukoencephalopathy (PML), pulmonary fibrosis, pulmonary hemorrhage, pulmonary infiltrate, respiratory distress, respiratory failure, skin cancer (new onset or exacerbation), Stevens-Johnson syndrome, thrombocytopenia (autoimmune), thrombocytopenic purpura (autoimmune), toxic epidermal necrolysis, trilineage bone marrow aplasia, trilineage bone marrow hypoplasia, urate crystalluria, wrist drop

Also observed: Neurologic syndrome characterized by cortical blindness, coma, and paralysis [36% at doses >96 mg/m^2 for 5-7 days; <0.2% at doses <125 mg/m^2/cycle (onset of neurologic symptoms may be delayed for 3-4 weeks)]

Drug Interactions

Avoid Concomitant Use

Avoid concomitant use of Fludarabine with any of the following: Natalizumab; Pentostatin; Vaccines (Live)

Increased Effect/Toxicity

Fludarabine may increase the levels/effects of: Leflunomide; Natalizumab; Pentostatin; Vaccines (Live)

The levels/effects of Fludarabine may be increased by: Pentostatin; Trastuzumab

Decreased Effect

Fludarabine may decrease the levels/effects of: Vaccines (Inactivated); Vaccines (Live)

The levels/effects of Fludarabine may be decreased by: Echinacea

Ethanol/Nutrition/Herb Interactions Ethanol: Avoid ethanol (due to GI irritation).

Storage/Stability

I.V.: Store intact vials under refrigeration at 2°C to 8°C (36°F to 46°F). Reconstituted vials are stable for 16 days at room temperature of 15°C to 30°C (59°F to 86°F) or refrigerated, although the manufacturer recommends use within 8 hours. Solutions diluted in saline or dextrose are stable for 48 hours at room temperature or under refrigeration.

◄   Tablet: Store at 25°C (77°F); excursions permitted to 15°C to 30°C (59°F to 86°F); should be kept within packaging until use.

Reconstitution Use appropriate precautions for handling and disposal. Reconstitute vials with SWI, NS, or D_5W to a concentration of 10-25 mg/mL. Standard I.V. dilution: 100-125 mL D_5W or NS.

Compatibility Stable in D_5W, NS, sterile water for injection.

Y-site administration: Compatible: Allopurinol, amifostine, amikacin, aminophylline, ampicillin, ampicillin/sulbactam, amsacrine, aztreonam, bleomycin, butorphanol, carboplatin, carmustine, cefazolin, cefepime, cefotaxime, cefotetan, ceftazidime, ceftizoxime, ceftriaxone, cefuroxime, cimetidine, cisplatin, clindamycin, co-trimoxazole, cyclophosphamide, cytarabine, dacarbazine, dactinomycin, dexamethasone sodium phosphate, diphenhydramine, doxorubicin, doxycycline, droperidol, etoposide, etoposide phosphate, famotidine, filgrastim, floxuridine, fluconazole, fluorouracil, furosemide, gemcitabine, gentamicin, granisetron, haloperidol lactate, heparin, hydrocortisone sodium succinate, hydromorphone, ifosfamide, imipenem/cilastatin, lorazepam, magnesium sulfate, mannitol, mechlorethamine, melphalan, meperidine, mesna, methotrexate, methylprednisolone sodium succinate, metoclopramide, mitoxantrone, morphine, multivitamins, nalbuphine, ondansetron, pentostatin, piperacillin, piperacillin/tazobactam, potassium chloride, promethazine, ranitidine, sodium bicarbonate, teniposide, thiotepa, ticarcillin/clavulanate, tobramycin, vancomycin, vinblastine, vincristine, vinorelbine, zidovudine. Incompatible: Acyclovir, amphotericin B, chlorpromazine, daunorubicin HCl, ganciclovir, hydroxyzine HCl, prochlorperazine edisylate.

Mechanism of Action Fludarabine inhibits DNA synthesis by inhibition of DNA polymerase and ribonucleotide reductase; also inhibits DNA primase and DNA ligase I

Pharmacodynamics/Kinetics

Distribution: V_d: 38-96 L/m^2; widely with extensive tissue binding

Protein binding: 2-fluoro-ara-A: ~19% to 29%

Metabolism: I.V.: Fludarabine phosphate is rapidly dephosphorylated in the plasma to 2-fluoro-ara-A (active metabolite), which subsequently enters tumor cells and is phosphorylated by deoxycytidine kinase to the active triphosphate derivative (2-fluoro-ara-ATP)

Bioavailability: Oral: 2-fluoro-ara-A: 50% to 65%

Half-life elimination: 2-fluoro-ara-A: ~20 hours

Time to peak, plasma: Oral: 1-2 hours

Excretion: Urine (60%, 23% as 2-fluoro-ara-A) within 24 hours

Dosage Details concerning dosing in combination regimens should also be consulted.

Oral: Adults: CLL: 40 mg/m^2 once daily for 5 days every 28 days

I.V.:

Children (unlabeled use):

Refractory acute leukemia: 10 mg/m^2 bolus over 15 minutes followed by continuous infusion of 30.5 mg/m^2/day for 5 days **or**

  10.5 mg/m^2 bolus over 15 minutes followed by 30.5 mg/m^2/day for 48 hours

Refractory solid tumors: 7 mg/m^2 bolus followed by 20 mg/m^2/day continuous infusion for 5 days

Adults:

CLL: 25 mg/m^2/day for 5 days every 28 days

Non-hodgkin's lymphoma, WM (unlabeled uses): 25 mg/m^2/day for 5 days every 28 days

Reduced-intensity conditioning regimens prior to allogeneic hematopoietic stem cell transplantation (unlabeled use): 120-150 mg/m^2 administered in divided doses over 4-5 days

Dosage adjustment for toxicity:

Hematologic or nonhematologic toxicity (other than neurotoxicity): Consider treatment delay or dosage reduction

Hemolysis: Discontinue treatment

Neurotoxicity: Consider treatment delay or discontinuation

Dosing in renal impairment:

FDA-approved labeling contains the following adjustment recommendations:

Adults:

Cl_{cr} 30-70 mL/minute: Administer 80% of dose

Cl_{cr} <30 mL/minute:

I.V.: Avoid use

Oral: Administer 50% of dose

Canadian labeling contains the following adjustment recommendations:

Cl_{cr} 30-70 mL/minute: Administer 50% of dose

Cl_{cr} <30 mL/minute: Use is contraindicated

The following guidelines have been used by some clinicians:

Aronoff, 2007:

Children:

Cl_{cr} 30-50 mL/minute: Administer 80% of dose

Cl_{cr} <30 mL/minute: Not recommended

Hemodialysis: Administer 25% of dose

Continuous ambulatory peritoneal dialysis (CAPD): Not recommended

Continuous renal replacement therapy (CRRT): Administer 80% of dose

Adults:

Cl_{cr} 10-50 mL/minute: Administer 75% of dose

Cl_{cr} <10 mL/minute: Administer 50% of dose

Hemodialysis: Administer after dialysis

Continuous ambulatory peritoneal dialysis (CAPD): Administer 50% of dose

Continuous renal replacement therapy (CRRT): Administer 75% of dose

Kintzel, 1995:

Cl_{cr} 46-60 mL/minute: Administer 80% of dose

Cl_{cr} 31-45 mL/minute: Administer 75% of dose

Cl_{cr} <30 mL/minute: Administer 65% of dose

Combination Regimens

Leukemia, acute lymphocytic: FIS-HAM on page 1322

Leukemia, acute myeloid:

FIS-HAM on page 1322

FLAG (AML) on page 1323

FLAG-IDA on page 1324

Leukemia, chronic lymphocytic:

Fludarabine-Cyclophosphamide (CLL) on page 1325

Fludarabine-Cyclophosphamide-Rituximab (CLL) on page 1327

Fludarabine-Rituximab (CLL) on page 1330

OFAR (CLL) on page 1381

Lymphoma, non-Hodgkin's:

Fludarabine-Cyclophosphamide-Mitoxantrone-Rituximab on page 1326

Fludarabine-Cyclophosphamide-Rituximab (NHL-Follicular) on page 1328

Fludarabine-Mitoxantrone on page 1328

Fludarabine-Mitoxantrone-Dexamethasone (NHL) on page 1328

Fludarabine-Mitoxantrone-Dexamethasone-Rituximab on page 1329

Fludarabine-Mitoxantrone-Rituximab on page 1330

Lymphoma, non-Hodgkin's (Mantle cell): Fludarabine-Cyclophosphamide (NHL-Mantle Cell) on page 1327

Administration

Oral: Tablet may be administered with or without food; should be swallowed whole with water; do not chew, break, or crush.

I.V.: Usually administered as a 30-minute infusion; continuous infusions are occasionally used

Monitoring Parameters CBC with differential, platelet count, AST, ALT, serum creatinine, serum albumin, uric acid; monitor for signs of infection and neurotoxicity

Dietary Considerations Tablet may be taken with or without food.

Emetic Potential

Oral: Low (10% to 30%)

I.V.: Very low (<10%)

Product Availability Fludarabine oral formulation (brand name pending): FDA approved December 2008; availability currently undetermined

Dosage Forms Excipient information presented when available (limited, particularly for generics); consult specific product labeling. [CAN] = Canadian brand name

Injection, powder for reconstitution, as phosphate: 50 mg

Fludara®: 50 mg

Injection, solution, as phosphate [preservative free]: 25 mg/mL (2 mL)

Tablet, as phosphate: 10 mg

Fludara® [CAN]: 10 mg

References

Aronoff GR, Bennett WM, Berns JS, et al, *Drug Prescribing in Renal Failure: Dosing Guidelines for Adults and Children*, 5th ed. Philadelphia, PA: American College of Physicians; 2007, p 99, 172.

Bacigalupo A, "Second EBMT Workshop on Reduced Intensity Allogeneic Hemopoietic Stem Cell Transplants (RI-HSCT)," *Bone Marrow Transplant*, 2002, 29(3):191-5.

Boogaerts MA, Van Hoof A, Catovsky D, et al, "Activity of Oral Fludarabine Phosphate in Previously Treated Chronic Lymphocytic Leukemia," *J Clin Oncol*, 2001, 19(22):4252-8.

Foran JM, Rohatiner AZ, Coiffier B, et al, "Multicenter Phase II Study of Fludarabine Phosphate for Patients With Newly Diagnosed Lymphoplasmacytoid Lymphoma, Waldenström's Macroglobulinemia, and Mantle-Cell Lymphoma," *J Clin Oncol*, 1999, 17(2):546-53.

Giralt S, Aleman A, Anagnostopoulos A, et al, "Fludarabine/Melphalan Conditioning for Allogeneic Transplantation in Patients With Multiple Myeloma," *Bone Marrow Transplant*, 2002, 30 (6):367-73.

Hagenbeek A, Eghbali H, Monfardini S, et al, "Phase III Intergroup Study of Fludarabine Phosphate Compared With Cyclophosphamide, Vincristine, and Prednisone Chemotherapy in Newly Diagnosed Patients With Stage III and IV Low-Grade Malignant Non-Hodgkin's Lymphoma," *J Clin Oncol*, 2006, 24(10):1590-6.

Johnson SA, "Clinical Pharmacokinetics of Nucleoside Analogues: Focus on Haematological Malignancies," *Clin Pharmacokinet*, 2000, 39(1):5-26.

Kintzel PE and Dorr RT, "Anticancer Drug Renal Toxicity and Elimination: Dosing Guidelines for Altered Renal Function," *Cancer Treat Rev*, 1995, 21(1):33-64.

Plosker GL and Figgitt DP, "Oral fludarabine," *Drugs*, 2003, 63(21):2317-23.

Plunkett W, Gandhi V, Huang P, et al, "Fludarabine: Pharmacokinetics, Mechanisms of Action, and Rationales for Combination Therapies," *Semin Oncol*, 1993, 20(5 Suppl 7):2-12.

Rossi JF, van Hoof A, de Boeck K, et al, "Efficacy and Safety of Oral Fludarabine Phosphate in Previously Untreated Patients With Chronic Lymphocytic Leukemia," *J Clin Oncol*, 2004, 22 (7):1260-7.

Schetelig J, Bornhauser M, Kiehl M, et al, "Reduced-Intensity Conditioning With Busulfan and Fludarabine With or Without Antithymocyte Globulin in HLA-Identical Sibling Transplantation - A Retrospective Analysis," *Bone Marrow Transplant*, 2004, 33(5):483-90.

Van Besien K, Devine S, Wickrema A, et al, "Regimen-Related Toxicity After Fludarabine-Melphalan Conditioning: A Prospective Study of 31 Patients With Hematologic Malignancies," *Bone Marrow Transplant*, 2003, 32(5):471-6.

◆ **Fludarabine Phosphate** see Fludarabine on page 492

◆ **5-Fluorocytosine** *see* Flucytosine *on page 490*

◆ **Fluorodeoxyuridine** *see* Floxuridine *on page 482*

◆ **Fluoroplex®** *see* Fluorouracil *on page 499*

Fluorouracil (flure oh YOOR a sil)

Medication Safety Issues

Sound-alike/look-alike issues:
  Carac® may be confused with Kuric™
  Fluorouracil may be confused with flucytosine
  Efudex® may be confused with Efidac (Efidac 24®), Eurax®

High alert medication: The Institute for Safe Medication Practices (ISMP) includes this medication among its list of drugs which have a heightened risk of causing significant patient harm when used in error.

International issues:
  Carac® may be confused with Carace® which is a brand name for lisinopril in Ireland and Great Britain

Related Information

  Fertility and Cancer Therapy *on page 1430*
  Management of Drug Extravasations *on page 1447*
  Oral Mucositis / Stomatitis *on page 1460*
  Safe Handling of Hazardous Drugs *on page 1517*

U.S. Brand Names Adrucil®; Carac®; Efudex®; Fluoroplex®; Fluorouracil® [DSC]

Index Terms 5-Fluorouracil; 5-FU; FU

Generic Available Yes: Injection, topical solution

Canadian Brand Names Efudex®

Pharmacologic Category Antineoplastic Agent, Antimetabolite (Pyrimidine Analog)

Use Treatment of carcinomas of the breast, colon, rectum, pancreas, or stomach; topically for the management of actinic or solar keratoses and superficial basal cell carcinomas

Unlabeled/Investigational Use Treatment of head and neck cancer, anal cancer, cervical cancer

Pregnancy Risk Factor D (injection); X (topical)

Lactation Excretion in breast milk unknown/not recommended

Labeled Contraindications Hypersensitivity to fluorouracil or any component of the formulation; dihydropyrimidine dehydrogenase (DPD) enzyme deficiency; pregnancy

Warnings/Precautions Hazardous agent - use appropriate precautions for handling and disposal. Use with caution in patients with impaired kidney or liver function. The drug should be discontinued if intractable vomiting or diarrhea, precipitous falls in leukocyte or platelet counts, stomatitis, hemorrhage, or myocardial ischemia occurs. Use with caution in patients who have had high-dose pelvic radiation or previous use of alkylating agents. Palmar-plantar erythrodysesthesia (hand-foot) syndrome has been associated with use. Safety and efficacy have not been established in pediatric patients.

Administration to patients with a genetic deficiency of dihydropyrimidine dehydrogenase (DPD) has been associated with increased toxicity following administration (diarrhea, neutropenia, and neurotoxicity). Systemic toxicity normally associated with parenteral administration has also been associated with topical use, particularly in patients with DPD. Discontinue if symptoms of ▶

◀ DPD occur. **[U.S. Boxed Warning]: Should be administered under the supervision of an experienced cancer chemotherapy physician.**

Avoid topical application to mucous membranes due to potential for local inflammation and ulceration. The use of occlusive dressings with topical preparations may increase the severity of inflammation in nearby skin areas. Avoid exposure to ultraviolet rays during and immediately following therapy.

Adverse Reactions Toxicity depends on route and duration of treatment

I.V.:
Cardiovascular: Angina, myocardial ischemia, nail changes
Central nervous system: Acute cerebellar syndrome, confusion, disorientation, euphoria, headache, nystagmus
Dermatologic: Alopecia, dermatitis, dry skin, fissuring, palmar-plantar erythrodysesthesia syndrome, pruritic maculopapular rash, photosensitivity, vein pigmentations
Gastrointestinal: Anorexia, bleeding, diarrhea, esophagopharyngitis, nausea, sloughing, stomatitis, ulceration, vomiting
Hematologic: Agranulocytosis, anemia, leukopenia, pancytopenia, thrombocytopenia
Myelosuppression:
Onset: 7-10 days
Nadir: 9-14 days
Recovery: 21-28 days
Local: Thrombophlebitis
Ocular: Lacrimation, lacrimal duct stenosis, photophobia, visual changes
Respiratory: Epistaxis
Miscellaneous: Anaphylaxis, generalized allergic reactions, nail loss

Topical: Note: Systemic toxicity normally associated with parenteral administration (including neutropenia, neurotoxicity, and gastrointestinal toxicity) has been associated with topical use particularly in patients with a genetic deficiency of dihydropyrimidine dehydrogenase (DPD).
Central nervous system: Headache, insomnia, irritability
Dermatologic: Alopecia, photosensitivity, pruritus, rash, scarring, telangiectasia
Gastrointestinal: Medicinal taste, stomatitis
Hematologic: Leukocytosis, thrombocytopenia
Local: Application site reactions: Allergic contact dermatitis, burning, crusting, dryness, edema, erosion, erythema, hyperpigmentation, irritation, pain, soreness, ulceration
Ocular: Eye irritation (burning, watering, sensitivity, stinging, itching)
Miscellaneous: Birth defects, herpes simplex, miscarriage

Drug Interactions

Avoid Concomitant Use
Avoid concomitant use of Fluorouracil with any of the following: Natalizumab; Vaccines (Live)

Increased Effect/Toxicity
Fluorouracil may increase the levels/effects of: Carvedilol; CYP2C9 Substrates (High risk); Leflunomide; Natalizumab; Phenytoin; Vaccines (Live); Vitamin K Antagonists

The levels/effects of Fluorouracil may be increased by: Gemcitabine; Leucovorin-Levoleucovorin; Sorafenib; Trastuzumab

Decreased Effect
Fluorouracil may decrease the levels/effects of: Vaccines (Inactivated); Vaccines (Live); Vitamin K Antagonists

The levels/effects of Fluorouracil may be decreased by: Echinacea; Sorafenib

Ethanol/Nutrition/Herb Interactions

Ethanol: Avoid ethanol (due to GI irritation).

Herb/Nutraceutical: Avoid black cohosh, dong quai in estrogen-dependent tumors.

Storage/Stability

Injection: Store intact vials at room temperature. Protect from light. Slight discoloration does not usually denote decomposition. If exposed to cold, a precipitate may form; **gentle** heating to 60°C will dissolve the precipitate without impairing the potency. Solutions in 50-1000 mL NS or D_5W, or undiluted solutions in syringes are stable for 72 hours at room temperature.

Topical: Store at controlled room temperature of 15°C to 30°C (59°F to 86°F).

Reconstitution Dilute in 50-1000 mL NS, D_5W, or bacteriostatic NS for infusion.

Compatibility Stable in D_5LR, D_5W, NS, bacteriostatic NS; **incompatible** with concentrations >25 mg/mL of fluorouracil and >2 mg/mL of leucovorin (precipitation occurs).

Y-site administration: Compatible: Allopurinol, amifostine, aztreonam, bleomycin, cefepime, cisplatin, cyclophosphamide, doxorubicin, doxorubicin liposome, etoposide phosphate, fludarabine, furosemide, gatifloxacin, gemcitabine, granisetron, heparin, hydrocortisone sodium succinate, leucovorin, linezolid, mannitol, melphalan, methotrexate, metoclopramide, mitomycin, paclitaxel, piperacillin/tazobactam, potassium chloride, propofol, sargramostim, teniposide, thiotepa, vinblastine, vincristine, vitamin B complex with C. **Incompatible:** Amphotericin B cholesteryl sulfate complex, droperidol, filgrastim, ondansetron, topotecan, vinorelbine.

Compatibility in syringe: Compatible: Bleomycin, cisplatin, cyclophosphamide, furosemide, heparin, leucovorin, methotrexate, metoclopramide, mitomycin, vinblastine, vincristine. **Incompatible:** Droperidol, epirubicin. **Variable (consult detailed reference):** Doxorubicin.

Compatibility when admixed: Compatible: Bleomycin, cyclophosphamide, cyclophosphamide with methotrexate, etoposide, floxuridine, hydromorphone, ifosfamide, methotrexate, mitoxantrone, vincristine. **Incompatible:** Carboplatin, cisplatin, cytarabine, diazepam, doxorubicin, fentanyl, leucovorin, metoclopramide, morphine.

Mechanism of Action A pyrimidine antimetabolite that interferes with DNA synthesis by blocking the methylation of deoxyuridylic acid; fluorouracil inhibits thymidylate synthetase (TS), or is incorporated into RNA. The reduced folate cofactor is required for tight binding to occur between the 5-FdUMP and TS.

Pharmacodynamics/Kinetics

Duration: ~3 weeks

Distribution: V_d: ~22% of total body water; penetrates extracellular fluid, CSF, and third space fluids (eg, pleural effusions and ascitic fluid)

Metabolism: Hepatic (90%); via a dehydrogenase enzyme; FU must be metabolized to be active

Bioavailability: <75%, erratic and undependable

Half-life elimination: Biphasic: Initial: 6-20 minutes; two metabolites, FdUMP and FUTP, have prolonged half-lives depending on the type of tissue

Excretion: Lung (large amounts as CO_2); urine (5% as unchanged drug) in 6 hours

◀ **Dosage** Adults:

Refer to individual protocols:

I.V. bolus: 500-600 mg/m^2 every 3-4 weeks **or** 425 mg/m^2 on days 1-5 every 4 weeks

Continuous I.V. infusion: 1000 mg/m^2/day for 4-5 days every 3-4 weeks **or** 2300-2600 mg/m^2 on day 1 every week **or**

300-400 mg/m^2/day **or**

225 mg/m^2/day for 5-8 weeks (with radiation therapy)

Actinic keratoses: Topical:

Carac™: Apply thin film to lesions once daily for up to 4 weeks, as tolerated

Efudex®: Apply to lesions twice daily for 2-4 weeks; complete healing may not be evident for 1-2 months following treatment

Fluoroplex®: Apply to lesions twice daily for 2-6 weeks

Superficial basal cell carcinoma: Topical: Efudex® 5%: Apply to affected lesions twice daily for 3-6 weeks; treatment may be continued for up to 10-12 weeks

Dosage adjustment for renal impairment: The FDA-approved labeling does not contain specific dosing adjustment guidelines; however, it is stated that extreme caution should be used in patients with renal impairment.

Hemodialysis: Administer dose following hemodialysis.

Aronoff (2007): Recommends that dosage adjustment is not needed in adult patients with Cl$_{cr}$ <50 mL/minute and patients receiving hemodialysis should be administered 50% of dose.

Dosage adjustment for hepatic impairment: The FDA-approved labeling does not contain specific dosing adjustment guidelines; however, it is stated that extreme caution should be used in patients with hepatic impairment. The following guidelines have been used by some clinicians:

Floyd, 2006: Bilirubin >5 mg/dL: Avoid use.

Koren, 1992: Hepatic impairment (degree not specified): Administer <50% of dose, then increase if toxicity does not occur.

Combination Regimens

◀ **Administration**

I.V.: I.V. bolus as a slow push or short (5-15 minutes) bolus infusion, or as a continuous infusion. Doses >1000 mg/m^2 are usually administered as a 24-hour infusion. Toxicity may be reduced by giving the drug as a constant infusion. Bolus doses may be administered by slow IVP or IVPB.

Topical: Apply 10 minutes after washing, rinsing, and drying the affected area. Apply using fingertip (wash hands immediately after application) or nonmetal applicator. Do not cover area with an occlusive dressing. Wash hands immediately after topical application of the 5% cream. Topical preparations are for external use only; not for ophthalmic, oral, or intravaginal use.

Monitoring Parameters CBC with differential and platelet count, renal function tests, liver function tests

Dietary Considerations Increase dietary intake of thiamine.

Additional Information Oncology Comment: An investigational uridine prodrug, vistonuridine, has been studied in a limited number of cases of fluorouracil overdose. Of 17 patients receiving vistonuridine beginning within 8-96 hours after fluorouracil overdose, all patients fully recovered (von Borstel, 2009); refer to Vistonuridine monograph.

Emetic Potential Low (10% to 30%)

Vesicant May be an irritant

Dosage Forms Excipient information presented when available (limited, particularly for generics); consult specific product labeling. [DSC] = Discontinued product

Cream, topical:

Carac®: 0.5% (30 g)

Efudex®: 5% (40 g)

Fluoroplex®: 1% (30 g) [contains benzyl alcohol]

Injection, solution: 50 mg/mL (10 mL, 20 mL, 50 mL, 100 mL)

Adrucil®: 50 mg/mL (10 mL, 50 mL, 100 mL)

Solution, topical: 2% (10 mL); 5% (10 mL)

Efudex®: 2% (10 mL, 25 mL) [DSC]; 5% (10 mL, 25 mL [DSC])

Fluorouracil®: 5% (10 mL) [DSC]

References

Aronoff GR, Bennett WM, Berns JS, et al, *Drug Prescribing in Renal Failure: Dosing Guidelines for Adults and Children*, 5th ed. Philadelphia, PA: American College of Physicians; 2007, p 100.

Curran CF and Luce JK, "Fluorouracil and Palmar-Plantar Erythrodysesthesia," *Ann Intern Med*, 1989, 111(10):858.

Diasio RB and Harris BE, "Clinical Pharmacology of 5-Fluorouracil," *Clin Pharmacokinet*, 1989, 16 (4):215-37.

Diasio RB and Johnson MR, "The Role of Pharmacogenetics and Pharmacogenomics in Cancer Chemotherapy With 5-Fluorouracil," *Pharmacology*, 2000, 61(3):199-203.

Floyd J, Mirza I, Sachs B, et al, "Hepatotoxicity of Chemotherapy," *Semin Oncol*, 2006, 33 (1):50-67.

Iyer L and Ratain MJ, "5-Fluorouracil Pharmacokinetics: Causes for Variability and Strategies for Modulation in Cancer Chemotherapy," *Cancer Invest*, 1999, 17(7):494-506.

Koren G, Beatty K, Seto A, et al, "The Effects of Impaired Liver Function on the Elimination of Antineoplastic Agents," *Ann Pharmacother*, 1992, 26(3):363-71.

Kuhn JG, "Fluorouracil and the New Oral Fluorinated Pyrimidines," *Ann Pharmacother*, 2001, 35 (2):217-27.

Milano G and Chamorey AL, "Clinical Pharmacokinetics of 5-Fluorouracil With Consideration of Chronopharmacokinetics," *Chronobiol Int*, 2002, 19(1):177-89.

Parker WB and Cheng YC, "Metabolism and Mechanism of Action of 5-Fluorouracil," *Pharmacol Ther*, 1990, 48(3):381-95.

Schilsky RL, "Biochemical and Clinical Pharmacology of 5-Fluorouracil," *Oncology*, 1998, 12(10 Suppl 7):13-8.

Trissel LA, Martinez JF, and Xu QA, "Incompatibility of Fluorouracil With Leucovorin Calcium or Levoleucovorin Calcium," *Am J Health Syst Pharm*, 1995, 52(7):710-5.

von Borstel R, O'Neil J, and Bamat M, "Vistonuridine: An Orally Administered, Life-Saving Antidote for 5-Fluorouracil (5FU) Overdose," *J Clin Oncol*, 2009, 27(15S):9616 [abstract from 2009 ASCO Annual Meeting].

♦ **Fluorouracil® [DSC]** *see* Fluorouracil *on page 499*

♦ **5-Fluorouracil** *see* Fluorouracil *on page 499*

Fluoxymesterone (floo oks i MES te rone)

Medication Safety Issues
Sound-alike/look-alike issues:
Halotestin® may be confused with Haldol®, haloperidol, halothane

Related Information
Safe Handling of Hazardous Drugs *on page 1517*

U.S. Brand Names Androxy™

Generic Available Yes

Pharmacologic Category Androgen

Use Replacement of endogenous testicular hormone; in females, palliative treatment of breast cancer

Unlabeled/Investigational Use Stimulation of erythropoiesis, angioneurotic edema

Restrictions C-III

Pregnancy Risk Factor X

Lactation Excretion in breast milk unknown/contraindicated

Labeled Contraindications Hypersensitivity to fluoxymesterone or any component of the formulation; serious cardiac disease; liver or kidney disease; pregnancy

Warnings/Precautions Prolonged use and/or high doses may cause peliosis hepatis or liver cell tumors which may not be apparent until liver failure or intra-abdominal hemorrhage develops. Discontinue in case of cholestatic hepatitis with jaundice or abnormal liver function tests. Use with caution in patients with breast cancer; may cause hypercalcemia by stimulating osteolysis. Use with caution in patients with diabetes mellitus; monitor carefully. Use with caution in patients with conditions influenced by edema (eg, cardiovascular disease, migraine, seizure disorder, renal impairment); may cause fluid retention. Discontinue with evidence of mild virilization in women. Use with caution in elderly. Use with caution in hepatic impairment. May accelerate bone maturation without producing compensatory gain in linear growth in children. In prepubertal children, perform radiographic examination of the hand and wrist every 6 months to determine the rate of bone maturation and to assess the effect of treatment on the epiphyseal centers. Product may contain tartrazine.

Adverse Reactions
>10%:
Male: Priapism
Female: Menstrual problems (amenorrhea), virilism, breast soreness
Cardiovascular: Edema
Dermatologic: Acne
1% to 10%:
Male: Prostatic carcinoma, hirsutism (increase in pubic hair growth), impotence, testicular atrophy
Cardiovascular: Edema
Gastrointestinal: GI irritation, nausea, vomiting
Genitourinary: Prostatic hyperplasia
Hepatic: Hepatic dysfunction

◀ <1%:

Male: Gynecomastia

Female: Amenorrhea

Hypercalcemia, leukopenia, polycythemia, hepatic necrosis, cholestatic hepatitis, hypersensitivity reactions

Drug Interactions

Avoid Concomitant Use There are no known interactions where it is recommended to avoid concomitant use.

Increased Effect/Toxicity

Fluoxymesterone may increase the levels/effects of: CycloSPORINE; Vitamin K Antagonists

Decreased Effect There are no known significant interactions involving a decrease in effect.

Storage/Stability Protect from light.

Mechanism of Action Synthetic androgenic anabolic hormone responsible for the normal growth and development of male sex hormones and development of male sex organs and maintenance of secondary sex characteristics; synthetic testosterone derivative with significant androgen activity; stimulates RNA polymerase activity resulting in an increase in protein production; increases bone development; halogenated derivative of testosterone with up to 5 times the activity of methyltestosterone

Pharmacodynamics/Kinetics

Absorption: Rapid

Protein binding: 98%

Metabolism: Hepatic; enterohepatic recirculation

Half-life elimination: 10-100 minutes

Excretion: Urine (90%)

Dosage Adults: Oral:

Male:

Hypogonadism: 5-20 mg/day

Delayed puberty: 2.5-20 mg/day for 4-6 months

Female: Inoperable breast carcinoma: 10-40 mg/day in divided doses for 1-3 months

Combination Regimens

Breast cancer: VATH on page 1418

Monitoring Parameters In prepubertal children, perform radiographic examination of the hand and wrist every 6 months

Test Interactions Decreased levels of thyroxine-binding globulin; decreased total T_4 serum levels; increased resin uptake of T_3 and T_4

Dosage Forms Excipient information presented when available (limited, particularly for generics); consult specific product labeling.

Tablet: 10 mg

Androxy™: 10 mg

♦ **5-Flurocytosine** *see* Flucytosine *on page* 490

Flutamide (FLOO ta mide)

Medication Safety Issues

Sound-alike/look-alike issues:

Flutamide may be confused with Flumadine®, thalidomide

Eulexin® may be confused with Edecrin®, Eurax®

Related Information

Safe Handling of Hazardous Drugs *on page 1517*

Index Terms 4'-Nitro-3'-Trifluoromethylisobutyrantide; Niftolid; NSC-147834; SCH 13521

Generic Available Yes

Canadian Brand Names Apo-Flutamide®; Euflex®; Eulexin®; Novo-Flutamide

Pharmacologic Category Antineoplastic Agent, Antiandrogen

Use Treatment of metastatic prostatic carcinoma in combination therapy with LHRH agonist analogues

Unlabeled/Investigational Use Female hirsutism

Pregnancy Risk Factor D

Lactation Excretion in breast milk unknown/not recommended

Labeled Contraindications Hypersensitivity to flutamide or any component of the formulation; severe hepatic impairment; pregnancy

Warnings/Precautions Hazardous agent - use appropriate precautions for handling and disposal. **[U.S. Boxed Warning]: Hospitalization and, rarely, death due to liver failure have been reported in patients taking flutamide.** Elevated serum transaminase levels, jaundice, hepatic encephalopathy, and acute hepatic failure have been reported. Product labeling states flutamide is not for use in women, particularly for non-life-threatening conditions. In some patients, the toxicity reverses after discontinuation of therapy. About 50% of the cases occur within the first 3 months of treatment. Serum transaminase levels should be measured prior to starting treatment, monthly for 4 months, and periodically thereafter. Liver function tests should be obtained at the first suggestion of liver dysfunction (nausea, vomiting, abdominal pain, fatigue, anorexia, "flu-like" symptoms, hyperbilirubinuria, jaundice, or right upper quadrant tenderness). Flutamide should be immediately discontinued any time a patient has jaundice, and/or an ALT level greater than twice the upper limit of normal. Flutamide should not be used in patients whose ALT values are greater than twice the upper limit of normal.

Patients with glucose-6 phosphate dehydrogenase deficiency or hemoglobin M disease or smokers are at risk of toxicities associated with aniline exposure, including methemoglobinemia, hemolytic anemia, and cholestatic jaundice. Monitor methemoglobin levels.

Adverse Reactions

>10%:

Endocrine & metabolic: Galactorrhea (9% to 42%), breast tenderness, gynecomastia, hot flashes, impotence, libido decreased, tumor flare

Gastrointestinal: Vomiting (11% to 12%), nausea

Hepatic: AST increased (transient; mild), LDH increased (transient; mild)

1% to 10%:

Cardiovascular: Hypertension (1%), edema

Central nervous system: Anxiety, confusion, depression, dizziness, drowsiness, headache, insomnia, nervousness

Dermatologic: Ecchymosis, photosensitivity, pruritus

Gastrointestinal: Upset stomach (4% to 6%), anorexia, appetite increased, constipation, diarrhea, indigestion

Hematologic: Anemia (6%), leukopenia (3%), thrombocytopenia (1%)

Neuromuscular & skeletal: Weakness (1%)

Miscellaneous: Herpes zoster

◄ <1%: Discoloration of urine (yellow), hepatic failure, hepatitis, hypersensitivity pneumonitis, jaundice, malignant breast neoplasm (male), MI, pulmonary embolism, sulfhemoglobinemia, thrombophlebitis

Drug Interactions

Metabolism/Transport Effects Substrate (major) of CYP1A2, 3A4; **Inhibits** CYP1A2 (weak)

Avoid Concomitant Use There are no known interactions where it is recommended to avoid concomitant use.

Increased Effect/Toxicity

The levels/effects of Flutamide may be increased by: CYP1A2 Inhibitors (Moderate); CYP1A2 Inhibitors (Strong); CYP3A4 Inhibitors (Moderate); CYP3A4 Inhibitors (Strong); Dasatinib

Decreased Effect

The levels/effects of Flutamide may be decreased by: CYP1A2 Inducers (Strong); CYP3A4 Inducers (Strong); Deferasirox; Herbs (CYP3A4 Inducers)

Ethanol/Nutrition/Herb Interactions

Food: No effect on bioavailability of flutamide.

Herb/Nutraceutical: St John's wort may decrease flutamide levels.

Storage/Stability Store at room temperature.

Mechanism of Action Nonsteroidal antiandrogen that inhibits androgen uptake or inhibits binding of androgen in target tissues

Pharmacodynamics/Kinetics

Absorption: Oral: Rapid and complete

Protein binding: Parent drug: 94% to 96%; 2-hydroxyflutamide: 92% to 94%

Metabolism: Extensively hepatic to more than 10 metabolites, primarily 2-hydroxyflutamide (active)

Half-life elimination: 5-6 hours (2-hydroxyflutamide)

Excretion: Primarily urine (as metabolites)

Dosage Oral: Adults:

Prostatic carcinoma: 250 mg 3 times/day; alternatively, once-daily doses of 0.5-1.5 g have been used (unlabeled dosing)

Female hirsutism (unlabeled use): 250 mg daily

Combination Regimens

Prostate cancer:

FL on page 1323

FZ on page 1340

Administration Usually administered orally in 3 divided doses. Contents of capsule may be opened and mixed with applesauce, pudding, or other soft foods. Mixing with a beverage is not recommended.

Monitoring Parameters Serum transaminase levels should be measured prior to starting treatment and should be repeated monthly for the first 4 months of therapy, and periodically thereafter. LFTs should be checked at the first sign or symptom of liver dysfunction (eg, nausea, vomiting, abdominal pain, fatigue, anorexia, flu-like symptoms, hyperbilirubinuria, jaundice, or right upper quadrant tenderness). Other parameters include tumor reduction, testosterone/estrogen, and phosphatase serum levels.

Dosage Forms Excipient information presented when available (limited, particularly for generics); consult specific product labeling.

Capsule: 125 mg

References

Goldspiel BR and Kohler DR, "Flutamide: An Antiandrogen for Advanced Prostate Cancer," *DICP Ann Pharmacother*, 1990, 24(6):616-23.

Labrie F, "Mechanism of Action and Pure Antiandrogenic Properties of Flutamide," *Cancer*, 1993, 72(12 Suppl):3816-27.

Luo S, Martel C, Chen C, "Daily Dosing With Flutamide or Casodex Exerts Maximal Antiandrogenic Activity," *Urology,* 1997, 50(6):913-9.

Moghetti P, Tosi F, Tosti A, et al, "Comparison of Spironolactone, Flutamide, and Finasteride Efficacy in the Treatment of Hirsutism: A Randomized, Double Blind, Placebo-Controlled Trial," *J Clin Endocrinol Metab,* 2000, 85(1):89-94.

Thrasher JB, Deeths J, and Bennett C, "Comparative Study of the Clinical Efficacy of Two Dosing Regimens of Flutamide," *Mol Urol,* 2000, 4(3):259-63.

◆ **Folinic Acid (error prone synonym)** *see* Leucovorin Calcium *on page 697*

◆ **Folotyn™** *see* Pralatrexate *on page 974*

Fondaparinux (fon da PARE i nuks)

Medication Safety Issues

High alert medication: The Institute for Safe Medication Practices (ISMP) includes this medication among its list of drugs which have a heightened risk of causing significant patient harm when used in error.

U.S. Brand Names Arixtra®

Index Terms Fondaparinux Sodium

Generic Available No

Canadian Brand Names Arixtra®

Pharmacologic Category Factor Xa Inhibitor

Use Prophylaxis of deep vein thrombosis (DVT) in patients undergoing surgery for hip replacement, knee replacement, hip fracture (including extended prophylaxis following hip fracture surgery), or abdominal surgery (in patients at risk for thromboembolic complications); treatment of acute pulmonary embolism (PE); treatment of acute DVT without PE

Note: Additional Canadian approvals (not approved in U.S.): Unstable angina or non-ST segment elevation myocardial infarction (UA/NSTEMI) for the prevention of death and subsequent MI; ST segment elevation MI (STEMI) for the prevention of death and myocardial reinfarction

Unlabeled/Investigational Use Prophylaxis of DVT in patients with a history of heparin-induced thrombocytopenia (HIT)

Pregnancy Risk Factor B

Lactation Excretion in breast milk unknown/use caution

Labeled Contraindications Hypersensitivity to fondaparinux or any component of the formulation; severe renal impairment (Cl_{cr} <30 mL/minute); body weight <50 kg (prophylaxis); active major bleeding; bacterial endocarditis; thrombocytopenia associated with a positive *in vitro* test for antiplatelet antibody in the presence of fondaparinux

Warnings/Precautions [U.S. Boxed Warning]: Patients with recent or anticipated neuraxial anesthesia (epidural or spinal anesthesia) are at risk of spinal or epidural hematoma and subsequent paralysis. Not to be used interchangeably (unit-for-unit) with heparin, low molecular weight heparins (LMWHs), or heparinoids. Use caution in patients with moderate renal dysfunction (Cl_{cr} 30-50 mL/minute); contraindicated in patients with Cl_{cr} <30 mL/minute. Discontinue if severe dysfunction or labile function develops.

Use caution in congenital or acquired bleeding disorders; active ulcerative or angiodysplastic gastrointestinal disease; hemorrhagic stroke; shortly after brain, spinal, or ophthalmologic surgery; or in patients taking platelet inhibitors. Risk of major bleeding may be increased if initial dose is administered earlier then recommended (initiation recommended at 6-8 hours following surgery). Discontinue agents that may enhance the risk of hemorrhage if possible. Although considered an insensitive measure of fondaparinux activity, there have been postmarketing reports of bleeding associated with elevated aPTT. ▶

Thrombocytopenia has occurred with administration, including reports of thrombocytopenia with thrombosis similar to heparin-induced thrombocytopenia. Monitor patients closely and discontinue therapy if platelets fall to <100,000/mm^3.

For subcutaneous administration; not for I.M. administration. Do not use interchangeably (unit for unit) with low molecular weight heparins, heparin, or heparinoids. Use caution in patients <50 kg who are being treated for DVT/PE; dosage reduction recommended. Contraindicated in patients <50 kg when used for prophylactic therapy. Use with caution in the elderly. The needle guard contains natural latex rubber. Safety and efficacy in pediatric patients have not been established.

The administration of fondaparinux is **not recommended** prior to and during primary PCI in patients with STEMI, due to an increased risk for guiding-catheter thrombosis. Patients with UA/NSTEMI or STEMI undergoing any PCI should not receive fondaparinux as the sole anticoagulant. Use of an anticoagulant with antithrombin activity (eg, unfractionated heparin) is recommended as adjunctive therapy to PCI even if prior treatment with fondaparinux (must take into account whether GP IIb/IIIa antagonists have been administered) (King, 2008).

Additional Canadian labeling warnings: Following sheath removal, fondaparinux therapy should not resume for at least 2 hours in patients with UA/NSTEMI and 3 hours in patients with STEMI. Avoid administration 24 hours before and 48 hours after coronary artery bypass graft (CABG) surgery.

Adverse Reactions As with all anticoagulants, bleeding is the major adverse effect. Hemorrhage may occur at any site. Risk appears increased by a number of factors including renal dysfunction, age (>75 years), and weight (<50 kg).

>10%:
  Central nervous system: Fever (4% to 14%)
  Gastrointestinal: Nausea (3% to 11%)
  Hematologic: Anemia (1% to 20%)

1% to 10%:
  Cardiovascular: Edema (9%), hypotension (4%), hypertension (2%), chest pain (1%), thrombosis PCI catheter (without heparin 1%)
  Central nervous system: Insomnia (4% to 5%), headache (2% to 5%), dizziness (4%), confusion (3%), pain (2%), anxiety (1%)
  Dermatologic: Rash (8%), purpura (4%), bullous eruption (3%), bruising (1%)
  Endocrine & metabolic: Hypokalemia (1% to 4%)
  Gastrointestinal: Constipation (5% to 9%), vomiting (1% to 6%), diarrhea (2% to 3%), dyspepsia (2%), abdominal pain (1%)
  Genitourinary: Urinary tract infection (2% to 4%), urinary retention (3%)
  Hematologic: Minor bleeding (2% to 4%), moderate thrombocytopenia (50,000-100,000/mm^3: 3%), hematoma (3%), major bleeding (1% to 3%), prothrombin decreased (1%), risk of major bleeding increased as high as 5% in patients receiving initial dose <6 hours following surgery
  Hepatic: ALT increased (≤3%), AST increased (≤2%)
  Local: Injection site reaction (bleeding, rash, pruritus)
  Neuromuscular & skeletal: Back pain (1%), leg pain (1%)
  Respiratory: Cough (2%), pneumonia (2%), epistaxis (1%)
  Miscellaneous: Wound drainage increased (5%)

<1%, postmarketing, and/or case reports: aPTT increased (associated with bleeding), heparin-induced thrombocytopenia (1 case report), hepatic dysfunction, severe thrombocytopenia (<50,000/mm^3)

Drug Interactions

Avoid Concomitant Use There are no known interactions where it is recommended to avoid concomitant use.

Increased Effect/Toxicity

Fondaparinux may increase the levels/effects of: Anticoagulants; Ibritumomab; Tositumomab and Iodine I 131 Tositumomab

The levels/effects of Fondaparinux may be increased by: Antiplatelet Agents; Dasatinib; Drotrecogin Alfa; Herbs (Anticoagulant/Antiplatelet Properties); Nonsteroidal Anti-Inflammatory Agents; Pentosan Polysulfate Sodium; Prostacyclin Analogues; Salicylates; Thrombolytic Agents

Decreased Effect There are no known significant interactions involving a decrease in effect.

Ethanol/Nutrition/Herb Interactions Herb/Nutraceutical: Avoid alfalfa, anise, bilberry, bladderwrack, bromelain, cat's claw, celery, coleus, cordyceps, dong quai, evening primrose oil, fenugreek, feverfew, garlic, ginger, ginkgo biloba, ginseng (American/Panax/Siberian), grapeseed, green tea, guggul, horse chestnut seed, horseradish, licorice, prickly ash, red clover, reishi, sweet clover, turmeric, white willow (all possess anticoagulant or antiplatelet activity and as such, may enhance the anticoagulant effects of fondaparinux).

Storage/Stability Store at 25°C (77°F); excursions permitted to 15°C to 30°C (59°F to 86°F).

Canadian labeling: For I.V. administration: Manufacturer recommends immediate use once diluted in NS, but is stable for up to 24 hours at 15°C to 30°C (59°F to 86°F).

Reconstitution Canadian labeling: For I.V. administration: May mix with 25 mL or 50 mL NS

Compatibility

Do not mix with other injections or infusions.

Canadian labeling: Stable in NS

Mechanism of Action Fondaparinux is a synthetic pentasaccharide that causes an antithrombin III-mediated selective inhibition of factor Xa. Neutralization of factor Xa interrupts the blood coagulation cascade and inhibits thrombin formation and thrombus development.

Pharmacodynamics/Kinetics

Absorption: SubQ: Rapid and complete

Distribution: V_d: 7-11 L; mainly in blood

Protein binding: ≥94% to antithrombin III

Bioavailability: SubQ: 100%

Half-life elimination: 17-21 hours; prolonged with worsening renal impairment

Time to peak: SubQ: 2-3 hours

Excretion: Urine (~77%, unchanged drug)

Dosage SubQ: Adults:

DVT prophylaxis: Adults ≥50 kg: 2.5 mg once daily. **Note:** Initiate dose after hemostasis has been established, 6-8 hours postoperatively.

DVT prophylaxis with history of HIT (unlabeled use): 2.5 mg once daily

Usual duration: 5-9 days (up to 10 days following abdominal surgery or up to 11 days following hip replacement or knee replacement)

Extended prophylaxis is recommended following hip fracture surgery (has been tolerated for up to 32 days total).

Acute DVT/PE treatment: **Note:** Start warfarin on the first treatment day and continue fondaparinux until INR is between 2 and 3 (usually 5-7 days) (Hirsh, 2008):

<50 kg: 5 mg once daily

50-100 kg: 7.5 mg once daily

>100 kg: 10 mg once daily

Usual duration: 5-9 days (has been administered up to 26 days)

Canadian labeling only: Adults:

UA/NSTEMI: SubQ: 2.5 mg once daily; initiate as soon as possible after diagnosis; treat for up to 8 days or until hospital discharge.

STEMI: I.V.: 2.5 mg once; subsequent doses: SubQ: 2.5 mg once daily; treat for up to 8 days or until hospital discharge

Dosage adjustment in renal impairment:

Cl_{cr} 30-50 mL/minute: Use caution

Cl_{cr} <30 mL/minute: Contraindicated

Administration Do **not** administer I.M.; for SubQ administration only. Do not mix with other injections or infusions. Do not expel air bubble from syringe before injection. Administer according to recommended regimen; early initiation (before 6 hours after surgery) has been associated with increased bleeding.

To convert from I.V. unfractionated heparin (UFH) infusion to SubQ fondaparinux (Nutescu, 2007): Calculate specific dose for fondaparinux based on indication, discontinue UFH, and begin fondaparinux within 1 hour

To convert from SubQ fondaparinux to I.V. UFH infusion (Nutescu, 2007): Discontinue fondaparinux; calculate specific dose for I.V. UFH infusion based on indication; omit heparin bolus/loading dose

For subQ fondaparinux dosed every 24 hours: Start I.V. UFH infusion 22-23 hours after last dose of fondaparinux

Canadian labeling only: STEMI patients: I.V. push or mixed in 25-50 mL of NS and infused over 2 minutes. Flush tubing with NS after infusion to ensure complete administration of fondaparinux. Infusion bag should not be mixed with other agents.

Monitoring Parameters Periodic monitoring of CBC, serum creatinine, occult blood testing of stools recommended. Anti-Xa activity of fondaparinux can be measured by the assay if fondaparinux is used as the calibrator. PT and aPTT are insensitive measures of fondaparinux activity.

Test Interactions International standards of heparin or LMWH are not the appropriate calibrators for antifactor Xa activity of fondaparinux.

Dosage Forms Excipient information presented when available (limited, particularly for generics); consult specific product labeling.

Injection, solution, as sodium [preservative free]: 2.5 mg/0.5 mL (0.5 mL); 5 mg/0.4 mL (0.4 mL); 7.5 mg/0.6 mL (0.6 mL); 10 mg/0.8 mL (0.8 mL) [prefilled syringe]

References

Bauer KA, "Fondaparinux Sodium: A Selective Inhibitor of Factor Xa," *Am J Health Syst Pharm*, 2001, 58(Suppl 2):14-7.

Buller HR, Davidson BL, Decousus H, et al, "Fondaparinux or Enoxaparin for the Initial Treatment of Symptomatic Deep Venous Thrombosis: A Randomized Trial," *Ann Intern Med*, 2004, 140 (11):867-73.

Buller HR, Davidson BL, Decousus H, et al, "Subcutaneous Fondaparinux Versus Intravenous Unfractionated Heparin in the Initial Treatment of Pulmonary Embolism," *N Engl J Med*, 2003, 349(18):1695-702.

Hassell K, "The Management of Patients With Heparin-Induced Thrombocytopenia Who Require Anticoagulation Therapy," *Chest*, 2005, 127(2 Suppl):1-8.

Hirsh J, Guyatt G, Albers GW, et al, "Executive Summary: American College of Chest Physicians Evidence-Based Clinical Practice Guidelines (8th Edition)," *Chest*, 2008, 133(6 Suppl):71-109.

Warkentin TE, Maurer BT, and Aster RH, "Heparin-Induced Thrombocytopenia Associated With Fondaparinux," *N Engl J Med*, 2007, 356(25):2653-55.

♦ **Fondaparinux Sodium** *see Fondaparinux on page 509*

♦ **5-Formyl Tetrahydrofolate** *see Leucovorin Calcium on page 697*

♦ **Fortaz®** *see Ceftazidime on page 196*

♦ **Fortical®** *see Calcitonin on page 165*

Fosaprepitant (fos a PRE pi tant)

Medication Safety Issues

Sound-alike/look-alike issues:

Fosaprepitant may be confused with aprepitant, fosamprenavir, fospropofol

Emend® for Injection (fosaprepitant) may be confused with Emend®
(aprepitant) which is an oral capsule formulation.

U.S. Brand Names Emend® for Injection

Index Terms Aprepitant Injection; Fosaprepitant Dimeglumine; L-758,298; MK
0517

Generic Available No

Pharmacologic Category Antiemetic; Substance P/Neurokinin 1 Receptor
Antagonist

Use Prevention of acute and delayed nausea and vomiting associated with
moderately- and highly-emetogenic chemotherapy (in combination with other
antiemetics)

Pregnancy Risk Factor B

Lactation Excretion in breast milk unknown/not recommended

Labeled Contraindications Hypersensitivity to fosaprepitant, aprepitant,
polysorbate 80, or any component of the formulation; concurrent use with
pimozide or cisapride

Warnings/Precautions Fosaprepitant is rapidly converted to aprepitant,
which has a high potential for drug interactions. Use caution with agents
primarily metabolized via CYP3A4; aprepitant is a 3A4 inhibitor. Effect on orally
administered 3A4 substrates is greater than those administered intravenously.
Use caution with hepatic impairment; has not been studied in patients with
severe hepatic impairment (Child-Pugh class C). Not intended for treatment of
existing nausea and vomiting or for chronic continuous therapy.

Adverse Reactions Adverse reactions reported with aprepitant and
fosaprepitant (as part of a combination chemotherapy regimen) occurring at
a higher frequency than standard therapy:

>10%:
Central nervous system: Fatigue (≤18%)
Gastrointestinal: Nausea (≤13%)
Neuromuscular & skeletal: Weakness (≤18%)
Miscellaneous: Hiccups (11%)

1% to 10%:
Central nervous system: Dizziness (≤7%), headache (≤3%)
Endocrine & metabolic: Dehydration (6%), hot flushing (3%)
Gastrointestinal: Diarrhea (≤10%), dyspepsia (≤8%), abdominal pain (5%),
stomatitis (≤5%), epigastric discomfort (4%), gastritis (4%), throat pain
(≤3%)
Hematologic: Neutropenia (≤9%)
Hepatic: ALT increased (≤6%), AST increased (≤3%)
Local: Injection site pain (8%), injection site induration (2%)
Renal: Proteinuria (≤7%), BUN increased (≤5%)

>0.5%: Acid reflux, acne, alkaline phosphatase increased, anemia, anxiety,
appetite decreased, arthralgia, back pain, candidiasis, confusion, conjunctivitis, cough, depression, diabetes mellitus, diaphoresis, DVT, dysphagia, ▶

dyspnea, dysuria, edema, eructation, erythrocyturia, flatulence, herpes simplex, hyper-/hypotension, hypokalemia, hyponatremia, leukocytes increased, leukocyturia, malaise, MI, muscle weakness, musculoskeletal pain, myalgia, nasal secretion, obstipation, palpitation, pelvic pain, peripheral neuropathy, pharyngitis, pneumonitis, pulmonary embolism, rash, renal insufficiency, respiratory infection, respiratory insufficiency, rigors, salivation increased, sensory neuropathy, septic shock, swallowing disorder, tachycardia, taste disturbance, tremor, urinary tract infection, vocal disturbance, weight loss, xerostomia

Postmarketing and/or case reports (with fosaprepitant or aprepitant): Albumin decreased, anaphylactic reaction, angioedema, bilirubin increased, bradycardia, disorientation, duodenal ulcer (perforating), dysarthria, enterocolitis, fever, glycosuria, hematoma, hyperglycemia, hypersensitivity reaction, hypoesthesia, hypothermia, hypovolemia, hypoxia, miosis, neutropenic sepsis, pneumonia, pruritus, sensory disturbance, sinus tachycardia, Stevens-Johnson syndrome, subileus, syncope, urticaria, visual acuity decreased, wheezing

Drug Interactions

Metabolism/Transport Effects **Substrate** of CYP1A2 (minor), 2C19 (minor), 3A4 (major); **Inhibits** CYP2C9 (weak), 2C19 (weak), 3A4 (moderate); **Induces** CYP2C9 (weak), 3A4 (weak)

Avoid Concomitant Use

Avoid concomitant use of Fosaprepitant with any of the following: Cisapride; Everolimus; Pimozide; Tolvaptan

Increased Effect/Toxicity

Fosaprepitant may increase the levels/effects of: Benzodiazepines (metabolized by oxidation); Cisapride; Colchicine; Corticosteroids (Systemic); CYP3A4 Substrates; Diltiazem; Eplerenone; Everolimus; FentaNYL; Halofantrine; Pimecrolimus; Pimozide; Ranolazine; Salmeterol; Saxagliptin; Tolvaptan

The levels/effects of Fosaprepitant may be increased by: Antifungal Agents (Azole Derivatives, Systemic); CYP3A4 Inhibitors (Moderate); CYP3A4 Inhibitors (Strong); Dasatinib; Diltiazem

Decreased Effect

Fosaprepitant may decrease the levels/effects of: Contraceptive (Progestins); Oral Contraceptive (Estrogens); Saxagliptin; Warfarin

The levels/effects of Fosaprepitant may be decreased by: CYP3A4 Inducers (Strong); Deferasirox; Herbs (CYP3A4 Inducers); Rifampin

Ethanol/Nutrition/Herb Interactions

Food: Aprepitant serum concentration may be increased when taken with grapefruit juice; avoid concurrent use.

Herb/Nutraceutical: Avoid St John's wort (may decrease aprepitant levels).

Storage/Stability Store intact vials at 2°C to 8°C (36°F to 46°F). Solutions diluted for infusion are stable for 24 hours at room temperature of ≤25°C (≤77°F).

Reconstitution Reconstitute with 5 mL of sodium chloride 0.9%, directing diluent down side of vial to avoid foaming. Add reconstituted contents of vial to 110 mL sodium chloride 0.9%, resulting in a final concentration of 1 mg/mL; gently invert bag to mix.

Compatibility Stable in sodium chloride 0.9%

Incompatible with solutions containing calcium (eg, lactated Ringer's solution, Hartmann's solution) or magnesium.

Mechanism of Action Fosaprepitant is a prodrug of aprepitant, which prevents acute and delayed vomiting by inhibiting the substance P/neurokinin 1 (NK1) receptor; augments the antiemetic activity of the 5-HT_3 receptor antagonist and corticosteroid activity and inhibits chemotherapy-induced emesis.

Pharmacodynamics/Kinetics

Distribution: Fosaprepitant: ~5 L; Aprepitant: V_d: ~70 L; crosses the blood brain barrier

Protein binding: Aprepitant: >95%

Metabolism:

Fosaprepitant: Hepatic and extrahepatic; rapidly converted to aprepitant (nearly complete conversion)

Aprepitant: Hepatic via CYP3A4 (major); CYP1A2 and CYP2C19 (minor); forms 7 weakly-active metabolites

Bioavailability: Fosaprepitant 115 mg I.V. is bioequivalent to aprepitant 125 mg orally.

Half-life elimination: Half-life elimination: Fosaprepitant: ~2 minutes; Aprepitant: ~9-13 hours

Time to peak, plasma: Fosaprepitant is converted to aprepitant within 30 minutes after the end of infusion

Excretion: Urine (57%); feces (45%)

Dosage I.V.: Adults: Prevention of chemotherapy-induced nausea/vomiting: 115 mg 30 minutes prior to chemotherapy on day 1 (followed by aprepitant 80 mg orally on days 2 and 3) in combination with other antiemetics

Dosage adjustment in renal impairment:

Mild, moderate, or severe impairment: No adjustment required

Dialysis-dependent end-stage renal disease (ESRD): No adjustment required

Dosage adjustment in hepatic impairment:

Child-Pugh class A and B: No adjustment required

Child-Pugh class C: Has not been evaluated

Administration Infuse over 15 minutes

Additional Information

Oncology Comment: Fosaprepitant is recommended in the National Comprehensive Cancer Network® (NCCN) Clinical Practice Guidelines in Oncology for Antiemesis (version 2.2009) for use on day 1 only in combination with a serotonin receptor antagonist and dexamethasone for chemotherapy with high emetic risk and for select moderately emetogenic regimens (carboplatin, cisplatin, doxorubicin, epirubicin, ifosfamide, irinotecan, or methotrexate). Either fosaprepitant 115 mg or aprepitant (125 mg orally) are administered on day 1; for day 2 and 3, patients should receive aprepitant 80 mg orally.

Dosage Forms Excipient information presented when available (limited, particularly for generics); consult specific product labeling.

Injection, powder for reconstitution:

Emend® for Injection: 115 mg [contains edetate disodium; lactose; polysorbate 80]

References

Cocquyt V, Van Belle S, Reinhardt RR, et al, "Comparison of L-758,298, a Prodrug for the Selective Neurokinin-1 Antagonist, L-754,030, With Ondansetron for the Prevention of Cisplatin-Induced Emesis," *Eur J Cancer*, 2001, 37(7):835-42.

Lasseter KC, Gambelle J, Jin B, et al, "Tolerability of Fosaprepitant and Bioequivalency to Aprepitant in Healthy Subjects," *J Clin Pharmacol*, 2007,47(7):834-40.

National Comprehensive Cancer Network® (NCCN), "Clinical Practice Guidelines in Oncology™: Antiemesis," Version 2.2009. Available at http://www.nccn.org/professionals/physician_gls/PDF/antiemesis.pdf.

Van Belle S, Lichinitser SR, Navari RM, et al," Prevention of Cisplatin-Induced Acute and Delayed Emesis by the Selective Neurokinin-1 Antagonists, L-758,298 and MK-869," *Cancer*, 2002, 94 (11):3032-41.

◆ **Fosaprepitant Dimeglumine** *see* Fosaprepitant *on page 513*

Foscarnet (fos KAR net)

U.S. Brand Names Foscavir® [DSC]

Index Terms PFA; Phosphonoformate; Phosphonoformic Acid

Generic Available Yes

Canadian Brand Names Foscavir®

Pharmacologic Category Antiviral Agent

Use Treatment of acyclovir-resistant mucocutaneous herpes simplex virus (HSV) infections in immunocompromised persons (eg, with advanced AIDS); treatment of CMV retinitis in persons with HIV

Unlabeled/Investigational Use Other CMV infections (eg, colitis, esophagitis, neurological disease); CMV prophylaxis for cancer patients receiving alemtuzumab therapy or allogeneic stem cell transplant

Pregnancy Risk Factor C

Lactation Excretion in breast milk unknown/contraindicated

Labeled Contraindications Hypersensitivity to foscarnet or any component of the formulation

Warnings/Precautions Hazardous agent - use appropriate precautions for handling and disposal. **[U.S. Boxed Warning]: Indicated only for immunocompromised patients with CMV retinitis and mucocutaneous acyclovir-resistant HSV infection. [U.S. Boxed Warning]: Renal impairment occurs to some degree in the majority of patients treated with foscarnet;** renal impairment may occur at any time and is usually reversible within 1 week following dose adjustment or discontinuation of therapy, however, several patients have died with renal failure within 4 weeks of stopping foscarnet; therefore, renal function should be closely monitored. To reduce the risk of nephrotoxicity and the potential to administer a relative overdose, always calculate the creatine clearance even if serum creatinine is within the normal range. Adequate hydration may reduce the risk of nephrotoxicity; the manufacturer makes specific recommendations regarding this (see Administration).

Imbalance of serum electrolytes or minerals occurs in at least 15% of patients (hypocalcemia, low ionized calcium, hyper/hypophosphatemia, hypomagnesemia, or hypokalemia). Correct electrolytes before initiating therapy. Use caution when administering other medications that cause electrolyte imbalances. Patients who experience signs or symptoms of an electrolyte imbalance should be assessed immediately. **[U.S. Boxed Warning]: Seizures related to plasma electrolyte/mineral imbalance may occur;** incidence has been reported in up to 10% of HIV patients. Risk factors for seizures include impaired baseline renal function, low total serum calcium, and underlying CNS conditions. May cause anemia and granulocytopenia. May cause genital/vascular tissue irritation/ulceration; adequately hydrate and administer only into vein with adequate blood flow to minimize risk. Foscarnet is deposited in teeth and bone of young, growing animals; it has adversely affected tooth enamel development in rats.

Adverse Reactions

>10%:

Central nervous system: Fever (65%), headache (26%)

Endocrine & metabolic: Hypokalemia (16% to 48%), hypocalcemia (15% to 30%), hypomagnesemia (15% to 30%), hypophosphatemia (8% to 26%)

Gastrointestinal: Nausea (47%), diarrhea (30%), vomiting (26%)

Hematologic: Anemia (33%), granulocytopenia (17%)

Renal: Abnormal renal function/decreased creatinine clearance (12%; without adequate hydration 33%)

1% to 10%:

Cardiovascular: Chest pain (1% to 5%), edema (1% to 5%), facial edema (1% to 5%), flushing (1% to 5%), hyper-/hypotension (1% to 5%), palpitation (1% to 5%), ECG changes (1% to 5%)

Central nervous system: Seizure (includes grand mal; 8%), anxiety (≥5%), confusion (≥5%), depression (≥5%), dizziness (≥5%), fatigue (≥5%), hypoesthesia (≥5%), malaise (≥5%), pain (≥5%), aggressiveness (1% to 5%), agitation (1% to 5%), amnesia (1% to 5%), aphasia (1% to 5%), ataxia (1% to 5%), coordination abnormal (1% to 5%), dementia (1% to 5%), EEG abnormal (1% to 5%), hallucination (1% to 5%), insomnia (1% to 5%), meningitis (1% to 5%), nervousness (1% to 5%), somnolence (1% to 5%), stupor (1% to 5%)

Dermatologic: Rash (≥5%), erythematous rash (1% to 5%), maculopapular rash (1% to 5%), pruritus (1% to 5%), seborrhea (1% to 5%), skin discoloration (1% to 5%), skin ulceration (1% to 5%)

Endocrine & metabolic: Hyperphosphatemia (6%), acidosis (1% to 5%), hyponatremia (1% to 5%)

Gastrointestinal: Abdominal pain (≥5%), anorexia (≥5%), constipation (1% to 5%), dyspepsia (1% to 5%), dysphasia (1% to 5%), flatulence (1% to 5%), melena (1% to 5%), pancreatitis (1% to 5%), rectal hemorrhage (1% to 5%), taste perversion (1% to 5%), ulcerative stomatitis (1% to 5%), weight loss (1% to 5%), xerostomia (1% to 5%)

Genitourinary: Dysuria (1% to 5%), nocturia (1% to 5%), urinary retention (1% to 5%)

Hematologic: Leukopenia (≥5%), lymphadenopathy (1% to 5%), thrombocytopenia (1% to 5%), thrombosis (1% to 5%)

Hepatic: Alkaline phosphatase increased (1% to 5%), ALT increased (1% to 5%), AST increased (1% to 5%), hepatic function abnormal (1% to 5%), LDH increased (1% to 5%)

Local: Injection site pain/inflammation (1% to 5%)

Neuromuscular & skeletal: Paresthesia (≥5%), involuntary muscle contractions (≥5%), rigors (≥5%), neuropathy (peripheral; ≥5%), weakness (≥5%), arthralgia (1% to 5%), back pain (1% to 5%), leg cramps (1% to 5%), myalgia (1% to 5%), tremor (1% to 5%)

Ocular: Vision abnormalities (≥5%), conjunctivitis (1% to 5%), eye pain (1% to 5%)

Renal: Acute renal failure (1% to 5%), albuminuria (1% to 5%), BUN increased (1% to 5%), polyuria (1% to 5%), urinary tract infection (1% to 5%)

Respiratory: Cough (≥5%), dyspnea (≥5%), bronchospasm (1% to 5%), hemoptysis (1% to 5%), pharyngitis (1% to 5%), pneumonia (1% to 5%), pneumothorax (1% to 5%), rhinitis (1% to 5%), sinusitis (1% to 5%), stridor (1% to 5%)

Miscellaneous: Diaphoresis (≥5%), sepsis (≥5%), infection (includes bacterial and fungal; ≥5%), flu-like syndrome (1% to 5%), malignancies (lymphoma/sarcoma 1% to 5%), thirst (1% to 5%)

◀ <1%, postmarketing, and/or case reports: Amylase increased, cardiac arrest, coma, creatine phosphokinase increased, dehydration, diabetes insipidus (usually nephrogenic), erythema multiforme, GGT increased muscle weakness, hematuria, hypoproteinemia, myopathy, myositis, neutropenia, pancytopenia, QT_c prolongation, renal calculus, rhabdomyolysis, Stevens-Johnson syndrome, syndrome of inappropriate antidiuretic hormone (SIADH), toxic epidermal necrolysis, ventricular arrhythmia, vesiculobullous eruptions

Drug Interactions

Avoid Concomitant Use

Avoid concomitant use of Foscarnet with any of the following: Artemether; Dronedarone; Lumefantrine; Nilotinib; Pimozide; QuiNINE; Tetrabenazine; Thioridazine; Ziprasidone

Increased Effect/Toxicity

Foscarnet may increase the levels/effects of: Dronedarone; Pimozide; QTc-Prolonging Agents; QuiNINE; Tetrabenazine; Thioridazine; Ziprasidone

The levels/effects of Foscarnet may be increased by: Alfuzosin; Artemether; Chloroquine; Ciprofloxacin; Gadobutrol; Lumefantrine; Nilotinib; QuiNINE

Decreased Effect There are no known significant interactions involving a decrease in effect.

Storage/Stability Foscarnet injection is a clear, colorless solution. Store intact bottles at room temperature of 15°C to 30°C (59°F to 86°F) and protect from temperatures >40°C and from freezing. Diluted solution is stable for 24 hours at room temperature or under refrigeration.

Reconstitution Foscarnet should be diluted in D_5W or NS. For peripheral line administration, foscarnet **must** be diluted to ≤12 mg/mL with D_5W or NS. For central line administration, foscarnet may be administered undiluted.

Compatibility Stable in D_5W, NS; **incompatible** with dextrose 30%, LR, TPN, and I.V. solutions containing calcium, magnesium, vancomycin.

Y-site administration: Compatible: Aldesleukin, amikacin, aminophylline, ampicillin, aztreonam, cefazolin, cefoperazone, cefoxitin, ceftazidime, ceftizoxime, ceftriaxone, cefuroxime, chloramphenicol, cimetidine, clindamycin, dexamethasone sodium phosphate, dopamine, erythromycin lactobionate, fluconazole, flucytosine, furosemide, gentamicin, heparin, hydrocortisone sodium succinate, hydromorphone, hydroxyzine, imipenem/cilastatin, metoclopramide, metronidazole, morphine, nafcillin, oxacillin, penicillin G potassium, phenytoin, piperacillin, ranitidine, ticarcillin/clavulanate, tobramycin. **Incompatible:** Acyclovir, amphotericin B, diazepam, digoxin, diphenhydramine, dobutamine, droperidol, ganciclovir, haloperidol, leucovorin, midazolam, pentamidine, prochlorperazine edisylate, promethazine. **Variable (consult detailed reference):** Co-trimoxazole, lorazepam, vancomycin.

Compatibility when admixed: Compatible: Potassium chloride.

Mechanism of Action Pyrophosphate analogue which acts as a noncompetitive inhibitor of many viral RNA and DNA polymerases as well as HIV reverse transcriptase. Similar to ganciclovir, foscarnet is a virostatic agent. Foscarnet does not require activation by thymidine kinase.

Pharmacodynamics/Kinetics

Distribution: V_d: ~0.5 L/kg; up to 28% of cumulative I.V. dose may be deposited in bone

Protein binding: 14% to 17%

Metabolism: Biotransformation does not occur

Half-life elimination: Elimination: ~3-4 hours; terminal: ~88 hours (due to bone deposition)

Excretion: Urine (≤28% as unchanged drug)

Dosage

CMV retinitis: I.V.:

Induction treatment: 60 mg/kg/dose every 8 hours **or** 90 mg/kg every 12 hours for 14-21 days

Maintenance therapy: 90-120 mg/kg/day as a single daily infusion

Herpes simplex infections (acyclovir-resistant): Induction: I.V.: 40 mg/kg/dose every 8-12 hours for 14-21 days

Therapy of CMV infection in cancer patients (unlabeled use): I.V.:

Prophylaxis: 60 mg/kg every 8-12 hours for 7 days, followed by 90-120 mg/kg daily until day 100 after HSCT

Pre-emptive treatment: 60 mg/kg every 12 hours for 14 days; if CMV still detectable, continue with 90 mg/kg daily for 5 days/week for 2 additional weeks

Treatment: 90 mg/kg every 12 hours for 2 weeks, followed by 120 mg/kg daily for ≥2 weeks

Dosage adjustment in renal impairment: Induction and maintenance dosing schedules based on creatinine clearance (mL/minute/kg): See tables below and on next page.

Induction Dosing of Foscarnet in Patients With Abnormal Renal Function

Cl_{cr} (mL/min/kg)	HSV Equivalent to 40 mg/kg q12h	HSV Equivalent to 40 mg/kg q8h	CMV Equivalent to 60 mg/kg q8h	CMV Equivalent to 90 mg/kg q12h
<0.4	Not recommended	Not recommended	Not recommended	Not recommended
≥0.4-0.5	20 mg/kg every 24 hours	35 mg/kg every 24 hours	50 mg/kg every 24 hours	50 mg/kg every 24 hours
>0.5-0.6	25 mg/kg every 24 hours	40 mg/kg every 24 hours	60 mg/kg every 24 hours	60 mg/kg every 24 hours
>0.6-0.8	35 mg/kg every 24 hours	25 mg/kg every 12 hours	40 mg/kg every 12 hours	80 mg/kg every 24 hours
>0.8-1.0	20 mg/kg every 12 hours	35 mg/kg every 12 hours	50 mg/kg every 12 hours	50 mg/kg every 12 hours
>1.0-1.4	30 mg/kg every 12 hours	30 mg/kg every 8 hours	45 mg/kg every 8 hours	70 mg/kg every 12 hours
>1.4	40 mg/kg every 12 hours	40 mg/kg every 8 hours	60 mg/kg every 8 hours	90 mg/kg every 12 hours

◀

Maintenance Dosing of Foscarnet in Patients With Abnormal Renal Function

Cl_cr (mL/min/kg)	CMV Equivalent to 90 mg/kg q24h	CMV Equivalent to 120 mg/kg q24h
<0.4	Not recommended	Not recommended
≥0.4-0.5	50 mg/kg every 48 hours	65 mg/kg every 48 hours
>0.5-0.6	60 mg/kg every 48 hours	80 mg/kg every 48 hours
>0.6-0.8	80 mg/kg every 48 hours	105 mg/kg every 48 hours
>0.8-1.0	50 mg/kg every 24 hours	65 mg/kg every 24 hours
>1.0-1.4	70 mg/kg every 24 hours	90 mg/kg every 24 hours
>1.4	90 mg/kg every 24 hours	120 mg/kg every 24 hours

Hemodialysis:

Foscarnet is highly removed by hemodialysis (up to ~38% in 2.5 hours HD with high-flux membrane)

Doses of 50 mg/kg/dose posthemodialysis have been found to produce similar serum concentrations as doses of 90 mg/kg twice daily in patients with normal renal function

Doses of 60-90 mg/kg/dose loading dose (posthemodialysis) followed by 45-60 mg/kg/dose posthemodialysis (3 times/week) with the monitoring of weekly plasma concentrations to maintain peak plasma concentrations in the range of 400-800 μMolar have been recommended by some clinicians

Continuous arteriovenous or venovenous hemodiafiltration effects: Dose as for Cl_cr 10-50 mL/minute

Administration Foscarnet is administered by intravenous infusion, using an infusion pump, at a rate not exceeding 1 mg/kg/minute. Undiluted (24 mg/mL) solution can be administered without further dilution when using a central venous catheter for infusion. For peripheral vein administration, the solution **must** be diluted to a final concentration **not to exceed** 12 mg/mL. The manufacturer recommends 750-1000 mL of NS or D_5W be administered prior to first infusion to establish diuresis. With subsequent infusions of 90-120 mg/kg, this volume would be repeated. If the dose were 40-60 mg/kg, then the volume could be reduced to 500 mL. After the first dose, the hydration fluid should be administered concurrently with foscarnet.

Monitoring Parameters 24-hour creatinine clearance at baseline and periodically thereafter. During induction therapy: Obtain complete blood counts, and electrolytes (including serum creatinine, calcium, magnesium, potassium and phosphorus) twice weekly and then one weekly during maintenance therapy. More frequent monitoring may be required in some patients. Check hydration status before and after infusion.

Additional Information CMV retinitis maintenance treatment may be discontinued if immune reconstitution occurs as a result of ART.

Dosage Forms Excipient information presented when available (limited, particularly for generics); consult specific product labeling. [DSC] = Discontinued product

Injection, solution, as sodium [preservative-free]: 24 mg/mL (250 mL, 500 mL)

Foscavir®: 24 mg/mL (500 mL) [DSC]

References

Aweeka FT, Jacobson MA, Martin-Munley S, et al, "Effect of Renal Disease and Hemodialysis on Foscarnet Pharmacokinetics and Dosing Recommendations," *J Acquir Immune Def Syndr Hum Retrovirol*, 1999, 20(4):350-7.

Chilukuri S and Rosen T, "Management of Acyclovir-Resistant Herpes Simplex Virus," *Dermatol Clin*, 2003, 21(2):311-20.

Deray G, Martinez F, Katlama C, et al, "Foscarnet Nephrotoxicity: Mechanism, Incidence and Prevention," *Am J Nephrol*, 1989, 9:316-21.

"Drugs for Non-HIV Viral Infections," *Med Lett Drugs Ther*, 1994, 36(919):27.

Jacobson MA, "Review of the Toxicities of Foscarnet," *J Acquir Immune Defic Syndr*, 1992, 5(Suppl 1):11-7.

Jayaweera DT, "Minimizing the Dosage-Limiting Toxicities of Foscarnet Induction Therapy," *Drug Saf*, 1997, 16(4):258-66.

Keating MR, "Antiviral Agents," *Mayo Clin Proc*, 1992, 67(2):160-78.

National Comprehensive Cancer Network (NCCN), "Clinical Practice Guidelines in Oncology™: Prevention and Treatment of Cancer-Related Infections," Version 1.2008. Available at http://www.nccn.org/professionals/physician_gls/PDF/infections.pdf.

♦ **Foscavir® [DSC]** *see* Foscarnet *on page 516*

♦ **Foscavir® (Can)** *see* Foscarnet *on page 516*

♦ **Fragmin®** *see* Dalteparin *on page 303*

♦ **FU** *see* Fluorouracil *on page 499*

♦ **5-FU** *see* Fluorouracil *on page 499*

♦ **FUDR** *see* Floxuridine *on page 482*

♦ **FUDR®** *see* Floxuridine *on page 482*

Fulvestrant (fool VES trant)

Related Information
Safe Handling of Hazardous Drugs *on page 1517*

U.S. Brand Names Faslodex®

Index Terms ICI-182,780; Zeneca 182,780; ZM-182,780

Generic Available No

Pharmacologic Category Antineoplastic Agent, Estrogen Receptor Antagonist

Use Treatment of hormone receptor positive metastatic breast cancer in postmenopausal women with disease progression following antiestrogen therapy

Pregnancy Risk Factor D

Lactation Excretion in breast milk unknown/contraindicated

Labeled Contraindications Hypersensitivity to fulvestrant or any component of the formulation; contraindications to I.M. injections (bleeding diatheses, thrombocytopenia, or therapeutic anticoagulation); pregnancy

Warnings/Precautions Hazardous agent - use appropriate precautions for handling and disposal. Use caution in hepatic impairment. Safety and efficacy have not been established in children.

Adverse Reactions
>10%:
Cardiovascular: Vasodilation (18%)
Central nervous system: Pain (19%), headache (15%)
Endocrine & metabolic: Hot flushes (19% to 24%)
Gastrointestinal: Nausea (26%), vomiting (13%), constipation (13%), diarrhea (12%), abdominal pain (12%)
Local: Injection site reaction (11%)
Neuromuscular & skeletal: Weakness (23%), bone pain (16%), back pain (14%)

Respiratory: Pharyngitis (16%), dyspnea (15%)

1% to 10%:

Cardiovascular: Edema (9%), chest pain (7%)

Central nervous system: Dizziness (7%), insomnia (7%), paresthesia (6%), fever (6%), depression (6%), anxiety (5%)

Dermatologic: Rash (7%)

Gastrointestinal: Anorexia (9%), weight gain (1% to 2%)

Genitourinary: Pelvic pain (10%), urinary tract infection (6%), vaginitis (2% to 3%)

Hematologic: Anemia (5%)

Neuromuscular & skeletal: Arthritis (3%)

Respiratory: Cough (10%)

Miscellaneous: Diaphoresis increased (5%)

<1%: Angioedema, hypersensitivity reactions, leukopenia, myalgia, thrombosis, urticaria, vaginal bleeding, vertigo

Drug Interactions

Metabolism/Transport Effects Substrate of CYP3A4 (minor)

Avoid Concomitant Use There are no known interactions where it is recommended to avoid concomitant use.

Increased Effect/Toxicity There are no known significant interactions involving an increase in effect.

Decreased Effect There are no known significant interactions involving a decrease in effect.

Storage/Stability Store under refrigeration at 2°C to 8°C (36°F to 46°F).

Mechanism of Action Steroidal compound which competitively binds to estrogen receptors on tumors and other tissue targets, producing a nuclear complex that decreases DNA synthesis and inhibits estrogen effects. Fulvestrant has no estrogen-receptor agonist activity. Causes down-regulation of estrogen receptors and inhibits tumor growth.

Pharmacodynamics/Kinetics

Duration: I.M.: Plasma levels maintained for at least 1 month

Distribution: V_d: 3-5 L/kg

Protein binding: 99%

Metabolism: Hepatic via multiple pathways (CYP3A4 substrate, relative contribution to metabolism unknown)

Bioavailability: Oral: Poor

Half-life elimination: ~40 days

Time to peak, plasma: I.M.: 7-9 days

Excretion: Feces (>90%); urine (<1%)

Dosage I.M.: Adults (postmenopausal women): 250 mg at 1-month intervals

Dosage adjustment in renal impairment: No adjustment required.

Dosage adjustment in hepatic impairment: Use in moderate-to-severe hepatic impairment has not been evaluated; use caution.

Administration I.M. injection into a relatively large muscle (ie, buttock); do not administer I.V., SubQ, or intra-arterially. May be administered as a single 5 mL injection or two concurrent 2.5 mL injections.

Dosage Forms Excipient information presented when available (limited, particularly for generics); consult specific product labeling.

Injection, solution:

Faslodex®: 50 mg/mL (2.5 mL, 5 mL) [contains alcohol, benzyl alcohol, benzyl stearate, castor oil]

References

Bundred N and Howell A, "Fulvestrant (Faslodex): Current Status in the Therapy of Breast Cancer," *Expert Rev Anticancer Ther*, 2002, 2(2):151-60.

Wardley AM, "Fulvestrant: A Review of Its Development, Preclinical and Clinical Data," *Int J Clin Pract*, 2002, 56(4):305-9.

◆ **Fungizone® (Can)** *see* Amphotericin B (Conventional) *on page 66*

◆ **Fusilev™** *see* LEVOleucovorin *on page 714*

Gallium Nitrate (GAL ee um NYE trate)

U.S. Brand Names Ganite™

Index Terms NSC-15200

Generic Available No

Pharmacologic Category Calcium-Lowering Agent

Use Treatment of symptomatic cancer-related hypercalcemia

Pregnancy Risk Factor C

Lactation Excretion in breast milk unknown/not recommended

Labeled Contraindications Hypersensitivity to gallium nitrate or any component of the formulation; severe renal dysfunction (serum creatinine >2.5 mg/dL)

Warnings/Precautions Hazardous agent - use appropriate precautions for handling and disposal. BUN and serum creatinine elevations have been observed with gallium nitrate use; monitor closely; discontinue with serum creatinine >2.5 mg/dL. **[U.S. Boxed Warning]: Concurrent administration with other nephrotoxic drugs (eg, aminoglycosides, amphotericin B) may increase the risk for renal insufficiency; discontinue gallium nitrate during treatment with nephrotoxic drugs.** Establish and maintain adequate hydration with normal saline. Urinary output of ≥2 L/day should be established prior to treatment initiation. Use with caution in patients where aggressive hydration may be poorly tolerated, such as in cardiovascular disease (HF or hypertension) and pulmonary disease. Therapy may result in mild-to-moderate hypocalcemia. Safety and efficacy in pediatric patients have not been established.

Adverse Reactions Frequency not always defined.

Cardiovascular: Edema (lower extremity), hypotension, tachycardia

Central nervous system: Coma, confusion, dreams, encephalopathy, fever, hallucinations, hypothermia, lethargy

Dermatologic: Rash

Endocrine & metabolic: Hypophosphatemia (up to 79%), serum bicarbonate decreased (40% to 50%), hypocalcemia (38%), respiratory alkalosis (mild)

Hematologic: Anemia, leukopenia

Gastrointestinal: Constipation, diarrhea, nausea, vomiting

Neuromuscular & skeletal: Paresthesia, positive Cvostek's sign

Ocular: Optic neuritis

Otic: Auditory acuity decreased (<1%), tinnitus (<1%), hearing decreased

Renal: BUN increased (13%), creatinine increased (13%), acute renal failure

Respiratory: Dyspnea, pleural effusion, pulmonary infiltrates, rales, rhonchi

Drug Interactions

Avoid Concomitant Use

Avoid concomitant use of Gallium Nitrate with any of the following: Aminoglycosides; Amphotericin B; Vancomycin

Increased Effect/Toxicity

The levels/effects of Gallium Nitrate may be increased by: Aminoglycosides; Amphotericin B; Vancomycin

◄ **Decreased Effect** There are no known significant interactions involving a decrease in effect.

Storage/Stability Store unopened vials (25 mg/mL) at room temperature of 20°C to 25°C (68°F to 77°F); not light sensitive. Solutions in 0.9% NaCl or D_5W are stable for 48 hours at room temperature or for 7 days under refrigeration at 2°C to 8°C (36°F to 46°F).

Reconstitution Dilute in 1000 mL NS (preferred) or D_5W for infusion.

Compatibility Stable in NS, D_5W.

Mechanism of Action Inhibits bone resorption by inhibiting osteoclast function. Gallium nitrate appears to be effective in parathyroid hormone-related protein (PTHrP) and non-PTHrP-associated hypercalcemia.

Pharmacodynamics/Kinetics

Onset of calcium lowering: Seen within 24-48 hours of beginning therapy, with normocalcemia achieved within 4-7 days of beginning therapy

Duration: Normocalcemia: 7-10 days

Bioavailability: Oral: 5%

Distribution: Tissue concentrations were determined postmortem in one patient and concentrations were higher in liver and kidney than in lung, skin, muscle, heart, and cervix tumor; in dogs, tissue gallium concentrations were higher in renal cortex, bone, bone marrow, small intestine, and liver than in skeletal muscle and brain

Half-life elimination: Alpha: 1.25 hours; Beta: ~24 hours

Elimination half-life varies with method of administration (72-115 hours with prolonged intravenous infusion versus 24 hours with bolus administration); long elimination half-life may be related to slow release from tissue such as bone

Excretion: Primarily renal with no prior metabolism in the liver or kidney

Dosage Note: Initiate I.V. hydration prior to treatment; maintain throughout treatment.

I.V.: Adults: 200 mg/m²/day for 5 days; duration may be shortened during a course if normocalcemia is achieved. If hypercalcemia is mild and with very few symptoms, 100 mg/m²/day may be used.

Dosage adjustment in renal impairment:

Serum creatinine >2.5 mg/dL: Contraindicated

Serum creatinine 2 to ≤2.5 mg/dL: No guidelines exist; frequent monitoring is recommended

Administration The manufacturer recommends continuous I.V. infusion over 24 hours.

Monitoring Parameters Renal function (BUN, serum creatinine); serum calcium (baseline, then daily); serum phosphorus (baseline, then twice weekly); fluid intake, urine output

Additional Information In addition to the hypocalcemic effect, gallium nitrate has also been studied for its antitumor effects. Gallium nitrate was studied at higher doses infused over 30 minutes every 2 weeks in bladder cancer and lymphoma (Einhorn, 2003; Straus, 2003). Rapid infusion rates and higher doses are associated with an increased risk of toxicity, including nephrotoxicity and gastrointestinal toxicity.

Dosage Forms Excipient information presented when available (limited, particularly for generics); consult specific product labeling.

Injection, solution [preservative free]:

Ganite™: 25 mg/mL (20 mL)

References

Cvitkovic F, Armand JP, Tubiana-Hulin M, et al, "Randomized, Double-Blind, Phase II Trial of Gallium Nitrate Compared With Pamidronate for Acute Control of Cancer-Related Hypercalcemia," *Cancer J*, 2006, 12(1):47-53.

Einhorn L, "Gallium Nitrate in the Treatment of Bladder Cancer," *Sem Oncol*, 2003, 30(2 Suppl 5):34-41.

Hortobagyi GN, "Novel Approaches to the Management of Bone Metastases," *Semin Oncol*, 2003, 30(5 Suppl 16):161-6.

Leyland-Jones B, "Pharmacokinetics and Therapeutic Index of Gallium Nitrate," *Semin Oncol*, 1991, 18(4 Suppl 5):16-20.

Leyland-Jones B, "Treatment of Cancer-Related Hypercalcemia: The Role of Gallium Nitrate," *Semin Oncol*, 2003, 30(2 Suppl 5):13-9.

Straus DJ, "Gallium Nitrate in the Treatment of Lymphoma", *Sem Oncol*, 2003, 30(2 Suppl 5):25-33.

◆ **Gamimune® N (Can)** *see* Immune Globulin (Intravenous) *on page* 627

◆ **Gammagard Liquid** *see* Immune Globulin (Intravenous) *on page* 627

◆ **Gammagard S/D** *see* Immune Globulin (Intravenous) *on page* 627

◆ **Gammaphos** *see* Amifostine *on page* 50

◆ **Gamunex®** *see* Immune Globulin (Intravenous) *on page* 627

Ganciclovir (gan SYE kloe veer)

Medication Safety Issues

Sound-alike/look-alike issues:

Cytovene® may be confused with Cytosar®, Cytosar-U®

Ganciclovir may be confused with acyclovir

Related Information

Safe Handling of Hazardous Drugs *on page* 1517

U.S. Brand Names Cytovene®; Vitrasert®; Zirgan™

Index Terms DHPG Sodium; GCV Sodium; Nordeoxyguanosine

Generic Available Yes: Capsule

Canadian Brand Names Cytovene®; Vitrasert®

Pharmacologic Category Antiviral Agent

Use

Parenteral: Treatment of CMV retinitis in immunocompromised individuals, including patients with acquired immunodeficiency syndrome; prophylaxis of CMV infection in transplant patients

Oral: Alternative to the I.V. formulation for maintenance treatment of CMV retinitis in immunocompromised patients, including patients with AIDS, in whom retinitis is stable following appropriate induction therapy and for whom the risk of more rapid progression is balanced by the benefit associated with avoiding daily I.V. infusions.

Implant: Treatment of CMV retinitis

Unlabeled/Investigational Use May be given in combination with foscarnet in patients who relapse after monotherapy with either drug

Pregnancy Risk Factor C

Lactation Excretion in breast milk unknown/contraindicated

Labeled Contraindications Hypersensitivity to ganciclovir, acyclovir, or any component of the formulation; absolute neutrophil count <500/mm^3; platelet count <25,000/mm^3

Warnings/Precautions Hazardous agent - use appropriate precautions for handling and disposal. **[U.S. Boxed Warning]: Granulocytopenia (neutropenia), anemia, and thrombocytopenia may occur.** Dosage adjustment or interruption of ganciclovir therapy may be necessary in patients with neutropenia and/or thrombocytopenia and patients with impaired renal function. **[U.S. Boxed Warning]: Animal studies have demonstrated carcinogenic and teratogenic effects, and inhibition of spermatogenesis;** contraceptive precautions for female and male patients need to be followed during and for at least 90 days after therapy with the drug; take care to administer only into veins with good blood flow. **[U.S. Boxed Warning]: Indicated only for treatment of CMV retinitis in the immunocompromised patient and CMV prevention in transplant patients at risk.**

Adverse Reactions

>10%:
  Central nervous system: Fever (38% to 48%)
  Dermatologic: Rash (15% oral, 10% I.V.)
  Gastrointestinal: Diarrhea (40%), nausea (25%), abdominal pain (17% to 19%), anorexia (15%), vomiting (13%)
  Hematologic: Leukopenia (30% to 40%), anemia (20% to 25%)

1% to 10%:
  Central nervous system: Neuropathy (8% to 9%), headache (4%), confusion
  Dermatologic: Pruritus (5%)
  Hematologic: Thrombocytopenia (6%), neutropenia with ANC <500/mm^3 (5% oral, 14% I.V.)
  Neuromuscular & skeletal: Paresthesia (6% to 10%), weakness (6%)
  Ocular: Retinal detachment (8% oral, 11% I.V.; relationship to ganciclovir not established)
  Miscellaneous: Sepsis (4% oral, 15% I.V.)

<1% (Limited to important or life-threatening): Alopecia, arrhythmia, ataxia, bronchospasm, coma, dyspnea, encephalopathy, exfoliative dermatitis, extrapyramidal symptoms, nervousness, pancytopenia, psychosis, seizure, alopecia, urticaria, eosinophilia, hemorrhage, Stevens-Johnson syndrome, torsade de pointes, renal failure, SIADH, visual loss

Drug Interactions

Avoid Concomitant Use

Avoid concomitant use of Ganciclovir with any of the following: Imipenem

Increased Effect/Toxicity

Ganciclovir may increase the levels/effects of: Imipenem; Mycophenolate; Reverse Transcriptase Inhibitors (Nucleoside); Tenofovir

The levels/effects of Ganciclovir may be increased by: Mycophenolate

Decreased Effect There are no known significant interactions involving a decrease in effect.

Storage/Stability Intact vials should be stored at room temperature and protected from temperatures >40°C. Reconstituted solution is stable for 12 hours at room temperature, however, conflicting data indicates that reconstituted solution is stable for 60 days under refrigeration (4°C). Stability of parenteral admixture at room temperature (25°C) and at refrigeration temperature (4°C) is 5 days.

Reconstitution Reconstitute powder with unpreserved sterile water not bacteriostatic water because parabens may cause precipitation. Dilute in 250-1000 mL D$_5$W or NS to a concentration ≤10 mg/mL for infusion.

Compatibility Stable in D$_5$W, LR, NS; **incompatible** with paraben preserved bacteriostatic water for injection (may cause precipitation).

Y-site administration: Compatible: Allopurinol, amphotericin B cholesteryl sulfate complex, cisplatin, cyclophosphamide, docetaxel, doxorubicin liposome, enalaprilat, etoposide phosphate, filgrastim, fluconazole, gatifloxacin, granisetron, linezolid, melphalan, methotrexate, paclitaxel, propofol, remifentanil, tacrolimus, teniposide, thiotepa. **Incompatible:** Aldesleukin, amifostine, amsacrine, aztreonam, cefepime, cytarabine, doxorubicin, fludarabine, foscarnet, gemcitabine, ondansetron, piperacillin/tazobactam, sargramostim, vinorelbine. **Variable (consult detailed reference):** Cisatracurium.

Mechanism of Action Ganciclovir is phosphorylated to a substrate which competitively inhibits the binding of deoxyguanosine triphosphate to DNA polymerase resulting in inhibition of viral DNA synthesis

Pharmacodynamics/Kinetics

Distribution: V_d: 15.26 L/1.73 m^2; widely to all tissues including CSF and ocular tissue

Protein binding: 1% to 2%

Bioavailability: Oral: Fasting: 5%; Following food: 6% to 9%; Following fatty meal: 28% to 31%

Half-life elimination: 1.7-5.8 hours; prolonged with renal impairment; End-stage renal disease: 5-28 hours

Excretion: Urine (80% to 99% as unchanged drug)

Dosage

CMV retinitis: Slow I.V. infusion (dosing is based on total body weight):
Children >3 months and Adults:
Induction therapy: 5 mg/kg/dose every 12 hours for 14-21 days followed by maintenance therapy
Maintenance therapy: 5 mg/kg/day as a single daily dose for 7 days/week or 6 mg/kg/day for 5 days/week

CMV retinitis: Oral: 1000 mg 3 times/day with food **or** 500 mg 6 times/day with food

Prevention of CMV disease in patients with advanced HIV infection and normal renal function: Oral: 1000 mg 3 times/day with food

Prevention of CMV disease in transplant patients: Same initial and maintenance dose as CMV retinitis except duration of initial course is 7-14 days, duration of maintenance therapy is dependent on clinical condition and degree of immunosuppression

Intravitreal implant: One implant for 5- to 8-month period; following depletion of ganciclovir, as evidenced by progression of retinitis, implant may be removed and replaced

Elderly: Refer to adult dosing; in general, dose selection should be cautious, reflecting greater frequency of organ impairment

Dosing adjustment in renal impairment:

I.V. (Induction):
Cl_{cr} 50-69 mL/minute: Administer 2.5 mg/kg/dose every 12 hours
Cl_{cr} 25-49 mL/minute: Administer 2.5 mg/kg/dose every 24 hours
Cl_{cr} 10-24 mL/minute: Administer 1.25 mg/kg/dose every 24 hours
Cl_{cr} <10 mL/minute: Administer 1.25 mg/kg/dose 3 times/week following hemodialysis

I.V. (Maintenance):
Cl_{cr} 50-69 mL/minute: Administer 2.5 mg/kg/dose every 24 hours
Cl_{cr} 25-49 mL/minute: Administer 1.25 mg/kg/dose every 24 hours
Cl_{cr} 10-24 mL/minute: Administer 0.625 mg/kg/dose every 24 hours
Cl_{cr} <10 mL/minute: Administer 0.625 mg/kg/dose 3 times/week following hemodialysis

Oral:
Cl_{cr} 50-69 mL/minute: Administer 1500 mg/day or 500 mg 3 times/day
Cl_{cr} 25-49 mL/minute: Administer 1000 mg/day or 500 mg twice daily
Cl_{cr} 10-24 mL/minute: Administer 500 mg/day
Cl_{cr} <10 mL/minute: Administer 500 mg 3 times/week following hemodialysis

◄ Hemodialysis effects: Dialyzable (50%) following hemodialysis; administer dose postdialysis. During peritoneal dialysis, dose as for Cl_{cr} <10 mL/minute. During continuous arteriovenous or venovenous hemofiltration, administer 2.5 mg/kg/dose every 24 hours.

Administration
Oral: Should be administered with food.
I.V.: Should not be administered by I.M., SubQ, or rapid IVP; administer by slow I.V. infusion over at least 1 hour

Monitoring Parameters CBC with differential and platelet count, serum creatinine, ophthalmologic exams

Dietary Considerations Sodium content of 500 mg vial: 46 mg

Product Availability
Zirgan™: FDA approved September 2009; availability expected in early 2010
Zirgan™ is an ophthalmic gel indicated for the treatment of acute herpetic keratitis.

Dosage Forms Excipient information presented when available (limited, particularly for generics); consult specific product labeling.
Capsule: 250 mg, 500 mg
Implant, intravitreal:
Vitrasert®: 4.5 mg [released gradually over 5-8 months]
Injection, powder for reconstitution, as sodium:
Cytovene®: 500 mg

References
"Drugs for Non-HIV Viral Infections," *Med Lett Drugs Ther*, 1994, 36(919):27.
Fletcher C, Sawchuk R, Chinnock B, et al, "Human Pharmacokinetics of the Antiviral Drug DHPG," *Clin Pharmacol Ther*, 1986, 40(3):281-6.
Goodrich JM, Bowden RA, Fisher L, et al, "Ganciclovir Prophylaxis to Prevent Cytomegalovirus Disease After Allogeneic Marrow Transplant," *Ann Intern Med*, 1993, 118(3):173-8.
Gudnason T, Belani KK, and Balfour HH Jr, "Ganciclovir Treatment of Cytomegalovirus Disease in Immunocompromised Children," *Pediatr Infect Dis J*, 1989, 8(7):436-40.
Lake KD, Fletcher CV, Love KR, et al, "Ganciclovir Pharmacokinetics During Renal Impairment," *Antimicrob Agents Chemother*, 1988, 32(12):1899-900.
Paul S and Dummer S, "Topics in Clinical Pharmacology, Ganciclovir," *Am J Med Sci*, 1992, 304 (4):272-7.
Sommadossi JP, Bevan R, Ling T, et al, "Clinical Pharmacokinetics of Ganciclovir in Patients With Normal and Impaired Renal Function," *Rev Infect Dis*, 1988, 10(Suppl 3):507-14.

◆ **Ganite™** *see* Gallium Nitrate *on page 523*

◆ **Garamycin® (Can)** *see* Gentamicin *on page 542*

◆ **Gardasil®** *see* Papillomavirus (Types 6, 11, 16, 18) Vaccine (Human, Recombinant) *on page 922*

◆ **G-CSF** *see* Filgrastim *on page 475*

◆ **G-CSF (PEG Conjugate)** *see* Pegfilgrastim *on page 929*

◆ **GCV Sodium** *see* Ganciclovir *on page 525*

◆ **GD-Celecoxib (Can)** *see* Celecoxib *on page 206*

Gefitinib (ge FI tye nib)
Medication Safety Issues
Sound-alike/look-alike issues:
Gefitinib may be confused with erlotinib

High alert medication: The Institute for Safe Medication Practices (ISMP) includes this medication among its list of drugs which have a heightened risk of causing significant patient harm when used in error.

Related Information
Safe Handling of Hazardous Drugs *on page 1517*

U.S. Brand Names IRESSA®

Index Terms NSC-715055; ZD1839

Generic Available No

Pharmacologic Category Antineoplastic Agent, Tyrosine Kinase Inhibitor

Use

U.S. labeling: Treatment of locally advanced or metastatic nonsmall cell lung cancer after failure of platinum-based and docetaxel therapies. Treatment is limited to patients who are benefiting or have benefited from treatment with gefitinib.

Note: Due to the lack of improved survival data from clinical trials of gefitinib, and in response to positive survival data with another EGFR inhibitor, physicians are advised to use other treatment options in advanced nonsmall cell lung cancer patients following one or two prior chemotherapy regimens when they are refractory/intolerant to their most recent regimen.

Canada labeling: Approved indication is limited to NSCLC patients with epidermal growth factor receptor (EGFR) expression status positive or unknown.

Restrictions As of September 15, 2005, distribution will be limited to patients enrolled in the Iressa Access Program. Under this program, access to gefitinib will be limited to the following groups:

Patients who are currently receiving and benefitting from gefitinib (IRESSA®)

Patients who have previously received and benefited from gefitinib (IRESSA®)

Previously-enrolled patients or new patients in non-Investigational New Drug (IND) clinical trials involving gefitinib (IRESSA®) if these protocols were approved by an IRB prior to June 17, 2005

New patients may also receive Iressa if the manufacturer (AstraZeneca) decides to make it available under IND, and the patients meet the criteria for enrollment under the IND

Additional information on the IRESSA® Access Program, including enrollment forms, may be obtained by calling AstraZeneca at 1-800-601-8933 or via the web at www.Iressa-access.com

Pregnancy Risk Factor D

Lactation Excretion in breast milk unknown/not recommended

Labeled Contraindications Hypersensitivity to gefitinib or any component of the formulation; pregnancy

Warnings/Precautions Hazardous agent - use appropriate precautions for handling and disposal. Rare, sometimes fatal, pulmonary toxicity (eg, alveolitis, interstitial pneumonia, pneumonitis) has occurred. Therapy should be interrupted in patients with acute onset or worsening pulmonary symptoms; discontinue gefitinib if interstitial pneumonitis is confirmed. Use caution in hepatic or severe renal impairment. May cause hepatic injury and elevation of transaminases; discontinue if elevations/changes are severe. Interruption of therapy may be required in patients with poorly tolerated diarrhea or adverse skin reactions. Eye pain should be promptly evaluated and therapy may be interrupted based on appropriate medical evaluation; may be reinitiated following resolution of symptoms and eye changes. Safety and efficacy in pediatric patients have not been established.

Adverse Reactions

>10%:

Dermatologic: Rash (43% to 54%), acne (25% to 33%), dry skin (13% to 26%)

Gastrointestinal: Diarrhea (48% to 76%), nausea (13% to 18%), vomiting (9% to 12%)

1% to 10%:

Cardiovascular: Peripheral edema (2%)

Dermatologic: Pruritus (8% to 9%)

Gastrointestinal: Anorexia (7% to 10%), weight loss (3% to 5%), mouth ulceration (1%)

Neuromuscular & skeletal: Weakness (4% to 6%)

Ocular: Amblyopia (2%), conjunctivitis (1%)

Respiratory: Dyspnea (2%), interstitial lung disease (1% to 2%)

<1%: Aberrant eyelash growth, angioedema, corneal erosion and membrane sloughing, epistaxis, erythema multiforme, eye pain, hematuria, hemorrhage, ocular hemorrhaging, ocular ischemia, pancreatitis, toxic epidermal necrolysis, urticaria

Postmarketing and/or case reports: CNS hemorrhage and death were reported in clinical trials of pediatric patients with primary CNS tumors

Drug Interactions

Metabolism/Transport Effects Substrate of CYP3A4 (major); **Inhibits** CYP2C19 (weak), 2D6 (weak)

Avoid Concomitant Use

Avoid concomitant use of Gefitinib with any of the following: Natalizumab; Vaccines (Live)

Increased Effect/Toxicity

Gefitinib may increase the levels/effects of: Leflunomide; Natalizumab; Topotecan; Vaccines (Live); Vitamin K Antagonists

The levels/effects of Gefitinib may be increased by: Antifungal Agents (Azole Derivatives, Systemic); CYP3A4 Inhibitors (Moderate); CYP3A4 Inhibitors (Strong); Dasatinib; Trastuzumab

Decreased Effect

Gefitinib may decrease the levels/effects of: Cardiac Glycosides; Vaccines (Inactivated); Vaccines (Live); Vitamin K Antagonists

The levels/effects of Gefitinib may be decreased by: CYP3A4 Inducers (Strong); Deferasirox; Echinacea; Herbs (CYP3A4 Inducers); Ranitidine; Rifamycin Derivatives

Ethanol/Nutrition/Herb Interactions Food: Grapefruit juice may increase serum gefitinib concentrations; St John's wort may decrease serum gefitinib concentrations.

Storage/Stability Store tablets at controlled room temperature of 20°C to 25°C (68°F to 77°F).

Mechanism of Action The mechanism of antineoplastic action is not fully understood. Gefitinib inhibits tyrosine kinases (TK) associated with transmembrane cell surface receptors found on both normal and cancer cells. One such receptor is epidermal growth factor receptor. TK activity appears to be vitally important to cell proliferation and survival.

Pharmacodynamics/Kinetics

Absorption: Oral: slow

Distribution: I.V.: 1400 L

Protein binding: 90%, albumin and alpha$_1$-acid glycoprotein

Metabolism: Hepatic, primarily via CYP3A4; forms metabolites

Bioavailability: 60%
Half-life elimination: I.V.: 48 hours
Time to peak, plasma: Oral: 3-7 hours
Excretion: Feces (86%); urine (<4%)

Dosage Note: In response to the lack of improved survival data from the ISEL trial, AstraZeneca has temporarily suspended promotion of this drug.

Oral: Adults: 250 mg/day; consider 500 mg/day in patients receiving effective CYP3A4 inducers (eg, rifampin, phenytoin)

Dosage adjustment in renal/hepatic impairment: No adjustment necessary

Dosage adjustment for toxicity: Consider interruption of therapy in any patient with evidence of pulmonary decompensation or severe hepatic injury; discontinuation may be required if toxicity is confirmed. Poorly tolerated diarrhea or adverse skin reactions may be managed by a brief interruption of therapy (up to 14 days), followed by reinitiation of therapy at 250 mg/day. Eye pain should be promptly evaluated and therapy may be interrupted based on appropriate medical evaluation; may be reinitiated following resolution of symptoms and eye changes.

Administration May administer with or without food.

For patients unable to swallow tablets or for administration via NG tube: Tablets may be dispersed in noncarbonated drinking water. Drop whole tablet (do not crush) into 1/2 glass of water; stir until tablet is dispersed (~10 minutes). Drink immediately. Rinse with 1/2 glass of water and drink.

Monitoring Parameters Periodic liver function tests (asymptomatic increases in liver enzymes have occurred)

Dietary Considerations Food does not affect gefitinib absorption.

Emetic Potential Very low (<10%)

Dosage Forms Excipient information presented when available (limited, particularly for generics); consult specific product labeling.
Tablet: 250 mg

References

Cohen EE, Rosen F, Stadler WM, et al, "Phase II Trial of ZD1839 in Recurrent or Metastatic Squamous Cell Carcinoma of the Head and Neck," *J Clin Oncol*, 2003, 21(10):1980-7.

Fukuoka M, Yano S, Giaccone G, et al, "Multi-Institutional Randomized Phase II Trial of Gefitinib for Previously Treated Patients With Advanced Non-Small-Cell Lung Cancer," *J Clin Oncol*, 2003, 21 (12):2237-46.

◆ **Gelclair®** *see* Mucosal Barrier Gel, Oral *on page 827*

Gemcitabine (jem SITE a been)

Medication Safety Issues

Sound-alike/look-alike issues:
Gemcitabine may be confused with gemtuzumab
Gemzar® may be confused with Zinecard®

High alert medication: The Institute for Safe Medication Practices (ISMP) includes this medication among its list of drugs which have a heightened risk of causing significant patient harm when used in error.

Related Information

Management of Drug Extravasations *on page 1447*
Safe Handling of Hazardous Drugs *on page 1517*

U.S. Brand Names Gemzar®

Index Terms Gemcitabine Hydrochloride

Generic Available No

Canadian Brand Names Gemzar®

Pharmacologic Category Antineoplastic Agent, Antimetabolite (Pyrimidine Analog)

Use Treatment of metastatic breast cancer; locally-advanced or metastatic nonsmall cell lung cancer (NSCLC) or pancreatic cancer; advanced, relapsed ovarian cancer

Unlabeled/Investigational Use Treatment of bladder cancer, cervical cancer, Hodgkin's disease, non-Hodgkin's lymphomas, small cell lung cancer, hepatobiliary cancers

Pregnancy Risk Factor D

Lactation Excretion in breast milk unknown/not recommended

Labeled Contraindications Hypersensitivity to gemcitabine or any component of the formulation; pregnancy

Warnings/Precautions Hazardous agent - use appropriate precautions for handling and disposal. Prolongation of the infusion time >60 minutes and more frequent than weekly dosing have been shown to increase toxicity. Gemcitabine can suppress bone marrow function (leukopenia, thrombocytopenia, and anemia); myelosuppression is usually the dose-limiting toxicity. Gemcitabine may cause fever in the absence of clinical infection. Pulmonary toxicity has occurred; discontinue if severe.

Hemolytic uremic syndrome has been reported; monitor for evidence of microangiopathic hemolysis (elevation of bilirubin or LDH, reticulocytosis, severe thrombocytopenia, and/or renal failure); use with caution in patients with pre-existing renal impairment. Serious hepatotoxicity has been reported. Use caution with hepatic impairment (history of cirrhosis, hepatitis, or alcoholism) or in patients with hepatic metastases; may lead to exacerbation of hepatic impairment. Use caution with concurrent radiation therapy; radiation toxicity has been reported with concurrent and nonconcurrent administration; may have radiosensitizing activity when gemcitabine and radiation therapy are given ≤7 days apart; optimum regimen for combination therapy has not been determined for all tumor types. Use caution in the elderly; clearance is affected by age. Efficacy in children has not been established

Adverse Reactions

>10%:

Cardiovascular: Peripheral edema (20%), edema (13%)

Central nervous system: Pain (10% to 48%), fever (30% to 41%), somnolence (5% to 11%)

Dermatologic: Rash (24% to 30%), alopecia (15% to 18%), pruritus (13%)

Gastrointestinal: Nausea/vomiting (64% to 71%; grades 3/4: 1% to 13%), constipation (10% to 31%), diarrhea (19% to 30%), stomatitis (10% to 14%)

Hematologic: Anemia (65% to 73%; grade 4: 1% to 3%), leukopenia (62% to 71%; grade 4: ≤1%), neutropenia (61% to 63%; grade 4: 6% to 7%), thrombocytopenia (24% to 47%; grade 4: ≤1%), hemorrhage (4% to 17%; grades 3/4: <1% to 2%); myelosuppression is the dose-limiting toxicity

Hepatic: Transaminases increased (67% to 78%; grades 3/4: 1% to 12%), alkaline phosphatase increased (55% to 77%; grades 3/4: 2% to 16%), bilirubin increased (13% to 26%; grades 3/4: <1% to 6%)

Renal: Proteinuria (10% to 45%; grades 3/4: <1%), hematuria (13% to 35%; grades 3/4: <1%), BUN increased (8% to 16%; grades 3/4: 0%)

Respiratory: Dyspnea (6% to 23%)

Miscellaneous: Flu-like syndrome (19%), infection (8% to 16%; grades 3/4: <1% to 2%)

1% to 10%:

Local: Injection site reactions (4%)

Neuromuscular & skeletal: Paresthesia (2% to 10%)

Renal: Creatinine increased (2% to 8%)

Respiratory: Bronchospasm (<2%)

<1%, postmarketing, and/or case reports (reported with single-agent use or with combination therapy, all reported rarely): Adult respiratory distress syndrome, anaphylactoid reaction, anorexia, arrhythmias, bullous skin eruptions, cellulitis, cerebrovascular accident, CHF, chills, cough, desquamation, diaphoresis, gangrene, GGT increased, headache, hemolytic uremic syndrome (HUS), hepatotoxic reaction (rare), hypertension, insomnia, interstitial pneumonitis, liver failure, malaise, MI, peripheral vasculitis, petechiae, pulmonary edema, pulmonary fibrosis, radiation recall, renal failure, respiratory failure, rhinitis, sepsis, supraventricular arrhythmia, weakness

Drug Interactions

Avoid Concomitant Use

Avoid concomitant use of Gemcitabine with any of the following: Natalizumab; Vaccines (Live)

Increased Effect/Toxicity

Gemcitabine may increase the levels/effects of: Bleomycin; Fluorouracil; Leflunomide; Natalizumab; Vaccines (Live); Vitamin K Antagonists

The levels/effects of Gemcitabine may be increased by: Trastuzumab

Decreased Effect

Gemcitabine may decrease the levels/effects of: Vaccines (Inactivated); Vaccines (Live); Vitamin K Antagonists

The levels/effects of Gemcitabine may be decreased by: Echinacea

Ethanol/Nutrition/Herb Interactions Ethanol: Avoid ethanol (due to GI irritation).

Storage/Stability Store intact vials at room temperature of 20°C to 25°C (68°F to 77°F). Reconstituted vials are stable for up to 35 days and infusion solutions diluted in 0.9% sodium chloride are stable up to 7 days at 23°C when protected from light; however, the manufacturer recommends use within 24 hours for both reconstituted vials and infusion solutions. Do not refrigerate.

Reconstitution Reconstitute the 200 mg vial with preservative free 0.9% NaCl 5 mL or the 1000 mg vial with preservative free 0.9% NaCl 25 mL. Resulting solution is 38 mg/mL. Dilute with 50-500 mL 0.9% sodium chloride injection or D_5W to concentrations as low as 0.1 mg/mL.

Compatibility Stable in D_5W, NS.

Y-site administration: Compatible: Amifostine, amikacin, aminophylline, ampicillin, ampicillin/sulbactam, aztreonam, bleomycin, bumetanide, buprenorphine, butorphanol, calcium gluconate, carboplatin, carmustine, cefazolin, cefotetan, cefoxitin, ceftazidime, ceftizoxime, ceftriaxone, cefuroxime, chlorpromazine, cimetidine, ciprofloxacin, cisplatin, clindamycin, co-trimoxazole, cyclophosphamide, cytarabine, dactinomycin, daunorubicin, dexamethasone sodium phosphate, dexrazoxane, diphenhydramine, dobutamine, docetaxel, dopamine, doxorubicin, doxycycline, droperidol, enalaprilat, etoposide, etoposide phosphate, famotidine, floxuridine, fluconazole, fludarabine, fluorouracil, gatifloxacin, gentamicin, granisetron, haloperidol, heparin, hydrocortisone sodium phosphate, hydrocortisone sodium succinate, hydromorphone, hydroxyzine, idarubicin, ifosfamide, leucovorin, linezolid, lorazepam, mannitol, meperidine, mesna, metoclopramide, metronidazole, minocycline, mitoxantrone, morphine, nalbuphine, netilmicin, ofloxacin, ondansetron, paclitaxel, plicamycin, potassium chloride, promethazine, ranitidine, sodium bicarbonate, streptozocin, teniposide, thiotepa, ticarcillin, ticarcillin/clavulanate, tobramycin, topotecan, vancomycin, vinblastine, vincristine, vinorelbine, zidovudine. **Incompatible:** Acyclovir, amphotericin B, cefoperazone, cefotaxime, furosemide, ganciclovir, imipenem/cilastatin, irinotecan, methotrexate, methylprednisolone sodium succinate, mitomycin, piperacillin, piperacillin/tazobactam, prochlorperazine edisylate.

Mechanism of Action A pyrimidine antimetabolite that inhibits DNA synthesis by inhibition of DNA polymerase and ribonucleotide reductase, specific for the S-phase of the cycle. Gemcitabine is phosphorylated intracellularly by deoxycytidine kinase to gemcitabine monophosphate, which is further phosphorylated to active metabolites gemcitabine diphosphate and gemcitabine triphosphate. Gemcitabine diphosphate inhibits DNA synthesis by inhibiting ribonucleotide reductase; gemcitabine triphosphate incorporates into DNA and inhibits DNA polymerase.

Pharmacodynamics/Kinetics

Distribution: Infusions <70 minutes: 50 L/m^2; Long infusion times: 370 L/m^2

Protein binding: Low

Metabolism: Metabolized intracellularly by nucleoside kinases to the active diphosphate (dFdCDP) and triphosphate (dFdCTP) nucleoside metabolites

Half-life elimination:

Gemcitabine: Infusion time ≤1 hour: 42-94 minutes; infusion time 3-4 hours: 4-10.5 hours

Metabolite (gemcitabine triphosphate), terminal phase: 1.7-19.4 hours

Time to peak, plasma: 30 minutes after completion of infusion

Excretion: Urine (92% to 98%; primarily as inactive uracil metabolite); feces (<1%)

Dosage Refer to individual protocols. **Note**: Prolongation of the infusion time >60 minutes and administration more frequently than once weekly have been shown to increase toxicity. I.V.:

Pancreatic cancer: Initial: 1000 mg/m^2 weekly for up to 7 weeks followed by 1 week rest; then weekly for 3 weeks out of every 4 weeks.

Dose adjustment: Patients who complete an entire cycle of therapy may have the dose in subsequent cycles increased by 25% as long as the absolute granulocyte count (AGC) nadir is >1500 x 10^6/L, platelet nadir is >100,000 x 10^6/L, and nonhematologic toxicity is less than WHO Grade 1. If the increased dose is tolerated (with the same parameters) the dose in subsequent cycles may again be increased by 20%.

Nonsmall cell lung cancer:

1000 mg/m^2 days 1, 8, and 15; repeat cycle every 28 days

or

1250 mg/m^2 days 1 and 8; repeat cycle every 21 days

Breast cancer: 1250 mg/m^2 days 1 and 8; repeat cycle every 21 days

Ovarian cancer: 1000 mg/m^2 days 1 and 8; repeat cycle every 21 days

Bladder cancer (unlabeled use):

I.V.: 1000 mg/m^2 once weekly for 3 weeks; repeat cycle every 4 weeks

Intravesicular instillation: 2000 mg (in 100 mL NS; retain for 1 hour) twice weekly for 3 weeks; repeat cycle every 4 weeks (for at least 2 cycles)

Dosing adjustment for toxicity:

Pancreatic cancer: Hematologic toxicity:

AGC ≥1000 x 10^6/L and platelet count ≥100,000 x 10^6/L: Administer 100% of full dose

AGC 500-999 x 10^6/L or platelet count 50,000-90,000 x 10^6/L: Administer 75% of full dose

AGC <500 x 10^6/L or platelet count <50,000 x 10^6/L: Hold dose

Nonsmall cell lung cancer:

Hematologic toxicity: Refer to guidelines for pancreatic cancer. Cisplatin dosage may also need adjusted.

Severe (grades 3 or 4) nonhematologic toxicity (except alopecia, nausea and vomiting): Hold or decrease dose by 50%.

Breast cancer:

Hematologic toxicity: Adjustments based on granulocyte and platelet counts on day 8:

AGC ≥1200 x 10^6/L and platelet count >75,000 x 10^6/L: Administer 100% of full dose

AGC 1000-1199 x 10^6/L or platelet count 50,000-75,000 x 10^6/L: Administer 75% of full dose

AGC 700-999 x 10^6/L and platelet count ≥50,000 x 10^6/L: Administer 50% of full dose

AGC <700 x 10^6/L or platelet count <50,000 x 10^6/L: Hold dose

Severe (grades 3 or 4) nonhematologic toxicity (except alopecia, nausea, and vomiting): Hold or decrease dose by 50%. Paclitaxel dose may also need adjusted.

Ovarian cancer:

Hematologic toxicity: Adjustments based on granulocyte and platelet counts on day 8:

AGC ≥1500 x 10^6/L and platelet count ≥100,000 x 10^6/L: Administer 100% of full dose

AGC 1000-1499 x 10^6/L and/or platelet count 75,000-99,999 x 10^6/L: Administer 50% of full dose

AGC <1000 x 10^6/L and/or platelet count <75,000 x 10^6/L: Hold dose

Severe (grades 3 or 4) nonhematologic toxicity (except nausea and vomiting): Hold or decrease dose by 50%. Carboplatin dose may also need adjusted.

Dose adjustment for subsequent cycles:

AGC < 500 x 10^6/L for >5 days, AGC <100 x 10^6/L for >3 days, febrile neutropenia, platelet count <25,000 x 10^6/L, cycle delay >1 week due to toxicity: Reduce gemcitabine to 800 mg/m^2 on days 1 and 8.

For recurrence of any of the above toxicities after initial dose reduction: Administer gemcitabine 800 mg/m^2 on day 1 only for the subsequent cycle

Dosing adjustment in renal impairment: The FDA-approved labeling does not contain dosing adjustment guidelines; use caution. Gemcitabine has not been studied in patients with significant renal dysfunction.

Dosing adjustment in hepatic impairment: The FDA-approved labeling does not contain dosing adjustment guidelines; use caution. Gemcitabine has not been studied in patients with significant hepatic dysfunction. The following guidelines have been used by some clinicians (Floyd, 2006): Serum bilirubin >1.6 mg/dL: Use starting dose of 800 mg/m^2

Combination Regimens

Biliary adenocarcinoma:

Gemcitabine-Capecitabine on page 1340
Gemcitabine-Cisplatin (Biliary Cancer) on page 1341
GEMOX (Biliary Cancer) on page 1347

Bladder cancer:

Gemcitabine-Carboplatin (Bladder Cancer) on page 1340
Gemcitabine-Cisplatin (Bladder Cancer) on page 1342
Gemcitabine-Docetaxel (Bladder Cancer) on page 1344

Administration Infuse over 30 minutes. **Note**: Prolongation of the infusion time >60 minutes has been shown to increase toxicity. Gemcitabine is being investigated in clinical trials for fixed dose rate (FDR) infusion administration at doses from 1000 mg/m^2 to 2200 mg/m^2 at a rate of 10 mg/m^2/minute. Prolonged infusion times increase the accumulation of the active metabolite, gemcitabine triphosphate. Patients who receive gemcitabine FDR experience more grade 3/4 hematologic toxicity.

Monitoring Parameters CBC with differential and platelet count (prior to each dose); hepatic and renal function (prior to initiation of therapy and periodically, thereafter); monitor electrolytes, including potassium, magnesium, and calcium (when in combination therapy with cisplatin)

Emetic Potential Low (10% to 30%)

Vesicant May be an irritant

Dosage Forms Excipient information presented when available (limited, particularly for generics); consult specific product labeling.

Injection, powder for reconstitution:
  Gemzar®: 200 mg, 1 g

References

Bredenfeld H, Franklin J, Nogova L, et al, "Severe Pulmonary Toxicity in Patients With Advanced-Stage Hodgkin's Disease Treated With a Modified Bleomycin, Doxorubicin, Cyclophosphamide, Vincristine, Procarbazine, Prednisone, and Gemcitabine (BEACOPP) Regimen is Probably Related to the Combination of Gemcitabine and Bleomycin: A Report of the German Hodgkin's Lymphoma Study Group," *J Clin Oncol*, 2004, 22(12):2424-9.

Correale P, Cerretani D, Marsili S, et al, "Gemcitabine Increases Systemic 5-Fluorouracil Exposure in Advanced Cancer Patients," *Eur J Cancer*, 2003, 39(11):1547-51.

Dalbagni G, Russo P, Bochner B, et al, "Phase II Trial of Intravesical Gemcitabine in Bacille Calmette-Guerin-Refractory Transitional Cell Carcinoma of the Bladder," *J Clin Oncol*, 2006, 24 (18):2729-34.

Floyd J, Mirza I, Sachs B, et al, "Hepatotoxicity of Chemotherapy," *Semin Oncol*, 2006, 33 (1):50-67.

Pfisterer J, Vergote I, Du Bois A, et al, "Combination Therapy with Gemcitabine and Carboplatin in Recurrent Ovarian Cancer," *Int J Gynecol Cancer*, 2005, 15 (Suppl 1):36-41.

Plunkett W, Huang P, Xu YZ, et al, "Gemcitabine: Metabolism, Mechanisms of Action, and Self-Potentiation," *Semin Oncol*, 1995, 22(4 Suppl 11):3-10.

Tempero M, Plunkett W, Ruiz Van Haperen V, "Randomized Phase II Comparison of Dose-Intense Gemcitabine: Thirty-Minute Infusion and Fixed Dose Rate Infusion in Patients With Pancreatic Adenocarcinoma," *J Clin Oncol*, 2003, 21(18):3402-8.

Xu Q, Zhang Y, and Trissel LA, "Physical and Chemical Stability of Gemcitabine Hydrochloride Solutions," *J Am Pharm Assoc*, 1999, 39(4):509-13.

♦ **Gemcitabine Hydrochloride** *see* Gemcitabine *on page 531*

Gemtuzumab Ozogamicin (gem TOO zoo mab oh zog a MY sin)

Medication Safety Issues
Sound-alike/look-alike issues:
Gemtuzumab may be confused with gemcitabine

High alert medication: The Institute for Safe Medication Practices (ISMP) includes this medication among its list of drug classes which have a heightened risk of causing significant patient harm when used in error.

Related Information
Management of Drug Extravasations *on page 1447*
Safe Handling of Hazardous Drugs *on page 1517*

U.S. Brand Names Mylotarg®

Index Terms CMA-676; NSC-720568

Generic Available No

Canadian Brand Names Mylotarg®

Pharmacologic Category Antineoplastic Agent, Monoclonal Antibody

Use Treatment of relapsed CD33 positive acute myeloid leukemia (AML) in patients ≥60 years of age who are not candidates for cytotoxic chemotherapy

Unlabeled/Investigational Use Salvage therapy for acute promyelocytic leukemia (APL), relapsed/ refractory CD33 positive acute myeloid leukemia in children and adults <60 years

Pregnancy Risk Factor D

Lactation Excretion in breast milk unknown/not recommended

Labeled Contraindications Hypersensitivity to gemtuzumab ozogamicin, calicheamicin derivatives, or any component of the formulation; patients with anti-CD33 antibody

Warnings/Precautions Hazardous agent - use appropriate precautions for handling and disposal.

[U.S. Boxed Warning]: Gemtuzumab has been associated with hepato-toxicity, including severe hepatic veno-occlusive disease (VOD). Symptoms of VOD include right upper quadrant pain, rapid weight gain, ascites, hepatomegaly, and bilirubin/transaminase elevations. Risk may be increased by combination chemotherapy, underlying hepatic disease, or hematopoietic stem cell transplant. Use with caution in patients with hepatic impairment; has not been studied in patients with serum bilirubin >2 mg/dL.

[U.S. Boxed Warning]: Severe hypersensitivity reactions (including anaphylaxis) and other infusion-related reactions may occur. Infusion-related events are common, generally reported to occur with the first dose after the end of the 2-hour intravenous infusion. These symptoms usually resolved after 2-4 hours with a supportive therapy of acetaminophen, diphenhydramine, and intravenous fluids. Other severe and potentially fatal infusion related pulmonary events (including dyspnea and hypoxia) have been reported infrequently. Symptomatic intrinsic lung disease or high peripheral blast counts ▶

may increase the risk of severe reactions. Fewer infusion-related events were observed after the second dose. Postinfusion reactions (may include fever, chills, hypotension, or dyspnea) may occur during the first 24 hours after administration. Consider discontinuation in patients who develop severe infusion-related reactions. In addition to infusion-related pulmonary events, gemtuzumab therapy is also associated with acute respiratory distress syndrome, pulmonary infiltrates, pleural effusion, noncardiogenic pulmonary edema, and pulmonary insufficiency.

[U.S. Boxed Warning]: Severe myelosuppression occurs in all patients at recommended dosages. Use caution in patients with renal impairment. Tumor lysis syndrome may occur as a consequence of leukemia treatment, adequate hydration and prophylactic allopurinol must be instituted prior to use. Other methods to lower WBC <30,000 cells/mm^3 may be considered (hydroxyurea or leukapheresis) to minimize the risk of tumor lysis syndrome, and/or severe infusion reactions. **[U.S. Boxed Warning]: Should be administered under the supervision of an experienced cancer chemotherapy physician. Should only be administered in facilities equipped to monitor and treat patients with leukemia. [U.S. Boxed Warning]: Safety and efficacy have not been established in combination with other chemotherapy agents,** in pediatric patients, or in patients with poor performance status. Gemtuzumab is not FDA-approved for use in children.

Adverse Reactions Adverse reactions reported for adults of all ages. **Note:** A postinfusion symptom complex (fever, chills, less commonly hypertension, and/or dyspnea) may occur within 24 hours of administration; the incidence of infusion-related events decreases with repeat administration.

>10%:
  Cardiovascular: Hypotension (20%), hypertension (16%), peripheral edema (14%)
  Central nervous system: Fever (82%), chills (66%), headache (37%), pain (18%), dizziness (12%), insomnia (12%)
  Dermatologic: Petechiae (19%), rash (18%)
  Endocrine & metabolic: Hypokalemia (26%)
  Gastrointestinal: Nausea (68%), vomiting (58%), abdominal pain (32%), diarrhea (32%), anorexia (25%), mucositis/stomatitis (25%), constipation (23%)
  Hematologic: Thrombocytopenia (grades 3/4: 49% to 99%; median recovery 36-51 days), neutropenia (grades 3/4: 98%; median recovery 40-51 days), leukopenia (grades 3/4: 46% to 96%), lymphopenia (grades 3/4: 94%), anemia/hemoglobin decreased (grades 3/4: 14% to 52%), neutropenic fever (17%), hemorrhage (11% to 13%)
  Hepatic: Hyperbilirubinemia (grades 3/4: 29%), veno-occlusive disease (1% to 20%; higher frequency in patients with prior history of or subsequent hematopoietic stem cell transplant), AST increased (grades 3/4: 18%), LDH increased (16%)
  Local: Local reaction (22%)
  Neuromuscular & skeletal: Weakness (36%), back pain (14%)
  Respiratory: Epistaxis (28%; grade 3/4: 3%), dyspnea (26%), cough (17%), pneumonia (13%; grades 3/4: 8%), pharyngitis (12%)
  Miscellaneous: Infection (grades 3/4: 30%), sepsis (26%; grades 3/4: 17%), cutaneous herpes simplex (21%)
1% to 10%:
  Cardiovascular: Tachycardia (10%), cerebral hemorrhage (2%)

Central nervous system: Depression (9%), anxiety (8%), intracranial hemorrhage (1%)

Dermatologic: Bruising (10%), pruritus (6%)

Endocrine & metabolic: Hyperglycemia (10%), hypocalcemia (10%), hypophosphatemia (8%) hypomagnesemia (6%)

Gastrointestinal: Dyspepsia (10%), gingival hemorrhage (9%), melena (1%)

Genitourinary: Vaginal hemorrhage (4%), vaginal bleeding (3%), hematuria (grade 3/4: 1%)

Hematologic: Disseminated intravascular coagulation (DIC) (1%)

Hepatic: ALT increased (grades 3/4: 9%), prothrombin time increased (grades 3/4: 9%), alkaline phosphatase increased (8%; grades 3/4: 4%), ascites (3%), PTT increased (grades 3/4: 2%)

Neuromuscular & skeletal: Arthralgia (10%), myalgia (6%)

Renal: Creatinine increased (2%)

Respiratory: Rhinitis (8%), hypoxia (5%)

<1%, postmarketing, and/or case reports: Acute respiratory distress syndrome, anaphylaxis, bradycardia, Budd-Chiari syndrome, gastrointestinal hemorrhage, hepatic failure, hepatosplenomegaly, hypersensitivity reactions, jaundice, neutropenic sepsis, noncardiogenic pulmonary edema, portal vain thrombosis, pulmonary hemorrhage, renal impairment, renal failure (including renal failure secondary to tumor lysis syndrome)

Drug Interactions

Avoid Concomitant Use
Avoid concomitant use of Gemtuzumab Ozogamicin with any of the following: Natalizumab; Vaccines (Live)

Increased Effect/Toxicity
Gemtuzumab Ozogamicin may increase the levels/effects of: Leflunomide; Natalizumab; Vaccines (Live)

The levels/effects of Gemtuzumab Ozogamicin may be increased by: Abciximab; Trastuzumab

Decreased Effect
Gemtuzumab Ozogamicin may decrease the levels/effects of: Vaccines (Inactivated); Vaccines (Live)

The levels/effects of Gemtuzumab Ozogamicin may be decreased by: Echinacea

Ethanol/Nutrition/Herb Interactions Ethanol: Avoid ethanol (due to GI irritation).

Storage/Stability Light sensitive; protect from light (including direct and indirect sunlight, and unshielded fluorescent light). The infusion container should be placed in a UV protectant bag immediately after preparation. Store intact vials under refrigeration at 2°C to 8°C (36°F to 46°F). Reconstituted solutions may be stored for up to 2 hours at room temperature or under refrigeration. Following dilution for infusion, solutions are stable for up to 16 hours at room temperature. Administration requires 2 hours; therefore, the maximum elapsed time from initial reconstitution to completion of infusion should be 20 hours.

Reconstitution Protect from light during preparation (and administration). Prepare in biologic safety hood with shielded fluorescent light; (some institutions prepare in a darkened room with the lights in the biologic safety cabinet turned off). Allow to warm to room temperature prior to reconstitution. Reconstitute vial with sterile water for injection to a concentration of 1 mg/mL. Dilute in 100 mL of 0.9% sodium chloride injection. Hazardous agent - use appropriate precautions for handling and disposal.

◄ **Compatibility** Stable in NS. **Incompatible** in D_5W and electrolyte-containing solutions. Infuse via a separate line.

Mechanism of Action Antibody to CD33 antigen, which is expressed on leukemic blasts in 80% of AML patients. Binds to the CD33 antigen, resulting in internalization of the antibody-antigen complex. Following internalization, the calicheamicin derivative is released inside the myeloid cell. The calicheamicin derivative binds to DNA resulting in double strand breaks and cell death. Pluripotent stem cells and nonhematopoietic cells are not affected.

Pharmacodynamics/Kinetics

Distribution: V_{ss}: Adults: Initial dose: 21 L; Repeat dose: 10 L

Half-life elimination: Total calicheamicin: Initial: 41-45 hours, Repeat dose: 60-64 hours; Unconjugated: 100-143 hours (no change noted in repeat dosing)

Time to peak, plasma: Immediate; higher concentrations observed after repeat dose

Dosage I.V.:

Children: **Note:** Patients should receive diphenhydramine (1 mg/kg) 1 hour prior to infusion and acetaminophen 15 mg/kg 1 hour prior to infusion and every 4 hours for 2 additional doses.

AML (unlabeled use): 4-9 mg/m^2 infused over 2 hours every 2 weeks for a total of 1-3 doses per treatment course. Patients received the second and third doses and/or dose escalation if no dose-limiting toxicities were observed. (**Note:** Higher incidences of liver toxicities were observed in children at the 9 mg/m^2 dose level.)

or

Children <3 years: 0.2 mg/kg infused over 2 hours every 2 weeks for a total of 2 doses

Children ≥3 years: 6 mg/m^2 infused over 2 hours every 2 weeks for a total of 2 doses

Adults: **Note:** Patients should receive diphenhydramine 50 mg orally and acetaminophen 650-1000 mg orally 1 hour prior to administration of each dose. Acetaminophen dosage should be repeated as needed every 4 hours for 2 additional doses. Pretreatment with methylprednisolone may ameliorate infusion-related symptoms.

AML:

≥60 years: 9 mg/m^2 infused over 2 hours. A full treatment course is a total of 2 doses administered with 14 days between doses. Full hematologic recovery is not necessary for administration of the second dose. There has been only limited experience with repeat courses of gemtuzumab ozogamicin.

<60 years (unlabeled use): 9 mg/m^2 infused over 2 hours. A full treatment course is a total of 2 doses administered with 14 days between doses.

APL (unlabeled use): 6 mg/m^2 infused over 2 hours. A full treatment course is a total of 2 doses administered with 15 days between doses.

Dosage adjustment with recent hematopoietic stem cell transplant (HSCT): Gemtuzumab use within 3-4 months of HSCT is associated with an increased risk of hepatic veno-occlusive disease, the National Comprehensive Cancer Network (NCCN) guidelines (AML, v.1.2009) recommend a 30% to 50% dosage reduction in this situation.

Dosage adjustment for toxicity:

Dyspnea or significant hypotension: Interrupt infusion; monitor

Anaphylaxis, pulmonary edema, acute respiratory distress syndrome: Strongly consider discontinuing treatment

Dosage adjustment in renal impairment: No recommendation (not studied)

Dosage adjustment in hepatic impairment: Use extra caution; has not been studied in patients with bilirubin >2 mg/dL

Combination Regimens

Leukemia, acute promyelocytic: Tretinoin-Arsenic Trioxide-Gemtuzumab (APL) on page 1411

Administration Do not administer as I.V. push or bolus. Administer via I.V. infusion, over at least 2 hours through a low protein-binding (0.2-1.2 micron) in-line filter. Protect from light during infusion. Premedicate with acetaminophen and diphenhydramine prior to each infusion.

Monitoring Parameters Monitor vital signs during the infusion and for 4 hours following the infusion. Monitor for signs/symptoms of postinfusion reaction. Monitor electrolytes, liver function, CBC with differential and platelets frequently. Monitor for signs and symptoms of hepatic veno-occlusssive disease (weight gain, right upper quadrant abdominal pain, hepatomegaly, ascites).

Test Interactions None known

Additional Information Oncology Comment: In addition to the FDA-approved indication, the National Comprehensive Cancer Network® (NCCN) Acute Myeloid Leukemia Guidelines (AML, v.1.2009) recommend gemtuzumab ozogamicin as salvage and/or post remission therapy for the treatment of acute promyelocytic leukemia (APL). Gemtuzumab has activity (single agent) in patients with persistent disease following postremission arsenic trioxide therapy in APL patients who are not candidates for allogeneic transplantation.

Emetic Potential Very low (<10%)

Dosage Forms Excipient information presented when available (limited, particularly for generics); consult specific product labeling.

Injection, powder for reconstitution [preservative free]:

Mylotarg®: 5 mg

References

Arceci RJ, Sande J, Lange B, et al, "Safety and Efficacy of Gemtuzumab Ozogamicin in Pediatric Patients With Advanced CD33+ Acute Myeloid Leukemia," *Blood*, 2005, 106(4):1183-8.

Brethon B, Auvrignon A, Galambrun C, et al, "Efficacy and Tolerability of Gemtuzumab Ozogamicin (Anti-CD33 Monoclonal Antibody, CMA-676, Mylotarg) in Children With Relapsed/Refractory Myeloid Leukemia," *BMC Cancer*, 2006, 6:172.

Buckwalter M, Dowell JA, Korth-Bradley J, et al, "Pharmacokinetics of Gemtuzumab Ozogamicin as a Single-Agent Treatment of Pediatric Patients With Refractory or Relapsed Acute Myeloid Leukemia," *J Clin Pharmacol*, 2004, 44(8):873-80.

Dowell JA, Korth-Bradley J, Liu H, et al, "Pharmacokinetics of Gemtuzumab Ozogamicin, an Antibody-Targeted Chemotherapy Agent for the Treatment of Patients With Acute Myeloid Leukemia in First Relapse," *J Clin Pharmacol*, 2001, (11):1206-14.

Larson RA, Boogaerts M, Estey E, et al, "Antibody-Targeted Chemotherapy of Older Patients With Acute Myeloid Leukemia in First Relapse Using Mylotarg (Gemtuzumab Ozogamicin)," *Leukemia*, 2002, 16(9):1627-36.

Larson RA, Sievers EL, Stadtmauer EA, et al, "Final Report of the Efficacy and Safety of Gemtuzumab Ozogamicin (Mylotarg) in Patients With CD33-Positive Acute Myeloid Leukemia in First Recurrence," *Cancer*, 2005, 104(7):1442-52.

Lo-Coco F, Cimino G, Breccia M, et al, "Gemtuzumab Ozogamicin (Mylotarg) as a Single Agent for Molecularly Relapsed Acute Promyelocytic Leukemia," *Blood*, 2004, 104(7):1995-9.

National Comprehensive Cancer Network® (NCCN), "Clinical Practice Guidelines in Oncology™: Acute Myeloid Leukemia," Version 1.2009. Available at http://www.nccn.org/professionals/physician_gls/PDF/aml.pdf.

Roman E, Cooney E, Harrison L, et al, "Preliminary Results of the Safety of Immunotherapy With Gemtuzumab Ozogamicin Following Reduced Intensity Allogeneic Stem Cell Transplant in Children With CD33+ Acute Myeloid Leukemia," *Clin Cancer Res*, 2005, 11(19 Pt 2):7164-70.

Sievers EL, Larson RA, Stadtmauer EA, et al, "Efficacy and Safety of Gemtuzumab Ozogamicin in Patients With CD33-Positive Acute Myeloid Leukemia in First Relapse," *J Clin Oncol*, 2001, 19 (13):3244-54.

Zwaan CM, Reinhardt D, Corbacioglu S, et al, "Gemtuzumab Ozogamicin: First Clinical Experiences in Children With Relapsed/Refractory Acute Myeloid Leukemia Treated on Compassionate-Use Basis," *Blood*, 2003, 101(10):3868-71.

- ◆ **Gemzar®** *see* Gemcitabine *on page* 531
- ◆ **Gen-Acyclovir (Can)** *see* Acyclovir *on page* 18
- ◆ **Gen-Bicalutamide (Can)** *see* Bicalutamide *on page* 147
- ◆ **Gen-Cyproterone (Can)** *see* Cyproterone *on page* 279
- ◆ **Gen-Fluconazole (Can)** *see* Fluconazole *on page* 485
- ◆ **Gengraf®** *see* CycloSPORINE *on page* 268
- ◆ **Gen-Hydroxyurea (Can)** *see* Hydroxyurea *on page* 589
- ◆ **Gen-Medroxy (Can)** *see* MedroxyPROGESTERone *on page* 739
- ◆ **Gen-Ondansetron (Can)** *see* Ondansetron *on page* 874
- ◆ **Gentak®** *see* Gentamicin *on page* 542

Gentamicin (jen ta MYE sin)

Medication Safety Issues

Sound-alike/look-alike issues:
Garamycin® may be confused with kanamycin, Terramycin®
Gentamicin may be confused with gentian violet, kanamycin, vancomycin

High alert medication: The Institute for Safe Medication Practices (ISMP) includes this medication (intrathecal administration) among its list of drug classes which have a heightened risk of causing significant patient harm when used in error.

U.S. Brand Names Gentak®; Gentasol™

Index Terms Gentamicin Sulfate

Generic Available Yes

Canadian Brand Names Alcomicin®; Diogent®; Garamycin®; Gentamicin Injection, USP; SAB-Gentamicin

Pharmacologic Category Antibiotic, Aminoglycoside; Antibiotic, Ophthalmic; Antibiotic, Topical

Use Treatment of susceptible bacterial infections, normally gram-negative organisms, including *Pseudomonas*, *Proteus*, *Serratia*, and gram-positive *Staphylococcus*; treatment of bone infections, respiratory tract infections, skin and soft tissue infections, as well as abdominal and urinary tract infections, and septicemia; treatment of infective endocarditis; used topically to treat superficial infections of the skin or ophthalmic infections caused by susceptible bacteria

Pregnancy Risk Factor C (ophthalmic, topical); D (injection)

Lactation Enters breast milk (small amounts)/use caution (AAP rates "compatible")

Labeled Contraindications Hypersensitivity to gentamicin or other aminoglycosides

Warnings/Precautions [U.S. Boxed Warning]: Aminoglycosides may cause neurotoxicity and/or nephrotoxicity; usual risk factors include pre-existing renal impairment, concomitant neuro-/nephrotoxic medications, advanced age and dehydration. Ototoxicity may be directly proportional to the amount of drug given and the duration of treatment; tinnitus or vertigo are indications of vestibular injury and impending hearing loss; renal damage is usually reversible. May cause neuromuscular blockade and respiratory paralysis; especially when given soon after anesthesia or muscle relaxants.

Not intended for long-term therapy due to toxic hazards associated with extended administration; use caution in pre-existing renal insufficiency, vestibular or cochlear impairment, myasthenia gravis, hypocalcemia, conditions which depress neuromuscular transmission. Dosage modification required in patients with impaired renal function. Prolonged use may result in fungal or bacterial superinfection, including *C. difficile*-associated diarrhea (CDAD) and pseudomembranous colitis; CDAD has been observed >2 months postantibiotic treatment.

Adverse Reactions

>10%:

Central nervous system: Neurotoxicity (vertigo, ataxia)

Neuromuscular & skeletal: Gait instability

Otic: Ototoxicity (auditory), ototoxicity (vestibular)

Renal: Nephrotoxicity, decreased creatinine clearance

1% to 10%:

Cardiovascular: Edema

Dermatologic: Skin itching, reddening of skin, rash

<1%: Agranulocytosis allergic reaction, anorexia, burning, drowsiness, dyspnea, enterocolitis erythema, granulocytopenia headache, LFTs increased, muscle cramps, nausea, photosensitivity, pseudomotor cerebri, salivation increased, stinging, thrombocytopenia, tremor, vomiting, weakness, weight loss

Drug Interactions

Avoid Concomitant Use

Avoid concomitant use of Gentamicin with any of the following: Gallium Nitrate

Increased Effect/Toxicity

Gentamicin may increase the levels/effects of: AbobotulinumtoxinA; Bisphosphonate Derivatives; CARBOplatin; Colistimethate; CycloSPORINE; Gallium Nitrate; Neuromuscular-Blocking Agents; OnabotulinumtoxinA; RimabotulinumtoxinB

The levels/effects of Gentamicin may be increased by: Amphotericin B; Capreomycin; CISplatin; Loop Diuretics; Nonsteroidal Anti-Inflammatory Agents; Vancomycin

Decreased Effect

Gentamicin may decrease the levels/effects of: Typhoid Vaccine

The levels/effects of Gentamicin may be decreased by: Penicillins

Storage/Stability Gentamicin is a colorless to slightly yellow solution which should be stored between 2°C to 30°C, but refrigeration is not recommended. I.V. infusion solutions mixed in NS or D_5W solution are stable for 24 hours at room temperature and refrigeration. Premixed bag: Manufacturer expiration date; remove from overwrap stability: 30 days.

Compatibility Stable in dextran 40, D_5W, $D_{10}W$, mannitol 20%, LR, NS; **incompatible** with fat emulsion 10%; **variable stability (consult detailed reference)** in peritoneal dialysis solution.

Y-site administration: Compatible: Acyclovir, alatrofloxacin, amifostine, amiodarone, amsacrine, atracurium, aztreonam, cefpirome, ciprofloxacin, cisatracurium, clarithromycin, cyclophosphamide, cytarabine, diltiazem, docetaxel, doxorubicin liposome, enalaprilat, esmolol, etoposide phosphate, famotidine, fluconazole, fludarabine, foscarnet, gatifloxacin, gemcitabine, granisetron, hydromorphone, IL-2, insulin (regular), labetalol, levofloxacin, linezolid, lorazepam, magnesium sulfate, melphalan, meperidine, meropenem, midazolam, morphine, multivitamins, ondansetron, paclitaxel, pancuronium, perphenazine, remifentanil, sargramostim, tacrolimus, teniposide, theophylline, thiotepa, tolazoline, vecuronium, vinorelbine, vitamin B complex with C, zidovudine. **Incompatible:** Allopurinol, amphotericin B cholesteryl sulfate complex, cefamandole, furosemide, heparin, hetastarch, idarubicin, indomethacin, iodipamide meglumine, phenytoin, propofol, warfarin. **Variable (consult detailed reference):** Filgrastim.

Compatibility in syringe: Compatible: Clindamycin, diatrizoate meglumine 52% and diatrizoate sodium 8%, diatrizoate sodium 60%, iohexol, iopamidol, iothalamate meglumine 60%, penicillin G sodium. **Incompatible:** Ampicillin, cefamandole, heparin. **Variable (consult detailed reference):** Ioxaglate meglumine 39.3% and ioxaglate sodium 19.6%.

Compatibility when admixed: Compatible: Atracurium, aztreonam, bleomycin, cefoxitin, cimetidine, chloroprocaine, ciprofloxacin, fluconazole, hexylcaine, lidocaine, lidocaine with epinephrine, mepivacaine, meropenem, metronidazole, metronidazole with sodium bicarbonate, ofloxacin, penicillin G sodium, piperocaine, procaine, ranitidine, verapamil. **Incompatible:** Amphotericin B, ampicillin, cefamandole, cefazolin with clindamycin, cefepime, heparin, nafcillin, ticarcillin. **Variable (consult detailed reference):** Cefotaxime, cefotetan, cefuroxime, clindamycin, cytarabine, dopamine, floxacillin, furosemide.

Mechanism of Action Interferes with bacterial protein synthesis by binding to 30S and 50S ribosomal subunits resulting in a defective bacterial cell membrane

Pharmacodynamics/Kinetics

Absorption:

Intramuscular: Rapid and complete

Oral: None

Distribution: Primarily into extracellular fluid (highly hydrophilic); high concentration in the renal cortex; minimal penetration to ocular tissues via I.V. route

V_d: Increased by edema, ascites, fluid overload; decreased with dehydration

Neonates: 0.4-0.6 L/kg

Children: 0.3-0.35 L/kg

Adults: 0.2-0.3 L/kg

Relative diffusion from blood into CSF: Minimal even with inflammation

CSF:blood level ratio: Normal meninges: Nil; Inflamed meninges: 10% to 30%

Protein binding: <30%

Half-life elimination:

Infants: <1 week: 3-11.5 hours; 1 week to 6 months: 3-3.5 hours

Adults: 1.5-3 hours; End-stage renal disease: 36-70 hours

Time to peak, serum: I.M.: 30-90 minutes; I.V.: 30 minutes after 30-minute infusion

Excretion: Urine (as unchanged drug)

Clearance: Directly related to renal function

Dosage Note: Dosage Individualization is **critical** because of the low therapeutic index.

Use of ideal body weight (IBW) for determining the mg/kg/dose appears to be more accurate than dosing on the basis of total body weight (TBW). In morbid obesity, dosage requirement may best be estimated using a dosing weight of IBW + 0.4 (TBW - IBW).

Initial and periodic plasma drug levels (eg, peak and trough with conventional dosing) should be determined, particularly in critically-ill patients with serious infections or in disease states known to significantly alter aminoglycoside pharmacokinetics (eg, cystic fibrosis, burns, or major surgery).

Usual dosage ranges:

Infants and Children <5 years: I.M., I.V.: 2.5 mg/kg/dose every 8 hours*

Children ≥5 years: I.M., I.V.: 2-2.5 mg/kg/dose every 8 hours*

*Note: Higher individual doses and/or more frequent intervals (eg, every 6 hours) may be required in selected clinical situations (cystic fibrosis) or serum levels document the need

Children and Adults:

Ophthalmic:

Ointment: Instill 1/2" (1.25 cm) 2-3 times/day to every 3-4 hours

Solution: Instill 1-2 drops every 2-4 hours, up to 2 drops every hour for severe infections

Topical: Apply 3-4 times/day to affected area

Adults:

I.M., I.V.:

Conventional: 1-2.5 mg/kg/dose every 8-12 hours; to ensure adequate peak concentrations early in therapy, higher initial dosage may be considered in selected patients when extracellular water is increased (edema, septic shock, postsurgical, or trauma)

Once daily: 4-7 mg/kg/dose once daily; some clinicians recommend this approach for all patients with normal renal function; this dose is at least as efficacious with similar, if not less, toxicity than conventional dosing

Intrathecal: 4-8 mg/day

Indication-specific dosing:

Neonates: I.V.:

Meningitis:

0-7 days of age: <2000 g: 2.5 mg/kg every 18-24 hours; >2000 g: 2.5 mg/kg every 12 hours

8-28 days of age: <2000 g: 2.5 mg/kg every 8-12 hours; >2000 g: 2.5 mg/kg every 8 hours

Children and Adults: I.M., I.V.:

Brucellosis: 240 mg (I.M.) daily or 5 mg/kg (I.V.) daily for 7 days; either regimen recommended in combination with doxycycline

Cholangitis: 4-6 mg/kg once daily with ampicillin

Diverticulitis (complicated): 1.5-2 mg/kg every 8 hours (with ampicillin and metronidazole)

Endocarditis: Treatment: 3 mg/kg/day in 1-3 divided doses

Meningitis:

Enterococcus sp or *Pseudomonas aeruginosa*: Loading dose 2 mg/kg, then 1.7 mg/kg/dose every 8 hours (administered with another bacteriocidal drug)

Listeria: 5-7 mg/kg/day (with penicillin) for 1 week

Pelvic inflammatory disease: Loading dose: 2 mg/kg, then 1.5 mg/kg every 8 hours

Alternate therapy: 4.5 mg/kg once daily

Plague *(Yersinia pestis):* Treatment: 5 mg/kg/day, followed by postexposure prophylaxis with doxycycline

Pneumonia, hospital- or ventilator-associated: 7 mg/kg/day (with antipseudomonal beta-lactam or carbapenem)

Synergy (for gram-positive infections): 3 mg/kg/day in 1-3 divided doses (with ampicillin)

Tularemia: 5 mg/kg/day divided every 8 hours for 1-2 weeks

Urinary tract infection: 1.5 mg/kg/dose every 8 hours

Dosing interval in renal impairment:

Conventional dosing:

Cl_{cr} ≥60 mL/minute: Administer every 8 hours

Cl_{cr} 40-60 mL/minute: Administer every 12 hours

Cl_{cr} 20-40 mL/minute: Administer every 24 hours

Cl_{cr} <20 mL/minute: Loading dose, then monitor levels

◀ High-dose therapy: Interval may be extended (eg, every 48 hours) in patients with moderate renal impairment (Cl_{cr} 30-59 mL/minute) and/or adjusted based on serum level determinations.

Hemodialysis: Dialyzable; removal by hemodialysis: 30% removal of aminoglycosides occurs during 4 hours of HD; administer dose after dialysis and follow levels

Removal by continuous ambulatory peritoneal dialysis (CAPD):

Administration via CAPD fluid:

Gram-negative infection: 4-8 mg/L (4-8 mcg/mL) of CAPD fluid

Gram-positive infection (eg, synergy): 3-4 mg/L (3-4 mcg/mL) of CAPD fluid

Administration via I.V., I.M. route during CAPD: Dose as for Cl_{cr} <10 mL/minute and follow levels

Removal via continuous arteriovenous or venovenous hemofiltration: Dose as for Cl_{cr} 10-40 mL/minute and follow levels

Dosing adjustment/comments in hepatic disease: Monitor plasma concentrations

Administration

I.M.: Administer by deep I.M. route if possible. Slower absorption and lower peak concentrations, probably due to poor circulation in the atrophic muscle, may occur following I.M. injection; in paralyzed patients, suggest I.V. route.

Ophthalmic: Administer any other ophthalmics 10 minutes before or after gentamicin preparations.

Some penicillins (eg, carbenicillin, ticarcillin, and piperacillin) have been shown to inactivate aminoglycosides *in vitro*. This has been observed to a greater extent with tobramycin and gentamicin, while amikacin has shown greater stability against inactivation. Concurrent use of these agents may pose a risk of reduced antibacterial efficacy *in vivo*, particularly in the setting of profound renal impairment. However, definitive clinical evidence is lacking. If combination penicillin/aminoglycoside therapy is desired in a patient with renal dysfunction, separation of doses (if feasible), and routine monitoring of aminoglycoside levels, CBC, and clinical response should be considered.

Monitoring Parameters Urinalysis, urine output, BUN, serum creatinine; hearing should be tested before, during, and after treatment; particularly in those at risk for ototoxicity or who will be receiving prolonged therapy (>2 weeks)

Some penicillin derivatives may accelerate the degradation of aminoglycosides *in vitro*. This may be clinically-significant for certain penicillin (ticarcillin, piperacillin, carbenicillin) and aminoglycoside (gentamicin, tobramycin) combination therapy in patients with significant renal impairment. Close monitoring of aminoglycoside levels is warranted.

Test Interactions

Some penicillin derivatives may accelerate the degradation of aminoglycosides *in vitro*, leading to a potential underestimation of aminoglycoside serum concentration.

Dietary Considerations Calcium, magnesium, potassium: Renal wasting may cause hypocalcemia, hypomagnesemia, and/or hypokalemia.

Dosage Forms Excipient information presented when available (limited, particularly for generics); consult specific product labeling. [DSC] = Discontinued product

Cream, topical: 0.1% (15 g, 30 g)

Infusion [premixed in NS]: 40 mg (50 mL); 60 mg (50 mL, 100 mL); 70 mg (50 mL); 80 mg (50 mL, 100 mL); 90 mg (100 mL); 100 mg (50 mL, 100 mL); 120 mg (100 mL)

Injection, solution: 10 mg/mL (6 mL, 8 mL, 10 mL)
Injection, solution: 40 mg/mL (2 mL, 20 mL)
Injection, solution [pediatric]: 10 mg/mL (2 mL)
Injection, solution [pediatric] [preservative free]: 10 mg/mL (2 mL)
Ointment, ophthalmic:
Gentak®: 0.3% [3 mg/g] (3.5 g)
Ointment, topical: 0.1% (15 g, 30 g)
Solution, ophthalmic: 0.3% (5 mL, 15 mL) [contains benzalkonium chloride]
Gentak®: 0.3% (5 mL; 15 mL [DSC]) [contains benzalkonium chloride]
Gentasol™: 0.3% (5 mL) [contains benzalkonium chloride]

References

Ahkee S, Smith R, and Ritter GW, "Once-Daily Aminoglycoside Dosing in Lower Respiratory Tract Infections," *Pharm Therapeut*, 1995, 20:226-34.

American Thoracic Society and Infectious Diseases Society of America, "Guidelines for the Management of Adults With Hospital-Acquired, Ventilator-Associated, and Healthcare-Associated Pneumonia," *Am J Respir Crit Care Med*, 2005, 171(4):388-416.

Edson RS and Terrell CL, "The Aminoglycosides," *Mayo Clin Proc*, 1999, 74(5):519-28.

Mann HJ, Fuhs DW, Awang R, et al, "Altered Aminoglycoside Pharmacokinetics in Critically Ill Patients With Sepsis," *Clin Pharm*, 1987, 6(2):148-53.

Matzke GR, Jameson JJ, and Halstenson CE, "Gentamicin Disposition in Young and Elderly Patients With Various Degrees of Renal Function," *J Clin Pharmacol*, 1987, 27(3):216-20.

McCormack JP and Jewesson PJ, "A Critical Re-Evaluation of the "Therapeutic Range" of Aminoglycosides," *Clin Infect Dis*, 1992, 14(1):320-39.

Nicolau DP, Freeman CD, Belliveau PP, et al, "Experience With a Once-Daily Aminoglycoside Program Administered to 2184 Adult Patients," *Antimicrob Agents Chemother*, 1995, 39(3):650-5.

Glucarpidase (gloo KAR pid ase)

Index Terms Carboxypeptidase-G2; CPDG2; CPG2; Voraxaze

Pharmacologic Category Antidote; Enzyme

Unlabeled/Investigational Use Rescue agent to reduce methotrexate toxicity in patients with delayed methotrexate elimination (in high-dose methotrexate [≥1 g/m^2] treatment), methotrexate-induced nephrotoxicity, or accidental intrathecal methotrexate overdose

Restrictions Investigational agent - not approved for use in the U.S.

Glucarpidase is available for intrathecal (IT) use through an Emergency Use IND. Information is available from BTG/Protherics Inc at 1-888-327-1027. For FDA Emergency Use IND information and procedures, refer to http://www.fda.gov/cder/cancer/singleIND.htm.

Glucarpidase is available for I.V. use under an Open-Label Treatment protocol. Information and participation requirements are available from AAI Pharma at 1-866-918-1731.

Warnings/Precautions Glucarpidase use for methotrexate toxicity due to delayed elimination should be accompanied with adequate hydration, urinary alkalinization, and concurrent leucovorin; hemodialysis may be required. Leucovorin is a substrate for glucarpidase and may compete with methotrexate for binding sites; protocols may require withholding concomitant leucovorin for 2-4 hours before and 1-2 hours after glucarpidase.

Glucarpidase use for intrathecal methotrexate overdose should be used in conjunction with immediate lumbar drainage; concurrent dexamethasone (4 mg I.V. every 6 hours for 4 doses) may minimize methotrexate-induced chemical arachnoiditis; leucovorin (100 mg I.V. every 6 hours for 4 doses) may prevent systemic methotrexate toxicity.

Adverse Reactions Frequency not defined.

Cardiovascular: Flushing

Central nervous system: Fever, head pressure

Dermatologic: Burning sensation (face and extremities), pruritus

Neuromuscular & skeletal: Tingling of fingers

Miscellaneous: Shaking, warmth

Reconstitution Reconstitute immediately prior to use.

Intrathecal: Reconstitute 2000 units with 12 mL preservative-free normal saline (Widemann, 2004)

I.V.: Reconstitute each 1000 units with 1 mL normal saline; prior to administration, further dilute with normal saline (Buchen, 2005)

Mechanism of Action Recombinant enzyme which rapidly hydrolyzes extracellular methotrexate into inactive metabolites, resulting in a rapid reduction of methotrexate concentrations

Pharmacodynamics/Kinetics

Distribution: V_{dss}: ~60-70 mL/kg

Half-life elimination: I.V.: Normal renal function: 9 hours; impaired renal function (Cl_{cr} <30 mL/minute): 10 hours

Dosage Children and Adults:

Intrathecal: intrathecal methotrexate overdose (unlabeled use): 2000 units as soon as possible after accidental overdose (Widemann, 2004)

I.V.: Methotrexate toxicity (unlabeled use): 50 units/kg (Buchen, 2005; Schwartz, 2007; Widemann, 1997); may require a second dose 24 hours later (Schwartz, 2007; Widemann, 1997)

Administration

I.V.: Infuse over 5 minutes

Intrathecal (for intrathecal methotrexate overdose): Glucarpidase was administered within 3-9 hours of accidental intrathecal methotrexate overdose in conjunction with lumbar drainage or ventriculolumbar perfusion (Widemann, 2004).

Monitoring Parameters Serum methotrexate levels, CBC with differential, bilirubin, ALT, AST, serum creatinine; evaluate for signs/symptoms of methotrexate toxicity

Test Interactions Methotrexate levels: Follow specific procedures for sample handling and processing; lack of glucarpidase inactivation may allow for continued methotrexate degradation within the sample; due to potential cross reactivity between methotrexate antibodies and DAMPA (inactive methotrexate metabolite) the FPIA assay may overestimate serum methotrexate concentrations and the HPLC assay is recommended for monitoring serum methotrexate concentrations (Buchen, 2005; Widemann, 1997).

References

Buchen S, Ngampolo D, Melton RG, et al, "Carboxypeptidase G2 Rescue in Patients With Methotrexate Intoxication and Renal Failure," Br J Cancer, 2005, 92(3):480-7.

Krause AS, Weihrauch MR, Bode U, et al, "Carboxypeptidase-G2 Rescue in Cancer Patients With Delayed Methotrexate Elimination After High-Dose Methotrexate Therapy," Leuk Lymphoma, 2002, 43(11):2139-43.

Phillips M, Smith W, Balan G, et al, "Pharmacokinetics of Glucarpidase in Subjects With Normal and Impaired Renal Function," J Clin Pharmacol, 2008, 48(3):279-84.

Schwartz S, Borner K, Muller K, et al, "Glucarpidase (Carboxypeptidase G2) Intervention in Adult and Elderly Cancer Patients With Renal Dysfunction and Delayed Methotrexate Elimination After High-Dose Methotrexate Therapy," Oncologist, 2007 12(11):1299-308.

Smith SW and Nelson LS, "Case Files of the New York City Poison Control Center: Antidotal Strategies for the Management of Methotrexate Toxicity," *J Med Toxicol*, 2008, 4(2):132-40.

Widemann BC, Balis FM, Murphy RF, et al, "Carboxypeptidase-G2, Thymidine, and Leucovorin Rescue in Cancer Patients With Methotrexate-Induced Renal Dysfunction," *J Clin Oncol*, 1997, 15(5):2125-34.

Widemann BC, Balis FM, Shalabi A, et al, "Treatment of Accidental Intrathecal Methotrexate Overdose With Intrathecal Carboxypeptidase G2," *J Natl Cancer Inst*, 2004, 96(20):1557-9.

◆ **GM-CSF** *see* Sargramostim *on page 1029*

◆ **GMD-Fluconazole (Can)** *see* Fluconazole *on page 485*

◆ **GnRH Agonist** *see* Histrelin *on page 570*

Goserelin (GOE se rel in)

Related Information
Safe Handling of Hazardous Drugs *on page 1517*

U.S. Brand Names Zoladex®

Index Terms D-Ser(Bu^t)^6,Azgly^{10}-LHRH; Goserelin Acetate; ICI-118630

Generic Available No

Canadian Brand Names Zoladex®; Zoladex® LA

Pharmacologic Category Antineoplastic Agent, Gonadotropin-Releasing Hormone Agonist; Gonadotropin Releasing Hormone Agonist

Use Treatment (including palliative treatment) of prostate cancer; palliative treatment of advanced breast cancer; treatment of endometriosis, including pain relief and reduction of endometriotic lesions; endometrial thinning agent as part of treatment for dysfunctional uterine bleeding

Pregnancy Risk Factor X (endometriosis, endometrial thinning); D (advanced breast cancer)

Lactation Excretion in breast milk unknown/not recommended

Labeled Contraindications Hypersensitivity to goserelin, GnRH, GnRH agonist analogues, or any component of the formulation; pregnancy (except if using for palliative treatment of advanced breast cancer)

Warnings/Precautions Hazardous agent - use appropriate precautions for handling and disposal. Allergic hypersensitivity reactions (including anaphylaxis) and antibody formation may occur; monitor. Transient worsening of signs and symptoms (tumor flare) may develop during the first few weeks of treatment. Urinary tract obstruction or spinal cord compression have been reported when used for prostate cancer; closely observe patients for weakness, paresthesias, and urinary tract obstruction in first few weeks of therapy. Decreased bone density has been reported in women and may be irreversible; use caution if other risk factors are present; evaluate and institute preventative treatment if necessary. Women of childbearing potential should not receive therapy until pregnancy has been excluded. Nonhormonal contraception is recommended during therapy and for 12 weeks after therapy is discontinued. Cervical resistance may be increased; use caution when dilating the cervix. The 3-month implant currently has no approved indications for use in women. Rare cases of pituitary apoplexy (frequently secondary to pituitary adenoma) have been observed with leuprolide administration (onset from 1 hour to usually <2 weeks); may present as sudden headache, vomiting, visual or mental status changes, and infrequently cardiovascular collapse; immediate medical attention required. Hyperglycemia has been reported in males and may manifest as diabetes or worsening of pre-existing diabetes. Decreased bioavailability may be observed when using the 3-month implant in obese patients. Monitor testosterone levels if desired clinical response is not observed. Safety and efficacy have not been established in pediatric patients.

◀ **Adverse Reactions** Percentages reported in males with prostatic carcinoma and females with endometriosis using the 1-month implant:

>10%:

Cardiovascular: Edema (peripheral [female 21%])

Central nervous system: Headache (female 32% to 75%; male 1% to 5%), emotional lability (female 60%), depression (female 54%; male 1% to 5%), pain (female 17%; male 8%), insomnia (female 11%; male 5%)

Dermatologic: Acne (female 42%), seborrhea (female 26%)

Endocrine & metabolic: Hot flashes (female 96%; male 62%), libido decreased (female 61%), sexual dysfunction (male 21%), breast atrophy (female 33%), breast enlargement (female 18%), erections decreased (18%), libido increased (female 12%)

Genitourinary: Vaginitis (75%), pelvic symptoms (female 18%), dyspareunia (female 14%), lower urinary symptoms (male 13%)

Neuromuscular & skeletal: Weakness (female 11%)

Miscellaneous: Diaphoresis (female 45%; male 6%); infection (female 13%)

1% to 10%:

Cardiovascular: Heart failure (male 5%), arrhythmia, cerebrovascular accident, hypertension, MI, peripheral vascular disorder, chest pain, palpitation, tachycardia, edema

Central nervous system: Lethargy (male 8%), dizziness (female 6%; male 5%), abnormal thinking, anxiety, chills, fever, malaise, migraine, nervousness, somnolence

Dermatologic: Hirsutism (female 7%), rash (female >1%; male 6%), alopecia, bruising, dry skin, pruritus, skin discoloration

Endocrine & metabolic: Breast pain (female 7%), breast swelling/tenderness (male 1% to 5%), dysmenorrhea, gout, hyperglycemia

Gastrointestinal: Anorexia (female >1%; male 5%), nausea (female 8%; male 5%), appetite increased, constipation, diarrhea, flatulence, dyspepsia, ulcer, vomiting, weight gain/loss, xerostomia

Genitourinary: Renal insufficiency, urinary frequency, urinary obstruction, urinary tract infection, vaginal hemorrhage

Hematologic: Anemia, hemorrhage

Local: Application site reaction (female 6%)

Neuromuscular & skeletal: Back pain (female 7%), arthralgia, bone mineral density decreased (female; ~4% decrease in 6 months; postmarketing reports in males), hypertonia, joint disorder, leg cramps, myalgia, paresthesia

Ocular: Amblyopia, dry eyes

Respiratory: Upper respiratory tract infection (male 7%), COPD (male 5%), pharyngitis (female 5%), bronchitis, cough, epistaxis, rhinitis, sinusitis

Miscellaneous: Allergic reaction, voice alteration (female 3%)

Postmarketing and/or case reports: ALT increased, anaphylaxis, AST increased, lipids increased, glucose tolerance decreased, hypersensitivity reactions, hypotension, ovarian cyst, pituitary apoplexy, psychotic disorders, urticaria

Drug Interactions

Avoid Concomitant Use There are no known interactions where it is recommended to avoid concomitant use.

Increased Effect/Toxicity There are no known significant interactions involving an increase in effect.

Decreased Effect

Goserelin may decrease the levels/effects of: Antidiabetic Agents

Storage/Stability Zoladex® should be stored at room temperature not to exceed 25°C (77°F). Protect from light. Should be dispensed in a lightproof bag.

Mechanism of Action Goserelin (a gonadotropin-releasing hormone [GnRH] analog) causes an initial increase in luteinizing hormone (LH) and follicle stimulating hormone (FSH), chronic administration of goserelin results in a sustained suppression of pituitary gonadotropins. Serum testosterone falls to levels comparable to surgical castration. The exact mechanism of this effect is unknown, but may be related to changes in the control of LH or down-regulation of LH receptors.

Pharmacodynamics/Kinetics Note: Data reported using the 1-month implant.

Absorption: SubQ: Rapid and can be detected in serum in 10 minutes; 3.6 mg: released slowly in first 8 days, then rapid and continuous release for 28 days

Distribution: V_d: Male: 44.1 L; Female: 20.3 L

Protein binding: 27%

Time to peak, serum: SubQ: Male: 12-15 days, Female: 8-22 days

Half-life elimination: SubQ: Male: ~4 hours, Female: ~2 hours; Renal impairment: Male: 12 hours

Excretion: Urine (>90%; 20% as unchanged drug)

Dosage SubQ: Adults:

Prostate cancer, palliative:

Monthly implant: 3.6 mg every 28 days

3-month implant: 10.8 mg every 12 weeks

Prostate cancer, treatment (in combination with flutamide and radiotherapy; begin 8 weeks prior to radiotherapy):

Combination monthly/3-month implant: 3.6 mg implant, followed in 28 days by 10.8 mg implant

Monthly implant (alternate dosing): 3.6 mg; repeated every 28 days for a total of 4 doses

Breast cancer: Monthly implant: 3.6 mg every 28 days

Endometriosis: Monthly implant: 3.6 mg every 28 days for 6 months

Endometrial thinning: Monthly implant: 3.6 mg every 28 days for 1 or 2 doses

Dosing adjustment in renal impairment: No adjustment is necessary

Dosing adjustment in hepatic impairment: No adjustment is necessary with moderate impairment; no data for severe impairment

Combination Regimens

Prostate cancer:

Bicalutamide-Goserelin on page 1234

FZ on page 1340

Administration SubQ: Administer into the anterior abdominal wall below the naval line every 28 days. Goserelin is an implant; therefore, do not attempt to eliminate air bubbles prior to injection.

Monitoring Parameters Bone mineral density, serum calcium

Prostate cancer: Weakness, paresthesias, and urinary tract obstruction in first few weeks of therapy; screen for diabetes

Test Interactions Interferes with pituitary gonadotropic and gonadal function tests during and for up to 12 weeks after discontinued

Additional Information If removal is necessary, implant may be located by ultrasound.

Dosage Forms Excipient information presented when available (limited, particularly for generics); consult specific product labeling.

Implant, subcutaneous:

Zoladex®:

3.6 mg [1-month implant packaged with 16-gauge hypodermic needle]
10.8 mg [3-month implant packaged with 14-gauge hypodermic needle]

References

Ahmann FR, Citrin DL, deHaan HA, et al, "Zoladex: A Sustained-Release, Monthly Luteinizing Hormone-Releasing Hormone Analog for the Treatment of Advanced Prostate Cancer," *J Clin Oncol*, 1987, 5(6):912-7.

Goldspiel BR and Kohler DR, "Goserelin Acetate Implant: A Depot Luteinizing Hormone-Releasing Hormone Analog for Advanced Prostate Cancer," *DICP*, 1991, 25(7-8):796-804.

◆ **Goserelin Acetate** *see* Goserelin *on page* 549

◆ **GR38032R** *see* Ondansetron *on page* 874

Granisetron (gra NI se tron)

Medication Safety Issues

Sound-alike/look-alike issues:

Granisetron may be confused with dolasetron, ondansetron, palonosetron

Related Information

Management of Chemotherapy-Induced Nausea and Vomiting *on page* 1434

U.S. Brand Names Granisol™; Kytril®; Sancuso®

Index Terms BRL 43694

Generic Available Yes

Canadian Brand Names Apo-Granisetron; Kytril®

Pharmacologic Category Antiemetic; Selective 5-HT$_3$ Receptor Antagonist

Use Prophylaxis of nausea and vomiting associated with emetogenic chemotherapy and radiation therapy; prophylaxis and treatment of post-operative nausea and vomiting (PONV)

Unlabeled/Investigational Use Breakthrough treatment of nausea and vomiting associated with chemotherapy

Pregnancy Risk Factor B

Lactation Excretion in breast milk unknown/use caution

Labeled Contraindications Hypersensitivity to granisetron or any component of the formulation

Warnings/Precautions Use with caution in patients with congenital long QT syndrome or other risk factors for QT prolongation (eg, medications known to prolong QT interval, electrolyte abnormalities, and cumulative high-dose anthracycline therapy). 5-HT$_3$ antagonists have been associated with a number of dose-dependent increases in ECG intervals (eg, PR, QRS duration, QT/QT$_c$, JT), usually occurring 1-2 hours after I.V. administration. In general, these changes are not clinically relevant, however, when used in conjunction with other agents that prolong these intervals, arrhythmia may occur. When used with agents that prolong the QT interval (eg, Class I and III antiarrhythmics), clinically relevant QT interval prolongation may occur resulting in torsade de pointes. I.V. formulations of 5-HT$_3$ antagonists have more association with ECG interval changes, compared to oral formulations.

For chemotherapy-related emesis, **granisetron should be used on a scheduled basis, not on an "as needed" (PRN) basis**, since data support the use of this drug in the prevention of nausea and vomiting and not in the rescue of nausea and vomiting. Granisetron should be used only in the first 24-48 hours of receiving chemotherapy or radiation. Data do not support any increased efficacy of granisetron in delayed nausea and vomiting.

Use with caution in patients allergic to other 5-HT$_3$ receptor antagonists; cross-reactivity has been reported. Routine prophylaxis for PONV is not recommended in patients where there is little expectation of nausea and vomiting postoperatively. In patients where nausea and vomiting must be avoided postoperatively, administer to all patients even when expected incidence of nausea and vomiting is low. Use caution following abdominal surgery or in chemotherapy-induced nausea and vomiting; may mask progressive ileus or gastric distention. Application site reactions, generally mild, have occurred with transdermal patch use; if skin reaction is severe or generalized, remove patch. Cover patch application site with clothing to protect from natural or artificial sunlight exposure while patch is applied and for 10 days following removal; granisetron may potentially be affected by natural or artificial sunlight. Do not apply patch to red, irritated, or damaged skin. Injection contains benzyl alcohol (1 mg/mL) and should not be used in neonates.

Adverse Reactions

>10%:

Central nervous system: Headache (3% to 21%; transdermal patch: 1%)

Gastrointestinal: Constipation (3% to 18%)

Neuromuscular & skeletal: Weakness (5% to 18%)

1% to 10%:

Cardiovascular: QT_c prolongation (1% to 3%), hypertension (1% to 2%)

Central nervous system: Pain (10%), fever (3% to 9%), dizziness (4% to 5%), insomnia (<2% to 5%), somnolence (1% to 4%), anxiety (2%), agitation (<2%), CNS stimulation (<2%)

Dermatologic: Rash (1%)

Gastrointestinal: Diarrhea (3% to 9%), abdominal pain (4% to 6%), dyspepsia (3% to 6%), taste perversion (2%)

Hepatic: Liver enzymes increased (5% to 6%)

Renal: Oliguria (2%)

Respiratory: Cough (2%)

Miscellaneous: Infection (3%)

<1%, postmarketing, and/or case reports: Agitation, allergic reactions; anaphylaxis (including hypotension, dyspnea, urticaria); angina, application site reactions (transdermal patch), arrhythmias, atrial fibrillation, extrapyramidal syndrome, hot flashes, hypotension, hypersensitivity, syncope

Drug Interactions

Metabolism/Transport Effects Substrate of CYP3A4 (minor)

Avoid Concomitant Use

Avoid concomitant use of Granisetron with any of the following: Apomorphine

Increased Effect/Toxicity

Granisetron may increase the levels/effects of: Apomorphine

Decreased Effect There are no known significant interactions involving a decrease in effect.

Storage/Stability

I.V.: Store at 15°C to 30°C (59°F to 86°F). Protect from light. Do not freeze vials. Stable when mixed in NS or D_5W for 7 days under refrigeration and for 3 days at room temperature.

Oral: Store tablet or oral solution at 15°C to 30°C (59°F to 86°F). Protect from light.

Transdermal patch: Store at 20°C to 25°C (68°F to 77°F). Keep patch in original packaging until immediately prior to use.

Compatibility Stable in $D_5^{1}/_2NS$, D_5NS, D_5W, NS, bacteriostatic water.

Y-site administration: Compatible: Acyclovir, allopurinol, amifostine, amikacin, aminophylline, amphotericin B cholesteryl sulfate complex, ampicillin, ampicillin/sulbactam, amsacrine, aztreonam, bleomycin, bumetanide, buprenorphine, butorphanol, calcium gluconate, carboplatin, carmustine, cefazolin, cefepime, cefotaxime, cefotetan, cefoxitin, ceftazidime, ceftizoxime, ceftriaxone, cefuroxime, chlorpromazine, cimetidine, ciprofloxacin, cisplatin, cladribine, clindamycin, co-trimoxazole, cyclophosphamide, cytarabine, dacarbazine, dactinomycin, daunorubicin, dexamethasone sodium phosphate, dexmedetomidine, diphenhydramine, dobutamine, docetaxel, dopamine, doxorubicin, doxorubicin liposome, doxycycline, droperidol, enalaprilat, etoposide, etoposide phosphate, famotidine, fenoldopam mesylate, filgrastim, floxuridine, fluconazole, fludarabine, fluorouracil, furosemide, gallium nitrate, ganciclovir, gatifloxacin, gemcitabine, gentamicin, haloperidol, heparin, hetastarch in lactated electrolytes, hydrocortisone sodium succinate, hydromorphone, hydroxyzine, idarubicin, ifosfamide, imipenem/cilastatin, leucovorin calcium, levoleucovorin, linezolid, lorazepam, magnesium sulfate, mechlorethamine, melphalan, meperidine, mesna, methotrexate, methylprednisolone sodium succinate, metoclopramide, metronidazole, mitomycin, mitoxantrone, morphine, nalbuphine, netilmicin, ofloxacin, paclitaxel, pemetrexed, piperacillin, piperacillin/tazobactam, potassium chloride, prochlorperazine edisylate, promethazine, propofol, ranitidine, sargramostim, sodium bicarbonate, streptozocin, teniposide, thiotepa, ticarcillin, ticarcillin/clavulanate, tobramycin, topotecan, vancomycin, vinblastine, vincristine, vinorelbine, zidovudine. **Incompatible:** Amphotericin B.

Compatibility in syringe: Compatible: Dexamethasone sodium phosphate, methylprednisolone sodium succinate.

Compatibility when admixed: Compatible: Dexamethasone sodium phosphate, methylprednisolone sodium succinate.

Mechanism of Action
Selective 5-HT$_3$-receptor antagonist, blocking serotonin, both peripherally on vagal nerve terminals and centrally in the chemoreceptor trigger zone

Pharmacodynamics/Kinetics
Duration: Oral, I.V.: Generally up to 24 hours

Absorption: Oral: Tablets and oral solution are bioequivalent; Transdermal patch: ~66% over 7 days

Distribution: V$_d$: 2-4 L/kg; widely throughout body

Protein binding: 65%

Metabolism: Hepatic via N-demethylation, oxidation, and conjugation; some metabolites may have 5-HT$_3$ antagonist activity

Half-life elimination: Oral: 6 hours; I.V.: 9 hours

Time to peak, plasma: Transdermal patch: Maximum systemic concentrations: ~48 hours after application (range: 24-168 hours)

Excretion: Urine (12% as unchanged drug, 48% to 49% as metabolites); feces (34% to 38% as metabolites)

Dosage
Oral: Adults:

Prophylaxis of chemotherapy-related emesis: 2 mg once daily up to 1 hour before chemotherapy or 1 mg twice daily; the first 1 mg dose should be given up to 1 hour before chemotherapy.

Prophylaxis of radiation therapy-associated emesis: 2 mg once daily given 1 hour before radiation therapy.

I.V.:

Children ≥2 years and Adults: Prophylaxis of chemotherapy-related emesis: Within U.S.: 10 mcg/kg/dose (maximum: 1 mg/dose) given 30 minutes prior to chemotherapy; for some drugs (eg, carboplatin, cyclophosphamide) with a later onset of emetic action, 10 mcg/kg every 12 hours may be necessary

Outside U.S.: 40 mcg/kg/dose (or 3 mg/dose); maximum: 9 mg/24 hours

Breakthrough: Granisetron has not been shown to be effective in terminating nausea or vomiting once it occurs and should not be used for this purpose.

Adults: PONV:

Prevention: 1 mg given undiluted over 30 seconds; the manufacturer recommends administration before induction of anesthesia or immediately before reversal of anesthesia. **Note:** The Society for Ambulatory Anesthesia (SAMBA) Guidelines recommend a dosage range of 0.35-1.5 mg administered at the end of surgery (Gan, 2007). However, doses ≤1 mg are generally used since doses >1 mg are not more effective. Of note, 5 mcg/kg (~0.35 mg in a 70 kg adult) has been shown to be effective; doses >5 mcg/kg were not more effective (Mikawa, 1997).

Treatment: 1 mg given undiluted over 30 seconds

Transdermal patch: Adults: Prophylaxis of chemotherapy-related emesis: Apply 1 patch at least 24 hours prior to chemotherapy; do not apply ≥48 hours before chemotherapy. Remove patch a minimum of 24 hours after chemotherapy completion. Maximum duration: Patch may be worn up to 7 days, depending on chemotherapy regimen duration.

Dosing interval in renal impairment: No dosage adjustment required.

Dosing interval in hepatic impairment: Kinetic studies in patients with hepatic impairment showed that total clearance was approximately halved, however, standard doses were very well tolerated, and dose adjustments are not necessary.

Administration

Oral: Doses should be given up to 1 hour prior to initiation of chemotherapy/radiation

I.V.: Administer I.V. push over 30 seconds or as a 5-10 minute-infusion

Prevention of PONV: Administer before induction of anesthesia or immediately before reversal of anesthesia.

Treatment of PONV: Administer undiluted over 30 seconds.

Transdermal (Sancuso®): Apply patch to clean, dry, intact skin on upper outer arm. Do not use on red, irritated or damaged skin. Remove patch from pouch immediately before application. Do not cut patch.

Dosage Forms Excipient information presented when available (limited, particularly for generics); consult specific product labeling. [DSC] = Discontinued product

Injection, solution: 1 mg/mL (1 mL, 4 mL)

Kytril®: 1 mg/mL (1 mL, 4 mL) [contains benzyl alcohol]

Injection, solution [preservative free]: 0.1 mg/mL (1 mL); 1 mg/mL (1 mL)

Kytril®: 0.1 mg/mL (1 mL)

Solution, oral:

Granisol™: 2 mg/10 mL (30 mL) [contains sodium benzoate; orange flavor]

Kytril®: 2 mg/10 mL (30 mL) [contains sodium benzoate; orange flavor] [DSC]

Tablet: 1 mg

Kytril®: 1 mg

Transdermal system, topical:

Sancuso®: 3.1 mg/24 hours (1s) [52 cm^2, total granisetron 34.3 mg]

References

Gan TJ, Meyer TA, Apfel CC, et al, "Society for Ambulatory Anesthesia Guidelines for the Management of Postoperative Nausea and Vomiting," *Anesth Analg*, 2007, 105(6):1615-28.

Gill D and Howell J, "Pharmacokinetics and Bioavailability of Transdermal Granisetron After a Six-Day Application of Three Patch Sizes, Compared to 2 mg Once-Daily Oral Dose of Granisetron for Five Days," *Support Care Cancer*, 2008, 16(6):619-756 [abstract from 2008 International MASCC/ISOO Symposium].

Kris MG, Hesketh PJ, Somerfield MR, et al, "American Society of Clinical Oncology Guideline for Antiemetics in Oncology: Update 2006," *J Clin Oncol*, 2006, 24(18):2932-47.

Mikawa K, Takao Y, Nishina K, et al, "Optimal Dose of Granisetron for Prophylaxis Against Postoperative Emesis After Gynecological Surgery,"*Anesth Analg*, 1997, 85(3):652-6.

Navari RM and Koeller JM, "Electrocardiographic and Cardiovascular Effects of the 5-Hydroxytryptamine₃ Receptor Antagonists," *Ann Pharmacother*, 2003, 37(9):1276-86.

Palmer R, "Efficacy and Safety of Granisetron (Kytril®) in Two Special Populations: Children and Adults With Impaired Hepatic Function," *Semin Oncol*, 1994, 21(3 Suppl 5):22-5.

◆ **Granisol™** *see* Granisetron *on page* 552

◆ **Granulocyte Colony Stimulating Factor** *see* Filgrastim *on page* 475

◆ **Granulocyte Colony Stimulating Factor (PEG Conjugate)** *see* Pegfilgrastim *on page* 929

◆ **Granulocyte-Macrophage Colony Stimulating Factor** *see* Sargramostim *on page* 1029

◆ **GW506U78** *see* Nelarabine *on page* 843

◆ **GW-1000-02** *see* Tetrahydrocannabinol and Cannabidiol *on page* 1090

◆ **GW572016** *see* Lapatinib *on page* 684

◆ **Gyne-Lotrimin® 3 [OTC]** *see* Clotrimazole *on page* 253

◆ **Gyne-Lotrimin® 7 [OTC]** *see* Clotrimazole *on page* 253

◆ **Haldol®** *see* Haloperidol *on page* 556

◆ **Haldol® Decanoate** *see* Haloperidol *on page* 556

Haloperidol (ha loe PER i dole)

Medication Safety Issues
Sound-alike/look-alike issues:

Haloperidol may be confused Halotestin®

Haldol® may be confused with Halcion®, Halenol®, Halog®, Halotestin®, Stadol®

Related Information
Management of Chemotherapy-Induced Nausea and Vomiting *on page 1434*

U.S. Brand Names Haldol®; Haldol® Decanoate

Index Terms Haloperidol Decanoate; Haloperidol Lactate

Generic Available Yes

Canadian Brand Names Apo-Haloperidol LA®; Apo-Haloperidol®; Haloperidol Injection, USP; Haloperidol Long Acting; Haloperidol-LA; Haloperidol-LA Omega; Novo-Peridol; Peridol; PMS-Haloperidol LA

Pharmacologic Category Antipsychotic Agent, Typical

Use Management of schizophrenia; control of tics and vocal utterances of Tourette's disorder in children and adults; severe behavioral problems in children

Unlabeled/Investigational Use Treatment of non-schizophrenia psychosis; may be used for the emergency sedation of severely-agitated or delirious patients; adjunctive treatment of ethanol dependence; antiemetic; psychosis/agitation related to Alzheimer's dementia

Pregnancy Risk Factor C

Lactation Enters breast milk/not recommended (AAP rates "of concern")

Labeled Contraindications Hypersensitivity to haloperidol or any component of the formulation; Parkinson's disease; severe CNS depression; coma

Warnings/Precautions [U.S. Boxed Warning]: Elderly patients with dementia-related psychosis treated with antipsychotics are at an increased risk of death compared to placebo. Most deaths appeared to be either cardiovascular (eg, heart failure, sudden death) or infectious (eg, pneumonia) in nature. Haloperidol is not approved for the treatment of dementia-related psychosis. Hypotension may occur, particularly with parenteral administration. Although the short-acting form (lactate) is used clinically, the I.V. use of the injection is not an FDA-approved route of administration; the decanoate form should never be administered intravenously.

May alter cardiac conduction and prolong QT interval; life-threatening arrhythmias have occurred with therapeutic doses of antipsychotics but risk may be increased with doses exceeding recommendations and/or intravenous administration (unlabeled route). Use caution or avoid use in patients with electrolyte abnormalities (eg, hypokalemia, hypomagnesemia), hypothyroidism, familial long QT syndrome, concomitant medications which may augment QT prolongation, or any underlying cardiac abnormality which may also potentiate risk. Monitor ECG closely for dose-related QT effects. Adverse effects of decanoate may be prolonged. Avoid in thyrotoxicosis. Myelosuppression (eg, leukopenia, agranulocytosis) has been observed with antipsychotic use; check blood counts periodically and discontinue at first signs of blood dyscrasias; use is contraindicated in patients with bone marrow suppression. May be sedating, use with caution in disorders where CNS depression is a feature. Effects may be potentiated when used with other sedative drugs or ethanol. Caution in patients with severe cardiovascular disease, predisposition to seizures, subcortical brain damage, or renal disease. Esophageal dysmotility and aspiration have been associated with antipsychotic use - use with caution in patients at risk of pneumonia (eg, Alzheimer's disease). Use associated with increased prolactin levels; clinical significance of hyperprolactinemia in patients with breast cancer or other prolactin-dependent tumors is unknown. May alter temperature regulation or mask toxicity of other drugs due to antiemetic effects. May cause orthostatic hypotension; use with caution in patients at risk of this effect or those who would tolerate transient hypotensive episodes (cerebrovascular disease, cardiovascular disease, or other medications which may predispose). Some tablets contain tartrazine. Antipsychotics have been associated with pigmentary retinopathy.

May cause anticholinergic effects (confusion, agitation, constipation, xerostomia, blurred vision, urinary retention). Therefore, they should be used with caution in patients with decreased gastrointestinal motility, urinary retention, BPH, xerostomia, or visual problems. Conditions which also may be exacerbated by cholinergic blockade include narrow-angle glaucoma and worsening of myasthenia gravis. Relative to other neuroleptics, haloperidol has a low potency of cholinergic blockade.

May cause extrapyramidal symptoms (EPS), including pseudoparkinsonism, acute dystonic reactions, akathisia, and tardive dyskinesia (risk of these reactions is high relative to other neuroleptics). Risk of dystonia (and possibly other EPS) may be greater with increased doses, use of conventional antipsychotics, males, and younger patients. May be associated with neuroleptic malignant syndrome (NMS). Use with caution in the elderly.

Adverse Reactions Frequency not defined.

Cardiovascular: Abnormal T waves with prolonged ventricular repolarization, arrhythmia, hyper-/hypotension, QT prolongation, sudden death, tachycardia, torsade de pointes

Central nervous system: Agitation, akathisia, altered central temperature regulation, anxiety, confusion, depression, drowsiness, dystonic reactions, euphoria, extrapyramidal reactions, headache, insomnia, lethargy, neuroleptic malignant syndrome (NMS), pseudoparkinsonian signs and symptoms, restlessness, seizure, tardive dyskinesia, tardive dystonia, vertigo

Dermatologic: Alopecia, contact dermatitis, hyperpigmentation, photosensitivity (rare), pruritus, rash

Endocrine & metabolic: Amenorrhea, breast engorgement, galactorrhea, gynecomastia, hyper-/hypoglycemia, hyponatremia, lactation, mastalgia, menstrual irregularities, sexual dysfunction

Gastrointestinal: Anorexia, constipation, diarrhea, dyspepsia, hypersalivation, nausea, vomiting, xerostomia

Genitourinary: Priapism, urinary retention

Hematologic: Cholestatic jaundice, obstructive jaundice

Ocular: Blurred vision

Respiratory: Bronchospasm, laryngospasm

Miscellaneous: Diaphoresis, heat stroke

Drug Interactions

Metabolism/Transport Effects Substrate of CYP1A2 (minor), 2D6 (major), 3A4 (major); **Inhibits** CYP2D6 (moderate), 3A4 (moderate)

Avoid Concomitant Use

Avoid concomitant use of Haloperidol with any of the following: Artemether; Dronedarone; Everolimus; Lumefantrine; Nilotinib; Pimozide; QuiNINE; Tetrabenazine; Thioridazine; Tolvaptan; Ziprasidone

Increased Effect/Toxicity

Haloperidol may increase the levels/effects of: Alcohol (Ethyl); Anticholinergics; ChlorproMAZINE; CNS Depressants; Colchicine; CYP2D6 Substrates; CYP3A4 Substrates; Dronedarone; Eplerenone; Everolimus; FentaNYL; Fesoterodine; Nebivolol; Pimecrolimus; Pimozide; QTc-Prolonging Agents; QuiNINE; Salmeterol; Saxagliptin; Tamoxifen; Tetrabenazine; Thioridazine; Tolvaptan; Ziprasidone

The levels/effects of Haloperidol may be increased by: Acetylcholinesterase Inhibitors (Central); Alfuzosin; Artemether; Chloroquine; ChlorproMAZINE; Ciprofloxacin; CYP2D6 Inhibitors (Moderate); CYP2D6 Inhibitors (Strong); CYP3A4 Inhibitors (Moderate); CYP3A4 Inhibitors (Strong); Darunavir; Gadobutrol; Lithium formulations; Lumefantrine; Nilotinib; Pramlintide; QuiNIDine; QuiNINE; Selective Serotonin Reuptake Inhibitors; Tetrabenazine

Decreased Effect

Haloperidol may decrease the levels/effects of: Amphetamines; Anti-Parkinson's Agents (Dopamine Agonist); Codeine; TraMADol

The levels/effects of Haloperidol may be decreased by: CarBAMazepine; CYP3A4 Inducers (Strong); Deferasirox; Herbs (CYP3A4 Inducers); Lithium formulations; Peginterferon Alfa-2b

Ethanol/Nutrition/Herb Interactions

Ethanol: Avoid ethanol (may increase CNS depression).

Herb/Nutraceutical: Avoid valerian, St John's wort, kava kava, gotu kola (may increase CNS depression).

Storage/Stability Protect oral dosage forms from light. Haloperidol lactate injection should be stored at controlled room temperature; do not freeze or expose to temperatures >40°C. Protect from light; exposure to light may cause discoloration and the development of a grayish-red precipitate over several weeks. Stability of standardized solutions is 38 days at room temperature (24°C).

Reconstitution Haloperidol lactate may be administered IVPB or I.V. infusion in D_5W solutions. NS solutions should not be used due to reports of decreased stability and incompatibility.

Standardized dose: 0.5-100 mg/50-100 mL D$_5$W.

Compatibility Stable in D$_5$W; **variable stability (consult detailed reference)** in D$_5$1/4NS, LR, 1/2NS, NS.

Y-site administration: Compatible: Amifostine, amsacrine, aztreonam, cimetidine, cisatracurium, cladribine, dobutamine, docetaxel, dopamine, doxorubicin liposome, etoposide phosphate, famotidine, filgrastim, fludarabine, gatifloxacin, gemcitabine, granisetron, lidocaine, linezolid, lorazepam, melphalan, midazolam, nitroglycerin, norepinephrine ondansetron, paclitaxel, phenylephrine, propofol, remifentanil, sufentanil, tacrolimus, teniposide, theophylline, thiotepa, vinorelbine. **Incompatible:** Allopurinol, amphotericin B cholesteryl sulfate complex, cefepime, fluconazole, foscarnet, heparin, piperacillin/tazobactam, sargramostim. **Variable (consult detailed reference):** Sodium nitroprusside.

Compatibility in syringe: Compatible: Hydromorphone, sufentanil. **Incompatible:** Diphenhydramine, heparin, hydroxyzine, ketorolac. **Variable (consult detailed reference):** Benztropine, cyclizine, diamorphine, morphine.

Mechanism of Action Haloperidol is a butyrophenone antipsychotic which blocks postsynaptic mesolimbic dopaminergic D$_1$ and D$_2$ receptors in the brain; depresses the release of hypothalamic and hypophyseal hormones; believed to depress the reticular activating system thus affecting basal metabolism, body temperature, wakefulness, vasomotor tone, and emesis

Pharmacodynamics/Kinetics

Onset of action: Sedation: I.M., I.V.: 30-60 minutes

Duration: Decanoate: 2-4 weeks

Distribution: V$_d$: 8-18 L/kg; crosses placenta; enters breast milk

Protein binding: 90%

Metabolism: Hepatic to inactive compounds

Bioavailability: Oral: 60%

Half-life elimination: 18 hours; Decanoate: ~1 day

Time to peak, serum: Oral: 2-6 hours; I.M.: 20 minutes; Decanoate: 7 days

Excretion: Urine (33% to 40% as metabolites) within 5 days; feces (15%)

Clearance: 550 ± 133 mL/minute

Dosage

Children: 3-12 years (15-40 kg): Oral:

Initial: 0.05 mg/kg/day or 0.25-0.5 mg/day given in 2-3 divided doses; increase by 0.25-0.5 mg every 5-7 days; maximum: 0.15 mg/kg/day

Usual maintenance:

Agitation or hyperkinesia: 0.01-0.03 mg/kg/day once daily

Nonpsychotic disorders: 0.05-0.075 mg/kg/day in 2-3 divided doses

Psychotic disorders: 0.05-0.15 mg/kg/day in 2-3 divided doses

Children 6-12 years: Sedation/psychotic disorders: I.M. (as lactate): 1-3 mg/dose every 4-8 hours to a maximum of 0.15 mg/kg/day; change over to oral therapy as soon as able

Adults:

Psychosis:

Oral: 0.5-5 mg 2-3 times/day; usual maximum: 30 mg/day

I.M. (as lactate): 2-5 mg every 4-8 hours as needed

I.M. (as decanoate): Initial: 10-20 times the daily oral dose administered at 4-week intervals

Maintenance dose: 10-15 times initial oral dose; used to stabilize psychiatric symptoms

Delirium in the intensive care unit (unlabeled use, unlabeled route):

I.V.: 2-10 mg; may repeat bolus doses every 20-30 minutes until calm achieved then administer 25% of the maximum dose every 6 hours; monitor ECG and QT_c interval

Intermittent I.V.: 0.03-0.15 mg/kg every 30 minutes to 6 hours

Oral: Agitation: 5-10 mg

Continuous intravenous infusion (100 mg/100 mL D_5W): Rates of 3-25 mg/hour have been used

Rapid tranquilization of severely-agitated patient (unlabeled use): Administer every 30-60 minutes:

Oral: 5-10 mg

I.M. (as lactate): 5 mg

Average total dose (oral or I.M.) for tranquilization: 10-20 mg

Elderly: Nonpsychotic patient, dementia behavior (unlabeled use): Initial: Oral: 0.25-0.5 mg 1-2 times/day; increase dose at 4- to 7-day intervals by 0.25-0.5 mg/day; increase dosing intervals (twice daily, 3 times/day, etc) as necessary to control response or side effects

Hemodialysis/peritoneal dialysis: Supplemental dose is not necessary

Administration The decanoate injectable formulation should be administered I.M. only, **do not administer decanoate I.V.** Dilute the oral concentrate with water or juice before administration. Avoid skin contact with oral suspension or solution; may cause contact dermatitis.

Monitoring Parameters Vital signs; lipid profile, fasting blood glucose/Hgb A_{1c}; BMI; mental status, abnormal involuntary movement scale (AIMS), extrapyramidal symptoms (EPS); ECG (with off-label intravenous administration)

Dosage Forms Excipient information presented when available (limited, particularly for generics); consult specific product labeling. [DSC] = Discontinued product

Note: Strength expressed as base.

Injection, oil, as decanoate: 50 mg/mL (1 mL, 5 mL); 100 mg/mL (1 mL, 5 mL)
Haldol® Decanoate: 50 mg/mL (1 mL; 5 mL [DSC]); 100 mg/mL (1 mL; 5 mL [DSC]) [contains benzyl alcohol, sesame oil]

Injection, solution, as lactate: 5 mg/mL (1 mL, 10 mL)
Haldol®: 5 mg/mL (1 mL)

Solution, oral concentrate, as lactate: 2 mg/mL (15 mL, 120 mL)

Tablet: 0.5 mg, 1 mg, 2 mg, 5 mg, 10 mg, 20 mg

References

Cole RM, Robinson F, Harvey L, et al, "Successful Control of Intractable Nausea and Vomiting Requiring Combined Ondansetron and Haloperidol in a Patient With Advanced Cancer," *J Pain Symptom Manage*, 1994, 9(1):48-50.

Di Salvo TG and O'Gara PT, "Torsade de Pointes Caused by High-Dose Intravenous Haloperidol in Cardiac Patients," *Clin Cardiol*, 1995, 18(5):285-90.

Gill SS, Bronskill SE, Normand SL, et al, "Antipsychotic Drug Use and Mortality in Older Adults With Dementia," *Ann Intern Med*, 2007, 146(11):775-86.

Neidhart JA, Gagen MM, Wilson HE, et al, "Comparative Trial of the Antiemetic Effects of THC and Haloperidol," *J Clin Pharmacol*, 1981, 21(8-9 Suppl):38-42.

Riker RR, Fraser GL, and Cox PM, "Continuous Infusion of Haloperidol Controls Agitation in Critically Ill Patients," *Crit Care Med*, 1994, 22(3):433-40.

Sharma ND, Rosman HS, Padhi ID, et al, "Torsades de Pointes Associated With Intravenous Haloperidol in Critically Ill Patients," *Am J Cardiol*, 1998, 81(2):238-40.

- ◆ **Haloperidol-LA Omega (Can)** *see* Haloperidol *on page 556*
- ◆ **Haloperidol Long Acting (Can)** *see* Haloperidol *on page 556*
- ◆ **Helixate® FS** *see* Antihemophilic Factor (Recombinant) *on page 93*
- ◆ **Hemofil M** *see* Antihemophilic Factor (Human) *on page 91*
- ◆ **Hemorrhoidal HC** *see* Hydrocortisone *on page 575*
- ◆ **Hemril®-30** *see* Hydrocortisone *on page 575*
- ◆ **Hepalean® (Can)** *see* Heparin *on page 561*
- ◆ **Hepalean® Leo (Can)** *see* Heparin *on page 561*
- ◆ **Hepalean®-LOK (Can)** *see* Heparin *on page 561*

Heparin (HEP a rin)

Medication Safety Issues

Sound-alike/look-alike issues:
Heparin may be confused with Hespan®

High alert medication: The Institute for Safe Medication Practices (ISMP) includes this medication among its list of drugs which have a heightened risk of causing significant patient harm when used in error.

Heparin sodium injection 10,000 units/mL and Hep-Lock U/P 10 units/mL have been confused with each other. Fatal medication errors have occurred between the two whose labels are both blue. **Never rely on color as a sole indicator to differentiate product identity.**

Heparin lock flush solution is intended only to maintain patency of I.V. devices and is **not** to be used for anticoagulant therapy.

Note: The 100 unit/mL concentration should not be used in neonates or infants <10 kg. The 10 unit/mL concentration may cause systemic anticoagulation in infants <1 kg who receive frequent flushes.

2009 National Patient Safety Goals: The Joint Commission on Accreditation of Healthcare Organizations requires healthcare organizations that provide anticoagulant therapy to have a process in place to reduce the risk of anticoagulant-associated patient harm. Patients receiving anticoagulants should receive individualized care through a defined process that includes standardized ordering, dispensing, administration, monitoring and education. This does not apply to routine short-term use of anticoagulants for prevention of venous thromboembolism when the expectation is that the patient's laboratory values will remain within or close to normal values (NPSG.03.05.01).

U.S. Brand Names Hep-Lock U/P; Hep-Lock®; HepFlush®-10

Index Terms Heparin Calcium; Heparin Lock Flush; Heparin Sodium

Generic Available Yes

Canadian Brand Names Hepalean®; Hepalean® Leo; Hepalean®-LOK

Pharmacologic Category Anticoagulant

Use Prophylaxis and treatment of thromboembolic disorders; as an anticoagulant for extracorporeal and dialysis procedures

Note: Heparin lock flush solution is intended only to maintain patency of I.V. devices and is **not** to be used for anticoagulant therapy.

Unlabeled/Investigational Use ST-elevation myocardial infarction (STEMI) - combination regimen of heparin (unlabeled dose), tenecteplase (half dose), and abciximab (full dose)

Pregnancy Risk Factor C

▶

Lactation Does not enter breast milk/compatible

Labeled Contraindications Hypersensitivity to heparin or any component of the formulation (unless a life-threatening situation necessitates use and use of an alternative anticoagulant is not possible); severe thrombocytopenia; uncontrolled active bleeding except when due to disseminated intravascular coagulation (DIC); suspected intracranial hemorrhage; not for I.M. use; not for use when appropriate blood coagulation tests cannot be obtained at appropriate intervals (applies to full-dose heparin only)

Warnings/Precautions Hypersensitivity reactions can occur. Only in life-threatening situations when use of an alternative anticoagulant is not possible should heparin be cautiously used in patients with a documented hyper-sensitivity reaction. Hemorrhage is the most common complication. Monitor for signs and symptoms of bleeding. Certain patients are at increased risk of bleeding. Risk factors for bleeding include bacterial endocarditis; congenital or acquired bleeding disorders; active ulcerative or angiodysplastic GI diseases; continuous GI tube drainage; severe uncontrolled hypertension; history of hemorrhagic stroke; or use shortly after brain, spinal, or ophthalmology surgery; patient treated concomitantly with platelet inhibitors; conditions associated with increased bleeding tendencies (hemophilia, vascular purpura); recent GI bleeding; thrombocytopenia or platelet defects; severe liver disease; hypertensive or diabetic retinopathy; or in patients undergoing invasive procedures including spinal tap or spinal anesthesia. Many concentrations of heparin are available ranging from 1 unit/mL to 20,000 units/mL. Clinicians **must** carefully examine each prefilled syringe or vial prior to use ensuring that the correct concentration is chosen; fatal hemorrhages have occurred related to heparin overdose especially in pediatric patients. A higher incidence of bleeding has been reported in patients >60 years of age, particularly women. They are also more sensitive to the dose. Discontinue heparin if hemorrhage occurs; severe hemorrhage or overdosage may require protamine.

May cause thrombocytopenia; monitor platelet count closely. Patients who develop HIT may be at risk of developing a new thrombus (heparin-induced thrombocytopenia and thrombosis [HITT]). Discontinue therapy and consider alternatives if platelets are <100,000/mm³ and/or thrombosis develops. HIT or HITT may be delayed and can occur up to several weeks after discontinuation of heparin. Osteoporosis may occur with prolonged use (>6 months) due to a reduction in bone mineral density. Monitor for hyperkalemia; can cause hyperkalemia by suppressing aldosterone production. Patients >60 years of age may require lower doses of heparin.

Some preparations contain benzyl alcohol as a preservative. In neonates, large amounts of benzyl alcohol (>100 mg/kg/day) have been associated with fatal toxicity (gasping syndrome). The use of preservative-free heparin is, therefore, recommended in neonates. Some preparations contain sulfite which may cause allergic reactions.

Heparin resistance may occur in patients with antithrombin deficiency, increased heparin clearance, elevations in heparin-binding proteins, elevations in factor VIII and/or fibrinogen; frequently encountered in patients with fever, thrombosis, thrombophlebitis, infections with thrombosing tendencies, MI, cancer, and in postsurgical patients; measurement of anticoagulant effects using antifactor Xa levels may be of benefit.

Adverse Reactions Frequency not defined.

Cardiovascular: Allergic vasospastic reaction (possibly related to thrombosis), chest pain, hemorrhagic shock, shock, thrombosis

Central nervous system: Chills, fever, headache

Dermatologic: Alopecia (delayed, transient), bruising (unexplained), cutaneous necrosis, dysesthesia pedis, erythematous plaques (case reports), eczema, urticaria, purpura

Endocrine & metabolic: Adrenal hemorrhage, hyperkalemia (suppression of aldosterone synthesis), ovarian hemorrhage, rebound hyperlipidemia on discontinuation

Gastrointestinal: Constipation, hematemesis, nausea, tarry stools, vomiting

Genitourinary: Frequent or persistent erection

Hematologic: Bleeding from gums, epistaxis, hemorrhage, ovarian hemorrhage, retroperitoneal hemorrhage, thrombocytopenia (see Note)

Hepatic: Liver enzymes increased

Local: Irritation, erythema, pain, hematoma, and ulceration have been rarely reported with deep SubQ injections; I.M. injection (not recommended) is associated with a high incidence of these effects

Neuromuscular & skeletal: Peripheral neuropathy, osteoporosis (chronic therapy effect)

Ocular: Conjunctivitis (allergic reaction), lacrimation

Renal: Hematuria

Respiratory: Asthma, bronchospasm (case reports), hemoptysis, pulmonary hemorrhage, rhinitis

Miscellaneous: Allergic reactions, anaphylactoid reactions, heparin resistance, hypersensitivity (including chills, fever, and urticaria)

Note: Thrombocytopenia has been reported to occur at an incidence between 0% and 30%. It is often of no clinical significance. However, immunologically mediated heparin-induced thrombocytopenia (HIT) has been estimated to occur in 1% to 2% of patients, and is marked by a progressive fall in platelet counts and, in some cases, thromboembolic complications (skin necrosis, pulmonary embolism, gangrene of the extremities, stroke or MI). For recommendations regarding platelet monitoring during heparin therapy, see Monitoring Parameters.

Drug Interactions

Avoid Concomitant Use

Avoid concomitant use of Heparin with any of the following: Corticorelin

Increased Effect/Toxicity

Heparin may increase the levels/effects of: Anticoagulants; Corticorelin; Drotrecogin Alfa; Ibritumomab; Tositumomab and Iodine I 131 Tositumomab

The levels/effects of Heparin may be increased by: Antiplatelet Agents; Aspirin; Dasatinib; Herbs (Anticoagulant/Antiplatelet Properties); Nonsteroidal Anti-Inflammatory Agents; Pentosan Polysulfate Sodium; Pentoxifylline; Prostacyclin Analogues; Salicylates; Thrombolytic Agents

Decreased Effect

The levels/effects of Heparin may be decreased by: Nitroglycerin

Ethanol/Nutrition/Herb Interactions Herb/Nutraceutical: Avoid cat's claw, dong quai, evening primrose, feverfew, red clover, horse chestnut, garlic, green tea, ginseng, ginkgo (all have additional antiplatelet activity).

Storage/Stability Heparin solutions are colorless to slightly yellow. Minor color variations do not affect therapeutic efficacy. Heparin should be stored at controlled room temperature. Protect from freezing and temperatures >40°C.

Stability at room temperature and refrigeration:
Prepared bag: 24 hours.
Premixed bag: After seal is broken. 4 days.
Out of overwrap stability: 30 days.

Reconstitution

Standard concentration/diluent: 25,000 units/500 mL D_5W (premixed). If preparing solution, mix thoroughly prior to administration.

Minimum volume: 250 mL D_5W.

Compatibility Stable in dextran 6% in dextrose, dextran 6% in NS, D_5LR, $D_5^{1}/_4NS$, $D_5^{1}/_2NS$, $D_{25}W$, fat emulsion 10%, $^{1}/_2NS$, NS, Ringer's injection; **variable stability (consult detailed reference)** in D_5NS, D_5W, $D_{10}W$, LR, peritoneal dialysis solutions, TPN.

Y-site administration: Compatible: Acyclovir, allopurinol, amifostine, aminophylline, ampicillin, ampicillin/sulbactam, anidulafungin, atracurium, atropine, aztreonam, bleomycin, calcium gluconate, cefazolin, cefotetan, ceftazidime, ceftriaxone, chlordiazepoxide, chlorpromazine, cimetidine, cisplatin, cladribine, clindamycin, cyanocobalamin, cyclophosphamide, cytarabine, daptomycin, dexmedetomidine, dexamethasone sodium phosphate, digoxin, diphenhydramine, docetaxel, dopamine, doxapram, doxorubicin liposome, edrophonium, enalaprilat, epinephrine, ertapenem, erythromycin lactobionate, esmolol, estrogens (conjugated), ethacrynate, etoposide phosphate, famotidine, fenoldopam, fentanyl, fluconazole, fludarabine, fluorouracil, foscarnet, furosemide, gemcitabine, granisetron, hetastarch in lactated electrolyte injection, hydralazine, hydrocortisone sodium succinate, hydromorphone, insulin (regular), isoproterenol, kanamycin, leucovorin calcium, lidocaine, linezolid, lorazepam, magnesium sulfate, melphalan, menadiol sodium diphosphate, meperidine, meropenem, methotrexate, methoxamine, methyldopate, methylergonovine, metoclopramide, metronidazole, micafungin, midazolam, milrinone, minocycline, mitomycin, morphine, nafcillin, neostigmine, nitroglycerin, norepinephrine, ondansetron, oxacillin, oxytocin, paclitaxel, pancuronium, pemetrexed, penicillin G potassium, pentazocine, phytonadione, piperacillin, piperacillin/tazobactam, potassium chloride, procainamide, prochlorperazine edisylate, propofol, propranolol, pyridostigmine, ranitidine, remifentanil, sargramostim, scopolamine, sodium bicarbonate, sodium nitroprusside, streptokinase, succinylcholine, tacrolimus, theophylline, thiopental, thiotepa, ticarcillin/clavulanate potassium, tigecycline, tirofiban, trimethobenzamide, trimethaphan camsylate, vasopressin, vecuronium, vinblastine, vincristine, warfarin, zidovudine. **Incompatible:** Alteplase, amiodarone, amphotericin B cholesteryl sulfate complex, amsacrine, ciprofloxacin, clarithromycin, diazepam, doxycycline, ergotamine, filgrastim, gatifloxacin, gentamicin, haloperidol lactate, idarubicin, isosorbide dinitrate, levofloxacin, methotrimeprazine, nesiritide, phenytoin, tobramycin, triflupromazine. **Variable (consult detailed reference):** Aldesleukin, antithymocyte globulin (rabbit), cisatracurium, dacarbazine, diltiazem, dobutamine, doxorubicin HCl, droperidol, drotrecogin alfa, fentanyl, labetalol, methylprednisolone sodium succinate, nicardipine, promethazine, quinidine gluconate, TPN, vancomycin, vinorelbine.

Compatibility in syringe: Compatible: Aminophylline, amphotericin B, ampicillin, atropine, bleomycin, buprenorphine, caffeine citrate, cefazolin, cefotaxime, cefoxitin, chloramphenicol, cisplatin, clindamycin, clonazepam, clonidine, cyclophosphamide, diatrizoate meglumine 52%, diatrizoate sodium 8%, diatrizoate sodium 60%, diazoxide, digoxin, dopamine, epinephrine, etomidate, fentanyl, floxacillin, fluorouracil, fosfomycin, furosemide, iohexol, iopamidol, iothalamate meglumine 60%, ioxaglate meglumine 39.3%, ioxaglate sodium 19.6%, leucovorin calcium, lidocaine, lincomycin, methotrexate, metoclopramide, mitomycin, nafcillin, naloxone, neostigmine, nitroglycerin, norepinephrine, pancuronium, penicillin G, pentoxifylline, phenobarbital, piperacillin, ranitidine, sodium nitroprusside, succinylcholine, tramadol, trimethoprim/sulfamethoxazole, verapamil, vincristine. **Incompatible:** Amikacin, amiodarone, chlorpromazine, diazepam, doxorubicin hydrochloride, droperidol, erythromycin, erythromycin lactobionate, gentamicin, haloperidol lactate, hydromorphone, kanamycin, meperidine, methotrimeprazine, midazolam, pantoprazole, pentazocine, promethazine, streptomycin, tobramycin, trifluromazine, vancomycin, warfarin. **Variable (consult detailed reference):** Cimetidine, dimenhydrinate, morphine, vinblastine.

Compatibility when admixed: Compatible: Aminophylline, amphotericin B, amphotericin B with hydrocortisone sodium succinate, ascorbic acid injection, bleomycin, calcium gluconate, cefepime, chloramphenicol, clindamycin, colistimethate, dimenhydrinate, dopamine, enalaprilat, esmolol, floxacillin, fluconazole, flumazenil, furosemide, hydromorphone, isoproterenol, lidocaine, lincomycin, magnesium sulfate, meropenem, methyldopate, methylprednisolone sodium succinate, nafcillin, norepinephrine, octreotide, potassium chloride, promazine, ranitidine, sodium bicarbonate, teicoplanin, verapamil, vitamin B complex, vitamin B complex with C. **Incompatible:** Alteplase, amikacin, atracurium, ciprofloxacin, cytarabine, daunorubicin hydrochloride, erythromycin lactobionate, gentamicin, hyaluronidase, kanamycin, levorphanol, meperidine, morphine, polymyxin B sulfate, promethazine, streptomycin. **Variable (consult detailed reference):** Ampicillin, antithymocyte globulin (rabbit), dobutamine, hydrocortisone sodium succinate, mitomycin, penicillin G potassium, penicillin G sodium, vancomycin.

Mechanism of Action Potentiates the action of antithrombin III and thereby inactivates thrombin (as well as activated coagulation factors IX, X, XI, XII, and plasmin) and prevents the conversion of fibrinogen to fibrin; heparin also stimulates release of lipoprotein lipase (lipoprotein lipase hydrolyzes triglycerides to glycerol and free fatty acids)

Pharmacodynamics/Kinetics

Onset of action: Anticoagulation: I.V.: Immediate; SubQ: ~20-30 minutes

Absorption: Oral, rectal: Erratic at best from these routes of administration; SubQ absorption is also erratic, but considered acceptable for prophylactic use

Distribution: Does not cross placenta; does not enter breast milk

Metabolism: Hepatic; may be partially metabolized in the reticuloendothelial system

Half-life elimination: Mean: 1.5 hours; Range: 1-2 hours; affected by obesity, renal function, hepatic function, malignancy, presence of pulmonary embolism, and infections

Excretion: Urine (small amounts as unchanged drug)

Dosage Note: Many concentrations of heparin are available ranging from 1 unit/mL to 20,000 units/mL. Carefully examine each prefilled syringe or vial prior to use ensuring that the correct concentration is chosen. Heparin lock flush solution is intended only to maintain patency of I.V. devices and is not to be used for anticoagulant therapy.

Children >1 year:

Prophylaxis for cardiac catheterization (arterial approach): I.V.: Bolus: 100-150 units/kg (Monagle, 2008)

Systemic heparinization:

Intermittent I.V.: Initial: 50-100 units/kg, then 50-100 units/kg every 4 hours (**Note:** Continuous I.V. infusion is preferred)

◀ I.V. infusion: Initial loading dose: 75 units/kg given over 10 minutes, then initial maintenance dose: 20 units/kg/hour; adjust dose to maintain aPTT of 60-85 seconds (assuming this reflects an antifactor Xa level of 0.35-0.7 units/mL); see table.

Pediatric Protocol For Systemic Heparin Adjustment

To be used after initial loading dose and maintenance I.V. infusion dose (see usual dosage listed above) to maintain aPTT of 60-85 seconds (assuming this reflects antifactor Xa level of 0.35-0.7 units/mL).

Obtain blood for aPTT 4 hours after heparin loading dose and 4 hours after every infusion rate change.

Obtain daily CBC and aPTT after aPTT is therapeutic.

aPTT (seconds)	Dosage Adjustment	Time to Repeat aPTT
<50	Give 50 units/kg bolus and increase infusion rate by 10%	4 h after rate change
50-59	Increase infusion rate by 10%	4 h after rate change
60-85	Keep rate the same	Next day
86-95	Decrease infusion rate by 10%	4 h after rate change
96-120	Hold infusion for 30 minutes and decrease infusion rate by 10%	4 h after rate change
>120	Hold infusion for 60 minutes and decrease infusion rate by 15%	4 h after rate change

Modified from Monagle P, Chalmers E, Chan A, et al, "Antithrombotic Therapy in Neonates and Children," *Chest*, 2008, 133(6 Suppl):887-968.

Adults:

Thromboprophylaxis (low-dose heparin): SubQ: 5000 units every 8-12 hours

Intermittent I.V.: Initial: 10,000 units, then 50-70 units/kg (5000-10,000 units) every 4-6 hours

I.V. infusion (weight-based dosing per institutional nomogram recommended):

Acute coronary syndromes:

STEMI: Fibrinolytic therapy:

Full-dose alteplase, reteplase, or tenecteplase with dosing as follows: Concurrent bolus of 60 units/kg (maximum: 4000 units), then 12 units/kg/hour (maximum: 1000 units/hour) as continuous infusion. Check aPTT every 4-6 hours; adjust to target of 1.5-2 times the upper limit of control (50-70 seconds in clinical trials); usual range 10-30 units/kg/hour. Duration of heparin therapy depends on concurrent therapy and the specific patient risks for systemic or venous thromboembolism.

Combination regimen (unlabeled): Half-dose tenecteplase (15-25 mg based on weight) and abciximab 0.25 mg/kg bolus then 0.125 mcg/kg/minute (maximum 10 mcg/minute) for 12 hours with heparin dosing as follows: Concurrent bolus of 40 units/kg (maximum 3000 units), then 7 units/kg/hour (maximum: 800 units/hour) as continuous infusion. Adjust to aPTT target of 50-70 seconds.

Percutaneous coronary intervention:

If no concurrent GPIIb/IIIa inhibitor: Initial bolus of 60-100 units/kg (target ACT 250-350 seconds)

or

If receiving GPIIb/IIIa inhibitor: Initial bolus of 50-70 units/kg (target ACT 200-250 seconds)

Treatment of unstable angina/non-ST-elevation myocardial infarction (NSTEMI): Initial bolus of 60 units/kg (maximum: 4000 units), followed by an initial infusion of 12 units/kg/hour (maximum: 1000 units/hour). The American College of Chest Physicians consensus conference has recommended dosage adjustments to correspond to a therapeutic range equivalent to heparin levels of 0.3-0.7 units/mL by antifactor Xa determinations.

Treatment of venous thromboembolism:

DVT/PE: I.V.: 80 units/kg (or 5000 units) I.V. push followed by continuous infusion of 18 units/kg/hour (or 1300 units/hour). The American College of Chest Physicians consensus conference has recommended dosage adjustments to correspond to a therapeutic range equivalent to heparin levels of 0.3-0.7 units/mL by antifactor Xa determinations.

DVT/PE: SubQ:

Monitored dosing regimen: Initial: 17,500 units or 250 units/kg then 250 units/kg every 12 hours. The American College of Chest Physicians consensus conference has recommended dosage adjustments to correspond to a therapeutic range equivalent to heparin levels of 0.3-0.7 units/mL by antifactor Xa determinations.

Unmonitored dosing regimen: Initial: 333 units/kg then 250 units/kg every 12 hours

Line flushing: When using daily flushes of heparin to maintain patency of single and double lumen central catheters, 10 units/mL is commonly used for younger infants (eg, <10 kg) while 100 units/mL is used for older infants, children, and adults. Capped PVC catheters and peripheral heparin locks require flushing more frequently (eg, every 6-8 hours). Volume of heparin flush is usually similar to volume of catheter (or slightly greater). Additional flushes should be given when stagnant blood is observed in catheter, after catheter is used for drug or blood administration, and after blood withdrawal from catheter.

Addition of heparin (0.5-3 unit/mL) to peripheral and central parenteral nutrition has not been shown to decrease catheter-related thrombosis. The final concentration of heparin used for TPN solutions may need to be decreased to 0.5 units/mL in small infants receiving larger amounts of volume in order to avoid approaching therapeutic amounts. Arterial lines are heparinized with a final concentration of 1 unit/mL.

Dosing adjustments in the elderly: Patients >60 years of age may have higher serum levels and clinical response (longer aPTTs) as compared to younger patients receiving similar dosages; lower dosages may be required

Administration SubQ: Inject in subcutaneous tissue only (not muscle tissue). Injection sites should be rotated (usually left and right portions of the abdomen, above iliac crest).

Do not administer I.M. due to pain, irritation, and hematoma formation; central venous catheters must be flushed with heparin solution when newly inserted, daily (at the time of tubing change), after blood withdrawal or transfusion, and after an intermittent infusion through an injectable cap. A volume of at least

10 mL of blood should be removed and discarded from a heparinized line before blood samples are sent for coagulation testing.

Monitoring Parameters Hemoglobin, hematocrit, signs of bleeding; fecal occult blood test; aPTT (or antifactor Xa activity levels) or ACT depending upon indication

Platelet counts should be routinely monitored when the risk of HIT is >0.1% (eg, receiving therapeutic dose heparin, postoperative antithrombotic prophylaxis), if the patient has received heparin or low molecular weight heparin (eg, enoxaparin) within the past 100 days, if preexposure history is uncertain, or if anaphylactoid reaction to heparin occurs. When the risk of HIT is <0.1% (eg, medical/obstetrical patients receiving heparin flushes), routine platelet count monitoring is not recommended (Hirsh, 2008).

For intermittent I.V. injections, aPTT is measured 3.5-4 hours after I.V. injection.

For SubQ injections, when used for treatment (eg, monitored dosing regimen), aPTT is measured 6 hours after injection.

Note: Continuous I.V. infusion is preferred over I.V. intermittent injections. For full-dose heparin (ie, nonlow-dose), the dose should be titrated according to aPTT results. For anticoagulation, an aPTT 1.5-2.5 times normal is usually desired. Because of variation among hospitals in the control aPTT values, nomograms should be established at each institution, designed to achieve aPTT values in the target range (eg, for a control aPTT of 30 seconds, the target range [1.5-2.5 times control] would be 45-75 seconds). Measurements should be made prior to heparin therapy, 6 hours (pediatric: 4 hours) after initiation, and 6 hours (pediatric: 4 hours) after any dosage change, and should be used to adjust the heparin infusion until the aPTT exhibits a therapeutic level. When two consecutive aPTT values are therapeutic, subsequent measurements may be made every 24 hours, and if necessary, dose adjustment carried out. In addition, a significant change in the patient's clinical condition (eg, recurrent ischemia, bleeding, hypotension) should prompt an immediate aPTT determination, followed by dose adjustment if necessary. In general, may increase or decrease infusion by 2-4 units/kg/hour dependent upon aPTT.

Heparin infusion dose adjustment: A number of dose-adjustment nomograms have been developed which target an aPTT range of 1.5-2.5 times control (Cruickshank, 1991; Flaker, 1994; Hull, 1992; Raschke, 1993). However, institution-specific and indication-specific nomograms should be consulted for dose adjustment. **Note:** aPTT values vary throughout the day with maximum values occurring during the night (Decousus, 1985).

Test Interactions Increased thyroxine (competitive protein binding methods); increased PT

Aprotinin significantly increases aPTT and celite Activated Clotting Time (ACT) which may not reflect the actual degree of anticoagulation by heparin. Kaolin-based ACTs are not affected by aprotinin to the same degree as celite ACTs. While institutional protocols may vary, a minimal celite ACT of 750 seconds or kaolin-ACT of 480 seconds is recommended in the presence of aprotinin. Consult the manufacturer's information on specific ACT test interpretation in the presence of aprotinin.

Dosage Forms Excipient information presented when available (limited, particularly for generics); consult specific product labeling.

Infusion, as sodium [premixed in NaCl 0.45%; porcine intestinal mucosa source]: 12,500 units (250 mL); 25,000 units (250 mL, 500 mL)

Infusion, as sodium [preservative free; premixed in D_5W; porcine intestinal mucosa source]: 10,000 units (100 mL) [contains sodium metabisulfite]; 12,500 units (250 mL) [contains sodium metabisulfite]; 20,000 units (500 mL) [contains sodium metabisulfite]; 25,000 units (250 mL, 500 mL) [contains sodium metabisulfite]

Infusion, as sodium [preservative free; premixed in NaCl 0.9%; porcine intestinal mucosa source]: 1000 units (500 mL); 2000 units (1000 mL)

Injection, solution, as sodium [lock flush preparation; porcine intestinal mucosa source; multidose vial]: 10 units/mL (1 mL, 10 mL, 30 mL) [contains parabens]; 100 units/mL (1 mL, 5 mL) [contains parabens]

Injection, solution, as sodium [lock flush preparation; porcine intestinal mucosa source; multidose vial]: 10 units/mL (10 mL, 30 mL); 100 units/mL (10 mL, 30 mL) [contains benzyl alcohol]

Hep-Lock®: 10 units/mL (1 mL, 2 mL, 10 mL, 30 mL); 100 units/mL (1 mL, 2 mL, 10 mL, 30 mL) [contains benzyl alcohol]

Injection, solution, as sodium [lock flush preparation; porcine intestinal mucosa source; prefilled syringe]: 10 units/mL (1 mL, 2 mL, 3 mL, 5 mL); 100 units/mL (1 mL, 2 mL, 3 mL, 5 mL) [contains benzyl alcohol]

Injection, solution, as sodium [preservative free; lock flush preparation; porcine intestinal mucosa source; prefilled syringe]: 1 unit/mL (2 mL, 3 mL, 5 mL); 2 units/mL (3 mL); 10 units/mL (2.5 mL, 3 mL, 5 mL, 10 mL); 100 units/mL (3 mL, 5 mL, 10 mL)

Injection, solution, as sodium [preservative free; lock flush preparation; porcine intestinal mucosa source; vial]:

HepFlush®-10: 10 units/mL (10 mL)

Hep-Lock U/P: 10 units/mL (1 mL); 100 units/mL (1 mL)

Injection, solution, as sodium [porcine intestinal mucosa source; multidose vial]: 1000 units/mL (1 mL, 10 mL, 30 mL) [contains benzyl alcohol]; 1000 units/mL (1 mL, 10 mL, 30 mL) [contains methylparabens]; 5000 units/mL (1 mL, 10 mL) [contains benzyl alcohol]; 5000 units/mL (1 mL) [contains methylparabens]; 10,000 units/mL (1 mL, 4 mL) [contains benzyl alcohol]; 10,000 units/mL (1 mL, 5 mL) [contains methylparabens]; 20,000 units/mL (1 mL) [contains methylparabens]

Injection, solution, as sodium [porcine intestinal mucosa source; prefilled syringe]: 5000 units/mL (1 mL) [contains benzyl alcohol]

Injection, solution, as sodium [preservative free; porcine intestinal mucosa source; prefilled syringe]: 10,000 units/mL (0.5 mL)

Injection, solution, as sodium [preservative free; porcine intestinal mucosa source; vial]: 1000 units/mL (2 mL); 2000 units/mL (5 mL); 2500 units/mL (10 mL)

References

Dager WE and White RH, "Pharmacotherapy of Heparin-Induced Thrombocytopenia," *Expert Opin Pharmacother*, 2003, 4(6):919-40.

Francis JL, Groce JB 3rd, and the Heparin Consensus Group, "Challenges in Variation and Response of Unfractionated Heparin," *Pharmacotherapy*, 2004, 24(8 Pt 2), 108-19.

Hirsh J, Guyatt G, Albers GW, et al, "Executive Summary: American College of Chest Physicians Evidence-Based Clinical Practice Guidelines (8th Edition)," *Chest*, 2008, 133(6 Suppl):71-109.

Hull RD, Raskob GE, Rosenbloom D, et al, "Optimal Therapeutic Level of Heparin Therapy in Patients with Venous Thromboembolism," *Arch Intern Med*, 1992, 152(8):1589-95.

Klerk CP, Smorenburg SM, and Buller HR, "Thrombosis Prophylaxis in Patient Populations With a Central Venous Catheter: A Systematic Review," *Arch Intern Med*, 2003, 163(16):1913-21.

Raschke RA, Reilly BM, Guidry JR, et al, "The Weight-Based Heparin Dosing Nomogram Compared With a "Standard Care" Nomogram: A Randomized Controlled Trial," *Ann Intern Med*, 1993, 119(9):874-81.

◀

Warkentin TE, Greinacher A, Koster A, et al, "Treatment and Prevention of Heparin-induced Thrombocytopenia: American College of Chest Physicians Evidence-Based Clinical Practice Guidelines (8th Edition)," *Chest*, 2008, 133(6 Suppl):340-80.

◆ **Heparin Calcium** *see* Heparin *on page* 561

◆ **Heparin Cofactor I** *see* Antithrombin III *on page* 96

◆ **Heparin Lock Flush** *see* Heparin *on page* 561

◆ **Heparin Sodium** *see* Heparin *on page* 561

◆ **HepFlush®-10** *see* Heparin *on page* 561

◆ **Hep-Lock®** *see* Heparin *on page* 561

◆ **Hep-Lock U/P** *see* Heparin *on page* 561

◆ **Herceptin®** *see* Trastuzumab *on page* 1136

◆ **Hexalen®** *see* Altretamine *on page* 48

◆ **Hexamethylmelamine** *see* Altretamine *on page* 48

◆ **HEXM** *see* Altretamine *on page* 48

◆ **High-Molecular-Weight Iron Dextran (DexFerrum®)** *see* Iron Dextran Complex *on page* 658

◆ **Histantil (Can)** *see* Promethazine *on page* 997

Histrelin (his TREL in)

Related Information
Safe Handling of Hazardous Drugs *on page* 1517

U.S. Brand Names Supprelin® LA; Vantas™

Index Terms GnRH Agonist; Histrelin Acetate; LH-RH Agonist

Generic Available No

Canadian Brand Names Vantas™

Pharmacologic Category Gonadotropin Releasing Hormone Agonist

Use Palliative treatment of advanced prostate cancer; treatment of children with central precocious puberty (CPP)

Pregnancy Risk Factor X

Lactation Excretion in breast milk unknown/contraindicated

Labeled Contraindications Hypersensitivity to histrelin acetate, GnRH, GnRH-agonist analogs, or any component of the formulation; pregnancy

Warnings/Precautions
CPP: Transient increases in estradiol serum levels (female) or testosterone levels (female and male) may occur during the first week of use. Worsening symptoms may occur, however, manifestations of puberty should decrease within 4 weeks. Safety and efficacy have not been established in children <2 years of age

Prostate cancer: Transient increases in testosterone serum levels occur during the first week of use (initial flare). Worsening symptoms such as bone pain, hematuria, neuropathy, ureteral or bladder outlet obstruction, and spinal cord compression have been reported. Spinal cord compression and ureteral obstruction may contribute to paralysis; close attention should be given during the first few weeks of therapy to both patients having metastatic vertebral lesions and/or urinary tract obstructions, and to any patients reporting weakness, paresthesias or poor urine output. Safety and efficacy have not been established in patients with hepatic dysfunction.

Adverse Reactions

CPP:

>10%: Local: Insertion site reaction (51%; includes bruising, discomfort, itching, pain, protrusion of implant area, soreness, swelling, tingling)

>2% to 10%:

Endocrine & metabolic: Metrorrhagia (4%)

Local: Keloid scar (6%), scar (6%), suture-related complication (6%), pain at the application site (4%), post procedural pain (4%)

≤2%: Amblyopia, breast tenderness, cold feeling, disease progression, dysmenorrhea, epistaxis, erythema, flu-like syndrome, gynecomastia, headache, infection at the implant site, menorrhagia, migraine, mood swings, pituitary adenoma, pruritus, weight increase

Prostate cancer:

>10%:

Endocrine & metabolic: Hot flashes (66%)

Local: Implant site reaction (6% to 14%; includes bruising, erythema, pain, soreness, swelling, tenderness)

2% to 10%:

Central nervous system: Fatigue (10%), headache (3%), insomnia (3%)

Endocrine & metabolic: Gynecomastia (4%), sexual dysfunction (4%), libido decreased (2%)

Gastrointestinal: Constipation (4%), weight gain (2%)

Genitourinary: Expected pharmacological consequence of testosterone suppression: Testicular atrophy (5%)

Renal: Renal impairment (5%)

<2%: Abdominal discomfort, alopecia, anemia, appetite increased, arthralgia, AST increased, back pain, bone density decreased, bone pain, breast pain, breast tenderness, cold feeling, contusion, craving food, creatinine increased, depression, diaphoresis, dizziness, dyspnea (exertional), dysuria, fluid retention, flushing, genital pruritus, hematoma, hematuria, hypercalcemia, hypercholesterolemia, hyperglycemia, irritability, LDH increased, lethargy, limb pain, liver disorder, malaise, muscle twitching, myalgia, nausea, neck pain, night sweats, palpitation, peripheral edema, prostatic acid phosphatase increased, pruritus, renal calculi, renal failure, stent occlusion, testosterone increased, tremor, urinary frequency, urinary retention, ventricular asystoles, weakness, weight loss

Drug Interactions

Avoid Concomitant Use There are no known interactions where it is recommended to avoid concomitant use.

Increased Effect/Toxicity

Histrelin may increase the levels/effects of: Vitamin K Antagonists

Decreased Effect

Histrelin may decrease the levels/effects of: Antidiabetic Agents; Cardiac Glycosides; Vitamin K Antagonists

Storage/Stability Supprelin® LA, Vantas™: Upon delivery, separate contents of implant carton. Store implant under refrigeration at 2°C to 8°C (36°F to 46°F), wrapped in the amber pouch for protection from light. Do not freeze. The implantation kit does not require refrigeration.

Mechanism of Action Potent inhibitor of gonadotropin secretion; continuous administration results in, after an initiation phase, the suppression of luteinizing hormone (LH), follicle-stimulating hormone (FSH), and a subsequent decrease in testosterone (females and males) and estrogen (premenopausal females). Additionally, in patients with CPP, linear growth velocity is slowed (improves chance of attaining predicted adult height).

◀ **Pharmacodynamics/Kinetics**

Onset of action: Prostate cancer: Chemical castration: 2-4 weeks; CPP: progression of sexual development stops and growth is decreased in ~1 month

Duration: 1 year

Distribution: Adults: V_d: ~58 L

Protein binding: Adults: 70% ± 9%

Metabolism: Hepatic via C-terminal dealkylation and hydrolysis

Bioavailability: Adults: 92%

Half-life elimination: Adults: Terminal: ~4 hours

Time to peak, serum: Adults: 12 hours

Dosage SubQ:

Children ≥2 years: CPP (Supprelin® LA): 50 mg implant surgically inserted every 12 months. Discontinue at the appropriate time for the onset of puberty.

Adults: Prostate cancer (Vantas™): 50 mg implant surgically inserted every 12 months

Elderly: See adult dosing

Dosage adjustment in renal impairment: Cl_{cr}: 15-60 mL/minute: Adjustment not needed

Administration SubQ: Surgical implantation into the inner portion of the upper arm requires the use of the implantation device provided. Use the patient's nondominant arm for placement. Removal must occur after 12 months; a replacement implant may be required. Palpate area of incision to locate implant for removal. If not readily palpated, ultrasound, CT or MRI may be used to locate implant; plain films are not recommended because the implant is not radiopaque.

Monitoring Parameters

CPP: LH, FSH, estradiol, or testosterone (after 1 month then every 6 months); height, bone age (every 6-12 months); tanner staging

Prostate cancer: LH and FSH levels, serum testosterone levels, prostate specific antigen (PSA), bone mineral density; weakness, paresthesias, and urinary tract obstruction (especially during first few weeks of therapy)

Test Interactions Results of diagnostic test of pituitary gonadotropic and gonadal functions may be affected during and after therapy

Dosage Forms Excipient information presented when available (limited, particularly for generics); consult specific product labeling.

Implant, subcutaneous:

Supprelin® LA: 50 mg (1) [releases ~65 mcg/day over 12 months; packaged with implantation kit]

Vantas™: 50 mg (1) [releases 50-60 mcg/day over 12 months; packaged with implantation kit]

References

Dineen MK, Tierney DS, Kuzma P, et al, "An Evaluation of the Pharmacokinetics and Pharmacodynamics of the Histrelin Implant for the Palliative Treatment of Prostate Cancer," *J Clin Pharmacol*, 2005, 45(11):1245-9.

Schlegel PN, Histrelin Study Group, "Efficacy and Safety of Histrelin Subdermal Implant in Patients With Advanced Prostate Cancer," *J Urol*, 2006, 175(4):1353-8.

◆ **Histrelin Acetate** *see* Histrelin *on page 570*

◆ **HMM** *see* Altretamine *on page 48*

◆ **HN₂** *see* Mechlorethamine *on page 736*

◆ **Horse Antihuman Thymocyte Gamma Globulin** *see* Antithymocyte Globulin (Equine) *on page 98*

◆ **HPV4** *see* Papillomavirus (Types 6, 11, 16, 18) Vaccine (Human, Recombinant) *on page 922*

◆ **HPV Vaccine** *see* Papillomavirus (Types 6, 11, 16, 18) Vaccine (Human, Recombinant) *on page 922*

◆ **Humanized IgG1 Anti-CD52 Monoclonal Antibody** *see* Alemtuzumab *on page 30*

◆ **Human Papillomavirus Vaccine** *see* Papillomavirus (Types 6, 11, 16, 18) Vaccine (Human, Recombinant) *on page 922*

◆ **Human Thyroid Stimulating Hormone** *see* Thyrotropin Alfa *on page 1103*

◆ **HXM** *see* Altretamine *on page 48*

Hyaluronidase (hye al yoor ON i dase)

Medication Safety Issues
Sound-alike/look-alike issues:
Wydase may be confused with Lidex®, Wyamine®

Related Information
Management of Drug Extravasations *on page 1447*

U.S. Brand Names Amphadase™; Hydase™; Hylenex™; Vitrase®

Generic Available No

Pharmacologic Category Enzyme

Use Increase the dispersion and absorption of other injected drugs; increase rate of absorption of parenteral fluids given by subcutaneous administration (hypodermoclysis)

Unlabeled/Investigational Use Management of drug extravasations; local anesthetic adjuvant in bupivacaine-lidocaine mixture for retrobulbar/peribulbar block

Pregnancy Risk Factor C

Lactation Excretion in breast milk unknown/use caution

Labeled Contraindications Hypersensitivity to hyaluronidase or any component of the formulation

Warnings/Precautions Do not inject in or around infected or inflamed areas; may spread localized infection. Should not be used for extravasation management of dopamine or alpha agonists, or to reduce swelling of bites or stings. Do not administer intravenously. Do not apply directly to the cornea. Discontinue if sensitization occurs.

Adverse Reactions
Frequency not defined:
Cardiovascular: Edema

Local: Injection site reactions

<1%: Allergic reactions, anaphylactic-like reactions (retrobulbar block or I.V. injections), angioedema, urticaria

Drug Interactions
Avoid Concomitant Use There are no known interactions where it is recommended to avoid concomitant use.

Increased Effect/Toxicity There are no known significant interactions involving an increase in effect.

Decreased Effect There are no known significant interactions involving a decrease in effect.

Storage/Stability
Amphadase™, Hydase™, Hylenex™: Store in refrigerator at 2°C to 8°C (35°F to 46°F); do not freeze.

Vitrase®: Store unopened vial in refrigerator at 2°C to 8°C (35°F to 46°F). After reconstitution, store at 20°C to 25°C (68°F to 77°F) and use within 6 hours.

Reconstitution Vitrase®: Add 6.2 mL of NaCl to vial (1000 units/mL). Further dilute with NaCl before administration.

For 50 units/mL, draw up 0.05 mL of hyaluronidase reconstituted solution (1000 units/mL) and add 0.95 mL of NaCl.

For 75 units/mL, draw up 0.075 mL of hyaluronidase reconstituted solution and add 0.925 mL of NaCl.

For 150 units/mL, draw up 0.15 mL of hyaluronidase reconstituted solution and add 0.85 mL of NaCl.

For 300 units/mL, draw up 0.3 mL of hyaluronidase reconstituted solution and add 0.7 mL of NaCl.

Compatibility Stable in dextran 6% in dextrose, dextran 6% in NS, D_5LR, $D_5^1/_4NS$, $D_5^1/_2NS$, D_5NS, D_5W, $D_{10}W$, LR, $^1/_2NS$, NS.

Compatibility in syringe: Compatible: Diatrizoate meglumine 34.3%, diatrizoate sodium 35%, iothalamate meglumine 60%, iothalamate sodium 80%, pentobarbital, thiopental. **Incompatible:** Hydromorphone. **Variable (consult detailed reference):** Diatrizoate meglumine 52%, diatrizoate sodium 8%, diatrizoate sodium 75%, iodipamide meglumine 52%.

Compatibility when admixed: Compatible: Amikacin, sodium bicarbonate. **Incompatible:** Benzodiazepines, epinephrine, furosemide, heparin, phenytoin.

Mechanism of Action Modifies the permeability of connective tissue through hydrolysis of hyaluronic acid, one of the chief components of tissue cement which offers resistance to diffusion of liquids through tissues; hyaluronidase increases both the distribution and absorption of locally injected substances.

Pharmacodynamics/Kinetics

Onset of action: SubQ: Immediate

Duration: 24-48 hours

Dosage Note: A preliminary skin test for hypersensitivity can be performed.

Skin test: Intradermal: 0.02 mL (3 units) of a 150 units/mL solution. Positive reaction consists of a wheal with pseudopods appearing within 5 minutes and persisting for 20-30 minutes with localized itching.

Hypodermoclysis: SubQ: Infants and Children: 150 units followed by subcutaneous isotonic fluid administration at a rate appropriate for age, weight, and clinical condition of the patient; 150 units facilitates absorption of >1000 mL of solution **or** add 15 units to each 100 mL of I.V. fluid to be administered subcutaneously

Premature Infants and Neonates: Volume of a single clysis should not exceed 25 mL/kg and the rate of administration should not exceed 2 mL/minute

Children <3 years (Amphadase™, Hydase™, Vitrase®): Volume of a single clysis should not exceed 200 mL

Children ≥3 years and Adults: Rate and volume of a single clysis should not exceed those used for infusion of I.V. fluids

Extravasation (unlabeled use): Adults: SubQ: Inject 1 mL of a 150 unit/mL solution (as 5-10 injections of 0.1-0.2 mL) into affected area; doses of 15-250 units have been reported. **Note:** Do not use for extravasation of pressor agents (eg, dopamine, norepinephrine).

Elderly: See adult dosing. Adjust dose carefully to individual patient.

Administration Do **not** administer I.V.

Additional Information

Amphadase™: pH: 6.8

Hydase™: pH: 6.9, osmolality: 275-305 mOsm

Hylenex™: pH: 7.4, osmolality: 290-350 mOsm

Vitrase®: pH: ~6.7

Dosage Forms Excipient information presented when available (limited, particularly for generics); consult specific product labeling.

Injection, powder for reconstitution:

Vitrase®: 6200 units [ovine derived; contains lactose]

Injection, solution:

Amphadase™: 150 units/mL (1 mL) [bovine derived; contains edetate disodium 1 mg, thimerosal ≤0.1 mg]

Injection, solution [preservative free]:

Hydase™: 150 units/mL (1 mL) [bovine derived; contains edetate disodium 1 mg]

Hylenex™: 150 units/mL (1 mL, 2 mL) [recombinant; contains human albumin and edetate disodium]

Vitrase®: 200 units/mL (2 mL) [ovine derived; contains lactose]

References

Albanell J and Baselga J, "Systemic Therapy Emergencies," *Semin Oncol*, 2000, 27(3):347-61.

Bertelli G, "Prevention and Management of Extravasation of Cytotoxic Drugs," *Drug Saf*, 1995, 12 (4):245-55.

Bertelli G, Dini D, Forno GB, et al, "Hyaluronidase as an Antidote to Extravasation of Vinca Alkaloids: Clinical Results," *J Cancer Res Clin Oncol*, 1994, 120(8):505-6.

Cochran ST, Bomyea K, and Kahn M, "Treatment of Iodinated Contrast Material Extravasation With Hyaluronidase," *Acad Radiol*, 2002, 9(Suppl 2):544-6.

Dorr RT, "Vinca Alkaloid Ulceration: Experimental Mouse Model and Effects of Local Antidotes," *Proc Am Soc Clin Oncol*, 1982, 1:428.

Elam EA, Dorr RT, Lagel KE, et al, "Cutaneous Ulceration Due to Contrast Extravasation. Experimental Assessment of Injury and Potential Antidotes," *Invest Radiol*, 1991, 26(1):13-6.

Kallio H, Paloheimo M, and Maunuksela EL, "Hyaluronidase as an Adjuvant in Bupivacaine-Lidocaine Mixture for Retrobulbar/Peribulbar Block," *Anesth Analg*, 2000, 91(4):934-7.

Kumar MM and Sprung J, "The Use of Hyaluronidase to Treat Mannitol Extravasation," *Anesth Analg*, 2003, 97(4):1199-200.

Raszka WV Jr, Kueser TK, Smith FR, et al, "The Use of Hyaluronidase in the Treatment of Intravenous Extravasation Injuries," *J Perinatol*, 19909, 10(2):146-9.

Sokol DK, Dahlmann A, and Dunn DW, "Hyaluronidase Treatment for Intravenous Phenytoin Extravasation," *J Child Neurol*, 1998, 13(5):246-7.

Zenk KE, "Hyaluronidase: An Antidote for Intravenous Extravasations," *CSHP Voice*, 1981, 66-8.

Zenk KE, "Management of Intravenous Extravasations," *Infusion*, 1981, 5:77-9.

Zenk KE, "Treating I.V. Extravasations With Hyaluronidase," *ASHP Signal*, 1986, 10:25,29.

♦ **Hycamptamine** *see* Topotecan *on page 1116*

♦ **Hycamtin®** *see* Topotecan *on page 1116*

♦ **Hycort™ (Can)** *see* Hydrocortisone *on page 575*

♦ **Hydase™** *see* Hyaluronidase *on page 573*

♦ **Hydeltra T.B.A.® (Can)** *see* PrednisoLONE *on page 977*

♦ **Hyderm (Can)** *see* Hydrocortisone *on page 575*

♦ **Hydrea®** *see* Hydroxyurea *on page 589*

Hydrocortisone (hye droe KOR ti sone)

Medication Safety Issues

Sound-alike/look-alike issues:

Hydrocortisone may be confused with hydrocodone, hydroxychloroquine, hydrochlorothiazide

Anusol® may be confused with Anusol-HC®, Aplisol®, Aquasol®

Anusol-HC® may be confused with Anusol®

Cortef® may be confused with Coreg®, Lortab®

Cortizone® may be confused with cortisone

HCT (occasional abbreviation for hydrocortisone) is an error-prone abbreviation (mistaken as hydrochlorothiazide)

Hytone® may be confused with Vytone®
Proctocort® may be confused with ProctoCream®
ProctoCream® may be confused with Proctocort®
Solu-Cortef® may be confused with Solu-Medrol®

International issues:

Hytone® may be confused with Hysone® [Australia]

Nutracort® may be confused with Nitrocor® which is a brand name of nitroglycerin in Chile and Italy

U.S. Brand Names Anucort-HC®; Anusol-HC®; Anusol® HC-1 [OTC]; Aquanil™ HC [OTC]; Beta-HC®; Caldecort® [OTC]; Cetacort® [DSC]; Colocort®; Cortaid® Intensive Therapy [OTC]; Cortaid® Maximum Strength [OTC]; Cortaid® Sensitive Skin [OTC]; Cortef®; Cortenema®; Corticool® [OTC]; Cortifoam®; Cortizone-10® Maximum Strength Cooling Relief [OTC]; Cortizone-10® Maximum Strength Easy Relief [OTC]; Cortizone-10® Maximum Strength Intensive Healing Formula [OTC]; Cortizone-10® Maximum Strength [OTC]; Cortizone-10® Plus Maximum Strength [OTC]; Cortizone-10® Quick Shot [OTC] [DSC]; Dermarest Dricort® [OTC]; Dermtex® HC [OTC]; Encort™; Hemril®-30; Hydro-Rx; HydroZone Plus [OTC]; Hytone® [DSC]; IvySoothe® [OTC]; Locoid Lipocream®; Locoid®; Nupercainal® Hydrocortisone Cream [OTC]; Nutracort®; Pandel®; Post Peel Healing Balm [OTC]; Preparation H® Hydrocortisone [OTC]; Procto-Kit™; Procto-Pak™; Proctocort®; ProctoCream® HC; Proctosert; Proctosol-HC®; Proctozone-HC™; Sarnol-HC [OTC]; Solu-Cortef®; Summer's Eve® SpecialCare™ Medicated Anti-Itch Cream [OTC] [DSC]; Texacort®; Tucks® Anti-Itch [OTC]; Westcort®

Index Terms A-hydroCort; Compound F; Cortisol; Hemorrhoidal HC; Hydrocortisone Acetate; Hydrocortisone Butyrate; Hydrocortisone Probutate; Hydrocortisone Sodium Succinate; Hydrocortisone Valerate

Generic Available Yes: Excludes acetate foam, butyrate cream and ointment, gel as base, otic drops as base, probutate cream, sodium succinate injection

Canadian Brand Names Aquacort®; Cortamed®; Cortef®; Cortenema®; Cortifoam™; Emo-Cort®; Hycort™; Hyderm; HydroVal®; Locoid®; Prevex® HC; Sarna® HC; Solu-Cortef®; Westcort®

Pharmacologic Category Corticosteroid, Rectal; Corticosteroid, Systemic; Corticosteroid, Topical

Use Management of adrenocortical insufficiency; relief of inflammation of corticosteroid-responsive dermatoses (low and medium potency topical corticosteroid); adjunctive treatment of ulcerative colitis

Unlabeled/Investigational Use Management of septic shock when blood pressure is poorly responsive to fluid resuscitation and vasopressor therapy

Pregnancy Risk Factor C

Lactation Enters breast milk/use caution

Labeled Contraindications Hypersensitivity to hydrocortisone or any component of the formulation; serious infections, except septic shock or tuberculous meningitis; viral, fungal, or tubercular skin lesions; I.M. administration contraindicated in idiopathic thrombocytopenia purpura

Rectal suspension: Systemic fungal infections; ileocolostomy during the immediate or early postoperative period

Warnings/Precautions Use with caution in patients with thyroid disease, hepatic impairment, renal impairment, heart failure, hypertension, diabetes, glaucoma, cataracts, myasthenia gravis, patients at risk for osteoporosis, patients at risk for seizures, or GI diseases (diverticulitis, peptic ulcer, ulcerative colitis) due to perforation risk. Use caution following acute MI (corticosteroids have been associated with myocardial rupture). Because of the risk of adverse effects, systemic corticosteroids should be used cautiously in the elderly in the smallest possible effective dose for the shortest duration. May affect growth velocity; growth should be routinely monitored in pediatric patients. Withdraw therapy with gradual tapering of dose.

May cause hypercorticism or suppression of hypothalamic-pituitary-adrenal (HPA) axis, particularly in younger children or in patients receiving high doses for prolonged periods. HPA axis suppression may lead to adrenal crisis. Withdrawal and discontinuation of a corticosteroid should be done slowly and carefully. Particular care is required when patients are transferred from systemic corticosteroids to inhaled products due to possible adrenal insufficiency or withdrawal from steroids, including an increase in allergic symptoms. Patients receiving >20 mg per day of prednisone (or equivalent) may be most susceptible. Fatalities have occurred due to adrenal insufficiency in asthmatic patients during and after transfer from systemic corticosteroids to aerosol steroids; aerosol steroids do not provide the systemic steroid needed to treat patients having trauma, surgery, or infections. Avoid use of topical preparations with occlusive dressings or on weeping or exudative lesions. Some dosage forms may contain benzyl alcohol which has been associated with "gasping syndrome" in neonates.

Acute myopathy has been reported with high dose corticosteroids, usually in patients with neuromuscular transmission disorders; may involve ocular and/or respiratory muscles; monitor creatine kinase; recovery may be delayed. Corticosteroid use may cause psychiatric disturbances, including depression, euphoria, insomnia, mood swings, and personality changes. Pre-existing psychiatric conditions may be exacerbated by corticosteroid use. Prolonged use of corticosteroids may also increase the incidence of secondary infection, mask acute infection (including fungal infections), prolong or exacerbate viral infections, or limit response to vaccines. Exposure to chickenpox should be avoided; corticosteroids should not be used to treat ocular herpes simplex. Corticosteroids should not be used for cerebral malaria or viral hepatitis. Close observation is required in patients with latent tuberculosis and/or TB reactivity; restrict use in active TB (only in conjunction with antituberculosis treatment). Prolonged treatment with corticosteroids has been associated with the development of Kaposi's sarcoma (case reports); if noted, discontinuation of therapy should be considered. High-dose corticosteroids should not be used to manage acute head injury.

Adverse Reactions

Systemic: Frequency not defined:

Cardiovascular: Edema, hypertension

Central nervous system: Delirium, euphoria, hallucinations, headache, insomnia, nervousness, pseudotumor cerebri, psychoses, seizure, vertigo

Dermatologic: Bruising, hyperpigmentation, skin atrophy

Endocrine & metabolic: Adrenal suppression, alkalosis, amenorrhea, Cushing's syndrome, diabetes mellitus, glucose intolerance, growth suppression, hyperglycemia, hyperlipidemia, hypokalemia, pituitary-adrenal axis suppression, sodium and water retention

Gastrointestinal: Abdominal distention, appetite increased, indigestion, nausea, pancreatitis, peptic ulcer, ulcerative esophagitis, vomiting

Hematologic: Leukocytosis (transient)

Neuromuscular & skeletal: Arthralgia, fractures, muscle weakness, osteoporosis

Ocular: Cataracts, glaucoma

Miscellaneous: Avascular necrosis, hypersensitivity reactions, infection, secondary malignancy

Topical:
>10%: Dermatologic: Eczema (12.5%)
1% to 10%: Dermatologic: Pruritus (6%), stinging (2%), dry skin (2%)
<1%: Allergic contact dermatitis, burning, dermal atrophy, folliculitis, HPA axis suppression, hypopigmentation; metabolic effects (hyperglycemia, hypokalemia); striae

Drug Interactions
Metabolism/Transport Effects Substrate of CYP3A4 (minor); **Induces** CYP3A4 (weak)

Avoid Concomitant Use
Avoid concomitant use of Hydrocortisone with any of the following: Natalizumab; Vaccines (Live)

Increased Effect/Toxicity
Hydrocortisone may increase the levels/effects of: Acetylcholinesterase Inhibitors; Amphotericin B; CycloSPORINE; Leflunomide; Loop Diuretics; Natalizumab; NSAID (COX-2 Inhibitor); NSAID (Nonselective); Thiazide Diuretics; Vaccines (Live); Warfarin

The levels/effects of Hydrocortisone may be increased by: Antifungal Agents (Azole Derivatives, Systemic); Aprepitant; Calcium Channel Blockers (Nondihydropyridine); CycloSPORINE; Estrogen Derivatives; Fluconazole; Fosaprepitant; Macrolide Antibiotics; Neuromuscular-Blocking Agents (Nondepolarizing); P-Glycoprotein Inhibitors; Quinolone Antibiotics; Salicylates; Trastuzumab

Decreased Effect
Hydrocortisone may decrease the levels/effects of: Antidiabetic Agents; Calcitriol; Corticorelin; Isoniazid; Salicylates; Vaccines (Inactivated); Vaccines (Live)

The levels/effects of Hydrocortisone may be decreased by: Aminoglutethimide; Antacids; Barbiturates; Bile Acid Sequestrants; Echinacea; Mitotane; P-Glycoprotein Inducers; Primidone; Rifamycin Derivatives

Ethanol/Nutrition/Herb Interactions
Ethanol: Avoid ethanol (may enhance gastric mucosal irritation).
Food: Hydrocortisone interferes with calcium absorption.
Herb/Nutraceutical: St John's wort may decrease hydrocortisone levels. Avoid cat's claw, echinacea (have immunostimulant properties).

Storage/Stability Store at controlled room temperature 20°C to 25°C (68°F to 77°F). Protect from light. Hydrocortisone sodium phosphate and hydrocortisone sodium succinate are clear, light yellow solutions which are heat labile.

Sodium succinate: After initial reconstitution, hydrocortisone sodium succinate solutions are stable for 3 days at room temperature or under refrigeration when protected from light. Stability of parenteral admixture (Solu-Cortef®) at room temperature (25°C) and at refrigeration temperature (4°C) is concentration-dependent:
Stability of concentration 1 mg/mL: 24 hours.
Stability of concentration 2 mg/mL to 60 mg/mL: At least 4 hours.

Reconstitution
Sodium succinate: Reconstitute 100 mg vials with bacteriostatic water (not >2 mL). Act-O-Vial (self-contained powder for injection plus diluent) may be reconstituted by pressing the activator to force diluent into the powder

compartment. Following gentle agitation, solution may be withdrawn via syringe through a needle inserted into the center of the stopper. May be administered (I.V. or I.M.) without further dilution.

Solutions for I.V. infusion: Reconstituted solutions may be added to an appropriate volume of compatible solution for infusion. Concentration should generally not exceed 1 mg/mL. However, in cases where administration of a small volume of fluid is desirable, 100-3000 mg may be added to 50 mL of D5W or NS (stability limited to 4 hours).

Compatibility

Hydrocortisone sodium phosphate: Stable in D5W, NS, fat emulsion 10%.

Y-site administration: Compatible: Allopurinol, amifostine, aztreonam, cefepime, cladribine, clarithromycin, docetaxel, etoposide, famotidine, filgrastim, fluconazole, fludarabine, gemcitabine, granisetron, melphalan, ondansetron, paclitaxel, piperacillin/tazobactam, teniposide, thiotepa, vinorelbine. **Incompatible:** Sargramostim.

Compatibility in syringe: Compatible: Metoclopramide. **Incompatible:** Doxapram.

Compatibility when admixed: Compatible: Amikacin, amphotericin B, amphotericin B with heparin, bleomycin, dacarbazine, metaraminol, sodium bicarbonate, verapamil. **Variable (consult detailed reference):** Mitoxantrone.

Hydrocortisone sodium succinate: Stable in dextran 6% in dextrose, dextran 6% in NS, D5LR, D5¼NS, D5½NS, D5NS, D5W, D10W, D20W, LR, ½NS, NS, fat emulsion 10%.

Y-site administration: Compatible: Acyclovir, allopurinol, amifostine, aminophylline, amphotericin B cholesteryl sulfate complex, ampicillin, amsacrine, argatroban, atracurium, atropine, aztreonam, betamethasone sodium phosphate, bivalirudin, calcium gluconate, cefepime, chlordiazepoxide, chlorpromazine, cisatracurium, cladribine, cyanocobalamin, cytarabine, dexamethasone sodium phosphate, digoxin, diphenhydramine, docetaxel, dopamine, doxorubicin liposome, droperidol, droperidol and fentanyl, edrophonium, enalaprilat, epinephrine, esmolol, estrogens (conjugated), ethacrynate sodium, etoposide, famotidine, fentanyl, filgrastim, fludarabine, fluorouracil, foscarnet, furosemide, gatifloxacin, gemcitabine, granisetron, heparin, hydralazine, inamrinone, insulin (regular), isoproterenol, kanamycin, lidocaine, linezolid, lorazepam, magnesium sulfate, melphalan, menadiol sodium diphosphate, meperidine, methoxamine, methylergonovine, minocycline, morphine, neostigmine, nicardipine, norepinephrine, ondansetron, oxacillin, oxytocin, paclitaxel, pancuronium, penicillin G potassium, pentazocine, phytonadione, piperacillin/tazobactam, procainamide, prochlorperazine edisylate, propofol, propranolol, pyridostigmine, remifentanil, scopolamine, sodium bicarbonate, succinylcholine, tacrolimus, teniposide, theophylline, thiotepa, trimethaphan camsylate, trimethobenzamide, vecuronium, vinorelbine. **Incompatible:** Ciprofloxacin, diazepam, ergotamine, idarubicin, midazolam, phenytoin, sargramostim. **Variable (consult detailed reference):** Diltiazem, methylprednisolone sodium succinate, promethazine.

Compatibility in syringe: Compatible: Diatrizoate meglumine 52%, diatrizoate sodium 8%, diatrizoate sodium 60%, iohexol, iopamidol, iothalamate meglumine 60%, ioxaglate meglumine 39.3%, ioxaglate sodium 19.6%, metoclopramide, thiopental. **Incompatible:** Doxapram.

Compatibility when admixed: Compatible: Amikacin, aminophylline, amphotericin B, calcium chloride, calcium gluconate, chloramphenicol, clindamycin, corticotropin, daunorubicin, diphenhydramine, dopamine, erythromycin lactobionate, floxacillin, lidocaine, magnesium sulfate, mephentermine, metronidazole, metronidazole with sodium bicarbonate, mitomycin, mitoxantrone, norepinephrine, penicillin G potassium, penicillin G sodium, piperacillin, polymyxin B sulfate, potassium chloride, procaine, sodium bicarbonate, theophylline, thiopental, vancomycin, verapamil, vitamin B complex with C. **Incompatible:** Aminophylline with cephalothin, bleomycin, colistimethate, ephedrine, hydralazine, nafcillin, pentobarbital, phenobarbital, prochlorperazine edisylate, promethazine. **Variable (consult detailed reference):** Amobarbital, ampicillin, cytarabine, dimenhydrinate, furosemide, heparin, kanamycin, metaraminol.

Mechanism of Action Decreases inflammation by suppression of migration of polymorphonuclear leukocytes and reversal of increased capillary permeability

Pharmacodynamics/Kinetics

Onset of action:
  Hydrocortisone acetate: Slow
  Hydrocortisone sodium succinate (water soluble): Rapid
Duration: Hydrocortisone acetate: Long
Absorption: Rapid by all routes, except rectally
Metabolism: Hepatic
Half-life elimination: Biologic: 8-12 hours
Excretion: Urine (primarily as 17-hydroxysteroids and 17-ketosteroids)

Dosage Dose should be based on severity of disease and patient response

Adrenal hyperplasia (congenital): Children: Oral: Initial: 10-20 mg/m^2/day in 3 divided doses; a variety of dosing schedules have been used.

  Note: Inconsistencies have occurred with liquid formulations; tablets may provide more reliable levels. Doses must be individualized by monitoring growth, bone age, and hormonal levels. Mineralocorticoid and sodium supplementation may be required based upon electrolyte regulation and plasma renin activity.

Adrenal insufficiency (acute): I.M., I.V.:
  Infants and young Children: Succinate: 1-2 mg/kg/dose bolus, then 25-150 mg/day in divided doses every 6-8 hours
  Older Children: Succinate: 1-2 mg/kg bolus then 150-250 mg/day in divided doses every 6-8 hours
  Adults: Succinate: 100 mg I.V. bolus, then 300 mg/day in divided doses every 8 hours or as a continuous infusion for 48 hours; once patient is stable change to oral, 50 mg every 8 hours for 6 doses, then taper to 30-50 mg/day in divided doses

Adrenal insufficiency (chronic): Adults: Oral: 20-30 mg/day

Anti-inflammatory or immunosuppressive:
  Infants and Children:
    Oral: 2.5-10 mg/kg/day **or** 75-300 mg/m^2/day every 6-8 hours
    I.M., I.V.: Succinate: 1-5 mg/kg/day **or** 30-150 mg/m^2/day divided every 12-24 hours
  Adolescents and Adults: Oral, I.M., I.V.: Succinate: 15-240 mg every 12 hours

Physiologic replacement: Children:
  Oral: 0.5-0.75 mg/kg/day **or** 20-25 mg/m^2/day every 8 hours
  I.M.: Succinate: 0.25-0.35 mg/kg/day **or** 12-15 mg/m^2/day once daily

Rheumatic diseases: Adults:
  Intralesional, intra-articular, soft tissue injection: Acetate:
    Large joints: 25 mg (up to 37.5 mg)
    Small joints: 10-25 mg
  Tendon sheaths: 5-12.5 mg
  Soft tissue infiltration: 25-50 mg (up to 75 mg)

Bursae: 25-37.5 mg

Ganglia: 12.5-25 mg

Septic shock (unlabeled use): I.V.: 50 mg every 6 hours (Annane, 2002; Marik, 2008). Taper slowly (for total of 11 days) and do not stop abruptly.

Note: Fludrocortisone is optional with use of hydrocortisone.

Shock: I.M., I.V.: Succinate:

Children: Initial: 50 mg/kg, then repeated in 4 hours and/or every 24 hours as needed

Adolescents and Adults: 500 mg to 2 g every 2-6 hours

Status asthmaticus: Children and Adults: I.V.: Succinate: 1-2 mg/kg/dose every 6 hours for 24 hours, then maintenance of 0.5-1 mg/kg every 6 hours

Stress dosing (surgery) in patients known to be adrenally-suppressed or on chronic systemic steroids: I.V.: Adults:

Minor stress (ie, inguinal herniorrhaphy): 25 mg/day for 1 day

Moderate stress (ie, joint replacement, cholecystectomy): 50-75 mg/day (25 mg every 8-12 hours) for 1-2 days

Major stress (pancreatoduodenectomy, esophagogastrectomy, cardiac surgery): 100-150 mg/day (50 mg every 8-12 hours) for 2-3 days

Dermatosis: Children >2 years and Adults: Topical: Apply to affected area 2-4 times/day (Buteprate: Apply once or twice daily). Therapy should be discontinued when control is achieved; if no improvement is seen, reassessment of diagnosis may be necessary.

Ulcerative colitis: Adults: Rectal: 10-100 mg 1-2 times/day for 2-3 weeks

Combination Regimens

Prostate cancer:

Estramustine + Docetaxel + Hydrocortisone on page 1314

Mitoxantrone + Hydrocortisone on page 1368

Administration

Oral: Administer with food or milk to decrease GI upset

Parenteral: Hydrocortisone sodium succinate may be administered by I.M. or I.V. routes

I.V. bolus: Dilute to 50 mg/mL and administer over 30 seconds or over 10 minutes for doses ≥500 mg

I.V. intermittent infusion: Dilute to 1 mg/mL and administer over 20-30 minutes

Topical: Apply a thin film to clean, dry skin and rub in gently

Monitoring Parameters Blood pressure, weight, serum glucose, and electrolytes

Dietary Considerations Systemic use of corticosteroids may require a diet with increased potassium, vitamins A, B_6, C, D, folate, calcium, zinc, phosphorus, and decreased sodium. Sodium content of 1 g (sodium succinate injection): 47.5 mg (2.07 mEq)

Additional Information Hydrocortisone base topical cream, lotion, and ointments in concentrations of 0.25%, 0.5%, and 1% may be OTC or prescription depending on the product labeling.

Dosage Forms Excipient information presented when available (limited, particularly for generics); consult specific product labeling. [DSC] = Discontinued product

Aerosol, rectal, as acetate:

Cortifoam®: 10% (15 g) [90 mg/applicator]

Cream, rectal, as acetate:

Nupercainal® Hydrocortisone Cream: 1% (30 g) [strength expressed as base]

◀ Cream, topical, as acetate: 0.5% (9 g, 30 g, 60 g) [available with aloe]; 1% (30 g, 454 g) [available with aloe]

Cream, topical, as base: 0.5% (30 g); 1% (1.5 g, 30 g, 114 g, 454 g); 2.5% (20 g, 30 g, 454 g)

Anusol-HC®: 2.5% (30 g) [contains benzyl alcohol]

Caldecort®: 1% (30 g) [contains aloe vera gel]

Cortaid® Intensive Therapy: 1% (60 g)

Cortaid® Maximum Strength: 1% (15 g, 30 g, 40 g, 60 g) [contains aloe vera gel and benzyl alcohol]

Cortaid® Sensitive Skin: 0.5% (15 g) [contains aloe vera gel]

Cortizone-10® Maximum Strength: 1% (15 g, 30 g, 60 g) [contains aloe]

Cortizone-10® Maximum Strength Intensive Healing Formula: 1% (28 g, 56 g) [contains aloe, benzyl alcohol]

Cortizone-10® Plus Maximum Strength: 1% (30 g, 60 g) [contains vitamins A, D, E and aloe]

Dermarest® Dricort®: 1% (15 g, 30 g)

HydroZone Plus, Proctocort®, Procto-Pak™: 1% (30 g)

Hytone®: 1% (30 g), 2.5% (30 g, 60 g) [DSC]

IvySoothe®: 1% (30 g) [contains aloe]

Post Peel Healing Balm: 1% (23 g)

Preparation H® Hydrocortisone: 1% (27 g) [contains sodium benzoate]

ProctoCream® HC: 2.5% (30 g) [contains benzyl alcohol]

Procto-Kit™: 1% (30 g) [packaged with applicator tips and finger cots]; 2.5% (30 g) [packaged with applicator tips and finger cots]

Proctosol-HC®, Proctozone-HC™: 2.5% (30 g)

Summer's Eve® SpecialCare™ Medicated Anti-Itch Cream: 1% (30 g) [DSC]

Cream, topical, as butyrate:

Locoid®: 0.1% (15 g, 45 g)

Locoid Lipocream®: 0.1% (15 g, 45 g)

Cream, topical, as probutate:

Pandel®: 0.1% (15 g, 45 g, 80 g)

Cream, topical, as valerate: 0.2% (15 g, 45 g, 60 g)

Westcort®: 0.2% (15 g, 45 g, 60 g)

Gel, topical, as base:

Corticool®: 1% (45 g)

Cortizone-10® Maximum Strength Cooling Relief: 1% (28 g) [contains aloe, ethanol 15%]

Injection, powder for reconstitution, as sodium succinate:

A-Hydrocort®: 100 mg [contains monobasic sodium phosphate 0.8 mg, anhydrous dibasic sodium phosphate 8.73 mg; strength expressed as base]

Solu-Cortef®: 100 mg, 250 mg, 500 mg, 1 g [diluent contains benzyl alcohol; strength expressed as base]

Lotion, topical, as base [spray]:

Cortizone-10® Maximum Strength Easy Relief: 1% (36 mL) [contains aloe, ethanol 45%]

Lotion, topical, as base: 1% (120 mL); 2.5% (60 mL)

Aquanil™ HC: 1% (120 mL)

Beta-HC®

Cetacort® [DSC]

HydroZone Plus: 1% (120 mL)

Hytone®: 2.5% (60 mL) [DSC]

Nutracort®: 1% (60 mL, 120 mL); 2.5% (60 mL, 120 mL)

Sarnol®-HC: 1% (60 mL)

Lotion, topical, as butyrate:

Locoid®: 0.1% (60 mL)

Ointment, topical, as acetate: 1% (30 g) [strength expressed as base; available with aloe]

Anusol® HC-1: 1% (21 g) [strength expressed as base]

Cortaid® Maximum Strength: 1% (15 g, 30 g) [strength expressed as base]

Ointment, topical, as base: 0.5% (30 g); 1% (30 g, 454 g); 2.5% (20 g, 30 g, 454 g)

Cortizone-10® Maximum Strength: 1% (30 g, 60 g)

Hytone®: 2.5% (30 g) [DSC]

Ointment, topical, as butyrate:

Locoid®: 0.1% (15 g, 45 g)

Ointment, topical, as valerate: 0.2% (15 g, 45 g, 60 g)

Westcort®: 0.2% (15 g, 45 g, 60 g)

Powder, for prescription compounding [micronized]:

Hydro-Rx: USP (10 g, 25 g, 50 g, 100 g)

Powder, for prescription compounding, as acetate [micronized]: USP (10 g, 25 g, 50 g)

Solution, topical, as base: 2.5% (30 mL)

Texacort®: 2.5% (30 mL) [contains ethanol 48%]

Solution, topical, as butyrate: 0.1% (20 mL, 60 mL)

Locoid®: 0.1% (20 mL, 60 mL) [contains alcohol 50%]

Solution, topical, as base [spray]:

Cortaid® Intensive Therapy: 1% (60 mL) [contains alcohol]

Cortizone-10® Quick Shot: 1% (44 mL) [contains benzyl alcohol] [DSC]

Dermtex® HC: 1% (52 mL) [contains menthol 1%]

Suppository, rectal, as acetate: 25 mg (12s [DSC]; 24s, 100s)

Anucort-HC®, Tucks® Anti-Itch: 25 mg (12s, 24s, 100s) [strength expressed as base; Anucort-HC® renamed Tucks® Anti-Itch]

Anusol-HC®, Proctosol-HC®: 25 mg (12s, 24s)

Encort™, Proctocort®: 30 mg (12s)

Hemril®-30, Proctosert: 30 mg (12s, 24s)

Suspension, rectal, as base: 100 mg/60 mL (1s, 7s)

Colocort®, Cortenema®: 100 mg/60 mL (1s, 7s)

Tablet, as base: 20 mg

Cortef®: 5 mg, 10 mg, 20 mg

References

Annane D, Sebille V, Charpentier C, et al, "Effect of Treatment With Low Doses of Hydrocortisone and Fludrocortisone on Mortality in Patients With Septic Shock," *JAMA*, 2002, 288(7):862-71.

Cooper MS and Stewart PM, "Corticosteroid Insufficiency in Acutely Ill Patients," *N Engl J Med*, 2003, 348(8):727-34.

Coursin DB and Wood KE, "Corticosteroid Supplementation for Adrenal Insufficiency," *JAMA*, 2002, 287(2):236-40.

Dellinger RP, Levy MM, Carlet JM, et al, "Surviving Sepsis Campaign: International Guidelines for Management of Severe Sepsis and Septic Shock: 2008," *Intensive Care Med*, 2008, 34(1):17-60. Available at http://www.survivingsepsis.org/system/files/images/2008_20International_20SSC_20Guidelines_1_.pdf

Goedert JJ, Vitale F, Lauria C, et al, "Risk Factors for Classical Kaposi's Sarcoma," *J Natl Cancer Inst*, 2002, 94(22):1712-8.

Hotchkiss RS and Karl IE, "The Pathophysiology and Treatment of Sepsis," *N Engl J Med*, 2003, 348(2):138-50.

Marik PE, Pastores SM, Annane D, et al, "Recommendations for the Diagnosis and Management of Corticosteroid Insufficiency in Critically Ill Adult Patients: Consensus Statements From an International Task Force by the American College of Critical Care Medicine," *Crit Care Med*, 2008, 36(6):1937-49.

Sprung CL, Annane D, Keh D, et al, "Hydrocortisone Therapy for Patients With Septic Shock," *N Engl J Med*, 2008, 358(2):111-24.

◆ **Hydrocortisone Acetate** *see* Hydrocortisone *on page 575*

◆ **Hydrocortisone Butyrate** *see* Hydrocortisone *on page 575*

◆ **Hydrocortisone Probutate** *see* Hydrocortisone *on page* 575

◆ **Hydrocortisone Sodium Succinate** *see* Hydrocortisone *on page* 575

◆ **Hydrocortisone Valerate** *see* Hydrocortisone *on page* 575

◆ **Hydromorph Contin® (Can)** *see* HYDROmorphone *on page* 584

◆ **Hydromorph-IR® (Can)** *see* HYDROmorphone *on page* 584

HYDROmorphone (hye droe MOR fone)

Medication Safety Issues

Sound-alike/look-alike issues:

Dilaudid® may be confused with Demerol®, Dilantin®

HYDROmorphone may be confused with morphine; significant overdoses have occurred when hydromorphone products have been inadvertently administered instead of morphine sulfate. Commercially available prefilled syringes of both products looks similar and are often stored in close proximity to each other. **Note:** Hydromorphone 1 mg oral is approximately equal to morphine 4 mg oral; hydromorphone 1 mg I.V. is approximately equal to morphine 5 mg I.V.

High alert medication: The Institute for Safe Medication Practices (ISMP) includes this medication among its list of drug classes which have a heightened risk of causing significant patient harm when used in error.

Dilaudid®, Dilaudid-HP®: Extreme caution should be taken to avoid confusing the highly-concentrated (Dilaudid-HP®) injection with the less-concentrated (Dilaudid®) injectable product.

Significant differences exist between oral and I.V. dosing. Use caution when converting from one route of administration to another.

U.S. Brand Names Dilaudid-HP®; Dilaudid®

Index Terms Dihydromorphinone; Hydromorphone Hydrochloride

Generic Available Yes: Excludes capsule, liquid, powder for injection

Canadian Brand Names Dilaudid-HP-Plus®; Dilaudid-HP®; Dilaudid-XP®; Dilaudid®; Dilaudid® Sterile Powder; Hydromorph Contin®; Hydromorph-IR®; Hydromorphone HP; Hydromorphone HP® 10; Hydromorphone HP® 20; Hydromorphone HP® 50; Hydromorphone HP® Forte; Hydromorphone Hydrochloride Injection, USP; PMS-Hydromorphone

Pharmacologic Category Analgesic, Opioid

Use Management of moderate-to-severe pain

Unlabeled/Investigational Use Antitussive

Restrictions C-II

Pregnancy Risk Factor C/D (prolonged use or high doses at term)

Lactation Excretion in breast milk unknown/not recommended

Labeled Contraindications Hypersensitivity to hydromorphone, any component of the formulation; acute or severe asthma, severe respiratory depression (in absence of resuscitative equipment or ventilatory support); severe CNS depression; pregnancy (prolonged use or high doses at term); obstetrical analgesia

Warnings/Precautions Use with caution in patients with hypersensitivity reactions to other phenanthrene derivative opioid agonists (codeine, hydrocodone, levorphanol, oxycodone, oxymorphone). Hydromorphone shares toxic potential of opiate agonists, including CNS depression and respiratory depression. Precautions associated with opiate agonist therapy should be observed. May cause CNS depression, which may impair physical or mental abilities; patients must be cautioned about performing tasks which require mental alertness (eg, operating machinery or driving). Myoclonus and seizures have been reported with high doses. Critical respiratory depression may occur, even at therapeutic dosages, particularly in elderly or debilitated patients or in patients with pre-existing respiratory compromise (hypoxia and/or hypercapnia). Use caution in COPD or other obstructive pulmonary disease. Use with caution in patients with hypersensitivity to other phenanthrene opiates, kyphoscoliosis, biliary tract disease, acute pancreatitis, morbid obesity, adrenocortical insufficiency, hypothyroidism, acute alcoholism, toxic psychoses, prostatic hyperplasia and/or urinary stricture, or severe liver or renal failure. Use extreme caution in patients with head injury, intracranial lesions, or elevated intracranial pressure; exaggerated elevation of ICP may occur (in addition, hydromorphone may complicate neurologic evaluation due to pupillary dilation and CNS depressant effects). Use with caution in patients with depleted blood volume or drugs which may exaggerate hypotensive effects (including phenothiazines or general anesthetics). May obscure diagnosis or clinical course of patients with acute abdominal conditions.

[U.S. Boxed Warning]: Hydromorphone has a high potential for abuse. Those at risk for opioid abuse include patients with a history of substance abuse or mental illness. Tolerance or drug dependence may result from extended use; however, concerns for abuse should not prevent effective management of pain. In general, abrupt discontinuation of therapy in dependent patients should be avoided.

An opioid-containing analgesic regimen should be tailored to each patient's needs and based upon the type of pain being treated (acute versus chronic), the route of administration, degree of tolerance for opioids (naive versus chronic user), age, weight, and medical condition. The optimal analgesic dose varies widely among patients. Doses should be titrated to pain relief/prevention. I.M. use may result in variable absorption and a lag time to peak effect.

Dosage form specific warnings:
  [U.S. Boxed Warning]: Dilaudid-HP®: Extreme caution should be taken to avoid confusing the highly-concentrated (Dilaudid-HP®) injection with the less-concentrated (Dilaudid®) injectable product. Dilaudid-HP® should only be used in patients who are opioid-tolerant.
  Controlled release: Capsules should only be used when continuous analgesia is required over an extended period of time. Controlled release products are not to be used on an "as needed" (PRN) basis.
  Some dosage forms contain trace amounts of sodium metabisulfite which may cause allergic reactions in susceptible individuals.

Adverse Reactions Frequency not defined.
Cardiovascular: Bradycardia, flushing of face, hyper-/hypotension, palpitation, peripheral vasodilation, syncope, tachycardia
Central nervous system: Agitation, chills, CNS depression, dizziness, drowsiness, dysphoria, euphoria, fatigue, hallucinations, headache, increased intracranial pressure, insomnia, lightheadedness, mental depression, nervousness, restlessness, sedation, seizure
Dermatologic: Pruritus, rash, urticaria
Endocrine & metabolic: Antidiuretic hormone release
Gastrointestinal: Anorexia, biliary tract spasm, constipation, diarrhea, nausea, paralytic ileus, stomach cramps, taste perversion, vomiting, xerostomia
Genitourinary: Ureteral spasm, urinary retention, urinary tract spasm, urination decreased
Hepatic: LFTs increased

▶

Local: Pain at injection site (I.M.), wheal/flare over vein (I.V.)

Neuromuscular & skeletal: Myoclonus, paresthesia, trembling, tremor, weakness

Ocular: Blurred vision, diplopia, miosis, nystagmus

Respiratory: Apnea, bronchospasm, dyspnea, laryngospasm, respiratory depression

Miscellaneous: Diaphoresis, histamine release, physical and psychological dependence

Drug Interactions

Avoid Concomitant Use There are no known interactions where it is recommended to avoid concomitant use.

Increased Effect/Toxicity

HYDROmorphone may increase the levels/effects of: Alcohol (Ethyl); Alvimopan; CNS Depressants; Desmopressin; Selective Serotonin Reuptake Inhibitors; Thiazide Diuretics

The levels/effects of HYDROmorphone may be increased by: Amphetamines; Antipsychotic Agents (Phenothiazines); Succinylcholine

Decreased Effect

HYDROmorphone may decrease the levels/effects of: Pegvisomant

The levels/effects of HYDROmorphone may be decreased by: Ammonium Chloride

Ethanol/Nutrition/Herb Interactions

Ethanol: Avoid ethanol (may increase CNS depression).

Herb/Nutraceutical: Avoid valerian, St John's wort, kava kava, gotu kola (may increase CNS depression).

Storage/Stability Store injection and oral dosage forms at 15°C to 30°C (59°F to 86°F). Protect tablets from light. A slightly yellowish discoloration has not been associated with a loss of potency.

Compatibility Stable in D_5LR, D_5W, $D_5^{1/2}NS$, D_5NS, LR, $^{1/2}NS$, NS.

Y-site administration: **Compatible:** Acyclovir, allopurinol, amifostine, amikacin, amsacrine, aztreonam, cefamandole, cefepime, cefoperazone, cefotaxime, cefoxitin, ceftazidime, ceftizoxime, cefuroxime, chloramphenicol, cisatracurium, cisplatin, cladribine, clindamycin, cyclophosphamide, cytarabine, diltiazem, dobutamine, docetaxel, dopamine, doxorubicin, doxorubicin liposome, doxycycline, epinephrine, erythromycin lactobionate, etoposide, famotidine, fentanyl, filgrastim, fludarabine, foscarnet, furosemide, gatifloxacin, gemcitabine, gentamicin, granisetron, heparin, kanamycin, labetalol, linezolid, lorazepam, magnesium sulfate, melphalan, methotrexate, metronidazole, midazolam, milrinone, morphine, nafcillin, nicardipine, nitroglycerin, norepinephrine, ondansetron, oxacillin, paclitaxel, penicillin G potassium, piperacillin, piperacillin/tazobactam, propofol, ranitidine, remifentanil, tacrolimus, teniposide, thiotepa, ticarcillin, tobramycin, trimethoprim/sulfamethoxazole, vancomycin, vecuronium, vinorelbine. **Incompatible:** Amphotericin B cholesteryl sulfate complex, diazepam, minocycline, phenobarbital, phenytoin, sargramostim, tetracycline, thiopental. **Variable (consult detailed reference):** Ampicillin, cefazolin.

Compatibility in syringe: **Compatible:** Albuterol, atropine, bupivacaine, ceftazidime, chlorpromazine, cimetidine, dimenhydrinate, diphenhydramine, fentanyl, glycopyrrolate, haloperidol, hydroxyzine, lorazepam, midazolam, pentazocine, pentobarbital, prochlorperazine mesylate, promethazine, ranitidine, scopolamine, thiethylperazine, trimethobenzamide. **Incompatible:** Ampicillin, diazepam, hyaluronidase, phenobarbital, phenytoin.

Variable (consult detailed reference): Cefazolin, dexamethasone sodium phosphate, ketorolac, prochlorperazine edisylate.

Compatibility when admixed: Compatible: Bupivacaine, fluorouracil, midazolam, ondansetron, promethazine, verapamil. **Incompatible:** Sodium bicarbonate, thiopental. **Variable (consult detailed reference):** Tetracaine.

Mechanism of Action Binds to opiate receptors in the CNS, causing inhibition of ascending pain pathways, altering the perception of and response to pain; causes cough supression by direct central action in the medulla; produces generalized CNS depression

Pharmacodynamics/Kinetics

Onset of action: Analgesic: Immediate release formulations:

Oral: 15-30 minutes; Peak effect: 30-60 minutes

I.V.: 5 minutes; Peak effect: 10-20 minutes

Duration: Immediate release formulations: Oral, I.V.: 4-5 hours

Absorption: I.M.: Variable and delayed

Distribution: V_d: 4 L/kg

Protein binding: ~8% to 19%

Metabolism: Hepatic via glucuronidation; to inactive metabolites

Bioavailability: 62%

Half-life elimination: Immediate release formulations: 1-3 hours

Excretion: Urine (primarily as glucuronide conjugates)

Dosage

Acute pain (moderate-to-severe): **Note:** These are guidelines and do not represent the maximum doses that may be required in all patients. Doses should be titrated to pain relief/prevention.

Children ≥6 months and <50 kg:

Oral: 0.03-0.08 mg/kg/dose every 3-4 hours as needed. **Note:** The American Pain Society recommends an initial dose of 0.06 mg/kg for severe pain in children.

I.V.: 0.015 mg/kg/dose every 3-6 hours as needed

Patient-controlled analgesia (PCA) (American Pain Society, 2008): **Note:** Opiate-naive: Consider lower end of dosing range:

Usual concentration: 0.2 mg/mL

Demand dose: Usual: 0.003-0.004 mg/kg/dose; range: 0.003-0.005 mg/kg/dose

Lockout interval: 6-10 minutes

Usual basal rate: 0-0.004 mg/kg/hour

Children >50 kg and Adults:

Oral: Initial: Opiate-naive: 2-4 mg every 3-6 hours as needed; elderly/debilitated patients may require lower doses; patients with prior opiate exposure may require higher initial doses; usual dosage range: 2-8 mg every 3-4 hours as needed. **Note:** The American Pain Society recommends an initial dose of 4-8 mg for severe pain in adults.

I.V.: Initial: Opiate-naive: 0.2-0.6 mg every 2-3 hours as needed; patients with prior opiate exposure may tolerate higher initial doses

Critically-ill patients (unlabeled dose): 0.7-2 mg (based on 70 kg patient) every 1-2 hours as needed. **Note:** More frequent dosing may be needed (eg, mechanically-ventilated patients).

Continuous infusion: Usual dosage range: 0.5-1 mg/hour (based on 70 kg patient) or 7-15 mcg/kg/hour

Patient-controlled analgesia (PCA): **Note:** Opiate-naive: Consider lower end of dosing range:

Usual concentration: 0.2 mg/mL

Demand dose: Usual: 0.1-0.2 mg; range: 0.05-0.4 mg

Lockout interval: 5-10 minutes

Epidural:
Bolus dose: 1-1.5 mg
Infusion concentration: 0.05-0.075 mg/mL
Infusion rate: 0.04-0.4 mg/hour
Demand dose: 0.15 mg
Lockout interval: 30 minutes
I.M., SubQ: **Note:** I.M. use may result in variable absorption and a lag time to peak effect.
Initial: Opiate-naive: 0.8-1 mg every 4-6 hours as needed; patients with prior opiate exposure may require higher initial doses; usual dosage range: 1-2 mg every 3-6 hours as needed
Rectal: 3 mg every 4-8 hours as needed

Chronic pain: Adults: Oral: **Note:** Patients taking opioids chronically may become tolerant and require doses higher than the usual dosage range to maintain the desired effect. Tolerance can be managed by appropriate dose titration. There is no optimal or maximal dose for hydromorphone in chronic pain. The appropriate dose is one that relieves pain throughout its dosing interval without causing unmanageable side effects.
Controlled release formulation (Hydromorph Contin®, not available in U.S.): 3-30 mg every 12 hours. **Note:** A patient's hydromorphone requirement should be established using prompt release formulations; conversion to long acting products may be considered when chronic, continuous treatment is required. Higher dosages should be reserved for use only in opioid-tolerant patients.

Antitussive (unlabeled use): Oral:
Children 6-12 years: 0.5 mg every 3-4 hours as needed
Children >12 years and Adults: 1 mg every 3-4 hours as needed

Dosing adjustment in hepatic impairment: Should be considered
Administration
Parenteral: May be given SubQ or I.M.; vial stopper contains latex
I.V.: For IVP, must be given slowly over 2-3 minutes (rapid IVP has been associated with an increase in side effects, especially respiratory depression and hypotension)
Oral: Hydromorph Contin®: Capsule should be swallowed whole; do not crush or chew; contents may be sprinkled on soft food and swallowed
Monitoring Parameters Pain relief, respiratory and mental status, blood pressure
Test Interactions Some quinolones may produce a false-positive urine screening result for opiates using commercially-available immunoassay kits. This has been demonstrated most consistently for levofloxacin and ofloxacin, but other quinolones have shown cross-reactivity in certain assay kits. Confirmation of positive opiate screens by more specific methods should be considered.
Additional Information Equianalgesic doses: Morphine 10 mg I.M. = hydromorphone 1.5 mg I.M.
Dosage Forms Excipient information presented when available (limited, particularly for generics); consult specific product labeling. [DSC] = Discontinued product; [CAN] = Canadian brand name
Capsule, controlled release:
Hydromorph Contin® [CAN]: 3 mg, 6 mg, 12 mg, 18 mg, 24 mg, 30 mg [not available in U.S.]

Injection, powder for reconstitution, as hydrochloride:
Dilaudid-HP®: 250 mg [contains sodium metabisulfite]

Injection, solution, as hydrochloride: 1 mg/mL (1 mL); 2 mg/mL (1 mL, 20 mL); 4 mg/mL (1 mL)
Dilaudid®: 1 mg/mL (1 mL); 2 mg/mL (1 mL; 20 mL [DSC]) [20 mL size contains edetate sodium; natural rubber/natural latex in packaging]; 4 mg/mL (1 mL) [contains sodium metabisulfite]
Dilaudid-HP®: 10 mg/mL (1 mL, 5 mL) [contains sodium metabisulfite]
Dilaudid-HP®: 10 mg/mL (50 mL) [contains sodium metabisulfite; natural rubber/natural latex in packaging]

Injection, solution, as hydrochloride [preservative free]: 10 mg/mL (1 mL, 5 mL, 50 mL)

Liquid, oral, as hydrochloride:
Dilaudid®: 1 mg/mL (480 mL) [contains sodium metabisulfite (may have trace amounts)]

Powder, for prescription compounding: 100% (15 grain)

Suppository, rectal, as hydrochloride: 3 mg
Dilaudid®: 3 mg (6s) [DSC]

Tablet, as hydrochloride: 2 mg, 4 mg, 8 mg
Dilaudid®: 2 mg, 4 mg, 8 mg [contains sodium metabisulfite (may have trace amounts)]

References

"Drugs for Pain," *Med Lett Drugs Ther*, 2000, 42(1085):73-8.

Jacobi J, Fraser GL, Coursin DB, et al, "Clinical Practice Guidelines for the Sustained Use of Sedatives and Analgesics in the Critically Ill Adult," *Crit Care Med*, 2002, 30(1):119-41. Available at: http://www.sccm.org/pdf/sedatives.pdf. Accessed August 2, 2003.

Levy MH, "Pharmacologic Treatment of Cancer Pain," *N Engl J Med*, 1996, 335(15):1124-32.

Lugo RD and Kern SE, "Pharmacokinetics of Opioids," *Management of Pain*, Lipman AG ed, Bethesda, MD: ASHP, 2004, 77.

"Principles of Analgesic Use in the Treatment of Acute Pain and Cancer Pain," 5th ed, Glenview, IL: American Pain Society, 2003.

◆ **Hydromorphone HP (Can)** *see* HYDROmorphone *on page 584*

◆ **Hydromorphone HP® 10 (Can)** *see* HYDROmorphone *on page 584*

◆ **Hydromorphone HP® 20 (Can)** *see* HYDROmorphone *on page 584*

◆ **Hydromorphone HP® 50 (Can)** *see* HYDROmorphone *on page 584*

◆ **Hydromorphone HP® Forte (Can)** *see* HYDROmorphone *on page 584*

◆ **Hydromorphone Hydrochloride** *see* HYDROmorphone *on page 584*

◆ **Hydromorphone Hydrochloride Injection, USP (Can)** *see* HYDROmorphone *on page 584*

◆ **Hydro-Rx** *see* Hydrocortisone *on page 575*

◆ **HydroVal® (Can)** *see* Hydrocortisone *on page 575*

◆ **Hydroxycarbamide** *see* Hydroxyurea *on page 589*

◆ **Hydroxydaunomycin Hydrochloride** *see* DOXOrubicin *on page 372*

◆ **Hydroxyldaunorubicin Hydrochloride** *see* DOXOrubicin *on page 372*

Hydroxyurea (hye droks ee yoor EE a)

Medication Safety Issues

Sound-alike/look-alike issues:
Hydroxyurea may be confused with hydrOXYzine

High alert medication: The Institute for Safe Medication Practices (ISMP) includes this medication among its list of drugs which have a heightened risk of causing significant patient harm when used in error.

International issues:
Hydrea® may be confused with Hydra® which is a brand name for isoniazid in Japan

Related Information
Safe Handling of Hazardous Drugs *on page 1517*

U.S. Brand Names Droxia®; Hydrea®; Mylocel™

Index Terms Hydroxycarbamide

Generic Available Yes: Capsule

Canadian Brand Names Apo-Hydroxyurea®; Gen-Hydroxyurea; Hydrea®; Mylan-Hydroxyurea

Pharmacologic Category Antineoplastic Agent, Antimetabolite

Use Treatment of melanoma, refractory chronic myelocytic leukemia (CML), relapsed and refractory metastatic ovarian cancer; radiosensitizing agent in the treatment of squamous cell head and neck cancer (excluding lip cancer); adjunct in the management of sickle cell patients who have had at least three painful crises in the previous 12 months (to reduce frequency of these crises and the need for blood transfusions)

Unlabeled/Investigational Use Treatment of HIV; treatment of psoriasis, treatment of hematologic conditions such as essential thrombocythemia, polycythemia vera, hypereosinophilia, and hyperleukocytosis due to acute leukemia; treatment of uterine, cervix and nonsmall cell lung cancers; radiosensitizing agent in the treatment of primary brain tumors

Pregnancy Risk Factor D

Lactation Enters breast milk/contraindicated

Labeled Contraindications Hypersensitivity to hydroxyurea or any component of the formulation; severe anemia; severe bone marrow suppression; WBC <2500/mm^3 or platelet count <100,000/mm^3 (neutrophils <2000/mm^3, platelets <80,000/mm^3, and hemoglobin <4.5 g/dL for sickle cell anemia); pregnancy

Warnings/Precautions Hazardous agent - use appropriate precautions for handling and disposal. Patients with a history of prior cytotoxic chemotherapy and radiation therapy are more likely to experience bone marrow depression. Patients with a history of radiation therapy are also at risk for exacerbation of post irradiation erythema. Megaloblastic erythropoiesis may be seen early in hydroxyurea treatment; plasma iron clearance may be delayed and the rate of utilization of iron by erythrocytes may be delayed. HIV-infected patients treated with hydroxyurea and antiretroviral agents (including didanosine) are at higher risk for potentially fatal pancreatitis, hepatotoxicity, hepatic failure, and severe peripheral neuropathy. **[U.S. Boxed Warning]: Hydroxyurea is mutagenic and clastogenic. Treatment of myeloproliferative disorders (polycythemia vera and thrombocythemia) with long-term hydroxyurea is associated with secondary leukemia**; it is unknown if this is drug-related or disease-related. Cutaneous vasculitic toxicities (vasculitic ulceration and gangrene) have been reported with hydroxyurea treatment, most often in patients with a history of or receiving concurrent interferon therapy; discontinue hydroxyurea and consider alternate cytoreductive therapy if cutaneous vasculitic toxicity develops. Use caution with renal dysfunction; may require dose reductions. **[U.S. Boxed Warning]: Should be administered under the supervision of a physician experienced in cancer chemotherapy or in the treatment of sickle cell anemia.**

Adverse Reactions Frequency not defined.
Cardiovascular: Edema
Central nervous system: Chills, disorientation, dizziness, drowsiness (dose-related), fever, hallucinations, headache, malaise, seizure

Dermatologic: Alopecia (rare), cutaneous vasculitic toxicities, dermatomyositis-like skin changes, dry skin, facial erythema, gangrene, hyperpigmentation, maculopapular rash, nail atrophy, nail pigmentation, peripheral erythema, scaling, skin atrophy, skin cancer, skin ulcer, vasculitis ulcerations, violet papules

Endocrine & metabolic: Hyperuricemia

Gastrointestinal: Anorexia, constipation, diarrhea, gastrointestinal irritation and mucositis, (potentiated with radiation therapy), nausea, pancreatitis, stomatitis, vomiting

Genitourinary: Dysuria (rare)

Hematologic: Myelosuppression (primarily leukopenia; onset: 24-48 hours; nadir: 10 days; recovery: 7 days after stopping drug; reversal of WBC count occurs rapidly but the platelet count may take 7-10 days to recover); thrombocytopenia and anemia, megaloblastic erythropoiesis, macrocytosis, hemolysis, serum iron decreased, persistent cytopenias, secondary leukemias (long-term use)

Hepatic: Hepatic enzymes increased, hepatotoxicity

Neuromuscular & skeletal: Peripheral neuropathy, weakness

Renal: BUN increased, creatinine increased

Respiratory: Acute diffuse pulmonary infiltrates (rare), dyspnea, pulmonary fibrosis (rare)

Drug Interactions
Avoid Concomitant Use
Avoid concomitant use of Hydroxyurea with any of the following: Natalizumab; Vaccines (Live)

Increased Effect/Toxicity
Hydroxyurea may increase the levels/effects of: Leflunomide; Natalizumab; Vaccines (Live)

The levels/effects of Hydroxyurea may be increased by: Didanosine; Trastuzumab

Decreased Effect
Hydroxyurea may decrease the levels/effects of: Vaccines (Inactivated); Vaccines (Live)

The levels/effects of Hydroxyurea may be decreased by: Echinacea

Storage/Stability Store at room temperature between 15°C and 30°C (59°F and 86°F).

Mechanism of Action Thought to interfere (unsubstantiated hypothesis) with synthesis of DNA, during the S phase of cell division, without interfering with RNA synthesis; inhibits ribonucleoside diphosphate reductase, preventing conversion of ribonucleotides to deoxyribonucleotides; cell-cycle specific for the S phase and may hold other cells in the G_1 phase of the cell cycle. In sickle cell anemia, hydroxyurea increases red blood cell (RBC) hemoglobin F levels, RBC water content, deformability of sickled cells, and alters adhesion of RBCs to endothelium.

Pharmacodynamics/Kinetics
Absorption: Readily (≥80%)

Distribution: Readily crosses blood-brain barrier; distributes into intestine, brain, lung, kidney tissues, effusions and ascites

Metabolism: 60% via hepatic and GI tract

Half-life elimination: 3-4 hours

Time to peak: 1-4 hours

Excretion: Urine (80%, 50% as unchanged drug, 30% as urea); exhaled gases (as CO_2)

Dosage Oral (refer to individual protocols): All doses should be based on ideal or actual body weight, whichever is less:

Children (unlabeled use):
No FDA-approved dosage regimens have been established; dosages of 1500-3000 mg/m^2 as a single dose in combination with other agents every 4-6 weeks have been used in the treatment of pediatric astrocytoma, medulloblastoma, and primitive neuroectodermal tumors
CML: Initial: 10-20 mg/kg/day once daily; adjust dose according to hematologic response

Adults: Dose should always be titrated to patient response and WBC counts; usual oral doses range from 10-30 mg/kg/day or 500-3000 mg/day; if WBC count falls to <2500 cells/mm^3, or the platelet count to <100,000/mm^3, therapy should be stopped for at least 3 days and resumed when values rise toward normal

Solid tumors:
Intermittent therapy: 80 mg/kg as a single dose every third day
Continuous therapy: 20-30 mg/kg/day given as a single dose/day
Concomitant therapy with irradiation: 80 mg/kg as a single dose every third day starting at least 7 days before initiation of irradiation
Resistant chronic myelocytic leukemia: Continuous therapy: 20-30 mg/kg once daily
HIV (unlabeled use; in combination with antiretroviral agents): 1000-1500 mg daily in a single dose or divided doses
Psoriasis (unlabeled use): 1000-1500 mg/day in a single dose or divided doses
Sickle cell anemia (moderate/severe disease): Initial: 15 mg/kg/day, increased by 5 mg/kg every 12 weeks if blood counts are in an acceptable range until the maximum tolerated dose of 35 mg/kg/day is achieved or the dose that does not produce toxic effects

Acceptable range:
Neutrophils ≥2500 cells/mm^3
Platelets ≥95,000/mm^3
Hemoglobin >5.3 g/dL, and
Reticulocytes ≥95,000/mm^3 if the hemoglobin concentration is <9 g/dL

Toxic range:
Neutrophils <2000 cells/mm^3
Platelets <80,000/mm^3
Hemoglobin <4.5 g/dL
Reticulocytes <80,000/mm^3 if the hemoglobin concentration is <9 g/dL
Monitor for toxicity every 2 weeks; if toxicity occurs, stop treatment until the bone marrow recovers; restart at 2.5 mg/kg/day less than the dose at which toxicity occurs; if no toxicity occurs over the next 12 weeks, then the subsequent dose should be increased by 2.5 mg/kg/day; reduced dosage of hydroxyurea alternating with erythropoietin may decrease myelotoxicity and increase levels of fetal hemoglobin in patients who have not been helped by hydroxyurea alone

Dosing adjustment in renal impairment:
The FDA-approved labeling recommends the following adjustment:
Sickle cell anemia: Cl$_{cr}$ <60 mL/minute or ESRD: Reduce initial dose to 7.5 mg/kg; titrate to response/avoidance of toxicity (refer to usual dosing).
Other indications: It is recommended to reduce the initial dose; however, no specific guidelines are available.

The following guidelines have been used by some clinicians:

Aronoff, 2007: Adults:

Cl_{cr} 10-50 mL/minute: Administer 50% of dose

Cl_{cr} <10 mL/minute: Administer 20% of dose

Hemodialysis: Administer dose after dialysis on dialysis days; supplemental dose is not necessary. Hydroxyurea is a low molecular weight compound with high aqueous solubility that may be freely dialyzable, however, clinical studies confirming this hypothesis have not been performed.

Continuous renal replacement therapy (CRRT): Administer 50% of dose

Kintzel, 1995:

Cl_{cr} 46-60 mL/minute: Administer 85% of dose

Cl_{cr} 31-45 mL/minute: Administer 80% of dose

Cl_{cr} <30 mL/minute: Administer 75% of dose

Dosing adjustment in hepatic impairment: Specific guidelines are not available for dosage adjustment in hepatic impairment. The FDA-approved labeling recommends closely monitoring for bone marrow toxicity in patients with hepatic impairment.

Combination Regimens

Brain tumors: 8 in 1 (Brain Tumors) on page 1221

Gestational trophoblastic tumor:

CHAMOCA (Modified Bagshawe Regimen) on page 1259

CHAMOMA (Bagshawe Regimen) on page 1261

Neuroblastoma: N4SE Protocol on page 1380

Retinoblastoma: 8 in 1 (Retinoblastoma) on page 1222

Administration Capsules may be opened and emptied into water (will not dissolve completely); observe proper handling procedures

Monitoring Parameters CBC with differential and platelets, renal function and liver function tests, serum uric acid

Sickle cell disease: Monitor for toxicity every 2 weeks. If toxicity occurs, stop treatment until the bone marrow recovers; restart at 2.5 mg/kg/day less than the dose at which toxicity occurs. If no toxicity occurs over the next 12 weeks, then the subsequent dose should be increased by 2.5 mg/kg/day. Reduced dosage of hydroxyurea alternating with erythropoietin may decrease myelotoxicity and increase levels of fetal hemoglobin in patients who have not been helped by hydroxyurea alone.

Acceptable range: Neutrophils ≥2500 cells/mm^3, platelets ≥95,000/mm^3, hemoglobin >5.3 g/dL, and reticulocytes ≥95,000/mm^3 if the hemoglobin concentration is <9 g/dL

Toxic range: Neutrophils <2000 cells/mm^3, platelets <80,000/mm^3, hemoglobin <4.5 g/dL, and reticulocytes <80,000/mm^3 if the hemoglobin concentration is <9 g/dL

Dietary Considerations In sickle cell patients, supplemental administration of folic acid is recommended; hydroxyurea may mask development of folic acid deficiency.

Additional Information Although I.V. use is reported, no parenteral product is commercially available in the U.S.

If WBC decreases to <2500/mm^3 or platelet count to <100,000/mm^3 (neutrophils <2000/mm^3 and platelets <80,000/mm^3 for patients with sickle cell anemia), interrupt therapy until values rise significantly toward normal. Treat anemia with whole blood replacement; do not interrupt therapy (for sickle cell anemia patients, withhold treatment for hemoglobin <4.5 g/dL until recovery to >5.3 g/dL). Adequate trial period to determine the antineoplastic effectiveness is 6 weeks. Almost all patients receiving hydroxyurea in clinical ▶

trials needed to have their medication stopped for a time to allow their low blood count to return to acceptable levels.

Emetic Potential Very low (<10%)

Dosage Forms Excipient information presented when available (limited, particularly for generics); consult specific product labeling.

Capsule: 500 mg

Droxia®: 200 mg, 300 mg, 400 mg

Hydrea®: 500 mg

Tablet:

Mylocel™: 1000 mg

References

Aronoff GR, Bennett WM, Berns JS, et al, *Drug Prescribing in Renal Failure: Dosing Guidelines for Adults and Children*, 5th ed. Philadelphia, PA: American College of Physicians; 2007, p 100.

Gwilt PR and Tracewell WG, "Pharmacokinetics and Pharmacodynamics of Hydroxyurea," *Clin Pharmacokinet*, 1998, 34(5):347-58.

Howard LW and Kennedy LD, "Hydroxyurea in the Treatment of Sickle-Cell Anemia," *Ann Pharmacother*, 1997, 31(11):1393-6.

Kintzel PE and Dorr RT, "Anticancer Drug Renal Toxicity and Elimination: Dosing Guidelines for Altered Renal Function," *Cancer Treat Rev*, 1995, 21(1):33-64.

Maier-Redelsperger M, de Montalembert M, Flahault A, et al, "Fetal Hemoglobin and F-Cell Responses to Long-Term Hydroxyurea Treatment in Young Sickle Cell Patients. The French Study Group on Sickle Cell Disease," *Blood*, 1998, 91(12):4472-9.

Yarboro JW, "Mechanism of Action of Hydroxyurea," *Semin Oncol*, 1992, 19(3 Suppl 9):1-10.

HydrOXYzine (hye DROKS i zeen)

Medication Safety Issues

Sound-alike/look-alike issues:

HydrOXYzine may be confused with hydrALAZINE, hydroxyurea

Atarax® may be confused with amoxicillin, Ativan®

Vistaril® may be confused with Restoril™, Versed, Zestril®

International issues:

Vistaril® may be confused with Vastarel® which is a brand name for trimetazidine in multiple international markets

Related Information

Management of Chemotherapy-Induced Nausea and Vomiting *on page 1434*

Management of Drug Extravasations *on page 1447*

U.S. Brand Names Vistaril®

Index Terms Hydroxyzine Hydrochloride; Hydroxyzine Pamoate

Generic Available Yes

Canadian Brand Names Apo-Hydroxyzine®; Atarax®; Hydroxyzine Hydrochloride Injection, USP; Novo-Hydroxyzin; PMS-Hydroxyzine; Vistaril®

Pharmacologic Category Antiemetic; Histamine H$_1$ Antagonist; Histamine H$_1$ Antagonist, First Generation

Use Treatment of anxiety; preoperative sedative; antipruritic

Unlabeled/Investigational Use Antiemetic; ethanol withdrawal symptoms

Pregnancy Risk Factor C

Lactation Excretion in breast milk unknown/not recommended

Labeled Contraindications Hypersensitivity to hydroxyzine or any component of the formulation; early pregnancy; SubQ, intra-arterial, or I.V. administration of injection

Warnings/Precautions Causes sedation, caution must be used in performing tasks which require alertness (eg, operating machinery or driving). Sedative effects of CNS depressants or ethanol are potentiated. SubQ, I.V., and intra-arterial administration are contraindicated since tissue damage, intravascular hemolysis, thrombosis, and digital gangrene can occur. Use with caution with

narrow-angle glaucoma, prostatic hyperplasia, bladder neck obstruction, asthma, or COPD.

Anticholinergic effects are not well tolerated in the elderly. Hydroxyzine may be useful as a short-term antipruritic, but it is not recommended for use as a sedative or anxiolytic in the elderly.

Adverse Reactions Frequency not defined.

Central nervous system: Dizziness, drowsiness, fatigue, hallucination, headache, nervousness, seizure

Dermatologic: Pruritus, rash, urticaria

Gastrointestinal: Xerostomia

Neuromuscular & skeletal: Involuntary movements, paresthesia, tremor

Ocular: Blurred vision

Respiratory: Thickening of bronchial secretions

Miscellaneous: Allergic reaction

Drug Interactions

Metabolism/Transport Effects Inhibits CYP2D6 (weak)

Avoid Concomitant Use There are no known interactions where it is recommended to avoid concomitant use.

Increased Effect/Toxicity

HydrOXYzine may increase the levels/effects of: Alcohol (Ethyl); Anticholinergics; CNS Depressants

The levels/effects of HydrOXYzine may be increased by: Pramlintide

Decreased Effect

HydrOXYzine may decrease the levels/effects of: Acetylcholinesterase Inhibitors (Central); Betahistine

The levels/effects of HydrOXYzine may be decreased by: Acetylcholinesterase Inhibitors (Central); Amphetamines

Ethanol/Nutrition/Herb Interactions

Ethanol: Avoid ethanol (may increase CNS depression).

Herb/Nutraceutical: Avoid valerian, St John's wort, kava kava, gotu kola (may increase CNS depression).

Storage/Stability Injection: Store at 15°C to 30°C. Protect from light.

Compatibility Compatibility in syringe: Compatible: Atropine, atropine with meperidine, butorphanol, chlorpromazine, cimetidine, codeine, diphenhydramine, doxapram, droperidol, fentanyl, fluphenazine, glycopyrrolate, hydromorphone, lidocaine, meperidine, methotrimeprazine, metoclopramide, midazolam, morphine, nalbuphine, oxymorphone, pentazocine, perphenazine, procaine, prochlorperazine edisylate, promazine, promethazine, scopolamine, sufentanil. **Incompatible:** Dimenhydrinate, haloperidol, ketorolac, pentobarbital, ranitidine.

Mechanism of Action Competes with histamine for H_1-receptor sites on effector cells in the gastrointestinal tract, blood vessels, and respiratory tract. Possesses skeletal muscle relaxing, bronchodilator, antihistamine, antiemetic, and analgesic properties.

Pharmacodynamics/Kinetics

Onset of action: Oral: 15-30 minutes

Duration: 4-6 hours

Absorption: Oral: Rapid

Metabolism: Forms metabolites

Half-life elimination: 3-7 hours

Time to peak: ~2 hours

Excretion: Urine

◀ **Dosage**
Children:
Preoperative sedation:
Oral: 0.6 mg/kg/dose
I.M.: 0.5-1 mg/kg/dose
Pruritus, anxiety: Oral:
<6 years: 50 mg daily in divided doses
≥6 years: 50-100 mg daily in divided doses
Adults:
Antiemetic (unlabeled use): I.M.: 25-100 mg/dose every 4-6 hours as needed
Anxiety: Oral, I.M.: 50-100 mg 4 times/day
Preoperative sedation:
Oral: 50-100 mg
I.M.: 25-100 mg
Pruritus: Oral, I.M.: 25 mg 3-4 times/day

Dosing interval in hepatic impairment: Change dosing interval to every 24 hours in patients with primary biliary cirrhosis
Administration Do not administer SubQ or intra-arterially. Administer I.M. deep in large muscle. With I.V. administration, extravasation can result in sterile abscess and marked tissue induration.
Monitoring Parameters Relief of symptoms, mental status, blood pressure
Dosage Forms Excipient information presented when available (limited, particularly for generics); consult specific product labeling. [DSC] = Discontinued product
Capsule, as pamoate: 25 mg, 50 mg, 100 mg
Vistaril®: 25 mg, 50 mg
Injection, solution, as hydrochloride: 25 mg/mL (1 mL); 50 mg/mL (1 mL, 2 mL, 10 mL)
Suspension, oral, as pamoate:
Vistaril®: 25 mg/5 mL (120 mL, 480 mL) [lemon flavor] [DSC]
Syrup, as hydrochloride: 10 mg/5 mL (120 mL, 480 mL)
Tablet, as hydrochloride: 10 mg, 25 mg, 50 mg

References
Simons FE, Simons KJ, and Frith EM, "The Pharmacokinetics and Antihistaminic of the H₁ Receptor Antagonist Hydroxyzine," *J Allergy Clin Immunol*, 1984, 73(1 Pt 1):69-75.
Simons FE, Watson WT, Chen XY, et al, "The Pharmacokinetics and Pharmacodynamics of Hydroxyzine in Patients With Primary Biliary Cirrhosis," *J Clin Pharmacol*, 1989, 29(9):809-15.
Simons KJ, Watson WT, Chen XY, et al, "Pharmacokinetic and Pharmacodynamic Studies of the H₁-Receptor Antagonist Hydroxyzine in the Elderly," *Clin Pharmacol Ther*, 1989, 45(1):9-14.

◆ **Hydroxyzine Hydrochloride** *see* HydrOXYzine *on page 594*
◆ **Hydroxyzine Hydrochloride Injection, USP (Can)** *see* HydrOXYzine *on page 594*
◆ **Hydroxyzine Pamoate** *see* HydrOXYzine *on page 594*
◆ **HydroZone Plus [OTC]** *see* Hydrocortisone *on page 575*
◆ **Hylenex™** *see* Hyaluronidase *on page 573*
◆ **HyperRHO™ S/D Full Dose** *see* Rhₒ(D) Immune Globulin *on page 1011*
◆ **HyperRHO™ S/D Mini Dose** *see* Rhₒ(D) Immune Globulin *on page 1011*
◆ **Hytone® [DSC]** *see* Hydrocortisone *on page 575*
◆ **I¹²³ Iobenguane** *see* Iobenguane I 123 *on page 649*
◆ **I-123 MIBG** *see* Iobenguane I 123 *on page 649*

Ibandronate (eye BAN droh nate)

U.S. Brand Names Boniva®

Index Terms Ibandronate Sodium; Ibandronic Acid

Generic Available No

Canadian Brand Names Bondronat®

Pharmacologic Category Bisphosphonate Derivative

Use Treatment and prevention of osteoporosis in postmenopausal females

Unlabeled/Investigational Use Hypercalcemia of malignancy; corticosteroid-induced osteoporosis; Paget's disease; reduce bone pain and skeletal complications from metastatic bone disease

Pregnancy Risk Factor C

Lactation Excretion in breast milk unknown/use caution

Labeled Contraindications Hypersensitivity to ibandronate or any component of the formulation; hypocalcemia; oral tablets are also contraindicated in patients unable to stand or sit upright for at least 60 minutes

Warnings/Precautions Hypocalcemia must be corrected before therapy initiation. Ensure adequate calcium and vitamin D intake. Bisphosphonate therapy has been associated with osteonecrosis, primarily of the jaw; this has been observed mostly in cancer patients, but also in patients with postmenopausal osteoporosis and other diagnoses. Most reported cases occurred after I.V. bisphosphonate therapy; however, cases have been reported following oral therapy. Dental exams and preventative dentistry should be performed prior to placing patients with risk factors on chronic bisphosphonate therapy. Invasive dental procedures should be avoided during treatment.

Infrequently, severe (and occasionally debilitating) bone, joint, and/or muscle pain have been reported during bisphosphonate treatment. The onset of pain ranged from a single day to several months. Consider discontinuing therapy in patients who experience severe symptoms; symptoms usually resolve upon discontinuation. Some patients experienced recurrence when rechallenged with same drug or another bisphosphonate; avoid use in patients with a history of these symptoms in association with bisphosphonate therapy.

Oral bisphosphonates may cause dysphagia, esophagitis, esophageal or gastric ulcer; risk may increase in patients unable to comply with dosing instructions; discontinue use if new or worsening symptoms develop. Intravenous bisphosphonates may cause transient decreases in serum calcium and have also been associated with renal toxicity.

Use not recommended with severe renal impairment (Cl_{cr} <30 mL/minute). Safety and efficacy have not been established in patients <18 years of age.

Adverse Reactions Percentages vary based on frequency of administration (daily vs monthly). Unless specified, percentages are reported with oral use.

>10%:

  Gastrointestinal: Dyspepsia (6% to 12%)

  Neuromuscular & skeletal: Back pain (4% to 14%)

1% to 10%:

  Cardiovascular: Hypertension (6% to 7%)

  Central nervous system: Headache (3% to 7%), dizziness (1% to 4%), insomnia (1% to 2%)

  Dermatologic: Rash (1% to 2%)

  Endocrine & metabolic: Hypercholesterolemia (5%)

  Gastrointestinal: Abdominal pain (5% to 8%), diarrhea (4% to 7%), nausea (5%), tooth disorder (4%), constipation (3% to 4%), vomiting (3%)

Genitourinary: Urinary tract infection (2% to 6%)

Hepatic: Alkaline phosphatase decreased (frequency not defined)

Local: Injection site reaction (<2%)

Neuromuscular & skeletal: Pain in extremity (1% to 8%), arthralgia (4% to 6%), myalgia (1% to 6%), joint disorder (4%), weakness (4%), muscle cramp (2%)

Respiratory: Bronchitis (3% to 10%), pneumonia (6%), pharyngitis/nasopharyngitis (3% to 4%), upper respiratory infection (2%)

Miscellaneous: Acute phase reaction (I.V. 10%; oral 3% to 9%), infection (4%), flu-like syndrome (1% to 4%), allergic reaction (3%)

Postmarketing and/or case reports: Anaphylaxis; angioedema; bronchospasm; esophageal cancer; hypocalcemia; incapacitating bone, joint, or muscle pain; iritis; ocular inflammation; osteonecrosis of the jaw; scleritis; uveitis

Drug Interactions

Avoid Concomitant Use There are no known interactions where it is recommended to avoid concomitant use.

Increased Effect/Toxicity

Ibandronate may increase the levels/effects of: Phosphate Supplements

The levels/effects of Ibandronate may be increased by: Aminoglycosides; Nonsteroidal Anti-Inflammatory Agents

Decreased Effect

The levels/effects of Ibandronate may be decreased by: Antacids; Calcium Salts; Iron Salts; Magnesium Salts

Ethanol/Nutrition/Herb Interactions

Ethanol: Avoid ethanol (may increase risk of osteoporosis).

Food: May reduce absorption; mean oral bioavailability is decreased up to 90% when given with food.

Storage/Stability Store at controlled room temperature of 25°C (77°F); excursions permitted to 15°C to 30°C (59°F to 86°F).

Mechanism of Action A bisphosphonate which inhibits bone resorption via actions on osteoclasts or on osteoclast precursors; decreases the rate of bone resorption, leading to an indirect increase in bone mineral density.

Pharmacodynamics/Kinetics

Distribution: Terminal V_d: 90 L; 40% to 50% of circulating ibandronate binds to bone

Protein binding: 85.7% to 99.5%

Metabolism: Not metabolized

Bioavailability: Oral: Reduced by 90% following standard breakfast

Half-life elimination:

Oral: 150 mg dose: Terminal: 37-157 hours

I.V.: Terminal: ~5-25 hours

Time to peak, plasma: Oral: 0.5-2 hours

Excretion: Urine (50% to 60% of absorbed dose, excreted as unchanged drug); feces (unabsorbed drug)

Dosage

Oral:

Treatment of postmenopausal osteoporosis: 2.5 mg once daily **or** 150 mg once a month

Prevention of postmenopausal osteoporosis: 2.5 once daily **or** 150 mg once a month

Metastatic bone disease (unlabeled use): 50 mg once daily

I.V.:

Treatment of postmenopausal osteoporosis: 3 mg every 3 months

Hypercalcemia of malignancy (unlabeled use): 2-4 mg over 2 hours

Metastatic bone disease (unlabeled use): 6 mg over 1 hour every 3-4 weeks

Dosage adjustment in renal impairment:

Mild or moderate impairment: Dosing adjustment not needed

Severe impairment (Cl_{cr} <30 mL/minute): Use not recommended

Dose adjustment in renal impairment for oncologic uses (unlabeled): Severe impairment (Cl_{cr} <30 mL/minute):

Oral: 50 mg once weekly

I.V.: 2 mg over 1 hour every 3-4 weeks

Dosage adjustment in hepatic impairment: Dosing adjustment not needed

Administration

Oral: Should be administered 60 minutes before the first food or drink of the day (other than water) and prior to taking any oral medications or supplements (eg, calcium, antacids, vitamins). Ibandronate should be taken in an upright position with a full glass (6-8 oz) of plain water and the patient should avoid lying down for 60 minutes to minimize the possibility of GI side effects. Mineral water with a high calcium content should be avoided. The tablet should be swallowed whole; do not chew or suck. Do not eat or drink anything (except water) for 60 minutes following administration of ibandronate.

Once-monthly dosing: The 150 mg tablet should be taken on the same date each month. In case of a missed dose, do not take two 150 mg tablets within the same week. If the next scheduled dose is 1-7 days away, wait until the next scheduled dose to take the tablet. If the next scheduled dose is >7 days away, take the dose the morning it is remembered, and then resume taking the once-monthly dose on the originally scheduled day.

I.V.: Administer as a 15-30 second bolus. Do not mix with calcium-containing solutions or other drugs. For osteoporosis, do not administer more frequently than every 3 months. Infuse over 1 hour for metastatic bone disease and over 2 hours for hypercalcemia of malignancy.

Monitoring Parameters Bone mineral density as measured by central dual-energy x-ray absorptiometry (DXA) of the hip or spine (at least every 2 years); serum creatinine prior to each I.V. dose

Test Interactions Bisphosphonates may interfere with diagnostic imaging agents such as technetium-99m-diphosphonate in bone scans.

Dietary Considerations Supplemental calcium or vitamin D may be required if dietary intake is not adequate; women >50 years of age should consume 1200-1500 mg/day of elemental calcium and 800-1000 int. units/day of vitamin D. Ibandronate tablet should be taken with a full glass (6-8 oz) of plain water, at least 60 minutes prior to any food, beverages, or medications. Mineral water with a high calcium content should be avoided.

Dosage Forms Excipient information presented when available (limited, particularly for generics); consult specific product labeling.

Injection, solution: 1 mg/mL (3 mL) [prefilled syringe]

Tablet: 2.5 mg [once-daily formulation]; 150 mg [once-monthly formulation]

References

Barrett J, Worth E, Bauss F, et al, "Ibandronate: A Clinical Pharmacological and Pharmacokinetic Update," *J Clin Pharmacol*, 2004, 44(9):951-65.

Hillner BE, Ingle JN, Chlebowski RT, et al, "American Society of Clinical Oncology 2003 Update on the Role of Bisphosphonates and Bone Health Issues in Women With Breast Cancer," *J Clin Oncol*, 2003, 21(21):4042-57.

Marx RE, Sawatari Y, Fortin M, et al, "Bisphosphonate-Induced Exposed Bone (Osteonecrosis/Osteopetrosis) of the Jaws: Risk Factors, Recognition, Prevention, and Treatment," *J Oral Maxillofac Surg*, 2005, 63(11):1567-75.

McCormack PL and Plosker GL, "Ibandronic Acid: A Review of its Use in the Treatment of Bone Metastases of Breast Cancer," *Drugs*, 2006, 66(5):711-28.

National Osteoporosis Foundation, "Clinician's Guide to Prevention and Treatment of Osteoporosis," Washington, DC, 2008. Available at http://www.nof.org

Tripathy D, Body JJ, and Bergstrom B, "Review of Ibandronate in the Treatment of Metastatic Bone Disease: Experience From Phase III Trials," *Clin Ther*, 2004, 26(12):1947-59.

Wysowski DK, "Reports of Esophageal Cancer With Oral Bisphosphonate Use," *N Engl J Med*, 2009, 360(1):89-90.

◆ **Ibandronate Sodium** *see* Ibandronate *on page* 597

◆ **Ibandronic Acid** *see* Ibandronate *on page* 597

Ibritumomab (ib ri TYOO mo mab)

Medication Safety Issues

High alert medication: The Institute for Safe Medication Practices (ISMP) includes this medication among its list of drug classes which have a heightened risk of causing significant patient harm when used in error.

Dosage maximum: Do not exceed the Y-90 Ibritumomab maximum allowable dose of 32 mCi, regardless of the patient's body weight.

Related Information

Management of Drug Extravasations *on page* 1447
Safe Handling of Hazardous Drugs *on page* 1517

U.S. Brand Names Zevalin®

Index Terms Ibritumomab Tiuxetan; IDEC-Y2B8; In-111 Ibritumomab; In-111 Zevalin; Y-90 Ibritumomab; Y-90 Zevalin

Generic Available No

Canadian Brand Names Zevalin®

Pharmacologic Category Antineoplastic Agent, Monoclonal Antibody; Radiopharmaceutical

Use Treatment of relapsed or refractory low-grade or follicular B-cell non-Hodgkin's lymphoma (NHL); treatment of follicular NHL in patients who achieve a response (partial or complete) to first-line chemotherapy

Pregnancy Risk Factor D

Lactation Excretion in breast milk unknown/not recommended

Labeled Contraindications There are no contraindications listed within the manufacturer's labeling.

Warnings/Precautions Hazardous agent - use appropriate precautions for handling and disposal. **[U.S. Boxed Warning]: Severe cutaneous and mucocutaneous skin reactions have been reported (with fatalities) in postmarketing experience. Discontinue all components of the therapeutic regimen in patients experiencing severe cutaneous or mucocutaneous skin reactions,** including erythema multiforme, Stevens-Johnson syndrome, toxic epidermal necrolysis, bullous dermatitis, and exfoliative dermatitis. Onset may occur within days to 4 months following infusion.

To be used as part of the Zevalin® therapeutic regimen (in combination with rituximab). **[U.S. Boxed Warning]: Do not exceed the Y-90 ibritumomab maximum allowable dose of 32 mCi; do not administer to patients with altered biodistribution (determined by imaging with In-111 ibritumomab).** Use should be reserved to physicians and other professionals qualified and experienced in the safe handling of radiopharmaceuticals, and in monitoring and emergency treatment of infusion reactions. The contents of the kit are not radioactive until radiolabeling occurs. During and after radiolabeling, adequate shielding should be used with this product, in accordance with institutional radiation safety practices.

[U.S. Boxed Warning]: Serious fatal infusion reactions may occur with the rituximab component of the therapeutic regimen; fatalities were associated with acute respiratory distress syndrome, hypoxia, pulmonary infiltrates, cardiogenic shock, MI, or ventricular fibrillation. Immediately stop infusion and discontinue in patients who develop severe infusion reactions. Reactions typically occur with the first rituximab infusion (onset within 30-120 minutes). Reactions may also include angioedema, bronchospasm, and urticaria. Less severe reactions may be managed by slowing or interrupting infusion.

[U.S. Boxed Warning]: Delayed, prolonged, and severe cytopenias (thrombocytopenia and neutropenia) are common. Do not administer to patients with ≥25% lymphoma marrow involvement, patients with impaired bone marrow reserve (eg, prior myeloablative treatment, platelet count <100,000/mm^3, neutrophil count <1500/mm^3, hypocellular marrow), or to patients with prior stem cell collection failure. Patients with mild baseline thrombocytopenia may experience higher incidences of severe neutropenia and thrombocytopenia; hemorrhage may occur due to thrombocytopenia; avoid concomitant use of medications interfering with coagulation or platelet function. Closely monitor patients for complications of cytopenias (eg, febrile neutropenia, hemorrhage) for up to 3 months after administration.

Secondary malignancies (acute myelogenous leukemia and/or myelodysplastic syndrome) have been reported following use; the median time to diagnosis (secondary malignancy) following ibritumomab treatment was 1.9 years (range: 0.4-6.3 years). Product contains albumin, which confers a theoretical risk of transmission of viral disease or Creutzfeldt-Jakob disease. The safety of immunization with live vaccines following ibritumomab therapy has not been studied; do not administer live viral vaccines to patients who have recently received ibritumomab treatment; the ability to generate a response to any vaccine after receiving treatment has not been studied. Safety and efficacy of repeated courses of the therapeutic regimen have not been established. Infusion site erythema and ulceration have been reported following extravasation; monitor infusion site; promptly terminate infusion with symptoms/signs of extravasation (restart in another limb). There is a case report of (delayed) erythema and ulceration, which is described as radiation necrosis following yttrium-90-ibritumomab extravasation (Williams, 2006). Delayed (up to 1 month) radiation injury has occurred in or near areas of lymphomatous involvement. Safety and efficacy have not been established in pediatric patients.

Adverse Reactions Severe, potentially life-threatening allergic reactions have occurred in association with infusions. Also refer to Rituximab monograph.

>10%:

Central nervous system: Fatigue (33%), chills (24%), fever (10% to 17%), pain (13%), headache (12%)

Gastrointestinal: Nausea (18% to 31%), abdominal pain (16% to 17%), vomiting (12%), diarrhea (9% to 11%)

Hematologic: Thrombocytopenia (62% to 95%; grades 3/4: 51% to 63%; nadir: 49-53 days), neutropenia (45% to 77%; grades 3/4: 41% to 60%; nadir: 61-62 days), anemia (22% to 61%; grades 3/4: 5% to 17%; nadir: 68-69 days), leukopenia (43%; grades 3/4: 36%), lymphopenia (26%; grades 3/4: 18%), myelosuppression (nadir: 7-9 weeks; duration: 22-35 days)

Neuromuscular & skeletal: Weakness (15% to 43%)

Respiratory: Nasopharyngitis (19%), dyspnea (14%), cough (10% to 11%)

Miscellaneous: Infection (29%; serious 1% to 5%)

1% to 10%:

Cardiovascular: Peripheral edema (8%), hypertension (7%), flushing (6%), hypotension (6%)

Central nervous system: Dizziness (7% to 10%), insomnia (5%), anxiety (4%)

Dermatologic: Pruritus (7% to 9%), rash (7% to 8%), petechiae (3% to 8%), bruising (7%), angioedema (5%; grades 3/4: <1%), urticaria (4%)

Gastrointestinal: Anorexia (8%), abdominal distension (5%), constipation (5%), dyspepsia (4%), melena (2%; life threatening in 1%), gastrointestinal hemorrhage (severe: 1%)

Genitourinary: Urinary tract infection (7%)

Hematologic: Secondary malignancies (1% to 6%; includes acute myelogenous leukemia and myelodysplastic syndrome), pancytopenia (severe: 2%)

Neuromuscular & skeletal: Myalgia (7% to 9%), back pain (8%), arthralgia (7%)

Respiratory: Throat irritation (10%), bronchitis (8%), rhinitis (6% to 8%), pharyngolaryngeal pain (7%), sinusitis (7%), bronchospasm (5%), epistaxis (3% to 5%), apnea (severe: 1%)

Miscellaneous: Flu-like syndrome (8%), night sweats (8%), diaphoresis (4%), HAMA antibody formation (4%), allergic reaction (2%), infusion reaction (severe: 1%), tumor pain (severe: 1%)

<1%: Anaphylactic reactions, arthritis, cerebral hemorrhage, cytogenetic abnormalities, encephalopathy, hematemesis, hemorrhage, hypersensitivity, meningioma (benign), pulmonary edema, pulmonary embolism, stroke (hemorrhagic), subdural hematoma, tachycardia, vaginal hemorrhage

Postmarketing and/or case reports: Cutaneous and mucocutaneous reactions (eg, erythema multiforme, Stevens-Johnson syndrome, toxic epidermal necrolysis, bullous dermatitis and exfoliative dermatitis); infusion site erythema/ulceration (following extravasation), radiation injury/complications (delayed; in tissues in or near areas of lymphomatous involvement); radiation necrosis (following yttrium-90-ibritumomab extravasation)

Drug Interactions

Avoid Concomitant Use

Avoid concomitant use of Ibritumomab with any of the following: Natalizumab; Vaccines (Live)

Increased Effect/Toxicity

Ibritumomab may increase the levels/effects of: Leflunomide; Natalizumab; Vaccines (Live); Vitamin K Antagonists

The levels/effects of Ibritumomab may be increased by: Anticoagulants; Antiplatelet Agents; Trastuzumab

Decreased Effect

Ibritumomab may decrease the levels/effects of: Cardiac Glycosides; Vaccines (Inactivated); Vaccines (Live); Vitamin K Antagonists

The levels/effects of Ibritumomab may be decreased by: Echinacea

Ethanol/Nutrition/Herb Interactions Herb/Nutraceutical: Avoid echinacea (may diminish therapeutic effect). Avoid cat's claw, dong quai, evening primrose, feverfew, garlic, ginger, ginkgo, red clover, horse chestnut, green tea, ginseng (all have antiplatelet activity).

Storage/Stability Store at 2°C to 8°C (36°F to 46°F); do not freeze. Administer Y-90 ibritumomab within 8 hours of radiolabeling and In-111 ibritumomab within 12 hours of radiolabeling.

Reconstitution To prepare radiolabeled injection, follow preparation guidelines provided by manufacturer.

Mechanism of Action Ibritumomab is a monoclonal antibody directed against the CD20 antigen found on B lymphocytes (normal and malignant). Ibritumomab binding induces apoptosis in B lymphocytes *in vitro*. It is combined with the chelator tiuxetan, which acts as a specific chelation site for either Indium-111 (In-111) or Yttrium-90 (Y-90). The monoclonal antibody acts as a delivery system to direct the radioactive isotope to the targeted cells, however, binding has been observed in lymphoid cells throughout the body and in lymphoid nodules in organs such as the large and small intestines. Indium-111 is a gamma-emitter used to assess biodistribution of ibritumomab, while Y-90 emits beta particles. Beta-emission induces cellular damage through the formation of free radicals (in both target cells and surrounding cells).

Pharmacodynamics/Kinetics

Duration: Beta cell recovery begins in ~12 weeks; generally in normal range within 9 months

Distribution: To lymphoid cells throughout the body and in lymphoid nodules in organs such as the large and small intestines, spleen, testes, and liver

Metabolism: Has not been characterized; the product of yttrium-90 radioactive decay is zirconium-90 (nonradioactive); Indium-111 decays to cadmium-111 (nonradioactive)

Half-life elimination: Y-90 ibritumomab: 30 hours; Indium-111 decays with a physical half-life of 67 hours; Yttrium-90 decays with a physical half-life of 64 hours

Excretion: A median of 7.2% of the radiolabeled activity was excreted in urine over 7 days

Dosage I.V.: Adults: **Note:** Premedication with oral acetaminophen 650 mg and diphenhydramine 50 mg is recommended prior to each rituximab infusion. Ibritumomab is administered **only** as part of the Zevalin® therapeutic regimen (a combined treatment regimen with rituximab). Allow at least 6 weeks, but no more than 12 weeks following first-line chemotherapy before treatment initiation; platelets should recover to ≥150,000/mm³ prior to treatment. The regimen consists of two steps:

Day 1:

Rituximab infusion: 250 mg/m² at an initial rate of 50 mg/hour. If hypersensitivity or infusion-related events do not occur, increase infusion in increments of 50 mg/hour every 30 minutes, to a maximum of 400 mg/hour. Stop rituximab and discontinue regimen for severe infusion reaction. For less severe infusion reactions, temporarily slow or interrupt; the infusion may be resumed at one-half the previous rate upon improvement of symptoms.

In-111 ibritumomab infusion: Within 4 hours of the completion of rituximab infusion, inject 5 mCi (1.6 mg total antibody dose) over 10 minutes.

Biodistribution of In-111 ibritumomab should be assessed by imaging at 48-72 hours postinjection. Optional additional imaging may be performed to resolve ambiguities. If biodistribution is not acceptable, the patient should not proceed to Step 2.

Day 7, 8, or 9:

Rituximab infusion: 250 mg/m² at an initial rate of 100 mg/hour (50 mg/hour if infusion-related events occurred with the first infusion). If hypersensitivity or infusion-related events do not occur, increase infusion in increments of

100 mg/hour every 30 minutes, to a maximum of 400 mg/hour, as tolerated (increase in 50 mg/hour increments if initial infusion rate was 50 mg/hour).

Y-90 ibritumomab infusion: Within 4 hours of the completion of rituximab infusion:

Platelet count ≥150,000 cells/mm^3: Inject 0.4 mCi/kg (14.8 MBq/kg actual body weight) over 10 minutes; maximum dose: 32 mCi (1184 MBq)

Platelet count between 100,000-149,000 cells/mm^3 (in relapsed or refractory patients): Inject 0.3 mCi/kg (11.1 MBq/kg actual body weight) over 10 minutes; maximum dose: 32 mCi (1184 MBq)

Platelet count <100,000 cells/mm^3: Do **not** administer

Maximum dose: The prescribed, measured, and administered dose of Y-90 ibritumomab must not exceed 32 mCi (1184 MBq), regardless of the patient's body weight

Administration

Rituximab: Administer the first infusion of rituximab at an initial rate of 50 mg/hour. If hypersensitivity or infusion-related events do not occur, escalate the infusion rate in 50 mg/hour increments every 30 minutes, to a maximum of 400 mg/hour. Immediately stop infusion for severe infusion reaction (discontinue ibritumomab regimen); less severe reactions may be managed by slowing or interrupting infusion. For less severe reactions, infusion may continue at one-half the previous rate upon improvement of patient symptoms. If infusion reaction did not occur in initial rituximab infusion, subsequent rituximab infusion can be administered at an initial rate of 100 mg/hour and increased in 100 mg/hour increments at 30-minute intervals, to a maximum of 400 mg/hour as tolerated. If infusion reaction occurred with initial rituximab infusion, initiate at 50 mg/hour with increases of 50 mg/hour increments.

In-111 and Y-90 ibritumomab: Inject slowly, over 10 minutes through a 0.22 micron low protein binding in-line filter (between syringe and infusion port). After injection, flush line with at least 10 mL normal saline. Y-90 ibritumomab: establish free-flowing I.V. line prior to administration. Avoid extravasation; if signs or symptoms of extravasation occur, stop infusion and restart in another limb.

Monitoring Parameters Patients must be monitored for infusion-related allergic reactions (typically within 30-120 minutes of administration). Monitor for extravasation during ibritumomab infusion. Obtain CBC with differential and platelet counts weekly. Platelet count must be obtained prior to Day 7, 8,or 9. Monitor for up to 3 months after use.

Biodistribution of In-111 ibritumomab should be assessed by imaging at 48-72 hours post injection. Optional additional imaging may be performed to resolve ambiguities. If biodistribution is altered, the patient should not proceed to Day 7, 8, or 9.

Additional Information Ibritumomab tiuxetan is produced in Chinese hamster ovary cell cultures. Kit is not radioactive. Radiolabeling of ibritumomab with Yttrium-90 and Indium-111 (not included in kit) must be performed by appropriate personnel in a specialized facility.

Vesicant May be an irritant; there is an isolated case report of (delayed) erythema and ulceration, which is described as radiation necrosis following yttrium-90-ibritumomab extravasation (Williams, 2006).

Dosage Forms Excipient information presented when available (limited, particularly for generics); consult specific product labeling.

Each kit contains 4 vials for preparation of either In-111 or Y-90 conjugate (as indicated on container label)

Injection, solution:

Zevalin®: 1.6 mg/mL (2 mL) [supplied with sodium acetate solution, formulation buffer vial (includes albumin 750 mg), and an empty reaction vial]

References

Czuczman MS, Emmanouilides C, Darif M, et al, "Treatment-Related Myelodysplastic Syndrome and Acute Myelogenous Leukemia in Patients Treated With Ibritumomab Tiuxetan Radioimmunotherapy," *J Clin Oncol*, 2007, 25(27):4285-92.

Gordon LI, Molina A, Witzig T, et al, "Durable Responses after Ibritumomab Tiuxetan Radioimmunotherapy for CD20+ B-Cell Lymphoma: Long-Term Follow-Up of a Phase 1/2 Study," *Blood*, 2004, 103(12):4429-31.

National Comprehensive Cancer Network® (NCCN), "Clinical Practice Guidelines in Oncology™: Non-Hodgkin's Lymphomas," Version 2.2009. Available at http://www.nccn.org/professionals/physician_gls/PDF/nhl.pdf

Williams G, Palmer MR, Parker JA, et al, "Extravasation of Therapeutic Yttrium-90-Ibritumomab Tiuxetan (Zevalin®): A Case Report," *Cancer Biother Radiopharm*, 2006, 21(2):101-5.

Witzig TE, Gordon LI, Cabanillas F, et al, "Randomized Controlled Trial of Yttrium-90-Labeled Ibritumomab Tiuxetan Radioimmunotherapy Versus Rituximab Immunotherapy for Patients With Relapsed or Refractory Low-Grade, Follicular, or Transformed B-Cell Non-Hodgkin's Lymphoma," *J Clin Oncol*, 2002, 20(10):2453-63.

Witzig TE, White CA, Gordon LI, et al, "Safety of Yttrium-90 Ibritumomab Tiuxetan Radioimmunotherapy for Relapsed Low-Grade, Follicular, or Transformed Non-Hodgkin's Lymphoma," *J Clin Oncol*, 2003, 21(7):1263-70.

Witzig TE, White CA, Wiseman GA, et al, "Phase I/II Trial of IDEC-Y2B8 Radioimmunotherapy for Treatment of Relapsed or Refractory CD20(+) B-Cell Non-Hodgkin's Lymphoma," *J Clin Oncol*, 1999, 17(12):3793-803.

◆ **Ibritumomab Tiuxetan** see Ibritumomab on page 600

◆ **ICI-182,780** see Fulvestrant on page 521

◆ **ICI-46474** see Tamoxifen on page 1072

◆ **ICI-118630** see Goserelin on page 549

◆ **ICI-176334** see Bicalutamide on page 147

◆ **ICI-D1033** see Anastrozole on page 85

◆ **ICI-D1694** see Raltitrexed on page 1005

◆ **ICL670** see Deferasirox on page 330

◆ **ICRF-187** see Dexrazoxane on page 357

◆ **Idamycin® (Can)** see IDArubicin on page 605

◆ **Idamycin PFS®** see IDArubicin on page 605

IDArubicin (eye da ROO bi sin)

Medication Safety Issues

Sound-alike/look-alike issues:

IDArubicin may be confused with DOXOrubicin, DAUNOrubicin, epirubicin

Idamycin PFS® may be confused with Adriamycin

High alert medication: The Institute for Safe Medication Practices (ISMP) includes this medication among its list of drugs which have a heightened risk of causing significant patient harm when used in error.

Related Information

Management of Drug Extravasations on page 1447

Safe Handling of Hazardous Drugs on page 1517

U.S. Brand Names Idamycin PFS®

Index Terms 4-Demethoxydaunorubicin; 4-DMDR; Idarubicin Hydrochloride; IDR; IMI 30; SC 33428

Generic Available Yes

Canadian Brand Names Idamycin®

Pharmacologic Category Antineoplastic Agent, Anthracycline; Antineoplastic Agent, Antibiotic

Use Treatment of acute myeloid leukemia (AML)

Unlabeled/Investigational Use Acute lymphocytic leukemia (ALL)

Pregnancy Risk Factor D

Lactation Excretion in breast milk unknown

Labeled Contraindications Hypersensitivity to idarubicin, other anthracyclines, or any component of the formulation; bilirubin >5 mg/dL; pregnancy

Warnings/Precautions Hazardous agent - use appropriate precautions for handling and disposal. **[U.S. Boxed Warning]: May cause myocardial toxicity (HF, arrhythmias or cardiomyopathies) and is more common in patients who have previously received anthracyclines or have pre-existing cardiac disease.** The risk of myocardial toxicity is also increased in patients with concomitant or prior mediastinal/pericardial irradiation, patients with anemia, bone marrow depression, infections, leukemic pericarditis or myocarditis. Monitor cardiac function during treatment.

[U.S. Boxed Warnings]: May cause severe myelosuppression; use caution in patients with pre-existing myelosuppression from prior treatment or radiation. Use caution with renal or hepatic impairment; may required dosage reductions. For I.V. administration only; may cause severe local tissue damage and necrosis if extravasation occurs. Rapid lysis of leukemic cells may lead to hyperuricemia. Systemic infections should be managed prior to initiation of treatment. **[U.S. Boxed Warning]: Should be administered under the supervision of an experienced cancer chemotherapy physician. Safety and efficacy in children have not been established.**

Adverse Reactions

>10%:

Cardiovascular: Transient ECG abnormalities (supraventricular tachycardia, S-T wave changes, atrial or ventricular extrasystoles); generally asymptomatic and self-limiting. CHF, dose related. The relative cardiotoxicity of idarubicin compared to doxorubicin is unclear. Some investigators report no increase in cardiac toxicity at cumulative oral idarubicin doses up to 540 mg/m^2; other reports suggest a maximum cumulative intravenous dose of 150 mg/m^2.

Central nervous system: Headache

Dermatologic: Alopecia (25% to 30%), radiation recall, skin rash (11%), urticaria

Gastrointestinal: Nausea, vomiting (30% to 60%); diarrhea (9% to 22%); stomatitis (11%); GI hemorrhage (30%)

Genitourinary: Discoloration of urine (darker yellow)

Hematologic: Myelosuppression, primarily leukopenia; thrombocytopenia and anemia. Effects are generally less severe with oral dosing.

Nadir: 10-15 days

Recovery: 21-28 days

Hepatic: Bilirubin and transaminases increased (44%)

1% to 10%:

Central nervous system: Seizure

Neuromuscular & skeletal: Peripheral neuropathy

<1%: Hyperuricemia

Drug Interactions

Avoid Concomitant Use

Avoid concomitant use of IDArubicin with any of the following: Natalizumab; Vaccines (Live)

Increased Effect/Toxicity

IDArubicin may increase the levels/effects of: Leflunomide; Natalizumab; Vaccines (Live)

The levels/effects of IDArubicin may be increased by: Bevacizumab; P-Glycoprotein Inhibitors; Taxane Derivatives; Trastuzumab

Decreased Effect

IDArubicin may decrease the levels/effects of: Cardiac Glycosides; Vaccines (Inactivated); Vaccines (Live)

The levels/effects of IDArubicin may be decreased by: Cardiac Glycosides; Echinacea; P-Glycoprotein Inducers

Storage/Stability Store intact vials of solution under refrigeration at 2°C to 8°C (36°F to 46°F). Protect from light. Solutions diluted in D_5W or NS for infusion are stable for 4 weeks at room temperature, protected from light. Syringe and IVPB solutions are stable for 72 hours at room temperature and 7 days under refrigeration.

Compatibility Stable in D_5NS, D_5W, LR, NS, sterile water for injection, **incompatible** with bacteriostatic water.

Y-site administration: Compatible: Amifostine, amikacin, aztreonam, cimetidine, cladribine, cyclophosphamide, cytarabine, diphenhydramine, droperidol, erythromycin lactobionate, etoposide phosphate, filgrastim, gemcitabine, granisetron, imipenem/cilastatin, magnesium sulfate, mannitol, melphalan, metoclopramide, potassium chloride, ranitidine, sargramostim, thiotepa, vinorelbine. **Incompatible:** Acyclovir, allopurinol, ampicillin/sulbactam, cefazolin, cefepime, ceftazidime, clindamycin, dexamethasone sodium phosphate, etoposide, fluorouracil, furosemide, gentamicin, heparin, hydrocortisone sodium succinate, lorazepam, meperidine, methotrexate, piperacillin/tazobactam, sodium bicarbonate, teniposide, vancomycin, vincristine.

Compatibility when admixed: Incompatible: Heparin.

Mechanism of Action Similar to doxorubicin and daunorubicin; inhibition of DNA and RNA synthesis by intercalation between DNA base pairs

Pharmacodynamics/Kinetics

Absorption: Oral: Variable (4% to 77%; mean: ~30%)

Distribution: V_d: 64 L/kg (some reports indicate 2250 L); extensive tissue binding; CSF

Protein binding: 94% to 97%

Metabolism: Hepatic to idarubicinol (pharmacologically active)

Half-life elimination: Oral: 14-35 hours; I.V.: 12-27 hours

Time to peak, serum: 1-5 hours

Excretion:

Oral: Urine (~5% of dose; 0.5% to 0.7% as unchanged drug, 4% as idarubicinol); hepatic (8%)

I.V.: Urine (13% as idarubicinol, 3% as unchanged drug); hepatic (17%)

Dosage Refer to individual protocols. I.V.:

Children: AML (unlabeled use): 10-12 mg/m^2/day for 3 days every 3 weeks

Adults:

AML induction: 12 mg/m^2/day for 3 days

AML consolidation: 10-12 mg/m^2/day for 2 days

◄ **Dosing adjustment in renal impairment:** The FDA-approved labeling does not contain specific dosing adjustment guidelines; however, it does reccomend that dosage reductions be made. Patients with S_{cr}: ≥2 mg/dL did not receive treatment in many clinical trials. The following guidelines have been used by some clinicians (Aronoff, 2007):

Children:

Cl_{cr} <50 mL/minute: Administer 75% of dose

Hemodialysis: Administer 75% of dose

Continuous ambulatory peritoneal dialysis (CAPD): Administer 75% of dose

Continuous renal replacement therapy (CRRT): Administer 75% of dose

Adults:

Cl_{cr} 10-50 mL/minute: Administer 75% of dose

Cl_{cr} <10 mL/minute: Administer 50% of dose

Hemodialysis/CAPD: Supplemental dose not needed

Dosing adjustment/comments in hepatic impairment:

Bilirubin 2.6-5 mg/dL: Administer 50% of dose

Bilirubin >5 mg/dL: Avoid use

Combination Regimens

Leukemia, acute myeloid:

7 + 3 (Idarubicin) on page 1221

FLAG-IDA on page 1324

Idarubicin, Cytarabine, Etoposide (ICE Protocol) on page 1357

Idarubicin-Cytarabine (High Dose)-Etoposide (AML) on page 1358

Leukemia, acute promyelocytic: Tretinoin-Idarubicin (APL) on page 1414

Administration Do not administer I.M. or SubQ; administer as slow push over 3-5 minutes, preferably into the side of a freely-running saline or dextrose infusion **or** as intermittent infusion over 10-15 minutes into a free-flowing I.V. solution of NS or D_5W; also occasionally administered as a bladder lavage.

Extravasation management: Topical cooling may be achieved using ice packs or cooling pad with circulating ice water. Cooling of site for 24 hours as tolerated by the patient. Elevate and rest extremity 24-48 hours, then resume normal activity as tolerated. Application of cold inhibits vesicant's cytotoxicity. **Application of heat can be harmful and is contraindicated.** If pain, erythema, and/or swelling persist beyond 48 hours, refer patient immediately to plastic surgeon for consultation and possible debridement.

Monitoring Parameters CBC with differential, platelet count, cardiac function, serum electrolytes, creatinine, uric acid, ALT, AST, bilirubin, signs of extravasation

Emetic Potential Moderate (30% to 90%)

Vesicant Yes; see Management of Drug Extravasations on page 1447.

Dosage Forms Excipient information presented when available (limited, particularly for generics); consult specific product labeling.

Injection, solution, as hydrochloride [preservative free] (Idamycin PFS®): 1 mg/mL (5 mL, 10 mL, 20 mL)

References

Aronoff GR, Bennett WM, Berns JS, et al, *Drug Prescribing in Renal Failure: Dosing Guidelines for Adults and Children,* 5th ed. Philadelphia, PA: American College of Physicians; 2007, p 100, 172.

Blijlevens NM, Donnelly JP, and de Pauw BE, "Prospective Evaluation of Gut Mucosal Barrier Injury Following Various Myeloablative Regimens for Haematopoietic Stem Cell Transplant," *Bone Marrow Transplant,* 2005, 35:707-11.

Ferrara F, Palmieri S, Annunziata M, et al, "Continuous Infusion Idarubicin and Oral Busulfan as Conditioning for Patients With Acute Myeloid Leukemia Aged Over 60 Years Undergoing Autologous Stem Cell Transplantation," *Bone Marrow Transplant,* 2004, 34(7):73-576.

Hollingshead LM and Faulds D, "Idarubicin: A Review of Its Pharmacodynamic and Pharmacokinetic Properties, and Therapeutic Potential in the Chemotherapy of Cancer," *Drugs*, 1991, 42(4):690-719.

Mengarelli A, Iori AP, Guglielmi C, et al, "Idarubicin Intensified BUCY2 Regimen in Allogeneic Unmanipulated Transplant for High-Risk Hematological Malignancies," *Leukemia*, 2000, 14 (12):2052-8.

◆ **Idarubicin Hydrochloride** *see* IDArubicin *on page 605*

◆ **IDEC-C2B8** *see* RiTUXimab *on page 1017*

◆ **IDEC-Y2B8** *see* Ibritumomab *on page 600*

◆ **IDR** *see* IDArubicin *on page 605*

◆ **Ifex® [DSC]** *see* Ifosfamide *on page 609*

◆ **Ifex® (Can)** *see* Ifosfamide *on page 609*

Ifosfamide (eye FOSS fa mide)

Medication Safety Issues

Sound-alike/look-alike issues:

Ifosfamide may be confused with cyclophosphamide

High alert medication: The Institute for Safe Medication Practices (ISMP) includes this medication among its list of drugs which have a heightened risk of causing significant patient harm when used in error.

Related Information

Management of Drug Extravasations *on page 1447*
Safe Handling of Hazardous Drugs *on page 1517*

U.S. Brand Names Ifex® [DSC]

Index Terms Isophosphamide; Z4942

Generic Available Yes

Canadian Brand Names Ifex®

Pharmacologic Category Antineoplastic Agent, Alkylating Agent; Antineoplastic Agent, Alkylating Agent (Nitrogen Mustard)

Use Treatment of testicular cancer

Unlabeled/Investigational Use Treatment of bladder cancer, cervical cancer, ovarian cancer, nonsmall cell lung cancer, small cell lung cancer, Hodgkin's and non-Hodgkin's lymphoma; acute lymphocytic leukemia; Ewing's sarcoma, osteosarcoma, and soft tissue sarcomas

Pregnancy Risk Factor D

Lactation Enters breast milk/not recommended

Labeled Contraindications Hypersensitivity to ifosfamide or any component of the formulation; patients with severely depressed bone marrow function

Warnings/Precautions Hazardous agent - use appropriate precautions for handling and disposal. **[U.S. Boxed Warning]: Urotoxic side effects, primarily hemorrhagic cystitis, may occur (dose-limiting toxicity).** Hydration (at least 2 L/day) and/or mesna administration will protect against hemorrhagic cystitis. **[U.S. Boxed Warning]: Severe bone marrow suppression may occur (dose-limiting toxicity);** use is contraindicated in patients with severely depressed bone marrow function. **[U.S. Boxed Warning]: May cause CNS toxicity, including confusion and coma;** usually reversible upon discontinuation of treatment. Encephalopathy, ranging from mild somnolence to hallucinations and/or coma may occur; risk factors may include hypoalbuminemia, renal dysfunction and prior history of ifosfamide-induced encephalopathy. Use with caution in patients with impaired renal function or those with compromised bone marrow reserve. May interfere with wound healing. **[U.S. Boxed Warning]: Should be administered under the** ▶

◄ **supervision of an experienced cancer chemotherapy physician.** Safety and efficacy in children have not been established.

Adverse Reactions

>10%:

Central nervous system: CNS toxicity or encephalopathy (10% to 30%; includes somnolence, agitation, confusion, delirium, hallucinations, depressive psychosis, incontinence, palsy, diplopia, aphasia, or coma)

Dermatologic: Alopecia (83%)

Endocrine & metabolic: Metabolic acidosis (31%)

Gastrointestinal: Nausea/vomiting (58%), may be more common with higher doses or bolus infusion

Hematologic: Myelosuppression (onset: 7-14 days; nadir: 21-28 days; recovery: 21-28 days), leukopenia (50% to ≤100%; grade 4: ≤50%), thrombocytopenia (20%; grades 3/4: 8%)

Renal: Hematuria (6% to 92%; grade 2 [gross hematuria]: 8% to 12%)

1% to 10%:

Central nervous system: Fever

Hepatic: Bilirubin increased (3%), liver dysfunction (3%), transaminases increased (3%)

Local: Phlebitis (2%)

Renal: Renal impairment (6%)

Miscellaneous: Infection (8%)

<1%, postmarketing, and/or case reports: Acidosis, acute renal failure, acute tubular necrosis, allergic reaction, anemia, anorexia, BUN increased, cardiotoxicity, chronic renal failure, coagulopathy, constipation, creatinine increased, dermatitis, diarrhea, Fanconi syndrome, fatigue, hyper-/hypotension, hyperpigmentation, malaise, nail banding/ridging, nonconvulsive status epilepticus, polyneuropathy, proteinuria, pulmonary fibrosis, renal rickets, renal tubular acidosis, salivation, SIADH, sterility, stomatitis

Drug Interactions

Metabolism/Transport Effects Substrate of CYP2A6 (major), 2B6 (minor), 2C8 (minor), 2C9 (minor), 2C19 (major), 3A4 (major); **Inhibits** CYP3A4 (weak); **Induces** CYP2C8 (weak), 2C9 (weak)

Avoid Concomitant Use

Avoid concomitant use of Ifosfamide with any of the following: Natalizumab; Vaccines (Live)

Increased Effect/Toxicity

Ifosfamide may increase the levels/effects of: Leflunomide; Natalizumab; Vaccines (Live); Vitamin K Antagonists

The levels/effects of Ifosfamide may be increased by: CYP2A6 Inhibitors (Moderate); CYP2A6 Inhibitors (Strong); CYP2C19 Inhibitors (Moderate); CYP2C19 Inhibitors (Strong); CYP3A4 Inhibitors (Moderate); CYP3A4 Inhibitors (Strong); Dasatinib; Trastuzumab

Decreased Effect

Ifosfamide may decrease the levels/effects of: Vaccines (Inactivated); Vaccines (Live); Vitamin K Antagonists

The levels/effects of Ifosfamide may be decreased by: CYP2A6 Inducers (Strong); CYP2C19 Inducers (Strong); CYP3A4 Inducers (Strong); Deferasirox; Echinacea; Herbs (CYP3A4 Inducers)

Ethanol/Nutrition/Herb Interactions Herb/Nutraceutical: St John's wort may decrease ifosfamide levels.

Storage/Stability Store intact vials of powder for injection at room temperature of 20°C to 25°C (68°F to 77°F). Store intact vials of solution under refrigeration at 2°C to 8°C (36°F to 46°F). Reconstituted solutions may be stored under refrigeration for up to 21 days. Solutions diluted for administration are stable for 7 days at room temperature and for 6 weeks under refrigeration.

Reconstitution Dilute powder with SWFI or bacteriostatic SWFI to a concentration of 50 mg/mL. Further dilution in 50-1000 mL D_5W or NS (to a final concentration of 0.6-20 mg/mL) is recommended for I.V. infusion.

Compatibility Stable in D_5LR, D_5NS, D_5W, LR, $\frac{1}{2}NS$, NS.

Y-site administration: Compatible: Allopurinol, amifostine, amphotericin B cholesteryl sulfate complex, aztreonam, doxorubicin liposome, etoposide phosphate, filgrastim, fludarabine, gatifloxacin, gemcitabine, granisetron, linezolid, melphalan, ondansetron, paclitaxel, piperacillin/tazobactam, propofol, sargramostim, sodium bicarbonate, teniposide, thiotepa, topotecan, vinorelbine. **Incompatible:** Cefepime, methotrexate.

Compatibility in syringe: Compatible: Epirubicin, mesna. **Incompatible:** Mesna with epirubicin.

Compatibility when admixed: Compatible: Carboplatin, carboplatin with etoposide, cisplatin, cisplatin with etoposide, epirubicin, etoposide, fluorouracil, mesna. **Incompatible:** Mesna with epirubicin.

Mechanism of Action Causes cross-linking of strands of DNA by binding with nucleic acids and other intracellular structures; inhibits protein synthesis and DNA synthesis

Pharmacodynamics/Kinetics Pharmacokinetics are dose dependent

Distribution: V_d: 5.7-49 L; does penetrate CNS, but not in therapeutic levels

Protein binding: Negligible

Metabolism: Hepatic to active metabolites isofosforamide mustard, 4-hydroxyifosfamide, acrolein, and inactive dichloroethylated and carboxy metabolites; acrolein is the agent implicated in development of hemorrhagic cystitis

Half-life elimination:

High dose (3800-5000 mg/m^2): ~15 hours

Lower dose (1600-2400 mg/m^2): ~7 hours

Excretion:

High dose (5000 mg/m^2): Urine (70% to 86%; 61% as unchanged drug)

Lower dose (1600-2400 mg/m^2): Urine (12% to 18% as unchanged drug)

Dosage Refer to individual protocols. To prevent bladder toxicity, ifosfamide should be given with the urinary protector mesna and hydration of at least 2 L of oral or I.V. fluid per day.

Children (unlabeled use): I.V.

1200-1800 mg/m^2/day for 3-5 days every 21-28 days **or**

5 g/m^2 once every 21-28 days **or**

3 g/m^2/day for 2 days every 21-28 days

Adults: I.V.:

Testicular cancer: 1200 mg/m^2/day for 5 days every 3 weeks

Dose ranges used in other cancers (unlabeled uses):

4000-5000 mg/m^2/day for 1 day every 14-28 days **or**

1000-3000 mg/m^2/day for 2-5 days every 21-28 days

Dosing adjustment in renal impairment: The FDA-approved labeling does not contain dosage adjustment guidelines (has not been studied). The following guidelines have been used by some clinicians:

Aronoff, 2007:

Cl_{cr} <10 mL/minute: Children and Adults: Administer 75% of dose

Hemodialysis:

Children: 1 g/m^2 followed by hemodialysis 6-8 hours later

Adults: No supplemental dose needed

Kintzel, 1995:
Cl$_{cr}$ 46-60 mL/minute: Administer 80% of dose
Cl$_{cr}$ 31-45 mL/minute: Administer 75% of dose
Cl$_{cr}$ <30 mL/minute: Administer 70% of dose

Dosing adjustment in hepatic impairment: The FDA-approved labeling does not contain dosage adjustment guidelines (has not been studied). The following guidelines have been used by some clinicians (Floyd, 2006):
Bilirubin >3 mg/dL: Administer 25% of dose

Combination Regimens

Breast cancer: ICE-T on page 1357
Cervical cancer: BIP on page 1235
Esophageal cancer: TIP on page 1407
Head and neck cancer: TIP on page 1407
Hepatoblastoma: IPA on page 1360
Lung cancer (small cell): VIP (Small Cell Lung Cancer) on page 1425
Lymphoma, Hodgkin's: VIM-D (Hodgkin's Lymphoma) on page 1420
Lymphoma, non-Hodgkin's:
ICE (Lymphoma, non-Hodgkin's) on page 1356
IMVP-16 on page 1358
IVAC on page 1361
MINE on page 1366
MINE-ESHAP on page 1367
RICE on page 1402
Lymphoma, non-Hodgkin's (Burkitt's): CODOX-M/IVAC on page 1278
Neuroblastoma:
CI (Neuroblastoma) on page 1263
HIPE-IVAD on page 1348
Osteosarcoma: ICE (Sarcoma) on page 1357
Sarcoma: VAC Alternating With IE (Ewing's Sarcoma) on page 1416
Soft tissue sarcoma:
AI on page 1225
ICE (Sarcoma) on page 1357
ICE-T on page 1357
IE on page 1358
MAID on page 1365
Testicular cancer:
Paclitaxel-Ifosfamide-Cisplatin on page 1389
VIP (Etoposide) (Testicular Cancer) on page 1424
VIP (Vinblastine) (Testicular Cancer) on page 1426

Administration Administer I.V. over 30 minutes to several hours or continuous I.V. over 5 days

Monitoring Parameters CBC with differential, hemoglobin, and platelet count, urine output, urinalysis (prior to each dose), liver function, and renal function tests

Emetic Potential Moderate (30% to 90%)

Vesicant May be an irritant

High Dose Considerations
High Dose I.V.: 7.5-16 g/m^2 in divided doses over several days; generally combined with other high-dose chemotherapy

Dosage Forms Excipient information presented when available (limited, particularly for generics); consult specific product labeling. [DSC] = Discontinued product
Injection, powder for reconstitution: 1 g
Ifex®: 1 g, 3 g [DSC]
Injection, solution: 50 mg/mL (20 mL, 60 mL)

References

Aronoff GR, Bennett WM, Berns JS, et al, *Drug Prescribing in Renal Failure: Dosing Guidelines for Adults and Children*, 5th ed. Philadelphia, PA: American College of Physicians; 2007, p 100, 172.

Brade WP, Herdrich K, Kachel-Fischer U, et al, "Dosing and Side-Effects of Ifosfamide Plus Mesna," *J Cancer Res Clin Oncol*, 1991, 117(Suppl 4):164-86.

David KA and Picus J, "Evaluating Risk Factors for the Development of Ifosfamide Encephalopathy," *Am J Clin Oncol*, 2005, 28(3):277-80.

Floyd J, Mirza I, Sachs B, et al, "Hepatotoxicity of Chemotherapy," *Semin Oncol*, 2006, 33 (1):50-67.

Furlanut M and Franceschi L, "Pharmacology of Ifosfamide," *Oncology*, 2003, 65 Suppl 2:2-6.

Kerbusch T, de Kraker J, Keizer HJ, et al, "Clinical Pharmacokinetics and Pharmacodynamics of Ifosfamide and its Metabolites," *Clin Pharmacokinet*, 2001, 40(1):41-62.

Kintzel PE and Dorr RT, "Anticancer Drug Renal Toxicity and Elimination: Dosing Guidelines for Altered Renal Function," *Cancer Treat Rev*, 1995, 21(1):33-64.

Lotz JP, Bouleuc C, Andre T, et al, "Tandem High-Dose Chemotherapy With Ifosfamide, Carboplatin, and Teniposide With Autologous Bone Marrow Transplantation for the Treatment of Poor Prognosis Common Epithelial Ovarian Carcinoma," *Cancer*, 1996, 77(12):2550-9.

Pelgrims J, DeVos F, Van den Brande J, et al, "Methylene Blue in the Treatment and Prevention of Ifosfamide-Induced Encephalopathy: Report of 12 Cases and a Review of the Literature," *Br J Cancer*, 2000, 82(2) 291-4.

Turner AR, Duong CD, and Good DJ, "Methylene Blue for the Treatment and Prophylaxis of Ifosfamide-Induced Encephalopathy," *Clin Pharmacokinet*, 2003, 15(7):435-9.

Wilson WH, Jain V, Bryant G, et al, "Phase I and II Study of High-Dose Ifosfamide, Carboplatin, and Etoposide With Autologous Bone Marrow Rescue in Lymphomas and Solid Tumors," *J Clin Oncol*, 1992, 10(11):1712-22.

◆ **IGIV** *see* Immune Globulin (Intravenous) *on page 627*

◆ **IGIVnex® (Can)** *see* Immune Globulin (Intravenous) *on page 627*

◆ **IL-2** *see* Aldesleukin *on page 25*

◆ **IL-11** *see* Oprelvekin *on page 880*

Imatinib (eye MAT eh nib)

Medication Safety Issues

Sound-alike/look-alike issues:

Imatinib may be confused with dasatinib, erlotinib, nilotinib, sorafenib, sunitinib

High alert medication: The Institute for Safe Medication Practices (ISMP) includes this medication among its list of drug classes which have a heightened risk of causing significant patient harm when used in error.

Related Information

Safe Handling of Hazardous Drugs *on page 1517*

U.S. Brand Names Gleevec®

Index Terms CGP-57148B; Glivec; Imatinib Mesylate; STI-571

Generic Available No

Canadian Brand Names Gleevec®

Pharmacologic Category Antineoplastic Agent, Tyrosine Kinase Inhibitor

Use Treatment of:

Gastrointestinal stromal tumors (GIST) kit-positive (CD117), including unresectable and/or metastatic malignant and adjuvant treatment following complete resection

Philadelphia chromosome-positive (Ph+) chronic myeloid leukemia (CML) in chronic phase (newly-diagnosed)

Ph+ CML in chronic phase in pediatric patients recurring following stem cell transplant or who are resistant to interferon-alpha therapy (**not** an approved use in Canada)

Ph+ CML in blast crisis, accelerated phase, or chronic phase after failure of interferon therapy

Ph+ acute lymphoblastic leukemia (ALL) (relapsed or refractory)

Aggressive systemic mastocytosis (ASM) without D816V c-Kit mutation (or c-Kit mutation status unknown)

Dermatofibrosarcoma protuberans (DFSP) (unresectable, recurrent and/or metastatic)

Hypereosinophilic syndrome (HES) and/or chronic eosinophilic leukemia (CEL)

Myelodysplastic/myeloproliferative disease (MDS/MPD) associated with platelet-derived growth factor receptor (PDGFR) gene rearrangements

Note: The following use is approved in Canada (not an approved indication in the U.S.):

Ph+ ALL induction therapy (newly diagnosed)

Unlabeled/Investigational Use Treatment of desmoid tumors (soft tissue sarcoma); post-stem cell transplant (allogeneic) follow-up treatment in CML

Pregnancy Risk Factor D

Lactation Enters breast milk/not recommended

Labeled Contraindications There are no contraindications listed within the FDA-approved manufacturer's labeling.

Canadian labeling: Hypersensitivity to imatinib or any component of the formulation

Warnings/Precautions Hazardous agent - use appropriate precautions for handling and disposal. Often associated with fluid retention, weight gain, and edema (probability increases with higher doses and age >65 years); occasionally leading to significant complications, including pleural effusion, pericardial effusion, pulmonary edema, and ascites. Use with caution in patients where fluid accumulation may be poorly tolerated, such as in cardiovascular disease (heart failure [HF] or hypertension) and pulmonary disease. Severe HF and left ventricular dysfunction (LVD) have been reported rarely, usually in patients with comorbidities and/or risk factors; carefully monitor patients with pre-existing cardiac disease or risk factors for HF. With initiation of imatinib treatment, cardiogenic shock and/or LVD have been reported in patients with hypereosinophilic syndrome and cardiac involvement (reversible with systemic steroids, circulatory support and temporary cessation of imatinib). Patients with high eosinophil levels and an abnormal echocardiogram or abnormal serum troponin level may benefit from prophylactic systemic steroids with the initiation of imatinib.

Severe bullous dermatologic reactions (including erythema multiforme and Stevens-Johnson syndrome) have been reported; reintroduction has been attempted following resolution. Successful resumption at a lower dose (with corticosteroids and/or antihistamine) has been described; however, some patients may experience recurrent reactions.

Hepatotoxicity may occur (may be severe); monitor; therapy interruption or dose reduction may be necessary. Transaminase and bilirubin elevations, and acute liver failure have been observed with imatinib in combination with chemotherapy. Use with caution in patients with pre-existing hepatic impairment; may require dosage adjustment. Use with caution in renal impairment; may require dosage adjustment.

May cause GI irritation, severe hemorrhage (grades 3 and 4; including gastrointestinal hemorrhage and/or tumor hemorrhage; hemorrhage incidence is higher in patients with GIST), or hematologic toxicity (anemia, neutropenia, and thrombocytopenia); median duration of neutropenia is 2-3 weeks; median duration of thrombocytopenia is 3-4 weeks. Hypothyroidism has been reported in thyroidectomy patients (receiving thyroid hormone replacement therapy) during imatinib therapy; monitor. Has been associated with development of opportunistic infections. Use with caution in patients receiving concurrent therapy with drugs which alter cytochrome P450 activity or require metabolism by these isoenzymes; avoid concomitant use of strong CYP3A4 inducers. Safety and efficacy in patients <2 years of age have not been established.

Adverse Reactions Note: Adverse reactions listed as a composite of data across many trials, except where noted for a specific cancer type.

>10%:

Cardiovascular: Edema/fluid retention (33% to 86%; grades 3/4: 3% to 13%; includes aggravated edema, anasarca, ascites, pericardial effusion, peripheral edema, pleural effusion, pulmonary edema and superficial edema); facial edema (DFSP 17%), chest pain (GIST ≤7%, CML 7% to 11%)

Central nervous system: Fatigue (29% to 75%), fever (13% to 41%), headache (19% to 37%), dizziness (10% to 19%), insomnia (10% to 19%), depression (≤15%), anxiety (7% to 12%), chills (≤11%)

Dermatologic: Rash (9% to 50%; grades 3/4: 1% to 9%), pruritus (8% to 19%), alopecia (GIST 10% to 15%)

Endocrine & metabolic: Hypokalemia (6% to 13%)

Gastrointestinal: Nausea (42% to 73%), diarrhea (25% to 59%), vomiting (23% to 58%), abdominal pain (6% to 57%), anorexia (≤36%), weight gain (5% to 32%), dyspepsia (11% to 27%), constipation (9% to 16%)

Hematologic: Hemorrhage (12% to 53%; grades 3/4: 2% to 19%), neutropenia (grade 3: 7% to 27%; grade 4: 3% to 48%), thrombocytopenia (grade 3: 1% to 31%; grade 4: <1% to 33%), anemia (grade 3: 1% to 42%; grade 4: 1% to 11%), leukopenia (GIST 5% to 20%)

Hepatic: ALT increased (≤17%; grade 3: 2% to 7%; grade 4: <3%), hepatotoxicity (6% to 12%; grades 3/4: 3% to 8%)

Neuromuscular & skeletal: Muscle cramps (16% to 62%), arthralgia (≤40%), joint pain (11% to 31%), myalgia (9% to 32%), weakness (≤21%), musculoskeletal pain (children 21%; adults 12% to 49%), rigors (10% to 12%), bone pain (≤11%)

Ocular: Periorbital edema (DFSP 33%; MPD 29%; GIST ≤47%), lacrimation increased (DFSP 25%; GIST ≤10%)

Renal: Serum creatinine increased (≤12%; grade 3: ≤3%; DFSP: grade 4: 8%)

Respiratory: Nasopharyngitis (10% to 31%), cough (11% to 27%), dyspnea (≤21%), upper respiratory tract infection (3% to 21%), pharyngolaryngeal pain (7% to 18%), rhinitis (DFSP 17%), pharyngitis (CML 10% to 15%), pneumonia (CML 4% to 13%), sinusitis (4% to 11%)

Miscellaneous: Night sweats (CML 13% to 17%), infection without neutropenia (GIST ≤17%), influenza (1% to 14%), diaphoresis (GIST ≤13%)

1% to 10%:

Cardiovascular: Flushing

Central nervous system: CNS/cerebral hemorrhage (≤9%), hypoesthesia

Dermatologic: Dry skin, erythema, photosensitivity reaction

Endocrine & metabolic: Hyperglycemia (≤10%), hypocalcemia (GIST ≤6%), albumin decreased (grade 3: ≤4%)

Gastrointestinal: Flatulence (≤10%), stomatitis/mucositis (≤10%), weight loss (≤10%), gastrointestinal hemorrhage (2% to 8%), abdominal distension, gastritis, gastroesophageal reflux, mouth ulceration, taste disturbance, xerostomia

Hematologic: Lymphopenia (GIST ≤10%), neutropenic fever, pancytopenia

Hepatic: Alkaline phosphatase increased (grade 3: ≤6%; grade 4: <1%), AST increased (grade 3: 2% to 4%; grade 4: ≤3%), bilirubin increased (grade 3: 1% to 4%; grade 4: ≤3%)

Neuromuscular & skeletal: Back pain (GIST ≤7%), limb pain (GIST ≤7%), peripheral neuropathy, joint swelling, paresthesia

Ocular: Blurred vision, conjunctival hemorrhage, conjunctivitis, dry eyes, eyelid edema

Respiratory: Epistaxis

<1%, postmarketing, and/or case reports (limited to important or life-threatening): Acute febrile neutropenic dermatosis (Sweet's syndrome), amylase increased, anaphylactic shock, angina, angioedema, aplastic anemia, arrhythmia, ascites, atrial fibrillation, avascular necrosis, blepharitis, breast enlargement, bullous eruption, cardiac arrest, cardiac failure, cardiac tamponade, cardiogenic shock, cataract, cellulitis, cerebral edema, cheilitis, CHF (severe), colitis, confusion, CPK increased, dehydration, diverticulitis, dysphagia, embolism, eosinophilia, erythema multiforme, esophagitis, exanthematous pustulosis (acute generalized), exfoliative dermatitis, fungal infection, gastric ulcer, gastroenteritis, gastrointestinal obstruction, gastrointestinal perforation, glaucoma, gout, hearing loss, hematoma, hematemesis, hematuria, hemolytic anemia, hemorrhagic corpus luteum, hemorrhagic ovarian cyst, hepatic failure, hepatic necrosis, hepatitis, herpes simplex, herpes zoster, hip osteonecrosis, hypercalcemia, hyperkalemia, hyperuricemia, hyper-/hypotension, hypomagnesemia, hyponatremia, hypophosphatemia, ileus, inflammatory bowel disease, interstitial lung disease, interstitial pneumonitis, intracranial pressure increased, jaundice, LDH increased, left ventricular dysfunction, leukocytoclastic vasculitis, libido decreased, lichen planus, lichenoid keratosis, lymphadenopathy, macular edema, melena, memory impairment, menorrhagia, MI, migraine, myopathy, optic neuritis, palpitation, pancreatitis, papilledema, pericarditis, petechiae, pleural effusion, pleuritic pain, pulmonary fibrosis, pulmonary hemorrhage, pulmonary hypertension, purpura, pustular rash, Raynaud's phenomenon, renal failure, respiratory failure, respiratory tract (lower) infection, retinal hemorrhage, rhabdomyolysis, sciatica, scleral hemorrhage, seizure, sepsis, sexual dysfunction, skin pigment changes, somnolence, Stevens-Johnson syndrome, syncope, tachycardia, thrombocythemia, thrombosis, tinnitus, toxic epidermal necrolysis, tremor, tumor hemorrhage (GIST), tumor necrosis, urinary tract infection, urticaria, vertigo, vesicular rash, vitreous hemorrhage

Drug Interactions

Metabolism/Transport Effects Substrate of CYP1A2 (minor), 2D6 (minor), 2C9 (minor), 2C19 (minor), 3A4 (major), **Inhibits** CYP2C9 (weak), 2D6 (moderate), 3A4 (strong)

Avoid Concomitant Use

Avoid concomitant use of Imatinib with any of the following: Alfuzosin; Dronedarone; Eplerenone; Everolimus; Halofantrine; Natalizumab; Nilotinib; Nisoldipine; Ranolazine; Rivaroxaban; Salmeterol; Silodosin; Thioridazine; Tolvaptan; Vaccines (Live)

Increased Effect/Toxicity

Imatinib may increase the levels/effects of: Acetaminophen; Alfuzosin; Almotriptan; Alosetron; Ciclesonide; Colchicine; CycloSPORINE; CYP2D6 Substrates; CYP3A4 Substrates; Dronedarone; Dutasteride; Eplerenone; Everolimus; FentaNYL; Fesoterodine; Halofantrine; Ixabepilone; Leflunomide; Maraviroc; Natalizumab; Nebivolol; Nilotinib; Nisoldipine; Paricalcitol; Pimecrolimus; Ranolazine; Rivaroxaban; Salmeterol; Saxagliptin; Silodosin;

Simvastatin; Sorafenib; Tadalafil; Tamoxifen; Thioridazine; Tolvaptan; Topotecan; Vaccines (Live); Vitamin K Antagonists; Warfarin

The levels/effects of Imatinib may be increased by: Antifungal Agents (Azole Derivatives, Systemic); CYP3A4 Inhibitors (Moderate); CYP3A4 Inhibitors (Strong); Dasatinib; Lansoprazole; P-Glycoprotein Inhibitors; Trastuzumab

Decreased Effect

Imatinib may decrease the levels/effects of: Cardiac Glycosides; Codeine; Prasugrel; TraMADol; Vaccines (Inactivated); Vaccines (Live); Vitamin K Antagonists

The levels/effects of Imatinib may be decreased by: CYP3A4 Inducers (Strong); Deferasirox; Echinacea; Peginterferon Alfa-2b; P-Glycoprotein Inducers; Rifamycin Derivatives; St Johns Wort

Ethanol/Nutrition/Herb Interactions

Ethanol: Avoid ethanol.

Food: Food may reduce gastrointestinal irritation. Avoid grapefruit juice (may increase imatinib plasma concentration).

Herb/Nutraceutical: Avoid St John's wort (may increase metabolism and decrease imatinib plasma concentration).

Storage/Stability Store at 25°C (77°F); excursions permitted between 15°C to 30°C (59°F to 86°F). Protect from moisture.

Mechanism of Action Inhibits Bcr-Abl tyrosine kinase, the constitutive abnormal gene product of the Philadelphia chromosome in chronic myeloid leukemia (CML). Inhibition of this enzyme blocks proliferation and induces apoptosis in Bcr-Abl positive cell lines as well as in fresh leukemic cells in Philadelphia chromosome positive CML. Also inhibits tyrosine kinase for platelet-derived growth factor (PDGF), stem cell factor (SCF), c-Kit, and cellular events mediated by PDGF and SCF.

Pharmacodynamics/Kinetics

Absorption: Rapid

Protein binding: Parent drug and metabolite: ~95% to albumin and alpha$_1$-acid glycoprotein

Metabolism: Hepatic via CYP3A4 (minor metabolism via CYP1A2, CYP2D6, CYP2C9, CYP2C19); primary metabolite (active): N-demethylated piperazine derivative (CGP74588); severe hepatic impairment (bilirubin >3-10 times ULN) increases AUC by 45% to 55% for imatinib and its active metabolite, respectively

Bioavailability: 98%

Half-life elimination: Adults: Parent drug: ~18 hours; N-desmethyl metabolite: ~40 hours; Children: Parent drug: ~15 hours

Time to peak: 2-4 hours

Excretion: Feces (68% primarily as metabolites, 20% as unchanged drug); urine (13% primarily as metabolites, 5% as unchanged drug)

Dosage Oral: **Note:** For concurrent use with a strong CYP3A4 enzyme-inducing agent (eg, rifampin, phenytoin), imatinib dosage should be increased by at least 50%. The optimal duration of therapy for CML is not yet determined, discontinuing treatment is not recommended after achieving remission due to the potential for relapse (NCCN CML guidelines v.2.2010).

Children ≥2 years: **Note:** May be administered once daily or in 2 divided doses.
Ph+ CML (chronic phase, recurrent or resistant): 260 mg/m^2/day

Ph+ CML (chronic phase, newly diagnosed): 340 mg/m^2/day; maximum: 600 mg/day

Adults: **Note:** Doses ≤600 mg should be administered once daily, 800 mg doses should be administered as 400 mg twice a day.

Ph+ CML:

Chronic phase: 400 mg once daily; may be increased to 600 mg/day, if tolerated, for disease progression, lack of hematologic response after 3 months, lack of cytogenetic response after 6-12 months, or loss of previous hematologic or cytogenetic response

Canadian labeling and NCCN CML guidelines (v.2.2010): Includes range up to 800 mg/day (400 mg twice daily)

Accelerated phase or blast crisis: 600 mg once daily; may be increased to 800 mg/day (400 mg twice daily), if tolerated, for disease progression, lack of hematologic response after 3 months, lack of cytogenetic response after 6-12 months, or loss of previous hematologic or cytogenetic response

Ph+ ALL (relapsed or refractory): 600 mg once daily

GIST (adjuvant treatment following complete resection): 400 mg once daily

GIST (unresectable and/or metastatic malignant): 400 mg once daily; may be increased up to 800 mg/day (400 mg twice daily), if tolerated, for disease progression. **Note:** Significant improvement (progression-free survival, objective response rate) was demonstrated in patients with KIT exon 9 mutation with 800 mg (versus 400 mg), although overall survival (OS) was not impacted. The higher dose did not demonstrate a difference in time to progression or OS patients with Kit exon 11 mutation or wild-type status (Debiec-Rychter, 2006; Heinrich, 2009).

ASM with eosinophilia: Initiate at 100 mg once daily; titrate up to a maximum of 400 mg once daily (if tolerated) for insufficient response to lower dose

ASM without D816V c-Kit mutation or c-Kit mutation status unknown: 400 mg once daily

DFSP: 400 mg twice daily

HES/CEL: 400 mg once daily

HES/CEL with FIP1L1-PDGFRα fusion kinase: Initiate at 100 mg once daily; titrate up to a maximum of 400 mg once daily (if tolerated) if insufficient response to lower dose

MDS/MPD: 400 mg once daily

Ph+ ALL (induction, newly diagnosed): *Canadian labeling (not an approved use in the U.S.):* 600 mg once daily

Dosage adjustment with concomitant strong CYP3A4 inducers: Avoid concomitant use of strong CYP3A4 inducers (eg, dexamethasone, carbamazepine, phenobarbital, phenytoin, rifampin); if concomitant use can not be avoided, increase imatinib dose by at least 50% with careful monitoring.

Dosage adjustment for renal impairment:

Recommendation in the FDA-approved labeling:

Mild impairment (Cl_{cr} 40-59 mL/minute): Maximum recommended dose: 600 mg

Moderate impairment (Cl_{cr} 20-39 mL/minute): Decrease recommended starting dose by 50%; dose may be increased as tolerated; maximum recommended dose: 400 mg

Severe impairment (Cl_{cr} <20 mL/minute): Use caution; a dose of 100 mg/day has been tolerated in severe impairment (Gibbons, 2008)

Canadian labeling recommendation:

Mild impairment (Cl_{cr} 40-59 mL/minute): Use caution; usual minimum recommended effective dose: 400 mg once daily; titrate to efficacy and tolerability

Moderate impairment (Cl_{cr} 20-39 mL/minute): Use caution; usual minimum recommended effective dose: 400 mg once daily; titrate to efficacy and tolerability; the use of 800 mg dose is not recommended

Severe impairment (Cl$_{cr}$ <20 mL/minute): Use is not recommended

Dosage adjustment for hepatic impairment:
Mild-to-moderate impairment: No adjustment necessary
Canadian labeling: GIST: Minimum effective dose: 400 mg once daily
Severe impairment:
   Manufacturer's FDA-approved labeling: Reduce dose by 25%
   Canadian labeling: GIST: 200 mg dose once daily with titration to 300 mg
   once daily in the absence of severe toxicity
   NCCN soft tissue sarcoma guidelines (v.2.2009): GIST: Reduce dose by
   25% to 50%

Dosage adjustment for hepatotoxicity (during therapy) or other non-hematologic adverse reactions: Withhold treatment until toxicity resolves; may resume if appropriate (depending on initial severity of adverse event)
NCCN soft tissue sarcoma guidelines (v.2.2009): GIST: Superficial edema:
   Manage with supportive care, diuretics, or dosage reduction

Hepatotoxicity (during therapy): If elevations of bilirubin >3 times upper limit of normal (ULN) or transaminases >5 times ULN occur, withhold treatment until bilirubin <1.5 times ULN and transaminases <2.5 times ULN. Resume treatment at a reduced dose as follows:
Children ≥2 years:
   If current dose 260 mg/m^2/day, reduce dose to 200 mg/m^2/day
   If current dose 340 mg/m^2/day, reduce dose to 260 mg/m^2/day
Adults:
   If current dose 400 mg, reduce dose to 300 mg
   If current dose 600 mg, reduce dose to 400 mg
   If current dose 800 mg, reduce dose to 600 mg

Dosage adjustment for hematologic adverse reactions:
Chronic phase CML (initial dose 400 mg/day in adults or 260-340 mg/m^2/day in children), ASM, MDS/MPD, and HES/CEL (initial dose 400 mg/day), or GIST (initial dose 400 mg): If ANC <1 x 10^9/L and/or platelets <50 x 10^9/L: Withhold until ANC ≥1.5 x 10^9/L and platelets ≥75 x 10^9/L; resume treatment at original starting dose. For recurrent neutropenia or thrombocytopenia, withhold until recovery, and reinstitute treatment at a reduced dose as follows:
Children ≥2 years:
   If initial dose 260 mg/m^2/day, reduce dose to 200 mg/m^2/day
   If initial dose 340 mg/m^2/day, reduce dose to 260 mg/m^2/day
Adults: If initial dose 400 mg, reduce dose to 300 mg
CML (accelerated phase or blast crisis) and PH+ ALL: Adults (initial dose 600 mg): If ANC <0.5 x 10^9/L and/or platelets <10 x 10^9/L, establish whether cytopenia is related to leukemia (bone marrow aspirate or biopsy). If unrelated to leukemia, reduce dose to 400 mg. If cytopenia persists for an additional 2 weeks, further reduce dose to 300 mg. If cytopenia persists for 4 weeks and is still unrelated to leukemia, withhold treatment until ANC ≥1 x 10^9/L and platelets ≥20 x 10^9/L, then resume treatment at 300 mg.
ASM associated with eosinophilia and HES/CEL with FIP1L1-PDGFRα fusion kinase (starting dose 100 mg/day): If ANC <1 x 10^9/L and/or platelets <50 x 10^9/L: Withhold until ANC ≥1.5 x 10^9/L and platelets ≥75 x 10^9/L; resume treatment at previous dose.
DFSP (initial dose 800 mg/day): If ANC <1 x 10^9/L and/or platelets <50 x 10^9/L, withhold until ANC ≥1.5 x 10^9/L and platelets ≥75 x 10^9/L; resume treatment at reduced dose of 600 mg/day. If depression in neutrophils or

platelets recurs, withhold until recovery, and reinstitute treatment with a further dose reduction to 400 mg/day.

Combination Regimens

Leukemia, acute lymphocytic: Hyper-CVAD + Imatinib on page 1348

Administration Should be administered with a meal and a large glass of water. Tablets may be dispersed in water or apple juice (using ~50 mL for 100 mg tablet, ~200 mL for 400 mg tablet); stir until dissolved and use immediately. For daily dosing ≥800 mg, the 400 mg tablets should be used in order to reduce iron exposure.

Monitoring Parameters CBC (weekly for first month, biweekly for second month, then periodically thereafter), liver function tests (at baseline and monthly or as clinically indicated; more frequently [at least weekly] in patients with moderate-to-severe hepatic impairment [Ramanathan, 2008]), renal function, serum electrolytes (including calcium, phosphorus, potassium and sodium levels); thyroid function tests (in thyroidectomy patients); fatigue, weight, and edema/fluid status; consider echocardiogram and serum troponin levels in patients with HES/CEL, and in patients with MDS/MPD or ASM with high eosinophil levels; in pediatric patients, also monitor serum glucose and albumin

Monitor for signs/symptoms of CHF in patients with at risk for cardiac failure or patients with pre-existing cardiac disease. In Canada, a baseline evaluation of left ventricular ejection fraction is recommended prior to initiation of imatinib therapy in all patients with known underlying heart disease or in elderly patients.

Dietary Considerations Should be taken with food and a large glass of water to decrease gastrointestinal irritation. Avoid grapefruit juice.

Additional Information Patients with HES/CEL, MDS/MPD or ASM with an abnormal echocardiogram or abnormal serum troponin level may benefit from prophylactic systemic steroids (1-2 mg/kg for 1-2 weeks) with the initiation of imatinib.

Emetic Potential Moderate (30% to 60%)

Dosage Forms Excipient information presented when available (limited, particularly for generics); consult specific product labeling.

Tablet:

Gleevec®: 100 mg; 400 mg

References

Atallah E, Durand JB, Kantarjian H, et al, "Congestive Heart Failure is a Rare Event in Patients Receiving Imatinib Therapy," *Blood*, 2007, 110(4):1233-7.

Ault P, Kantarjian H, O'Brien S, et al, "Pregnancy Among Patients with Chronic Myeloid Leukemia Treated with Imatinib," *J Clin Oncol*, 2006, 24(7):1204-8.

Berman E, Nicolaides M, Maki RG, et al, "Altered Bone and Mineral Metabolism in Patients Receiving Imatinib Mesylate," *N Engl J Med*, 2006, 354(19):2006-13.

Carpenter PA, Snyder DS, Flowers ME, et al, "Prophylactic Administration of Imatinib After Hematopoietic Cell Transplantation for High-Risk Philadelphia Chromosome-Positive Leukemia," *Blood*, 2007, 109(7):2791-3.

Debiec-Rychter M, Sciot R, Le Cesne A, et al, "KIT mutations and Dose Selection for Imatinib in Patients With Advanced Gastrointestinal Stromal Tumors," *Eur J Cancer*, 2006, 42(8):1093-103.

de Groot JW, Zonnenberg BA, Plukker JT, et al, "Imatinib Induces Hypothyroidism in Patients Receiving Levothyroxine," *Clin Pharmacol Ther*, 2005, 78(4):433-8.

DeMatteo R, Owzar K, Maki R, et al, "Adjuvant Imatinib Mesylate Increases Recurrence Free Survival (RFS) in Patients With Completely Resected Localized Primary Gastrointestinal Stromal Tumor (GIST): North American Intergroup Phase III Trial ACOSOG Z9001," *J Clin Oncol*, 2007, 28(18 Supp) [abstract 10079 from 2007 ASCO Annual Meeting].

Dewar AL, Farrugia AN, Condina MR, et al, "Imatinib as a Potential Antiresorptive Therapy for Bone Disease," *Blood*, 2006, 107(11):4334-7.

Droogendijk HJ, Kluin-Nelemans HJ, van Doormaal JJ, et al, "Imatinib Mesylate in the Treatment of Systemic Mastocytosis: A Phase II Trial," *Cancer*, 2006, 107(2):345-51

Druker BJ, Sawyers CL, Kantarjian H, et al, "Activity of a Specific Inhibitor of the BCR-ABL Tyrosine Kinase in the Blast Crisis of Chronic Myeloid Leukemia and Acute Lymphoblastic Leukemia With the Philadelphia Chromosome," *N Engl J Med*, 2001, 344(14):1038-42.

Druker BJ, Talpaz M, Resta DJ, et al, "Efficacy and Safety of a Specific Inhibitor of the BCR-ABL Tyrosine Kinase in Chronic Myeloid Leukemia," *N Engl J Med*, 2001, 344(14):1031-7.

Gibbons J, Egorin MJ, Ramanathan RK, et al, "Phase I and Pharmacokinetic Study of Imatinib Mesylate in Patients With Advanced Malignancies and Varying Degrees of Renal Dysfunction: A Study by the National Cancer Institute Organ Dysfunction Working Group," *J Clin Oncol*, 2008, 26 (4):570-6.

Gotlib J, Cools J, Malone JM 3rd, et al, "The FIP1L1-PDGFRalpha Fusion Tyrosine Kinase in Hypereosinophilic Syndrome and Chronic Eosinophilic Leukemia: Implications for Diagnosis, Classification, and Management," *Blood*, 2004, 103(8):2879-91.

Heinrich MC, Owzar K, Corless CL, et al, "Correlation of Kinase Genotype and Clinical Outcome in the North American Intergroup Phase III Trial of Imatinib Mesylate for Treatment of Advanced Gastrointestinal Stromal Tumor: CALGB 150105 Study by Cancer and Leukemia Group B and Southwest Oncology Group," *J Clin Oncol*, 2008, 26(33):5360-7.

Hess G, Bunjes D, Siegert W, et al, "Sustained Complete Molecular Remissions After Treatment With Imatinib-Mesylate in Patients With Failure After Allogeneic Stem Cell Transplantation for Chronic Myelogenous Leukemia: Results of a Prospective Phase II Open-Label Multicenter Study," *J Clin Oncol*, 2005, 23(30):7583-93.

Kantarjian H, Sawyers CL, Hochhaus A, et al, "Hematologic and Cytogenetic Responses to Imatinib Mesylate in Chronic Myelogenous Leukemia," *N Engl J Med*, 2002, 346:645-52.

Kerkela R, Grazette L, Yacobi R, et al, "Cardiotoxicity of the Cancer Therapeutic Agent Imatinib Mesylate," *Nat Med*, 2006, 12(8):908-16.

Larson RA, Druker BJ, Guilhot F, et al, "Imatinib Pharmacokinetics and its Correlation With Response and Safety in Chronic-Phase Chronic Myeloid Leukemia: A Subanalysis of the IRIS Study," *Blood*, 2008, 111(8):4022-8.

McArthur GA, Demetri GD, van Oosterom A, et al, "Molecular and Clinical Analysis of Locally Advanced Dermatofibrosarcoma Protuberans Treated with Imatinib: Imatinib Target Exploration Consortium Study B2225," *J Clin Oncol*, 2005, 23(4):866-73.

National Comprehensive Cancer Network (NCCN)® "Practice Guidelines in Oncology™: Chronic Myelogenous Leukemia Version 2.2010." Available at http://www.nccn.org/professionals/ physician_gls/PDF/cml.pdf.

National Comprehensive Cancer Network (NCCN)®."Practice Guidelines in Oncology™: Soft Tissue Sarcoma Version 2.2009." Available at http://www.nccn.org/professionals/physician_gls/ PDF/sarcoma.pdf

Ottmann OG, Wassmann B, Pfeifer H, et al, "Imatinib Compared With Chemotherapy as Front-Line Treatment of Elderly Patients With Philadelphia Chromosome-Positive Acute Lymphoblastic Leukemia (Ph+ALL)," *Cancer*, 2007, 109(10):2068-76.

Pye SM, Cortes J, Ault P, et al, "The Effects of Imatinib on Pregnancy Outcome," *Blood*, 2008, 111 (12):5505-8.

Ramanathan RK, Egorin MJ, Takimoto CH, et al, "Phase I and Pharmacokinetic Study of Imatinib Mesylate in Patients With Advanced Malignancies and Varying Degrees of Liver Dysfunction: A Study by the National Cancer Institute Organ Dysfunction Working Group," *J Clin Oncol*, 2008, 26 (4):563-9.

Thomas DA, Faderl S, Cortes J, et al, "Treatment of Philadelphia Chromosome-Positive Acute Lymphocytic Leukemia With Hyper-CVAD and Imatinib Mesylate," *Blood*, 2004, 103 (12):4396-407.

Yanada M, Takeuchi J, Sugiura I, et al, "High Complete Remission Rate and Promising Outcome by Combination of Imatinib and Chemotherapy for Newly Diagnosed BCR-ABL-Positive Acute Lymphoblastic Leukemia: A Phase II Study by the Japan Adult Leukemia Study Group," *J Clin Oncol*, 2006, 24(3):460-6.

Imipenem and Cilastatin (i mi PEN em & sye la STAT in)

Medication Safety Issues
Sound-alike/look-alike issues:
Imipenem may be confused with ertapenem, meropenem
Primaxin® may be confused with Premarin®, Primacor®

U.S. Brand Names Primaxin®

Index Terms Imipemide

Generic Available No

Canadian Brand Names Primaxin®; Primaxin® I.V.

Pharmacologic Category Antibiotic, Carbapenem

Use Treatment of lower respiratory tract, urinary tract, intra-abdominal, gynecologic, bone and joint, skin and skin structure, and polymicrobic infections as well as bacterial septicemia and endocarditis. Antibacterial activity includes resistant gram-negative bacilli (*Pseudomonas aeruginosa* and *Enterobacter* sp), gram-positive bacteria (methicillin-sensitive *Staphylococcus aureus* and *Streptococcus* sp) and anaerobes.

Unlabeled/Investigational Use Hepatic abscess; neutropenic fever; melioidosis

Pregnancy Risk Factor C

Lactation Enters breast milk/use caution

Labeled Contraindications Hypersensitivity to imipenem/cilastatin or any component of the formulation
I.M. formulation (due to lidocaine diluent) additional contraindications: Hypersensitivity to amide-type anesthetics; severe shock or heart block

Warnings/Precautions Dosage adjustment required in patients with impaired renal function; elderly patients often require lower doses (adjust carefully to renal function). Prolonged use may result in fungal or bacterial superinfection, including *C. difficile*-associated diarrhea (CDAD) and pseudomembranous colitis; CDAD has been observed >2 months postantibiotic treatment. Has been associated with CNS adverse effects, including confusional states and seizures (myoclonic); use with caution in patients with a history of seizures or hypersensitivity to beta-lactams (including penicillins and cephalosporins); patients with impaired renal function are at increased risk of seizures if not properly dose adjusted. Not recommended in pediatric CNS infections due to seizure potential. Serious hypersensitivity reactions, including anaphylaxis, have been reported (some without a history of previous allergic reactions to beta-lactams). Doses for I.M. administration are mixed with lidocaine; consult information on lidocaine for associated warnings/precautions. Two different imipenem/cilastatin products are available; due to differences in formulation, the I.V. and I.M. preparations **cannot** be interchanged. Safety and efficacy of I.M. administration in children <12 years of age have not been established.

Adverse Reactions Adverse reactions reported with use for both I.V. and I.M. formulations in adults, except where noted.
1% to 10%:
Cardiovascular: Tachycardia (infants 2%; adults <1%)
Central nervous system: Seizure (infants 6%; adults <1%)
Dermatologic: Rash (≤1%, children 2%)
Gastrointestinal: Nausea (1% to 2%), diarrhea (children 3% to 4%; adults 1% to 2%), vomiting (≤2%)
Genitourinary: Oliguria/anuria (infants 2%; adults <1%)
Local: Phlebitis/thrombophlebitis (3%), pain at I.M. injection site (1.2%)
<1%, postmarketing and/or case reports: Abdominal pain, abnormal urinalysis, acute renal failure, alkaline phosphatase increased, anaphylaxis, anemia,

angioneurotic edema, asthenia, bilirubin increased, bone marrow depression, BUN/creatinine increased, candidiasis, confusion, cyanosis, dizziness, drug fever, dyspnea, encephalopathy, eosinophilia, erythema multiforme, fever, flushing, gastroenteritis, glossitis, hallucinations, headache, hearing loss, hematocrit decreased, hemoglobin decreased, hemolytic anemia, hemorrhagic colitis, hepatitis (including fulminant onset), hepatic failure, hyperchloremia, hyperhidrosis, hyperkalemia, hypersensitivity, hyperventilation, hyponatremia, hypotension, injection site erythema, jaundice, lactate dehydrogenase increased, leukocytosis, leukopenia, myoclonus, neutropenia (including agranulocytosis), palpitation, pancytopenia, paresthesia, pharyngeal pain, polyarthralgia, polyuria, positive Coombs' test, prothrombin time increased, pruritus, pruritus vulvae, pseudomembranous colitis, psychic disturbances, rash, resistant *P. aeruginosa*, salivation increased, somnolence, staining of teeth, Stevens-Johnson syndrome, taste perversion, thoracic spine pain, thrombocythemia, thrombocytopenia, tinnitus, tongue/ tooth discoloration, tongue papillar hypertrophy, toxic epidermal necrolysis, transaminases increased, tremor, urine discoloration, urticaria, vertigo

Drug Interactions

Avoid Concomitant Use

Avoid concomitant use of Imipenem and Cilastatin with any of the following: Ganciclovir

Increased Effect/Toxicity

The levels/effects of Imipenem and Cilastatin may be increased by: Ganciclovir; Uricosuric Agents

Decreased Effect

Imipenem and Cilastatin may decrease the levels/effects of: Typhoid Vaccine; Valproic Acid

Storage/Stability Imipenem/cilastatin powder for injection should be stored at <25°C (77°F).

I.M.: The I.M. suspension should be used within 1 hour of reconstitution.

I.V.: Reconstituted I.V. solutions are stable for 4 hours at room temperature and 24 hours when refrigerated. Do not freeze.

Reconstitution

I.M.: Prepare 500 mg vial with 2 mL 1% lidocaine (do not use lidocaine with epinephrine). The I.V. formulation does not form a stable suspension in lidocaine and cannot be used to prepare an I.M dose.

I.V.: Prior to use, dilute dose into 100-250 mL of an appropriate solution. Imipenem is inactivated at acidic or alkaline pH. Final concentration should not exceed 5 mg/mL. The I.M. formulation is not buffered and cannot be used to prepare I.V. solutions.

Compatibility I.V. formulation:

Variable stability (consult detailed reference) in D_5W, D_5LR, $D_51/4NS$, $D_51/2NS$, D_5NS, $D_{10}W$, mannitol 2.5%, mannitol 5%, mannitol 10%, NS, TPN.

Y-site administration: Compatible: Acyclovir, amifostine, aztreonam, cefepime, cisatracurium, diltiazem, docetaxel, famotidine, fludarabine, foscarnet, gatifloxacin, granisetron, idarubicin, insulin (regular), linezolid, melphalan, methotrexate, ondansetron, propofol, remifentanil, tacrolimus, teniposide, thiotepa, vinorelbine, zidovudine. **Incompatible:** Allopurinol, amphotericin B cholesteryl sulfate complex, etoposide phosphate, fluconazole, gemcitabine, lorazepam, meperidine, midazolam, sargramostim, sodium bicarbonate. **Variable (consult detailed reference):** Filgrastim, TPN.

Mechanism of Action Inhibits bacterial cell wall synthesis by binding to one or more of the penicillin binding proteins (PBPs); which in turn inhibits the final transpeptidation step of peptidoglycan synthesis in bacterial cell walls, thus inhibiting cell wall biosynthesis. Bacteria eventually lyse due to ongoing activity of cell wall autolytic enzymes (autolysins and murein hydrolases) while cell wall assembly is arrested. Cilastatin prevents renal metabolism of imipenem by competitive inhibition of dehydropeptidase along the brush border of the renal tubules.

Pharmacodynamics/Kinetics

Absorption: I.M.: Imipenem: 60% to 75%; cilastatin: 95% to 100%

Distribution: Rapidly and widely to most tissues and fluids including sputum, pleural fluid, peritoneal fluid, interstitial fluid, bile, aqueous humor, and bone; highest concentrations in pleural fluid, interstitial fluid, and peritoneal fluid; low concentrations in CSF

Protein binding: Imipenem: 20%; cilastatin: 40%

Metabolism: Imipenem is metabolized in the kidney by dehydropeptidase I; cilastatin prevents imipenem metabolism by this enzyme; cilastatin is partially metabolized renally

Half-life elimination: I.V.: Both drugs: 60 minutes; prolonged with renal impairment; I.M.: Imipenem: 2-3 hours

Time to peak: I.M.: 3.5 hours

Excretion: Both drugs: Urine (~70% as unchanged drug)

Dosage

Usual dosage ranges: Note: Dosage based on **imipenem** content:

Neonates ≤3 months and weight ≥1500 g: Non-CNS infections: I.V.:

<1 week: 25 mg/kg every 12 hours

1-4 weeks: 25 mg/kg every 8 hours

4 weeks to 3 months: 25 mg/kg every 6 hours

Children >3 months: Non-CNS infections: I.V.: 15-25 mg/kg every 6 hours; maximum dosage: Susceptible infections: 2 g/day; moderately-susceptible organisms: 4 g/day

Adults:

I.M.: 500-750 mg every 12 hours; maximum: 1500 mg/day

I.V.: Weight ≥70 kg: 250-1000 mg every 6-8 hours; maximum: 4 g/day. **Note:** For adults weighing <70 kg, refer to Dosing Adjustment in Renal Impairment:

Indication-specific dosing: Note: Doses based on imipenem content. I.M. administration is not intended for severe or life-threatening infections (eg, septicemia, endocarditis, shock), UTI, bone/joint or polymicrobic infections:

Children: I.V.:

Burkholderia mallei (melioidosis) (unlabeled use): 20 mg/kg every 8 hours for 10 days

Cystic fibrosis: Doses up to 90 mg/kg/day have been used

Adults:

Burkholderia mallei (melioidosis) (unlabeled use): I.V.: 20 mg/kg (up to 1 g) every 6-8 hours for 10 days

Intra-abdominal infections:

I.V.: Mild infection: 250-500 mg every 6 hours; severe: 500 mg every 6 hours

I.M.: Mild-to-moderate infection: 750 mg every 12 hours

Liver abscess (unlabeled use): I.V.: 500 mg every 6 hours for 2-3 weeks, then appropriate oral therapy for a total of 4-6 weeks

Lower respiratory tract, skin/skin structure, gynecologic infections: I.M.: Mild/moderate: 500-750 mg every 12 hours

Mild infection: Note: Rarely a suitable option in mild infections; normally reserved for moderate-severe cases:

I.M.: 500 mg every 12 hours

I.V.:

Fully-susceptible organisms: 250 mg every 6 hours

Moderately-susceptible organisms: 500 mg every 6 hours

Moderate infection:

I.M.: 750 mg every 12 hours

I.V.:

Fully-susceptible organisms: 500 mg every 6-8 hours

Moderately-susceptible organisms: 500 mg every 6 hours or 1 g every 8 hours

Neutropenic fever (unlabeled use): I.V.: 500 mg every 6 hours

***Pseudomonas* infections:** I.V.: 500 mg every 6 hours; **Note:** Higher doses may be required based on organism sensitivity.

Severe infection: I.V.:

Fully-susceptible organisms: 500 mg every 6 hours

Moderately-susceptible organisms: 1 g every 6-8 hours

Maximum daily dose should not exceed 50 mg/kg or 4 g/day, whichever is lower

Urinary tract infection: I.V.:

Uncomplicated: 250 mg every 6 hours

Complicated: 500 mg every 6 hours

Dosage adjustment in renal impairment: I.V.: **Note:** Adjustments have not been established for I.M. dosing:

Patients with a Cl_{cr} ≤5 mL/minute/1.73 m^2 should not receive imipenem/cilastatin unless hemodialysis is instituted within 48 hours.

Patients weighing <30 kg with impaired renal function should not receive imipenem/cilastatin.

Hemodialysis: Use the dosing recommendation for patients with a Cl_{cr} 6-20 mL/minute; administer dose after dialysis session and every 12 hours thereafter

Peritoneal dialysis: Dose as for Cl_{cr} 6-20 mL/minute

Continuous renal replacement therapy (CRRT): Drug clearance is highly dependent on the method of renal replacement, filter type, and flow rate. Appropriate dosing requires close monitoring of pharmacologic response, signs of adverse reactions due to drug accumulation, as well as drug levels in relation to target trough (if appropriate). The following are general recommendations only (based on dialysate flow/ultrafiltration rates of 1 L/hour) and should not supersede clinical judgment:

CVVH: 250 mg every 6 hours or 500 mg every 8 hours

CVVHD/CVVHDF: 250 mg every 6 hours or 500 mg every 6-8 hours

Note: Data suggest that 500 mg every 12 hours may provide sufficient T>MIC to cover organisms with MIC values ≤2 mg/L; however, a higher dose of 500 mg every 6 hours is recommended for resistant organisms (particularly *Pseudomonas*) with MIC ≥4 mg/L (Fish, 2005).

Dosage adjustment in hepatic impairment: Hepatic dysfunction may further impair cilastatin clearance; consider decreasing the dosing frequency.

See table on next page.

▶

Imipenem and Cilastatin Dosage in Renal Impairment

Reduced I.V. Dosage Regimen Based on Creatinine Clearance (mL/minute/1.73 m²) and/or Body Weight <70 kg					
	Body Weight (kg)				
	≥70	60	50	40	30
Total daily dose for normal renal function: 1 g/day					
Cl$_{cr}$ ≥71	250 mg q6h	250 mg q8h	125 mg q6h	125 mg q6h	125 mg q8h
Cl$_{cr}$ 41-70	250 mg q8h	125 mg q6h	125 mg q6h	125 mg q8h	125 mg q8h
Cl$_{cr}$ 21-40	250 mg q12h	250 mg q12h	125 mg q8h	125 mg q12h	125 mg q12h
Cl$_{cr}$ 6-20	250 mg q12h	125 mg q12h	125 mg q12h	125 mg q12h	125 mg q12h
Total daily dose for normal renal function: 1.5 g/day					
Cl$_{cr}$ ≥71	500 mg q8h	250 mg q6h	250 mg q6h	250 mg q8h	125 mg q6h
Cl$_{cr}$ 41-70	250 mg q6h	250 mg q8h	250 mg q8h	125 mg q6h	125 mg q8h
Cl$_{cr}$ 21-40	250 mg q8h	250 mg q8h	250 mg q12h	125 mg q8h	125 mg q8h
Cl$_{cr}$ 6-20	250 mg q12h	250 mg q12h	250 mg q12h	125 mg q12h	125 mg q12h
Total daily dose for normal renal function: 2 g/day					
Cl$_{cr}$ ≥71	500 mg q6h	500 mg q8h	250 mg q6h	250 mg q6h	250 mg q8h
Cl$_{cr}$ 41-70	500 mg q8h	250 mg q6h	250 mg q6h	250 mg q8h	125 mg q6h
Cl$_{cr}$ 21-40	250 mg q6h	250 mg q8h	250 mg q8h	250 mg q12h	125 mg q8h
Cl$_{cr}$ 6-20	250 mg q12h	250 mg q12h	250 mg q12h	250 mg q12h	125 mg q12h
Total daily dose for normal renal function: 3 g/day					
Cl$_{cr}$ ≥71	1000 mg q8h	750 mg q8h	500 mg q6h	500 mg q8h	250 mg q6h
Cl$_{cr}$ 41-70	500 mg q6h	500 mg q8h	500 mg q8h	250 mg q6h	250 mg q8h
Cl$_{cr}$ 21-40	500 mg q8h	500 mg q8h	250 mg q6h	250 mg q8h	250 mg q8h
Cl$_{cr}$ 6-20	500 mg q12h	500 mg q12h	250 mg q12h	250 mg q12h	250 mg q12h
Total daily dose for normal renal function: 4 g/day					
Cl$_{cr}$ ≥71	1000 mg q6h	1000 mg q8h	750 mg q8h	500 mg q8h	500 mg q8h
Cl$_{cr}$ 41-70	750 mg q8h	750 mg q8h	500 mg q6h	500 mg q8h	250 mg q6h
Cl$_{cr}$ 21-40	500 mg q6h	500 mg q8h	500 mg q8h	250 mg q6h	250 mg q8h
Cl$_{cr}$ 6-20	500 mg q12h	500 mg q12h	500 mg q12h	250 mg q12h	250 mg q12h

Administration

I.M.: **Note:** I.M. administration is not intended for severe or life-threatening infections (eg, septicemia, endocarditis, shock). Administer by deep injection into a large muscle (gluteal or lateral thigh). **Only the I.M. formulation can be used for I.M. administration.**

I.V.: Do not administer I.V. push. Infuse doses ≤500 mg over 20-30 minutes; infuse doses ≥750 mg over 40-60 minutes. **Only the I.V. formulation can be used for I.V. administration.**

Monitoring Parameters Periodic renal, hepatic, and hematologic function tests; monitor for signs of anaphylaxis during first dose

Test Interactions Interferes with urinary glucose determination using Clinitest®

Dietary Considerations Sodium content of 500 mg injection:

I.M.: 32 mg (1.4 mEq)

I.V.: 37.5 mg (1.6 mEq)

Dosage Forms Excipient information presented when available (limited, particularly for generics); consult specific product labeling.

Injection, powder for reconstitution [I.M.]:

Primaxin®: Imipenem 500 mg and cilastatin 500 mg [contains sodium 32 mg (1.4 mEq)]

Injection, powder for reconstitution [I.V.]:

Primaxin®: Imipenem 250 mg and cilastatin 250 mg [contains sodium 18.8 mg (0.8 mEq)]; imipenem 500 mg and cilastatin 500 mg [contains sodium 37.5 mg (1.6 mEq)]

References

American Thoracic Society and Infectious Diseases Society of America, "Guidelines for the Management of Adults With Hospital-Acquired, Ventilator-Associated, and Healthcare-Associated Pneumonia," *Am J Respir Crit Care Med*, 2005, 171(4):388-416.

Balfour JA, Bryson HM, and Brogden RN, "Imipenem/Cilastatin: An Update of Its Antibacterial Activity, Pharmacokinetics, and Therapeutic Efficacy in the Treatment of Serious Infections," *Drugs*, 1996, 51(1):99-136.

Hughes WT, Armstrong D, Bodey GP, et al, "2002 Guidelines for the Use of Antimicrobial Agents in Neutropenic Patients With Cancer," *Clin Infect Dis*, 2002, 34(6):730-51.

◆ **ImmuCyst® (Can)** *see* BCG Vaccine *on page 128*

Immune Globulin (Intravenous) (i MYUN GLOB yoo lin, IN tra VEE nus)

Medication Safety Issues

Sound-alike/look-alike issues:

Gamimune® N may be confused with CytoGam®

Immune globulin (intravenous) may be confused with hepatitis B immune globulin

U.S. Brand Names Carimune® NF; Flebogamma®; Gammagard Liquid; Gammagard S/D; Gamunex®; Octagam®; Privigen™

Index Terms IGIV; IV Immune Globulin; IVIG; Panglobulin

Generic Available No

Canadian Brand Names Gamimune® N; Gammagard Liquid; Gammagard S/D; Gamunex®; IGIVnex®; Privigen™

Pharmacologic Category Blood Product Derivative; Immune Globulin

Use

Treatment of primary immunodeficiency syndromes (congenital agammaglobulinemia, severe combined immunodeficiency syndromes [SCIDS], common variable immunodeficiency, X-linked immunodeficiency, Wiskott-Aldrich syndrome) (Carimune® NF, Flebogamma®, Gammagard Liquid, Gammagard S/D, Gamunex®, Octagam®, Privigen™)

Treatment of immune (idiopathic) thrombocytopenic purpura (ITP) (Carimune® NF, Gammagard S/D, Gamunex®, Privigen™)

Treatment of chronic inflammatory demyelinating polyneuropathy (CIDP) (Gamunex®)

Prevention of coronary artery aneurysms associated with Kawasaki disease (in combination with aspirin) (Gammagard S/D)

◄ Prevention of bacterial infection in B-cell chronic lymphocytic leukemia (CLL) (Gammagard S/D)

Unlabeled/Investigational Use Prevention of serious bacterial infections among HIV-infected children with hypogammaglobulinemia (IgG <400 mg/dL) (CDC guidelines); hematopoietic stem cell transplantation (HSCT), to prevent bacterial infections among allogeneic recipients with severe hypogammaglobulinemia (IgG <400 mg/dL) at <100 days post transplant (CDC guidelines); fetal-neonatal alloimmune thrombocytopenia; Guillain-Barré syndrome; pregnancy-associated ITP; prevention of gastroenteritis in children; multiple sclerosis (relapsing, remitting when other therapies cannot be used); hemolytic disease of the newborn; HIV-associated thrombocytopenia; acquired hypogammaglobulinemia secondary to malignancy; myasthenia gravis; refractory dermatomyositis/polymyositis

Pregnancy Risk Factor C

Lactation Excretion in breast milk unknown

Labeled Contraindications Hypersensitivity to immune globulin or any component of the formulation; selective IgA deficiency; hyperprolinemia (Privigen™)

Warnings/Precautions [U.S. Boxed Warning]: Acute renal dysfunction (increased serum creatinine, oliguria, acute renal failure, osmotic nephrosis) can rarely occur; usually within 7 days of use (more likely with products stabilized with sucrose). Use with caution in the elderly, patients with renal disease, diabetes mellitus, volume depletion, sepsis, paraproteinemia, and nephrotoxic medications due to risk of renal dysfunction. In patients at risk of renal dysfunction, the rate of infusion and concentration of solution should be minimized. discontinue if renal function deteriorates. High-dose regimens (1000 mg/kg for 1-2 days) are not recommended for individuals with fluid overload or where fluid volume may be of concern. Hypersensitivity and anaphylactic reactions can occur; immediate treatment (including epinephrine 1:1000) should be available; product of human plasma; may potentially contain infectious agents which could transmit disease. Screening of donors, as well as testing and/or inactivation or removal of certain viruses, reduces the risk. Infections thought to be transmitted by this product should be reported to the manufacturer. Aseptic meningitis may occur with high doses (≥2 g/kg); syndrome usually appears within several hours to 2 days following treatment; usually resolves within several days after IVIG is discontinued; patients with a migraine history may be at higher risk for AMS.

Intravenous immune globulin has been associated with antiglobulin hemolysis; monitor for signs of hemolytic anemia. Patients should be adequately hydrated prior to initiation of therapy. Hyperproteinemia, increased serum viscosity and hyponatremia may occur; distinguish hyponatremia from pseudohyponatremia to prevent volume depletion and further increase in serum viscosity. Use caution in patients with a history of thrombotic events or a history of atherosclerosis or cardiovascular disease or patients with known/suspected hyperviscosity; there is clinical evidence of a possible association between thrombotic events and administration of intravenous immune globulin. Consider a baseline assessment of blood viscosity in patients at risk for hyperviscosity. For intravenous administration only. Patients should be monitored for adverse events during and after the infusion. Stop administration with signs of infusion reaction (fever, chills, nausea, vomiting, and rarely shock). Risk may be increased with initial treatment, when switching brands of immune globulin, and with treatment interruptions of >8 weeks. Monitor for transfusion-related acute lung injury (TRALI); noncardiogenic pulmonary edema has been reported with intravenous immune globulin use. TRALI is characterized by severe respiratory distress, pulmonary edema, hypoxemia, and fever (in the presence of normal left ventricular function) and usually occurs within 1-6 hours after infusion. Response to live vaccinations may be impaired. Some products may contain maltose, which may result in falsely-elevated blood glucose readings. Some products may contain sucrose. Some products may contain sorbitol; do not use in patients with fructose intolerance. Privigen™ contains the stabilizer L-proline and is contraindicated in patients with hyperprolinemia. Packaging of some products may contain natural latex/natural rubber.

Adverse Reactions Frequency not defined.

Cardiovascular: Chest tightness, edema, flushing of the face, hyper-/hypotension, palpitation, tachycardia

Central nervous system: Anxiety, aseptic meningitis syndrome, chills, dizziness, drowsiness, fatigue, fever, headache, irritability, lethargy, light-headedness, malaise, migraine, pain

Dermatologic: Bruising, petechiae, pruritus, purpura, rash, urticaria

Gastrointestinal: Abdominal cramps, abdominal pain, diarrhea, discomfort, dyspepsia, nausea, sore throat, vomiting

Hematologic: Anemia, autoimmune hemolytic anemia, hematocrit decreased, hemolysis (mild), hemorrhage, thrombocytopenia

Hepatic: Bilirubin increased, LDH increased, liver function test increased

Local: Pain or irritation at the infusion site

Neuromuscular & skeletal: Arthralgia, back or hip pain, leg cramps, muscle cramps, myalgia, neck pain, weakness

Otic: Ear pain

Renal: Acute renal failure, acute tubular necrosis, anuria, BUN increased, creatinine increased, oliguria, proximal tubular nephropathy, osmotic nephrosis

Respiratory: Asthma aggravated, bronchitis, cough, dyspnea, epistaxis, nasal congestion, pharyngeal pain, pharyngitis, rhinitis, rhinorrhea, sinus headache, sinusitis, upper respiratory infection, wheezing

Miscellaneous: Anaphylaxis, diaphoresis, flu-like syndrome, hypersensitivity reactions, infusion reaction

Postmarketing and/or case reports: Apnea, ARDS, autoimmune pure red cell aplasia (PRCA) exacerbation, bronchopneumonia, bronchospasm, bullous dermatitis, cardiac arrest, chest pain, coma, Coombs' test positive, cyanosis, epidermolysis, erythema multiforme, hepatic dysfunction, hypoxemia, leukopenia, loss of consciousness, pancytopenia, papular rash, pulmonary edema, pulmonary embolism, rigors, seizure, Stevens-Johnson syndrome, thromboembolism, transfusion-related acute lung injury (TRALI), tremor, vascular collapse

Drug Interactions

Avoid Concomitant Use There are no known interactions where it is recommended to avoid concomitant use.

Increased Effect/Toxicity There are no known significant interactions involving an increase in effect.

Decreased Effect

Immune Globulin (Intravenous) may decrease the levels/effects of: Vaccines (Live)

Storage/Stability Stability is dependent upon the manufacturer and brand. Do not freeze.

Carimune® NF: Prior to reconstitution, store at or below 30°C (86°F). Following reconstitution, store under refrigeration. Begin infusion within 24 hours.

Flebogamma®: Store at 2°C to 25°C (36°F to 77°F).

Gammagard Liquid: Prior to use, store at 2°C to 8°C (36°F to 46°F) for up to 36 months. May store at room temperature of 25°C (77°F) within the first 24 months of manufacturing. Storage time at room temperature varies with length of time previously refrigerated; refer to product labeling for details.

Gammagard S/D: Store at ≤25°C (≤77°F).

Gamunex®: May be stored for up to 36 months at 2°C to 8°C (36°F to 46°F); may be stored at ≤25°C (≤77°F) for up to 6 months.

Octagam®: Store at 2°C to 25°C (36°F to 77°F).

Privigen™: Store at ≤25°C (≤77°F); do not freeze (do not use if previously frozen). Protect from light.

Reconstitution Dilution is dependent upon the manufacturer and brand. Gently swirl; do not shake; avoid foaming. Do not mix products from different manufacturers together. Discard unused portion of vials.

Carimune® NF: Reconstitute with NS, D_5W, or SWFI.

Flebogamma®: Dilution is not recommended.

Gammagard Liquid: May dilute in D_5W only.

Gammagard S/D: Reconstitute with SWFI.

Gamunex®:Dilute in D_5W only.

Privigen™: If necessary to further dilute, D_5W may be used.

Compatibility Stable (variable/product dependent) in D_5W, $D_{15}W$, $D_5\frac{1}{4}NS$; **variable stability (consult detailed reference)** in TPN.

Y-site administration: Compatible: Fluconazole, sargramostim.

Mechanism of Action Replacement therapy for primary and secondary immunodeficiencies; interference with F_c receptors on the cells of the reticuloendothelial system for autoimmune cytopenias and ITP; possible role of contained antiviral-type antibodies

Pharmacodynamics/Kinetics

Onset of action: I.V.: Provides immediate antibody levels

Duration: Immune effect: 3-4 weeks (variable)

Distribution: V_d: 0.09-0.13 L/kg

Intravascular portion (primarily): Healthy subjects: 41% to 57%; Patients with congenital humoral immunodeficiencies: ~70%

Half-life elimination: IgG (variable among patients): Healthy subjects: 14-24 days; Patients with congenital humoral immunodeficiencies: 26-40 days; hypermetabolism associated with fever and infection have coincided with a shortened half-life

Dosage Approved doses and regimens may vary between brands; check manufacturer guidelines. **Note:** Some clinicians dose IVIG on ideal body weight or an adjusted ideal body weight in morbidly-obese patients.

Children: I.V.: Pediatric HIV, prevention of infection (CDC guidelines): 400 mg/kg every 2-4 weeks

Children and Adults: I.V.:

Primary immunodeficiency disorders: **Note:** Adjust dose/frequency based desired IgG levels and clinical response:

General dosing range: 200-800 mg/kg per month

Carimune® NF: 200 mg/kg every 4 weeks. May increase dose to 300 mg/kg every 4 weeks or may increase frequency based on patient response.

Flebogamma®, Gammagard Liquid, Gammagard S/D, Gamunex®, Octagam®: 300-600 mg/kg every 3-4 weeks; adjusted based on dosage and interval in conjunction with monitored serum IgG concentrations

Privigen™: 200-800 mg/kg every 3-4 weeks; adjusted based on dosage and interval in conjunction with monitored serum IgG concentrations

B-cell chronic lymphocytic leukemia (CLL) (Gammagard S/D): 400 mg/kg/dose every 3-4 weeks

Immune (idiopathic) thrombocytopenic purpura (ITP):

Carimune® NF:

Acute: 400 mg/kg/day for 2-5 days

Chronic: 400 mg/kg as needed to maintain platelet count ≥30,000/mm³ or to control significant bleeding; may increase dose if needed (range: 800-1000 mg/kg)

Gammagard S/D: 1000 mg/kg; adjust additional doses based on patient response or platelet count. Up to 3 separate doses may be administered on alternate days if required.

Gamunex®: 1000 mg/kg/day for 1-2 days, **or** 400 mg/kg/day for 5 days

Privigen™: 1000 mg/kg/day for 2 consecutive days

Chronic inflammatory demyelinating polyneuropathy (CIDP): Gamunex®: Loading dose: 2000 mg/kg divided over 2-4 consecutive days; Maintenance: 1000 mg/kg/day for 1 day every 3 weeks **or** 500 mg/kg/day for 2 consecutive days every 3 weeks

Kawasaki disease: Initiate IVIG therapy within 10 days of disease onset: Must be used in combination with aspirin: 80-100 mg/kg/day in 4 divided doses for 14 days; when fever subsides, dose aspirin at 3-5 mg/kg once daily for ≥6-8 weeks

AHA guidelines: 2000 mg/kg as a single dose

Gammagard S/D: 1000 mg/kg as a single dose administered over 10 hours, **or** 400 mg/kg/day for 4 days. Begin within 7 days of onset of fever.

Unlabeled uses:

Acquired hypogammaglobulinemia secondary to malignancy (unlabeled use): Adults: 400 mg/kg/dose every 3 weeks; reevaluate every 4-6 months

Guillain-Barré syndrome (unlabeled use): Children and Adults: Various regimens have been used, including:

400 mg/kg/day for 5 days

or

2000 mg/kg in divided doses administered over 2 days

Hematopoietic stem cell transplantation with hypogammaglobulinemia (CDC guidelines):

Children: 400 mg/kg per month; increase dose or frequency to maintain IgG levels >400 mg/dL

Adolescents and Adults: 500 mg/kg/week

HIV-associated thrombocytopenia (unlabeled use): Adults: 1000 mg/kg/day for 2 days

Multiple sclerosis (relapsing-remitting, when other therapies cannot be used) (unlabeled use): Adults: 1000 mg/kg per month, with or without an induction of 400 mg/kg/day for 5 days

Myasthenia gravis (severe exacerbation) (unlabeled use): Adults: Total dose of 2000 mg/kg over 2-5 days

Refractory dermatomyositis (unlabeled use): Adults: 2000 mg/kg per month administered over 2-5 days

Refractory polymyositis (unlabeled use): Adults: 2000 mg/kg per course administered over 2-5 days

Dosing adjustment/comments in renal impairment: Cl_{cr} <10 mL/minute: Avoid use; in patients at risk of renal dysfunction, consider infusion at a rate less than maximum.

Administration I.V. infusion over 2-24 hours; for initial treatment, a lower concentration and/or a slower rate of infusion should be used. Initial rate of administration and titration is specific to each IVIG product. Consult specific product prescribing information for detailed recommendations. Administer in separate infusion line from other medications; if using primary line, flush with saline prior administration. Refrigerated product should be warmed to room temperature prior to infusion. Some products require filtration; refer to individual product labeling. Antecubital veins should be used, especially with concentrations ≥10% to prevent injection site discomfort. Decrease dose, rate and/or concentration of infusion in patients who may be at risk of renal failure. Decreasing the rate or stopping the infusion may help relieve some adverse effects (flushing, changes in pulse rate, changes in blood pressure). Epinephrine should be available during administration.

Monitoring Parameters Renal function, urine output, hemoglobin and hematocrit, platelets (in patients with ITP); infusion-related adverse reactions, anaphylaxis, signs and symptoms of hemolysis; blood viscosity (in patients at risk for hyperviscosity); presence of antineutrophil antibodies (if TRALI is suspected)

Test Interactions Octagam® contains maltose. Falsely-elevated blood glucose levels may occur when glucose monitoring devices and test strips utilizing the glucose dehydrogenase pyrroloquinolinequinone (GDH-PQQ) based methods are used. Glucose monitoring devices and test strips which utilize the glucose-specific method are recommended. Passively-transferred antibodies may yield false-positive serologic testing results; may yield false-positive direct and indirect Coombs' test.

Dietary Considerations Octagam® contains sodium 30 mmol/L

Dosage Forms Excipient information presented when available (limited, particularly for generics); consult specific product labeling.

Injection, powder for reconstitution [preservative free, nanofiltered]:
  Carimune® NF: 3 g, 6 g, 12 g [contains sucrose]

Injection, powder for reconstitution [preservative free, solvent detergent-treated]:
  Gammagard S/D: 2.5 g, 5 g, 10 g [stabilized with human albumin, glycine, glucose, and polyethylene glycol; packaging may contain natural latex/natural rubber]

Injection, solution [preservative free; solvent detergent-treated]:
  Gammagard Liquid: 10% (10 mL, 25 mL, 50 mL, 100 mL, 200 mL) [latex free, sucrose free; stabilized with glycine]
  Octagam®: 5% (20 mL, 50 mL, 100 mL, 200 mL) [sucrose free; contains sodium 30 mmol/L and maltose]

Injection, solution [preservative free]
  Flebogamma®: 5% (10 mL, 50 mL, 100 mL, 200 mL) [contains polyethylene glycol and sorbitol]
  Gamunex®: 10% (10 mL, 25 mL, 50 mL, 100 mL, 200 mL) [caprylate/chromatography purified]
  Privigen™: 10% (50 mL, 100 mL, 200 mL) [sucrose free]

References
Anderson D, Ali K, Blanchette V, et al, "Guidelines on the Use of Intravenous Immune Globulin for Hematologic Conditions," *Transfus Med Rev*, 2007, 21(2 Suppl 1):9-56.

ASHP Commission on Therapeutics, "ASHP Therapeutic Guidelines for Intravenous Immune Globulin," *Am J Hosp Pharm*, 1992, 49(3):652-4.

Blanchette VS, Luke B, Andrew M, et al, "A Prospective Randomized Trial of High-Dose Intravenous Immune Globulin G Therapy, Oral Prednisone Therapy, and No Therapy in Childhood Acute Immune Thrombocytopenic Purpura," *J Pediatr*, 1993, 123(6):989-95.

British Committee for Standards in Haematology General Haematology Task Force, "Guidelines for the Investigation and Management of Idiopathic Thrombocytopenic Purpura in Adults, Children and in Pregnancy," *Br J Haematol*, 2003, 120(4):574-96.

Centers for Disease Control and Prevention, "Guidelines for Preventing Opportunistic Infections Among Hematopoietic Stem Cell Transplant Recipients: Recommendations of CDC, the Infectious Disease Society of America, and the American Society of Blood and Marrow Transplantation," *MMWR Recomm Rep*, 2000, 49(RR-10):1-125.

Dalakas MC, "Intravenous Immunoglobulin In Autoimmune Neuromuscular Diseases," *JAMA*, 2004, 291(19):2367-75.

Eijkhout HW, van Der Meer JW, Kallenberg CG, et al, "The Effect of Two Different Dosages of Intravenous Immunoglobulin on the Incidenceof Recurrent Infections In Patients With Primary Hypogammaglobulinemia. A Randomized, Double-Blind, Multicenter Crossover Trial," *Ann Intern Med*, 2001, 135(3):165-74.

Feasby T, Banwell B, Benstead T, et al, "Guidelines on the Use of Intravenous Immune Globulin for Neurologic Conditions," *Transfus Med Rev*, 2007, 21(2 Suppl 1):57-107.

Gottstein R and Cooke RW, "Systematic Review of Intravenous Immunoglobulin in Haemolytic Disease of the Newborn," *Arch Dis Child Fetal Neonatal Ed*, 2003, 88(1):F6-10.

Gurcan HM and Ahmed AR, "Efficacy of Various Intravenous Immunoglobulin Therapy Protocols in Autoimmune and Chronic Inflammatory Disorders," *Ann Pharmacother*, 2007, 41(5):812-23.

Hilgartner MW and Bussel J, "Use of Intravenous Gamma Globulin for the Treatment of Autoimmune Neutropenia of Childhood and Autoimmune Hemolytic Anemia," *Am J Med*, 1987, 83(4A):25-9.

Hughes RA, Bouche P, Cornblath DR, et al, "European Federation of Neurological Societies/Peripheral Nerve Society Guideline on Management of Chronic Inflammatory Demyelinating Polyradiculoneuropathy: Report of a Joint Task Force of the European Federation of Neurological Societies and the Peripheral Nerve Society," *Eur J Neurol*, 2006, 13(4):326-32.

Hughes RA, Wijdicks EF, Barohn R, et al, "Practice Parameter: Immunotherapy for Guillain-Barré Syndrome: Report of the Quality Standards Subcommittee of the American Academy of Neurology," *Neurology*, 2003, 61(6):736-40.

Newburger JW, Takahashi M, Gerber MA, et al, "Diagnosis, Treatment, and Long-Term Management of Kawasaki Disease: A Statement for Health Professionals From the Committee on Rheumatic Fever, Endocarditis, and Kawasaki Disease, Council on Cardiovascular Disease in the Young, American Heart Association," *Pediatrics*, 2004, 114(6):1708-33.

Skvaril F and Gardi A, "Differences Among Available Immunoglobulin Preparations for Intravenous Use," *Pediatr Infect Dis J*, 1988, 7:543-48.

"University Hospital Consortium Expert Panel for Off-Label Use of Polyvalent Intravenously Administered Immunoglobulin Preparations Consensus Statement," *JAMA*, 1995, 273 (23):1865-70.

van Schaik IN, Winer JB, de Haan R, et al, "Intravenous Immunoglobulin for Chronic Inflammatory Demyelinating Polyradiculoneuropathy: A Systematic Review," *Lancet Neurol*, 2002, 1(8):491-8.

Immune Globulin (Subcutaneous)

(i MYUN GLOB yoo lin sub kyoo TAY nee us)

U.S. Brand Names Vivaglobin®

Index Terms Immune Globulin Subcutaneous (Human); SCIG

Generic Available No

Pharmacologic Category Blood Product Derivative; Immune Globulin

Use Treatment of primary immune deficiency (PID)

Pregnancy Risk Factor C

Lactation Excretion in breast milk unknown/use caution

Labeled Contraindications Hypersensitivity to immune globulin or any component of the formulation; history of anaphylactic or severe systemic reaction to immune globulin preparations; selective IgA deficiency with known antibody against IgA

Warnings/Precautions For subcutaneous administration only; not for I.V. use. Hypersensitivity reactions and anaphylactic reactions can occur; use caution with initial treatment, when switching brands of immune globulin, and with treatment interruptions of >8 weeks. Patients should be monitored for adverse events during and after the first infusion. Stop infusion with signs of infusion reaction (fever, chills, nausea, vomiting, and rarely shock); medications for the treatment of hypersensitivity reactions should be available for immediate use. Use caution with IgA deficiency; sensitization to IgA may cause anaphylactic reaction. Product of human plasma; may potentially contain infectious agents which could transmit disease. Screening of donors, as well as testing and/or inactivation or removal of certain viruses, reduces the risk. Infections thought to be transmitted by this product should be reported to the manufacturer. Safety and effectiveness for children <2 years of age have not been established.

Adverse Reactions Adverse reactions can be expected to be similar to those experienced with other immune globulin products; percentages are reported as adverse events per patient; injection site reactions decreased with subsequent infusions

>10%:
  Central nervous system: Headache (32% to 48%), fever (3% to 25%)
  Dermatologic: Rash (6% to 17%)
  Gastrointestinal: Gastrointestinal disorder (5% to 37%), nausea (11% to 18%), sore throat (17%)
  Local: Injection site reactions (swelling, redness, itching; 92%)
  Miscellaneous: Allergic reaction (11%)
1% to 10%:
  Cardiovascular: Tachycardia (3%)
  Central nervous system: Pain (10%)
  Dermatologic: Skin disorder (3%)
  Gastrointestinal: Diarrhea (10%)
  Genitourinary: Urine abnormality (3%)
  Neuromuscular & skeletal: Weakness (5%)
  Respiratory: Cough (10%)
<1%: Abdominal pain, dyspnea, nervousness

Drug Interactions

  Avoid Concomitant Use There are no known interactions where it is recommended to avoid concomitant use.

  Increased Effect/Toxicity There are no known significant interactions involving an increase in effect.

  Decreased Effect
  Immune Globulin (Subcutaneous) may decrease the levels/effects of:
  Vaccines (Live)

Storage/Stability Store at 2°C to 8°C (36°F to 46°F); do not freeze. Do not shake. Store in original box until ready to use. Allow vial(s) to reach room temperature prior to use. The appearance of immune globulin (subcutaneous) may vary from colorless to light brown; do not use if cloudy or contains precipitate.

Compatibility Do not mix with other products.

Mechanism of Action Immune globulin replacement therapy of IgG antibodies against bacteria and viral agents.

Pharmacodynamics/Kinetics
  Bioavailability: 73% (compared to I.V.)
  Time to peak, plasma: 2.5 days

Dosage Note: Consider premedicating with acetaminophen and diphenhydramine.

  SubQ infusion: Children ≥2 years and Adults: 100-200 mg/kg weekly (maximum rate: 20 mL/hour; doses >15 mL should be divided between sites); adjust the dose over time to achieve desired clinical response or target IgG levels

  Conversion from I.V. to SubQ: Multiply previous I.V. dose by 1.37, then divide into a weekly regimen by dividing by the previous I.V. dosing interval (eg, if the dosing interval was every 3 weeks, divide by 3); adjust the dose over time to achieve desired clinical response or target IgG levels. SubQ infusion administration should begin 1 week after the last I.V. dose.

Administration Subcutaneous: Initial dose should be administered in a healthcare setting capable of providing monitoring and treatment in the event of hypersensitivity. Using aseptic technique, follow the infusion device manufacturer's instructions for filling the reservoir and preparing the pump. Remove air from administration set and needle by priming. Inject via infusion pump into the abdomen, thigh, upper arm, and/or lateral hip. The maximum rate is 20 mL/hour and maximum volume per injection site is 15 mL (doses >15 mL should be divided and infused into several sites). Select the number of required infusion sites; multiple concurrent injection sites may be achieved with the use of Y-site connection tubing; injection sites must be at least 2 inches apart. After the sites are clean and dry, insert subcutaneous needle and prime administration set. Attach sterile needle to administration set, gently pull back on the syringe to assure a blood vessel has not been inadvertently accessed. Repeat for each injection site; infuse following instructions for the infusion device. Rotate the site(s) weekly. Treatment may be transitioned to the home/home care setting in the absence of adverse reactions.

Monitoring Parameters Infusion-related adverse reactions, anaphylaxis, IgG levels, clinical response

Test Interactions Passively-transferred antibodies may yield false-positive serologic testing results; may yield false-positive direct and indirect Coombs' test

Additional Information Serum IgG levels may be drawn at any time. Subcutaneous weekly treatments provide more constant levels rather than the more pronounced peak and trough patterns observed with I.V. monthly immune globulin treatments.

Dosage Forms Excipient information presented when available (limited, particularly for generics); consult specific product labeling.
Injection, solution [preservative free]: IgG 160 mg/mL (3 mL, 10 mL, 20 mL)

References
Chapel HM, Spickett GP, Ericson D, et al, "The Comparison of the Efficacy and Safety of Intravenous Versus Subcutaneous Immunoglobulin Replacement Therapy," *J Clin Immunol*, 2000, 20(2):94-100.
Gardulf A, Hammerstrom L, and Smith CI, "Home Treatment of Hypogammaglobulinaemia With Subcutaneous Gammaglobulin by Rapid Infusion," *Lancet*, 1991, 338(8760):162-6.
Stiehm ER, Casillas AM, Finkelstein JZ, et al, "Slow Subcutaneous Human Intravenous Immunoglobulin in the Treatment of Antibody Immunodeficiency: Use of an Old Method With a New Product," *J Allergy Clin Immunol*, 1998, 101(6):848-9.

InFLIXimab (in FLIKS e mab)
Medication Safety Issues
Sound-alike/look-alike issues:
Remicade® may be confused with Renacidin®, Rituxan®
InFLIXimab may be confused with riTUXimab
U.S. Brand Names Remicade®

Index Terms Avakine; Infliximab, Recombinant

Generic Available No

Canadian Brand Names Remicade®

Pharmacologic Category Antirheumatic, Disease Modifying; Gastrointestinal Agent, Miscellaneous; Immunosuppressant Agent; Monoclonal Antibody; Tumor Necrosis Factor (TNF) Blocking Agent

Use

Treatment of moderately- to severely-active rheumatoid arthritis (with methotrexate)

Treatment of moderately- to severely-active Crohn's disease with inadequate response to conventional therapy (to reduce signs/symptoms and induce and maintain clinical remission) or to reduce the number of draining enterocutaneous and rectovaginal fistulas and maintain fistula closure

Treatment of psoriatic arthritis (to reduce signs/symptoms of active arthritis and inhibit progression of structural damage and improve physical function)

Treatment of chronic severe plaque psoriasis

Treatment of active ankylosing spondylitis (reduce signs/symptoms)

Treatment of moderately- to severely-active ulcerative colitis with inadequate response to conventional therapy (reduce signs/symptoms and induce and maintain clinical remission, mucosal healing and eliminate corticosteroid use)

Unlabeled/Investigational Use Acute graft-versus-host disease (GVHD)

Pregnancy Risk Factor B

Lactation Excretion in breast milk unknown/not recommended

Labeled Contraindications Hypersensitivity to infliximab, murine proteins or any component of the formulation; doses >5 mg/kg in patients with moderate or severe congestive heart failure (NYHA Class III/IV)

Canadian labeling: Additional contraindications (not in U.S. labeling): Severe infections (eg, sepsis, abscesses, tuberculosis, and opportunistic infections)

Warnings/Precautions [U.S. Boxed Warning]: Patients receiving infliximab are at increased risk for serious infections which may result in hospitalization and/or fatality; infections usually developed in patients receiving concomitant immunosuppressive agents (eg, methotrexate or corticosteroids) and may present as disseminated (rather than local) disease. Active tuberculosis (or reactivation of latent tuberculosis), invasive fungal (including aspergillosis, blastomycosis, candidiasis, coccidioidomycosis, histoplasmosis, and pneumocystosis) and bacterial, viral or other opportunistic infections have been reported in patients receiving TNF-blocking agents, including infliximab. Monitor closely for signs/symptoms of infection. Discontinue for serious infection or sepsis. Consider risks versus benefits prior to use in patients with a history of chronic or recurrent infection. Consider empiric antifungal therapy in patients who are at risk for invasive fungal infection and develop severe systemic illness. Other opportunistic infections (eg, invasive fungal infections, listeriosis, *Pneumocystis*) have occurred during therapy. Caution should be exercised when considering the use in patients with conditions that predispose them to infections (eg, diabetes) or residence/travel from areas of endemic mycoses (blastomycosis, coccidioidomycosis, histoplasmosis), or with latent or localized infections. Do not give with clinically important active infection. Patients who develop a new infection while undergoing treatment should be monitored closely. Serious infections were reported when used in combination with anakinra or etanercept; concurrent use of infliximab and anakinra is not recommended.

[U.S. Boxed Warning]: Infliximab treatment has been associated with active tuberculosis (may be disseminated or extrapulmonary) or reactivation of latent infections; evaluate patients for tuberculosis risk factors and latent tuberculosis infection (with a tuberculin skin test) prior to and during therapy; treatment of latent tuberculosis should be initiated before use. Patients with initial negative tuberculin skin tests should receive continued monitoring for tuberculosis throughout treatment. Most cases of reactivation have been reported within the first 3-6 months of treatment. Caution should be exercised when considering the use of infliximab in patients who have been exposed to tuberculosis.

Patients should be brought up to date with all immunizations before initiating therapy. Live vaccines should not be given concurrently; there is no data available concerning secondary transmission of live vaccines in patients receiving therapy. Rare reactivation of hepatitis B virus (HBV) has occurred in chronic virus carriers; use with caution; evaluate prior to initiation and during treatment.

[U.S. Boxed Warning]: Hepatosplenic T-cell lymphoma has been reported in patients with Crohn's disease or ulcerative colitis treated with infliximab and concurrent or prior azathioprine or mercaptopurine use, usually reported in adolescent and young adult males. The impact of infliximab on the development and course of malignancies is not fully defined, but may be dose dependent. As compared to the general population, an increased risk of lymphoma has been noted in clinical trials; however, rheumatoid arthritis alone has been previously associated with an increased rate of lymphoma. Use caution in patients with a history of COPD, higher rates of malignancy were reported in COPD patients treated with infliximab. Psoriasis patients with a history of phototherapy had a higher incidence of nonmelanoma skin cancers.

Severe hepatic reactions (including hepatitis, jaundice, acute hepatic failure, and cholestasis) have been reported during treatment; discontinue with jaundice or marked increase in liver enzymes (≥5 times ULN). Use caution with heart failure; if a decision is made to use with heart failure, monitor closely and discontinue if exacerbated or new symptoms occur. Doses >5 mg/kg should not be administered in patients with moderate-to-severe heart failure (NYHA Class III/IV). Use caution with history of hematologic abnormalities; hematologic toxicities (eg, leukopenia, neutropenia, thrombocytopenia, pancytopenia) have been reported; discontinue if significant abnormalities occur. Autoimmune antibodies and a lupus-like syndrome have been reported. If antibodies to double-stranded DNA are confirmed in a patient with lupus-like symptoms, infliximab should be discontinued. Rare cases of optic neuritis and demyelinating disease (including multiple sclerosis, systemic vasculitis, and Guillain-Barré syndrome) have been reported; use with caution in patients with pre-existing or recent onset CNS demyelinating disorders, or seizures; discontinue if significant CNS adverse reactions develop.

Acute infusion reactions may occur. Hypersensitivity reaction may occur within 2 hours of infusion. Medication and equipment for management of hypersensitivity reaction should be available for immediate use. Interruptions and/or reinstitution at a slower rate may be required (consult protocols). Pretreatment may be considered, and may be warranted in all patients with prior infusion reactions. Serum sickness-like reactions have occurred; may be associated with a decreased response to treatment. Efficacy was not established in a study to evaluate infliximab use in juvenile rheumatoid arthritis. Safety and efficacy for use in pediatric plaque psoriasis or pediatric ulcerative colitis have not been established. **Note:** For use in Crohn's disease: Safety and efficacy have not been established in children <6 years of age (U.S. labeling) and in children <9 years of age (Canadian labeling).

Adverse Reactions Although profile is similar, frequency of adverse effects may vary with disease state. Except where noted, percentages reported in adults with rheumatoid arthritis:

>10%:

Central nervous system: Headache (18%)

Gastrointestinal: Nausea (21%), diarrhea (12%), abdominal pain (12%; Crohn's 26%)

Hepatic: ALT increased (risk increased with concomitant methotrexate)

Respiratory: Upper respiratory tract infection (32%), sinusitis (14%), cough (12%), pharyngitis (12%)

Miscellaneous: Development of antinuclear antibodies (~50%), infection (36%), infusion reactions (20%; severe <1%), development of antibodies to double-stranded DNA (17%); Crohn's patients with fistulizing disease: Development of new abscess (15%)

5% to 10%:

Cardiovascular: Hypertension (7%)

Central nervous system: Fatigue (9%), pain (8%), fever (7%)

Dermatologic: Rash (1% to 10%), pruritus (7%)

Gastrointestinal: Dyspepsia (10%)

Genitourinary: Urinary tract infection (8%)

Neuromuscular & skeletal: Arthralgia (1% to 8%), back pain (8%)

Respiratory: Bronchitis (10%), rhinitis (8%), dyspnea (6%)

Miscellaneous: Moniliasis (5%)

<5%: Abscess, adult respiratory distress syndrome, allergic reaction, anemia, arrhythmia, basal cell carcinoma, biliary pain, bradycardia, brain infarction, breast cancer, cardiac arrest, cellulitis, cholecystitis, cholelithiasis, circulatory failure, confusion, constipation, dehydration, delayed hypersensitivity (plaque psoriasis), diaphoresis increased, dizziness, edema, gastrointestinal hemorrhage, heart failure, hemolytic anemia, hepatitis, hypersensitivity reactions, hypotension, ileus, intervertebral disk herniation, intestinal obstruction, intestinal perforation, intestinal stenosis, leukopenia, lupus-like syndrome, lymphadenopathy, lymphoma, malignancies, meningitis, menstrual irregularity, MI, myalgia, neuritis, pancreatitis, pancytopenia, peripheral neuropathy, peritonitis, pleural effusion, pleurisy, proctalgia, pulmonary edema, pulmonary embolism, renal calculus, renal failure, respiratory insufficiency, seizure, sepsis, serum sickness, suicide attempt, syncope, tachycardia, tendon disorder, thrombocytopenia, thrombophlebitis (deep), ulceration

The following adverse events were reported in children with Crohn's disease and were found more frequently in children than adults:

>10%:

Hepatic: Liver enzymes increased (18%; ≥5 times ULN: 1%)

Hematologic: Anemia (11%)

Miscellaneous: Infections (56%; more common with every 8-week versus every 12-week infusions)

1% to 10%:

Central nervous system: Flushing (9%)

Gastrointestinal: Blood in stool (10%)

Hematologic: Leukopenia (9%), neutropenia (7%)

Neuromuscular & skeletal: Bone fracture (7%)

Respiratory: Respiratory tract allergic reaction (6%)

Miscellaneous: Viral infection (8%), bacterial infection (6%), antibodies to infliximab (3%)

Postmarketing and/or case reports (adults or children): Agranulocytosis, anaphylactic reactions, anaphylactic shock, angina, angioedema, autoimmune hepatitis, bronchospasm, central demyelinating disorders (eg, multiple sclerosis, optic neuritis); cholestasis, drug-induced lupus-like syndrome, erythema multiforme, heart failure (worsening), hepatitis B reactivation, hepatocellular damage, hepatosplenic T-cell lymphoma (HSTCL), Hodgkin's disease, idiopathic thrombocytopenia purpura, interstitial fibrosis, interstitial pneumonitis, jaundice, laryngeal/pharyngeal edema, latent tuberculosis reactivation, leukemias, liver failure, liver function tests increased, neuropathy, numbness, opportunistic infection, pericardial effusion, peripheral demyelinating disorders (eg, Guillain-Barré syndrome, chronic inflammatory demyelinating polyneuropathy, multifocal motor neuropathy); pneumonia, psoriasis (including new onset, palmoplantar, pustular, or exacerbation), seizure, Stevens-Johnson syndrome, thrombotic thrombocytopenia purpura, taste abnormal, tingling, toxic epidermal necrolysis, transverse myelitis, tuberculosis, urticaria, vasculitis (systemic and cutaneous)

Drug Interactions

Avoid Concomitant Use

Avoid concomitant use of InFLIXimab with any of the following: Abatacept; Anakinra; Canakinumab; Certolizumab Pegol; Natalizumab; Rilonacept; Vaccines (Live)

Increased Effect/Toxicity

InFLIXimab may increase the levels/effects of: Abatacept; Anakinra; Canakinumab; Certolizumab Pegol; Leflunomide; Natalizumab; Rilonacept; Vaccines (Live)

The levels/effects of InFLIXimab may be increased by: Abciximab; Trastuzumab

Decreased Effect

InFLIXimab may decrease the levels/effects of: Vaccines (Inactivated); Vaccines (Live)

The levels/effects of InFLIXimab may be decreased by: Echinacea

Ethanol/Nutrition/Herb Interactions Herb/Nutraceutical: Avoid echinacea (may diminish the therapeutic effect of infliximab).

Storage/Stability Store vials at 2°C to 8°C (36°F to 46°F); do not freeze.

Reconstitution Reconstitute vials with 10 mL sterile water for injection. Swirl vial gently to dissolve powder; do not shake. Allow solution to stand for 5 minutes. Total dose of reconstituted product should be further diluted to 250 mL of 0.9% sodium chloride injection to a final concentration of 0.4-4 mg/mL. Infusion of dose should begin within 3 hours of preparation.

Compatibility Do not infuse with other agents.

Mechanism of Action Infliximab is a chimeric monoclonal antibody that binds to human tumor necrosis factor alpha (TNFα), thereby interfering with endogenous TNFα activity. Elevated TNFα levels have been found in involved tissues/fluids of patients with rheumatoid arthritis, ankylosing spondylitis, psoriatic arthritis, plaque psoriasis, Crohn's disease and ulcerative colitis. Biological activities of TNFα include the induction of proinflammatory cytokines (interleukins), enhancement of leukocyte migration, activation of neutrophils and eosinophils, and the induction of acute phase reactants and tissue ▶

degrading enzymes. Animal models have shown TNFα expression causes polyarthritis, and infliximab can prevent disease as well as allow diseased joints to heal.

Pharmacodynamics/Kinetics

Onset of action: Crohn's disease: ~2 weeks

Distribution: V_d: 3-6 L

Half-life elimination: 7-12 days

Dosage I.V.: **Note:** Premedication with antihistamines (H_1-antagonist and/or H_2-antagonist), acetaminophen and/or corticosteroids may be considered to prevent and/or manage infusion-related reactions:

Children: U.S. labeling ≥6 years, Canadian labeling ≥9 years: Crohn's disease: 5 mg/kg at 0, 2, and 6 weeks, followed by a maintenance dose of 5 mg/kg every 8 weeks; if no response by week 14, consider discontinuing therapy

Adults:

Crohn's disease: Induction regimen: 5 mg/kg at 0, 2, and 6 weeks, followed by 5 mg/kg every 8 weeks thereafter; dose may be increased to 10 mg/kg in patients who respond but then lose their response. If no response by week 14, consider discontinuing therapy.

Psoriatic arthritis (with or without methotrexate): 5 mg/kg at 0, 2, and 6 weeks, then every 8 weeks

Rheumatoid arthritis (in combination with methotrexate therapy): 3 mg/kg at 0, 2, and 6 weeks, then every 8 weeks thereafter; doses have ranged from 3-10 mg/kg intravenous infusion repeated at 4- to 8-week intervals

Ankylosing spondylitis: 5 mg/kg at 0, 2, and 6 weeks, followed by 5 mg/kg every 6 weeks thereafter

Plaque psoriasis: 5 mg/kg at 0, 2, and 6 weeks, then every 8 weeks thereafter

Ulcerative colitis: 5 mg/kg at 0, 2, and 6 weeks, followed by 5 mg/kg every 8 weeks thereafter

Acute GVHD (unlabeled use): 10 mg/kg weekly for up to 8 weeks (median 4 weeks of treatment)

Dosage adjustment with CHF: Weigh risk versus benefits for individual patient:

NYHA Class III or IV: ≤5 mg/kg

Dosage adjustment in renal impairment: No specific adjustment is recommended

Dosage adjustment in hepatic impairment: No specific adjustment is recommended

Administration Infuse over at least 2 hours; do not infuse with other agents; use in-line low protein binding filter (≤1.2 micron). Temporarily discontinue or decrease infusion rate with infusion-related reactions. Antihistamines (H_1-antagonist and/or H_2-antagonist), acetaminophen and/or corticosteroids may be used to manage reactions. Infusion may be reinitiated at a lower rate upon resolution of mild-to-moderate symptoms.

Canadian labeling (not approved in U.S. labeling): Infusion of doses ≤6 mg/kg over not less than 1 hour may be considered in patients treated for rheumatoid arthritis who have initially tolerated 3 infusions each over 2 hours. Safety of shortened infusion has not been studied with doses >6 mg/kg.

Guidelines for the treatment and prophylaxis of infusion reactions: (Note: Limited to dosages used in Crohn's; prospective information on other indications/dosing such as in GVHD are not available).

A protocol for the treatment of acute infusion reactions, as well as prophylactic therapy for repeat infusions, has been published (Cheifetz, 2003).

Treatment of infusion reactions: Medications for the treatment of hypersensitivity reactions should be available for immediate use. For mild reactions, the rate of infusion should be decreased to 10 mL/hour. Following appropriate symptomatic treatment (eg, acetaminophen and diphenhydramine, monitor vital signs every 10 minutes until normal. After 20 minutes, the infusion may be increased at 15-minute intervals, as tolerated (initial increase to 20 mL/hour, then 40 mL/hour, then 80 mL/hour to completion). For moderate reactions, the infusion should be stopped or slowed with administration of appropriate symptomatic treatment. Monitor vital signs every 5 minutes until normal. After 20 minutes, the infusion may be reinstituted at 10 mL/hour; then increased at 15-minute intervals, as tolerated (initial increase 20 mL/hour, then 40 mL/hour, then 80 mL/hour to completion). For severe reactions, the infusion should be stopped with administration of appropriate symptomatic treatment (eg, hydrocortisone/methylprednisolone and epinephrine) and frequent monitoring of vitals (consult institutional policies, if available). If patient stabilizes, may reinstitute infusion as per moderate reaction protocol.

Prophylaxis of infusion reactions: Premedication with acetaminophen and diphenhydramine 90 minutes prior to infusion may be considered in all patients with prior infusion reactions, and in patients with severe reactions corticosteroid administration is recommended. Steroid dosing may be oral (prednisone 50 mg orally for 3 doses over a 24-hour period prior to infusion) or intravenous (a single dose of hydrocortisone 100 mg or methylprednisolone 20-40 mg administered 20 minutes prior to the infusion). On initiation of the infusion, a test dose (infusion at 10 mL/hour for 15 minutes) may be considered. If tolerated, for patients with mild reactions, the infusion may be completed over 3 hours. For patients with prior moderate-to-severe reactions, the infusion may be increased at 15-minute intervals, as tolerated, to completion (initial increase 20 mL/hour, then 40 mL/hour, then 80 mL/hour, then 100 mL/hour, and finally 125 mL/hour [only for prior moderate reactions] to completion). A maximum rate of 100 mL/hour is recommended in patients who experienced prior severe reactions. In patients with cutaneous flushing, aspirin may be considered (Becker, 2004).

Monitoring Parameters During infusion, if reaction is noted, monitor vital signs every 10 minutes until normal. Follow-up monitoring includes monitoring for improvement of symptoms; signs of infection; LFTs (discontinue if >5 times ULN); place and read PPD before initiation. Psoriasis patients with history of phototherapy should be monitored for nonmelanoma skin cancer.

Dosage Forms Excipient information presented when available (limited, particularly for generics); consult specific product labeling.

Injection, powder for reconstitution [preservative free]:

Remicade®: 100 mg [contains sucrose 500 mg and polysorbate 80]

References

Bongartz T, Sutton AJ, Sweeting MJ, et al, "Anti-TNF Antibody Therapy In Rheumatoid Arthritis and the Risk of Serious Infections and Malignancies: Systematic Review and Meta-Analysis of Rare Harmful Effects in Randomized Controlled Trials," *JAMA*, 2006, 295(19):2275-85.

Buch MH, Bryer D, Lindsay S, et al, "Shortening Infusion Times for Infliximab Administration," *Rheumatology (Oxford)*, 2006, 45(4):485-6.

Carpenter PA and Sanders JE, "Steroid-Refractory Graft-vs-Host Disease: Past, Present and Future," *Pediatr Transplant.* 2003, 7(Suppl 3):19-31.

Cheifetz A, Smedley M, Martin S, et al, "The Incidence and Management of Infusion Reactions to Infliximab: A Large Center Experience," *Am J Gastroenterol*, 2003, 98(6):1315-24.

Couriel D, Saliba R, Hicks K, et al, "Tumor Necrosis Factor-Alpha Blockade for the Treatment of Acute GVHD," *Blood*, 2004, 104(3):649-54.

Klotz U, Teml A, and Schwab M, "Clinical Pharmacokinetics and Use of Infliximab," *Clin Pharmacokinet*, 2007, 45(8):645-60.

Thayu M, Markowitz JE, Mamula P, et al, "Hepatosplenic T-Cell Lymphoma in an Adolescent Patient After Immunomodulator and Biologic Therapy for Crohn Disease," *J Pediatr Gastroenterol Nutr*, 2005, 40(2):220-2.

Van Vollenhoven RF, Gullstrom E, and Klareskog L, "Feasibility of 1 Hour Infliximab Infusions," *Ann Rheum Dis*, 2005, 64(4):654.

◆ **Infliximab, Recombinant** *see* InFLIXimab *on page 635*

◆ **Infufer® (Can)** *see* Iron Dextran Complex *on page 658*

◆ **Infumorph® 200** *see* Morphine Sulfate *on page 816*

◆ **Infumorph® 500** *see* Morphine Sulfate *on page 816*

◆ **α-2-interferon** *see* Interferon Alfa-2b *on page 642*

◆ **Interferon Alfa-2b (PEG Conjugate)** *see* Peginterferon Alfa-2b *on page 931*

Interferon Alfa-2b (in ter FEER on AL fa too bee)

Medication Safety Issues

Sound-alike/look-alike issues:

Interferon alfa-2b may be confused with interferon alfa-2a, interferon alfa-n3, pegylated interferon alfa-2b

Intron® A may be confused with PEG-Intron®

International issues:

Interferon alfa-2b may be confused with interferon alpha multi-subtype which is available in international markets

Related Information

Safe Handling of Hazardous Drugs *on page 1517*

U.S. Brand Names Intron® A

Index Terms INF-alpha 2; Interferon Alpha-2b; rLFN-α2; α-2-interferon

Generic Available No

Canadian Brand Names Intron® A

Pharmacologic Category Interferon

Use

Patients ≥1 year of age: Chronic hepatitis B

Patients ≥3 years of age: Chronic hepatitis C (in combination with ribavirin)

Patients ≥18 years of age: Condyloma acuminata, chronic hepatitis B, chronic hepatitis C, hairy cell leukemia, malignant melanoma, AIDS-related Kaposi's sarcoma, follicular non-Hodgkin's lymphoma

Unlabeled/Investigational Use AIDS-related thrombocytopenia, cutaneous ulcerations of Behçet's disease, neuroendocrine tumors (including carcinoid syndrome and islet cell tumor), cutaneous T-cell lymphoma, desmoid tumor, lymphomatoid granulomatosis, hepatitis D, chronic myelogenous leukemia (CML), non-Hodgkin's lymphomas (other than follicular lymphoma, see approved use), multiple myeloma, renal cell carcinoma, West Nile virus

Pregnancy Risk Factor C / X in combination with ribavirin

Lactation Enters breast milk/not recommended (AAP rates "compatible")

Labeled Contraindications Hypersensitivity to interferon alfa or any component of the formulation; decompensated liver disease; autoimmune hepatitis

Warnings/Precautions Hazardous agent - use appropriate precautions for handling and disposal.

[U.S. Boxed Warning]: May cause or aggravate fatal or life-threatening autoimmune disorders, neuropsychiatric symptoms (including depression and/or suicidal thoughts/behaviors), ischemic, and/or infectious disorders; discontinue treatment for persistent severe or worsening symptoms.

Neuropsychiatric disorders: May cause severe psychiatric adverse events (eg, depression, psychosis, mania, suicidal behavior/ideation) in patients with and without previous psychiatric symptoms, avoid use in patients with pre-existing psychiatric condition, severe psychiatric disorder or history of severe depression; careful neuropsychiatric monitoring is required during and for 6 months after therapy. Suicidal ideation or attempts may occur more frequently in pediatric patients when compared to adults. Discontinue in patients developing severe depression or psychiatric disorders. Higher doses in elderly patients, or diseases other than hairy cell leukemia, may result in increased CNS toxicity.

Hepatic disease: May cause hepatotoxicity; monitor closely if abnormal liver function tests develop. A transient increase in ALT (≥2 times baseline) may occur in patients treated with interferon alfa-2b for chronic hepatitis B. Therapy generally may continue; monitor. Worsening and potentially fatal liver disease, including jaundice, hepatic encephalopathy, and hepatic failure have been reported in patients receiving interferon alfa for chronic hepatitis B and C with decompensated liver disease, autoimmune hepatitis, history of autoimmune disease, and immunosuppressed transplant recipients; avoid use in these patients. Chronic hepatitis B or C patients with a history of autoimmune disease or who are immunosuppressed transplant recipients should not receive interferon alfa-2b. Discontinue treatment (if appropriate) in any patient developing signs or symptoms of liver failure.

Bone marrow suppression: Causes bone marrow suppression, including potentially severe cytopenias, and very rarely, aplastic anemia. Discontinue treatment for severe neutropenia (ANC <500/mm^3) or thrombocytopenia (platelets <25,000/mm^3). Hemolytic anemia (hemoglobin <10 g/dL) was observed when combined with ribavirin; anemia occurred within 1-2 weeks of initiation of therapy. Use caution in patients with pre-existing myelosuppression and in patients with concomitant medications which cause myelosuppression.

Autoimmune disorders: Avoid use in patients with history of autoimmune disorders; development of autoimmune disorders (thrombocytopenia, vasculitis, Raynaud's disease, rheumatoid arthritis, lupus erythematosus and rhabdomyolysis) has been associated with use. Monitor closely; consider discontinuing. Worsening of psoriasis and sarcoidosis (and the development of new sarcoidosis) have been reported; use caution.

Cardiovascular disease/coagulation disorders: Use caution and monitor closely in patients with cardiovascular disease (ischemic or thromboembolic), arrhythmias, hypertension, and in patients with a history of MI or prior therapy with cardiotoxic drugs. Patients with pre-existing cardiac disease and/or advanced cancer should have baseline and periodic ECGs. May cause hypotension (during administration or delayed), arrhythmia, tachycardia, cardiomyopathy (~2% in AIDS-related Kaposi's Sarcoma patients) and/or MI. Hemorrhagic cerebrovascular events have been observed with therapy. Use caution in patients with coagulation disorders.

Endocrine disorders: Thyroid disorders (possibly reversible) have been reported; use caution in patients with pre-existing thyroid disease. Discontinue use in patients who cannot maintain normal ranges with thyroid medication. Diabetes mellitus has been reported; discontinue if cannot effectively manage with medication. Use caution in patients with a history of diabetes mellitus, particularly if prone to DKA. Hypertriglyceridemia has been reported; discontinue if severe, and/or combined with symptoms of pancreatitis.

Pulmonary disease: Pulmonary infiltrates, pneumonitis and pneumonia have been reported with interferon alfa therapy; occurs more frequently in patients being treated for chronic hepatitis C. Patients with fever, cough, dyspnea or other respiratory symptoms should be evaluated with a chest x-ray; monitor closely and consider discontinuing treatment with evidence of impaired pulmonary function. Use with caution in patients with a history of pulmonary disease.

Ophthalmic disorders: Decreased/loss of vision, macular edema, optic neuritis, retinal hemorrhages, cotton wool spots, papilledema, and retinal artery or vein thrombosis have occurred (or been aggravated) in patients receiving alpha interferons. Use caution in patients with pre-existing eye disorders; monitor closely; discontinue with new or worsening ophthalmic disorders.

Commonly associated with fever and flu-like symptoms; rule out other causes/ infection with persistent fever; use with caution in patients with debilitating conditions. Acute hypersensitivity reactions have been reported. Do not treat patients with visceral AIDS-related Kaposi's sarcoma associated with rapidly-progressing or life-threatening disease. Some formulations contain albumin, which may carry a remote risk of viral transmission. Due to differences in dosage, patients should not change brands of interferons without the concurrence of their healthcare provider. Safety and efficacy in children <1 year of age have not been established.

Adverse Reactions Note: In a majority of patients, a flu-like syndrome (fever, chills, tachycardia, malaise, myalgia, headache), occurs within 1-2 hours of administration; may last up to 24 hours and may be dose limiting.

>10%:

Cardiovascular: Chest pain (≤28%)

Central nervous system: Fatigue (8% to 96%), fever (34% to 94%), headache (21% to 62%), chills (≤54%), depression (3% to 40%; grades 3/4: 2%), somnolence (≤33%), dizziness (≤24%), irritability (≤22%), pain (≤18%), amnesia (≤14%), concentration impaired (≤14%), malaise (≤14%), confusion (≤12%), insomnia (≤12%)

Dermatologic: Alopecia (≤38%), rash (≤25%), pruritus (≤11%)

Endocrine & metabolic: Amenorrhea (≤12%)

Gastrointestinal: Anorexia (1% to 69%), nausea, (17% to 66%), diarrhea (2% to 45%), vomiting (2% to 32%), xerostomia (≤28%), taste alteration (≤24%), abdominal pain (1% to 23%), constipation (≤14%), gingivitis (≤14%), weight loss (<1% to 13%)

Hematologic: Neutropenia (≤92%; grade 4: 1% to 4%), leukopenia (≤68%), anemia (≤32%), thrombocytopenia (≤15%)

Hepatic: AST increased (≤63%; grades 3/4: 14%), ALT increased (≤15%), pain (upper right quadrant: up to 15%); alkaline phosphatase increased (≤13%)

Local: Injection site reaction (≤20%)

Neuromuscular & skeletal: Myalgia (28% to 75%), weakness (≤63%), rigors (≤42%), paresthesia (1% to 21%), skeletal pain (≤21%), arthralgia (≤19%), back pain (≤19%)

Renal: BUN increased (≤12%)

Respiratory: Dyspnea (≤34%), cough (≤31%), pharyngitis (≤31%), sinusitis (≤21%)

Miscellaneous: Flu-like syndrome (≤79%), diaphoresis (1% to 21%), moniliasis (≤17%)

5% to 10%:

Cardiovascular: Edema (≤10%), hypertension (≤9%)

Central nervous system: Hypoesthesia (≤10%), anxiety (≤9%), vertigo (≤8%), agitation (≤7%)

Dermatologic: Dry skin (≤10%), dermatitis (≤8%), purpura (≤5%)

Endocrine & metabolic: Libido decreased (≤5%)

Gastrointestinal: Loose stools (≤10%), dyspepsia (≤8%)

Genitourinary: Urinary tract infection (≤5%)

Renal: Polyuria (≤10%), serum creatinine increased (≤6%)

Respiratory: Bronchitis (≤10%), nasal congestion (≤10%), epistaxis (≤7%)

Miscellaneous: Infection (≤7%), herpes virus infections (≤5%)

<5%, postmarketing, and/or case reports (limited to important or life-threatening):

Cardiovascular: Angina, arrhythmia, arteritis, atrial fibrillation, bradycardia, cardiac failure, cardiomegaly, cardiomyopathy, coronary artery disorder, ejection fraction decreased, extrasystoles, flushing, heart valve disorder, hypotension, MI, palpitation, peripheral ischemia, polyarteritis, Raynaud's disease, syncope, tachycardia, thrombosis, vasculitis

Central nervous system: Nervousness (≤3%), aggression, alcohol intolerance, aphasia, ataxia, Bell's palsy, coma, extrapyramidal disorder, hallucination, hypothermia, mania, migraine, neurosis, paranoia, psychosis, stroke, suicidal attempt/ideation, seizure

Dermatologic: Angioedema, cellulitis, dermatitis lichenoides, eczema, epidermal necrolysis, erythema, erythema multiforme, erythematous rash, folliculitis, hirsutism, lipoma, maculopapular rash, photosensitivity, psoriasis, psoriasis exacerbation, sebaceous cyst, Stevens-Johnson syndrome, toxic epidermal necrolysis, urticaria

Endocrine & metabolic: Dehydration, diabetes mellitus, goiter, hot flashes, hypercalcemia, hyperglycemia, hyper-/hypothyroidism, hypertriglyceridemia, mastitis, menorrhagia, sexual dysfunction

Gastrointestinal: Colitis, dysphasia, esophagitis, gastritis, gastrointestinal hemorrhage, mucositis, pancreatitis, rectal bleeding/hemorrhage, stomatitis, ulcerative stomatitis

Genitourinary: Cystitis, dysuria, incontinence, impotence, leukorrhea, nocturia, pelvic pain, uterine bleeding

Hematologic: Aplastic anemia (rarely), granulocytopenia, hemolytic anemia, hypochromic anemia, lymphopenia, lymphadenitis, lymphadenopathy, lymphocytosis, pure red cell aplasia, thrombocytopenia purpura (idiopathic and thrombotic)

Hepatic: Ascites, biliary pain, bilirubinemia, hepatic encephalopathy, hepatic failure, hepatitis, hepatotoxicity, jaundice, lactate dehydrogenase increased (up to 1%), liver function test abnormal

Local: Injection site necrosis

Neuromuscular & skeletal: Arthritis, carpal tunnel syndrome, hyporeflexia, leg cramps, muscle atrophy, myositis, neuralgia, neuropathy, rhabdomyolysis, rheumatoid arthritis, spondylitis, tendonitis, tremor

Ocular: Blurred vision, conjunctivitis, cotton wool spots, macular edema, nystagmus, optic neuritis, papilledema, photophobia, retinal artery thrombosis, retinal vein thrombosis

Otic: Hearing impairment, hearing loss

Renal: Albuminuria, hematuria, nephrotic syndrome, proteinuria, renal failure, renal insufficiency

Respiratory: Asthma, bronchoconstriction, bronchospasm, cyanosis, hemoptysis, hypoventilation, pleural effusion, pneumonitis, pneumothorax, pulmonary embolism, pulmonary fibrosis, respiratory insufficiency, upper respiratory tract infection, wheezing

Miscellaneous: Abscess, acute hypersensitivity reaction, allergic reactions, anaphylaxis, fungal infection, lupus erythematosus, sarcoidosis, sarcoidosis exacerbation, sepsis

Drug Interactions

Metabolism/Transport Effects Inhibits CYP1A2 (weak)

Avoid Concomitant Use There are no known interactions where it is recommended to avoid concomitant use.

Increased Effect/Toxicity

Interferon Alfa-2b may increase the levels/effects of: Aldesleukin; Ribavirin; Theophylline Derivatives; Zidovudine

Decreased Effect There are no known significant interactions involving a decrease in effect.

Storage/Stability Store powder and solution for injection (vials and pens) under refrigeration at 2°C to 8°C (36°F to 46°F); do not freeze.

Powder for injection: Following reconstitution, should be used immediately, but may be stored under refrigeration for up to 24 hours.

Prefilled pens: After first use, discard unused portion after 4 weeks.

Reconstitution The manufacturer recommends reconstituting vial with the diluent provided (SWFI). To prepare solution for infusion, further dilute appropriate dose in NS 100 mL. Final concentration should be ≥10 million units/100 mL.

Compatibility Stable in LR, NS; **incompatible** with D_5W.

Mechanism of Action Following activation, multiple effects can be detected including induction of gene transcription. Inhibits cellular growth, alters the state of cellular differentiation, interferes with oncogene expression, alters cell surface antigen expression, increases phagocytic activity of macrophages, and augments cytotoxicity of lymphocytes for target cells

Pharmacodynamics/Kinetics

Distribution: V_d: 31 L; but has been noted to be much greater (370-720 L) in leukemia patients receiving continuous infusion IFN; IFN does not penetrate the CSF

Metabolism: Primarily renal

Bioavailability: I.M.: 83%; SubQ: 90%

Half-life elimination: I.V.: ~2 hours; I.M., SubQ: ~2-3 hours

Time to peak, serum: I.M., SubQ: ~3-12 hours

Dosage Details concerning dosing in combination regimens should also be consulted. **Note:** Withhold treatment for ANC <500/mm^3 or platelets <25,000/mm^3. Consider premedication with acetaminophen prior to administration to reduce the incidence of some adverse reactions. Not all dosage forms and strengths are appropriate for all indications; refer to product labeling for details.

Children 1-17 years: Chronic hepatitis B: SubQ: 3 million units/m^2 3 times/week for 1 week; then 6 million units/m^2 3 times/week; maximum: 10 million units 3 times/week; total duration of therapy 16-24 weeks

Children ≥3 years: Chronic hepatitis C: In combination with ribavirin

Adults:

Hairy cell leukemia: I.M., SubQ: 2 million units/m^2 3 times/week for up to 6 months (may continue treatment with continued treatment response)

Lymphoma (follicular): SubQ: 5 million units 3 times/week for up to 18 months

Malignant melanoma: Induction: 20 million units/m^2 I.V. for 5 consecutive days per week for 4 weeks, followed by maintenance dosing of 10 million units/m^2 SubQ 3 times/week for 48 weeks

AIDS-related Kaposi's sarcoma: I.M., SubQ: 30 million units/m^2 3 times/week

Chronic hepatitis B: I.M., SubQ: 5 million units/day or 10 million units 3 times/week for 16 weeks

Chronic hepatitis C: I.M., SubQ: 3 million units 3 times/week for 16 weeks. In patients with normalization of ALT at 16 weeks, continue treatment for 18-24 months; consider discontinuation if normalization does not occur at 16 weeks. **Note:** May be used in combination therapy with ribavirin in previously untreated patients or in patients who relapse following alpha interferon therapy.

Condyloma acuminata: Intralesionally: 1 million units/lesion (maximum: 5 lesions/treatment) 3 times/week (on alternate days) for 3 weeks; may administer a second course at 12-16 weeks

Dosage adjustment in renal impairment: Combination therapy with ribavirin (hepatitis C) should not be used in patients with reduced renal function (Cl$_{cr}$ <50 mL/minute).

Dosage adjustment for toxicity: Manufacturer-recommended adjustments, listed according to indication:

Lymphoma (follicular):

Neutrophils >1000/mm^3 to <1500/mm^3: Reduce dose by 50%; may re-escalate to starting dose when neutrophils return to >1500/mm^3

Severe toxicity (neutrophils <1000/mm^3 or platelets <50,000/mm^3): Temporarily withhold

AST >5 times ULN or serum creatinine >2 mg/dL: Permanently discontinue

Hairy cell leukemia, chronic hepatitis C: Severe toxicity: Reduce dose by 50% or temporarily withhold and resume with 50% dose reduction; permanently discontinue if persistent or recurrent severe toxicity is noted

Chronic hepatitis B:

WBC <1500/mm^3, granulocytes <750/mm^3, or platelet count <50,000/mm^3, or other laboratory abnormality or severe adverse reaction: Reduce dose by 50%; may re-escalate to starting dose upon resolution of hematologic toxicity. Discontinue for persistent intolerance.

WBC <1000/mm^3, granulocytes <500/mm^3, or platelet count <25,000/mm^3: Permanently discontinue

Kaposi sarcoma: Severe toxicity: Reduce dose by 50% or temporarily withhold; may resume at reduced dose with toxicity resolution; permanently discontinue for persistent/recurrent toxicities

Malignant melanoma:

Severe toxicity (neutrophils >250/mm^3 to <500/mm^3 or ALT/AST >5-10 times ULN): Temporarily withhold; resume with a 50% dose reduction when adverse reaction abates

Neutrophils <250/mm^3, ALT/AST >10 times ULN, or severe/persistent adverse reactions: Permanently discontinue

◄ ## Combination Regimens

Head and neck cancer: PFL + IFN on page 1395

Leukemia, acute lymphocytic: Hyper-CVAD (Leukemia, Acute Lymphocytic) on page 1349

Lymphoma, non-Hodgkin's: Fludarabine-Mitoxantrone-Dexamethasone-Rituximab on page 1329

Melanoma:

BOLD + Interferon on page 1235

Cisplatin-Dacarbazine-Interferon Alfa-2b-Aldesleukin on page 1266

CVD-Interleukin-Interferon (Melanoma) on page 1282

Renal cell cancer:

Bevacizumab-Interferon Alfa (RCC) on page 1232

Interleukin 2-Interferon Alfa-2 on page 1359

Interleukin 2 (Low Dose)-Interferon Alfa 2b on page 1359

Administration

I.M.: Administer in evening (if possible)

I.V.: Infuse over ~20 minutes

SubQ: Suggested for those who are at risk for bleeding or are thrombocytopenic. Rotate SubQ injection site. Administer in evening (if possible). Patient should be well hydrated. Reconstitute with recommended amount of SWFI and agitate gently; do not shake. **Note:** Different vial strengths require different amounts of diluent. Not every dosage form is appropriate for every indication; refer to manufacturer's labeling.

Monitoring Parameters Baseline chest x-ray, ECG; CBC with differential and platelets (baseline and routinely during treatment), liver function tests, serum creatinine, electrolytes, triglycerides, thyroid function tests (baseline and periodically during treatment); weight; ophthalmic exam (baseline and periodic, or with new ocular symptoms); patients with pre-existing cardiac abnormalities or in advanced stages of cancer should have ECGs taken before and during treatment

Emetic Potential

>10,000 units/m^2: Moderate (30% to 90%)

5,000-10,000 units/m^2: Low (10% to 30%)

Dosage Forms Excipient information presented when available (limited, particularly for generics); consult specific product labeling.

Injection, powder for reconstitution [preservative free]:

Intron® A: 10 million int. units; 18 million int. units; 50 million int. units [contains human albumin]

Injection, solution:

Intron® A: 6 million int. units/mL (3 mL); 10 million int. units/1 mL (2.5 mL) [contains edetate disodium, polysorbate 80]

Intron® A: 3 million int. units/0.2 mL (1.2 mL) [contains edetate disodium, polysorbate 80; delivers 6 doses of 0.2 mL each; 18 million int. units total per pen]

Intron® A: 5 million int. units/0.2 mL (1.2 mL) [contains edetate disodium, polysorbate 80; delivers 6 doses of 0.2 mL each; 30 million int. units total per pen]

Intron® A: 10 million int. units/0.2 mL (1.2 mL) [contains edetate disodium, polysorbate 80; delivers 6 doses of 0.2 mL each; 60 million int. units total per pen]

References

Legha SS, "The Role of Interferon Alfa in the Treatment of Metastatic Melanoma," *Semin Oncol*, 1997, 24(1 Suppl 4):24-31.

Musselman DL, Lawson DH, Gumnick JF, et al, "Paroxetine for the Prevention of Depression Induced by High-Dose Interferon Alfa," *N Engl J Med*, 2001, 344(13):961-6.

♦ **Interferon Alpha-2b** *see* Interferon Alfa-2b *on page 642*

♦ **Interleukin-2** *see* Aldesleukin *on page 25*

♦ **Interleukin-11** *see* Oprelvekin *on page 880*

♦ **Intrapleural Talc** *see* Talc (Sterile) *on page 1071*

♦ **Intron® A** *see* Interferon Alfa-2b *on page 642*

Iobenguane I 123 (eye oh BEN gwane eye one TWEN tee three)

U.S. Brand Names AdreView™

Index Terms 123 Meta-Iodobenzlyguanidine Sulfate; 123I-Metaiodobenzyl-guanidine (MIBG); I-123 MIBG; I^{123} Iobenguane; Iobenguane Sulfate I 123

Generic Available No

Pharmacologic Category Radiopharmaceutical

Use As an adjunct to other diagnostic tests, in the detection of primary or metastatic pheochromocytoma or neuroblastoma

Pregnancy Risk Factor C

Lactation Excretion in breast milk unknown/not recommended

Labeled Contraindications Hypersensitivity to iobenguane or any component of the formulation

Warnings/Precautions Radiopharmaceutical; use appropriate precautions for handling, disposal and minimizing exposure to patients and healthcare personnel. Use under supervision of experienced personnel. Hypersensitivity reactions have been reported. Use extreme caution in patients with iodine or iodine-contrast agent hypersensitivity. Appropriate equipment and emergency medications should be available during use. Use with caution in patients with hypertension; may increase blood pressure and heart rate. Use with caution in patients with severe renal impairment; safety and efficacy have not been established. Patients with severe renal impairment may have delayed elimination, therefore, decreasing quality of images. Not dialyzable. If possible, discontinue medications that inhibit norepinephrine uptake prior to iobenguane I 123 administration; allow at least 5 half-lives to elapse. These medications may interfere with the uptake of iobenguane I 123 in neuroendocrine tumors leading to false-negative results. Administer thyroid blocking medications (eg, potassium iodide oral solution, potassium perchlorate) at least 1 hour prior to administration; long-term risk for thyroid neoplasia can occur from failure to block thyroid uptake of iodine 123. Patients should be adequately hydrated prior to dosing instruct patients to void frequently for 48 hours following administration to decrease radiation exposure. Contains benzyl alcohol which has been associated with "gasping syndrome" in neonates. Safety and efficacy have not been established in infants <1 month of age.

Adverse Reactions <1%, postmarketing, and/or case reports: Dizziness, flushing, hypersensitivity (rare), injection site hemorrhage, pruritus, rash

Drug Interactions

Avoid Concomitant Use

Avoid concomitant use of Iobenguane I 123 with any of the following: Alpha2-Agonists; Antidepressants (Selective Norepinephrine Reuptake Inhibitor); Cocaine; Methyldopa; Reserpine; Selective Serotonin Reuptake Inhibitors; Serotonin/Norepinephrine Reuptake Inhibitors; Sympathomimetics; Tricyclic Antidepressants

Increased Effect/Toxicity There are no known significant interactions involving an increase in effect.

Decreased Effect

The levels/effects of Iobenguane I 123 may be decreased by: Alpha2-Agonists; Antidepressants (Selective Norepinephrine Reuptake Inhibitor);

Cocaine; Methyldopa; Reserpine; Selective Serotonin Reuptake Inhibitors; Serotonin/Norepinephrine Reuptake Inhibitors; Sympathomimetics; Tricyclic Antidepressants

Storage/Stability Store at controlled room temperature of 20°C to 25°C (68°F to 77°F). Should be stored in original lead container or adequate radiation shield.

Mechanism of Action Iobenguane is structurally similar to norepinephrine and therefore is taken up and stored in adrenergic tissue such as adrenal medulla, heart, liver, lungs, salivary glands, and spleen. Iobenguane is bound to radioactive iodine in order to obtain organ and tissue images.

Pharmacodynamics/Kinetics

Distribution: Increased in adrenergically innervated tissues (eg, heart, salivary glands, adrenal medulla)

Metabolism: Has not been characterized

Half-life elimination: Iodine 123: 13.2 hours

Excretion: Urine (70 % to 90%) within 4 days (normal renal function); feces <1%

Dosage Note: Thyroid protective agents (SSKI, Lugol's solution or potassium iodide), should be given at least 1 hour prior to administration. Perform whole body planar scintigraphy imaging 18-30 hours after Iobenguane I 123 administration.

Radioimaging: I.V.:

Children 1 month to 16 years and <70 kg: Dose according to body weight; see table.

Children <16 years and ≥70 kg: 10 mCi (370 MBq)

Children ≥16 years and Adults: 10 mCi (370 MBq)

Iobenguane I 123 Pediatric Dosing by Body Weight

(Children 1 Month to 16 Years and <70 kg)

Weight (kg)	mCi Dose	MBq Dose
3	1	37
4	1.4	52
6	1.9	70
8	2.3	85.1
10	2.7	99.9
12	3.2	118.4
14	3.6	133.2
16	4	148
18	4.4	162.8
20	4.6	170.2
22	5	185
24	5.3	196.1
26	5.6	207.2
28	5.8	214.6
30	6.2	229.4
32	6.5	240.5
34	6.8	251.6
36	7.1	262.7

Iobenguane I 123 Pediatric Dosing by Body Weight *(continued)*

Weight (kg)	mCi Dose	MBq Dose
38	7.3	270.1
40	7.6	281.2
42	7.8	288.6
44	8	296
46	8.2	303.4
48	8.5	314.5
50	8.8	325.6
52-54	9	333
56-58	9.2	340.4
60-62	9.6	355.2
64-66	9.8	362.6
68	9.9	366.3

Administration Administer intravenously over 1-2 minutes. May flush with NS to ensure full delivery of dose. Prior to administration, a thyroid-protective agent should be started. Ensure adequate hydration before and after treatment.

Monitoring Parameters Pulse and blood pressure prior to administration and intermittently for 30 minutes following; monitor for hypersensitivity reaction

Dietary Considerations Some dietary sources of iodine include cow's milk and dairy products, fish, seaweed, eggs, chocolate, and iodized salt.

Dosage Forms Excipient information presented when available (limited, particularly for generics); consult specific product labeling.
Injection, solution:
AdreView™: Iobenguane sulfate 0.08 mg and I 123 74 MBq (2 mCi) per mL (5 mL) [contains benzyl alcohol]

◆ **Iobenguane Sulfate I 123** *see* Iobenguane I 123 *on page 649*

◆ **Iodine I 131 Tositumomab and Tositumomab** *see* Tositumomab and Iodine I 131 Tositumomab *on page 1123*

◆ **Iquix®** *see* Levofloxacin *on page 707*

◆ **IRESSA®** *see* Gefitinib *on page 528*

Irinotecan (eye rye no TEE kan)

Medication Safety Issues
High alert medication: The Institute for Safe Medication Practices (ISMP) includes this medication among its list of drug classes which have a heightened risk of causing significant patient harm when used in error.

Related Information
Management of Chemotherapy-Induced Nausea and Vomiting *on page 1434*
Management of Drug Extravasations *on page 1447*
Safe Handling of Hazardous Drugs *on page 1517*

U.S. Brand Names Camptosar®

Index Terms Camptothecin-11; CPT-11

Generic Available Yes

Canadian Brand Names Camptosar®; Irinotecan Hydrochloride Trihydrate

Pharmacologic Category Antineoplastic Agent, Camptothecin; Antineoplastic Agent, Natural Source (Plant) Derivative

Use Treatment of metastatic carcinoma of the colon or rectum

Unlabeled/Investigational Use Nonsmall cell lung cancer, small cell lung cancer, cervical cancer, gastric cancer, pancreatic cancer, brain tumors

Pregnancy Risk Factor D

Lactation Excretion in breast milk unknown/not recommended

Labeled Contraindications Hypersensitivity to irinotecan or any component of the formulation; concurrent use of ketoconazole, St John's wort

Warnings/Precautions Hazardous agent - use appropriate precautions for handling and disposal. Severe hypersensitivity reactions have occurred.

Patients with diarrhea should be carefully monitored and treated promptly. **[U.S. Boxed Warning]: Severe diarrhea may be dose-limiting and potentially fatal; two severe (life-threatening) forms of diarrhea may occur.** Early diarrhea occurs during or within 24 hours of receiving irinotecan and is characterized by cholinergic symptoms (eg, increased salivation, diaphoresis, abdominal cramping); it is usually responsive to atropine. Late diarrhea occurs more than 24 hours after treatment which may lead to dehydration, electrolyte imbalance, or sepsis; it should be promptly treated with loperamide. Colitis, complicated by ulceration, bleeding, ileus, and infection has been reported.

[U.S. Boxed Warning]: May cause severe myelosuppression. Deaths due to sepsis following severe myelosuppression have been reported. Therapy should be temporarily discontinued if neutropenic fever occurs or if the absolute neutrophil count is <1000/mm^3. The dose of irinotecan should be reduced if there is a clinically significant decrease in the total WBC (<200/mm^3), neutrophil count (<1500/mm^3), hemoglobin (<8 g/dL), or platelet count (<100,000/mm^3). Routine administration of a colony-stimulating factor is generally not necessary, but may be considered for patients experiencing significant neutropenia.

Patients with even modest elevations in total serum bilirubin levels (1-2 mg/dL) have a significantly greater likelihood of experiencing first-course grade 3 or 4 neutropenia than those with bilirubin levels that were <1 mg/dL. Patients with abnormal glucuronidation of bilirubin, such as those with Gilbert's syndrome, may also be at greater risk of myelosuppression when receiving therapy with irinotecan. Use caution when treating patients with known hepatic dysfunction or hyperbilirubinemia. Dosage adjustments should be considered.

Patients homozygous for the UGT1A1*28 allele are at increased risk of neutropenia; initial one-level dose reduction should be considered for both single-agent and combination regimens. Heterozygous carriers of the UGT1A1*28 allele may also be at increased risk; however, most patients have tolerated normal starting doses.

Renal impairment and acute renal failure have been reported, possibly due to dehydration secondary to diarrhea. Patients with bowel obstruction should not be treated with irinotecan until resolution of obstruction. Use caution in patients who previously received pelvic/abdominal radiation, elderly patients with comorbid conditions, or baseline performance status of 2; close monitoring and dosage adjustments are recommended. Contains sorbitol; do not use in patients with hereditary fructose intolerance. **[U.S. Boxed Warning]: Should be administered under the supervision of an experienced cancer chemotherapy physician.** Except as part of a clinical trial, use in combination with fluorouracil and leucovorin "Mayo Clinic" regimen is not recommended. Increased toxicity has also been noted in patients with a baseline performance status of 2 in other combination regimens containing irinotecan, leucovorin, and fluorouracil.

Adverse Reactions Frequency of adverse reactions reported for single-agent use of irinotecan only.

>10%:

Cardiovascular: Vasodilation (9% to 11%)

Central nervous system: Cholinergic toxicity (47% - includes rhinitis, increased salivation, miosis, lacrimation, diaphoresis, flushing and intestinal hyperperistalsis); fever (44% to 45%), pain (23% to 24%), dizziness (15% to 21%), insomnia (19%), headache (17%), chills (14%)

Dermatologic: Alopecia (46% to 72%), rash (13% to 14%)

Endocrine & metabolic: Dehydration (15%)

Gastrointestinal: Diarrhea, late (83% to 88%; grade 3/4: 6% to 31%), diarrhea, early (43% to 51%; grade 3/4: 6% to 22%), nausea (70% to 86%), abdominal pain (57% to 68%), vomiting (62% to 67%), cramps (57%), anorexia (44% to 55%), constipation (30% to 32%), mucositis (30%), weight loss (30%), flatulence (12%), stomatitis (12%)

Hematologic: Anemia (60% to 97%; grades 3/4: 5% to 22%), leukopenia (63% to 96%, grades 3/4: 14% to 28%), thrombocytopenia (96%, grades 3/4: 1% to 4%), neutropenia (30% to 96%; grades 3/4: 14% to 31%)

Hepatic: Bilirubin increased (84%), alkaline phosphatase increased (13%)

Neuromuscular & skeletal: Weakness (69% to 76%), back pain (14%)

Respiratory: Dyspnea (22%), cough (17% to 20%), rhinitis (16%)

Miscellaneous: Diaphoresis (16%), infection (14%)

1% to 10%:

Cardiovascular: Edema (10%), hypotension (6%), thromboembolic events (5%)

Central nervous system: Somnolence (9%), confusion (3%)

Gastrointestinal: Abdominal fullness (10%), dyspepsia (10%)

Hematologic: Neutropenic fever (grades 3/4: 2% to 6%), hemorrhage (grades 3/4: 1% to 5%), neutropenic infection (grades 3/4: 1% to 2%)

Hepatic: AST increased (10%), ascites and/or jaundice (grades 3/4: 9%)

Respiratory: Pneumonia (4%)

<1%, postmarketing, and/or case reports: ALT increased, amylase increased, anaphylactoid reaction, anaphylaxis, angina, arterial thrombosis, bleeding, bradycardia, cardiac arrest, cerebral infarct, cerebrovascular accident, circulatory failure, colitis, deep thrombophlebitis, dysrhythmia, embolus, gastrointestinal bleeding, gastrointestinal obstruction, hepatomegaly, hiccups, hyperglycemia, hypersensitivity, hyponatremia, ileus, interstitial lung disease, intestinal perforation, ischemic colitis, lipase increased, lymphocytopenia, megacolon, MI, muscle cramps, myocardial ischemia, pancreatitis, paresthesia, peripheral vascular disorder, pulmonary embolus, pulmonary toxicity (dyspnea, fever, reticulonodular infiltrates on chest x-ray); renal failure (acute), renal impairment, syncope, thrombophlebitis, thrombosis, typhlitis, ulceration, ulcerative colitis, vertigo

Note: In limited pediatric experience, dehydration (often associated with severe hypokalemia and hyponatremia) was among the most significant grade 3/4 adverse events, with a frequency up to 29%. In addition, grade 3/4 infection was reported in 24%.

Drug Interactions

Metabolism/Transport Effects Substrate (major) of CYP2B6, 3A4

Avoid Concomitant Use

Avoid concomitant use of Irinotecan with any of the following: Atazanavir; Natalizumab; St Johns Wort; Vaccines (Live)

◄ **Increased Effect/Toxicity**
Irinotecan may increase the levels/effects of: Leflunomide; Natalizumab; Vaccines (Live)

The levels/effects of Irinotecan may be increased by: Antifungal Agents (Azole Derivatives, Systemic); Atazanavir; Bevacizumab; CYP2B6 Inhibitors (Moderate); CYP2B6 Inhibitors (Strong); CYP3A4 Inhibitors (Moderate); CYP3A4 Inhibitors (Strong); Dasatinib; Eltrombopag; P-Glycoprotein Inhibitors; Sorafenib; Trastuzumab

Decreased Effect
Irinotecan may decrease the levels/effects of: Vaccines (Inactivated); Vaccines (Live)

The levels/effects of Irinotecan may be decreased by: CarBAMazepine; CYP2B6 Inducers (Strong); CYP3A4 Inducers (Strong); Deferasirox; Echinacea; P-Glycoprotein Inducers; PHENobarbital; Phenytoin; St Johns Wort

Ethanol/Nutrition/Herb Interactions Herb/Nutraceutical: Avoid St John's wort (decreases the efficacy of irinotecan).

Storage/Stability Store intact vials of injection at room temperature of 15°C to 30°C (59°F to 86°F). Protect from light. Solutions diluted in NS may precipitate if refrigerated. Solutions diluted in D_5W are stable for 24 hours at room temperature or 48 hours under refrigeration at 2°C to 8°C. Do not freeze.

Reconstitution Dilute in 250-500 mL D_5W or NS to a final concentration of 0.12-2.8 mg/mL. Due to the relatively acidic pH, irinotecan appears to be more stable in D_5W than NS.

Compatibility Stable in D_5W, NS.
Y-site administration: Compatible: Leucovorin; **Incompatible:** Gemcitabine.
Compatibility when admixed: Incompatible: Methylprednisolone sodium succinate.

Mechanism of Action Irinotecan and its active metabolite (SN-38) bind reversibly to topoisomerase I-DNA complex preventing religation of the cleaved DNA strand. This results in the accumulation of cleavable complexes and double-strand DNA breaks. As mammalian cells cannot efficiently repair these breaks, cell death consistent with S-phase cell cycle specificity occurs, leading to termination of cellular replication.

Pharmacodynamics/Kinetics
Distribution: V_d: 33-150 L/m^2
Protein binding, plasma: Predominantly albumin; Parent drug: 30% to 68%, SN-38 (active metabolite): ~95%
Metabolism: Primarily hepatic to SN-38 (active metabolite) by carboxylesterase enzymes; SN-38 undergoes conjugation by UDP- glucuronosyl transferase 1A1 (UGT1A1) to form a glucuronide metabolite. Conversion of irinotecan to SN-38 is decreased and glucuronidation of SN-38 is increased patients who smoke cigarettes, resulting in lower levels of the metabolite and overall decreased systemic exposure. SN-38 is increased by UGT1A1*28 polymorphism (10% of North Americans are homozygous for UGT1A1*28 allele). The lactones of both irinotecan and SN-38 undergo hydrolysis to inactive hydroxy acid forms.
Half-life elimination: SN-38: Mean terminal: 10-20 hours
Time to peak: SN-38: Following 90-minute infusion: ~1 hour
Excretion: Within 24 hours: Urine: Irinotecan (11% to 20%), metabolites (SN-38 <1%, SN-38 glucuronide, 3%)

Dosage I.V. (Refer to individual protocols): **Note:** A reduction in the starting dose by one dose level should be considered for patients ≥65 years of age, prior pelvic/abdominal radiotherapy, performance status of 2, homozygosity for UGT1A1*28 allele, or increased bilirubin (dosing for patients with a bilirubin >2 mg/dL cannot be recommended based on lack of data per manufacturer).

Single-agent therapy:

125 mg/m^2 over 90 minutes on days 1, 8, 15, and 22 of a 6-week treatment cycle

Adjusted dose level -1: 100 mg/m^2

Adjusted dose level -2: 75 mg/m^2

Once-every-3-week regimen: 350 mg/m^2 over 90 minutes, once every 3 weeks

Adjusted dose level -1: 300 mg/m^2

Adjusted dose level -2: 250 mg/m^2

Depending on the patient's ability to tolerate therapy, doses should be adjusted in increments of 25-50 mg/m^2. Irinotecan doses may range from 50-150 mg/m^2 for the weekly regimen. Patients may be dosed as low as 200 mg/m^2 (in 50 mg/m^2 decrements) for the once-every-3-week regimen.

Combination therapy with fluorouracil and leucovorin: Six-week (42-day) cycle:

Regimen 1: 125 mg/m^2 over 90 minutes on days 1, 8, 15, and 22; to be given in combination with bolus leucovorin and fluorouracil (leucovorin administered immediately following irinotecan; fluorouracil immediately following leucovorin)

Adjusted dose level -1: 100 mg/m^2

Adjusted dose level -2: 75 mg/m^2

Regimen 2: 180 mg/m^2 over 90 minutes on days 1, 15, and 29; to be given in combination with infusional leucovorin and bolus/infusion fluorouracil (leucovorin administered immediately following irinotecan; fluorouracil immediately following leucovorin)

Adjusted dose level -1: 150 mg/m^2

Adjusted dose level -2: 120 mg/m^2

Note: For all regimens: It is recommended that new courses begin only after the granulocyte count recovers to ≥1500/mm^3, the platelet count recovers to ≥100,000/mm^3, and treatment-related diarrhea has fully resolved. Treatment should be delayed 1-2 weeks to allow for recovery from treatment-related toxicities. If the patient has not recovered after a 2-week delay, consideration should be given to discontinuing irinotecan.

Dosing adjustment in renal impairment: Effects have not been evaluated; not recommended for use in patients on dialysis

Dosing adjustment in hepatic impairment: The manufacturer recommends that no change in dosage or administration be made for patients with liver metastases and normal hepatic function.

Consideration may be given to starting irinotecan at a lower dose (eg, 100 mg/m^2) if bilirubin is 1-2 mg/dL; for total serum bilirubin elevations >2 mg/dL, specific recommendations are not available in the FDA labeling. The following guidelines have been used by some clinicians:

Bilirubin 1.5-3 mg/dL: Administer 75% of dose (Floyd, 2006).

Dosage adjustment for toxicities: It is recommended that new courses begin only after the granulocyte count recovers to ≥1500/mm^3, the platelet counts recovers to ≥100,000/mm^3, and treatment-related diarrhea has fully resolved. Depending on the patient's ability to tolerate therapy, doses should be adjusted in increments of 25-50 mg/m^2. Treatment should be delayed 1-2 weeks to allow for recovery from treatment-related toxicities. If the patient has not recovered after a 2-week delay, consideration should be given to discontinuing irinotecan. See tables on the following pages.

Single-Agent Schedule: Recommended Dosage Modifications[1]

Toxicity NCI Grade[2] (Value)	During a Cycle of Therapy	At Start of Subsequent Cycles of Therapy (After Adequate Recovery), Compared to Starting Dose in Previous Cycle[1]	
	Weekly	Weekly	Once Every 3 Weeks
No toxicity	Maintain dose level	↑ 25 mg/m^2 up to a maximum dose of 150 mg/m^2	Maintain dose level
Neutropenia			
1 (1500-1999/mm^3)	Maintain dose level	Maintain dose level	Maintain dose level
2 (1000-1499/mm^3)	↓ 25 mg/m^2	Maintain dose level	Maintain dose level
3 (500-999/mm^3)	Omit dose until resolved to ≤ grade 2, then ↓ 25 mg/m^2	↓ 25 mg/m^2	↓ 50 mg/m^2
4 (<500/mm^3)	Omit dose until resolved to ≤ grade 2, then ↓ 50 mg/m^2	↓ 50 mg/m^2	↓ 50 mg/m^2
Neutropenic Fever (grade 4 neutropenia and ≥ grade 2 fever)	Omit dose until resolved, then ↓ 50 mg/m^2	↓ 50 mg/m^2	↓ 50 mg/m^2
Other Hematologic Toxicities	Dose modifications for leukopenia, thrombocytopenia, and anemia during a course of therapy and at the start of subsequent courses of therapy are also based on NCI toxicity criteria and are the same as recommended for neutropenia above.		
Diarrhea			
1 (2-3 stools/day > pretreatment)	Maintain dose level	Maintain dose level	Maintain dose level
2 (4-6 stools/day > pretreatment)	↓ 25 mg/m^2	Maintain dose level	Maintain dose level
3 (7-9 stools/day > pretreatment)	Omit dose until resolved to ≤ grade 2, then ↓ 25 mg/m^2	↓ 25 mg/m^2	↓ 50 mg/m^2
4 (≥10 stools/day > pretreatment)	Omit dose until resolved to ≤ grade 2, then ↓ 50 mg/m^2	↓ 50 mg/m^2	↓ 50 mg/m^2
Other Nonhematologic Toxicities[3]			
1	Maintain dose level	Maintain dose level	Maintain dose level
2	↓ 25 mg/m^2	↓ 25 mg/m^2	↓ 50 mg/m^2
3	Omit dose until resolved to ≤ grade 2, then ↓ 25 mg/m^2	↓ 25 mg/m^2	↓ 50 mg/m^2
4	Omit dose until resolved to ≤ grade 2, then ↓ 50 mg/m^2	↓ 50 mg/m^2	↓ 50 mg/m^2

[1]All dose modifications should be based on the worst preceding toxicity.

[2]National Cancer Institute Common Toxicity Criteria (version 1.0).

[3]Excludes alopecia, anorexia, asthenia.

Combination Schedules: Recommended Dosage Modifications[1]

Toxicity NCI[2] Grade (Value)	During a Cycle of Therapy	At the Start of Subsequent Cycles of Therapy (After Adequate Recovery), Compared to the Starting Dose in the Previous Cycle[1]
No toxicity	Maintain dose level	Maintain dose level
Neutropenia		
1 (1500-1999/mm³)	Maintain dose level	Maintain dose level
2 (1000-1499/mm³)	↓ 1 dose level	Maintain dose level
3 (500-999/mm³)	Omit dose until resolved to ≤ grade 2, then ↓ 1 dose level	↓ 1 dose level
4 (<500/mm³)	Omit dose until resolved to ≤ grade 2, then ↓ 2 dose levels	↓ 2 dose levels
Neutropenic Fever (grade 4 neutropenia and ≥ grade 2 fever)	Omit dose until resolved, then ↓ 2 dose levels	
Other Hematologic Toxicities	Dose modifications for leukopenia or thrombocytopenia during a course of therapy and at the start of subsequent courses of therapy are also based on NCI toxicity criteria and are the same as recommended for neutropenia above.	
Diarrhea		
1 (2-3 stools/day > pretreatment)	Delay dose until resolved to baseline, then give same dose	Maintain dose level
2 (4-6 stools/day > pretreatment)	Omit dose until resolved to baseline, then ↓ 1 dose level	Maintain dose level
3 (7-9 stools/day > pretreatment)	Omit dose until resolved to baseline, then ↓ by 1 dose level	↓ 1 dose level
4 (≥10 stools/day > pretreatment)	Omit dose until resolved to baseline, then ↓ 2 dose levels	↓ 2 dose levels
Other Nonhematologic Toxicities[3]		
1	Maintain dose level	Maintain dose level
2	Omit dose until resolved to ≤ grade 1, then ↓ 1 dose level	Maintain dose level
3	Omit dose until resolved to ≤ grade 2, then ↓ 1 dose level	↓ 1 dose level
4	Omit dose until resolved to ≤ grade 2, then ↓ 2 dose levels	↓ 2 dose levels
Mucositis and/or stomatitis	Decrease only 5-FU, not irinotecan	Decrease only 5-FU, not irinotecan

[1]All dose modifications should be based on the worst preceding toxicity.

[2]National Cancer Institute Common Toxicity Criteria (version 1.0).

[3]Excludes alopecia, anorexia, asthenia.

Combination Regimens

Brain tumors: Bevacizumab-Irinotecan (Glioblastoma) on page 1233
Colorectal cancer:
  Bevacizumab-Irinotecan-Fluorouracil-Leucovorin on page 1233
  Cetuximab (Biweekly)-Irinotecan on page 1255
  Cetuximab-Irinotecan on page 1258
  Fluorouracil-Leucovorin-Irinotecan (Saltz Regimen) on page 1333
  FOIL (Colorectal Cancer) on page 1335

FOLFOXIRI (Colorectal Cancer) on page 1338
FU-LV-CPT-11 on page 1338
Esophageal cancer: Irinotecan-Cisplatin (Esophageal Cancer) on page 1360
Pancreatic cancer:
FOLFIRINOX (Pancreatic Cancer) on page 1336
Gemcitabine-Irinotecan on page 1345
Lung cancer, small cell: Cisplatin-Irinotecan (Small Cell Lung Cancer) on page 1272

Administration Administer by I.V. infusion, usually over 90 minutes.

Monitoring Parameters CBC with differential, platelet count, and hemoglobin with each dose; bilirubin, electrolytes (with severe diarrhea); bowel movements and hydration status; monitor infusion site for signs of inflammation and avoid extravasation

Dietary Considerations Contains sorbitol; do not use in patients with hereditary fructose intolerance

Additional Information Patients who are homozygous for the UGT1A1*28 allele are at increased risk for neutropenia; a decreased dose is recommended. Clinical research of patients who are heterozygous for UGT1A1*28 have been variable for increased neutropenic risk and such patients have tolerated normal starting doses. An FDA-approved test (Invader® Molecular Assay) is available for clinical determination of UGT phenotype.

The recommended regimen to manage late diarrhea is loperamide 4 mg orally at onset of late diarrhea, followed by 2 mg every 2 hours (or 4 mg every 4 hours at night) until 12 hours have passed without a bowel movement. If diarrhea recurs, then repeat administration. Loperamide should not be used for more than 48 consecutive hours.

Emetic Potential Moderate (30% to 90%)

Vesicant May be an irritant

Dosage Forms Excipient information presented when available (limited, particularly for generics); consult specific product labeling.

Injection, solution, as hydrochloride: 20 mg/mL (2 mL, 5 mL, 25 mL)

Camptosar®: 20 mg/mL (2 mL, 5 mL) [contains sorbitol 45 mg/mL]

References

Floyd J, Mirza I, Sachs B, et al, "Hepatotoxicity of Chemotherapy," *Semin Oncol*, 2006, 33 (1):50-67.

Marsh S and McLeod HL, "Pharmacogenetics of Irinotecan Toxicity," *Pharmacogenomics*, 2004, 5 (7):835-43.

Mathijssen RH, van Alphen RJ, Verweij J, et al, "Clinical Pharmacokinetics and Metabolism of Irinotecan (CPT-11)," *Clin Cancer Res*, 2001, 7(8):2182-94.

Toffoli G, Cecchin E, Corona G, et al, "The Role of UGT1A1*28 Polymorphism in the Pharmacodynamics and Pharmacokinetics of Irinotecan in Patients With Metastatic Colorectal Cancer," *J Clin Oncol*, 2006, 24(19):3061-8.

Walker SE, Law S, and Puodziunas A, "Simulation of Y-Site Compatibility of Irinotecan and Leucovorin at Room Temperature in 5% Dextrose in Water in 3 Different Containers," *Can J Hosp Pharm*, 2005, 58(4): 212-22.

van der Bol JM, Mathijssen RH, Loos WJ, et al, "Cigarette Smoking and Irinotecan Treatment: Pharmacokinetic Interaction and Effects on Neutropenia," *J Clin Oncol*, 2007, 25(19):2719-26.

◆ **Irinotecan Hydrochloride Trihydrate (Can)** see Irinotecan on page 651

◆ **Iron Dextran** see Iron Dextran Complex on page 658

Iron Dextran Complex (EYE ern DEKS tran KOM pleks)

Medication Safety Issues

Sound-alike/look-alike issues:

Dexferrum® may be confused with Desferal®

Iron dextran complex may be confused with ferumoxytol

U.S. Brand Names Dexferrum®; INFeD®

Index Terms High-Molecular-Weight Iron Dextran (DexFerrum®); Imferon; Iron Dextran; Low-Molecular-Weight Iron Dextran (INFeD®)

Generic Available No

Canadian Brand Names Dexiron™; Infufer®

Pharmacologic Category Iron Salt

Use Treatment of iron deficiency in patients in whom oral administration is infeasible or ineffective

Unlabeled/Investigational Use Cancer-/chemotherapy-associated anemia

Pregnancy Risk Factor C

Lactation Enters breast milk/use caution

Labeled Contraindications Hypersensitivity to iron dextran or any component of the formulation; any anemia not associated with iron deficiency

Warnings/Precautions [U.S. Boxed Warning]: Deaths associated with parenteral administration following anaphylactic-type reactions have been reported (use only where resuscitation equipment and personnel are available). A test dose should be administered to all patients prior to the first therapeutic dose. Fatal reactions have occurred even in patients who tolerated the test dose. Monitor patients for signs/symptoms of anaphylactic reactions during any iron dextran administration. A history of drug allergy (including multiple drug allergies) and/or the concomitant use of an ACE inhibitor may increase the risk of anaphylactic-type reactions. Adverse events (including life-threatening) associated with iron dextran usually occur with the high-molecular-weight formulation (Dexferrum®), compared to low-molecular-weight (INFeD®) (Chertow, 2006). Delayed (1-2 days) infusion reaction (including arthralgia, back pain, chills, dizziness, and fever) may occur with large doses (eg, total dose infusion) of I.V. iron dextran; usually subsides within 3-4 days. Delayed reaction may also occur (less commonly) with I.M. administration; subsiding within 3-7 days. Use with caution in patients with a history of significant allergies, asthma, serious hepatic impairment, pre-existing cardiac disease (may exacerbate cardiovascular complications), and rheumatoid arthritis (may exacerbate joint pain and swelling). Avoid use during acute kidney infection.

In patients with chronic kidney disease (CKD) requiring iron supplementation, the I.V. route is preferred for hemodialysis patients; either oral iron or I.V. iron may be used for nondialysis and peritoneal dialysis CKD patients. In patients with cancer-related anemia (either due to cancer or chemotherapy-induced) requiring iron supplementation, the I.V. route is superior to oral therapy; I.M. administration is not recommended for parenteral iron supplementation.

[U.S. Boxed Warning]: Use only in patients where the iron deficient state is not amenable to oral iron therapy. Discontinue oral iron prior to initiating parenteral iron therapy. Exogenous hemosiderosis may result from excess iron stores; patients with refractory anemias and/or hemoglobinopathies may be prone to iron overload with unwarranted iron supplementation. Anemia in the elderly is often caused by "anemia of chronic disease" or associated with inflammation rather than blood loss. Iron stores are usually normal or increased, with a serum ferritin >50 ng/mL and a decreased total iron binding capacity. I.V. administration of iron dextran is often preferred over I.M. in the elderly secondary to a decreased muscle mass and the need for daily injections. Intramuscular injections of iron-carbohydrate complexes may have a risk of delayed injection site tumor development. Iron dextran products differ in chemical characteristics. The high-molecular-weight formulation

(Dexferrum®) and the low-molecular-weight formulation (INFeD®) are not clinically interchangeable. Not recommended in children <4 months of age. Intramuscular iron dextran use in neonates may be associated with an increased incidence of gram-negative sepsis.

Adverse Reactions Frequency not defined. **Note:** Adverse event risk is reported to be higher with the high-molecular-weight iron dextran formulation.

Cardiovascular: Arrhythmia, bradycardia, cardiac arrest, chest pain, chest tightness, cyanosis, flushing, hyper-/hypotension, shock, syncope, tachycardia

Central nervous system: Chills, disorientation, dizziness, fever, headache, malaise, seizure, unconsciousness, unresponsiveness

Dermatologic: Pruritus, purpura, rash, urticaria

Gastrointestinal: Abdominal pain, diarrhea, nausea, taste alteration, vomiting

Genitourinary: Discoloration of urine

Hematologic: Leukocytosis, lymphadenopathy

Local: Injection site reactions (cellulitis, inflammation, pain, phlebitis, soreness, swelling), muscle atrophy/fibrosis (with I.M. injection), skin/tissue staining (at the site of I.M. injection), sterile abscess

Neuromuscular & skeletal: Arthralgia, arthritis/arthritis exacerbation, back pain, myalgia, paresthesia, weakness

Respiratory: Bronchospasm, dyspnea, respiratory arrest, wheezing

Renal: Hematuria

Miscellaneous: Anaphylactic reactions (sudden respiratory difficulty, cardiovascular collapse), diaphoresis

Postmarketing and/or case reports: Angioedema, tumor formation (at former injection site)

Drug Interactions

Avoid Concomitant Use

Avoid concomitant use of Iron Dextran Complex with any of the following: Dimercaprol

Increased Effect/Toxicity

The levels/effects of Iron Dextran Complex may be increased by: Dimercaprol

Decreased Effect There are no known significant interactions involving a decrease in effect.

Storage/Stability Store at controlled room temperature.

Reconstitution Solutions for infusion should be diluted in 250-1000 mL NS.

Compatibility Stable in D_5W, NS; **variable stability (consult detailed reference)** in TPN.

Compatibility when admixed: Compatible: Cyanocobalamin, netilmicin.

Mechanism of Action The released iron, from the plasma, eventually replenishes the depleted iron stores in the bone marrow where it is incorporated into hemoglobin

Pharmacodynamics/Kinetics

Onset of action: I.V.: Serum ferritin peak: 7-9 days after dose

Absorption:

I.M.: 50% to 90% is promptly absorbed, balance is slowly absorbed over month

I.V.: Uptake of iron by the reticuloendothelial system appears to be constant at about 10-20 mg/hour

Excretion: Urine and feces via reticuloendothelial system

Dosage I.M. (INFeD®; Z-track method should be used for I.M. injection), I.V. (Dexferrum®, INFeD®):

A 0.5 mL test dose (0.25 mL in infants) should be given prior to starting iron dextran therapy; total dose should be divided into a daily schedule for I.M., total dose may be given as a single continuous infusion. Individual doses of ≤2 mL may be administered daily until calculated total dose is received.

Iron-deficiency anemia:

Children 5-15 kg: Should not normally be given in the first 4 months of life:

Dose (mL) = 0.0442 (desired hemoglobin - observed hemoglobin) x W + (0.26 x W)

Desired hemoglobin: Usually 12 g/dL

W = Total body weight in kg

Children >15 kg and Adults:

Dose (mL) = 0.0442 (desired hemoglobin - observed hemoglobin) x LBW + (0.26 x LBW)

Desired hemoglobin: Usually 14.8 g/dL

LBW = Lean body weight in kg

Iron replacement therapy for blood loss: Replacement iron (mg) = blood loss (mL) x hematocrit

Maximum daily dosage: Manufacturer's labeling: **Note:** Replacement of larger estimated iron deficits may be achieved by serial administration of smaller incremental dosages. Daily dosages should be limited to:

Children:

<5 kg: 25 mg iron (0.5 mL)

5-10 kg: 50 mg iron (1 mL)

Children ≥10 kg and Adults: 100 mg iron (2 mL)

Total dose infusion (unlabeled): The entire dose (estimated iron deficit) may be diluted and administered as a one-time I.V. infusion.

Cancer-/chemotherapy-associated anemia (NCCN guidelines v.2.2010) (unlabeled use): Adults: I.V.: Test dose: 25 mg slow I.V. push, followed 1 hour later by 100 mg over 5 minutes; larger doses (unlabeled), up to total dose infusion (over several hours) may be administered. Low-molecular-weight iron dextran preferred.

Administration Note: Test dose: A test dose should be given on the first day of therapy; patient should be observed for 1 hour for hypersensitivity reaction, then the remaining dose (dose minus test dose) should be given. Resuscitation equipment and trained personnel should be available. An uneventful test dose does not ensure an anaphylactic-type reaction will not occur during administration of the therapeutic dose.

I.M. (INFeD®): Use Z-track technique (displacement of the skin laterally prior to injection); injection should be deep into the upper outer quadrant of buttock; alternate buttocks with subsequent injections. Administer test dose at same recommended site using the same technique.

I.V.: Test dose should be given gradually over at least 30 seconds (INFeD®) or 5 minutes (Dexferrum®). Subsequent dose(s) may be administered by I.V. bolus undiluted at a rate not to exceed 50 mg/minute or diluted in 250-1000 mL NS and infused over 1-6 hours (initial 25 mL should be given slowly and patient should be observed for allergic reactions); avoid dilutions with dextrose (increased incidence of local pain and phlebitis)

Monitoring Parameters Hemoglobin, hematocrit, reticulocyte count, serum ferritin, serum iron, TIBC; monitor for anaphylaxis/hypersensitivity reaction (during test dose and therapeutic dose)

Test Interactions May cause falsely elevated values of serum bilirubin and falsely decreased values of serum calcium. Residual iron dextran may remain in reticuloendothelial cells; may affect accuracy of examination of bone marrow iron stores. Bone scans with 99m Tc-labeled bone seeking agents may show reduced bony uptake, marked renal activity, and excess blood pooling and soft tissue accumulation following I.V. iron dextran infusion or with high serum ferritin levels. Following I.M. iron dextran, bone scans with 99m Tc-diphosphonate may show dense activity in the buttocks.

Dosage Forms Excipient information presented when available (limited, particularly for generics); consult specific product labeling.

Note: Strength expressed as elemental iron

Injection, solution:

Dexferrum®: 50 mg/mL (1 mL, 2 mL) [high-molecular-weight iron dextran]

INFeD®: 50 mg/mL (2 mL) [low-molecular-weight iron dextran]

References

Auerbach M, Ballard H, Trout JR, et al, "Intravenous Iron Optimizes the Response to Recombinant Human Erythropoietin in Cancer Patients With Chemotherapy-Associated Anemia: A Multicenter, Open-Label, Randomized Trial," *J Clin Oncol,* 2004, 22(7):1301-7.

Chertow GM, Mason PD, Vaage-Nilsen O, et al, "Update on Adverse Drug Events Associated With Parenteral Iron," *Nephrol Dial Transplant,* 2006, 21(2):378-82.

National Comprehensive Cancer Network® (NCCN), "Practice Guidelines in Oncology™: Cancer-and Chemotherapy-Induced Anemia Version 2.2009." Available at http://www.nccn.org/professionals/physician_gls/PDF/anemia.pdf

National Kidney Foundation, "KDOQI Clinical Practice Guidelines and Clinical Practice Recommendations for Anemia in Chronic Kidney Disease," available at http://www.kidney.org/professionals/KDOQI/guidelines_anemia/cpr32.htm and http://www.kidney.org/professionals/KDOQI/guidelines_anemia/ped32.htm.

Rizzo JD, Somerfield MR, Hagerty LK, et al, "American Society of Hematology/American Society of Clinical Oncology 2007 Clinical Practice Guideline Update on the Use of Epoetin and Darbepoetin," *Blood,* 2008, 111(1):25-41.

Iron Sucrose (EYE ern SOO krose)

Medication Safety Issues

Sound-alike/look-alike issues:

Iron sucrose may be confused with ferumoxytol

U.S. Brand Names Venofer®

Generic Available No

Canadian Brand Names Venofer®

Pharmacologic Category Iron Salt

Use Treatment of iron-deficiency anemia in chronic renal failure, including nondialysis-dependent patients (with or without erythropoietin therapy) and dialysis-dependent patients receiving erythropoietin therapy

Unlabeled/Investigational Use Cancer-/chemotherapy-associated anemia

Pregnancy Risk Factor B

Lactation Excretion in breast milk unknown/use caution

Labeled Contraindications Hypersensitivity to iron sucrose or any component of the formulation; evidence of iron overload; anemia not caused by iron deficiency

Warnings/Precautions Hypersensitivity reactions, including rare postmarketing anaphylactic and anaphylactoid reactions, have been reported. Hypotension has been reported frequently in hemodialysis-dependent patients. Hypotension has also been reported in peritoneal dialysis and nondialysis patients. Hypotension may be related to total dose or rate of administration (avoid rapid I.V. injection), follow recommended guidelines. Withhold iron in the presence of tissue iron overload; periodic monitoring of hemoglobin, hematocrit, serum ferritin, and transferrin saturation is recommended.

Adverse Reactions

>10%:

Cardiovascular: Hypotension (1% to 7%; 39% in hemodialysis patients; may be related to total dose or rate of administration), peripheral edema (2% to 13%)

Central nervous system: Headache (3% to 13%)

Gastrointestinal: Nausea (1% to 15%)

Neuromuscular & skeletal: Muscle cramps (1% to 3%; 29% in hemodialysis patients)

1% to 10%:

Cardiovascular: Hypertension (6% to 8%), edema (1% to 7%), chest pain (1% to 6%), murmur (<1% to 3%), heart failure

Central nervous system: Dizziness (1% to 10%), fatigue (2% to 5%), fever (1% to 3%)

Dermatologic: Pruritus (1% to 7%), rash (≤1%)

Endocrine & metabolic: Gout (2% to 7%), hypoglycemia (<1% to 4%), hyperglycemia (3% to 4%), fluid overload (1% to 3%)

Gastrointestinal: Diarrhea (1% to 10%), vomiting (3% to 9%), taste perversion (1% to 9%), peritoneal infection (≤8%), constipation (1% to 7%), abdominal pain (1% to 4%), positive fecal occult blood (1% to 3%)

Genitourinary: Urinary tract infection (≤1%)

Local: Injection site reaction (2% to 4%), catheter site infection (≤4%)

Neuromuscular & skeletal: Muscle pain (1% to 7%), extremity pain (3% to 6%), arthralgia (1% to 4%), weakness (1% to 3%), back pain (1% to 3%)

Ocular: Conjunctivitis (<1% to 3%)

Otic: Ear pain (1% to 7%)

Respiratory: Dyspnea (1% to 10%), pharyngitis (<1% to 7%), cough (1% to 7%), sinusitis (1% to 4%), nasopharyngitis (≤3%), upper respiratory infection (1% to 3%), nasal congestion (1%), rhinitis (≤1%)

Miscellaneous: Graft complication (1% to 10%), sepsis

<1%, postmarketing, and/or case reports: Anaphylactoid reactions, anaphylactic shock, bronchospasm (with dyspnea), collapse, facial rash, hypersensitivity (including wheezing), hypoesthesia, loss of consciousness, necrotizing enterocolitis (reported in premature infants, no causal relationship established), seizure, urticaria

Drug Interactions

Avoid Concomitant Use

Avoid concomitant use of Iron Sucrose with any of the following: Dimercaprol

Increased Effect/Toxicity

The levels/effects of Iron Sucrose may be increased by: Dimercaprol

Decreased Effect There are no known significant interactions involving a decrease in effect.

Storage/Stability Store vials at controlled room temperature of 25°C (77°F); do not freeze. Following dilution, solutions are stable for 48 hours at room temperature or under refrigeration.

Reconstitution May be administered via the dialysis line as an undiluted solution or by diluting 100 mg (5 mL) in a maximum of 100 mL normal saline. Doses ≥200 mg should be diluted in a maximum of 250 mL normal saline.

Compatibility Do not mix with other medications.

Mechanism of Action Iron sucrose is dissociated by the reticuloendothelial system into iron and sucrose. The released iron increases serum iron concentrations and is incorporated into hemoglobin.

◀ **Pharmacodynamics/Kinetics**

Distribution: V_{dss}: Healthy adults: 7.9 L

Metabolism: Dissociated into iron and sucrose by the reticuloendothelial system

Half-life elimination: Healthy adults: 6 hours

Excretion: Healthy adults: Urine (5%) within 24 hours

Dosage Doses expressed in mg of **elemental** iron. **Note:** Test dose: Product labeling does not indicate need for a test dose in product-naive patients.

Children ≥2 years (unlabeled use): Iron-deficiency anemia in chronic renal disease (hemodialysis-dependent patients): I.V.:

Correction: 1 mg/kg/dose per dialysis session (maximum: 100 mg)

Maintenance therapy: 0.3 mg/kg/dose per dialysis session (maximum: 100 mg). **Note:** Dosing based on limited data from a study (Leijn, 2004); study used only 14 patients (2-14 years of age) with ESRD on hemodialysis. Study initially used an iron repletion dose of 3 mg/kg/dose per dialysis session which resulted in possible iron overload (ferritin >400 mcg/L); protocol dose subsequently lowered to 1 mg/kg/dose per dialysis session which resulted in a gradual increase in ferritin levels >100 mcg/L; maintenance therapy resulted in median ferritin levels between 193-250 mcg/L.

Adults:

Iron-deficiency anemia in chronic renal disease: I.V.:

Hemodialysis-dependent patient: 100 mg over 2-5 minutes administered 1-3 times/week during dialysis; administer no more than 3 times/week to a cumulative total dose of 1000 mg (10 doses); may continue to administer at lowest dose necessary to maintain target hemoglobin, hematocrit, and iron storage parameters

Peritoneal dialysis-dependent patient: Slow intravenous infusion at the following schedule: Two infusions of 300 mg each over 1½ hours 14 days apart followed by a single 400 mg infusion over 2½ hours 14 days later (total cumulative dose of 1000 mg in 3 divided doses)

Nondialysis-dependent patient: 200 mg slow injection (over 2-5 minutes) on 5 different occasions within a 14-day period. Total cumulative dose: 1000 mg in 14-day period. **Note:** Dosage has also been administered as two infusions of 500 mg in a maximum of 250 mL 0.9% NaCl infused over 3.5-4 hours on day 1 and day 14 (limited experience)

Cancer-/chemotherapy-associated anemia (unlabeled use): I.V. infusion: 200 mg over 1 hour; maximum 300-400 mg/infusion. Repeat dose every 2-3 weeks. Test doses (25 mg slow I.V. push) are recommended in patients with iron dextran hypersensitivity or those with other drug allergies (NCCN guidelines, v.2.2010)

Elderly: Insufficient data to identify differences between elderly and other adults; use caution

Administration Not for rapid I.V. injection; inject slowly over 2-5 minutes. Can be administered through dialysis line. Do not mix with other medications or parenteral nutrient solutions.

Slow I.V. injection: May administer undiluted by slow I.V. injection (100 mg over 2-5 minutes in hemodialysis-dependent patients **or** 200 mg over 2-5 minutes in nondialysis-dependent patients)

Infusion: Dilute 100 mg in maximum of 100 mL 0.9% NaCl; infuse over at least 15 minutes; 300 mg/250 mL should be infused over at least 1½ hours; 400 mg/250 mL should be infused over at least 2½ hours; 500 mg/250 mL should be infused over at least 3½ hours.

Monitoring Parameters Hematocrit, hemoglobin, serum ferritin, transferrin, percent transferrin saturation, TIBC; takes about 4 weeks of treatment to see increased serum iron and ferritin, and decreased TIBC. Serum iron concentrations should be drawn 48 hours after last dose.

Dosage Forms Excipient information presented when available (limited, particularly for generics); consult specific product labeling.

Injection, solution [preservative free]:

Venofer®: 20 mg of elemental iron/mL (5 mL, 10 mL)

References

American College of Obstetricians and Gynecologists, "ACOG Practice Bulletin No. 95: Anemia in Pregnancy," *Obstet Gynecol*, 2008, 112(1):201-7.

Aronoff GR, Bennett WM, Blumenthal S, et al, "Iron Sucrose in Hemodialysis Patients: Safety of Replacement and Maintenance Regimens," *Kidney Int*, 2004, 66(3):1193-8.

Baker WF Jr, "Iron Deficiency in Pregnancy, Obstetrics, and Gynecology," *Hematol Oncol Clin North Am*, 2000, 14(5):1061-77.

Goodnough LT, Skikne B, and Brugnara C, "Erythropoietin, Iron, and Erythropoiesis," *Blood*, 2000, 96(3):823-33.

Leijn E, Monnens LA, and Cornelissen EA, "Intravenous Iron Supplementation in Children on Hemodialysis," *J Nephrol*, 2004, 17(3):423-6.

National Kidney Foundation, "KDOQI Clinical Practice Guidelines and Clinical Practice Recommentaions for Anemia in Chronic Kidney Disease," *Am J Kidney Dis*, 2007, 50 (3):529-30. Available at http://www.kidney.org/professionals/kdoqi/pdf/KDOQI_finalPDF.pdf or http://www.kidney.org/professionals/KDOQI.

"Recommendations to Prevent and Control Iron Deficiency in the United States. Centers for Disease Control and Prevention," *MMWR Recomm Rep*, 1998, 47(RR-3):1-29.

Van Damme-Lombaerts R and Herman J, "Erythropoietin Treatment In Children With Renal Failure," *Prediatr Nephrol*, 1999, 13(2):148-52.

♦ **Isonipecaine Hydrochloride** *see* Meperidine *on page 750*

♦ **Isophosphamide** *see* Ifosfamide *on page 609*

♦ **Isopto® Carpine** *see* Pilocarpine *on page 956*

Isosulfan Blue (eye soe SUL fan bloo)

U.S. Brand Names Lymphazurin™

Generic Available No

Pharmacologic Category Contrast Agent

Use Adjunct to lymphography for visualization of the lymphatic system; sentinel node identification

Pregnancy Risk Factor C

Lactation Excretion in breast milk is unknown/use caution

Labeled Contraindications Hypersensitivity to isosulfan, triphenylmethane, or any component of the formulation

Warnings/Precautions Hypersensitivity reactions, including anaphylactic reactions (rare), may occur; appropriate equipment and emergency medications should be available during use. Competent personnel and emergency facilities should be available during and for at least 60 minutes after administration, since severe delayed reactions may occur. Risk likely higher risk in patients with history of asthma, allergies, drug reactions, including previous sensitivity to triphenylmethane dyes. Peripheral oxygenation measurements may be falsely depressed due to discoloration of serum caused by isosulfan blue; (peak interference 30 minutes after administration; minimal effect by 4 hours postdose); direct determination of arterial blood gases (ABG) may be required. Methemoglobin levels via ABG may be falsely elevated; co-oximetry may be required to accurately assess. Safety and efficacy have not been established in children.

Adverse Reactions

1% to 10%:

Dermatologic: Pruritus (2%; affecting hands, abdomen and neck)

Local: Administration site swelling (2%)

Miscellaneous: Hypersensitivity reactions (2%)

Postmarketing and/or case reports: Anaphylaxis; body fluid discoloration (urine, serum; may lead to falsely low oximetry readings); skin discoloration (including blue urticaria)

Drug Interactions

Avoid Concomitant Use There are no known interactions where it is recommended to avoid concomitant use.

Increased Effect/Toxicity There are no known significant interactions involving an increase in effect.

Decreased Effect There are no known significant interactions involving a decrease in effect.

Storage/Stability Store at room temperature. Avoid prolonged exposure to elevated temperatures.

Compatibility Compatibility in syringe: Incompatible: Local anesthetics (eg, lidocaine)

Mechanism of Action Following subcutaneous administration, isosulfan blue binds to interstitial proteins; these proteins/extracellular fluids are drained by the regional lymphatic system, resulting in concentration of the dye within the lymph. Bright blue coloration imparted by the dye permits delineation of the vessels against the surrounding tissue.

Pharmacodynamics/Kinetics

Absorption: 34% absorbed in 30 minutes; 69% and 100% in 1 and 24 hours, respectively

Protein binding: ~50%

Excretion: Urine (10%; as unchanged drug); feces (~90%; via biliary excretion)

Dosage SubQ: Adults: Inject 0.5 mL into 3 interdigital spaces of each extremity per study; maximum: 3 mL (30 mg)

Administration SubQ: Single patient use only; do not mix with local anesthetics (in same syringe)

Test Interactions Peripheral oxygenation measurements may be falsely depressed (peak interference 30 minutes after administration; minimal effect by 4 hours postdose). Methemoglobin levels via arterial blood gas analyzer may be falsely elevated.

Additional Information May cause blue discoloration of urine for 24 hours.

Dosage Forms Excipient information presented when available (limited, particularly for generics); consult specific product labeling.

Injection, solution [preservative-free]:

Lymphazurin™: 1% (5 mL)

References

Hoskin RW and Granger R, "Intraoperative Decrease in Pulse Oximeter Readings Following Injection of Isosulfan Blue," *Can J Anesth*, 2001, 48(1):38-40.

Kern KA, "Sentinel Lymph Node Mapping in Breast Cancer Using Subareolar Injection of Blue Dye," *J Am Coll Surg*, 1999, 189(6):539-45.

Sadiq TS, Burns WW, Taber DJ et al, "Blue Urticaria: A Previously Unreported Adverse Event Associated With Isosulfan Blue," *Arch Surg*, 2001, 136(12): 1433-5.

Sprung J, Tully MJ, and Ziser A, "Anaphylactic Reactions to Isosulfan Blue Dye During Sentinel Node Lymphadenectomy for Breast Cancer," *Anesth Analg*, 2003, 96(4):1051-3.

Itraconazole (i tra KOE na zole)

Medication Safety Issues

Sound-alike/look-alike issues:

Itraconazole may be confused with fluconazole

Sporanox® may be confused with Suprax®, Topamax®

U.S. Brand Names Sporanox®

Generic Available Yes: Capsule

Canadian Brand Names Sporanox®

Pharmacologic Category Antifungal Agent, Oral

Use

Oral capsules: Treatment of susceptible fungal infections in immunocompromised and immunocompetent patients including blastomycosis and histoplasmosis; indicated for aspergillosis (in patients intolerant/refractory to amphotericin B), and onychomycosis of the toenail and fingernail (in non-immunocompromised patients)

Oral solution: Treatment of oral and esophageal candidiasis

Pregnancy Risk Factor C

Lactation Enters breast milk/not recommended

Labeled Contraindications Hypersensitivity to itraconazole (use caution in patients with a history of hypersensitivity to other azoles), any component of the formulation; concurrent administration with cisapride, dofetilide, ergot derivatives, levomethadyl, lovastatin, midazolam (oral), nisoldipine, pimozide, quinidine, simvastatin, or triazolam; treatment of onychomycosis (or other non-life-threatening indications) in patients with evidence of ventricular dysfunction, heart failure (HF) or a history of HF; treatment of onychomycosis in patients who are pregnant or intend on becoming pregnant

Warnings/Precautions [U.S. Boxed Warning]: Negative inotropic effects have been observed following intravenous administration. Discontinue or reassess use if signs or symptoms of HF (heart failure) occur during treatment. [U.S. Boxed Warning]: Not recommended for treatment of onychomycosis in patients with ventricular dysfunction or a history of HF. HF has been reported, particularly in patients receiving a total daily oral dose of 400 mg. Use with caution in patients with risk factors for HF (COPD, renal failure, edematous disorders, ischemic or valvular disease). Discontinue if signs or symptoms of HF or neuropathy occur during treatment. [U.S. Boxed Warning]: Serious cardiovascular adverse events including, QT prolongation, ventricular tachycardia, torsade de pointes, cardiac arrest and/or sudden death have been observed due to increased cisapride, pimozide, quinidine or levomethadyl concentrations induced by itraconazole; concurrent use contraindicated. Additionally, the following drugs metabolized by the CYP 3A4 isoenzyme system are also contraindicated: Ergot derivatives, lovastatin, midazolam (oral), simvastatin, and triazolam.

Calcium channel blockers (CCBs) may cause additive negative inotropic effects when used concurrently with itraconazole. Itraconazole may also inhibit the metabolism of CCBs. Use caution with concurrent use of itraconazole and CCBs due to an increased risk of HF. Concurrent use of itraconazole and nisoldipine is contraindicated.

Use with caution in patients with renal impairment. Rare cases of serious hepatotoxicity (including liver failure and death) have been reported (including some cases occurring within the first week of therapy); hepatotoxicity was reported in some patients without pre-existing liver disease or risk factors. Use with caution in patients with pre-existing hepatic impairment; monitor liver function closely and dosage adjustment may be warranted. Not recommended for use in patients with active liver disease, elevated liver enzymes, or prior hepatotoxic reactions to other drugs unless the expected benefit exceeds the risk of hepatotoxicity. Transient or permanent hearing loss has been reported. Quinidine (a contraindicated drug) was used concurrently in several of these cases. Hearing loss usually resolves after discontinuation, but may persist in some patients.

Large differences in itraconazole pharmacokinetic parameters have been observed in cystic fibrosis patients receiving the solution; if a patient with cystic fibrosis does not respond to therapy, alternate therapies should be considered. Due to differences in bioavailability, oral capsules and oral solution cannot be used interchangeably. Only the oral solution has proven efficacy for oral and esophageal candidiasis. Initiation of treatment with oral solution is not recommended in patients at immediate risk for systemic candidiasis (eg, patients with severe neutropenia).

Adverse Reactions

>10%: Gastrointestinal: Nausea (11%), diarrhea (3% to 11%)

1% to 10%:

Cardiovascular: Edema (4%), hypertension (3%), chest pain (3%)

Central nervous system: Fever (3% to 7%), headache (4%), fatigue (2% to 3%), dizziness (2%), depression (2%)

Dermatologic: Rash (4% to 9%), pruritus (3%)

Endocrine & metabolic: Hypokalemia (2%)

Gastrointestinal: Vomiting (5% to 7%), abdominal pain (2% to 6%), constipation (2%)

Hepatic: LFTs abnormal (3%)

Respiratory: Rhinitis (5% to 9%), cough (4%), dyspnea (2%), pneumonia (2%), sinusitis (2%), sputum increased (2%)

Miscellaneous: Diaphoresis increased (3%)

<2%, postmarketing, and/or case reports: Adrenal insufficiency, albuminuria, allergic reactions, alopecia, anaphylactoid reactions, anaphylaxis, angioedema, anorexia, arrhythmia, arthralgia, asthenia, blurred vision, diplopia, dysgeusia, dyspepsia, dysphagia, erythema multiforme, exfoliative dermatitis, flatulence, gastritis, gynecomastia, hearing loss, heart failure, hematuria, hepatic failure, hepatitis, hepatotoxicity, hepatitis, hot flashes, hypertriglyceridemia, hypoesthesia, impotence, insomnia, leukocytoclastic dermatitis, leukopenia, libido decreased, malaise, menstrual disorders, myalgia, neutropenia, paresthesia, peripheral neuropathy, photosensitivity, pollakiuria, pulmonary edema, pharyngitis, rigors, serum sickness, somnolence, Stevens-Johnson syndrome, stomatitis ulcerative, thrombocytopenia, taste perversion, tinnitus, toxic epidermal necrolysis, urinary incontinence, urticaria, vasculitis

Drug Interactions

Metabolism/Transport Effects Substrate of CYP3A4 (major); **Inhibits** CYP3A4 (strong)

Avoid Concomitant Use

Avoid concomitant use of Itraconazole with any of the following: Alfuzosin; Cisapride; Conivaptan; Dabigatran Etexilate; Dofetilide; Dronedarone; Eplerenone; Ergot Derivatives; Everolimus; Halofantrine; Nilotinib; Nisoldipine; Pimozide; QuiNIDine; Ranolazine; Rivaroxaban; Salmeterol; Silodosin; Tolvaptan; Topotecan

Increased Effect/Toxicity

Itraconazole may increase the levels/effects of: Alfentanil; Alfuzosin; Almotriptan; Alosetron; Aprepitant; Benzodiazepines (metabolized by oxidation); Bosentan; BusPIRone; Busulfan; Calcium Channel Blockers; CarBAMazepine; Cardiac Glycosides; Ciclesonide; Cilostazol; Cisapride; Colchicine; Conivaptan; Corticosteroids (Orally Inhaled); Corticosteroids (Systemic); CycloSPORINE; CYP3A4 Substrates; Dabigatran Etexilate; Docetaxel; Dofetilide; Dronedarone; Dutasteride; Eletriptan; Eplerenone; Ergot Derivatives; Erlotinib; Eszopiclone; Everolimus; FentaNYL; Fesoterodine; Fexofenadine; Fosaprepitant; Gefitinib; Halofantrine; HMG-CoA Reductase Inhibitors; Imatinib; Irinotecan; Ixabepilone; Losartan; Macrolide Antibiotics; Maraviroc; Methadone; Nilotinib; Nisoldipine; Paliperidone; Paricalcitol; P-Glycoprotein Substrates; Phenytoin; Phosphodiesterase 5 Inhibitors; Pimecrolimus; Pimozide; Protease Inhibitors; QuINIDine; Ramelteon; Ranolazine; Repaglinide; Rifamycin Derivatives; Rivaroxaban; Salmeterol; Saxagliptin; Silodosin; Sirolimus; Solifenacin; Sorafenib; Sunitinib; Tacrolimus; Tadalafil; Temsirolimus; Tolterodine; Tolvaptan; Topotecan; Trimetrexate; VinBLAStine; VinCRIStine; Vitamin K Antagonists; Ziprasidone; Zolpidem

The levels/effects of Itraconazole may be increased by: Grapefruit Juice; Macrolide Antibiotics; Protease Inhibitors

Decreased Effect

Itraconazole may decrease the levels/effects of: Amphotericin B; Prasugrel; Saccharomyces boulardii

The levels/effects of Itraconazole may be decreased by: Antacids; CYP3A4 Inducers (Strong); Deferasirox; Didanosine; Efavirenz; H2-Antagonists; Herbs (CYP3A4 Inducers); Phenytoin; Proton Pump Inhibitors; Rifamycin Derivatives; Sucralfate

Ethanol/Nutrition/Herb Interactions

Food:

Capsules: Absorption enhanced by food and possibly by gastric acidity. Cola drinks have been shown to increase the absorption of the capsules in patients with achlorhydria or those taking H_2-receptor antagonists or other gastric acid suppressors. Avoid grapefruit juice.

Solution: Food decreases the bioavailability and increases the time to peak concentration.

Herb/Nutraceutical: St John's wort may decrease itraconazole levels.

Storage/Stability

Capsule: Store at room temperature, 15°C to 25°C (59°F to 77°F). Protect from light and moisture.

Oral solution: Store at ≤25°C (77°F); do not freeze.

Mechanism of Action Interferes with cytochrome P450 activity, decreasing ergosterol synthesis (principal sterol in fungal cell membrane) and inhibiting cell membrane formation

Pharmacodynamics/Kinetics

Absorption: Requires gastric acidity; capsule better absorbed with food, solution better absorbed on empty stomach

Distribution: V_d (average): 796 ± 185 L or 10 L/kg; highly lipophilic and tissue concentrations are higher than plasma concentrations. The highest concentrations: adipose, omentum, endometrium, cervical and vaginal mucus, and skin/nails. Aqueous fluids (eg, CSF and urine) contain negligible amounts.

Protein binding, plasma: 99.8%; metabolite hydroxy-itraconazole: 99.5%

Metabolism: Extensively hepatic via CYP3A4 into >30 metabolites including hydroxy-itraconazole (major metabolite); appears to have *in vitro* antifungal activity. Main metabolic pathway is oxidation; may undergo saturation metabolism with multiple dosing.

Bioavailability: Variable, ~55% (oral solution) in 1 small study; **Note:** Oral solution has a higher degree of bioavailability (149% ± 68%) relative to oral capsules; should not be interchanged

Half-life elimination: Oral: Single dose: ~21 hours, steady state: 64 hours; Cirrhosis (single dose): 37 hours (range 20-54 hours)

Time to peak, plasma: Capsules: 3-5 hours; Oral solution: 2-3 hours

Excretion: Urine (<0.03% active drug, 40% as inactive metabolites); feces (~3% to 18%)

Dosage Oral:

Usual dosage ranges:

Children: Efficacy and safety have not been established; a small number of patients 3-16 years of age have been treated with 100 mg/day for systemic fungal infections with no serious adverse effects reported. A dose of 5 mg/kg once daily was used in a pharmacokinetic study using the oral solution in patients 6 months to 12 years; duration of study was 2 weeks.

Adults: 100-400 mg/day; doses >200 mg/day are given in 2 divided doses; length of therapy varies from 1 day to >6 months depending on the condition and mycological response

Indication-specific dosing:

Adults:

Aspergillosis, invasive (salvage therapy): Duration of therapy should be a minimum of 6-12 weeks or throughout period of immunosuppression: Oral: 200-400 mg/day; **Note:** 2008 IDSA guidelines recommend 600 mg/day for 3 days, followed by 400 mg/day

Appropriate use: Itraconazole should **NOT** be used for voriconazole-refractory aspergillosis since the same antifungal and/or resistance mechanism(s) may be shared by both agents. Itraconazole oral solution and capsule formulations are not bioequivalent or interchangeable. Due to variable bioavailability of oral preparations, therapeutic drug monitoring advisable.

Aspergillosis, allergic (ABPA, sinusitis): 200 mg/day; may be used in conjunction with corticosteroids

Blastomycosis: 200 mg 3 times/day for 3 days, then 200 mg twice daily for 6-12 months; in moderately-severe to severe infection, therapy should be initiated with ~2 weeks of amphotericin B (Chapman, 2008)

Brain abscess: Cerebral phaeohyphomycosis (dematiaceous): 200 mg twice daily for at least 6 months with amphotericin

Candidiasis:

Oropharyngeal: Oral solution: 200 mg once daily for 1-2 weeks; in patients unresponsive or refractory to fluconazole: 100 mg twice daily (clinical response expected in 1-2 weeks)

Esophageal: Oral solution: 100-200 mg once daily for a minimum of 3 weeks; continue dosing for 2 weeks after resolution of symptoms

Coccidioidomycosis: 200 mg twice daily

Histoplasmosis: 200 mg 3 times/day for 3 days, then 200 mg twice daily (or once daily in mild-moderate disease) for 6-12 weeks in mild-moderate disease or ≥12 months in progressive disseminated or chronic cavitary pulmonary histoplasmosis; in moderately-severe to severe infection, therapy should be initiated with ~2 weeks of a lipid formation of amphotericin B (Wheat, 2007)

Long-term suppression therapy: 200 mg/day (AIDS*info* guidelines, 2008)

Meningitis:

Coccidioides: 400-800 mg/day

Coccidioides, HIV-positive (unlabeled use): 200 mg 3 times/day for 3 days, then 200 mg twice daily; maintenance: 200 mg twice daily life-long (AIDS*info* guidelines, 2008)

Appropriate use: Fluconazole is preferred for meningeal infections.

Onychomycosis: 200 mg once daily for 12 consecutive weeks; alternative "pulse-dosing" may be considering for fingernail involvement only: 200 mg twice daily for 1 week; repeat 1-week course after 3-week off-time

Penicilliosis, HIV-positive (unlabeled use): 200 mg twice daily for 8-10 weeks (in severely-ill patients, initiate therapy with 2 weeks of amphotericin B); maintenance: 200 mg/day (*AIDSinfo* guidelines, 2008)

Pneumonia:

Coccidioides: Mild-to-moderate: 200 mg twice daily

Coccidioides, HIV-positive (focal pneumonia): 200 mg 3 times/day for 3 days, then 200 mg twice daily (AIDS*info* guidelines, 2008)

Protothecal infection: 200 mg once daily for 2 months

Sporotrichosis:

Lymphocutaneous: 100-200 mg/day for 3-6 months

Osteoarticular and pulmonary: 200 mg twice daily for 1-2 years (may use amphotericin B initially for stabilization)

Dosing adjustment in renal impairment: The FDA-approved labeling states to use with caution in patients with renal impairment. The following guidelines have been used by some clinicians:

Aronoff, 2007:

Cl_{cr} >10 mL/minute: No adjustment recommended

Cl_{cr} <10 mL/minute: Administer 50% of normal dose

Continuous renal replacement therapy (CRRT)/hemodialysis: 200 mg every 12 hours for 4 doses, then 200 mg every 24 hours (Heintz, 2009)

Hemodialysis: Not dialyzable

Dosing adjustment in hepatic impairment: Use caution in patients with hepatic impairment

Administration Doses >200 mg/day are given in 2 divided doses; do not administer with antacids. Capsule and oral solution formulations are not bioequivalent and thus are not interchangeable. Capsule absorption is best if taken with food, therefore, it is best to administer itraconazole after meals; solution should be taken on an empty stomach. When treating oropharyngeal and esophageal candidiasis, solution should be swished vigorously in mouth, then swallowed.

Monitoring Parameters Liver function in patients with pre-existing hepatic dysfunction, and in all patients being treated for longer than 1 month; serum concentrations particularly for oral therapy (due to erratic bioavailability with capsule formulation); renal function

Dietary Considerations

Capsule: Administer with food.

Solution: Take without food, if possible.

Additional Information Due to potential toxicity, the manufacturer recommends confirmation of diagnosis testing of nail specimens prior to treatment of onychomycosis.

◀ **Dosage Forms** Excipient information presented when available (limited, particularly for generics); consult specific product labeling.

Capsule: 100 mg

Sporanox®: 100 mg

Solution, oral:

Sporanox®: 100 mg/10 mL (150 mL) [cherry flavor]

References

Aronoff GR, Bennett WM, Berns JS, et al, *Drug Prescribing in Renal Failure: Dosing Guidelines for Adults and Children*, 5th ed. Philadelphia, PA: American College of Physicians; 2007.

Chapman SW, Dismukes WE, Proia LA, et al, "Clinical Practice Guidelines for the Management of Blastomycosis: 2008 Update by the Infectious Diseases Society of America," *Clin Infect Dis*, 2008, 46(12):1801-12.

Cowie F, Meller ST, Cushing P, et al, "Chemoprophylaxis for Pulmonary Aspergillosis During Intensive Chemotherapy," *Arch Dis Child*, 1994, 70(2):136-8.

Denning DW, Lee JY, Hostetler JS, et al, "NIAID Mycoses Study Group Multicenter Trial of Oral Itraconazole Therapy for Invasive Aspergillosis," *Am J Med*, 1994, 97(2):135-44.

Jennings TS and Hardin TC, "Treatment of Aspergillosis With Itraconazole," *Ann Pharmacother*, 1993, 27(10):1206-11.

Kintzel PE, Rollins CJ, Yee WJ, et al, "Low Itraconazole Serum Concentrations Following Administration of Itraconazole Suspension to Critically Ill Allogenic Bone Marrow Transplant Recipients," *Ann Pharmacother*, 1995, 29(2):140-3.

Terrell CL, "Antifungal Agents. Part II. The Azoles," *Mayo Clin Proc*, 1999, 74(1):78-100.

Tobon AM, Franco L, Espinal D, et al, "Disseminated Histoplasmosis in Children: The Role of Itraconazole Therapy," *Pediatr Infect Dis J*, 1996; 15:1002-8.

Walsh TJ, Anaissie EJ, Denning DW, et al, "Treatment of Aspergillosis: Clinical Practice Guidelines of the Infectious Diseases Society of America," *Clin Infect Dis*, 2008, 46(3):327-60.

Wheat J, Hafner R, Korzun AH, et al, "Itraconazole Treatment of Disseminated Histoplasmosis in Patients With the Acquired Immunodeficiency Syndrome," *Am J Med*, 1995, 98(4):336-42.

♦ **IVIG** *see* Immune Globulin (Intravenous) *on page* 627

♦ **IV Immune Globulin** *see* Immune Globulin (Intravenous) *on page* 627

♦ **IvySoothe® [OTC]** *see* Hydrocortisone *on page* 575

Ixabepilone (ix ab EP i lone)

Medication Safety Issues

High alert medication: The Institute for Safe Medication Practices (ISMP) includes this medication among its list of drug classes which have a heightened risk of causing significant patient harm when used in error.

Related Information

Management of Chemotherapy-Induced Nausea and Vomiting *on page* 1434

Safe Handling of Hazardous Drugs *on page* 1517

U.S. Brand Names Ixempra®

Index Terms Azaepothilone B; BMS-247550; Epothilone B Lactam

Generic Available No

Pharmacologic Category Antineoplastic Agent, Antimicrotubular; Antineoplastic Agent, Epothilone B Analog

Use Treatment of metastatic or locally-advanced breast cancer (refractory or resistant)

Pregnancy Risk Factor D

Lactation Excretion in breast milk unknown/not recommended

Labeled Contraindications History of severe hypersensitivity to Cremophor® EL or its derivatives (eg, polyoxyethylated castor oil); neutrophil count <1500/mm^3 or platelet count <100,000/mm^3; combination therapy with ixabepilone and capecitabine in patients with AST or ALT >2.5 times ULN or bilirubin >1 times ULN

Warnings/Precautions Hazardous agent - use appropriate precautions for handling and disposal. **[U.S. Boxed Warning]: Due to increased risk of**

toxicity and neutropenia-related mortality, combination therapy with capecitabine is contraindicated in patients with AST or ALT >2.5 times ULN or bilirubin >1 times ULN. Use (as monotherapy) is not recommended if AST or ALT >10 times ULN or bilirubin >3 times ULN; use caution in patients with AST or ALT >5 times ULN. Toxicities and serious adverse reactions are increased (in mono- and combination therapy) with hepatic dysfunction; dosage reductions are necessary. Diluent contains Cremophor® EL, which is associated with hypersensitivity reactions; use is contraindicated in patients with a history of severe hypersensitivity to Cremophor® EL or its derivatives. Medications for the treatment of reaction should be available for immediate use; reactions may also be managed with a reduction of infusion rate. Premedicate with an H_1- and H_2-antagonist 1 hour prior to infusion; patients who experience hypersensitivity (eg, bronchospasm, dyspnea, flushing, rash) should also be premedicated with a corticosteroid for all subsequent cycles if treatment is continued.

Dose-dependent myelosuppression, particularly neutropenia, may occur with mono- or combination therapy. Neutropenic fever and infection have been reported with use. The risk for neutropenia is increased with hepatic dysfunction, especially when used in combination with capecitabine. Severe neutropenia and/or thrombocytopenia may require dosage adjustment and/or treatment delay. Peripheral (sensory and motor) neuropathy occurs commonly; may require dose reductions, treatment delays or discontinuation. Usually occurs during the first 3 cycles. Use with caution in patients with pre-existing neuropathy. Patients with diabetes may have an increased risk for severe peripheral neuropathy. Use with caution in patients with a history of cardiovascular disease; the incidence of MI, ventricular dysfunction, and supraventricular arrhythmias is higher when ixabepilone is used in combination with capecitabine (as compared to capecitabine alone). Consider discontinuing ixabepilone in patients who develop cardiac ischemia or impaired cardiac function.

Avoid concurrent use with strong CYP3A4 inhibitors (eg, itraconazole, ketoconazole, voriconazole, clarithromycin, telithromycin, nefazodone, ampre-navir, atazanavir, delavirdine, indinavir, nelfinavir, ritonavir, saquinavir); dosage reductions are recommended if concurrent use cannot be avoided; allow ~1 week to elapse prior to adjusting ixabepilone dose upward after a strong CYP3A4 inhibitor is discontinued. Avoid strong CYP3A4 inducers (eg, dexamethasone, phenytoin, carbamazepine, rifampin, phenobarbital); may decrease the ixabepilone levels. Due to the ethanol content in the diluent, may cause cognitive impairment; patients must be cautioned about performing tasks which require mental alertness (eg, operating machinery or driving). Toxicities or serious adverse events with combination therapy may be increased in the elderly. Safety and efficacy have not been established in children.

Adverse Reactions

Percentages reported with monotherapy:

>10%:

Central nervous system: Headache (11%)

Dermatologic: Alopecia (48%)

Gastrointestinal: Nausea (42%), vomiting (29%), mucositis/stomatitis (29%), diarrhea (22%), anorexia (19%), constipation (16%), abdominal pain (13%)

Hematologic: Leukopenia (36%; grade 4: 13%), neutropenia (31%; grade 4: 23%)

Neuromuscular & skeletal: Peripheral neuropathy (~75%; grades 3/4: 14%; median onset: cycle 4), sensory neuropathy (62%; grades 3/4: 14%), weakness (56%), myalgia/arthralgia (49%), musculoskeletal pain (20%)

1% to 10%:

Cardiovascular: Edema (9%), hot flush (6%), chest pain (5%)

Central nervous system: Fever (8%), pain (8%), dizziness (7%), insomnia (5%)

Dermatologic: Nail disorder (9%), rash (9%), palmar-plantar erythrodysesthesia/hand-and-foot syndrome (8%), pruritus (6%), skin exfoliation (2%), hyperpigmentation (2%)

Endocrine & metabolic: Dehydration (2%)

Gastrointestinal: Gastroesophageal reflux disease (6%), taste perversion (6%), weight loss (6%)

Hematologic: Anemia (6%; grade 4: 2%), neutropenic fever (3%; grade 3: 3%), thrombocytopenia (5%; grade 4: 2%)

Neuromuscular & skeletal: Motor neuropathy (10%; grade 3: 1%)

Ocular: Lacrimation increased (4%)

Respiratory: Dyspnea (9%), upper respiratory tract infection (6%), cough (2%)

Miscellaneous: Hypersensitivity (5%; grade 3: 1%), infection (5%)

Mono- and combination therapy: <1%, postmarketing, and/or case reports (limited to important or life-threatening): Alkaline phosphatase increased, angina, atrial flutter, autonomic neuropathy, cardiomyopathy, cerebral hemorrhage, coagulopathy, colitis, embolism, dysphagia, enterocolitis, erythema multiforme, gastrointestinal hemorrhage, gastroparesis, GGT increased, hemorrhage, hepatic failure (acute), hypokalemia, hyponatremia, hypotension, hypovolemia, hypovolemic shock, hypoxia, ileus, interstitial pneumonia, jaundice, left ventricular dysfunction, metabolic acidosis, MI, nephrolithiasis, neutropenic infection, orthostatic hypotension, pneumonia, pneumonitis, pulmonary edema (acute), renal failure, respiratory failure, sepsis, septic shock, supraventricular arrhythmia, syncope, thrombosis, transaminases increased, trismus, urinary tract infection, vasculitis

Drug Interactions

Metabolism/Transport Effects Substrate of CYP3A4 (major)

Avoid Concomitant Use There are no known interactions where it is recommended to avoid concomitant use.

Increased Effect/Toxicity

The levels/effects of Ixabepilone may be increased by: CYP3A4 Inhibitors (Moderate); CYP3A4 Inhibitors (Strong); Dasatinib

Decreased Effect

The levels/effects of Ixabepilone may be decreased by: CYP3A4 Inducers (Strong); Deferasirox; Herbs (CYP3A4 Inducers)

Ethanol/Nutrition/Herb Interactions

Food: Avoid grapefruit juice (may increase plasma concentrations of ixabepilone).

Herb/Nutraceutical: Avoid St John's wort (may decrease ixabepilone levels).

Storage/Stability Store intact vials under refrigeration at 2°C to 8°C (36°F to 46°F); protect from light. Reconstituted solution (in the vial) is stable for 1 hour at room temperature; infusion solution diluted in appropriate solution for infusion is stable for 6 hours at room temperature if a pH range of 6-9 is maintained.

Reconstitution Allow to reach room temperature for ~30 minutes prior to reconstitution. Diluent vial may contain a white precipitate which should dissolve upon reaching room temperature. **Reconstitute only with the**

provided diluent. Dilute the 15 mg vial with 8 mL and the 45 mg vial with 23.5 mL (using provided diluent) to a concentration of 2 mg/mL (contains overfill). Gently swirl and invert vial until dissolved completely. Prior to administration, further dilute using a non-DEHP container (eg, glass, polypropylene or polyolefin), to a final concentration of 0.2-0.6 mg/mL in ~250 mL lactated Ringer's, adjusted sodium chloride 0.9% (pH adjusted prior to ixabepilone addition with 2 mEq sodium bicarbonate per 250-500 mL sodium chloride) or PLASMA-LYTE A Injection pH 7.4®. Mix thoroughly. Use appropriate precautions for handling and disposal.

Compatibility Stable in lactated Ringer's injection, adjusted sodium chloride 0.9% (pH adjusted with sodium bicarbonate); PLASMA-LYTE A Injection pH 7.4®.

Mechanism of Action Epothilone B analog; binds to the beta-tubulin subunit of the microtubule, stabilizing microtubular promoting tubulin polymerization and stabilizing microtubular function, thus arresting the cell cycle (at the G2/M phase) and inducing apoptosis. Activity in taxane-resistant cells has been demonstrated.

Pharmacodynamics/Kinetics

Distribution: >1000 L/m^2

Protein binding: 67% to 77%

Metabolism: Extensively hepatic, via CYP3A4; >30 metabolites (inactive) formed

Half-life elimination: ~52 hours

Time to peak, plasma: At the end of infusion (3 hours)

Excretion: Feces (65%; 2% as unchanged drug); urine (21%; 6% as unchanged drug)

Dosage Details concerning dosing in combination regimens should also be consulted. **Note:** Premedicate with an H$_1$-antagonist (eg, oral diphenhydramine 50 mg) and H$_2$-antagonist (eg, oral ranitidine 150-300 mg) 1 hour prior to infusion. Patients with a history of hypersensitivity should also be premedicated with corticosteroids (orally 1 hour before or I.V. 30 minutes before infusion). Body surface area (BSA) is capped at a maximum of 2.2 m^2.

I.V.: Adults: Breast cancer (metastatic or locally advanced): 40 mg/m^2/dose over 3 hours every 3 weeks (maximum dose: 88 mg) either as monotherapy or in combination with capecitabine

Dosage adjustment with concurrent strong CYP3A4 inhibitor: If concurrent use can not be avoided, reduce ixabepilone dose to 20 mg/m^2. When a strong CYP3A4 inhibitor is discontinued, allow ~1 week to elapse prior to adjusting ixabepilone dose upward.

Ixabepilone dosage adjustments for toxicity for monotherapy or combination therapy:

Hematologic:

Neutrophils <500/mm^3 for ≥7 days: Reduce dose by 20%

Neutropenic fever: Reduce dose by 20%

Platelets <25,000/mm^3 (or <50,000/mm^3 with bleeding): Reduce dose by 20%

Nonhematologic:

Neuropathy:

Grade 2 (moderate) for ≥7 days: Reduce dose by 20%

Grade 3 (severe) for <7 days: Reduce dose by 20%

Grade 3 (severe or disabling) for ≥7 days: Discontinue treatment

Grade 3 toxicity (severe; other than neuropathy): Reduce dose by 20%

Grade 3 arthralgia/myalgia or fatigue (transient): Continue at current dose

▶

Grade 3 hand-foot syndrome: Continue at current dose

Grade 4 toxicity (disabling): Discontinue treatment

Note: Adjust dosage at the start of a cycle are based on toxicities (hematologic and nonhematologic) from the previous cycle; delay new cycles until neutrophils have recovered to ≥1500/mm^3, platelets have recovered to ≥100,000/mm^3 and nonhematologic toxicities have resolved or improved to at least grade 1. If toxicities persist despite initial dose reduction, reduce dose an additional 20%.

Capecitabine dosage adjustments for toxicity in combination therapy with ixabepilone:

Hematologic:

Neutrophils <500/mm^3 for ≥7 days or neutropenic fever: Hold for concurrent diarrhea or stomatitis until neutrophils recover to >1000/mm^3, then continue at same dose

Platelets <25,000/mm^3 (or <50,000/mm^3 with bleeding): Hold for concurrent diarrhea or stomatitis until platelets recover to >50,000/mm^3, then continue at same dose

Nonhematologic: Refer to Capecitabine monograph.

Dosage adjustment in renal impairment: Pharmacokinetics (monotherapy) are not affected in patients with mild-to-moderate renal insufficiency (Cl$_{cr}$ >30 mL/minute); monotherapy has not been studied in patients with serum creatinine >1.5 times ULN. Combination therapy with capecitabine has not been studied in patients with Cl$_{cr}$ <50 mL/minute.

Dosage adjustment in hepatic impairment:

Ixabepilone monotherapy (initial cycle; adjust doses for subsequent cycles based on toxicity):

AST and ALT ≤2.5 times ULN and bilirubin ≤1 times ULN: No adjustment necessary

AST or ALT ≤10 times ULN and bilirubin ≤1.5 times ULN: Reduce dose to 32 mg/m^2

AST and ALT ≤10 times ULN and bilirubin >1.5 - ≤3 times ULN: Reduce dose to 20-30 mg/m^2 (initiate treatment at 20 mg/m^2, may escalate up to a maximum of 30 mg/m^2 in subsequent cycles if tolerated)

AST or ALT >10 times ULN or bilirubin >3 times ULN: Use is not recommended

Combination therapy of ixabepilone with capecitabine:

AST and ALT ≤2.5 times ULN and bilirubin ≤1 times ULN: No adjustment necessary

AST or ALT >2.5 times ULN or bilirubin >1 times ULN: Use is contraindicated

Combination Regimens

Breast cancer: Ixabepilone-Capecitabine on page 1361

Administration I.V.: Infuse over 3 hours. Use non-DEHP administration set (eg, polyethylene); filter with a 0.2-1.2 micron inline filter.

Monitoring Parameters CBC with differential; hepatic function (ALT, AST, bilirubin); monitor for hypersensitivity, neuropathy

Dietary Considerations Avoid grapefruit juice (may increase plasma concentrations of ixabepilone).

Emetic Potential Low (10% to 30%)

Dosage Forms Excipient information presented when available (limited, particularly for generics); consult specific product labeling.

Injection, powder for reconstitution:
Ixempra®: 15 mg, 45 mg [packaged with diluent; diluent contains alcohol and purified polyoxyethylated castor oil (Cremophor® EL)]

References

Dendurali N, Low JA, Lee JJ, et al, "Phase II Trial of Ixabepilone, an Epothilone B Analog, in Patients With Metastatic Breast Cancer Previously Untreated With Taxanes," *J Clin Oncol*, 2007, 25(23):3421-7.

Lee JJ, Low JA, Croarkin E, et al, "Changes in Neurologic Function Tests May Predict Neurotoxicity Caused by Ixabepilone," *J Clin Oncol*, 2006, 24(13):2084-91.

Low JA, Wedam SB, Lee JJ, et al, "Phase II Clinical Trial of Ixabepilone (BMS-247550), an Epothilone B Analog, in Metastatic and Locally Advanced Breast Cancer," *J Clin Oncol*, 2005, 23 (12):2726-34.

Mani S, McDid H, Hamilton A, et al, "Phase I and Clinical Pharmacokinetic Study of BMS-247550, a Novel Derivative of Epothilone B,in Solid Tumors," *Clin Cancer Res*, 2004, 10(4):1289-98.

National Comprehensive Cancer Network® (NCCN), "Clinical Practice Guidelines in Oncology™: Breast Cancer," Version 1.2009. Available at http://www.nccn.org/professionals/physician_gls/PDF/breast.pdf.

Perez EA, Lerzo G, Pivot X, et al, "Efficacy and Safety of Ixabepilone (BMS-247550), in a Phase II Study of Patients With Advanced Breast Cancer Resistant to an Anthracycline, a Taxane and Capecitabine," *J Clin Oncol*, 2007, 25(23):3407-14.

Roche H, Yelle L, Cognetti F, et al, "Phase II Clinical Trial of Ixabepilone (BMS-247550), an Epothilone B Analog, as First Line Therapy in Patients With Metastatic Breast Cancer Previously Treated With Anthracycline Chemotherapy," *J Clin Oncol*, 2007, 25(23):3415-20.

Takimoto CH, Liu PY, Lenz H, et al, "A Phase I Pharmacokinetic (PK) Study of the Epothilone B Analogue, Ixabepilone (BMS-247550) in Patients (pts) With Advanced Malignancies and Varying Degrees of Hepatic Impairment: A SWOG Early Therapeutics Committee and NCI Organ Dysfunction Working Group Trial," *J Clin Oncol*, 2006, 24(18S):2004 [abstract from 2006 ASCO Annual Meeting Proceedings]

Thomas ES, Gomez HL, Li RK, et al, "Ixabepilone Plus Capecitabine for Metastatic Breast Cancer Progressing After Anthracycline and Taxane Treatment," *J Clin Oncol*, 2007, 25(33):5210-7.

Thomas E, Tabernero J, Fornier M, et al, "Phase II Clinical Trial of Ixabepilone (BMS-247550), an Epothilone B Analog, in Patients With Taxane-Resistant Metastatic Breast Cancer," *J Clin Oncol*, 2007, 25(23):3399-406.

♦ **Ixempra®** see Ixabepilone on page 672

♦ **JAMP-Ondansetron (Can)** see Ondansetron on page 874

♦ **Kadian®** see Morphine Sulfate on page 816

♦ **Keoxifene Hydrochloride** see Raloxifene on page 1002

♦ **Kepivance®** see Palifermin on page 908

Ketoconazole (kee toe KOE na zole)

Medication Safety Issues

Sound-alike/look-alike issues:

Kuric™ may be confused with Carac®

Nizoral® may be confused with Nasarel®, Neoral®, Nitrol®

U.S. Brand Names Extina®; Kuric™; Nizoral®; Nizoral® A-D [OTC]; Xolegel®

Generic Available Yes: Cream, shampoo, tablet

Canadian Brand Names Apo-Ketoconazole®; Ketoderm®; Novo-Ketoconazole; Xolegel®

Pharmacologic Category Antifungal Agent, Oral; Antifungal Agent, Topical

Use

Systemic: Treatment of susceptible fungal infections, including candidiasis, oral thrush, blastomycosis, histoplasmosis, paracoccidioidomycosis, coccidioidomycosis, chromomycosis, candiduria, chronic mucocutaneous candidiasis, as well as certain recalcitrant cutaneous dermatophytoses

Topical:

Cream: Treatment of tinea corporis, tinea cruris, tinea versicolor, cutaneous candidiasis, seborrheic dermatitis

Foam, gel: Treatment of seborrheic dermatitis

Shampoo: Treatment of dandruff, seborrheic dermatitis, tinea versicolor

Unlabeled/Investigational Use Tablet: Treatment of prostate cancer (androgen synthesis inhibitor)

Pregnancy Risk Factor C

Lactation Enters breast milk/not recommended

Labeled Contraindications Hypersensitivity to ketoconazole or any component of the formulation; CNS fungal infections (due to poor CNS penetration); coadministration with ergot derivatives, cisapride, or triazolam is contraindicated due to risk of potentially fatal cardiac arrhythmias

Warnings/Precautions [U.S. Boxed Warning]: Ketoconazole has been associated with hepatotoxicity, including some fatalities; use with caution in patients with impaired hepatic function and perform periodic liver function tests. **[U.S. Boxed Warning]: Concomitant use with cisapride is contraindicated due to the occurrence of ventricular arrhythmias.** High doses of ketoconazole may depress adrenocortical function. Cases of hypersensitivity reactions (including rare cases of anaphylaxis) have been reported.

Topical: Formulations may contain sulfites. Avoid exposure of gel to open flames during or immediately after application. Use of shampoo may remove curl from permanently wavy hair, cause hair discoloration, and changes in hair texture; avoid contact with eyes. Foam formulation contains alcohol and propane/butane; do not expose to open flame or smoking during or immediately after application; do not puncture or incinerate container.

Adverse Reactions

Oral:

1% to 10%:

Dermatologic: Pruritus (2%)

Gastrointestinal: Nausea/vomiting (3% to 10%), abdominal pain (1%)

<1%: Bulging fontanelles, chills, depression, diarrhea, dizziness, fever, gynecomastia, headache, hemolytic anemia, hepatotoxicity, impotence, leukopenia, photophobia, somnolence, thrombocytopenia

Topical cream/gel: Allergic reaction, contact dermatitis (possibly related to sulfites or propylene glycol), facial swelling, headache, impetigo, local burning, ocular irritation, paresthesia, pruritus, severe irritation, stinging (~5%)

Topical foam: Application site burning (10%), application site reaction (6%), contact sensitization, dryness, erythema, pruritus, rash

Shampoo: Abnormal hair texture, alopecia, application site reaction, burning sensation, contact dermatitis, hair discoloration, hair loss increased (<1%), hypersensitivity, irritation (<1%), itching, mild dryness of skin, oiliness/dryness of hair, pruritus, rash, scalp pustules, urticaria

Drug Interactions

Metabolism/Transport Effects Substrate of CYP3A4 (major); **Inhibits** CYP1A2 (strong), 2A6 (moderate), 2B6 (weak), 2C8 (weak), 2C9 (strong), 2C19 (moderate), 2D6 (moderate), 3A4 (strong)

Avoid Concomitant Use

Avoid concomitant use of Ketoconazole with any of the following: Alfuzosin; Cisapride; Clopidogrel; Conivaptan; Dabigatran Etexilate; Dofetilide; Dronedarone; Eplerenone; Everolimus; Halofantrine; Nilotinib; Nisoldipine; Pimozide; QuiNIDine; Ranolazine; Rivaroxaban; Salmeterol; Silodosin; Thioridazine; Tolvaptan; Topotecan

Increased Effect/Toxicity

Ketoconazole may increase the levels/effects of: Alfentanil; Alfuzosin; Aliskiren; Almotriptan; Alosetron; Aprepitant; Bendamustine;

Benzodiazepines (metabolized by oxidation); Bosentan; BusPIRone; Busulfan; Calcium Channel Blockers; CarBAMazepine; Cardiac Glycosides; Carvedilol; Ciclesonide; Cilostazol; Cinacalcet; Cisapride; Colchicine; Conivaptan; Corticosteroids (Orally Inhaled); Corticosteroids (Systemic); CycloSPORINE; CYP1A2 Substrates; CYP2A6 Substrates; CYP2C19 Substrates; CYP2C9 Substrates (High risk); CYP2D6 Substrates; CYP3A4 Substrates; Dabigatran Etexilate; Docetaxel; Dofetilide; Dronedarone; Dutasteride; Eletriptan; Eplerenone; Erlotinib; Eszopiclone; Everolimus; FentaNYL; Fesoterodine; Fexofenadine; Fosaprepitant; Gefitinib; Halofantrine; HMG-CoA Reductase Inhibitors; Imatinib; Irinotecan; Ixabepilone; Losartan; Macrolide Antibiotics; Maraviroc; Methadone; Nebivolol; Nilotinib; Nisoldipine; Paricalcitol; P-Glycoprotein Substrates; Phenytoin; Phosphodiesterase 5 Inhibitors; Pimecrolimus; Pimozide; Praziquantel; Protease Inhibitors; Proton Pump Inhibitors; QuiNIDine; Ramelteon; Ranolazine; Repaglinide; Rifamycin Derivatives; Rivaroxaban; Salmeterol; Saxagliptin; Silodosin; Sirolimus; Solifenacin; Sorafenib; Sunitinib; Tacrolimus; Tadalafil; Tamoxifen; Temsirolimus; Thioridazine; Tolterodine; Tolvaptan; Topotecan; Trimetrexate; Vitamin K Antagonists; Ziprasidone; Zolpidem

The levels/effects of Ketoconazole may be increased by: Grapefruit Juice; Macrolide Antibiotics; Protease Inhibitors

Decreased Effect

Ketoconazole may decrease the levels/effects of: Amphotericin B; Clopidogrel; Codeine; Prasugrel; Saccharomyces boulardii; TraMADol

The levels/effects of Ketoconazole may be decreased by: Antacids; CYP3A4 Inducers (Strong); Deferasirox; Didanosine; H2-Antagonists; Herbs (CYP3A4 Inducers); Phenytoin; Proton Pump Inhibitors; Rifamycin Derivatives; Sucralfate

Ethanol/Nutrition/Herb Interactions

Food: Ketoconazole peak serum levels may be prolonged if taken with food.

Herb/Nutraceutical: St John's wort may decrease ketoconazole levels.

Storage/Stability

Cream: Store at <25°C (<77°F).

Foam: Store at 20°C to 25°C (68°F to 77°F). Do not refrigerate. Do not store in direct sunlight. Contents are flammable.

Gel: Store at 15°C to 30°C (59°F to 86°F).

Shampoo:

Nizoral®: Store at ≤25°C (≤77°F). Protect from light.

Nizoral® A-D:Store between 2°C to 30°C (35°F to 86°F); protect from freezing. Protect from light.

Tablet: Store at 15°C to 25°C (59°F to 77°F).

Mechanism of Action Alters the permeability of the cell wall by blocking fungal cytochrome P450; inhibits biosynthesis of triglycerides and phospholipids by fungi; inhibits several fungal enzymes that results in a build-up of toxic concentrations of hydrogen peroxide; also inhibits androgen synthesis

Pharmacodynamics/Kinetics

Absorption: Oral: Rapid (~75%); Shampoo: None; Gel: Minimal

Distribution: Well into inflamed joint fluid, saliva, bile, urine, breast milk, sebum, cerumen, feces, tendons, skin and soft tissue, and testes; crosses blood-brain barrier poorly; only negligible amounts reach CSF

Protein binding: 93% to 96%

Metabolism: Partially hepatic via CYP3A4 to inactive compounds

Bioavailability: Decreases as gastric pH increases

Half-life elimination: Biphasic: Initial: 2 hours; Terminal: 8 hours

Time to peak, serum: 1-2 hours

Excretion: Feces (57%); urine (13%)

Dosage

Oral:

Fungal infections:

Children ≥2 years: 3.3-6.6 mg/kg/day as a single dose for 1-2 weeks for candidiasis, for at least 4 weeks in recalcitrant dermatophyte infections, and for up to 6 months for other systemic mycoses

Adults: 200-400 mg/day as a single daily dose for durations as stated above

Prostate cancer (unlabeled use): Adults: 400 mg 3 times/day

Shampoo:

Seborrheic dermatitis (ketoconazole 1%): Children ≥12 years and Adults: Apply twice weekly for up to 8 weeks with at least 3 days between each shampoo

Tinea versicolor (ketoconazole 2%): Adults: Apply to damp skin, lather, leave on 5 minutes, and rinse (one application should be sufficient)

Topical:

Tinea infections: Adults: Cream: Rub gently into the affected area once daily. Duration of treatment: Tinea corporis, cruris: 2 weeks; tinea pedis: 6 weeks

Seborrheic dermatitis: Children ≥12 years and Adults:

Cream: Rub gently into the affected area twice daily for 4 weeks or until clinical response is noted

Foam: Apply to affected area twice daily for 4 weeks

Gel: Rub gently into the affected area once daily for 2 weeks

Dosing adjustment in renal impairment: Hemodialysis: Not dialyzable (0% to 5%)

Dosing adjustment in hepatic impairment: Dose reductions should be considered in patients with severe liver disease

Combination Regimens

Prostate cancer:

Doxorubicin + Ketoconazole on page 1296

Doxorubicin + Ketoconazole/Estramustine + Vinblastine on page 1296

Administration

Oral: Administer oral tablets 2 hours prior to antacids to prevent decreased absorption due to the high pH of gastric contents.

Cream, foam, gel, and shampoo are for external use only. Avoid exposure to flame or smoking immediately following application of gel or foam; do not apply directly to hands.

Monitoring Parameters Liver function tests

Dietary Considerations Tablet: May be taken with food or milk to decrease GI adverse effects.

Dosage Forms Excipient information presented when available (limited, particularly for generics); consult specific product labeling.

Aerosol, topical [foam]:

Extina®: 2% (50 g, 100 g)

Cream, topical: 2% (15 g, 30 g, 60 g)

Kuric™: 2%: (75 g)

Gel, topical:

Xolegel®: 2% (15 g, 45 g) [contains dehydrated alcohol 34%]

Shampoo, topical: 1% (120 mL), 2% (120 mL)

Nizoral®: 2% (120 mL)

Nizoral® A-D: 1% (120 mL, 210 mL)

Tablet: 200 mg

Extemporaneous Preparations A 20 mg/mL suspension may be made by pulverizing twelve 200 mg ketoconazole tablets to a fine powder; add 40 mL Ora-Plus® in small portions with thorough mixing; incorporate Ora-Sweet® to make a final volume of 120 mL and mix thoroughly; refrigerate (no stability information is available)

Allen LV, "Ketoconazole Oral Suspension," *US Pharm*, 1993, 18(2):98-9, 101.

References

Herrod HG, "Chronic Mucocutaneous Candidiasis in Childhood and Complications of non-*Candida* Infection: A Report of the Pediatric Immunodeficiency Collaborative Study Group," *J Pediatr*, 1990, 116(3):377-82.

Janssen PA and Symoens JE, "Hepatic Reactions During Ketoconazole Treatment," *Am J Med*, 1983, 74(1B):80-5.

Lyman CA and Walsh TJ, "Systemically Administered Antifungal Agents. A Review of Their Clinical Pharmacology and Therapeutic Applications," *Drugs*, 1992, 44(1):9-35.

Small EJ, Halabi S, Dawson NA, et al, "Antiandrogen Withdrawal Alone or in Combination With Ketoconazole in Androgen-Independent Prostate Cancer Patients: A Phase III Trial (CALGB 9583)," *J Clin Oncol*, 2004, 22(6):1025-33.

Trachtenberg J and Pont A, "Ketoconazole Therapy for Advanced Prostate Cancer," *Lancet*, 1984, (8400):433-5.

♦ **Ketoderm® (Can)** see Ketoconazole on page 677

♦ **Khloditan** see Mitotane on page 807

♦ **Kidrolase® (Can)** see Asparaginase on page 111

♦ **Kogenate® (Can)** see Antihemophilic Factor (Recombinant) on page 93

♦ **Kogenate® FS** see Antihemophilic Factor (Recombinant) on page 93

♦ **Konakion (Can)** see Phytonadione on page 953

♦ **Koāte®-DVI** see Antihemophilic Factor (Human) on page 91

♦ **Kuric™** see Ketoconazole on page 677

♦ **Kytril®** see Granisetron on page 552

♦ **L-758,298** see Fosaprepitant on page 513

♦ **L 754030** see Aprepitant on page 104

♦ **Ladakamycin** see AzaCITIDine on page 117

♦ **L-AmB** see Amphotericin B (Liposomal) on page 74

Lanreotide (lan REE oh tide)

Medication Safety Issues

Sound-alike/look-alike issues:

Somatuline® may be confused with somatropin, SUMAtriptan

International issues:

Somatuline® may be confused with Soma® which is a brand name for carisoprodol in the U.S.

U.S. Brand Names Somatuline® Depot

Index Terms Lanreotide Acetate

Canadian Brand Names Somatuline® Autogel®

Pharmacologic Category Somatostatin Analog

Use Long-term treatment of acromegaly in patients who are not candidates for or are unresponsive to surgery and/or radiotherapy

Canadian labeling: Also approved in Canada for relief of symptoms of acromegaly

Pregnancy Risk Factor C

Lactation

Excretion into breast milk unknown/not recommended

Labeled Contraindications
There are no contraindications listed in the manufacturer's labeling.

Canadian labeling contraindications: Hypersensitivity to lanreotide, somatostatin (or related peptides), or any component of the formulation; complicated, untreated lithiasis of the bile ducts

Warnings/Precautions Inhibition of insulin and glucagon secretion may affect glucose regulation, leading to hyper-/hypoglycemia, especially in patients with diabetes. Monitor serum glucose levels with the initiation of therapy and with dosage changes; dose adjustments in antidiabetic medications may be necessary. May reduce gall bladder motility, leading to cholelithiasis (may be dose- or duration-related); monitor. **Note:** In Canada, ultrasonography is recommended when initiating therapy and periodically thereafter. Slight decreases in thyroid function have been observed during therapy; may require monitoring of thyroid function tests.

Bradycardia, sinus bradycardia and hypertension have been observed with therapy; use with caution in patients with preexisting cardiac disease. Patients without preexisting cardiac disease may experience a decrease in heart rate though not to the level of bradycardia. Concurrent use with cyclosporine may lead to decreased levels of cyclosporine; monitor cyclosporine levels during therapy. Use with caution in patients with renal and hepatic impairment; lower doses are recommended at therapy initiation in patients with moderate-to-severe impairment. The packaging (needle cover) may contain latex. Safety and efficacy have not been established in children. **Note:** In Canada, safety and efficacy have not been established in children <16 years of age.

Adverse Reactions
>10%:
  Cardiovascular: Bradycardia (5% to 18%)
  Gastrointestinal: Diarrhea (26% to 65%; dose related), abdominal pain (7% to 19%; dose related), flatulence (≤14%; dose related), nausea (11%), weight loss (5% to 11%)
  Hematologic: Anemia (3% to 14%)
  Hepatic: Cholelithiasis/gall bladder sludge (2% to 20%)
  Local: Injection site reaction (6% to 22%; induration 5%; pain 4%; mass 2%)
1% to 10%:
  Cardiovascular: Hypertension (5%), sinus bradycardia (3%)
  Central nervous system: Headache (7%)
  Endocrine & metabolic: Hyper-/hypoglycemia/diabetes (7%)
  Gastrointestinal: Constipation (8%), vomiting (7%), loose stools (6%)
  Neuromuscular & skeletal: Arthralgia (7%)
<1%, postmarketing, and/or case reports: Allergic skin reaction, aortic valve regurgitation, dysautonomia, injection site pruritus, mitral valve regurgitation, steatorrhea

Drug Interactions
Avoid Concomitant Use There are no known interactions where it is recommended to avoid concomitant use.

Increased Effect/Toxicity
Lanreotide may increase the levels/effects of: Codeine; Hypoglycemic Agents; Pegvisomant

The levels/effects of Lanreotide may be increased by: Herbs (Hypoglycemic Properties)

Decreased Effect
Lanreotide may decrease the levels/effects of: CycloSPORINE

Ethanol/Nutrition/Herb Interactions Herb/Nutraceutical: Avoid hypoglycemic herbs, including alfalfa, aloe, bilberry, bitter melon, burdock, celery, damiana, fenugreek, garcinia, garlic, ginger, ginseng, gymnema, marshmallow, and stinging nettle (may enhance the hypoglycemic effect of lanreotide).

Storage/Stability Store under refrigeration 2°C to 8°C (36°F to 46°F). Protect from light. Allow to reach room temperature by removing sealed pouch from refrigerator 30 minutes prior to administration; keep in sealed pouch until just prior to administration.

Mechanism of Action Synthetic octapeptide analogue of somatostatin which is a peptide inhibitor of multiple endocrine, neuroendocrine, and exocrine mechanisms. Displays a greater affinity for somatostatin type 2 (SSTR2) and type 5 (SSTR5) receptors found in pituitary gland, pancreas, and growth hormone (GH) secreting neoplasms of pituitary gland and a lesser affinity for somatostatin receptors 1, 3, and 4. Reduces GH secretion and also reduces the levels of insulin-like growth factor 1.

Pharmacodynamics/Kinetics

Distribution: V_{ss}: ~0.2 L/kg

Protein binding: 79% to 83%

Metabolism: Extensively within GI tract after biliary excretion

Bioavailability: 69% to 83%

Half-life, elimination: 23-36 days

Time to peak, plasma: Mean: 7-12 hours

Excretion: Urine (<1% to 5% as unchanged drug); feces (<0.5% as unchanged drug)

Dosage SubQ: Note: Differences in U.S. and Canadian labeled dosing:

U.S. labeling: Adults: Acromegaly: 90 mg once every 4 weeks for 3 months; after initial 90 days of therapy, adjust dose based on clinical response of patient, growth hormone (GH) levels, and/or insulin-like growth factor 1 (IGF-1) levels as follows:

GH ≤1 ng/mL, IGF-1 normal, symptoms stable:60 mg once every 4 weeks

GH >1-2.5 ng/mL, IGF-1 normal, symptoms stable: 90 mg once every 4 weeks

GH >2.5 ng/mL, IGF-1 elevated and/or uncontrolled symptoms: 120 mg once every 4 weeks

Canadian labeling: Children ≥16 years and Adults: Acromegaly: 90 mg once every 4 weeks for 3 months; after initial 90 days of therapy, adjust dose based on clinical response of patient, growth hormone (GH) levels, and/or insulin-like growth factor 1 (IGF-1) levels as follows:

GH = 1 ng/mL, IGF-1 normal, symptoms stable: 60 mg once every 4 weeks

GH >1-2.5 ng/mL, IGF-1 normal, symptoms stable: 90 mg once every 4 weeks

GH >2.5 ng/mL, IGF-1 elevated and/or uncontrolled symptoms: 120 mg once every 4 weeks

Dosing adjustment in renal impairment:

U.S. labeling: Moderate-to-severe impairment: Recommended starting dose: 60 mg

Canadian labeling: No adjustment is necessary

Dosing adjustment in hepatic impairment:

U.S. labeling: Moderate-to-severe impairment: Recommended starting dose: 60 mg

Canadian labeling: No adjustment is necessary

Administration Administer by deep subcutaneous injection into superior outer quadrant of buttocks. Do not fold skin. Alternate injection sites.

◀ **Monitoring Parameters** Serum GH, IGF-1, glucose levels, thyroid function (where clinically indicated); heart rate, gall bladder ultrasonography (prior to initiation and periodically during therapy)

Dosage Forms Excipient information presented when available (limited, particularly for generics); consult specific product labeling. [CAN] = Canadian brand name

Injection, solution:

Somatuline® Autogel® [CAN]: 60 mg/ 0.3 mL (0.3 mL); 90 mg/ 0.3 mL (0.3 mL); 120 mg/0.5 mL (0.5 mL) [packaging contains natural rubber/natural latex]

Somatuline® Depot: 60 mg/~0.4 mL (~0.4 mL); 90 mg/~0.4 mL (~0.4 mL); 120 mg/~0.5 mL (~0.5 mL) [packaging contains natural rubber/natural latex]

References

Caron P, Beckers A, Cullen DR, et al, "Efficacy of the New Long-Acting Formulation of Lanreotide (Lanreotide Autogel) in the Management of Acromegaly," *J Clin Endocrinol Metab,* 2002, 87 (1):99-104.

Rasmussen E, Eriksson B, Oberg K, et al, "Selective Effects of Somatostatin Analogs on Human Drug-Metabolizing Enzymes," *Clin Pharmacol Ther,* 1998, 64(2):150-9.

◆ **Lanreotide Acetate** see Lanreotide on page *681*

◆ **Lanvis® (Can)** see Thioguanine on page *1098*

Lapatinib (la PA ti nib)

Medication Safety Issues

Sound-alike/look-alike issues:

Lapatinib may be confused with dasatinib, erlotinib, imatinib

High alert medication: The Institute for Safe Medication Practices (ISMP) includes this medication among its list of drug classes which have a heightened risk of causing significant patient harm when used in error.

Related Information

Management of Chemotherapy-Induced Nausea and Vomiting *on page 1434*
Safe Handling of Hazardous Drugs *on page 1517*

U.S. Brand Names Tykerb®

Index Terms GW572016; Lapatinib Ditosylate

Generic Available No

Canadian Brand Names Tykerb®

Pharmacologic Category Antineoplastic Agent, Tyrosine Kinase Inhibitor; Epidermal Growth Factor Receptor (EGFR) Inhibitor

Use Treatment (in combination with capecitabine) of HER2/neu overexpressing advanced or metastatic breast cancer, in patients who have received prior therapy (with an anthracycline, a taxane, and trastuzumab)

Restrictions Lapatinib is available **only** at specialty pharmacies through a restricted-access program, Tykerb® CARES. Information is available at www.tykerbcares.com or 1-866-489-5372.

Pregnancy Risk Factor D

Lactation Excretion in breast milk unknown/not recommended

Labeled Contraindications There are no contraindications listed within the manufacturer's labeling.

Warnings/Precautions Hazardous agent - use appropriate precautions for handling and disposal.

Decreases in left ventricular ejection fraction (LVEF) have been reported; baseline and periodic LVEF evaluations are recommended; interrupt therapy or decrease dose with with decreased LVEF ≥ grade 2 or LVEF < LLN.

QT$_c$ prolongation has been observed; use caution in patients with a history of QT$_c$ prolongation or with medications known to prolong the QT interval; a baseline and periodic 12-lead ECG should be considered; correct electrolyte (potassium, calcium and magnesium) abnormalities prior to and during treatment. Use caution in patients with a history of or predisposed (prior treatment with anthracyclines, chest wall irradiation) to left ventricular dysfunction. Interstitial lung disease (ILD) and pneumonitis have been reported (with lapatinib monotherapy and with combination chemotherapy); discontinue therapy for grade 3 (or higher) pulmonary symptoms indicative of ILD or pneumonitis (eg, dyspnea, dry cough).

[U.S. Boxed Warning]: Hepatotoxicity (ALT or AST >3 times ULN and total bilirubin >1.5 times ULN) has been reported with lapatinib; may be severe and/or fatal. Onset of hepatotoxicity may occur within days to several months after treatment initiation; monitor; discontinue with severe changes in liver function; do not retreat. Use caution in patients with hepatic dysfunction. Dose reductions should be considered in patients with severe (Child-Pugh class C) hepatic impairment. Avoid concurrent use with strong CYP3A4 inhibitors or inducers; if concomitant therapy cannot be avoided, lapatinib dosage adjustments should be considered. May cause diarrhea (may be severe); manage with antidiarrheal agents; severe diarrhea may require hydration, electrolytes, or interruption of therapy. Safety and efficacy have not been established in children.

Adverse Reactions Percentages reported for combination chemotherapy.
>10%:
   Central nervous system: Fatigue (10% to 18%)
   Dermatologic: Palmar-plantar erythrodysesthesia (hand-and-foot syndrome) (53%; grade 3: 12%), rash (28%)
   Gastrointestinal: Diarrhea (65%; grade 3: 13%; grade 4: 1%), nausea (44%), vomiting (26%), abdominal pain (15%), mucosal inflammation (15%), stomatitis (14%), dyspepsia (11%)
   Hematologic: Anemia (56%; grade 3: <1%), neutropenia (22%; grade 3: 3%; grade 4: <1%), thrombocytopenia (18%; grade 3: <1%)
   Hepatic: AST increased (49%; grade 3: 2%; grade 4: <1%), total bilirubin increased (45%; grade 3: 4%), ALT increased (37%; grade 3: 2%)
   Neuromuscular & skeletal: Limb pain (12%), back pain (11%)
   Respiratory: Dyspnea (12%)
1% to 10%:
   Cardiovascular: LVEF decreased (grade 2: 2%; grade 3: <1%)
   Central nervous system: Insomnia (10%)
   Dermatologic: Dry skin (10%)
<1%, postmarketing, and/or case reports: Hepatotoxicity, interstitial lung disease, pneumonitis, Prinzmetal's angina, QT$_c$ prolongation

Drug Interactions
   Metabolism/Transport Effects Substrate of CYP2C8 (minor), 3A4 (major), P-glycoprotein (P-gp, ABCB1); **Inhibits** CYP2C8, 3A4
   Avoid Concomitant Use
      Avoid concomitant use of Lapatinib with any of the following: Artemether; Dabigatran Etexilate; Dronedarone; Everolimus; Lumefantrine; Nilotinib; Pimozide; QuiNINE; Silodosin; Tetrabenazine; Thioridazine; Tolvaptan; Topotecan; Ziprasidone
   Increased Effect/Toxicity
      Lapatinib may increase the levels/effects of: Colchicine; CYP2C8 Substrates (High risk); CYP3A4 Substrates; Dabigatran Etexilate; Dronedarone; Eplerenone; Everolimus; FentaNYL; P-Glycoprotein Substrates;

Pimecrolimus; Pimozide; QTc-Prolonging Agents; QuiNINE; Rivaroxaban; Salmeterol; Saxagliptin; Silodosin; Tetrabenazine; Thioridazine; Tolvaptan; Topotecan; Ziprasidone

The levels/effects of Lapatinib may be increased by: Alfuzosin; Artemether; Chloroquine; Ciprofloxacin; CYP3A4 Inhibitors (Moderate); CYP3A4 Inhibitors (Strong); Gadobutrol; Lumefantrine; Nilotinib; P-Glycoprotein Inhibitors; QuiNINE

Decreased Effect

The levels/effects of Lapatinib may be decreased by: CYP3A4 Inducers (Strong); Deferasirox; Herbs (CYP3A4 Inducers); P-Glycoprotein Inducers

Ethanol/Nutrition/Herb Interactions

Food: Systemic exposure of lapatinib is increased when administered with food (AUC three- to fourfold higher). Avoid grapefruit juice (may increase the levels/effects of lapatinib).

Herb/Nutraceutical: Avoid St John's wort (may increase metabolism and decrease lapatinib concentrations).

Storage/Stability Store at room temperature of 25°C (77°F); excursions permitted between 15°C and 30°C (59°F and 86°F).

Mechanism of Action Tyrosine kinase (dual kinase) inhibitor; inhibitor of EGFR (ErbB1) and HER2 (ErbB2) by reversibly binding to tyrosine kinase, blocking phosphorylation and activation of downstream second messengers (Erk1/2 and Akt), regulating cellular proliferation and survival in ErbB- and ErbB2-expressing tumors.

Pharmacodynamics/Kinetics

Absorption: Incomplete and variable

Protein binding: >99% to albumin and alpha$_1$-acid glycoprotein

Metabolism: Hepatic; extensive via CYP3A4 and 3A5, and to a lesser extent via CYP2C19 and 2C8 to oxidized metabolites

Half-life elimination: ~24 hours

Time to peak, plasma: 3-6 hours

Excretion: Feces (27% as unchanged drug; range 3% to 67%); urine (<2%)

Dosage Details concerning dosing in combination regimens should also be consulted. **Note:** Dose reductions are likely to be needed when lapatinib is administered concomitantly with a strong CYP3A4 inhibitor (an alternate medication for CYP3A4 enzyme inhibitors should be investigated first).

Oral: Adults: 1250 mg once daily (in combination with capecitabine)

Dosage adjustment for concomitant CYP3A4 inhibitors/inducers:

CYP3A4 inhibitors: Dose reductions are likely to be needed when lapatinib is administered concomitantly with a strong CYP3A4 inhibitor (an alternate medication for CYP3A4 enzyme inhibitors should be investigated first); in the event that lapatinib must be administered concomitantly with a potent enzyme inhibitor, consider reducing lapatinib to 500 mg once daily with careful monitoring. (When a strong CYP3A4 inhibitor is discontinued; allow ~1 week to elapse prior to adjusting the lapatinib dose upward.)

CYP3A4 inducers: Concomitant administration with CYP3A4 inducers may require increased lapatinib doses (alternatives to the enzyme-inducing agent should be utilized first); consider titrating gradually up to 4500 mg/day, with careful monitoring. (If the strong CYP3A4 enzyme inducer is discontinued, reduce the lapatinib dose to the indicated dose.)

Dosage adjustment for toxicity:

Cardiac toxicity: Discontinue treatment for decreased LVEF ≥ grade 2 or LVEF < LLN; may be restarted after 2 weeks at 1000 mg once daily if LVEF recovers to normal and patient is asymptomatic

Other toxicities: Withhold for any toxicity (other than cardiac) ≥ grade 2 until toxicity resolves to ≤ grade 1; reduce dosage to 1000 mg once daily for persistent toxicity

Dosage adjustment in renal impairment: Not studied in renal dysfunction, however, due to the minimal renal elimination (<2%), dosage adjustments for renal dysfunction may not be necessary.

Dosage adjustment in hepatic impairment: Severe hepatic impairment (Child-Pugh Class C): Consider a dose reduction to 750 mg once daily.

Combination Regimens

Breast cancer: Capecitabine + Lapatinib on page 1245

Administration Administer once daily, on an empty stomach, 1 hour before or 1 hour after a meal. Take at the same time each day; dividing doses is not recommended.

Monitoring Parameters LVEF (baseline and periodic), CBC with differential, liver function tests, including transaminases, bilirubin, and alkaline phosphatase (baseline and every 4-6 weeks during treatment); electrolytes including calcium, potassium, magnesium; monitor for fluid retention; ECG monitoring if at risk for QT_c prolongation; symptoms of ILD

Dietary Considerations Take on an empty stomach, 1 hour before or 1 hour after a meal. (**Note:** For combination with capecitabine treatment, capecitabine should be taken with food, or within 30 minutes after a meal.)

Additional Information Oncology Comment: The National Comprehensive Cancer Network (NCCN) breast cancer guidelines list lapatinib (in combination with capecitabine) as an option for the treatment of HER2-positive breast cancer in patients who are refractory to anthracycline, taxane, and trastuzumab treatment. In a randomized phase III study (Geyer, 2006) of lapatinib plus capecitabine versus capecitabine alone in HER2-positive advanced breast cancer, the addition of lapatinib was associated with a 51% reduction in the risk of disease progression in heavily pretreated patients. Lapatinib shows activity in HER2-positive metastatic breast cancer that has progressed after trastuzumab treatment.

Emetic Potential Low (10% to 30%)

Dosage Forms Excipient information presented when available (limited, particularly for generics); consult specific product labeling.

Tablet:

Tykerb®: 250 mg

References

Burris HA 3rd, Hurwitz HI, Dees EC, et al, "Phase I Safety, Pharmacokinetics, and Clinical Activity Study of Lapatinib (GW572016), a Reversible Dual Inhibitor of Epidermal Growth Factor Receptor Tyrosine Kinases, in Heavily Pretreated Patients with Metastatic Carcinomas," *J Clin Oncol*, 2005, 23(23):5305-13.

Geyer CE, Forster J, Lindquist D, et al "Lapatinib Plus Capecitabine for HER2-Positive Advanced Breast Cancer," *N Engl J Med*, 2006, 355(26):2733-43.

National Comprehensive Cancer Network (NCCN), "Clinical Practice Guidelines in Oncology™: Breast Cancer Version 2.2008." Available at http://www.nccn.org/professionals/physician_gls/PDF/breast.pdf

Spector NL, Xia W, Burris H 3rd, et al, "Study of the Biologic Effects of Lapatinib, a Reversible Inhibitor of ErbB1 and ErbB2 Tyrosine Kinases, on Tumor Growth and Survival Pathways in Patients with Advanced Malignancies," *J Clin Oncol*, 2005, 23(11):2502-12.

♦ **Lapatinib Ditosylate** *see* Lapatinib *on page* 684

♦ **Largactil® (Can)** *see* ChlorproMAZINE *on page* 220

♦ **L-asparaginase** *see* Asparaginase *on page* 111

♦ **L-asparaginase with Polyethylene Glycol** *see* Pegaspargase *on page* 925

♦ **LDP-341** *see* Bortezomib *on page* 155

Lenalidomide (le na LID oh mide)

Medication Safety Issues

Sound-alike/look-alike issues:
Lenalidomide may be confused with thalidomide

High alert medication: The Institute for Safe Medication Practices (ISMP) includes this medication among its list of drug classes which have a heightened risk of causing significant patient harm when used in error.

Related Information

Safe Handling of Hazardous Drugs on page 1517

U.S. Brand Names Revlimid®

Index Terms CC-5013; IMid-1

Generic Available No

Canadian Brand Names Revlimid®

Pharmacologic Category Angiogenesis Inhibitor; Antineoplastic Agent; Immunomodulator, Systemic

Use Treatment of myelodysplastic syndrome (MDS) in patients with deletion 5q (del 5q) cytogenetic abnormality with transfusion-dependent anemia; treatment of multiple myeloma

Unlabeled/Investigational Use Treatment of mantle cell lymphoma; systemic amyloidosis (light chain); lower risk myelodysplastic syndrome (MDS) in transfusion-dependent patients without deletion 5q (del 5q); relapsed or refractory chronic lymphocytic leukemia (CLL)

Restrictions Lenalidomide is approved for marketing in the U.S. only under a Food and Drug Administration (FDA) approved, restricted distribution program called RevAssist^{SM} (www.REVLIMID.com or 1-888-423-5436). In Canada, distribution is restricted through RevAid^{SM} (www.RevAid.ca or 1-888-738-2431). Physicians, pharmacies, and patients must be registered; a maximum 28-day supply may be dispensed; a new prescription is required each time it is filled; pregnancy testing is required for females of childbearing potential.

Pregnancy Risk Factor X

Lactation Excretion in breast milk unknown/not recommended

Labeled Contraindications Hypersensitivity to lenalidomide or any component of the formulation; pregnancy or women capable of becoming pregnant

Canadian labeling: Additional contraindications (not in U.S. labeling): Platelet count <50,000/mm³; hypersensitivity to thalidomide; breast-feeding women

Warnings/Precautions Hazardous agent - use appropriate precautions for handling and disposal. **[U.S. Boxed Warning]: Hematologic toxicity (neutropenia and thrombocytopenia) occurs in a majority of patients (grade 3/4: 80%)** and may require dose reductions and/or delays; the use of blood product support and/or growth factors may be needed. **[U.S. Boxed Warning]: Lenalidomide has been associated with a significant increase in risk for thrombosis and embolism in multiple myeloma patients treated with combination therapy. Deep vein thrombosis (DVT) and pulmonary embolism (PE) have occurred;** monitor for signs and symptoms of thromboembolism (shortness of breath, chest pain, or arm or leg swelling) and seek prompt medical attention with development of these symptoms. Use caution in renal impairment; may experience an increased rate of toxicities. The NCCN multiple myeloma guidelines (v2.2009) recommend anticoagulant prophylaxis when used in combination with dexamethasone. Anticoagulant prophylaxis should be individualized and selected based on the venous thromboembolism risk of the combination treatment regimen, using the safest and easiest to administer (Palumbo, 2008).

Angioedema, Stevens-Johnson syndrome (SJS), and toxic epidermal necrolysis (TEN) have been reported; may be fatal. Consider interrupting or discontinuing treatment with grade 2 or 3 skin rash; discontinue and do not reinitiate treatment with grade 4 rash, exfoliative or bullous rash, or for suspected SJS or TEN. Patients with a history of grade 4 rash with thalidomide should not receive lenalidomide. Discontinue treatment with angioedema. Use caution in renal impairment; may experience an increased rate of toxicities (due to reduced clearance and increased half-life); initial dosage adjustments are recommended for moderate-to-severe and dialysis-dependent renal impairment. Patients with a high tumor burden may be at risk for tumor lysis syndrome.

[U.S. Boxed Warning]: Lenalidomide is an analogue of thalidomide (a human teratogen) and could potentially cause birth defects in humans; avoid pregnancy while taking lenalidomide. Distribution is restricted; physicians, pharmacists, and patients must be registered with the RevAssist^SM program. Patients should be advised not to donate blood during therapy and for 4 weeks following completion of therapy. May cause dizziness or fatigue; caution patients about performing tasks which require mental alertness (eg, operating machinery or driving). Formulation contains lactose; avoid use in patients with Lapp lactase deficiency, glucose-galactose malabsorption, or glucose intolerance. Lenalidomide should only be prescribed to patients (male and female) who can understand and comply with the conditions of the RevAssist^SM program. Safety and effectiveness in children <18 years of age have not been established (if used in patients between 12-18 years of age, the parent or legal guardian must agree to ensure compliance with the RevAssist^SM program).

Adverse Reactions

>10%:

Cardiovascular: Peripheral edema (8% to 21%)

Central nervous system: Fatigue (31% to 38%), insomnia (10% to 32%), fever (21% to 23%), dizziness (20% to 21%), headache (20%)

Dermatologic: Pruritus (42%), rash (16% to 36%; grades 3/4: 7%), dry skin (14%)

Endocrine & metabolic: Hyperglycemia (15%), hypokalemia (11%)

Gastrointestinal: Diarrhea (29% to 49%), constipation (24% to 39%), nausea (22% to 24%), weight loss (18%), dyspepsia (14%), anorexia (10% to 14%), taste perversion (6% to 13%), abdominal pain (8% to 12%)

Genitourinary: Urinary tract infection (11%)

Hematologic: Thrombocytopenia (17% to 62%; grades 3/4: 10% to 50%; onset [MDS]: 28 days [range 8-290 days]; recovery [MDS]: 22 days [range: 5-224 days]), neutropenia (28% to 59%; grades 3/4: 21% to 53%; onset [MDS]: 42 days [range 14-411 days]; recovery [MDS]: 17 days [range: 2-170 days]), anemia (12% to 24%; grades 3/4: 6% to 8%); myelosuppression is dose-dependent and reversible with treatment interruption and/or dose reduction

Neuromuscular & skeletal: Muscle cramp (18% to 30%), weakness (15% to 23%), arthralgia (10% to 22%), back pain (15% to 21%), tremor (20%), paresthesia (12%), limb pain (11%)

Ocular: Blurred vision (15%)

Respiratory: Nasopharyngitis (23%), cough (15% to 20%), dyspnea (7% to 20%), pharyngitis (16%), epistaxis (15%), upper respiratory infection (14% to 15%), pneumonia (11% to 12%)

◄ 1% to 10%:

Cardiovascular: Edema (10%), deep vein thrombosis (≤8%; grades 3/4: 7%), hypertension (6%), chest pain (5%), palpitation (5%), atrial fibrillation (grades 3/4: 3%), syncope (grade 3: 1%)

Central nervous system: Hypoesthesia (7%), pain (7%), depression (5%)

Dermatologic: Bruising (5% to 8%), cellulitis (5%), erythema (5%)

Endocrine & metabolic: Hypothyroidism (7%), hypomagnesemia (6%), hypocalcemia (grades 3/4: 4%)

Gastrointestinal: Vomiting (10%), xerostomia (7%), loose stools (6%)

Genitourinary: Dysuria (7%)

Hematologic: Leukopenia (8%; grade 3/4: 4% to 5%), febrile neutropenia (5%; grades 3/4: 4%), granulocytopenia (grades 3/4: 2%), lymphopenia (grade 3: 2%), pancytopenia (grades 3/4: 2%)

Hepatic: ALT increased (8%)

Neuromuscular & skeletal: Myalgia (9%), rigors (6%), neuropathy (peripheral 5%)

Respiratory: Sinusitis (8%), rhinitis (7%), bronchitis (6%), pulmonary embolism (≤3%; grades 3/4: 1% to 2%), respiratory distress (grades 3/4: 2%), hypoxia (grades 3/4: 1%), pleural effusion (grades 3/4: 1%), pneumonitis (grades 3/4: 1%), pulmonary hypertension (grades 3/4: 1%)

Miscellaneous: Night sweats (8%), diaphoresis increased (7%), sepsis (grades 3/4: 3%)

<1%, postmarketing, and/or case reports (limited to important or life-threatening): Acute febrile neutrophilic dermatosis, acute leukemia, acute myeloid leukemia (AML), adrenal insufficiency, angina, angioedema, aortic disorder, aphasia, atrial flutter, azotemia, bacteremia, Basedow's disease, biliary obstruction, blindness, bone marrow depression, bradycardia, brain edema, C-reactive protein decreased, cardiac arrest, cardiac failure, cardiogenic shock, cardiomyopathy, cardiopulmonary arrest, cellulitis, cerebellar infarction, cerebral infarction, cerebrovascular accident, CHF, cholecystitis, chondrocalcinosis, chronic obstructive airway disease, circulatory collapse, coagulopathy, colonic polyp, dehydration, delirium, delusion, diabetes mellitus, diabetic ketoacidosis, diverticulitis, dysphagia, encephalitis, erythema multiforme, Fanconi syndrome, gait abnormal, gastritis, gastroenteritis, gastrointestinal hemorrhage, gout, hematuria, hemoglobin decreased, hemolysis, hemolytic anemia, hemorrhage, hepatic failure, hepatitis, herpesvirus infection, hyperbilirubinemia, hypernatremia, hypersensitivity, hypoglycemia, hypotension, infection, INR increased, interstitial lung disease, intestinal perforation, intracranial hemorrhage, intracranial venous sinus thrombosis, irritable bowel syndrome, ischemia, ischemic colitis, leukoencephalopathy, liver failure, liver function tests abnormal, lung cancer, lung infiltration, lymphoma, melena, MI, migraine, myocardial ischemia, myopathy, neutropenic sepsis, orthostatic hypotension, pancreatitis, performance status decreased, peripheral ischemia, phlebitis, post procedural hemorrhage, pseudomembraneous colitis, pulmonary edema, rectal hemorrhage, refractory anemia, renal calculus, renal failure, renal mass, renal tubular necrosis, respiratory failure, septic shock, serum creatinine increased, skin desquamation, small bowel obstruction, somnolence, spinal cord compression, splenic infarction, Stevens-Johnson syndrome, stomatitis, subarachnoid hemorrhage, supraventricular arrhythmia, tachyarrhythmia, thrombophlebitis, thrombosis, toxic epidermal necrolysis, toxic hepatitis, transient ischemic attack, troponin I increased, urinary retention, urosepsis, urticaria, ventricular dysfunction, wheezing

Drug Interactions

Avoid Concomitant Use

Avoid concomitant use of Lenalidomide with any of the following: Abatacept; Anakinra; Canakinumab; Certolizumab Pegol; Natalizumab; Rilonacept; Vaccines (Live)

Increased Effect/Toxicity

Lenalidomide may increase the levels/effects of: Abatacept; Anakinra; Canakinumab; Certolizumab Pegol; Leflunomide; Natalizumab; Rilonacept; Vaccines (Live)

The levels/effects of Lenalidomide may be increased by: Dexamethasone; Trastuzumab

Decreased Effect

Lenalidomide may decrease the levels/effects of: Vaccines (Inactivated); Vaccines (Live)

The levels/effects of Lenalidomide may be decreased by: Echinacea

Ethanol/Nutrition/Herb Interactions Herb/Nutraceutical: Avoid echinacea (has immunostimulant properties; consider therapy modifications).

Storage/Stability Store at controlled room temperature of 25°C (77°F); excursions permitted to 15°C and 30°C (59°F and 86°F).

Mechanism of Action Immunomodulatory, antiangiogenic, and antineoplastic characteristics via multiple mechanisms. Selectively inhibits secretion of proinflammatory cytokines (potent inhibitor of tumor necrosis factor-alpha secretion); enhances cell-mediated immunity by stimulating proliferation of anti-CD3 stimulated T cells (resulting in increased IL-2 and interferon gamma secretion); inhibits trophic signals to angiogenic factors in cells. Inhibits the growth of myeloma cells by inducing cell cycle arrest and cell death.

Pharmacodynamics/Kinetics

Absorption: Rapid

Protein binding: ~30%

Half-life elimination: ~3 hours; moderate-to-severe renal impairment: ~9 hours; hemodialysis patients: ~13.5 hours

Time, to peak, plasma: Healthy volunteers: ~0.6-1.5 hours; Myeloma patients: 0.5-4 hours

Excretion: Urine (~67% as unchanged drug)

Hemodialysis effect: ~40% of a dose is removed in a single dialysis session

Dosage Oral:

Adults:

Multiple myeloma: 25 mg once daily for 21 days of a 28-day treatment cycle (in combination with dexamethasone)

Myelodysplastic syndrome (MDS) with deletion 5q: 10 mg once daily

Myelodysplastic syndrome (MDS), lower risk, without deletion 5q (unlabeled use): 10 mg once daily (Raza, 2008)

Elderly: Refer to adult dosing; due to the potential for decreased renal function in the elderly, select dose carefully and closely monitor renal function

Dosage adjustment in renal impairment: Hemodialysis: ~40% of a dose is removed in a single dialysis session.

◀ *Recommended adjustment in the FDA-approved labeling:*
  MDS:
   Cl_{cr} ≥60 mL/minute: No adjustment required
   Cl_{cr} 30-59 mL/minute: 5 mg once daily
   Cl_{cr} <30 mL/minute (nondialysis dependent): 5 mg every 48 hours
   Cl_{cr} <30 mL/minute (dialysis dependent): 5 mg 3 times/week (administer following each dialysis)
  Multiple myeloma:
   Cl_{cr} ≥60 mL/minute: No adjustment required
   Cl_{cr} 30-59 mL/minute: 10 mg once daily
   Cl_{cr} <30 mL/minute (nondialysis dependent): 15 mg every 48 hours
   Cl_{cr} <30 mL/minute (dialysis dependent): 5 mg once daily (administer after dialysis on dialysis days)
Recommended adjustment in Canadian labeling:
  MDS:
   Cl_{cr} ≥50 mL/minute: No adjustment required
   Cl_{cr} 30-49 mL/minute: 5 mg once daily
   Cl_{cr} <30 mL/minute (nondialysis dependent): 5 mg every 48 hours
   Cl_{cr} <30 mL/minute (dialysis dependent): 5 mg 3 times/week (administer following each dialysis)
  Multiple myeloma:
   Cl_{cr} ≥50 mL/minute: No adjustment required
   Cl_{cr} 30-49 mL/minute: 10 mg once daily
   Cl_{cr} <30 mL/minute (nondialysis dependent): 15 mg every 48 hours
   Cl_{cr} <30 mL/minute (dialysis dependent): 5 mg once daily (administer following each dialysis)

Dosage adjustment for NONHEMATOLOGIC toxicities:
  Dermatologic toxicities:
   Skin rash, grade 2 or 3: Consider interrupting or discontinuing treatment
   Angioedema, grade 4 rash, exfoliative or bullous rash, or suspected Stevens-Johnson syndrome or toxic epidermal necrolysis: Discontinue treatment
  Other toxicities in multiple myeloma: For additional treatment-related grade 3/4 toxicities, hold treatment and restart at next lower dose level when toxicity has resolved to ≤ grade 2.

Dosage adjustment for HEMATOLOGIC toxicities:
Adjustment for thrombocytopenia in MDS:
  Thrombocytopenia developing within 4 weeks of beginning treatment at 10 mg/day:
   Baseline platelets ≥100,000/mm³:
    If platelets <50,000/mm³: Hold treatment
    When platelets return to ≥50,000/mm³: Resume treatment at 5 mg/day
   Baseline platelets <100,000/mm³:
    If platelets fall to 50% of baseline: Hold treatment
    If baseline ≥60,000/mm³ and platelet level returns to ≥50,000/mm³: Resume at 5 mg/day
    If baseline <60,000/mm³ and platelet level returns to ≥30,000/mm³: Resume at 5 mg/day
  Thrombocytopenia developing after 4 weeks of beginning treatment at 10 mg/day:
   Platelets <30,000/mm³ **or** <50,000/mm³ with platelet transfusions: Hold treatment
   Platelets ≥30,000/mm³ (without hemostatic failure): Resume at 5 mg/day

Thrombocytopenia developing with treatment at 5 mg/day:
Platelets <30,000/mm³ **or** <50,000/mm³ with platelet transfusions: Hold treatment
Platelets ≥30,000/mm³ (without hemostatic failure): Resume at 5 mg every other day

Adjustment for neutropenia in MDS:

Neutropenia developing within 4 weeks of beginning treatment at 10 mg/day:
For baseline absolute neutrophil count (ANC) ≥1000/mm³:
ANC <750/mm³: Hold treatment
When ANC returns to ≥1000/mm³: Resume at 5 mg/day
For baseline absolute neutrophil count (ANC) <1000/mm³:
ANC <500/mm³: Hold treatment
When ANC returns to ≥500/mm³: Resume at 5 mg/day
Neutropenia developing after 4 weeks of beginning treatment at 10 mg/day:
ANC <500/mm³ for ≥7 days or associated with fever: Hold treatment
When ≥500/mm³: Resume at 5 mg/day
Neutropenia developing with treatment at 5 mg/day:
ANC <500/mm³ for ≥7 days or associated with fever: Hold treatment
When ≥500/mm³: Resume at 5 mg every other day

Adjustment for thrombocytopenia in multiple myeloma:

Platelets <30,000/mm³: Hold treatment, check CBC weekly
When platelets ≥30,000/mm³: Resume at 15 mg daily
Additional occurrence of platelets <30,000/mm³: Hold treatment
When platelets ≥30,000/mm³: Resume treatment at 5 mg below previous dose; do not dose below 5 mg daily

Adjustment for neutropenia in multiple myeloma:

ANC <1000/mm³: Hold treatment, add G-CSF, check CBC weekly
When ≥1000/mm³ (with neutropenia as only toxicity): Resume at 25 mg/day
When ≥1000/mm³ (with additional toxicities): Resume at 15 mg/day
Additional occurrence of ANC <1000/mm³: Hold treatment
When ≥1000/mm³: Resume treatment at 5 mg below previous dose; do not dose below 5 mg daily.

Combination Regimens

Multiple myeloma:
Lenalidomide-Dexamethasone on page 1362
Lenalidomide-Dexamethasone (Low Dose) on page 1362

Administration Administer with water. Swallow capsule whole; do not break, open, or chew.

Monitoring Parameters CBC with differential (MDS: weekly for first 8 weeks; multiple myeloma: every 2 weeks for the first 3 months), then monthly thereafter; serum creatinine, liver function tests, thyroid function tests; ECG when clinically indicated; monitor for signs and symptoms of thromboembolism or tumor lysis syndrome

Women of childbearing potential: Pregnancy test 10-14 days **and** 24 hours prior to initiating therapy, weekly during the first 4 weeks of treatment, then every 2-4 weeks through 4 weeks after therapy discontinued

Additional Information Pregnancy tests are required prior to beginning therapy, throughout treatment and during therapy interruptions for all women of childbearing age. The pregnancy test must be verified by the prescriber and the pharmacist prior to dispensing. Effective contraception with at least two reliable forms of contraception (IUD, hormonal contraception, tubal ligation or partner's vasectomy plus latex condom, diaphragm, or cervical cap) should be used for 4 weeks prior to beginning therapy, during therapy, and for 4 weeks

◀ following discontinuance of therapy. Women who have undergone a hysterectomy or have been postmenopausal for at least 24 consecutive months are the only exception. Do not prescribe, administer, or dispense to women of childbearing age or males who may have intercourse with women of childbearing age unless both female and male are capable of complying with contraceptive measures. Even males who have undergone vasectomy must acknowledge these risks in writing, and must use a latex condom during any sexual contact with women of childbearing age. Oral and written warnings concerning contraception and the hazards of thalidomide must be conveyed to females and males and they must acknowledge their understanding in writing. Parents or guardians must consent and sign acknowledgment for patients 12-18 years of age following therapy. A maximum 28-day supply should be dispensed.

Emetic Potential Very low (<10%)

Dosage Forms Excipient information presented when available (limited, particularly for generics); consult specific product labeling.

Capsule:
Revlimid®: 5 mg, 10 mg, 15 mg, 25 mg

References

Barlogie B, Shaughnessy J, Tricot G, et al, "Treatment of Multiple Myeloma," *Blood*, 2004, 103 (1):20-32.

Chanan-Khan A, Miller KC, Musial L, et al, "Clinical Efficacy of Lenalidomide in Patients With Relapsed or Refractory Chronic Lymphocytic Leukemia: Results of a Phase II Study," *J Clin Oncol*, 2006, 24(34):5343-9.

Chen N, Lau H, Kong L, et al, "Pharmacokinetics of Lenalidomide in Subjects With Various Degrees of Renal Function," *J Clin Oncol*, 2007, 25(18S):2520 [abstract from ASCO Annual Meeting Proceedings, Part I]

Dimopoulos M, Spencer A, Attal M, et al, "Lenalidomide Plus Dexamethasone for Relapsed or Refractory Multiple Myeloma," *N Engl J Med*, 2007, 357(21):2123-32.

Ferrajoli A, Lee BN, Schlette EJ, et al, "Lenalidomide Induces Complete and Partial Remissions in Patients With Relapsed and Refractory Chronic Lymphocytic Leukemia," *Blood*, 2008, 111(11):5291-7.

Kyle RA and Rajkumar SV, "Multiple Myeloma," *N Engl J Med*, 2004, 351(18):1860-73.

List A, Dewald G, Bennett J, et al, "Lenalidomide in Myelodysplastic Syndrome With Chromosome 5q Deletion," *N Engl J Med*, 2006, 355(14):1456-65.

National Comprehensive Cancer Network® (NCCN), "Clinical Practice Guidelines in Oncology™: Multiple Myeloma," Version 2.2009. Available at http://www.nccn.org/professionals/physician_gls/PDF/myeloma.pdf.

National Comprehensive Cancer Network® (NCCN), "Clinical Practice Guidelines in Oncology™: Myelodysplastic Syndromes," Version 2.2009. Available at http://www.nccn.org/professionals/physician_gls/PDF/mds.pdf

National Comprehensive Cancer Network® (NCCN), "Clinical Practice Guidelines in Oncology™: Non-Hodgkin's Lymphomas," Version 1.2009. Available at http://www.nccn.org/professionals/physician_gls/PDF/nhl.pdf

Palumbo A, Rajkumar SV, Dimopoulos MA, et al, "Prevention of Thalidomide- and Lenalidomide-Associated Thrombosis in Myeloma," *Leukemia*, 2008, 22(2): 414-23.

Rajkumar SV, Hayman SR, Lacy MQ, et al, "Combination Therapy With Lenalidomide Plus Dexamethasone (Rev/Dex) for Newly Diagnosed Myeloma," *Blood*, 2005, 106(13):4050-3.

Raza A, Reeves JA, Feldman JA, et al, "Phase 2 Study of Lenalidomide in Transfusion-Dependent, Low-Risk, and Intermediate-1 Risk Myelodysplastic Syndromes With Karyotypes Other than Deletion 5q," *Blood*, 2008, 111(1):86-93.

Richardson PG, Schlossman RL, Weller E, et al, "Immunomodulatory Drug CC-5013 Overcomes Drug Resistance and Is Well Tolerated in Patients With Relapsed Multiple Myeloma," *Blood*, 2002, 100(9):3063-7.

Weber DM, Chen C, Niesvizky R, et al, "Lenalidomide Plus Dexamethasone for Relapsed Multiple Myeloma in North America," *N Engl J Med*, 2007, 357(21):2133-42.

Letrozole (LET roe zole)

Medication Safety Issues

Sound-alike/look-alike issues:
Femara® may be confused with Famvir®, femhrt®, Provera®

Letrozole may be confused with anastrozole

Related Information

Safe Handling of Hazardous Drugs *on page 1517*

U.S. Brand Names Femara®

Index Terms CGS-20267

Generic Available No

Canadian Brand Names Femara®

Pharmacologic Category Antineoplastic Agent, Aromatase Inhibitor

Use For use in postmenopausal women in the adjuvant treatment of hormone receptor positive early breast cancer, extended adjuvant treatment of early breast cancer after 5 years of tamoxifen, advanced breast cancer with disease progression following antiestrogen therapy, hormone receptor positive or hormone receptor unknown, locally-advanced, or metastatic breast cancer

Unlabeled/Investigational Use Treatment of ovarian (epithelial) cancer, endometrial cancer

Pregnancy Risk Factor D

Lactation Excretion in breast milk unknown/use caution

Labeled Contraindications Hypersensitivity to letrozole or any component of the formulation; women of premenopausal endocrine status

Warnings/Precautions Hazardous agent - use appropriate precautions for handling and disposal. Use caution with hepatic impairment; dose adjustment may be required. Increases in transaminases ≥5 times the upper limit of normal and in bilirubin ≥1.5 times the upper limit of normal were most often, but not always, associated with metastatic liver disease. May cause dizziness, fatigue, and somnolence; patients should be cautioned before performing tasks which require mental alertness (eg, operating machinery or driving). May increase total serum cholesterol. May cause decreases in bone mineral density. Safety and efficacy have not been established in children.

Adverse Reactions

>10%:

Cardiovascular: Edema (7% to 18%)

Central nervous system: Headache (4% to 20%), dizziness (2% to 14%), fatigue (6% to 13%)

Endocrine & metabolic: Hot flashes (5% to 50%), hypercholesterolemia (3% to 16%)

Gastrointestinal: Nausea (9% to 17%), constipation (2% to 11%), weight gain (2% to 11%)

Neuromuscular & skeletal: Weakness (4% to 34%), bone pain (22%), arthralgia (8% to 22%), arthritis (7% to 21%), back pain (5% to 18%)

Respiratory: Dyspnea (6% to 18%), cough (5% to 13%)

Miscellaneous: Diaphoresis (≤24%), night sweats (14%)

2% to 10%:

Cardiovascular: Chest pain (3% to 8%), hypertension (5% to 8%), peripheral edema (5%)

Central nervous system: Insomnia (6% to 7%), pain (5%), somnolence (2% to 3%), depression (<5%), anxiety (<5%), vertigo (<5%)

Dermatologic: Rash (4% to 5%), alopecia (<5%), pruritus (1% to 2%)

Endocrine & metabolic: Breast pain (7%), hypercalcemia (<5%)

Gastrointestinal: Diarrhea (5% to 8%), vomiting (3% to 7%), weight loss (7%), abdominal pain (5% to 6%), anorexia (3% to 5%), dyspepsia (3% to 4%)

Genitourinary: Urinary tract infection (6%), vaginal bleeding (5%), vaginal dryness (5%), vaginal hemorrhage (5%), vaginal irritation (4%)

Hepatic: Transaminases increased (≤3%)

Neuromuscular & skeletal: Limb pain (10%), myalgia (6% to 7%), bone fractures (≤6%), bone mineral density decreased/osteoporosis (2% to 7%)

Renal: Renal disorder (5%)

Respiratory: Pleural effusion (<5%)

Miscellaneous: Infection (7%), flu (6%), viral infection (5% to 6%)

<2%, postmarketing, and/or case reports: Anaphylactic reaction, angina, angioedema, appetite increase, arterial thrombosis, bilirubin increased, blurred vision, cardiac ischemia, cardiac failure, cataract, coronary artery disease, dry skin, dysesthesia, endometrial cancer, endometrial proliferation disorder, erythema multiforme, eye irritation, fever, hemiparesis, hemorrhagic stroke, hepatitis, hypoesthesia, irritability, leukopenia, lymphopenia, MI, memory impairment, nervousness, palpitations, paresthesia, portal vein thrombosis, pulmonary embolism, secondary malignancy, stomatitis, tachycardia, taste disturbance, thirst, thrombocytopenia, thrombophlebitis, thromboembolic event, thrombotic stroke, toxic epidermal necrolysis, transient ischemic attack, urinary frequency increased, urticaria, vaginal discharge, venous thrombosis, xerostomia

Drug Interactions

Metabolism/Transport Effects Substrate (minor) of CYP2A6, 3A4; **Inhibits** CYP2A6 (strong), 2C19 (weak)

Avoid Concomitant Use There are no known interactions where it is recommended to avoid concomitant use.

Increased Effect/Toxicity

Letrozole may increase the levels/effects of: CYP2A6 Substrates

Decreased Effect

The levels/effects of Letrozole may be decreased by: Tamoxifen

Storage/Stability Store at room temperature of 25°C (77°F); excursions permitted to 15°C to 30°C (59°F to 86°F).

Mechanism of Action Nonsteroidal competitive inhibitor of the aromatase enzyme system which binds to the heme group of aromatase, a cytochrome P450 enzyme which catalyzes conversion of androgens to estrogens (specifically, androstenedione to estrone and testosterone to estradiol). This leads to inhibition of the enzyme and a significant reduction in plasma estrogen (estrone, estradiol and estrone sulfate) levels. Does not affect synthesis of adrenal or thyroid hormones, aldosterone, or androgens.

Pharmacodynamics/Kinetics

Absorption: Rapid and well absorbed; not affected by food

Distribution: V_d: ~1.9 L/kg

Protein binding, plasma: Weak

Metabolism: Hepatic via CYP3A4 and 2A6 to an inactive carbinol metabolite

Half-life elimination: Terminal: ~2 days

Time to steady state, plasma: 2-6 weeks

Excretion: Urine (90%; 6% as unchanged drug, 75% as glucuronide carbinol metabolite, 9% as unidentified metabolites)

Dosage Oral: Adults: Females:

Breast cancer: 2.5 mg once daily

Ovarian (epithelial) cancer (unlabeled use): 2.5 mg once daily (Ramirez, 2008)

Elderly: No dosage adjustments required

Dosage adjustment in renal impairment: No dosage adjustment is required in patients with renal impairment if Cl_{cr} ≥10 mL/minute

Dosage adjustment in hepatic impairment:
Mild-to-moderate impairment (Child-Pugh class A and B): No adjustment recommended

Severe impairment (Child-Pugh class C) and cirrhosis: 2.5 mg every other day

Administration Administer with or without food.

Monitoring Parameters Monitor periodically during therapy: Complete blood counts, thyroid function tests; serum electrolytes, cholesterol, transaminases, and creatinine; blood pressure; bone density

Dietary Considerations May be taken without regard to meals. Calcium and vitamin D supplementation are recommended.

Dosage Forms Excipient information presented when available (limited, particularly for generics); consult specific product labeling.
Tablet:
Femara®: 2.5 mg

References

Buzdar AU, Robertson JF, Eiermann W, et al, "An Overview of the Pharmacology and Pharmacokinetics of the Newer Generation Aromatase Inhibitors Anastrozole, Letrozole, and Exemestane," Cancer, 2002, 95(9):2006-16.

Coates AS, Keshaviah A, Thurlimann B, et al, "Five Years of Letrozole Compared With Tamoxifen as Initial Adjuvant Therapy for Postmenopausal Women With Endocrine-Responsive Early Breast Cancer: Update of Study BIG 1-98," J Clin Oncol, 2007, 25(5):486-92.

National Comprehensive Cancer Network (NCCN)®, "Clinical Practice Guidelines in Oncology™: Breast Cancer," Version 1.2009. Available at http://www.nccn.org/professionals/physician_gls/PDF/breast.pdf

National Comprehensive Cancer Network (NCCN)®, "Clinical Practice Guidelines in Oncology™: Ovarian Cancer," Version 2.2009. Available at http://www.nccn.org/professionals/physician_gls/PDF/ovarian.pdf

National Comprehensive Cancer Network (NCCN)®, "Clinical Practice Guidelines in Oncology™: Uterine Neoplasms," Version 2.2009. Available at http://www.nccn.org/professionals/physician_gls/PDF/uterine.pdf

Ramirez PT, Schmeler EM, Milam MR, et al, "Efficacy of Letrozole in the Treatment of Recurrent Platinum- and Taxane-Resistant High-Grade Cancer of the Ovary or Peritoneum," Gynecol Oncol, 2008, 110(1):56-9.

Smith IE and Dowsett M, "Aromatase Inhibitors in Breast Cancer," N Engl J Med, 2003, 348 (24):2431-42.

Thurlimann B, Keshaviah A, Coates AS, et al, "A Comparison of Letrozole and Tamoxifen in Postmenopausal Women with Early Breast Cancer," N Engl J Med, 2005, 353(26):2747-57.

Winer EP, Hudis C, Burstein HJ, et al, "American Society of Clinical Oncology Technology Assessment on the Use of Aromatase Inhibitors as Adjuvant Therapy for Postmenopausal Women With Hormone Receptor-Positive Breast Cancer: Status Report 2004," J Clin Oncol, 2005, 23(3):619-29.

Leucovorin Calcium (loo koe VOR in KAL see um)

Medication Safety Issues

Sound-alike/look-alike issues:
Leucovorin may be confused with Leukeran®, Leukine®, LEVOleucovorin
Folinic acid may be confused with folic acid
Folinic acid is an error prone synonym and should not be used

Index Terms 5-Formyl Tetrahydrofolate; Calcium Leucovorin; Citrovorum Factor; Folinic Acid (error prone synonym)

Generic Available Yes

Pharmacologic Category Antidote; Chemotherapy Modulating Agent; Rescue Agent (Chemotherapy); Vitamin, Water Soluble

Use Antidote for folic acid antagonists (methotrexate, trimethoprim, pyrimethamine) and rescue therapy following high-dose methotrexate; in combination with fluorouracil in the treatment of colon cancer; treatment of megaloblastic anemias when folate is deficient as in infancy, sprue, pregnancy, and nutritional deficiency when oral folate therapy is not possible

Pregnancy Risk Factor C

Lactation Excretion in breast milk unknown/use caution

Labeled Contraindications Pernicious anemia or vitamin B_{12}-deficient megaloblastic anemias

Warnings/Precautions When used for the treatment of accidental folic acid antagonist overdose, administer as soon as possible. When used for methotrexate rescue therapy, methotrexate serum concentrations should be monitored to determine dose and duration of leucovorin therapy. Dose may need increased or administration prolonged in situations where methotrexate excretion may be delayed (eg, ascites, pleural effusion, renal insufficiency, inadequate hydration). Combination of leucovorin and sulfamethoxazole-trimethoprim for the acute treatment of PCP in patients with HIV infection has been reported to cause increased rates of treatment failure. Leucovorin may increase the toxicity of 5-fluorouracil; dose of 5-fluorouracil may need decreased.

Powder for injection: When doses >10 mg/m^2 are required, reconstitute using sterile water for injection, not a solution containing benzyl alcohol.

Injection: Due to calcium content, do not administer I.V. solutions at a rate >160 mg/ minute. Not intended for intrathecal use.

Adverse Reactions Frequency not defined. Toxicities (especially gastro-intestinal toxicity) of fluorouracil is higher when used in combination with leucovorin.

Dermatologic: Rash, pruritus, erythema, urticaria

Hematologic: Thrombocytosis

Respiratory: Wheezing

Miscellaneous: Allergic reactions, anaphylactoid reactions

Drug Interactions

Avoid Concomitant Use

Avoid concomitant use of Leucovorin Calcium with any of the following: Raltitrexed

Increased Effect/Toxicity

Leucovorin Calcium may increase the levels/effects of: Capecitabine; Fluorouracil

Decreased Effect

Leucovorin Calcium may decrease the levels/effects of: PHENobarbital; Phenytoin; Primidone; Raltitrexed; Trimethoprim

Storage/Stability

Powder for injection: Store at room temperature of 25°C (77°F). Protect from light. Solutions reconstituted with bacteriostatic water for injection U.S.P., must be used within 7 days. Solutions reconstituted with SWFI must be used immediately. Parenteral admixture is stable for 24 hours stored at room temperature (25°C) and for 4 days when stored under refrigeration (4°C).

Solution for injection: Prior to dilution, store vials under refrigeration at 2°C to 8°C (36°F to 46°F). Protect from light.

Tablet: Store at room temperature of 15°C to 30°C (59°F to 86°F).

Reconstitution Powder for injection: Reconstitute with SWFI or BWFI; dilute in 100-1000 mL NS, D_5W for infusion. When doses >10 mg/m^2 are required, reconstitute using sterile water for injection, not a solution containing benzyl alcohol.

Compatibility Stable in $D_{10}NS$, D_5W, $D_{10}W$, LR, sterile water for injection, bacteriostatic water, bacteriostatic NS; **variable stability (consult detailed reference)** in NS.

Y-site administration: Compatible: Amifostine, aztreonam, bleomycin, cefepime, cisplatin, cladribine, cyclophosphamide, docetaxel, doxorubicin, doxorubicin liposome, etoposide phosphate, filgrastim, fluconazole, fluorouracil, furosemide, gatifloxacin, gemcitabine, granisetron, heparin, irinotecan, linezolid, methotrexate, metoclopramide, mitomycin, piperacillin/tazobactam, tacrolimus, teniposide, thiotepa, vinblastine, vincristine. **Incompatible:** Amphotericin B cholesteryl sulfate complex, droperidol, foscarnet, sodium bicarbonate.

Compatibility in syringe: Compatible: Bleomycin, cisplatin, cyclophosphamide, doxorubicin, fluorouracil, furosemide, heparin, methotrexate, metoclopramide, mitomycin, vinblastine, vincristine. **Incompatible:** Droperidol.

Compatibility when admixed: Compatible: Cisplatin, cisplatin with floxuridine, floxuridine. **Incompatible:** Concentrations >2 mg/mL of leucovorin and >25 mg/mL of fluorouracil.

Mechanism of Action A reduced form of folic acid, leucovorin supplies the necessary cofactor blocked by methotrexate, enters the cells via the same active transport system as methotrexate. Stabilizes the binding of 5-dUMP and thymidylate synthetase, enhancing the activity of fluorouracil.

Methanol toxicity treatment: Formic acid (methanol's toxic metabolite) is normally metabolized to carbon dioxide and water by 10-formyltetrahydrofolate dehydrogenase after being bound to tetrahydrofolate. Administering a source of tetrahydrofolate may aid the body in eliminating formic acid.

Pharmacodynamics/Kinetics

Absorption: Oral, I.M.: Well absorbed

Metabolism: Intestinal mucosa and hepatically to 5-methyl-tetrahydrofolate (5MTHF; active)

Bioavailability: Saturable at oral doses >25 mg; 25 mg (97%), 50 mg (75%), 100 mg (37%)

Half-life elimination: ~4-8 hours

Time to peak: Oral: ~2 hours; I.V.: Total folates: 10 minutes; 5MTHF: ~1 hour

Excretion: Urine (primarily); feces

Dosage

Children and Adults:

Treatment of folic acid antagonist overdosage: Oral: 5-15 mg/day

Folate-deficient megaloblastic anemia: I.M.: ≤1 mg/day

High-dose methotrexate-rescue dose: Initial: Oral, I.M., I.V.: 15 mg (~10 mg/m²); start 24 hours after beginning methotrexate infusion; continue every 6 hours for 10 doses, until methotrexate level is <0.05 micromole/L. Adjust dose as follows:

Normal methotrexate elimination: Oral, I.M., I.V.: 15 mg every 6 hours

Delayed early methotrexate elimination: I.V.: 150 mg every 3 hours until methotrexate level is <1 micromole/L, then 15 mg every 3 hours until methotrexate level is <0.05 micromole/L

Adults:

Colorectal cancer (also refer to Combination Regimens):

I.V.: 200 mg/m² over at least 3 minutes (used in combination with fluorouracil 370 mg/m²)

or

I.V.: 20 mg/m² (used in combination with fluorouracil 425 mg/m²)

Pemetrexed toxicity (unlabeled dose): I.V.: 100 mg/m² once, followed by 50 mg/m² every 6 hours for 8 days was used in clinical trial for CTC grade 4 leukopenia ≥3 days; CTC grade 4 neutropenia ≥3 days; immediately for CTC grade 4 thrombocytopenia, bleeding associated with grade 3 thrombocytopenia, or grade 3 or 4 mucositis

◀ **Combination Regimens**

Osteosarcoma:
HDMTX on page 1348
MTX-CDDPAdr on page 1374
POG-8651 on page 1396
Pancreatic cancer: FOLFIRINOX (Pancreatic Cancer) on page 1336

Administration Due to calcium content, do not administer I.V. solutions at a rate >160 mg/ minute.

Refer to individual protocols. Should be administered I.M., I.V. push, or I.V. infusion (15 minutes to 2 hours). Leucovorin should not be administered concurrently with methotrexate. It is commonly initiated 24 hours after the start of methotrexate. Toxicity to normal tissues may be irreversible if leucovorin is not initiated by ~40 hours after the start of methotrexate.

As a rescue after folate antagonists: Administer by I.V. bolus, I.M., or orally.

Do not administer orally in the presence of nausea or vomiting. Doses >25 mg should be administered parenterally.

In combination with fluorouracil: Fluorouracil activity, the fluorouracil is usually given after, or at the midpoint, of the leucovorin infusion. Leucovorin is usually administered by I.V. bolus injection or short (10-120 minutes) I.V. infusion. Other administration schedules have been used; refer to individual protocols.

Monitoring Parameters

High-dose methotrexate therapy: Plasma methotrexate concentration; leucovorin is continued until the plasma methotrexate level <0.05 micromole/L. With 4- to 6-hour high-dose methotrexate infusions, plasma drug values in excess of 50 and 1 micromole/L at 24 and 48 hours after starting the infusion, respectively, are often predictive of delayed methotrexate clearance.

Fluorouracil therapy: CBC with differential and platelets, liver function tests, electrolytes

Dietary Considerations Solutions for injection contain calcium 0.004 mEq per leucovorin 1 mg

Dosage Forms Excipient information presented when available (limited, particularly for generics); consult specific product labeling. **Note:** Strength expressed as base

Injection, powder for reconstitution: 50 mg, 100 mg, 200 mg, 350 mg

Injection, solution [preservative free]: 10 mg/mL (50 mL)

Tablet: 5 mg, 10 mg, 15 mg, 25 mg

References

Hansen RM, "Systemic Therapy in Metastatic Colorectal Cancer," *Arch Intern Med*, 1990, 150 (11):2265-9.

Jolivet J, "Role of Leucovorin Dosing and Administration Schedule," *Eur J Cancer*, 1995, 31A (7-8):1311-5.

Machover D, "A Comprehensive Review of 5-Fluorouracil and Leucovorin in Patients With Metastatic Colorectal Carcinoma," *Cancer*, 1997, 80(7):1179-87.

McGuire BW, Sia LL, Leese PT, et al, "Pharmacokinetics of Leucovorin Calcium After Intravenous, Intramuscular, and Oral Administration," *Clin Pharm*, 1988, 7(1):52-8.

Rustum YM, "Modulation of Fluoropyrimidines by Leucovorin: Rationale and Status," *J Surg Oncol Suppl*, 1991, 2:116-23.

Trissel LA, Martinez JF, and Xu QA, "Incompatibility of Fluorouracil With Leucovorin Calcium or Levoleucovorin Calcium," *Am J Health Syst Pharm*, 1995, 52(7):710-5.

Walker SE, Law S, and Puodziunas A, "Simulation of Y-Site Compatibility of Irinotecan and Leucovorin at Room Temperature in 5% Dextrose in Water in 3 Different Containers," *Can J Hosp Pharm*, 2005, 58(4): 212-22.

◆ **Leukeran®** *see* Chlorambucil *on page 216*

◆ **Leukine®** *see* Sargramostim *on page 1029*

Leuprolide (loo PROE lide)

Medication Safety Issues

Sound-alike/look-alike issues:

Lupron® may be confused with Nuprin®

Lupron Depot®-3 Month may be confused with Lupron Depot-Ped®

Related Information

Safe Handling of Hazardous Drugs *on page 1517*

U.S. Brand Names Eligard®; Lupron Depot-Ped®; Lupron Depot®; Lupron®

Index Terms Abbott-43818; Leuprolide Acetate; Leuprorelin Acetate; TAP-144

Generic Available Yes: Injection (solution)

Canadian Brand Names Eligard®; Lupron®; Lupron® Depot®

Pharmacologic Category Antineoplastic Agent, Gonadotropin-Releasing Hormone Agonist; Gonadotropin Releasing Hormone Agonist

Use Palliative treatment of advanced prostate cancer; management of endometriosis; treatment of anemia caused by uterine leiomyomata (fibroids); central precocious puberty

Unlabeled/Investigational Use Treatment of breast cancer; infertility; prostatic hyperplasia

Pregnancy Risk Factor X

Lactation Excretion in breast milk unknown/contraindicated

Labeled Contraindications Hypersensitivity to leuprolide, GnRH, GnRH-agonist analogs, or any component of the formulation; undiagnosed abnormal vaginal bleeding; pregnancy; breast-feeding

Lupron Depot®-4 month (30 mg) is not indicated for use in women

Eligard® is contraindicated in women and children

Warnings/Precautions Hazardous agent - use appropriate precautions for handling and disposal. Transient increases in testosterone serum levels occur at the start of treatment. Tumor flare, bone pain, neuropathy, urinary tract obstruction, and spinal cord compression have been reported when used for prostate cancer; closely observe patients for weakness, paresthesias, hematuria, and urinary tract obstruction in first few weeks of therapy. Observe patients with metastatic vertebral lesions or urinary obstruction closely. Exacerbation of endometriosis or uterine leiomyomata may occur initially. Decreased bone density has been reported when used for ≥6 months; use caution in patients with additional risk factors for bone loss (eg, chronic alcohol use, corticosteroid therapy). In patients with prostate cancer, androgen deprivation therapy may increase the risk for cardiovascular disease, diabetes, insulin resistance, obesity, alterations in lipids, and fractures. Use caution in patients with a history of psychiatric illness; alteration in mood, memory impairment, and depression have been associated with use. Rare cases of pituitary apoplexy (frequently secondary to pituitary adenoma) have been observed with leuprolide administration (onset from 1 hour to usually <2 weeks); may present as sudden headache, vomiting, visual or mental status changes, and infrequently cardiovascular collapse; immediate medical attention required. Females treated for precocious puberty may experience menses or spotting during the first 2 months of treatment; notify healthcare provider if bleeding continues after the second month.

Some dosage forms may contain benzyl alcohol which has been associated with "gasping syndrome" in neonates; patients with benzyl alcohol allergy may demonstrate a hypersensitivity reaction (usually local) in the form of erythema and induration at the injection site. Vehicle used in injectable (polylactide-co-glycolide microspheres) has rarely been associated with retinal artery occlusion in patients with abnormal arteriovenous anastomosis.

Adverse Reactions

Children:

2% to 10%:

Central nervous system: Pain (2%)

Dermatologic: Acne (2%), rash (2% including erythema multiforme), seborrhea (2%)

Genitourinary: Vaginitis (2%), vaginal bleeding (2%), vaginal discharge (2%)

Local: Injection site reaction (5%)

<2%: Alopecia, body odor, cervix disorder, dysphagia, emotional lability, epistaxis, fever, gingivitis, gynecomastia, headache, nausea, nervousness, peripheral edema, personality disorder, sexual maturity accelerated, skin striae, somnolence, syncope, urinary incontinence, vasodilation, vomiting, weight gain

Adults:

Note: For prostate cancer treatment, an initial rise in serum testosterone concentrations may cause "tumor flare" or worsening of symptoms, including bone pain, neuropathy, hematuria, or ureteral or bladder outlet obstruction during the first 2 weeks. Similarly, an initial increase in estradiol levels, with a temporary worsening of symptoms, may occur in women treated with leuprolide.

Delayed release formulations:

10%:

Cardiovascular: Edema (≤14%)

Central nervous system: Headache (≤65%), pain (<2% to 33%), depression (≤31%), insomnia (≤31%), fatigue (≤17%), dizziness/vertigo (≤16%)

Dermatologic: Skin reaction (≤12%)

Endocrine & metabolic: Hot flashes (25% to 98%), testicular atrophy (≤20%), hyperlipidemia (≤12%), libido decreased (≤11%)

Gastrointestinal: Nausea/vomiting (≤25%), bowel function altered (≤14%), weight gain/loss (≤13%)

Genitourinary: Vaginitis (11% to 28%), urinary disorder (13% to 15%)

Local: Injection site burning/stinging (transient: ≤35%)

Neuromuscular & skeletal: Weakness (≤18%), joint disorder (≤12%)

Miscellaneous: Flu-like syndrome (≤12%)

1% to 10% (limited to important or life-threatening):

Cardiovascular: Angina (<5%), arrhythmia (<5%), atrial fibrillation (<5%), bradycardia (<5%), CHF (<5%), deep thrombophlebitis (<5%), hyper-/hypotension (<5%), palpitation (<5%), syncope (<5%), tachycardia (<5%)

Central nervous system: Nervousness (≤8%), anxiety (≤6%), confusion (<5%), delusions (<5%), dementia (<5%), fever (<5%), seizure (<5%)

Dermatologic: Acne (≤10%), alopecia (≤5%), bruising (≤5%), cellulitis (<5%), pruritus (≤3%), hirsutism (<2%), rash (<2%)

Endocrine & metabolic: Dehydration (≤8%), gynecomastia (≤7%), breast tenderness/pain (≤6%), bicarbonate decreased (≥5%), hyper-/hypocholesterolemia (≥5%), hyperglycemia (≥5%), hyperphosphatemia (≥5%), hyperuricemia (≥5%), hypoalbuminemia (≥5%), hypoproteinemia (≥5%), lactation (<5%), testicular pain (≤4%), menstrual disorder (<2%)

Gastrointestinal: Dysphagia (<5%), gastrointestinal hemorrhage (<5%), intestinal obstruction (<5%), ulcer (<5%), gastroenteritis/colitis (≤3%), diarrhea (≤2%), constipation (≤2%)

Genitourinary: Prostatic acid phosphatase increased/decreased (≥5%), urine specific gravity increased/decreased (≥5%), impotence (≤5%), balanitis (<5%), incontinence (<5%), penile/testis disorder (<5%), urinary tract infection (<5%), nocturia (≤4%), polyuria (2% to 4%), bladder spasm

(<2%), dysuria (<2%), erectile dysfunction (<2%), hematuria (<2%), urinary retention (<2%), urinary urgency (<2%)

Hematologic: Eosinophilia (≥5%), leukopenia (≥5%), platelets increased (≥5%), anemia

Hepatic: Liver function tests abnormal (≥5%), partial thromboplastin time increased (≥5%), prothrombin time increased (≥5%), hepatomegaly (<5%)

Local: Injection site pain (2% to 5%), injection site erythema (1% to 3%)

Neuromuscular & skeletal: Myalgia (≤8%), paresthesia (≤8%), neuropathy (<5%), paralysis (<5%), pathologic fracture (<5%), bone pain (<2%)

Renal: BUN increased (≥5%), creatinine increased (≥5%)

Respiratory: Emphysema (<5%), epistaxis (<5%), hemoptysis (<5%), pleural effusion (<5%), pulmonary edema (<5%), dyspnea (≤2%)

Miscellaneous: Diaphoresis (≤5%), allergic reaction (<5%), infection (5%), lymphadenopathy (<5%)

Immediate release formulation:

>10%:

Cardiovascular: ECG changes/ischemia (19%), peripheral edema (12%)

Central nervous system: Pain (13%)

Endocrine & metabolic: Hot flashes (55%)

1% to 10% (limited to important or life-threatening):

Cardiovascular: Hypertension (8%), murmur (3%), thrombosis/phlebitis (2%), CHF (1%), angina, arrhythmia, MI, syncope

Central nervous system: Headache (7%), insomnia (7%), dizziness/light-headedness (5%), anxiety, depression, fatigue, fever, nervousness

Dermatologic: Dermatitis (5%), alopecia, bruising, itching, lesions, pigmentation

Endocrine & metabolic: Gynecomastia/breast tenderness/pain (7%), testicular size decreased (7%), diabetes, hypercalcemia, hypoglycemia, libido decreased, thyroid enlarged

Gastrointestinal: Constipation (7%), anorexia (6%), nausea/vomiting (5%), diarrhea, dysphagia, gastrointestinal bleeding, peptic ulcer, rectal polyps

Genitourinary: Urinary frequency/urgency (6%), impotence (4%), urinary tract infection (3%), bladder spasm, dysuria, incontinence, testicular pain, urinary obstruction

Hematologic: Anemia (5%)

Local: Injection site reaction

Neuromuscular & skeletal: Weakness (10%), bone pain (5%), peripheral neuropathy

Ocular: Blurred vision

Renal: Hematuria (6%), BUN increased, creatinine increased

Respiratory: Dyspnea (2%), cough, pneumonia, pulmonary embolus, pulmonary fibrosis

Miscellaneous: Infection, inflammation

Children and Adults: *Any formulations:* Postmarketing and/or case reports (limited to important or life-threatening): Anaphylactic/anaphylactoid reactions, asthmatic reactions, bone density decreased; fibromyalgia-like symptoms (arthralgia/myalgia, headaches, GI distress); hemoptysis, hepatic dysfunction, hypokalemia, hypoproteinemia, injection site induration/abscess, MI, pelvic fibrosis, penile swelling, photosensitivity; pituitary apoplexy (cardiovascular collapse, mental status altered, ophthalmoplegia, sudden headache, visual changes, vomiting); prostate pain, pulmonary embolism, pulmonary infiltrate, spinal fracture/paralysis, stroke, tenosynovitis-like symptoms, thrombocytopenia, transient ischemia attack, uric acid increased, urticaria, WBC increased

Drug Interactions

Avoid Concomitant Use There are no known interactions where it is recommended to avoid concomitant use.

Increased Effect/Toxicity There are no known significant interactions involving an increase in effect.

Decreased Effect

Leuprolide may decrease the levels/effects of: Antidiabetic Agents

Storage/Stability

Lupron®: Lupron®: Store below 25°C (77°F). Protect from light and store vial in carton until use. Do not freeze.

Eligard®: Store at 2°C to 8°C (36°F to 46°C). Allow to reach room temperature prior to using; once mixed, must be administered within 30 minutes.

Lupron Depot® may be stored at room temperature of 15°C to 30°C (59°F to 86°F). Upon reconstitution, the suspension does not contain a preservative and should be used immediately.

Reconstitution

Eligard®: Packaged in two syringes; one contains the Atrigel® polymer system and the second contains leuprolide acetate powder; follow package instructions for mixing

Lupron Depot®: Reconstitute only with diluent provided

Mechanism of Action Leuprolide, is an agonist of luteinizing hormone-releasing hormone (LHRH). Acting as a potent inhibitor of gonadotropin secretion; continuous administration results in suppression of ovarian and testicular steroidogenesis due to decreased levels of LH and FSH with subsequent decrease in testosterone (male) and estrogen (female) levels. In males, testosterone levels are reduced to below castrate levels. Leuprolide may also have a direct inhibitory effect on the testes, and act by a different mechanism not directly related to reduction in serum testosterone.

Pharmacodynamics/Kinetics

Onset of action: Following transient increase, testosterone suppression occurs in ~2-4 weeks of continued therapy

Distribution: Males: V_d: 27 L

Protein binding: 43% to 49%

Metabolism: Major metabolite, pentapeptide (M-1)

Bioavailability: Oral: None; SubQ: 94%

Excretion: Urine (<5% as parent and major metabolite)

Dosage

Children: Precocious puberty (consider discontinuing by age 11 for females and by age 12 for males):

SubQ (Lupron®): Initial: 50 mcg/kg/day (per manufacturer, doses of 20-45 mcg/kg/day have also been reported); titrate dose upward by 10 mcg/kg/day if down-regulation is not achieved. **Note:** Higher mg/kg doses may be required in younger children.

I.M. (Lupron Depot-Ped®): 0.3 mg/kg/dose given every 28 days (minimum dose: 7.5 mg)

≤25 kg: 7.5 mg

>25-37.5 kg: 11.25 mg

>37.5 kg: 15 mg

Titrate dose upward in increments of 3.75 mg every 4 weeks if down-regulation is not achieved.

Adults:
Advanced prostate cancer:
SubQ:
Eligard®: 7.5 mg monthly **or** 22.5 mg every 3 months **or** 30 mg every 4 months **or** 45 mg every 6 months
Lupron®: 1 mg/day

I.M.:
Lupron Depot®: 7.5 mg/dose given monthly (every 28-33 days) **or**
Lupron Depot®-3: 22.5 mg every 3 months **or**
Lupron Depot®-4: 30 mg every 4 months

Breast cancer, premenopausal ovarian ablation (unlabeled use; Boccardo, 1999): I.M.:
Lupron Depot®: 3.75 mg every 28 days **or**
Lupron Depot®-3: 11.25 mg every 3 months

Endometriosis: I.M.: Initial therapy may be with leuprolide alone or in combination with norethindrone; if retreatment for an additional 6 months is necessary, norethindrone should be used. Retreatment is not recommended for longer than one additional 6-month course.
Lupron Depot®: 3.75 mg/month for up to 6 months **or**
Lupron Depot®-3: 11.25 mg every 3 months for up to 2 doses (6 months total duration of treatment)

Uterine leiomyomata (fibroids): I.M. (in combination with iron):
Lupron Depot®: 3.75 mg/month for up to 3 months **or**
Lupron Depot®-3: 11.25 mg as a single injection

Combination Regimens

Prostate cancer:
Bicalutamide-Leuprolide on page 1234
FL on page 1323

Administration

I.M.: Lupron Depot®: Vary injection site periodically
SubQ:
Eligard®: Vary injection site; choose site with adequate subcutaneous tissue (eg, abdomen, upper buttocks)
Lupron®: Vary injection site; if an alternate syringe from the syringe provided is required, insulin syringes should be used

Monitoring Parameters Bone mineral density

Precocious puberty: GnRH testing (blood LH and FSH levels), measurement of bone age every 6-12 months, testosterone in males and estradiol in females; Tanner staging
Prostatic cancer: LH and FSH levels, serum testosterone (2-4 weeks after initiation of therapy), PSA; weakness, paresthesias, and urinary tract obstruction in first few weeks of therapy. Screen for diabetes and cardiovascular risk prior to initiating treatment.

Test Interactions Interferes with pituitary gonadotropic and gonadal function tests during and up to 3 months after monthly administration of leuprolide therapy.

Additional Information

Eligard® Atrigel®: A nongelatin-based, biodegradable, polymer matrix

Oncology Comment: Guidelines from the American Society of Clinical Oncology (ASCO) for hormonal management of advanced prostate cancer which is androgen-sensitive (Loblaw, 2007) recommend either orchiectomy or luteinizing hormone-releasing hormone (LHRH) agonists as initial treatment for androgen deprivation.

Dosage Forms Excipient information presented when available (limited, particularly for generics); consult specific product labeling. [DSC] = Discontinued product

Injection, solution, as acetate: 5 mg/mL (2.8 mL)
Lupron®: 5 mg/mL (2.8 mL) [contains benzyl alcohol]
Lupron®: 5 mg/mL (2.8 mL) [contains benzyl alcohol; packaged with syringes and alcohol swabs] [DSC]

Injection, powder for reconstitution, as acetate [depot formulation]:
Eligard®:
7.5 mg [released over 1 month; contains polylactide-co-glycolide]
22.5 mg [released over 3 months; contains polylactide-co-glycolide]
30 mg [released over 4 months; contains polylactide-co-glycolide]
45 mg [released over 6 months; contains polylactide-co-glycolide]
Lupron Depot®: 3.75 mg, 7.5 mg [released over 1 month; contains polysorbate 80, polylactide-co-glycolide]
Lupron Depot®-3 Month: 11.25 mg, 22.5 mg [released over 3 months; contains polysorbate 80, polylactide-co-glycolide]
Lupron Depot®-4 Month: 30 mg [released over 4 months; contains polysorbate 80, polylactide-co-glycolide]
Lupron Depot-Ped®: 7.5 mg, 11.25 mg, 15 mg [released over 1 month; contains polysorbate 80, polylactide-co-glycolide]

References

Adjuvant Breast Cancer Trials Collaborative Group, "Ovarian Ablation or Suppression in Premenopausal Early Breast Cancer: Results From the International Adjuvant Breast Cancer Ovarian Ablation or Suppression Randomized Trial," *J Natl Cancer Inst*, 2007, 99(7):516-25.

Boccardo F, Rubagotti A, Amoroso D, et al, "Endocrinological and Clinical Evaluation of Two Depot Formulations of Leuprolide Acetate in Pre- and Perimenopausal Breast Cancer Patients," *Cancer Chemother Pharmacol*, 1999, 43(6):461-6.

Crawford ED, Eisenberger MA, McLeod DG, et al, "A Controlled Trial of Leuprolide With and Without Flutamide in Prostatic Carcinoma," *N Engl J Med*, 1989, 321(7):419-24.

Kavanagh JJ, Roberts W, Townsend P, et al, "Leuprolide Acetate in the Treatment of Refractory or Persistent Epithelial Ovarian Cancer," *J Clin Oncol*, 1989, 7(1):115-8.

Keating NL, O'Malley AJ, and Smith MR, "Diabetes and Cardiovascular Disease During Androgen Deprivation Therapy for Prostate Cancer," *J Clin Oncol*, 2006, 24(27):4448-56.

Loblaw DA, Virgo KS, Nam R, et al, "Initial Hormonal Management of Androgen-Sensitive Metastatic, Recurrent, or Progressive Prostate Cancer: 2006 Update of an American Society of Clinical Oncology Practice Guideline," *J Clin Oncol*, 2007, 25(12):1596-605.

National Comprehensive Cancer Network® (NCCN), "Clinical Practice Guidelines in Oncology™: Breast Cancer," Version 1.2009. Available at http://www.nccn.org/professionals/physician_gls/PDF/breast.pdf.

National Comprehensive Cancer Network® (NCCN), "Clinical Practice Guidelines in Oncology™: Ovarian Cancer," Version 2.2009. Available at http://www.nccn.org/professionals/physician_gls/PDF/ovarian.pdf

National Comprehensive Cancer Network® (NCCN), "Clinical Practice Guidelines in Oncology™: Prostate Carcinoma," Version 2.2009. Available at http://www.nccn.org/professionals/physician_gls/PDF/prostate.pdf

Levofloxacin (lee voe FLOKS a sin)

Medication Safety Issues

Sound-alike/look-alike issues:
Levaquin® may be confused with Levoxyl®, Levsin/SL®, Lovenox®

Levofloxacin may be confused with levetiracetam, levodopa, levothyroxine

U.S. Brand Names Iquix®; Levaquin®; Quixin®

Generic Available No

Canadian Brand Names Apo-Levofloxacin®; CO Levofloxacin; Levaquin®; Mylan-Levofloxacin; Novo-Levofloxacin; PMS-Levofloxacin; Sandoz-Levofloxacin

Pharmacologic Category Antibiotic, Quinolone; Respiratory Fluoroquinolone

Use

Systemic: Treatment of community-acquired pneumonia, including multidrug resistant strains of *S. pneumoniae* (MDRSP); nosocomial pneumonia; chronic bronchitis (acute bacterial exacerbation); acute bacterial sinusitis; prostatitis, urinary tract infection (uncomplicated or complicated); acute pyelonephritis; skin or skin structure infections (uncomplicated or complicated); reduce incidence or disease progression of inhalational anthrax (postexposure)

Ophthalmic: Treatment of bacterial conjunctivitis caused by susceptible organisms (Quixin® 0.5% ophthalmic solution); treatment of corneal ulcer caused by susceptible organisms (Iquix® 1.5% ophthalmic solution)

Unlabeled/Investigational Use Diverticulitis, enterocolitis (*Shigella* spp.), epididymitis (nongonococcal), gonococcal infections, Legionnaires' disease, peritonitis, PID

Note: As of April 2007, the CDC no longer recommends the use of fluoroquinolones for the treatment of gonococcal disease.

Pregnancy Risk Factor C

Lactation Enters breast milk/not recommended

Labeled Contraindications Hypersensitivity to levofloxacin, any component of the formulation, or other quinolones

Warnings/Precautions

Systemic: [U.S. Boxed Warning]: There have been reports of tendon inflammation and/or rupture with quinolone antibiotics; risk may be increased with concurrent corticosteroids, organ transplant recipients, and in patients >60 years of age. Rupture of the Achilles tendon sometimes requiring surgical repair has been reported most frequently; but other tendon sites (eg, rotator cuff, biceps) have also been reported. Strenuous physical activity, rheumatoid arthritis, and renal impairment may be an independent risk factor for tendonitis. Discontinue at first sign of tendon inflammation or pain. May occur even after discontinuation of therapy. Use with caution in patients with rheumatoid arthritis; may increase risk of tendon rupture. Systemic use is only recommended in children <18 years of age for the prevention of inhalational anthrax (postexposure); increased incidence of musculoskeletal disorders (eg, arthralgia, tendon rupture) has been observed in children; CNS stimulation may occur (tremor, restlessness, confusion, and very rarely hallucinations or seizures). Potential for seizures, although very rare, may be increased with concomitant NSAID therapy. Use with caution in individuals at risk of seizures, with known or suspected CNS disorders or renal dysfunction. Avoid excessive sunlight and take precautions to limit exposure (eg, loose fitting clothing, sunscreen); may cause moderate-to-severe phototoxicity reactions. Discontinue use if photosensitivity occurs.

Rare cases of torsade de pointes have been reported in patients receiving levofloxacin. Use caution in patients with known prolongation of QT interval, bradycardia, hypokalemia, hypomagnesemia, or in those receiving concurrent therapy with Class Ia or Class III antiarrhythmics.

Severe hypersensitivity reactions, including anaphylaxis, have occurred with quinolone therapy. Reactions may present as typical allergic symptoms after a single dose, or may manifest as severe idiosyncratic dermatologic, vascular, pulmonary, renal, hepatic, and/or hematologic events, usually after multiple doses. Prompt discontinuation of drug should occur if skin rash or other symptoms arise. Prolonged use may result in fungal or bacterial superinfection, including *C. difficile*-associated diarrhea (CDAD) and pseudomembranous colitis; CDAD has been observed >2 months postantibiotic treatment. Peripheral neuropathies have been linked to levofloxacin use; discontinue if numbness, tingling, or weakness develops. Quinolones may exacerbate myasthenia gravis. Unrelated to hypersensitivity, severe hepatotoxicity (including acute hepatitis and fatalities) has been reported. Elderly patients may be at greater risk. Discontinue therapy immediately if signs and symptoms of hepatitis occur. Hemolytic reactions may (rarely) occur with quinolone use in patients with latent or actual G6PD deficiency.

Fluoroquinolones have been associated with the development of serious, and sometimes fatal, hypoglycemia, most often in elderly diabetics, but also in patients without diabetes. This occurred most frequently with gatifloxacin (no longer available systemically) but may occur at a lower frequency with other quinolones.

Ophthalmic solution: For topical use only. Do not inject subconjunctivally or introduce into anterior chamber of the eye. Contact lenses should not be worn during treatment for bacterial conjunctivitis. Safety and efficacy in children <1 year of age (Quixin®) or <6 years of age (Iquix®) have not been established. **Note:** Indications for ophthalmic solutions are product concentration-specific and should not be used interchangeably.

Adverse Reactions

1% to 10%:

Cardiovascular: Chest pain (1%), edema (1%)

Central nervous system: Headache (6%), insomnia (4%), dizziness (3%), fatigue (1%), pain (1%)

Dermatologic: Rash (2%), pruritus (1%)

Gastrointestinal: Taste disturbance (8% to 10% [ophthalmic]), nausea (7%), diarrhea (5%), constipation (3%), abdominal pain (2%), dyspepsia (2%), vomiting (2%)

Genitourinary: Vaginitis (1%)

Local: Injection site reaction (1%)

Ocular (with ophthalmic solution use): Decreased vision (transient), foreign body sensation, transient ocular burning, ocular pain or discomfort, photophobia

Respiratory: Pharyngitis (4%), dyspnea (1%)

Miscellaneous: Moniliasis (1%)

<1%, postmarketing, and/or case reports (limited to important or life-threatening):

Systemic: Acute renal failure, agitation, agranulocytosis; allergic reaction (including anaphylaxis, angioedema, pneumonitis rash, pneumonitis, and serum sickness); anaphylactoid reaction, arrhythmia (including atrial/ventricular tachycardia/fibrillation and torsade de pointes), aplastic anemia, arthralgia, ascites, bradycardia, bronchospasm, carcinoma, cardiac failure, cholecystitis, cholelithiasis, confusion, depression, EEG abnormalities, encephalopathy, eosinophilia, erythema multiforme, GI hemorrhage, granulocytopenia, hallucination, heart block, hemolytic anemia, hemoptysis, hepatic failure (some fatal), hepatitis, hyper-/hypoglycemia, hyperkalemia, hyperkinesias, hyper-/hypotension, infection, INR increased, intestinal obstruction, intracranial hypertension, involuntary muscle contractions, jaundice, leukocytosis, leukopenia, leukorrhea, lymphadenopathy, MI, migraine, multiple organ failure, myalgia, nephritis (interstitial), palpitation, pancreatitis, pancytopenia, paralysis, paresthesia, peripheral neuropathy, photosensitivity (<0.1%), pleural effusion, pneumonitis, postural hypotension, prothrombin time increased/decreased, pseudomembranous colitis, psychosis, pulmonary edema, pulmonary embolism, purpura, QT_c prolongation, respiratory depression, rhabdomyolysis, seizure, skin disorder, somnolence, speech disorder, Stevens-Johnson syndrome, stupor, suicide attempt/ideation, syncope, tendonitis, tendon rupture, tongue edema, toxic epidermal necrolysis, transaminases increased, thrombocythemia, thrombocytopenia, tremor, urticaria, WBC abnormality

Ophthalmic solution: Allergic reaction, lid edema, ocular dryness, ocular itching

Drug Interactions

Avoid Concomitant Use

Avoid concomitant use of Levofloxacin with any of the following: Artemether; Dronedarone; Lumefantrine; Nilotinib; Pimozide; QuiNINE; Tetrabenazine; Thioridazine; Ziprasidone

Increased Effect/Toxicity

Levofloxacin may increase the levels/effects of: Corticosteroids (Systemic); Dronedarone; Pimozide; QTc-Prolonging Agents; QuiNINE; Sulfonylureas; Tetrabenazine; Thioridazine; Vitamin K Antagonists; Ziprasidone

The levels/effects of Levofloxacin may be increased by: Alfuzosin; Artemether; Chloroquine; Ciprofloxacin; Gadobutrol; Insulin; Lumefantrine; Nilotinib; Nonsteroidal Anti-Inflammatory Agents; Probenecid; QuiNINE

Decreased Effect

Levofloxacin may decrease the levels/effects of: Mycophenolate; Sulfonylureas; Typhoid Vaccine

The levels/effects of Levofloxacin may be decreased by: Antacids; Calcium Salts; Didanosine; Iron Salts; Magnesium Salts; Quinapril; Sevelamer; Sucralfate; Zinc Salts

Storage/Stability

Solution for injection:

Vial: Store at room temperature. Protect from light. Diluted solution is stable for 72 hours when stored at room temperature; stable for 14 days when stored under refrigeration. When frozen, stable for 6 months; do not refreeze. Do not thaw in microwave or by bath immersion.

Premixed: Store at ≤25°C (77°F); do not freeze. Brief exposure to 40°C (104°F) does not affect product. Protect from light.

Tablet, oral solution: Store at 25°C (77°F); excursions permitted to 15°C to 30°C (59°F to 86°F).

Ophthalmic solution: Store at 15°C to 25°C (59°F to 77°F).

Reconstitution Solution for injection: Single-use vials must be further diluted in compatible solution to a final concentration of 5 mg/mL prior to infusion.

Compatibility Stable in D₅LR, D₅NS, D₅¹/₂NS with 0.15% KCl, D₅W, NS, Plasma-Lyte® 56/5% dextrose, sodium lactate (M/6); **incompatible** with mannitol 20%, sodium bicarbonate 5%.

Y-site administration: Compatible: Amikacin, aminophylline, ampicillin, bivalirudin, caffeine citrate, cefotaxime, cimetidine, clindamycin, daptomycin, dexamethasone sodium phosphate, dobutamine, dopamine, epinephrine, fenoldopam, fentanyl, gentamicin, isoproterenol, lidocaine, linezolid, lorazepam, metoclopramide, morphine, oxacillin, pancuronium, penicillin G sodium, phenobarbital, phenylephrine, sodium bicarbonate, vancomycin. **Incompatible:** Acyclovir, alprostadil, azithromycin, drotrecogin alfa, furosemide, heparin, indomethacin, lansoprazole, nitroglycerin, propofol, sodium nitroprusside. **Variable (consult detailed reference):** Insulin (regular).

Mechanism of Action As the S (-) enantiomer of the fluoroquinolone, ofloxacin, levofloxacin, inhibits DNA-gyrase in susceptible organisms thereby inhibits relaxation of supercoiled DNA and promotes breakage of DNA strands. DNA gyrase (topoisomerase II), is an essential bacterial enzyme that maintains the superhelical structure of DNA and is required for DNA replication and transcription, DNA repair, recombination, and transposition.

Pharmacodynamics/Kinetics

Absorption: Rapid and complete

Distribution: V_d: 74-112 L; CSF concentrations ~15% of serum levels; high concentrations are achieved in prostate, lung, and gynecological tissues, sinus, saliva

Protein binding: ~24% to 38%; primarily to albumin

Metabolism: Minimally hepatic

Bioavailability: ~99%

Half-life elimination: ~6-8 hours

Time to peak, serum: Oral: 1-2 hours

Excretion: Urine (~87% as unchanged drug, <5% as metabolites); feces (<4%)

Dosage Note: Sequential therapy (intravenous to oral) may be instituted based on prescriber's discretion.

Usual dosage range:

Children ≥1 year: Ophthalmic: 1-2 drops every 2-6 hours

Adults:

Ophthalmic: 1-2 drops every 2-6 hours

Oral, I.V.: 250-500 mg every 24 hours; severe or complicated infections: 750 mg every 24 hours

Indication-specific dosing:

Children ≥1 year and Adults: Ophthalmic:

Conjunctivitis (0.5% ophthalmic solution):

Treatment day 1 and day 2: Instill 1-2 drops into affected eye(s) every 2 hours while awake, up to 8 times/day

Treatment day 3 through day 7: Instill 1-2 drops into affected eye(s) every 4 hours while awake, up to 4 times/day

Children ≥6 years and Adults: Ophthalmic:

Corneal ulceration (1.5% ophthalmic solution):

Treatment day 1 through day 3: Instill 1-2 drops into affected eye(s) every 30 minutes to 2 hours while awake and 4-6 hours after retiring

Treatment day 4 through completion: Instill 1-2 drops into affected eye(s) every 1-4 hours while awake

Children ≥6 months and Adults: Oral, I.V.:

Anthrax (inhalational, postexposure):

≤50 kg: 8 mg/kg every 12 hours for 60 days (do not exceed 250 mg/dose), beginning as soon as possible after exposure

>50 kg and Adults: 500 mg every 24 hours for 60 days, beginning as soon as possible after exposure

Adults: Oral, I.V.:

Chronic bronchitis (acute bacterial exacerbation): 500 mg every 24 hours for at least 7 days

Diverticulitis, peritonitis (unlabeled use): 750 mg every 24 hours for 7-10 days; use adjunctive metronidazole therapy

◄ **Dysenteric enterocolitis, *Shigella* spp. (unlabeled use):** 500 mg every 24 hours for 3-5 days

Epididymitis, nongonococcal (unlabeled use): 500 mg once daily for 10 days

Gonococcal infection (unlabeled use):

Cervicitis, urethritis: 250 mg for one dose with azithromycin or doxycycline; **Note:** As of April 2007, the CDC no longer recommends the use of fluoroquinolones for the treatment of uncomplicated gonococcal disease.

Disseminated infection: 250 mg I.V. once daily; 24 hours after symptoms improve may change to 500 mg orally every 24 hours to complete total therapy of 7 days; **Note:** As of April 2007, the CDC no longer recommends the use of fluoroquinolones for the treatment of more serious gonococcal disease, unless no other options exist and susceptibility can be confirmed via culture.

Pelvic inflammatory disease (unlabeled use): 500 mg once daily for 14 days with or without adjunctive metronidazole; **Note:** The CDC recommends use only if standard cephalosporin therapy is not feasible and community prevalence of quinolone-resistant gonococcal organisms is low. Culture sensitivity must be confirmed.

Pneumonia:

Community-acquired: 500 mg every 24 hours for 7-14 days or 750 mg every 24 hours for 5 days (efficacy of 5-day regimen for MDRSP not established)

Nosocomial: 750 mg every 24 hours for 7-14 days

Prostatitis (chronic bacterial): 500 mg every 24 hours for 28 days

Sinusitis (acute bacterial): 500 mg every 24 hours for 10-14 days or 750 mg every 24 hours for 5 days

Skin and skin structure infections:

Uncomplicated: 500 mg every 24 hours for 7-10 days

Complicated: 750 mg every 24 hours for 7-14 days

Traveler's diarrhea (unlabeled use): 500 mg for one dose

Urinary tract infections:

Uncomplicated: 250 mg once daily for 3 days

Complicated, including pyelonephritis: 250 mg once daily for 10 days **or** 750 mg once daily for 5 days

Dosing adjustment in renal impairment:

Normal renal function dosing of 750 mg/day:

Cl_{cr} 20-49 mL/minute: Administer 750 mg every 48 hours

Cl_{cr} 10-19 mL/minute: Administer 750 mg initial dose, followed by 500 mg every 48 hours

Hemodialysis/CAPD: Administer 750 mg initial dose, followed by 500 mg every 48 hours

Normal renal function dosing of 500 mg/day:

Cl_{cr} 20-49 mL/minute: Administer 500 mg initial dose, followed by 250 mg every 24 hours

Cl_{cr} 10-19 mL/minute: Administer 500 mg initial dose, followed by 250 mg every 48 hours

Hemodialysis/CAPD: Administer 500 mg initial dose, followed by 250 mg every 48 hours

Normal renal function dosing of 250 mg/day:

Cl_{cr} 20-49 mL/minute: No dosage adjustment required

Cl_{cr} 10-19 mL/minute: Administer 250 mg every 48 hours (except in uncomplicated UTI, where no dosage adjustment is required)

Hemodialysis/CAPD: No information available

CRRT: **Note:** Clearance dependent on filter type, flow rates, and other variables.

CVVH/CVVHD/CVVHDF: Alternative recommendations exist:

500 mg every 48 hours **or**

250 mg every 24 hours (**Note:** This regimen has been shown to be equivalent to 500 mg/day in normal renal function. Appropriateness of this regimen for target dosing equal to 750 mg/day is not known.)

Administration

Oral: Tablets may be administered without regard to meals. Oral solution should be administered 1 hour before or 2 hours after meals. Maintain adequate hydration of patient to prevent crystalluria.

I.V.: Infuse 250-500 mg I.V. solution over 60 minutes; infuse 750 mg I.V. solution over 90 minutes. Too rapid of infusion can lead to hypotension. Avoid administration through an intravenous line with a solution containing multivalent cations (eg, magnesium, calcium). Maintain adequate hydration of patient to prevent crystalluria.

Monitoring Parameters Evaluation of organ system functions (renal, hepatic, ophthalmologic, and hematopoietic) is recommended periodically during therapy; the possibility of crystalluria should be assessed; WBC and signs of infection

Test Interactions Some quinolones may produce a false-positive urine screening result for opiates using commercially-available immunoassay kits. This has been demonstrated most consistently for levofloxacin and ofloxacin, but other quinolones have shown cross-reactivity in certain assay kits. Confirmation of positive opiate screens by more specific methods should be considered.

Dietary Considerations Tablets may be taken without regard to meals. Oral solution should be administered on an empty stomach (1 hour before or 2 hours after a meal). Take 2 hours before or 2 hours after multiple vitamins, antacids, or other products containing magnesium, aluminum, iron, or zinc.

Dosage Forms Excipient information presented when available (limited, particularly for generics); consult specific product labeling. [DSC] = Discontinued product

Infusion, premixed in D_5W [preservative free]:

Levaquin®: 250 mg (50 mL); 500 mg (100 mL); 750 mg (150 mL)

Injection, solution [preservative free]:

Levaquin®: 25 mg/mL (20 mL, 30 mL)

Solution, ophthalmic [drops]:

Iquix®: 1.5% (5 mL)

Quixin®: 0.5% (5 mL) [contains benzalkonium chloride]

Solution, oral:

Levaquin®: 25 mg/mL (480 mL) [contains benzyl alcohol, propylene glycol]

Tablet, oral:

Levaquin®: 250 mg, 500 mg, 750 mg [DSC]

Levaquin® Leva-Pak: 750 mg (5s) [DSC]

References

American Thoracic Society and Infectious Diseases Society of America, "Guidelines for the Management of Adults With Hospital-Acquired, Ventilator-Associated, and Healthcare-Associated Pneumonia," *Am J Respir Crit Care Med*, 2005, 171(4):388-416.

Nicolle LN, Bradley S, Colgan R et al, "Infectious Disease Society of America Guidelines for the Diagnosis and Treatment of Asymptomatic Bacteriuria in Adults," *Clinical Infectious Diseases*, 2005, 40:643-54.

◀
North DS, Fish DN, and Redington JJ, "Levofloxacin, A Second-Generation Fluoroquinolone," *Pharmacotherapy*, 1998, 18(5):915-35.

Szarfman A, Chen M, and Blum MD, "More on Fluoroquinolone Antibiotics and Tendon Rupture," *N Engl J Med*, 1995, 332(3):193.

◆ **Levo-folinic Acid** *see* LEVOleucovorin *on page 714*

LEVOleucovorin (lee voe loo koe VOR in)

Medication Safety Issues

Sound-alike/look-alike issues:

LEVOleucovorin may be confused with leucovorin calcium, Leukeran®, Leukine®

U.S. Brand Names Fusilev™

Index Terms 6S-leucovorin; Calcium Levoleucovorin; L-leucovorin; Levo-folinic Acid; Levo-leucovorin; Levoleucovorin Calcium Pentahydrate; S-leucovorin

Generic Available No

Pharmacologic Category Antidote; Rescue Agent (Chemotherapy)

Use Rescue agent after high-dose methotrexate therapy in osteosarcoma; antidote for impaired methotrexate elimination and for inadvertent overdosage of folic acid antagonists

Unlabeled/Investigational Use Treatment of colorectal cancer (in combination with fluorouracil)

Pregnancy Risk Factor C

Lactation Excretion in breast milk unknown/use caution

Labeled Contraindications History of prior allergic reaction to folic acid or leucovorin (folinic acid)

Warnings/Precautions For I.V. administration only; do not administer intrathecally. Due to calcium content, do not administer I.V. solutions at a rate >160 mg levoleucovorin/minute. Levoleucovorin is not approved for and should not be used to treat pernicious anemia or megaloblastic anemias secondary to vitamin B_{12} deficiency; improper use may induce hematologic remission with progressive neurologic manifestations. Methotrexate serum concentrations should be monitored to determine dose and duration of levoleucovorin therapy; dose may need to be increased or administration prolonged in situations where methotrexate excretion may be delayed (eg, ascites, pleural effusion, renal insufficiency, inadequate hydration). When used for the treatment of accidental folic acid antagonist overdose, administer as soon as possible.

The toxicity of fluorouracil is enhanced by leucovorin and levoleucovorin. Deaths due to severe enterocolitis, diarrhea, and dehydration have been reported in elderly patients receiving weekly leucovorin in combination with fluorouracil. Concomitant use of leucovorin and sulfamethoxazole-trimethoprim for the acute treatment of PCP in patients with HIV infection has been associated with increased rates of treatment failure and morbidity; may also occur with levoleucovorin.

Adverse Reactions Note: Adverse reactions reported with levoleucovorin following high-dose methotrexate treatment.

>10%: Gastrointestinal: Stomatitis (38%), vomiting (38%), nausea (19%)

1% to 10%:

Central nervous system: Confusion (6%)

Dermatologic: Dermatitis (6%)

Gastrointestinal: Diarrhea (6%), dyspepsia (6%), taste perversion (6%), typhlitis (6%)

Neuromuscular & skeletal: Neuropathy (6%)

Renal: Renal function abnormal (6%)

Respiratory: Dyspnea (6%)

<1%, postmarketing, and/or case reports: Pruritus, rash, rigors, temperature changes

Drug Interactions

Avoid Concomitant Use

Avoid concomitant use of LEVOleucovorin with any of the following: Raltitrexed

Increased Effect/Toxicity

LEVOleucovorin may increase the levels/effects of: Capecitabine; Fluorouracil

Decreased Effect

LEVOleucovorin may decrease the levels/effects of: PHENobarbital; Phenytoin; Primidone; Raltitrexed; Trimethoprim

Storage/Stability Prior to reconstitution, store intact vials at 25°C (77°F); excursions permitted up to 15°C to 30°C (59°F to 86°F). Protect from light. Reconstituted solutions in the vial and further diluted for infusion in NS are stable for 12 hours at room temperature. Solutions further diluted for infusion in D_5W are stable for 4 hours at room temperature.

Reconstitution Reconstitute the 50 mg vial with 5.3 mL NS (preservative free) to a concentration of 10 mg/mL. Do not use if solution appears cloudy or contains a precipitate. May further dilute for infusion in NS or D_5W to a final concentration of 0.5-5 mg/mL.

Compatibility Stable in NS, D_5W

Mechanism of Action Levoleucovorin counteracts the toxic (and therapeutic) effects of folic acid antagonists (eg, methotrexate) which act by inhibiting dihydrofolate reductase. Levoleucovorin is the levo isomeric and pharmacologic active form of leucovorin (levoleucovorin does not require reduction by dihydrofolate reductase). A reduced derivative of folic acid, leucovorin supplies the necessary cofactor blocked by methotrexate, enters the cells via the same active transport system as methotrexate.

Leucovorin enhances the activity (and toxicity) of fluorouracil by stabilizing the binding of 5-dUMP and thymidylate synthetase.

Pharmacodynamics/Kinetics

Metabolism: Converted to the active reduced form of folate, 5-methyl-tetrahydrofolate (5-methyl-THF; active)

Half-life elimination: 15 mg: 5-7 hours; 300 mg: elimination half life: 16-30 hours

Time to peak, serum: I.V.: 0.9 hours

Dosage Note: Levoleucovorin is dosed at **one-half** the usual dose of the racemic form (leucovorin calcium):

High-dose methotrexate rescue: Children and Adults: I.V.: Usual dose: 7.5 mg (~5 mg/m²) every 6 hours for 10 doses, beginning 24 hours after the start of the methotrexate infusion (based on a methotrexate dose of 12 g/m² I.V. over 4 hours). Levoleucovorin (and hydration and urinary alkalinization) should be continued and/or adjusted until the methotrexate level is <0.05 micromolar (5 x 10^{-8} M) as follows:

Normal methotrexate elimination (serum methotrexate levels ~10 micromolar at 24 hours post administration, 1 micromolar at 48 hours and <0.2 micromolar at 72 hours post infusion): 7.5 mg I.V. every 6 hours for 10 doses

Delayed late methotrexate elimination (serum methotrexate levels >0.2 micromolar at 72 hours and >0.05 micromolar at 96 hours post methotrexate infusion): Continue 7.5 mg I.V. every 6 hours until methotrexate level is <0.05 micromolar

Delayed early methotrexate elimination and/or evidence of acute renal injury (serum methotrexate level ≥50 micromolar at 24 hours, ≥5 micromolar at 48 hours or a doubling or more of the serum creatinine level at 24 hours post methotrexate infusion): 75 mg I.V. every 3 hours until methotrexate level is <1 micromolar, followed by 7.5 mg I.V. every 3 hours until methotrexate level is <0.05 micromolar

Significant clinical toxicity in the presence of less severe abnormalities in methotrexate elimination or renal function (as described above): Extend levoleucovorin treatment for an additional 24 hours (total of 14 doses) in subsequent treatment cycles.

Delayed methotrexate elimination due to third space fluid accumulation, renal insufficiency, or inadequate hydration: May require higher levoleucovorin doses or prolonged administration.

Methotrexate overdose (inadvertent): Children and Adults: I.V.: 7.5 mg (~5 mg/m^2) every 6 hours; continue until the methotrexate level is <0.01 micromolar (10^{-8} M). Initiate treatment as soon as possible after methotrexate overdose. Increase the levoleucovorin dose to 50 mg/m^2 I.V. every 3 hours if the 24 hour serum creatinine has increased 50% over baseline, or if the 24-hour methotrexate level is >5 micromolar (5×10^{-6} M), or if the 48-hour methotrexate level is >0.9 micromolar (9×10^{-7} M); continue levoleucovorin until the methotrexate level is <0.01 micromolar (10^{-8} M). Hydration (3 L/day) and urinary alkalinization (with sodium bicarbonate) should also be maintained.

Treatment of colorectal cancer (in combination with fluorouracil; unlabeled use): Adults: I.V.: Levoleucovorin is dosed at **one-half** the usual dose of the racemic form (leucovorin)

Administration For I.V. use only; do not administer intrathecally. Due to calcium content, do not administer I.V. solutions at a rate >160 mg/minute.

For colorectal cancer (unlabeled use): Levoleucovorin has been administered as I.V. push and as I.V. infusion over 2 hours in clinical trials.

Monitoring Parameters High-dose methotrexate therapy: Serum methotrexate and creatinine levels at least once daily. Monitor fluid and electrolyte status in patients with delayed methotrexate elimination (likely to experience renal toxicity).

Dosage Forms Excipient information presented when available (limited, particularly for generics); consult specific product labeling.

Note: Strength expressed as base.

Injection, powder for reconstitution:

Fusilev™: 50 mg

References

Comella P, De Vita F, Mancarella S, et al, "Biweekly Irinotecan or Raltitrexed Plus 6S-Leucovorin and Bolus 5-Fluorouracil in Advanced Colorectal Carcinoma: A Southern Italy Cooperative Oncology Group Phase II-III Randomized Trial," *Ann Oncol*, 2000, 11(10):1323-33.

Goorin A, Strother D, Poplack D, et al, "Safety and Efficacy of l-leucovorin Rescue Following High-Dose Methotrexate for Osteosarcoma," *Med Pediatr Oncol*, 1995, 24(6):362-7.

Hempel G, Lingg R, and Boos J, "Interactions of Carboxypeptidase G2 With 6S-Leucovorin and 6R-Leucovorin *in vitro*: Implications for the Application in Case of Methotrexate Intoxications," *Cancer Chemother Pharmacol*, 2005, 55(4):347-53.

Jaffe N, Jorgensen K, Robertson R, et al, "Substitution of l-leucovorin for d,l-leucovorin in the Rescue from High-Dose Methotrexate Treatment in Patients With Osteosarcoma," *Anticancer Drugs*, 1993, 4(5):559-64.

Labianca R, Casciini S, Frontini L, et al, "High-Versus Low-Dose Levo-Leucovorin as a Modulator of 5-Fluorouracil in Advanced Colorectal Cancer: A 'GISCAD' Phase III Study," *Ann Oncol*, 1997, 8(2):169-74.

Mader RM, Steger GG, Rizovsky B, et al, "Pharmacokinetics of Rac-Leucovorin vs [S]-Leucovorin in Patients With Advanced Gastrointestinal Cancer," *Br J Clin Pharmacol*, 1994, 37(3):243-8.

Scheithauer W, Kornek G, Marczell A, et al, "Fluorouracil Plus Racemic Leucovorin Versus Fluorouracil Combined With the Pure L-Isomer of Leucovorin for the Treatment of Advanced Colorectal Cancer: A Randomized Phase III Study," *J Clin Oncol*, 1997, 15(3):908-14.

Tournigand C, Cervantes A, Figer A, et al, "OPTIMOX1: A Randomized Study of FOLFOX4 or FOLFOX7 With Oxaliplatin in a Stop-and-Go Fashion in Advanced Colorectal Cancer–A GERCOR Study," *J Clin Oncol*, 2006, 24(3):394-400.

◆ **Levo-leucovorin** *see* LEVOleucovorin *on page 714*

◆ **Levoleucovorin Calcium Pentahydrate** *see* LEVOleucovorin *on page 714*

Levorphanol (lee VOR fa nole)

Medication Safety Issues

High alert medication: The Institute for Safe Medication Practices (ISMP) includes this medication among its list of drug classes which have a heightened risk of causing significant patient harm when used in error.

U.S. Brand Names Levo-Dromoran®

Index Terms Levorphan Tartrate; Levorphanol Tartrate

Generic Available Yes: Tablet

Pharmacologic Category Analgesic, Opioid

Use Relief of moderate-to-severe pain; preoperative sedation/analgesia; management of chronic pain (eg, cancer) requiring opoid therapy

Restrictions C-II

Pregnancy Risk Factor B/D (prolonged use or high doses at term)

Lactation Excretion in breast milk unknown/not recommended

Labeled Contraindications Hypersensitivity to levorphanol or any component of the formulation; pregnancy (prolonged use or high doses at term)

Warnings/Precautions An opioid-containing analgesic regimen should be tailored to each patient's needs and based upon the type of pain being treated (acute versus chronic), the route of administration, degree of tolerance for opioids (naive versus chronic user), age, weight, and medical condition. The optimal analgesic dose varies widely among patients. Doses should be titrated to pain relief/prevention.

May cause CNS depression, which may impair physical or mental abilities; patients must be cautioned about performing tasks which require mental alertness (eg, operating machinery or driving). Effects may be potentiated when used with other sedative drugs or ethanol. Use with caution in patients with hypersensitivity reactions to other phenanthrene derivative opioid agonists (morphine, hydrocodone, hydromorphone, oxycodone, oxymorphone); respiratory diseases including asthma, emphysema, COPD, hypothyroidism, head trauma, morbid obesity, adrenal insufficiency, prostatic hyperplasia/urinary stricture, or severe liver or renal insufficiency. Use with caution in patients with biliary tract dysfunction; acute pancreatitis may cause constriction of sphincter of Oddi. Some preparations contain sulfites which may cause allergic reactions. May be habit-forming. May cause hypotension; use with caution in patients with depleted blood volume or drugs which may exaggerate hypotensive effects (including phenothiazines or general anesthetics). May obscure diagnosis or clinical course of patients with acute abdominal conditions. Concurrent use of agonist/antagonist analgesics may precipitate ▶

withdrawal symptoms and/or reduced analgesic efficacy in patients following prolonged therapy with mu opioid agonists. Abrupt discontinuation following prolonged use may also lead to withdrawal symptoms. Elderly and debilitated patients may be particularly susceptible to the adverse effects of narcotics. Safety and efficacy have not been established in children.

Adverse Reactions Frequency not defined.

Cardiovascular: Palpitation, hypotension, bradycardia, peripheral vasodilation, cardiac arrest, shock, tachycardia

Central nervous system: CNS depression, fatigue, drowsiness, dizziness, nervousness, headache, restlessness, anorexia, malaise, confusion, coma, convulsion, insomnia, amnesia, mental depression, hallucinations, paradoxical CNS stimulation, intracranial pressure increased

Dermatologic: Pruritus, urticaria, rash

Endocrine & metabolic: Antidiuretic hormone release

Gastrointestinal: Nausea, vomiting, dyspepsia, stomach cramps, xerostomia, constipation, abdominal pain, dry mouth, biliary tract spasm, paralytic ileus

Genitourinary: Decreased urination, urinary tract spasm, urinary retention

Local: Pain at injection site

Neuromuscular & skeletal: Weakness

Ocular: Miosis, diplopia

Respiratory: Respiratory depression, apnea, hypoventilation, cyanosis

Miscellaneous: Histamine release, physical and psychological dependence

Drug Interactions

Avoid Concomitant Use There are no known interactions where it is recommended to avoid concomitant use.

Increased Effect/Toxicity

Levorphanol may increase the levels/effects of: Alcohol (Ethyl); Alvimopan; CNS Depressants; Desmopressin; Selective Serotonin Reuptake Inhibitors; Thiazide Diuretics

The levels/effects of Levorphanol may be increased by: Amphetamines; Antipsychotic Agents (Phenothiazines); Succinylcholine

Decreased Effect

Levorphanol may decrease the levels/effects of: Pegvisomant

The levels/effects of Levorphanol may be decreased by: Ammonium Chloride

Ethanol/Nutrition/Herb Interactions

Ethanol: Avoid or limit ethanol (may increase CNS depression). Watch for sedation.

Herb/Nutraceutical: Avoid valerian, St John's wort, kava kava, gotu kola (may increase CNS depression).

Storage/Stability Store at room temperature; do not freeze.

Compatibility

Y-site administration: Compatible: Propofol.

Compatibility in syringe: Compatible: Glycopyrrolate.

Compatibility when admixed: Incompatible: Aminophylline, ammonium chloride, amobarbital, chlorothiazide, heparin, pentobarbital, phenobarbital, phenytoin, sodium bicarbonate, thiopental.

Mechanism of Action Levorphanol tartrate is a synthetic opioid agonist that is classified as a morphinan derivative. Opioids interact with stereospecific opioid receptors in various parts of the central nervous system and other tissues. Analgesic potency parallels the affinity for these binding sites. These drugs do not alter the threshold or responsiveness to pain, but the perception of pain.

Pharmacodynamics/Kinetics
Onset of action: Oral: 10-60 minutes
Duration: 4-8 hours
Metabolism: Hepatic
Half-life elimination: 11-16 hours
Excretion: Urine (as inactive metabolite)

Dosage Adults: **Note:** These are guidelines and do not represent the maximum doses that may be required in all patients. Doses should be titrated to pain relief/prevention.

Acute pain (moderate-to-severe):
Oral: Initial: Opiate-naive: 2 mg every 6-8 hours as needed; patients with prior opiate exposure may require higher initial doses; usual dosage range: 2-4 mg every 6-8 hours as needed
I.M., SubQ: Initial: Opiate-naive: 1 mg every 6-8 hours as needed; patients with prior opiate exposure may require higher initial doses; usual dosage range: 1-2 mg every 6-8 hours as needed
Slow I.V.: Initial: Opiate-naive: Up to 1 mg/dose every 3-6 hours as needed; patients with prior opiate exposure may require higher initial doses
Chronic pain: Patients taking opioids chronically may become tolerant and require doses higher than the usual dosage range to maintain the desired effect. Tolerance can be managed by appropriate dose titration. **There is no optimal or maximal dose for levorphanol in chronic pain. The appropriate dose is one that relieves pain throughout its dosing interval without causing unmanageable side effects.**
Premedication: I.M., SubQ: 1-2 mg/dose 60-90 minutes prior to surgery; older or debilitated patients usually require less drug

Dosing adjustment in hepatic disease: Reduction is necessary in patients with liver disease

Administration I.V.: Inject 3 mg over 4-5 minutes

Monitoring Parameters Pain relief, respiratory and mental status, blood pressure

Dosage Forms Excipient information presented when available (limited, particularly for generics); consult specific product labeling.
Injection, solution, as tartrate: 2 mg/mL (1 mL, 10 mL)
Tablet, as tartrate: 2 mg

References
"Drugs for Pain," *Med Lett Drugs Ther,* 2000, 42(1085):73-8.
"Principles of Analgesic Use in the Treatment of Acute Pain and Chronic Cancer Pain," 5th ed, Glenview, IL: American Pain Society, 2003.

♦ **Levorphanol Tartrate** *see* Levorphanol *on page 717*

♦ **Levorphan Tartrate** *see* Levorphanol *on page 717*

♦ **Levulan® Kerastick®** *see* Aminolevulinic Acid *on page 60*

♦ **LH-RH Agonist** *see* Histrelin *on page 570*

Lidocaine and Prilocaine (LYE doe kane & PRIL oh kane)

U.S. Brand Names EMLA®; Oraqix®
Index Terms Prilocaine and Lidocaine
Generic Available Yes: Cream
Canadian Brand Names EMLA®
Pharmacologic Category Local Anesthetic
Use Topical anesthetic for use on normal intact skin to provide local analgesia for minor procedures such as I.V. cannulation or venipuncture; has also been used for painful procedures such as lumbar puncture and skin graft harvesting;

for superficial minor surgery of genital mucous membranes and as an adjunct for local infiltration anesthesia in genital mucous membranes.

Pregnancy Risk Factor B

Lactation Lidocaine enters breast milk/use caution

Labeled Contraindications Hypersensitivity to amide-type anesthetic agents; hypersensitivity to any component of the formulation selected; application on mucous membranes or broken or inflamed skin; infants <1 month of age if gestational age is <37 weeks; infants <12 months of age receiving therapy with methemoglobin-inducing agents; children with congenital or idiopathic methemoglobinemia, or in children who are receiving medications associated with drug-induced methemoglobinemia (eg, acetaminophen [overdosage], benzocaine, chloroquine, dapsone, nitrofurantoin, nitroglycerin, nitroprusside, phenazopyridine, phenelzine, phenobarbital, phenytoin, quinine, sulfonamides)

Warnings/Precautions Use with caution in patients with severe hepatic impairment. Use with caution in the debilitated or acutely ill patients and the elderly. Use with caution in patients receiving class I and III antiarrhythmic drugs, since systemic absorption occurs and synergistic toxicity is possible. Although the incidence of systemic adverse reactions with EMLA® is very low, caution should be exercised, particularly when applying over large areas and leaving on for longer than 2 hours. Avoid use on open wounds or near the eyes.

Adverse Reactions Frequency not defined.

Cardiovascular: Hypotension, angioedema

Central nervous system: Shock

Dermatologic: Hyperpigmentation, erythema, itching, rash, burning, urticaria

Genitourinary: Blistering of foreskin (rare)

Local: Burning, stinging, edema

Respiratory: Bronchospasm

Miscellaneous: Alteration in temperature sensation, hypersensitivity reactions

Drug Interactions

Metabolism/Transport Effects Lidocaine: **Substrate** of CYP1A2 (minor), 2A6 (minor), 2B6 (minor), 2C9 (minor), 2D6 (major), 3A4 (major); **Inhibits** CYP1A2 (strong), 2D6 (strong), 3A4 (moderate)

Avoid Concomitant Use There are no known interactions where it is recommended to avoid concomitant use.

Increased Effect/Toxicity There are no known significant interactions involving an increase in effect.

Decreased Effect There are no known significant interactions involving a decrease in effect.

Storage/Stability Store at room temperature.

Mechanism of Action Local anesthetic action occurs by stabilization of neuronal membranes and inhibiting the ionic fluxes required for the initiation and conduction of impulses

Pharmacodynamics/Kinetics

EMLA®:

Onset of action: 1 hour

Peak effect: 2-3 hours

Duration: 1-2 hours after removal

Absorption: Related to duration of application and area where applied

3-hour application: 3.6% lidocaine and 6.1% prilocaine

24-hour application: 16.2% lidocaine and 33.5% prilocaine

See individual agents.

Dosage Although the incidence of systemic adverse effects with EMLA® is very low, caution should be exercised, particularly when applying over large areas and leaving on for >2 hours

Children (intact skin): EMLA® should **not** be used in neonates with a gestation age <37 weeks nor in infants <12 months of age who are receiving treatment with methemoglobin-inducing agents

Dosing is based on child's age and weight:

Age 0-3 months or <5 kg: Apply a maximum of 1 g over no more than 10 cm^2 of skin; leave on for no longer than 1 hour

Age 3 months to 12 months and >5 kg: Apply no more than a maximum 2 g total over no more than 20 cm^2 of skin; leave on for no longer than 4 hours

Age 1-6 years and >10 kg: Apply no more than a maximum of 10 g total over no more than 100 cm^2 of skin; leave on for no longer than 4 hours.

Age 7-12 years and >20 kg: Apply no more than a maximum 20 g total over no more than 200 cm^2 of skin; leave on for no longer than 4 hours.

Note: If a patient greater than 3 months old does not meet the minimum weight requirement, the maximum total dose should be restricted to the corresponding maximum based on patient weight.

Adults (intact skin):

EMLA® cream and EMLA® anesthetic disc: A thick layer of EMLA® cream is applied to intact skin and covered with an occlusive dressing, or alternatively, an EMLA® anesthetic disc is applied to intact skin

Minor dermal procedures (eg, I.V. cannulation or venipuncture): Apply 2.5 g of cream (1/2 of the 5 g tube) over 20-25 cm of skin surface area, or 1 anesthetic disc (1 g over 10 cm^2) for at least 1 hour. **Note:** In clinical trials, 2 sites were usually prepared in case there was a technical problem with cannulation or venipuncture at the first site.

Major dermal procedures (eg, more painful dermatological procedures involving a larger skin area such as split thickness skin graft harvesting): Apply 2 g of cream per 10 cm^2 of skin and allow to remain in contact with the skin for at least 2 hours.

Adult male genital skin (eg, pretreatment prior to local anesthetic infiltration): Apply a thick layer of cream (1 g/10 cm^2) to the skin surface for 15 minutes. Local anesthetic infiltration should be performed immediately after removal of EMLA® cream.

Note: Dermal analgesia can be expected to increase for up to 3 hours under occlusive dressing and persist for 1-2 hours after removal of the cream

Adult females: Genital mucous membranes: Minor procedures (eg, removal of condylomata acuminata, pretreatment for local anesthetic infiltration): Apply 5-10 g (thick layer) of cream for 5-10 minutes

Periodontal gel (Oraqix®): Adults: Apply on gingival margin around selected teeth using the blunt-tipped applicator included in package. Wait 30 seconds, then fill the periodontal pockets using the blunt-tipped applicator until gel becomes visible at the gingival margin. Wait another 30 seconds before starting treatment. Maximum recommended dose: One treatment session: 5 cartridges (8.5 g)

Administration For external use only. Avoid application to open wounds or near the eyes. In small infants and children, observe patient to prevent accidental ingestion of cream, disc, or dressing. Choose two application sites available for intravenous access. Apply a thick layer (2.5 g/site ~1/2 of a 5 g tube) of cream to each designated site of intact skin. Cover each site with the occlusive dressing (Tegaderm®). Mark the time on the dressing. **Allow at least 1 hour for optimum therapeutic effect.** Remove the dressing and wipe off

◀ excess EMLA® cream (gloves should be worn). **Smaller areas of treatment are recommended for debilitated patients.**

Dosage Forms Excipient information presented when available (limited, particularly for generics); consult specific product labeling.

Cream, topical: Lidocaine 2.5% and prilocaine 2.5% (5 g, 30 g)

EMLA®: Lidocaine 2.5% and prilocaine 2.5% (5 g, 30 g) [each packaged with Tegaderm® dressings]

Disc, topical: Lidocaine 2.5% and prilocaine 2.5% per disc (2s, 10s) [each 1 g disc is 10 cm^2]

Gel, periodontal:

Oraqix®: Lidocaine 2.5% and prilocaine 2.5% (1.7 g)

References

Broadman LM, Soliman IE, Hannallah RS, et al, "Analgesic Efficacy of Eutectic Mixture of Local Anesthetics (EMLA®) vs Intradermal Infiltration Prior to Venous Cannulation in Children," *Am J Anaesthesiol*, 1987, 34:S56.

Halperin DL, Koren G, Attias D, et al, "Topical Skin Anesthesia for Venous Subcutaneous Drug Reservoir and Lumbar Puncture in Children," *Pediatrics*, 1989, 84(2):281-4.

Robieux I, Kumar R, Radhakrishnan S, et al, "Assessing Pain and Analgesia With a Lidocaine-Prilocaine Emulsion in Infants and Toddlers During Venipuncture," *J Pediatr*, 1991, 118(6):971-3.

◆ **Lilly CT-3231** see Vindesine on page 1180

Linezolid (li NE zoh lid)

Medication Safety Issues

Sound-alike/look-alike issues:

Zyvox® may be confused with Ziox™, Zosyn®, Zovirax®

U.S. Brand Names Zyvox®

Generic Available No

Canadian Brand Names Zyvoxam®

Pharmacologic Category Antibiotic, Oxazolidinone

Use Treatment of vancomycin-resistant *Enterococcus faecium* (VRE) infections, nosocomial pneumonia caused by *Staphylococcus aureus* including MRSA or *Streptococcus pneumoniae* (including multidrug-resistant strains [MDRSP]), complicated and uncomplicated skin and skin structure infections (including diabetic foot infections without concomitant osteomyelitis), and community-acquired pneumonia caused by susceptible gram-positive organisms

Pregnancy Risk Factor C

Lactation Excretion in breast milk unknown/use caution

Labeled Contraindications Hypersensitivity to linezolid or any other component of the formulation; concurrent use or within 2 weeks of MAO inhibitors; patients with uncontrolled hypertension, pheochromocytoma, thyrotoxicosis, and/or taking sympathomimetics (eg, pseudoephedrine), vasopressive agents (eg, epinephrine, norepinephrine), or dopaminergic agents (eg, dopamine, dobutamine) unless closely monitored for increased blood pressure; patients with carcinoid syndrome and/or taking SSRIs, tricyclic antidepressants, serotonin 5-HT$_{1B,1D}$ receptor agonists, meperidine, or buspirone unless closely monitored for sign/symptoms of serotonin syndrome

Warnings/Precautions Myelosuppression has been reported and may be dependent on duration of therapy (generally >2 weeks of treatment); use with caution in patients with pre-existing myelosuppression, in patients receiving other drugs which may cause bone marrow suppression, or in chronic infection (previous or concurrent antibiotic therapy). Weekly CBC monitoring is recommended. Discontinue linezolid in patients developing myelosuppression (or in whom myelosuppression worsens during treatment).

Lactic acidosis has been reported with use. Linezolid exhibits mild MAO inhibitor properties and has the potential to have the same interactions as other MAO inhibitors; use with caution and monitor closely in patients with uncontrolled hypertension, pheochromocytoma, carcinoid syndrome, or untreated hyperthyroidism; use is contraindicated in the absence of close monitoring. Symptoms of agitation, confusion, hallucinations, hyper-reflexia, myoclonus, shivering, and tachycardia may occur with concomitant proserotonergic drugs (eg, SSRIs/SNRIs or triptans) or agents which reduce linezolid's metabolism; concurrent use with these medications is contraindicated unless patient is closely monitored for signs/symptoms of serotonin syndrome. Unnecessary use may lead to the development of resistance to linezolid; consider alternatives before initiating outpatient treatment.

Peripheral and optic neuropathy (with vision loss) has been reported and may occur primarily with extended courses of therapy >28 days; any symptoms of visual change or impairment warrant immediate ophthalmic evaluation and possible discontinuation of therapy. Seizures have been reported; use with caution in patients with a history of seizures. Prolonged use may result in fungal or bacterial superinfection, including *C. difficile*-associated diarrhea (CDAD) and pseudomembranous colitis; CDAD has been observed >2 months postantibiotic treatment.

Due to inconsistent concentrations in the CSF, empiric use in pediatric patients with CNS infections is not recommended by the manufacturer; however, there are multiple case reports describing successful treatment of documented VRE and *Staphylococcus aureus* CNS and shunt infections in the literature. Oral suspension contains phenylalanine.

Adverse Reactions Percentages as reported in adults; frequency similar in pediatric patients

>10%:

Central nervous system: Headache (<1% to 11%)

Gastrointestinal: Diarrhea (3% to 11%)

1% to 10%:

Central nervous system: Insomnia (3%), dizziness (≤2%), fever (2%)

Dermatologic: Rash (2%)

Gastrointestinal: Nausea (3% to 10%), vomiting (1% to 4%), pancreatic enzymes increased (≤4%), constipation (2%), taste alteration (1% to 2%), tongue discoloration (≤1%), oral moniliasis (≤1%), pancreatitis

Genitourinary: Vaginal moniliasis (1% to 2%)

Hematologic: Hemoglobin decreased (1% to 7%), thrombocytopenia (≤3%), anemia, leukopenia, neutropenia; **Note:** Myelosuppression (including anemia, leukopenia, pancytopenia, and thrombocytopenia; may be more common in patients receiving linezolid for >2 weeks)

Hepatic: Abnormal LFTs (≤10%), bilirubin increased (≤1%)

Renal: BUN increased (≤2%)

Miscellaneous: Fungal infection (0.1% to 2%), lactate dehydrogenase increased (<1% to 2%)

<1% or frequency not defined: Blurred vision, *C. difficile*-related complications, creatinine increased, dyspepsia, hypertension, localized abdominal pain, pruritus

Postmarketing and/or case reports: Anaphylaxis, angioedema, bullous skin disorders, lactic acidosis, peripheral neuropathy, optic neuropathy, seizures, serotonin syndrome (with concurrent use of other serotonergic agents), Stevens-Johnson syndrome, vision loss

Drug Interactions

Avoid Concomitant Use

Avoid concomitant use of Linezolid with any of the following: Alpha-/Beta-Agonists (Indirect-Acting); Alpha1-Agonists; Alpha2-Agonists (Ophthalmic); Amphetamines; Anilidopiperidine Opioids; Atomoxetine; BuPROPion; BusPIRone; CarBAMazepine; Cyclobenzaprine; Dexmethylphenidate; Dextromethorphan; MAO Inhibitors; Maprotiline; Meperidine; Methyldopa; Methylphenidate; Mirtazapine; Propoxyphene; Selective Serotonin Reuptake Inhibitors; Serotonin 5-HT1D Receptor Agonists; Serotonin/Norepinephrine Reuptake Inhibitors; Sibutramine; Tapentadol; Tetrabenazine; Tricyclic Antidepressants

Increased Effect/Toxicity

Linezolid may increase the levels/effects of: Alpha-/Beta-Agonists (Direct-Acting); Alpha-/Beta-Agonists (Indirect-Acting); Alpha1-Agonists; Alpha2-Agonists (Ophthalmic); Amphetamines; Antihypertensives; Atomoxetine; Beta2-Agonists; BuPROPion; Dexmethylphenidate; Dextromethorphan; Lithium; Meperidine; Methyldopa; Methylphenidate; Mirtazapine; Orthostasis Producing Agents; Rauwolfia Alkaloids; Selective Serotonin Reuptake Inhibitors; Serotonin 5-HT1D Receptor Agonists; Serotonin Modulators; Serotonin/Norepinephrine Reuptake Inhibitors; Tricyclic Antidepressants

The levels/effects of Linezolid may be increased by: Altretamine; Anilidopiperidine Opioids; BusPIRone; CarBAMazepine; COMT Inhibitors; Cyclobenzaprine; Levodopa; MAO Inhibitors; Maprotiline; Propoxyphene; Sibutramine; Tapentadol; Tetrabenazine; TraMADol

Decreased Effect There are no known significant interactions involving a decrease in effect.

Ethanol/Nutrition/Herb Interactions

Ethanol: Avoid ethanol (based on CNS depressant effects and potential tyramine content)

Food: Concurrent ingestion of foods rich in tyramine may cause sudden and severe high blood pressure (hypertensive crisis). Avoid tyramine-containing foods with MAO-Is. Food's freshness is also an important concern; improperly stored or spoiled food can create an environment where tyramine concentrations may increase.

Herb/Nutraceutical: Avoid supplements containing caffeine, tyrosine, tryptophan or phenylalanine. Ingestion of large quantities may increase the risk of severe side effects (eg, hypertensive reactions, serotonin syndrome).

Storage/Stability

Infusion: Store at 25°C (77°F). Protect from light. Keep infusion bags in overwrap until ready for use. Protect infusion bags from freezing.

Oral suspension: Following reconstitution, store at 25°C (77°F). Use reconstituted suspension within 21 days. Protect from light.

Tablet: Store at 25°C (77°F). Protect from light; protect from moisture.

Reconstitution Oral suspension: Reconstitute with 123 mL of distilled water (in 2 portions); shake vigorously. Concentration is 100 mg/5 mL. Prior to administration mix gently by inverting bottle; do not shake.

Compatibility Stable in D_5W, LR, NS

Y-site administration: Compatible: Acyclovir, alfentanil, amikacin, aminophylline, ampicillin, ampicillin sulbactam, aztreonam, bretylium, buprenorphine, butorphanol, calcium gluconate, carboplatin, cefazolin, cefotetan, cefoxitin, ceftazidime, ceftizoxime, ceftriaxone, cefuroxime, cimetidine, ciprofloxacin, cisatracurium, cisplatin, clindamycin, cyclophosphamide, cyclosporine, cytarabine, dexamethasone, dexmedetomidine, $D_5$1/2 NS, D_5NS, digoxin, diphenhydramine, dobutamine, dopamine, doxorubicin, doxycycline, droperidol, enalaprilat, Esmolol, etoposide phosphate, famotidine, fenoldopam, fentanyl, fluconazole, fluorouracil, furosemide, ganciclovir, gemcitabine, gentamicin, granisetron, haloperidol, heparin, hydrocortisone sodium succinate, hydromorphone, hydroxyzine, ifosfamide, imipenem, labetalol, leucovorin, levofloxacin, lidocaine, lorazepam, magnesium sulfate, mannitol, meperidine, meropenem, mesna, methotrexate, methylprednisolone sodium succinate, metoclopramide, metronidazole, midazolam, mitoxantrone, morphine, nalbuphine, naloxone, nicardipine, nitroglycerin, ofloxacin, ondansetron, paclitaxel, pentobarbital, phenobarbital, piperacillin (tazobactam), potassium chloride, prochlorperazine, promethazine, propranolol, ranitidine remifentanil, sodium bicarbonate, sufentanil, theophylline, tobramycin, vancomycin, vecuronium, verapamil, vincristine, zidovudine. **Incompatible:** Amphotericin B, chlorpromazine, diazepam, erythromycin, pentamidine, phenytoin, sulfamethoxazole/trimethoprim.

Compatibility when admixed: Compatible: Aztreonam, cefazolin, ceftazidime, ciprofloxacin, gentamicin, levofloxacin, ofloxacin, tobramycin. **Incompatible:** Ceftriaxone, erythromycin, sulfamethoxazole/trimethoprim.

Mechanism of Action Inhibits bacterial protein synthesis by binding to bacterial 23S ribosomal RNA of the 50S subunit. This prevents the formation of a functional 70S initiation complex that is essential for the bacterial translation process. Linezolid is bacteriostatic against enterococci and staphylococci and bactericidal against most strains of streptococci.

Pharmacodynamics/Kinetics

Absorption: Rapid and extensive

Distribution: V_{dss}: Adults: 40-50 L

Protein binding: Adults: 31%

Metabolism: Hepatic via oxidation of the morpholine ring, resulting in two inactive metabolites (aminoethoxyacetic acid, hydroxyethyl glycine); does not involve CYP

Bioavailability: Oral: ~100%

Half-life elimination: Children ≥1 week (full-term) to 11 years: 1.5-3 hours; Adults: 4-5 hours

Time to peak: Adults: Oral: 1-2 hours

Excretion: Urine (30% as parent drug, 50% as metabolites); feces (9% as metabolites)

Nonrenal clearance: ~65%; increased in children ≥1 week to 11 years

Dosage

Oral, I.V.:

VRE infections including concurrent bacteremia:

Preterm neonates (<34 weeks gestational age): 10 mg/kg every 12 hours; neonates with a suboptimal clinical response can be advanced to 10 mg/kg every 8 hours. By day 7 of life, all neonates should receive 10 mg/kg every 8 hours.

Infants (excluding preterm neonates <1 week) and Children ≤11 years: 10 mg/kg every 8 hours for 14-28 days

Children ≥12 years and Adults: 600 mg every 12 hours for 14-28 days

MRSA: Adults: 600 mg every 12 hours

Nosocomial pneumonia, complicated skin and skin structure infections, community acquired pneumonia including concurrent bacteremia: Oral, I.V.:

Preterm neonates (<34 weeks gestational age): 10 mg/kg every 12 hours; neonates with a suboptimal clinical response can be advanced to 10 mg/kg every 8 hours. By day 7 of life, all neonates should receive 10 mg/kg every 8 hours.

Infants (excluding preterm neonates <1 week) and Children ≤11 years: 10 mg/kg every 8 hours for 10-14 days

Children ≥12 years and Adults: 600 mg every 12 hours for 10-14 days

Uncomplicated skin and skin structure infections: Oral:

Preterm neonates (<34 weeks gestational age): 10 mg/kg every 12 hours; neonates with a suboptimal clinical response can be advanced to 10 mg/kg every 8 hours. By day 7 of life, all neonates should receive 10 mg/kg every 8 hours.

Infants (excluding preterm neonates <1 week) and Children <5 years: 10 mg/kg every 8 hours for 10-14 days

Children 5-11 years: 10 mg/kg every 12 hours for 10-14 days

Children ≥12-18 years: 600 mg every 12 hours for 10-14 days

Adults: 400 mg every 12 hours for 10-14 days

Note: 400 mg dose is recommended in the product labeling; however, 600 mg dose is commonly employed clinically

Elderly: No dosage adjustment required

Dosage adjustment in renal impairment: No adjustment is recommended. The two primary metabolites may accumulate in patients with renal impairment but the clinical significance is unknown. Weigh the risk of accumulation of metabolites versus the benefit of therapy. Monitor for hematopoietic (eg, anemia, leukopenia, thrombocytopenia) and neuropathic (eg, peripheral neuropathy) adverse events when administering for extended periods. Both linezolid and the two metabolites are eliminated by dialysis. Linezolid should be given after hemodialysis.

Continuous renal replacement therapy (CRRT): No adjustment needed.

Dosage adjustment in hepatic impairment: No dosage adjustment required for mild-to-moderate hepatic insufficiency (Child-Pugh Class A or B). Use in severe hepatic insufficiency has not been adequately evaluated.

Administration

I.V.: Administer intravenous infusion over 30-120 minutes. Do not mix or infuse with other medications. When the same intravenous line is used for sequential infusion of other medications, flush line with D_5W, NS, or LR before and after infusing linezolid. The yellow color of the injection may intensify over time without affecting potency.

Oral suspension: Invert gently to mix prior to administration, do not shake.

Monitoring Parameters Weekly CBC and platelet counts, particularly in patients at increased risk of bleeding, with pre-existing myelosuppression, on concomitant medications that cause bone marrow suppression, in those who require >2 weeks of therapy, or in those with chronic infection who have received previous or concomitant antibiotic therapy; visual function with extended therapy (≥3 months) or in patients with new onset visual symptoms, regardless of therapy length

Dietary Considerations Take with or without food. Avoid consuming large amounts of tyramine-containing foods/beverages. Some examples include aged or matured cheese, air-dried or cured meats (including sausages and salamis), fava or broad bean pods, tap/draft beers, Marmite concentrate, sauerkraut, soy sauce and other soybean condiments.

Suspension contains 20 mg phenylalanine per teaspoonful. Sodium content: 0.1 mEq/tablet; 0.4 mEq/5 mL; 1.7 mEq/100 mL infusion; 3.3 mEq/200 mL infusion; 5 mEq/300 mL infusion

Dosage Forms Excipient information presented when available (limited, particularly for generics); consult specific product labeling.

Infusion [premixed]:

Zyvox®: 200 mg (100 mL) [contains sodium 1.7 mEq]; 600 mg (300 mL) [contains sodium 5 mEq]

Powder for oral suspension:

Zyvox®: 20 mg/mL (150 mL) [contains phenylalanine 20 mg/5 mL, sodium benzoate, and sodium 0.4 mEq/5 mL; orange flavor]

Tablet:

Zyvox®: 600 mg [contains sodium 0.1 mEq/tablet]

References

Bain KT and Wittbrodt ET, "Linezolid for the Treatment of Resistant Gram-Positive Cocci," *Ann Pharmacother*, 2001, 35(5):566-75.

Mandell LA, Wunderink RG, Anzueto A, et al, "Infectious Diseases Society of America/American Thoracic Society Consensus Guidelines on the Management of Community-Acquired Pneumonia in Adults," *Clin Infect Dis*, 2007, 44(Suppl 2):27-72.

Perry CM and Jarvis B, "Linezolid: A Review of Its Use in the Management of Serious Gram-Positive Infections," *Drugs*, 2001, 61(4):525-51.

Roberts JA and Lipman J, "Antibacterial Dosing in Intensive Care: Pharmacokinetics, Degree of Disease and Pharmacodynamics of Sepsis," *Clin Pharmacokinet*, 2006, 45(8):755-73.

Shulman KI and Walker SE, "A Reevaluation of Dietary Restrictions for Irreversible Monoamine Oxidase Inhibitors," *Psychiatr Ann*, 2001, 31(6):378-84.

Shulman KI and Walker SE, "Refining the MAOI Diet: Tyramine Content of Pizzas and Soy Products," *J Clin Psychiatry*, 1999, 60(3):191-3.

Walker SE, Shulman KI, Tailor SA, et al, "Tyramine Content of Previously Restricted Foods in Monoamine Oxidase Inhibitor Diets," *J Clin Psychopharmacol*, 1996, 16(5):383-8.

♦ **Liposomal DAUNOrubicin** see DAUNOrubicin Citrate (Liposomal) *on page 319*

♦ **Liposomal DOXOrubicin** see DOXOrubicin (Liposomal) *on page 379*

♦ **L-leucovorin** see LEVOleucovorin *on page 714*

♦ **LM3100** see Plerixafor *on page 965*

♦ **Locoid®** see Hydrocortisone *on page 575*

♦ **Locoid Lipocream®** see Hydrocortisone *on page 575*

♦ **L-OHP** see Oxaliplatin *on page 882*

Lomustine (loe MUS teen)

Medication Safety Issues

Sound-alike/look-alike issues:

Lomustine may be confused with bendamustine, carmustine

High alert medication: The Institute for Safe Medication Practices (ISMP) includes this medication among its list of drug classes which have a heightened risk of causing significant patient harm when used in error.

Lomustine should only be administered as a single dose once every 6 weeks; serious errors have occurred when lomustine was inadvertently administered daily.

Related Information

Safe Handling of Hazardous Drugs *on page 1517*

U.S. Brand Names CeeNU®

Index Terms CCNU; Lomustinum

Generic Available No

Canadian Brand Names CeeNU®

Pharmacologic Category Antineoplastic Agent; Antineoplastic Agent, Alkylating Agent; Antineoplastic Agent, Alkylating Agent (Nitrosourea)

Use Treatment of primary and metastatic brain tumors (after surgery and/or radiation therapy); treatment of relapsed or refractory Hodgkin's disease (as part of a combination chemotherapy regimen)

◀ **Unlabeled/Investigational Use** Treatment of gastric cancer, metastatic melanoma

Pregnancy Risk Factor D

Lactation Enters breast milk/not recommended

Labeled Contraindications Hypersensitivity to lomustine or any component of the formulation

Warnings/Precautions Hazardous agent - use appropriate precautions for handling and disposal. **[U.S. Boxed Warnings]: Cumulative and delayed bone marrow suppression, particularly thrombocytopenia and leukopenia, commonly occur; may lead to bleeding and overwhelming infections in an already compromised patient.** Do not administer courses more frequently than every 6 weeks due to delayed myelotoxicity. Use with caution in patients with depressed platelet, leukocyte, or erythrocyte counts. Because bone marrow toxicity is cumulative, dose adjustments should be based on nadir counts from prior dose.

May cause delayed pulmonary toxicity (infiltrates and/or fibrosis); usually related to cumulative doses >1100 mg/m^2; may be delayed (has been reported up to 17 years after childhood administration in combination with radiation therapy); patients with baseline below 70% of predicted forced vital capacity or carbon monoxide diffusing capacity are in increased risk. Long-term use may be associated with the development of secondary malignancies. Reversible hepatotoxicity (transaminase, alkaline phosphatase and bilirubin elevations) has been reported; use with caution in patients with hepatic impairment. Kidney damage has been observed and azotemia, decreased kidney size and renal failure have been reported with long-term use; use with caution in patients with renal impairment; may require dosage adjustment. **[U.S. Boxed Warning]: Should be administered under the supervision of an experienced cancer chemotherapy physician.**

Adverse Reactions

>10%:

Gastrointestinal: Nausea and vomiting, (onset: 3-6 hours after oral administration; duration: <24 hours)

Hematologic: Myelosuppression (dose-limiting, delayed, cumulative); leukopenia (65%; nadir: 5-6 weeks; recovery 6-8 weeks); thrombocytopenia (nadir: 4 weeks; recovery 5-6 weeks)

Frequency not defined: Acute leukemia, alkaline phosphatase increased, alopecia, anemia, ataxia, azotemia (progressive), bilirubin increased, blindness, bone marrow dysplasia, disorientation, dysarthria, hepatotoxicity, kidney size decreased, lethargy, optic atrophy, pulmonary fibrosis, pulmonary infiltrates, renal damage, renal failure, stomatitis, transaminases increased, visual disturbances

Drug Interactions

Metabolism/Transport Effects Substrate of CYP2D6 (major); **Inhibits** CYP2D6 (weak), 3A4 (weak)

Avoid Concomitant Use

Avoid concomitant use of Lomustine with any of the following: Natalizumab; Vaccines (Live)

Increased Effect/Toxicity

Lomustine may increase the levels/effects of: Leflunomide; Natalizumab; Vaccines (Live)

The levels/effects of Lomustine may be increased by: CYP2D6 Inhibitors (Moderate); CYP2D6 Inhibitors (Strong); Darunavir; Trastuzumab

Decreased Effect

Lomustine may decrease the levels/effects of: Vaccines (Inactivated); Vaccines (Live)

The levels/effects of Lomustine may be decreased by: Echinacea; Peginterferon Alfa-2b

Ethanol/Nutrition/Herb Interactions Ethanol: Avoid ethanol (due to GI irritation).

Storage/Stability Store at room temperature of 25°C (77°F); excursions permitted to 15°C to 30°C (59°F to 86°F).

Mechanism of Action Inhibits DNA and RNA synthesis via carbamylation of DNA polymerase, alkylation of DNA, and alteration of RNA, proteins, and enzymes

Pharmacodynamics/Kinetics

Duration: Marrow recovery: ~5-8 weeks

Absorption: Complete

Distribution: Crosses blood-brain barrier to a greater degree than BCNU; CNS concentrations are ≥50% of plasma concentrations

Metabolism: Rapidly hepatic via hydroxylation producing at least two active metabolites; enterohepatically recycled

Half-life elimination: Parent drug: 16-24 hours; Active metabolite: 16-48 hours

Time to peak, serum: Active metabolite: ~3 hours

Excretion: Urine (~50%, as metabolites); feces (<5%); expired air (<10%)

Dosage Note: Repeat courses should only be administered after adequate recovery of leukocytes to >4000/mm^3 and platelets to >100,000/mm^3. Details concerning dosage in combination regimens should also be consulted.

Oral:

Children and Adults: Brain tumors, Hodgkin's lymphoma: 130 mg/m^2 as a single dose once every 6 weeks (dosage reductions may be recommended for combination chemotherapy regimens)

Compromised marrow function: Reduce dose to 100 mg/m^2 as a single.dose once every 6 weeks

Dosing adjustment (based on nadir) for subsequent cycles:

Leukocytes >3000/mm^3, platelets >75,000/mm^3: No adjustment required

Leukocytes 2000-2999/mm^3, platelets 25,000-74,999/mm^3: Administer 70% of prior dose

Leukocytes <2000/mm^3, platelets <25,000/mm^3: Administer 50% of prior dose

Dosage adjustment in renal impairment: The FDA-approved labeling does not contain renal dosing adjustment guidelines. The following guidelines have been used by some clinicians:

Aronoff, 2007: Adults:

Cl_{cr} 10-50 mL/minute: Administer 75% of dose

Cl_{cr} <10 mL/minute: Administer 25% to 50% of dose

Hemodialysis: Supplemental dose is not necessary

Continuous ambulatory peritoneal dialysis (CAPD): Administer 25% to 50% of dose

Kintzel, 1995:

Cl_{cr} 46-60 mL/minute: Administer 75% of normal dose

Cl_{cr} 31-45 mL/minute: Administer 70% of normal dose

Cl_{cr} ≤30 mL/minute: Avoid use

Dosage adjustment in hepatic impairment: The FDA-approved labeling does not contain hepatic adjustment guidelines; lomustine is hepatically metabolized and caution should be used in patients with hepatic dysfunction.

◄ **Combination Regimens**
Brain tumors:
8 in 1 (Brain Tumors) on page 1221
PCV (Brain Tumor Regimen) on page 1392
POC on page 1396
Gastric cancer: FAMe on page 1320
Lymphoma, Hodgkin's disease: CAD/MOPP/ABV on page 1242
Melanoma:
BOLD on page 1235
BOLD + Interferon on page 1235
BOLD (Melanoma) on page 1237
Retinoblastoma: 8 in 1 (Retinoblastoma) on page 1222

Administration Oral: Administer with fluids on an empty stomach; no food or drink for 2 hours after administration. Administering on an empty stomach will reduce the incidence of nausea and vomiting. Standard antiemetics may be administered if needed. Varying strengths of capsules may be required to obtain necessary dose.

Do not break capsules; use appropriate precautions (eg, gloves) when handling; avoid exposure to broken capsules.

Monitoring Parameters CBC with differential and platelet count (for at least 6 weeks after dose), hepatic and renal function tests (periodic), pulmonary function tests (baseline and periodic)

Dietary Considerations Should be taken with fluids on an empty stomach; no food or drink for 2 hours after administration to decrease nausea.

Emetic Potential Moderate (30% to 90%)

Dosage Forms Excipient information presented when available (limited, particularly for generics); consult specific product labeling.
Capsule:
CeeNU® 10 mg, 40 mg, 100 mg

References

Aronoff GR, Bennett WM, Berns JS, et al, *Drug Prescribing in Renal Failure: Dosing Guidelines for Adults and Children*, 5th ed. Philadelphia, PA: American College of Physicians; 2007, p 101.

Cullinan SA, Moertel CG, Wieand HS, et al, "Controlled Evaluation of Three Drug Combination Regimens Versus Fluorouracil Alone for the Therapy of Advanced Gastric Cancer. North Central Cancer Treatment Group," *J Clin Oncol*, 1994, 12(2):412-6.

Federico M, Luminari S, Iannitto E, et al, "ABVD Compared With BEACOPP Compared With CEC for the Initial Treatment of Patients With Advanced Hodgkin's Lymphoma: Results From the HD2000 Gruppo Italiano per lo Studio dei Linfomi Trial," *J Clin Oncol*, 2009, 27(5):805-11.

Kintzel PE and Dorr RT, "Anticancer Drug Renal Toxicity and Elimination: Dosing Guidelines for Altered Renal Function," *Cancer Treat Rev*, 1995, 21(1):33-64.

Lakhani S, Selby P, Bliss JM, et al, "Chemotherapy for Malignant Melanoma: Combinations and High Doses Produce More Responses Without Survival Benefit," *Br J Cancer*, 1990, 61(2):330-4.

Lee FY, Workman P, Roberts JT, et al, "Clinical Pharmacokinetics or Oral CCNU (Lomustine)," *Cancer Chemother Pharmacol*, 1985, 14(2):125-31.

Medical Research Council Brain Tumor Working Party, "Randomized Trial of Procarbazine, Lomustine, and Vincristine in the Adjuvant Treatment of High-Grade Astrocytoma: A Medical Research Council Trial," *J Clin Oncol*, 2001, 19(2):509-18.

National Comprehensive Cancer Network® (NCCN), "Clinical Practice Guidelines in Oncology™: Central Nervous System Cancers," Version 1.2009. Available at http://www.nccn.org/professionals/physician_gls/PDF/cns.pdf

Pendergrass TW, Milstein JM, Geyer JR, et al, "Eight Drugs in One Day Chemotherapy for Brain Tumors: Experience in 107 Children and Rationale for Preradiation Chemotherapy," *J Clin Oncol*, 1987, 5(8):1221-31.

◆ **Lomustinum** *see* Lomustine *on page* 727

LORazepam (lor A ze pam)

Medication Safety Issues

Sound-alike/look-alike issues:

LORazepam may be confused with ALPRAZolam, clonazePAM, diazepam, Lovaza®, temazepam, zolpidem

Ativan® may be confused with Ambien®, Atarax®, Atgam®, Avitene®

Injection dosage form contains propylene glycol. Monitor for toxicity when administering continuous lorazepam infusions.

Related Information

Management of Chemotherapy-Induced Nausea and Vomiting *on page 1434*

U.S. Brand Names Ativan®; Lorazepam Intensol™

Generic Available Yes

Canadian Brand Names Apo-Lorazepam®; Ativan®; Lorazepam Injection, USP; Novo-Lorazepam; Nu-Loraz; PHL-Lorazepam; PMS-Lorazepam; Riva-Lorazepam

Pharmacologic Category Benzodiazepine

Use

Oral: Management of anxiety disorders or short-term (≤4 months) relief of the symptoms of anxiety or anxiety associated with depressive symptoms

I.V.: Status epilepticus, amnesia, sedation

Unlabeled/Investigational Use Ethanol detoxification; insomnia; psychogenic catatonia; partial complex seizures; agitation (I.V.); antiemetic adjunct

Restrictions C-IV

Pregnancy Risk Factor D

Lactation Enters breast milk/not recommended (AAP rates "of concern")

Labeled Contraindications Hypersensitivity to lorazepam or any component of the formulation (cross-sensitivity with other benzodiazepines may exist); acute narrow-angle glaucoma; sleep apnea (parenteral); intra-arterial injection of parenteral formulation; severe respiratory insufficiency (except during mechanical ventilation)

Warnings/Precautions Use with caution in elderly or debilitated patients, patients with hepatic disease (including alcoholics) or renal impairment. Use with caution in patients with respiratory disease (COPD or sleep apnea) or limited pulmonary reserve, or impaired gag reflex. Initial doses in elderly or debilitated patients should be at the lower end of the dosing range. May worsen hepatic encephalopathy.

Causes CNS depression (dose-related) resulting in sedation, dizziness, confusion, or ataxia which may impair physical and mental capabilities. Patients must be cautioned about performing tasks which require mental alertness (eg, operating machinery or driving). Use with caution in patients receiving other CNS depressants or psychoactive agents. Effects with other sedative drugs or ethanol may be potentiated. Benzodiazepines have been associated with falls and traumatic injury and should be used with extreme caution in patients who are at risk of these events (especially the elderly).

Lorazepam may cause anterograde amnesia. Paradoxical reactions, including hyperactive or aggressive behavior have been reported with benzodiazepines, particularly in adolescent/pediatric or psychiatric patients. Does not have analgesic, antidepressant, or antipsychotic properties.

Use caution in patients with depression, particularly if suicidal risk may be present. Pre-existing depression may worsen or emerge during therapy. Not recommended for use in primary depressive or psychotic disorders. Use with caution in patients with a history of drug dependence, alcoholism, or significant personality disorders. Benzodiazepines have been associated with dependence and acute withdrawal symptoms on discontinuation or reduction in dose. Acute withdrawal, including seizures, may be precipitated after administration of flumazenil to patients receiving long-term benzodiazepine therapy.

As a hypnotic agent, should be used only after evaluation of potential causes of sleep disturbance. Failure of sleep disturbance to resolve after 7-10 days may indicate psychiatric or medical illness. A worsening of insomnia or the emergence of new abnormalities of thought or behavior may represent unrecognized psychiatric or medical illness and requires immediate and careful evaluation.

Parenteral formulation of lorazepam contains polyethylene glycol which has resulted in toxicity during high-dose and/or longer-term infusions. Parenteral formulation also contains propylene glycol (PG); may be associated with dose-related toxicity and can occur ≥48 hours after initiation of lorazepam. Limited data suggest increased risk of PG accumulation at doses of ≥6 mg/hour for 48 hours or more (Nelson, 2008). Consider monitoring for signs of toxicity which may include acute renal failure, lactic acidosis, and/or osmol gap. In high-risk patients requiring higher doses/extended treatment durations, use of enteral delivery of lorazepam tablets may be beneficial (Jacobi, 2002). Also contains benzyl alcohol; avoid in neonates.

Safety and efficacy have not been established in children <12 years of age.

Adverse Reactions

>10%:

Central nervous system: Sedation

Respiratory: Respiratory depression

1% to 10%:

Cardiovascular: Hypotension

Central nervous system: Akathisia, amnesia, ataxia, confusion, depression, disorientation, dizziness, headache

Dermatologic: Dermatitis, rash

Gastrointestinal: Changes in appetite, nausea, weight gain/loss

Neuromuscular & skeletal: Weakness

Ocular: Visual disturbances

Respiratory: Apnea, hyperventilation, nasal congestion

<1% or frequency not defined: Asthenia, blood dyscrasias, disinhibition, euphoria, fatigue, increased salivation, menstrual irregularities, physical and psychological dependence (with prolonged use), reflex slowing, polyethylene glycol or propylene glycol poisoning (prolonged I.V. infusion), suicidal ideation, seizure, vertigo

Drug Interactions

Avoid Concomitant Use There are no known interactions where it is recommended to avoid concomitant use.

Increased Effect/Toxicity

LORazepam may increase the levels/effects of: Alcohol (Ethyl); Clozapine; CNS Depressants; Methotrimeprazine; Phenytoin

The levels/effects of LORazepam may be increased by: Loxapine; Methotrimeprazine; Probenecid; Valproic Acid

Decreased Effect

The levels/effects of LORazepam may be decreased by: Theophylline Derivatives; Yohimbine

Ethanol/Nutrition/Herb Interactions

Ethanol: Avoid or limit ethanol (may increase CNS depression).

Herb/Nutraceutical: Avoid valerian, St John's wort, kava kava, gotu kola (may increase CNS depression).

Storage/Stability

I.V.: Intact vials should be refrigerated. Protect from light. Do not use discolored or precipitate-containing solutions. May be stored at room temperature for up to 60 days. Parenteral admixture is stable at room temperature (25°C) for 24 hours.

Tablet: Store at room temperature.

Reconstitution

Injection: Dilute with equal volume of compatible diluent (D_5W, NS, SWI).

Infusion: Use 2 mg/mL injectable vial to prepare; there may be deceased stability when using 4 mg/mL vial. Dilute ≤1 mg/mL and mix in glass bottle. Precipitation may develop. Can also be administered undiluted via infusion.

Compatibility Variable stability (consult detailed reference) in D_5W, LR, NS.

Y-site administration: Compatible: Acyclovir, alatrofloxacin, albumin, allopurinol, amifostine, amikacin, amphotericin B cholesteryl sulfate complex, amsacrine, atracurium, bumetanide, cefepime, cefotaxime, ciprofloxacin, cisatracurium, cisplatin, cladribine, clonidine, co-trimoxazole, cyclophosphamide, cytarabine, dexamethasone sodium phosphate, diltiazem, dobutamine, docetaxel, dopamine, doxorubicin, doxorubicin liposome, epinephrine, erythromycin lactobionate, etomidate, etoposide phosphate, famotidine, fentanyl, filgrastim, fluconazole, fludarabine, fosphenytoin, furosemide, gatifloxacin, gemcitabine, gentamicin, granisetron, haloperidol, heparin, hydrocortisone sodium succinate, hydromorphone, ketanserin, labetalol, levofloxacin, linezolid, melphalan, methotrexate, metronidazole, midazolam, milrinone, morphine, nicardipine, nitroglycerin, norepinephrine, paclitaxel, pancuronium, piperacillin, piperacillin/tazobactam, potassium chloride, propofol, ranitidine, remifentanil, tacrolimus, teniposide, thiotepa, vancomycin, vecuronium, vinorelbine, zidovudine. Incompatible: Aldesleukin, aztreonam, floxacillin, idarubicin, imipenem/cilastatin, omeprazole, ondansetron, sargramostim, sufentanil. Variable (consult detailed reference): Foscarnet, thiopental, TPN.

Compatibility in syringe: Compatible: Cimetidine, hydromorphone. Incompatible: Sufentanil. Variable (consult detailed reference): Ranitidine.

Compatibility when admixed: Incompatible: Buprenorphine, dexamethasone sodium phosphate with diphenhydramine and metoclopramide.

Mechanism of Action Binds to stereospecific benzodiazepine receptors on the postsynaptic GABA neuron at several sites within the central nervous system, including the limbic system, reticular formation. Enhancement of the inhibitory effect of GABA on neuronal excitability results by increased neuronal membrane permeability to chloride ions. This shift in chloride ions results in hyperpolarization (a less excitable state) and stabilization.

Pharmacodynamics/Kinetics

Onset of action:

Hypnosis: I.M.: 20-30 minutes

Sedation: I.V.: 5-20 minutes

Anticonvulsant: I.V.: 5 minutes, oral: 30-60 minutes

Duration: 6-8 hours

Absorption: Oral, I.M.: Prompt

Distribution:
V_d: Neonates: 0.76 L/kg, Adults: 1.3 L/kg; crosses placenta; enters breast milk

Protein binding: 85%; free fraction may be significantly higher in elderly

Metabolism: Hepatic to inactive compounds

Bioavailability: Oral: 90%

Half-life elimination: Neonates: 40.2 hours; Older children: 10.5 hours; Adults: 12.9 hours; Elderly: 15.9 hours; End-stage renal disease: 32-70 hours

Time to peak: Oral: 2 hours

Excretion: Urine; feces (minimal)

Dosage

Antiemetic (unlabeled use):
Children 2-15 years: I.V.: 0.05 mg/kg (up to 2 mg/dose) prior to chemotherapy

Adults: Oral, I.V. (**Note:** May be administered sublingually; not a labeled route): 0.5-2 mg every 4-6 hours as needed

Anxiety and sedation (unlabeled in children except for oral use in children >12 years):
Infants and Children: Oral, I.M., I.V.: Usual: 0.05 mg/kg/dose (range: 0.02-0.09 mg/kg) every 4-8 hours

I.V.: May use smaller doses (eg, 0.01-0.03 mg/kg) and repeat every 20 minutes, as needed to titrate to effect

Adults: Oral: 1-10 mg/day in 2-3 divided doses; usual dose: 2-6 mg/day in divided doses

Elderly: 0.5-4 mg/day; initial dose not to exceed 2 mg

Insomnia: Adults: Oral: 2-4 mg at bedtime

Preoperative: Adults:
I.M.: 0.05 mg/kg administered 2 hours before surgery (maximum: 4 mg/dose)

I.V.: 0.044 mg/kg 15-20 minutes before surgery (usual maximum: 2 mg/dose)

Preprocedural anxiety (dental use): Adults: Oral: 1-2 mg 1 hour before procedure

Operative amnesia: Adults: I.V.: Up to 0.05 mg/kg (maximum: 4 mg/dose)

Sedation (preprocedure): Infants and Children (unlabeled):
Oral, I.M., I.V.: Usual: 0.05 mg/kg (range: 0.02-0.09 mg/kg)

I.V.: May use smaller doses (eg, 0.01-0.03 mg/kg) and repeat every 20 minutes, as needed to titrate to effect

Status epilepticus: I.V.:
Infants and Children (unlabeled): 0.05-0.1 mg/kg (maximum: 4 mg/dose) slow I.V. (maximum rate: 2 mg/minute); may repeat every 10-15 minutes as needed (Hegenbarth, 2008; Sabo-Graham, 1998)

Adults: 4 mg/dose slow I.V. (maximum rate: 2 mg/minute); may repeat in 10-15 minutes; usual maximum dose: 8 mg

Rapid tranquilization of agitated patient (administer every 30-60 minutes): Adults:
Oral: 1-2 mg

I.M.: 0.5-1 mg

Average total dose for tranquilization: Oral, I.M.: 4-8 mg

Agitation in the ICU patient (unlabeled): Adults:
I.V.: 0.02-0.06 mg/kg every 2-6 hours

I.V. infusion: 0.01-0.1 mg/kg/hour

Concurrent use of probenecid or valproic acid: Reduce lorazepam dose by 50%

Dosage adjustment in renal impairment: I.V.: Risk of propylene glycol toxicity. Monitor closely if using for prolonged periods of time or at high doses.

Dosage adjustment in hepatic impairment: Use cautiously.

Administration May be administered by I.M., I.V., or orally

I.M.: Should be administered deep into the muscle mass

I.V.: Do not exceed 2 mg/minute or 0.05 mg/kg over 2-5 minutes; dilute I.V. dose with equal volume of compatible diluent (D$_5$W, NS, SWI). Avoid intra-arterial administration. Monitor I.V. site for extravasation.

Monitoring Parameters Respiratory and cardiovascular status, blood pressure, heart rate, symptoms of anxiety

Clinical signs of propylene glycol toxicity (for continuous high-dose and/or long duration intravenous use): Serum creatinine, BUN, serum lactate, osmol gap

Additional Information Oral doses >0.09 mg/kg produced increased ataxia without increased sedative benefit vs lower doses; preferred anxiolytic when I.M. route needed. Abrupt discontinuation after sustained use (generally >10 days) may cause withdrawal symptoms.

Dosage Forms Excipient information presented when available (limited, particularly for generics); consult specific product labeling. [DSC] = Discontinued product

Injection, solution: 2 mg/mL (1 mL, 10 mL); 4 mg/mL (1 mL, 10 mL)

Ativan®: 2 mg/mL (1 mL; 10 mL [DSC]); 4 mg/mL (1 mL, 10 mL) [contains benzyl alcohol, polyethylene glycol 400, and propylene glycol]

Injection, solution [preservative free]: 2 mg/mL (1 mL); 4 mg/mL (1 mL)

Solution, oral [concentrate]: 2 mg/mL (30 mL)

Lorazepam Intensol™: 2 mg/mL (30 mL) [ethanol free, sugar free, dye free; contains propylene glycol]

Tablet: 0.5 mg, 1 mg, 2 mg

Ativan®: 0.5 mg

Ativan®: 1 mg, 2 mg [scored]

References

Ameer B and Greenblatt DJ, "Lorazepam: A Review of Its Clinical Pharmacological Properties and Therapeutic Uses," *Drugs*, 1981, 21(3):162-200.

Bishop JF, Olver IN, Wolf MM, et al, "Lorazepam: A Randomized, Double-Blind, Crossover Study of a New Antiemetic in Patients Receiving Cytotoxic Chemotherapy and Prochlorperazine," *J Clin Oncol*, 1984, 2(5):691-5.

Buzdar AU, Esparza L, Natale R, et al, "Lorazepam-Enhancement of the Antiemetic Efficacy of Dexamethasone and Promethazine. A Placebo-Controlled Study," *Am J Clin Oncol*, 1994, 17 (5):417-21.

Greenblatt DJ, Allen MD, Locniskar A, et al, "Lorazepam Kinetics in the Elderly," *Clin Pharmacol Ther*, 1979, 26(1):103-13.

Laszlo J, Clark RA, Hanson DC, et al, "Lorazepam in Cancer Patients Treated With Cisplatin: A Drug Having Antiemetic, Amnesic, and Anxiolytic Effects," *J Clin Oncol*, 1985, 3(6):864-9.

Malik IA, Khan WA, Qazilbash M, et al, "Clinical Efficacy of Lorazepam in Prophylaxis of Anticipatory, Acute, and Delayed Nausea and Vomiting Induced by High Doses of Cisplatin. A Prospective Randomized Trial," *Am J Clin Oncol*, 1995, 18(2):170-5.

Mechlorethamine (me klor ETH a meen)

Medication Safety Issues

High alert medication: The Institute for Safe Medication Practices (ISMP) includes this medication among its list of drugs which have a heightened risk of causing significant patient harm when used in error.

Related Information

Fertility and Cancer Therapy *on page* 1430
Management of Drug Extravasations *on page* 1447
Safe Handling of Hazardous Drugs *on page* 1517

U.S. Brand Names Mustargen®

Index Terms Chlorethazine; Chlorethazine Mustard; HN_2; Mechlorethamine Hydrochloride; Mustine; Nitrogen Mustard; NSC-762

Generic Available No

Canadian Brand Names Mustargen®

Pharmacologic Category Antineoplastic Agent, Alkylating Agent (Nitrogen Mustard)

Use Hodgkin's disease; non-Hodgkin's lymphoma; intracavitary injection for treatment of metastatic tumors; pleural and other malignant effusions; topical treatment of mycosis fungoides

Pregnancy Risk Factor D

Lactation Excretion in breast milk unknown/not recommended

Labeled Contraindications Hypersensitivity to mechlorethamine or any component of the formulation; pre-existing profound myelosuppression or infection

Warnings/Precautions [U.S. Boxed Warnings]: Hazardous agent - use appropriate precautions for handling and disposal. Avoid contact with skin or eyes; avoid exposure during pregnancy. Mechlorethamine is a potent vesicant; if extravasation occurs, severe tissue damage (leading to ulceration and necrosis) and pain may occur. Sodium thiosulfate should be available for treatment of extravasation. May cause lymphopenia, granulocytopenia, thrombocytopenia and anemia. Hyperuricemia may occur, especially with lymphomas; ensure adequate hydration. **[U.S. Boxed Warning]: Should be administered under the supervision of an experienced cancer chemotherapy physician.**

Adverse Reactions
>10%:
  Dermatologic: Alopecia; hyperpigmentation of veins; contact and allergic dermatitis (50% with topical use)
  Endocrine & metabolic: Chromosomal abnormalities, delayed menses, oligomenorrhea, amenorrhea, impaired spermatogenesis
  Gastrointestinal: Nausea and vomiting (almost 100%), onset may be within minutes of drug administration
  Genitourinary: Azoospermia
  Hematologic: Myelosuppression, leukopenia, and thrombocytopenia
    Onset: 4-7 days
    Nadir: 14 days
    Recovery: 21 days
1% to 10%:
  Central nervous system: Fever
  Gastrointestinal: Diarrhea, anorexia, metallic taste
  Otic: Tinnitus
<1%: Vertigo, rash, hemolytic anemia, hepatotoxicity, weakness, peripheral neuropathy

Drug Interactions
Avoid Concomitant Use
  Avoid concomitant use of Mechlorethamine with any of the following: Natalizumab; Vaccines (Live)
Increased Effect/Toxicity
  Mechlorethamine may increase the levels/effects of: Leflunomide; Natalizumab; Vaccines (Live)

  The levels/effects of Mechlorethamine may be increased by: Trastuzumab
Decreased Effect
  Mechlorethamine may decrease the levels/effects of: Vaccines (Inactivated); Vaccines (Live)

  The levels/effects of Mechlorethamine may be decreased by: Echinacea
Ethanol/Nutrition/Herb Interactions Ethanol: Avoid ethanol (due to GI irritation).
Storage/Stability Store intact vials at room temperature. Solution is stable for only 15-60 minutes after dilution
Reconstitution Must be prepared immediately before use. Dilute powder with 10 mL SWI to a final concentration of 1 mg/mL. May be diluted in up to 100 mL NS for intracavitary or topical administration.
Compatibility Stable in sterile water for injection; **incompatible** with D$_5$W; **variable stability (consult detailed reference)** in NS.
  Y-site administration: **Compatible:** Amifostine, aztreonam, filgrastim, fludarabine, granisetron, melphalan, ondansetron, sargramostim, teniposide, vinorelbine. **Incompatible:** Allopurinol, cefepime.
  Compatibility when admixed: **Incompatible:** Methohexital.
Mechanism of Action Bifunctional alkylating agent that inhibits DNA and RNA synthesis via formation of carbonium ions; cross-links strands of DNA, causing miscoding, breakage, and failure of replication; produces interstrand and intrastrand cross-links in DNA resulting in miscoding, breakage, and failure

of replication. Although not cell phase-specific *per se*, mechlorethamine effect is most pronounced in the S phase, and cell proliferation is arrested in the G_2 phase.

Pharmacodynamics/Kinetics

Duration: Unchanged drug is undetectable in blood within a few minutes

Absorption: Intracavitary administration: Incomplete secondary to rapid deactivation by body fluids

Metabolism: Rapid hydrolysis and demethylation, possibly in plasma

Half-life elimination: <1 minute

Excretion: Urine (50% as metabolites, <0.01% as unchanged drug)

Dosage Refer to individual protocols.

Children and Adults: I.V.: 6 mg/m^2 on days 1 and 8 of a 28-day cycle (MOPP regimen)

Adults:

I.V.: 0.4 mg/kg **or** 12-16 mg/m^2 for one dose **or** divided into 0.1 mg/kg/day for 4 days, repeated at 4- to 6-week intervals

Intracavitary: 0.2-0.4 mg/kg (10-20 mg) as a single dose; may be repeated if fluid continues to accumulate.

Intrapericardially: 0.2-0.4 mg/kg as a single dose; may be repeated if fluid continues to accumulate.

Topical: 0.01% to 0.02% solution, lotion, or ointment

Hemodialysis: Not removed; supplemental dosing is not required.

Peritoneal dialysis: Not removed; supplemental dosing is not required.

Combination Regimens

Brain tumors:

MOP on page 1369

MOPP (Medulloblastoma) on page 1373

Lymphoma, Hodgkin's:

CAD/MOPP/ABV on page 1242

MOPP (Lymphoma, Hodgkin's Disease) on page 1372

MOPP/ABV Hybrid on page 1372

MOPP/ABVD on page 1369

MVPP on page 1380

Stanford V Regimen on page 1403

Administration I.V. as a slow push through the side of a freely-flowing saline or dextrose solution. Due to the limited stability of the drug, and the increased risk of phlebitis and venous irritation and blistering with increased contact time, infusions of the drug are not recommended.

Mechlorethamine may cause extravasation. Use within 1 hour of preparation. Avoid extravasation since mechlorethamine is a potent vesicant.

Monitoring Parameters CBC with differential, hemoglobin, and platelet count

Emetic Potential Very high (>90%)

Vesicant Yes; see Management of Drug Extravasations on page 1447.

High Dose Considerations

High Dose I.V.: 0.3-2 mg/kg

Dosage Forms Excipient information presented when available (limited, particularly for generics); consult specific product labeling.

Injection, powder for reconstitution, as hydrochloride: 10 mg

References

Bonadonna G, Valagussa P, and Santoro A, "Alternating Non-Cross-Resistant Combination Chemotherapy or MOPP in Stage IV Hodgkin's Disease. A Report of 8-Year Results," *Ann Intern Med*, 1986, 104(6):739-46.

DeVita VT, Serpick A, and Carbone PP, "Combination Chemotherapy in the Treatment of Advanced Hodgkin's Disease," *Ann Intern Med*, 1970, 73:881-95.

Dorr RT, Soble M, and Alberts DS, "Efficacy of Sodium Thiosulfate as a Local Antidote to Mechlorethamine Skin Toxicity in the Mouse," *Cancer Chemother Pharmacol*, 1988, 22 (4):299-302.

Price NM, Hoppe RT, and Deneau DG, "Ointment Based Mechlorethamine Treatment for Mycosis Fungoides," *Cancer*, 1983, 52:2214-9.

Taylor JR, Halprin KM, Levine V, et al, "Mechlorethamine Hydrochloride Solutions and Ointments," *Arch Dermatol*, 1980, 116:783-5.

Vonderheid EC, "Topical Mechlorethamine Chemotherapy: Considerations on its Use in Mycosis Fungoides," *Int J Dermatol*, 1984, 23(3):180-6.

◆ **Mechlorethamine Hydrochloride** *see* Mechlorethamine *on page 736*

◆ **Medrol®** *see* MethylPREDNISolone *on page 782*

◆ **Medrol Dose Pack** *see* MethylPREDNISolone *on page 782*

MedroxyPROGESTERone (me DROKS ee proe JES te rone)

Medication Safety Issues

Sound-alike/look-alike issues:

Depo-Provera® may be confused with depo-subQ provera 104™

depo-subQ provera 104™ may be confused with Depo-Provera®

MedroxyPROGESTERone may be confused with hydroxyprogesterone, methylPREDNISolone, methylTESTOSTERone

Provera® may be confused with Covera®, Femara®, Parlodel®, Premarin®, Proscar®, Prozac®

The injection dosage form is available in different formulations. Carefully review prescriptions to assure the correct formulation and route of administration.

Related Information

Safe Handling of Hazardous Drugs *on page 1517*

U.S. Brand Names Depo-Provera®; Depo-Provera® Contraceptive; depo-subQ provera 104™; Provera®

Index Terms Acetoxymethylprogesterone; Medroxyprogesterone Acetate; Methylacetoxyprogesterone; MPA

Generic Available Yes

Canadian Brand Names Alti-MPA; Apo-Medroxy®; Depo-Prevera®; Depo-Provera®; Gen-Medroxy; Novo-Medrone; Provera-Pak; Provera®

Pharmacologic Category Contraceptive; Progestin

Use Secondary amenorrhea or abnormal uterine bleeding due to hormonal imbalance; reduction of endometrial hyperplasia in nonhysterectomized postmenopausal women receiving conjugated estrogens; prevention of pregnancy; management of endometriosis-associated pain

Unlabeled/Investigational Use Treatment of endometrial carcinoma

Pregnancy Risk Factor X

Lactation Enters breast milk/compatible

Labeled Contraindications Hypersensitivity to medroxyprogesterone or any component of the formulation; history of or current thrombophlebitis or venous thromboembolic disorders (including DVT, PE); cerebral vascular disease; severe hepatic dysfunction or disease; carcinoma of the breast or genital organs, undiagnosed vaginal bleeding; missed abortion, diagnostic test for pregnancy, pregnancy

Warnings/Precautions [U.S. Boxed Warning]: **Prolonged use of medroxyprogesterone contraceptive injection may result in a loss of bone mineral density (BMD).** Loss is related to the duration of use, and may not be completely reversible on discontinuation of the drug. The impact on peak bone mass in adolescents should be considered in treatment decisions. **[U.S. Boxed Warning]: Long-term use (ie, >2 years) should be limited to**

situations where other birth control methods are inadequate. Consider other methods of birth control in women with (or at risk for) osteoporosis.

Use caution with cardiovascular disease or dysfunction. MPA used in combination with estrogen may increase the risks of hypertension, myocardial infarction (MI), stroke, pulmonary emboli (PE), and deep vein thrombosis; incidence of these effects was shown to be significantly increased in postmenopausal women using conjugated equine estrogens (CEE) in combination with MPA. MPA in combination with estrogens should not be used to prevent coronary heart disease. Use with caution in patients with diabetes mellitus; may cause glucose intolerance.

The risk of dementia may be increased in postmenopausal women; increased incidence was observed in women ≥65 years of age taking MPA in combination with CEE. An increased risk of invasive breast cancer was observed in postmenopausal women using MPA in combination with CEE. An increase in abnormal mammograms has also been reported with estrogen and progestin therapy.

Discontinue pending examination in cases of sudden partial or complete vision loss, sudden onset of proptosis, diplopia, or migraine; discontinue permanently if papilledema or retinal vascular lesions are observed on examination. Use with caution in patients with diseases that may be exacerbated by fluid retention (including asthma, epilepsy, migraine, diabetes, or renal dysfunction). Use caution with history of depression. Whenever possible, progestins in combination with estrogens should be discontinued at least 4-6 weeks prior to surgeries associated with an increased risk of thromboembolism or during periods of prolonged immobilization. Progestins used in combination with estrogen should be used for shortest duration possible consistent with treatment goals. Conduct periodic risk:benefit assessments. Not for use prior to menarche.

Adverse Reactions Adverse effects as reported with any dosage form; percent ranges presented are noted with the MPA contraceptive injection:

>5%:
  Central nervous system: Dizziness, headache, nervousness
  Endocrine & metabolic: Libido decreased, menstrual irregularities (includes bleeding, amenorrhea, or both)
  Gastrointestinal: Abdominal pain/discomfort, weight changes (average: 3-5 pounds after 1 year, 8 pounds after 2 years)
  Neuromuscular & skeletal: Weakness

1% to 5%:
  Cardiovascular: Edema
  Central nervous system: Depression, fatigue, insomnia, irritability, pain
  Dermatologic: Acne, alopecia, rash
  Endocrine & metabolic: Anorgasmia, breast pain, hot flashes
  Gastrointestinal: Bloating, nausea
  Genitourinary: Cervical smear abnormal, leukorrhea, menometrorrhagia, menorrhagia, pelvic pain, urinary tract infection, vaginitis, vaginal infection, vaginal hemorrhage
  Local: Injection site atrophy, injection site reaction, injection site pain
  Neuromuscular & skeletal: Arthralgia, backache, leg cramp
  Respiratory: Respiratory tract infections

<1%: Allergic reaction, anemia, angioedema, appetite changes, asthma, axillary swelling, blood dyscrasia, body odor, breast cancer, breast changes, cervical cancer, chest pain, chills, chloasma, convulsions, deep vein thrombosis, diaphoresis, drowsiness, dry skin, dysmenorrhea, dyspareunia,

dyspnea, facial palsy, fever, galactorrhea, genitourinary infections, glucose tolerance decreased, hirsutism, hoarseness, jaundice, lack of return to fertility, lactation decreased, libido increased, melasma, nipple bleeding, osteoporosis, paralysis, paresthesia, pruritus, pulmonary embolus, rectal bleeding, scleroderma, sensation of pregnancy, somnolence, syncope, tachycardia, thirst, thrombophlebitis, uterine hyperplasia, vaginal cysts, varicose veins; residual lump, sterile abscess, or skin discoloration at the injection site

Postmarketing and/or case reports: Anaphylaxis, anaphylactoid reactions, bone mineral density decreased, osteoporotic fractures

Drug Interactions

Metabolism/Transport Effects Substrate of CYP3A4 (major); Induces CYP3A4 (weak)

Avoid Concomitant Use

Avoid concomitant use of MedroxyPROGESTERone with any of the following: Acitretin; Griseofulvin

Increased Effect/Toxicity

The levels/effects of MedroxyPROGESTERone may be increased by: Herbs (Progestogenic Properties)

Decreased Effect

MedroxyPROGESTERone may decrease the levels/effects of: Saxagliptin; Vitamin K Antagonists

The levels/effects of MedroxyPROGESTERone may be decreased by: Acitretin; Aminoglutethimide; Aprepitant; Artemether; Barbiturates; Bosentan; CarBAMazepine; CYP3A4 Inducers (Strong); Deferasirox; Fosaprepitant; Griseofulvin; Phenytoin; Rifamycin Derivatives; St Johns Wort; Topiramate

Ethanol/Nutrition/Herb Interactions

Ethanol: Avoid ethanol (may increase risk of osteoporosis).

Food: Bioavailability of the oral tablet is increased when taken with food; half-life is unchanged.

Herb/Nutraceutical: St John's wort may diminish the therapeutic effect of progestin contraceptives (contraceptive failure is possible).

Storage/Stability Store at controlled room temperature.

Mechanism of Action Inhibits secretion of pituitary gonadotropins, which prevents follicular maturation and ovulation; causes endometrial thinning

Pharmacodynamics/Kinetics

Absorption: Oral: Well absorbed; I.M.: Slow

Protein binding: 86% to 90% primarily to albumin; does not bind to sex hormone-binding globulin

Metabolism: Extensively hepatic via hydroxylation and conjugation; forms metabolites

Time to peak: Oral: 2-4 hours

Half-life elimination: Oral: 12-17 hours; I.M. (Depo-Provera® Contraceptive): 50 days; SubQ: ~40 days

Excretion: Urine

Dosage

Adolescents and Adults:

Amenorrhea: Oral: 5-10 mg/day for 5-10 days

Abnormal uterine bleeding: Oral: 5-10 mg for 5-10 days starting on day 16 or 21 of cycle

Contraception:

Depo-Provera® Contraceptive: I.M.: 150 mg every 3 months

depo-subQ provera 104™: SubQ: 104 mg every 3 months (every 12-14 weeks)

Endometriosis (depo-subQ provera 104™): SubQ: 104 mg every 3 months (every 12-14 weeks)

Adults:

Endometrial carcinoma (unlabeled use) (Depo-Provera®): I.M.: 400-1000 mg/week

Accompanying cyclic estrogen therapy, postmenopausal: Oral: 5-10 mg for 12-14 consecutive days each month, starting on day 1 or day 16 of the cycle; lower doses may be used if given with estrogen continuously throughout the cycle

Dosing adjustment in hepatic impairment: Use is contraindicated with severe impairment. Consider lower dose or less frequent administration with mild-to-moderate impairment. Use of the contraceptive injection has not been studied in patients with hepatic impairment; consideration should be given to not readminister if jaundice develops

Administration

I.M.: Depo-Provera® Contraceptive: Administer first dose during the first 5 days of menstrual period, or within the first 5 days postpartum if not breast-feeding, or at the sixth week postpartum if breast-feeding exclusively. Shake vigorously prior to administration. Administer by deep I.M. injection in the gluteal or deltoid muscle.

SubQ: depo-subQ provera 104™: Administer first dose during the first 5 days of menstrual period, or at the sixth week postpartum if breast-feeding. Shake vigorously prior to administration. Administer by SubQ injection in the upper thigh or abdomen; avoid boney areas and the umbilicus. Administer over 5-7 seconds. Do not rub the injection area. When switching from combined hormonal contraceptives (estrogen plus progestin), the first injection should be within 7 days after the last active pill, or removal of patch or ring. If switching from the I.M. to SubQ formulation, the next dose should be given within the prescribed dosing period for the I.M. injection.

Monitoring Parameters Before starting therapy, a physical exam with reference to the breasts and pelvis are recommended, including a Papanicolaou smear. Exam may be deferred if appropriate prior to administration of MPA contraceptive injection; pregnancy should be ruled out prior to use. Monitor patient closely for loss of vision; sudden onset of proptosis, diplopia, or migraine; signs and symptoms of thromboembolic disorders; signs or symptoms of depression; glucose in patients with diabetes; or blood pressure.

Test Interactions

The following tests may be decreased: Steroid levels (plasma and urinary), gonadotropin levels, SHBG concentration, T_3 uptake

The following tests may be increased: Protein-bound iodine, butanol extractable protein-bound iodine, Factors II, VII, VIII, IX, X

Pathologist should be advised of estrogen/progesterone therapy when specimens are submitted.

Dietary Considerations Ensure adequate calcium and vitamin D intake when used for the prevention of pregnancy

Dosage Forms Excipient information presented when available (limited, particularly for generics); consult specific product labeling.

Injection, suspension, as acetate: 150 mg/mL (1 mL)

Depo-Provera®: 400 mg/mL (2.5 mL)

Depo-Provera® Contraceptive: 150 mg/mL (1 mL) [prefilled syringe or vial]

depo-subQ provera 104™: 104 mg/0.65 mL (0.65 mL) [prefilled syringe]

Tablet, as acetate: 2.5 mg, 5 mg, 10 mg
Provera®: 2.5 mg, 5 mg, 10 mg

♦ **Medroxyprogesterone Acetate** *see* MedroxyPROGESTERone *on page 739*

♦ **Megace®** *see* Megestrol *on page 743*

♦ **Megace® ES** *see* Megestrol *on page 743*

♦ **Megace® OS (Can)** *see* Megestrol *on page 743*

Megestrol (me JES trole)

Medication Safety Issues

Sound-alike/look-alike issues:
Megace® may be confused with Reglan®
Megestrol may be confused with mesalamine

Related Information

Safe Handling of Hazardous Drugs *on page 1517*

U.S. Brand Names Megace®; Megace® ES

Index Terms 5071-1DL(6); Megestrol Acetate; NSC-71423

Generic Available Yes: Excludes Megace® ES

Canadian Brand Names Apo-Megestrol®; Megace®; Megace® OS; Nu-Megestrol

Pharmacologic Category Antineoplastic Agent, Hormone; Appetite Stimulant; Progestin

Use Palliative treatment of breast and endometrial carcinoma; treatment of anorexia, cachexia, or unexplained significant weight loss in patients with AIDS

Pregnancy Risk Factor D (tablet) / X (suspension)

Lactation Enters breast milk/not recommended

Labeled Contraindications Hypersensitivity to megestrol or any component of the formulation; pregnancy (suspension)

Warnings/Precautions Hazardous agent - use appropriate precautions for handling and disposal. May suppress hypothalamic-pituitary-adrenal (HPA) axis during chronic administration; consider the possibility of adrenal suppression in any patient receiving or being withdrawn from chronic therapy when signs/symptoms suggestive of hypoadrenalism are noted (during stress or in unstressed state). Laboratory evaluation and replacement/stress doses of rapid-acting glucocorticoid should be considered. New-onset diabetes and exacerbation of pre-existing diabetes have been reported with long-term use. Use with caution in patients with a history of thromboembolic disease. Vaginal bleeding or discharge may occur in females. Megace® ES suspension is not equivalent to other formulations on a mg per mg basis; Megace® ES suspension 625 mg/5 mL is equivalent to megestrol acetate suspension 800 mg/20 mL. Safety and efficacy in children have not been established.

Adverse Reactions

Frequency not always defined.

Cardiovascular: Hypertension (≤8%), cardiomyopathy (1% to 3%), chest pain (1% to 3%), edema (1% to 3%), palpitation (1% to 3%), peripheral edema (1% to 3%), heart failure

Central nervous system: Headache (≤10%), insomnia (≤6%), fever (1% to 6%), pain (≤6%, similar to placebo), abnormal thinking (1% to 3%), confusion (1% to 3%), depression (1% to 3%), hypoesthesia (1% to 3%), seizure (1% to 3%), mood changes, malaise, lethargy

Dermatologic: Rash (2% to 12%), alopecia (1% to 3%), pruritus (1% to 3%), vesiculobullous rash (1% to 3%)

Endocrine & metabolic: Hyperglycemia (≤6%), gynecomastia (1% to 3%), adrenal insufficiency, amenorrhea, breakthrough bleeding, cervical erosion and secretions (changes), breast tenderness increased, Cushing's syndrome, diabetes, glucose intolerance, HPA axis suppression, hot flashes, hypercalcemia, menstrual flow changes, spotting, vaginal bleeding pattern changes

Gastrointestinal: Diarrhea (6% to 15%, similar to placebo), flatulence (≤10%), vomiting (≤6%), nausea (≤5%), dyspepsia (≤4%), abdominal pain (1% to 3%), constipation (1% to 3%), salivation increased (1% to 3%), xerostomia (1% to 3%), weight gain (not attributed to edema or fluid retention)

Genitourinary: Impotence (4% to 14%), decreased libido (≤5%), urinary incontinence (1% to 3%), urinary tract infection (1% to 3%), urinary frequency (≤2%)

Hematologic: Anemia (≤5%), leukopenia (1% to 3%)

Hepatic: Hepatomegaly (1% to 3%), LDH increased (1% to 3%), cholestatic jaundice, hepatotoxicity

Neuromuscular & skeletal: Weakness (2% to 6%), neuropathy (1% to 3%), paresthesia (1% to 3%), carpal tunnel syndrome

Ocular: Amblyopia (1% to 3%)

Renal: Albuminuria (1% to 3%)

Respiratory: Dyspnea (1% to 3%), cough (1% to 3%), pharyngitis (1% to 3%), pneumonia (≤2%), hyperpnea

Miscellaneous: Diaphoresis (1% to 3%), herpes infection (1% to 3%), infection (1% to 3%), moniliasis (1% to 3%), tumor flare

Postmarketing and/or case reports: Thromboembolic phenomena (including deep vein thrombosis, pulmonary embolism, thrombophlebitis)

Drug Interactions

Avoid Concomitant Use
Avoid concomitant use of Megestrol with any of the following: Dofetilide

Increased Effect/Toxicity
Megestrol may increase the levels/effects of: Dofetilide

The levels/effects of Megestrol may be increased by: Herbs (Progestogenic Properties)

Decreased Effect
The levels/effects of Megestrol may be decreased by: Aminoglutethimide

Ethanol/Nutrition/Herb Interactions Herb/Nutraceutical: Avoid herbs with progestogenic properties (eg, bloodroot, chasteberry, damiana, oregano, and yucca); may enhance the adverse/toxic effect of megestrol.

Storage/Stability
Suspension: Store at 15°C to 25°C (59°F to 77°F); protect from heat.

Tablet: Store at 25°C (77°F); excursions permitted to 15°C to 30°C (59°F to 86°F); protect from heat (temperatures >40°C [>104°F])

Mechanism of Action A synthetic progestin with antiestrogenic properties which disrupt the estrogen receptor cycle. Megestrol interferes with the normal estrogen cycle and results in a lower LH titer. May also have a direct effect on the endometrium. Megestrol is an antineoplastic progestin thought to act through an antileutenizing effect mediated via the pituitary. May stimulate appetite by antagonizing the metabolic effects of catabolic cytokines.

Pharmacodynamics/Kinetics
Absorption: Well absorbed orally

Metabolism: Hepatic (to free steroids and glucuronide conjugates)

Half-life elimination: 13-105 hours

Time to peak, serum: 1-3 hours

Excretion: Urine (57% to 78%; 5% to 8% as metabolites); feces (8% to 30%)

Dosage Adults: Oral: **Note:** Megace® ES suspension is not equivalent to other formulations on a mg-per-mg basis:

Tablet: Females (refer to individual protocols):

Breast carcinoma: 40 mg 4 times/day

Endometrial carcinoma: 40-320 mg/day in divided doses; use for 2 months to determine efficacy; maximum doses used have been up to 800 mg/day

Suspension: Males/Females: HIV-related cachexia:

Megace®: Initial dose: 800 mg/day; daily doses of 400 and 800 mg/day were found to be clinically effective

Megace® ES: 625 mg/day

Dosing adjustment in renal impairment: No data available; however, the urinary excretion of megestrol acetate administered in doses of 4-90 mg ranged from 57% to 78% within 10 days

Administration Megestrol acetate (Megace®) oral suspension is compatible with water, orange juice, apple juice, or Sustacal H.C. for immediate consumption. Shake suspension well before use.

Monitoring Parameters Observe for signs of thromboembolic phenomena; blood pressure, weight; serum glucose

Test Interactions Altered thyroid and liver function tests

Dosage Forms Excipient information presented when available (limited, particularly for generics); consult specific product labeling.

Suspension, oral, as acetate: 40 mg/mL (10 mL, 20 mL, 240 mL, 480 mL)

Megace®: 40 mg/mL (240 mL) [contains ethanol 0.06% and sodium benzoate; lemon-lime flavor]

Megace® ES: 125 mg/mL (150 mL) [contains ethanol 0.06% and sodium benzoate; lemon-lime flavor]

Tablet, as acetate: 20 mg, 40 mg

References

Fietkau R, Riepl M, Kettner H, et al, "Supportive Use of Megestrol Acetate in Patients With Head and Neck Cancer During Radio(Chemo)Therapy," *Eur J Cancer,* 1997, 33(1):75-9.

Lentz SS, Brady MF, Major FJ, et al, "High-Dose Megestrol Acetate in Advanced or Recurrent Endometrial Carcinoma: A Gynecologic Oncology Group Study," *J Clin Oncol,* 1996, 14 (2):357-61.

Strang P, "The Effect of Megestrol Acetate on Anorexia, Weight Loss and Cachexia in Cancer and AIDS Patients," *Anticancer Res,* 1997, 17(1B):657-62.

◆ **Megestrol Acetate** *see* Megestrol *on page 743*

Melphalan (MEL fa lan)

Medication Safety Issues

Sound-alike/look-alike issues:

Melphalan may be confused with Mephyton®, Myleran®

Alkeran® may be confused with Alferon®, Leukeran®, Myleran®

High alert medication: The Institute for Safe Medication Practices (ISMP) includes this medication among its list of drugs which have a heightened risk of causing significant patient harm when used in error.

Related Information

Fertility and Cancer Therapy *on page 1430*

Hematopoietic Stem Cell Transplantation *on page 1501*

Management of Drug Extravasations *on page 1447*

Oral Mucositis / Stomatitis *on page 1460*

Safe Handling of Hazardous Drugs *on page 1517*

U.S. Brand Names Alkeran®

Index Terms L-PAM; L-Sarcolysin; Phenylalanine Mustard

Generic Available No

Canadian Brand Names Alkeran®

Pharmacologic Category Antineoplastic Agent, Alkylating Agent

Use Palliative treatment of multiple myeloma and nonresectable epithelial ovarian carcinoma

Unlabeled/Investigational Use Treatment of neuroblastoma, rhabdomyosarcoma, breast cancer, Hodgkin's disease; part of an induction regimen for marrow and stem cell transplantation

Pregnancy Risk Factor D

Lactation Excretion in breast milk unknown/not recommended

Labeled Contraindications Hypersensitivity to melphalan or any component of the formulation; severe bone marrow suppression; patients whose disease was resistant to prior melphalan therapy; pregnancy

Warnings/Precautions Hazardous agent - use appropriate precautions for handling and disposal. **[U.S. Boxed Warning]: Is potentially mutagenic, leukemogenic,** and carcinogenic. Suppresses ovarian function and produces amenorrhea; may also cause testicular suppression. **[U.S. Boxed Warning]: Bone marrow suppression is common.** Use with caution in patients with prior bone marrow suppression, impaired renal function (consider dose reduction), or who have received prior chemotherapy or irradiation. Toxicity to immunosuppressives is increased in elderly; start with lowest recommended adult doses. Signs of infection, such as fever and WBC rise, may not occur. Lethargy and confusion may be more prominent signs of infection. **[U.S. Boxed Warning]: Hypersensitivity has been reported with I.V. administration** and oral melphalan; may occur after multiple treatment cycles. **[U.S. Boxed Warning]: Should be administered under the supervision of an experienced cancer chemotherapy physician.** Safety and efficacy in children have not been established.

Adverse Reactions

>10%:

Gastrointestinal: Vomiting (oral low-dose: <10%; I.V.: 30% to 90%)

Hematologic: Myelosuppression, leukopenia (onset 7 days; nadir 14-35 days; recovery 28-56 days), thrombocytopenia (onset 7 days; nadir 14-35 days; recovery 28-56 days)

Miscellaneous: Secondary malignancy (<2% to 20%; cumulative dose and duration dependent)

1% to 10%: Miscellaneous: Hypersensitivity (I.V.: 2%)

Infrequent, frequency undefined, postmarketing, and/or case reports: Agranulocytosis, allergic reactions, alopecia, amenorrhea, anaphylaxis, anemia, bladder irritation, bone marrow failure (irreversible), diarrhea, hemolytic anemia, hemorrhagic cystitis, hemorrhagic necrotic enterocolitis, hepatic veno-occlusive disease (I.V. melphalan), hepatitis, interstitial pneumonitis, jaundice, nausea, ovarian suppression, pruritus, pulmonary fibrosis, radiation myelopathy, rash, secondary carcinoma, secondary leukemia, secondary myeloproliferative syndrome, SIADH, skin hypersensitivity, skin necrosis, skin ulceration (injection site), skin vesiculation, sterility, stomatitis, testicular suppression, transaminases increased, vasculitis

Drug Interactions

Avoid Concomitant Use

Avoid concomitant use of Melphalan with any of the following: Nalidixic Acid; Natalizumab; Vaccines (Live)

Increased Effect/Toxicity

Melphalan may increase the levels/effects of: CycloSPORINE; Leflunomide; Natalizumab; Vaccines (Live); Vitamin K Antagonists

The levels/effects of Melphalan may be increased by: Nalidixic Acid; Trastuzumab

Decreased Effect

Melphalan may decrease the levels/effects of: Cardiac Glycosides; Vaccines (Inactivated); Vaccines (Live); Vitamin K Antagonists

The levels/effects of Melphalan may be decreased by: Echinacea

Ethanol/Nutrition/Herb Interactions

Ethanol: Avoid ethanol (due to GI irritation).

Food: Food interferes with oral absorption.

Storage/Stability

Tablet: Store in refrigerator at 2°C to 8°C (36°F to 46°F). Protect from light.

Injection: Store at room temperature (15°C to 30°C). Protect from light. Reconstituted solution is chemically and physically stable for at least 90 minutes when stored at 25°C (77°F). Diluted solution is physically and chemically stable for at least 60 minutes at 25°C (77°F).

Reconstitution Injection must be prepared fresh. **The time between reconstitution/dilution and administration of parenteral melphalan must be kept to a minimum (manufacturer recommends <60 minutes) because reconstituted and diluted solutions are unstable.** Dissolve powder initially with 10 mL of diluent to a concentration of 5 mg/mL. Shake vigorously to dissolve. **Immediately** dilute dose in 250-500 mL NS to a concentration of 0.1-0.45 mg/mL.

Compatibility Incompatible with D_5W, LR; **variable stability (consult detailed reference)** in NS.

Y-site administration: Compatible: Acyclovir, amikacin, aminophylline, ampicillin, aztreonam, bleomycin, bumetanide, buprenorphine, butorphanol, calcium gluconate, carboplatin, carmustine, cefazolin, cefepime, cefoperazone, cefotaxime, cefotetan, ceftazidime, ceftizoxime, ceftriaxone, cefuroxime, cimetidine, cisplatin, clindamycin, co-trimoxazole, cyclophosphamide, cytarabine, dacarbazine, dactinomycin, daunorubicin, dexamethasone sodium phosphate, diphenhydramine, doxorubicin, doxycycline, droperidol, enalaprilat, etoposide, famotidine, floxuridine, fluconazole, fludarabine, fluorouracil, furosemide, ganciclovir, gentamicin, granisetron, haloperidol, heparin, hydrocortisone sodium phosphate, hydrocortisone sodium succinate, hydromorphone, hydroxyzine, idarubicin, ifosfamide, imipenem/cilastatin, lorazepam, mannitol, mechlorethamine, meperidine, mesna, methotrexate, methylprednisolone sodium succinate, metoclopramide, metronidazole, minocycline, mitomycin, mitoxantrone, morphine, nalbuphine, netilmicin, ondansetron, pentostatin, piperacillin, plicamycin, potassium chloride, prochlorperazine edisylate, promethazine, ranitidine, sodium bicarbonate, streptozocin, teniposide, thiotepa, ticarcillin, ticarcillin/clavulanate, tobramycin, vancomycin, vinblastine, vincristine, vinorelbine, zidovudine. **Incompatible:** Amphotericin B, chlorpromazine.

Mechanism of Action Alkylating agent which is a derivative of mechlorethamine that inhibits DNA and RNA synthesis via formation of carbonium ions; cross-links strands of DNA; acts on both resting and rapidly dividing tumor cells.

Pharmacodynamics/Kinetics

Absorption: Oral: Variable and incomplete

Distribution: V_d: 0.5-0.6 L/kg throughout total body water

Protein binding: 60% to 90%; primarily to albumin, 20% to α_1-acid glycoprotein

Metabolism: Hepatic; chemical hydrolysis to monohydroxymelphalan and dihydroxymelphalan

Bioavailability: Unpredictable; 61% ± 26%, decreasing with repeated doses

Half-life elimination: Terminal: I.V.: 1.5 hours; oral: 1-1.25 hours

Time to peak, serum: ~1-2 hours

Excretion: Oral: Feces (20% to 50%); urine (10% to 30% as unchanged drug)

Dosage Refer to individual protocols.

Oral: Dose should always be adjusted to patient response and weekly blood counts:

Children (unlabeled use): 4-20 mg/m^2/day for 1-21 days

Adults:

Multiple myeloma (multiple regimens have been employed): **Note:** Response is gradual; may require repeated courses to realize benefit:

6 mg daily for 2-3 weeks initially, followed by up to 4 weeks rest, then a maintenance dose of 2 mg daily as hematologic recovery begins **or**

10 mg daily for 7-10 days; institute 2 mg daily maintenance dose after WBC >4000 cells/mm^3 and platelets >100,000 cells/mm^3 (~4-8 weeks); titrate maintenance dose to hematologic response **or**

0.15 mg/kg/day for 7 days, with a 2-6 week rest, followed by a maintenance dose of ≤0.05 mg/kg/day as hematologic recovery begins **or**

0.25 mg/kg/day for 4 days (or 0.2 mg/kg/day for 5 days); repeat at 4- to 6-week intervals as ANC and platelet counts return to normal

Ovarian carcinoma: 0.2 mg/kg/day for 5 days, repeat every 4-5 weeks.

I.V.:

Children (unlabeled use):

Pediatric rhabdomyosarcoma: 10-35 mg/m^2/dose every 21-28 days

High-dose melphalan with bone marrow transplantation for neuroblastoma: I.V.: 100-220 mg/m^2 as a single dose or divided into 2-5 daily doses. Infuse over 20-60 minutes.

Adults: Multiple myeloma: 16 mg/m^2 administered at 2-week intervals for 4 doses, then administer at 4-week intervals after adequate hematologic recovery.

Dosing adjustment in renal impairment: The FDA-approved labeling contains the following adjustment recommendations based on route of administration:

Oral: Moderate-to-severe renal impairment: Consider a reduced dose initially

I.V.: BUN >30 mg/dL: Reduce dose by up to 50%

The following guidelines have been used by some clinicians:

Aronoff, 2007 (route of administration not specified): Adults:

Cl$_{cr}$ 10-50 mL/minute: Administer 75% of dose

Cl$_{cr}$ <10 mL/minute: Administer 50% of dose

Hemodialysis: Administer dose after hemodialysis

Continuous ambulatory peritoneal dialysis (CAPD): Administer 50% of dose

Continuous renal replacement therapy (CRRT): Administer 75% of dose

Kintzel, 1995:

Oral: Adjust dose in the presence of hematologic toxicity

I.V.:

Cl$_{cr}$ 46-60 mL/minute: Administer 85% of normal dose

Cl$_{cr}$ 31-45 mL/minute: Administer 75% of normal dose

Cl$_{cr}$ <30 mL/minute: Administer 70% of normal dose

Dosing adjustment in hepatic impairment: Melphalan is hepatically metabolized; however, dosage adjustment does not appear to be necessary (King, 2001).

Combination Regimens

Gestational trophoblastic tumor:
CHAMOCA (Modified Bagshawe Regimen) on page 1259
CHAMOMA (Bagshawe Regimen) on page 1261

Lymphoma, Hodgkin's disease:
CAD/MOPP/ABV on page 1242
mini-BEAM on page 1367

Multiple myeloma:
Bortezomib-Melphalan-Prednisone on page 1240
Bortezomib-Melphalan-Prednisone-Thalidomide on page 1241
M-2 on page 1364
Melphalan-Prednisone-Thalidomide on page 1365
MP (Multiple Myeloma) on page 1374
VBMCP on page 1419

Administration

Oral: Administer on an empty stomach (1 hour prior to or 2 hours after meals)

Parenteral: Due to limited stability, complete administration of I.V. dose should occur within 60 minutes of reconstitution

I.V. infusion: Infuse over 15-20 minutes

I.V. bolus:

Central line: I.V. bolus doses of 17-200 mg/m^2 (reconstituted and not diluted) have been infused over 2-20 minutes

Peripheral line: I.V. bolus doses of 2-23 mg/m^2 (reconstituted and not diluted) have been infused over 1-4 minutes

Monitoring Parameters CBC with differential and platelet count, serum electrolytes, serum uric acid

Test Interactions False-positive Coombs' test [direct]

Dietary Considerations Should be taken on an empty stomach (1 hour prior to or 2 hours after meals).

Emetic Potential

>50 mg/m^2: Moderate (30% to 90%)

Oral, low dose: Very low (<10%)

Vesicant May be an irritant

High Dose Considerations

Comments Saline-based hydration (100-125 mg/m^2/hour) preceding (2-4 hours), during, and following (6-12 hours) administration reduces risk of drug precipitation in renal tubules. Hydrolysis causes loss of 1% melphalan injection per 10 minutes. Infusion of admixture must be completed within 100 minutes of preparation to deliver ordered dose. Reconstitute dose to 5 mg/mL in diluent provided by manufacturer. Dose may be infused via central or peripheral venous access without further dilution to minimize volume of infusion.

High Dose I.V.: 100-240 mg/m^2 administered as a single dose or divided into 2-4 daily doses. Maximum dose as a single agent: 200-400 mg/m^2. Maximum dose with total body irradiation (TBI): 110-140 mg/m^2; other high-dose chemotherapeutic drugs: 100-180 mg/m^2. Generally infused over 20-60 minutes.

Unique Toxicities

Cardiovascular: Atrial fibrillation, left ventricular heart failure

Dermatologic: Alopecia

Gastrointestinal: Mucositis (severity increases with Cl_{cr} ≤40 mL/minute; pretreatment with amifostine or glutamine may decrease mucositis), nausea and vomiting (moderate), diarrhea

Hematologic: Myelosuppression, secondary leukemia

Renal: Increased serum creatinine and azotemia possible without adequate hydration

Rare side effects: Abnormal LFTs, atrial fibrillation, interstitial pneumonitis, secondary leukemia, SIADH, vasculitis

Dosage Forms Excipient information presented when available (limited, particularly for generics); consult specific product labeling.

Injection, powder for reconstitution: 50 mg [diluent contains ethanol and propylene glycol]

Tablet: 2 mg

References

Alberts DS, Chang SY, Chen HS, et al, "Oral Melphalan Kinetics," *Clin Pharmacol Ther*, 1979, 26 (6):737-45.

Aronoff GR, Bennett WM, Berns JS, et al, *Drug Prescribing in Renal Failure: Dosing Guidelines for Adults and Children*, 5th ed. Philadelphia, PA: American College of Physicians; 2007, p 100.

Berg SL, Grisell DL, DeLaney TF, et al, "Principles of Treatment of Pediatric Solid Tumors," *Pediatr Clin North Am*, 1991, 38(2):249-67.

Kellie SJ and Kingston JE, "Ovarian Failure After High-Dose Melphalan in Adolescents," *Lancet*, 1987, 1(8547):1425.

King PD and Perry MC, "Hepatotoxicity of Chemotherapy," *Oncologist*, 2001, 6(2):162-76.

Kintzel PE and Dorr RT, "Anticancer Drug Renal Toxicity and Elimination: Dosing Guidelines for Altered Renal Function," *Cancer Treat Rev*, 1995, 21(1):33-64.

Kyle RA and Rajkumar SV, "Multiple Myeloma," *N Engl J Med*, 2004, 351(18):1860-73.

National Comprehensive Cancer Network (NCCN), "Clinical Practice Guidelines in Oncology™: Antiemesis," Version 1.2008. Available at http://www.nccn.org/professionals/physician_gls/PDF/antiemesis.pdf.

Pole JG, Casper J, Elfenbein G, et al, "High-Dose Chemoradiotherapy Supported by Marrow Infusions for Advanced Neuroblastoma: A Pediatric Oncology Group Study," *J Clin Oncol*, 1991, 9(1):152-8.

Schroeder H, Pinkerton CR, Powles RL, et al, "High-Dose Melphalan and Total Body Irradiation With Autologous Marrow Rescue in Childhood Acute Lymphoblastic Leukemia After Relapse," *Bone Marrow Transplant*, 1991, 7(1):11-15.

Seddon BM, Cassoni AM, Galloway MJ, et al, "Fatal Radiation Myelopathy After High-Dose Busulfan and Melphalan Chemotherapy and Radiotherapy for Ewing's Sarcoma: A Review of the Literature and Implications for Practice," *Clin Oncol*, 2005, 17(5):385-90.

Meperidine (me PER i deen)

Medication Safety Issues

Avoid the use of meperidine for pain control, especially in elderly and renally-compromised patients because of the risk of neurotoxicity (Institute for Safe Medication Practices [ISMP], 2007; American Pain Society, 2008)

Sound-alike/look-alike issues:

Meperidine may be confused with meprobamate

Demerol® may be confused with Demulen®, Desyrel®, dicumarol, Dilaudid®, Dymelor®, Pamelor®

High alert medication: The Institute for Safe Medication Practices (ISMP) includes this medication among its list of drug classes which have a heightened risk of causing significant patient harm when used in error.

U.S. Brand Names Demerol®

Index Terms Isonipecaine Hydrochloride; Meperidine Hydrochloride; Pethidine Hydrochloride

Generic Available Yes

Canadian Brand Names Demerol®

Pharmacologic Category Analgesic, Opioid

Use Management of moderate-to-severe pain; adjunct to anesthesia and preoperative sedation

Unlabeled/Investigational Use Reduce postoperative shivering; reduce rigors from amphotericin B (conventional)

Restrictions C-II

Pregnancy Risk Factor C/D (prolonged use or high doses at term)

Lactation Enters breast milk/contraindicated (AAP rates "compatible")

Labeled Contraindications Hypersensitivity to meperidine or any component of the formulation; use with or within 14 days of MAO inhibitors; pregnancy (prolonged use or high doses near term)

Warnings/Precautions Oral meperidine is not recommended for acute/chronic pain management. Meperidine should not be used for acute/cancer pain because of the risk of neurotoxicity. Normeperidine (an active metabolite and CNS stimulant) may accumulate and precipitate anxiety, tremors, or seizures; risk increases with CNS or renal dysfunction, prolonged use (>48 hours), and cumulative dose (>600 mg/24 hours). The Institute for Safe Medication Practice recommends avoiding the use of meperidine for pain control, especially in the elderly and renally-impaired (ISMP, 2007).

May cause CNS depression, which may impair physical or mental abilities; patients must be cautioned about performing tasks which require mental alertness (eg, operating machinery or driving). Effects may be potentiated when used with other sedative drugs or ethanol. Use only with extreme caution (if at all) in patients with head injury or increased intracranial pressure (ICP). Use caution with pulmonary, hepatic, or renal disorders, supraventricular tachycardias, acute abdominal conditions, hypothyroidism, toxic psychosis, kyphoscoliosis, morbid obesity, Addison's disease, BPH, or urethral stricture. Use with caution in patients with biliary tract dysfunction; acute pancreatitis may cause constriction of sphincter of Oddi. May cause hypotension; use with caution in patients with depleted blood volume or drugs which may exaggerate hypotensive effects (including phenothiazines or general anesthetics).

An opioid-containing analgesic regimen should be tailored to each patient's needs and based upon the type of pain being treated (acute versus chronic), the route of administration, degree of tolerance for opioids (naive versus chronic user), age, weight, and medical condition. The optimal analgesic dose varies widely among patients. Some preparations contain sulfites which may cause allergic reaction. Tolerance or drug dependence may result from extended use. Healthcare provider should be alert to problems of abuse, misuse, and diversion. Concurrent use of agonist/antagonist analgesics may precipitate withdrawal symptoms and/or reduced analgesic efficacy in patients following prolonged therapy with mu opioid agonists. Abrupt discontinuation following prolonged use may also lead to withdrawal symptoms. Avoid use in the elderly.

Adverse Reactions Frequency not defined.

Cardiovascular: Hypotension

Central nervous system: Fatigue, drowsiness, dizziness, nervousness, headache, restlessness, malaise, confusion, mental depression, hallucinations, paradoxical CNS stimulation, increased intracranial pressure, seizure (associated with metabolite accumulation), serotonin syndrome

Dermatologic: Rash, urticaria

Gastrointestinal: Nausea, vomiting, constipation, anorexia, stomach cramps, xerostomia, biliary spasm, paralytic ileus, sphincter of Oddi spasm

Genitourinary: Ureteral spasms, decreased urination

Local: Pain at injection site

Neuromuscular & skeletal: Weakness

Respiratory: Dyspnea

Miscellaneous: Anaphylaxis, histamine release, hypersensitivity reactions, physical and psychological dependence

◄ **Drug Interactions**

Metabolism/Transport Effects Substrate (minor) of CYP2B6, 2C19, 3A4

Avoid Concomitant Use

Avoid concomitant use of Meperidine with any of the following: MAO Inhibitors; Sibutramine

Increased Effect/Toxicity

Meperidine may increase the levels/effects of: Alcohol (Ethyl); Alvimopan; CNS Depressants; Desmopressin; Selective Serotonin Reuptake Inhibitors; Serotonin Modulators; Thiazide Diuretics

The levels/effects of Meperidine may be increased by: Amphetamines; Antipsychotic Agents (Phenothiazines); Barbiturates; MAO Inhibitors; Protease Inhibitors; Sibutramine; Succinylcholine

Decreased Effect

Meperidine may decrease the levels/effects of: Pegvisomant

The levels/effects of Meperidine may be decreased by: Ammonium Chloride; Phenytoin; Protease Inhibitors

Ethanol/Nutrition/Herb Interactions

Ethanol: Avoid or limit ethanol (may increase CNS depression). Watch for sedation.

Herb/Nutraceutical: Avoid valerian, St John's wort, kava kava, gotu kola (may increase CNS depression).

Storage/Stability Meperidine injection should be stored at room temperature; do not freeze. Protect from light. Protect oral dosage forms from light.

Compatibility Stable in dextran 6% in dextrose, dextran 6% in NS, D$_5$LR, D$_5$¼NS, D$_5$½NS, D$_5$NS, D$_5$W, D$_{10}$W, LR, ½NS, NS.

Y-site administration: **Compatible:** Amifostine, amikacin, ampicillin, ampicillin/sulbactam, atenolol, aztreonam, bumetanide, cefamandole, cefazolin, cefotaxime, cefotetan, cefoxitin, ceftazidime, ceftizoxime, ceftriaxone, cefuroxime, chloramphenicol, cisatracurium, cladribine, clindamycin, cotrimoxazole, dexamethasone sodium phosphate, diltiazem, diphenhydramine, dobutamine, docetaxel, dopamine, doxycycline, droperidol, erythromycin lactobionate, etoposide phosphate, famotidine, filgrastim, fluconazole, fludarabine, gatifloxacin, gemcitabine, gentamicin, granisetron, heparin, hydrocortisone sodium succinate, insulin (regular), kanamycin, labetalol, lidocaine, linezolid, magnesium sulfate, melphalan, methyldopate, methylprednisolone sodium succinate, metoclopramide, metoprolol, metronidazole, ondansetron, oxacillin, oxytocin, paclitaxel, penicillin G potassium, piperacillin, piperacillin/tazobactam, potassium chloride, propofol, propranolol, ranitidine, remifentanil, sargramostim, teniposide, thiotepa, ticarcillin, ticarcillin/clavulanate, tobramycin, vancomycin, verapamil, vinorelbine. **Incompatible:** Allopurinol, amphotericin B cholesteryl sulfate complex, cefepime, cefoperazone, doxorubicin liposome, idarubicin, imipenem/cilastatin, minocycline. **Variable (consult detailed reference):** Acyclovir, furosemide, nafcillin.

Compatibility in syringe: **Compatible:** Atropine, atropine with hydroxyzine, atropine with promethazine, butorphanol, chlorpromazine, cimetidine, dimenhydrinate, diphenhydramine, droperidol, fentanyl, glycopyrrolate, hydroxyzine, ketamine, metoclopramide, midazolam, ondansetron, pentazocine, pentazocine with perphenazine, perphenazine, prochlorperazine edisylate, promazine, promethazine, ranitidine, scopolamine. **Incompatible:** Heparin, morphine, pentobarbital.

Compatibility when admixed: **Compatible:** Cefazolin, dobutamine, metoclopramide, ondansetron, scopolamine, succinylcholine, triflupromazine, verapamil. **Incompatible:** Aminophylline, amobarbital, floxacillin, furosemide, heparin, morphine, phenobarbital, phenytoin, thiopental. **Variable (consult detailed reference):** Sodium bicarbonate.

Mechanism of Action Binds to opiate receptors in the CNS, causing inhibition of ascending pain pathways, altering the perception of and response to pain; produces generalized CNS depression

Pharmacodynamics/Kinetics

Onset of action: Analgesic: Oral, SubQ: 10-15 minutes; I.V.: ~5 minutes
Peak effect: SubQ.: ~1 hour; Oral: 2 hours

Duration: Oral, SubQ: 2-4 hours

Absorption: I.M.: Erratic and highly variable

Distribution: Crosses placenta; enters breast milk

Protein binding: 65% to 75%

Metabolism: Hepatic; hydrolyzed to meperidinic acid (inactive) or undergoes N-demethylation to normeperidine (active; has 1/2 the analgesic effect and 2-3 times the CNS effects of meperidine)

Bioavailability: ~50% to 60%; increased with liver disease

Half-life elimination:
Parent drug: Terminal phase: Adults: 2.5-4 hours, Liver disease: 7-11 hours
Normeperidine (active metabolite): 15-30 hours; can accumulate with high doses (>600 mg/day) or with decreased renal function

Excretion: Urine (as metabolites)

Dosage Note: The American Pain Society (2008) and ISMP (2007) do not recommend meperidine's use as an analgesic.

Children: Pain: Oral, I.M., I.V., SubQ: 1-1.5 mg/kg/dose every 3-4 hours as needed; 1-2 mg/kg as a single dose preoperative medication may be used; maximum 100 mg/dose (**Note:** Oral route is not recommended for acute pain.)

Adults: Pain:
Oral: Initial: Opiate-naive: 50 mg every 3-4 hours as needed; usual dosage range: 50-150 mg every 2-4 hours as needed (manufacturers recommendation; oral route is not recommended for acute pain)
I.M., SubQ: Initial: Opiate-naive: 50-75 mg every 3-4 hours as needed; patients with prior opiate exposure may require higher initial doses
Slow I.V.: Initial: 5-10 mg every 5 minutes as needed
Preoperatively: 50-100 mg given 30-90 minutes before the beginning of anesthesia

Note: If use in acute pain (in patients without renal or CNS disease) cannot be avoided, treatment should be limited to ≤48 hours and doses should not exceed 600 mg/24 hours.

Elderly:
Oral: 50 mg every 4 hours
I.M.: 25 mg every 4 hours

Dosing adjustment in renal impairment: Avoid use in renal impairment
Dosing adjustment/comments in hepatic disease: Increased narcotic effect in cirrhosis; reduction in dose more important for oral than I.V. route

Administration

Solution for injection: Meperidine may be administered I.M., SubQ, or I.V.; I.V. push should be administered slowly, use of a 10 mg/mL concentration has been recommended. For continuous I.V. infusions, a more dilute solution (eg, 1 mg/mL) should be used.

Oral solution: Administer solution in 1/2 glass of water; undiluted solution may exert topical anesthetic effect on mucous membranes

◀ **Monitoring Parameters** Pain relief, respiratory and mental status, blood pressure; observe patient for excessive sedation, CNS depression, seizures, respiratory depression

Test Interactions Increased amylase (S), increased BSP retention, increased CPK (I.M. injections)

Dosage Forms Excipient information presented when available (limited, particularly for generics); consult specific product labeling. [DSC] = Discontinued product

Injection, solution, as hydrochloride [ampul]: 25 mg/0.5 mL (0.5 mL); 25 mg/mL (1 mL); 50 mg/mL (1 mL, 1.5 mL, 2 mL); 75 mg/mL (1 mL); 100 mg/mL (1 mL)

Injection, solution, as hydrochloride [prefilled syringe]: 25 mg/mL (1 mL); 50 mg/mL (1 mL); 75 mg/mL (1 mL); 100 mg/mL (1 mL)

Injection, solution, as hydrochloride [for PCA pump]: 10 mg/mL (30 mL, 50 mL [DSC], 60 mL)

Injection, solution, as hydrochloride [vial]: 25 mg/mL (1 mL); 50 mg/mL (1 mL, 30 mL); 75 mg/mL (1 mL); 100 mg/mL (1 mL, 20 mL) [may contain sodium metabisulfite]

Solution, oral, as hydrochloride: 50 mg/5 mL (500 mL)

Tablet, as hydrochloride: 50 mg, 100 mg

Demerol®: 50 mg, 100 mg

References

Cole TB, Sprinkle RH, Smith SJ, et al, "Intravenous Narcotic Therapy for Children With Severe Sickle Cell Pain Crisis," *Am J Dis Child*, 1986, 140(12):1255-9.

Institute for Safe Medication Practice, "High Alert Medication Feature: Reducing Patient Harm From Opiates," *ISMP Medication Safety Alert*, February 22, 2007. Available online at http://www.ismp.org/Newsletters/acutecare/articles/20070222.asp.

Jacobi J, Fraser GL, Coursin DB, et al, "Clinical Practice Guidelines for the Sustained Use of Sedatives and Analgesics in the Critically Ill Adult," *Crit Care Med*, 2002, 30(1):119-41. Available at: http://www.sccm.org/pdf/sedatives.pdf. Accessed August 2, 2003.

"Principles of Analgesic Use in the Treatment of Acute Pain and Chronic Cancer Pain," 5th ed, Glenview, IL: American Pain Society, 2003.

◆ **Meperidine Hydrochloride** see Meperidine on page 750

◆ **Mephyton®** see Phytonadione on page 953

◆ **Mercaptoethane Sulfonate** see Mesna on page 758

Mercaptopurine (mer kap toe PYOOR een)

Medication Safety Issues

Sound-alike/look-alike issues:

Mercaptopurine may be confused with methotrexate

Purinethol® may be confused with propylthiouracil

High alert medication: The Institute for Safe Medication Practices (ISMP) includes this medication among its list of drugs which have a heightened risk of causing significant patient harm when used in error.

To avoid potentially serious dosage errors, the terms "6-mercaptopurine" or "6-MP" should be avoided; use of these terms has been associated with sixfold overdosages.

Azathioprine is metabolized to mercaptopurine; concurrent use of these commercially-available products has resulted in profound myelosuppression.

Related Information

Safe Handling of Hazardous Drugs on page 1517

U.S. Brand Names Purinethol®

Index Terms 6-Mercaptopurine (error-prone abbreviation); 6-MP (error-prone abbreviation); NSC-755

Generic Available Yes

Canadian Brand Names Purinethol®

Pharmacologic Category Antineoplastic Agent, Antimetabolite; Immuno-suppressant Agent

Use Treatment (maintenance and induction) of acute lymphoblastic leukemia (ALL)

Unlabeled/Investigational Use Steroid-sparing agent for corticosteroid-dependent Crohn's disease (CD) and ulcerative colitis (UC); maintenance of remission in CD; fistulizing Crohn's disease

Pregnancy Risk Factor D

Lactation Enters breast milk/contraindicated

Labeled Contraindications Hypersensitivity to mercaptopurine or any component of the formulation; patients whose disease showed prior resistance to mercaptopurine or thioguanine; severe liver disease, severe bone marrow suppression; pregnancy

Warnings/Precautions Hazardous agent - use appropriate precautions for handling and disposal. Consider adjusting dosage in patients with renal impairment or hepatic failure; use with caution in patients with prior bone marrow suppression. Toxicity to immunosuppressives is increased in elderly. Start with lowest recommended adult doses. Signs of infection, such as fever and WBC rise, may not occur. Lethargy and confusion may be more prominent signs of infection. Use caution with other hepatotoxic drugs or in dosages >2.5 mg/kg/day; hepatotoxicity may occur. Patients with genetic deficiency of thiopurine methyltransferase (TPMT) or concurrent therapy with drugs which may inhibit TPMT (eg, olsalazine) or xanthine oxidase (eg, allopurinol) may be sensitive to myelosuppressive effects. Azathioprine is metabolized to mercaptopurine; concomitant use may result in profound myelosuppression and should be avoided. Immune response to vaccines may be diminished.

To avoid potentially serious dosage errors, the terms "6-mercaptopurine" or "6-MP" should be avoided; use of these terms has been associated with sixfold overdosages.

Adverse Reactions

>10%:

Hematologic: Myelosuppression; leukopenia, thrombocytopenia, anemia
Onset: 7-10 days
Nadir: 14-16 days
Recovery: 21-28 days

Hepatic: Intrahepatic cholestasis and focal centralobular necrosis (40%), characterized by hyperbilirubinemia, increased alkaline phosphatase and AST, jaundice, ascites, encephalopathy; more common at doses >2.5 mg/kg/day. Usually occurs within 2 months of therapy but may occur within 1 week, or be delayed up to 8 years.

1% to 10%:

Central nervous system: Drug fever

Dermatologic: Hyperpigmentation, rash

Endocrine & metabolic: Hyperuricemia

Gastrointestinal: Anorexia, diarrhea, mucositis, nausea, pancreatitis, stomach pain, stomatitis, vomiting

Renal: Renal toxicity

<1%: Alopecia, dry and scaling rash, glossitis, oligospermia, tarry stools, eosinophilia

Drug Interactions

Avoid Concomitant Use

Avoid concomitant use of Mercaptopurine with any of the following: Febuxostat; Natalizumab; Vaccines (Live)

Increased Effect/Toxicity

Mercaptopurine may increase the levels/effects of: Leflunomide; Natalizumab; Vaccines (Live); Vitamin K Antagonists

The levels/effects of Mercaptopurine may be increased by: 5-ASA Derivatives; Allopurinol; AzaTHIOprine; Febuxostat; Trastuzumab

Decreased Effect

Mercaptopurine may decrease the levels/effects of: Vaccines (Inactivated); Vaccines (Live); Vitamin K Antagonists

The levels/effects of Mercaptopurine may be decreased by: Echinacea

Storage/Stability Store at room temperature of 15°C to 25°C (59°F to 77°F). Protect from moisture.

Mechanism of Action Purine antagonist which inhibits DNA and RNA synthesis; acts as false metabolite and is incorporated into DNA and RNA, eventually inhibiting their synthesis; specific for the S phase of the cell cycle

Pharmacodynamics/Kinetics

Absorption: Variable and incomplete (16% to 50%)

Distribution: V_d = total body water; CNS penetration is poor

Protein binding: 19%

Metabolism: Hepatic and in GI mucosa; hepatically via xanthine oxidase and methylation via TPMT to sulfate conjugates, 6-thiouric acid, and other inactive compounds; first-pass effect

Half-life elimination (age dependent): Children: 21 minutes; Adults: 47 minutes

Time to peak, serum: ~2 hours

Excretion: Urine (46% as mercaptopurine and metabolites)

Dosage Oral (refer to individual protocols):

Children: ALL:
  Induction: 2.5-5 mg/kg/day **or** 70-100 mg/m²/day given once daily
  Maintenance: 1.5-2.5 mg/kg/day **or** 50-75 mg/m²/day given once daily

Adults:
  ALL:
    Induction: 2.5-5 mg/kg/day (100-200 mg)
    Maintenance: 1.5-2.5 mg/kg/day **or** 80-100 mg/m²/day given once daily
  Reduction of steroid use in CD or UC, maintenance of remission in CD or fistulizing disease (unlabeled uses): Initial: 50 mg daily; may increase by 25 mg/day every 1-2 weeks as tolerated to target dose of 1-1.5 mg/kg/day

Dosage adjustment with concurrent allopurinol: Reduce mercaptopurine dosage to ¼ to ⅓ the usual dose.

Dosage adjustment in TPMT-deficiency: Not established; substantial reductions are generally required only in homozygous deficiency.

Elderly: Due to renal decline with age, start with lower recommended doses for adults

Note: In ALL, administration in the evening (vs morning administration) may lower the risk of relapse.

Dosing adjustment in renal impairment: The FDA-approved labeling recommends starting with reduced doses in patients with renal impairment to avoid accumulation; however, specific guidelines are not available. The following guidelines have been used by some clinicians (Aronoff, 2007):

Children:
  Cl_{cr} <50 mL/minute: Administer every 48 hours
  Hemodialysis: Administer every 48 hours
  Continuous ambulatory peritoneal dialysis (CAPD): Administer every 48 hours
  Continuous renal replacement therapy (CRRT): Administer every 48 hours

Dosing adjustment in hepatic impairment: The FDA-approved labeling recommends considering a reduced dose in patients with hepatic impairment; however, specific guidelines are not available.

Combination Regimens

Leukemia, acute lymphocytic:
Leukemia, acute promyelocytic:

Administration Preferably on an empty stomach (1 hour before or 2 hours after meals)

Monitoring Parameters CBC with differential and platelet count, liver function tests, uric acid, urinalysis; TPMT genotyping may identify individuals at risk for toxicity

For use as immunomodulatory therapy in CD or UC, monitor CBC with differential weekly for 1 month, then biweekly for 1 month, followed by monitoring every 1-2 months throughout the course of therapy. LFTs should be assessed every 3 months.

Dietary Considerations Should not be administered with meals.

Emetic Potential Very low (<10%)

Dosage Forms Excipient information presented when available (limited, particularly for generics); consult specific product labeling.

Tablet [scored]: 50 mg

Extemporaneous Preparations A 50 mg/mL oral suspension can be prepared by crushing thirty 50 mg tablets in a mortar, and then mixing in a small amount of vehicle (a 1:1 combination of methylcellulose 1% and syrup) to create a uniform paste. Add a sufficient quantity of vehicle to make 30 mL of suspension. Label "shake well." Room temperature stability is 14 days.

Dressman JB and Poust RI, "Stability of Allopurinol and Five Antineoplastics in Suspension," *Am J Hosp Pharm*, 1983, 40:616-8.

Nahata MC, Morosco RS, and Hipple TF, 4th ed, *Pediatric Drug Formulations*, Cincinnati, OH: Harvey Whitney Books Co, 2000.

References

Aronoff GR, Bennett WM, Berns JS, et al, *Drug Prescribing in Renal Failure: Dosing Guidelines for Adults and Children*, 5th ed. Philadelphia, PA: American College of Physicians; 2007, p 173.

Kaplan HG, "Use of Cancer Chemotherapy in the Elderly," *Drug Treatment in the Elderly*, Vestal RE, ed, Boston, MA: ADIS Health Science Press, 1984, 338-49.

Lennard L, "The Clinical Pharmacology of 6-Mercaptopurine," *Eur J Clin Pharmacol*, 1992, 43 (4):329-39.

Lichtenstein GR, Abreu MT, Cohen R, et al, "American Gastroenterological Association Institute Medical Position Statement on Corticosteroids, Immunomodulators, and Infliximab in Inflammatory Bowel Disease," *Gastroenterology*, 2006, 130(3):935-9.

Sandborn WJ, "A Review of Immune Modifier Therapy for Inflammatory Bowel Disease: Azathioprine, 6-mercaptopurine, Cyclosporine, and Methotrexate," *Am J Gastroenterol*, 1996, 91(3):423-33.

Van Scoik KG, Johnson CA, and Porter WR, "The Pharmacology and Metabolism of the Thiopurine Drugs 6-Mercaptopurine and Azathioprine," *Drug Metab Rev*, 1985, 16(1-2):157-74.

◆ **6-Mercaptopurine (error-prone abbreviation)** *see* Mercaptopurine *on page 754*

◆ **M-Eslon® (Can)** *see* Morphine Sulfate *on page 816*

Mesna (MES na)

U.S. Brand Names Mesnex®

Index Terms Mercaptoethane Sulfonate; Sodium 2-Mercaptoethane Sulfonate

Generic Available Yes: Solution for injection

Canadian Brand Names Mesnex®; Uromitexan

Pharmacologic Category Antidote; Uroprotectant

Use Preventative agent to reduce the incidence of ifosfamide-induced hemorrhagic cystitis

Unlabeled/Investigational Use Preventative agent to reduce the incidence of cyclophosphamide-induced hemorrhagic cystitis with high-dose cyclophosphamide

Pregnancy Risk Factor B

Lactation Excretion in breast milk unknown/not recommended

Labeled Contraindications Hypersensitivity to mesna or other thiol compounds, or any component of the formulation

Warnings/Precautions Examine morning urine specimen for hematuria prior to ifosfamide or cyclophosphamide treatment; if hematuria (>50 RBC/HPF) develops, reduce the ifosfamide/cyclophosphamide dose or discontinue the drug; will not prevent or alleviate other toxicities associated with ifosfamide or cyclophosphamide and will not prevent hemorrhagic cystitis in all patients. Mesna will not reduce the risk of thrombocytopenia-related hematuria. Allergic reactions have been reported; symptoms ranged from mild hypersensitivity to systemic anaphylactic reactions and may include fever, hypotension, and/or tachycardia; patients with autoimmune disorders receiving cyclophosphamide and mesna may be at increased risk. Patients should receive adequate hydration during treatment. I.V. formulation contains benzyl alcohol; do not use in neonates or infants (associated with "gasping syndrome").

Adverse Reactions

Mesna alone (frequency not defined):

Cardiovascular: Flushing

Central nervous system: Dizziness, fever, headache, hyperesthesia, somnolence

Dermatologic: Rash

Gastrointestinal: Anorexia, constipation, diarrhea, flatulence, nausea, taste alteration/bad taste (with oral administration), vomiting

Local: Injection site reactions

Neuromuscular: Arthralgia, back pain, rigors

Ocular: Conjunctivitis

Respiratory: Cough, pharyngitis, rhinitis

Miscellaneous: Flu-like syndrome

Mesna alone or in combination: Postmarketing and/or case reports: Allergic reaction, anaphylactic reaction, hypersensitivity, hyper-/hypotension, injection site erythema, injection site pain, limb pain, malaise, myalgia, platelets decreased, ST-segment increased, tachycardia, tachypnea, transaminases increased

Drug Interactions

Avoid Concomitant Use There are no known interactions where it is recommended to avoid concomitant use.

Increased Effect/Toxicity There are no known significant interactions involving an increase in effect.

Decreased Effect There are no known significant interactions involving a decrease in effect.

Storage/Stability Store intact vials and tablets at room temperature of 20°C to 25°C (68°F to 77°F). Opened multidose vials may be stored and used for use to 8 days after opening. Solutions diluted for infusion are stable for at least 24 hours at room temperature. Solutions in plastic syringes are stable for 9 days under refrigeration, or at room or body temperature. Solutions of mesna and ifosfamide in lactated Ringer's are stable for 7 days in a PVC ambulatory infusion pump reservoir. Solutions of mesna (0.5-3.2 mg/mL) and cyclophosphamide (1.8-10.8 mg/mL) in D_5W are stable for 48 hours refrigerated or 6 hours at room temperature (Menard, 2003). Mesna injection is stable for at least 7 days when diluted 1:2 or 1:5 with grape- and orange-flavored syrups or 11:1 to 1:100 in carbonated beverages for oral administration.

Reconstitution Dilute in 50-1000 mL D_5W, NS, $D_5^1/4$NS, $D_5^1/3$NS, $D_5^1/2$NS, or lactated Ringer's (the manufacturer recommends a final concentration of 20 mg/mL).

Compatibility Stable in $D_5^1/4$NS, $D_5^1/3$NS, $D_5^1/2$NS, D_5W, LR, NS.

Y-site administration: Compatible: Allopurinol, amifostine, aztreonam, caspofungin, cefepime, cladribine, cytarabine, docetaxel, doxorubicin liposome, etoposide phosphate, filgrastim, fludarabine, gallium nitrate, gemcitabine, granisetron, ifosfamide, melphalan, methotrexate, micafungin, ondansetron, oxaliplatin, paclitaxel, pemetrexed, piperacillin/tazobactam, sargramostim, sodium bicarbonate, teniposide, thiotepa, vinorelbine. **Incompatible:** Amphotericin B cholesteryl sulfate complex, fenoldopam, lansoprazole, quinupristin-dalfopristin.

Compatibility in syringe: Compatible: Ifosfamide. **Incompatible:** Ifosfamide with epirubicin.

Compatibility when admixed: Compatible: Hydroxyzine HCl, ifosfamide. **Incompatible:** Carboplatin, cisplatin, ifosfamide with epirubicin, ondansetron. **Variable (consult detailed reference):** Cyclophosphamide.

Mechanism of Action In blood, mesna is oxidized to dimesna which in turn is reduced in the kidney back to mesna, supplying a free thiol group which binds to and inactivates acrolein, the urotoxic metabolite of ifosfamide and cyclophosphamide

Pharmacodynamics/Kinetics

Distribution: No tissue penetration

Protein binding: 69% to 75%

Metabolism: Rapidly oxidized intravascularly to mesna disulfide (dimesna); dimesna is reduced in renal tubules back to mesna following glomerular filtration

Bioavailability: Oral: 45% to 79%

Half-life elimination:

I.V.: Mesna: ~22 minutes; Dimesna: ~70 minutes

I.V. followed by oral: 1-8 hours

Time to peak, plasma: 2-3 hours

Excretion: Urine (18% to 32% as mesna; 33% as dimesna)

Dosage

Children and Adults: **Note:** Details concerning dosing in combination regimens should also be consulted. Mesna dosing schedule should be repeated each day ifosfamide is received. If ifosfamide dose is adjusted, the mesna dose should also be modified to maintain the mesna-to-ifosfamide ratio.

I.V.: Prevention of ifosfamide-induced hemorrhagic cystitis:

Short infusion standard-dose ifosfamide (<2.5 g/m^2/day): Mesna dose is equal to 60% of the ifosfamide dose given in 3 divided doses (0, 4, and 8 hours after the start of ifosfamide)

◀ Continuous infusion standard-dose ifosfamide (<2.5 g/m^2/day): ASCO guidelines: Mesna dose (as an I.V. bolus) is equal to 20% of the ifosfamide dose, followed by a continuous infusion of mesna at 40% of the ifosfamide dose, continue mesna infusion for 12-24 hours after completion of ifosfamide infusion (Hensley, 2008)

High-dose ifosfamide (>2.5 g/m^2/day): ASCO guidelines: Evidence for use is inadequate; more frequent and prolonged mesna administration regimens may be required.

I.V. followed by oral (for ifosfamide doses ≤2 g/m^2/day): Mesna dose is equal to 100% of the ifosfamide dose, given as 20% of the ifosfamide dose I.V. at hour 0, followed by 40% of the ifosfamide dose given orally 2- and 6 hours after start of ifosfamide

Combination Regimens

Breast cancer: ICE-T on page 1357

Cervical cancer: BIP on page 1235

Esophageal cancer: TIP on page 1407

Head and neck cancer: TIP on page 1407

Leukemia, acute lymphocytic:
  Hyper-CVAD + Imatinib on page 1348
  Hyper-CVAD (Leukemia, Acute Lymphocytic) on page 1349

Lung cancer (small cell): VIP (Small Cell Lung Cancer) on page 1425

Lymphoma, Hodgkin's: VIM-D (Hodgkin's Lymphoma) on page 1420

Lymphoma, non-Hodgkin's:
  ICE (Lymphoma, non-Hodgkin's) on page 1356
  IMVP-16 on page 1358
  IVAC on page 1361
  MINE on page 1366
  MINE-ESHAP on page 1367
  RICE on page 1402

Lymphoma, non-Hodgkin's (Burkitt's): CODOX-M/IVAC on page 1278

Lymphoma, non-Hodgkin's (Mantle cell): Hyper-CVAD + Rituximab on page 1356

Multiple myeloma: Hyper-CVAD (Multiple Myeloma) on page 1355

Neuroblastoma:
  CI (Neuroblastoma) on page 1263
  HIPE-IVAD on page 1348

Osteosarcoma: ICE (Sarcoma) on page 1357

Soft tissue sarcoma:
  AI on page 1225
  ICE (Sarcoma) on page 1357
  ICE-T on page 1357
  IE on page 1358
  MAID on page 1365

Testicular cancer:
  Paclitaxel-Ifosfamide-Cisplatin on page 1389
  VIP (Etoposide) (Testicular Cancer) on page 1424
  VIP (Vinblastine) (Testicular Cancer) on page 1426

Administration

Oral: Administer orally in tablet formulation or parenteral solution diluted in water, milk, juice, or carbonated beverages; patients who vomit within 2 hours after taking oral mesna should repeat the dose or receive I.V. mesna

I.V.: Administer by short (15-30 minutes) infusion or continuous infusion (maintain continuous infusion for 12-24 after completion of ifosfamide infusion) (Hensley, 2008)

Monitoring Parameters Urinalysis

Test Interactions False-positive urinary ketones with Multistix® or Labstix®

Additional Information Oncology Comment: Guidelines from the American Society of Clinical Oncology (ASCO) for the use of chemotherapy and radiotherapy protectants (Hensley, 2008 [update]; Schuchter, 2002) recommend mesna to decrease the incidence of ifosfamide-induced urotoxicity associated with short infusion and continuous infusion standard-dose ifosfamide (<2.5 g/m^2/day). Although evidence is inadequate regarding mesna's uroprotective effects in high-dose ifosfamide (>2.5 g/m^2/day), the guidelines suggest more frequent and prolonged mesna administration times may be required. For prevention high-dose cyclophosphamide-induced urotoxicity (associated with stem cell transplantation), the guidelines recommend mesna in conjunction with saline diuresis (or forced saline diuresis alone).

Emetic Potential When administered orally, the unpleasant taste may result in vomiting.

Dosage Forms Excipient information presented when available (limited, particularly for generics); consult specific product labeling.

Injection, solution: 100 mg/mL (10 mL) [contains benzyl alcohol]

Mesnex®: 100 mg/mL (10 mL) [contains benzyl alcohol]

Tablet:

Mesnex®: 400 mg

References

Goren MP, "Oral Administration of Mesna With Ifosfamide,"*Semin Oncol,* 1996, 23(3 Suppl 6):91-6.

Goren MP, "Oral Mesna: A Review," *Semin Oncol,* 1992, 19(6 Suppl 12):65-71.

Hensley ML, Hagerty KL, Kewalramani T, et al, "American Society of Clinical Oncology 2008 Clinical Practice Guideline Update: Use of Chemotherapy and Radiotherapy Protectants," *J Clin Oncol,* 2008, 27(1):127-45.

Khaw SL, Downie PA, Waters KD, et al, "Adverse Hypersensitivity Reactions to Mesna as Adjunctive Therapy for Cyclophosphamide," *Pediatr Blood Cancer,* 2007, 49(3):341-3.

Mace JR, Keohan ML, Bernardy H, et al, "Crossover Randomized Comparison of Intravenous Versus Intravenous/Oral Mesna in Soft Tissue Sarcoma Treated With High-Dose Ifosfamide," *Clin Cancer Res,* 2003, 9(16 Pt 1):5829-34.

Menard C, Bourguignon C, Schlatter J, et al, "Stability of Cyclophosphamide and Mesna Admixtures in Polyethylene Infusion Bags," *Ann Pharmacother,* 2003, 37(12):1789-92.

Schuchter LM, Hensley ML, Meropol NJ, et al, "2002 Update of Recommendations for the Use of Chemotherapy and Radiotherapy Protectants: Clinical Practice Guidelines of the American Society of Clinical Oncology," *J Clin Oncol,* 2002, 20(12):2895-903.

Siu LL and Moore MJ, "Use of Mesna to Prevent Ifosfamide-Induced Urotoxicity," *Support Care Cancer,* 1998, 6(2):144-54.

Methadone (METH a done)

Medication Safety Issues

Sound-alike/look-alike issues:

Methadone may be confused with dexmethylphenidate, Mephyton®, methylphenidate, Metadate® CD, and Metadate® ER

High alert medication: The Institute for Safe Medication Practices (ISMP) includes this medication among its list of drug classes which have a heightened risk of causing significant patient harm when used in error.

◀ **U.S. Brand Names** Dolophine®; Methadone Diskets®; Methadone Intensol™; Methadose®

Index Terms Methadone Hydrochloride

Generic Available Yes

Canadian Brand Names Metadol-D™; Metadol™

Pharmacologic Category Analgesic, Opioid

Use Management of moderate-to-severe pain; detoxification and maintenance treatment of opioid addiction as part of an FDA-approved program

Restrictions C-II

When used for treatment of opioid addiction: May only be dispensed in accordance with guidelines established by the Substance Abuse and Mental Health Services Administration's (SAMHSA) Center for Substance Abuse Treatment (CSAT). Regulations regarding methadone use may vary by state and/or country. Obtain advice from appropriate regulatory agencies and/or consult with pain management/palliative care specialists.

Note: Regulatory Exceptions to the General Requirement to Provide Opioid Agonist Treatment (per manufacturer's labeling):
1. During inpatient care, when the patient was admitted for any condition other than concurrent opioid addiction, to facilitate the treatment of the primary admitting diagnosis.
2. During an emergency period of no longer than 3 days while definitive care for the addiction is being sought in an appropriately licensed facility.

Pregnancy Risk Factor C/D (prolonged use or high doses at term)

Lactation Enters breast milk/not recommended (AAP rates "compatible")

Labeled Contraindications Hypersensitivity to methadone or any component of the formulation; respiratory depression (in the absence of resuscitative equipment or in an unmonitored setting); acute bronchial asthma or hypercarbia; paralytic ileus; concurrent use of selegiline

Warnings/Precautions An opioid-containing analgesic regimen should be tailored to each patient's needs and based upon the type of pain being treated (acute versus chronic), the route of administration, degree of tolerance for opioids (naive versus chronic user), age, weight, and medical condition. The optimal analgesic dose varies widely among patients. Doses should be titrated to pain relief/prevention. Patients maintained on stable doses of methadone may need higher and/or more frequent doses in case of acute pain (eg, postoperative pain, physical trauma). Methadone is ineffective for the relief of anxiety.

[U.S. Boxed Warning]: May prolong the QT_c interval and increase risk for torsade de pointes. Patients should be informed of the potential arrhythmia risk, evaluated for any history of structural heart disease, arrhythmia, syncope, and for existence of potential drug interactions including drugs that possess QT_c interval-prolonging properties, promote hypokalemia, hypomagnesemia, or hypocalcemia, or reduce elimination of methadone (eg, CYP3A4 inhibitors). Obtain baseline ECG for all patients and risk stratify according to QT_c interval (see Monitoring Parameters). Use with caution in patients at risk for QT_c prolongation, with medications known to prolong the QT_c interval, promote electrolyte depletion, or inhibit CYP3A4, or history of conduction abnormalities. QT_c interval prolongation and torsade de pointes may be associated with doses >100 mg/day, but have also been observed with lower doses. May cause severe hypotension; use caution with severe volume depletion or other conditions which may compromise maintenance of normal blood pressure. Use caution with cardiovascular disease or patients predisposed to dysrhythmias.

[U.S. Boxed Warning]: May cause respiratory depression. Use caution in patients with respiratory disease or pre-existing respiratory conditions (eg, severe obesity, asthma, COPD, sleep apnea, CNS depression). Because the respiratory effects last longer than the analgesic effects, slow titration is required. Use extreme caution during treatment initiation, dose titration and conversion from other opioid agonists. Incomplete cross tolerance may occur; patients tolerant to other mu opioid agonists may not be tolerant to methadone. Abrupt cessation may precipitate withdrawal symptoms.

May cause CNS depression, which may impair physical or mental abilities. Patients must be cautioned about performing tasks which require mental alertness (eg, operating machinery or driving). Effects with other sedative drugs or ethanol may be potentiated. Use with caution in patients with depression or suicidal tendencies, or in patients with a history of drug abuse. Tolerance or psychological and physical dependence may occur with prolonged use.

Use with caution in patients with head injury or increased intracranial pressure. May obscure diagnosis or clinical course of patients with acute abdominal conditions. Elderly may be more susceptible to adverse effects (eg, CNS, respiratory, gastrointestinal). Decrease initial dose and use caution in the elderly or debilitated; with hyper/hypothyroidism, morbid obesity, adrenal insufficiency, prostatic hyperplasia, or urethral stricture; or with severe renal or hepatic failure. Use with caution in patients with biliary tract dysfunction; acute pancreatitis may cause constriction of sphincter of Oddi. Safety and efficacy have not been established in children. **[U.S. Boxed Warning]: For oral administration only;** excipients to deter use by injection are contained in tablets.

[U.S. Boxed Warning]: When used for treatment of narcotic addiction: May only be dispensed by opioid treatment programs certified by the Substance Abuse and Mental Health Services Administration (SAMHSA) and certified by the designated state authority. Exceptions include inpatient treatment of other conditions and emergency period (not >3 days) while definitive substance abuse treatment is being sought.

Adverse Reactions Frequency not defined. During prolonged administration, adverse effects may decrease over several weeks; however, constipation and sweating may persist.

Cardiovascular: Arrhythmia, bigeminal rhythms, bradycardia, cardiac arrest, cardiomyopathy, ECG changes, edema, extrasystoles, faintness, flushing, heart failure, hypotension, palpitation, peripheral vasodilation, phlebitis, orthostatic hypotension, QT interval prolonged, shock, syncope, tachycardia, torsade de pointes, T-wave inversion, ventricular fibrillation, ventricular tachycardia,

Central nervous system: Agitation, confusion, disorientation, dizziness, drowsiness, dysphoria, euphoria, hallucination, headache, insomnia, light-headedness, sedation, seizure

Dermatologic: Hemorrhagic urticaria, pruritus, rash, urticaria

Endocrine & metabolic: Antidiuretic effect, amenorrhea, hypokalemia, hypomagnesemia, libido decreased

Gastrointestinal: Abdominal pain, anorexia, biliary tract spasm, constipation, glossitis, nausea, stomach cramps, vomiting, weight gain, xerostomia

Genitourinary: Impotence, urinary retention or hesitancy

Hematologic: Thrombocytopenia (reversible, reported in patients with chronic hepatitis)

Neuromuscular & skeletal: Weakness

Local: I.M./SubQ injection: Erythema, pain, swelling; I.V. injection: Hemorrhagic urticaria (rare), pruritus, urticaria, rash

Ocular: Miosis, visual disturbances

Respiratory: Pulmonary edema, respiratory depression, respiratory arrest

Miscellaneous: Death, diaphoresis, physical and psychological dependence

Drug Interactions

Metabolism/Transport Effects Substrate of CYP2C9 (minor), 2C19 (minor), 2D6 (minor), 3A4 (major); **Inhibits** CYP2D6 (moderate), 3A4 (weak)

Avoid Concomitant Use

Avoid concomitant use of Methadone with any of the following: Artemether; Dronedarone; Lumefantrine; Nilotinib; Pimozide; QuiNINE; Tetrabenazine; Thioridazine; Ziprasidone

Increased Effect/Toxicity

Methadone may increase the levels/effects of: Alcohol (Ethyl); Alvimopan; CNS Depressants; CYP2D6 Substrates; Desmopressin; Dronedarone; Fesoterodine; Nebivolol; Pimozide; QTc-Prolonging Agents; QuiNINE; Selective Serotonin Reuptake Inhibitors; Tamoxifen; Tetrabenazine; Thiazide Diuretics; Thioridazine; Zidovudine; Ziprasidone

The levels/effects of Methadone may be increased by: Alfuzosin; Amphetamines; Antifungal Agents (Azole Derivatives, Systemic); Antipsychotic Agents (Phenothiazines); Artemether; Chloroquine; Ciprofloxacin; CYP3A4 Inhibitors (Moderate); CYP3A4 Inhibitors (Strong); Gadobutrol; Lumefantrine; Nilotinib; Protease Inhibitors; QuiNINE; Selective Serotonin Reuptake Inhibitors; Succinylcholine

Decreased Effect

Methadone may decrease the levels/effects of: Codeine; Didanosine; Pegvisomant; TraMADol

The levels/effects of Methadone may be decreased by: Ammonium Chloride; Barbiturates; CarBAMazepine; CYP3A4 Inducers (Strong); Deferasirox; Etravirine; Herbs (CYP3A4 Inducers); Phenytoin; Reverse Transcriptase Inhibitors (Non-Nucleoside); Rifamycin Derivatives

Ethanol/Nutrition/Herb Interactions

Ethanol: Avoid ethanol (may increase CNS effects). Watch for sedation.

Herb/Nutraceutical: Avoid St John's wort (may decrease methadone levels; may increase CNS depression). Avoid valerian, kava kava, gotu kola (may increase CNS depression). Methadone is metabolized by CYP3A4 in the intestines; avoid concurrent use of grapefruit juice.

Storage/Stability

Injection: Store at controlled room temperature of 15°C to 30°C (59°F to 86°F). Protect from light.

Oral concentrate, oral solution, tablet: Store at controlled room temperature of 15°C to 30°C (59°F to 86°F).

Compatibility Stable in NS.

Mechanism of Action Binds to opiate receptors in the CNS, causing inhibition of ascending pain pathways, altering the perception of and response to pain; produces generalized CNS depression

Pharmacodynamics/Kinetics

Onset of action: Oral: Analgesic: 0.5-1 hour; Parenteral: 10-20 minutes

Peak effect: Parenteral: 1-2 hours; Oral: continuous dosing: 3-5 days

Duration of analgesia: Oral: 4-8 hours, increases to 22-48 hours with repeated doses

Distribution: V_{dss}: 1-8 L/kg

Protein binding: 85% to 90%

Metabolism: Hepatic; N-demethylation primarily via CYP3A4, CYP2B6, and CYP2C19 to inactive metabolites

Bioavailability: Oral: 36% to 100%

Half-life elimination: 8-59 hours; may be prolonged with alkaline pH, decreased during pregnancy

Time to peak, plasma: 1-7.5 hours

Excretion: Urine (<10% as unchanged drug); increased with urine pH <6

Dosage Regulations regarding methadone use may vary by state and/or country. Obtain advice from appropriate regulatory agencies and/or consult with pain management/palliative care specialists. **Note:** These are guidelines and do not represent the maximum doses that may be required in all patients. Methadone accumulates with repeated doses and dosage may need reduction after 3-5 days to prevent CNS depressant effects. Some patients may benefit from every 8-12 hour dosing interval for chronic pain management. Doses should be titrated to appropriate effects.

Children (unlabeled use):

Pain (analgesia):

Oral: Initial: 0.1-0.2 mg/kg 4-8 hours initially for 2-3 doses, then every 6-12 hours as needed. Dosing interval may range from 4-12 hours during initial therapy; decrease in dose or frequency may be required (~days 2-5) due to accumulation with repeated doses (maximum dose: 5-10 mg)

I.V.: 0.1 mg/kg every 4-8 hours initially for 2-3 doses, then every 6-12 hours as needed. Dosing interval may range from 4-12 hours during initial therapy; decrease in dose or frequency may be required (~days 2-5) due to accumulation with repeated doses (maximum dose: 5-8 mg)

Iatrogenic narcotic dependency: Oral: General guidelines: Initial: 0.05-0.1 mg/kg/dose every 6 hours; increase by 0.05 mg/kg/dose until withdrawal symptoms are controlled; after 24-48 hours, the dosing interval can be lengthened to every 12-24 hours; to taper dose, wean by 0.05 mg/kg/day; if withdrawal symptoms recur, taper at a slower rate

Adults:

Acute pain (moderate-to-severe):

Oral: Opioid-naive: Initial: 2.5-10 mg every 8-12 hours; more frequent administration may be required during initiation to maintain adequate analgesia. Dosage interval may range from 4-12 hours, since duration of analgesia is relatively short during the first days of therapy, but increases substantially with continued administration.

Chronic pain (opioid-tolerant): **Conversion from oral morphine to oral methadone: Note:** 1) There is not a linear relationship when converting to methadone from oral morphine. The higher the daily morphine equivalent dose the more potent methadone is, and 2) conversion to methadone is more of a process than a calculation. Patient response to methadone needs to be monitored closely throughout the process of the conversion.

Daily oral morphine dose <100 mg: Estimated daily oral methadone dose: 20% to 30% of total daily morphine dose

Daily oral morphine dose 100-300 mg: Estimated daily oral methadone dose: 10% to 20% of total daily morphine dose

Daily oral morphine dose 300-600 mg: Estimated daily oral methadone dose: 8% to 12% of total daily morphine dose

Daily oral morphine dose 600-1000 mg: Estimated daily oral methadone dose: 5% to 10% of total daily morphine dose.

Daily oral morphine dose >1000 mg: Estimated daily oral methadone dose: <5% of total daily morphine dose.

Note: The total daily methadone dose should then be divided to reflect the intended dosing schedule.

Or, per American Pain Society:

Daily oral morphine or equivalent dose per day <90 mg: Estimated daily oral methadone dose: 25% of total daily morphine dose

Daily oral morphine or equivalent dose per day 90-300 mg: Estimated daily oral methadone dose: 12% of total daily morphine dose

Daily oral morphine or equivalent dose per day >300 mg: Estimated daily oral methadone dose: 8% of total daily morphine dose

Note: The estimated total daily methadone dose should then be divided by 3 and administered every 8 hours.

I.V.: Manufacturers labeling: Initial: 2.5-10 mg every 8-12 hours in opioid-naive patients; titrate slowly to effect; may also be administered by SubQ or I.M. injection

Conversion from oral methadone to parenteral methadone dose: Initial dose: Parenteral:Oral ratio: 1:2 (eg, 5 mg parenteral methadone equals 10 mg oral methadone)

Detoxification: Oral:

Initial: A single dose of 20-30 mg is generally sufficient to suppress symptoms. Should not exceed 30 mg; lower doses should be considered in patients with low tolerance at initiation (eg, absence of opioids ≥5 days); an additional 5-10 mg of methadone may be provided if withdrawal symptoms have not been suppressed or if symptoms reappear after 2-4 hours; total daily dose on the first day should not exceed 40 mg, unless the program physician documents in the patient's record that 40 mg did not control opiate abstinence symptoms.

Maintenance: Titrate to a dosage which attenuates craving, blocks euphoric effects of other opiates, and tolerance to sedative effect of methadone. Usual range: 80-120 mg/day (titration should occur cautiously)

Withdrawal: Dose reductions should be <10% of the maintenance dose, every 10-14 days

Detoxification (short-term): Oral:

Initial: Titrate to ~40 mg/day in divided doses to achieve stabilization, may continue 40 mg dose for 2-3 days

Maintenance: Titrate to a dosage which prevents/attenuates euphoric effects of self-administered opioids, reduces drug craving, and withdrawal symptoms are prevented for 24 hours.

Withdrawal: Requires individualization. Decrease daily or every other day, keeping withdrawal symptoms tolerable; hospitalized patients may tolerate a 20% reduction/day; ambulatory patients may require a slower reduction

Dosage adjustment during pregnancy: Methadone dose may need to be increased, or the dosing interval decreased; use should be reserved for cases where the benefits clearly outweigh the risks

Dosage adjustment for toxicity:

QT_c *>450-499 msecs:* Monitor QT_c more frequently

QT_c *≥500 msecs:* Consider discontinuation or reducing methadone dose

Dosage adjustment in renal impairment: Cl_{cr} <10 mL/minute: Administer 50% to 75% of normal dose

Dosage adjustment in hepatic impairment: Avoid in severe liver disease

Administration Oral dose for detoxification and maintenance may be administered in fruit juice or water. Dispersible tablet should not be chewed or swallowed; add to liquid and allow to dissolve before administering. May rinse if residual remains.

Monitoring Parameters Obtain baseline ECG (evaluate QT_c interval), within 30 days of initiation, and then annually for all patients receiving methadone. Increase ECG monitoring if patient receiving >100 mg/day or if unexplained syncope or seizure occurs while on methadone (Krantz, 2008).

If before or at anytime during therapy:

QT_c >450-499 msecs: Discuss potential risks and benefits; monitor QT_c more frequently

QT_c ≥500 msecs: Consider discontinuation or reducing methadone dose **or** eliminate factors promoting QT_c prolongation (eg, potassium-wasting drugs) **or** use alternative therapy (eg, buprenorphine)

Pain relief, respiratory and mental status, blood pressure

Test Interactions Some quinolones may produce a false-positive urine screening result for opiates using commercially-available immunoassay kits. This has been demonstrated most consistently for levofloxacin and ofloxacin, but other quinolones have shown cross-reactivity in certain assay kits. Confirmation of positive opiate screens by more specific methods should be considered.

Dosage Forms Excipient information presented when available (limited, particularly for generics); consult specific product labeling. [DSC] = Discontinued product

Injection, solution, as hydrochloride: 10 mg/mL (20 mL)

Solution, oral, as hydrochloride: 5 mg/5 mL (500 mL); 10 mg/5 mL (500 mL) [contains alcohol 8%; citrus flavor]

Solution, oral, as hydrochloride [concentrate]: 10 mg/mL (946 mL)

Methadone Intensol™: 10 mg/mL (30 mL) [dye free, sugar free; contains sodium benzoate; unflavored]

Methadose®: 10 mg/mL (1000 mL) [contains propylene glycol; cherry flavor]

Methadose®: 10 mg/mL (1000 mL) [dye free, sugar free; contains sodium benzoate; unflavored]

Tablet, as hydrochloride: 5 mg, 10 mg

Dolophine®: 5 mg, 10 mg

Methadose®: 5 mg, 10 mg [DSC]

Tablet, dispersible, as hydrochloride: 40 mg

Methadose®: 40 mg

Methadone Diskets®: 40 mg [orange-pineapple flavor]

References

Department of Health and Human Services: Substance Abuse and Mental Health Services Administration, "Opioid Drugs in Maintenance and Detoxification of Opiate Addiction; Final Rule," *Fed Regist*, 2001, 66(11): 4075-102.

Gazelle G and Fine PG, "Methadone for the Treatment of Pain #75," *J Palliat Med*, 2003, 6 (4):620-1.

Lauriault G, LeBelle MJ, Lodge BA, et al, "Stability of Methadone in Four Vehicles for Oral Administration," *Am J Hosp Pharm*, 1991, 48(6):1252-6.

"Principles of Analgesic Use in the Treatment of Acute Pain and Chronic Cancer Pain," 5th ed, Glenview, IL: American Pain Society, 2003.

◆ **Methadone Diskets®** *see* Methadone *on page* 761

◆ **Methadone Hydrochloride** *see* Methadone *on page* 761

◆ **Methadone Intensol™** *see* Methadone *on page* 761

◆ **Methadose®** *see* Methadone *on page* 761

Methotrexate (meth oh TREKS ate)

Medication Safety Issues

Sound-alike/look-alike issues:

Methotrexate may be confused with mercaptopurine, methylPREDNISolone sodium succinate, metolazone, metroNIDAZOLE, mitoxantrone, pralatrexate

MTX is an error-prone abbreviation (mistaken as mitoxantrone)

High alert medication: The Institute for Safe Medication Practices (ISMP) includes this medication among its list of drugs which have a heightened risk of causing significant patient harm when used in error.

Errors have occurred (resulting in death) when methotrexate was administered as "daily" dose instead of the recommended "weekly" dose.

International issues:

Trexall™ may be confused with Truxal® which is a brand name for chlorprothixene in Belgium

Trexall™ may be confused with Trexol® which is a brand name for tramadol in Mexico

Related Information

Hematopoietic Stem Cell Transplantation *on page 1501*
Oral Mucositis / Stomatitis *on page 1460*
Safe Handling of Hazardous Drugs *on page 1517*

U.S. Brand Names Rheumatrex®; Trexall™

Index Terms Amethopterin; Methotrexate Sodium; Methotrexatum; MTX (error-prone abbreviation)

Generic Available Yes

Canadian Brand Names Apo-Methotrexate®; ratio-Methotrexate

Pharmacologic Category Antineoplastic Agent, Antimetabolite (Antifolate); Antirheumatic, Disease Modifying

Use

Oncology-related uses: Treatment of trophoblastic neoplasms (gestational choriocarcinoma, chorioadenoma destruens and hydatidiform mole), acute lymphocytic leukemia (ALL), meningeal leukemia, breast cancer, head and neck cancer (epidermoid), cutaneous T-Cell lymphoma (advanced mycosis fungoides), lung cancer (squamous cell and small cell), advanced non-Hodgkin's lymphomas (NHL), osteosarcoma

Nononcology uses: Treatment of psoriasis (severe, recalcitrant, disabling) and severe rheumatoid arthritis (RA), including polyarticular-course juvenile rheumatoid arthritis (JRA)

Unlabeled/Investigational Use Treatment and maintenance of remission in Crohn's disease; ectopic pregnancy; dermatomyositis; bladder cancer, central nervous system tumors (including nonleukemic meningeal cancers), acute promyelocytic leukemia (maintenance treatment), soft tissue sarcoma (desmoid tumors)

Pregnancy Risk Factor X (psoriasis, rheumatoid arthritis)

Lactation Enters breast milk/contraindicated

Labeled Contraindications Hypersensitivity to methotrexate or any component of the formulation; breast-feeding

Additional contraindications for patients with psoriasis or rheumatoid arthritis: Pregnancy, alcoholism, alcoholic liver disease or other chronic liver disease, immunodeficiency syndrome (overt or laboratory evidence); pre-existing blood dyscrasias (eg, bone marrow hypoplasia, leukopenia, thrombocytopenia, significant anemia)

Warnings/Precautions Hazardous agent - use appropriate precautions for handling and disposal.

[U.S. Boxed Warning]: Methotrexate has been associated with acute (elevated transaminases) and potentially fatal chronic (fibrosis, cirrhosis) hepatotoxicity. Risk is related to cumulative dose and prolonged exposure. Monitor closely (with liver function tests, including serum albumin) for liver toxicities. Liver enzyme elevations may be noted, but may not be predictive of hepatic disease in long term treatment for psoriasis (but generally is predictive in rheumatoid arthritis [RA] treatment). With long-term use, liver biopsy may show histologic changes, fibrosis or cirrhosis; periodic liver biopsy is recommended with long-term use for psoriasis and for persistent abnormal liver function tests with RA; discontinue methotrexate with moderate-to-severe change in liver biopsy. Ethanol abuse, obesity, advanced age, and diabetes may increase the risk of hepatotoxic reactions. Use caution with preexisting liver impairment; may require dosage reduction. Use caution when used with other hepatotoxic agents (azathioprine, retinoids, sulfasalazine). **[U.S. Boxed Warning]: Methotrexate elimination is reduced in patients with ascites;** may require dose reduction or discontinuation. Monitor closely for toxicity.

[U.S. Boxed Warning]: May cause renal damage leading to acute renal failure, especially with high-dose methotrexate; monitor renal function and methotrexate levels closely, maintain adequate hydration and urinary alkalinization. Use caution in osteosarcoma patients treated with high-dose methotrexate in combination with nephrotoxic chemotherapy (eg, cisplatin). **[U.S. Boxed Warning]: Methotrexate elimination is reduced in patients with renal impairment;** may require dose reduction or discontinuation; monitor closely for toxicity. **[U.S. Boxed Warning]: Tumor lysis syndrome may occur in patients with high tumor burden;** use appropriate prevention and treatment.

[U.S. Boxed Warning]: May cause potentially life-threatening pneumonitis (may occur at any time during therapy and at any dosage); monitor closely for pulmonary symptoms, particularly dry, nonproductive cough. Other potential symptoms include fever, dyspnea, hypoxemia, or pulmonary infiltrate. **[U.S. Boxed Warning]: Methotrexate elimination is reduced in patients with pleural effusions;** may require dose reduction or discontinuation. Monitor closely for toxicity.

[U.S. Boxed Warning]: Bone marrow suppression may occur, resulting in anemia, aplastic anemia, pancytopenia, leukopenia, neutropenia, and/or thrombocytopenia. Use caution in patients with pre-existing bone marrow suppression. Discontinue therapy in RA or psoriasis if a significant decrease in hematologic components is noted. **[U.S. Boxed Warning]: Use of low dose methotrexate has been associated with the development of malignant lymphomas;** may regress upon discontinuation of therapy; treat lymphoma appropriately if regression is not induced by cessation of methotrexate.

[U.S. Boxed Warning]: Diarrhea and ulcerative stomatitis may require interruption of therapy; death from hemorrhagic enteritis or intestinal perforation has been reported. Use with caution in patients with peptic ulcer disease, ulcerative colitis.

May cause neurotoxicity including seizures (usually in pediatric ALL patients), leukoencephalopathy (usually with concurrent cranial irradiation) and stroke-like encephalopathy (usually with high-dose regimens). Chemical arachnoiditis (headache, back pain, nuchal rigidity, fever), myelopathy and chronic leukoencephalopathy may result from intrathecal administration.

[U.S. Boxed Warning]: Any dose level or route of administration may cause severe and potentially fatal dermatologic reactions, including toxic epidermal necrolysis, Stevens-Johnson syndrome, exfoliative dermatitis, skin necrosis, and erythema multiforme. Radiation dermatitis and sunburn may be precipitated by methotrexate administration. Psoriatic lesions may be worsened by concomitant exposure to ultraviolet radiation.

[U.S. Boxed Warning]: Concomitant administration with NSAIDs may cause severe bone marrow suppression, aplastic anemia, and GI toxicity. Do not administer NSAIDs prior to or during high dose methotrexate therapy; may increase and prolong serum methotrexate levels. Doses used for psoriasis may still lead to unexpected toxicities; use caution when administering NSAIDs or salicylates with lower doses of methotrexate for RA. Methotrexate may increase the levels and effects of mercaptopurine; may require dosage adjustments. Vitamins containing folate may decrease response to systemic methotrexate; folate deficiency may increase methotrexate toxicity. **[U.S. Boxed Warning]: Concomitant methotrexate administration with radiotherapy may increase the risk of soft tissue necrosis and osteonecrosis.**

[U.S. Boxed Warnings]: Should be administered under the supervision of a physician experienced in the use of antimetabolite therapy; serious and fatal toxicities have occurred at all dose levels. Immune suppression may lead to potentially fatal opportunistic infections. For rheumatoid arthritis and psoriasis, immunosuppressive therapy should only be used when disease is active and less toxic, traditional therapy is ineffective. Methotrexate formulations and/or diluents containing preservatives should not be used for intrathecal or high-dose therapy. May cause fetal death or congenital abnormalities; do not use for psoriasis or RA treatment in pregnant women. May cause impairment of fertility, oligospermia, and menstrual dysfunction. Toxicity from methotrexate or any immunosuppressive is increased in the elderly. Methotrexate injection may contain benzyl alcohol and should not be used in neonates.

Adverse Reactions Note: Adverse reactions vary by route and dosage. Hematologic and/or gastrointestinal toxicities may be common at dosages used in chemotherapy; these reactions are much less frequent when used at typical dosages for rheumatic diseases.

>10%:
  Central nervous system (with I.T. administration or very high-dose therapy):
    Arachnoiditis: Acute reaction manifested as severe headache, nuchal rigidity, vomiting, and fever; may be alleviated by reducing the dose
    Subacute toxicity: 10% of patients treated with 12-15 mg/m^2 of I.T. methotrexate may develop this in the second or third week of therapy; consists of motor paralysis of extremities, cranial nerve palsy, seizure, or coma. This has also been seen in pediatric cases receiving very high-dose I.V. methotrexate.
    Demyelinating encephalopathy: Seen months or years after receiving methotrexate; usually in association with cranial irradiation or other systemic chemotherapy
  Dermatologic: Reddening of skin

Endocrine & metabolic: Hyperuricemia, defective oogenesis or spermatogenesis

Gastrointestinal: Ulcerative stomatitis, glossitis, gingivitis, nausea, vomiting, diarrhea, anorexia, intestinal perforation, mucositis (dose dependent; appears in 3-7 days after therapy, resolving within 2 weeks)

Hematologic: Leukopenia, myelosuppression (nadir: 7-10 days), thrombocytopenia

Renal: Renal failure, azotemia, nephropathy

Respiratory: Pharyngitis

1% to 10%:

Cardiovascular: Vasculitis

Central nervous system: Dizziness, malaise, encephalopathy, seizure, fever, chills

Dermatologic: Alopecia, rash, photosensitivity, depigmentation or hyper-pigmentation of skin

Endocrine & metabolic: Diabetes

Genitourinary: Cystitis

Hematologic: Hemorrhage

Hepatic: Cirrhosis and portal fibrosis have been associated with chronic methotrexate therapy; acute elevation of liver enzymes are common after high-dose methotrexate, and usually resolve within 10 days.

Neuromuscular & skeletal: Arthralgia

Ocular: Blurred vision

Renal: Renal dysfunction: Manifested by an abrupt rise in serum creatinine and BUN and a fall in urine output; more common with high-dose methotrexate, and may be due to precipitation of the drug.

Respiratory: Pneumonitis: Associated with fever, cough, and interstitial pulmonary infiltrates; treatment is to withhold methotrexate during the acute reaction; interstitial pneumonitis has been reported to occur with an incidence of 1% in patients with RA (dose 7.5-15 mg/week)

<1% (Limited to important or life-threatening): Acute neurologic syndrome (at high dosages - symptoms include confusion, hemiparesis, transient blind-ness, and coma); anaphylaxis, alveolitis, cognitive dysfunction (has been reported at low dosage), decreased resistance to infection, erythema multiforme, hepatic failure, leukoencephalopathy (especially following craniospinal irradiation or repeated high-dose therapy), lymphoproliferative disorders, osteonecrosis and soft tissue necrosis (with radiotherapy), pericarditis, plaque erosions (psoriasis), seizure (more frequent in pediatric patients with ALL), Stevens-Johnson syndrome, thromboembolism

Drug Interactions

Avoid Concomitant Use

Avoid concomitant use of Methotrexate with any of the following: Acitretin; Natalizumab; Vaccines (Live)

Increased Effect/Toxicity

Methotrexate may increase the levels/effects of: CycloSPORINE; Lefluno-mide; Natalizumab; Vaccines (Live); Vitamin K Antagonists

The levels/effects of Methotrexate may be increased by: Acitretin; Ciprofloxacin; CycloSPORINE; Eltrombopag; Nonsteroidal Anti-Inflammatory Agents; Penicillins; P-Glycoprotein Inhibitors; Proton Pump Inhibitors; Salicylates; Sulfonamide Derivatives; Trastuzumab; Trimethoprim; Uricosuric Agents

Decreased Effect

Methotrexate may decrease the levels/effects of: Cardiac Glycosides; Sapropterin; Vaccines (Inactivated); Vaccines (Live); Vitamin K Antagonists

The levels/effects of Methotrexate may be decreased by: Bile Acid Sequestrants; Echinacea; P-Glycoprotein Inducers

Ethanol/Nutrition/Herb Interactions

Ethanol: Avoid ethanol (may be associated with increased liver injury).

Food: Methotrexate peak serum levels may be decreased if taken with food. Milk-rich foods may decrease methotrexate absorption. Folate may decrease drug response.

Herb/Nutraceutical: Avoid echinacea (has immunostimulant properties).

Storage/Stability Store tablets and intact vials at room temperature (15°C to 25°C). Protect from light. Solution diluted in D_5W or NS is stable for 24 hours at room temperature (21°C to 25°C). Reconstituted solutions with a preservative may be stored under refrigeration for up to 3 months, and up to 4 weeks at room temperature. Intrathecal dilutions are stable at room temperature for 7 days, but it is generally recommended that they be used within 4-8 hours.

Reconstitution Dilute powder with D_5W or NS to a concentration ≤25 mg/mL (20 mg and 50 mg vials) and 50 mg/mL (1 g vial). Intrathecal solutions may be reconstituted to 2.5-5 mg/mL with NS, D_5W, lactated Ringer's, or Elliott's B solution. **Use preservative free preparations for intrathecal or high-dose administration.**

Compatibility Stable in D_5NS, D_5W, NS.

Y-site administration: Compatible: Allopurinol, amifostine, amphotericin B cholesteryl sulfate complex, asparaginase, aztreonam, bleomycin, cefepime, ceftriaxone, cimetidine, cisplatin, cyclophosphamide, cytarabine, daunorubicin HCl, diphenhydramine, doxorubicin HCl, doxorubicin liposome, etoposide, etoposide phosphate, famotidine, filgrastim, fludarabine, fluorouracil, furosemide, gallium nitrate, ganciclovir, granisetron, heparin, hydromorphone, imipenem/cilastatin, leucovorin calcium, linezolid, lorazepam, melphalan, mesna, methylprednisolone sodium succinate, metoclopramide, mitomycin, morphine, ondansetron, oxacillin, oxaliplatin, paclitaxel, piperacillin/tazobactam, prochlorperazine edisylate, ranitidine, sargramostim, teniposide, thiotepa, vinblastine, vincristine, vinorelbine. **Incompatible:** Chlorpromazine, gemcitabine, idarubicin, ifosfamide, midazolam, nalbuphine, promethazine, propofol. **Variable (consult detailed reference):** Dexamethasone sodium phosphate, droperidol, vancomycin.

Compatibility in syringe: Compatible: Bleomycin, cisplatin, cyclophosphamide, doxapram, doxorubicin HCl, fluorouracil, furosemide, heparin sodium, leucovorin calcium, mitomycin, vinblastine, vincristine. **Incompatible:** Droperidol. **Variable (consult detailed reference):** Metoclopramide.

Compatibility when admixed: Compatible: Cyclophosphamide, cyclophosphamide with fluorouracil, cytarabine, fluorouracil, hydroxyzine HCl, ondansetron, sodium bicarbonate, vincristine. **Incompatible:** Bleomycin.

Mechanism of Action Methotrexate is a folate antimetabolite that inhibits DNA synthesis. Methotrexate irreversibly binds to dihydrofolate reductase, inhibiting the formation of reduced folates, and thymidylate synthetase, resulting in inhibition of purine and thymidylic acid synthesis. Methotrexate is cell cycle specific for the S phase of the cycle.

The MOA in the treatment of rheumatoid arthritis is unknown, but may affect immune function. In psoriasis, methotrexate is thought to target rapidly proliferating epithelial cells in the skin.

In Crohn's disease, it may have immune modulator and anti-inflammatory activity.

Pharmacodynamics/Kinetics

Onset of action: Antirheumatic: 3-6 weeks; additional improvement may continue longer than 12 weeks

Absorption: Oral: Rapid; well absorbed at low doses (<30 mg/m²), incomplete after large doses; I.M.: Complete

Distribution: Penetrates slowly into 3rd space fluids (eg, pleural effusions, ascites), exits slowly from these compartments (slower than from plasma); crosses placenta; small amounts enter breast milk; sustained concentrations retained in kidney and liver

Protein binding: 50%

Metabolism: <10%; degraded by intestinal flora to DAMPA by carboxypeptidase; hepatic aldehyde oxidase converts methotrexate to 7-OH methotrexate; polyglutamates are produced intracellularly and are just as potent as methotrexate; their production is dose- and duration-dependent and they are slowly eliminated by the cell once formed

Half-life elimination: Low dose: 3-10 hours; High dose: 8-12 hours

Time to peak, serum: Oral: 1-2 hours; I.M.: 30-60 minutes

Excretion: Urine (44% to 100%); feces (small amounts)

Dosage Details concerning dosing in combination regimens should also be consulted.

Note: Doses between 100-500 mg/m² **may require** leucovorin rescue. Doses >500 mg/m² **require** leucovorin rescue: Oral, I.M., I.V.: Leucovorin 10-15 mg/m² every 6 hours for 8 or 10 doses, starting 24 hours after the start of methotrexate infusion. Continue until the methotrexate level is ≤0.1 micromolar (10^{-7} M). Some clinicians continue leucovorin until the methotrexate level is <0.05 micromolar (5×10^{-8} M) or 0.01 micromolar (10^{-8} M).

If the 48-hour methotrexate level is >1 micromolar (10^{-6} M) or the 72-hour methotrexate level is >0.2 micromolar (2×10^{-7} M): I.V., I.M, Oral: Leucovorin 100 mg/m² every 6 hours until the methotrexate level is ≤0.1 micromolar (10^{-7} M). Some clinicians continue leucovorin until the methotrexate level is <0.05 micromolar (5×10^{-8} M) or 0.01 micromolar (10^{-8} M).

Children:

Dermatomyositis (unlabeled use): Oral: 15-20 mg/m²/week as a single dose once weekly **or** 0.3-1 mg/kg/dose once weekly

Juvenile rheumatoid arthritis: Oral, I.M.: 10 mg/m² once weekly, then 5-15 mg/m²/week as a single dose **or** as 3 divided doses given 12 hours apart

Antineoplastic dosage range:

Oral, I.M.: 7.5-30 mg/m²/week **or** every 2 weeks

I.V.: 10-18,000 mg/m² bolus dosing **or** continuous infusion over 6-42 hours

Pediatric solid tumors (high-dose): I.V.:

<12 years: 12-25 g/m²

≥12 years: 8 g/m²

Acute lymphocytic leukemia (intermediate-dose): I.V.: Loading: 100 mg/m² bolus dose, followed by 900 mg/m²/day infusion over 23-41 hours.

Meningeal leukemia: I.T.: 6-12 mg/dose based on age:

<1 year: 6 mg/dose

1 year: 8 mg/dose

2 years: 10 mg/dose

≥3 years: 12 mg/dose

Adults: I.V.: Range is wide from 30-40 mg/m^2/week to 100-12,000 mg/m^2 with leucovorin rescue

Trophoblastic neoplasms:
   Oral, I.M.: 15-30 mg/day for 5 days; repeat in 7 days for 3-5 courses
   I.V.: 11 mg/m^2 days 1 through 5 every 3 weeks

Head and neck cancer: Oral, I.M., I.V.: 25-50 mg/m^2 once weekly

Mycosis fungoides (cutaneous T-cell lymphoma): Oral, I.M.: Initial (early stages):
   5-50 mg once weekly **or**
   15-37.5 mg twice weekly

Breast cancer: I.V.: 30-60 mg/m^2 days 1 and 8 every 3-4 weeks

Lymphoma, non-Hodgkin's: I.V.:
   30 mg/m^2 days 3 and 10 every 3 weeks **or**
   120 mg/m^2 day 8 and 15 every 3-4 weeks **or**
   200 mg/m^2 day 8 and 15 every 3 weeks **or**
   400 mg/m^2 every 4 weeks for 3 cycles **or**
   1 g/m^2 every 3 weeks **or**
   1.5 g/m^2 every 4 weeks

Meningeal leukemia: I.T.: Usual dose: 12 mg/dose

Osteosarcoma: I.V.: 8-12 g/m^2 weekly for 2-4 weeks

Rheumatoid arthritis: Oral: 7.5 mg once weekly **or** 2.5 mg every 12 hours for 3 doses/week, not to exceed 20 mg/week

Psoriasis:
   Oral: 2.5-5 mg/dose every 12 hours for 3 doses given weekly **or**
   Oral, I.M.: 10-25 mg/dose given once weekly

Bladder cancer (unlabeled use): I.V.:
   30 mg/m^2 day 1 and 8 every 3 weeks **or**
   30 mg/m^2 day 1, 15, and 22 every 4 weeks

Ectopic pregnancy (unlabeled use): I.M.:
   Single-dose regimen: Methotrexate 50 mg/m^2 on day 1; Measure serum hCG levels on days 4 and 7; if needed, repeat dose on day 7 (Barnhart 2009)
   Two-dose regimen: Methotrexate 50 mg/m^2 on day 1; Measure serum hCG levels on day 4 and administer a second dose of methotrexate 50 mg/m^2; Measure serum hCG levels on day 7 and if needed, administer a third dose of 50 mg/m^2 (Barnhart 2009)
   Multidose regimen: Methotrexate 1 mg/kg on day 1; leucovorin 0.1 mg/kg I.M. on day 2; measure serum hCG on day 2; methotrexate 1mg/kg on day 3; leucovorin 0.1 mg/kg on day 4; measure serum hCG on day 4; continue up to a total of 4 courses based on hCG concentrations (Barnhart 2009)

Active Crohn's disease (unlabeled use): Induction of remission: I.M., SubQ: 15-25 mg once weekly; remission maintenance: 15 mg once weekly
   Note: Oral dosing has been reported as effective but oral absorption is highly variable. If patient relapses after a switch to oral, may consider returning to injectable.

Nonleukemic meningeal cancer (unlabeled uses): I.T.: 10-12 mg/dose twice weekly for 4 weeks, then weekly for 4 weeks, then monthly (NCCN CNS cancer guidelines v.2.2009) **or** 12 mg/dose twice weekly for 4 weeks, then weekly for 4 doses, then monthly for 4 doses (Glantz, 1998) **or** 10 mg twice weekly for 4 weeks, then weekly for 1 month, then every 2 weeks for 2 months (Glantz, 1999)

Elderly: Rheumatoid arthritis/psoriasis: Oral: Initial: 5-7.5 mg/week, not to exceed 20 mg/week

Dosing adjustment in renal impairment: The FDA-approved labeling does not contain dosage adjustment guidelines. The following guidelines have been used by some clinicians:

Cl_{cr} 61-80 mL/minute: Administer 75% of dose

Cl_{cr} 51-60 mL/minute: Administer 70% of dose

Cl_{cr} 10-50 mL/minute: Administer 30% to 50% of dose

Cl_{cr} <10 mL/minute: Avoid use

Hemodialysis: Not dialyzable (0% to 5%); supplemental dose is not necessary

Peritoneal dialysis effects: Supplemental dose is not necessary

CAVH effects: Unknown

Aronoff, 2007:
  Children:
    Cl_{cr} 10-50 mL/minute: Administer 50% of dose
    Cl_{cr} <10 mL/minute: Administer 30% of dose
    Hemodialysis: Administer 30% of dose
    Continuous ambulatory peritoneal dialysis (CAPD): Administer 30% of dose
    Continuous renal replacement therapy (CRRT): Administer 50% of dose
  Adults:
    Cl_{cr} 10-50 mL/minute: Administer 50% of dose
    Cl_{cr} <10 mL/minute: Avoid use
    Hemodialysis: Administer 50% of dose
    Continuous renal replacement therapy (CRRT): Administer 50% of dose

Kintzel, 1995:
  Cl_{cr} 46-60 mL/minute: Administer 65% of normal dose
  Cl_{cr} 31-45 mL/minute: Administer 50% of normal dose
  Cl_{cr} <30 mL/minute: Avoid use

Dosage adjustment in hepatic impairment: The FDA-approved labeling does not contain dosage adjustment guidelines. The following guidelines have been used by some clinicians (Floyd, 2006):

Bilirubin 3.1-5 mg/dL **or** transaminases >3 times ULN: Administer 75% of dose

Bilirubin >5 mg/dL: Avoid use

Combination Regimens

Bladder cancer:
  CMV on page 1277
  M-VAC (Bladder Cancer) on page 1375
Breast cancer:
  CMF on page 1275
  CMF-IV on page 1276
  CMFP on page 1276
  CMFVP (Cooper Regimen, VPCMF) on page 1276
  Dox-CMF (Sequential) on page 1295
  MF on page 1366
  M-VAC (Breast Cancer) on page 1378
Cervical Cancer: M-VAC (Cervical Cancer) on page 1379
Endometrial cancer: M-VAC (Endometrial Cancer) on page 1379
Gastric cancer: FAMTX on page 1321
Gestational trophoblastic tumor:
  CHAMOCA (Modified Bagshawe Regimen) on page 1259
  CHAMOMA (Bagshawe Regimen) on page 1261
  EMA/CO on page 1301
  EP/EMA on page 1304

◄ Head and neck cancer:
Leukemia, acute lymphocytic:
Leukemia, acute promyelocytic:
Lymphoma, non-Hodgkin's:
Osteosarcoma:

Administration Methotrexate may be administered I.M., I.V., or I.T.; I.V. administration may be as slow push, short bolus infusion, or 24- to 42-hour continuous infusion

Specific dosing schemes vary, but high dose should be followed by leucovorin calcium to prevent toxicity; refer to Leucovorin Calcium monograph on page 697

Monitoring Parameters

Patients with psoriasis or RA: CBC with differential and platelets (baseline and monthly); serum creatinine (baseline and every 1-2 months), LFTs (baseline and every 1-2 months); chest x-ray (baseline); pulmonary function test (if methotrexate-induced lung disease suspected); liver biopsy (psoriasis patients: baseline and each 1-1.5 g cumulative dose interval; RA: baseline [if persistent abnormal baseline LFTs, history of alcoholism, or chronic hepatitis B or C] and with LFT or serum albumin abnormality)

Patients with cancer: Baseline and frequently during treatment: CBC with differential and platelets, serum creatinine, LFTs; chest x-ray (baseline); methotrexate levels and urine pH (with high-dose therapy); pulmonary function test (if methotrexate-induced lung disease suspected)

Ectopic pregnancy (unlabeled use): Prior to therapy, measure serum hCG, CBC with differential, liver function tests, serum creatinine. Serum hCG concentrations should decrease between treatment days 4 and 7. If hCG decreases by >15%, additional courses are not needed however, continue to measure hCG weekly until no longer detectable. If <15% decrease is observed, repeat dose per regimen (Barnhart 2009).

Dietary Considerations

Sodium content of 100 mg injection: 20 mg (0.86 mEq)

Sodium content of 100 mg (low sodium) injection: 15 mg (0.65 mEq)

Additional Information Oncology Comment: Methotrexate overexposure: The investigational rescue agent, glucarpidase, is an enzyme which rapidly hydrolyzes extracellular methotrexate into inactive metabolites, resulting in a rapid reduction of methotrexate concentrations. Glucarpidase is available for intrathecal (IT) use through an Emergency Use IND and for I.V. use under an Open-Label Treatment protocol. Refer to Glucarpidase monograph.

Emetic Potential

≥ 250 mg/m^2: Moderate (30% to 90%)

50-250 mg/m^2: Low (10% to 30%)

≤ 50 mg/m^2: Very low (<10%)

Oral: Very low (<10%)

Dosage Forms

Excipient information presented when available (limited, particularly for generics); consult specific product labeling.

Injection, powder for reconstitution: 1 g

Injection, solution: 25 mg/mL (2 mL, 10 mL) [contains benzyl alcohol]

Injection, solution [preservative free]: 25 mg/mL (2 mL, 4 mL, 8 mL, 10 mL, 40 mL)

Tablet: 2.5 mg

Trexall™: 5 mg, 7.5 mg, 10 mg, 15 mg

Tablet [dose pack]: 2.5 mg (4 cards with 2, 3, 4, 5, or 6 tablets each)

Rheumatrex®: 2.5 mg (4 cards with 2, 3, 4, 5, or 6 tablets each)

References

"American Academy of Pediatrics Committee on Drugs. The Transfer of Drugs and Other Chemicals Into Human Milk," *Pediatrics*, 2001, 108(3):776-89.

Aronoff GR, Bennett WM, Berns JS, et al, *Drug Prescribing in Renal Failure: Dosing Guidelines for Adults and Children*, 5th ed. Philadelphia, PA: American College of Physicians; 2007, p 101.

Azzarelli A, Gronchi A, Bertulli R, et al, "Low-Dose Chemotherapy With Methotrexate and Vinblastine for Patients With Advanced Aggressive Fibromatosis," *Cancer*, 2001, 92(5):1259-64.

Barnhart KT, "Clinical Practice. Ectopic Pregnancy," *N Engl J Med*, 2009, 361(4):379-87.

Egan LJ, Sandborn WJ, Tremaine WJ, et al, "A Randomized Dose-Response and Pharmacokinetic Study of Methotrexate for Refractory Inflammatory Crohn's Disease and Ulcerative Colitis," *Aliment Pharmacol Ther*, 1999, 13(12):1597-604.

Evans WE, Pratt CB, Taylor RH, et al, "Pharmacokinetic Monitoring of High-Dose Methotrexate: Early Recognition of High-Risk Patients," *Cancer Chemother Pharmacol*, 1979, 3:161-6.

Feagan BG, Fedorak RN, Irvine EJ, et al, "A Comparison of Methotrexate With Placebo for the Maintenance of Remission in Crohn's Disease. North American Crohn's Study Group Investigators," *N Engl J Med*, 2000, 342(22):1627-32.

Floyd J, Mirza I, Sachs B, et al, "Hepatotoxicity of Chemotherapy," *Semin Oncol*, 2006, 33 (1):50-67.

Glantz MJ, Cole BF, Recht L, Akerley W, et al, "High-Dose Intravenous Methotrexate for Patients With Nonleukemic Leptomeningeal Cancer: Is Intrathecal Chemotherapy Necessary?" *J Clin Oncol*, 1998, 16(4):1561-7.

Glantz MJ, Jaeckle KA, Chamberlain MC, et al, "A Randomized Controlled Trial Comparing Intrathecal Sustained-Release Cytarabine (DepoCyt) to Intrathecal Methotrexate in Patients With Neoplastic Meningitis from Solid Tumors," *Clin Cancer Res*, 1999, 5(11):3394-402.

Grem JL, King SA, Wittes RE, et al, "The Role of Methotrexate in Osteosarcoma," *J Natl Cancer Inst*, 1988, 80(9):626-55.

Jolivet J, Cowan KH, Curt GA, et al, "The Pharmacology and Clinical Use of Methotrexate," *N Engl J Med*, 1983, 309(18):1094-104.

Kintzel PE and Dorr RT, "Anticancer Drug Renal Toxicity and Elimination: Dosing Guidelines for Altered Renal Function," *Cancer Treat Rev*, 1995, 21(1):33-64.

National Comprehensive Cancer Network® (NCCN), "Clinical Practice Guidelines in Oncology™: Central Nervous System Cancers," Version 2.2009. Available at http://www.nccn.org/professionals/physician_gls/PDF/cns.pdf

Ortega JJ, Madero L, Martin G, et al, "Treatment With All-*Trans* Retinoic Acid and Anthracycline Monochemotherapy for Children With Acute Promyelocytic Leukemia: A Multicenter Study by the PETHEMA Group," *J Clin Oncol*, 2005, 23(30):7632-40.

Sanz MA, Martin G, Gonzalez M, et al, "Risk-Adapted Treatment of Acute Promyelocytic Leukemia With All-*Trans*-Retinoic Acid and Anthracycline Monochemotherapy: A Multicenter Study by the PETHEMA Group," *Blood*, 2004, 103(4):1237-43.

Schwartz S, Borner K, Muller K, et al, "Glucarpidase (Carboxypeptidase G2) Intervention in Adult and Elderly Cancer Patients With Renal Dysfunction and Delayed Methotrexate Elimination After High-Dose Methotrexate Therapy," *Oncologist*, 2007 12(11):1299-308.

Seeber BE and Barnhart KT, "Suspected Ectopic Pregnancy," *Obstet Gynecol*, 2006, 107(2 Pt 1):399-413.

Treon SP and Chabner BA, "Concepts in Use of High-Dose Methotrexate Therapy," *Clin Chem*, 1996, 42(8 Pt 2):1322-9.

Sternberg CN, de Mulder PH, Schornagel JH, et al, "Randomized Phase III Trial of High-Dose-Intensity Methotrexate, Vinblastine, Doxorubicin, and Cisplatin (MVAC) Chemotherapy and Recombinant Human Granulocyte Colony-Stimulating Factor Versus Classic MVAC in Advanced Urothelial Tract Tumors: European Organization for Research and Treatment of Cancer Protocol No. 30924," *J Clin Oncol*, 2001, 19(10):2638-46.

Widemann BC, Balis FM, Murphy RF, et al, "Carboxypeptidase-G2, Thymidine, and Leucovorin Rescue in Cancer Patients With Methotrexate-Induced Renal Dysfunction," *J Clin Oncol*, 1997, 15(5):2125-34.

Widemann BC, Balis FM, Shalabi A, et al, "Treatment of Accidental Intrathecal Methotrexate Overdose With Intrathecal Carboxypeptidase G2," *J Natl Cancer Inst*, 2004, 96(20):1557-9.

◆ **Methotrexate Sodium** see Methotrexate on page 768

◆ **Methotrexatum** see Methotrexate on page 768

◆ **Methylacetoxyprogesterone** see MedroxyPROGESTERone on page 739

Methylene Blue (METH i leen bloo)

Medication Safety Issues Due to potential toxicity (hemolytic anemia), do not use methylene blue to color enteral feedings to detect aspiration.

Generic Available Yes

Pharmacologic Category Antidote

Use Antidote for cyanide poisoning and drug-induced methemoglobinemia, indicator dye

Unlabeled/Investigational Use Treatment/prevention of ifosfamide-induced encephalopathy; topically, in conjunction with polychromatic light to photo-inactivate viruses such as herpes simplex; alone or in combination with vitamin C for the management of chronic urolithiasis

Pregnancy Risk Factor C

Labeled Contraindications Hypersensitivity to methylene blue or any component of the formulation; intraspinal injection; renal insufficiency

Warnings/Precautions Do not inject SubQ or intrathecally; use with caution in young patients and in patients with G6PD deficiency; continued use can cause profound anemia. At high doses or in patients with G6PD-deficiency and infants, methylene blue may catalyze the oxidation of ferrous iron in hemoglobin to ferric iron causing paradoxical methemoglobinemia; monitor methemoglobin concentrations regularly during administration. Methylene blue should not be added to enteral feeding products (Durfee, 2006; Wessel, 2005); safety and efficacy have not been established.

Adverse Reactions Frequency not defined.

Cardiovascular: Hypertension, precordial pain

Central nervous system: Dizziness, mental confusion, headache, fever

Dermatologic: Staining of skin

Gastrointestinal: Fecal discoloration (blue-green), nausea, vomiting, abdominal pain

Genitourinary: Discoloration of urine (blue-green), bladder irritation

Hematologic: Anemia

Miscellaneous: Diaphoresis

Drug Interactions

Avoid Concomitant Use There are no known interactions where it is recommended to avoid concomitant use.

Increased Effect/Toxicity There are no known significant interactions involving an increase in effect.

Decreased Effect There are no known significant interactions involving a decrease in effect.

Mechanism of Action Weak germicide in low concentrations, hastens the conversion of methemoglobin to hemoglobin; has opposite effect at high concentrations by converting ferrous ion of reduced hemoglobin to ferric ion to form methemoglobin; in cyanide toxicity, it combines with cyanide to form cyanmethemoglobin preventing the interference of cyanide with the cytochrome system

Pharmacodynamics/Kinetics

Onset of action: Reduction of methemoglobin: I.V.: 30-60 minutes

Absorption: Oral: 53% to 97%

Excretion: Urine and feces

Dosage

Children and Adults: Methemoglobinemia: I.V.: 1-2 mg/kg or 25-50 mg/m^2 over several minutes; may be repeated in 1 hour if necessary

Adults: Ifosfamide-induced encephalopathy (unlabeled use): **Note:** Treatment may not be necessary; encephalopathy may improve spontaneously: I.V.:

Prevention: 50 mg every 6-8 hours

Treatment: 50 mg as a single dose or every 4-8 hours until symptoms resolve

Administration I.V.: Administer undiluted by direct I.V. injection over several minutes. For the treatment of ifosfamide-induced encephalopathy, methylene blue may be administered either undiluted as a slow I.V. push over at least 5 minutes or diluted in 50 mL NS or D$_5$W and infused over at least 5 minutes. Consider concomitant dextrose administration, especially in patients who are hypoglycemic, to ensure efficacy of methylene blue.

Monitoring Parameters Arterial blood gases; cardiac monitoring (patients with pre-existing pulmonary and/or cardiac disease); CBC; methemoglobin levels (co-oximetry yields a direct and accurate measure of methemoglobin levels); pulse oximeter (will not provide accurate measurement of oxygenation when methemoglobin levels are >35%); renal function; signs and symptoms of methemoglobinemia such as pallor, cyanosis, nausea, muscle weakness, dizziness, confusion, agitation, dyspnea and tachycardia; transcutaneous O$_2$ saturation

Additional Information Skin stains may be removed using a hypochlorite solution.

Dosage Forms Excipient information presented when available (limited, particularly for generics); consult specific product labeling.

Injection, solution: 10 mg/mL (1 mL, 10 mL)

References

Albert M, Lessin MS, and Gilchrist BF, "Methylene Blue: Dangerous Dye for Neonates," J Pediatr Surg, 2003, 38(8):1244-5.

David KA and Picus J, "Evaluating Risk Factors for the Development of Ifosfamide Encephalopathy," Am J Clin Oncol, 2005, 28(3):277-80.

Durfee SM, Gallagher-Allred C, Pasquale JA, "Standards for Specialized Nutrition Support for Adult Residents of Long-Term Care Facilities," Nutr Clin Pract, 2006, 21(1):96-104.

Maloney JP, Ryan TA, Brasel KJ, et al, "Food Dye Use in Enteral Feedings: A Review and a Call for a Moratorium," *Nutr Clin Pract*, 2002, 17(3):169-81.

Patel PN, "Methylene Blue for Management of Ifosfamide-Induced Encephalopathy," *Ann Pharmacother*, 2006, 40(2):299-303.

Pelgrims J, DeVos F, Van den Brande J, et al, "Methylene Blue in the Treatment and Prevention of Ifosfamide-Induced Encephalopathy: Report of 12 Cases and a Review of the Literature," *Br J Cancer*, 2000, 82(2) 291-4.

Sills M and Zinkham W, "Methylene Blue-Induced Heinz Body Hemolytic Anemia," *Arch Pediatr Adolesc Med*, 1994, 148(3):306-10.

Turner AR, Duong CD, and Good DJ, "Methylene Blue for the Treatment and Prophylaxis of Ifosfamide-Induced Encephalopathy," *Clin Oncol (R Coll Radiol)*, 2003, 15(7):435-9.

Wessel J, Balint J, Crill C, et al, "Standards for Specialized Nutrition Support: Hospitalized Pediatric Patients," *Nutr Clin Pract*, 2005, 20(1):103-116.

Zulian GB, Tullen E, and Maton B, "Methylene Blue for Ifosfamide-Associated Encephalopathy," *N Engl J Med*, 1995, 332(18):1239-40.

♦ **Methylmorphine** *see* Codeine *on page* 256

Methylnaltrexone (meth il nal TREKS one)

Medication Safety Issues
Sound-alike/look-alike issues:
Methylnaltrexone may be confused with naltrexone

U.S. Brand Names Relistor™

Index Terms Methylnaltrexone Bromide; N-methylnaltrexone Bromide

Generic Available No

Canadian Brand Names Relistor™

Pharmacologic Category Gastrointestinal Agent, Miscellaneous; Opioid Antagonist, Peripherally-Acting

Use Treatment of opioid-induced constipation in patients with advanced illness receiving palliative care with inadequate response to conventional laxative regimens

Pregnancy Risk Factor B

Lactation Excretion in breast milk unknown/use caution

Labeled Contraindications Known or suspected mechanical bowel obstruction

Warnings/Precautions Discontinue treatment for severe or persistent diarrhea. Use with caution in patients with renal impairment; dosage adjustment recommended for severe renal impairment (Cl_{cr} <30 mL/minute). Has not been studied in patients with end-stage renal impairment requiring dialysis. Discontinue methylnaltrexone if opioids are discontinued. Use has not been studied in patients with peritoneal catheters. Use beyond 4 months has not been studied. Safety and efficacy have not been established in children.

Adverse Reactions
>10%: Gastrointestinal: Abdominal pain (29%), flatulence (13%), nausea (12%)

1% to 10%:
Central nervous system: Dizziness (7%)
Gastrointestinal: Diarrhea (6%)

<1%, postmarketing, and/or case reports: Abdominal cramps, body temperature increased, muscle spasm, syncope

Drug Interactions
Metabolism/Transport Effects Inhibits CYP2D6 (weak)

Avoid Concomitant Use There are no known interactions where it is recommended to avoid concomitant use.

Increased Effect/Toxicity There are no known significant interactions involving an increase in effect.

Decreased Effect

The levels/effects of Methylnaltrexone may be decreased by: Peginterferon Alfa-2b

Storage/Stability Store intact vials at room temperature of 20°C to 25°C (68°F to 77°F); excursions permitted to 15°C to 30°C (59°F to 86°F); do not freeze. Protect from light. Solution for injection is stable in a syringe for 24 hours at room temperature (protection from light during this 24 hours is not necessary).

Mechanism of Action An opioid receptor antagonist which blocks opioid binding at the mu receptor, methylnaltrexone is a quaternary derivative of naltrexone with ability to cross the blood-brain barrier restricted. It therefore functions as a peripheral acting opioid antagonist, including actions on the gastrointestinal tract to inhibit opioid-induced decreased gastrointestinal motility and delay in gastrointestinal transit time, decreasing opioid-induced constipation. Does not affect opioid analgesic effects or induce opioid withdrawal symptoms.

Pharmacodynamics/Kinetics

Onset of action: Usually within 30-60 minutes (in responding patients)

Absorption: SubQ: Rapid

Distribution: V_{ss}: 1.1 L/kg

Protein binding: 11% to 15%

Metabolism: Metabolized to methyl-6-naltrexol isomers, methylnaltrexone sulfate. and other minor metabolites

Half-life elimination: Terminal: ~8 hours

Time to peak, plasma: SubQ: 30 minutes

Excretion: Urine (~50%, primarily as unchanged drug); feces (<50%, primarily as unchanged drug)

Dosage SubQ: Adults: Opioid-induced constipation: Dosing is according to body weight: Administer 1 dose every other day as needed; maximum: 1 dose/24 hours

<38 kg: 0.15 mg/kg (round dose up to nearest 0.1 mL of volume)

38 to <62 kg: 8 mg

62-114 kg: 12 mg

>114 kg: 0.15 mg/kg (round dose up to nearest 0.1 mL of volume)

Dosage adjustment in renal impairment:

Mild-to-moderate renal impairment: No adjustment required

Severe renal impairment (Cl_{cr} <30 mL/minute): Administer 50% of normal dose

End-stage renal impairment (dialysis-dependent): Has not been studied

Dosage adjustment in hepatic impairment:

Mild-to-moderate hepatic impairment (Child-Pugh class A and B): No adjustment required

Severe hepatic impairment: Has not been studied

Administration SubQ: Administer subcutaneously into upper arm, abdomen, or thigh. Rotate injection site. Do not use tender, bruised, red, or hard areas.

Additional Information In some clinical trials, patients who received methylnaltrexone were on a palliative opioid therapy equivalent to a mean daily oral morphine dose of 172 mg, at a stable dose for ≥3 days. Constipation was defined as <3 bowel movements/week or no bowel movement for >2 days. Patients maintained their regular laxative regimen for at least 3 days prior to treatment and throughout the study.

◀ **Dosage Forms** Excipient information presented when available (limited, particularly for generics); consult specific product labeling.

Injection, solution:

Relistor™: 12 mg/0.6 mL (0.6 mL) [contains edetate calcium disodium]

References

Portenoy RK, Thomas J, Moehl Boatwright ML, et al, "Subcutaneous Methylnaltrexone for the Treatment of Opioid-Induced Constipation in Patients With Advanced Illness: A Double-Blind Randomized, Parallel Group, Dose-Ranging Study," *J Pain Symptom Manage*, 2008, 35 (5):458-68.

Thomas J, "Opioid-Induced Bowel Dysfunction," *J Pain Symptom Manage*, 2008, 35(1):103-13.

Thomas J, Karver S, Cooney GA, et al, "Methylnaltrexone for Opioid-Induced Constipation in Advanced Illness," *N Engl J Med*, 2008, 358(22):2332-43.

Yuan CS, "Methylnaltrexone Mechanisms of Action and Effects on Opioid Bowel Dysfunction and Other Opioid Adverse Effects," *Ann Pharmacother*, 2007, 41(6):984-93.

♦ **Methylnaltrexone Bromide** see Methylnaltrexone on page 780

♦ **Methylphytyl Napthoquinone** see Phytonadione on page 953

MethylPREDNISolone (meth il pred NIS oh lone)

Medication Safety Issues

Sound-alike/look-alike issues:

MethylPREDNISolone may be confused with medroxyPROGESTERone, methotrexate, predniSONE

Depo-Medrol® may be confused with Solu-Medrol®

Medrol® may be confused with Mebaral®

Solu-Medrol® may be confused with Depo-Medrol®, salmeterol, Solu-Cortef®

International issues:

Medor® may be confused with Medral® which is a brand name for omeprazole in Mexico

Related Information

Hematopoietic Stem Cell Transplantation on page 1501

U.S. Brand Names A-Methapred®; Depo-Medrol®; Medrol®; Solu-Medrol®

Index Terms 6-α-Methylprednisolone; A-Methapred; Medrol Dose Pack; Methylprednisolone Acetate; Methylprednisolone Sodium Succinate; Solumedrol

Generic Available Yes

Canadian Brand Names Depo-Medrol®; Medrol®; Methylprednisolone Acetate; Solu-Medrol®

Pharmacologic Category Corticosteroid, Systemic

Use Primarily as an anti-inflammatory or immunosuppressant agent in the treatment of a variety of diseases including those of hematologic, allergic, inflammatory, neoplastic, and autoimmune origin. Prevention and treatment of graft-versus-host disease following allogeneic bone marrow transplantation.

Lactation Enters breast milk/use caution

Labeled Contraindications Hypersensitivity to methylprednisolone or any component of the formulation; systemic fungal infection (except intra-articular injection in localized joint conditions); administration of live virus vaccines. methylprednisolone formulations containing benzyl alcohol preservative are contraindicated in infants; I.M. administration in idiopathic thrombocytopenia purpura; intrathecal administration of methylprednisolone acetate suspension

Warnings/Precautions Use with caution in patients with thyroid disease, hepatic impairment, renal impairment, cardiovascular disease, diabetes, glaucoma, cataracts, myasthenia gravis, patients at risk for osteoporosis, patients at risk for seizures, or GI diseases (diverticulitis, peptic ulcer, ulcerative colitis) due to perforation risk. Not recommended for the treatment of optic neuritis; may increase frequency of new episodes. Use caution following acute MI (corticosteroids have been associated with myocardial rupture). Cardiomegaly and congestive heart failure have been reported following concurrent use of amphotericin B and hydrocortisone for the management of fungal infections.

Because of the risk of adverse effects, systemic corticosteroids should be used cautiously in the elderly in the smallest possible effective dose for the shortest duration. May affect growth velocity; growth should be routinely monitored in pediatric patients. Withdraw therapy with gradual tapering of dose.

May cause hypercorticism or suppression of hypothalamic-pituitary-adrenal (HPA) axis, particularly in younger children or in patients receiving high doses for prolonged periods. HPA axis suppression may lead to adrenal crisis. Withdrawal and discontinuation of a corticosteroid should be done slowly and carefully. Particular care is required when patients are transferred from systemic corticosteroids to inhaled products due to possible adrenal insufficiency or withdrawal from steroids, including an increase in allergic symptoms. Patients receiving >20 mg per day of prednisone (or equivalent) may be most susceptible. Fatalities have occurred due to adrenal insufficiency in asthmatic patients during and after transfer from systemic corticosteroids to aerosol steroids; aerosol steroids do not provide the systemic steroid needed to treat patients having trauma, surgery, or infections.

Acute myopathy has been reported with high dose corticosteroids, usually in patients with neuromuscular transmission disorders; may involve ocular and/or respiratory muscles; monitor creatine kinase; recovery may be delayed. Corticosteroid use may cause psychiatric disturbances, including depression, euphoria, insomnia, mood swings, and personality changes. Pre-existing psychiatric conditions may be exacerbated by corticosteroid use. Prolonged use of corticosteroids may also increase the incidence of secondary infection, cause activation of latent infections, mask acute infection (including fungal infections), prolong or exacerbate viral or parasitic infections, or limit response to vaccines. Exposure to chickenpox or measles should be avoided; corticosteroids should not be used to treat ocular herpes simplex. Corticosteroids should not be used for cerebral malaria or viral hepatitis. Close observation is required in patients with latent tuberculosis and/or TB reactivity; restrict use in active TB (only in conjunction with antituberculosis treatment). Amebiasis should be ruled out in any patient with recent travel to tropic climates or unexplained diarrhea prior to initiation of corticosteroids. Prolonged treatment with corticosteroids has been associated with the development of Kaposi's sarcoma (case reports); discontinuation may result in clinical improvement.

High-dose corticosteroids should not be used to manage acute head injury. Rare cases of anaphylactoid reactions have been observed in patients receiving corticosteroids. Dermal and/or subdermal skin depression may occur at the site of methylprednisolone acetate injection. Avoid injection or leakage into the dermis. Some dosage forms contain benzyl alcohol which has been associated with "gasping syndrome" in neonates.

Adverse Reactions Frequency not defined.

Cardiovascular: Arrhythmias, bradycardia, cardiac arrest, cardiomegaly, circulatory collapse, congestive heart failure, edema, fat embolism, hypertension, hypertrophic cardiomyopathy in premature infants, myocardial rupture (post MI), syncope, tachycardia, thromboembolism, vasculitis

◀ Central nervous system: Delirium, depression, emotional instability, euphoria, hallucinations, headache, intracranial pressure increased, insomnia, malaise, mood swings, nervousness, neuritis, personality changes, psychic disorders, pseudotumor cerebri (usually following discontinuation), seizure, vertigo

Dermatologic: Acne, allergic dermatitis, alopecia, dry scaly skin, ecchymoses, edema, erythema, hirsutism, hyper-/hypopigmentation, hypertrichosis, impaired wound healing, petechiae, rash, skin atrophy, sterile abscess, skin test reaction impaired, striae, urticaria

Endocrine & metabolic: Adrenal suppression, amenorrhea, carbohydrate intolerance increased, Cushing's syndrome, diabetes mellitus, fluid retention, glucose intolerance, growth suppression (children), hyperglycemia, hyperlipidemia, hypokalemia, hypokalemic alkalosis, menstrual irregularities, negative nitrogen balance, pituitary-adrenal axis suppression, protein catabolism, sodium and water retention

Gastrointestinal: Abdominal distention, appetite increased, bowel/bladder dysfunction (after intrathecal administration), gastrointestinal hemorrhage, gastrointestinal perforation, nausea, pancreatitis, peptic ulcer, perforation of the small and large intestine, ulcerative esophagitis, vomiting, weight gain

Hematologic: Leukocytosis (transient)

Hepatic: Hepatomegaly, transaminases increased

Local: Postinjection flare (intra-articular use), thrombophlebitis

Neuromuscular & skeletal: Arthralgia, arthropathy, aseptic necrosis (femoral and humoral heads), fractures, muscle mass loss, muscle weakness, myopathy (particularly in conjunction with neuromuscular disease or neuromuscular-blocking agents), neuropathy, osteoporosis, parasthesia, tendon rupture, vertebral compression fractures, weakness

Ocular: Cataracts, exophthalmoses, glaucoma, intraocular pressure increased

Renal: Glycosuria

Respiratory: Pulmonary edema

Miscellaneous: Abnormal fat disposition, anaphylactoid reaction, anaphylaxis, angioedema, avascular necrosis, diaphoresis, hiccups, hypersensitivity reactions, infections, secondary malignancy

Drug Interactions

Metabolism/Transport Effects Substrate of CYP3A4 (major); **Inhibits** CYP2C8 (weak), 3A4 (weak)

Avoid Concomitant Use

Avoid concomitant use of MethylPREDNISolone with any of the following: Natalizumab; Vaccines (Live)

Increased Effect/Toxicity

MethylPREDNISolone may increase the levels/effects of: Acetylcholinesterase Inhibitors; Amphotericin B; CycloSPORINE; Leflunomide; Loop Diuretics; Natalizumab; NSAID (COX-2 Inhibitor); NSAID (Nonselective); Thiazide Diuretics; Vaccines (Live); Warfarin

The levels/effects of MethylPREDNISolone may be increased by: Antifungal Agents (Azole Derivatives, Systemic); Aprepitant; Calcium Channel Blockers (Nondihydropyridine); CycloSPORINE; Estrogen Derivatives; Fluconazole; Fosaprepitant; Macrolide Antibiotics; Neuromuscular-Blocking Agents (Nondepolarizing); Quinolone Antibiotics; Salicylates; Trastuzumab

Decreased Effect

MethylPREDNISolone may decrease the levels/effects of: Antidiabetic Agents; Calcitriol; Corticorelin; Isoniazid; Salicylates; Vaccines (Inactivated); Vaccines (Live)

The levels/effects of MethylPREDNISolone may be decreased by: Amino-glutethimide; Antacids; Barbiturates; Bile Acid Sequestrants; Echinacea; Mitotane; Primidone; Rifamycin Derivatives

Ethanol/Nutrition/Herb Interactions

Ethanol: Avoid ethanol (may increase gastric mucosal irritation).

Food: Methylprednisolone interferes with calcium absorption. Limit caffeine.

Herb/Nutraceutical: St John's wort may decrease methylprednisolone levels. Avoid cat's claw, echinacea (have immunostimulant properties).

Storage/Stability Intact vials of methylprednisolone sodium succinate should be stored at controlled room temperature of 20°C to 25°C (68°F to 77°F). Protect from light. Reconstituted solutions of methylprednisolone sodium succinate should be stored at room temperature of 20°C to 25°C (68°F to 77°F) and used within 48 hours. Stability of parenteral admixture at room temperature (25°C) and at refrigeration temperature (4°C) is 48 hours.

Reconstitution

Standard diluent (Solu-Medrol®): 40 mg/50 mL D_5W; 125 mg/50 mL D_5W.

Minimum volume (Solu-Medrol®): 50 mL D_5W.

Compatibility Incompatible with $D_5{}^1/_2NS$; **variable stability (consult detailed reference)** in D_5NS, D_5W, LR, NS.

Y-site administration: Compatible: Acyclovir, amifostine, amiodarone, amphotericin B cholesteryl sulfate complex, aztreonam, cefepime, cisplatin, cladribine, cyclophosphamide, cytarabine, dopamine, doxorubicin, doxorubicin liposome, enalaprilat, famotidine, fludarabine, gatifloxacin, granisetron, heparin, inamrinone, linezolid, melphalan, meperidine, methotrexate, metronidazole, midazolam, morphine, piperacillin/tazobactam, remifentanil, sodium bicarbonate, tacrolimus, teniposide, theophylline, thiotepa, topotecan. **Incompatible:** Allopurinol, amsacrine, ciprofloxacin, docetaxel, etoposide phosphate, filgrastim, gemcitabine, ondansetron, paclitaxel, propofol, sargramostim, vinorelbine. **Variable (consult detailed reference):** Cisatracurium, diltiazem, heparin with hydrocortisone sodium succinate, potassium chloride, vitamin B complex with C.

Compatibility in syringe: Compatible: Diatrizoate meglumine 52% and diatrizoate sodium 8%, diatrizoate sodium 60%, granisetron, iohexol, iopamidol, iothalamate meglumine 60%, ioxaglate meglumine 39.3% and ioxaglate sodium 19.6%, metoclopramide. **Incompatible:** Doxapram.

Compatibility when admixed: Compatible: Chloramphenicol, cimetidine, clindamycin, dopamine, granisetron, heparin, norepinephrine, penicillin G potassium, ranitidine, theophylline, verapamil. **Incompatible:** Calcium gluconate, glycopyrrolate, insulin (regular), metaraminol, nafcillin, penicillin G sodium. **Variable (consult detailed reference):** Aminophylline, amphotericin B, cytarabine.

Mechanism of Action In a tissue-specific manner, corticosteroids regulate gene expression subsequent to binding specific intracellular receptors and translocation into the nucleus. Corticosteroids exert a wide array of physiologic effects including modulation of carbohydrate, protein, and lipid metabolism and maintenance of fluid and electrolyte homeostasis. Moreover cardiovascular, immunologic, musculoskeletal, endocrine, and neurologic physiology are influenced by corticosteroids. Decreases inflammation by suppression of migration of polymorphonuclear leukocytes and reversal of increased capillary permeability.

Pharmacodynamics/Kinetics

Onset of action: Peak effect (route dependent): Oral: 1-2 hours; I.M.: 4-8 days; Intra-articular: 1 week; methylprednisolone sodium succinate is highly soluble and has a rapid effect by I.M. and I.V. routes

Duration (route dependent): Oral: 30-36 hours; I.M.: 1-4 weeks; Intra-articular: 1-5 weeks; methylprednisolone acetate has a low solubility and has a sustained I.M. effect

Distribution: V_d: 0.7-1.5 L/kg

Half-life elimination: 3-3.5 hours; reduced in obese

Excretion: Clearance: Reduced in obese

Dosage Dosing should be based on the lesser of ideal body weight or actual body weight

Only sodium succinate may be given I.V.; methylprednisolone sodium succinate is highly soluble and has a rapid effect by I.M. and I.V. routes. Methylprednisolone acetate has a low solubility and has a sustained I.M. effect.

Children:

Acute spinal cord injury: I.V. (sodium succinate): 30 mg/kg over 15 minutes, followed in 45 minutes by a continuous infusion of 5.4 mg/kg/hour for 23 hours

Anti-inflammatory or immunosuppressive: Oral, I.M., I.V. (sodium succinate): 0.5-1.7 mg/kg/day **or** 5-25 mg/m^2/day in divided doses every 6-12 hours; "Pulse" therapy: 15-30 mg/kg/dose over ≥30 minutes given once daily for 3 days

Asthma exacerbations, including status asthmaticus (emergency medical care or hospital doses) (NIH Asthma Guidelines, NAEPP, 2007): Children <12 years: Oral, I.V.: 1-2 mg/kg/day in 2 divided doses (maximum: 60 mg/day) until peak expiratory flow is 70% of predicted or personal best

Lupus nephritis: I.V. (sodium succinate): 30 mg/kg over ≥30 minutes every other day for 6 doses

Status asthmaticus: I.V. (sodium succinate): Previous NAEPP guidelines still encountered in clinical practice: Loading dose: 2 mg/kg/dose, then 0.5-1 mg/kg/dose every 6 hours for up to 5 days; **Note:** See new dosing guidelines for asthma exacerbations above.

Adults: **Only sodium succinate may be given I.V.;** methylprednisolone sodium succinate is highly soluble and has a rapid effect by I.M. and I.V. routes. Methylprednisolone acetate has a low solubility and has a sustained I.M. effect.

Acute spinal cord injury: I.V. (sodium succinate): 30 mg/kg over 15 minutes, followed in 45 minutes by a continuous infusion of 5.4 mg/kg/hour for 23 hours

Allergic conditions: Oral: Tapered-dosage schedule:

Day 1: 24 mg on day 1 administered as 8 mg before breakfast, 4 mg after lunch, 4 mg after supper, and 8 mg at bedtime **OR** 24 mg as a single dose or divided into 2 or 3 doses upon initiation (regardless of time of day)

Day 2: 20 mg on day 2 administered as 4 mg before breakfast, 4 mg after lunch, 4 mg after supper, and 8 mg at bedtime

Day 3: 16 mg on day 3 administered as 4 mg before breakfast, 4 mg after lunch, 4 mg after supper, and 4 mg at bedtime

Day 4: 12 mg on day 4 administered as 4 mg before breakfast, 4 mg after lunch, and 4 mg at bedtime

Day 5: 8 mg on day 5 administered as 4 mg before breakfast and 4 mg at bedtime

Day 6: 4 mg on day 6 administered as 4 mg before breakfast

Anti-inflammatory or immunosuppressive:

Oral: 2-60 mg/day in 1-4 divided doses to start, followed by gradual reduction in dosage to the lowest possible level consistent with maintaining an adequate clinical response.

I.M. (sodium succinate): 10-80 mg/day once daily

I.M. (acetate): 10-80 mg every 1-2 weeks

I.V. (sodium succinate): 10-40 mg over a period of several minutes and repeated I.V. or I.M. at intervals depending on clinical response; when high dosages are needed, give 30 mg/kg over a period ≥30 minutes and may be repeated every 4-6 hours for 48 hours.

Dermatitis, acute severe: I.M. (acetate): 80-120 mg as a single dose

Dermatitis, chronic: I.M. (acetate): 40-120 mg every 5-10 days

Status asthmaticus: I.V. (sodium succinate): Loading dose: 2 mg/kg/dose, then 0.5-1 mg/kg/dose every 6 hours for up to 5 days

Lupus nephritis: High-dose "pulse" therapy: I.V. (sodium succinate): 1 g/day for 3 days

Aplastic anemia: I.V. (sodium succinate): 1 mg/kg/day or 40 mg/day (whichever dose is higher), for 4 days. After 4 days, change to oral and continue until day 10 or until symptoms of serum sickness resolve, then rapidly reduce over approximately 2 weeks.

Pneumocystis pneumonia in AIDS patients: I.V.: 30 mg twice daily for 5 days, then 30 mg once daily for 5 days, then 15 mg once daily for 11 days

Intra-articular (acetate): Administer every 1-5 weeks.

Large joints: 20-80 mg

Small joints: 4-10 mg

Intralesional (acetate): 20-60 mg every 1-5 weeks

Combination Regimens

Brain tumors: 8 in 1 (Brain Tumors) on page 1221

Leukemia, acute lymphocytic: Hyper-CVAD (Leukemia, Acute Lymphocytic) on page 1349

Lymphoma, non-Hodgkin's: ESHAP on page 1312

Retinoblastoma: 8 in 1 (Retinoblastoma) on page 1222

Administration

Oral: Administer after meals or with food or milk

Parenteral: Methylprednisolone sodium succinate may be administered I.M. or I.V.; I.V. administration may be IVP over one to several minutes or IVPB or continuous I.V. infusion. **Acetate salt should not be given I.V.**

I.V.: Succinate:

Low dose: ≤1.8 mg/kg or ≤125 mg/dose: I.V. push over 3-15 minutes

Moderate dose: ≥2 mg/kg or 250 mg/dose: I.V. over 15-30 minutes

High dose: 15 mg/kg or ≥500 mg/dose: I.V. over ≥30 minutes

Doses >15 mg/kg or ≥1 g: Administer over 1 hour

Do **not** administer high-dose I.V. push; hypotension, cardiac arrhythmia, and sudden death have been reported in patients given high-dose methylprednisolone I.V. push (>0.5 g over <10 minutes); intermittent infusion over 15-60 minutes; maximum concentration: I.V. push 125 mg/mL

I.M.: Acetate: Avoid injection into the deltoid muscle due to a high incidence of subcutaneous atrophy. Do not inject into areas that have evidence of acute local infection.

Monitoring Parameters Blood pressure, blood glucose, electrolytes

Test Interactions Interferes with skin tests

Dietary Considerations Should be taken after meals or with food or milk; need diet rich in pyridoxine, vitamin C, vitamin D, folate, calcium, phosphorus, and protein.

Sodium content of 1 g sodium succinate injection: 2.01 mEq; 53 mg of sodium succinate salt is equivalent to 40 mg of methylprednisolone base

Methylprednisolone acetate: Depo-Medrol®

Methylprednisolone sodium succinate: Solu-Medrol®

Additional Information Sodium content of 1 g sodium succinate injection: 2.01 mEq; 53 mg of sodium succinate salt is equivalent to 40 mg of methylprednisolone base

Methylprednisolone acetate: Depo-Medrol®

Methylprednisolone sodium succinate: Solu-Medrol®

Dosage Forms Excipient information presented when available (limited, particularly for generics); consult specific product labeling.

Injection, powder for reconstitution, as sodium succinate: 40 mg, 125 mg, 500 mg, 1 g [strength expressed as base]

A-Methapred®: 40 mg, 125 mg [strength expressed as base]

Solu-Medrol®: 40 mg, 125 mg, 500 mg, 1 g, 2 g [contains benzyl alcohol (in diluent); strength expressed as base]

Solu-Medrol®: 500 mg, 1 g [strength expressed as base]

Injection, suspension, as acetate: 40 mg/mL (1 mL, 5 mL, 10 mL); 80 mg/mL (1 mL, 5 mL)

Depo-Medrol®: 20 mg/mL (5 mL); 40 mg/mL (5 mL, 10 mL); 80 mg/mL (5 mL) [contains benzyl alcohol, polysorbate 80]

Depo-Medrol®: 40 mg/mL (1 mL); 80 mg/mL (1 mL)

Tablet, oral: 4 mg

Medrol®: 2 mg, 4 mg, 8 mg, 16 mg, 32 mg

Tablet, oral [dose-pack]: 4 mg (21s) [scored]

Medrol® Dosepak™: 4 mg (21s) [scored]

References

Annane D, Sebille V, Charpentier C, et al, "Effect of Treatment With Low Doses of Hydrocortisone and Fludrocortisone on Mortality in Patients With Septic Shock," *JAMA*, 2002, 288(7):862-71.

Cooper MS and Stewart PM, "Corticosteroid Insufficiency in Acutely Ill Patients," *N Engl J Med*, 2003, 348(8):727-34.

Coursin DB and Wood KE, "Corticosteroid Supplementation for Adrenal Insufficiency," *JAMA*, 2002, 287(2):236-40.

Dellinger RP, Levy MM, Carlet JM, et al, "Surviving Sepsis Campaign: International Guidelines for Management of Severe Sepsis and Septic Shock: 2008," *Intensive Care Med*, 2008, 34(1):17-60. Available at http://www.survivingsepsis.org/system/files/images/2008_20International_20SSC_20Guidelines_1_.pdf

Goedert JJ, Vitale F, Lauria C, et al, "Risk Factors for Classical Kaposi's Sarcoma," *J Natl Cancer Inst*, 2002, 94(22):1712-8.

Hotchkiss RS and Karl IE, "The Pathophysiology and Treatment of Sepsis," *N Engl J Med*, 2003, 348(2):138-50.

Sprung CL, Annane D, Keh D, et al, "Hydrocortisone Therapy for Patients With Septic Shock," *N Engl J Med*, 2008, 358(2):111-24.

Steinberg KP, Hudson LD, Goodman RB, et al, "Efficacy and Safety of Corticosteroids for Persistent Acute Respiratory Distress Syndrome. National Heart, Lung and Blood Institute Acute Respiratory Distress Syndrome (ARDS) Clinical Trials Network," *N Engl J Med*, 2006, 354 (16):1671-84.

Tornatore KM, Logue G, Venuto RC, et al, "Pharmacokinetics of Methylprednisolone in Elderly and Young Healthy Males," *J Am Geriatr Soc*, 1994, 42(10):1118-22.

◆ **6-α-Methylprednisolone** *see* MethylPREDNISolone *on page 782*

◆ **Methylprednisolone Acetate** *see* MethylPREDNISolone *on page 782*

◆ **Methylprednisolone Sodium Succinate** *see* MethylPREDNISolone *on page 782*

Metoclopramide (met oh KLOE pra mide)

Medication Safety Issues

Sound-alike/look-alike issues:

Metoclopramide may be confused with metolazone, metoprolol, metroNIDAZOLE

Reglan® may be confused with Megace®, Regonol®, Renagel®

Related Information
Management of Chemotherapy-Induced Nausea and Vomiting *on page 1434*

U.S. Brand Names Reglan®

Generic Available Yes

Canadian Brand Names Apo-Metoclop®; Metoclopramide Hydrochloride Injection; Metoclopramide Omega; Nu-Metoclopramide; PMS-Metoclopramide

Pharmacologic Category Antiemetic; Gastrointestinal Agent, Prokinetic

Use
Oral: Symptomatic treatment of diabetic gastroparesis; gastroesophageal reflux

I.V., I.M.: Symptomatic treatment of diabetic gastroparesis; postpyloric placement of enteral feeding tubes; prevention and/or treatment of nausea and vomiting associated with chemotherapy, or postsurgery; to stimulate gastric emptying and intestinal transit of barium during radiological examination of the stomach/small intestine

Pregnancy Risk Factor B

Lactation Enters breast milk/use caution

Labeled Contraindications Hypersensitivity to metoclopramide or any component of the formulation; GI obstruction, perforation or hemorrhage; pheochromocytoma; history of seizures or concomitant use of other agents likely to increase extrapyramidal reactions

Warnings/Precautions [U.S. Boxed Warning]: May cause tardive dyskinesia, which is often irreversible; duration of treatment and total cumulative dose are associated with an increased risk. Therapy durations >12 weeks should be avoided (except in rare cases following risk:benefit assessment). Risk appears to be increased in the elderly, women, and diabetics; however, it is not possible to predict which patients will develop tardive dyskinesia. Therapy should be discontinued in any patient if signs/symptoms of tardive dyskinesia appear.

May cause extrapyramidal symptoms, generally manifested as acute dystonic reactions within the initial 24-48 hours of use. Risk of these reactions is increased at higher doses, and in pediatric patients, and adults <30 years of age. Pseudoparkinsonism (eg, bradykinesia, tremor, rigidity) may also occur (usually within first 6 months of therapy) and is generally reversible following discontinuation. Use with caution or avoid in patients with Parkinson's disease. Use caution in the elderly; may have increased risk of tardive dyskinesia, particularly older women. Neuroleptic malignant syndrome (NMS) has been reported (rarely) with metoclopramide.

May cause transient increase in serum aldosterone; use caution in patients who are at risk of fluid overload (HF, cirrhosis). Use caution in patients with hypertension or following surgical anastomosis/closure. Use caution with a history of mental illness; has been associated with depression. Abrupt discontinuation may (rarely) result in withdrawal symptoms (dizziness, headache, nervousness). Use caution and adjust dose in renal impairment. Patients with NADH-cytochrome b5 reductase deficiency are at increased risk of methemoglobinemia and/or sulfhemoglobinemia. Neonates may have an increased risk of methemoglobinemia due to decreased levels of NADH-cytochrome b5 reductase deficiency and prolonged clearance of metoclopramide.

Adverse Reactions Frequency not always defined.
Cardiovascular: AV block, bradycardia, HF, fluid retention, flushing (following high I.V. doses), hyper-/hypotension, supraventricular tachycardia

Central nervous system: Drowsiness (~10% to 70%; dose related), acute dystonic reactions (<1% to 25%; dose and age related), fatigue (~10%), lassitude (~10%), restlessness (~10%), akathisia, confusion, depression, dizziness, hallucinations (rare), headache, insomnia, neuroleptic malignant syndrome (rare), Parkinsonian-like symptoms, suicidal ideation, seizure, tardive dyskinesia

Dermatologic: Angioneurotic edema (rare), rash, urticaria

Endocrine & metabolic: Amenorrhea, galactorrhea, gynecomastia, hyper-prolactinemia, impotence

Gastrointestinal: Diarrhea, nausea

Genitourinary: Incontinence, urinary frequency

Hematologic: Agranulocytosis, leukopenia, neutropenia, porphyria

Hepatic: Hepatotoxicity (rare)

Ocular: Visual disturbance

Respiratory: Bronchospasm, laryngeal edema (rare), laryngospasm (rare)

Miscellaneous: Allergic reactions, methemoglobinemia, sulfhemoglobinemia

Drug Interactions

Metabolism/Transport Effects Substrate (minor) of CYP1A2, 2D6; **Inhibits** CYP2D6 (weak)

Avoid Concomitant Use There are no known interactions where it is recommended to avoid concomitant use.

Increased Effect/Toxicity

Metoclopramide may increase the levels/effects of: CycloSPORINE; Sertraline; Venlafaxine

Decreased Effect

Metoclopramide may decrease the levels/effects of: Anti-Parkinson's Agents (Dopamine Agonist); Posaconazole

The levels/effects of Metoclopramide may be decreased by: Peginterferon Alfa-2b

Ethanol/Nutrition/Herb Interactions Ethanol: Avoid ethanol (may increase CNS depression).

Storage/Stability

Injection: Store intact vial at controlled room temperature; injection is photosensitive and should be protected from light during storage; parenteral admixtures in D_5W or NS are stable for at least 24 hours and do not require light protection if used within 24 hours.

Tablet: Store at controlled room temperature.

Compatibility Stable in $D_5^{1/2}NS$, D_5W, mannitol 20%, LR, NS; **variable stability (consult detailed reference)** in TPN.

Y-site administration: Compatible: Acyclovir, aldesleukin, amifostine, aztreonam, bleomycin, caffeine citrate, ciprofloxacin, cisatracurium, cisplatin, cladribine, clarithromycin, cyclophosphamide, cytarabine, diltiazem, docetaxel, doxorubicin, droperidol, etoposide phosphate, famotidine, filgrastim, fluconazole, fludarabine, fluorouracil, foscarnet, gatifloxacin, gemcitabine, granisetron, heparin, hetastarch in lactated electrolyte injection, idarubicin, leucovorin, levofloxacin, linezolid, melphalan, meperidine, meropenem, methotrexate, mitomycin, morphine, ondansetron, paclitaxel, palonosetron, piperacillin/tazobactam, remifentanil, sargramostim, sufentanil, tacrolimus, teniposide, thiotepa, topotecan, vinblastine, vincristine, vinorelbine, zidovudine. **Incompatible:** Allopurinol, amphotericin B cholesteryl sulfate complex, amsacrine, cefepime, doxorubicin liposome, furosemide, pantoprazole, propofol. **Variable (consult detailed reference):** TPN.

Compatibility in syringe: Compatible: Aminophylline, ascorbic acid injection, atropine, benztropine, bleomycin, butorphanol, chlorpromazine, cisplatin, cyclophosphamide, cytarabine, dexamethasone sodium phosphate, diamorphine, dimenhydrinate, diphenhydramine, doxorubicin, droperidol, fentanyl, fluorouracil, heparin, hydrocortisone sodium phosphate, hydroxyzine, insulin (regular), leucovorin, lidocaine, magnesium sulfate, meperidine, methotrimeprazine, methylprednisolone sodium succinate, midazolam, mitomycin, morphine, ondansetron, pentazocine, perphenazine, prochlorperazine edisylate, promazine, promethazine, ranitidine, scopolamine, sufentanil, vinblastine, vincristine, vitamin B complex with C. **Incompatible:** Ampicillin, calcium gluconate, chloramphenicol, furosemide, penicillin G potassium, sodium bicarbonate. **Variable (consult detailed reference):** Methotrexate.

Compatibility when admixed: Compatible: Cimetidine, clindamycin, meperidine, meropenem, morphine, multivitamins, potassium acetate, potassium chloride, potassium phosphate, verapamil. **Incompatible:** Dexamethasone sodium phosphate with lorazepam and diphenhydramine, erythromycin lactobionate, floxacillin, fluorouracil, furosemide.

Mechanism of Action Blocks dopamine receptors and (when given in higher doses) also blocks serotonin receptors in chemoreceptor trigger zone of the CNS; enhances the response to acetylcholine of tissue in upper GI tract causing enhanced motility and accelerated gastric emptying without stimulating gastric, biliary, or pancreatic secretions; increases lower esophageal sphincter tone

Pharmacodynamics/Kinetics

Onset of action: Oral: 30-60 minutes; I.V.: 1-3 minutes; I.M.: 10-15 minutes

Duration: Therapeutic: 1-2 hours, regardless of route

Absorption: Oral: Rapid

Distribution: V_d: ~3.5 L/kg

Protein binding: ~30%

Bioavailability: Oral: Range: 65% to 95%

Half-life elimination: Normal renal function: Children: ~4 hours; Adults: 5-6 hours (may be dose dependent)

Time to peak, serum: Oral: 1-2 hours

Excretion: Urine (~85%)

Dosage

Children:

Gastroesophageal reflux (unlabeled use): Oral: 0.1-0.2 mg/kg/dose 4 times/day

Antiemetic (chemotherapy-induced emesis) (unlabeled): I.V.: 1-2 mg/kg 30 minutes before chemotherapy and every 2-4 hours (maximum: 5 doses/day); pretreatment with diphenhydramine will decrease risk of extrapyramidal reactions to this dosage

Postpyloric feeding tube placement: I.V.:

<6 years: 0.1 mg/kg as a single dose

6-14 years: 2.5-5 mg as a single dose

>14 years: Refer to adult dosing.

Adults:

Gastroesophageal reflux: Oral: 10-15 mg/dose up to 4 times/day 30 minutes before meals or food and at bedtime; single doses of 20 mg are occasionally needed prior to provoking situations. Treatment >12 weeks has not been evaluated and is not recommended.

Diabetic gastroparesis:

Oral: 10 mg 30 minutes before each meal and at bedtime for 2-8 weeks

I.M., I.V. (for severe symptoms): 10 mg over 1-2 minutes; 10 days of I.V. therapy may be necessary before symptoms are controlled to allow transition to oral administration

Chemotherapy-induced emesis prophylaxis: I.V.: 1-2 mg/kg 30 minutes before chemotherapy and repeated every 2 hours for 2 doses, then every 3 hours for 3 doses (manufacturer labeling); pretreatment with diphenhydramine will decrease risk of extrapyramidal reactions

Alternate dosing: **Note:** Metoclopramide is considered an antiemetic with a low therapeutic index; use is generally reserved for agents with low emetogenic potential or in patients intolerant/refractory to first-line antiemetics.

Low-risk chemotherapy (unlabeled): I.V., Oral: 10-40 mg prior to dose, then every 4-6 hours as needed (NCCN Antiemesis guidelines, v.4.2009)

Breakthrough treatment (unlabeled): I.V., Oral: 10-40 mg every 4-6 hours (NCCN Antiemesis guidelines, v.4.2009)

Delayed-emesis prophylaxis (unlabeled): Oral: 20-40 mg/dose (or 0.5 mg/kg/dose) 2-4 times/day for 3-4 days (in combination with dexamethasone [ASCO guidelines, 2006])

Refractory or intolerant to antiemetics with a higher therapeutic index (unlabeled; Hesketh, 2008):

I.V.: 1-2 mg/kg/dose before chemotherapy and repeat 2 hours after chemotherapy

Oral: 0.5 mg/kg every 6 hours on days 2-4

Postoperative nausea and vomiting prophylaxis: I.M.: 10-20 mg near end of surgery

Postpyloric feeding tube placement, radiological exam: I.V.: 10 mg as a single dose

Elderly: Initial: Dose at the lower end of the recommended range. Refer to adult dosing.

Dosing adjustment in renal impairment: Cl_{cr} <40 mL/minute: Administer at 50% of normal dose

Hemodialysis: Not dialyzable (0% to 5%); supplemental dose is not necessary

Administration Injection solution may be given I.M., direct I.V. push, short infusion (15-30 minutes), or continuous infusion; lower doses (≤10 mg) of metoclopramide can be given I.V. push undiluted over 1-2 minutes; higher doses (>10 mg) to be diluted in 50 mL of compatible solution (preferably NS) and given IVPB over at least 15 minutes; continuous SubQ infusion and rectal administration have been reported. **Note:** Rapid I.V. administration may be associated with a transient (but intense) feeling of anxiety and restlessness, followed by drowsiness.

Monitoring Parameters Dystonic reactions; signs of hypoglycemia in patients using insulin and those being treated for gastroparesis; agitation, and confusion

Test Interactions Increased aminotransferase [ALT/AST] (S), increased amylase (S)

Dosage Forms Excipient information presented when available (limited, particularly for generics); consult specific product labeling.

Injection, solution [preservative free]: 5 mg/mL (2 mL)

Reglan®: 5 mg/mL (2 mL, 10 mL, 30 mL)

Solution, oral: 5 mg/5 mL (10 mL, 480 mL)

Tablet: 5 mg, 10 mg

Reglan®: 5 mg, 10 mg

References

Bruera E, Seifert L, Watanabe S, et al, "Chronic Nausea in Advanced Cancer Patients: A Retrospective Assessment of a Metoclopramide-Based Antiemetic Regimen," *J Pain Symptom Manage*, 1996, 11(3):147-53.

Harrington RA, Hamilton CW, Brogden RN, et al, "Metoclopramide. An Updated Review of Its Pharmacological Properties and Clinical Use," *Drugs*, 1983, 25(5):451-94.

McGovern EM, Grevel J, and Bryson SM, "Pharmacokinetics of High-Dose Metoclopramide in Cancer Patients," *Clin Pharmacokinet*, 1986, 11(6):415-24.

National Comprehensive Cancer Network (NCCN), "Clinical Practice Guidelines in Oncology™: Antiemesis," Version 1.2008. Available at http://www.nccn.org/professionals/physician_gls/PDF/antiemesis.pdf.

◆ **Metoclopramide Hydrochloride Injection (Can)** *see* Metoclopramide *on page* 788

◆ **Metoclopramide Omega (Can)** *see* Metoclopramide *on page* 788

◆ **MetroCream®** *see* MetroNIDAZOLE *on page* 793

◆ **MetroGel®** *see* MetroNIDAZOLE *on page* 793

◆ **Metrogel® (Can)** *see* MetroNIDAZOLE *on page* 793

◆ **MetroGel-Vaginal®** *see* MetroNIDAZOLE *on page* 793

◆ **MetroLotion®** *see* MetroNIDAZOLE *on page* 793

MetroNIDAZOLE (met roe NYE da zole)

Medication Safety Issues

Sound-alike/look-alike issues:

MetroNIDAZOLE may be confused with meropenem, metFORMIN, methotrexate

U.S. Brand Names Flagyl®; Flagyl® 375; Flagyl® ER; MetroCream®; MetroGel-Vaginal®; MetroGel®; MetroLotion®; Noritate®; Vandazole®

Index Terms Metronidazole Hydrochloride

Generic Available Yes: Capsule, cream, gel, infusion, lotion, tablet

Canadian Brand Names Apo-Metronidazole®; Flagyl®; Florazole® ER; MetroCream®; Metrogel®; Nidagel™; Noritate®; Trikacide

Pharmacologic Category Amebicide; Antibiotic, Miscellaneous; Antibiotic, Topical; Antiprotozoal, Nitroimidazole

Use Treatment of susceptible anaerobic bacterial and protozoal infections in the following conditions: Amebiasis, symptomatic and asymptomatic trichomoniasis; skin and skin structure infections; CNS infections; intra-abdominal infections (as part of combination regimen); systemic anaerobic infections; treatment of antibiotic-associated pseudomembranous colitis (AAPC), bacterial vaginosis; as part of a multidrug regimen for *H. pylori* eradication to reduce the risk of duodenal ulcer recurrence

Topical: Treatment of inflammatory lesions and erythema of rosacea

Unlabeled/Investigational Use Crohn's disease

Pregnancy Risk Factor B (may be contraindicated in 1st trimester)

Lactation Enters breast milk/not recommended (AAP rates "of concern")

Labeled Contraindications Hypersensitivity to metronidazole, nitroimidazole derivatives, or any component of the formulation; pregnancy (1st trimester - found to be carcinogenic in rats)

Warnings/Precautions Use with caution in patients with liver impairment due to potential accumulation, blood dyscrasias; history of seizures, CHF, or other sodium retaining states; reduce dosage in patients with severe liver impairment, CNS disease, and consider dosage reduction in longer-term therapy with severe renal failure (Cl_{cr} <10 mL/minute); if *H. pylori* is not eradicated in patients being treated with metronidazole in a regimen, it should be assumed that metronidazole-resistance has occurred and it should not again be used; seizures and neuropathies have been reported especially with increased doses and chronic treatment; if this occurs, discontinue therapy. **[U.S. Boxed Warning]: Possibly carcinogenic based on animal data.** Prolonged use may result in fungal or bacterial superinfection, including *C. difficile*-associated diarrhea (CDAD) and pseudomembranous colitis; CDAD has been observed >2 months postantibiotic treatment.

Adverse Reactions

Systemic: Frequency not defined:

Cardiovascular: Flattening of the T-wave, flushing

Central nervous system: Ataxia, confusion, coordination impaired, dizziness, fever, headache, insomnia, irritability, seizure, vertigo

Dermatologic: Erythematous rash, urticaria

Endocrine & metabolic: Disulfiram-like reaction, dysmenorrhea, libido decreased

Gastrointestinal: Nausea (~12%), anorexia, abdominal cramping, constipation, diarrhea, furry tongue, glossitis, proctitis, stomatitis, unusual/metallic taste, vomiting, xerostomia

Genitourinary: Cystitis, darkened urine (rare), dysuria, incontinence, polyuria, vaginitis

Hematologic: Neutropenia (reversible), thrombocytopenia (reversible, rare)

Neuromuscular & skeletal: Peripheral neuropathy, weakness

Respiratory: Nasal congestion, rhinitis, sinusitis, pharyngitis

Miscellaneous: Flu-like syndrome, moniliasis

Topical: Frequency not defined:

Central nervous system: Headache

Dermatologic: Burning, contact dermatitis, dryness, erythema, irritation, pruritus, rash

Gastrointestinal: Unusual/metallic taste, nausea, constipation

Local: Local allergic reaction

Neuromuscular & skeletal: Tingling/numbness of extremities

Ocular: Eye irritation

Vaginal:

>10%: Genitourinary: Vaginal discharge (12%)

1% to 10%:

Central nervous system: Headache (5%), dizziness (2%)

Gastrointestinal: Gastrointestinal discomfort (7%), nausea and/or vomiting (4%), unusual/metallic taste (2%), diarrhea (1%)

Genitourinary: Vaginitis (10%), vulva/vaginal irritation (9%), pelvic discomfort (3%)

Hematologic: WBC increased (2%)

<1%: Abdominal bloating, abdominal gas, darkened urine, depression, fatigue, itching, rash, thirst, xerostomia

Drug Interactions

Metabolism/Transport Effects Inhibits CYP2C9 (weak), 3A4 (moderate)

Avoid Concomitant Use

Avoid concomitant use of MetroNIDAZOLE with any of the following: Amprenavir; Everolimus; Tolvaptan

Increased Effect/Toxicity

MetroNIDAZOLE may increase the levels/effects of: Alcohol (Ethyl); Amprenavir; Busulfan; Calcineurin Inhibitors; Colchicine; CYP3A4 Substrates; Eplerenone; Everolimus; FentaNYL; Halofantrine; Pimecrolimus; Ranolazine; Salmeterol; Saxagliptin; Tipranavir; Tolvaptan; Vitamin K Antagonists

The levels/effects of MetroNIDAZOLE may be increased by: Disulfiram; Mebendazole

Decreased Effect

MetroNIDAZOLE may decrease the levels/effects of: Mycophenolate; Typhoid Vaccine

Ethanol/Nutrition/Herb Interactions

Ethanol: The manufacturer recommends to avoid all ethanol or any ethanol-containing drugs (may cause disulfiram-like reaction characterized by flushing, headache, nausea, vomiting, sweating, or tachycardia).

Food: Peak antibiotic serum concentration lowered and delayed, but total drug absorbed not affected.

Storage/Stability

Injection: Should be stored at 15°C to 30°C and protected from light. Product may be refrigerated but crystals may form. Crystals redissolve on warming to room temperature. Prolonged exposure to light will cause a darkening of the product. However, short-term exposure to normal room light does not adversely affect metronidazole stability. Direct sunlight should be avoided. Stability of parenteral admixture at room temperature (25°C): Out of overwrap stability: 30 days.

Cream, topical gel, lotion: Store at controlled room temperature of 20°C to 25°C (68°C to 77°C).

Vaginal gel: Store at controlled room temperature of 15°C to 30°C (59°C to 86°C).

Reconstitution Standard diluent: 500 mg/100 mL NS.

Compatibility Stable in D_5W, NS.

Y-site administration: Compatible: Acyclovir, allopurinol, amiodarone, amifostine, cefepime, cisatracurium, clarithromycin, cyclophosphamide, diltiazem, docetaxel, dopamine, doxorubicin liposome, enalaprilat, esmolol, etoposide phosphate, fluconazole, foscarnet, gatifloxacin, gemcitabine, granisetron, heparin, hydromorphone, labetalol, linezolid, lorazepam, magnesium sulfate, melphalan, meperidine, methylprednisolone sodium succinate, midazolam, morphine, perphenazine, piperacillin/tazobactam, remifentanil, sargramostim, tacrolimus, teniposide, theophylline, thiotepa, vinorelbine. Incompatible: Amphotericin B cholesteryl sulfate complex, aztreonam, filgrastim, meropenem, warfarin.

Compatibility when admixed: Compatible: Amikacin, aminophylline, ampicillin, cefazolin, cefotaxime, cefoxitin, ceftazidime, ceftizoxime, ceftriaxone, cefuroxime, chloramphenicol, ciprofloxacin, clindamycin, disopyramide, floxacillin, fluconazole, gentamicin, heparin, hydrocortisone sodium succinate, multivitamins, netilmicin, penicillin G potassium, tobramycin. Incompatible: Aztreonam, dopamine, meropenem. Variable (consult detailed reference): Cefamandole, cefepime.

Mechanism of Action After diffusing into the organism, interacts with DNA to cause a loss of helical DNA structure and strand breakage resulting in inhibition of protein synthesis and cell death in susceptible organisms

Pharmacodynamics/Kinetics

Absorption: Oral: Well absorbed; Topical: Concentrations achieved systemically after application of 1 g topically are 10 times less than those obtained after a 250 mg oral dose

Distribution: To saliva, bile, seminal fluid, breast milk, bone, liver, and liver abscesses, lung and vaginal secretions; crosses placenta and blood-brain barrier

CSF:blood level ratio: Normal meninges: 16% to 43%; Inflamed meninges: 100%

Protein binding: <20%

Metabolism: Hepatic (30% to 60%)

Half-life elimination: Neonates: 25-75 hours; Others: 6-8 hours, prolonged with hepatic impairment; End-stage renal disease: 21 hours

Time to peak, serum: Oral: Immediate release: 1-2 hours

Excretion: Urine (20% to 40% as unchanged drug); feces (6% to 15%)

◀ **Dosage**

Infants and Children:

Amebiasis: Oral: 35-50 mg/kg/day in divided doses every 8 hours for 10 days

Trichomoniasis: Oral: 15-30 mg/kg/day in divided doses every 8 hours for 7 days

Anaerobic infections:

Oral: 15-35 mg/kg/day in divided doses every 8 hours

I.V.: 30 mg/kg/day in divided doses every 6 hours

Clostridium difficile (antibiotic-associated colitis): Oral: 20 mg/kg/day divided every 6 hours

Maximum dose: 2 g/day

Adults:

Anaerobic infections (diverticulitis, intra-abdominal, peritonitis, cholangitis, or abscess): Oral, I.V.: 500 mg every 6-8 hours, not to exceed 4 g/day

Acne rosacea: Topical:

0.75%: Apply and rub a thin film twice daily, morning and evening, to entire affected areas after washing. Significant therapeutic results should be noticed within 3 weeks. Clinical studies have demonstrated continuing improvement through 9 weeks of therapy.

1%: Apply thin film to affected area once daily

Amebiasis: Oral: 500-750 mg every 8 hours for 5-10 days

Antibiotic-associated pseudomembranous colitis: Oral: 250-500 mg 3-4 times/day for 10-14 days

Note: Due to the emergence of a new strain of *C. difficile*, some clinicians recommend converting to oral vancomycin therapy if the patient does not show a clear clinical response after 2 days of metronidazole therapy.

Giardiasis: 500 mg twice daily for 5-7 days

Helicobacter pylori eradication: Oral: 250-500 mg with meals and at bedtime for 14 days; requires combination therapy with at least one other antibiotic and an acid-suppressing agent (proton pump inhibitor or H_2 blocker)

Bacterial vaginosis or vaginitis due to *Gardnerella, Mobiluncus*:

Oral: 500 mg twice daily (regular release) or 750 mg once daily (extended release tablet) for 7 days

Vaginal: 1 applicatorful (~37.5 mg metronidazole) intravaginally once or twice daily for 5 days; apply once in morning and evening if using twice daily, if daily, use at bedtime

Trichomoniasis: Oral: 250 mg every 8 hours for 7 days **or** 375 mg twice daily for 7 days **or** 2 g as a single dose

Elderly: Use lower end of dosing recommendations for adults, do not administer as a single dose

Dosing adjustment in renal impairment: Cl_{cr} <10 mL/minute, but not on dialysis: Recommendations vary: To reduce possible accumulation in patients receiving multiple doses, consider reduction to 50% of dose or every 12 hours; **Note:** Dosage reduction is unnecessary in short courses of therapy. Clinical recommendations and practice vary. Some references do not recommend reduction at any level of renal impairment (Lamp, 1999).

Hemodialysis: Extensively removed by hemodialysis and peritoneal dialysis (50% to 100%); dosage reduction not recommended; administer full dose posthemodialysis

Peritoneal dialysis: Dose as for Cl_{cr} <10 mL/minute

Continuous arteriovenous or venovenous hemofiltration: Administer usual dose

Dosing adjustment/comments in hepatic disease: Unchanged in mild liver disease; reduce dosage in severe liver disease

Administration

Oral: May be taken with food to minimize stomach upset. Extended release tablets should be taken on an empty stomach (1 hour before or 2 hours after meals).

Topical: No disulfiram-like reactions have been reported after **topical** application, although metronidazole can be detected in the blood. Apply to clean, dry skin. Cosmetics may be used after application (wait at least 5 minutes after using lotion).

Test Interactions May interfere with AST, ALT, triglycerides, glucose, and LDH testing

Dietary Considerations Take on an empty stomach. Drug may cause GI upset; if GI upset occurs, take with food. Extended release tablets should be taken on an empty stomach (1 hour before or 2 hours after meals). Sodium content of 500 mg (I.V.): 322 mg (14 mEq). The manufacturer recommends that ethanol be avoided during treatment and for 3 days after therapy is complete.

Dosage Forms Excipient information presented when available (limited, particularly for generics); consult specific product labeling.

Capsule, oral: 375 mg
  Flagyl® 375: 375 mg
Cream, topical: 0.75% (45 g)
  MetroCream®: 0.75% (45 g) [contains benzyl alcohol]
  Noritate®: 1% (60 g)
Gel, topical: 1% (45 g)
  MetroGel®: 1% (60 g) [60 g tube also packaged in a kit with Cetaphil® skin cleanser]
Gel, vaginal: 0.75% (70 g)
  MetroGel-Vaginal®, Vandazole®: 0.75% (70 g)
Infusion [premixed iso-osmotic sodium chloride solution]: 500 mg (100 mL)
Lotion, topical: 0.75% (60 mL)
  MetroLotion®: 0.75% (60 mL) [contains benzyl alcohol]
Tablet, oral: 250 mg, 500 mg
  Flagyl®: 250 mg, 500 mg
Tablet, extended release, oral:
  Flagyl® ER: 750 mg

Extemporaneous Preparations A 20 mg/mL oral suspension can be prepared by crushing ten 250 mg tablets in a mortar, and then adding 10 mL purified water USP to create a uniform paste. Add a small quantity of syrup, then transfer to a graduate and add a sufficient quantity of syrup to make 125 mL. Label "shake well" and "refrigerate." Refrigerated stability is 10 days.

Irwin DB, Dupuis LL, Prober CG, et al, "The Acceptability, Stability, and Relative Bioavailability of an Extemporaneous Metronidazole Suspension," *Can J Hosp Pharm*, 1987, 40:42-6.

Nahata MC, Morosco RS, and Hipple TF, 4th ed, *Pediatric Drug Formulations*, Cincinnati, OH: Harvey Whitney Books Co, 2000.

References

Bartlett JG and Perl TM, "The New *Clostridium difficile*- What Does it Mean?" *N Engl J Med*, 2005, 353(23):2503-5.

Belliveau PP, Nightingale CH, and Quintilani R, "Stability of Cefotaxime Sodium and Metronidazole in 0.9% Sodium Chloride Injection or in Ready-to-Use Metronidazole Bags," *Am J Health Syst Pharm*, 1995, 52(14):1561-3.

Brodgen RN, Heel RC, Speight TM, et al, "Metronidazole in Anaerobic Infections: A Review of Its Activity, Pharmacokinetics and Therapeutic Use," *Drugs*, 1978, 16(5):387-417.

Fekety R and Shah AB, "Diagnosis and Treatment of *Clostridium difficile* Colitis," *JAMA*, 1993, 269 (1):71-5.

Freeman CD, Klutman NE, and Lamp KC, "Metronidazole. A Therapeutic Review and Update," *Drugs*, 1997, 54(5):679-708.

Kelly CP, Pothoulakis C, and LaMont JT, "*Clostridium difficile* Colitis," *N Engl J Med*, 1994, 330 (4):257-62.

Lam S and Bank S, "Hepatotoxicity Caused by Metronidazole Overdose," *Ann Intern Med*, 1995, 122(10):803.

Lamp KC, Freeman CD, Klutman NE, et al, "Pharmacokinetics and Pharmacodynamics of the Nitroimidazole Antimicrobials," *Clin Pharmacokinet*, 1999, 36(5):353-73.

Lorber B, "Update in Infectious Diseases," *Ann Intern Med*, 2006, 145:356-7.

Ludwig E, Csiba A, Magyar T, et al, "Age-Associated Pharmacokinetic Changes of Metronidazole," *Int J Clin Pharmacol Ther Toxicol*, 1983, 21(2):87-91.

Ralph ED, "Clinical Pharmacokinetics of Metronidazole," *Clin Pharmacokinet*, 1983, 8:43-62.

◆ **Metronidazole Hydrochloride** *see* MetroNIDAZOLE *on page* 793

◆ **Miacalcin®** *see* Calcitonin *on page* 165

◆ **Miacalcin® NS (Can)** *see* Calcitonin *on page* 165

Micafungin (mi ka FUN gin)

U.S. Brand Names Mycamine®

Index Terms Micafungin Sodium

Generic Available No

Canadian Brand Names Mycamine®

Pharmacologic Category Antifungal Agent, Parenteral; Echinocandin

Use Treatment of esophageal candidiasis; *Candida* prophylaxis in patients undergoing hematopoietic stem cell transplant (HSCT); treatment of candidemia, acute disseminated candidiasis, and other *Candida* infections (peritonitis and abscesses)

Unlabeled/Investigational Use Treatment of infections due to *Aspergillus* spp; prophylaxis of HIV-related esophageal candidiasis

Pregnancy Risk Factor C

Lactation Excretion in breast milk unknown/use caution

Labeled Contraindications Hypersensitivity to micafungin, other echinocandins, or any component of the formulation

Warnings/Precautions Anaphylactic reactions, including shock, have been reported. New onset or worsening hepatic failure has been reported; use caution in pre-existing mild-moderate hepatic impairment; safety in severe liver failure has not been evaluated. Hemolytic anemia and hemoglobinuria have been reported. Increased BUN, serum creatinine, renal dysfunction, and/or acute renal failure has been reported; use with caution in patients with pre-existing renal impairment and monitor closely. Safety and efficacy in pediatric patients have not been established.

Adverse Reactions Percentages reflect incidence across all approved indications (prophylaxis and treatment); however, in general, a higher frequency of adverse reactions was observed in studies with HSCT patients.

>10%:

Central nervous system: Fever (20%), headache (16%)

Endocrine & metabolic: Hypokalemia (18%), hypomagnesemia (13%)

Gastrointestinal: Diarrhea (23%), nausea (22%), vomiting (22%), mucosal inflammation (14%), constipation (11%)

Hematologic: Thrombocytopenia (15%), neutropenia (14%)

1% to 10%:

Cardiovascular: Hypotension (9%), tachycardia (8%), hypertension (7%), peripheral edema (7%), phlebitis (6%), edema (5%)

Central nervous system: Insomnia (10%), anxiety (6%), fatigue (6%)

Dermatologic: Rash (9%), pruritus (6%)

Endocrine & metabolic: Hypocalcemia (7%), hyperglycemia (6%)

Gastrointestinal: Abdominal pain (10%), anorexia (6%), dyspepsia (6%)

Hematologic: Anemia (10%), febrile neutropenia (6%)

Hepatic: AST increased (6%), ALT increased (5%), serum alkaline phosphatase increased (5%)

Neuromuscular & skeletal: Rigors (9%), back pain (5%)

Respiratory: Cough (8%), dyspnea (6%), epistaxis (6%)

Miscellaneous: Bacteremia (6%), sepsis (5%)

<1%, postmarketing and/or case reports, or frequency not defined: Acidosis, acute renal failure, anuria, apnea, arrhythmia, arthralgia, atrial fibrillation, BUN increased, cardiac arrest, coagulopathy, creatinine increased, cyanosis, deep vein thrombosis, delirium, hypoxia, encephalopathy, erythema multiforme, facial edema, hemoglobinuria, hemolysis, hemolytic anemia, hepatic dysfunction, hepatic failure, hepatocellular damage, hepatomegaly, hiccups, hyperbilirubinemia, hyponatremia, hypoxia, infection, injection site necrosis, injection site thrombosis, intracranial hemorrhage, jaundice, MI, mucosal inflammation, oliguria, pancytopenia, pneumonia, pulmonary embolism, renal impairment, renal tubular necrosis, seizure, shock, skin necrosis, thrombotic thrombocytopenia purpura, thrombophlebitis, urticaria, vasodilatation, WBC decreased

Drug Interactions

Metabolism/Transport Effects Substrate of CYP3A4 (minor); **Inhibits** CYP3A4 (weak)

Avoid Concomitant Use There are no known interactions where it is recommended to avoid concomitant use.

Increased Effect/Toxicity There are no known significant interactions involving an increase in effect.

Decreased Effect

Micafungin may decrease the levels/effects of: Saccharomyces boulardii

Storage/Stability Store at controlled room temperature of 25°C (77°F). Reconstituted and diluted solutions are stable for 24 hours at room temperature. Protect from light.

Reconstitution Aseptically add 5 mL of NS (preservative-free) to each 50 or 100 mg vial. Swirl to dissolve; do not shake. Further dilute 50-150 mg in 100 mL NS. Protect from light. Alternatively, D_5W may be used for reconstitution and dilution.

Compatibility Do not mix or coinfuse with other intravenous solutions.

Mechanism of Action Concentration-dependent inhibition of 1,3-beta-D-glucan synthase resulting in reduced formation of 1,3-beta-D-glucan, an essential polysaccharide comprising 30% to 60% of *Candida* cell walls (absent in mammalian cells); decreased glucan content leads to osmotic instability and cellular lysis

Pharmacodynamics/Kinetics

Distribution: 0.28-0.5 L/kg

Protein binding: >99%; primarily to albumin

Metabolism: Hepatic; forms M-1 (catechol) and M-2 (methoxy) metabolites (activity unknown)

Half-life elimination: 11-21 hours

Excretion: Primarily feces (71%); urine (<15%)

Dosage I.V.: Adults:

Candidemia, acute disseminated candidiasis, and *Candida* peritonitis and abscesses: 100 mg daily; mean duration of therapy (from clinical trials) was 15 days (range: 10-47 days)

▶

Esophageal candidiasis: 150 mg daily; mean duration of therapy (from clinical trials) was 15 days (range: 10-30 days)

Prophylaxis of *Candida* infection in hematopoietic stem cell transplantation: 50 mg daily

Dosing adjustment in renal impairment: No adjustment required

Dosing adjustment in hepatic impairment: No dosage adjustment required for moderate hepatic impairment (Child-Pugh score 7-9). Patients with severe hepatic dysfunction have not been studied.

Administration For intravenous use only; infuse over 1 hour. Flush line with NS prior to administration.

Monitoring Parameters Liver function tests

Dosage Forms Excipient information presented when available (limited, particularly for generics); consult specific product labeling.

Injection, powder for reconstitution, as sodium [preservative-free]:

Mycamine®: 50 mg, 100 mg [contains lactose]

References

Pappas PG, Rotstein CM, Betts RF, et al, "Micafungin vVersus Caspofungin for Treatment of Candidemia and Other Forms of Invasive Candidiasis," *Clin Infect Dis*, 2007, 45(7):883-93.

Pettengell K, Mynhardt J, Kluyts T, et al, "Successful Treatment of Oesophageal Candidiasis by Micafungin: A Novel Systemic Antifungal Agent," *Aliment Pharmacol Ther*, 2004, 20(4):475-81.

Yokote T, Akioka T, Oka S, et al, "Successful Treatment With Micafungin of Invasive Pulmonary Aspergillosis in Acute Myeloid Leukemia, With Renal Failure Due to Amphotericin B Therapy," *Ann Hematol*, 2004, 83(1):64-6.

◆ **Micafungin Sodium** see Micafungin on page 798

◆ **MICRhoGAM®** see Rh₀(D) Immune Globulin on page 1011

◆ **Mifeprex®** see Mifepristone on page 800

Mifepristone (mi FE pris tone)

Medication Safety Issues

Sound-alike/look-alike issues:

Mifeprex® may be confused with Mirapex®

Mifepristone may be confused with misoprostol

High alert medication: The Institute for Safe Medication Practices (ISMP) includes this medication among its list of drug classes which have a heightened risk of causing significant patient harm when used in error.

Related Information

Safe Handling of Hazardous Drugs on page 1517

U.S. Brand Names Mifeprex®

Index Terms RU-38486; RU-486

Generic Available No

Pharmacologic Category Abortifacient; Antineoplastic Agent, Hormone Antagonist; Antiprogestin

Use Medical termination of intrauterine pregnancy, through day 49 of pregnancy. Patients may need treatment with misoprostol and possibly surgery to complete therapy

Unlabeled/Investigational Use Treatment of unresectable meningioma; has been studied in the treatment of breast cancer, ovarian cancer, and adrenal cortical carcinoma

Restrictions Investigators wishing to obtain the agent for use in oncology patients must apply for a patient-specific IND from the FDA. Mifepristone will be supplied only to licensed physicians who sign and return a "Prescriber's Agreement." Distribution of mifepristone will be subject to specific requirements imposed by the distributor. Mifepristone will **not** be available to the public through licensed pharmacies.

Not available in Canada

Pregnancy Risk Factor X

Lactation Excretion in breast milk unknown/contraindicated

Labeled Contraindications Hypersensitivity to mifepristone, misoprostol, other prostaglandins, or any component of the formulation; chronic adrenal failure; porphyrias; hemorrhagic disorder or concurrent anticoagulant therapy; pregnancy termination >49 days; intrauterine device (IUD) in place; ectopic pregnancy or undiagnosed adnexal mass; concurrent long-term corticosteroid therapy; inadequate or lack of access to emergency medical services; inability to understand effects and/or comply with treatment

Warnings/Precautions [U.S. Boxed Warning]: Patient must be instructed of the treatment procedure and expected effects. A signed agreement form must be kept in the patient's file. Physicians may obtain patient agreement forms, physician enrollment forms, and medical consultation directly from Danco Laboratories at 1-877-432-7596. Adverse effects (including blood transfusions, hospitalization, ongoing pregnancy, and other major complications) must be reported in writing to the medication distributor. To be administered only by physicians who can date pregnancy, diagnose ectopic pregnancies, provide access to surgical abortion (if needed), and can provide access to emergency care. Medication will be distributed directly to these physicians following signed agreement with the distributor. Must be administered under supervision by the qualified physician. Pregnancy is dated from day 1 of last menstrual period (presuming a 28-day cycle, ovulation occurring midcycle). Pregnancy duration can be determined using menstrual history and clinical examination. Ultrasound should be used if an ectopic pregnancy is suspected or if duration of pregnancy is uncertain. Ultrasonography may not identify all ectopic pregnancies, and healthcare providers should be alert for signs and symptoms which may be related to undiagnosed ectopic pregnancy in any patient who receives mifepristone

[U.S. Boxed Warning]: Patients should be counseled to seek medical attention in cases of excessive bleeding. Bleeding occurs and should be expected (average 9-16 days, may be ≥30 days). In some cases, bleeding may be prolonged and heavy, potentially leading to hypovolemic shock; the manufacturer cites soaking through two thick sanitary pads per hour for two consecutive hours as an example of excessive bleeding. Bleeding may require blood transfusion (rare), curettage, saline infusions, and/or vasoconstrictors. Use caution in patients with severe anemia. Confirmation of pregnancy termination by clinical exam or ultrasound must be made 14 days following treatment. Manufacturer recommends surgical termination of pregnancy when medical termination fails or is not complete. Prescriber should determine in advance whether they will provide such care themselves or through other providers. Preventative measures to prevent rhesus immunization must be taken prior to surgical abortion. Prescriber should also give the patient clear instructions on whom to call and what to do in the event of an emergency following administration of mifepristone.

[U.S. Boxed Warning]: Bacterial infections have been reported following use of this product. In rare cases, these infections may be serious and/or fatal, with septic shock as a potential complication. A causal relationship has not been established. Sustained fever, abdominal pain, or pelvic tenderness should prompt evaluation; however, healthcare professionals are warned that atypical presentations of serious infection without these symptoms have also been noted. Patients presenting with nausea, vomiting, diarrhea, or weakness,

◄ with or without abdominal pain or fever, should be evaluated for serious bacterial infection when symptoms occur >24 hours after taking misoprostol. Treatment with antibiotics, including coverage for anaerobic bacteria (eg, *Clostridium sordellii*) should be initiated. **[U.S. Boxed Warning]: Patients undergoing treatment with mifepristone should be instructed to bring their Medication Guide with them when an obtaining treatment from an emergency room or healthcare provider that did not prescribe the medication initially in order to identify that they are undergoing a medical abortion.**

Safety and efficacy have not been established for use in women with chronic cardiovascular, hypertensive, hepatic, respiratory, or renal disease, insulin-dependent diabetes mellitus, severe anemia, or heavy smokers. Women >35 years of age and smokers (>10 cigarettes/day) were excluded from clinical trials. Safety and efficacy in pediatric patients have not been established.

Adverse Reactions Vaginal bleeding and uterine cramping are expected to occur when this medication is used to terminate a pregnancy; 90% of women using this medication for this purpose also report adverse reactions. Bleeding or spotting occurs in most women for a period of 9-16 days. Up to 8% of women will experience some degree of bleeding or spotting for 30 days or more. In some cases, bleeding may be prolonged and heavy, potentially leading to hypovolemic shock.

>10%:
  Central nervous system: Headache (2% to 31%), dizziness (1% to 12%)
  Gastrointestinal: Abdominal pain (cramping) (96%), nausea (43% to 61%), vomiting (18% to 26%), diarrhea (12% to 20%)
  Genitourinary: Uterine cramping (83%)
1% to 10%:
  Cardiovascular: Syncope (1%)
  Central nervous system: Fatigue (10%), fever (4%), insomnia (3%), anxiety (2%), fainting (2%)
  Gastrointestinal: Dyspepsia (3%)
  Genitourinary: Uterine hemorrhage (5%), vaginitis (3%), pelvic pain (2%), endometriosis/salpingitis/pelvic inflammatory disease (1%)
  Hematologic: Decreased hemoglobin >2 g/dL (6%), anemia (2%), leukorrhea (2%)
  Neuromuscular & skeletal: Back pain (9%), rigors (3%), leg pain (2%), weakness (2%)
  Respiratory: Sinusitis (2%)
  Miscellaneous: Viral infection (4%)
<1%: Significant ALT/AST, alkaline phosphatase, and GT changes have been reported rarely
Postmarketing and/or case reports: Adult respiratory distress syndrome (ADRS), allergic reaction including urticaria and hives, bacterial infection (including an ectopic bacteria such as *Clostridium sordellii*), Crohn's disease (exacerbation), disseminated intravascular coagulopathy (DIC), dyspnea, hematometra, hypotension, lightheadedness, loss of consciousness, MI, pancreatitis (acute), pelvic infection, postabortal infection, QT prolongation, ruptured ectopic pregnancy, sepsis, septic shock, sickle cell crisis (exacerbation), tachycardia, toxic shock syndrome

In trials for unresectable meningioma, the most common adverse effects included fatigue, hot flashes, gynecomastia or breast tenderness, hair thinning, and rash. In premenopausal women, vaginal bleeding may be seen shortly after beginning therapy and cessation of menses is common. Thyroiditis and effects related to antiglucocorticoid activity have also been noted.

Drug Interactions

Metabolism/Transport Effects Substrate of CYP3A4 (minor); **Inhibits** CYP2D6 (weak), 3A4 (weak)

Avoid Concomitant Use There are no known interactions where it is recommended to avoid concomitant use.

Increased Effect/Toxicity There are no known significant interactions involving an increase in effect.

Decreased Effect There are no known significant interactions involving a decrease in effect.

Ethanol/Nutrition/Herb Interactions

Food: Do not take with grapefruit juice; grapefruit juice may inhibit mifepristone metabolism leading to increased levels.

Herb/Nutraceutical: Avoid St John's wort (may induce mifepristone metabolism, leading to decreased levels).

Storage/Stability Store at room temperature of 25°C (77°F).

Mechanism of Action Mifepristone, a synthetic steroid, competitively binds to the intracellular progesterone receptor, blocking the effects of progesterone. When used for the termination of pregnancy, this leads to contraction-inducing activity in the myometrium. In the absence of progesterone, mifepristone acts as a partial progesterone agonist. Mifepristone also has weak antiglucocorticoid and antiandrogenic properties; it blocks the feedback effect of cortisol on corticotropin secretion.

Pharmacodynamics/Kinetics

Absorption: Oral: rapid

Protein binding: 98% to albumin and α_1-acid glycoprotein

Metabolism: Hepatic via CYP3A4 to three metabolites (may possess some antiprogestin and antiglucocorticoid activity)

Bioavailability: Oral: 69%

Half-life elimination: Terminal: 18 hours following a slower phase where 50% eliminated between 12-72 hours

Time to peak: Oral: 90 minutes

Excretion: Feces (83%); urine (9%)

Dosage Oral:

Adults:

Termination of pregnancy: Treatment consists of three office visits by the patient; the patient must read medication guide and sign patient agreement prior to treatment:

Day 1: 600 mg (three 200 mg tablets) taken as a single dose under physician supervision

Day 3: Patient must return to the healthcare provider 2 days following administration of mifepristone; unless abortion has occurred (confirmed using ultrasound or clinical examination): 400 mcg (two 200 mcg tablets) of misoprostol; patient may need treatment for cramps or gastrointestinal symptoms at this time

Day 14: Patient must return to the healthcare provider ~14 days after administration of mifepristone; confirm complete termination of pregnancy by ultrasound or clinical exam. Surgical termination is recommended to manage treatment failures.

Meningioma (unlabeled use): Refer to individual protocols. The dose used in meningioma is usually 200 mg/day, continued based on toxicity and response.

Elderly: Safety and efficacy have not been established

◄ **Dosage adjustment in renal impairment:** Safety and efficacy have not been established

Dosage adjustment in hepatic impairment: Safety and efficacy have not been established; use with caution due to CYP3A4 metabolism

Monitoring Parameters Clinical exam and/or ultrasound to confirm complete termination of pregnancy; hemoglobin, hematocrit, and red blood cell count in cases of heavy bleeding. Consider CBC in any patient who reports nausea, vomiting, or diarrhea and weakness with or without abdominal pain, and without fever or other signs of infection more than 24 hours after administration of misoprostol.

Test Interactions hCG levels will not be useful to confirm pregnancy termination until at least 10 days following mifepristone treatment

Additional Information Medication will be distributed directly to qualified physicians following signed agreement with the distributor, Danco Laboratories. It will not be available through pharmacies. Major adverse reactions (hospitalization, blood transfusion, ongoing pregnancy, etc) should be reported to Danco Laboratories.

Dosage Forms Excipient information presented when available (limited, particularly for generics); consult specific product labeling.

Tablet: 200 mg

References
Grumberg SM, Weiss MH, Spitz IM, et al, "Treatment of Unresectable Meningiomas With the Antiprogesterone Agent Mifepristone," *J Neurosurg*, 1991, 74(6):861-6.

Perrault D, Eisenhauer EA, Pritchard KI, et al, "Phase II Study of the Progesterone Antagonist Mifepristone in Patients With Untreated Metastatic Breast Carcinoma: A National Cancer Institute of Canada Clinical Trials Group Study," *J Clin Oncol*, 1996, 14(10):2709-12.

Rocereto TF, Saul HM, Aikins JA, et al, "Phase II Study of Mifepristone (RU486) in Refractory Ovarian Cancer," *Gynecol Oncol*, 2000, 77(3):429-32.

Spitz IM and Bardin CW, "Mifepristone (RU486) - A Modulator of Progestin and Glucocorticoid Action," *N Engl J Med*, 1993, 329(6):404-12.

◆ **Millipred™** *see* PrednisoLONE *on page 977*

◆ **Minirin® (Can)** *see* Desmopressin *on page 344*

◆ **Mint-Ciprofloxacin (Can)** *see* Ciprofloxacin *on page 228*

◆ **MINT-Ondansetron (Can)** *see* Ondansetron *on page 874*

Mitomycin (mye toe MYE sin)

Medication Safety Issues

Sound-alike/look-alike issues:

Mitomycin may be confused with mithramycin, mitotane, mitoxantrone

High alert medication: The Institute for Safe Medication Practices (ISMP) includes this medication among its list of drugs which have a heightened risk of causing significant patient harm when used in error.

Related Information

Management of Drug Extravasations *on page 1447*

Safe Handling of Hazardous Drugs *on page 1517*

Index Terms Mitomycin-C; Mitomycin-X; MTC

Generic Available Yes

Canadian Brand Names Mutamycin®

Pharmacologic Category Antineoplastic Agent, Antibiotic

Use Treatment of adenocarcinoma of stomach or pancreas

Unlabeled/Investigational Use Treatment of bladder cancer; prevention of excess scarring in glaucoma filtration procedures in patients at high risk of bleb failure

Pregnancy Risk Factor D

Lactation Enters breast milk/contraindicated

Labeled Contraindications Hypersensitivity to mitomycin or any component of the formulation; thrombocytopenia; coagulation disorders, increased bleeding tendency; pregnancy

Warnings/Precautions Hazardous agent - use appropriate precautions for handling and disposal. **[U.S. Boxed Warning]: May cause bone marrow suppression (thrombocytopenia and leukopenia);** monitor for infections. Use with caution in patients who have received radiation therapy or in the presence of hepatobiliary dysfunction; reduce dosage in patients who are receiving radiation therapy simultaneously. Monitor for renal toxicity; do not administer if serum creatinine is >1.7 mg/dL. **[U.S. Boxed Warning]: Hemolytic-uremic syndrome, potentially fatal, has been reported;** is correlated with total dose (single doses ≥60 mg or cumulative doses ≥50 mg/m²) and total duration of therapy (>5-11 months). Bladder fibrosis/contraction has been reported with intravesical administration. **Mitomycin is a potent vesicant, may cause ulceration, necrosis, cellulitis, and tissue sloughing if infiltrated.** Shortness of breath and bronchospasm have been reported in patients receiving vinca alkaloids in combination with or after mitomycin; may be managed with bronchodilators, steroids and/or oxygen. Safety and efficacy in children have not been established. **[U.S. Boxed Warning]: Should be administered under the supervision of an experienced cancer chemotherapy physician.**

Adverse Reactions

>10%:

  Cardiovascular: CHF (3% to 15%) (doses >30 mg/m²)

  Central nervous system: Fever (14%)

  Dermatologic: Alopecia, nail banding/discoloration

  Gastrointestinal: Nausea, vomiting and anorexia (14%)

  Hematologic: Anemia (19% to 24%); myelosuppression, common, dose limiting, delayed

  Onset: 3 weeks

  Nadir: 4-6 weeks

  Recovery: 6-8 weeks

1% to 10%:

  Dermatologic: Rash

  Gastrointestinal: Stomatitis

  Neuromuscular: Paresthesia

  Renal: Creatinine increased (2%)

  Respiratory: Interstitial pneumonitis, infiltrates, dyspnea, cough (7%)

<1%: Malaise, pruritus, extravasation reactions, hemolytic uremic syndrome, renal failure, bladder fibrosis/contraction (intravesical administration)

Drug Interactions

Avoid Concomitant Use

Avoid concomitant use of Mitomycin with any of the following: Natalizumab; Vaccines (Live)

Increased Effect/Toxicity

Mitomycin may increase the levels/effects of: Leflunomide; Natalizumab; Vaccines (Live)

The levels/effects of Mitomycin may be increased by: Antineoplastic Agents (Vinca Alkaloids); P-Glycoprotein Inhibitors; Trastuzumab

Decreased Effect

Mitomycin may decrease the levels/effects of: Vaccines (Inactivated); Vaccines (Live)

The levels/effects of Mitomycin may be decreased by: Echinacea; P-Glycoprotein Inducers

Ethanol/Nutrition/Herb Interactions Herb/Nutraceutical: Avoid black cohosh, dong quai in estrogen-dependent tumors.

Storage/Stability Store intact vials at controlled room temperature. Mitomycin solution is stable for 7 days at room temperature and 14 days when refrigerated if protected from light. Solution of 0.5 mg/mL in a syringe is stable for 7 days at room temperature and 14 days when refrigerated and protected from light.

Further dilution to 20-40 mcg/mL:

In normal saline: Stable for 12 hours at room temperature.

In sodium lactate: Stable for 24 hours at room temperature.

Reconstitution Dilute powder with SWFI or 0.9% sodium chloride to a concentration of 0.5-1 mg/mL.

Compatibility Stable in LR; **variable stability (consult detailed reference)** in D_5W, NS.

Y-site administration: Compatible: Amifostine, bleomycin, cisplatin, cyclophosphamide, doxorubicin, droperidol, fluorouracil, furosemide, granisetron, heparin, leucovorin, melphalan, methotrexate, metoclopramide, ondansetron, teniposide, thiotepa, vinblastine, vincristine. **Incompatible:** Aztreonam, cefepime, etoposide phosphate, filgrastim, gemcitabine, piperacillin/tazobactam, sargramostim, topotecan, vinorelbine.

Compatibility in syringe: Compatible: Bleomycin, cisplatin, cyclophosphamide, doxorubicin, droperidol, fluorouracil, furosemide, heparin, leucovorin, methotrexate, metoclopramide, vinblastine, vincristine.

Compatibility when admixed: Compatible: Dexamethasone sodium phosphate, hydrocortisone sodium succinate. **Incompatible:** Bleomycin. **Variable (consult detailed reference):** Heparin.

Mechanism of Action Acts like an alkylating agent and produces DNA cross-linking (primarily with guanine and cytosine pairs); cell-cycle nonspecific; inhibits DNA and RNA synthesis; degrades preformed DNA, causes nuclear lysis and formation of giant cells. While not phase-specific *per se*, mitomycin has its maximum effect against cells in late G and early S phases.

Pharmacodynamics/Kinetics

Distribution: V_d: 22 L/m^2; high drug concentrations found in kidney, tongue, muscle, heart, and lung tissue; probably not distributed into the CNS

Metabolism: Hepatic

Half-life elimination: 23-78 minutes; Terminal: 50 minutes

Excretion: Urine (<10% as unchanged drug), with elevated serum concentrations

Dosage Refer to individual protocols. Children (unlabeled use) and Adults:

Single agent therapy: I.V.: 20 mg/m^2 every 6-8 weeks

Combination therapy: I.V.: 10 mg/m^2 every 6-8 weeks

Bladder carcinoma (unlabeled use): Intravesicular instillation (unapproved route): 20-40 mg instilled into the bladder and retained for 3 hours up to 3 times/week for up to 20 procedures per course

Glaucoma surgery (unlabeled use): 0.2-0.5 mg (0.2-0.5 mg/mL solution)

Dosage adjustment in renal impairment: The FDA-approved labeling states to avoid use in patients with serum creatine >1.7 mg/dL, but offers no other dosage adjustment guidelines. The following guidelines have been used by some clinicians (Aronoff, 2007): Adults:

Cl_{cr} <10 mL/minute: Administer 75% of dose

Continuous ambulatory peritoneal dialysis (CAPD): Administer 75% of dose

Dosage adjustment in hepatic impairment: Although some mitomycin may be excreted in the bile, no specific guidelines regarding dosage adjustment in hepatic impairment are available.

Combination Regimens

Anal cancer: Fluorouracil-Mitomycin (Anal Cancer) on page 1335
Breast cancer:
  Mitomycin-Vinblastine on page 1367
  VM on page 1426
Gastric cancer: FAM on page 1319
Pancreatic cancer: FAM on page 1319

Administration

I.V.: Administer slow I.V. push or by slow (15-30 minute) infusion via a freely-running dextrose or saline infusion. Consider using a central venous catheter.
Intravesicular (unlabeled route): Instill into bladder for up to 3 hours (rotate patient every 15-30 minutes)
Glaucoma surgery (unlabeled route): Apply to pledget and place in contact with surgical wound for 2-5 minutes (doses and techniques may vary)

Monitoring Parameters Platelet count, CBC with differential, hemoglobin, prothrombin time, renal and pulmonary function tests

Emetic Potential Low (10% to 30%)

Vesicant Yes; see Management of Drug Extravasations on page 1447.

Dosage Forms Excipient information presented when available (limited, particularly for generics); consult specific product labeling.
Injection, powder for reconstitution: 5 mg, 20 mg, 40 mg

References

Aronoff GR, Bennett WM, Berns JS, et al, *Drug Prescribing in Renal Failure: Dosing Guidelines for Adults and Children*, 5th ed. Philadelphia, PA: American College of Physicians; 2007, p 101.
Bradner WT, "Mitomycin C: A Clinical Update," *Cancer Treat Rev*, 2001, 27(1):35-50.
Gandolfi SA, Vecchi M and Braccio L, "Decrease of Intraocular Pressure After Subconjunctival Injection of Mitomycin in Human Glaucoma," *Arch Ophthalmol*, 1995, 113(5):582-5.
Gibson NW, Phillips RM, and Ross D, "Mitomycin C," *Cancer Chemother Biol Response Modif*, 1994, 15:51-7.
Rodriguez JA, Ferrari C, and Hernandez GA, "Intraoperative Application of Topical Mitomycin C 0.05% for Pterygium Surgery," *Bol Asoc Med P R*, 2004, 96(2):100-2.
Verweij J and Pinedo HM, "Mitomycin C: Mechanism of Action, Usefulness and Limitations," *Anticancer Drugs*, 1990, 1(1):5-13.
Wilkins M, Indar A, and Wormald R, "Intra-Operative Mitomycin C for Glaucoma Surgery," *Cochrane Database Syst Rev*, 2001, (1):CD002897.

◆ **Mitomycin-X** *see* Mitomycin *on page 804*

◆ **Mitomycin-C** *see* Mitomycin *on page 804*

Mitotane (MYE toe tane)

Medication Safety Issues

Sound-alike/look-alike issues:
  Mitotane may be confused with mitomycin, mitoxantrone

High alert medication: The Institute for Safe Medication Practices (ISMP) includes this medication among its list of drug classes which have a heightened risk of causing significant patient harm when used in error.

Related Information

Safe Handling of Hazardous Drugs *on page 1517*

U.S. Brand Names Lysodren®

Index Terms Chloditan; Chlodithane; Khloditan; Mytotan; o,p'-DDD; Ortho, para-DDD

Generic Available No

Canadian Brand Names Lysodren®

Pharmacologic Category Antineoplastic Agent, Miscellaneous

Use Treatment of inoperable adrenocortical carcinoma

Unlabeled/Investigational Use Treatment of Cushing's syndrome

Pregnancy Risk Factor C

Lactation Excretion in breast milk unknown/not recommended

Labeled Contraindications Hypersensitivity to mitotane or any component of the formulation

Warnings/Precautions Hazardous agent - use appropriate precautions for handling and disposal. Patients treated with mitotane may develop adrenal insufficiency; steroid replacement with glucocorticoid, and sometimes mineralocorticoid, is necessary. It has been recommended that steroid replacement therapy be initiated at the start of therapy, rather than waiting for evidence of adrenal insufficiency. **[U.S. Boxed Warning]: Because the primary action of mitotane is through adrenal suppression, discontinue mitotane temporarily with onset of shock or severe trauma; administer appropriate steroid coverage.** Because mitotane can increase the metabolism of exogenous steroids, higher than usual replacement steroid doses may be required. Surgically remove tumor tissues from metastatic masses prior to initiation of treatment; rapid cytotoxic effect may cause tumor hemorrhage. Observe patients for neurotoxicity with long-term (>2 years) use. Use caution with hepatic impairment; metabolism may be decreased. Other CNS adverse effects, including lethargy, sedation, and vertigo may occur; patients must be cautioned about performing tasks which require mental alertness (eg, operating machinery or driving). The manufacturer recommends initiating treatment within a hospital environment until a stabilized dose is achieved. Continue treatment as long as clinical benefit (maintenance of clinical status or metastatic lesion growth slowing) is observed. Clinical benefit is usually observed within 3 months at maximum tolerated dose, although 10% of patients may require more than 3 months for benefit. Continuous treatment at the maximum tolerated dose is generally the best approach. Some patients have been treated intermittently, restarting when severe symptoms reappear, although often response is no longer observed after 3 or 4 courses of intermittent treatment. **[U.S. Boxed Warnings]: Should be administered under the supervision of an experienced cancer chemotherapy physician.** Safety and efficacy in children have not been established.

Adverse Reactions The majority of adverse events are dose-dependent.

>10%:

Central nervous system: CNS depression (32%), lethargy/somnolence (25%), dizziness/vertigo (15%)

Dermatologic: Skin rash (15%)

Gastrointestinal: Anorexia (24%), nausea (39%), vomiting (37%), diarrhea (13%)

Neuromuscular & skeletal: Weakness (12%)

1% to 10%:

Central nervous system: Headache (5%), confusion (3%)

Neuromuscular & skeletal: Muscle tremor (3%)

<1%, postmarketing, and/or case reports: Aches (generalized), adrenal insufficiency, albuminuria, anemia, ataxia, autoimmune hepatitis, bleeding time prolonged, blurred vision, cataract, diplopia, flushing, GGT increased, gynecomastia, hematuria, hemorrhagic cystitis, hormone binding globulins increased, hypercholesterolemia, hyperpyrexia, hypertension, hypertriglyceridemia, lens opacity, leukopenia, macular edema, memory decreased, mucositis, myalgia, neuropathy, orthostatic hypotension, primary

hypogonadism, protein bound iodine decreased, thrombocytopenia, thyroid function tests altered, toxic retinopathy, transaminases increased

Drug Interactions

Avoid Concomitant Use There are no known interactions where it is recommended to avoid concomitant use.

Increased Effect/Toxicity

Mitotane may increase the levels/effects of: Vitamin K Antagonists

The levels/effects of Mitotane may be increased by: MAO Inhibitors

Decreased Effect

Mitotane may decrease the levels/effects of: Corticosteroids (Systemic); Vitamin K Antagonists

The levels/effects of Mitotane may be decreased by: Potassium-Sparing Diuretics

Ethanol/Nutrition/Herb Interactions Ethanol: Avoid ethanol (may increase CNS depression).

Storage/Stability Store at room temperature of 25°C (77°F); excursions permitted to 15°C to 30°C (59°F to 86°F).

Mechanism of Action Adrenolytic agent which causes adrenal cortical atrophy; affects mitochondria in adrenal cortical cells and decreases production of cortisol; also alters the peripheral metabolism of steroids

Pharmacodynamics/Kinetics

Absorption: Oral: ~5% to 40%

Distribution: Stored mainly in fat tissue but is found in all body tissues

Metabolism: Hepatic and other tissues

Half-life elimination: 18-159 days

Time to peak, serum: 3-5 hours

Excretion: Urine (~10%, as metabolites); feces (1% to 17%, as metabolites)

Dosage Oral:

Adrenocortical carcinoma:

Children (unlabeled use): 1-2 g/day in divided doses, increasing gradually to a maximum of 5-7 g/day

Adults: Start at 2-6 g/day in 3-4 divided doses, then increase incrementally to 9-10 g/day in 3-4 divided doses (maximum tolerated range: 2-16 g/day, usually 9-10 g/day; maximum dose studied: 18-19 g/day)

Cushing's syndrome (unlabeled use): Adults: Initial dose: 500 mg 3 times/day; maximum dose 3000 mg 3 times/day (Biller, 2008)

Dosing adjustment for toxicity:

Severe side effects: Reduce dose until achieve a maximum tolerated dose

Significant neuropsychiatric adverse effects: Withhold treatment for at least 1 week and restart at a lower dose (Allolio, 2006)

Dosing adjustment in hepatic impairment: Dose may need to be decreased in patients with liver disease

Administration Oral: Administer in 3-4 divided doses/day. Do not crush tablets; wear gloves when handling; avoid exposure to crushed or broken tablets.

Monitoring Parameters Adrenal function; neurologic assessments (including behavioral) at regular intervals with chronic (>2 years) use

Dosage Forms Excipient information presented when available (limited, particularly for generics); consult specific product labeling.

Tablet [scored]:

Lysodren®: 500 mg

References

Allolio B and Fassnacht M, "Clinical Review: Adrenocortical Carcinoma: Clinical Update," *J Clin Endocrinol Metab*, 2006, 91(6):2027-37.

Biller BM, Grossman AB, Stewart PM, et al, "Treatment of Adrenocorticotropin-Dependent Cushing's Syndrome: A Consensus Statement," *J Clin Endocrinol Metab*, 2008, 93(7):2454-62.

Boscaro M, Barzon L, Fallo F, et al, "Cushing's Syndrome," *Lancet*, 2001, 357(9258):783-91.

De Leon DD, Lange BJ, Walterhouse D, et al, "Long-Term (15 years) Outcome in an Infant with Metastatic Adrenocortical Carcinoma," *J Clin Endocrinol Metab*, 2002, 87(10):4452-6.

National Comprehensive Cancer Network® (NCCN) "Practice Guidelines in Oncology™: Neuroendocrine Tumors," Version 1.2008. Available at http://www.nccn.org/professionals/physician_gls/PDF/neuroendocrine.pdf

Newell-Price J, Bertagna X, Grossman AB, et al, "Cushing's Syndrome," *Lancet*, 2006, 367 (9522):1605-17.

Rodriguez-Galindo C, Figueiredo BC, Zambetti GP, et al, "Biology, Clinical Characteristics, and Management of Adrenocortical Tumors in Children," *Pediatr Blood Cancer*, 2005, 45(3):265-73.

Terzolo M, Angeli A, Fassnacht M, et al, "Adjuvant Mitotane Treatment for Adrenal Carcinoma," *N Engl J Med*, 2007, 356(23): 2372-80.

Mitoxantrone (mye toe ZAN trone)

Medication Safety Issues

Sound-alike/look-alike issues:

Mitoxantrone may be confused with methotrexate, mitomycin, mitotane, Mutamycin®

High alert medication: The Institute for Safe Medication Practices (ISMP) includes this medication among its list of drug classes which have a heightened risk of causing significant patient harm when used in error.

Related Information

Hematopoietic Stem Cell Transplantation *on page 1501*

Management of Drug Extravasations *on page 1447*

Safe Handling of Hazardous Drugs *on page 1517*

U.S. Brand Names Novantrone®

Index Terms CL-232315; DHAD; DHAQ; Dihydroxyanthracenedione; Dihydroxyanthracenedione Dihydrochloride; Mitoxantrone Dihydrochloride; Mitoxantrone HCl; Mitoxantrone Hydrochloride; Mitozantrone

Generic Available Yes

Canadian Brand Names Mitoxantrone Injection®; Novantrone®

Pharmacologic Category Antineoplastic Agent, Anthracenedione

Use Treatment of acute nonlymphocytic leukemias (ANLL [includes myelogenous, promyelocytic, monocytic and erythroid leukemias]); advanced hormone-refractory prostate cancer; secondary progressive or relapsing-remitting multiple sclerosis (MS)

Unlabeled/Investigational Use Treatment of Hodgkin's lymphoma, non-Hodgkin's lymphomas (NHL), acute lymphocytic leukemia (ALL), myelodysplastic syndrome, breast cancer, pediatric acute leukemias, pediatric sarcoma; part of a conditioning regimen for autologous hematopoietic stem cell transplantation (HSCT)

Pregnancy Risk Factor D

Lactation Enters breast milk/not recommended

Labeled Contraindications Hypersensitivity to mitoxantrone or any component of the formulation

Warnings/Precautions Hazardous agent - use appropriate precautions for handling and disposal.

[U.S. Boxed Warning]: Usually should not be administered if baseline neutrophil count <1500 cells/mm³ (except for treatment of ANLL). Monitor blood counts and monitor for infection due to neutropenia. Treatment may lead to severe myelosuppression; use with caution in patients with pre-existing myelosuppression.

[U.S. Boxed Warning]: May cause myocardial toxicity and potentially-fatal heart failure (HF); risk increases with cumulative dosing. Effects may occur during therapy or may be delayed (months or years after completion of therapy). Predisposing factors for mitoxantrone-induced cardiotoxicity include prior anthracycline or anthracenedione therapy, prior cardiovascular disease, concomitant use of cardiotoxic drugs, and mediastinal/pericardial irradiation, although may also occur in patients without risk factors. Prior to therapy initiation, evaluate all patients for cardiac-related signs/symptoms, including history, physical exam, and ECG; and evaluate baseline left ventricular ejection fraction (LVEF) with echocardiogram or multigated radionuclide angiography (MUGA) or MRI. Not recommended for use in MS patients when LVEF <50%, or baseline LVEF below the lower limit of normal (LLN). Evaluate for cardiac signs/ symptoms (by history, physical exam, and ECG) and evaluate LVEF (using same method as baseline LVEF) in MS patients prior to each dose and if signs/symptoms of HF develop. Use in MS should be limited to a cumulative dose of ≤140 mg/m^2, and discontinued if LVEF falls below LLN or a significant decrease in LVEF is observed; decreases in LVEF and HF have been observed in patients with MS who have received cumulative doses <100 mg/m^2. Patients with MS should undergo annual LVEF evaluation following discontinuation of therapy to monitor for delayed cardiotoxicity.

[U.S. Boxed Warnings]: For I.V. administration only, into a free-flowing I.V.; may cause severe local tissue damage if extravasation occurs; do not administer subcutaneously, intramuscularly, or intra-arterially. Do not administer intrathecally; may cause serious and permanent neurologic damage. Extravasation resulting in burning, erythema, pain, swelling and skin discoloration (blue) has been reported; extravasation may result in tissue necrosis and require debridement for skin graft. May cause urine, saliva, tears, and sweat to turn blue-green for 24 hours postinfusion. Whites of eyes may have blue-green tinge. **[U.S. Boxed Warning]: Has been associated with the development of secondary acute myelogenous leukemia in both patients with cancer and with MS.**

[U.S. Boxed Warning]: Should be administered under the supervision of a physician experienced in cancer chemotherapy agents. Dosage should be reduced in patients with impaired hepatobiliary function (clearance is reduced); not for treatment of multiple sclerosis in patients with concurrent hepatic impairment. Not for treatment of primary progressive multiple sclerosis. Rapid lysis of tumor cells may lead to hyperuricemia. Safety and efficacy in children have not been established.

Adverse Reactions Includes events reported with any indication; incidence varies based on treatment, dose, and/or concomitant medications

>10%:

Cardiovascular: Edema (10% to 30%), arrhythmia (3% to 18%), cardiac function changes (≤18%), ECG changes (≤11%)

Central nervous system: Fever (6% to 78%), pain (8% to 41%), fatigue (≤39%), headache (6% to 13%)

Dermatologic: Alopecia (20% to 61%), nail bed changes (≤11%), petechiae/ bruising (6% to 11%)

Endocrine & metabolic: Menstrual disorder (26% to 61%), amenorrhea (28% to 53%), hyperglycemia (10% to 31%)

Gastrointestinal: Nausea (26% to 76%), vomiting (6% to 72%), diarrhea (14% to 47%), mucositis (10% to 29%; onset: ≤1 week), stomatitis (8% to 29%; onset: ≤1 week), anorexia (22% to 25%), weight gain/loss (13% to 17%), constipation (10% to 16%), GI bleeding (2% to 16%), abdominal pain (9% to 15%), dyspepsia (5% to 14%)

Genitourinary: Urinary tract infection (7% to 32%), abnormal urine (5% to 11%)

Hematologic: Neutropenia (79% to 100%; onset: ≤3 weeks; grade 4: 23% to 54%), leukopenia (9% to 100%), lymphopenia (72% to 95%), anemia/hemoglobin decreased (5% to 75%) thrombocytopenia (33% to 39%; grades 3/4: 3% to 4%), neutropenic fever (≤11%)

Hepatic: Alkaline phosphatase increased (≤37%), transaminases increased (5% to 20%), GGT increased (3% to 15%)

Neuromuscular & skeletal: Weakness (≤24%)

Renal: BUN increased (≤22%), creatinine increased (≤13%), hematuria (≤11%)

Respiratory: Upper respiratory tract infection (7% to 53%), pharyngitis (≤19%), dyspnea (6% to 18%), cough (5% to 13%)

Miscellaneous: Infection (4% to 60%), sepsis (ANLL 31% to 34%), fungal infection (9% to 15%)

1% to 10%:

Cardiovascular: CHF (≤5%), ischemia (≤5%), LVEF decreased (≤5%), hypertension (≤4%)

Central nervous system: Chills (≤5%), anxiety (5%), depression (5%), seizure (2% to 4%)

Dermatologic: Cutaneous mycosis (≤10%), skin infection (≤5%)

Endocrine & metabolic: Hypocalcemia (10%), hypokalemia (7% to 10%), hyponatremia (9%), menorrhagia (7%)

Gastrointestinal: Aphthosis (≤10%)

Genitourinary: Impotence (≤7%), sterility (≤5%)

Hematologic: Granulocytopenia (6%), hemorrhage (5% to 6%)

Hepatic: Jaundice (3% to 7%)

Neuromuscular & skeletal: Back pain (6% to 8%), myalgia (≤5%), arthralgia (≤5%)

Ocular: Conjunctivitis (≤5%), blurred vision (≤3%)

Renal: Renal failure (≤8%), proteinuria (≤6%)

Respiratory: Rhinitis (10%), pneumonia (≤9%), sinusitis (≤6%)

Miscellaneous: Systemic infection (≤10%), diaphoresis (≤9%), development of secondary leukemia (~1% to 2%)

<1% or frequency not defined: Allergic reaction, anaphylactoid reactions, anaphylaxis, chest pain, dehydration; extravasation at injection site (may result in burning, erythema, pain, skin discoloration, swelling, or tissue necrosis); interstitial pneumonitis (with combination chemotherapy), hyperuricemia, hypotension, phlebitis at the infusion site, rash, sclera discoloration (blue), tachycardia, urine discoloration (blue-green), urticaria

Drug Interactions

Metabolism/Transport Effects Inhibits CYP3A4 (weak)

Avoid Concomitant Use

Avoid concomitant use of Mitoxantrone with any of the following: Natalizumab; Vaccines (Live)

Increased Effect/Toxicity

Mitoxantrone may increase the levels/effects of: Leflunomide; Natalizumab; Vaccines (Live)

The levels/effects of Mitoxantrone may be increased by: Trastuzumab

Decreased Effect

Mitoxantrone may decrease the levels/effects of: Vaccines (Inactivated); Vaccines (Live)

The levels/effects of Mitoxantrone may be decreased by: Echinacea

Ethanol/Nutrition/Herb Interactions Herb/Nutraceutical: Avoid echinacea (may diminish the immunosuppressant effect).

Storage/Stability Store intact vials at 15°C to 25°C (59°F to 77°F); do not freeze. Opened vials may be stored at room temperature for 7 days or under refrigeration for up to 14 days. Solutions diluted for administration are stable for 7 days at room temperature or under refrigeration, although the manufacturer recommends immediate use.

Reconstitution Dilute in at least 50 mL of NS or D_5W.

Compatibility Stable in D_5NS, D_5W, NS.

Y-site administration: Compatible: Allopurinol, amifostine, cladribine, etoposide, etoposide phosphate, filgrastim, fludarabine, gemcitabine, granisetron, linezolid, melphalan, ondansetron, oxaliplatin, sargramostim, teniposide, thiotepa, vinorelbine. **Incompatible:** Amphotericin B cholesteryl sulfate complex, aztreonam, cefepime, doxorubicin liposome, paclitaxel, pemetrexed, piperacillin/tazobactam, propofol.

Compatibility when admixed: Compatible: Cyclophosphamide, cytarabine, etoposide, fluorouracil, hydrocortisone sodium succinate, potassium chloride. **Incompatible:** Heparin.

Mechanism of Action Related to the anthracyclines, mitoxantrone intercalates into DNA resulting in cross-links and strand breaks; binds to nucleic acids and inhibits DNA and RNA synthesis by template disordering and steric obstruction; replication is decreased by binding to DNA topoisomerase II and seems to inhibit the incorporation of uridine into RNA and thymidine into DNA; active throughout entire cell cycle (cell-cycle nonspecific)

Pharmacodynamics/Kinetics

Absorption: Oral: Poor

Distribution: V_d: 14 L/kg; V_{dss}: >1000 L/m^2; distributes extensively into tissue (pleural fluid, kidney, thyroid, liver, heart) and red blood cells

Protein binding: >95%, 76% to 78% to albumin

Metabolism: Hepatic; pathway not determined

Half-life elimination: Terminal: 23-215 hours (median: ~75 hours); may be prolonged with hepatic impairment

Excretion: Feces (25%); urine (6% to 11%; 65% as unchanged drug)

Dosage Details concerning dosing in combination regimens should also be consulted. I.V.:

Acute nonlymphocytic leukemias:

Children ≤2 years (unlabeled use): 0.4 mg/kg/day once daily for 3-5 days

Children >2 years (unlabeled use): 8-12 mg/m^2/day once daily for 5 days

Adults:

Induction: 12 mg/m^2 once daily for 3 days (in combination with cytarabine); for incomplete response, may repeat at 12 mg/m^2 once daily for 2 days

Consolidation: 12 mg/m^2 once daily for 2 days, repeat in 4 weeks

Multiple sclerosis: Adults: 12 mg/m^2 every 3 months (maximum lifetime cumulative dose: 140 mg/m^2; discontinue use with LVEF <50% or clinically significant reduction in LVEF)

Prostate cancer (advanced, hormone-refractory): Adults: 12-14 mg/m^2 every 3 weeks (in combination with corticosteroids)

Non-Hodgkin's lymphoma (unlabeled use): Adults: 8-10 mg/m^2 every 21-28 days (as part of a combination chemotherapy regimen)

◄ Solid tumors (unlabeled use):
Children: 18-20 mg/m^2 every 3-4 weeks **or** 5-8 mg/m^2 every week
Adults: 12-14 mg/m^2 every 3-4 weeks (maximum total: 80-120 mg/m^2)
Stem cell transplantation, autologous (unlabeled use): Adults: 60 mg/m^2 4-5 days prior to autografting (in combination with other chemotherapeutic agent[s]) (Oyan, 2006; Tarella, 2001)

Dosing adjustment for toxicity:
ANLL patients: Severe or life-threatening nonhematologic toxicity: Withhold treatment until toxicity resolves
MS patients:
Neutrophils <1500/mm^3: Use is not recommended
Signs/symptoms of HF: Evaluate for cardiac signs/symptoms and LVEF
LVEF <50% or baseline LVEF below the lower limit of normal (LLN): Use is not recommended

Dosing adjustment in renal impairment: Safety and efficacy have not been established
Hemodialysis: Supplemental dose is not necessary
Peritoneal dialysis: Supplemental dose is not necessary
Elderly: Clearance is decreased in elderly patients; use with caution

Dosing adjustment in hepatic impairment: Official dosage adjustment recommendations have not been established. Clearance is reduced in hepatic dysfunction; patients with severe hepatic dysfunction (bilirubin >3.4 mg/dL) have an AUC of 3 times greater than patients with normal hepatic function. Consider dose adjustments. **Note:** MS patients with hepatic impairment should not receive mitoxantrone.

Combination Regimens
Breast cancer:
CNF on page 1277
NFL on page 1381
Leukemia, acute lymphocytic: FIS-HAM on page 1322
Leukemia, acute myeloid:
7 + 3 (Mitoxantrone) on page 1221
EMA 86 on page 1300
FIS-HAM on page 1322
MV on page 1375
Leukemia, acute promyelocytic: Tretinoin-Idarubicin (APL) on page 1414
Lymphoma, Hodgkin's: VIM-D (Hodgkin's Lymphoma) on page 1420
Lymphoma, non-Hodgkin's:
CNOP on page 1277
Fludarabine-Cyclophosphamide-Mitoxantrone-Rituximab on page 1326
Fludarabine-Mitoxantrone on page 1328
Fludarabine-Mitoxantrone-Dexamethasone (NHL) on page 1328
Fludarabine-Mitoxantrone-Dexamethasone-Rituximab on page 1329
Fludarabine-Mitoxantrone-Rituximab on page 1330
MINE on page 1366
MINE-ESHAP on page 1367
Prostate cancer:
Mitoxantrone + Hydrocortisone on page 1368
Mitoxantrone-Prednisone (Prostate Cancer) on page 1368

Administration Irritant (is considered a vesicant by some institutions). For I.V. administration only; do not administer intrathecally, subcutaneously, intra-muscularly or intra-arterially. Must be diluted prior to use. Avoid extravasation; may cause severe local tissue damage if extravasation occurs. Usually administered as a short I.V. infusion over 5-15 minutes; do not infuse over less then 3 minutes. High doses for bone marrow transplant (unlabeled use) are usually given as 1- to 4-hour infusions.

Monitoring Parameters CBC with differential, serum uric acid (for leukemia treatment), liver function tests; for the treatment of multiple sclerosis, obtain pregnancy test; monitor injection site for extravasation

Cardiac monitoring: Prior to initiation, evaluate all patients for cardiac-related signs/symptoms, including history, physical exam, and ECG; evaluate baseline and periodic left ventricular ejection fraction (LVEF) with echocardiogram or multigated radionuclide angiography (MUGA) or MRI. In patients with MS, evaluate for cardiac signs/symptoms (by history, physical exam, and ECG) and evaluate LVEF (using same method as baseline LVEF) prior to each dose and if signs/symptoms of HF develop. Patients with MS should undergo annual LVEF evaluation following discontinuation of therapy to monitor for delayed cardiotoxicity.

Emetic Potential Low (10% to 30%)

Vesicant Yes; see Management of Drug Extravasations on page 1447.

High Dose Considerations

Comments Extensive pretreatment with anthracyclines increases risk of cardiac toxicity.

High Dose I.V.: 24-60 mg/m^2 as a single dose; duration of infusion is 1-4 hours; total doses of 75-90 mg/m^2 have been used. Generally used in combination with other high-dose chemotherapeutic drugs.

Unique Toxicities

Cardiovascular: Bradycardia (infusion-related), heart failure

Dermatologic: Alopecia

Gastrointestinal: Severe mucositis, skin discoloration

Dosage Forms Excipient information presented when available (limited, particularly for generics); consult specific product labeling. [DSC] = Discontinued product

Injection, solution [concentrate; preservative free]: 2 mg/mL (10 mL, 12.5 mL, 15 mL, 20 mL)

Novantrone®: 2 mg/mL (10 mL, 15 mL [DSC])

References

Donelli MG, Zuchetti M, Munzone E, et al, "Pharmacokinetics of Anticancer Agents in Patients With Impaired Liver Function," *Eur J Cancer,* 1998, 34(1):33-46.

Ehninger G, Schuler U, Proksch B, et al, "Pharmacokinetics and Metabolism of Mitoxantrone. A Review,"*Clin Pharmacokinet,* 1990, 18(5):365-80.

Faulds D, Balfour JA, Chrisp P, et al, "Mitoxantrone. A Review of Its Pharmacodynamic and Pharmacokinetic Properties, and Therapeutic Potential in the Chemotherapy of Cancer," *Drugs,* 1991, 41(3):400-49.

National Comprehensive Cancer Network® (NCCN), "Clinical Practice Guidelines in Oncology™: Non-Hodgkin's Lymphomas," Version 1.2009. Available at http://www.nccn.org/professionals/physician_gls/PDF/nhl.pdf

Oyan B, Koc Y, Ozdemir E, et al, "High Dose Sequential Chemotherapy and Autologous Stem Cell Transplantation in Patients With Relapsed/Refractory Lymphoma," *Leuk Lymphoma,* 2006, 47 (8):1545-52.

Scott LJ and Figgitt DP, "Mitoxantrone: A Review of its Use in Multiple Sclerosis," *CNS Drugs,* 2004, 18(6):379-96.

Tarella C, Zallio F, Caracciolo D, et al, "High-Dose Mitoxantrone + Melphalan (MITO/L-PAM) as Conditioning Regimen Supported by Peripheral Blood Progenitor Cell (PBPC) Autograft in 113 Lymphoma Patients: High Tolerability With Reversible Cardiotoxicity," *Leukemia,* 2001, 15 (2):256-63.

Weiss M, Maslak P, Feldman E, et al, "Cytarabine With High-Dose Mitoxantrone Induces Rapid Complete Remissions in Adult Acute Lymphoblastic Leukemia Without the Use of Vincristine or Prednisone," *J Clin Oncol,* 1996, 14(9):2480-5.

Wiseman LR and Spencer CM, "Mitoxantrone. A Review of its Pharmacology and Clinical Efficacy in the Management of Hormone-Resistant Advanced Prostate Cancer," *Drugs Aging*, 1997, 10 (6):473-85.

- ◆ **Mitoxantrone Dihydrochloride** *see* Mitoxantrone *on page 810*
- ◆ **Mitoxantrone HCl** *see* Mitoxantrone *on page 810*
- ◆ **Mitoxantrone Hydrochloride** *see* Mitoxantrone *on page 810*
- ◆ **Mitoxantrone Injection® (Can)** *see* Mitoxantrone *on page 810*
- ◆ **Mitozantrone** *see* Mitoxantrone *on page 810*
- ◆ **MK 0517** *see* Fosaprepitant *on page 513*
- ◆ **MK 869** *see* Aprepitant *on page 104*
- ◆ **MLN341** *see* Bortezomib *on page 155*
- ◆ **MMF** *see* Mycophenolate *on page 831*
- ◆ **MOAB ABX-EGF** *see* Panitumumab *on page 919*
- ◆ **MOAB C225** *see* Cetuximab *on page 211*
- ◆ **MoAb CD52** *see* Alemtuzumab *on page 30*
- ◆ **Moi-Stir® [OTC]** *see* Saliva Substitute *on page 1027*
- ◆ **Monarc-M™** *see* Antihemophilic Factor (Human) *on page 91*
- ◆ **Monoclate-P®** *see* Antihemophilic Factor (Human) *on page 91*
- ◆ **Monoclonal Antibody** *see* Muromonab-CD3 *on page 827*
- ◆ **Monoclonal Antibody ABX-EGF** *see* Panitumumab *on page 919*
- ◆ **Monoclonal Antibody Campath-1H** *see* Alemtuzumab *on page 30*
- ◆ **Monoclonal Antibody CD52** *see* Alemtuzumab *on page 30*
- ◆ **Mononine®** *see* Factor IX *on page 449*
- ◆ **Morphine HP® (Can)** *see* Morphine Sulfate *on page 816*
- ◆ **Morphine LP® Epidural (Can)** *see* Morphine Sulfate *on page 816*

Morphine Sulfate (MOR feen SUL fate)

Medication Safety Issues

Sound-alike/look-alike issues:

Morphine may be confused with HYDROmorphone

Morphine sulfate may be confused with magnesium sulfate

MS Contin® may be confused with Oxycontin®

MSO_4 and MS are error-prone abbreviations (mistaken as magnesium sulfate)

Avinza® may be confused with Evista®, Invanz®

Roxanol™ may be confused with OxyFast®, Roxicet™, Roxicodone®

High alert medication: The Institute for Safe Medication Practices (ISMP) includes this medication (I.V. formulation) among its list of drug classes which have a heightened risk of causing significant patient harm when used in error.

Use care when prescribing and/or administering morphine solutions. These products are available in different concentrations. Always prescribe dosage in mg; **not** by volume (mL).

Use caution when selecting a morphine formulation for use in neurologic infusion pumps (eg, Medtronic delivery systems). The product should be appropriately labeled as "preservative-free" and suitable for intraspinal use via continuous infusion. In addition, the product should be formulated in a pH range that is compatible with the device operation specifications.

Significant differences exist between oral and I.V. dosing. Use caution when converting from one route of administration to another.

U.S. Brand Names Astramorph/PF™; Avinza®; DepoDur®; Duramorph®; Infumorph® 200; Infumorph® 500; Kadian®; MS Contin®; Oramorph® SR; Roxanol™

Index Terms MS (error-prone abbreviation and should not be used); MSO₄ (error-prone abbreviation and should not be used)

Generic Available Yes: Excludes capsule, controlled release tablet, sustained release tablet, extended release liposomal suspension for injection

Canadian Brand Names Doloral; Kadian®; M-Eslon®; M.O.S.-SR®; M.O.S.-Sulfate®; M.O.S.® 10; M.O.S.® 20; M.O.S.® 30; Morphine HP®; Morphine LP® Epidural; MS Contin®; MS-IR®; Novo-Morphine SR; PMS-Morphine Sulfate SR; ratio-Morphine; ratio-Morphine SR; Statex®; Zomorph®

Pharmacologic Category Analgesic, Opioid

Use Relief of moderate-to-severe acute and chronic pain; relief of pain of myocardial infarction; relief of dyspnea of acute left ventricular failure and pulmonary edema; preanesthetic medication

DepoDur®: Epidural (lumbar) single-dose management of surgical pain

Infumorph®: Used in continuous microinfusion devices for intrathecal or epidural administration in treatment of intractable chronic pain

Controlled, extended, or sustained release products: Only intended/indicated for use when repeated doses for an extended period of time are required. The 100 mg and 200 mg tablets or capsules of Kadian®, MS Contin®, and morphine sulfate controlled-release tablets and the 60 mg, 90 mg, and 120 mg capsules of Avinza® should only be used in opioid-tolerant patients.

Restrictions C-II

Pregnancy Risk Factor C/D (prolonged use or high doses at term)

Lactation Enters breast milk/use caution (AAP rates "compatible")

Labeled Contraindications Note: Some contraindications are product specific. For details, please see detailed product prescribing information.

Hypersensitivity to morphine sulfate or any component of the formulation; severe respiratory depression (without resuscitative equipment); acute or severe asthma; known or suspected paralytic ileus; sustained release products are not recommended with gastrointestinal obstruction or in acute/postoperative pain; pregnancy (prolonged use or high doses at term). Oral solutions contraindicated in patients with heart failure due to chronic lung disease, cardiac arrhythmias, head injuries, brain tumors, acute alcoholism, deliriums tremens, seizure disorders, Injectable solution contraindicated during labor when a premature birth is anticipated. Some products contraindicated in patients with head injuries or increased intracranial pressure. DepoDur® contraindicated in circulatory shock and upper airway obstruction. MS Contin® and Kadian® contraindicated in patients with hypercarbia. Some immediate release formulations (tablets and solution) contraindicated in post biliary tract surgery, suspected surgical abdomen, surgical anastomosis, MAO inhibitor use (concurrent or within 14 days), general CNS depression.

Warnings/Precautions An opioid-containing analgesic regimen should be tailored to each patient's needs and based upon the type of pain being treated (acute versus chronic), the route of administration, degree of tolerance for opioids (naive versus chronic user), age, weight, and medical condition. The optimal analgesic dose varies widely among patients. Doses should be titrated to pain relief/prevention. When used as an epidural injection, monitor for delayed sedation. **[U.S. Boxed Warning]: Healthcare provider should be alert to problems of abuse, misuse, and diversion.**

◀

May cause respiratory depression; use with caution in patients (particularly elderly or debilitated) with impaired respiratory function, morbid obesity, adrenal insufficiency, prostatic hyperplasia, urinary stricture, renal impairment, or severe hepatic dysfunction and in patients with hypersensitivity reactions to other phenanthrene derivative opioid agonists (codeine, hydrocodone, hydromorphone, levorphanol, oxycodone, oxymorphone). Use with caution in patients with biliary tract dysfunction; acute pancreatitis may cause constriction of sphincter of Oddi. Some preparations contain sulfites which may cause allergic reactions; infants <3 months of age are more susceptible to respiratory depression, use with caution and generally in reduced doses in this age group.

May cause CNS depression, which may impair physical or mental abilities; patients must be cautioned about performing tasks which require mental alertness (eg, operating machinery or driving). Effects may be potentiated when used with other sedative drugs or ethanol. May cause hypotension in patients with acute myocardial infarction, volume depletion, or concurrent drug therapy which may exaggerate vasodilation. Use with extreme caution in patients with head injury, intracranial lesions, or elevated intracranial pressure; exaggerated elevation of ICP may occur. May cause seizures if high doses are used; use with caution in patients with seizure disorders. Tolerance or drug dependence may result from extended use. Concurrent use of agonist/antagonist analgesics may precipitate withdrawal symptoms and/or reduced analgesic efficacy in patients following prolonged therapy with mu opioid agonists. Abrupt discontinuation following prolonged use may also lead to withdrawal symptoms. Elderly may be particularly susceptible to adverse effects of narcotics. May obscure diagnosis or clinical course of patients with acute abdominal conditions.

Extended or sustained-release formulations:

[U.S. Boxed Warning]: Extended or sustained release dosage forms should not be crushed or chewed. Controlled-, extended-, or sustained-release products are not intended for "as needed (PRN)" use. **MS Contin® 100 or 200 mg tablets and Kadian® 100 mg or 200 mg capsules are for use only in opioid-tolerant patients.** Avinza®, Kadian®, MS Contin®: **[U.S. Boxed Warning]: Indicated for the management of moderate-to-severe pain when around the clock pain control is needed for an extended time period.**

[U.S. Boxed Warning]: Avinza®: Do not administer with alcoholic beverages or ethanol-containing products, which may disrupt extended-release characteristic of product.

Injections: Note: Products are designed for administration by specific routes (I.V., intrathecal, epidural). Use caution when prescribing, dispensing, or administering to use formulations only by intended route(s).

[U.S. Boxed Warning]: Duramorph®: Due to the risk of severe and/or sustained cardiopulmonary depressant effects of Duramorph® must be administered in a fully equipped and staffed environment. Naloxone injection should be immediately available. Patient should remain in this environment for at least 24 hours following the initial dose.

[U.S. Boxed Warning]: Intrathecal dosage is usually 1/10 that of epidural dosage.

Infumorph® solutions are **for use in microinfusion devices only**; not for I.V., I.M., or SubQ administration, or for single-dose administration.

When used as an epidural injection, monitor for delayed sedation.

DepoDur®: **For lumbar administration only.** Intrathecal administration has resulted in prolonged respiratory depression. Freezing may adversely affect modified-release mechanism of drug; check freeze indicator within carton prior to administration.

Adverse Reactions Note: Individual patient differences are unpredictable, and percentage may differ in acute pain (surgical) treatment. Reactions may be dose, formulation, and/or route dependent.

Frequency not defined:
Cardiovascular: Circulatory depression, flushing, shock
Central nervous system: Physical and psychological dependence, sedation
Endocrine & metabolic: Antidiuretic hormone release
>10%:
Cardiovascular: Bradycardia, hypotension
Central nervous system: Drowsiness (9% to 48%; tolerance usually develops to drowsiness with regular dosing for 1-2 weeks), dizziness (6% to 20%), fever (<3% to >10%), confusion, headache (following epidural or intrathecal use)
Dermatologic: Pruritus (may be dose related)
Gastrointestinal: Xerostomia (78%), constipation (9% to 40%; tolerance develops very slowly if at all), nausea (7% to 28%; tolerance usually develops to nausea and vomiting with chronic use), vomiting
Genitourinary: Urinary retention (16%; may be prolonged, up to 20 hours, following epidural or intrathecal use)
Hematologic: Anemia (following intrathecal use)
Local: Pain at injection site
Neuromuscular & skeletal: Weakness
Respiratory: Oxygen saturation decreased
Miscellaneous: Histamine release
1% to 10%:
Cardiovascular: Atrial fibrillation (<3%), chest pain (<3%), edema, hypertension, palpitation, peripheral edema, syncope, tachycardia, vasodilation
Central nervous system: Amnesia, agitation, anxiety, apathy, ataxia, chills, coma, delirium, depression, dream abnormalities, euphoria, false sense of well being, hallucination, hypoesthesia, insomnia, lethargy, malaise, nervousness, restlessness, seizure, slurred speech, somnolence, vertigo
Dermatologic: Dry skin, rash, urticaria
Endocrine & metabolic: Gynecomastia (<3%), hypokalemia, hyponatremia, libido decreased
Gastrointestinal: Abdominal distension, abdominal pain, anorexia, biliary colic, diarrhea, dyspepsia, dysphagia, flatulence, gastroenteritis, GERD, GI irritation, paralytic ileus, rectal disorder, taste perversion, weight loss
Genitourinary: Bladder spasm, dysuria, ejaculation abnormal, impotence, urination decreased
Hematologic: Leukopenia (<3%), thrombocytopenia (<3%), hematocrit decreased
Hepatic: Liver function tests increased
Neuromuscular & skeletal: Arthralgia, back pain, bone pain, foot drop, gait abnormalities, paresthesia, rigors, skeletal muscle rigidity, tremor
Ocular: Amblyopia, conjunctivitis, eye pain, vision problems/disturbance
Renal: Oliguria

Respiratory: Asthma, atelectasis, dyspnea, hiccups, hypercapnia, hypoxia, pulmonary edema (noncardiogenic), respiratory depression, rhinitis

Miscellaneous: Diaphoresis, flu-like syndrome, infection, thirst, voice alteration, withdrawal syndrome

<1%, postmarketing, and/or case reports: Amenorrhea, anaphylaxis, apnea, biliary tract spasm, blurred vision, bronchospasm, cardiac arrest, cough reflex decreased, dehydration, diplopia, disorientation, hemorrhagic urticaria, intestinal obstruction, intracranial pressure increased, laryngospasm, menstrual irregularities, miosis, myoclonus, nystagmus, paradoxical CNS stimulation, respiratory arrest, sepsis, urinary tract spasm, thermal dysregulation, toxic psychoses

Drug Interactions

Metabolism/Transport Effects Substrate of CYP2D6 (minor)

Avoid Concomitant Use There are no known interactions where it is recommended to avoid concomitant use.

Increased Effect/Toxicity

Morphine Sulfate may increase the levels/effects of: Alcohol (Ethyl); Alvimopan; CNS Depressants; Desmopressin; Selective Serotonin Reuptake Inhibitors; Thiazide Diuretics

The levels/effects of Morphine Sulfate may be increased by: Amphetamines; Antipsychotic Agents (Phenothiazines); Succinylcholine

Decreased Effect

Morphine Sulfate may decrease the levels/effects of: Pegvisomant; Trovafloxacin

The levels/effects of Morphine Sulfate may be decreased by: Ammonium Chloride; Peginterferon Alfa-2b; Rifamycin Derivatives

Ethanol/Nutrition/Herb Interactions

Ethanol: Avoid ethanol, including alcoholic beverages or ethanol-containing products (may increase CNS depression).

Avinza®: Alcoholic beverages or ethanol-containing products may disrupt extended-release formulation resulting in rapid release of entire morphine dose.

Food: Administration of oral morphine solution with food may increase bioavailability (ie, a report of 34% increase in morphine AUC when morphine oral solution followed a high-fat meal). The bioavailability of Avinza®, Oramorph SR®, or Kadian® does not appear to be affected by food.

Herb/Nutraceutical: Avoid valerian, St John's wort, kava kava, gotu kola (may increase CNS depression).

Storage/Stability

Capsule, sustained release (Avinza®, Kadian®): Store at 25°C (77°F); excursions permitted to 15°C to 30°C (59°F to 86°F). Protect from light and moisture.

Injection: Store at controlled room temperature of 20°C to 25°C (68°F to 77°F); do not freeze. Protect from light. Degradation depends on pH and presence of oxygen; relatively stable in pH ≤4; darkening of solutions indicate degradation.

DepoDur®: Store under refrigeration at 2°C to 8°C (36°F to 46°F); keep vials in carton during refrigeration; do not freeze. Check freeze indicator before administration; do not administer if bulb is pink or purple. May store at room temperature for up to 30 days in sealed, unopened vials. Gently invert to suspend particles prior to removal from vial. Once vial is opened, use within 4 hours.

Oral solution: Store at controlled room temperature of 25°C (68°F to 77°F); do not freeze.

Suppositories: Store at controlled room temperature 25°C (77°F). Protect from light.

Tablet, extended release: Store at controlled room temperature of 25°C (77°F).

Tablet, immediate release: Store at controlled room temperature of 25°C (77°F). Protect from moisture.

Reconstitution Usual concentration for continuous I.V. infusion: 0.1-1 mg/mL in D_5W. DepoDur® may be diluted in preservative-free NS to a volume of 5 mL.

Compatibility Stable in dextran 6% in dextrose, dextran 6% in NS, D_5LR, $D_5^{1/4}NS$, $D_5^{1/2}NS$, D_5NS, D_5W, $D_{10}W$, LR, $^{1/2}NS$, NS; **variable stability (consult detailed reference)** in TPN.

Y-site administration: Compatible: Allopurinol, amifostine, amikacin, aminophylline, amiodarone, ampicillin, ampicillin/sulbactam, amsacrine, atenolol, atracurium, aztreonam, bumetanide, calcium chloride, cefamandole, cefazolin, cefoperazone, cefotaxime, cefotetan, cefoxitin, ceftazidime, ceftizoxime, ceftriaxone, cefuroxime, chloramphenicol, cisatracurium, cisplatin, cladribine, clindamycin, co-trimoxazole, cyclophosphamide, cytarabine, dexamethasone sodium phosphate, digoxin, diltiazem, dobutamine, docetaxel, dopamine, doxorubicin, doxycycline, enalaprilat, epinephrine, erythromycin lactobionate, esmolol, etomidate, etoposide phosphate, famotidine, fentanyl, filgrastim, fluconazole, fludarabine, foscarnet, gatifloxacin, gemcitabine, gentamicin, granisetron, heparin, hydrocortisone sodium succinate, hydromorphone, IL-2, insulin (regular), kanamycin, labetalol, levofloxacin, lidocaine, linezolid, lorazepam, magnesium sulfate, melphalan, meropenem, methotrexate, methyldopate, methylprednisolone sodium succinate, metoclopramide, metoprolol, metronidazole, midazolam, milrinone, nafcillin, nicardipine, nitroglycerin, norepinephrine, ondansetron, oxacillin, oxytocin, paclitaxel, pancuronium, penicillin G potassium, piperacillin, piperacillin/tazobactam, potassium chloride, propofol, propranolol, ranitidine, remifentanil, sodium bicarbonate, sodium nitroprusside, tacrolimus, teniposide, thiotepa, ticarcillin, ticarcillin/clavulanate, tobramycin, vancomycin, vecuronium, vinorelbine, vitamin B complex with C, warfarin, zidovudine. **Incompatible:** Alatrofloxacin, amphotericin B cholesteryl sulfate complex, cefepime, doxorubicin liposome, minocycline, sargramostim. **Variable (consult detailed reference):** Acyclovir, furosemide, thiopental, TPN.

Compatibility in syringe: Compatible: Atropine, bupivacaine, bupivacaine with clonidine, butorphanol, cimetidine, dimenhydrinate, diphenhydramine, droperidol, fentanyl, glycopyrrolate, hydroxyzine, ketamine, ketamine with lidocaine, metoclopramide, midazolam, milrinone, ondansetron, pentazocine, perphenazine, promazine, ranitidine, scopolamine. **Incompatible:** Meperidine, thiopental. **Variable (consult detailed reference):** Chlorpromazine, haloperidol, heparin, pentobarbital, prochlorperazine edisylate, promethazine.

Compatibility when admixed: Compatible: Alteplase, atracurium, baclofen, bupivacaine, dobutamine, fluconazole, furosemide, ketamine, meropenem, metoclopramide, ondansetron, succinylcholine, verapamil. **Incompatible:** Aminophylline, amobarbital, chlorothiazide, fluorouracil, heparin, meperidine, phenobarbital, phenytoin, sodium bicarbonate, thiopental.

DepoDur®: Do not mix with other medications.

Mechanism of Action Binds to opiate receptors in the CNS, causing inhibition of ascending pain pathways, altering the perception of and response to pain; produces generalized CNS depression

Pharmacodynamics/Kinetics

Onset of action (patient dependent; dosing must be individualized): Oral (immediate release): ~30 minutes; I.V.: 5-10 minutes

Duration (patient dependent; dosing must be individualized): Pain relief:
Immediate release formulations: 4 hours
Extended release capsule and tablet: 8-24 hours (formulation dependent)
Extended release epidural injection (DepoDur®): >48 hours

Absorption: Variable

Distribution: V_d: 3-4 L/kg; binds to opioid receptors in the CNS and periphery (eg, GI tract)

Protein binding: 30% to 35%

Metabolism: Hepatic via conjugation with glucuronic acid primarily to morphine-6-glucuronide (active analgesic) morphine-3-glucuronide (inactive as analgesic); minor metabolites include morphine-3-6-diglucuronide; other minor metabolites include normorphine (active) and morphine 3-ethereal sulfate

Bioavailability: Oral: 17% to 33% (first-pass effect limits oral bioavailability; oral:parenteral effectiveness reportedly varies from 1:6 in opioid naive patients to 1:3 with chronic use)

Half-life elimination: Adults: 2-4 hours (immediate release forms)

Time to peak, plasma: Avinza®: 30 minutes (maintained for 24 hours); Kadian®: ~10 hours; Oramorph® SR: ~4 hours

Excretion: Urine (primarily as morphine-3-glucuronide, ~2% to 12% excreted unchanged); feces (~7% to 10%). It has been suggested that accumulation of morphine-6-glucuronide might cause toxicity with renal insufficiency. All of the metabolites (ie, morphine-3-glucuronide, morphine-6-glucuronide, and normorphine) have been suggested as possible causes of neurotoxicity (eg, myoclonus).

Dosage Note: These are guidelines and do not represent the doses that may be required in all patients. Doses and dosage intervals should be titrated to pain relief/prevention.

Children >6 months and <50 kg: Acute pain (moderate-to-severe):

Oral (immediate release formulations): 0.15-0.3 mg/kg every 3-4 hours as needed. **Note:** The American Pain Society recommends an initial dose of 0.3 mg/kg for children with severe pain.

I.M., I.V.: 0.1-0.2 mg/kg every 3-4 hours as needed

I.V. infusion: Range: 10-60 mcg/kg/hour

Patient-controlled analgesia (PCA) (American Pain Society, 2008): **Note:** Opiate-naive: Consider lower end of dosing range:
Usual concentration: 1 mg/mL
Demand dose: Usual: 0.02 mg/kg/dose; range: 0.01-0.03 mg/kg/dose
Lockout interval: 6-8 minutes
Usual basal rate: 0-0.03 mg/kg/hour

Adults:

Acute pain (moderate-to-severe):

Oral (immediate release formulations): Opiate-naive: Initial: 10 mg every 4 hours as needed; patients with prior opiate exposure may require higher initial doses: usual dosage range: 10-30 mg every 4 hours as needed

I.M., SubQ: **Note:** Repeated SubQ administration causes local tissue irritation, pain, and induration.
Initial: Opiate-naive: 5-10 mg every 4 hours as needed; patients with prior opiate exposure may require higher initial doses; usual dosage range: 5-20 mg every 4 hours as needed

Rectal: 10-20 mg every 3-4 hours

I.V.: Initial: Opiate-naive: 2.5-5 mg every 3-4 hours; patients with prior opiate exposure may require higher initial doses. **Note:** Repeated doses (up to every 5 minutes if needed) in small increments (eg, 1-4 mg) may be preferred to larger and less frequent doses.

Acute myocardial infarction, analgesia (ACC/AHA 2004 guidelines): Initial management: 2-4 mg, give 2-8 mg every 5-15 minutes as needed.

Critically-ill patients (unlabeled dose): 0.7-10 mg (based on 70 kg patient) **or** 0.01-0.15 mg/kg every 1-2 hours as needed. **Note:** More frequent dosing may be needed (eg, mechanically-ventilated patients).

I.V., SubQ continuous infusion: 0.8-10 mg/hour; usual range: Up to 80 mg/hour

Continuous infusion: Usual dosage range: 5-35 mg/hour (based on 70 kg patient) **or** 0.07-0.5 mg/kg/hour

Patient-controlled analgesia (PCA): **Note:** Opiate-naive: Consider lower end of dosing range:

Usual concentration: 1 mg/mL

Demand dose: Usual: 1 mg; range: 0.5-2.5 mg

Lockout interval: 5-10 minutes

Intrathecal (I.T.): **Note: Must be preservative-free.** Administer with extreme caution and in reduced dosage to geriatric or debilitated patients. I.T. dose is usually 1/10 that of epidural dosage.

Opioid-naive: 0.2-1 mg/dose (may provide adequate relief for up to 24 hours); repeat doses are **not** recommended. **Note:** The American Pain Society recommends 0.1-0.3 mg/dose; adjust dose for age, injection site, and patient's medical condition and degree of opioid tolerance.

Continuous microinfusion (Infumorph®): Initial: 0.2-1 mg/day

Opioid-tolerant: 1-10 mg/day

Continuous microinfusion (Infumorph®): Initial: 1-10 mg/day, titrate to effect; usual maximum is ~20 mg/day

Epidural: Pain management: **Note: Must be preservative-free.** Administer with extreme caution and in reduced dosage to geriatric or debilitated patients. Vigilant monitoring is particularly important in these patients.

Single-dose (Astromorph/PF™, Duramorph®): Initial: 5 mg, if pain relief not achieved in 1 hour, careful administration of 1-2 mg at intervals sufficient to assess effectiveness may be given; maximum: 10 mg/24 hours (single doses may provide adequate relief for up to 24 hours)

Infusion: Bolus dose: 1-6 mg; infusion rate: 0.1-0.2 mg/hour; maximum dose: 10 mg/24 hours.

Note: The American Pain Society recommends 1-6 mg/dose as a single dose or an infusion of 0.1-1 mg/hour; adjust dose for age, injection site, and patient's medical condition and degree of opioid tolerance.

Continuous microinfusion (Infumorph®):

Opioid-naive: Initial: 0.2-1 mg/day

Opioid-tolerant: Initial: 1-10 mg/day, titrate to effect; usual maximum is ~20 mg/day

Surgical anesthesia: Epidural: Single-dose (extended release, DepoDur®):
Lumbar epidural only; not recommended in patients <18 years of age:

Cesarean section: 10 mg (after clamping umbilical cord)

Lower abdominal/pelvic surgery: 10-15 mg

Major orthopedic surgery of lower extremity: 15 mg

For DepoDur®: To minimize the pharmacokinetic interaction resulting in higher peak serum concentrations of morphine, administer the test dose of the local anesthetic at least 15 minutes prior to DepoDur® administration. Use of DepoDur® with epidural local anesthetics has not been studied.

◀

Other medications should not be administered into the epidural space for at least 48 hours after administration of DepoDur®.

Note: Some patients may benefit from a 20 mg dose; however, the incidence of adverse effects may be increased.

Chronic pain: Note: Patients taking opioids chronically may become tolerant and require doses higher than the usual dosage range to maintain the desired effect. Tolerance can be managed by appropriate dose titration. There is no optimal or maximal dose for morphine in chronic pain. The appropriate dose is one that relieves pain throughout its dosing interval without causing unmanageable side effects.

Oral: Controlled-, extended-, or sustained-release formulations: A patient's morphine requirement should be established using prompt-release formulations. Conversion to long-acting products may be considered when chronic, continuous treatment is required. Higher dosages should be reserved for use only in opioid-tolerant patients.

Capsules, extended release (Avinza®): Daily dose administered once daily (for best results, administer at same time each day)

Capsules, sustained release (Kadian®): Daily dose administered once daily or in 2 divided doses daily (every 12 hours)

Tablets, controlled release (MS Contin®), sustained release (Oramorph SR®), or extended release: Daily dose divided and administered every 8 or every 12 hours

Elderly or debilitated patients: Use with caution; may require dose reduction

Dosing adjustment in renal impairment:

Cl_{cr} 10-50 mL/minute: Children and Adults: Administer at 75% of normal dose

Cl_{cr} <10 mL/minute: Children and Adults: Administer at 50% of normal dose

Intermittent HD:

Children: Administer 50% of normal dose

Adults: No dosage adjustment necessary

Peritoneal dialysis: Children: Administer 50% of normal dose

CRRT: Children and Adults: Administer 75% of normal dose, titrate

Dosing adjustment/comments in hepatic disease: Unchanged in mild liver disease; substantial extrahepatic metabolism may occur; excessive sedation may occur in cirrhosis

Administration

Oral: Do not crush controlled release drug product, swallow whole. Kadian® and Avinza® can be opened and sprinkled on applesauce; do not crush or chew the beads. Contents of Kadian® capsules may be opened and sprinkled over 10 mL water and flushed through prewetted 16F gastrostomy tube; do not administer Kadian® through nasogastric tube.

I.V.: When giving morphine I.V. push, it is best to first dilute with sterile water or NS for a final concentration of 1-2 mg/mL and then administer slowly.

Epidural: Use preservative-free solutions

Epidural, extended release liposomal suspension (DepoDur®): Intended for lumbar administration only. Thoracic administration has not been studied. May be administered undiluted or diluted up to 5 mL total volume in preservative-free NS. Do not use an in-line filter during administration. Not for I.V., I.M., or intrathecal administration.

Resedation may occur following epidural administration; this may be delayed ≥48 hours in patients receiving extended-release (DepoDur®) injections.

Administration of an epidural test dose (lidocaine 1.5% and epinephrine 1:200,000) may affect the release of morphine from the liposomal preparation. Delaying the dose for an interval of at least 15 minutes following the test dose minimizes this pharmacokinetic interaction. Except for a test dose, other epidural local anesthetics or medications should not be administered epidurally before or after this product for a minimum of 48 hours.

Intrathecal: Use preservative-free solutions

Monitoring Parameters Pain relief, respiratory and mental status, blood pressure

Astromorph/PF™, Duramorph®, Infumorph®: Patients should be observed in a fully-equipped and staffed environment for at least 24 hours following initiation, and as appropriate for the first several days after catheter implantation.

DepoDur®: Patient should be monitored for at least 48 hours following administration.

Test Interactions Some quinolones may produce a false-positive urine screening result for opiates using commercially-available immunoassay kits. This has been demonstrated most consistently for levofloxacin and ofloxacin, but other quinolones have shown cross-reactivity in certain assay kits. Confirmation of positive opiate screens by more specific methods should be considered.

Dietary Considerations Morphine may cause GI upset; take with food if GI upset occurs. Be consistent when taking morphine with or without meals.

Dosage Forms Excipient information presented when available (limited, particularly for generics); consult specific product labeling. [DSC] = Discontinued product; [CAN] = Canadian brand name

Capsule, extended release, oral:
Avinza®: 30 mg, 45 mg, 60 mg, 75 mg, 90 mg, 120 mg
Kadian®: 10 mg, 20 mg, 30 mg, 50 mg, 60 mg, 80 mg, 100 mg, 200 mg
Infusion [premixed in D_5W]: 1 mg/mL (100 mL, 250 mL)
Injection, extended release liposomal suspension [lumbar epidural injection, preservative free]:
DepoDur®: 10 mg/mL (1 mL, 1.5 mL)
Injection, solution: 1 mg/mL (10 mL); 2 mg/mL (1 mL); 4 mg/mL (1 mL); 5 mg/mL (1 mL); 8 mg/mL (1 mL); 10 mg/0.7 mL (0.7 mL); 10 mg/mL (1 mL, 10 mL); 15 mg/mL (1 mL, 20 mL); 25 mg/mL (4 mL, 10 mL, 20 mL, 40 mL, 50 mL, 100 mL, 250 mL); 50 mg/mL (20 mL, 40 mL, 50 mL) [some preparations contain sodium metabisulfite]
Injection, solution [epidural, intrathecal, or I.V. infusion; preservative free]:
Astramorph/PF™: 0.5 mg/mL (2 mL, 10 mL); 1 mg/mL (2 mL, 10 mL)
Duramorph®: 0.5 mg/mL (10 mL); 1 mg/mL (10 mL)
Injection, solution [epidural or intrathecal infusion via microinfusion device; preservative free]:
Infumorph® 200: 10 mg/mL (20 mL)
Infumorph® 500: 25 mg/mL (20 mL)
Injection, solution [for PCA pump]: 1 mg/mL (30 mL; 50 mL [DSC]); 5 mg/mL (30 mL; 50 mL [DSC])
Injection, solution [for PCP pump, preservative free]: 1 mg/mL (30 mL)
Injection, solution [preservative free]: 0.5 mg/mL (10 mL); 1 mg/mL (10 mL); 25 mg/mL (10 mL)
Solution, oral: 10 mg/5 mL (5 mL, 100 mL, 500 mL)
Doloral [CAN]: 1 mg/mL (10 mL, 250 mL, 500 mL); 5 mg/mL (10 mL, 250 mL, 500 mL) [not available in U.S.]
Solution, oral [concentrate]: 5 mg/0.25 mL (0.25 mL) [DSC]; 10 mg/0.5 mL (0.5 mL) [DSC]; 20 mg/mL (1 mL [DSC], 15 ml, 30 mL, 120 mL, 240 mL)
Roxanol™: 20 mg/mL (30 mL, 120 mL); 100 mg/5 mL (240 mL)
Suppository, rectal: 5 mg (12s), 10 mg (12s), 20 mg (12s), 30 mg (12s)

▶

Tablet, oral: 10 mg [DSC], 15 mg, 30 mg

Tablet, controlled release, oral: 15 mg, 30 mg, 60 mg, 100 mg, 200 mg
  MS Contin®: 15 mg, 30 mg, 60 mg, 100 mg, 200 mg

Tablet, extended release, oral: 15 mg, 30 mg, 60 mg, 100 mg, 200 mg

Tablet, sustained release, oral:
  Oramorph® SR: 15 mg, 30 mg, 60 mg, 100 mg

References

Antman EM, Anbe SC, Alpert JS, et al, "ACC/AHA Guidelines for the Management of Patients With ST-Elevation Myocardial Infarction - Executive Summary: A Report of the American College of Cardiology/American Heart Association Task Force on Practice Guidelines (Writing Committee to Revise the 1999 Guidelines for the Management of Patients With Acute Myocardial Infarction)," *Circulation*, 2004, 110(5):588-636. Available at: http://www.circulationaha.org/cgi/content/full/110/5/588. Last accessed October 26, 2004.

Aronoff GR, Bennett WM, Berns JS, et al, *Drug Prescribing in Renal Failure: Dosing Guidelines for Adults and Children*, 5th ed. Philadelphia, PA: American College of Physicians; 2007.

Berde C, Ablin A, Glazer J, et al, "American Academy of Pediatrics Report of the Subcommittee on Disease-Related Pain in Childhood Cancer," *Pediatrics*, 1990, 86(5 Pt 2):818-25.

Dampier CD, Setty BN, Logan J, et al, "Intravenous Morphine Pharmacokinetics in Pediatric Patients With Sickle Cell Disease," *J Pediatr*, 1995, 126(3):461-7.

Friedrichsdorf SJ and Kang TI, "The Management of Pain in Children With Life-Limiting Illness," *Pediatr Clin N Am*, 2007, 54(5):645-72.

Gerber N and Apseloff G, "Death From a Morphine Infusion During a Sickle Cell Crisis," *J Pediatr*, 1993, 123(2):322-5.

Glare PA and Walsh TD, "Clinical Pharmacokinetics of Morphine," *Ther Drug Monit*, 1991, 13 (1):1-23.

Golianu B, Krane EJ, Galloway KS, et al, "Pediatric Acute Pain Management," *Pediatr Clin North Am*, 2000, 47(3):559-87.

Jacobi J, Fraser GL, Coursin DB, et al, "Clinical Practice Guidelines for the Sustained Use of Sedatives and Analgesics in the Critically Ill Adult," *Crit Care Med*, 2002, 30(1):119-41. Available at: http://www.sccm.org/pdf/sedatives.pdf. Accessed August 2, 2003.

Kaiko RF, "Age and Morphine Analgesia in Cancer Patients With Postoperative Pain," *Clin Pharmacol Ther*, 1980, 28(6):823-6.

Mignault GG, Latreille J, Viguie F, et al, "Control of Cancer-Related Pain With MS Contin: A Comparison Between 12-Hourly and 8-Hourly Administration," *J Pain Symptom Manage*, 1995, 10(6):416-22.

American Pain Society, *Principles of Analgesic Use in the Treatment of Acute Pain and Chronic Cancer Pain*, 5th ed, Glenview, IL: American Pain Society, 2003.

◆ **M.O.S.® 10 (Can)** *see* Morphine Sulfate *on page* 816

◆ **M.O.S.® 20 (Can)** *see* Morphine Sulfate *on page* 816

◆ **M.O.S.® 30 (Can)** *see* Morphine Sulfate *on page* 816

◆ **M.O.S.-SR® (Can)** *see* Morphine Sulfate *on page* 816

◆ **M.O.S.-Sulfate® (Can)** *see* Morphine Sulfate *on page* 816

◆ **Mouthkote® [OTC]** *see* Saliva Substitute *on page* 1027

◆ **Mozobil™** *see* Plerixafor *on page* 965

◆ **MPA** *see* MedroxyPROGESTERone *on page* 739

◆ **MPA** *see* Mycophenolate *on page* 831

◆ **6-MP (error-prone abbreviation)** *see* Mercaptopurine *on page* 754

◆ **MS Contin®** *see* Morphine Sulfate *on page* 816

◆ **MS (error-prone abbreviation and should not be used)** *see* Morphine Sulfate *on page* 816

◆ **MS-IR® (Can)** *see* Morphine Sulfate *on page* 816

◆ **MSO₄ (error-prone abbreviation and should not be used)** *see* Morphine Sulfate *on page* 816

◆ **MTC** *see* Mitomycin *on page* 804

◆ **MTX (error-prone abbreviation)** *see* Methotrexate *on page* 768

Mucosal Barrier Gel, Oral (myoo KOH sul BAR ee er GEL, OR al)

U.S. Brand Names Gelclair®

Index Terms Mucosal Bioadherent Gel

Pharmacologic Category Gastrointestinal Agent, Miscellaneous

Use Management of oral mucosal pain caused by oral mucositis/stomatitis (resulting from chemotherapy or radiation therapy), irritation due to oral surgery, traumatic ulcers caused by braces/ill-fitting dentures or disease, diffuse aphthous ulcers (canker sores)

Labeled Contraindications Hypersensitivity to any component of the formulation

Warnings/Precautions Patients should avoid eating or drinking for a minimum of 1 hour following treatment. Consult a physician if no improvement is seen after 7 days of use.

Adverse Reactions Postmarketing and/or case reports: Burning sensation in the mouth, mild inflammation and stinging of the oral cavity

Storage/Stability Store at room temperature away from direct sunlight. The gel may become thicker and darker over time; however, this has not been shown to affect its safety or efficacy.

Mechanism of Action Mechanical action for the management and relief of pain by adhering to the mucosal surface of mouth forming a protective film over the irritated areas and lesions

Dosage Oral: Adults: Mucosal protection: Gargle and spit the mixture of 1 single-use packet (15 mL) and water 3 times daily, or as needed. See Administration for specific dilution and administration instructions. May be used undiluted if water is unavailable.

Administration Pour the contents of a single-use packet (15 mL) into a glass and mix with 1 tablespoon of water. May dilute with an additional 1-2 tablespoons of water to achieve desired thickness. Stir well and use immediately. Mixture should be rinsed around the mouth for a minimum of 1 minute (as long as possible) to coat the tongue, palate, throat, inside of cheeks, and all oral tissue thoroughly. Mixture should be gargled and spit out. Accidental ingestion is not expected to cause adverse effects. The gel may become thicker and darker over time; however, this has not been shown to affect its safety or efficacy. Any packet that is not intact should not be used. **Note:** Studies have instructed patients to use 30-60 minutes prior to meals to gain maximum benefit (Barber, 2007; Hita-Iglesias, 2006)

Monitoring Parameters Consult a physician if improvement is not seen after 7 days of use.

Dosage Forms Excipient information presented when available (limited, particularly for generics); consult specific product labeling.

Gel, oral [concentrate]:

Gelclair®: 15 mL/packet (15s) [contains benzalkonium chloride, castor oil, propylene glycol, and sodium benzoate]

References

Barber C, Powell R, Ellis A, et al, "Comparing Pain Control and Ability to Eat and Drink With Standard Therapy vs Gelclair: A Preliminary, Double Centre, Randomized Controlled Trial on Patients With Radiotherapy-Induced Oral Mucositis," *Support Care Cancer*, 2007, 15(4):427-40.

Hita-Iglesias P, Torres-Lagares D, and Gutiérrez-Pérez JL, "Evaluation of the Clinical Behavior of a Polyvinylpyrrolidone and Sodium Hyalunorate gel (Gelclair) in Patients Subjected to Surgical Treatment With CO2 Laser," *Int J Oral Maxillofac Surg*, 2006, 35(6):514-7.

♦ **Mucosal Bioadherent Gel** *see* Mucosal Barrier Gel, Oral *on page* 827

Muromonab-CD3 (myoo roe MOE nab see dee three)

U.S. Brand Names Orthoclone OKT® 3

◀ **Index Terms** Monoclonal Antibody; OKT3

Generic Available No

Canadian Brand Names Orthoclone OKT® 3

Pharmacologic Category Immunosuppressant Agent

Use Treatment of acute allograft rejection in renal transplant patients; treatment of acute hepatic, and kidney rejection episodes resistant to conventional treatment

Unlabeled/Investigational Use Treatment of acute pancreas rejection episodes resistant to conventional treatment

Pregnancy Risk Factor C

Lactation Excretion in breast milk unknown/contraindicated

Labeled Contraindications Hypersensitivity to OKT3 or any murine product; patients with uncompensated heart failure or uncontrolled hypertension, in fluid overload or those with >3% weight gain within 1 week prior to start of OKT3; mouse antibody titers >1:1000; history of seizures; known or suspected pregnancy; breast-feeding

Warnings/Precautions It is imperative, especially prior to the first few doses, that there be no clinical evidence of volume overload, uncontrolled hypertension, or uncompensated heart failure, including a clear chest x-ray and weight restriction of ≤3% above the patient's minimum weight during the week prior to injection.

Risk of development of lymphoproliferative disorders (particularly of the skin) is increased. May result in an increased susceptibility to infection; dosage of concomitant immunosuppressants should be reduced during OKT3 therapy; cyclosporine should be decreased to 50% usual maintenance dose and maintenance therapy resumed about 4 days before stopping OKT3.

Severe pulmonary edema has occurred in patients with fluid overload. Seizures, encephalopathy, cerebral edema, aseptic meningitis, and headache have been reported following muromonab-CD3. Contraindicated for use in patients with a history of seizures or those who are predisposed to seizures. Arterial, venous, and capillary thrombosis of allografts and other vascular beds have been reported with use; use with caution in patients with history of thrombosis or underlying vascular disease.

[U.S. Boxed Warning]: Anaphylactic and anaphylactoid reactions may occur after administration of any dose of muromonab-CD3; acute hypersensitivity reactions may be characterized by cardiovascular collapse, cardiorespiratory arrest, loss of consciousness, shock, tachycardia, tingling, angioedema, airway obstruction, bronchospasm, dyspnea, urticaria, and pruritus. These reactions may be difficult to differentiate from the cytokine release syndrome associated with use; however, hypersensitivity reactions are more likely to occur within the first 10 minutes after administration. Cytokine release syndrome may occur in a significant proportion of patients following the first couple of doses of muromonab-CD3; symptoms usually begin 30-60 minutes after administration of dose and may persist for several hours; symptoms range from a mild, self-limiting "flu-like reaction" to severe, life-threatening shock-like reaction. Patients at higher risk for serious complications include those with unstable angina, recent MI or ischemic heart disease, heart failure, pulmonary edema, COPD, intravascular volume overload or depletion, cerebrovascular disease, patients with advanced symptomatic vascular disease or neuropathy, history of seizures, and septic shock. Pretreatment with corticosteroids may decrease serum levels of cytokines and manifestations of the syndrome, but it is not known if this decreases organ damage and sequelae associated with it.

Cardiopulmonary resuscitation may be needed. If the patient's temperature is >37.8°C, reduce before administering OKT3. **[U.S. Boxed Warning]: Should be administered under the supervision of a physician experienced in immunosuppressive therapy in a facility appropriate for monitoring and resuscitation.**

Adverse Reactions Note: Signs and symptoms of cytokine release syndrome (characterized by pyrexia, chills, dyspnea, nausea, vomiting, chest pain, diarrhea, tremor, wheezing, headache, tachycardia, rigor, hypertension, pulmonary edema and/or other cardiorespiratory manifestations) occurs in a significant proportion of patients following the first couple of doses of muromonab-CD3. See Warnings/Precautions. Additionally, some patients have experienced immediate hypersensitivity reactions to muromonab-CD3 (characterized by cardiovascular collapse, cardiorespiratory arrest, loss of consciousness, hypotension/shock, tachycardia, tingling, angioedema (including laryngeal, pharyngeal, or facial edema), airway obstruction, bronchospasm, dyspnea, urticaria, and/or pruritus) upon initial exposure and re-exposure.

>10%:

Cardiovascular: Tachycardia (26%), hypotension (25%), hypertension (19%), edema (12%)

Central nervous system: Pyrexia (77%), chills (43%), headache (28%)

Dermatologic: Rash (14%; erythematous 2%)

Gastrointestinal: Diarrhea (37%), nausea (32%), vomiting (25%)

Respiratory: Dyspnea (16%)

1% to 10%:

Cardiovascular: Chest pain (9%), vasodilation (7%), arrhythmia (4%), bradycardia (4%), vascular occlusion (2%)

Central nervous system: Fatigue (9%), confusion (6%), dizziness (6%), lethargy (6%), pain trunk (6%), malaise (5%), nervousness (5%), depression (3%), somnolence (2%), meningitis (1%), seizure (1%)

Dermatologic: Pruritus (7%)

Gastrointestinal: Gastrointestinal pain (7%), abdominal pain (6%), anorexia (4%)

Hematologic: Leukopenia (7%), anemia (2%), thrombocytopenia (2%), leukocytosis (1%)

Neuromuscular & skeletal: Weakness (10%), arthralgia (7%), myalgia (1%), tremor (14%)

Ocular: Photophobia (1%)

Otic: Tinnitus (1%)

Renal: Renal dysfunction (3%)

Respiratory: Abnormal chest sound (10%), hyperventilation (7%), wheezing (6%), respiratory congestion (4%), pulmonary edema (2%), hypoxia (1%), pneumonia (1%)

Miscellaneous: Diaphoresis (7%), infections (various)

<1%: ALT increased, AST increased, angina, anuria, apnea, cardiac arrest, coagulation disorder, coma, conjunctivitis, encephalopathy, epilepsy, GI hemorrhage, hallucinations, hearing decreased, heart failure, hepatitis, hypotonia, lymphadenopathy, lymphopenia, MI, mood changes, neoplasms (various), oliguria, paranoia, pneumonitis, psychosis, shock, thrombosis

◄ **Drug Interactions**
Avoid Concomitant Use
Avoid concomitant use of Muromonab-CD3 with any of the following:
Natalizumab; Vaccines (Live)
Increased Effect/Toxicity
Muromonab-CD3 may increase the levels/effects of: Leflunomide; Natalizumab; Vaccines (Live)

The levels/effects of Muromonab-CD3 may be increased by: Trastuzumab
Decreased Effect
Muromonab-CD3 may decrease the levels/effects of: Vaccines (Inactivated); Vaccines (Live)

The levels/effects of Muromonab-CD3 may be decreased by: Echinacea
Storage/Stability Refrigerate; do not freeze. Do not shake. Stable in Becton Dickinson syringe for 16 hours at room temperature or refrigeration.
Mechanism of Action Reverses graft rejection by binding to T cells and interfering with their function by binding T-cell receptor-associated CD3 glycoprotein
Pharmacodynamics/Kinetics
Duration: 7 days after discontinuation
Time to peak: Steady-state: Trough: 3-14 days
Dosage I.V. (refer to individual protocols):
Children <30 kg: 2.5 mg/day once daily for 7-14 days
Children >30 kg: 5 mg/day once daily for 7-14 days
   OR
Children <12 years: 0.1 mg/kg/day once daily for 10-14 days
Children ≥12 years and Adults: 5 mg/day once daily for 10-14 days
Hemodialysis: Molecular size of OKT3 is 150,000 daltons; not dialyzed by most standard dialyzers; however, may be dialyzed by high flux dialysis; OKT3 will be removed by plasmapheresis; administer following dialysis treatments
Peritoneal dialysis: Significant drug removal is unlikely based on physiochemical characteristics

Note: Suggested prevention/treatment of muromonab-CD3 first-dose effects (grouped by adverse reaction):
Severe pulmonary edema:
 • Effective prevention or palliation: Clear chest x-ray within 24 hours preinjection; weight restriction to ≤3% gain over 7days preinjection
 • Supportive treatment: Prompt intubation and oxygenation; 24 hours close observation
Fever, chills:
 • Effective prevention or palliation: 15 mg/kg methylprednisolone sodium succinate 1 hour preinjection; fever reduction to <37.8°C (100°F) 1 hour preinjection; acetaminophen (1 g orally) and diphenhydramine(50 mg orally) 1 hour preinjection
 • Supportive treatment: Cooling blanket; acetaminophen as needed
Respiratory effects:
 • Effective prevention or palliation: 100 mg hydrocortisone sodium succinate 30 minutes postinjection
 • Supportive treatment: Additional 100 mg hydrocortisone sodium succinate as needed for wheezing; if respiratory distress, give epinephrine 1:1000 (0.3 mL SubQ)

Administration **Not for I.M. administration.** Filter each dose through a low protein-binding 0.22 micron filter (Millex GV) before administration; administer I.V. push over <1 minute at a final concentration of 1 mg/mL

Children and Adults:

Methylprednisolone sodium succinate 15 mg/kg I.V. administered prior to first muromonab-CD3 administration and I.V. hydrocortisone sodium succinate 50-100 mg given 30 minutes after administration are strongly recommended to decrease the incidence of reactions to the first dose

Patient temperature should not exceed 37.8°C (100°F) at time of administration

Monitoring Parameters Chest x-ray, weight gain, CBC with differential, temperature, vital signs (blood pressure, temperature, pulse, respiration); immunologic monitoring of T cells, serum levels of OKT3

Dietary Considerations Injection solution contains sodium 43 mg/5 mL.

Dosage Forms Excipient information presented when available (limited, particularly for generics); consult specific product labeling.

Injection, solution: 1 mg/mL (5 mL) [contains polysorbate 80]

References

Hooks MA, Wade CS, and Millikan WJ Jr, "Muromonab CD-3: A Review of Its Pharmacology, Pharmacokinetics, and Clinical Use in Transplantation," *Pharmacotherapy*, 1991, 11(1):26-37.

Niaudet P, Murcia I, Jean G, et al, "A Comparative Trial of OKT3 and Antilymphocyte Serum in the Preventive Treatment of Rejection After Kidney Transplantation in Children," *Ann Pediatr (Paris)*, 1990, 37(2):83-5.

Ross SJ, "Immunologic Monitoring of OKT3 Therapy," *Transplantation Pharm Newslet*, 1995:2-5.

◆ **Mustargen®** see Mechlorethamine on page 736

◆ **Mustine** see Mechlorethamine on page 736

◆ **Mutamycin® (Can)** see Mitomycin on page 804

◆ **Mycamine®** see Micafungin on page 798

◆ **Mycelex®** see Clotrimazole on page 253

Mycophenolate (mye koe FEN oh late)

Related Information

Hematopoietic Stem Cell Transplantation on page 1501
Safe Handling of Hazardous Drugs on page 1517

U.S. Brand Names CellCept®; Myfortic®

Index Terms MMF; MPA; Mycophenolate Mofetil; Mycophenolate Sodium; Mycophenolic Acid

Generic Available Yes: Capsule, tablet

Canadian Brand Names CellCept®; Myfortic®

Pharmacologic Category Immunosuppressant Agent

Use Prophylaxis of organ rejection concomitantly with cyclosporine and corticosteroids in patients receiving allogeneic renal (CellCept®, Myfortic®), cardiac (CellCept®), or hepatic (CellCept®) transplants

Unlabeled/Investigational Use Treatment of rejection in liver transplant patients unable to tolerate tacrolimus or cyclosporine due to neurotoxicity; mild rejection in heart transplant patients; treatment of moderate-severe psoriasis; treatment of proliferative lupus nephritis; treatment of myasthenia gravis; prevention and treatment of graft-versus-host disease (GVHD)

Pregnancy Risk Factor D

Lactation Excretion in breast milk unknown/not recommended

Labeled Contraindications Hypersensitivity to mycophenolate mofetil, mycophenolic acid, mycophenolate sodium, or any component of the ▶

formulation; intravenous formulation is contraindicated in patients who are allergic to polysorbate 80

Warnings/Precautions Hazardous agent - use appropriate precautions for handling and disposal. **[U.S. Boxed Warning]: Risk for infection and development of lymphoma and skin malignancy is increased.** Opportunistic infections, sepsis, and/or fatal infections may occur with immunosuppressive therapy. Patients should be monitored appropriately. Instruct patients to limit exposure to sunlight/UV light and give supportive treatment should these conditions occur. Pure red cell aplasia (PRCA) or progressive multifocal leukoencephalopathy (PML) may occur rarely, particularly in immunosuppressed patients or those receiving immunosuppressant therapy; monitor for signs of PRCA (anemia, fatigue, lethargy, pallor, dyspnea) or PML (neurologic impairment, apathy, ataxia, cognitive deficiencies, confusion, and hemiparesis); may require dosage reduction or discontinuation of therapy. Neutropenia (including severe neutropenia) may occur, requiring dose reduction or interruption of treatment (risk greater from day 31-180 posttransplant). Use caution with active peptic ulcer disease; may be associated with gastric or duodenal ulcers, GI bleeding and/or perforation. Use caution in renal impairment as toxicity may be increased; may require dosage adjustment in severe impairment.

[U.S. Boxed Warning]: Mycophenolate is associated with an increased risk of congenital malformations and spontaneous abortions when used during pregnancy. Females of childbearing potential should have a negative pregnancy test within 1 week prior to beginning therapy. Two reliable forms of contraception should be used beginning 4 weeks prior to, during, and for 6 weeks after therapy. Because mycophenolate mofetil has demonstrated teratogenic effects in rats and rabbits, tablets should not be crushed, and capsules should not be opened or crushed. Avoid inhalation or direct contact with skin or mucous membranes of the powder contained in the capsules and the powder for oral suspension. Caution should be exercised in the handling and preparation of solutions of intravenous mycophenolate. Avoid skin contact with the intravenous solution and reconstituted suspension. If such contact occurs, wash thoroughly with soap and water, rinse eyes with plain water.

Theoretically, use should be avoided in patients with the rare hereditary deficiency of hypoxanthine-guanine phosphoribosyltransferase (such as Lesch-Nyhan or Kelley-Seegmiller syndrome). Intravenous solutions should be given over at least 2 hours; never administer intravenous solution by rapid or bolus injection. **[U.S. Boxed Warning]: Should be administered under the supervision of a physician experienced in immunosuppressive therapy.**

Note: CellCept® and Myfortic® dosage forms should not be used interchangeably due to differences in absorption. Some dosage forms may contain phenylalanine.

Adverse Reactions As reported in adults following oral dosing of CellCept® alone in renal, cardiac, and hepatic allograft rejection studies. In general, lower doses used in renal rejection patients had less adverse effects than higher doses. Rates of adverse effects were similar for each indication, except for those unique to the specific organ involved. The type of adverse effects observed in pediatric patients was similar to those seen in adults; abdominal pain, anemia, diarrhea, fever, hypertension, infection, pharyngitis, respiratory tract infection, sepsis, and vomiting were seen in higher proportion; lymphoproliferative disorder was the only type of malignancy observed.

Percentages of adverse reactions were similar in studies comparing CellCept® to Myfortic® in patients following renal transplant.

>20%:

Cardiovascular: Hypertension (28% to 77%), hypotension (up to 33%), peripheral edema (27% to 64%), edema (27% to 28%), chest pain (26%), tachycardia (20% to 22%)

Central nervous system: Pain (31% to 76%), headache (16% to 54%), insomnia (41% to 52%), fever (21% to 52%), dizziness (up to 29%), anxiety (28%)

Dermatologic: Rash (up to 22%)

Endocrine & metabolic: Hyperglycemia (44% to 47%), hypercholesterolemia (41%), hypomagnesemia (up to 39%), hypokalemia (32% to 37%), hypocalcemia (up to 30%), hyperkalemia (up to 22%)

Gastrointestinal: Abdominal pain (25% to 63%), nausea (20% to 55%), diarrhea (31% to 51%), constipation (19% to 41%), vomiting (33% to 34%), anorexia (up to 25%), dyspepsia (22%)

Genitourinary: Urinary tract infection (37%)

Hematologic: Leukopenia (23% to 46%), anemia (26% to 43%; hypochromic 25%), leukocytosis (22% to 40%), thrombocytopenia (24% to 38%)

Hepatic: Liver function tests abnormal (up to 25%), ascites (24%)

Neuromuscular & skeletal: Back pain (35% to 47%), weakness (35% to 43%), tremor (24% to 34%), paresthesia (21%)

Renal: Creatinine increased (up to 39%), BUN increased (up to 35%)

Respiratory: Dyspnea (31% to 37%), respiratory tract infection (22% to 37%), pleural effusion (34%), cough (31%), lung disorder (22% to 30%), sinusitis (26%)

Miscellaneous: Infection (18% to 27%), *Candida* (17% to 22%), herpes simplex (10% to 21%)

3% to <20%:

Cardiovascular: Angina, arrhythmia, arterial thrombosis, atrial fibrillation, atrial flutter, bradycardia, cardiac arrest, cardiac failure, CHF, extrasystole, facial edema, hypervolemia, pallor, palpitation, pericardial effusion, peripheral vascular disorder, postural hypotension, supraventricular extrasystoles, supraventricular tachycardia, syncope, thrombosis, vasodilation, vasospasm, venous pressure increased, ventricular extrasystole, ventricular tachycardia

Central nervous system: Agitation, chills with fever, confusion, convulsion, delirium, depression, emotional lability, hallucinations, hypoesthesia, malaise, nervousness, psychosis, somnolence, thinking abnormal, vertigo

Dermatologic: Acne, alopecia, bruising, cellulitis, hirsutism, petechia, pruritus, skin carcinoma, skin hypertrophy, skin ulcer, vesiculobullous rash

Endocrine & metabolic: Acidosis, Cushing's syndrome, dehydration, diabetes mellitus, gout, hypercalcemia, hyperlipemia, hyperphosphatemia, hyperuricemia, hypochloremia, hypoglycemia, hyponatremia, hypoproteinemia, hypothyroidism, parathyroid disorder, weight gain/loss

Gastrointestinal: Abdomen enlarged, dry mouth, dysphagia, esophagitis, flatulence, gastritis, gastroenteritis, gastrointestinal hemorrhage, gastrointestinal moniliasis, gingivitis, gum hyperplasia, ileus, melena, mouth ulceration, oral moniliasis, stomach disorder, stomatitis

Genitourinary: Impotence, nocturia, pelvic pain, prostatic disorder, scrotal edema, urinary frequency, urinary incontinence, urinary retention, urinary tract disorder

Hematologic: Coagulation disorder, hemorrhage, neutropenia, pancytopenia, polycythemia, prothrombin time increased, thromboplastin increased

Hepatic: Alkaline phosphatase increased, alkalosis, bilirubinemia, cholangitis, cholestatic jaundice, GGT increased, hepatitis, jaundice, liver damage, transaminases increased

Local: Abscess

Neuromuscular & skeletal: Arthralgia, hypertonia, joint disorder, leg cramps, myalgia, myasthenia, neck pain, neuropathy, osteoporosis

Ocular: Amblyopia, cataract, conjunctivitis, eye hemorrhage, lacrimation disorder, vision abnormal

Otic: Deafness, ear disorder, ear pain, tinnitus

Renal: Albuminuria, creatinine increased, dysuria, hematuria, hydronephrosis, kidney failure, kidney tubular necrosis, oliguria

Respiratory: Apnea, asthma, atelectasis, bronchitis, epistaxis, hemoptysis, hiccup, hyperventilation, hypoxia, respiratory acidosis, lung edema, pharyngitis, pneumonia, pneumothorax, pulmonary hypertension, respiratory moniliasis, rhinitis, sputum increased, voice alteration

Miscellaneous: *Candida* (mucocutaneous 16% to 18%), CMV viremia/syndrome (12% to 14%), CMV tissue invasive disease (6% to 11%), herpes zoster cutaneous disease (4% to 10%), cyst, diaphoresis, flu-like syndrome, fungal dermatitis, healing abnormal, hernia, ileus infection, lactic dehydrogenase increased, peritonitis, pyelonephritis, sepsis, thirst

Postmarketing and/or case reports: Atypical mycobacterial infection, colitis, gastrointestinal perforation, gastrointestinal ulcers, infectious endocarditis, interstitial lung disorder, intestinal villous atrophy, meningitis, pancreatitis, progressive multifocal leukoencephalopathy, pulmonary fibrosis (fatal), pure red cell aplasia, tuberculosis

Drug Interactions

Avoid Concomitant Use

Avoid concomitant use of Mycophenolate with any of the following: Cholestyramine Resin; Natalizumab; Rifamycin Derivatives; Vaccines (Live)

Increased Effect/Toxicity

Mycophenolate may increase the levels/effects of: Acyclovir-Valacyclovir; Ganciclovir-Valganciclovir; Leflunomide; Natalizumab; Vaccines (Live)

The levels/effects of Mycophenolate may be increased by: Acyclovir-Valacyclovir; Ganciclovir-Valganciclovir; Probenecid; Trastuzumab

Decreased Effect

Mycophenolate may decrease the levels/effects of: Oral Contraceptive (Estrogens); Oral Contraceptive (Progestins); Vaccines (Inactivated); Vaccines (Live)

The levels/effects of Mycophenolate may be decreased by: Antacids; Cholestyramine Resin; CycloSPORINE; Echinacea; Magnesium Salts; MetroNIDAZOLE; Penicillins; Proton Pump Inhibitors; Quinolone Antibiotics; Rifamycin Derivatives; Sevelamer

Ethanol/Nutrition/Herb Interactions

Food: Decreases C_{max} of MPA by 40% following CellCept® administration and 33% following Myfortic® use; the extent of absorption is not changed

Herb/Nutraceutical: Avoid cat's claw, echinacea (have immunostimulant properties)

Storage/Stability

Capsules: Store at room temperature of 15°C to 30°C (59°F to 86°F).

Tablets: Store at room temperature of 15°C to 30°C (59°F to 86°F). Protect from moisture and light.

Oral suspension: Store powder for oral suspension at room temperature of 15°C to 30°C (59°F to 86°F). Once reconstituted, the oral solution may be stored at room temperature or under refrigeration. Do not freeze. The mixed suspension is stable for 60 days.

Injection: Store intact vials at room temperature 15°C to 30°C (59°F to 86°F). Store solutions at 15°C to 30°C (59°F to 86°F). Begin infusion within 4 hours of reconstitution.

Reconstitution

Oral suspension: Should be constituted prior to dispensing to the patient and **not** mixed with any other medication. Add 47 mL of water to the bottle and shake well for ~1 minute. Add another 47 mL of water to the bottle and shake well for an additional minute. Final concentration is 200 mg/mL of mycophenolate mofetil.

I.V.: Reconstitute the contents of each vial with 14 mL of 5% dextrose injection; dilute the contents of a vial with 5% dextrose in water to a final concentration of 6 mg mycophenolate mofetil per mL. **Note:** Vial is vacuum-sealed; if a lack of vacuum is noted during preparation, the vial should not be used.

Compatibility Stable in D_5W.

Mechanism of Action MPA exhibits a cytostatic effect on T and B lymphocytes. It is an inhibitor of inosine monophosphate dehydrogenase (IMPDH) which inhibits *de novo* guanosine nucleotide synthesis. T and B lymphocytes are dependent on this pathway for proliferation.

Pharmacodynamics/Kinetics

Onset of action: Peak effect: Correlation of toxicity or efficacy is still being developed, however, one study indicated that 12-hour AUCs >40 mcg/mL/hour were correlated with efficacy and decreased episodes of rejection

T_{max}: Oral: MPA:
CellCept®: 1-1.5 hours
Myfortic®: 1.5-2.75 hours

Absorption: AUC values for MPA are lower in the early post-transplant period versus later (>3 months) post-transplant period. The extent of absorption in pediatrics is similar to that seen in adults, although there was wide variability reported.
Oral: Myfortic®: 93%

Distribution:
CellCept®: MPA: Oral: 4 L/kg; I.V.: 3.6 L/kg
Myfortic®: MPA: Oral: 54 L (at steady state); 112 L (elimination phase)

Protein binding: MPA: >98%, MPAG 82%

Metabolism: Hepatic and via GI tract; CellCept® is completely hydrolyzed in the liver to mycophenolic acid (MPA; active metabolite); enterohepatic recirculation of MPA may occur; MPA is glucuronidated to MPAG (inactive metabolite)

Bioavailability: Oral: CellCept®: 94%; Myfortic®: 72%

Half-life elimination:
CellCept®: MPA: Oral: 18 hours; I.V.: 17 hours
Myfortic®: MPA: Oral: 8-16 hours; MPAG: 13-17 hours

Excretion:
CellCept®: MPA: Urine (<1%), feces (6%); MPAG: Urine (87%)
Myfortic®: MPA: Urine (3%), feces; MPAG: Urine (>60%)

Dosage

Children: Renal transplant: Oral:
CellCept® suspension: 600 mg/m²/dose twice daily; maximum dose: 1 g twice daily

Alternatively, may use solid dosage forms according to BSA as follows:
BSA 1.25-1.5 m²: 750 mg capsule twice daily
BSA >1.5 m²: 1 g capsule or tablet twice daily

Myfortic®: 400 mg/m^2/dose twice daily; maximum dose: 720 mg twice daily

    BSA <1.19 m^2: Use of this formulation is not recommended

    BSA 1.19-1.58 m^2: 540 mg twice daily (maximum: 1080 mg/day)

    BSA >1.58 m^2: 720 mg twice daily (maximum: 1440 mg/day)

Adults: **Note:** May be used I.V. for up to 14 days; transition to oral therapy as soon as tolerated.

Renal transplant:

  CellCept®:

    Oral: 1 g twice daily. Doses >2 g/day are not recommended.

    I.V.: 1 g twice daily

  Myfortic®: Oral: 720 mg twice daily (1440 mg/day)

Cardiac transplantation:

  Oral (CellCept®): 1.5 g twice daily

  I.V. (CellCept®): 1.5 g twice daily

Hepatic transplantation:

  Oral (CellCept®): 1.5 g twice daily

  I.V. (CellCept®): 1 g twice daily

Myasthenia gravis (unlabeled use): Oral (CellCept®): 1 g twice daily (range 1-3 g/day)

Elderly: Dosage is the same as younger patients, however, dosing should be cautious due to possibility of increased hepatic, renal or cardiac dysfunction; elderly patients may be at an increased risk of certain infections, gastrointestinal hemorrhage, and pulmonary edema, as compared to younger patients

Dosing adjustment for toxicity (neutropenia): Neutropenia (ANC <1.3 x 10^3/μL): Dosing should be interrupted or the dose reduced, appropriate diagnostic tests performed and patients managed appropriately

Dosing adjustment in renal impairment:

Renal transplant: GFR <25 mL/minute/1.73 m^2 in patients outside the immediate post-transplant period:

  CellCept®: Doses of >1 g administered twice daily should be avoided; patients should also be carefully observed; no dose adjustments are needed in renal transplant patients experiencing delayed graft function postoperatively

  Myfortic®: No dose adjustments are needed in renal transplant patients experiencing delayed graft function postoperatively; however, monitor carefully for potential concentration dependent adverse events

Cardiac or liver transplant: No data available; mycophenolate may be used in cardiac or hepatic transplant patients with severe chronic renal impairment if the potential benefit outweighs the potential risk

Hemodialysis: Not removed; supplemental dose is not necessary

Peritoneal dialysis: Supplemental dose is not necessary

Dosage adjustment in hepatic impairment: No dosage adjustment is recommended for renal patients with severe hepatic parenchymal disease; however, it is not currently known whether dosage adjustments are necessary for hepatic disease with other etiologies

Administration

Oral dosage formulations (tablet, capsule, suspension) should be administered on an empty stomach to avoid variability in MPA absorption. The oral solution may be administered via a nasogastric tube (minimum 8 French, 1.7 mm interior diameter); oral suspension should not be mixed with other medications. Delayed release tablets should not be crushed, cut, or chewed.

Intravenous solutions should be administered over at least 2 hours (either peripheral or central vein); do **not** administer intravenous solution by rapid or bolus injection.

Monitoring Parameters Complete blood count (weekly for first month, twice monthly during months 2 and 3, then monthly thereafter through the first year); renal and liver function; signs and symptoms of infection; pregnancy test (prior to initiation in females of childbearing potential)

Dietary Considerations Oral dosage formulations should be taken on an empty stomach to avoid variability in MPA absorption. However, in stable renal transplant patients, may be administered with food if necessary. Oral suspension contains 0.56 mg phenylalanine/mL; use caution if administered to patients with phenylketonuria.

Dosage Forms Excipient information presented when available (limited, particularly for generics); consult specific product labeling.

Capsule, oral, as mofetil: 250 mg
CellCept®: 250 mg
Injection, powder for reconstitution, as mofetil hydrochloride:
CellCept®: 500 mg [contains polysorbate 80]
Powder for suspension, oral, as mofetil:
CellCept®: 200 mg/mL (175 mL) [contains phenylalanine 0.56 mg/mL; mixed fruit flavor]
Tablet, oral, as mofetil: 500 mg
CellCept®: 500 mg [may contain ethyl alcohol]
Tablet, delayed release, as mycophenolic acid:
Myfortic®: 180 mg, 360 mg [formulated as a sodium salt]

References

Gabardi S, Tran JL, and Clarkson MR, "Enteric-Coated Mycophenolate Sodium," *Ann Pharmacother*, 2003, 37(11):1685-93.

Shaw LM, Sollinger HW, Halloran P, et al, "Mycophenolate Mofetil: A Report of the Consensus Panel," *Ther Drug Monit*, 1995, 17(6):690-9.

Vogelsang GB, and Arai S, "Mycophenolate Mofetil for the Prevention and Treatment of Graft-Versus-Host Disease Following Stem Cell Transplantation: Preliminary Findings," *Bone Marrow Transplant*, 2001, 27(12):1255-62.

◆ **Mylotarg®** *see* Gemtuzumab Ozogamicin *on page 537*

◆ **Mytotan** *see* Mitotane *on page 807*

Nabilone (NA bi lone)

Related Information

Management of Chemotherapy-Induced Nausea and Vomiting *on page 1434*

U.S. Brand Names Cesamet™

Generic Available No

Canadian Brand Names Cesamet™

Pharmacologic Category Antiemetic

Use Treatment of refractory nausea and vomiting associated with cancer chemotherapy

Restrictions C-II

Pregnancy Risk Factor C

Lactation Excretion in breast milk unknown/not recommended

Labeled Contraindications Hypersensitivity to nabilone, cannabinoids, tetrahydrocannabinol, or any component of the formulation

Warnings/Precautions May affect CNS function; use with caution in the elderly and those with pre-existing CNS depression. May cause additive CNS effects with sedatives, hypnotics, or other psychoactive agents; patients must be cautioned about performing tasks which require mental alertness (eg, operating machinery or driving). Use caution with current or previous history of mental illness; cannabinoid use may reveal symptoms of psychiatric disorders. Psychiatric adverse reactions may persist for up to 3 days after discontinuing treatment. Has potential for abuse and or dependence, use caution in patients with substance abuse history or potential. May cause tachycardia and orthostatic hypotension; use caution with cardiovascular disease. Safety and efficacy in children have not been established.

Adverse Reactions

>10%:

Central nervous system: Drowsiness (52% to 66%), dizziness (59%), vertigo (52% to 59%), euphoria (11% to 38%), ataxia (13% to 14%), depression (14%), concentration decreased (12%), sleep disturbance (11%)

Gastrointestinal: Xerostomia (22% to 36%)

Ocular: Visual disturbance (13%)

1% to 10%:

Cardiovascular: Hypotension (8%)

Central nervous system: Dysphoria (9%), headache (6% to 7%), sedation (3%), depersonalization (2%), disorientation (2%)

Gastrointestinal: Anorexia (8%), nausea (4%), appetite increased (2%)

Neuromuscular & skeletal: Weakness (8%)

<1%, postmarketing, or frequency not reported: Abdominal pain, abnormal dreams, akathisia, allergic reaction, amblyopia, anemia, anhydrosis, anxiety, apathy, aphthous ulcer, arrhythmia, back pain, cerebral vascular accident, chest pain, chills, constipation, cough, diaphoresis, diarrhea, dyspepsia, dyspnea, dystonia, emotional disorder, emotional lability, epistaxis, equilibrium dysfunction, eye irritation, fatigue, fever, flushing, gastritis, hallucinations, hot flashes, hyperactivity, hypertension, infection, insomnia, irritation, joint pain, leukopenia, lightheadedness, malaise, memory disturbance, mood swings, mouth irritation, muscle pain, nasal congestion, neck pain, nervousness, neurosis (phobic), numbness, orthostatic hypotension, pain, palpitation, panic disorder, paranoia, paresthesia, perception disturbance, pharyngitis, photophobia, photosensitivity, polyuria, pruritus, psychosis (toxic), pupil dilation, rash, seizure, sinus headache, speech disorder, stupor, syncope,

tachycardia, taste perversion, thirst, thought disorder, tinnitus, tremor, urination decreased, urinary retention, vomiting, wheezing, withdrawal, xerophthalmia

Drug Interactions

Avoid Concomitant Use There are no known interactions where it is recommended to avoid concomitant use.

Increased Effect/Toxicity

Nabilone may increase the levels/effects of: Alcohol (Ethyl); CNS Depressants; Methotrimeprazine; Sympathomimetics

The levels/effects of Nabilone may be increased by: Anticholinergic Agents; Cocaine; Methotrimeprazine

Decreased Effect There are no known significant interactions involving a decrease in effect.

Ethanol/Nutrition/Herb Interactions Ethanol: Avoid ethanol (may increase CNS depression).

Storage/Stability Store at room temperature between 15°C and 30°C (59°F and 86°F).

Mechanism of Action Not fully characterized; antiemetic activity may be due to effect on cannabinoid receptors (CB1) within the central nervous system.

Pharmacodynamics/Kinetics

Absorption: Rapid and complete

Distribution: ~12.5 L/kg

Metabolism: To several active metabolites by oxidation and stereospecific enzyme reduction; CYP450 enzymes may also be involved

Half-life elimination: Parent compound: 2 hours; Metabolites: 35 hours

Time to peak, serum: Within 2 hours

Excretion: Feces (~60%); renal (~24%)

Dosage Refer to individual protocols. Oral:

Children >4 years (unlabeled use):

<18 kg: 0.5 mg twice daily

18-30 kg: 1 mg twice daily

>30 kg: 1 mg 3 times/day

Adults: 1-2 mg twice daily (maximum: 6 mg divided in 3 doses daily)

Dosage adjustment in renal impairment: No adjustment required.

Administration Initial dose should be given 1-3 hours before chemotherapy; may be given 2-3 times a day during the entire chemotherapy course and for up to 48 hours after the last dose of chemotherapy; a dose of 1-2 mg the night before chemotherapy may be useful.

Monitoring Parameters Blood pressure, heart rate; signs and symptoms of excessive use, abuse, or misuse

Emetic Potential Very low (<10%)

Dosage Forms Excipient information presented when available (limited, particularly for generics); consult specific product labeling.

Capsule:

Cesamet™: 1 mg

References

Dupuis LL and Nathan PC, "Options for the Prevention and Management of Acute Chemotherapy-Induced Nausea and Vomiting in Children," *Pediatr Drug*, 2003, 5(9):597-613.

Tramer MR, Carroll D, Campbell FA, et al, "Cannabinoids for Control of Chemotherapy Induced Nausea and Vomiting: Quantitative Systematic Review," *BMJ*, 2001, 323(7303):16-21.

◆ **nab-Paclitaxel** *see* Paclitaxel (Protein Bound) *on page 904*

Nafcillin (naf SIL in)

Related Information
Management of Drug Extravasations *on page 1447*

Index Terms
Ethoxynaphthamido Penicillin Sodium; Nafcillin Sodium; Nallpen; Sodium Nafcillin

Generic Available
Yes

Canadian Brand Names
Nallpen®; Unipen®

Pharmacologic Category
Antibiotic, Penicillin

Use
Treatment of infections such as osteomyelitis, septicemia, endocarditis, and CNS infections caused by susceptible strains of staphylococci species

Pregnancy Risk Factor
B

Lactation
Enters breast milk/use caution

Labeled Contraindications
Hypersensitivity to nafcillin, or any component of the formulation, or penicillins; premixed injection may contain corn-derived dextrose and its use is contraindicated in patients with allergy to corn-related products

Warnings/Precautions
Serious and occasionally severe or fatal hypersensitivity (anaphylactoid) reactions have been reported in patients on penicillin therapy, especially with a history of beta-lactam hypersensitivity, history of sensitivity to multiple allergens, or previous IgE-mediated reactions (eg, anaphylaxis, angioedema, urticaria). Use with caution in asthmatic patients. Extravasation of I.V. infusions should be avoided. Modification of dosage is necessary in patients with both severe renal and hepatic impairment. Elimination rate will be slow in neonates. Prolonged use may result in fungal or bacterial superinfection, including *C. difficile*-associated diarrhea (CDAD) and pseudomembranous colitis; CDAD has been observed >2 months postantibiotic treatment.

Adverse Reactions
Frequency not defined.

Central nervous system: Neurotoxicity (high doses)

Gastrointestinal: Pseudomembranous colitis

Hematologic: Agranulocytosis, bone marrow depression, neutropenia

Local: Inflammation, pain, phlebitis, skin sloughing, swelling, and thrombophlebitis at the injection site; oxacillin (less likely to cause phlebitis) is often preferred in pediatric patients; tissue necrosis with sloughing (SubQ extravasation)

Renal: Interstitial nephritis (rare), renal tubular damage (rare)

Miscellaneous: Anaphylaxis, hypersensitivity reactions (immediate and delayed; general incidence of 1% to 10% for penicillins), serum sickness

Drug Interactions

Metabolism/Transport Effects
Induces CYP3A4 (strong)

Avoid Concomitant Use
Avoid concomitant use of Nafcillin with any of the following: Dronedarone; Everolimus; Nilotinib; Ranolazine; Tolvaptan

Increased Effect/Toxicity
Nafcillin may increase the levels/effects of: Methotrexate

The levels/effects of Nafcillin may be increased by: Uricosuric Agents

Decreased Effect
Nafcillin may decrease the levels/effects of: Calcium Channel Blockers; CycloSPORINE; CYP3A4 Substrates; Dronedarone; Everolimus; Maraviroc; Mycophenolate; Nilotinib; Oral Contraceptive (Estrogens); Ranolazine; Saxagliptin; Sorafenib; Tadalafil; Tolvaptan; Typhoid Vaccine; Vitamin K Antagonists

The levels/effects of Nafcillin may be decreased by: Fusidic Acid; Tetracycline Derivatives

Storage/Stability

Premixed infusions: Store in a freezer at -20°C (4°F). Thaw at room temperature or under refrigeration only. Thawed bags are stable for 21 days under refrigeration or 72 hours at room temperature. Do not refreeze.

Vials: Reconstituted parenteral solution is stable for 3 days at room temperature and 7 days when refrigerated or 12 weeks when frozen. For I.V. infusion in NS or D_5W, solution is stable for 24 hours at room temperature and 96 hours when refrigerated.

Compatibility Stable in dextran 40 10% in dextrose, D_5LR, D_5¼NS, D_5½NS, D_5NS, D_5W, D_{10}NS, D_{10}W, LR, NS; **variable stability (consult detailed reference)** in peritoneal dialysis solution, TPN.

Y-site administration: Compatible: Acyclovir, atropine, cyclophosphamide, diazepam, enalaprilat, esmolol, famotidine, fentanyl, fluconazole, foscarnet, heparin, hydromorphone, magnesium sulfate, morphine, nicardipine, perphenazine, propofol, theophylline, zidovudine. **Incompatible:** Droperidol, fentanyl and droperidol, insulin (regular), labetalol, midazolam, nalbuphine, pentazocine, verapamil. **Variable (consult detailed reference):** Diltiazem, meperidine, TPN, vancomycin.

Compatibility in syringe: Compatible: Cimetidine, heparin.

Compatibility when admixed: Compatible: Chloramphenicol, chlorothiazide, dexamethasone sodium phosphate, diphenhydramine, ephedrine, heparin, hydroxyzine, lidocaine, potassium chloride, prochlorperazine edisylate, sodium bicarbonate, sodium lactate. **Incompatible:** Ascorbic acid injection, aztreonam, bleomycin, cytarabine, gentamicin, hydrocortisone sodium succinate, methylprednisolone sodium succinate, promazine. **Variable (consult detailed reference):** Aminophylline, verapamil, vitamin B complex with C.

Mechanism of Action Interferes with bacterial cell wall synthesis during active multiplication, causing cell wall death and resultant bactericidal activity against susceptible bacteria

Pharmacodynamics/Kinetics

Distribution: Widely distributed; CSF penetration is poor but enhanced by meningeal inflammation

Protein binding: ~90%; primarily to albumin

Metabolism: Primarily hepatic; undergoes enterohepatic recirculation

Half-life elimination:

Neonates: <3 weeks: 2.2-5.5 hours; 4-9 weeks: 1.2-2.3 hours

Children 3 months to 14 years: 0.75-1.9 hours

Adults: Normal renal/hepatic function: 30-60 minutes

Time to peak, serum: I.M.: 30-60 minutes

Excretion: Primarily feces; urine (10% to 30% as unchanged drug)

Dosage

Usual dosage range:

Neonates: I.M., I.V.:

1200-2000 g, <7 days: 50 mg/kg/day divided every 12 hours

>2000 g, <7 days: 75 mg/kg/day divided every 8 hours

1200-2000 g, ≥7 days: 75 mg/kg/day divided every 8 hours

>2000 g, ≥7 days: 100-140 mg/kg/day divided every 6 hours

Children:

I.M.: 25 mg/kg twice daily

I.V.: 50-200 mg/kg/day in divided doses every 4-6 hours (maximum: 12 g/day)

Adults:
I.M.: 500 mg every 4-6 hours
I.V.: 500-2000 mg every 4-6 hours
Indication-specific dosing:
Children:
Mild-to-moderate infections: I.M., I.V.: 50-100 mg/kg/day in divided doses every 6 hours
Severe infections: I.M., I.V.: 100-200 mg/kg/day in divided doses every 4-6 hours (maximum dose: 12 g/day)
Staphylococcal endocarditis: I.V.:
Native valve: 200 mg/kg/day in divided doses every 4-6 hours for 6 weeks
Prosthetic valve: 200 mg/kg/day in divided doses every 4-6 hours for ≥6 weeks (use with rifampin and gentamicin)
Adults: I.V.:
Endocarditis: MSSA:
Native valve: 12 g/24 hours in 4-6 divided doses for 6 weeks
Prosthetic valve: 12 g/24 hours in 6 divided doses for ≥6 weeks (use with rifampin and gentamicin)
Joint:
Bursitis, septic: 2 g every 4 hours
Prosthetic: 2 g every 4-6 hours with rifampin for 6 weeks
***Staphylococcus aureus,* methicillin-susceptible infections, including brain abscess, empyema, erysipelas, mastitis, myositis, orbital cellulitis, osteomyelitis, pneumonia, splenic abscess, toxic shock, urinary tract (perinephric abscess):** 2 g every 4 hours

Dosing adjustment in renal impairment: Not necessary unless renal impairment is in the setting of concomitant hepatic impairment
Dialysis: Not dialyzable (0% to 5%) via hemodialysis; supplemental dosage not necessary with hemo- or peritoneal dialysis or continuous arteriovenous or venovenous hemofiltration
Dosing adjustment in hepatic impairment: In patients with both hepatic and renal impairment, modification of dosage may be necessary; no data available.
Administration
I.M.: Rotate injection sites
I.V.: Vesicant. Administer around-the-clock to promote less variation in peak and trough serum levels; infuse over 30-60 minutes

Extravasation management: Use cold packs. Hyaluronidase: Add 1 mL NS to 150 unit vial to make 150 units/mL of concentration; mix 0.1 mL of above with 0.9 mL NS in 1 mL syringe to make final concentration = 15 units/mL.
Monitoring Parameters Baseline and periodic CBC with differential; periodic urinalysis, BUN, serum creatinine, AST and ALT; observe for signs and symptoms of anaphylaxis during first dose
Test Interactions Positive Coombs' test (direct), false-positive urinary and serum proteins; may inactivate aminoglycosides *in vitro*
Dietary Considerations Premixed injection may contain corn-derived dextrose and its use is contraindicated in patients with allergy to corn-related products. Sodium content of 1 g: 76.6 mg (3.33 mEq).
Emetic Potential Very low (<10%)
Vesicant Yes; see Management of Drug Extravasations on page 1447.
Dosage Forms Excipient information presented when available (limited, particularly for generics); consult specific product labeling.
Infusion [premixed iso-osmotic dextrose solution]: 1 g (50 mL); 2 g (100 mL)
Injection, powder for reconstitution, as sodium: 1 g, 2 g, 10 g

References

Donowitz GR and Mandell GL, "Beta-Lactam Antibiotics," *N Engl J Med*, 1988, 318(7):419-26 and 318(8):490-500.
Wright AJ, "The Penicillins," *Mayo Clin Proc*, 1999, 74(3):290-307.

◆ **Nafcillin Sodium** *see* Nafcillin *on page* 840

◆ **Nallpen** *see* Nafcillin *on page* 840

◆ **Nallpen® (Can)** *see* Nafcillin *on page* 840

◆ **Nanoparticle Albumin-Bound Paclitaxel** *see* Paclitaxel (Protein Bound) *on page* 904

◆ **Natulan® (Can)** *see* Procarbazine *on page* 989

◆ **Navelbine®** *see* Vinorelbine *on page* 1181

◆ **NebuPent®** *see* Pentamidine *on page* 944

Nelarabine (nel AY re been)

Medication Safety Issues

High alert medication: The Institute for Safe Medication Practices (ISMP) includes this medication among its list of drugs which have a heightened risk of causing significant patient harm when used in error.

Related Information

Safe Handling of Hazardous Drugs *on page* 1517

U.S. Brand Names Arranon®

Index Terms 2-Amino-6-Methoxypurine Arabinoside; 506U78; GW506U78

Generic Available No

Canadian Brand Names Atriance™

Pharmacologic Category Antineoplastic Agent, Antimetabolite

Use Treatment of relapsed or refractory T-cell acute lymphoblastic leukemia (ALL) and T-cell lymphoblastic lymphoma

Pregnancy Risk Factor D

Lactation Excretion in breast milk unknown/not recommended

Labeled Contraindications Hypersensitivity to nelarabine or any component of the formulation

Warnings/Precautions Hazardous agent - use appropriate precautions for handling and disposal. **[U.S. Boxed Warning]: Neurotoxicity is the dose-limiting toxicity;** observe closely for signs and symptoms of neurotoxicity (somnolence, confusion, convulsions, ataxia, paresthesia, hypoesthesia, coma, status epilepticus, craniospinal demyelination, or ascending neuropathy). Risk of neurotoxicity may increase in patients with concurrent or previous intrathecal chemotherapy or history of craniospinal irradiation. Appropriate measures must be taken to prevent hyperuricemia and tumor lysis syndrome; use extreme caution in patients with increased uric acid, gout, and history of uric acid stones; monitor, consider allopurinol and hydrate accordingly. Bone marrow suppression is common. Avoid administration of live vaccines. Use caution in patients with renal impairment; ara-G clearance may be reduced with renal dysfunction. Use caution with severe hepatic impairment; risk of adverse reactions may be higher with hepatic dysfunction.

[U.S. Boxed Warning]: Should be administered under the supervision of an experienced cancer chemotherapy physician.

Adverse Reactions Note: Pediatric adverse reactions fell within a range similar to adults except where noted.

>10%:

Cardiovascular: Peripheral edema (15%), edema (11%)

Central nervous system: Fatigue (50%), fever (23%), somnolence (7% to 23%; grades 2-4: 1% to 6%), dizziness (21%; grade 2: 8% adults), headache (15% to 17%; grades 2-4: 4% to 8%), hypoesthesia (6% to 17%; grades 2-4: children 5%, adults 12%), pain (11%)

Dermatologic: Petechiae (12%)

Endocrine & metabolic: Hypokalemia (11%)

Gastrointestinal: Nausea (41%), diarrhea (22%), vomiting (10% to 22%), constipation (21%)

Hematologic: Anemia (95% to 99%; grade 4: 10% to 14%), neutropenia (81% to 94%; grade 4: children 62%, adults 49%), thrombocytopenia (86% to 88%; grade 4: 22% to 32%), leukopenia (38%; grade 4: 7%), febrile neutropenia (12%; grade 4: 1%)

Hepatic: Transaminases increased (12%)

Neuromuscular & skeletal: Peripheral neuropathy (12% to 21%; grades 2-4: 11% to 14%), weakness (6% to 17%; grade 4: 1%), paresthesia (4% to 15%; grades 2-4: 3% to 4%), myalgia (13%)

Respiratory: Cough (25%), dyspnea (7% to 20%)

1% to 10%:

Cardiovascular: Hypotension (8%), tachycardia (8%), chest pain (5%)

Central nervous system: Ataxia (2% to 9%; grades 2-4: children 1%, adults 8%), confusion (8%), insomnia (7%), depressed level of consciousness (6%; grades 2-4: 2%), depression (6%), seizure (grade 3: 1% adults; grade 4: 6% children), motor dysfunction (4%; grades 2-4: 2%), amnesia (3%; grades 2-4: 1%), balance disorder (2%; grades 2-4: 1%), nerve paralysis (2%), sensory loss (1% to 2%), aphasia (1%), cerebral hemorrhage (1%), coma (1%), encephalopathy (1%), hemiparesis (1%), hydrocephalus (1%), lethargy (1%), leukoencephalopathy (1%), loss of consciousness (1%), mental impairment (1%), neuropathic pain (1%), nerve palsy (1%), nystagmus (1%), paralysis (1%), sciatica (1%), sensory disturbance (1%), speech disorder (1%), demyelination, ascending peripheral neuropathy

Endocrine & Metabolic: Hypocalcemia (8%), dehydration (7%), hyper-/hypoglycemia (6%), hypomagnesemia (6%)

Gastrointestinal: Abdominal pain (9%), anorexia (9%), stomatitis (8%), abdominal distension (6%), taste perversion (3%)

Hepatic: Albumin decreased (10%), bilirubin increased (10%), AST increased (6%)

Neuromuscular & skeletal: Arthralgia (9%), back pain (8%), muscle weakness (8%), rigors (8%), limb pain (7%), abnormal gait (6%), noncardiac chest pain (5%), tremor (4% to 5%; grades 2-4: 2% to 3%), dysarthria (1%), hyporeflexia (1%), hypertonia (1%), incoordination (1%)

Ocular: Blurred vision (4%)

Renal: Creatinine increased (6%)

Respiratory: Pleural effusion (10%), epistaxis (8%), pneumonia (8%), sinusitis (7%), wheezing (5%), sinus headache (1%)

Miscellaneous: Infection (5% to 9%)

Postmarketing and/or case reports: Tumor lysis syndrome

Drug Interactions

Avoid Concomitant Use

Avoid concomitant use of Nelarabine with any of the following: Natalizumab; Vaccines (Live)

Increased Effect/Toxicity
Nelarabine may increase the levels/effects of: Leflunomide; Natalizumab; Vaccines (Live)

The levels/effects of Nelarabine may be increased by: Trastuzumab
Decreased Effect
Nelarabine may decrease the levels/effects of: Vaccines (Inactivated); Vaccines (Live)

The levels/effects of Nelarabine may be decreased by: Echinacea

Storage/Stability Store unopened vials at 15°C to 30°C (59°F to 86°F). Stable in plastic or glass containers for up to 8 hours at room temperature.

Reconstitution Reconstitution is not required; the appropriate dose should be added to empty plastic bag or glass container.

Compatibility Stable in sodium chloride 0.45%.

Mechanism of Action Nelarabine, a prodrug of ara-G, is demethylated by adenosine deaminase to ara-G and then converted to ara-GTP. Ara-GTP is incorporated into the DNA of the leukemic blasts, leading to inhibition of DNA synthesis and inducing apoptosis. Ara-GTP appears to accumulate at higher levels in T-cells, which correlates to clinical response.

Pharmacodynamics/Kinetics
Distribution: V_{ss}:
  Nelarabine: Children: ~213 L/m^2; Adults: ~197 L/m^2
  Ara-G: Children: ~50 L/m^2; Adults: ~33 L/m^2
Protein binding: Nelarabine and ara-G: <25%
Metabolism: Hepatic; demethylated by adenosine deaminase to form ara-G (active); also hydrolyzed to form methylguanine. Both ara-G and methylguanine metabolized to guanine. Guanine is deaminated into xanthine, which is further oxidized to form uric acid, which is then oxidized to form allantoin.
Half-life elimination: Nelarabine: 30 minutes; ara-G: 3 hours
Time to peak: Ara-G: 3-25 hours
Excretion: Urine (nelarabine 7%, ara-G 27%) within 24 hours of infusion on day 1

Dosage I.V.: T-cell ALL, T-cell lymphoblastic lymphoma:
Children: 650 mg/m^2/day on days 1 through 5; repeat every 21 days
Adults: 1500 mg/m^2/day on days 1, 3, and 5; repeat every 21 days

Dosage adjustment for toxicity:
  Neurologic toxicity ≥ grade 2: Discontinue treatment.
  Hematologic or other (non-neurologic) toxicity: Consider treatment delay.

Dosage adjustment in renal impairment:
Cl_{cr} ≥50 mL/minute: No adjustment recommended
Cl_{cr} <50 mL/minute: Safety has not been established
Cl_{cr} <30 mL/minute: Closely monitor

Dosage adjustment in hepatic impairment: Safety has not been established; closely monitor with severe impairment (bilirubin >3 mg/dL)

Administration Adequate I.V. hydration recommended to prevent tumor lysis syndrome; allopurinol may be used if hyperuricemia is anticipated.
Children: Infuse over 1 hour daily for 5 consecutive days
Adults: Infuse over 2 hours on days 1, 3, and 5

Monitoring Parameters Closely monitor for neurologic toxicity (severe somnolence, seizure, peripheral neuropathy, confusion, ataxia, paresthesia, hypoesthesia, coma, or craniospinal demyelination); signs and symptoms of tumor lysis syndrome; hydration status; CBC with platelet counts, liver and kidney function

◀ **Emetic Potential** Very low (<10%)

Dosage Forms Excipient information presented when available (limited, particularly for generics); consult specific product labeling. [CAN] = Canadian brand name

Injection, solution:

Arranon®: 5 mg/mL (50 mL)

Atriance™ [CAN]: 5 mg/ml (50 mL)

References

Berg SL, Blaney SM, Devidas M, et al, "Phase II Study of Nelarabine (Compound 506U78) in Children and Young Adults With Refractory T-Cell Malignancies: A Report from the Children's Oncology Group," *J Clin Oncol*, 2005, 23(15):3376-82.

Gandhi V, Plunkett W, Weller S, et al, "Evaluation of the Combination of Nelarabine and Fludarabine in Leukemias: Clinical Response, Pharmacokinetics, and Pharmacodynamics in Leukemia Cells," *J Clin Oncol*, 2001, 19(8):2142-52.

Kisor DF, "Nelarabine: A Nucleoside Analog With Efficacy in T-Cell and Other Leukemias," *Ann Pharmacother*, 2005, 39(6):1056-63.

Kurtzberg J, Ernst TJ, Keating MJ, et al, "Phase I Study of 506U78 Administered on a Consecutive 5-Day Schedule in Children and Adults With Refractory Hematologic Malignancies," *J Clin Oncol*, 2005, 23(15):3396-403.

◆ **Neoral®** see CycloSPORINE on page 268

◆ **Neosar** see Cyclophosphamide on page 260

◆ **Neulasta®** see Pegfilgrastim on page 929

◆ **Neumega®** see Oprelvekin on page 880

◆ **Neupogen®** see Filgrastim on page 475

◆ **Nexavar®** see Sorafenib on page 1042

◆ **Niastase® (Can)** see Factor VIIa (Recombinant) on page 446

◆ **Nidagel™ (Can)** see MetroNIDAZOLE on page 793

◆ **Niftolid** see Flutamide on page 506

◆ **Nilandron®** see Nilutamide on page 851

Nilotinib (nye LOE ti nib)

Medication Safety Issues

Sound-alike/look-alike issues:

Nilotinib may be confused with imatinib, nilutamide

High alert medication: The Institute for Safe Medication Practices (ISMP) includes this medication among its list of drug classes which have a heightened risk of causing significant patient harm when used in error.

Related Information

Management of Chemotherapy-Induced Nausea and Vomiting on page 1434

Safe Handling of Hazardous Drugs on page 1517

U.S. Brand Names Tasigna®

Index Terms AMN107; Nilotinib Hydrochloride Monohydrate

Generic Available No

Canadian Brand Names Tasigna®

Pharmacologic Category Antineoplastic Agent, Tyrosine Kinase Inhibitor

Use Treatment of Philadelphia chromosome-positive chronic myelogenous leukemia (Ph+ CML) in chronic and accelerated phase (refractory or intolerant to prior therapy, including imatinib)

Pregnancy Risk Factor D

Lactation Excretion in breast milk unknown/not recommended

Labeled Contraindications Use in patients with hypokalemia, hypomagnesemia, or long QT syndrome

Warnings/Precautions Hazardous agent - use appropriate precautions for handling and disposal. **[U.S. Boxed Warning]: May prolong the QT interval; sudden deaths have been reported. Use in patients with hypokalemia, hypomagnesemia, or long QT syndrome is contraindicated. Correct electrolyte imbalance prior to initiating therapy. Monitor ECG and QT$_c$ (baseline, at 7 days, with dose change, and periodically). Avoid the use of QT-prolonging agents and strong CYP3A4 inhibitors.** Concurrent use with other drugs which may prolong QT interval may increase the risk of potentially-fatal arrhythmias. Concurrent use with CYP3A4 inhibitors/inducers is not recommended; dosage adjustments are recommended if concurrent use cannot be avoided. Sudden deaths appear to be related to dose-dependent ventricular repolarization abnormalities. Prolonged QT interval may result in torsade de pointes, which may cause syncope, seizure, and/or death. Patients with uncontrolled or significant cardiovascular disease were excluded from studies.

[U.S. Boxed Warning]: Use with caution in patients with hepatic impairment; dosage reduction recommended. Nilotinib metabolism is primarily hepatic; carefully monitor for QT prolongation. May cause hepatotoxicity, including dose-limiting elevations in bilirubin, transaminases, and alkaline phosphatase; monitor liver function.

Reversible myelosuppression, including grades 3 and 4 thrombocytopenia, neutropenia, and anemia may occur; may require dose reductions and/or treatment delay. **[U.S. Boxed Warning]: Administer on an empty stomach, at least 1 hour before and 2 hours after food.** Use with caution in patients with a history of pancreatitis, may cause dose-limiting elevations of serum lipase and amylase; monitor. Capsules contain lactose; do not use with galactose intolerance, severe lactase deficiency, or glucose-galactose malabsorption syndromes. Safety and efficacy have not been established in children.

Adverse Reactions Frequency not always defined.

>10%:

Cardiovascular: Peripheral edema (11%)

Central nervous system: Headache (21% to 31%), fatigue (16% to 28%), fever (14% to 24%)

Dermatologic: Rash (28% to 33%), pruritus (20% to 29%)

Endocrine & metabolic: Hyperglycemia (grades 3 & 4: 4% to 11%)

Gastrointestinal: Nausea (18% to 31%), diarrhea (19% to 22%), constipation (18% to 21%), vomiting (10% to 21%), lipase increased (grades 3/4: 15% to 17%), abdominal pain (11% to 13%)

Hematologic: Neutropenia (grades 3/4: 28% to 37%; median duration: 15 days), thrombocytopenia (grade 3: 7% to 11%; grade 4: 17% to 30%; median duration: 22 days), anemia (grades 3/4: 8% to 23%)

Neuromuscular & skeletal: Arthralgia (16% to 18%), limb pain (13% to 16%), myalgia (14%), weakness (12% to 14%), muscle spasm (11% to 14%), bone pain (11% to 13%), back pain (10% to 12%)

Respiratory: Cough (13% to 17%), nasopharyngitis (11% to 16%), dyspnea (8% to 11%)

1% to 10%:

Cardiovascular: Flushing, hypertension, palpitation, QT interval prolonged

Central nervous system: Dizziness, dysphonia, insomnia, vertigo

Dermatologic: Alopecia, dry skin, eczema, erythema, hyperhidrosis, urticaria

Endocrine & metabolic: Hypophosphatemia (grades 3/4: 10%), hypokalemia (grades 3/4: 1% to 5%), hyperkalemia (grades 3/4: 3% to 4%), hypocalcemia (grades 3/4: 1% to 4%), hyponatremia (grades 3/4: 3%), albumin decreased (grades 3/4: 1%), hypomagnesemia

Gastrointestinal: Abdominal discomfort, amylase increased, anorexia, dyspepsia, flatulence, pancreatitis (≤1%)

Hematologic: Neutropenic fever, pancytopenia

Hepatic: Hyperbilirubinemia (grades 3/4: 9% to 10%), ALT increased (grades 3/4: 2% to 4%), alkaline phosphatase increased (grades 3/4: 1% to 3%), AST increased (grades 3/4: 1%), GGT increased

Neuromuscular & skeletal: Musculoskeletal pain, paresthesia

Respiratory: Dyspnea (exertional), pleural effusion (≤1%)

Miscellaneous: Night sweats

<1%, postmarketing, and/or case reports (limited to important or life-threatening): Angina, atrial fibrillation, blurred vision, bradycardia, brain edema, bruising, BUN increased, candidiasis, cardiac failure, cardiac flutter, cardiac murmur, cardiomegaly, chest pain, confusion, coronary artery disease, creatinine elevated, depression, diabetes mellitus, diplopia, dysuria, epistaxis, erectile dysfunction, erythema nodosum, exfoliative rash, extrasystoles, eye hemorrhage, facial edema, gastroenteritis, gastrointestinal hemorrhage, gastrointestinal ulcer perforation, gynecomastia, hematemesis, hematoma, hematuria, hemorrhagic shock, hepatitis, hepatomegaly, hepatotoxicity, herpes simplex, hypercalcemia, hyper-/hypothyroidism, hyperphosphatemia, hypertensive crisis, hypoglycemia, hypotension, influenza-like illness, interstitial lung disease, intracranial hemorrhage, jaundice, joint swelling, lactic dehydrogenase increased, leukocytosis, loss of consciousness, melena, MI, migraine, mouth ulceration, optic neuritis, papilledema, pericardial effusion, pericarditis, periorbital edema, peripheral neuropathy, petechiae, pneumonia, pulmonary edema, pulmonary hypertension, renal failure, retroperitoneal hemorrhage, sepsis, stomatitis, subileus, thrombocytosis, thrombosis, thyroiditis, troponin increased, ulcerative esophagitis, urinary tract infection, ventricular dysfunction, visual acuity decreased

Drug Interactions

Metabolism/Transport Effects Substrate of CYP3A4 (major), P-glycoprotein (P-gp, ABCB1); **Inhibits** CYP3A4, 2C8, 2C9, 2D6, UGT1A1, P-glycoprotein (P-gp, ABCB1); **Induces** CYP2B6, 2C8, 2C9

Avoid Concomitant Use

Avoid concomitant use of Nilotinib with any of the following: Artemether; CYP3A4 Inducers (Strong); CYP3A4 Inhibitors (Strong); Dabigatran Etexilate; Dronedarone; Lumefantrine; Natalizumab; Pimozide; QTc-Prolonging Agents; QuiNINE; Silodosin; Tetrabenazine; Thioridazine; Topotecan; Vaccines (Live); Ziprasidone

Increased Effect/Toxicity

Nilotinib may increase the levels/effects of: Carvedilol; Colchicine; CYP2C8 Substrates (High risk); CYP2C9 Substrates (High risk); CYP2D6 Substrates; Dabigatran Etexilate; Dronedarone; Fesoterodine; Leflunomide; Natalizumab; Nebivolol; P-Glycoprotein Substrates; Pimozide; QTc-Prolonging Agents; QuiNINE; Rivaroxaban; Silodosin; Tamoxifen; Tetrabenazine; Thioridazine; Topotecan; Vaccines (Live); Vitamin K Antagonists; Ziprasidone

The levels/effects of Nilotinib may be increased by: Alfuzosin; Artemether; Chloroquine; Ciprofloxacin; CYP3A4 Inhibitors (Moderate); CYP3A4 Inhibitors (Strong); Gadobutrol; Lumefantrine; QuiNINE; Trastuzumab

Decreased Effect

Nilotinib may decrease the levels/effects of: Cardiac Glycosides; Codeine; TraMADol; Vaccines (Inactivated); Vaccines (Live); Vitamin K Antagonists

The levels/effects of Nilotinib may be decreased by: CYP3A4 Inducers (Strong); Deferasirox; Echinacea; Herbs (CYP3A4 Inducers)

Ethanol/Nutrition/Herb Interactions Herb/Nutraceutical: Avoid St John's wort (may decrease nilotinib levels). Administration with grapefruit juice may result in increased concentrations of nilotinib and potentiate QT prolongation.

Storage/Stability Store at 25°C (77°F); excursions permitted to 15°C to 30°C (59°F to 86°F).

Mechanism of Action Selective tyrosine kinase inhibitor that targets BCR-ABL kinase, c-KIT and platelet derived growth factor receptor (PDGFR); does not have activity against the SRC family. Inhibits BCR-ABL mediated proliferation of leukemic cell lines by binding to the ATP-binding site of BCR-ABL and inhibiting tyrosine kinase activity. Nilotinib has activity in imatinib-resistant BCR-ABL kinase mutations.

Pharmacodynamics/Kinetics

Protein binding: ~98%

Metabolism: Hepatic; oxidation and hydroxylation, via CYP3A4 to primarily inactive metabolites

Bioavailability: Increased 82% when administered 30 minutes after a high-fat meal

Half-life elimination: ~15-17 hours

Time to peak: 3 hours

Excretion: Feces (93%; 69% as parent drug)

Dosage Oral: Adults: Ph+ CML: 400 mg twice daily (continue treatment until disease progression or unacceptable toxicity)

Dosage adjustment for concomitant CYP3A4 inhibitors/inducers:

CYP3A4 inhibitors: The concomitant use of a strong CYP3A4 inhibitor with nilotinib is not recommended. If a strong CYP3A4 inhibitor is required, interruption of nilotinib treatment is recommended; if therapy cannot be interrupted and concurrent use can not be avoided, consider reducing the nilotinib dose by 50%, to 400 mg once daily, with careful monitoring, especially of the QT interval. When a strong CYP3A4 inhibitor is discontinued, allow a washout period prior to adjusting nilotinib dose upward.

CYP3A4 inducers: The concomitant use of a strong CYP3A4 inducer with nilotinib is not recommended. If a strong CYP3A4 inducer is required, the nilotinib dose may need to be increased, with careful monitoring. When the strong CYP3A4 inducer is discontinued, reduce nilotinib to the indicated dose.

Dosage adjustment in renal impairment: Not studied in patients with serum creatinine >1.5 times ULN, however, nilotinib and its metabolites have minimal renal excretion; dosage adjustments for renal dysfunction may not be needed.

Dosage adjustment in hepatic impairment:

At treatment initiation: Consider alternative therapy; if alternative therapy not possible adjust as follows:

Mild-to-moderate impairment (Child-Pugh class A or B): Initial: 400 mg in the morning and 200 mg in the evening daily; may increase to 400 mg twice daily based on patient tolerability

Severe impairment (Child-Pugh class C): Initial: 200 mg twice daily; may increase to 400 mg in the morning and 200 mg in the evening daily; then further increase to 400 mg twice daily based on patient tolerability

For hepatotoxicity during treatment:
If bilirubin >3 times ULN (≥ grade 3): Withhold treatment, monitor bilirubin, resume treatment at 400 mg once daily when bilirubin returns to ≤1.5 times ULN (≤ grade 1)

If ALT or AST >5 times ULN (≥ grade 3): Withhold treatment, monitor transaminases, resume treatment at 400 mg once daily when ALT or AST returns to ≤2.5 times ULN (≤ grade 1)

Dosage adjustment for hematologic toxicity:
ANC <1000/mm^3 and/or platelets <50,000/mm^3: Withhold treatment, monitor blood counts

If ANC >1000/mm^3 and platelets >50,000/mm^3 within 2 weeks: Continue at 400 mg twice daily

If ANC <1000/mm^3 and/or platelets <50,000/mm^3 for >2 weeks: Reduce dose to 400 mg once daily

Dosage adjustment for nonhematologic toxicity:
Amylase or lipase ≥2 times ULN (≥ grade 3): Withhold treatment, monitor serum amylase or lipase, resume treatment at 400 mg once daily when lipase or amylase returns to ≤1.5 times ULN (≤ grade 1)

Clinically-significant moderate or severe nonhematologic toxicity: Withhold treatment, upon resolution of toxicity, resume at 400 mg once daily; may escalate back to 400 mg twice daily if clinically appropriate.

Dosage adjustment for QT prolongation: Note: Repeat ECG ~7 days after any dosage adjustment.
QT$_c$ >480 msec: Withhold treatment, monitor and correct potassium and magnesium levels.
If QT$_c$F returns to <450 msec and to within 20 msec of baseline within 2 weeks: Resume at 400 mg twice daily

If QT$_c$F returns to 450-480 msec for >2 weeks: Reduce dose to 400 mg once daily

If QT$_c$F >480 msec after dosage reduction to 400 mg once daily, discontinue therapy.

Administration Administer twice daily, ~12 hours apart. Swallow capsules whole with water. Administer on an empty stomach, at least 1 hour before or 2 hours after food.

Monitoring Parameters CBC with differential (every 2 weeks for first 2 months, then monthly); electrolytes (including potassium and magnesium; baseline and periodic); hepatic function (ALT/AST, bilirubin, alkaline phosphatase; baseline and periodic); serum lipase (baseline and monthly or as clinically indicated); bone marrow assessments; ECG and QT$_c$ (baseline, 7 days after treatment initiation or dosage adjustments, and periodically thereafter)

Dietary Considerations The bioavailability of nilotinib is increased with food. Take on an empty stomach, at least 1 hour before or 2 hours after food. Avoid grapefruit juice.

Additional Information If clinically indicated, may be administered in combination with hematopoietic growth factors (eg, erythropoietin, filgrastim) and with hydroxyurea or anagrelide.

Emetic Potential Low (10% to 30%)

Dosage Forms Excipient information presented when available (limited, particularly for generics); consult specific product labeling.
Capsule:
Tasigna®: 200 mg

References

Kantarjian HM, Giles F, Gattermann N, et al, "Nilotinib (Formerly AMN107), a Highly Selective Bcr-Abl Tyrosine Kinase Inhibitor, is Effective in Patients With Philadelphia Chromosome-Positive Chronic Myelogenous Leukemia in Chronic Phase Following Imatinib Resistance and Intolerance," *Blood*, 2007, 110(10):3540-6.

Kantarjian H, Giles F, Wunderle L, et al, "Nilotinib in Imatinib-Resistant CML and Philadelphia Chromosome-Positive ALL," *N Engl J Med*, 2006, 354(24):2542-51.

National Comprehensive Cancer Network® (NCCN) "Practice Guidelines in Oncology: Chronic Myelogenous Leukemia Version 2.2010." Available at http://www.nccn.org/professionals/physician_gls/PDF/cml.pdf

Weisberg E, Manley P, Mestan J, et al, "AMN107 (Nilotinib): A Novel and Selective Inhibitor of BCR-ABL," *Br J Cancer*, 2006, 94(12):1765-9.

◆ **Nilotinib Hydrochloride Monohydrate** *see* Nilotinib *on page* 846

◆ **Nilstat (Can)** *see* Nystatin *on page* 855

Nilutamide (ni LOO ta mide)

Medication Safety Issues
Sound-alike/look-alike issues:
Nilutamide may be confused with nilotinib

Related Information
Safe Handling of Hazardous Drugs *on page* 1517

U.S. Brand Names Nilandron®

Index Terms NSC-684588; RU-23908

Generic Available No

Canadian Brand Names Anandron®

Pharmacologic Category Antiandrogen; Antineoplastic Agent, Antiandrogen

Use Treatment of metastatic prostate cancer

Pregnancy Risk Factor C

Lactation Not indicated for use in women

Labeled Contraindications Hypersensitivity to nilutamide or any component of the formulation; severe hepatic impairment; severe respiratory insufficiency

Warnings/Precautions Hazardous agent - use appropriate precautions for handling and disposal. **[U.S. Boxed Warning]: Interstitial pneumonitis has been reported in 2% of patients exposed to nilutamide.** Patients typically experienced progressive exertional dyspnea, and possibly cough, chest pain and fever. X-rays showed interstitial or alveolo-interstitial changes. The suggestive signs of pneumonitis most often occurred within the first 3 months of nilutamide treatment.

Hepatitis or marked increases in liver enzymes leading to drug discontinuation occurred in 1% of nilutamide patients. Rare cases of elevated hepatic enzymes followed by death have been reported.

Thirteen percent to 57% of patients receiving nilutamide reported a delay in adaptation to the dark, ranging from seconds to a few minutes. This effect sometimes does not abate as drug treatment is continued. Caution patients who experience this effect about driving at night or through tunnels. This effect can be alleviated by wearing tinted glasses.

Adverse Reactions
>10%:
Central nervous system: Headache, insomnia
Endocrine & metabolic: Hot flashes (30% to 67%), gynecomastia (10%)
Gastrointestinal: Nausea (mild - 10% to 32%), abdominal pain (10%), constipation, anorexia
Genitourinary: Testicular atrophy (16%), libido decreased
Hepatic: Transaminases increased (8% to 13%; transient)

Ocular: Impaired dark adaptation (13% to 57%), usually reversible with dose reduction, may require discontinuation of the drug in 1% to 2% of patients

Respiratory: Dyspnea (11%)

1% to 10%:

Cardiovascular: Chest pain, edema, heart failure, hypertension, syncope

Central nervous system: Dizziness, drowsiness, fever, malaise, hypoesthesia, depression

Dermatologic: Pruritus, alopecia, dry skin, rash

Endocrine & metabolic: Disulfiram-like reaction (hot flashes, rash) (5%)

Gastrointestinal: Vomiting, diarrhea, dyspepsia, GI hemorrhage, melena, weight loss, xerostomia

Genitourinary: Hematuria, nocturia

Hematologic: Anemia

Hepatic: Hepatitis (1%)

Neuromuscular & skeletal: Arthritis, paresthesia

Ocular: Chromatopsia (9%), abnormal vision (6% to 7%), cataracts, photophobia

Respiratory: Interstitial pneumonitis (2% - typically exertional dyspnea, cough, chest pain, and fever; most often occurring within the first 3 months of treatment); rhinitis

Miscellaneous: Diaphoresis, flu-like syndrome

<1%, postmarketing, and/or case reports: Aplastic anemia

Drug Interactions

Metabolism/Transport Effects Substrate of CYP2C19 (major); **Inhibits** CYP2C19 (weak)

Avoid Concomitant Use There are no known interactions where it is recommended to avoid concomitant use.

Increased Effect/Toxicity

The levels/effects of Nilutamide may be increased by: CYP2C19 Inhibitors (Moderate); CYP2C19 Inhibitors (Strong)

Decreased Effect

The levels/effects of Nilutamide may be decreased by: CYP2C19 Inducers (Strong)

Ethanol/Nutrition/Herb Interactions

Ethanol: Avoid ethanol. Up to 5% of patients may experience a systemic reaction (flushing, hypotension, malaise) when combined with nilutamide.

Herb/Nutraceutical: St John's wort may decrease nilutamide levels.

Storage/Stability Store at room temperature of 15°C to 30°C (59°F to 86°F). Protect from light.

Mechanism of Action Nonsteroidal antiandrogen that inhibits androgen uptake or inhibits binding of androgen in target tissues. It specifically blocks the action of androgens by interacting with cytosolic androgen receptor F sites in target tissue

Pharmacodynamics/Kinetics

Absorption: Rapid and complete

Protein binding: 72% to 85%

Metabolism: Hepatic, forms active metabolites

Half-life elimination: Terminal: 23-87 hours; Metabolites: 35-137 hours

Excretion: Urine (up to 78% at 120 hours; <1% as unchanged drug); feces (1% to 7%)

Dosage Refer to individual protocols.

Adults: Oral: 300 mg daily for 30 days starting the same day or day after surgical castration, then 150 mg/day

Monitoring Parameters Obtain a chest x-ray if a patient reports dyspnea; if there are findings suggestive of interstitial pneumonitis, discontinue treatment with nilutamide. Measure serum hepatic enzyme levels at baseline and at regular intervals (3 months); if transaminases increase over 2-3 times the upper limit of normal, discontinue treatment. Perform appropriate laboratory testing at the first symptom/sign of liver injury (eg, jaundice, dark urine, fatigue, abdominal pain or unexplained GI symptoms).

Dietary Considerations May be taken without regard to food.

Dosage Forms Excipient information presented when available (limited, particularly for generics); consult specific product labeling.

Tablet: 150 mg

References

Bertagna C, DeGery A, Hucher M, et al, "Efficacy of the Combination of Nilutamide Plus Orchidectomy in Patients With Metastatic Prostatic Cancer, A Meta-Analysis of Seven Randomized Double-Blind Trials (1056 Patients)," *Br J Urol*, 1994, 73(4):396-402.

Creaven PJ, Pendyala L, and Tremblay D, "Pharmacokinetics and Metabolism of Nilutamide," *Urology*, 1991, 37(2 Suppl):13-9.

Dijkman GA, Janknegt RA, De Reijke TM, et al, "Long-Term Efficacy and Safety of Nilutamide Plus Castration in Advanced Prostate Cancer, and the Significance of Early Prostate Specific Antigen Normalization. International Anandron Study Group," *J Urol*, 1997, 158(1):160-3.

Dole EJ and Holdsworth MT, "Nilutamide: An Antiandrogen for the Treatment of Prostate Cancer," *Ann Pharmacother*, 1997, 31(1):65-75.

Du Plessis DJ, "Castration Plus Nilutamide vs Castration Plus Placebo in Advanced Prostate Cancer. A Review, *Urology*, 1991, 37(2 Suppl):20-4.

Harris MG, Coleman SG, Faulds D, et al, "Nilutamide. A Review of Its Pharmacodynamic and Pharmacokinetic Properties, and Therapeutic Efficacy in Prostate Cancer," *Drugs Aging*, 1993, 3 (1):9-25.

Pendyala L, Creaven PJ, Huben R, et al, "Pharmacokinetics of Anandron in Patients With Advanced Carcinoma of the Prostate," *Cancer Chemother Pharmacol*, 1988, 22(1):69-76.

- Novo-Hydroxyzin (Can) *see* HydrOXYzine *on page 594*
- Novo-Ketoconazole (Can) *see* Ketoconazole *on page 677*
- Novo-Levofloxacin (Can) *see* Levofloxacin *on page 707*
- Novo-Lorazepam (Can) *see* LORazepam *on page 731*
- Novo-Medrone (Can) *see* MedroxyPROGESTERone *on page 739*
- Novo-Morphine SR (Can) *see* Morphine Sulfate *on page 816*
- Novo-Ofloxacin (Can) *see* Ofloxacin *on page 863*
- Novo-Olanzapine (Can) *see* OLANZapine *on page 869*
- Novo-Ondansetron (Can) *see* Ondansetron *on page 874*
- Novo-Peridol (Can) *see* Haloperidol *on page 556*
- Novo-Prednisolone (Can) *see* PrednisoLONE *on page 977*
- Novo-Prednisone (Can) *see* PredniSONE *on page 982*
- Novo-Purol (Can) *see* Allopurinol *on page 37*
- Novo-Raloxifene (Can) *see* Raloxifene *on page 1002*
- NovoSeven [DSC] *see* Factor VIIa (Recombinant) *on page 446*
- NovoSeven® RT *see* Factor VIIa (Recombinant) *on page 446*
- Novo-Tamoxifen (Can) *see* Tamoxifen *on page 1072*
- Novo-Trimel (Can) *see* Sulfamethoxazole and Trimethoprim *on page 1051*
- Novo-Trimel D.S. (Can) *see* Sulfamethoxazole and Trimethoprim *on page 1051*
- Noxafil® *see* Posaconazole *on page 970*
- Nplate™ *see* Romiplostim *on page 1024*
- NSC-750 *see* Busulfan *on page 160*
- NSC-755 *see* Mercaptopurine *on page 754*
- NSC-762 *see* Mechlorethamine *on page 736*
- NSC-13875 *see* Altretamine *on page 48*
- NSC-15200 *see* Gallium Nitrate *on page 523*
- NSC-63878 *see* Cytarabine *on page 281*
- NSC-71423 *see* Megestrol *on page 743*
- NSC-89199 *see* Estramustine *on page 426*
- NSC-105014 *see* Cladribine *on page 244*
- NSC-106977 (*Erwinia*) *see* Asparaginase *on page 111*
- NSC-109229 (*E. coli*) *see* Asparaginase *on page 111*
- NSC-125066 *see* Bleomycin *on page 151*
- NSC-127716 *see* Decitabine *on page 327*
- NSC-147834 *see* Flutamide *on page 506*
- NSC-169780 *see* Dexrazoxane *on page 357*
- NSC-218321 *see* Pentostatin *on page 949*
- NSC-241240 *see* CARBOplatin *on page 178*
- NSC-245467 *see* Vindesine *on page 1180*
- NSC-249992 *see* Amsacrine *on page 79*
- NSC-312887 *see* Fludarabine *on page 492*
- NSC606869 *see* Clofarabine *on page 250*
- NSC-613795 *see* Sargramostim *on page 1029*

- ◆ **NSC-614629** *see* Filgrastim *on page 475*
- ◆ **NSC-628503** *see* Docetaxel *on page 361*
- ◆ **NSC-644468** *see* Deferoxamine *on page 334*
- ◆ **NSC-671663** *see* Octreotide *on page 857*
- ◆ **NSC-681239** *see* Bortezomib *on page 155*
- ◆ **NSC-683864** *see* Temsirolimus *on page 1083*
- ◆ **NSC-684588** *see* Nilutamide *on page 851*
- ◆ **NSC-688097** *see* Trastuzumab *on page 1136*
- ◆ **NSC-697732** *see* DAUNOrubicin Citrate (Liposomal) *on page 319*
- ◆ **NSC-701852** *see* Vorinostat *on page 1193*
- ◆ **NSC-706363** *see* Arsenic Trioxide *on page 107*
- ◆ **NSC-712807** *see* Capecitabine *on page 173*
- ◆ **NSC-714371** *see* Dalteparin *on page 303*
- ◆ **NSC-715055** *see* Gefitinib *on page 528*
- ◆ **NSC-720568** *see* Gemtuzumab Ozogamicin *on page 537*
- ◆ **NSC-722848** *see* Oprelvekin *on page 880*
- ◆ **NSC-724223** *see* Epoetin Alfa *on page 412*
- ◆ **NSC-724577** *see* Anagrelide *on page 83*
- ◆ **NSC-724772** *see* Sorafenib *on page 1042*
- ◆ **NSC-725961** *see* Pegfilgrastim *on page 929*
- ◆ **NSC-729969** *see* Darbepoetin Alfa *on page 308*
- ◆ **N-trifluoroacetyladriamycin-14-valerate** *see* Valrubicin *on page 1160*
- ◆ **Nu-Acyclovir (Can)** *see* Acyclovir *on page 18*
- ◆ **Nu-Cotrimox (Can)** *see* Sulfamethoxazole and Trimethoprim *on page 1051*
- ◆ **Nu-Loraz (Can)** *see* LORazepam *on page 731*
- ◆ **Nu-Megestrol (Can)** *see* Megestrol *on page 743*
- ◆ **Nu-Metoclopramide (Can)** *see* Metoclopramide *on page 788*
- ◆ **Numoisyn™** *see* Saliva Substitute *on page 1027*
- ◆ **Nupercainal® Hydrocortisone Cream [OTC]** *see* Hydrocortisone *on page 575*
- ◆ **Nu-Prochlor (Can)** *see* Prochlorperazine *on page 992*
- ◆ **Nutracort®** *see* Hydrocortisone *on page 575*
- ◆ **Nyaderm (Can)** *see* Nystatin *on page 855*
- ◆ **Nyamyc™** *see* Nystatin *on page 855*

Nystatin (nye STAT in)

Medication Safety Issues

Sound-alike/look-alike issues:

Nystatin may be confused with HMG-CoA reductase inhibitors (also known as "statins"; eg, atorvastatin, fluvastatin, lovastatin, pitavastatin, pravastatin, rosuvastatin, simvastatin), Nilstat®, Nitrostat®

Nilstat may be confused with Nitrostat®, nystatin

Related Information

Oral Mucositis / Stomatitis *on page 1460*

U.S. Brand Names Bio-Statin®; Mycostatin®; Nyamyc™; Nystat-Rx®; Nystop®; Paddock Nystatin™; Pedi-Dri®

Generic Available Yes: Cream, ointment, powder, suspension, tablet

◄ **Canadian Brand Names** Candistatin®; Nilstat; Nyaderm; PMS-Nystatin

Pharmacologic Category Antifungal Agent, Oral Nonabsorbed; Antifungal Agent, Topical; Antifungal Agent, Vaginal

Use Treatment of susceptible cutaneous, mucocutaneous, and oral cavity fungal infections normally caused by the *Candida* species

Pregnancy Risk Factor B/C (oral)

Lactation Does not enter breast milk/compatible (not absorbed orally)

Labeled Contraindications Hypersensitivity to nystatin or any component of the formulation

Adverse Reactions

Frequency not defined: Dermatologic: Contact dermatitis, Stevens-Johnson syndrome

1% to 10%: Gastrointestinal: Diarrhea, nausea, stomach pain, vomiting

<1%: Hypersensitivity reactions

Drug Interactions

Avoid Concomitant Use There are no known interactions where it is recommended to avoid concomitant use.

Increased Effect/Toxicity There are no known significant interactions involving an increase in effect.

Decreased Effect

Nystatin may decrease the levels/effects of: Saccharomyces boulardii

Storage/Stability

Vaginal insert: Store in refrigerator. Protect from temperature extremes, moisture, and light.

Oral tablet, ointment, topical powder, and oral suspension: Store at controlled room temperature 15°C to 25°C (59°F to 77°F).

Mechanism of Action Binds to sterols in fungal cell membrane, changing the cell wall permeability allowing for leakage of cellular contents

Pharmacodynamics/Kinetics

Onset of action: Symptomatic relief from candidiasis: 24-72 hours

Absorption: Topical: None through mucous membranes or intact skin; Oral: Poorly absorbed

Excretion: Feces (as unchanged drug)

Dosage

Oral candidiasis:

Suspension (swish and swallow orally):

Premature infants: 100,000 units 4 times/day

Infants: 200,000 units 4 times/day or 100,000 units to each side of mouth 4 times/day

Children and Adults: 400,000-600,000 units 4 times/day

Powder for compounding: Children and Adults: 1/8 teaspoon (500,000 units) to equal approximately 1/2 cup of water; give 4 times/day

Mucocutaneous infections: Children and Adults: Topical: Apply 2-3 times/day to affected areas; very moist topical lesions are treated best with powder

Intestinal infections: Adults: Oral: 500,000-1,000,000 units every 8 hours

Vaginal infections: Adults: Vaginal tablets: Insert 1 tablet/day at bedtime for 2 weeks

Administration Suspension: Shake well before using. Should be swished about the mouth and retained in the mouth for as long as possible (several minutes) before swallowing.

Dosage Forms Excipient information presented when available (limited, particularly for generics); consult specific product labeling. [DSC] = Discontinued product

Capsule:
  Bio-Statin®: 500,000 units, 1 million units
Cream: 100,000 units/g (15 g, 30 g)
  Mycostatin®: 100,000 units/g (30 g)
Ointment, topical: 100,000 units/g (15 g, 30 g)
Powder, for prescription compounding: 50 million units (10 g); 150 million units (30 g); 500 million units (100 g); 2 billion units (400 g)
  Nystat-Rx®: 50 million units (10 g); 150 million units (30 g); 500 million units (100 g); 1 billion units (190 g); 2 billion units (350 g)
Powder, for prescription compounding: 50 million units (10 g); 150 million units (30 g); 500 million units (100 g); 1 billion units (190 g); 2 billion units (350 g)
  Bio-Statin®: 2 billion units (30 g)
Powder for suspension, oral [preservative free]:
  Paddock Nystatin™: 50 million units (10 g); 150 million units (30 g); 500 million units (100 g); 2 billion units (400 g) [sugar free]
Powder, topical:
  Mycostatin®: 100,000 units/g (15 g) [contains talc] [DSC]
  Nyamyc™: 100,000 units/g (15 g, 30 g) [contains talc]
  Nystop®: 100,000 units/g (15 g, 30 g, 60 g) [contains talc]
  Pedi-Dri®: 100,000 units/g (56.7 g) [contains talc]
Suspension, oral: 100,000 units/mL (5 mL, 60 mL, 480 mL)
Tablet: 500,000 units
Tablet, vaginal: 100,000 units (15s) [packaged with applicator]

References

Dismukes WE, Wade JS, Lee JY, et al, "A Randomized, Double-Blind Trial of Nystatin Therapy for the Candidiasis Hypersensitivity Syndrome," *N Engl J Med*, 1990, 323(25):1717-23.

Epstein JB, Vickars L, Spinelli J, et al, "Efficacy of Chlorhexidine and Nystatin Rinses in Prevention of Oral Complications in Leukemia and Bone Marrow Transplantation," *Oral Surg Oral Med Oral Pathol*, 1992, 73(6):682-9.

Meunier-Carpentier F, "Symposium on Infectious Complications of Neoplastic Disease (Part II). Chemoprophylaxis of Fungal Infections," *Am J Med*, 1984, 76(4):652-6.

Poland JM, "Oral Thrush in the Oncologic Patient. Therapy Must Be Tailored," *Am J Hosp Care* 1987, 4(5):30-2.

◆ **Nystat-Rx®** see Nystatin on page 855

◆ **Nystop®** see Nystatin on page 855

◆ **Oasis®** see Saliva Substitute on page 1027

◆ **Octagam®** see Immune Globulin (Intravenous) on page 627

◆ **Octostim® (Can)** see Desmopressin on page 344

Octreotide (ok TREE oh tide)

Medication Safety Issues
Sound-alike/look-alike issues:
  Sandostatin® may be confused with Sandimmune®, Sandostatin LAR®, sargramostim, simvastatin

U.S. Brand Names Sandostatin LAR®; Sandostatin®

Index Terms NSC-671663; Octreotide Acetate

Generic Available Yes: Injection solution (excludes depot formulation)

Canadian Brand Names Octreotide Acetate Injection; Octreotide Acetate Omega; Sandostatin LAR®; Sandostatin®

Pharmacologic Category Antidiarrheal; Antidote; Somatostatin Analog

Use Control of symptoms in patients with metastatic carcinoid and vasoactive intestinal peptide-secreting tumors (VIPomas); treatment of acromegaly

Unlabeled/Investigational Use Secretory diarrhea (AIDS-associated [including *Cryptosporidiosis*], chemotherapy-induced, graft-versus-host disease (GVHD) induced, and postgastrectomy dumping syndrome); control of bleeding of esophageal varices; second-line treatment for thymic malignancies; Cushing's syndrome (ectopic); insulinomas; small bowel fistulas; pancreatic tumors; gastrinoma; Zollinger-Ellison syndrome; congenital hyperinsulinism; hypothalamic obesity; treatment of hypoglycemia secondary to sulfonylurea poisoning

Pregnancy Risk Factor B

Lactation Excretion in breast milk unknown/use caution

Labeled Contraindications Hypersensitivity to octreotide or any component of the formulation

Warnings/Precautions May impair gallbladder function; monitor patients for cholelithiasis. Use with caution in patients with renal and/or hepatic impairment; dosage adjustment is required in patients receiving dialysis and in patients with established cirrhosis. Somatostatin analogs may affect glucose regulation. In type I diabetes, severe hypoglycemia may occur; in type II diabetes or patients without diabetes, hyperglycemia may occur. Insulin and other hypoglycemic medication requirements may change. Do not use depot formulation for the treatment of sulfonylurea-induced hypoglycemia. Bradycardia, conduction abnormalities, and arrhythmia have been observed in acromegalic and carcinoid syndrome patients; use caution with CHF or concomitant medications that alter heart rate or rhythm. Cardiovascular medication requirements may change. Octreotide may enhance the adverse/toxic effects of other QT_c-prolonging agents. May alter absorption of dietary fats; monitor for pancreatitis. May reduce excessive fluid loss in patients with conditions that cause such loss; monitor for elevations in zinc levels in such patients that are maintained on total parenteral nutrition (TPN). Chronic treatment has been associated with abnormal Schillings test; monitor vitamin B_{12} levels. Suppresses secretion of TSH; monitor for hypothyroidism. Therapy may restore fertility; females of childbearing potential should use adequate contraception. Dosage adjustment may be necessary in the elderly; significant increases in elimination half-life have been observed in older adults. Vehicle used in depot injection (polylactide-co-glycolide microspheres) has rarely been associated with retinal artery occlusion in patients with abnormal arteriovenous anastomosis.

Adverse Reactions Adverse reactions vary by route of administration and dosage form. Frequency of cardiac, endocrine, and gastrointestinal adverse reactions was generally higher in acromegalics.

>16%:
  Cardiovascular: Sinus bradycardia (19% to 25%), chest pain (≤20%; non-depot formulations)
  Central nervous system: Fatigue (1% to 32%), headache (6% to 30%), malaise (16% to 20%), fever (16% to 20%), dizziness (5% to 20%)
  Dermatologic: Pruritus (≤18%)
  Endocrine & metabolic: Hyperglycemia (2% to 27%)
  Gastrointestinal: Abdominal pain (5% to 61%), loose stools (5% to 61%), nausea (5% to 61%), diarrhea (34% to 58%), flatulence (≤38%), cholelithiasis (13% to 38%; length of therapy dependent), biliary sludge (24%; length of therapy dependent), constipation (9% to 21%), vomiting (4% to 21%), biliary duct dilatation (12%)
  Local: Injection site pain (2% to 50%; dose and formulation related)
  Neuromuscular & skeletal: Back pain (1% to 27%), arthropathy (8% to 19%), myalgia (≤18%)
  Respiratory: Upper respiratory infection (10% to 23%), dyspnea (≤20%; non-depot formulations)

Miscellaneous: Antibodies to octreotide (up to 25%; no efficacy change), flu symptoms (1% to 20%)

5% to 15%:

Cardiovascular: Hypertension (≤13%), conduction abnormalities (9% to 10%), arrhythmia (3% to 9%), palpitation, peripheral edema

Central nervous system: Pain (4% to 15%), anxiety, confusion, hypoesthesia, insomnia

Dermatologic: Rash (15%; depot formulation), alopecia (≤13%)

Endocrine & metabolic: Hypothyroidism (≤12%; non-depot formulations), goiter (≤8%; non-depot formulations)

Gastrointestinal: Anorexia, cramping, tenesmus (4% to 6%), dyspepsia (4% to 6%), steatorrhea (4% to 6%), feces discoloration (4% to 6%)

Hematologic: Anemia (≤15%; non-depot formulations: <1%)

Neuromuscular & skeletal: Arthralgia, myalgia, paresthesia, rigors, weakness

Otic: Earache

Renal: Renal calculus

Respiratory: Cough, pharyngitis, sinusitis, rhinitis

Miscellaneous: Allergy, diaphoresis

1% to 4%:

Cardiovascular: Angina, cardiac failure, edema, flushing, hematoma, phlebitis

Central nervous system: Abnormal gait, amnesia, depression, dysphonia, hallucinations, nervousness, neuralgia, somnolence, vertigo

Dermatologic: Acne, bruising, cellulitis

Endocrine & metabolic: Hypoglycemia (2% to 4%), hypokalemia, hypoproteinemia, gout, cachexia, breast pain, impotence

Gastrointestinal: Colitis, diverticulitis, dysphagia, fat malabsorption, gastritis, gastroenteritis, gingivitis, glossitis, melena, stomatitis, taste perversion, xerostomia

Genitourinary: Incontinence, pollakuria (non-depot formulations), urinary tract infection

Local: Injection site hematoma

Neuromuscular & skeletal: Hyperkinesia, hypertonia, joint pain, neuropathy, tremor

Ocular: Blurred vision, visual disturbance

Otic: Tinnitus

Renal: Albuminuria, renal abscess

Respiratory: Bronchitis, epistaxis

Miscellaneous: Bacterial infection, cold symptoms, moniliasis

<1%, postmarketing, and/or case reports (limited to important or life-threatening): Anaphylactic shock, anaphylactoid reaction, aneurysm, aphasia, appendicitis, arthritis, ascending cholangitis, ascites, atrial fibrillation, basal cell carcinoma, Bell's palsy, biliary obstruction, breast carcinoma, cardiac arrest, cerebral vascular disorder, CHF, cholestatic hepatitis, CK increased, creatinine increased, deafness, diabetes insipidus, diabetes mellitus, facial edema, fatty liver, galactorrhea, gallbladder polyp, GI bleeding, GI hemorrhage, GI ulcer, glaucoma, gynecomastia, hearing loss, hematuria, hemiparesis, hemorrhoids, hepatitis, hyperesthesia, hypertensive reaction, hypoadrenalism, intestinal obstruction, intracranial hemorrhage, intraocular pressure increased, ischemia, jaundice, joint effusion, lactation, LFTs increased, libido decreased, malignant hyperpyrexia, menstrual irregularities, MI, migraine, nephrolithiasis, neuritis, orthostatic hypotension, pancreatitis, pancytopenia, paresis, petechiae, pituitary apoplexy, pleural effusion, pneumonia, pneumothorax, pulmonary embolism, pulmonary hypertension, pulmonary nodule, Raynaud's syndrome, rectal bleeding, renal failure, renal

insufficiency, retinal vein thrombosis, scotoma, seizure, status asthmaticus, suicide attempt, syncope, tachycardia, thrombocytopenia, thrombophlebitis, thrombosis, urticaria, visual field defect, weight loss, wheal/erythema

Drug Interactions

Avoid Concomitant Use

Avoid concomitant use of Octreotide with any of the following: Artemether; Dronedarone; Lumefantrine; Nilotinib; Pimozide; QuiNINE; Tetrabenazine; Thioridazine; Ziprasidone

Increased Effect/Toxicity

Octreotide may increase the levels/effects of: Codeine; Dronedarone; Hypoglycemic Agents; Pegvisomant; Pimozide; QTc-Prolonging Agents; QuiNINE; Tetrabenazine; Thioridazine; Ziprasidone

The levels/effects of Octreotide may be increased by: Alfuzosin; Artemether; Chloroquine; Ciprofloxacin; Gadobutrol; Herbs (Hypoglycemic Properties); Lumefantrine; Nilotinib; QuiNINE

Decreased Effect

Octreotide may decrease the levels/effects of: CycloSPORINE

Ethanol/Nutrition/Herb Interactions

Herb/Nutraceutical: Avoid hypoglycemic herbs, including alfalfa, aloe, bilberry, bitter melon, burdock, celery, damiana, fenugreek, garcinia, garlic, ginger, ginseng (American), gymnema, marshmallow, and stinging nettle (may enhance the hypoglycemic effect of octreotide).

Storage/Stability

Solution: Octreotide is a clear solution and should be stored at refrigerated temperatures between 2°C and 8°C (36°F and 46°F). Protect from light. May be stored at room temperature of 20°C to 30°C (70°F and 86°F) for up to 14 days when protected from light. Stability of parenteral admixture is stable in NS for 96 hours at room temperature (25°C) and in D_5W for 24 hours. Discard multidose vials within 14 days after initial entry.

Suspension: Prior to dilution, store at refrigerated temperatures between 2°C and 8°C (36°F and 46°F) and protect from light. Depot drug product kit may be at room temperature for 30-60 minutes prior to use. Use suspension immediately after preparation.

Compatibility Solution: Stable in D_5W, NS; **incompatible** with fat emulsion 10%; **variable stability** in TPN (The manufacturer states that octreotide solution is not compatible in TPN solutions due to the formation of a glycosyl octreotide conjugate which may have decreased activity; other sources give it limited compatibility.)

Y-site administration: Incompatible: Micafungin. **Variable (consult detailed reference):** Pantoprazole, TPN.

Compatibility when admixed: Compatible: Heparin. **Incompatible:** Pantoprazole.

Mechanism of Action Mimics natural somatostatin by inhibiting serotonin release, and the secretion of gastrin, VIP, insulin, glucagon, secretin, motilin, and pancreatic polypeptide. Decreases growth hormone and IGF-1 in acromegaly. Octreotide provides more potent inhibition of growth hormone, glucagon, and insulin as compared to endogenous somatostatin. Also suppresses LH response to GnRH, secretion of thyroid-stimulating hormone and decreases splanchnic blood flow.

Pharmacodynamics/Kinetics

Duration: SubQ: 6-12 hours

Absorption: SubQ: Rapid and complete; I.M. (depot formulation): Released slowly (via microsphere degradation in the muscle)

Distribution: V_d: 14 L (13-30 L in acromegaly)

Protein binding: 65%, mainly to lipoprotein (41% in acromegaly)

Metabolism: Extensively hepatic

Bioavailability: SubQ: 100%; I.M: 60% to 63% of SubQ dose

Half-life elimination: 1.7-1.9 hours; Increased in elderly patients; Cirrhosis: Up to 3.7 hours; Fatty liver disease: Up to 3.4 hours; Renal impairment: Up to 3.1 hours

Time to peak, plasma: SubQ: 0.4 hours (0.7 hours acromegaly); I.M.: 1 hour

Excretion: Urine (32% as unchanged drug)

Dosage

Acromegaly: Adults:

SubQ, I.V.: Initial: 50 mcg 3 times/day; titrate to achieve growth hormone levels <5 ng/mL or IGF-I (somatomedin C) levels <1.9 units/mL in males and <2.2 units/mL in females. Usual effective dose 100-200 mcg 3 times/day; range 300-1500 mcg/day. **Note:** Should be withdrawn yearly for a 4-week interval (8 weeks for depot injection) in patients who have received irradiation. Resume if levels increase and signs/symptoms recur.

I.M. depot injection: Patients must be stabilized on subcutaneous octreotide for at least 2 weeks before switching to the long-acting depot. Upon switch: 20 mg I.M. intragluteally every 4 weeks for 3 months, then the dose may be modified based upon response.

Dosage adjustment for acromegaly: After 3 months of depot injections, the dosage may be continued or modified as follows:

GH ≤1 ng/mL, IGF-1 normal, and symptoms controlled: Reduce octreotide LAR® to 10 mg I.M. every 4 weeks

GH ≤2.5 ng/mL, IGF-1 normal, and symptoms controlled: Maintain octreotide LAR® at 20 mg I.M. every 4 weeks

GH >2.5 ng/mL, IGF-1 elevated, and/or symptoms uncontrolled: Increase octreotide LAR® to 30 mg I.M. every 4 weeks

Note: Patients not adequately controlled at a dose of 30 mg may increase dose to 40 mg every 4 weeks. Dosages >40 mg are not recommended.

Carcinoid tumors: Adults:

SubQ, I.V.: Initial 2 weeks: 100-600 mcg/day in 2-4 divided doses; usual range 50-750 mcg/day (some patients may require up to 1500 mcg/day)

I.M. depot injection: Patients must be stabilized on subcutaneous octreotide for at least 2 weeks before switching to the long-acting depot. Upon switch: 20 mg I.M. intragluteally every 4 weeks for 2 months, then the dose may be modified based upon response.

Note: Patients should continue to receive their SubQ injections for the first 2 weeks at the same dose in order to maintain therapeutic levels (some patients may require 3-4 weeks of continued SubQ injections). Patients who experience periodic exacerbations of symptoms may require temporary SubQ injections in addition to depot injections (at their previous SubQ dosing regimen) until symptoms have resolved.

Dosage adjustment: See dosing adjustment for VIPomas.

VIPomas: Adults:

SubQ, I.V.: Initial 2 weeks: 200-300 mcg/day in 2-4 divided doses; titrate dose based on response/tolerance. Range: 150-750 mcg/day (doses >450 mcg/day are rarely required)

I.M. depot injection: Patients must be stabilized on subcutaneous octreotide for at least 2 weeks before switching to the long-acting depot. Upon switch: 20 mg I.M. intragluteally every 4 weeks for 2 months, then the dose may be modified based upon response.

Note: Patients receiving depot injection should continue to receive their SubQ injections for the first 2 weeks at the same dose in order to maintain therapeutic levels (some patients may require 3-4 weeks of continued SubQ injections). Patients who experience periodic exacerbations of symptoms may require temporary SubQ injections in addition to depot injections (at their previous SubQ dosing regimen) until symptoms have resolved.

Dosage adjustment for carcinoid tumors and VIPomas: After 2 months of depot injections, the dosage may be continued or modified as follows:

Increase to 30 mg I.M. every 4 weeks if symptoms are inadequately controlled

Decrease to 10 mg I.M. every 4 weeks, for a trial period, if initially responsive to 20 mg dose

Dosage >30 mg is not recommended

Congenital hyperinsulinism (unlabeled use): Infants and Children: SubQ: Doses of 3-40 mcg/kg/day have been used

Diarrhea (unlabeled use):

Infants and Children: I.V., SubQ: Doses of 1-10 mcg/kg every 12 hours have been used in children beginning at the low end of the range and increasing by 0.3 mcg/kg/dose at 3-day intervals. Suppression of growth hormone (animal data) is of concern when used as long-term therapy.

Adults: I.V.: Initial: 50-100 mcg every 8 hours; increase by 100 mcg/dose at 48-hour intervals; maximum dose: 500 mcg every 8 hours

Esophageal varices bleeding (unlabeled use): Adults: I.V. bolus: 25-50 mcg followed by continuous I.V. infusion of 25-50 mcg/hour

Hypoglycemia in sulfonylurea poisoning (unlabeled use): Note: SubQ is the preferred route of administration; repeat dosing, dose escalation, or initiation of a continuous infusion may be required in patients who experience recurrent hypoglycemia. Duration of treatment may exceed 24 hours. Optimal care decisions should be made based upon patient-specific details:

Children: SubQ: 1-1.5 mcg/kg; repeat in 6-12 hours as needed based upon blood glucose concentrations

Adults:

SubQ: 50-100 mcg; repeat in 6-12 hours as needed based upon blood glucose concentrations

I.V.: Doses up to 100-125 mcg/hour have been used successfully

Elderly: Elimination half-life is increased by 46% and clearance is decreased by 26%; dose adjustment may be required. Dosing should generally begin at the lower end of dosing range.

Dosage adjustment in renal impairment:

Nondialysis-dependent renal impairment: No dosage adjustment required

Dialysis-dependent renal impairment: Depot injection: Initial dose: 10 mg I.M. every 4 weeks; titrate based upon response (clearance is reduced by ~50%)

Dosage adjustment in hepatic impairment: Patients with established cirrhosis of the liver: Depot injection: Initial dose: 10 mg I.M. every 4 weeks; titrate based upon response

Administration

Regular injection formulation (do not use if solution contains particles or is discolored): Administer SubQ or I.V.; I.V. administration may be IVP, IVPB, or continuous I.V. infusion (unlabeled route):

IVP should be administered undiluted over 3 minutes

IVPB should be administered over 15-30 minutes

Continuous I.V. infusion rates have ranged from 25-50 mcg/hour for the treatment of esophageal variceal bleeding (unlabeled route/use); continuous I.V. infusion rates of 100-125 mcg/hour have been used for the treatment of sulfonylurea-induced hypoglycemia (unlabeled use).

SubQ: Use the concentration with smallest volume to deliver dose to reduce injection site pain. Rotate injection site; may bring to room temperature prior to injection.

Depot formulation: Administer I.M. intragluteal (avoid deltoid administration); alternate gluteal injection sites to avoid irritation. Do not administer Sandostatin LAR® intravenously or subcutaneously; must be administered immediately after mixing.

Monitoring Parameters

Acromegaly: Growth hormone, somatomedin C (IGF-1)

Carcinoid: 5-HIAA, plasma serotonin and plasma substance P

VIPomas: Vasoactive intestinal peptide

Chronic therapy: Thyroid function (baseline and periodic), vitamin B_{12} level, blood glucose, cardiac function (heart rate, ECG), zinc level (patients with excessive fluid loss maintained on TPN)

Dietary Considerations Schedule injections between meals to decrease GI effects. May alter absorption of dietary fats.

Dosage Forms Excipient information presented when available (limited, particularly for generics); consult specific product labeling.

Injection, microspheres for suspension, as acetate [depot formulation]:
Sandostatin LAR®: 10 mg, 20 mg, 30 mg [contains polylactide-co-glycolide; packaged with diluent and syringe]

Injection, solution, as acetate: 0.2 mg/mL (5 mL); 1 mg/mL (5 mL)
Sandostatin®: 0.2 mg/mL (5 mL); 1 mg/mL (5 mL)

Injection, solution, as acetate [preservative free]: 0.05 mg/mL (1 mL); 0.1 mg/mL (1 mL); 0.5 mg/mL (1 mL)
Sandostatin®: 0.05 mg/mL (1 mL); 0.1 mg/mL (1 mL); 0.5 mg/mL (1 mL)

References

Baillie-Johnson HR, "Octreotide in the Management of Treatment-Related Diarrhoea," *Anticancer Drugs*, 1996, 7(Suppl 1):11-5.

Corley DA, Cello JP, Adkisson W, et al, "Octreotide for Acute Esophageal Variceal Bleeding: A Meta-analysis," *Gastroenterology*, 2001, 120(4):946-54.

Erstad BL, "Octreotide for Acute Variceal Bleeding," *Ann Pharmacother*, 2001, 35(5):618-26.

Heikenen JB, Pohl JF, Werlin SL, et al, "Octreotide in Pediatric Patients," *J Pediatr Gastroenterol Nutr*, 2002, 35(5):600-9.

Hejna M, Schmidinger M, and Raderer M, "The Clinical Role of Somatostatin Analogues as Antineoplastic Agents: Much Ado About Nothing?" *Ann Oncol*, 2002, 13(5):653-68.

Jenkins SA, "Somatostatin in Acute Bleeding Oesophageal Varices. Clinical Evidence," *Drugs*, 1992, 44(Suppl 2):36-55.

Pollak M, "The Potential Role of Somatostatin Analogues in Breast Cancer Treatment," *Yale J Biol Med*, 1997, 70(5-6):535-9.

Tassiopoulos AK, Baum G, and Halverson JD, "Small Bowel Fistulas," *Surg Clin North Am*, 1996, 76(5):1175-81

von Werder K, Muller OA, and Stalla GK, "Somatostatin Analogs in Ectopic Corticotropin Production," *Metabolism*, 1996, 45(8 Suppl 1):129-31.

◆ **Octreotide Acetate** *see* Octreotide *on page 857*

◆ **Octreotide Acetate Injection (Can)** *see* Octreotide *on page 857*

◆ **Octreotide Acetate Omega (Can)** *see* Octreotide *on page 857*

◆ **Ocuflox®** *see* Ofloxacin *on page 863*

Ofloxacin (oh FLOKS a sin)

Medication Safety Issues

Sound-alike/look-alike issues:
Floxin® may be confused with Flexeril®
Ocuflox® may be confused with Occlusal®-HP, Ocufen®

International issues:

Floxin® may be confused with Flogen® which is a brand name for naproxen in Mexico

Floxin® may be confused with Fluoxin® which is a brand name for fluoxetine in the Czech Republic and Romania

Floxin® may be confused with Flexin® which is a brand name for orphenadrine in Israel and indomethacin in Great Britain

U.S. Brand Names Floxin®; Ocuflox®

Index Terms Floxin Otic Singles

Generic Available Yes

Canadian Brand Names Apo-Ofloxacin®; Apo-Oflox®; Floxin®; Novo-Ofloxacin; Ocuflox®; PMS-Ofloxacin

Pharmacologic Category Antibiotic, Quinolone

Use

Quinolone antibiotic for the treatment of acute exacerbations of chronic bronchitis, community-acquired pneumonia, skin and skin structure infections (uncomplicated), urethral and cervical gonorrhea (acute, uncomplicated), urethritis and cervicitis (nongonococcal), mixed infections of the urethra and cervix, pelvic inflammatory disease (acute), cystitis (uncomplicated), urinary tract infections (complicated), prostatitis

Note: As of April 2007, the CDC no longer recommends the use of fluoroquinolones for the treatment of gonococcal disease.

Ophthalmic: Treatment of superficial ocular infections involving the conjunctiva or cornea due to strains of susceptible organisms

Otic: Otitis externa, chronic suppurative otitis media, acute otitis media

Unlabeled/Investigational Use Epididymitis (nongonococcal), leprosy, Traveler's diarrhea

Pregnancy Risk Factor C

Lactation Enters breast milk/not recommended (AAP rates "compatible")

Labeled Contraindications Hypersensitivity to ofloxacin or other members of the quinolone group, such as nalidixic acid, oxolinic acid, cinoxacin, norfloxacin, and ciprofloxacin; hypersensitivity to any component of the formulation

Warnings/Precautions [U.S. Boxed Warning]: There have been reports of tendon inflammation and/or rupture with quinolone antibiotics; risk may be increased with concurrent corticosteroids, organ transplant recipients, and in patients >60 years of age. Rupture of the Achilles tendon sometimes requiring surgical repair has been reported most frequently; but other tendon sites (eg, rotator cuff, biceps) have also been reported. Strenuous physical activity, rheumatoid arthritis, and renal impairment are an independent risk factor for tendonitis. Discontinue at first sign of tendon inflammation or pain. May occur even after discontinuation of therapy. Use with caution in patients with rheumatoid arthritis; may increase risk of tendon rupture. Use with caution in patients with epilepsy or other CNS diseases which could predispose seizures; potential for seizures, although very rare, may be increased with concomitant NSAID therapy. Tremor, restlessness, confusion, and very rarely hallucinations or seizures may occur; use with caution in patients with known or suspected CNS disorder. Discontinue in patients who experience significant CNS adverse effects (eg, dizziness, hallucinations, suicidal ideations or actions). Use with caution in patients with renal or hepatic impairment. Peripheral neuropathies have been linked to ofloxacin use; discontinue if numbness, tingling, or weakness develops.

Fluoroquinolones have been associated with the development of serious, and sometimes fatal, hypoglycemia, most often in elderly diabetics, but also in patients without diabetes. This occurred most frequently with gatifloxacin (no longer available systemically) but may occur at a lower frequency with other quinolones.

Rare cases of torsade de pointes have been reported in patients receiving ofloxacin and other quinolones. Risk may be minimized by avoiding use in patients with known prolongation of the QT interval, bradycardia, hypokalemia, hypomagnesemia, cardiomyopathy, or in those receiving concurrent therapy with Class Ia or Class III antiarrhythmics.

Severe hypersensitivity reactions, including anaphylaxis, have occurred with quinolone therapy. Reactions may present as typical allergic symptoms after a single dose, or may manifest as severe idiosyncratic dermatologic, vascular, pulmonary, renal, hepatic, and/or hematologic events, usually after multiple doses. Prompt discontinuation of drug should occur if skin rash or other symptoms arise. Prolonged use may result in fungal or bacterial superinfection, including *C. difficile*-associated diarrhea (CDAD) and pseudomembranous colitis; CDAD has been observed >2 months postantibiotic treatment. Quinolones may exacerbate myasthenia gravis. Avoid excessive sunlight and take precautions to limit exposure (eg, loose fitting clothing, sunscreen); may cause moderate-to-severe phototoxicity reactions. Discontinue use if photosensitivity occurs. Since ofloxacin is ineffective in the treatment of syphilis and may mask symptoms, all patients should be tested for syphilis at the time of gonorrheal diagnosis and 3 months later. Hemolytic reactions may (rarely) occur with quinolone use in patients with latent or actual G6PD deficiency. Safety and efficacy have not been established in children.

Adverse Reactions
Systemic:
1% to 10%:

Cardiovascular: Chest pain (1% to 3%)

Central nervous system: Headache (1% to 9%), insomnia (3% to 7%), dizziness (1% to 5%), fatigue (1% to 3%), somnolence (1% to 3%), sleep disorders (1% to 3%), nervousness (1% to 3%), pyrexia (1% to 3%)

Dermatologic: Rash/pruritus (1% to 3%)

Gastrointestinal: Diarrhea (1% to 4%), vomiting (1% to 4%), GI distress (1% to 3%), abdominal cramps (1% to 3%), flatulence (1% to 3%), abnormal taste (1% to 3%), xerostomia (1% to 3%), appetite decreased (1% to 3%), nausea (3% to 10%), constipation (1% to 3%)

Genitourinary: Vaginitis (1% to 5%), external genital pruritus in women (1% to 3%)

Ocular: Visual disturbances (1% to 3%)

Respiratory: Pharyngitis (1% to 3%)

Miscellaneous: Trunk pain

<1%, postmarketing, and/or case reports (limited to important or life-threatening): Anaphylaxis reactions, anxiety, blurred vision, chills, cognitive change, cough, depression, dream abnormality, ecchymosis, edema, erythema nodosum, euphoria, extremity pain, hallucinations, hearing acuity decreased, hepatic dysfunction, hepatic failure (some fatal), hepatitis, hyper-/hypoglycemia, hypertension, interstitial nephritis, lightheadedness, malaise, myasthenia gravis exacerbation, palpitation, paresthesia, peripheral neuropathy, photophobia, photosensitivity, pneumonitis, psychotic reactions, rhabdomyolysis, seizure, Stevens-Johnson syndrome, syncope, tendonitis and tendon rupture, thirst, tinnitus, torsade de pointes, Tourette's syndrome,

toxic epidermal necrolysis, vasculitis, vasodilation, vertigo, weakness, weight loss

Ophthalmic: Frequency not defined:
Central nervous system: Dizziness
Gastrointestinal: Nausea
Ocular: Blurred vision, burning, chemical conjunctivitis/keratitis, discomfort, dryness, edema, eye pain, foreign body sensation, itching, photophobia, redness, stinging, tearing

Otic:
>10%: Local: Application site reaction (<1% to 17%)
1% to 10%:
Central nervous system: Dizziness (≤1%), vertigo (≤1%)
Dermatologic: Pruritus (1% to 4%), rash (1%)
Gastrointestinal: Taste perversion (7%)
Neuromuscular & skeletal: Paresthesia (1%)
<1% (Limited to important or life-threatening): Diarrhea, fever, headache, hearing loss (transient), hypertension, nausea, otorrhagia, tinnitus, tremor, vomiting, xerostomia
Postmarketing and/case reports: Transient neuropsychiatric disturbances

Drug Interactions

Metabolism/Transport Effects Inhibits CYP1A2 (strong)

Avoid Concomitant Use There are no known interactions where it is recommended to avoid concomitant use.

Increased Effect/Toxicity
Ofloxacin may increase the levels/effects of: Bendamustine; Corticosteroids (Systemic); CYP1A2 Substrates; Sulfonylureas; Theophylline Derivatives; Vitamin K Antagonists

The levels/effects of Ofloxacin may be increased by: Insulin; Nonsteroidal Anti-Inflammatory Agents; Probenecid

Decreased Effect
Ofloxacin may decrease the levels/effects of: Mycophenolate; Sulfonylureas; Typhoid Vaccine

The levels/effects of Ofloxacin may be decreased by: Antacids; Calcium Salts; Didanosine; Iron Salts; Magnesium Salts; Quinapril; Sevelamer; Sucralfate; Zinc Salts

Ethanol/Nutrition/Herb Interactions

Food: Ofloxacin average peak serum concentrations may be decreased by 20% if taken with food.
Herb/Nutraceutical: Avoid dong quai, St John's wort (may also cause photosensitization).

Storage/Stability

Ophthalmic and otic solution: Store between 15°C to 25°C (59°F to 77°F).
Otic Singles™: Store between 15°C to 30°C (59°F to 86°F). Store in pouch to protect from light.
Tablet: Store below 30°C (86°F).

Mechanism of Action Ofloxacin is a DNA gyrase inhibitor. DNA gyrase is an essential bacterial enzyme that maintains the superhelical structure of DNA. DNA gyrase is required for DNA replication and transcription, DNA repair, recombination, and transposition; bactericidal

Pharmacodynamics/Kinetics

Absorption: Well absorbed; food causes only minor alterations
Distribution: V_d: 2.4-3.5 L/kg

Protein binding: 32%

Bioavailability: Oral: 98%

Half-life elimination: Biphasic: 4-5 hours and 20-25 hours (accounts for <5%); prolonged with renal impairment

Excretion: Primarily urine (as unchanged drug)

Dosage

Usual dosage range:

Children ≥6 months: Otic: 5 drops daily

Children >1 year: Ophthalmic: 1-2 drops every 30 minutes to 4 hours initially, decreasing to every 4-6 hours

Children >12 years: Otic: 10 drops once or twice daily

Adults:

Ophthalmic: 1-2 drops every 30 minutes to 4 hours initially, decreasing to every 4-6 hours

Oral: 200-400 mg every 12 hours

Otic: 10 drops once or twice daily

Indication-specific dosing:

Children 6 months to 13 years: Otic:

Otitis externa: Instill 5 drops (or the contents of 1 single-dose container) into affected ear(s) once daily for 7 days

Children 1-12 years: Otic:

Acute otitis media with tympanostomy tubes: Instill 5 drops (or the contents of 1 single-dose container) into affected ear(s) twice daily for 10 days

Children >1 year and Adults: Ophthalmic:

Conjunctivitis: Instill 1-2 drops in affected eye(s) every 2-4 hours for the first 2 days, then use 4 times/day for an additional 5 days

Corneal ulcer: Instill 1-2 drops every 30 minutes while awake and every 4-6 hours after retiring for the first 2 days; beginning on day 3, instill 1-2 drops every hour while awake for 4-6 additional days; thereafter, 1-2 drops 4 times/day until clinical cure.

Children >12 years and Adults: Otic:

Otitis media, chronic suppurative with perforated tympanic membranes: Instill 10 drops (or the contents of 2 single-dose containers) into affected ear twice daily for 14 days

Children ≥13 years and Adults: Otic:

Otitis externa: Instill 10 drops (or the contents of 2 single-dose containers) into affected ear(s) once daily for 7 days

Adults: Oral:

Cervicitis/urethritis:

Nongonococcal: 300 mg every 12 hours for 7 days

Gonococcal (acute, uncomplicated): 400 mg as a single dose; **Note:** As of April 2007, the CDC no longer recommends the use of fluoroquinolones for the treatment of uncomplicated gonococcal disease.

Chronic bronchitis (acute exacerbation), community-acquired pneumonia, skin and skin structure infections (uncomplicated): 400 mg every 12 hours for 10 days

Epididymitis, nongonococcal (unlabeled use): 300 mg twice daily for 10 days

Leprosy (unlabeled use): 400 mg once daily

Pelvic inflammatory disease (acute): 400 mg every 12 hours for 10-14 days with or without metronidazole; **Note:** The CDC recommends use only if standard cephalosporin therapy is not feasible and community prevalence of quinolone-resistant gonococcal organisms is low. Culture sensitivity must be confirmed.

Prostatitis:
  Acute: 400 mg for 1 dose, then 300 mg twice daily for 10 days
  Chronic: 200 mg every 12 hours for 6 weeks
Traveler's diarrhea (unlabeled use): 300 mg twice daily for 3 days
UTI:
  Uncomplicated: 200 mg every 12 hours for 3-7 days
  Complicated: 200 mg every 12 hours for 10 days

Dosing adjustment/interval in renal impairment: Adults: Oral: After a normal initial dose, adjust as follows:
  Cl_{cr} 20-50 mL/minute: Administer usual dose every 24 hours
  Cl_{cr} <20 mL/minute: Administer half the usual dose every 24 hours
Continuous arteriovenous or venovenous hemodiafiltration effects: Administer 300 mg every 24 hours

Dosing adjustment in hepatic impairment: Severe impairment: Maximum dose: 400 mg/day

Administration

Ophthalmic: For ophthalmic use only; avoid touching tip of applicator to eye or other surfaces.

Oral: Do not take within 2 hours of food or any antacids which contain zinc, magnesium, or aluminum.

Otic: Prior to use, warm solution by holding container in hands for 1-2 minutes. Patient should lie down with affected ear upward and medication instilled. Pump tragus 4 times to ensure penetration of medication. Patient should remain in this position for 5 minutes.

Test Interactions Some quinolones may produce a false-positive urine screening result for opiates using commercially-available immunoassay kits. This has been demonstrated most consistently for levofloxacin and ofloxacin, but other quinolones have shown cross-reactivity in certain assay kits. Confirmation of positive opiate screens by more specific methods should be considered.

Dosage Forms Excipient information presented when available (limited, particularly for generics); consult specific product labeling. [DSC] = Discontinued product

Solution, ophthalmic [drops]: 0.3% (5 mL, 10 mL)
  Ocuflox®: 0.3% (5 mL) [contains benzalkonium chloride]
Solution, otic [drops]: 0.3% (5 mL, 10 mL)
  Floxin®: 0.3% (5 mL, 10 mL) [contains benzalkonium chloride]
  Floxin® Otic Singles™: 0.3% (0.25 mL) [contains benzalkonium chloride; packaged as 2 single-dose containers per pouch, 10 pouches per carton, total net volume 5 mL] [DSC]
Tablet: 200 mg, 300 mg, 400 mg

References

Abramowicz M, "Antimicrobial Prophylaxis in Surgery," *Medical Letter on Drugs and Therapeutics, Handbook of Antimicrobial Therapy,* 16th ed, New York, NY: Medical Letter, 2002.

Centers for Disease Control and Prevention, "Sexually Transmitted Diseases Treatment Guidelines, 2006," *MMWR,* 2006, 55(RR-11): 1-94.

Jacobs MR, Felmingham D, Appelbaum PC, et al, "The Alexander Project 1998-2000: Susceptibility of Pathogens Isolated From Community-Acquired Respiratory Tract Infection to Commonly Used Antimicrobial Agents," *J Antimicrob Chemother,* 2003, 52(2):229-46.

Khaliq Y and Zhanel GG, "Fluoroquinolone-Associated Tendinopathy: A Critical Review of the Literature," *Clin Infect Dis,* 2003, 36(11):1404-10.

Monk JP and Campoli-Richards DM, "Ofloxacin. A Review of Its Antibacterial Activity, Pharmacokinetic Properties, and Therapeutic Use," *Drugs,* 1987, 33(4):346-91.

Thalhammer F, Kletzmayr J, El Menyawi I, et al, "Ofloxacin Clearance During Hemodialysis: A Comparison of Polysulfone and Cellulose Acetate Hemodialyzers," *Am J Kidney Dis,* 1998, 32 (4):642-5.

◆ **OKT3** *see* Muromonab-CD3 *on page 827*

OLANZapine (oh LAN za peen)

Medication Safety Issues
Sound-alike/look-alike issues:
OLANZapine may be confused with olsalazine, QUEtiapine
Zyprexa® may be confused with Celexa®, Reprexain®, Zestril®, Zyrtec®
Zyprexa® Zydis® may be confused with Zelapar™

Related Information
Management of Chemotherapy-Induced Nausea and Vomiting *on page 1434*

U.S. Brand Names Zyprexa®; Zyprexa® IntraMuscular; Zyprexa® Zydis®

Index Terms LY170053; Zyprexa Zydis

Generic Available No

Canadian Brand Names Novo-Olanzapine; PMS-Olanzapine; Zyprexa®; Zyprexa® Zydis®

Pharmacologic Category Antimanic Agent; Antipsychotic Agent, Atypical

Use Treatment of the manifestations of schizophrenia; treatment of acute or mixed mania episodes associated with bipolar I disorder (as monotherapy or in combination with lithium or valproate); maintenance treatment of bipolar disorder; acute agitation (patients with schizophrenia or bipolar mania); in combination with fluoxetine for treatment-resistant or bipolar I depression

Unlabeled/Investigational Use Treatment of psychosis/schizophrenia in children or adolescents; chronic pain; prevention of chemotherapy-associated delayed nausea or vomiting; psychosis/agitation related to Alzheimer's dementia

Pregnancy Risk Factor C

Lactation Enters breast milk/not recommended

Labeled Contraindications Hypersensitivity to olanzapine or any component of the formulation

Warnings/Precautions [U.S. Boxed Warning]: **Elderly patients with dementia-related psychosis treated with antipsychotics are at an increased risk of death compared to placebo.** Most deaths appeared to be either cardiovascular (eg, heart failure, sudden death) or infectious (eg, pneumonia) in nature. In addition, an increased incidence of cerebrovascular effects (eg, transient ischemic attack, stroke) has been reported in studies of placebo-controlled trials of olanzapine in elderly patients with dementia-related psychosis. Olanzapine is not approved for the treatment of dementia-related psychosis.

Moderate to highly sedating, use with caution in disorders where CNS depression is a feature; patients must be cautioned about performing tasks which require mental alertness (eg, operating machinery or driving). Use caution in patients with cardiac disease. Use with caution in Parkinson's disease, predisposition to seizures, or severe hepatic or renal disease. Life-threatening arrhythmias have occurred with therapeutic doses of some neuroleptics. May induce orthostatic hypotension; use caution with history of cardiovascular disease, hemodynamic instability, prior myocardial infarction, or ischemic heart disease. Increases in cholesterol and triglycerides have been noted. Use with caution in patients with pre-existing abnormal lipid profile. Esophageal dysmotility and aspiration have been associated with antipsychotic use; use with caution in patients at risk of aspiration pneumonia. May increase prolactin levels; clinical significance of hyperprolactinemia in patients with breast cancer or other prolactin-dependent tumors is unknown. Significant weight gain (>7% of baseline weight) may occur; monitor waist circumference ▶

and BMI. Impaired core body temperature regulation may occur; caution with strenuous exercise, heat exposure, dehydration, and concomitant medication possessing anticholinergic effects.

May cause anticholinergic effects; use with caution in patients with decreased gastrointestinal motility, urinary retention, BPH, xerostomia, or narrow-angle glaucoma. Relative to other neuroleptics, olanzapine has a moderate potency of cholinergic blockade. May cause extrapyramidal symptoms (EPS), although risk of these reactions is lower relative to other neuroleptics. Risk of dystonia (and probably other EPS) may be greater with increased doses, use of conventional antipsychotics, males, and younger patients. May be associated with neuroleptic malignant syndrome (NMS). May cause extreme and life-threatening hyperglycemia; use with caution in patients with diabetes or other disorders of glucose regulation; monitor. Olanzapine levels may be lower in patients who smoke; the manufacturer does not require dosage adjustments, although dosage adjustments may be considered.

The possibility of a suicide attempt is inherent in psychotic illness or bipolar disorder; use caution in high-risk patients during initiation of therapy. Prescriptions should be written for the smallest quantity consistent with good patient care. Safety and efficacy in pediatric patients have not been established.

Intramuscular administration: Patients should remain recumbent if drowsy/dizzy until hypotension, bradycardia, and/or hypoventilation has been ruled out. Concurrent use of I.M./I.V. benzodiazepines is not recommended (fatalities have been reported, though causality not determined).

Adverse Reactions

>10%:
  Central nervous system: Somnolence (6% to 39% dose dependent), extrapyramidal symptoms (15% to 32% dose dependent), insomnia (up to 12%), dizziness (4% to 18%)
  Gastrointestinal: Dyspepsia (7% to 11%), constipation (9% to 11%), weight gain (5% to 6%, has been reported as high as 40%), xerostomia (9% to 22% dose dependent)
  Neuromuscular & skeletal: Weakness (2% to 20% dose dependent)
  Miscellaneous: Accidental injury (12%)
1% to 10%:
  Cardiovascular: Postural hypotension (1% to 5%), tachycardia (up to 3%), peripheral edema (up to 3%), chest pain (up to 3%), hyper-/hypotension (up to 2%)
  Central nervous system: Personality changes (8%), speech disorder (7%), fever (up to 6%), abnormal dreams, euphoria, amnesia, delusions, emotional lability, mania, schizophrenia
  Dermatologic: Bruising (up to 5%)
  Endocrine & metabolic: Cholesterol increased (4%), prolactin increased
  Gastrointestinal: Nausea (up to 9% dose dependent), appetite increased (3% to 6%), vomiting (up to 4%), flatulence, salivation increased, thirst
  Genitourinary: Incontinence (up to 2%), UTI (up to 2%), vaginitis
  Hepatic: ALT increased (2%)
  Local: Injection site pain (I.M. administration)
  Neuromuscular & skeletal: Tremor (1% to 7% dose dependent), abnormal gait (6%), back pain (up to 5%), joint/extremity pain (up to 5%), akathisia (3% to 5% dose dependent), hypertonia (up to 3%), articulation impairment (up to 2%), falling (particularly in older patients), joint stiffness, paresthesia, twitching

Ocular: Amblyopia (up to 3%), conjunctivitis

Respiratory: Rhinitis (up to 7%), cough (up to 6%), pharyngitis (up to 4%), dyspnea

Miscellaneous: Dental pain, diaphoresis, flu-like syndrome

<1%, postmarketing, and/or case reports (limited to important or life-threatening): Acidosis, akinesia, albuminuria, anaphylactoid reaction, anemia, angioedema, apnea, arteritis, asthma, ataxia, atelectasis, atrial fibrillation, AV block, cerebrovascular accident, coma, confusion, congestive heart failure, deafness, diabetes mellitus, diabetic acidosis, diabetic coma, dyskinesia, dysphagia, dystonia, dysuria, encephalopathy, facial paralysis, glaucoma, gynecomastia, heart arrest, heart block, heart failure, hematuria, hemoptysis, hemorrhage (eye, rectal, subarachnoid, vaginal), hepatitis, hyper-/hypoglycemia, hyper-/hypokalemia, hyperlipemia, hyper-/hyponatremia, hyperuricemia, hyper-/hypoventilation, hypoesthesia, hypokinesia, hypoproteinemia, hypoxia, jaundice, ileus, ketosis, leukocytosis (eosinophilia), leukopenia, liver damage (cholestatic or mixed), liver fatty deposit, lung edema, lymphadenopathy, menstrual irregularities, migraine, myasthenia, myopathy, neuralgia, neuroleptic malignant syndrome, neuropathy, neutropenia, osteoporosis, pancreatitis, paralysis, priapism, pulmonary embolus, rhabdomyolysis, seizure, stridor, stroke, sudden death, suicide attempt, syncope, tardive dyskinesia, thrombocythemia, thrombocytopenia, tongue edema, transient ischemic attack, venous thrombotic events, vomiting, withdrawal syndrome

Drug Interactions

Metabolism/Transport Effects Substrate of CYP1A2 (major), 2D6 (minor); **Inhibits** CYP1A2 (weak), 2C9 (weak), 2C19 (weak), 2D6 (weak), 3A4 (weak)

Avoid Concomitant Use There are no known interactions where it is recommended to avoid concomitant use.

Increased Effect/Toxicity

OLANZapine may increase the levels/effects of: Alcohol (Ethyl); Anticholinergics; CNS Depressants; Methotrimeprazine

The levels/effects of OLANZapine may be increased by: Acetylcholinesterase Inhibitors (Central); CYP1A2 Inhibitors (Moderate); CYP1A2 Inhibitors (Strong); Fluvoxamine; LamoTRIgine; Lithium formulations; Methotrimeprazine; Pramlintide; Tetrabenazine

Decreased Effect

OLANZapine may decrease the levels/effects of: Amphetamines; Anti-Parkinson's Agents (Dopamine Agonist)

The levels/effects of OLANZapine may be decreased by: CYP1A2 Inducers (Strong); Lithium formulations; Peginterferon Alfa-2b

Ethanol/Nutrition/Herb Interactions

Ethanol: Avoid ethanol (may increase CNS depression).

Herb/Nutraceutical: Avoid dong quai, St John's wort (may also cause photosensitization). Avoid kava kava, gotu kola, valerian, St John's wort (may increase CNS depression).

Storage/Stability

Injection, powder for reconstitution: Store at room temperature 15°C to 30°C (59°F to 86°F); do not freeze. Protect from light.

Tablet and orally-disintegrating tablet: Store at room temperature of 15°C to 30°C (59°F to 86°F). Protect from light and moisture.

Reconstitution Injection, powder for reconstitution: Reconstitute 10 mg vial with 2.1 mL SWFI. Resulting solution is ~5 mg/mL. Use immediately (within 1 hour) following reconstitution. Discard any unused portion.

◀ **Mechanism of Action** Olanzapine is a second generation thienobenzodiazepine antipsychotic which displays potent antagonism of serotonin $5-HT_{2A}$ and $5-HT_{2C}$, dopamine D_{1-4}, histamine H_1 and alpha$_1$-adrenergic receptors. Olanzapine shows moderate antagonism of $5-HT_3$ and muscarinic M_{1-5} receptors, and weak binding to GABA-A, BZD, and beta-adrenergic receptors. Although the precise mechanism of action in schizophrenia and bipolar disorder is not known, the efficacy of olanzapine is thought to be mediated through combined antagonism of dopamine and serotonin type 2 receptor sites.

Pharmacodynamics/Kinetics

Absorption:

I.M.: Rapidly absorbed

Oral: Well absorbed; not affected by food; tablets and orally-disintegrating tablets are bioequivalent

Distribution: V_d: Extensive, 1000 L

Protein binding, plasma: 93% bound to albumin and alpha$_1$-glycoprotein

Metabolism: Highly metabolized via direct glucuronidation and cytochrome P450 mediated oxidation (CYP1A2, CYP2D6); 40% removed via first pass metabolism

Bioavailability: >57%

Half-life elimination: 21-54 hours; ~1.5 times greater in elderly

Time to peak, plasma: Maximum plasma concentrations after I.M. administration are 5 times higher than maximum plasma concentrations produced by an oral dose.

I.M.: 15-45 minutes

Oral: ~6 hours

Excretion: Urine (57%, 7% as unchanged drug); feces (30%)

Clearance: 40% increase in olanzapine clearance in smokers; 30% decrease in females

Dosage

Children: Schizophrenia/bipolar disorder (unlabeled use): Oral: Initial: 2.5 mg/day; titrate as necessary to 20 mg/day (0.12-0.29 mg/kg/day)

Adults:

Agitation (acute, associated with bipolar I mania or schizophrenia): I.M.: Initial dose: 5-10 mg (a lower dose of 2.5 mg may be considered when clinical factors warrant); additional doses (2.5-10 mg) may be considered; however, 2-4 hours should be allowed between doses to evaluate response (maximum total daily dose: 30 mg, per manufacturer's recommendation)

Bipolar I acute mixed or manic episodes: Oral:

Monotherapy: Initial: 10-15 mg once daily; increase by 5 mg/day at intervals of not less than 24 hours. Maintenance: 5-20 mg/day; recommended maximum dose: 20 mg/day.

Combination therapy (with lithium or valproate): Initial: 10 mg once daily; dosing range: 5-20 mg/day; recommended maximum dose: 20 mg/day.

Depression associated with bipolar disorder (in combination with fluoxetine): Oral: Initial: 5 mg in the evening; adjust as tolerated to usual range of 5-12.5 mg/day. See **"Note."**

Schizophrenia: Oral: Initial: 5-10 mg once daily (increase to 10 mg once daily within 5-7 days); thereafter, adjust by 5 mg/day at 1-week intervals, up to a recommended maximum of 20 mg/day. Maintenance: 10-20 mg once daily. Doses of 30-50 mg/day have been used; however, doses >10 mg/day have not demonstrated better efficacy, and safety and efficacy of doses >20 mg/day have not been evaluated.

Treatment-resistant depression (in combination with fluoxetine): Oral: Initial: 5 mg in the evening; adjust as tolerated to usual range of 5-12.5 mg/day. See **"Note."**

Note: When using individual components of fluoxetine with olanzapine rather than fixed dose combination product (Symbyax®), approximate dosage correspondence is as follows:

Olanzapine 2.5 mg + fluoxetine 20 mg = Symbyax® 3/25

Olanzapine 5 mg + fluoxetine 20 mg = Symbyax® 6/25

Olanzapine 12.5 mg + fluoxetine 20 mg = Symbyax® 12/25

Olanzapine 5 mg + fluoxetine 50 mg = Symbyax® 6/50

Olanzapine 12.5 mg + fluoxetine 50 mg = Symbyax® 12/50

Prevention of chemotherapy-associated delayed nausea or vomiting (unlabeled use; in combination with a corticosteroid and serotonin [$5HT_3$] antagonist): Oral: 10 mg once daily for 3-5 days, beginning on day 1 of chemotherapy **or** 5 mg once daily for 2 days before chemotherapy, followed by 10 mg once daily (beginning on the day of chemotherapy) for 3-8 days

Elderly: Oral, I.M.: Consider lower starting dose of 2.5-5 mg/day for elderly or debilitated patients; may increase as clinically indicated and tolerated with close monitoring of orthostatic blood pressure

Psychosis/agitation related to Alzheimer's dementia (unlabeled use): Initial: 1.25-5 mg/day; if necessary, gradually increase as tolerated not to exceed 10 mg/day

Dosage adjustment in renal impairment: No adjustment required. Not removed by dialysis.

Dosage adjustment in hepatic impairment: Dosage adjustment may be necessary, however, there are no specific recommendations. Monitor closely.

Administration

Injection: For I.M. administration only; do not administer injection intravenously; inject slowly, deep into muscle. If dizziness and/or drowsiness are noted, patient should remain recumbent until examination indicates postural hypotension and/or bradycardia are not a problem. Concurrent use of I.M/ I.V. benzodiazepines is not recommended (fatalities have been reported, though causality not determined).

Tablet: May be administered with or without food.

Orally-disintegrating: Remove from foil blister by peeling back (do not push tablet through the foil); place tablet in mouth immediately upon removal; tablet dissolves rapidly in saliva and may be swallowed with or without liquid. May be administered with or without food/meals.

Monitoring Parameters Vital signs; fasting lipid profile and fasting blood glucose/Hgb A_{1c} (prior to treatment, at 3 months, then annually); periodic assessment of hepatic transaminases (in patients with hepatic disease); BMI, personal/family history of obesity, waist circumference; orthostatic blood pressure; mental status, abnormal involuntary movement scale (AIMS), extrapyramidal symptoms (EPS). Weight should be assessed prior to treatment, at 4 weeks, 8 weeks, 12 weeks, and then at quarterly intervals. Consider titrating to a different antipsychotic agent for a weight gain ≥5% of the initial weight.

Dietary Considerations Tablets may be taken with or without food. Zyprexa® Zydis®: 5 mg tablet contains phenylalanine 0.34 mg; 10 mg tablet contains phenylalanine 0.45 mg; 15 mg tablet contains phenylalanine 0.67 mg; 20 mg tablet contains phenylalanine 0.9 mg.

Dosage Forms Excipient information presented when available (limited, particularly for generics); consult specific product labeling.

Injection, powder for reconstitution:
Zyprexa® IntraMuscular: 10 mg [contains lactose 50 mg]
Tablet, oral:
Zyprexa®: 2.5 mg, 5 mg, 7.5 mg, 10 mg, 15 mg, 20 mg
Tablet, orally disintegrating:
Zyprexa® Zydis®:
5 mg [contains phenylalanine 0.34 mg/tablet]
10 mg [contains phenylalanine 0.45 mg/tablet]
15 mg [contains phenylalanine 0.67 mg/tablet]
20 mg [contains phenylalanine 0.9 mg/tablet]

References

American Diabetes Association; American Psychiatric Association; American Association of Clinical Endocrinologists; North American Association for the Study of Obesity, "Consensus Development Conference on Antipsychotic Drugs and Obesity and Diabetes," *Diabetes Care*, 2004, 27(2):596-601.

Duggal HS, Gates C, and Pathak PC, "Olanzapine-Induced Neutropenia: Mechanism and Treatment," *J Clin Psychopharmacol*, 2004, 24(2):234-5.

Gorski ED and Willis KC, "Report of Three Cases Studied With Olanzapine for Chronic Pain," *J Pain*, 2003, 4:166-8.

Khojainova N, Santiago-Palma J, Kornick C, et al, "Olanzapine in the Management of Cancer Pain," *J Pain Symptom Manage*, 2002, 23(4):346-50.

Navari RM, Einhorn LH, Loehrer PJ, et al, "A Phase II Trial of Olanzapine, Dexamethasone, and Palonosetron for the Prevention of Chemotherapy-Induced Nausea and Vomiting: A Hoosier Oncology Group Study," *Support Care Cancer*, 2007, 15(11):1285-91.

Navari RM, Einhorn LH, Passik SD, et al, "A Phase II Trial of Olanzapine for the Prevention of Chemotherapy-Induced Nausea and Vomiting: A Hoosier Oncology Group Study," *Support Care Cancer*, 2005, 13(7):529-34.

Passick SD, Navari RM, Jung SH, et al, "A Phase I Trial of Olanzapine (Zyprexa) for the Prevention of Delayed Emesis in Cancer Patients: A Hoosier Oncology Group Study," *Cancer Invest*, 2004, 22(3):383-8.

Thangadurai P, Jyothi KS, Gopalakrishman R, et al, "Reversible Neutropenia With Olanzapine Following Clozapine-Induced Neutropenia," *Am J Psychiatry*, 2006, 163(7):1298.

Thinn SS, Liew E, May AL, et al, "Reversible Delayed Onset Olanzapine-Associated Leukopenia and Neutropenia in a Clozapine-Naive Patient on Concomitant Depot Antipsychotic," *J Clin Psychopharmacol*, 2007, 27(4):394-5.

♦ **Omnipred™** *see* PrednisoLONE *on page 977*

♦ **Oncaspar®** *see* Pegaspargase *on page 925*

♦ **Oncotice™ (Can)** *see* BCG Vaccine *on page 128*

♦ **Oncovin** *see* VinCRIStine *on page 1174*

Ondansetron (on DAN se tron)

Medication Safety Issues

Sound-alike/look-alike issues:
Ondansetron may be confused with dolasetron, granisetron, palonosetron
Zofran® may be confused with Zantac®, Zosyn®

Related Information

Management of Chemotherapy-Induced Nausea and Vomiting *on page 1434*

U.S. Brand Names Zofran®; Zofran® ODT

Index Terms GR38032R; Ondansetron Hydrochloride

Generic Available Yes

Canadian Brand Names Apo-Ondansetron®; DOM-Ondansetron; Gen-Ondansetron; JAMP-Ondansetron; MINT-Ondansetron; Mylan-Ondansetron; Novo-Ondansetron; Ondansetron Injection; Ondansetron-Omega; PHL-Ondansetron; PMS-Ondansetron; RAN-Ondansetron; ratio-Ondansetron; Sandoz-Ondansetron; Zofran®; Zofran® ODT

Pharmacologic Category Antiemetic; Selective 5-HT$_3$ Receptor Antagonist

Use Prevention of nausea and vomiting associated with moderately- to highly-emetogenic cancer chemotherapy; radiotherapy; prevention of postoperative nausea and vomiting (PONV); treatment of PONV if no prophylactic dose of ondansetron received

Unlabeled/Investigational Use Hyperemesis gravidarum; breakthrough treatment of nausea and vomiting associated with chemotherapy

Pregnancy Risk Factor B

Lactation Excretion in breast milk unknown/use caution

Labeled Contraindications Hypersensitivity to ondansetron, other selective 5-HT$_3$ antagonists, or any component of the formulation

Warnings/Precautions Ondansetron should be used on a scheduled basis, not on an "as needed" (PRN) basis, since data support the use of this drug only in the prevention of nausea and vomiting (due to antineoplastic therapy) and not in the rescue of nausea and vomiting. Ondansetron should only be used in the first 24-48 hours of chemotherapy. Data do not support any increased efficacy of ondansetron in delayed nausea and vomiting. Does not stimulate gastric or intestinal peristalsis; may mask progressive ileus and/or gastric distension. Use with caution in patients allergic to other 5-HT$_3$ receptor antagonists; cross-reactivity has been reported.

Use with caution in patients with congenital long QT syndrome or other risk factors for QT prolongation (eg, medications known to prolong QT interval, electrolyte abnormalities, and cumulative high-dose anthracycline therapy). 5-HT$_3$ antagonists have been associated with a number of dose-dependent increases in ECG intervals (eg, PR, QRS duration, QT/QT$_c$, JT), usually occurring 1-2 hours after I.V. administration. In general, these changes are not clinically relevant, however, when used in conjunction with other agents that prolong these intervals, arrhythmia may occur. When used with agents that prolong the QT interval (eg, Class I and III antiarrhythmics), clinically relevant QT interval prolongation may occur resulting in torsade de pointes. I.V. formulations of 5-HT$_3$ antagonists have more association with ECG interval changes, compared to oral formulations.

Orally-disintegrating tablets contain phenylalanine. Safety and efficacy for children <1 month of age have not been established.

Adverse Reactions Note: Percentages reported in adult patients.

>10%:

Central nervous system: Headache (9% to 27%), malaise/fatigue (9% to 13%)

Gastrointestinal: Constipation (6% to 11%)

1% to 10%:

Central nervous system: Drowsiness (8%), fever (2% to 8%), dizziness (4% to 7%), anxiety (6%), cold sensation (2%)

Dermatologic: Pruritus (2% to 5%), rash (1%)

Gastrointestinal: Diarrhea (2% to 7%)

Genitourinary: Gynecological disorder (7%), urinary retention (5%)

Hepatic: ALT increased (1% to 5%), AST increased (1% to 5%)

Local: Injection site reaction (4%; pain, redness, burning)

Neuromuscular & skeletal: Paresthesia (2%)

Respiratory: Hypoxia (9%)

<1%: Anaphylaxis, angina, bronchospasm, ECG changes, extrapyramidal symptoms, grand mal seizure, hypokalemia, tachycardia, vascular occlusive events

Postmarketing and/or case reports: Anaphylactoid reactions, angioedema, arrhythmia, blindness (transient/following infusion; lasting ≤48 hours), blurred vision (transient/following infusion), bradycardia, cardiopulmonary arrest, dyspnea, dystonic reaction, electrocardiographic alterations (second-degree heart block and ST-segment depression), flushing, hiccups, hypersensitivity reaction, hypotension, laryngeal edema, laryngospasm, oculogyric crisis, palpitation, premature ventricular contractions (PVC), QT interval increased, shock, stridor, supraventricular tachycardia, syncope, urticaria, ventricular arrhythmia

Drug Interactions

Metabolism/Transport Effects Substrate of CYP1A2 (minor), 2C9 (minor), 2D6 (minor), 2E1 (minor), 3A4 (major); **Inhibits** CYP1A2 (weak), 2C9 (weak), 2D6 (weak)

Avoid Concomitant Use

Avoid concomitant use of Ondansetron with any of the following: Apomorphine

Increased Effect/Toxicity

Ondansetron may increase the levels/effects of: Apomorphine

The levels/effects of Ondansetron may be increased by: P-Glycoprotein Inhibitors

Decreased Effect

The levels/effects of Ondansetron may be decreased by: CYP3A4 Inducers (Strong); Deferasirox; Herbs (CYP3A4 Inducers); Peginterferon Alfa-2b; P-Glycoprotein Inducers; Rifamycin Derivatives

Ethanol/Nutrition/Herb Interactions

Food: Food increases the extent of absorption. The C_{max} and T_{max} do not change much.

Herb/Nutraceutical: St John's wort may decrease ondansetron levels.

Storage/Stability

Oral solution: Store between 15°C and 30°C (59°F and 86°F). Protect from light.

Premixed bag: Store between 2°C and 30°C (36°F and 86°F). Protect from light.

Tablet: Store between 2°C and 30°C (36°F and 86°F).

Vial: Store between 2°C and 30°C (36°F and 86°F). Protect from light. Stable when mixed in D_5W or NS for 48 hours at room temperature.

Reconstitution Prior to I.V. infusion, dilute in 50 mL D_5W or NS.

Compatibility Stable in $D_51/2NS$, D_5NS, D_5W, mannitol 10%, LR, NS, sodium chloride 3%; do not mix injection with alkaline solutions.

Y-site administration: Compatible: Alatrofloxacin, aldesleukin, amifostine, amikacin, aztreonam, bleomycin, carboplatin, carmustine, cefazolin, cefotaxime, cefoxitin, ceftazidime, ceftizoxime, cefuroxime, chlorpromazine, cimetidine, cisatracurium, cisplatin, cladribine, clindamycin, cyclophosphamide, cytarabine, dacarbazine, dactinomycin, daunorubicin, dexamethasone sodium phosphate, diphenhydramine, docetaxel, dopamine, doxorubicin, doxorubicin liposome, doxycycline, droperidol, etoposide, etoposide phosphate, famotidine, filgrastim, floxuridine, fluconazole, fludarabine, gatifloxacin, gemcitabine, gentamicin, haloperidol, heparin, hydrocortisone sodium phosphate, hydrocortisone sodium succinate, hydromorphone, hydroxyzine, ifosfamide, imipenem/cilastatin, linezolid, magnesium sulfate, mannitol, mechlorethamine, melphalan, meperidine, mesna, methotrexate, metoclopramide, mitomycin, mitoxantrone, morphine, paclitaxel, paclitaxel with ranitidine, pentostatin, piperacillin/tazobactam, potassium chloride, prochlorperazine edisylate, promethazine, ranitidine, remifentanil, sodium acetate, streptozocin, teniposide, thiotepa, ticarcillin, ticarcillin/clavulanate, topotecan, vancomycin, vinblastine, vincristine, vinorelbine, zidovudine. **Incompatible:** Acyclovir, allopurinol, aminophylline, amphotericin B, amphotericin B cholesteryl sulfate complex, ampicillin, ampicillin/sulbactam, amsacrine, cefepime, cefoperazone, furosemide, ganciclovir, lorazepam, methylprednisolone sodium succinate, piperacillin, sargramostim, sodium bicarbonate. **Variable (consult detailed reference):** Fluorouracil, meropenem.

Mechanism of Action Selective 5-HT$_3$-receptor antagonist, blocking serotonin, both peripherally on vagal nerve terminals and centrally in the chemoreceptor trigger zone

Pharmacodynamics/Kinetics

Onset of action: ~30 minutes

Distribution: V$_d$: Children: 1.7-3.7 L/kg; Adults: 2.2-2.5 L/kg

Protein binding, plasma: 70% to 76%

Metabolism: Extensively hepatic via hydroxylation, followed by glucuronide or sulfate conjugation; CYP1A2, CYP2D6, and CYP3A4 substrate; some demethylation occurs

Bioavailability: Oral: 56% to 71%; Rectal: 58% to 74%

Half-life elimination: Children <15 years: 2-7 hours; Adults: 3-6 hours
Mild-to-moderate hepatic impairment: Adults: 12 hours
Severe hepatic impairment (Child-Pugh C): Adults: 20 hours

Time to peak: Oral: ~2 hours

Excretion: Urine (44% to 60% as metabolites, 5% to 10% as unchanged drug); feces (~25%)

Dosage Note: Studies in adults have shown a single daily dose of 8-12 mg I.V. or 8-24 mg orally to be as effective as mg/kg dosing, and should be considered for **all** patients whose mg/kg dose exceeds 8-12 mg I.V.; oral solution and ODT formulations are bioequivalent to corresponding doses of tablet formulation

Children:

I.V.:

Prevention of chemotherapy-induced emesis: 6 months to 18 years: 0.15 mg/kg/dose administered 30 minutes prior to chemotherapy, 4 and 8 hours after the first dose **or** 0.45 mg/kg/day as a single dose

Prevention of postoperative nausea and vomiting: 1 month to 12 years:
≤40 kg: 0.1 mg/kg as a single dose
>40 kg: 4 mg as a single dose

Oral: Prevention of chemotherapy-induced emesis:

4-11 years: 4 mg 30 minutes before chemotherapy; repeat 4 and 8 hours after initial dose, then 4 mg every 8 hours for 1-2 days after chemotherapy completed

≥12 years: Refer to adult dosing.

Adults:

I.V.:

Prevention of chemotherapy-induced emesis:
0.15 mg/kg 3 times/day beginning 30 minutes prior to chemotherapy **or**
0.45 mg/kg once daily **or**
8-10 mg 1-2 times/day **or**
24 mg or 32 mg once daily

Treatment of hyperemesis gravidum (unlabeled use): 8 mg administered over 15 minutes every 12 hours **or** 1 mg/hour infused continuously for up to 24 hours

I.M., I.V.: Postoperative nausea and vomiting (PONV): 4 mg as a single dose approximately 30 minutes before the end of anesthesia (see Note below) or as treatment if vomiting occurs after surgery (Gan, 2007).

Note: The manufacturer recommends administration immediately before induction of anesthesia; however, this has been shown not to be as effective as administration at the end of surgery (Sun, 1997). Repeat doses given in response to inadequate control of nausea/vomiting from preoperative doses are generally ineffective.

Oral:

Chemotherapy-induced emesis:

Highly-emetogenic agents/single-day therapy: 24 mg given 30 minutes prior to the start of therapy

Moderately-emetogenic agents: 8 mg every 12 hours beginning 30 minutes before chemotherapy, continuously for 1-2 days after chemotherapy completed

Total body irradiation: 8 mg 1-2 hours before daily each fraction of radiotherapy

Single high-dose fraction radiotherapy to abdomen: 8 mg 1-2 hours before irradiation, then 8 mg every 8 hours after first dose for 1-2 days after completion of radiotherapy

Daily fractionated radiotherapy to abdomen: 8 mg 1-2 hours before irradiation, then 8 mg 8 hours after first dose for each day of radiotherapy

Postoperative nausea and vomiting: 16 mg given 1 hour prior to induction of anesthesia

Treatment of hyperemesis gravidum (unlabeled use): 8 mg every 12 hours

Elderly: No dosing adjustment required

Dosage adjustment in renal impairment: No dosing adjustment required

Dosage adjustment in hepatic impairment: Severe liver disease (Child-Pugh C): Maximum daily dose: 8 mg

Administration

Oral: Oral dosage forms should be administered 30 minutes prior to chemotherapy; 1-2 hours before radiotherapy; 1 hour prior to the induction of anesthesia.

Orally-disintegrating tablets: Do not remove from blister until needed. Peel backing off the blister, do not push tablet through. Using dry hands, place tablet on tongue and allow to dissolve. Swallow with saliva.

I.M.: Should be administered undiluted.

I.V.:

IVPB: Dilute in 50 mL D_5W or NS. Infuse over 15-30 minutes; 24-hour continuous infusions have been reported, but are rarely used.

Chemotherapy-induced nausea and vomiting: Give first dose 30 minutes prior to beginning chemotherapy.

I.V. push: Prevention of postoperative nausea and vomiting: Single doses may be administered I.V. injection over 2-5 minutes as undiluted solution.

Monitoring Parameters Closely monitor patients <4 months of age

Dietary Considerations Take without regard to meals.

Orally-disintegrating tablet contains <0.03 mg phenylalanine

Dosage Forms Excipient information presented when available (limited, particularly for generics); consult specific product labeling. [DSC] = Discontinued product

Infusion, premixed in D_5 [preservative free]: 32 mg (50 mL)

Zofran®: 32 mg (50 mL) [DSC]

Injection, solution: 2 mg/mL (2 mL, 20 mL)

Zofran®: 2 mg/mL (2 mL, 20 mL)

Injection, solution [preservative free]: 2 mg/mL (2 mL)

Solution, oral: 4 mg/5 mL (50 mL)

Zofran®: 4 mg/5 mL (50 mL) [contains sodium benzoate; strawberry flavor]

Tablet: 4 mg; 8 mg

Zofran®: 4 mg; 8 mg

Tablet, orally disintegrating: 4 mg; 8 mg

Zofran® ODT: 4 mg, 8 mg [each strength contains phenylalanine <0.03 mg/ tablet; strawberry flavor]

Extemporaneous Preparations A 0.8 mg/mL syrup may be made by crushing ten 8 mg tablets; flaking of the tablet coating occurs. Mix thoroughly with 50 mL of the suspending vehicle, Ora-Plus® (Paddock), in 5 mL increments. Add sufficient volume of any of the following syrups: Cherry syrup USP, Syrpalta® (Humco), Ora-Sweet® (Paddock), or Ora-Sweet® Sugar-Free (Paddock) to make a final volume of 100 mL. Stability is 42 days refrigerated.

Trissel LA, "Trissel's Stability of Compounded Formulations," American Pharmaceutical Association, 1996.

Rectal suppositories: Calibrate a suppository mold for the base being used. Determine the displacement factor (DF) for ondansetron for the base being used (Fattibase® = 1.1; Polybase® = 0.6). Weigh the ondansetron tablet. Divide the tablet weight by the DF. Subtract the weight of base displaced from the calculated weight of base required for each suppository. Grind the ondansetron tablets to a fine powder in a mortar. Weigh out the appropriate weight of suppository base. Melt the base over a water bath (<55°C). Add the ondansetron powder to the suppository base and mix well. Pour the mixture into the suppository mold and cool. Stable for at least 30 days under refrigeration.

Allen LV, "Ondansetron Suppositories," *US Pharm*, 20(7):84-6.

References

American College of Obstetrics and Gynecology, ACOG (American College of Obstetrics and Gynecology) Practice Bulletin: "Nausea and Vomiting of Pregnancy," *Obstet Gynecol*, 2004, 103 (4):803-14.

Kris MG, Hesketh PJ, Somerfield MR, et al, "American Society of Clinical Oncology Guideline for Antiemetics in Oncology: Update 2006," *J Clin Oncol*, 2006, 24(18):2932-47.

Levichek Z, Atanackovic G, Oepkes D, et al, "Nausea and Vomiting of Pregnancy. Evidence-Based Treatment Algorithm," *Can Fam Physician*, 2002, 48:267-8, 277.

Navari RM and Koeller JM, "Electrocardiographic and Cardiovascular Effects of the 5-Hydroxytryptamine₃ Receptor Antagonists," *Ann Pharmacother*, 2003, 37(9):1276-86.

Roila F and Del Favero A, "Ondansetron Clinical Pharmacokinetics," *Clin Pharmacokinet*, 1995, 29 (2):95-109.

Siu SS, Yip SK, Cheung CW, et al, "Treatment of Intractable Hyperemesis Gravidarum by Ondansetron," *Eur J Obstet Gynecol Reprod Biol*, 2002, 105(1):73-4.

♦ **Ondansetron Hydrochloride** *see* Ondansetron *on page 874*

♦ **Ondansetron Injection (Can)** *see* Ondansetron *on page 874*

♦ **Ondansetron-Omega (Can)** *see* Ondansetron *on page 874*

♦ **Onsolis™** *see* FentaNYL *on page 458*

♦ **ONTAK®** *see* Denileukin Diftitox *on page 340*

♦ **Onxol®** *see* Paclitaxel *on page 898*

♦ **Opana®** *see* Oxymorphone *on page 894*

♦ **Opana® ER** *see* Oxymorphone *on page 894*

♦ **o,p'-DDD** *see* Mitotane *on page 807*

♦ **Ophtho-Tate® (Can)** *see* PrednisoLONE *on page 977*

Oprelvekin (oh PREL ve kin)

Medication Safety Issues

Sound-alike/look-alike issues:

Oprelvekin may be confused with aldesleukin, Proleukin®

Neumega® may be confused with Neulasta®, Neupogen®

U.S. Brand Names Neumega®

Index Terms IL-11; Interleukin-11; NSC-722848; Recombinant Human Interleukin-11; Recombinant Interleukin-11; rhIL-11; rIL-11

Generic Available No

Pharmacologic Category Biological Response Modulator; Human Growth Factor

Use Prevention of severe thrombocytopenia; reduce the need for platelet transfusions following myelosuppressive chemotherapy

Pregnancy Risk Factor C

Lactation Excretion in breast milk unknown/not recommended

Labeled Contraindications Hypersensitivity to oprelvekin or any component of the formulation

Warnings/Precautions [U.S. Boxed Warning]: Allergic or hypersensitivity reactions, including anaphylaxis have been reported. May occur with the first or with subsequent doses. Permanently discontinue in any patient developing an allergic reaction. May cause serious fluid retention; use cautiously in patients with conditions where expansion of plasma volume should be avoided (eg, left ventricular dysfunction, HF, hypertension). Closely monitor fluid and electrolytes in patient on chronic diuretic therapy; severe hypokalemia contributing to sudden death have been reported in these patients. Arrhythmia, pulmonary edema, and cardiac arrest have been reported; use in patients with a history of atrial arrhythmia only if the potential benefit exceeds possible risks. Patients experiencing arrhythmia may be at risk for stroke; use caution in patients with a history of transient ischemic attack or stroke. Ventricular arrhythmia has also been reported, occurring within 2-7 days of treatment initiation. Use caution in patients with conduction defects, respiratory disease; history of thromboembolic problems; pre-existing pericardial effusions or ascites. Use with caution in hepatic or renal dysfunction. Not indicated following myeloablative chemotherapy; increased toxicities were reported when used following myeloablative therapy. Efficacy has not been established with chemotherapy regimens >5 days duration or with regimens associated with delayed myelosuppression (eg, nitrosoureas, mitomycin C). Safety and efficacy have not been established with chronic administration. Papilledema, more frequently associated with use in children, has occurred; use caution in patients with pre-existing papilledema or with tumors involving the central nervous system. Papilledema is dose limiting. Patients experiencing oprelvekin-related papilledema may be at risk for visual acuity changes, including blurred vision or blindness. Although used in children in clinical trials, safety and efficacy have not been established in pediatric patients.

Adverse Reactions

>10%:

Cardiovascular: Tachycardia (children 84%; adults 20%), edema (59%), palpitation (14%), cardiomegaly (children 21%), vasodilation (19%), syncope (13%), atrial arrhythmia (12%)

Central nervous system: Headache (41%), dizziness (38%), fever (36%), insomnia (33%), fatigue (30%)

Dermatologic: Rash (25%)

Endocrine & metabolic: Fluid retention

Gastrointestinal: Nausea/vomiting (77%), diarrhea (43%), oral moniliasis (14%)

Hematologic: Anemia (dilutional); appears within 3 days of initiation of therapy, resolves in about 1 week after cessation of oprelvekin

Neuromuscular & skeletal: Weakness (severe 14%), arthralgia, periostitis (children 11%)

Ocular: Conjunctival injection/redness/swelling (children 57%; adults 19%), papilledema (children 16%; adults 1%)

Respiratory: Dyspnea (48%), rhinitis (42%), cough (29%), pharyngitis (25%)

1% to 10%:

Gastrointestinal: Weight gain (5%)

Respiratory: Pleural effusion (10%)

Postmarketing and/or case reports: Allergic reaction, amblyopia, anaphylaxis/anaphylactoid reactions, blindness, blurred vision, capillary leak syndrome, CHF, dehydration, exfoliative dermatitis, eye hemorrhage, facial edema, fibrinogen increased, fluid overload, hypoalbuminemia, hypocalcemia, hypotension, injection site reactions (dermatitis, pain, discoloration), optic neuropathy, paresthesia, pericardial effusion, pulmonary edema, renal failure, skin discoloration, stroke, ventricular arrhythmia

Drug Interactions

Avoid Concomitant Use There are no known interactions where it is recommended to avoid concomitant use.

Increased Effect/Toxicity There are no known significant interactions involving an increase in effect.

Decreased Effect There are no known significant interactions involving a decrease in effect.

Storage/Stability Store vials under refrigeration between 2°C to 8°C (36°F to 46°F); do not freeze. Protect from light. Use reconstituted oprelvekin within 3 hours of reconstitution and store in the vial at either 2°C to 8°C (36°F to 46°F) or room temperature of ≤25°C (77°F). Do not freeze or shake reconstituted solution.

Reconstitution Reconstitute to a final concentration of 5 mg/mL with SWFI; swirl gently, do not shake.

Mechanism of Action Oprelvekin is a growth factor which stimulates multiple stages of megakaryocytopoiesis and thrombopoiesis, resulting in proliferation of megakaryocyte progenitors and megakaryocyte maturation, or increased platelet production.

Pharmacodynamics/Kinetics

Bioavailability: >80%

Half-life elimination: Terminal: 5-9 hours

Time to peak, serum: 1-6 hours

Excretion: Urine (primarily as metabolites)

Dosage SubQ: Administer first dose ~6-24 hours after the end of chemotherapy. Discontinue at least 48 hours before beginning the next cycle of chemotherapy.

Children (unlabeled use): 75-100 mcg/kg once daily for 10-21 days (until postnadir platelet count ≥50,000 cells/µL)

Note: A safe and effective dose for use in children has not been established by the manufacturer.

Adults: 50 mcg/kg once daily for ~10-21 days (until postnadir platelet count ≥50,000 cells/µL)

◄ **Dosage adjustment in renal impairment:** Cl_{cr} <30 mL/minute: 25 mcg/kg once daily

Administration Subcutaneously in the abdomen, thigh, hip, or upper arm.

Monitoring Parameters Monitor electrolytes and fluid balance during therapy; obtain a CBC at regular intervals during therapy; monitor platelet counts until adequate recovery has occurred

Test Interactions Decrease in hemoglobin concentration, serum concentration of albumin and other proteins (result of expansion of plasma volume)

Dosage Forms Excipient information presented when available (limited, particularly for generics); consult specific product labeling.

Injection, powder for reconstitution:

Neumega®: 5 mg [packaged with diluent]

References

Du X and Williams DA, "Interleukin-11: Review of Molecular, Cell Biology, and Clinical Use," *Blood*, 1997, 89(11):3897-908.

Gordon MS, "Thrombopoietic Activity of Recombinant Human Interleukin 11 in Cancer Patients Receiving Chemotherapy," *Cancer Chemother Pharmacol*, 1996, 38 (Suppl):96-8.

Tepler I, Elias L, Smith JW 2d, et al, "A Randomized Placebo-Controlled Trial of Recombinant Human Interleukin-11 in Cancer Patients With Severe Thrombocytopenia Due to Chemotherapy," *Blood*, 1996, 87(9):3607-14.

Teramura M, Kobayashi S, Yoshinaga K, et al, "Effect of Interleukin 11 on Normal and Pathological Thrombopoiesis," *Cancer Chemother Pharmacol*, 1996, 38 (Suppl):99-102.

Oxaliplatin (ox AL i pla tin)

Medication Safety Issues

Sound-alike/look-alike issues:

Oxaliplatin may be confused with Aloxi®, carboplatin, cisplatin

High alert medication: The Institute for Safe Medication Practices (ISMP) includes this medication among its list of drug classes which have a heightened risk of causing significant patient harm when used in error.

Related Information

Management of Drug Extravasations *on page 1447*

Safe Handling of Hazardous Drugs *on page 1517*

U.S. Brand Names Eloxatin®

Index Terms Diaminocyclohexane Oxalatoplatinum; L-OHP; Oxalatoplatin; Oxalatoplatinum

Generic Available Yes: Injection solution

Canadian Brand Names Eloxatin®

Pharmacologic Category Antineoplastic Agent, Alkylating Agent; Antineoplastic Agent, Platinum Analog

Use Treatment of stage III colon cancer (adjuvant) and advanced colorectal cancer

Unlabeled/Investigational Use Treatment of esophageal cancer, gastric cancer, hepatobiliary cancer, non-Hodgkin's lymphoma, ovarian cancer, pancreatic cancer, testicular cancer

Pregnancy Risk Factor D

Lactation Excretion in breast milk unknown/not recommended

Labeled Contraindications Hypersensitivity to oxaliplatin, other platinum-containing compounds, or any component of the formulation

Canadian labeling: Additional contraindications (not in U.S. labeling): Pregnancy, breast-feeding; severe renal impairment (Cl_{cr} <30 mL/minute)

Warnings/Precautions Hazardous agent - use appropriate precautions for handling and disposal. **[U.S. Boxed Warning]: Anaphylactic/anaphylactoid reactions may occur within minutes of oxaliplatin administration; symptoms may be managed with epinephrine, corticosteroids, and antihistamines.** Grade 3 or 4 hypersensitivity has been observed. Allergic reactions may occur with any cycle and may include bronchospasm (rare), erythema, hypotension (rare), pruritus, rash, and/or urticaria.

Two different types of peripheral sensory neuropathy may occur: First, an acute (within first 2 days), reversible (resolves within 14 days), with primarily peripheral symptoms that are often exacerbated by cold (may include pharyngolaryngeal dysesthesia); may recur with subsequent doses; avoid mucositis prophylaxis with ice chips during oxaliplatin infusion. Secondly, a more persistent (>14 days) presentation that often interferes with daily activities (eg, writing, buttoning, swallowing), these symptoms may improve in some patients upon discontinuing treatment.

May cause pulmonary fibrosis; withhold treatment for unexplained pulmonary symptoms (eg, crackles, dyspnea, nonproductive cough, pulmonary infiltrates) until interstitial lung disease or pulmonary fibrosis are excluded. Hepatotoxicity (including rare cases of hepatitis and hepatic failure) has been reported. Liver biopsy has revealed peliosis, nodular regenerative hyperplasia, sinusoidal alterations, perisinusoidal fibrosis, and veno-occlusive lesions; the presence of hepatic vascular disorders (including veno-occlusive disease) should be considered, especially in individuals developing portal hypertension or who present with increased liver function tests. Use caution with renal dysfunction; increased toxicity may occur. When administered as sequential infusions, taxane derivatives (docetaxel, paclitaxel) should be administered before platinum derivatives (carboplatin, cisplatin, oxaliplatin) to limit myelosuppression and enhance efficacy. Concomitant use with 5-FU may increase risk for adverse hematologic or GI effects. Elderly patients are more sensitive to some adverse events including diarrhea, dehydration, hypokalemia, leukopenia, fatigue and syncope. Safety and efficacy in children have not been established.

Adverse Reactions Percentages reported with monotherapy.
>10%:
Central nervous system: Fatigue (61%), fever (25%), pain (14%), headache (13%), insomnia (11%)
Gastrointestinal: Nausea (64%), diarrhea (46%), vomiting (37%), abdominal pain (31%), constipation (31%), anorexia (20%), stomatitis (14%)
Hematologic: Anemia (64%; grades 3/4: 1%), thrombocytopenia (30%; grades 3/4: 3%), leukopenia (13%)

Hepatic: AST increased (54%; grades 3/4: 4%), ALT increased (36%; grades 3/4: 1%), total bilirubin increased (13%; grades 3/4: 5%)

Neuromuscular & skeletal: Peripheral neuropathy (may be dose limiting; 76% to 92%; acute 65%; grades 3/4: 5%; persistent 43%; grades 3/4: 3%), back pain (11%)

Respiratory: Dyspnea (13%), cough (11%)

1% to 10%:

Cardiovascular: Edema (10%), chest pain (5%), peripheral edema (5%), flushing (3%), thromboembolism (2%)

Central nervous system: Dizziness (7%)

Dermatologic: Rash (5%), alopecia (3%), hand-foot syndrome (1%)

Endocrine & metabolic: Dehydration (5%), hypokalemia (3%)

Gastrointestinal: Dyspepsia (7%), taste perversion (5%), flatulence (3%), mucositis (2%), gastroesophageal reflux (1%), dysphagia (acute 1% to 2%)

Genitourinary: Dysuria (1%)

Hematologic: Neutropenia (7%)

Local: Injection site reaction (9%; redness/swelling/pain)

Neuromuscular & skeletal: Rigors (9%), arthralgia (7%)

Ocular: Abnormal lacrimation (1%)

Renal: Serum creatinine increased (5% to 10%)

Respiratory: URI (7%), rhinitis (6%), epistaxis (2%), pharyngitis (2%), pharyngolaryngeal dysesthesia (grades 3/4: 1% to 2%)

Miscellaneous: Allergic reactions (3%); hypersensitivity (includes urticaria, pruritus, facial flushing, shortness of breath, bronchospasm, diaphoresis, hypotension, syncope: grades 3/4: 2% to 3%); hiccup (2%)

<1%, postmarketing, and/or case reports (reported with mono- and combination therapy): Acute renal failure, alkaline phosphatase increased, anaphylactic/anaphylactoid reactions, anaphylactic shock, angioedema, aphonia, ataxia, colitis, cranial nerve palsies, deep tendon reflex loss, deafness, diplopia, dysarthria, dysphonia, eosinophilic pneumonia, extravasation (including necrosis), fasciculations, gait abnormal, hematuria, hemolysis, hemolytic anemia (immuno-allergic), hemolytic uremia syndrome, hemorrhage, hepatic failure, hepatitis, hepatotoxicity, hypertension, hypomagnesemia, hypoxia, ileus, INR increased, interstitial lung diseases, interstitial nephritis (acute), intestinal obstruction, intracerebral bleeding, Lhermittes' sign, metabolic acidosis, muscle spasm, myoclonus, neutropenic fever, neutropenic sepsis, nodular regenerative hyperplasia, optic neuritis, pancreatitis, peliosis, prothrombin time increased, ptosis, rectal hemorrhage, rhabdomyolysis, seizure, sepsis, thrombocytopenia (immuno-allergic), trigeminal neuralgia, tubular necrosis (acute), veno-occlusive liver disease (sinusoidal obstruction syndrome and perisinusoidal fibrosis), visual disturbance (acuity decreased, field disturbance, transient loss)

Drug Interactions

Avoid Concomitant Use

Avoid concomitant use of Oxaliplatin with any of the following: Natalizumab; Vaccines (Live)

Increased Effect/Toxicity

Oxaliplatin may increase the levels/effects of: Leflunomide; Natalizumab; Taxane Derivatives; Topotecan; Vaccines (Live); Vitamin K Antagonists

The levels/effects of Oxaliplatin may be increased by: Trastuzumab

Decreased Effect

Oxaliplatin may decrease the levels/effects of: Cardiac Glycosides; Vaccines (Inactivated); Vaccines (Live); Vitamin K Antagonists

The levels/effects of Oxaliplatin may be decreased by: Echinacea

Storage/Stability Store intact vials at room temperature of 25°C (77°F); excursions permitted to 15°C to 30°C (59°F to 86°F); do not freeze. Protect concentrated solution from light (store in original outer carton). According to the manufacturer, solutions diluted for infusion are stable up to 6 hours at room temperature of 20°C to 25°C (68°F to 77°F) or up to 24 hours under refrigeration at 2°C to 8°C (36°F to 46°F). Oxaliplatin solution diluted with D_5W to a final concentration of 0.7 mg/mL (polyolefin container) has been shown to retain >90% of it's original concentration for up to 30 days when stored at room temperature or refrigerated; artificial light did not affect the concentration (Andre, 2007). As this study did not examine sterility, refrigeration would be preferred to limit microbial growth. Solutions diluted for infusion do not require protection from light.

Reconstitution Do not prepare using a chloride-containing solution such as NaCl due to rapid conversion to monochloroplatinum, dichloroplatinum, and diaquoplatinum; all highly reactive in sodium chloride (Takimoto, 2007). Use appropriate precautions for handling and disposal. Do not use needles or administration sets containing aluminum during preparation.

Aqueous solution: Dilution with D_5W (250 or 500 mL) is required prior to administration.

Lyophilized powder [CAN; not available in U.S.]: Use only water for injection or D_5W to reconstitute powder. To obtain final concentration of 5 mg/mL add 10 mL of diluent to 50 mg vial or 20 mL diluent to 100 mg vial. Gently swirl vial to dissolve powder. Dilution with D_5W (250 or 500 mL) is required prior to administration. Discard unused portion of vial.

Compatibility Incompatible with alkaline solutions (eg, fluorouracil) and chloride-containing solutions. Flush infusion line with D_5W prior to, and following, administration of concomitant medications via same I.V. line.

Y-site administration: Compatible: Allopurinol, aminophylline, bumetanide, buprenorphine, butorphanol, calcium gluconate, carboplatin, chlorpromazine, cimetidine, cyclophosphamide, dexamethasone, diphenhydramine, dobutamine, docetaxel, dolasetron, dopamine, doxorubicin, droperidol, enalaprilat, epirubicin, etoposide phosphate, famotidine, fentanyl, furosemide, gemcitabine, granisetron, haloperidol lactate, heparin, hydrocortisone sodium succinate, hydromorphone, hydroxyzine, ifosfamide, irinotecan, leucovorin calcium, lorazepam, magnesium sulfate, mannitol, meperidine, mesna, methotrexate, methylprednisolone sodium succinate, metoclopramide, mitoxantrone, morphine, nalbuphine, ondansetron, paclitaxel, palonosetron, potassium chloride, prochlorperazine, promethazine, ranitidine, sodium bicarbonate, theophylline, topotecan, verapamil, vincristine, vinorelbine. **Incompatible:** Diazepam.

Mechanism of Action Oxaliplatin, a platinum derivative, is an alkylating agent. Following intracellular hydrolysis, the platinum compound binds to DNA forming cross-links which inhibit DNA replication and transcription, resulting in cell death. Cytotoxicity is cell-cycle nonspecific.

Pharmacodynamics/Kinetics

Distribution: V_d: 440 L

Protein binding: >90% primarily albumin and gamma globulin (irreversible binding to platinum)

Metabolism: Nonenzymatic (rapid and extensive), forms active and inactive derivatives

Half-life elimination: Terminal: 391 hours

Excretion: Urine (~54%); feces (~2%)

◀ **Dosage** Details concerning dosing in combination regimens should also be consulted. Delay dosage in subsequent cycles until recovery of neutrophils ≥1.5 x 10^9/L and platelets ≥75 x 10^9/L. I.V.:

Adults:

Advanced colorectal cancer: 85 mg/m^2 every 2 weeks until disease progression or unacceptable toxicity (in combination with fluorouracil/leucovorin)

Stage III colon cancer (adjuvant): 85 mg/m^2 every 2 weeks for 12 cycles (in combination with fluorouracil/leucovorin)

Colon/colorectal cancer (unlabeled doses or combinations): 85 mg/m^2/dose on days 1, 15, and 29 of an 8-week treatment cycle in combination with fluorouracil/leucovorin (Kuebler, 2007) **or** 85 mg/m^2 every 2 weeks in combination with fluorouracil/leucovorin/irinotecan (Falcone, 2007) **or** 130 mg/m^2 every 3 weeks in combination with capecitabine (Cassidy, 2008)

Esophageal/gastric cancers (unlabeled use; as part of a combination chemotherapy regimen): 85 mg/m^2 every 2 weeks (Al-Batran, 2008) **or** 130 mg/m^2 every 3 weeks (Cunningham, 2008) **or**
Gastric cancer: 100 mg/m^2 every 2 weeks (Louvet, 2002)

Hepatobiliary cancer (unlabeled use; as part of a combination chemotherapy regimen): 100 mg/m^2 every 2 weeks (Andre, 2004) **or** 130 mg/m^2 every 3 weeks (Nehls, 2008)

Non-Hodgkin's lymphoma (unlabeled use; as part of a combination chemotherapy regimen): 25 mg/m^2/day for 4 days every 4 weeks (Tsimberidou, 2008) **or** 100 mg/m^2 every 3 weeks (Lopez, 2008; Rodriguez, 2007) **or** 130 mg/m^2 every 3 weeks (Chau, 2001)

Ovarian cancer (unlabeled use): 130 mg/m^2 every 3 weeks (Dieras, 2002; Piccart, 2000)

Pancreatic cancer (unlabeled use; as part of a combination chemotherapy regimen): 85 mg/m^2 every 2 weeks (Conroy, 2005) **or** 100 mg/m^2 every 2 weeks (Louvet, 2005) **or** 110-130 mg/m^2 every 3 weeks (Xiong, 2008)

Testicular cancer (unlabeled use; in combination with gemcitabine): 130 mg/m^2 every 3 weeks (Kollmannsberger, 2004; Pectasides, 2004)

Elderly: No dosing adjustment recommended

Dosage adjustments for toxicity: Acute toxicities: Longer infusion times (up to 6 hours) may mitigate acute toxicities.

Neurosensory events:

Persistent (>7 days) grade 2 neurosensory events: Consider oxaliplatin dose reduction if symptoms do not resolve:

Adjuvant treatment of stage III colon cancer: Reduce dose to 75 mg/m^2

Advanced colorectal cancer: Reduce dose to 65 mg/m^2

Consider withholding oxaliplatin for grade 2 neuropathy lasting >7 days despite dose reduction.

Persistent grade 3 neurosensory events: Consider discontinuing oxaliplatin

Other toxicities (grade 3/4 gastrointestinal toxicity, grade 4 neutropenia, or grade 3/4 thrombocytopenia): After recovery from toxicity, oxaliplatin dose reductions are recommended:

Adjuvant treatment of stage III colon cancer: Reduce dose to 75 mg/m^2; delay next dose until neutrophils recover to ≥1500/mm^3 and platelets recover to ≥75,000/mm^3

Advanced colorectal cancer: Reduce dose to 65 mg/m^2; delay next dose until neutrophils recover to ≥1500/mm^3 and platelets recover to ≥75,000/mm^3

Dosage adjustment in renal impairment: The FDA-approved labeling does not contain renal dosing adjustment guidelines. Oxaliplatin is primarily eliminated renally; in patients with Cl_{cr} <30 mL/minute, the AUC is increased ~190%. Oxaliplatin use has been studied in 25 patients with renal dysfunction; treatment was well-tolerated in patients with mild-to-moderate impairment (Cl_{cr} 20-59 mL/minute), suggesting that dose reduction is not necessary in this patient population (Takimoto, 2003). Patients with severe renal impairment (Cl_{cr} <20 mL/minute) have not been adequately studied; consider omitting dose or changing chemotherapy regimen if Cl_{cr} <20 mL/minute.

Note: Canadian labeling: Use in patients with Cl_{cr} <30 mL/minute is contraindicated in Canadian labeling.

Dosage adjustment in hepatic impairment: Mild, moderate, or severe hepatic impairment: Dosage adjustment not necessary (Doroshow, 2003; Synold, 2007)

Combination Regimens

Biliary adenocarcinoma:
CAPOX (Biliary Cancer) on page 1246
GEMOX (Biliary Cancer) on page 1347
Colorectal cancer:
Bevacizumab-Oxaliplatin-Fluorouracil-Leucovorin on page 1233
CAPOX (Colorectal Cancer) on page 1246
Cetuximab-FOLFOX4 on page 1257
FLOX (Nordic FLOX) on page 1324
FOIL (Colorectal Cancer) on page 1335
FOLFOX 1 on page 1336
FOLFOX 2 on page 1336
FOLFOX 3 on page 1337
FOLFOX 4 on page 1337
FOLFOX 6 on page 1337
FOLFOX 7 on page 1338
FOLFOXIRI (Colorectal Cancer) on page 1338
Esophageal cancer:
Epirubicin-Oxaliplatin-Capecitabine on page 1306
Epirubicin-Oxaliplatin-Fluorouracil (Esophageal Cancer) on page 1306
Fluorouracil-Leucovorin-Oxaliplatin (Gastric/Esophageal Cancer) on page 1334
Oxaliplatin-Fluorouracil (Esophageal Cancer) on page 1384
Gastric cancer:
Epirubicin-Oxaliplatin-Capecitabine on page 1306
Fluorouracil-Leucovorin-Oxaliplatin (Gastric Cancer) on page 1334
Fluorouracil-Leucovorin-Oxaliplatin (Gastric/Esophageal Cancer) on page 1334
Leukemia, chronic lymphocytic: OFAR (CLL) on page 1381
Lymphoma, non-Hodgkin's:
Cisplatin-Cytarabine-Dexamethasone (NHL Regimen) on page 1265
Gemcitabine-Oxaliplatin-Rituximab (NHL) on page 1345
Oxaliplatin-Cytarabine-Dexamethasone (NHL Regimen) on page 1383
Ovarian caner: Docetaxel-Oxaliplatin (Ovarian Cancer) on page 1292
Pancreatic cancer:
CAPOX (Pancreatic Cancer) on page 1247
FOLFIRINOX (Pancreatic Cancer) on page 1336
Gemcitabine-Oxaliplatin (Pancreatic Cancer) on page 1345
Testicular cancer: GEMOX (Testicular Cancer) on page 1347

◀ **Administration** Administer as I.V. infusion over 2-6 hours. Flush infusion line with D_5W prior to administration of any concomitant medication. Patients should receive an antiemetic premedication regimen. Avoid mucositis prophylaxis with ice chips during oxaliplatin infusion (may exacerbate acute neurological symptoms).

Monitoring Parameters CBC with differential, blood chemistries (including serum creatinine, ALT, AST and bilirubin); INR and prothrombin time (in patients on oral anticoagulant therapy); signs of neuropathy, hypersensitivity, and/or respiratory effects

Additional Information Cold temperature may exacerbate acute neuropathy. Do not use ice for mucositis prophylaxis.

Emetic Potential Moderate (30% to 90%)

Vesicant Yes; see Management of Drug Extravasations on page 1447.

Cool compress may be used for immediate management of extravasation, with consideration of potential for peripheral neuropathy exacerbated by cold. Warm compresses will avoid peripheral neuropathy, however, while possibly increasing drug removal through local vasodilation, may increase cellular uptake and injury.

Dosage Forms Excipient information presented when available (limited, particularly for generics); consult specific product labeling. [CAN] = Canadian availability; not available in U.S.

Injection, solution [preservative free; concentrate]: 5 mg/mL (10 mL, 20 mL)

Eloxatin®: 5 mg/mL (10 mL, 20 mL, 40 mL)

Injection, powder for reconstitution [preservative free]:

Eloxatin® [CAN]: 50 mg [contains lactose], 100 mg [contains lactose] [not available in U.S.]

References

Al-Batran SE, Hartmann JT, Probst S, et al, "Phase III Trial in Metastatic Gastroesophageal Adenocarcinoma With Fluorouracil, Leucovorin Plus Either Oxaliplatin or Cisplatin: A Study of the Arbeitsgemeinschaft Internistische Onkologie," *J Clin Oncol*, 2008, 26(9):1435-42.

Andre P, Cisternino S, Roy AL, et al, "Stability of Oxaliplatin in Infusion Bags Containing 5% Dextrose Injection," *Am J Health Syst Pharm*, 2007, 64(18):1950-4.

Andre T, Boni C, Mounedji-Boudiaf L, et al, "Oxaliplatin, Fluorouracil, and Leucovorin as Adjuvant Treatment for Colon Cancer," *N Engl J Med*, 2004, 350(23):2343-51.

Andre T, Boni C, Navarro M, et al, "Improved Overall Survival With Oxaliplatin, Fluorouracil, and Leucovorin as Adjuvant Treatment in Stage II or III Colon Cancer in the MOSAIC Trial," *J Clin Oncol*, 2009 [epub ahead of print]

Andre T, Tournigand C, Rosmorduc O, et al, "Gemcitabine Combined With Oxaliplatin (GEMOX) in Advanced Biliary Tract Adenocarcinoma: A GERCOR Study," *Ann Oncol*, 2004, 15(9):1339-43.

Bertheault-Cvitkovic F, Jami A, Ithzaki M, et al, "Biweekly Intensified Ambulatory Chronomodulated Chemotherapy With Oxaliplatin, Fluorouracil, and Leucovorin in Patients With Metastatic Colorectal Cancer," *J Clin Oncol*, 1996, 14(11):2950-8.

Cassidy J, Clarke S, Díaz-Rubio E, et al, "Randomized Phase III Study of Capecitabine Plus Oxaliplatin Compared With Fluorouracil/Folinic Acid Plus Oxaliplatin as First-Line Therapy for Metastatic Colorectal Cancer," *J Clin Oncol*, 2008, 26(12):2006-12.

Chau I, Webb A, Cunningham D, et al, "An Oxaliplatin-Based Chemotherapy in Patients With Relapsed or Refractory Intermediate and High-Grade Non-Hodgkin's Lymphoma," *Br J Haematol*, 2001, 115(4):786-92.

Conroy T, Paillot B, François E, et al, "Irinotecan Plus Oxaliplatin and Leucovorin-Modulated Fluorouracil in Advanced Pancreatic Cancer – A Groupe Tumeurs Digestives of the Federation Nationale des Centres de Lutte Contre le Cancer Study," *J Clin Oncol*, 2005, 23(6):1228-36.

Cunningham D, Starling N, Rao S, et al, "Capecitabine and Oxaliplatin for Advanced Esophagogastric Cancer," *N Engl J Med*, 2008, 358(1):36-46.

de Lemos ML and Walisser S, "Management of Extravasation of Oxaliplatin," *J Oncol Pharm Pract*, 2005, 11(4):159-62.

Dieras V, Bougnoux P, Petit T, et al, "Multicentre Phase II Study of Oxaliplatin as a Single-Agent in Cisplatin/Carboplatin +/- Taxane-Pretreated Ovarian Cancer Patients," *Ann Oncol*, 2002, 13 (2):258-66.

Doroshow JH, Synold TW, Gandara D, et al, "Pharmacology of Oxaliplatin in Solid Tumor Patients With Hepatic Dysfunction: A Preliminary Report of the National Cancer Institute Organ Dysfunction Working Group," *Semin Oncol*, 2003, 30(4 Suppl 15):14-9.

Falcone A, Ricci S, Brunetti I, et al, "Phase III Trial of Infusional Fluorouracil, Leucovorin, Oxaliplatin, and Irinotecan (FOLFOXIRI) Compared With Infusional Fluorouracil, Leucovorin, and Irinotecan (FOLFIRI) as First-Line Treatment for Metastatic Colorectal Cancer: The Gruppo Oncologico Nord Ovest," *J Clin Oncol*, 2007, 25(13):1670-6.

Khushalani NI, Leichman CG, Proulx G, et al, "Oxaliplatin in Combination with Protracted-Infusion Fluorouracil and Radiation: Report of a Clinical Trial for Patients With Esophageal Cancer," *J Clin Oncol*, 2002, 20(12):2844-50.

Kollmannsberger C, Beyer J, Liersch R, et al, "Combination Chemotherapy With Gemcitabine Plus Oxaliplatin in Patients With Intensively Pretreated or Refractory Germ Cell Cancer: A Study of the German Testicular Cancer Study Group," *J Clin Oncol*, 2004, 22(1):108-14.

KueblerJP, Wieand HS, O'Connell MJ, et al, "Oxaliplatin Combined With Weekly Bolus Fluorouracil and Leucovorin as Surgical Adjuvant Chemotherapy for Stage II and III Colon Cancer: Results From NSABP C-07," *J Clin Oncol*, 2007, 25(16):2198-204.

López A, Gutiérrez A, Palacios A, et al, "GEMOX-R Regimen is a Highly Effective Salvage Regimen in Patients With Refractory/Relapsing Diffuse Large-Cell Lymphoma: A Phase II Study," *Eur J Haematol*, 2008, 80(2):127-32.

Louvet C, André T, Tigaud JM, et al, "Phase II Study of Oxaliplatin, Fluorouracil, and Folinic Acid in Locally Advanced or Metastatic Gastric Cancer Patients," *J Clin Oncol*, 2002, 20(23):4543-8.

Louvet C, Labianca R, Hammel P, et al, "Gemcitabine in Combination With Oxaliplatin Compared With Gemcitabine Alone in Locally Advanced or Metastatic Pancreatic Cancer: Results of a GERCOR and GISCAD Phase III Trial," *J Clin Oncol*, 2005, 23(15):3509-16.

Nehls O, Oettle H, Hartmann JT, et al, "Capecitabine Plus Oxaliplatin as First-Line Treatment in Patients With Advanced Biliary System Adenocarcinoma: A Prospective Multicentre Phase II Trial," *Br J Cancer*, 2008, 98(2):309-15.

Pectasides D, Pectasides M, Farmakis D, et al, "Gemcitabine and Oxaliplatin (GEMOX) in Patients With Cisplatin-Refractory Germ Cell Tumors: A Phase II Study," *Ann Oncol*, 2004, 15(3):493-7.

Piccart MJ, Green JA, Lacave AJ, et al, "Oxaliplatin or Paclitaxel in Patients With Platinum-Pretreated Advanced Ovarian Cancer: A Randomized Phase II Study of the European Organization for Research and Treatment of Cancer Gynecology Group," *J Clin Oncol*, 2000, 18(6):1193-202.

Rodríguez J, Gutierrez A, Palacios A, et al, "Rituximab, Gemcitabine and Oxaliplatin: An Effective Regimen in Patients With Refractory and Relapsing Mantle Cell Lymphoma," *Leuk Lymphoma*, 2007, 48(11):2172-8.

Synold TW, Takimoto CH, Doroshow JH, et al, "Dose-Escalating and Pharmacologic Study of Oxaliplatin in Adult Cancer Patients With Impaired Hepatic Function: A National Cancer Institute Organ Dysfunction Working Group Study," *Clin Cancer Res*, 2007, 13(12):3660-6.

Takimoto CH, Graham MA, Lockwood G, et al, "Oxaliplatin Pharmacokinetics and Pharmacodynamics in Adult Cancer patients With Impaired Renal Function," *Clin Cancer Res*, 2007, 13 (16):4832-9.

Takimoto CH, Remick SC, Sharma S, et al, "Dose-Escalating and Pharmacological Study of Oxaliplatin in Adult Cancer Patients With Impaired Renal Function: A National Cancer Institute Organ Dysfunction Working Group Study," *J Clin Oncol*, 2003, 21(14):2664-72.

Trissel LA, Saenz CA, Ingram DS, et al, "Compatibility Screening of Oxaliplatin During Simulated Y-Site Administration With Other Drugs," *J Oncol Pharm Practice*, 2002, 8(1):33-7.

Tsimberidou AM, Wierda WG, Plunkett W, et al, "Phase I-II Study of Oxaliplatin, Fludarabine, Cytarabine, and Rituximab Combination Therapy in Patients With Richter's Syndrome or Fludarabine-Refractory Chronic Lymphocytic Leukemia," *J Clin Oncol*, 2008, 26(2):196-203.

Xiong HQ, Varadhachary GR, Blais JC, et al, "Phase 2 Trial of Oxaliplatin Plus Capecitabine (XELOX) as Second-Line Therapy for Patients With Advanced Pancreatic Cancer," *Cancer*, 2008, 113(8):2046-52.

OxyCODONE (oks i KOE done)

Medication Safety Issues

Sound-alike/look-alike issues:

OxyCODONE may be confused with HYDROcodone, OxyContin®, oxymorphone

OxyContin® may be confused with MS Contin®, oxybutynin, oxycodone

OxyFast® may be confused with Roxanol™

Roxicodone® may be confused with Roxanol™

◀ **High alert medication:** The Institute for Safe Medication Practices (ISMP) includes this medication among its list of drug classes which have a heightened risk of causing significant patient harm when used in error.

U.S. Brand Names ETH-Oxydose™ [DSC]; OxyContin®; OxyIR®; Roxicodone®

Index Terms Dihydrohydroxycodeinone; Oxycodone Hydrochloride

Generic Available Yes

Canadian Brand Names Oxy.IR®; OxyContin®; PMS-Oxycodone; Supeudol®

Pharmacologic Category Analgesic, Opioid

Use Management of moderate-to-severe pain, normally used in combination with nonopioid analgesics

OxyContin® is indicated for around-the-clock management of moderate-to-severe pain when an analgesic is needed for an extended period of time.

Restrictions C-II

Pregnancy Risk Factor B/D (prolonged use or high doses at term)

Lactation Enters breast milk/use caution

Labeled Contraindications Hypersensitivity to oxycodone or any component of the formulation; significant respiratory depression; hypercarbia; acute or severe bronchial asthma; OxyContin® is also contraindicated in paralytic ileus (known or suspected); pregnancy (prolonged use or high doses at term)

Warnings/Precautions May cause CNS depression, which may impair physical or mental abilities; patients must be cautioned about performing tasks which require mental alertness (eg, operating machinery or driving). Effects may be potentiated when used with other sedative drugs or ethanol. Use with caution in patients with hypersensitivity reactions to other phenanthrene derivative opioid agonists (morphine, hydrocodone, hydromorphone, levor-phanol, oxymorphone), respiratory diseases including asthma, emphysema, or COPD. Use with caution in pancreatitis or biliary tract disease, acute alcoholism (including delirium tremens), morbid obesity, adrenocortical insufficiency, history of seizure disorders, CNS depression/coma, kyphosco-liosis (or other skeletal disorder which may alter respiratory function), hypothyroidism (including myxedema), prostatic hyperplasia, urethral stricture, and toxic psychosis. May obscure diagnosis or clinical course of patients with acute abdominal conditions.

Use with caution in the elderly, debilitated, severe hepatic or renal function. Hemodynamic effects (hypotension, orthostasis) may be exaggerated in patients with hypovolemia, concurrent vasodilating drugs, or in patients with head injury. Respiratory depressant effects and capacity to elevate CSF pressure may be exaggerated in presence of head injury, other intracranial lesion, or pre-existing intracranial pressure.

Use the oral concentrate formulation with caution in patients with latex sensitivity; dropper dispenser contains dry, natural rubber. Concurrent use of agonist/antagonist analgesics may precipitate withdrawal symptoms and/or reduced analgesic efficacy in patients following prolonged therapy with mu opioid agonists. Abrupt discontinuation following prolonged use may also lead to withdrawal symptoms.

[U.S. Boxed Warning]: Healthcare provider should be alert to problems of abuse, misuse, and diversion. Tolerance or drug dependence may result from extended use.

Controlled-release formulations:

[U.S. Boxed Warning]: OxyContin® is not intended for use as an "as needed" analgesic or for immediately-postoperative pain management (should be used postoperatively only if the patient has received it prior to surgery or if severe, persistent pain is anticipated). **[U.S. Boxed Warning]: Do NOT crush, break, or chew controlled-release tablets;** 60 mg, 80 mg, and 160 mg strengths are for use only in opioid-tolerant patients.

Adverse Reactions

>10%:

Central nervous system: Somnolence (23% to 24%), dizziness (13% to 16%)

Dermatologic: Pruritus (12% to 13%)

Gastrointestinal: Nausea (23% to 27%), constipation (23% to 26%), vomiting (12% to 14%)

1% to 10%:

Cardiovascular: Postural hypotension (1% to 5%)

Central nervous system: Headache (7% to 8%), abnormal dreams (1% to 5%), anxiety (1% to 5%), chills (1% to 5%), confusion (1% to 5%), euphoria (1% to 5%), fever (1% to 5%), insomnia (1% to 5%), nervousness (1% to 5%), thought abnormalities (1% to 5%)

Dermatologic: Rash (1% to 5%)

Gastrointestinal: Xerostomia (6% to 7%), abdominal pain (1% to 5%), anorexia (1% to 5%), diarrhea (1% to 5%), dyspepsia (1% to 5%), gastritis (1% to 5%)

Neuromuscular & skeletal: Weakness (6% to 7%), twitching (1% to 5%)

Respiratory: Dyspnea (1% to 5%), hiccups (1% to 5%)

Miscellaneous: Diaphoresis (5% to 6%)

<1% (Limited to important or life-threatening): Agitation, amenorrhea, amnesia, anaphylaxis, anaphylactoid reaction, appetite increased, chest pain, cough, dehydration, depression, dysphagia, dysuria, edema, emotional lability, eructation, exfoliative dermatitis, facial edema, hallucinations, hematuria, histamine release, hyperkinesia, hypoesthesia, hyponatremia, hypotonia, ileus, impotence, intracranial pressure increased, libido decreased, malaise, migraine, paradoxical CNS stimulation, paralytic ileus, paresthesia, pharyngitis, physical dependence, polyuria, psychological dependence, seizure, SIADH, speech disorder, ST segment depression, stomatitis, stupor, syncope, tablet in stool (OxyContin®), taste perversion, thirst, tinnitus, tremor, urinary retention, urticaria, vasodilation, vertigo, vision change, voice alteration, withdrawal syndrome

Drug Interactions

Metabolism/Transport Effects Substrate (minor) of CYP2D6, 3A

Avoid Concomitant Use There are no known interactions where it is recommended to avoid concomitant use.

Increased Effect/Toxicity

OxyCODONE may increase the levels/effects of: Alcohol (Ethyl); Alvimopan; CNS Depressants; Desmopressin; Selective Serotonin Reuptake Inhibitors; Thiazide Diuretics

The levels/effects of OxyCODONE may be increased by: Amphetamines; Antipsychotic Agents (Phenothiazines); Succinylcholine

Decreased Effect

OxyCODONE may decrease the levels/effects of: Pegvisomant

The levels/effects of OxyCODONE may be decreased by: Ammonium Chloride

◀ **Ethanol/Nutrition/Herb Interactions**
 Ethanol: Avoid ethanol (may increase CNS depression).
 Food: When taken with a high-fat meal, peak concentration is 25% greater following a single OxyContin® 160 mg tablet as compared to two 80 mg tablets.
 Herb/Nutraceutical: Avoid valerian, St John's wort, kava kava, gotu kola (may increase CNS depression).
Storage/Stability Store at 15°C to 30°C (59°F to 86°F). Protect from light.
Mechanism of Action Binds to opiate receptors in the CNS, causing inhibition of ascending pain pathways, altering the perception of and response to pain; produces generalized CNS depression

Pharmacodynamics/Kinetics
 Onset of action: Pain relief: 10-15 minutes
  Peak effect: 0.5-1 hour
 Duration: Immediate release: 3-6 hours; Controlled release: ≤12 hours
 Distribution: V_d: 2.6 L/kg; distributed to skeletal muscle, liver, intestinal tract, lungs, spleen, brain, and breast milk
 Protein binding: ~45%
 Metabolism: Hepatically via CYP3A4 to noroxycodone (has weak analgesic), noroxymorphone, and alpha- and beta-noroxycodol. CYP2D6 mediated metabolism produces oxymorphone (has analgesic activity; low plasma concentrations), alpha- and beta-oxymorphol.
 Bioavailability: Controlled release, immediate release: 60% to 87%
 Half-life elimination: Immediate release: 2-3 hours; controlled release: ~5 hours
 Excretion: Urine (~19% as parent; >64% as metabolites)

Dosage Oral:
 Children: Immediate release:
  6-12 years: 1.25 mg every 6 hours as needed
  >12 years: 2.5 mg every 6 hours as needed
 Adults:
  Immediate release: 5 mg every 6 hours as needed
  Controlled release:
   Opioid naive: 10 mg every 12 hours
   Concurrent CNS depressants: Reduce usual dose by 1/3 to 1/2
   Conversion from transdermal fentanyl: For each 25 mcg/hour transdermal dose, substitute 10 mg controlled release oxycodone every 12 hours; should be initiated 18 hours after the removal of the transdermal fentanyl patch
   Currently on opioids: Use standard conversion chart to convert daily dose to oxycodone equivalent. Divide daily dose in 2 (for twice-daily dosing, usually every 12 hours) and round down to nearest dosage form.
   Note: 60 mg, 80 mg, or 160 mg tablets are for use **only** in opioid-tolerant patients. Special safety considerations must be addressed when converting to OxyContin® doses ≥160 mg every 12 hours. Dietary caution must be taken when patients are initially titrated to 160 mg tablets. Using different strengths to obtain the same daily dose is equivalent (eg, four 40 mg tablets, two 80 mg tablets, one 160 mg tablet); all produce similar blood levels.
  Multiplication factors for converting the daily dose of current oral opioid to the daily dose of oral oxycodone:
   Current opioid mg/day dose x factor = Oxycodone mg/day dose
    Codeine mg/day oral dose **x 0.15** = Oxycodone mg/day dose
    Hydrocodone mg/day oral dose **x 0.9** = Oxycodone mg/day dose
    Hydromorphone mg/day oral dose **x 4** = Oxycodone mg/day dose

Levorphanol mg/day oral dose **x** 7.5 = Oxycodone mg/day dose
Meperidine mg/day oral dose **x** 0.1 = Oxycodone mg/day dose
Methadone mg/day oral dose **x** 1.5 = Oxycodone mg/day dose
Morphine mg/day oral dose **x** 0.5 = Oxycodone mg/day dose
Note: Divide the oxycodone mg/day dose into the appropriate dosing interval for the specific form being used.

Dosing adjustment in hepatic impairment: Reduce dosage in patients with severe liver disease

Administration Do not crush, break, or chew controlled-release tablets; 60 mg, 80 mg, and 160 mg tablets are for use **only** in opioid-tolerant patients. Do not administer OxyContin® 160 mg tablet with a high-fat meal. Controlled release tablets are not indicated for rectal administration; increased risk of adverse events due to better rectal absorption.

Monitoring Parameters Pain relief, respiratory and mental status, blood pressure

Test Interactions Some quinolones may produce a false-positive urine screening result for opiates using commercially-available immunoassay kits. This has been demonstrated most consistently for levofloxacin and ofloxacin, but other quinolones have shown cross-reactivity in certain assay kits. Confirmation of positive opiate screens by more specific methods should be considered.

Dietary Considerations Instruct patient to avoid high-fat meals when taking OxyContin® 160 mg tablets.

Additional Information Prophylactic use of a laxative should be considered. OxyContin® 60 mg, 80 mg, and 160 mg tablets are for use in opioid-tolerant patients only.

Dosage Forms Excipient information presented when available (limited, particularly for generics); consult specific product labeling. [DSC] = Discontinued product

Capsule, immediate release, as hydrochloride: 5 mg
  OxyIR®: 5 mg
Liquid, oral, as hydrochloride [concentrate]:
  Roxicodone®: 20 mg/mL (30 mL) [contains sodium benzoate]
Solution, oral, as hydrochloride: 5 mg/5 mL (500 mL)
  Roxicodone®: 5 mg/5 mL (5 mL, 500 mL) [contains ethanol]
Solution, oral, as hydrochloride [concentrate]: 20 mg/mL (30 mL)
  ETH-Oxydose™: 20 mg/mL (1 mL, 30 mL) [contains sodium benzoate; berry flavor] [DSC]
Tablet, as hydrochloride: 5 mg, 10 mg, 15 mg, 20 mg, 30 mg
  Roxicodone®: 5 mg, 15 mg, 30 mg
Tablet, controlled release, as hydrochloride:
  OxyContin®: 10 mg, 15 mg, 20 mg, 30 mg, 40 mg, 60 mg, 80 mg
Tablet, extended release, as hydrochloride: 10 mg, 20 mg, 40 mg, 80 mg [DSC]

References

Kalso E and Vainio A, "Morphine and Oxycodone Hydrochloride in the Management of Cancer Pain," *Clin Pharmacol Ther*, 1990, 47(5):639-46.

♦ **Oxycodone Hydrochloride** *see* OxyCODONE *on page 889*

♦ **OxyContin®** *see* OxyCODONE *on page 889*

♦ **OxyIR®** *see* OxyCODONE *on page 889*

♦ **Oxy.IR® (Can)** *see* OxyCODONE *on page 889*

Oxymorphone (oks i MOR fone)

Medication Safety Issues

Sound-alike/look-alike issues:

Oxymorphone may be confused with oxycodone, oxymetholone

High alert medication: The Institute for Safe Medication Practices (ISMP) includes this medication among its list of drug classes which have a heightened risk of causing significant patient harm when used in error.

U.S. Brand Names Opana®; Opana® ER

Index Terms Oxymorphone Hydrochloride

Generic Available No

Pharmacologic Category Analgesic, Opioid

Use

Parenteral: Management of moderate-to-severe pain

Oral, regular release: Management of moderate-to-severe pain

Oral, extended release: Management of moderate-to-severe pain in patients requiring around-the-clock opioid treatment for an extended period of time

Restrictions C-II

Pregnancy Risk Factor C/D (prolonged use or high doses at term)

Lactation Excretion in breast milk unknown/use caution

Labeled Contraindications Hypersensitivity to oxymorphone, other morphine analogs (phenanthrene derivatives), or any component of the formulation; paralytic ileus (known or suspected); increased intracranial pressure; moderate-to-severe hepatic impairment; severe respiratory depression (unless in monitored setting with resuscitative equipment); acute/severe bronchial asthma; hypercarbia; pregnancy (prolonged use or high doses at term).

Note: Injection formulation is also contraindicated in the treatment of upper airway obstruction and pulmonary edema due to a chemical respiratory irritant.

Warnings/Precautions An opioid-containing analgesic regimen should be tailored to each patient's needs and based upon the type of pain being treated (acute versus chronic), the route of administration, degree of tolerance for opioids (naive versus chronic user), age, weight, and medical condition. The optimal analgesic dose varies widely among patients. Doses should be titrated to pain relief/prevention.

May cause CNS depression, which may impair physical or mental abilities; patients must be cautioned about performing tasks which require mental alertness (eg, operating machinery or driving). Effects may be potentiated when used with other sedative drugs or ethanol. Use with caution in patients with hypersensitivity reactions to other phenanthrene-derivative opioid agonists (codeine, hydrocodone, hydromorphone, levorphanol, oxycodone). May cause respiratory depression. Use extreme caution in patients with COPD or other chronic respiratory conditions characterized by hypoxia, hypercapnia, or diminished respiratory reserve (myxedema, cor pulmonale, kyphoscoliosis, obstructive sleep apnea, severe obesity). Use with caution in patients (particularly elderly or debilitated) with impaired respiratory function, adrenal disease, morbid obesity, thyroid dysfunction, prostatic hyperplasia, or renal impairment. Use caution in mild hepatic dysfunction; use is contraindicated in moderate-to-severe hepatic impairment. Use only with extreme caution (if at all) in patients with head injury or increased intracranial pressure (ICP); potential to elevate ICP and/or blunt papillary response may be greatly exaggerated in these patients. Use with caution in biliary tract disease or acute pancreatitis (may cause constriction of sphincter of Oddi). May obscure diagnosis or clinical course of patients with acute abdominal conditions.

Oxymorphone shares the toxic potential of opiate agonists and usual precautions of opiate agonist therapy should be observed; may cause hypotension in patients with acute myocardial infarction, volume depletion, or concurrent drug therapy which may exaggerate vasodilation. The elderly may be particularly susceptible to adverse effects of narcotics. Safety and efficacy have not been established in children <18 years of age.

[U.S. Boxed Warning]: Healthcare provider should be alert to problems of abuse, misuse, and diversion. Tolerance or drug dependence may result from extended use. Use caution in patients with a history of drug dependence or abuse. Abrupt discontinuation may precipitate withdrawal syndrome.

Extended release formulation:

[U.S. Boxed Warnings]: Opana® ER is an extended release oral formulation of oxymorphone and is not suitable for use as an "as needed" analgesic. Tablets should not be broken, chewed, dissolved, or crushed; tablets should be swallowed whole. Opana® ER is intended for use in long-term, continuous management of moderate-to-severe chronic pain. It is not indicated for use in the immediate postoperative period (12-24 hours). **[U.S. Boxed Warning]: The coingestion of ethanol or ethanol-containing medications with Opana® ER may result in accelerated release of drug from the dosage form, abruptly increasing plasma levels, which may have fatal consequences.**

Adverse Reactions Frequency not defined.
Cardiovascular: Bradycardia, cardiac shock, flushing, hypotension, orthostatic hypotension, palpitation, peripheral vasodilation, shock, tachycardia
Central nervous system: Agitation, amnesia, anorexia, anxiety, CNS depression, coma, confusion, convulsion, dizziness, drowsiness, dysphoria, euphoria, fatigue, fever, hallucinations, headache, insomnia, intracranial pressure increased, malaise, mental depression, mental impairment, nervousness, restlessness, paradoxical CNS stimulation
Dermatologic: Pruritus, urticaria, rash
Endocrine & metabolic: Antidiuretic hormone release, weight loss
Gastrointestinal: Abdominal pain, appetite depression, biliary tract spasm, constipation, dehydration, dry mouth, dyspepsia, flatulence, nausea, paralytic ileus, stomach cramps, vomiting, xerostomia
Genitourinary: Urination decreased, urinary retention, urinary tract spasm
Local: Pain/reaction at injection site
Neuromuscular & skeletal: Weakness
Ocular: Blurred vision, diplopia, miosis
Renal: Oliguria
Respiratory: Apnea, bronchospasm, cyanosis, dyspnea, hypoventilation, laryngeal edema, laryngeal spasm, respiratory depression
Miscellaneous: Diaphoresis, histamine release, physical and psychological dependence

Drug Interactions
Avoid Concomitant Use There are no known interactions where it is recommended to avoid concomitant use.
Increased Effect/Toxicity
Oxymorphone may increase the levels/effects of: Alcohol (Ethyl); Alvimopan; CNS Depressants; Desmopressin; Selective Serotonin Reuptake Inhibitors; Thiazide Diuretics

The levels/effects of Oxymorphone may be increased by: Amphetamines; Antipsychotic Agents (Phenothiazines); Succinylcholine

Decreased Effect

Oxymorphone may decrease the levels/effects of: Pegvisomant

The levels/effects of Oxymorphone may be decreased by: Ammonium Chloride

Ethanol/Nutrition/Herb Interactions

Ethanol: Avoid ethanol (may increase CNS depression). Ethanol ingestion with extended-release tablets is specifically contraindicated due to possible accelerated release and potentially fatal overdose.

Food: When taken orally with a high-fat meal, peak concentration is 38% to 50% greater. Both immediate-release and extended-release tablets should be taken 1 hour before or 2 hours after eating.

Herb/Nutraceutical: Avoid valerian, St John's wort, kava kava, gotu kola (may increase CNS depression).

Storage/Stability Injection solution, tablet: Store at 15°C to 30°C (59°F to 86°F).

Compatibility Compatibility in syringe: Compatible: Glycopyrrolate, hydroxyzine, ranitidine.

Mechanism of Action Oxymorphone hydrochloride (Numorphan®) is a potent narcotic analgesic with uses similar to those of morphine. The drug is a semisynthetic derivative of morphine (phenanthrene derivative) and is closely related to hydromorphone chemically (Dilaudid®).

Pharmacodynamics/Kinetics

Onset of action: Parenteral: 5-10 minutes

Duration: Analgesic: Parenteral: 3-6 hours

Distribution: V_d: I.V.: 1.94-4.22 L/kg

Protein binding: 10% to 12%

Metabolism: Hepatic via glucuronidation to active and inactive metabolites

Bioavailability: Oral: 10%

Half-life elimination: Oral: Immediate release: 7-9 hours; Extended release: 9-11 hours

Excretion: Urine (<1% as unchanged drug); feces

Dosage Adults: **Note:** Dosage must be individualized.

I.M., SubQ: Initial: 1-1.5 mg; may repeat every 4-6 hours as needed

Labor analgesia: I.M.: 0.5-1 mg

I.V.: Initial: 0.5 mg

Oral:

Immediate release:

Opioid-naive: 10-20 mg every 4-6 hours as needed. Initial dosages as low as 5 mg may be considered in selected patients and/or patients with renal impairment. Dosage adjustment should be based on level of analgesia, side effects, and pain intensity. Initiation of therapy with initial dose >20 mg is **not** recommended.

Note: The American Pain Society recommends an initial dose of 5-10 mg for adult patients with severe pain.

Currently on stable dose of parenteral oxymorphone: ~10 times the daily parenteral requirement. The calculated amount should be divided and given in 4-6 equal doses.

Currently on other opioids: Use standard conversion chart to convert daily dose to oxymorphone equivalent. Generally start with 1/2 the calculated daily oxymorphone dosage and administered in divided doses every 4-6 hours.

Extended release (Opana® ER):

Opioid-naive: Initial: 5 mg every 12 hours. Supplemental doses of immediate-release oxymorphone may be used as "rescue" medication as dosage is titrated.

Note: Continued requirement for supplemental dosing may be used to titrate the dose of extended-release continuous therapy. Adjust therapy incrementally, by 5-10 mg every 12 hours at intervals of every 3-7 days. Ideally, basal dosage may be titrated to generally mild pain or no pain with the regular use of fewer than 2 supplemental doses per 24 hours.

Currently on stable dose of parenteral oxymorphone: Approximately 10 times the daily parenteral requirement. The calculated amount should be given in 2 divided doses (every 12 hours).

Currently on opioids: Use conversion chart (see Note below) to convert daily dose to oxymorphone equivalent. Generally start with 1/2 the calculated daily oxymorphone dosage. Divide daily dose in 2 (for every 12-hour dosing) and round down to nearest dosage form. **Note:** Per manufacturer, the following approximate oral dosages are equivalent to oxymorphone 10 mg:

Hydrocodone 20 mg
Oxycodone 20 mg
Methadone 20 mg
Morphine 30 mg

Conversion of stable dose of immediate-release oxymorphone to extended-release oxymorphone: Administer 1/2 of the daily dose of immediate-release oxymorphone (Opana®) as the extended-release formulation (Opana® ER) every 12 hours

Elderly: Initiate dosing at the lower end of the dosage range

Dosing adjustment in renal impairment: Cl_{cr} <50 mL/minute: Reduce initial dosage of oral formulations (bioavailability increased 57% to 65%). Begin therapy at lowest dose and titrate carefully.

Dosing adjustment in hepatic impairment: Generally, contraindicated for use in patients with moderate-to-severe liver disease. Initiate with lowest possible dose and titrate slowly in mild impairment.

Administration Administer immediate release and extended release tablets 1 hour before or 2 hours after eating. Opana® ER tablet should be swallowed; do not break, crush, or chew.

Monitoring Parameters Respiratory rate, heart rate, blood pressure, CNS activity

Test Interactions Some quinolones may produce a false-positive urine screening result for opiates using commercially-available immunoassay kits. This has been demonstrated most consistently for levofloxacin and ofloxacin, but other quinolones have shown cross-reactivity in certain assay kits. Confirmation of positive opiate screens by more specific methods should be considered. May cause elevation in amylase (due to constriction of the sphincter of Oddi).

Dietary Considerations Immediate release and extended release tablets should be taken 1 hour before or 2 hours after eating.

Dosage Forms Excipient information presented when available (limited, particularly for generics); consult specific product labeling.
Injection, solution, as hydrochloride:
Opana®: 1 mg/mL (1 mL)
Tablet, as hydrochloride:
Opana®: 5 mg, 10 mg

Tablet, extended release, as hydrochloride:
Opana®: ER: 5 mg, 7.5 mg, 10 mg, 15 mg, 20 mg, 30 mg, 40 mg

References

Gabrail NY, Dvergsten C, and Ahdieh H, "Establishing the Dosage Equivalency of Oxymorphone Extended Release and Oxycodone Controlled Release in Patients With Cancer Pain: A Randomized Controlled Study," *Curr Med Res Opin*, 2004, 20(6):911-8.

"Principles of Analgesic Use in the Treatment of Acute Pain and Chronic Cancer Pain," 5th ed, Glenview, IL: American Pain Society, 2003.

◆ **Oxymorphone Hydrochloride** *see* Oxymorphone *on page 894*

◆ **P32** *see* Chromic Phosphate P 32 *on page 224*

◆ **Pacis™ (Can)** *see* BCG Vaccine *on page 128*

Paclitaxel (pac li TAKS el)

Medication Safety Issues

Sound-alike/look-alike issues:
Paclitaxel may be confused with paroxetine, Paxil®
Paclitaxel (conventional) may be confused with paclitaxel (protein-bound)
Taxol® may be confused with Abraxane®, Paxil®, Taxotere®

High alert medication: The Institute for Safe Medication Practices (ISMP) includes this medication among its list of drugs which have a heightened risk of causing significant patient harm when used in error.

Related Information

Management of Drug Extravasations *on page 1447*
Safe Handling of Hazardous Drugs *on page 1517*

U.S. Brand Names Onxol®; Taxol® [DSC]

Generic Available Yes

Canadian Brand Names Abraxane® For Injectable Suspension; Apo-Paclitaxel®; Taxol®

Pharmacologic Category Antineoplastic Agent, Antimicrotubular; Antineoplastic Agent, Natural Source (Plant) Derivative; Antineoplastic Agent, Taxane Derivative

Use Treatment of breast, nonsmall cell lung, and ovarian cancers; treatment of AIDS-related Kaposi's sarcoma (KS)

Unlabeled/Investigational Use Treatment of bladder, cervical, small cell lung, and head and neck cancers; treatment of (unknown primary) adenocarcinoma

Pregnancy Risk Factor D

Lactation Excretion in breast milk unknown/contraindicated

Labeled Contraindications Hypersensitivity to paclitaxel, Cremophor® EL (polyoxyethylated castor oil), or any component of the formulation

Warnings/Precautions Hazardous agent - use appropriate precautions for handling and disposal. **[U.S. Boxed Warning]: Severe hypersensitivity reactions have been reported;** premedication may minimize this effect. Stop infusion and do not rechallenge for severe hypersensitivity reactions (hypotension requiring treatment, dyspnea requiring bronchodilators, angioedema, urticaria). Minor hypersensitivity reactions (flushing, skin reactions, dyspnea, hypotension, or tachycardia) do not require interruption of treatment. **[U.S. Boxed Warning]: Bone marrow suppression is the dose-limiting toxicity; do not administer if baseline absolute neutrophil count (ANC) is <1500 cells/mm³ (<1000 cells/mm³ for patients with AIDS-related KS);** reduce future doses by 20% for severe neutropenia (<500 cells/mm³ for 7 days or more) and consider the use of supportive therapy, including growth factor treatment.

Use extreme caution with hepatic dysfunction (myelotoxicity may be worsened); dose reductions are recommended. Peripheral neuropathy may occur; patients with pre-existing neuropathies from chemotherapy or coexisting conditions (eg, diabetes mellitus) may be at a higher risk; reduce dose by 20% for severe neuropathy. Paclitaxel formulations contain dehydrated alcohol; may cause adverse CNS effects. Infusion-related hypotension, bradycardia, and/or hypertension may occur; frequent monitoring of vital signs is recommended, especially during the first hour of the infusion. Rare but severe conduction abnormalities have been reported; conduct cardiac monitoring during subsequent infusions for these patients. When administered as sequential infusions, taxane derivatives (docetaxel, paclitaxel) should be administered before platinum derivatives (carboplatin, cisplatin) to limit myelosuppression. Elderly patients have an increased risk of toxicity (neutropenia, neuropathy). **[U.S. Boxed Warning]: Should be administered under the supervision of an experienced cancer chemotherapy physician.** Safety and efficacy in children have not been established.

Adverse Reactions Percentages reported with single-agent therapy. **Note:** Myelosuppression is dose related, schedule related, and infusion-rate dependent (increased incidences with higher doses, more frequent doses, and longer infusion times) and, in general, rapidly reversible upon discontinuation.

>10%:
Cardiovascular: Flushing (28%), ECG abnormal (14% to 23%), edema (21%), hypotension (4% to 12%)
Dermatologic: Alopecia (87%), rash (12%)
Gastrointestinal: Nausea/vomiting (52%), diarrhea (38%), mucositis (17% to 35%; grades 3/4: up to 3%), stomatitis (15%; most common at doses >390 mg/m^2), abdominal pain (with intraperitoneal paclitaxel)
Hematologic: Neutropenia (78% to 98%; grade 4: 14% to 75%; onset 8-10 days, median nadir 11 days, recovery 15-21 days), leukopenia (90%; grade 4: 17%), anemia (47% to 90%; grades 3/4: 2% to 16%), thrombocytopenia (4% to 20%; grades 3/4: 1% to 7%), bleeding (14%)
Hepatic: Alkaline phosphatase increased (22%), AST increased (19%)
Local: Injection site reaction (erythema, tenderness, skin discoloration, swelling; 13%)
Neuromuscular & skeletal: Peripheral neuropathy (42% to 70%; grades 3/4: up to 7%), arthralgia/myalgia (60%), weakness (17%)
Renal: Creatinine increased (observed in KS patients only: 18% to 34%; severe: 5% to 7%)
Miscellaneous: Hypersensitivity reaction (31% to 45%; grades 3/4: up to 2%), infection (15% to 30%)

1% to 10%:
Cardiovascular: Bradycardia (3%), tachycardia (2%), hypertension (1%), rhythm abnormalities (1%), syncope (1%), venous thrombosis (1%)
Dermatologic: Nail changes (2%)
Hematologic: Febrile neutropenia (2%)
Hepatic: Bilirubin increased (7%)
Respiratory: Dyspnea (2%)

<1%, postmarketing, and/or case reports: Anaphylaxis, ataxia, atrial fibrillation, AV block, back pain, cardiac conduction abnormalities, cellulitis, CHF, chills, conjunctivitis, dehydration, enterocolitis, extravasation recall, hepatic encephalopathy, hepatic necrosis, induration, intestinal obstruction, intestinal perforation, interstitial pneumonia, ischemic colitis, lacrimation increased, maculopapular rash, malaise, MI, necrotic changes and ulceration following extravasation, neuroencephalopathy, neutropenic enterocolitis, ototoxicity

(tinnitus and hearing loss), pancreatitis, paralytic ileus, phlebitis, pruritus, pulmonary embolism, pulmonary fibrosis, radiation recall, radiation pneumonitis, pruritus, renal insufficiency, seizure, skin exfoliation, skin fibrosis, skin necrosis, Stevens-Johnson syndrome, supraventricular tachycardia, toxic epidermal necrolysis, ventricular tachycardia (asymptomatic), visual disturbances (scintillating scotomata)

Drug Interactions

Metabolism/Transport Effects Substrate (major) of CYP2C8, 3A4; **Induces** CYP3A4 (weak)

Avoid Concomitant Use

Avoid concomitant use of Paclitaxel with any of the following: Natalizumab; Vaccines (Live)

Increased Effect/Toxicity

Paclitaxel may increase the levels/effects of: Antineoplastic Agents (Anthracycline); DOXOrubicin; Leflunomide; Natalizumab; Trastuzumab; Vaccines (Live); Vinorelbine

The levels/effects of Paclitaxel may be increased by: CYP2C8 Inhibitors (Moderate); CYP2C8 Inhibitors (Strong); CYP2C9 Inhibitors (Moderate); CYP2C9 Inhibitors (Strong); CYP3A4 Inhibitors (Moderate); CYP3A4 Inhibitors (Strong); Dasatinib; Deferasirox; P-Glycoprotein Inhibitors; Platinum Derivatives; Trastuzumab

Decreased Effect

Paclitaxel may decrease the levels/effects of: Saxagliptin; Vaccines (Inactivated); Vaccines (Live)

The levels/effects of Paclitaxel may be decreased by: CYP2C8 Inducers (Highly Effective); CYP2C9 Inducers (Highly Effective); CYP3A4 Inducers (Strong); Deferasirox; Echinacea; Herbs (CYP3A4 Inducers); Peginterferon Alfa-2b; P-Glycoprotein Inducers; Trastuzumab

Ethanol/Nutrition/Herb Interactions Herb/Nutraceutical: Avoid black cohosh, dong quai in estrogen-dependent tumors. Avoid valerian, St John's wort (may decrease paclitaxel levels), kava kava, gotu kola (may increase CNS depression).

Storage/Stability Store intact vials at room temperature of 20°C to 25°C (68°F to 77°F). Protect from light. Solutions in D_5W and NS are stable for up to 3 days at room temperature (25°C).

Paclitaxel should be dispensed in either glass or non-PVC containers (eg, Excel™/PAB™). Use **nonpolyvinyl** (non-PVC) tubing (eg, polyethylene) to minimize leaching. Formulated in a vehicle known as Cremophor® EL (polyoxyethylated castor oil). Cremophor® EL has been found to leach the plasticizer DEHP from polyvinyl chloride infusion bags or administration sets. Contact of the undiluted concentrate with plasticized polyvinyl chloride (PVC) equipment or devices is not recommended.

Reconstitution Dilute in 250-1000 mL D_5W, D_5LR, D_5NS, or NS to a concentration of 0.3-1.2 mg/mL. Chemotherapy dispensing devices (eg, Chemo Dispensing Pin™) should not be used to withdraw paclitaxel from the vial.

Compatibility Stable in D_5W, D_5LR, D_5NS, NS.

Y-site administration: Compatible: Acyclovir, amikacin, aminophylline, ampicillin/sulbactam, bleomycin, butorphanol, calcium chloride, carboplatin, cefepime, cefotetan, ceftazidime, ceftriaxone, cimetidine, cisplatin, cladribine, cyclophosphamide, cytarabine, dacarbazine, dexamethasone sodium phosphate, diphenhydramine, doxorubicin, droperidol, etoposide, etoposide phosphate, famotidine, floxuridine, fluconazole, fluorouracil, furosemide, ganciclovir, gatifloxacin, gemcitabine, gentamicin, granisetron, haloperidol, heparin, hydrocortisone sodium phosphate, hydrocortisone sodium succinate, hydromorphone, ifosfamide, linezolid, lorazepam, magnesium sulfate, mannitol, meperidine, mesna, methotrexate, metoclopramide, morphine, nalbuphine, ondansetron, ondansetron with ranitidine, pentostatin, potassium chloride, prochlorperazine edisylate, propofol, ranitidine, sodium bicarbonate, thiotepa, topotecan, vancomycin, vinblastine, vincristine, zidovudine. **Incompatible:** Amphotericin B, amphotericin B cholesteryl sulfate complex, chlorpromazine, doxorubicin liposome, hydroxyzine, methylprednisolone sodium succinate, mitoxantrone.

Compatibility when admixed: Compatible: Carboplatin, doxorubicin. **Variable (consult detailed reference):** Cisplatin.

Mechanism of Action Paclitaxel promotes microtubule assembly by enhancing the action of tubulin dimers, stabilizing existing microtubules, and inhibiting their disassembly, interfering with the late G_2 mitotic phase, and inhibiting cell replication. In addition, the drug can distort mitotic spindles, resulting in the breakage of chromosomes. Paclitaxel may also suppress cell proliferation and modulate immune response.

Pharmacodynamics/Kinetics

Distribution:

V_d: Widely distributed into body fluids and tissues; affected by dose and duration of infusion

V_{dss}:

1- to 6-hour infusion: 67.1 L/m^2
24-hour infusion: 227-688 L/m^2

Protein binding: 89% to 98%

Metabolism: Hepatic via CYP2C8 and 3A4; forms metabolites (primarily 6α-hydroxypaclitaxel)

Half-life elimination:

1- to 6-hour infusion: Mean (beta): 6.4 hours
3-hour infusion: Mean (terminal): 13.1-20.2 hours
24-hour infusion: Mean (terminal): 15.7-52.7 hours

Excretion: Feces (~70%, 5% as unchanged drug); urine (14%)

Clearance: Mean: Total body: After 1- and 6-hour infusions: 5.8-16.3 L/hour/m^2; After 24-hour infusions: 14.2-17.2 L/hour/m^2

Dosage Premedication with dexamethasone (20 mg orally or I.V. at 12 and 6 hours **or** 14 and 7 hours before the dose; reduce dexamethasone dose to 10 mg orally with advanced HIV disease), diphenhydramine (50 mg I.V. 30-60 minutes prior to the dose), and cimetidine, famotidine, or ranitidine (I.V. 30-60 minutes prior to the dose) is recommended.

Adults: I.V.: Refer to individual protocols

Ovarian carcinoma: 135-175 mg/m^2 over 3 hours every 3 weeks **or**
135 mg/m^2 over 24 hours every 3 weeks **or**
50-80 mg/m^2 over 1-3 hours weekly **or**
1.4-4 mg/m^2/day continuous infusion for 14 days every 4 weeks

Metastatic breast cancer: 175-250 mg/m^2 over 3 hours every 3 weeks **or**
50-80 mg/m^2 weekly **or**
1.4-4 mg/m^2/day continuous infusion for 14 days every 4 weeks

Nonsmall cell lung carcinoma: 135 mg/m^2 over 24 hours every 3 weeks

AIDS-related Kaposi's sarcoma: 135 mg/m^2 over 3 hours every 3 weeks **or**
100 mg/m^2 over 3 hours every 2 weeks

Intraperitoneal (unlabeled route): Ovarian carcinoma: 60 mg/m^2 on day 8 of a 21-day treatment cycle for 6 cycles, in combination with I.V. paclitaxel and ▶

intraperitoneal cisplatin. **Note:** Administration of intraperitoneal paclitaxel should include the standard paclitaxel premedication regimen.

Dosage modification for toxicity (solid tumors, including ovary, breast, and lung carcinoma): Courses of paclitaxel should not be repeated until the the neutrophil count is ≥1500 cells/mm^3 and the platelet count is ≥100,000 cells/mm^3; reduce dosage by 20% for patients experiencing severe peripheral neuropathy or severe neutropenia (neutrophil <500 cells/mm^3 for a week or longer)

Dosage modification for immunosuppression in advanced HIV disease: Paclitaxel should not be given to patients with HIV if the baseline or subsequent neutrophil count is <1000 cells/mm^3. Additional modifications include: Reduce dosage of dexamethasone in premedication to 10 mg orally; reduce dosage by 20% in patients experiencing severe peripheral neuropathy or severe neutropenia (neutrophil <500 cells/mm^3 for a week or longer); initiate concurrent hematopoietic growth factor (G-CSF) as clinically indicated

Dosage adjustment in renal impairment: There are no FDA-approved labeling guidelines for dosage adjustment in patients with renal impairment. Aronoff (2007) recommends no dosage adjustment necessary for adults with Cl$_{cr}$ <50 mL/minute.

Dosage adjustment in hepatic impairment: Note: The FDA-approved labeling recommendations are based upon the patient's first course of therapy where the usual dose would be 135 mg/m^2 dose over 24 hours or the 175 mg/m^2 dose over 3 hours in patients with normal hepatic function. Dosage in subsequent courses should be based upon individual tolerance. Adjustments for other regimens are not available.

24-hour infusion:

Transaminases <2 times upper limit of normal (ULN) and bilirubin level ≤1.5 mg/dL: 135 mg/m^2

Transaminases 2-<10 times ULN and bilirubin level ≤1.5 mg/dL: 100 mg/m^2

Transaminases <10 times ULN and bilirubin level 1.6-7.5 mg/dL: 50 mg/m^2

Transaminases ≥10 times ULN **or** bilirubin level >7.5 mg/dL: Avoid use

3-hour infusion:

Transaminases <10 times ULN and bilirubin level ≤1.25 times ULN: 175 mg/m^2

Transaminases <10 times ULN and bilirubin level 1.26-2 times ULN: 135 mg/m^2

Transaminases <10 times ULN and bilirubin level 2.01-5 times ULN: 90 mg/m^2

Transaminases ≥10 times ULN **or** bilirubin level >5 times ULN: Avoid use

Combination Regimens

Administration

I.V.: Infuse over 1-96 hours. When administered as sequential infusions, taxane derivatives should be administered before platinum derivatives (cisplatin, carboplatin) to limit myelosuppression and to enhance efficacy.

Premedication with dexamethasone (20 mg orally or I.V. at 12 and 6 hours **or** 14 and 7 hours before the dose; reduce to 10 mg with advanced HIV disease), diphenhydramine (50 mg I.V. 30-60 minutes prior to the dose), and cimetidine 300 mg, famotidine 20 mg, or ranitidine 50 mg (I.V. 30-60 minutes prior to the dose) is recommended.

Administer I.V. infusion over 1-24 hours; infuse through a 0.22 micron in-line filter and nonsorbing administration set.

Intraperitoneal: 1- to 2-hour infusion

Monitoring Parameters CBC with differential; monitor for hypersensitivity reactions, vital signs (frequently during the first hour of infusion), continuous cardiac monitoring (patients with conduction abnormalities)

Additional Information Sensory neuropathy is almost universal at doses >250 mg/m^2; motor neuropathy is uncommon at doses <250 mg/m^2. Myopathic effects are common with doses >200 mg/m^2, generally occur within 2-3 days of treatment, and resolve over 5-6 days. Intraperitoneal administration of paclitaxel is associated with a higher incidence of chemotherapy related toxicity.

Emetic Potential Low (10% to 30%)

Vesicant No; the drug is an irritant. See Management of Drug Extravasations on page 1447.

High Dose Considerations

Comments Glutamine may decrease mucositis

High Dose I.V.: 250-775 mg/m^2; generally combined with other high-dose chemotherapy; maximum dose as single agent: 825 mg/m^2

Dosage Forms Excipient information presented when available (limited, particularly for generics); consult specific product labeling. [DSC] = Discontinued product

Injection, solution: 6 mg/mL (5 mL, 16.7 mL, 25 mL, 50 mL) [contains ethanol and purified Cremophor® EL (polyoxyethylated castor oil)]

Onxol®: 6 mg/mL (5 mL, 25 mL, 50 mL) [contains ethanol and purified Cremophor® EL (polyoxyethylated castor oil)]

Taxol®: 6 mg/mL (5 mL, 16.7 mL, 25 mL, 50 mL) [contains ethanol and purified Cremophor® EL (polyoxyethylated castor oil)] [DSC]

References

Armstrong DK, Bundy B, Wenzel L, et al, "Intraperitoneal Cisplatin and Paclitaxel in Ovarian Cancer," *N Engl J Med*, 2006, 354(1):34-43.

Aronoff GR, Bennett WM, Berns JS, et al, *Drug Prescribing in Renal Failure: Dosing Guidelines for Adults and Children*, 5th ed. Philadelphia, PA: American College of Physicians; 2007, p 101.

Holmes FA, "Paclitaxel Combination Therapy in the Treatment of Metastatic Breast Cancer: A Review," *Semin Oncol*, 1996, 23(5 Suppl 11):46-56.

Miller K, Wang M, Gralow J, et al, "Paclitaxel Plus Bevacizumab Versus Paclitaxel Alone for Metastatic Breast Cancer," *N Engl J Med*, 2007, 357(26):2666-76.

Rowinsky EK, "The Taxanes: Dosing and Scheduling Considerations," *Oncology*, 1997, 11(3 Suppl 2):7-19.

Seetalarom K, Kudelka AP, Verschraegen CF, et al, "Taxanes in Ovarian Cancer Treatment," *Curr Opin Obstet Gynecol*, 1997, 9(1):14-20.

Sonnichsen DS and Relling MV, "Clinical Pharmacokinetics of Paclitaxel," *Clin Pharmacokinet*, 1994, 27(4):256-69.

Spencer CM and Faulds D, "Paclitaxel. A Review of Its Pharmacodynamic and Pharmacokinetic Properties and Therapeutic Potential in the Treatment of Cancer," *Drugs*, 1994, 48(5):794-847.

◆ **Paclitaxel, Albumin-Bound** *see* Paclitaxel (Protein Bound) *on page 904*

Paclitaxel (Protein Bound) (pac li TAKS el PROE teen bownd)

Medication Safety Issues

Sound-alike/look-alike issues:

Paclitaxel (protein bound) may be confused with paclitaxel (conventional)

Abraxane® may be confused with Paxil®, Taxol®, Taxotere®

High alert medication: The Institute for Safe Medication Practices (ISMP) includes this medication among its list of drug classes which have a heightened risk of causing significant patient harm when used in error.

Related Information

Management of Drug Extravasations *on page 1447*

Safe Handling of Hazardous Drugs *on page 1517*

U.S. Brand Names Abraxane®

Index Terms ABI-007; Albumin-Bound Paclitaxel; Albumin-Stabilized Nanoparticle Paclitaxel; nab-Paclitaxel; Nanoparticle Albumin-Bound Paclitaxel; Paclitaxel, Albumin-Bound; Protein-Bound Paclitaxel

Generic Available No

Pharmacologic Category Antineoplastic Agent, Antimicrotubular; Antineoplastic Agent, Natural Source (Plant) Derivative; Antineoplastic Agent, Taxane Derivative

Use Treatment of refractory (metastatic) or relapsed (within 6 months of adjuvant therapy) breast cancer

Unlabeled/Investigational Use Treatment of advanced nonsmall cell lung cancer (NSCLC)

Pregnancy Risk Factor D

Lactation Excretion in breast milk unknown/not recommended

Labeled Contraindications Patients with baseline neutrophils <1500/mm³

Warnings/Precautions Hazardous agent - use appropriate precautions for handling and disposal.

[U.S. Boxed Warning]: Paclitaxel (protein-bound) is not interchangeable with other forms of paclitaxel, including Cremophor®-based or unbound paclitaxel.

[U.S. Boxed Warning]: Bone marrow suppression, primarily neutropenia, may occur; monitor peripheral blood counts frequently. Baseline neutrophils should be ≥1500/mm³ for administration. Hematologic toxicity is dose-dependent and dose-limiting. Neutrophils should recover to >1500/mm³ and platelets should recover to >100,000/mm³ prior to the next treatment cycle. For severe neutropenia, dose reductions may be recommended for subsequent cycles. When administered as sequential infusions, taxane derivatives (docetaxel, paclitaxel) should be administered before platinum derivatives (carboplatin, cisplatin) to limit myelosuppression. Dose-related, cumulative sensory neuropathy is common (may require dosage modification); severe sensory neuropathy may occur. Prior therapy with neurotoxic agents may influence the frequency and severity of neurologic toxicity. Rare postmarketing cases of severe hypersensitivity have been reported; do not rechallenge after severe hypersensitivity reaction. Use has not been studied in patients with a prior hypersensitivity reaction to conventional paclitaxel or albumin.

Use with caution in patients with hepatic impairment; monitor closely; the risk of toxicities is increased. Reduced initial dosages are recommended for moderate and severe hepatic impairment; use is not recommended in patients with AST >10 times ULN or bilirubin >5 times ULN. Has not been studied in renal impairment; patients with serum creatinine >2 mg/dL were excluded from clinical trials.

[U.S. Boxed Warning]: Should be administered under the supervision of an experienced cancer chemotherapy physician. Product contains albumin, which confers a theoretical risk of transmission of viral disease or Creutzfeldt-Jakob disease. May cause fatigue, lethargy, malaise or weakness; caution patients about performing tasks which require mental alertness (eg, operating machinery or driving). Safety and efficacy in children have not been established.

Adverse Reactions

>10%:

Cardiovascular: ECG abnormal (60%; 35% in patients with a normal baseline)

Dermatologic: Alopecia (90%)

Gastrointestinal: Nausea (30%; grades 3/4: 3%), diarrhea (27%; grades 3/4: <1%), vomiting (18%; grades 3/4: 4%)

Hematologic: Neutropenia (80%; grade 4: 9%), anemia (33%; grades 3/4: 1%), myelosuppression (dose-related)

Hepatic: AST increased (39%), alkaline phosphatase increased (36%), GGT increased (grades 3/4: 14%)

Neuromuscular & skeletal: Sensory neuropathy (71%; grades 3/4: 10%; dose dependent; cumulative), weakness (47%; severe 8%), myalgia/arthralgia (44%)

Ocular: Vision disturbance (13%; severe [keratitis, blurred vision]: 1%)

Renal: Creatinine increased (11%; severe 1%)

Respiratory: Dyspnea (12%)

Miscellaneous: Infection (24%; primarily included oral candidiasis, respiratory tract infection, and pneumonia)

1% to 10%:

Cardiovascular: Edema /fluid retention (10%), hypotension (5%), cardiovascular events (grades 3/4: 3%; included chest pain, cardiac arrest, supraventricular tachycardia, thrombosis, pulmonary thromboembolism, pulmonary emboli, and hypertension)

Gastrointestinal: Mucositis (7%; grades 3/4: <1%)

Hematologic: Bleeding (2%), neutropenic fever (2%), thrombocytopenia (2%; grades 3/4: <1%)

Hepatic: Bilirubin increased (7%)

Neuromuscular & skeletal: Peripheral neuropathy (grade 3: 10%)

Respiratory: Cough (7%)

Miscellaneous: Hypersensitivity reaction (4%, includes chest pain, dyspnea, flushing, hypotension; severe: <1%)

<1%, postmarketing, and/or case reports: Arrhythmia, bradycardia, cardiac ischemia, cerebrovascular attack, cranial nerve palsies, embolism, erythema, hand-foot syndrome (in patients previously exposed to capecitabine), injection site reaction (mild), maculopapular rash, MI, motor neuropathy, nail discoloration, nail pigmentation changes, optic nerve damage (rare), photosensitivity reaction, pneumothorax, pruritus, radiation recall, rash (generalized), stroke, thrombosis, transient ischemic attack, vocal cord paresis

Adverse reactions reported with paclitaxel, which may occur with paclitaxel (protein bound): Autonomic neuropathy, cellulitis, conjunctivitis, extravasation recall, hepatic encephalopathy, hepatic necrosis, induration, intestinal obstruction, intestinal perforation, interstitial pneumonia, ischemic colitis, lacrimation increased, lung fibrosis, neutropenic enterocolitis (typhlitis), optic nerve damage (persistent), pancreatitis, paralytic ileus, phlebitis, pulmonary embolism, radiation pneumonitis with concurrent radiation therapy, skin exfoliation, skin fibrosis, skin necrosis, Stevens-Johnson syndrome, toxic epidermal necrolysis

Drug Interactions

Metabolism/Transport Effects Substrate (major) of CYP2C8, 2C9, 3A4; **Induces** CYP3A4 (weak)

Avoid Concomitant Use

Avoid concomitant use of Paclitaxel (Protein Bound) with any of the following: Natalizumab; Vaccines (Live)

Increased Effect/Toxicity

Paclitaxel (Protein Bound) may increase the levels/effects of: Antineoplastic Agents (Anthracycline); DOXOrubicin; Leflunomide; Natalizumab; Vaccines (Live); Vinorelbine; Vitamin K Antagonists

The levels/effects of Paclitaxel (Protein Bound) may be increased by: CYP2C8 Inhibitors (Moderate); CYP2C8 Inhibitors (Strong); CYP3A4 Inhibitors (Moderate); CYP3A4 Inhibitors (Strong); Dasatinib; Deferasirox; P-Glycoprotein Inhibitors; Platinum Derivatives; Trastuzumab

Decreased Effect

Paclitaxel (Protein Bound) may decrease the levels/effects of: Cardiac Glycosides; Saxagliptin; Vaccines (Inactivated); Vaccines (Live); Vitamin K Antagonists

The levels/effects of Paclitaxel (Protein Bound) may be decreased by: CYP2C8 Inducers (Highly Effective); CYP3A4 Inducers (Strong); Deferasirox; Echinacea; Herbs (CYP3A4 Inducers); P-Glycoprotein Inducers

Ethanol/Nutrition/Herb Interactions Herb/Nutraceutical: Avoid St John's wort (may decrease paclitaxel levels). Avoid echinacea. Avoid black cohosh, dong quai in estrogen-dependent tumors.

Storage/Stability Store intact vial at room temperature of 20°C to 25°C (68°F to 77°F) and protect from bright light. Reconstituted solution may be stored under refrigeration 2°C to 8°C (36°F to 46°F) for up to 8 hours, although the manufacturer recommends immediate use. The solution for administration is stable for up to 8 hours at room temperature and ambient light.

Reconstitution Use appropriate precautions for handling and disposal. Reconstitute vial with 20 mL NS to a concentration of 5 mg/mL. Add NS slowly, directing it along inside vial wall; allow vial to sit for 5 minutes, then gently swirl for 2 minutes; avoid foaming. Place dose without further dilution into an empty sterile container. **Note:** Use of DEHP-free containers or administration sets is not necessary. **Do not use an in-line filter.**

Compatibility Stable in NS. Formulation contains albumin; do not mix with other drugs.

Mechanism of Action Albumin-bound paclitaxel nanoparticle formulation. Paclitaxel promotes microtubule assembly by enhancing the action of tubulin dimers, stabilizing existing microtubules, and inhibiting their disassembly, interfering with the late G_2 mitotic phase, and inhibiting cell replication. May also distort mitotic spindles, resulting in the breakage of chromosomes. Paclitaxel may also suppress cell proliferation and modulate immune response.

Pharmacodynamics/Kinetics

Distribution: V_d: 632 L/m^2 (extensive extravascular distribution and/or tissue binding)

Protein binding: 89% to 98%

Metabolism: Hepatic primarily via CYP2C8 to 6-alpha-hydroxypaclitaxel; also to minor metabolites via CYP3A4

Half-life elimination: Terminal: 27 hours

Excretion: Feces (~20%); urine (4% as unchanged drug, <1% as metabolites)

Dosage I.V.: Adults:

Breast cancer: 260 mg/m^2 every 3 weeks

Breast cancer (weekly treatment; unlabeled schedule): 100-150 mg/m^2 on days 1, 8, and 15 of a 28-day cycle (Gradishar, 2009)

NSCLC (unlabeled use): 260 mg/m^2 every 3 weeks (Green, 2006) **or** 125 mg/m^2 on days 1, 8, and 15 of a 28-day cycle (Rizvi, 2008)

Dosage adjustment for toxicity:

Severe neutropenia (<500 cells/mm^3) ≥1 week: Reduce dose to 220 mg/m^2 for subsequent courses

Recurrent severe neutropenia: Reduce dose to 180 mg/m^2

Sensory neuropathy

Grade 1 or 2: Dosage adjustment generally not required

Grade 3: Hold treatment until resolved to grade 1 or 2, then resume with reduced dose for all subsequent cycles

Severe sensory neuropathy: Reduce dose to 220 mg/m^2 for subsequent courses

Recurrent severe sensory neuropathy: Reduce dose to 180 mg/m^2

Dosage adjustment in renal impairment: Has not been studied; patients with serum creatinine >2 mg/dL were excluded from clinical trials

Dosage adjustment in hepatic impairment: Every-3-week breast cancer regimen:

Mild impairment (AST <10 times ULN and bilirubin ≤1.25 times ULN): No adjustment required

Moderate impairment (AST <10 times ULN and bilirubin 1.26-2 times ULN): Reduce dose to 200 mg/m^2

Severe impairment:

AST <10 times ULN and bilirubin 2.01-5 times ULN: Reduce dose to 130 mg/m^2; may increase up to 200 mg/m^2 in subsequent cycles (based on individual tolerance)

AST >10 times ULN or bilirubin >5 times ULN: Use is not recommended

Administration I.V.: Administer over 30 minutes; do not use an in-line filter. Monitor infusion site; avoid extravasation. When given on a weekly (unlabeled) schedule, infusions were administered over ~30 minutes (Gradishar, 2009; Rizvi, 2008).

Monitoring Parameters CBC, BP (during infusion), baseline ECG; hepatic function; monitor infusion site

Emetic Potential Low (10% to 30%)

Vesicant May be an irritant

High Dose Considerations

Comments Glutamine may decrease mucositis.

Dosage Forms Excipient information presented when available (limited, particularly for generics); consult specific product labeling.

Injection, powder for reconstitution:

Abraxane®: 100 mg [contains albumin (human)]

References

Gradishar WJ, Krasnojon D, Cheporov S, et al, "Significantly Longer Progression-Free Survival With nab-paclitaxel Compared With Docetaxel as First-Line Therapy for Metastatic Breast Cancer," *J Clin Oncol*, 2009, 27(22):3611-9.

Gradishar WJ, Tjulandin S, Davidson N, et al, "Phase III Trial of Nanoparticle Albumin-Bound Paclitaxel Compared With Polyethylated Castor Oil-Based Paclitaxel in Women With Breast Cancer," *J Clin Oncol*, 2005, 23(31):7794-803.

Green MR, Manikhas GM, Orlov S, et al, "Abraxane®, a Novel Cremophor®-Free, Albumin-Bound Particle Form of Paclitaxel for the Treatment of Advanced Non-Small-Cell Lung Cancer," *Ann Oncol*, 2006, 17(8):1263-8.

Ibrahim NK, Samuels B, Page R, et al, "Multicenter Phase II Trial of ABI-007, an Albumin-Bound Paclitaxel, in Women With Metastatic Breast Cancer," *J Clin Oncol*, 2005, 23(25):6019-26.

National Comprehensive Cancer Network® (NCCN), "Clinical Practice Guidelines in Oncology™: Breast Cancer," Version 1, 2009. Available at http://www.nccn.org/professionals/physician_gls/PDF/breast.pdf.

National Comprehensive Cancer Network (NCCN)®, Clinical Practice Guidelines in Oncology™: Non-Small Cell Lung Cancer," Version 2, 2009. Available at: http://www.nccn.org/professionals/physician_gls/PDF/nscl.pdf.

Nyman DW, Campbell KJ, Hersh E, et al, "Phase I and Pharmacokinetics Trial of ABI-007, a Novel Nanoparticle Formulation of Paclitaxel in Patients With Advanced Nonhematologic Malignancies," *J Clin Oncol*, 2005, 23(31):7785-93.

Rizvi NA, Riely GJ, Azzoli CG, et al, "Phase I/II Trial of Weekly Intravenous 130-nm Albumin-Bound Paclitaxel as Initial Chemotherapy in Patients With Stage IV Non-Small-Cell Lung Cancer," *J Clin Oncol*, 2008, 26(4):639-43.

◆ **Paddock Nystatin™** *see* Nystatin *on page 855*

Palifermin (pal ee FER min)

Related Information

Oral Mucositis / Stomatitis *on page 1460*

U.S. Brand Names Kepivance®

Index Terms AMJ 9701; rhKGF; rhu Keratinocyte Growth Factor; rHu-KGF

Generic Available No

Pharmacologic Category Keratinocyte Growth Factor

Use Decrease the incidence and severity of severe oral mucositis associated with hematologic malignancies in patients receiving myelotoxic therapy requiring hematopoietic stem cell support

Pregnancy Risk Factor C

Lactation Excretion in breast milk unknown/use caution

Labeled Contraindications Hypersensitivity to palifermin, *E. coli*-derived proteins, or any component of the formulation

Warnings/Precautions Edema, erythema, pruritus, rash, oral/perioral dysesthesia, taste alteration, tongue discoloration, and tongue thickening may occur; instruct patients to report mucocutaneous effects. Safety and efficacy have not been established with nonhematologic malignancies; effect on the growth of nonhematopoietic human tumors is not known. Palifermin has been shown to enhance epithelial tumor cell lines *in vitro*. Palifermin should be administered prior to and following, but not with, chemotherapy. If administered during or within 24 hours of (before or after) chemotherapy, palifermin may increase the severity and duration of mucositis due to the increased sensitivity of rapidly-dividing epithelial cells. Safety and efficacy have not been established in children.

Adverse Reactions

>10%:

Cardiovascular: Edema (28%), hypertension (7% to 14%)

Central nervous system: Fever (39%); pain (16%); dysesthesia (oral hyperesthesia, hypoesthesia, and paresthesia 12%)

Dermatologic: Rash (62%; grade 3: 3%), pruritus (35%), erythema (32%)

Gastrointestinal: Serum amylase increased (grades 3/4: 38%), mouth/tongue discoloration or thickness (17%), taste alteration (16%), serum lipase increased (grades 3/4: 11%)

Renal: Proteinuria (17%)

Respiratory: Cough (32%), rhinitis (16%)

1% to 10%:

Neuromuscular & skeletal: Arthralgia (10%)

Miscellaneous: Antibody formation (2%)

<1%, postmarketing, and/or case reports: Flexural hyperpigmentation

Drug Interactions

Avoid Concomitant Use There are no known interactions where it is recommended to avoid concomitant use.

Increased Effect/Toxicity There are no known significant interactions involving an increase in effect.

Decreased Effect There are no known significant interactions involving a decrease in effect.

Storage/Stability Store intact vials under refrigeration at 2°C to 8°C (36°F to 46°F). Protect from light. Reconstituted vials are stable for up to 72 hours refrigerated and should not be used if left at room temperature >2 hours (data on file). The product labeling, however, indicates that reconstituted vials are stable for up to 24 hours refrigerated and should not be used if left at room temperature >1 hour. Protect reconstituted solution from light. Do not freeze reconstituted product.

Reconstitution To reconstitute, slowly add 1.2 mL SWFI, to a final concentration of 5 mg/mL. Swirl gently; do not shake or vigorously agitate. Do not filter during preparation or administration.

Compatibility Incompatible: Heparin.

Mechanism of Action Palifermin is a recombinant keratinocyte growth factor (KGF) produced in *E. coli*. Endogenous KGF is produced by mesenchymal cells in response to epithelial tissue injury. KGF binds to the KGF receptor resulting in proliferation, differentiation and migration of epithelial cells in multiple tissues, including (but not limited to) the tongue, buccal mucosa, esophagus, and salivary gland.

Pharmacodynamics/Kinetics

Onset of action: Epithelial cell proliferation (dose-dependent): 48 hours

Half-life elimination: 4.5 hours (range: 3.3-5.7 hours)

Dosage I.V.: Adults: 60 mcg/kg/day for 3 consecutive days before and after myelotoxic therapy; total of 6 doses

Note: Administer first 3 doses prior to myelotoxic therapy, with the 3rd dose given 24-48 hours before therapy begins. The last 3 doses should be administered after myelotoxic therapy, with the first of these doses after but on the same day as hematopoietic stem cell infusion and at least 4 days after the most recent dose of palifermin.

Dosage adjustment in renal impairment: No adjustment necessary

Administration Administer by I.V. bolus. If heparin is used to maintain the patency of the I.V. line, flush line with saline prior to and after palifermin administration. Do not administer palifermin during or within 24 hours before or after chemotherapy. Allow solution to reach room temperature prior to administration; do not use if at room temperature >1 hour. Do not filter.

Additional Information Oncology Comment: The Multinational Association of Supportive Care in Cancer and the International Society for Oral Oncology (MASCC/ISOO) guidelines for the prevention and treatment of mucositis recommend palifermin (at the FDA-approved dose) for the prevention of oral mucositis in patients with hematologic malignancies who are receiving high-dose chemotherapy and total body irradiation with autologous stem cell transplantation (Keefe, 2007).

Guidelines from the American Society of Clinical Oncology (ASCO) for the use of chemotherapy and radiotherapy protectants (Hensley, 2008) recommend the use of palifermin to decrease the incidence of severe mucositis in patients undergoing autologous stem-cell transplantation with a total body irradiation (TBI) conditioning regimen. According to the ASCO guidelines, data are insufficient to recommend palifermin when the conditioning regimen is chemotherapy only. Palifermin may be considered in patients undergoing myeloablative allogeneic stem-cell transplantation with a TBI conditioning regimen, however data are again insufficient to recommend palifermin when the conditioning regimen is chemotherapy only. Due to a lack of appropriate data, the guidelines also do not recommend palifermin use in non-stem-cell transplantation treatment regimens or for use when treating solid tumors.

Dosage Forms Excipient information presented when available (limited, particularly for generics); consult specific product labeling.

Injection, powder for reconstitution [preservative free]:

Kepivance®: 6.25 mg [contains mannitol 50 mg, sucrose 25 mg]

References

Gillespie B, Zia-Amirhosseini P, Salfi M, et al, "Effect of Renal Function on the Pharmacokinetics of Palifermin," *J Clin Pharmacol*, 2006, 46(12):1460-8.

Hensley ML, Hagerty KL, Kewalramani T, et al, "American Society of Clinical Oncology 2008 Clinical Practice Guideline Update: Use of Chemotherapy and Radiotherapy Protectants," *J Clin Oncol*, 2009, 27(1): 127-45.

Keefe DM, Schubert MM, Elting LS, et al, "Updated Clinical Practice Guidelines for the Prevention and Treatment of Mucositis," *Cancer*, 2007, 109(5):820-31.

Meropol NJ, Somer RA, Gutheil J, et al, "Randomized Phase I Trial of Recombinant Human Keratinocyte Growth Factor Plus Chemotherapy: Potential Role as Mucosal Protectant," *J Clin Oncol*, 2003, 21(8):1452-8.

Sibelt LA, Aboosy M, van der Velden WJ, et al, "Palifermin-Induced Flexural Hyperpigmentation: A Clinical and Histological Study of Five Cases," *Br J Dermatol*, 2008, 159(5):1200-3.

Spielberger R, Stiff P, Bensinger W, et al, "Palifermin for Oral Mucositis After Intensive Therapy for Hematologic Cancers," *N Engl J Med*, 2004, 351(25):2590-8.

Palonosetron (pal oh NOE se tron)

Medication Safety Issues

Sound-alike/look-alike issues:

Aloxi® may be confused with Eloxatin®, oxaliplatin

Palonosetron may be confused with dolasetron, granisetron, ondansetron

Related Information

Management of Chemotherapy-Induced Nausea and Vomiting *on page 1434*

U.S. Brand Names Aloxi®

Index Terms Palonosetron Hydrochloride; RS-25259; RS-25259-197

Generic Available No

Pharmacologic Category Antiemetic; Selective 5-HT$_3$ Receptor Antagonist

Use

I.V.: Prevention of chemotherapy-associated nausea and vomiting; indicated for prevention of acute (highly-emetogenic therapy) as well as acute and delayed (moderately-emetogenic therapy) nausea and vomiting; prevention of postoperative nausea and vomiting (PONV)

Oral: Prevention of chemotherapy-associated nausea and vomiting (moderately-emetogenic therapy)

Pregnancy Risk Factor B

Lactation Excretion in breast milk unknown/not recommended

Labeled Contraindications Hypersensitivity to palonosetron or any component of the formulation

Warnings/Precautions Hypersensitivity has been observed rarely with I.V. palonosetron. Use caution in patients allergic to other 5-HT$_3$ receptor antagonists; cross-reactivity is possible. Some selective 5-HT$_3$ receptor antagonists have been associated with dose-dependent increases in ECG intervals (eg, PR, QRS duration, QT/QT$_c$, JT), usually occurring 1-2 hours after I.V. administration. In general, these changes are not clinically relevant, however, when these agents are used in conjunction with other agents that prolong these intervals, arrhythmia may occur. When used with agents that prolong the QT interval (eg, Class I and III antiarrhythmics), clinically relevant QT interval prolongation could result in torsade de pointes. A number of trials have shown that 5-HT$_3$ antagonists produce QT interval prolongation to variable degrees. Use with caution in patients at risk of QT prolongation and/or ventricular arrhythmia. Reduction in heart rate may also occur with the 5-HT$_3$ antagonists. Use with caution in patients with congenital long QT syndrome or other risk factors for QT prolongation (eg, medications known to prolong QT interval, electrolyte abnormalities, and cumulative high dose anthracycline therapy).

Not intended for treatment of nausea and vomiting or for chronic continuous therapy. **For chemotherapy, should be used on a scheduled basis, not on an "as needed" (PRN) basis,** since data support the use of this drug only in the prevention of nausea and vomiting (due to antineoplastic therapy) and not in the rescue of nausea and vomiting. For PONV, may use for low expectation of PONV if it is essential to avoid nausea and vomiting in the postoperative period; use is not recommended if there is little expectation of nausea and vomiting. Safety and efficacy in children have not been established.

Adverse Reactions Adverse events may vary according to indication. In general, adverse reactions similar between I.V. and oral dosage forms.

◄ 1% to 10%:

Cardiovascular: QT prolongation (chemotherapy-associated <1%; PONV 1% to 5%), bradycardia (chemotherapy-associated 1%; PONV 4%), hypotension (≤1%), sinus bradycardia (≤1%), tachycardia (nonsustained) (≤1%)

Central nervous system: Headache (chemotherapy-associated 4% to 9%; PONV 3%), anxiety (1%), dizziness (≤1%), fatigue (≤1%)

Dermatologic: Pruritus (≤1%)

Endocrine & metabolic: Hyperkalemia (1%)

Gastrointestinal: Constipation (1% to 5%), diarrhea (≤1%), flatulence (≤1%)

Genitourinary: Urinary retention (≤1%)

Hepatic: ALT increased (≤1%; transient), AST increased (≤1%; transient)

Neuromuscular & skeletal: Weakness (1%)

<1%, postmarketing, and/or case reports: Abdominal pain, abnormal taste, allergic dermatitis, alopecia, amblyopia, anemia, anorexia, appetite decreased, arrhythmia, arthralgia, atrioventricular block (first and second degree), bilirubin increased (transient), chills, dyspepsia, dyspnea, edema (generalized), electrolyte fluctuations, epistaxis, erythema, euphoric mood, extrasystoles, eye irritation/edema, fever, flu-like syndrome, gastritis, glycosuria, hiccups, hot flash, hyperglycemia, hypersensitivity (rare), hypersomnia, hypertension, hypokalemia, hypoventilation, injection site reactions (burning/discomfort/induration/pain; rare), insomnia, intestinal hypomotility, joint stiffness, laryngospasm, metabolic acidosis, motion sickness, myalgia, myocardial ischemia, pain in extremities, paresthesia, platelets decreased, rash, salivation increased, sinus arrhythmia, sinus tachycardia, sinusitis, somnolence, supraventricular extrasystoles, tinnitus, T-wave amplitude decreased, vein discoloration, vein distention, ventricular extrasystoles, xerostomia

Drug Interactions

Metabolism/Transport Effects Substrate (minor) of CYP1A2, 2D6, 3A4

Avoid Concomitant Use

Avoid concomitant use of Palonosetron with any of the following: Apomorphine

Increased Effect/Toxicity

Palonosetron may increase the levels/effects of: Apomorphine

Decreased Effect

The levels/effects of Palonosetron may be decreased by: Peginterferon Alfa-2b

Storage/Stability

Capsule: Store at room temperature of 25°C (77°F); excursions permitted to 15°C to 30°C (59°F to 86°F). Protect from light.

Injection: Store intact vials at room temperature of 20°C to 25°C (68°F to 77°F); excursions permitted to 15°C to 30°C (59°F to 86°F); do not freeze. Protect from light. Solutions of 5 mcg/mL and 30 mcg/mL in NS, D_5W, $D_51/2NS$, and D_5LR injection are stable for 48 hours at room temperature and 14 days under refrigeration (Trissel, 2004).

Compatibility Stable in D_5W, NS, $D_51/2NS$, and D_5LR.

Y-site administration: Compatible: Atropine, carboplatin, cisplatin, cyclophosphamide, dacarbazine, docetaxel, doxorubicin, epirubicin, famotidine, fentanyl, fluorouracil, gemcitabine, heparin, hydromorphone, ifosfamide, irinotecan, lidocaine, lorazepam, meperidine, metoclopramide, midazolam, morphine, oxaliplatin, paclitaxel, potassium chloride, promethazine, sufentanil, topotecan. **Incompatible:** Methylprednisolone

Compatibility in syringe: Compatible: Dexamethasone

Compatibility when admixed: Compatible: Dexamethasone

Mechanism of Action Selective 5-HT$_3$ receptor antagonist, blocking serotonin, both on vagal nerve terminals in the periphery and centrally in the chemoreceptor trigger zone

Pharmacodynamics/Kinetics

Absorption: Oral: Well absorbed

Distribution: V$_d$: 8.3 ± 2.5 L/kg

Protein binding: ~62%

Metabolism: ~50% metabolized via CYP enzymes (and likely other pathways) to relatively inactive metabolites (N-oxide-palonosetron and 6-S-hydroxy-palonosetron); CYP1A2, 2D6, and 3A4 contribute to its metabolism

Bioavailability: Oral: 97%

Half-life elimination: I.V.: Terminal: ~40 hours; Oral: 29-45 hours (healthy patients), 38-62 hours (cancer patients)

Time to peak, plasma: Oral: 3-7 hours (healthy patients); ~5 hours (cancer patients)

Excretion: Urine (80% to 93%, 40% as unchanged drug); feces (5% to 8%)

Dosage Adults:

Chemotherapy-associated nausea and vomiting:

I.V.: 0.25 mg 30 minutes prior to the start of chemotherapy administration

Oral: 0.5 mg 1 hour prior to the start of chemotherapy

Breakthrough: Palonosetron has not been shown to be effective in terminating nausea or vomiting once it occurs and should not be used for this purpose.

PONV: I.V.: 0.075 mg immediately prior to anesthesia induction

Elderly: No dosage adjustment necessary

Dosage adjustment in renal/hepatic impairment: No dosage adjustment necessary

Administration

I.V.: Flush I.V. line with NS prior to and following administration.

Chemotherapy-associated nausea and vomiting: Infuse over 30 seconds, 30 minutes prior to the start of chemotherapy

PONV: Infuse over 10 seconds immediately prior to anesthesia induction

Oral: May administer with or without meals.

Dietary Considerations Capsule: May be taken with or without meals.

Product Availability Aloxi® capsules: FDA approved August 2008; anticipated availability currently undetermined

Dosage Forms Excipient information presented when available (limited, particularly for generics); consult specific product labeling.

Capsule:

Aloxi®: 0.5 mg

Injection, solution:

Aloxi®: 0.05 mg/mL (1.5 mL, 5 mL) [contains edetate disodium]

References

Aapro MS, Grunberg SM, Manikhas GM, et al, "A Phase III, Double-Blind, Randomized Trial of Palonosetron Compared With Ondansetron in Preventing Chemotherapy-Induced Nausea and Vomiting Following Highly Emetogenic Chemotherapy," *Ann Oncol*, 2006, 17(9):1441-9.

Boccia RV, Gonzalez EF, Pluzanska AG, et al, "Palonosetron (PALO), Administered Orally or Intravenously (IV), Plus Dexamethasone for Prevention of Chemotherapy-Induced Nausea and Vomiting (CINV)," *J Clin Oncol*, 2008, 26(Supp) [abstract 20608 from 2008 ASCO Annual Meeting].

Eisenberg P, Figueroa-Vadillo J, Zamora R, et al, "Improved Prevention of Moderately Emetogenic Chemotherapy-Induced Nausea and Vomiting With Palonosetron, a Pharmacologically Novel 5-HT3 Receptor Antagonist: Results of a Phase III, Single-Dose Trial Versus Dolasetron," *Cancer*, 2003, 98(11):2473-82.

Eisenberg P, MacKintosh FR, Ritch P, et al, "Efficacy, Safety and Pharmacokinetics of Palonosetron in Patients Receiving Highly Emetogenic Cisplatin-Based Chemotherapy: A Dose-Ranging Clinical Study," *Ann Oncol*, 2004, 15(2):330-7.

Gralla R, Lichinister M, Van Der Vegt S, et al, "Palonosetron Improves Prevention of Chemotherapy-Induced Nausea and Vomiting Following Moderately Emetogenic Chemotherapy: Results of a Double-Blind Randomized Phase III Trial Comparing Single Doses of Palonosetron With Ondansetron," *Ann Oncol*, 2003, 14(10):1570-7.

Kris MG, Hesketh PJ, Somerfield MR, et al, "American Society of Clinical Oncology Guideline for Antiemetics in Oncology: Update 2006," *J Clin Oncol*, 2006, 24(18):2932-47.

Kupiec TC, Trusley C, Ben M, et al, "Physical and Chemical Stability of Palonosetron Hydrochloride With Five Common Parenteral Drugs During Simulated Y-Site Administration," *Am J Health-Syst Pharm*, 2008, 65(18):1735-9.

National Comprehensive Cancer Network (NCCN), "Clinical Practice Guidelines in Oncology™: Antiemesis," Version 3, 2009. Available at http://www.nccn.org/professionals/physician_gls/PDF/antiemesis.pdf.

Trissel LA, Trusley C, Ben M, et al, "Physical and Chemical Stability of Palonosetron Hydrochloride With Five Opiate Agonists During Simulated Y-Site Administration," *Am J Health-Syst Pharm*, 2007, 64 (11):1209-13.

Trissel LA and Xu QA, "Physical and Chemical Stability of Palonosetron HCl in 4 Infusion Solutions," *Ann Pharmacother*, 2004, 38(10):1608-11.

Trissel LA and Zhang Y, "Compatibility and Stability of Aloxi (Palonosetron Hydrochloride) Admixed With Dexamethasone Sodium Phosphate," *Intl J Pharm Compounding*, 2004, 8(5):398-403.

Trissel LA and Zhang Y, "Palonosetron HCl Compatibility and Stability with Doxorubicin HCl and Epirubicin HCl During Simulated Y-Site Administration," *Ann Pharmacother*, 2005, 39(2):280-3.

Xu QA, and Trissel LA, "Compatibility of Palonosetron With Cyclophosphamide and With Ifosfamide During Simulated Y-site Administration," *Am J Health Syst Pharm*, 2005, 62 (19):1998-2000.

◆ **Palonosetron Hydrochloride** *see* Palonosetron *on page* 911

Pamidronate (pa mi DROE nate)

Medication Safety Issues

Sound-alike/look-alike issues:

Aredia® may be confused with Adriamycin, Meridia®

Pamidronate may be confused with papaverine

International issues:

Linoten® [Spain] may be confused with Lidopen® which is a brand name for lidocaine in the U.S.

Related Information

Safe Handling of Hazardous Drugs *on page* 1517

U.S. Brand Names Aredia®

Index Terms Pamidronate Disodium

Generic Available Yes

Canadian Brand Names Aredia®; Pamidronate Disodium Omega; Pamidronate Disodium®; PMS-Pamidronate; Rhoxal-pamidronate

Pharmacologic Category Antidote; Bisphosphonate Derivative

Use Treatment of moderate or severe hypercalcemia associated with malignancy; treatment of osteolytic bone lesions associated with multiple myeloma or metastatic breast cancer; moderate-to-severe Paget's disease of bone

Unlabeled/Investigational Use Treatment of pediatric osteoporosis, treatment of osteogenesis imperfecta; treatment of symptomatic bone metastases of thyroid cancer; prevention of bone loss associated with androgen deprivation treatment in prostate cancer

Pregnancy Risk Factor D

Lactation Excretion in breast milk unknown/use caution

Labeled Contraindications Hypersensitivity to pamidronate, other bisphosphonates, or any component of the formulation

Warnings/Precautions Bisphosphonate therapy has been associated with osteonecrosis, primarily of the jaw; this has been observed mostly in cancer patients, but also in patients with postmenopausal osteoporosis and other diagnoses. Most reported cases occurred after I.V. bisphosphonate therapy; however, cases have been reported following oral therapy. Literature suggests an increased incidence of ONJ in cancer patients of certain tumor types such as multiple myeloma and advanced breast cancer. Dental exams and preventative dentistry should be performed prior to placing patients with risk factors, including any cancer patient, on chronic bisphosphonate therapy. Good oral hygiene should be maintained and invasive dental procedures should be avoided during treatment.

Infrequently, severe (and occasionally debilitating) musculoskeletal (bone, joint, and/or muscle) pain have been reported during bisphosphonate treatment. The onset of pain ranged from a single day to several months. Consider discontinuing therapy in patients who experience severe symptoms; symptoms usually resolve upon discontinuation. Some patients experienced recurrence when rechallenged with same drug or another bisphosphonate; avoid use in patients with a history of these symptoms in association with bisphosphonate therapy.

Initial or single doses have been associated with renal deterioration, progressing to renal failure and dialysis. Withhold pamidronate treatment (until renal function returns to baseline) in patients with evidence of renal deterioration. Glomerulosclerosis (focal segmental) with or without nephrotic syndrome has also been reported. Longer infusion times (>2 hours) may reduce the risk for renal toxicity, especially in patients with pre-existing renal insufficiency. Single pamidronate doses should not exceed 90 mg. Patients with serum creatinine >3 mg/dL were not studied in clinical trials; limited data is available in patients with Cl_{cr} <30 mL/minute. Evaluate serum creatinine prior to each treatment. For the treatment of bone metastases, use is not recommended in patients with severe renal impairment; for renal impairment in indications other than bone metastases, use clinical judgment to determine if benefits outweigh potential risks.

Use has been associated with asymptomatic electrolyte abnormalities (including hypophosphatemia, hypokalemia, hypomagnesemia, and hypocalcemia). Rare cases of symptomatic hypocalcemia, including tetany have been reported. Patients with a history of thyroid surgery may have relative hypoparathyroidism; predisposing them to pamidronate-related hypocalcemia. Leukopenia has been observed with oral pamidronate and monitoring of white blood cell counts is suggested. Patients with pre-existing anemia, leukopenia, or thrombocytopenia should be closely monitored during the first 2 weeks of treatment.

According to the American Society of Clinical Oncology (ASCO) guidelines for bisphosphonates in multiple myeloma, treatment with pamidronate is not recommended for asymptomatic (smoldering) or indolent myeloma or with solitary plasmacytoma (Kyle, 2007). The National Comprehensive Cancer Network® (NCCN) multiple myeloma guidelines (v.2.2009) also do not recommend pamidronate use in stage 1 or smoldering disease, unless part of a clinical trial.

Adequate hydration is required during treatment (urine output ~2 L/day); avoid overhydration, especially in patients with heart failure. Vein irritation and thrombophlebitis may occur with infusions. Women of childbearing potential ▶

should be advised to use effective contraception and avoid becoming pregnant during therapy.

Adverse Reactions Note: Actual percentages may vary by indication; treatment for multiple myeloma is associated with higher percentage.

>10%:

Central nervous system: Fever (18% to 39%), fatigue (≤37%), headache (≤26%), insomnia (≤22%)

Endocrine & metabolic: Hypophosphatemia (≤18%), hypokalemia (4% to 18%), hypomagnesemia (4% to 12%), hypocalcemia (≤12%)

Gastrointestinal: Nausea (≤54%), vomiting (≤36%), anorexia (≤26%), abdominal pain (≤23%), dyspepsia (≤23%)

Genitourinary: Urinary tract infection (≤19%)

Hematologic: Anemia (≤43%), granulocytopenia (≤20%)

Local: Infusion site reaction (≤18%; includes induration, pain, redness and swelling)

Neuromuscular & skeletal: Myalgia (≤26%), weakness (≤22%), arthralgia (≤14%), osteonecrosis of the jaw (cancer patients: 1% to 11%)

Renal: Serum creatinine increased (≤19%)

Respiratory: Dyspnea (≤30%), cough (≤26%), upper respiratory tract infection (≤24%), sinusitis (≤16%), pleural effusion (≤11%)

1% to 10%:

Cardiovascular: Atrial fibrillation (≤6%), hypertension (≤6%), syncope (≤6%), tachycardia (≤6%), atrial flutter (≤1%), cardiac failure (≤1%), edema (≤1%)

Central nervous system: Somnolence (≤6%), psychosis (≤4%)

Endocrine & metabolic: Hypothyroidism (≤6%)

Gastrointestinal: Constipation (≤6%), gastrointestinal hemorrhage (≤6%), diarrhea (≤1%), stomatitis (≤1%)

Hematologic: Leukopenia (≤4%), neutropenia (≤1%), thrombocytopenia (≤1%)

Neuromuscular & skeletal: Back pain (≤5%), bone pain (≤5%)

Renal: Uremia (≤4%)

Respiratory: Rales (≤6%), rhinitis (≤6%)

Miscellaneous: Moniliasis (≤6%)

<1%, postmarketing, and/or case reports: Acute renal failure, adult respiratory distress syndrome, allergic reaction, anaphylactic shock, angioedema, bronchospasm, CHF, confusion, conjunctivitis, electrolyte/mineral abnormality, episcleritis, fluid overload, flu-like syndrome, focal segmental glomerulosclerosis (including collapsing variant), hallucinations (visual), hematuria, herpes virus reactivation, hyperkalemia, hypernatremia, hypotension, injection site phlebitis/thrombophlebitis, interstitial pneumonitis, iridocyclitis, iritis, joint and/or muscle pain (sometimes severe and/or incapacitating), left ventricular failure, lymphocytopenia, malaise, nephrotic syndrome, osteonecrosis (other than jaw), paresthesia, pruritus, rash, renal deterioration, renal failure, scleritis, seizure, tetany, uveitis, xanthopsia

Drug Interactions

Avoid Concomitant Use There are no known interactions where it is recommended to avoid concomitant use.

Increased Effect/Toxicity

Pamidronate may increase the levels/effects of: Phosphate Supplements

The levels/effects of Pamidronate may be increased by: Aminoglycosides; Nonsteroidal Anti-Inflammatory Agents; Thalidomide

Decreased Effect There are no known significant interactions involving a decrease in effect.

Storage/Stability

Powder for reconstitution: Store below 30°C (86°F). The reconstituted solution is stable for 24 hours stored under refrigeration at 2°C to 8°C (36°F to 46°F). Solution for injection: Store at 20°C to 25°C (68°f to 77°F).

Pamidronate solution for infusion is stable at room temperature for up to 24 hours.

Reconstitution Powder for injection: Reconstitute by adding 10 mL of SWFI to each vial of lyophilized pamidronate disodium powder, the resulting solution will be 30 mg/10 mL or 90 mg/10 mL.

Pamidronate may be further diluted in 250-1000 mL of 0.45% or 0.9% sodium chloride or 5% dextrose. (The manufacturer recommends dilution in 1000 mL for hypercalcemia of malignancy, 500 mL for Paget's disease and bone metastases of myeloma, and 250 mL for bone metastases of breast cancer.)

Compatibility Incompatible with calcium-containing infusion solutions such as Ringer's injection.

Mechanism of Action A bisphosphonate which inhibits bone resorption via actions on osteoclasts or on osteoclast precursors. Does not appear to produce any significant effects on renal tubular calcium handling and is poorly absorbed following oral administration (high oral doses have been reported effective); therefore, I.V. therapy is preferred.

Pharmacodynamics/Kinetics

Onset of action: 24-48 hours

Peak effect: Maximum: 5-7 days

Absorption: Poor; pharmacokinetic studies lacking

Metabolism: Not metabolized

Half-life elimination: 21-35 hours

Excretion: Biphasic; urine (30% to 62% as unchanged drug; lower in patients with renal dysfunction) within 120 hours

Dosage Dilute prior to administration and infuse intravenously slowly over at least 2 hours. Single doses should not exceed 90 mg. I.V.: Adults:

Hypercalcemia of malignancy:

Moderate cancer-related hypercalcemia (corrected serum calcium: 12-13.5 mg/dL): 60-90 mg, as a single dose over 2-24 hours

Severe cancer-related hypercalcemia (corrected serum calcium: >13.5 mg/dL): 90 mg, as a single dose over 2-24 hours

A period of 7 days should elapse before the use of second course; repeat infusions every 2-3 weeks have been suggested, however, could be administered every 2-3 months according to the degree of and of severity of hypercalcemia and/or the type of malignancy.

Osteolytic bone lesions with multiple myeloma: 90 mg over 2-4 hours monthly or every 3-4 weeks

Osteolytic bone lesions with metastatic breast cancer: 90 mg over 2 hours repeated every 3-4 weeks

Paget's disease: 30 mg over 4 hours daily for 3 consecutive days

Prevention of androgen deprivation-induced osteoporosis (unlabeled use): 60 mg over 2 hours every 3 months (Smith, 2001) **or** 90 mg as a single dose over 3-4 hours (Diamond, 2001)

Elderly: Begin at lower end of adult dosing range.

Dosing adjustment in renal impairment: Safety and efficacy have not been established in patients with serum creatinine >5 mg/dL; studies are limited in multiple myeloma patients with serum creatinine ≥3 mg/dL

◀ *Manufacturer recommends the following guidelines:*
   Treatment of bone metastases: Use is not recommended in patients with severe renal impairment.
   Renal impairment in indications other than bone metastases: Use clinical judgment to determine if benefits outweigh potential risks.
   Multiple myeloma: American Society of Clinical Oncology (ASCO) guidelines (Kyle, 2007):
   Pre-existing renal impairment: Consider a reduced initial dose
   Severe renal impairment (serum creatinine >3 mg/dL **or** Cl_{cr} <30 mL/minute) and extensive bone disease: 90 mg over 4-6 hours
   Albuminuria >500 mg/24 hours (unexplained): Withhold dose until returns to baseline, then recheck every 3-4 weeks; consider reinitiating at a dose not to exceed 90 mg every 4 weeks and with a longer infusion time of at least 4 hours

Dosing adjustment in renal toxicity: In patients with bone metastases, treatment should be withheld for deterioration in renal function (increase of serum creatinine ≥0.5 mg/dL in patients with normal baseline or ≥1.0 mg/dL in patients with abnormal baseline). Resumption of therapy may be considered when serum creatinine returns to within 10% of baseline.

Dosage adjustment in hepatic impairment: No adjustment required in patients with mild-to-moderate hepatic impairment; not studied in patients with severe hepatic impairment.

Administration I.V. infusion over 2-24 hours. Longer infusion times (>2 hours) may reduce the risk for renal toxicity, especially in patients with pre-existing renal insufficiency. The manufacturer recommends infusing over 2-24 hours for hypercalcemia of malignancy; over 2 hours for osteolytic bone lesions with metastatic breast cancer; and over 4 hours for Paget's disease and for osteolytic bone lesions with multiple myeloma. The ASCO guidelines for bisphosphonate use in multiple myeloma recommend infusing pamidronate over at least 2 hours; if therapy is withheld due to renal toxicity, infuse over at least 4 hours upon reintroduction of treatment after renal recovery.

Monitoring Parameters Serum creatinine (prior to each treatment); serum electrolytes, including calcium, phosphate, magnesium and potassium; CBC with differential; monitor for hypocalcemia for at least 2 weeks after therapy; dental exam and preventative dentistry prior to therapy for patients at risk of osteonecrosis, including all cancer patients; patients with pre-existing anemia, leukopenia, or thrombocytopenia should be closely monitored during the first 2 weeks of treatment; in addition, monitor urine every 3-6 months for albuminuria in multiple myeloma patients

Test Interactions Bisphosphonates may interfere with diagnostic imaging agents such as technetium-99m-diphosphonate in bone scans.

Dietary Considerations Multiple myeloma or metastatic bone lesions from solid tumors or Paget's disease: Take adequate daily calcium and vitamin D supplement

Dosage Forms Excipient information presented when available (limited, particularly for generics); consult specific product labeling.
   Injection, powder for reconstitution, as disodium: 30 mg, 90 mg
      Aredia®: 30 mg, 90 mg
   Injection, solution, as disodium: 3 mg/mL (10 mL); 6 mg/mL (10 mL); 9 mg/mL (10 mL)
   Injection, solution, as disodium [preservative free]: 3 mg/mL (10 mL)

References
Bamias A, Kastritis E, Bamia C, et al, "Osteonecrosis of the Jaw in Cancer After Treatment With Bisphosphonates: Incidence and Risk Factors," *J Clin Oncol*, 2005, 23(34):8580-7.

Diamond TH, Winters J, Smith A, et al, "The Antiosteoporotic Efficacy of Intravenous Pamidronate in Men With Prostate Carcinoma Receiving Combined Androgen Blockade: A Double Blind, Randomized, Placebo-Controlled Crossover Study," *Cancer*, 2001, 92(6):1444-50.

Durie BG, Katz M, and Crowley J, "Osteonecrosis of the Jaw and Bisphosphonate," *N Engl J Med*, 2005, 353(1):99-102.

Glorieux FH, Bishop NH, Plotkin H, et al, "Cyclic Administration of Pamidronate in Children With Severe Osteogenesis Imperfecta," *N Engl J Med*, 1998, 339(14):947-52.

Hillner BE, Ingel JN, Chlebowski RT, et al, "American Society of Clinical Oncology 2003 Update on the Role of Bisphosphonates and Bone Health Issues in Women With Breast Cancer," *J Clin Oncol*, 2003, 21(21):4042-57.

Kyle RA, Yee GC, Somerfield MR, et al, "American Society of Clinical Oncology 2007 Clinical Practice Guideline Update on the Role of Bisphosphonates in Multiple Myeloma," *J Clin Oncol*, 2007, 25(17):2464-72.

Lteif AN and Zimmerman D, "Bisphosphonates for Treatment of Childhood Hypercalcemia," *Pediatrics*, 1998, 102(4 Pt 1):990-3.

Maerevoet M, Martin C, and Duck L, "Osteonecrosis of the Jaw and Bisphosphonates," *N Engl J Med*, 2005, 353(1):99-102.

McMahon RE, Bouquot JE, Glueck CJ, et al, "Osteonecrosis: A Multifactorial Etiology," *J Oral Maxillofac Surg*, 2004, 62(7):904-5.

National Comprehensive Cancer Network® (NCCN), "Clinical Practice Guidelines in Oncology™: Multiple Myeloma," Version 2.2009. Available at http://www.nccn.org/professionals/physician_gls/PDF/myeloma.pdf.

National Comprehensive Cancer Network® (NCCN), "Clinical Practice Guidelines in Oncology™: Thyroid Carcinoma," Version 1.2008. Available at http://www.nccn.org/professionals/physicians_gls/PDF/thyroid.pdf.

Ralston SH, Gallacher SJ, Patel U, et al, "Cancer-Associated Hypercalcemia: Morbidity and Mortality, Clinical Experience in 126 Treated Patients," *Ann Intern Med*, 1990, 112(7):499-504.

Rauch F and Glorieux FH, "Osteogenesis Imperfecta," *Lancet*, 2004, 363(9418):1377-85.

Smith MR, McGovern FJ, Zietman AL, et al, "Pamidronate to Prevent Bone Loss During Androgen-Deprivation Therapy For Prostate Cancer," *N Engl J Med*, 2001, 345(13):948-55.

Tarassoff P and Csermak K, "Avascular Necrosis of the Jaws: Risk Factors in Metastatic Cancer Patients," *J Oral Maxillofac Surg*, 2003, 61(10):1238-9.

Panitumumab (pan i TOOM yoo mab)

U.S. Brand Names Vectibix®

Index Terms ABX-EGF; MOAB ABX-EGF; Monoclonal Antibody ABX-EGF; rHuMAb-EGFr

Generic Available No

Canadian Brand Names Vectibix®

Pharmacologic Category Antineoplastic Agent, Monoclonal Antibody; Epidermal Growth Factor Receptor (EGFR) Inhibitor

Use Monotherapy in treatment of refractory metastatic colorectal cancer

Note: Subset analyses (retrospective) in metastatic colorectal cancer trials have not shown a benefit with EGFR inhibitor treatment in patients whose tumors have codon 12 or 13 *KRAS* mutations; use is not recommended in these patients.

Pregnancy Risk Factor C

Lactation Excretion in breast milk unknown/not recommended

Labeled Contraindications There are no contraindications listed in manufacturer's labeling.

Warnings/Precautions [U.S. Boxed Warning]: Dermatologic toxicities have been reported in ~90% of patients (severe in 12% of patients); may include dermatitis acneiform, pruritus, erythema, rash, skin exfoliation, paronychia, dry skin and skin fissures. Severe skin toxicities may be complicated by infection, sepsis, or abscesses. The median time to development of skin (or ocular) toxicity was 2 weeks, with resolution ~7 weeks after discontinuation. Withhold treatment (and monitor) for severe or life-threatening dermatologic toxicities; may require dose reduction or permanent discontinuation. The severity of dermatologic toxicity is predictive for response; grades 2-4 skin toxicity correlates with improved progression free survival and overall survival, compared to grade 1 skin toxicity (Peeters, 2009; Van Cutsem, 2007). Patients should minimize sunlight exposure; may exacerbate skin reactions. Gastric mucosal, ocular and nail toxicities have also been reported.

[U.S. Boxed Warning]: Severe infusion reactions (anaphylactic reaction, bronchospasm, fever, chills, and hypotension) have been reported in ~1% of patients. Discontinue infusion for severe reactions; permanently discontinue in patients with persistent severe infusion reactions. Appropriate medical support for the management of infusion reactions should be readily available. Mild-to-moderate infusion reactions are managed by slowing the infusion rate.

Pulmonary fibrosis has been reported (rarely); permanently discontinue treatment if interstitial lung disease, pneumonitis or lung infiltrates develop. Use caution with lung disease; patients with underlying lung disease were excluded from clinical trials. May cause diarrhea; the incidence and severity of chemotherapy-induced diarrhea and other toxicities (rash, electrolyte abnormalities, stomatitis) is increased with combination chemotherapy; acute renal failure resulting from severe diarrhea and dehydration has also been observed in patients receiving panitumumab with combination chemotherapy. In addition to increased toxicity, studies using panitumumab in combination with chemotherapy (with or without bevacizumab) resulted in decreased progression-free survival compared to regimens without panitumumab; therefore, panitumumab is not indicated for use in combination with chemotherapy. Electrolyte depletion may occur during treatment and after treatment is discontinued; monitor for hypomagnesemia and hypocalcemia during treatment and for at least 8 weeks after completion. Patients with colorectal cancer with tumors with a codon 12 or 13 *KRAS* mutation are unlikely to benefit from EGFR inhibitor therapy and should not receive panitumumab treatment. Safety and efficacy in children have not been established.

Adverse Reactions

>10%:

Cardiovascular: Peripheral edema (12%)

Central nervous system: Fatigue (26%)

Dermatologic: Skin toxicity (90%; grades 3/4: 14% to 16%), erythema (65%; grades 3/4: 5%), acneiform rash (57%; grades 3/4: 7%), pruritus (57%; grades 3/4: 2%), exfoliation (25%; grades 3/4: 2%), paronychia (25%), rash (22%; grades 3/4: 1%), fissures (20%; grades 3/4: 1%), acne (13%; grades 3/4: 1%)

Endocrine & metabolic: Hypomagnesemia (38%; grades 3/4: 4%)

Gastrointestinal: Abdominal pain (25%), nausea (23%), diarrhea (21%; grades 3/4: 2%), constipation (21%), vomiting (19%)

Respiratory: Cough (14%)

1% to 10%:

Dermatologic: Dry skin (10%), nail disorder (other than paronychia: 9%)

Gastrointestinal: Stomatitis (7%), mucositis (6%)

Ocular: Eyelash growth (6%), conjunctivitis (4%), ocular hyperemia (3%), lacrimation increased (2%), eye/eye lid irritation (1%)

Miscellaneous: Antibody formation (≤5%), infusion reactions (3%; grades 3/4: 1%)

<1%, postmarketing, and/or case reports: Abscess, allergic reaction, anaphylactoid reaction, angioedema, chills, dyspnea, fever, hypocalcemia, hypoxia, pulmonary embolism, pulmonary fibrosis, pulmonary infiltrate, sepsis, septic death

Drug Interactions

Avoid Concomitant Use There are no known interactions where it is recommended to avoid concomitant use.

Increased Effect/Toxicity There are no known significant interactions involving an increase in effect.

Decreased Effect There are no known significant interactions involving a decrease in effect.

Storage/Stability Store unopened vials under refrigeration at 2°C to 8°C (36°F to 46°F). Do not freeze; do not shake; protect from light. Preparations in infusion containers are stable for 24 hours under refrigeration at 2°C to 8°C (36°F to 46°F) or for 6 hours at room temperature (do not freeze).

Reconstitution Dilute in 100-150 mL of normal saline to a final concentration of ≤10 mg/mL. Do not shake, invert gently to mix.

Mechanism of Action Recombinant human IgG2 monoclonal antibody which binds specifically to the epidermal growth factor receptor (EGFR, HER1, c-ErbB-1) and competitively inhibits the binding of epidermal growth factor (EGF) and other ligands. Binding to the EGFR blocks phosphorylation and activation of intracellular tyrosine kinases, resulting in inhibition of cell survival, growth, proliferation and transformation. EGFR signal transduction results in *KRAS* wild-type activation; cells with *KRAS* mutations appear to be unaffected by EGFR inhibition.

Pharmacodynamics/Kinetics Half-life elimination: ~7.5 days (range: 4-11 days)

Dosage I.V.: Adults: Metastatic colorectal cancer: 6 mg/kg every 2 weeks
Dosing adjustment for toxicity:

Infusion reactions, mild-to-moderate (grade 1 or 2): Reduce the infusion rate by 50% for the duration of infusion

Infusion reactions, severe (grade 3 or 4): Immediately and permanently discontinue treatment

Dermatologic toxicity (≥grade 3, or intolerable): Withhold treatment; if skin toxicity does not improve to ≤grade 2 within 1 month, permanently discontinue. If skin toxicity improves to ≤grade 2 within 1 month (with patient missing ≤2 doses), resume treatment at 50% of the original dose. Dose may be increased in increments of 25% of the original dose (up to 6 mg/kg) if skin toxicities do not recur. For recurrent skin toxicity, permanently discontinue.

Dosage adjustment in renal impairment: Has not been studied

Dosage adjustment in hepatic impairment: Has not been studied

Administration I.V.: Doses ≤1000 mg, infuse over 1 hour; doses >1000 mg, infuse over 90 minutes; reduce infusion rate by 50% for mild-to-moderate infusion reactions (grades 1 and 2); discontinue for severe infusion reactions (grades 3 and 4). Administer through a low protein-binding 0.2 or 0.22 micrometer in-line filter. Flush with NS before and after infusion.

Monitoring Parameters *KRAS* genotyping of tumor tissue. Monitor serum electrolytes, including magnesium and calcium (periodically during and for at least 8 weeks after therapy). Monitor vital signs and temperature before, during, and after infusion. Monitor for skin toxicity.

Additional Information Oncology Comment: The National Comprehensive Cancer Network® (NCCN) guidelines for colon cancer (v.2.2009) and the American Society of Clinical Oncology (ASCO) provisional clinical opinion (Allegra, 2009) recommend genotyping tumor tissue for *KRAS* mutation in all patients with metastatic colorectal cancer (genotyping may be done on archived specimens). Patients with known codon 12 or 13 *KRAS* gene mutations are unlikely to respond to EGFR inhibitors and should not receive panitumumab. Favorable progression-free survival and higher response rates have been demonstrated with panitumumab in patients with *KRAS* wild-type; patients with the *KRAS* mutation did not respond to panitumumab (Amado, 2008). Because EGFR testing in colorectal tumors does not correlate with response, the NCCN guidelines do not recommend routine EGFR testing in colorectal cancer. Severity of dermatologic toxicity associated with panitumumab is predictive for response; grades 2-4 skin toxicity correlates with improved progression free survival and overall survival, compared to patients with grade 1 skin toxicity (Van Cutsem, 2007). The association between dermatologic toxicity and progression free survival was not noted in patients with *KRAS* mutation (Peeters, 2009). The NCCN guidelines do not recommend the use of panitumumab after failure of cetuximab therapy.

Dosage Forms Excipient information presented when available (limited, particularly for generics); consult specific product labeling.

Injection, solution [preservative free]:
    Vectibix®: 20 mg/mL (5 mL, 10 mL, 20 mL)

References

Allegra CJ, Jessup JM, Somerfield MR, et al, "American Society of Clinical Oncology Provisional Clinical Opinion: Testing for *KRAS* Gene Mutations in Patients With Metastatic Colorectal Carcinoma to Predict Response to Anti-Epidermal Growth Factor Receptor Monoclonal Antibody Therapy, " *J Clin Oncol*, 2009, 27(12):2091-6.

Amado RG, Wolf M, Peeters M, et al, "Wild-Type KRAS is Required for Panitumumab Efficacy in Patients With Metastatic Colorectal Cancer," *J Clin Oncol*, 2008, 26(10):1626-34.

National Comprehensive Cancer Network (NCCN), "Clinical Practice Guidelines in Oncology™: Colon Cancer," Version 2, 2009. Accessible at http://www.nccn.org/professionals/physician_gls/PDF/colon.pdf

Peeters M, Siena S, Van Cutsem E, et al, "Association of Progression-Free Survival, Overall Survival, and Patient-Reported Outcomes by Skin Toxicity and KRAS Status in Patients Receiving Panitumumab Monotherapy," *Cancer*, 2009, 115(7):1544-54.

Rowinsky EK, Schwartz GH, Gollob JA, et al, "Safety, Pharmacokinetics, and Activity of ABX-EGF, a Fully Human Anti-Epidermal Growth Factor Receptor Monoclonal Antibody in Patients with Metastatic Renal Cell Cancer," *J Clin Oncol*, 2004, 22(15):3003-15.

Segaert S and Van Cutsem E, "Clinical Signs, Pathophysiology and Management of Skin Toxicity During Therapy With Epidermal Growth Factor Receptor Inhibitors," *Ann Oncol*, 2005, 16(9):1425-33.

Van Cutsem E, Peeters M, Siena S, et al, "Open-Label Phase III Trial of Panitumumab Plus Best Supportive Care Compared With Best Supportive Care Alone in Patients With Chemotherapy-Refractory Metastatic Colorectal Cancer," *J Clin Oncol*, 2007, 25(13): 1658-64.

◆ **Panretin®** *see* Alitretinoin *on page 36*

Papillomavirus (Types 6, 11, 16, 18) Vaccine (Human, Recombinant)

(pap ih LO ma VYE rus typs six e LEV en SIX teen AYE teen vak SEEN YU man ree KOM be nant)

U.S. Brand Names Gardasil®

Index Terms HPV Vaccine; HPV4; Human Papillomavirus Vaccine; Papillomavirus Vaccine, Recombinant; Quadrivalent Human Papillomavirus Vaccine

Generic Available No

Canadian Brand Names Gardasil®

Pharmacologic Category Vaccine, Inactivated (Viral)

Use Females ≥9 years and ≤26 years of age: Prevention of cervical, vulvar, and vaginal cancer, genital warts, cervical adenocarcinoma *in situ*, and vulvar, vaginal, or cervical intraepithelial neoplasia caused by human papillomavirus (HPV) types 6, 11, 16, 18

The Advisory Committee on Immunization Practices (ACIP) recommends routine vaccination for females 11-12 years of age; catch-up vaccination is recommended for females 13-26 years of age

Unlabeled/Investigational Use Prevention of cervical, vulvar, and vaginal cancer, genital warts, cervical adenocarcinoma *in situ*, and vulvar, vaginal, or cervical intraepithelial neoplasia caused by human papillomavirus (HPV) types 6, 11, 16, 18 in women 26-45 years of age

Pregnancy Risk Factor B

Lactation Excretion in breast milk unknown/use caution

Labeled Contraindications Hypersensitivity to papillomavirus recombinant vaccine or any component of the formulation

Warnings/Precautions Immediate treatment for anaphylactoid reaction should be available during vaccine use. There is no evidence that individuals already infected with HPV will be protected; those already infected with 1 or more HPV types were protected from disease in the remaining HPV types. Not for the treatment of active disease; will not protect against diseases not caused by human papillomavirus (HPV) vaccine types 6, 11, 16, and 18. May administer with mild concurrent febrile illness; consider deferring vaccination with serious illness. Immunocompromised patients may have a reduced response to vaccination. Administered I.M., therefore use caution in patients at risk for bleeding. The entire 3-dose regimen should be completed for maximum efficacy. Not recommended for use during pregnancy. Syncope may occur following vaccination and may be associated with tonic-clonic movements or other seizure-like activity; observe for 15 minutes following administration. Safety and efficacy in girls <9 years of age have not been established. Safety and efficacy have not been established in males. Product may contain yeast. In order to maximize vaccination rates, the ACIP recommends simultaneous administration of all age-appropriate vaccines (live or inactivated) for which a person is eligible at a single clinic visit, unless contraindications exist.

Adverse Reactions All serious adverse reactions must be reported to the U.S. Department of Health and Human Services (DHHS) Vaccine Adverse Event Reporting System (VAERS) 1-800-822-7967.

>10%:

Central nervous system: Fever (13%)

Local: Injection site: Pain (84%), swelling (25%), erythema (25%)

1% to 10%:

Central nervous system: Dizziness (4%), malaise (1%), insomnia (1%)

Gastrointestinal: Nausea (7%), diarrhea (4%), vomiting (2%), toothache (2%)

Local: Injection site: Bruising (3%), pruritus (3%)

Neuromuscular & skeletal: Arthralgia (1%)

Respiratory: Cough (2%), nasal congestion (1%)

<1%, postmarketing, and/or case reports: Anaphylactic/anaphylactoid reaction, appendicitis, arrhythmia, arthritis, asthma, autoimmune hemolytic anemia and other autoimmune diseases, bronchospasm, chills, DVT, fatigue, gastroenteritis, Guillain-Barré syndrome, headache, hypersensitivity reaction, hyperthyroidism, JRA, lymphadenopathy, motor neuron disease, myalgia, pancreatitis, paralysis, pelvic inflammatory disease, pulmonary embolus, RA,

renal failure (acute), seizure, sepsis, syncope (may result in falls with injury or be associated with tonic-clonic movements), transverse myelitis, urticaria, weakness

Drug Interactions

Avoid Concomitant Use There are no known interactions where it is recommended to avoid concomitant use.

Increased Effect/Toxicity There are no known significant interactions involving an increase in effect.

Decreased Effect

The levels/effects of Papillomavirus (Types 6, 11, 16, 18) Vaccine (Human, Recombinant) may be decreased by: Immunosuppressants

Storage/Stability Store at 2°C to 8°C (36°F to 46°F); do not freeze. Protect from light. May be stored at temperatures ≤25°C (≤77°F) for a total time of ≤72 hours.

Mechanism of Action Contains inactive human papillomavirus (HPV) proteins HPV 6 L1, HPV 11 L1, HPV 16 L1, and HPV 18 L1 which produce neutralizing antibodies to prevent cervical cancer, cervical adenocarcinoma, cervical, vaginal and vulvar neoplasia and genital warts caused by HPV.

Dosage I.M.: Females: Children ≥9 years and Adults ≤26 years: 0.5 mL followed by 0.5 mL at 2 and 6 months after initial dose

CDC recommended immunization schedule: Administer first dose to females at age 11-12 years; begin series in females aged 13-26 years if not previously vaccinated. Minimum interval between first and second doses is 4 weeks; the minimum interval between first and third doses is 24 weeks.

Administration Shake suspension well before use. Inject I.M. into the deltoid region of the upper arm or higher anterolateral thigh area. Observe for syncope for 15 minutes following administration.

Administration with other vaccines:

Papillomavirus (Types 6, 11, 16, 18) Recombinant vaccine with other inactivated vaccines: May be given simultaneously or at any interval between doses.

Papillomavirus (Types 6, 11, 16, 18) Recombinant vaccine with live vaccines: May be given simultaneously or at any interval between doses

Vaccine administration with antibody-containing products: Papillomavirus (Types 6, 11, 16, 18) Recombinant vaccine may be given simultaneously at different sites or at any interval between doses. Examples of antibody-containing products include I.M. and I.V. immune globulin, hepatitis B immune globulin, tetanus immune globulin, varicella zoster immune globulin, rabies immune globulin, whole blood, packed red cells, plasma, and platelet products

For patients at risk of hemorrhage following intramuscular injection, the ACIP recommends "it should be administered intramuscularly if, in the opinion of the physician familiar with the patients bleeding risk, the vaccine can be administered with reasonable safety by this route. If the patient receives antihemophilia or other similar therapy, intramuscular vaccination can be scheduled shortly after such therapy is administered. A fine needle (23 gauge or smaller) can be used for the vaccination and firm pressure applied to the site (without rubbing) for at least 2 minutes. The patient should be instructed concerning the risk of hematoma from the injection."

Monitoring Parameters Gynecologic screening exam, papillomavirus test; screening for cervical cancer should continue per current guidelines following vaccination; observe for syncope/fainting for ~15 minutes after administration of vaccine. If seizure-like activity associated with syncope occurs, maintain patient in supine or Trendelenburg position to re-establish adequate cerebral perfusion.

Additional Information Federal law requires that the date of administration, the vaccine manufacturer, lot number of vaccine, and the administering person's name, title and address be entered into the patient's permanent medical record. Ideally, administration of vaccine should occur prior to potential HPV exposure. Benefits of vaccine decrease once infected with ≥1 of the HPV vaccine types.

Dosage Forms Excipient information presented when available (limited, particularly for generics); consult specific product labeling.

Injection, suspension [preservative free]:

Gardasil®: HPV 6 L1 protein 20 mcg, HPV 11 L1 protein 40 mcg, HPV 16 L1 protein 40 mcg, and HPV 18 L1 protein 20 mcg per 0.5 mL (0.5 mL) [contains aluminum, polysorbate 80; manufactured using *S. cerevisiae* (baker's yeast)]

References

Centers for Disease Control, "General Recommendations on Immunization. Recommendations of the Advisory Committee on Immunization Practices (ACIP)," *MMWR Recomm Rep*, 2006, 55 (RR-15):1-48.

Centers for Disease Control and Prevention, "Quadrivalent Human Papillomavirus Vaccine. Recommendations of the Advisory Committee on Immunization Practices (ACIP)," *MMWR Recomm Rep*, 2007, 56(RR-2):1-24.

FUTURE II Study Group, "Quadrivalent Vaccine Against Human Papillomavirus to Prevent High-Grade Cervical Lesions," *N Engl J Med*, 2007, 356(19):1915-27.

Koutsky LA, Ault KA, Wheeler CM, et al, "A Controlled Trial of a Human Papillomavirus Type 16 Vaccine," *N Engl J Med*, 2002, 347(21):1645-51.

Mao C, Koutsky LA, Ault KA, et al, "Efficacy of Human Papillomavirus-16 Vaccine to Prevent Cervical Intraepithelial Neoplasia: A Randomized Controlled Trial," *Obstet Gynecol*, 2006, 107 (1):18-27.

Muñoz N, Manalastas R Jr, Pitisuttithum P, et al, "Safety, Immunogenicity, and Efficacy of Quadrivalent Human Papillomavirus (Types 6, 11, 16, 18) Recombinant Vaccine in Women Aged 24-45 Years: A Randomised, Double-Blind Trial," *Lancet*, 2009, 373(9679):1949-57.

National Advisory Committee on Immunization (NACI), "Statement on Human Papillomavirus Vaccine. An Advisory Committee Statement (ACS)," *Can Commun Dis Rep*, 2007, 33(ACS-2):1-31.

Saslow D, Castle PE, Cox JT, et al, "American Cancer Society Guideline for Human Papillomavirus (HPV) Vaccine Use to Prevent Cervical Cancer and Its Precursors," *CA Cancer J Clin*, 2007, 57 (1):7-28.

◆ **Papillomavirus Vaccine, Recombinant** *see* Papillomavirus (Types 6, 11, 16, 18) Vaccine (Human, Recombinant) *on page 922*

◆ **Paraplatin-AQ (Can)** *see* CARBOplatin *on page 178*

◆ **PDX** *see* Pralatrexate *on page 974*

◆ **Pediapred®** *see* PrednisoLONE *on page 977*

◆ **Pedi-Dri®** *see* Nystatin *on page 855*

◆ **PEG-L-asparaginase** *see* Pegaspargase *on page 925*

◆ **PEG-ASP** *see* Pegaspargase *on page 925*

◆ **PEG-asparaginase** *see* Pegaspargase *on page 925*

Pegaspargase (peg AS par jase)

Medication Safety Issues

Sound-alike/look-alike issues:

Oncaspar® may be confused with Elspar®

Pegaspargase may be confused with asparaginase

High alert medication: The Institute for Safe Medication Practices (ISMP) includes this medication among its list of drugs which have a heightened risk of causing significant patient harm when used in error.

Related Information

Safe Handling of Hazardous Drugs *on page 1517*

U.S. Brand Names Oncaspar®

Index Terms L-asparaginase with Polyethylene Glycol; PEG-ASP; PEG-asparaginase; PEG-L-asparaginase; PEGLA; Polyethylene Glycol-L-asparaginase

Generic Available No

Pharmacologic Category Antineoplastic Agent, Miscellaneous

Use Treatment of acute lymphocytic leukemia (ALL); treatment of ALL with previous hypersensitivity to native L-asparaginase

Pregnancy Risk Factor C

Lactation Excretion in breast milk unknown/not recommended

Labeled Contraindications History of serious allergic reactions to pegaspargase; history of any of the following with prior L-asparaginase treatment: pancreatitis, serious hemorrhagic events, serious thrombosis

Warnings/Precautions Hazardous agent - use appropriate precautions for handling and disposal. Serious allergic reactions may occur; discontinue in patients with serious allergic reaction. Observe patients for at least 1 hour after administration; immediate treatment for hypersensitivity reactions should be available during administration. Pegaspargase is indicated for use in patients who have had hypersensitivity reactions to native L-asparaginase; however, in one study, 32% of patients with a history of allergic reaction to *E. coli* asparaginase products also experienced allergic reaction to pegaspargase.

Serious thrombotic events, including sagittal sinus thrombosis may occur; discontinue with serious thrombotic event. Pancreatitis may occur; promptly evaluate patients with abdominal pain; discontinue if pancreatitis occurs during treatment. May cause glucose intolerance; irreversible in some cases; use with caution in patients with hyperglycemia, or diabetes. Coagulopathy has been reported; monitor coagulation parameters; severe or symptomatic coagulopathy may require treatment with fresh-frozen plasma; use with caution in patients with underlying coagulopathy. Reversible hepatotoxicity (hyperbilirubinemia and liver enzyme elevation) may occur; use with caution in patients with hepatic dysfunction or concomitant hepatotoxic medications. Use cautiously in patients with previous hematologic complications from asparaginase.

Adverse Reactions

>5%:

Cardiovascular: Edema

Central nervous system: Fever, malaise

Dermatologic: Rash

Gastrointestinal: Nausea, vomiting

Hematologic: Coagulopathy (7%; grades 3/4: 2%)

Hepatic: Transaminases increased (11%; grades 3/4: 3%)

Miscellaneous: Allergic reactions (including bronchospasm, chills, dyspnea, edema, erythema, hypotension, rash, swelling, urticaria; no prior asparaginase hypersensitivity: 1% to 10%; grades 3/4: 2%; prior asparaginase hypersensitivity: 32%; grades 3/4: 8%)

1% to 5%:

Cardiovascular: Hypotension, peripheral edema, tachycardia, thrombosis (4%)

Central nervous system: Chills, CNS thrombosis (2% to 4%; grades 3/4: 3%), CNS hemorrhage (2%), headache, seizure

Dermatologic: Lip edema, urticaria

Endocrine & metabolic: Hyperglycemia (3% to 5%; grades 3/4: ≤5%), hyperuricemia, hypoglycemia, hypoproteinemia

Gastrointestinal: Abdominal pain, anorexia, diarrhea, pancreatitis (1% to 2%; grades 3/4: 2%)

Hematologic: Anticoagulant effect decreased, disseminated intravascular coagulation (DIC), fibrinogen decreased, hemolytic anemia, leukopenia, pancytopenia, thrombocytopenia, thromboplastin increased, myelosuppression

Hepatic: Liver function tests abnormal (grades 3/4: 5%), hyperbilirubinemia (grades 3/4: 2%), jaundice

Local: Injection site hypersensitivity, pain or reaction

Neuromuscular & skeletal: Arthralgia, limb pain, myalgia, paresthesia

Respiratory: Dyspnea

Miscellaneous: Anaphylactic reactions, night sweats

<1%, postmarketing, and/or case reports (limited to important or life-threatening): Abnormal renal function, alopecia, amylase increased, anemia, antithrombin III decreased, ascites, bacteremia, bone pain, bronchospasm, bruising, BUN increased, chest pain, coagulation time increased, colitis, coma, confusion, constipation, cough, creatinine increased, dizziness, DVT, emotional lability, endocarditis, epistaxis, excessive thirst, face edema, fatigue, fatty liver deposits, gastrointestinal pain, hematuria, hemorrhagic cystitis, hepatomegaly, hyperammonemia, hypertension, hypoalbuminemia, hyponatremia, lipase increased, liver failure, metabolic acidosis, mucositis, petechial rash, proteinuria, prothrombin time increased, purpura, renal failure, sagittal sinus thrombosis, sepsis, septic shock, subacute bacterial endocarditis, superficial venous thrombosis, uric acid nephropathy

Drug Interactions

Avoid Concomitant Use

Avoid concomitant use of Pegaspargase with any of the following: Natalizumab; Vaccines (Live)

Increased Effect/Toxicity

Pegaspargase may increase the levels/effects of: Leflunomide; Natalizumab; Vaccines (Live)

The levels/effects of Pegaspargase may be increased by: Trastuzumab

Decreased Effect

Pegaspargase may decrease the levels/effects of: Vaccines (Inactivated); Vaccines (Live)

The levels/effects of Pegaspargase may be decreased by: Echinacea

Storage/Stability Refrigerate at 2°C to 8°C (36°F to 46°F); do not freeze. Do not use product if it is known to have been frozen. Do not use vial if stored at room temperature for >48 hours. Avoid excessive agitation; do not shake. Do not use if cloudy, discolored, or if precipitate is present. Solutions for infusion should be refrigerated immediately after aseptic preparation and administered within 24 hours of preparation (data on file).

Reconstitution I.V.: Dilute in 100 mL NS or D_5W; stable for 48 hours at room temperature.

Compatibility Stable in NS, D_5W.

Mechanism of Action Pegaspargase is a modified version of asparaginase. Leukemic cells, especially lymphoblasts, require exogenous asparagine; normal cells can synthesize asparagine. Asparaginase contains L-asparaginase amidohydrolase type EC-2 which inhibits protein synthesis by deaminating asparagine to aspartic acid and ammonia in the plasma and extracellular fluid and therefore deprives tumor cells of the amino acid for protein synthesis. Asparaginase is cycle-specific for the G_1 phase of the cell cycle.

Pharmacodynamics/Kinetics

Onset: Asparagine depletion: I.M.: Within 4 days

Duration: Asparagine depletion: I.M.: ~21 days; I.V. (in asparaginase naive adults): 2-4 weeks

Absorption: I.M.: Slow

Distribution: I.M.: Children: 1.5 L/m^2; I.V.: Adults (asparaginase naive): 2.4 L/m^2

Metabolism: Systemically degraded

Half-life elimination: I.M.: ~5.5-6 days; unaffected by age, renal or hepatic function; half life decreased to 1.8-3.2 days in patients with previous hypersensitivity to native L-asparaginase; I.V.: Adults (asparaginase naive): 7 days

Time to peak: I.M.: 3-4 days

Excretion: Urine (trace amounts)

Dosage Details concerning dosing in combinations regimens should also be consulted.

Children and Adults: I.M., I.V.: 2500 units/m^2 (as part of a combination chemotherapy regimen), do not administer more frequently than every 14 days

Hemodialysis, peritoneal dialysis: Significant drug removal is unlikely based on physiochemical characteristics

Combination Regimens

Leukemia, acute lymphocytic: Hyper-CVAD (Leukemia, Acute Lymphocytic) on page 1349

Administration Have available appropriate agents for maintenance of an adequate airway and treatment of a hypersensitivity reaction (antihistamine, epinephrine, oxygen, I.V. corticosteroids). Be prepared to treat anaphylaxis at each administration.

I.M.: Must only be administered as a deep intramuscular injection into a large muscle. Do not exceed 2 mL per injection site; use multiple injection sites for I.M. injection volume >2 mL.

I.V.: Administer over 1-2 hours through a running I.V. infusion line; **do not administer I.V. push.**

Monitoring Parameters Vital signs during administration, CBC with differential, platelets, amylase, liver enzymes, fibrinogen, PT, PTT (coagulation parameters [baseline and periodic]), renal function tests, urine glucose, blood glucose; monitor for onset of abdominal pain; observe for allergic reaction (for 1 hour after administration)

Emetic Potential Very low (<10%)

Dosage Forms Excipient information presented when available (limited, particularly for generics); consult specific product labeling.

Injection, solution [preservative free]:

Oncaspar®: 750 int. units/mL (5 mL)

References

Abshire TC, Pollock BH, Billett AL, et al, "Weekly Polyethylene Glycol Conjugated L-Asparaginase Compared With Biweekly Dosing Produces Superior Induction Remission Rates in Childhood Relapsed Acute Lymphoblastic Leukemia: A Pediatric Oncology Group Study," *Blood*, 2000, 96 (5):1709-15.

Avramis VI, Sencer S, Periclou AP, et al, "A Randomized Comparison of Native *Escherichia Coli* Asparaginase and Polyethylene Glycol Conjugated Asparaginase for Treatment of Children With Newly Diagnosed Standard-Risk Acute Lymphoblastic Leukemia: A Children's Cancer Group Study," *Blood*, 2002, 99(6):1986-94.

Avramis VI and Spence SA, "Clinical Pharmacology of Asparaginases in the United States: Asparaginase Population Pharmacokinetic and Pharmacodynamic (PK-PD) Models (NONMEM) in Adult and Pediatric Patients," *J Pediatr Hematol Oncol*, 2007, 29(4):239-47.

Douer D, Yampolsky H, Cohen LJ, et al, "Pharmacodynamics and Safety of Intravenous Pegaspargase During Remission Induction in Adults Aged 55 Years or Younger With Newly Diagnosed Acute Lymphoblastic Leukemia," *Blood*, 2007, 109(7):2744-50.

Pegfilgrastim (peg fil GRA stim)

Medication Safety Issues

Sound-alike/look-alike issues:

Neulasta® may be confused with Neumega®, Neupogen®, and Lunesta®

U.S. Brand Names Neulasta®

Index Terms G-CSF (PEG Conjugate); Granulocyte Colony Stimulating Factor (PEG Conjugate); NSC-725961; Pegylated G-CSF; SD/01

Generic Available No

Canadian Brand Names Neulasta®

Pharmacologic Category Colony Stimulating Factor

Use To decrease the incidence of infection, by stimulation of granulocyte production, in patients with nonmyeloid malignancies receiving myelosuppressive therapy associated with a significant risk of febrile neutropenia

Pregnancy Risk Factor C

Lactation Excretion in breast milk unknown/use caution

Labeled Contraindications Hypersensitivity to pegfilgrastim, filgrastim, or any component of the formulation

Warnings/Precautions Do not use pegfilgrastim in the period 14 days before to 24 hours after administration of cytotoxic chemotherapy because of the potential sensitivity of rapidly dividing myeloid cells to cytotoxic chemotherapy. Benefit has not been demonstrated with regimens under a two-week duration. Administration on the same day as chemotherapy is not recommended (NCCN Myeloid Growth Factor Guidelines, v.1.2009). Pegfilgrastim can potentially act as a growth factor for any tumor type, particularly myeloid malignancies. Caution should be exercised in the usage of pegfilgrastim in any malignancy with myeloid characteristics. Tumors of nonhematopoietic origin may have surface receptors for pegfilgrastim. Pegfilgrastim has not been evaluated with patients receiving radiation therapy, or with chemotherapy associated with delayed myelosuppression (nitrosoureas, mitomycin C). Safety and efficacy have not been evaluated for peripheral blood progenitor cell (PBPC) mobilization.

Allergic-type reactions (anaphylaxis, angioedema, erythema, skin rash, urticaria) have occurred primarily with the initial dose and may recur (possibly delayed) after discontinuation; close follow up for several days and permanent discontinuation are recommended for severe reactions. Rare cases of splenic rupture have been reported; patients must be instructed to report left upper quadrant pain or shoulder tip pain. Acute respiratory distress syndrome (ARDS) has been associated with use; evaluate patients with pulmonary symptoms such as fever, lung infiltrates, or respiratory distress; discontinue or withhold pegfilgrastim if ARDS occurs. May precipitate sickle cell crises in patients with sickle cell disease; carefully evaluate potential risks and benefits. The packaging (needle cover) contains latex. The 6 mg fixed dose should not be used in infants, children, and adolescents weighing <45 kg.

Adverse Reactions

>10%:

Cardiovascular: Peripheral edema (12%)

Central nervous system: Headache (16%)

◄

Gastrointestinal: Vomiting (13%)

Neuromuscular & skeletal: Bone pain (31% to 57%), myalgia (21%), arthralgia (16%), weakness (13%)

1% to 10%:

Gastrointestinal: Constipation (10%)

Miscellaneous: Antibody formation (1% to 6%)

<1%, postmarketing, and/or case reports: Acute respiratory distress syndrome (ARDS), allergic reaction, anaphylaxis, erythema, fever, flushing, hyperleukocytosis, hypoxia, injection site reactions (erythema, induration, pain), leukocytosis, rash, sickle cell crisis, splenic rupture, Sweet's syndrome (acute febrile dermatosis), urticaria. Cytopenias resulting from an antibody response to exogenous growth factors have been reported on rare occasions in patients treated with other recombinant growth factors.

Drug Interactions

Avoid Concomitant Use There are no known interactions where it is recommended to avoid concomitant use.

Increased Effect/Toxicity There are no known significant interactions involving an increase in effect.

Decreased Effect There are no known significant interactions involving a decrease in effect.

Storage/Stability Store under refrigeration 2°C to 8°C (36°F to 46°F); do not freeze. If inadvertently frozen, allow to thaw in refrigerator; discard if frozen more than one time. Protect from light. Do not shake. Allow to reach room temperature prior to injection. May be kept at room temperature for up to 48 hours.

Mechanism of Action Stimulates the production, maturation, and activation of neutrophils, pegfilgrastim activates neutrophils to increase both their migration and cytotoxicity. Pegfilgrastim has a prolonged duration of effect relative to filgrastim and a reduced renal clearance.

Pharmacodynamics/Kinetics Half-life elimination: SubQ: Adults: 15-80 hours; Children (100 mcg/kg dose): ~20-30 hours (range: up to 68 hours)

Dosage SubQ: **Note:** Do not administer in the period between 14 days before and 24 hours after administration of cytotoxic chemotherapy. According to the NCCN guidelines, efficacy has been demonstrated with every-2-week chemotherapy regimens, however, benefit has not been demonstrated with regimens under a two-week duration (NCCN Myeloid Growth Factor Guidelines, v.1.2009)

Children (unlabeled dose): 100 mcg/kg (maximum dose: 6 mg) once per chemotherapy cycle, beginning 24-72 hours after completion of chemotherapy

Adolescents >45 kg and Adults: 6 mg once per chemotherapy cycle, beginning 24-72 hours after completion of chemotherapy

Dosage adjustment in renal impairment: No adjustment necessary

Administration Administer subcutaneously. Do not use 6 mg fixed dose in infants, children, or adolescents <45 kg. Engage/activate needle guard following use to prevent accidental needlesticks.

Monitoring Parameters Complete blood count (with differential) and platelet count should be obtained prior to chemotherapy. Leukocytosis (white blood cell counts 100,000/mm^3) has been observed in <1% of patients receiving pegfilgrastim. Monitor platelets and hematocrit regularly. Evaluate fever, pulmonary infiltrates, and respiratory distress; evaluate for left upper abdominal pain, shoulder tip pain, or splenomegaly. Monitor for sickle cell crisis (in patients with sickle cell anemia).

Test Interactions May interfere with bone imaging studies; increased hematopoietic activity of the bone marrow may appear as transient positive bone imaging changes

Dosage Forms Excipient information presented when available (limited, particularly for generics); consult specific product labeling.

Injection, solution [preservative free]:

Neulasta®: 10 mg/mL (0.6 mL) [prefilled syringe; needle cover contains latex]

References

Andre N, Kababri ME, Bertrand P, et al, "Safety and Efficacy of Pegfilgrastim in Children With Cancer Receiving Myelosuppressive Chemotherapy," *Anticancer Drugs*, 2007, 18(3):277-81.

Andre N, Milano E, Rome A, et al, "Safety of Pegfilgrastim in Children", *Ann Pharmacother*, 2008, 42(2):290.

Fox E, Jayaprakash N, Widemann BC, et al, "Randomized Trial and Pharmacokinetic Study of Pegfilgrastim vs. Filgrastim in Children and Young Adults With Newly Diagnosed Sarcoma Treated With Dose Intensive Chemotherapy," *J Clin Oncol*, 2006, 24(18S):9020 [abstract from 2006 ASCO Annual Meeting Proceedings, Part I]

Holmes FA, O'Shaughnessy JA, Vukelja S, et al, "Blinded, Randomized, Multicenter Study to Evaluate Single Administration Pegfilgrastim Once Per Cycle Versus Daily Filgrastim as an Adjunct to Chemotherapy in Patients With High-Risk Stage II or Stage III/IV Breast Cancer," *J Clin Oncol*, 2002, 20(3): 727-31.

Kuendgen A, Fenk R, Bruns I, et al, "Splenic Rupture Following Administration of Pegfilgrastim in a Patient With Multiple Myeloma Undergoing Autologous Peripheral Stem Cell Transplantation," *Bone Marrow Transplant*, 2006, 38(1):69-70.

National Comprehensive Cancer Network® (NCCN), "Clinical Practice Guidelines in Oncology™: Myeloid Growth Factors," Version 1.2008. Available at http://www.nccn.org/professionals/physician_gls/PDF/myeloid_growth.pdf.

Smith TJ, Khatcheressian J, Lyman GH, et al, "2006 Update of Recommendations for the Use of White Blood Cell Growth Factors: An Evidence-Based Clinical Practice Guideline," *J Clin Oncol*, 2006, 24(19):3187-205.

Wolff AC, Jones RJ, Davidson NE, et al, "Myeloid Toxicity in Breast Cancer in Patients Receiving Adjuvant Chemotherapy With Pegfilgrastim Support," *J Clin Oncol*, 2006, 24(15):2392-4.

Peginterferon Alfa-2b (peg in ter FEER on AL fa too bee)

Medication Safety Issues

Sound-alike/look-alike issues:

Peginterferon alfa-2b may be confused with interferon alfa-2a, interferon alfa-2b, interferon alfa-n3, peginterferon alfa-2a

PegIntron™ may be confused with Intron® A

International issues:

Peginterferon alfa-2b may be confused with interferon alpha multi-subtype which is available in international markets

U.S. Brand Names PegIntron™; PegIntron™ Redipen®

Index Terms Interferon Alfa-2b (PEG Conjugate); Pegylated Interferon Alfa-2b

Generic Available No

Canadian Brand Names PegIntron™

Pharmacologic Category Interferon

Use Treatment of chronic hepatitis C (in combination with ribavirin) in patients who have never received alfa interferons and have compensated liver disease; treatment of chronic hepatitis C (as monotherapy) in adult patients with compensated liver disease who have never received alfa interferons

Unlabeled/Investigational Use Treatment of advanced melanoma

Pregnancy Risk Factor C / X in combination with ribavirin

Lactation Excretion in breast milk unknown/not recommended

Labeled Contraindications Hypersensitivity (including urticaria, angioedema, bronchoconstriction, anaphylaxis, Stevens Johnson syndrome and toxic epidermal necrolysis) to interferons, or any component of the formulation; autoimmune hepatitis; decompensated liver disease (Child-Pugh score >6, classes B and C) in cirrhotic chronic hepatitis C patients (prior to or during treatment)

Combination therapy with peginterferon alfa-2b and ribavirin is also contra-indicated in pregnancy, women who may become pregnant, males with pregnant partners; hemoglobinopathies (eg, thalassemia major, sickle-cell anemia); renal dysfunction (Cl_{cr} <50 mL/minute)

Warnings/Precautions Hazardous agent - use appropriate precautions for handling and disposal.

[U.S. Boxed Warning]: May cause or aggravate fatal or life-threatening autoimmune disorders, neuropsychiatric symptoms (including depression and/or suicidal thoughts/behaviors), infectious disorders, ischemic disorders, and/or hemorrhagic cerebrovascular events; discontinue treatment for persistent severe or worsening symptoms.

Neuropsychiatric disorders: Neuropsychiatric effects may occur in patients with and without a history of psychiatric disorder; addiction relapse, aggression, depression, homicidal ideation and suicidal behavior/ideation have been observed with peginterferon alfa-2b; bipolar disorder, hallucinations, mania, and psychosis have been observed with other alfa interferons. Use with extreme caution in patients with a history of psychiatric disorders, including depression. Monitor all patients for evidence of depression; patients who develop psychiatric disorders should be monitored during and for 6 months after completion of therapy; discontinue treatment if psychiatric symptoms persist, worsen, or if suicidal behavior develops. Higher doses may be associated with the development of encephalopathy (higher risk in elderly patients).

Bone marrow suppression: Causes bone marrow suppression, including potentially severe cytopenias; alfa interferons may (rarely) cause aplastic anemia. Use with caution in patients who are chronically immunosuppressed, with low peripheral blood counts or myelosuppression, including concurrent use of myelosuppressive therapy. Use with caution in patients with an increased risk for severe anemia (eg, spherocytosis, history of GI bleeding). Dosage modification may be necessary for hematologic toxicity. Combination therapy with ribavirin may potentiate the neutropenic effects of alfa interferons. When used in combination with ribavirin, an increased incidence of anemia was observed when using ribavirin weight-based dosing, as compared to flat-dose ribavirin.

Hepatic disease: Discontinue treatment immediately with hepatic decompensation (Child Pugh score >6). Patients with chronic hepatitis C (CHC) with cirrhosis receiving peginterferon alfa-2b are at risk for hepatic decompensation. CHC patients coinfected with human immunodeficiency virus (HIV) are at increased risk for hepatic decompensation when receiving highly active antiretroviral therapy (HAART); monitor closely. A transient increase in ALT (2-5 times above baseline) which is not associated with deterioration of liver function may occur with peginterferon alfa-2b use; therapy generally may continue with monitoring.

Gastrointestinal disorders: Pancreatitis has been observed with alfa interferon therapy; discontinue therapy if known or suspected pancreatitis develops. Ulcerative or hemorrhagic/ischemic colitis has been observed with alfa interferons; discontinue therapy if signs of colitis (abdominal pain, bloody diarrhea, fever) develop.

Autoimmune disorders: Thyroiditis, thrombotic thrombocytopenic purpura, idiopathic thrombocytopenic purpura, rheumatoid arthritis, interstitial nephritis, systemic lupus erythematosus, and psoriasis have been reported with therapy; use with caution in patients with autoimmune disorders.

Cardiovascular disease: Use with caution in patients with cardiovascular disease or a history of cardiovascular disease; hypotension, arrhythmia, tachycardia, cardiomyopathy, angina pectoris and MI have been observed with treatment. Patients with pre-existing cardiac abnormalities should have baseline ECGs prior to combination treatment with ribavirin; patients with a history of significant or unstable cardiac disease should not receive combination treatment with ribavirin.

Endocrine disorders: Diabetes mellitus, hyperglycemia, and thyroid disorders have been reported; discontinue peginterferon alfa-2b if cannot be effectively managed with medication. Use caution in patients with a history of diabetes mellitus, particularly if prone to DKA. Use with caution in patients with thyroid disorders; may cause or aggravate hyper- or hypothyroidism.

Pulmonary disease: May cause or aggravate dyspnea, pulmonary infiltrates, pneumonia, bronchiolitis obliterans, interstitial pneumonitis and sarcoidosis which may result in respiratory failure; may recur upon rechallenge with treatment; monitor closely.

Ophthalmic disorders: Ophthalmologic disorders (including decreased/loss of vision, macular edema, retinal hemorrhages, optic neuritis, papilledema, cotton wool spots, and retinal artery or vein thrombosis) have occurred with peginterferon alfa-2b and/or with other alfa interferons. Prior to start of therapy, ophthalmic exams are recommended for all patients; patients with diabetic or hypertensive retinopathy should have periodic ophthalmic exams during treatment. Discontinue treatment with new or worsening ophthalmic disorder.

[U.S. Boxed Warning]: Combination treatment with ribavirin may cause birth defects and/or fetal mortality (avoid pregnancy in females and female partners of male patients); hemolytic anemia (which may worsen cardiac disease), genotoxicity, mutagenicity, and may possibly be carcinogenic. Interferon therapy is commonly associated with flu-like symptoms, including fever; rule out other causes/infection with persistent or high fever. Acute hypersensitivity reactions and cutaneous reactions have been reported (rarely) with alfa interferons; prompt discontinuation is recommended; transient rashes do not require interruption of therapy. Hypertriglyceridemia has been reported with use; discontinue if severe (triglycerides >1000 mg/dL), particularly if combined with symptoms of pancreatitis. Use with caution in patients with renal impairment (Cl_{cr} <50 mL/minute); monitor closely; dosage adjustments are recommended with monotherapy in patients with moderate-to-severe impairment; do not use combination therapy with ribavirin in adult patients renal dysfunction (Cl_{cr} <50 mL/minute); discontinue if serum creatinine >2 mg/dL in children. Serum creatinine increases have been reported in patients with renal insufficiency. Use with caution in the elderly; the potential adverse effects may be more pronounced in the elderly. Dental/periodontal disorders have been reported with combination therapy; dry mouth may affect teeth and mucous membranes; instruct patients to brush teeth twice daily; encourage regular dental exams.

Combination therapy with ribavirin is preferred over monotherapy for the treatment of chronic hepatitis C (combination therapy provides a better ▶

response). Safety and efficacy have not been established in patients who have received organ transplants, are coinfected with HIV or hepatitis B, or received treatment for >1 year. Patients with significant bridging fibrosis or cirrhosis, genotype 1 infection or who have not responded to prior therapy, including previous pegylated interferon treatment are less likely to benefit from combination therapy with peginterferon alfa-2b and ribavirin. Growth velocity (height and weight) was decreased in children on combination treatment with ribavirin, particularly during the first 6 months of treatment. **[U.S. Boxed Warning]: Combination therapy with ribavirin is contraindicated in pregnancy.** Due to differences in dosage, patients should not change brands of interferon.

Adverse Reactions Note: Percentages reported for adults receiving monotherapy unless noted:

>10%:

Central nervous system: Headache (56%), fatigue (52%), depression (16% to 29%; may be severe), anxiety/emotional liability/irritability (28%), insomnia (23%), fever (22%), dizziness (12%)

Dermatologic: Alopecia (22%), pruritus (12%), dry skin (11%)

Gastrointestinal: Nausea (26%), anorexia (20%), diarrhea (18%), abdominal pain (8% to 15%), weight loss (11%)

Hematologic: Neutropenia (6% to 70%; grade 4: 1%), thrombocytopenia (7% to 20%; grades 3/4: <4%), anemia (in combination with ribavirin: 12% to 47%)

Local: Injection site inflammation/reaction (23% to 47%)

Neuromuscular & skeletal: Myalgia (54%), weakness (52%), musculoskeletal pain (28%), arthralgia (23%), rigors (23%)

Miscellaneous: Viral infection (11%)

>1% to 10%:

Cardiovascular: Chest pain (6%), flushing (6%)

Central nervous system: Concentration impaired (10%), malaise (7%), nervousness (4%), agitation (2%), suicidal behavior (ideation/attempt/ suicide ≤2%)

Dermatologic: Rash (6%)

Endocrine & metabolic: Hypothyroidism (5%), menstrual disorder (4%), hyperthyroidism (3%)

Gastrointestinal: Vomiting (7%), dyspepsia (6%), xerostomia (6%), constipation (1%)

Hepatic: Transaminases increased (10%; transient), hepatomegaly (6%)

Local: Injection site pain (2% to 3%)

Ocular: Conjunctivitis (4%), blurred vision (2%)

Respiratory: Pharyngitis (10%), cough (8%), sinusitis (7%), dyspnea (4%), rhinitis (2%)

Miscellaneous: Diaphoresis (6%), neutralizing antibodies (2%)

≤1%, postmarketing, and/or case reports (limited to important or life-threatening): Abscess, addiction (drug) relapse, aggressive behavior, anaphylaxis, angina, angioedema, aphthous stomatitis, aplastic anemia, arrhythmia, autoimmune thrombocytopenia (with or without purpura), bacterial infection, bronchiolitis obliterans, bronchoconstriction, cardiac arrest, cardiomyopathy, cellulitis, cerebral hemorrhage, cerebral ischemia, cotton wool spots, cytopenia, diabetes mellitus, drug overdose, emphysema, encephalopathy, erythema multiforme, fungal infection, gastroenteritis, gout, hallucinations, hearing impairment/loss, hemorrhagic colitis, homicidal ideation, hyperglycemia, hyper-/hypotension, hypersensitivity reactions, hypertriglyceridemia, injection site necrosis, interstitial nephritis, interstitial pneumonia, ischemic colitis, leukopenia, loss of consciousness, lupus-like syndrome, macular edema, memory loss, MI, migraine, myositis, nerve palsy (facial/oculomotor), optic neuritis, palpitation, pancreatitis, papilledema, paresthesia, pericardial effusion, peripheral neuropathy, phototoxicity, pleural effusion, pneumonia, pneumonitis, polyneuropathy, psoriasis, psychosis, pulmonary infiltrates, pure red cell aplasia, renal insufficiency, renal failure, retinal artery or vein thrombosis, retinal hemorrhage, retinal ischemia, rhabdomyolysis, rheumatoid arthritis, sarcoidosis, seizure, sepsis, serum creatinine increased, Stevens-Johnson syndrome, supraventricular arrhythmia, systemic lupus erythematosus, tachycardia, thrombotic thrombocytopenic purpura, thyroiditis, toxic epidermal necrolysis, transient ischemic attack, ulcerative colitis, urticaria, vasculitis, vertigo, vision decrease/loss, visual acuity decreased, Vogt-Koyanagi-Harada syndrome

Drug Interactions

Metabolism/Transport Effects Inhibits CYP1A2 (weak)

Avoid Concomitant Use There are no known interactions where it is recommended to avoid concomitant use.

Increased Effect/Toxicity

Peginterferon Alfa-2b may increase the levels/effects of: Aldesleukin; Ribavirin; Theophylline Derivatives; Zidovudine

Decreased Effect

Peginterferon Alfa-2b may decrease the levels/effects of: CYP2C9 Substrates (High risk); CYP2D6 Substrates

Ethanol/Nutrition/Herb Interactions Ethanol: Avoid use in patients with hepatitis C virus.

Storage/Stability Prior to reconstitution, store Redipen™ at 2°C to 8°C (36°F to 46°F). Store vials at 25°C (77°F); excursions permitted to 15°C to 30°C (59°F to 86°F). Once reconstituted each product should be used immediately or may be stored for ≤24 hours at 2°C to 8°C (36°F to 46°F); do not freeze. Products do not contain preservative.

Reconstitution

Redipen™: Hold cartridge upright and press the two halves together until there is a "click". Gently invert to mix; do not shake.

Vial: Add 0.7 mL of sterile water for injection, USP (supplied diluent) to the vial. Gently swirl. Do not re-enter vial after dose removed. Discard unused reconstituted portion; do not reuse.

Compatibility Do not mix with any other medicines.

Mechanism of Action Alpha interferons are a family of proteins, produced by nucleated cells, that have antiviral, antiproliferative, and immune-regulating activity. There are 16 known subtypes of alpha interferons. Interferons interact with cells through high affinity cell surface receptors. Following activation, multiple effects can be detected including induction of gene transcription. Inhibits cellular growth, alters the state of cellular differentiation, interferes with oncogene expression, alters cell surface antigen expression, increases phagocytic activity of macrophages, and augments cytotoxicity of lymphocytes for target cells.

Pharmacodynamics/Kinetics

Bioavailability: Increases with chronic dosing

Half-life elimination: ~40 hours (range: 22-60 hours)

Time to peak: 15-44 hours

Excretion: Urine (30%)

Dosage SubQ:

Children ≥3 years: Chronic hepatitis C:

Manufacturer labeling: Combination therapy with ribavirin: 60 mcg/m^2 once weekly (in combination with ribavirin 15 mg/kg/day in 2 divided doses);

Note: Children who reach their 18th birthday during treatment should remain on the pediatric regimen. Treatment duration is 48 weeks for genotype 1, 24 weeks for genotypes 2 and 3. Discontinue combination therapy in patients with HCV (genotype 1) at 12 weeks if HCV-RNA decreases <2 log (compared to pretreatment) or if detectable HCV-RNA at 24 weeks.

American Association for the Study of Liver Diseases (AASLD) guideline recommendations (Ghany, 2009): Children 2-17 years: Treatment of choice: **Peginterferon alfa-2b** 60 mcg/m^2 once weekly in combination with oral ribavirin 15 mg/kg/day for 48 weeks

Adults:

Chronic hepatitis C: Administer dose once weekly; **Note:** Treatment duration is 48 weeks for genotype 1, 24 weeks for genotypes 2 and 3, or 48 weeks for patients who previously failed therapy (regardless of genotype). Discontinue in patients with HCV (genotype 1) after 12 weeks if HCV RNA decreases <2 log (compared to pretreatment) or if detectable HCV RNA at 24 weeks.

Monotherapy: Initial: 1 mcg/kg/week
≤45 kg: 40 mcg once weekly
46-56 kg: 50 mcg once weekly
57-72 kg: 64 mcg once weekly
73-88 kg: 80 mcg once weekly
89-106 kg: 96 mcg once weekly
107-136 kg: 120 mcg once weekly
137-160 kg: 150 mcg once weekly

Combination therapy with ribavirin: Initial: 1.5 mcg/kg/week
<40 kg: 50 mcg once weekly (with ribavirin 800 mg/day)
40-50 kg: 64 mcg once weekly (with ribavirin 800 mg/day)
51-60 kg: 80 mcg once weekly (with ribavirin 800 mg/day)
61-65 kg: 96 mcg once weekly (with ribavirin 800 mg/day)
66-75 kg: 96 mcg once weekly (with ribavirin 1000 mg/day)
76-80 kg: 120 mcg once weekly (with ribavirin 1000 mg/day)
81-85 kg: 120 mcg once weekly (with ribavirin 1200 mg/day)
86-105 kg: 150 mcg once weekly (with ribavirin 1200 mg/day)
>105 kg: 1.5 mcg/kg once weekly (with ribavirin 1400 mg/day)

Note: *American Association for the Study of Liver Diseases (AASLD) guidelines recommendation:* Adults with chronic HCV infection: Treatment of choice: Ribavirin plus **peginterferon**; clinical condition and ability of patient to tolerate therapy should be evaluated to determine length and/or likely benefit of therapy. Recommended treatment duration (AASLD guidelines): Genotypes 1,4: 48 weeks; Genotypes 2,3: 24 weeks; Coinfection with HIV: 48 weeks.

Advanced melanoma (unlabeled use): 6 mcg/kg weekly for 8 weeks, followed by 3 mcg/kg weekly for up to a total of 5 years (Bottomley, 2009; Eggermont, 2008).

Elderly: May require dosage reduction based upon renal dysfunction, but no established guidelines are available.

Dosage adjustment for toxicity: For serious adverse reaction during treatment, modify dosage or discontinue; discontinue for persistent serious adverse reaction:

Adults:

Dosage reduction for peginterferon alfa-2b monotherapy:
≤45 kg: 20 mcg once weekly
46-56 kg: 25 mcg once weekly

57-72 kg: 30 mcg once weekly
73-88 kg: 40 mcg once weekly
89-106 kg: 50 mcg once weekly
107-136 kg: 64 mcg once weekly
≥137 kg: 80 mcg once weekly

Dosage reduction for peginterferon alfa-2b combination therapy:
<40 kg: 35 mcg once weekly; may further reduce to 20 mcg once weekly if needed

40-50 kg: 45 mcg once weekly; may further reduce to 25 mcg once weekly if needed

51-60 kg: 50 mcg once weekly; may further reduce to 30 mcg once weekly if needed

61-75 kg: 64 mcg once weekly; may further reduce to 35 mcg once weekly if needed

76-85 kg: 80 mcg once weekly; may further reduce to 45 mcg once weekly if needed

86-104 kg: 96 mcg once weekly; may further reduce to 50 mcg once weekly if needed

105-125 kg: 108 mcg once weekly; may further reduce to 64 mcg once weekly if needed

>125 kg: 135 mcg once weekly; may further reduce to 72 mcg once weekly if needed

Dosage adjustment for depression (severity based upon DSM-IV criteria):
Mild depression: No dosage adjustment required; evaluate once weekly by visit/phone call. If depression remains stable, continue weekly visits. If depression improves, resume normal visit schedule. For worsening depression, see "Moderate depression" below.

Moderate depression:
Children: Decrease peginterferon alfa-2b dose to 40 mcg/m^2/week, may further decrease to 20 mcg/m^2/week if needed
Adults:
Peginterferon alfa-2b combination therapy: Decrease peginterferon alfa-2b dose to 1 mcg/kg once weekly; may further reduce to 0.5 mcg/kg once weekly if needed
Peginterferon alfa-2b monotherapy: Decrease peginterferon alfa-2b dose to 0.5 mcg/kg once weekly

Note: Evaluate once weekly with an office visit at least every other week. If depression remains stable, consider psychiatric evaluation and continue with reduced dosing. If symptoms improve and remain stable for 4 weeks, resume normal visit schedule; continue reduced dosing or return to normal dose. For worsening depression, see "Severe depression" below.

Severe depression: Discontinue peginterferon alfa-2b and ribavirin permanently. Obtain immediate psychiatric consultation.

Dosage adjustment in hematologic toxicity:
Children:
Hemoglobin decrease ≥2 g/dL in any 4-week period in patients with preexisting cardiac disease: Monitor and evaluate weekly
Hemoglobin <10 g/dL: Decrease ribavirin dose to 12 mg/kg/day; may further reduce to 8 mg/kg/day
WBC <1.5 x 10^9/L, neutrophils <0.75 x 10^9/L, or platelets <70 x 10^9/L: Reduce peginterferon alfa-2b dose to 40 mcg/m^2/week; may further reduce to 20 mcg/m^2/week.
Hemoglobin <8.5 g/dL, WBC <1.0 x 10^9/L, neutrophils <0.5 x 10^9/L, or platelets <50 x 10^9/L: Permanently discontinue peginterferon alfa-2b and ribavirin

Adults:
  Hemoglobin decrease >2 g/dL in any 4-week period and stable cardiac disease: Decrease peginterferon alfa-2b dose by 50%; decrease ribavirin dose by 200 mg/day. Hemoglobin <12 g/dL after dose reductions: Permanently discontinue both peginterferon alfa-2b and ribavirin.
  Hemoglobin <10 g/dL in patients with cardiac disease: Reduce peginterferon alfa-2b dose by 50%; decrease ribavirin dose by 200 mg/day (patients receiving 1400 mg/day should decrease dose by 400 mg/day); may further reduce ribavirin dose by additional 200 mg/day if needed
  WBC <1.5 x 10^9/L, neutrophils <0.75 x 10^9/L, or platelets <50 x 10^9/L:
    Peginterferon alfa-2b combination therapy: Reduce peginterferon alfa-2b dose to 1 mcg/kg once weekly; may further reduce dose to 0.5 mcg/kg once weekly if needed
    Peginterferon alfa-2b monotherapy: Reduce peginterferon alfa-2b dose to 0.5 mcg/kg once weekly
  Hemoglobin <8.5 g/dL, WBC <1.0 x 10^9/L, neutrophils <0.5 x 10^9/L, or platelets <25 x 10^9/L: Permanently discontinue peginterferon alfa-2b and ribavirin.

Dosage adjustment in renal impairment:
  Peginterferon alfa-2b monotherapy:
    Cl_{cr} 30-50 mL/minute: Reduce dose by 25%
    Cl_{cr} 10-29 mL/minute: Reduce dose by 50%
    Hemodialysis: Reduce dose by 50%
    Discontinue use if renal function declines during treatment.
  Peginterferon alfa-2b combination with ribavirin:
    Children: Serum creatinine >2 mg/dL: Discontinue treatment
    Adults: Cl_{cr} <50 mL/minute: Combination therapy with ribavirin is not recommended
Dosage adjustment in hepatic impairment: Contraindicated in decompensated liver disease
Administration For SubQ administration; rotate injection site; thigh, outer surface of upper arm, and abdomen are preferred injection sites; do not inject near navel or waistline; patients who are thin should only use thigh or upper arm. Do not inject into bruised, infected, irritated, red, or scarred skin.
Monitoring Parameters Baseline and periodic TSH, hematology (including hemoglobin, CBC with differential, platelets), chemistry (including LFTs) testing, renal function, triglycerides. Clinical studies tested as follows: CBC (including hemoglobin, WBC, and platelets) and chemistries (including liver function tests and uric acid) measured at weeks 1, 2, 4, 6, and 8, and then every 4 weeks; TSH measured every 12 weeks during treatment.

Serum HCV RNA levels (pretreatment, 12- and 24 weeks after therapy initiation, 24 weeks after completion of therapy). **Note:** Discontinuation of therapy may be considered after 12 weeks in patients with HCV (genotype 1) who fail to achieve an early virologic response (EVR) (defined as ≥2-log decrease in HCV RNA compared to pretreatment) or after 24 weeks with detectable HCV RNA. Treat patients with HCV (genotypes 2,3) for 24 weeks (if tolerated) and then evaluate HCV RNA levels (Ghany, 2009).

Evaluate for depression and other psychiatric symptoms before and after initiation of therapy; baseline ophthalmic eye examination; periodic ophthalmic exam in patients with diabetic or hypertensive retinopathy; baseline echocardiogram in patients with cardiac disease; serum glucose or Hb A_{1c} (for patients with diabetes mellitus). In combination therapy with ribavirin, pregnancy tests (for women of childbearing age who are receiving treatment or who have male partners who are receiving treatment), continue monthly up to 6 months after discontinuation of therapy.

Dosage Forms Excipient information presented when available (limited, particularly for generics); consult specific product labeling.

Injection, powder for reconstitution [preservative free]:

PegIntron™: 50 mcg, 80 mcg, 120 mcg, 150 mcg [contains polysorbate 80 and sucrose]

PegIntron™ Redipen®: 50 mcg, 80 mcg, 120 mcg, 150 mcg [contains polysorbate 80 and sucrose]

References

Bottomley A, Coens C, Suciu S, et al, "Adjuvant Therapy With Pegylated Interferon Alfa-2b Versus Observation in Resected Stage III Melanoma: A Phase III Randomized Controlled Trial of Health-Related Quality of Life and Symptoms by the European Organisation for Research and Treatment of Cancer Melanoma Group," *J Clin Oncol*, 2009 [epub ahead of print]

Bukowski RM, Tendler C, Cutler D, et al, "Treating Cancer With PEG Intron: Pharmacokinetic Profile and Dosing Guidelines for an Improved Interferon-Alpha-2b Formulation," *Cancer*, 2002, 95(2):389-96.

Eggermont AM, Suciu S, Santinami M, et al, "EORTC18991: Long-Term Adjuvant Pegylated Interferon-Alpha2b (PEG-IFN) Compared to Observation in Resected Stage III Melanoma, Final Results of a Randomized Phase III Trial," *J Clin Onc*, 2007, 25(18S):8504 [abstract from 2007 Proceedings of ASCO Annual Meeting].

Eggermont AM, Suciu S, Santinami M, et al, "Adjuvant Therapy With Pegylated Interferon Alfa-2b Versus Observation Alone in Resected Stage III Melanoma: Final Results of EORTC 18991, A Randomised Phase III Trial," *Lancet*, 2008, 372(9633):117-26

Ghany MG, Strader DB, Thomas DL, et al, "Diagnosis, Management And Treatment Of Hepatitis C: An Update," *Hepatology*, 2009, 49(4):1335-74.

Zeuzem S, Feinman SV, Rasenack J, et al, "Peginterferon Alfa-2a in Patients With Chronic Hepatitis C," *N Engl J Med*, 2000, 343:1666-72.

Pemetrexed (pem e TREKS ed)

Medication Safety Issues

Sound-alike/look-alike issues:

Methotrexate may be confused with pralatrexate

High alert medication: The Institute for Safe Medication Practices (ISMP) includes this medication among its list of drug classes which have a heightened risk of causing significant patient harm when used in error.

Related Information

Safe Handling of Hazardous Drugs *on page 1517*

U.S. Brand Names Alimta®

Index Terms LY231514; Pemetrexed Disodium

Generic Available No

Canadian Brand Names Alimta®

Pharmacologic Category Antineoplastic Agent, Antimetabolite; Antineoplastic Agent, Antimetabolite (Antifolate)

Use Treatment of unresectable malignant pleural mesothelioma (in combination ▶

with cisplatin); treatment of locally advanced or metastatic nonsquamous nonsmall cell lung cancer (NSCLC; as initial treatment in combination with cisplatin, as single-agent maintenance treatment after 4 cycles of initial platinum-based doublet therapy, and single-agent treatment after prior chemotherapy)

Unlabeled/Investigational Use Treatment of bladder cancer (metastatic), cervical cancer, thymic malignancies

Pregnancy Risk Factor D

Lactation Excretion in breast milk unknown/not recommended

Labeled Contraindications Severe hypersensitivity to pemetrexed or any component of the formulation

Warnings/Precautions Hazardous agent - use appropriate precautions for handling and disposal. May cause bone marrow suppression (anemia, neutropenia, thrombocytopenia and/or pancytopenia); may require dose reductions in subsequent cycles. Prophylactic folic acid and vitamin B_{12} supplements are necessary to reduce hematologic and gastrointestinal toxicity and infection; initiate supplementation 1 week before the first dose of pemetrexed. Pretreatment with corticosteroids (dexamethasone or equivalent) reduces the incidence and severity of cutaneous reactions. Effects of third space fluid on drug disposition is unknown; consider draining effusion(s) prior to treatment. Use caution with hepatic dysfunction not due to metastases; may require dose adjustment.

The manufacturer does not recommend use in patients with Cl_{cr} <45 mL/minute. Decreased renal function results in increased toxicity. Use caution in patients receiving concurrent nephrotoxins; may result in delayed pemetrexed clearance. NSAIDs may reduce the clearance of pemetrexed; pemetrexed and ibuprofen (up to 1600 mg/day) may be administered in patients with Cl_{cr} ≥80 mL/minute; use with caution in patients with Cl_{cr} 45-79 mL/minute. Patients with Cl_{cr} 45-79 mL/minute should avoid NSAIDs with short elimination half-lives (eg, indomethacin, ketoprofen, ketorolac) for 2 days before, the day of, and 2 days following a dose of pemetrexed; all patients should avoid NSAIDs with long half-lives (eg, nabumetone, naproxen, oxaprozin, piroxicam) for 5 days before, the day of, and 2 days following a dose of pemetrexed. Safety and efficacy in children have not been established. Not indicated for use in patients with squamous cell NSCLC.

Adverse Reactions Note: Reported for single-agent therapy in patients who received folate and B_{12} supplementation.

>10%:
  Central nervous system: Fatigue (25% to 34%; dose-limiting)
  Dermatologic: Rash/desquamation (10% to 14%)
  Gastrointestinal: Nausea (19% to 31%), anorexia (19% to 22%), vomiting (9% to 16%), stomatitis (7% to 15%), diarrhea (5% to 13%)
  Hematologic: Anemia (15% to 19%; grades 3/4: 3% to 4%), leukopenia (6% to 12%; grades 3/4: 2% to 4%), neutropenia (6% to 11%; grades 3/4: 3% to 5%; nadir: 8-10 days; recovery: 12-17 days; dose-limiting)
  Respiratory: Pharyngitis (15%)
1% to 10%:
  Cardiovascular: Edema (1% to 5%)
  Central nervous system: Fever (1% to 8%)
  Dermatologic: Pruritus (1% to 7%), alopecia (1% to 6%), erythema multiforme (≤5%)
  Gastrointestinal: Constipation (1% to 6%), weight loss (1%), abdominal pain (≤5%)

Hematologic: Thrombocytopenia (1% to 8%; grades 3/4: 2%; dose-limiting), febrile neutropenia (grades 3/4: 2%)

Hepatic: ALT increased (8% to 10%; grades 3/4: ≤2%), AST increased (7% to 8%; grades 3/4: ≤1%)

Neuromuscular & skeletal: Sensory neuropathy (≤9%), motor neuropathy (≤5%)

Ocular: Conjunctivitis (≤5%), lacrimation increased (≤5%)

Renal: Creatinine increased/creatinine clearance decreased (1% to 5%)

Miscellaneous: Allergic reaction/hypersensitivity (≤5%), infection (≤5%)

<1%, postmarketing, and/or case reports (single-agent or combination therapy): Arrhythmia, chest pain, colitis, dehydration, hypertension, GGT increased, interstitial pneumonitis, pancytopenia, radiation recall (median onset: 6 days; range: 1-35 days), renal failure, supraventricular arrhythmia, thrombosis/embolism

Drug Interactions

Avoid Concomitant Use There are no known interactions where it is recommended to avoid concomitant use.

Increased Effect/Toxicity

The levels/effects of Pemetrexed may be increased by: NSAID (Nonselective)

Decreased Effect There are no known significant interactions involving a decrease in effect.

Ethanol/Nutrition/Herb Interactions Lower ANC nadirs occur in patients with elevated baseline cystathionine or homocysteine concentrations. Levels of these substances can be reduced by folic acid and vitamin B_{12} supplementation.

Storage/Stability Store intact vials at room temperature of 25°C (77°F); excursions permitted to 15°C to 30°C (59°F to 86°F). Reconstituted solution in NS and infusion solutions (in D_5W or NS) are stable for 24 hours when refrigerated at 2°C to 8°C (36°F to 46°F) or stored at room temperature of 15°C to 30°C (59°F to 86°F). Concentrations at 25 mg/mL are stable in polypropylene syringes for 2 days at room temperature (23°C) (Zhang, 2005).

Reconstitution Reconstitute with NS (preservative free); add 4.2 mL to the 100 mg vial and 20 mL to the 500 mg vial, resulting in a 25 mg/mL concentration. Gently swirl. Solution may be colorless to green-yellow. Further dilute in 100 mL NS for infusion; may also dilute in D_5W (Zhang, 2006), although the manufacturer recommends NS. Use appropriate precautions for handling and disposal.

Compatibility Stable in D_5W (Zhang, 2006), NS; physically **incompatible** with calcium-containing products, including Ringer's and lactated Ringer's injection.

Y-site administration: Compatible: Acyclovir, amifostine, amikacin sulfate, aminophylline, ampicillin sodium, ampicillin sodium-sulbactam sodium, aztreonam, bumetanide, buprenorphine hydrochloride, butorphanol tartrate, carboplatin, ceftizoxime sodium, ceftriaxone sodium, cefuroxime sodium, cimetidine hydrochloride, cisplatin, clindamycin phosphate, co-trimoxazole, cyclophosphamide, cytarabine, dexamethasone sodium phosphate, dexrazoxane, diphenhydramine hydrochloride, docetaxel, dopamine hydrochloride, enalaprilat, famotidine, fluconazole, fluorouracil, ganciclovir sodium, granisetron hydrochloride, haloperidol lactate, heparin sodium, hydromorphone hydrochloride, hydroxyzine hydrochloride, ifosfamide, leucovorin calcium, lorazepam, mannitol, meperidine hydrochloride, mesna, methylprednisolone sodium succinate, metoclopramide hydrochloride, morphine sulfate, paclitaxel, potassium chloride, promethazine hydrochloride, ranitidine hydrochloride, sodium bicarbonate, ticarcillin disodium, ticarcillin disodiumclavulanate potassium, vancomycin hydrochloride, vinblastine sulfate, vincristine sulfate, zidovudine. **Incompatible:** Amphotericin B, calcium gluconate, cefazolin sodium, cefotaxime sodium, cefotetan disodium, cefoxitin sodium, ceftazidime, chlorpromazine hydrochloride, ciprofloxacin, dobutamine hydrochloride, doxorubicin hydrochloride, doxycycline hyclate, droperidol, gemcitabine hydrochloride, gentamicin sulfate, irinotecan hydrochloride, metronidazole, minocycline hydrochloride, mitoxantrone hydrochloride, nalbuphine hydrochloride, ondansetron hydrochloride, prochlorperazine edisylate, tobramycin sulfate, topotecan hydrochloride.

Mechanism of Action Antifolate; disrupts folate-dependent metabolic processes. Inhibits thymidylate synthase (TS), dihydrofolate reductase (DHFR), glycinamide ribonucleotide formyltransferase (GARFT), and aminoimidazole carboxamide ribonucleotide formyltransferase (AICARFT), the enzymes involved in folate metabolism and DNA synthesis, resulting in inhibition of purine and thymidine nucleotide and protein synthesis.

Pharmacodynamics/Kinetics

Duration: V_{dss}: 16.1 L

Protein binding: ~73% to 81%

Metabolism: Minimal

Half-life elimination: Normal renal function: 3.5 hours; Cl_{cr} 40-59 mL/minute: 5.3-5.8 hours

Excretion: Urine (70% to 90% as unchanged drug)

Dosage Details concerning dosing in combination regimens should also be consulted. **Note:** Start vitamin supplements 1 week before initial pemetrexed dose: Folic acid 350-1000 mcg/day orally (must be taken at least 5 out of 7 days prior to treatment initiation; continue during treatment and for 21 days after last pemetrexed dose) and vitamin B_{12} 1000 mcg I.M. during the week prior to treatment initiation and then every 3 cycles. Give dexamethasone 4 mg orally twice daily for 3 days, beginning the day before treatment to minimize cutaneous reactions. New treatment cycles should not begin unless ANC ≥1500/mm^3, platelets ≥100,000/mm^3, and Cl_{cr} ≥45 mL/minute.

I.V.: Adults:

Malignant pleural mesothelioma: 500 mg/m^2 on day 1 of each 21-day cycle (in combination with cisplatin)

Nonsmall cell lung cancer:

Initial treatment: 500 mg/m^2 on day 1 of each 21-day cycle (in combination with cisplatin)

Maintenance or second-line treatment: 500 mg/m^2 on day 1 of each 21-day cycle (as a single-agent)

Bladder cancer (unlabeled use): 500 mg/m^2 on day 1 of each 21-day cycle (Sweeney, 2006)

Dosage adjustments for toxicities:

Toxicity: Discontinue if patient develops grade 3 or 4 toxicity after two dose reductions or immediately if grade 3 or 4 neurotoxicity develops

Hematologic toxicity: Upon recovery, reinitiate therapy

Nadir ANC <500/mm^3 and nadir platelets ≥50,000/mm^3: Reduce dose to 75% of previous dose of pemetrexed (and cisplatin)

Nadir platelets <50,000/mm^3 **without bleeding** (regardless of nadir ANC): Reduce dose to 75% of previous dose of pemetrexed (and cisplatin)

Nadir platelets <50,000/mm^3 **with bleeding** (regardless of nadir ANC): Reduce dose to 50% of previous dose of pemetrexed (and cisplatin)

Nonhematologic toxicity ≥grade 3 (excluding neurotoxicity): Withhold treatment until recovery to baseline; upon recovery, reinitiate therapy as follows:

Grade 3 or 4 toxicity (excluding mucositis): Reduce dose to 75% of previous dose of pemetrexed (and cisplatin)

Grade 3 or 4 diarrhea or any diarrhea requiring hospitalization: Reduce dose to 75% of previous dose of pemetrexed (and cisplatin)

Grade 3 or 4 mucositis: Reduce pemetrexed dose to 50% of previous dose (continue cisplatin at 100% of previous dose)

Neurotoxicity:

Grade 0-1: Continue pemetrexed at 100% of previous dose (and cisplatin)

Grade 2: Continue pemetrexed at 100% of previous dose; reduce cisplatin dose to 50% of previous dose

Dosage adjustment in renal impairment:

Cl_{cr} 45 to <80 mL/minute with concurrent NSAID use: Use with caution

Cl_{cr} ≥45 mL/minute: No dosage adjustment required.

Cl_{cr} <45 mL/minute: No dosage adjustment guidelines are available; manufacturer recommends not using the drug.

Dosage adjustment in hepatic impairment: Grade 3 (5.1-20 times ULN) **or** 4 (>20 times ULN) transaminase elevation: Reduce pemetrexed dose to 75% of previous dose (and cisplatin)

Combination Regimens

Bladder cancer: Pemetrexed (Bladder Cancer Regimen) on page 1393

Lung cancer (nonsmall cell): Pemetrexed-Cisplatin (NSCLC) on page 1394

Malignant pleural mesothelioma:

Cisplatin-Pemetrexed (Mesothelioma) on page 1273

Pemetrexed-Carboplatin (Mesothelioma) on page 1394

Administration I.V.: Infuse over 10 minutes.

Monitoring Parameters CBC with differential and platelets (before each dose; monitor for nadir and recovery); serum creatinine, BUN, total bilirubin, ALT, AST (periodic)

Dietary Considerations Initiate folic acid supplementation 1 week before first dose of pemetrexed, continue for full course of therapy, and for 21 days after last dose. Institute vitamin B_{12} 1 week before the first dose; administer every 9 weeks thereafter.

Emetic Potential Low (10% to 30%)

Dosage Forms Excipient information presented when available (limited, particularly for generics); consult specific product labeling.

Injection, powder for reconstitution:

Alimta®: 100 mg, 500 mg

References

Belani CP, Brodowicz T, Ciuleanu T, et al, "Maintenance Pemetrexed (Pem) Plus Best Supportive Care (BSC) Versus Placebo (Plac) Plus BSC: A Randomized Phase III Study in Advanced Non-Small Cell Lung Cancer (NSCLC), *J Clin Oncol*, 27(18S):CRA8000 [abstract from 2009 ASCO Annual Meeting].

Goldman ID and Zhao R, "Molecular, Biochemical, and Cellular Pharmacology of Pemetrexed," *Semin Oncol*, 2002, 29(6 Suppl 18):3-17.

Hanna N, Shepherd FA, Fossella FV, et al, "Randomized Phase III Trial of Pemetrexed Versus Docetaxel in Patients With Non-Small-Cell Lung Cancer Previously Treated With Chemotherapy," *J Clin Oncol*, 2004, 22(9):1589-97.

Manegold C, "Pemetrexed (Alimta, MTA, Multitargeted Antifolate, LY231514) for Malignant Pleural Mesothelioma," *Semin Oncol*, 2003, 30(4 Suppl 10):32-6.

Mita AC, Sweeney CJ, Baker SD, et al, "Phase I and Pharmacokinetic Study of Pemetrexed Administered Every 3 Weeks to Advanced Cancer Patients With Normal and Impaired Renal Function," *J Clin Oncol*, 2006, 24(4):552-62.

National Comprehensive Cancer Network (NCCN)®, "Clinical Practice Guidelines in Oncology™: Bladder Cancer," Version1.2009. Available at http://www.nccn.org/professionals/physician_gls/PDF/bladder.pdf

National Comprehensive Cancer Network (NCCN)®, "Clinical Practice Guidelines in Oncology™: Cervical Cancer," Version 1.2009. Available at: http://www.nccn.org/professionals/physician_gls/PDF/cervical.pdf

National Comprehensive Cancer Network (NCCN)®, "Clinical Practice Guidelines in Oncology™: Non-Small Cell Lung Cancer," Version 2.2009. Available at: http://www.nccn.org/professionals/physician_gls/PDF/nscl.pdf

National Comprehensive Cancer Network (NCCN)®, "Clinical Practice Guidelines in Oncology™: Thymic Malignancies," Version 2.2009. Available at: http://www.nccn.org/professionals/physician_gls/PDF/thymic.pdf

Scagliotti GV, Parikh P, von Pawel J, et al, "Phase III Study Comparing Cisplatin Plus Gemcitabine With Cisplatin Plus Pemetrexed in Chemotherapy-Naive Patients With Advanced-Stage Non-Small-Cell Lun Cancer," *J Clin Oncol*, 2008, 26(21):3543-51.

Sweeney CJ, Roth BJ, Kabbinavar FF, et al, "Phase II Study of Pemetrexed for Second-Line Treatment of Transitional Cell Cancer of the Urothelium," *J Clin Oncol*, 2006, 24(21):3451-7.

Sweeney CJ, Takimoto CH, Latz JE, et al, "Two Drug Interaction Studies Evaluating the Pharmacokinetics and Toxicity of Pemetrexed When Coadministered with Aspirin or Ibuprofen in Patients with Advanced Cancer," *Clin Cancer Res*, 2006, 12(2):536-42.

Trissel LA, Saenz CA, Ogundele AB, et al, "Physical Compatibility of Pemetrexed Disodium With Other Drugs During Simulated Y-Site Administration," *Am J Health Syst Pharm*, 2004, 61 (21):2289-93.

Zhang Y and Trissel LA, "Physical and Chemical Stability of Pemetrexed in Infusion Solutions," *Ann Pharmacother*, 2006, 40(6):1082-5.

Zhang Y and Trissel LA, "Physical and Chemical Stability of Pemetrexed Solutions in Plastic Syringes," *Ann Pharmacother*, 2005, 39(12):2026-8.

◆ **Pemetrexed Disodium** *see* Pemetrexed *on page* 939

◆ **Pentahydrate** *see* Sodium Thiosulfate *on page* 1040

◆ **Pentam®-300** *see* Pentamidine *on page* 944

Pentamidine (pen TAM i deen)

Related Information
Safe Handling of Hazardous Drugs *on page* 1517

U.S. Brand Names NebuPent®; Pentam®-300

Index Terms Pentamidine Isethionate

Generic Available No

Pharmacologic Category Antibiotic, Miscellaneous; Antiprotozoal

Use Treatment and prevention of pneumonia caused by *Pneumocystis jiroveci* pneumonia (PCP)

Unlabeled/Investigational Use Treatment of African trypanosomiasis, cutaneous leishmaniasis, and amebic meningoencephalitis

Pregnancy Risk Factor C

Lactation Excretion in breast milk unknown/not recommended

Labeled Contraindications Hypersensitivity to pentamidine isethionate or any component of the formulation

Warnings/Precautions Severe hypotension (some fatalities) has been observed (even after a single dose); may occur with either I.V. or I.M administration, although more common with rapid I.V. administration; monitor blood pressure during (and after) infusion. Use with caution in patients with pre-existing cardiovascular disease; hyper-/hypotension and arrhythmia, including ventricular tachycardia have been reported.

Use with caution in patients with diabetes mellitus or hypocalcemia; hyper-/hypoglycemia and pancreatic islet cell necrosis with hyperinsulinemia has been reported. Symptoms may occur months after therapy; monitor blood glucose daily on therapy and periodically thereafter. Use with caution in patients with a history of pancreatic disease or elevated amylase/lipase levels; acute pancreatitis (with fatality) has been reported. Concurrent use with other bone marrow suppressants may increase the risk for myelotoxicity; use with caution in patients with current evidence and/or prior history of hematologic disorders; anemia, leukopenia and/or thrombocytopenia have been reported. Use with caution in patients with hepatic or renal disease. Concurrent use with other nephrotoxic drugs may increase the risk for nephrotoxicity. Stevens-Johnson syndrome has been reported with use. Avoid extravasation; may cause tissue ulceration, necrosis, and/or sloughing; if extravasation occurs, treat symptomatically. Assess catheter position before and during infusion.

Aerosolized pentamidine may induce bronchospasm or cough, especially in patients with a smoking or asthma history (an inhaled bronchodilator prior to pentamidine may ameliorate symptoms). Use appropriate precautions to minimize exposure to healthcare personnel; refer to individual institutional policy. Acute PCP may develop despite aerosolized pentamidine prophylaxis. Although rare, extrapulmonary PCP disease may occur and has been associated with aerosolized pentamidine.

Adverse Reactions Aerosol:

>10%:

Central nervous system: Fatigue (66%), fever (51%), dizziness/lightheadedness (45%)

Gastrointestinal: Appetite decreased (50%)

Respiratory: Cough (1% to 63%), dyspnea (48%), wheezing (32%)

Miscellaneous: Infection (15%)

1% to 10%:

Central nervous system: Headache

Gastrointestinal: Diarrhea, nausea, oral candida, taste alteration

Hematologic: Anemia

Respiratory: Bronchitis, chest pain, pharyngitis, sinusitis, upper respiratory tract infection

Miscellaneous: Herpes infection, influenza, night sweats**Injection:**

>10%:

Local: Local reactions at I.M. injection site (11%; includes sterile abscess, necrosis, pain, induration)

Renal: Renal function impaired (29%), creatinine increased (24%)

1% to 10%:

Cardiovascular: Hypotension (5%)

Central nervous system: Confusion/hallucinations (2%)

Dermatologic: Rash (3%)

Endocrine & metabolic: Hypoglycemia (6%)

Gastrointestinal: Nausea/anorexia (6%), taste alteration (2%)

Hematologic: Leukopenia (10%), thrombocytopenia (3%), anemia (1%)

Hepatic: Liver function tests increased (9%)

Renal: Azotemia (9%), BUN increased (7%)

Aerosol or injection: <1%, postmarketing, and/or case reports (limited to important or life-threatening): Abdominal pain, allergic reaction, anaphylaxis, anxiety, arthralgia, asthma, blepharitis, blurred vision, bronchitis, bronchospasm, cardiac arrhythmia, central venous line related sepsis, cerebrovascular accident, chest tightness, chills, clotting time prolonged, CMV infection, colitis, confusion, congestion (chest, nasal), conjunctivitis, cough, cryptococcal meningitis, cyanosis, defibrination, depression, dermatitis, desquamation, diabetes mellitus, diabetic ketoacidosis, diarrhea, dizziness, drowsiness, dyspepsia, dyspnea, emotional lability, eosinophilia, erythema, esophagitis, extrapulmonary pneumocystosis, extravasation (tissue ulceration, necrosis, and/or sloughing), facial edema, flank pain, gait unsteady, gagging, gingivitis, headache, hearing loss, hematochezia, hematuria, hemoptysis, hepatic dysfunction, hepatitis, hepatomegaly, histoplasmosis, hyperglycemia, hyperkalemia, hypersalivation, hypertension, hyperventilation, hypesthesia, hypocalcemia, hypomagnesemia, incontinence, insomnia, laryngitis, laryngospasm, leg edema, melena, memory loss, nephritis, nervousness, neuralgia, neuropathy, neutropenia, night sweats, palpitation, pancreatitis, pancytopenia, paranoia, paresthesia, peripheral neuropathy, phlebitis, pleuritis, pneumonitis (eosinophilic or interstitial), pneumothorax, pruritus, rales, renal dysfunction, renal failure, rhinitis, seizure, splenomegaly, Stevens-Johnson syndrome, ST segment abnormal, syncope, syndrome of inappropriate antidiuretic hormone (SIADH), tachycardia, tachypnea, temperature abnormal, torsade de pointes, tremor, vasodilation, vasculitis, ventricular tachycardia, vertigo, vomiting, urticaria, xerostomia

Drug Interactions

Metabolism/Transport Effects Substrate of CYP2C19 (major); **Inhibits** CYP2C8/9 (weak), 2C19 (weak), 2D6 (weak), 3A4 (weak)

Avoid Concomitant Use

Avoid concomitant use of Pentamidine with any of the following: Artemether; Dronedarone; Lumefantrine; Nilotinib; Pimozide; QuiNINE; Tetrabenazine; Thioridazine; Ziprasidone

Increased Effect/Toxicity

Pentamidine may increase the levels/effects of: Dronedarone; Pimozide; QTc-Prolonging Agents; QuiNINE; Tetrabenazine; Thioridazine; Ziprasidone

The levels/effects of Pentamidine may be increased by: Alfuzosin; Artemether; Chloroquine; Ciprofloxacin; CYP2C19 Inhibitors (Moderate); CYP2C19 Inhibitors (Strong); Gadobutrol; Lumefantrine; Nilotinib; QuiNINE

Decreased Effect

Pentamidine may decrease the levels/effects of: Typhoid Vaccine

The levels/effects of Pentamidine may be decreased by: CYP2C19 Inducers (Strong)

Ethanol/Nutrition/Herb Interactions Ethanol: Avoid ethanol (may increase CNS depression or aggravate hypoglycemia).

Storage/Stability Store intact vials at 20°C to 25°C (68°F to 77°F); protect from light. Do not use sodium chloride for initial reconstitution (sodium chloride will cause precipitation).

Aerosol: The manufacturer recommends the use of freshly prepared solutions for inhalation; however, may be stored for up to 48 hours in the vial at room temperature if protected from light.

Injection: Reconstituted solution is stable for 48 hours in the vial at room temperature and protected from light. Solutions for injection (1-2.5 mg/mL) in D_5W are stable for at least 24 hours at room temperature. Store at room temperature to avoid crystallization.

Reconstitution Do not use sodium chloride for initial reconstitution (sodium chloride will cause precipitation).

Aerosol: Reconstitute with 6 mL SWFI. Do not mix with other nebulizer solutions.

Injection: I.M.: Reconstitute with 3 mL SWFI; I.V.: Reconstitute with 3-5 mL SWFI or D_5W; the manufacturer recommends further dilution in 50-250 mL D_5W; however, stability with further dilution in NS has also been documented.

Compatibility Stable in D_5W, NS (do not use NS for initial reconstitution)

Y-site administration: Compatible: Diltiazem, zidovudine. **Incompatible:** Aldesleukin, cefazolin, cefotaxime, cefoxitin, ceftazidime, ceftriaxone, fluconazole, foscarnet, linezolid.

Mechanism of Action Interferes with RNA/DNA, phospholipids and protein synthesis, through inhibition of oxidative phosphorylation and/or interference with incorporation of nucleotides and nucleic acids into RNA and DNA, in protozoa

Pharmacodynamics/Kinetics

Absorption: I.M.: Well absorbed; Inhalation: Limited systemic absorption

Distribution: V_{dss}: I.V.: 286-1356 L; I.M.: 1658-3790 L

Half-life elimination: I.V.: 5-8 hours; I.M.: 7-11 hours; may be prolonged with severe renal impairment

Excretion: Urine (I.V.: ≤12% as unchanged drug)

Dosage

Children:

PCP:

FDA-approved labeling: Children >4 months: Treatment: I.M., I.V.: 4 mg/kg once daily for 14-21 days

CDC recommendation:

Prevention (children ≥5 years): Inhalation: 300 mg/dose monthly via Respirgard® II nebulizer

Treatment: I.V.: 3-4 mg/kg once daily for 21 days

AIDS*info* guidelines (2009):

Prevention: Children ≥5 years: Inhalation: 300 mg/dose monthly via Respirgard® II nebulizer

Treatment: I.V.: 4 mg/kg once daily, if clinical improvement may change to atovaquone after 7-10 days

PCP prevention in pediatric oncology patients (age <5 years, intolerant to trimethoprim-sulfamethoxazole; unlabeled use): 4 mg/kg I.V. once monthly (Kim, 2008; Prasad, 2007)

Cutaneous leishmaniasis (unlabeled use; CDC recommendation): I.M., I.V.: 2-3 mg/kg once daily or every second day for 4-7 doses

Trypanosomiasis (unlabeled use; CDC recommendation): I.M.: 4 mg/kg once daily for 7 days

Adults:

PCP:

FDA-approved labeling:

Prevention: Inhalation: 300 mg every 4 weeks via Respirgard® II nebulizer

Treatment: I.M., I.V.: 4 mg/kg once daily for 14-21 days

CDC recommendation:

Prevention: Inhalation: 300 mg monthly via Respirgard® II nebulizer

Treatment: I.V.: 3-4 mg/kg once daily for 21 days

AIDS*info* guidelines (2009):

Prevention: Inhalation: 300 mg/dose monthly via Respirgard® II nebulizer

Treatment: I.V.: 4 mg/kg once daily, 3 mg/kg may be used by some clinicians

Cutaneous leishmaniasis (unlabeled use; CDC recommendation): I.M., I.V.: 2-3 mg/kg once daily or every second day for 4-7 doses

Trypanosomiasis (unlabeled use; CDC recommendation): I.M.: 4 mg/kg once daily for 7 days

Dosing adjustment in renal impairment: I.V.: The FDA-approved labeling recommends that caution should be used in patients with renal impairment; however, no specific dosage adjustment guidelines are available. The following guidelines have been used by some clinicians (Aronoff, 2007):

Children:
Cl_{cr} >30 mL/minute: No adjustment required
Cl_{cr} 10-30 mL/minute: Administer 4 mg/kg every 36 hours
Cl_{cr} <10 mL/minute and peritoneal dialysis: Administer 4 mg/kg every 48 hours
Hemodialysis: Administer 4 mg/kg every 48 hours, after dialysis on dialysis days

Adults:
Cl_{cr} ≥10 mL/minute: No adjustment required
Cl_{cr} <10 mL/minute: Administer 4 mg/kg every 24-36 hours

Administration Do not use NS to reconstitute.
Inhalation: Deliver via Respirgard® II nebulizer until nebulizer is emptied (30-45 minutes). Use appropriate precautions to minimize exposure to healthcare personnel; refer to individual institutional policy.
I.V.: Infuse slowly over 60-120 minutes. Avoid extravasation; assess catheter position before and during infusion.
I.M.: Administer deep I.M.

Monitoring Parameters Liver function tests, renal function tests, blood glucose, serum potassium and calcium, CBC and platelets; ECG, blood pressure

Vesicant Ulceration, tissue necrosis and/or sloughing have been reported with extravasation

Dosage Forms Excipient information presented when available (limited, particularly for generics); consult specific product labeling.
Injection, powder for reconstitution, as isethionate [preservative free]:
Pentam®-300: 300 mg
Powder for solution, for nebulization, as isethionate [preservative free]:
NebuPent®: 300 mg

References

Aronoff GR, Bennett WM, Berns JS, et al, *Drug Prescribing in Renal Failure: Dosing Guidelines for Adults and Children*, 5th ed. Philadelphia, PA: American College of Physicians; 2007, p 73, 160.

Centers for Disease Control and Prevention, "Amebic Meningoencephalitis, Primary and Granulomatous." Available at http://www.dpd.cdc.gov/dpdx/HTML/PDF_Files/MedLetter/AmebicMeningoencephalitis.pdf. Last accessed September 15, 2009.

Centers for Disease Control, "Guidelines for Prevention and Treatment of Opportunistic Infections Among HIV-Exposed and HIV-Infected Children," *MMWR Recomm Rep*, 2009, 58(RR-11):1-176. Available at http://aidsinfo.nih.gov/contentfiles/Pediatric_OI.pdf

Centers for Disease Control, "Guidelines for Prevention and Treatment of Opportunistic Infections in HIV-Infected Adults and Adolescents," *MMWR Recomm Rep*, 2009, 58(RR-4):1-194. Available at http://www.cdc.gov/mmwr/pdf/rr/rr5804.pdf

Centers for Disease Control and Prevention, "Leishmania." Available at http://www.dpd.cdc.gov/dpdx/HTML/PDF_Files/MedLetter/Leishmania.pdf. Last accessed September 15, 2009.

Centers for Disease Control and Prevention, "*Pneumocystis jiroveci* (formerly *carinii*) Pneumonia (PCP)." Available at http://www.dpd.cdc.gov/dpdx/HTML/PDF_Files/MedLetter/Pneumocystis_jiroveci.pdf. Last accessed September 15, 2009.

Centers for Disease Control and Prevention, "Trypanosomiasis." Available at http://www.dpd.cdc.gov/dpdx/HTML/PDF_Files/MedLetter/Trypanosomiasis.pdf. Last accessed September 15, 2009.

Conte JE Jr, "Pharmacokinetics of Intravenous Pentamidine in Patients With Normal Renal Function or Receiving Hemodialysis," *J Infect Dis*, 1991, 163(1):169-75.

Ito S and Koren G, "Estimation of Fetal Risk From Aerosolized Pentamidine in Pregnant Healthcare Workers," *Chest*, 1994, 106(5):1460-2.

Kim SY, Dabb AA, Glenn DJ, et al, "Intravenous Pentamidine is Effective as Second Line Pneumocystis Pneumonia Prophylaxis in Pediatric Oncology Patients," *Pediatr Blood Cancer*, 2008, 50(4):779-83.

Monk JP and Benfield P, "Inhaled Pentamidine. An Overview of Its Pharmacological Properties and a Review of Its Therapeutic Use in *Pneumocystis carinii* Pneumonia," *Drugs*, 1990, 39(5):741-56.

National Comprehensive Cancer Network® (NCCN), "Clinical Practice Guidelines in Oncology™: Prevention and Treatment of Cancer-Related Infections," Version 2.2009. Available at http://www.nccn.org/professionals/physician_gls/PDF/infections.pdf.

Prasad P, Nania JJ, and Shankar SM, "Pneumocystis Pneumonia in Children Receiving Chemotherapy," *Pediatr Blood Cancer*, 2008, 50(4):896-8.

Sattler FR, Cowan R, Nielsen DM, et al, " Trimethoprim-Sulfamethoxazole Compared With Pentamidine for Treatment of *Pneumocystis carinii* Pneumonia in the Acquired Immunodeficiency Syndrome," *Ann Intern Med*, 1988, 109(4):280-7.

Singh G, el-Gadi SM, and Sparks RA, "Pancreatitis Associated With Aerosolized Pentamidine," *Genitourin Med*, 1995, 71(2):130-1.

♦ **Pentamidine Isethionate** *see* Pentamidine *on page 944*

Pentostatin (pen toe STAT in)

Medication Safety Issues

Sound-alike/look-alike issues:

Pentostatin may be confused with pentamidine, pentosan

High alert medication: The Institute for Safe Medication Practices (ISMP) includes this medication among its list of drug classes which have a heightened risk of causing significant patient harm when used in error.

International issues:

Nipent® may be confused with Nipin® which is a brand name for nifedipine in Italy and Singapore

Related Information

Safe Handling of Hazardous Drugs *on page 1517*

U.S. Brand Names Nipent®

Index Terms 2'-Deoxycoformycin; Co-Vidarabine; dCF; Deoxycoformycin; NSC-218321

Generic Available Yes

Canadian Brand Names Nipent®

Pharmacologic Category Antineoplastic Agent, Antibiotic; Antineoplastic Agent, Antimetabolite (Purine Antagonist)

Use Treatment of hairy cell leukemia

Unlabeled/Investigational Use Treatment of cutaneous T-cell lymphoma, chronic lymphocytic leukemia (CLL), and acute and chronic graft-versus-host-disease (GVHD)

Pregnancy Risk Factor D

Lactation Excretion in breast milk unknown/not recommended

Labeled Contraindications Hypersensitivity to pentostatin or any component of the formulation

Warnings/Precautions Hazardous agent - use appropriate precautions for handling and disposal. **[U.S. Boxed Warnings]: Severe renal, liver, pulmonary and CNS toxicities have occurred with doses higher than recommended; do not exceed the recommended dose. Do not administer concurrently with fludarabine; concomitant use has resulted in serious or fatal pulmonary toxicity.** Bone marrow suppression may occur, primarily early in treatment; if neutropenia persists beyond early cycles, evaluate for disease status. In patients who present with infections prior to treatment, infections should be resolved, if possible, prior to initiation of treatment; treatment should be temporarily withheld for active infections during therapy. Use cautiously in patients with renal dysfunction (the half-life is prolonged); appropriate dosing guidelines in renal insufficiency have not been determined. May cause elevations (reversible) in liver function tests. Withhold treatment for CNS toxicity or severe rash. Fatal pulmonary edema and hypotension have been reported in patients treated with pentostatin in combination with carmustine, etoposide, or high-dose cyclophosphamide as part of a myeloablative regimen for bone marrow transplant. **[U.S. Boxed Warning]: Should be administered** ▶

◀ **under the supervision of an experienced cancer chemotherapy physician.** Safety and efficacy in children have not been established.

Adverse Reactions

>10%:

Central nervous system: Fever (42% to 46%), fatigue (29% to 42%), pain (8% to 20%), chills (11% to 19%), headache (13% to 17%), CNS toxicity (1% to 11%)

Dermatologic: Rash (26% to 43%), pruritus (10% to 21%), skin disorder (4% to 17%)

Gastrointestinal: Nausea/vomiting (22% to 63%), diarrhea (15% to 17%), anorexia (13% to 16%), abdominal pain (4% to 16%), stomatitis (5% to 12%)

Hematologic: Myelosuppression (nadir: 7 days; recovery: 10-14 days), leukopenia (22% to 60%), anemia (8% to 35%), thrombocytopenia (6% to 32%)

Hepatic: Transaminases increased (2% to 19%)

Neuromuscular & skeletal: Myalgia (11% to 19%), weakness (10% to 12%)

Respiratory: Cough (17% to 20%), upper respiratory infection (13% to 16%), rhinitis (10% to 11%), dyspnea (8% to 11%)

Miscellaneous: Infection (7% to 36%), allergic reaction (2% to 11%)

1% to 10%:

Cardiovascular: Chest pain (3% to 10%), facial edema (3% to 10%), hypotension (3% to 10%), peripheral edema (3% to 10%), angina (<3%), arrhythmia (<3%), AV block (<3%), bradycardia (<3%), cardiac arrest (<3%), deep thrombophlebitis (<3%), heart failure (<3%), hypertension (<3%), pericardial effusion (<3%), sinus arrest (<3%), syncope (<3%), tachycardia (<3%), vasculitis (<3%), ventricular extrasystoles (<3%)

Central nervous system: Anxiety (3% to 10%), confusion (3% to 10%), depression (3% to 10%), dizziness (3% to 10%), insomnia (3% to 10%), nervousness (3% to 10%), somnolence (3% to 10%), abnormal dreams/thinking (<3%), amnesia (<3%), ataxia (<3%), emotional lability (<3%), encephalitis (<3%), hallucination (<3%), hostility (<3%), meningism (<3%), neuritis (<3%), neurosis (<3%), seizure (<3%), vertigo (<3%)

Dermatologic: Cellulitis (6%), furunculosis (4%), dry skin (3% to 10%), urticaria (3% to 10%), acne (<3%), alopecia (<3%), eczema (<3%), petechial rash (<3%), photosensitivity (<3%), abscess (2%)

Endocrine & metabolic: Amenorrhea (<3%), hypercalcemia (<3%), hyponatremia (<3%), gout (<3%), libido decreased/loss (<3%)

Gastrointestinal: Dyspepsia (3% to 10%) flatulence (3% to 10%), gingivitis (3% to 10%), constipation (<3%), dysphagia (<3%), glossitis (<3%), ileus (<3%), taste perversion (<3%), oral moniliasis (2%)

Genitourinary: Urinary tract infection (3%), impotence (<3%)

Hematologic: Agranulocytosis (3% to 10%), hemorrhage (3% to 10%), acute leukemia (<3%), aplastic anemia (<3%), hemolytic anemia (<3%)

Local: Phlebitis (<3%)

Neuromuscular & skeletal: Arthralgia (3% to 10%), paresthesia (3% to 10%), arthritis (<3%), dysarthria (<3%), hyperkinesia (<3%), neuralgia (<3%), neuropathy (<3%), paralysis (<3%), twitching (<3%), osteomyelitis (1%)

Ocular: Conjunctivitis (4%), amblyopia (<3%), eyes nonreactive (<3%), lacrimation disorder (<3%), photophobia (<3%), retinopathy (<3%), vision abnormal (<3%), watery eyes (<3%), xerophthalmia (<3%)

Otic: Deafness (<3%), earache (<3%), labyrinthitis (<3%), tinnitus (<3%)

Renal: Creatinine increased (3% to 10%), nephropathy (<3%), renal failure (<3%), renal insufficiency (<3%), renal function abnormal (<3%), renal stone (<3%)

Respiratory: Pharyngitis (8% to 10%), sinusitis (6%), pneumonia (5%), asthma (3% to 10%), bronchitis (3%), bronchospasm (<3%), laryngeal edema (<3%), pulmonary embolus (<3%)

Miscellaneous: Diaphoresis (8% to 10%), herpes zoster (8%), viral infection (≤8%), bacterial infection (5%), herpes simplex (4%), sepsis (3%), flu-like syndrome (<3%)

<1%, postmarketing, and/or case reports: Dysuria, fungal infection (skin), hematuria, lethargy, pulmonary edema, pulmonary toxicity (fatal; in combination with fludarabine), uveitis/vision loss

Drug Interactions

Avoid Concomitant Use

Avoid concomitant use of Pentostatin with any of the following: Fludarabine; Natalizumab; Pegademase Bovine; Vaccines (Live)

Increased Effect/Toxicity

Pentostatin may increase the levels/effects of: Cyclophosphamide; Fludarabine; Leflunomide; Natalizumab; Vaccines (Live)

The levels/effects of Pentostatin may be increased by: Fludarabine; Trastuzumab

Decreased Effect

Pentostatin may decrease the levels/effects of: Pegademase Bovine; Vaccines (Inactivated); Vaccines (Live)

The levels/effects of Pentostatin may be decreased by: Echinacea; Pegademase Bovine

Storage/Stability Store intact vials under refrigeration at 2°C to 8°C (36°F to 46°F); reconstituted vials, or further dilutions, are stable at room temperature for 8 hours in D_5W or 48 hours in NS.

Reconstitution Reconstitute with 5 mL SWFI to a concentration of 2 mg/mL. The solution may be further diluted in 25-50 mL NS or D_5W for infusion.

Compatibility Stable in LR, NS; **variable stability (consult detailed reference)** in D_5W.

Y-site administration: Compatible: Fludarabine, melphalan, ondansetron, paclitaxel, sargramostim.

Mechanism of Action Pentostatin is a purine antimetabolite that inhibits adenosine deaminase, preventing the deamination of adenosine to inosine. Accumulation of deoxyadenosine (dAdo) and deoxyadenosine 5′-triphosphate (dATP) results in a reduction of purine metabolism and DNA synthesis and cell death.

Pharmacodynamics/Kinetics

Distribution: I.V.: V_d: 36.1 L (20.1 L/m^2); rapidly to body tissues

Protein binding: ~4%

Half-life elimination:

Distribution half-life: 11-85 minutes

Terminal: 3-7 hours

Renal impairment (Cl$_{cr}$ <50 mL/minute): 4-18 hours

Excretion: Urine (~50% to 96%) within 24 hours (30% to 90% as unchanged drug)

Dosage I.V.: Adults (refer to individual protocols):

Hairy cell leukemia: 4 mg/m^2 every 2 weeks

CLL (unlabeled use): 4 mg/m^2 weekly for 3 weeks, then every 2 weeks

Cutaneous T-cell lymphoma (unlabeled use): 3.75-5 mg/m^2 daily for 3 days every 3 weeks

Acute GVHD (unlabeled use): 1.5 mg/m^2 daily for 3 days; may repeat after 2 weeks if needed

◀ Chronic GVHD (unlabeled use): 4 mg/m² every 2 weeks for 12 doses; then 4 mg/m² every 3-4 weeks (if still improving)

Dosage adjustment in renal impairment: The FDA-approved labeling does not contain renal dosage adjustment guidelines; use with caution in patients with Cl_{cr} <60 mL/minute. Two patients with Cl_{cr} 50-60 mL/minute achieved responses when treated with 2 mg/m²/dose. The following guidelines have been used by some clinicians:

Kintzel, 1995:

Cl_{cr} 46-60 mL/minute: Administer 70% of dose

Cl_{cr} 31-45 mL/minute: Administer 60% of dose

Cl_{cr} <30 mL/minute: Consider use of alternative drug

Lathia, 2002:

Cl_{cr} 40-59 mL/minute: Administer 3 mg/m²/dose

Cl_{cr} 20-39 mL/minute: Administer 2 mg/m²/dose

Combination Regimens

Leukemia, chronic lymphocytic:

PCR on page 1391

Pentostatin-Cyclophosphamide on page 1394

Administration Administer I.V. 20- to 30-minute infusion or I.V. bolus over 5 minutes. Hydrate with 500-1000 mL fluid prior to infusion and 500 mL after infusion.

Monitoring Parameters CBC with differential, platelet count, liver function, serum uric acid, renal function (creatinine clearance), bone marrow evaluation

Emetic Potential Low (10% to 30%)

Dosage Forms Excipient information presented when available (limited, particularly for generics); consult specific product labeling.

Injection, powder for reconstitution [preservative free]: 10 mg [contains mannitol 50 mg]

Nipent®: 10 mg [contains mannitol 50 mg]

References

al-Razzak LA, Benedetti AE, Waugh WN, et al, "Chemical Stability of Pentostatin (NSC-218321), a Cytotoxic and Immunosuppressant Agent," *Pharm Res*, 1990, 7(5):452-60.

Bolanos-Meade J, Jacobsohn DA, Margolis J, et al, "Pentostatin in Steroid-Refractory Acute Graft-Versus-Host Disease," *J Clin Oncol*, 2005, 23(12):2661-8.

Dillman RO, Mick R and McIntyre OR, "Pentostatin in Chronic Lymphocytic Leukemia: A Phase II Trial of Cancer and Leukemia Group B," *J Clin Oncol*, 1989, 7(4):433-8.

Grever MR, Siaw MFE, Jacob WF, et al, "The Biochemical and Clinical Consequences of 2'-Deoxycoformycin in Refractory Lymphoproliferative Malignancy," *Blood*, 1981, 57(3):406-17.

Jacobsohn DA, Chen AR, Zahurak M, et al, "Phase II Study of Pentostatin in Patients With Corticosteroid-Refractory Chronic Graft-Versus-Host Disease," *J Clin Oncol*, 2007, 25 (27):4255-61.

Kintzel PE and Dorr RT, "Anticancer Drug Renal Toxicity and Elimination: Dosing Guidelines for Altered Renal Function," *Cancer Treat Rev*, 1995, 21(1):33-64.

Kurzrock R, Pilat S, and Duvic M, "Pentostatin Therapy of T-Cell Lymphomas With Cutaneous Manifestations," *J Clin Oncol*, 1999, 17(10):3117-21.

Lathia C, Fleming GF, Meyer M, et al, "Pentostatin Pharmacokinetics and Dosing Recommendations in Patients With Mild Renal Impairment," *Cancer Chemother Pharmacol*, 2002, 50(2):121-6.

Margolis J and Grever MR, "Pentostatin (Nipent): A Review of Potential Toxicity and its Management," *Semin Oncol*, 2000, 27(2 Suppl 5):9-14.

Tsimberidou AM, Giles F, Duvic M, et al, "Phase II Study of Pentostatin in Advanced T-Cell Lymphoid Malignancies: Update of an M.D. Anderson Cancer Center Series," *Cancer*, 2004, 100 (2):342-9.

◆ **Periactin** see Cyproheptadine on page 277

◆ **Peridol (Can)** see Haloperidol on page 556

◆ **Pethidine Hydrochloride** see Meperidine on page 750

- ♦ **PFA** *see* Foscarnet *on page 516*
- ♦ **Pharmorubicin® (Can)** *see* Epirubicin *on page 408*
- ♦ **Phenadoz™** *see* Promethazine *on page 997*
- ♦ **Phenergan®** *see* Promethazine *on page 997*
- ♦ **Phenylalanine Mustard** *see* Melphalan *on page 745*
- ♦ **PHL-Anagrelide (Can)** *see* Anagrelide *on page 83*
- ♦ **PHL-Bicalutamide (Can)** *see* Bicalutamide *on page 147*
- ♦ **PHL-Ciprofloxacin (Can)** *see* Ciprofloxacin *on page 228*
- ♦ **PHL-Fluconazole (Can)** *see* Fluconazole *on page 485*
- ♦ **PHL-Lorazepam (Can)** *see* LORazepam *on page 731*
- ♦ **PHL-Ondansetron (Can)** *see* Ondansetron *on page 874*
- ♦ **Phosphocol® P 32** *see* Chromic Phosphate P 32 *on page 224*
- ♦ **Phosphonoformate** *see* Foscarnet *on page 516*
- ♦ **Phosphonoformic Acid** *see* Foscarnet *on page 516*
- ♦ **Phosphorus p32** *see* Chromic Phosphate P 32 *on page 224*
- ♦ **Photofrin®** *see* Porfimer *on page 967*
- ♦ **Phylloquinone** *see* Phytonadione *on page 953*
- ♦ **Phytomenadione** *see* Phytonadione *on page 953*

Phytonadione (fye toe na DYE one)

Medication Safety Issues

Sound-alike/look-alike issues:

Mephyton® may be confused with melphalan, methadone

U.S. Brand Names Mephyton®

Index Terms Methylphytyl Napthoquinone; Phylloquinone; Phytomenadione; Vitamin K_1

Generic Available Yes

Canadian Brand Names AquaMEPHYTON®; Konakion; Mephyton®

Pharmacologic Category Vitamin, Fat Soluble

Use Prevention and treatment of hypoprothrombinemia caused by coumarin derivative-induced or other drug-induced vitamin K deficiency, hypoprothrombinemia caused by malabsorption or inability to synthesize vitamin K; hemorrhagic disease of the newborn

Unlabeled/Investigational Use Treatment of hypoprothrombinemia caused by anticoagulant rodenticides

Pregnancy Risk Factor C

Lactation Enters breast milk/use caution (AAP rates "compatible")

Labeled Contraindications Hypersensitivity to phytonadione or any component of the formulation

Warnings/Precautions [U.S. Boxed Warning]: Severe reactions resembling hypersensitivity (eg, anaphylaxis) reactions have occurred rarely during or immediately after I.V. administration. Allergic reactions have also occurred with I.M. and SubQ injections; oral administration is the safest. In obstructive jaundice or with biliary fistulas concurrent administration of bile salts is necessary. Manufacturers recommend the SubQ route over other parenteral routes. SubQ is less predictable when compared to the oral route. The American College of Chest Physicians recommends the I.V. route in patients with serious or life-threatening bleeding secondary to warfarin. The I.V. route should be restricted to emergency situations where oral phytonadione cannot be used. Efficacy is delayed regardless of route of administration; patient management may require other treatments in the interim. Administer a dose that will quickly lower the INR into a safe range without causing resistance to warfarin. High phytonadione doses may lead to warfarin resistance for at least one week. Use caution in newborns especially premature infants; hemolysis, jaundice and hyperbilirubinemia have been reported with larger than recommended doses. Some dosage forms contain benzyl alcohol which has been associated with "gasping syndrome" in premature infants. In liver disease, if initial doses do not reverse coagulopathy then higher doses are unlikely to have any effect. Ineffective in hereditary hypoprothrombinemia. Use caution with renal dysfunction (including premature infants). Injectable products may contain aluminum; may result in toxic levels following prolonged administration. Product may contain polysorbate 80.

Adverse Reactions Parenteral administration: Frequency not defined.

Cardiovascular: Cyanosis, flushing, hypotension

Central nervous system: Dizziness

Dermatologic: Scleroderma-like lesions

Endocrine & metabolic: Hyperbilirubinemia (newborn; greater than recommended doses)

Gastrointestinal: Abnormal taste

Local: Injection site reactions

Respiratory: Dyspnea

Miscellaneous: Anaphylactoid reactions, diaphoresis, hypersensitivity reactions

Drug Interactions

Avoid Concomitant Use There are no known interactions where it is recommended to avoid concomitant use.

Increased Effect/Toxicity There are no known significant interactions involving an increase in effect.

Decreased Effect

Phytonadione may decrease the levels/effects of: Vitamin K Antagonists

The levels/effects of Phytonadione may be decreased by: Mineral Oil; Orlistat

Storage/Stability

Injection: Store at 15°C to 30°C (59°F to 86°F). **Note:** Store Hospira product at 20°C to 25°C (68°F to 77°F).

Oral: Store tablets at 15°C to 30°C (59°F to 86°F). Protect from light.

Reconstitution Dilute injection solution in preservative-free NS, D_5W, or D_5NS.

Mechanism of Action Promotes liver synthesis of clotting factors (II, VII, IX, X); however, the exact mechanism as to this stimulation is unknown. Menadiol is a water soluble form of vitamin K; phytonadione has a more rapid and prolonged effect than menadione; menadiol sodium diphosphate (K_4) is half as potent as menadione (K_3).

Pharmacodynamics/Kinetics

Onset of action: Increased coagulation factors: Oral: 6-10 hours; I.V.: 1-2 hours

Peak effect: INR values return to normal: Oral: 24-48 hours; I.V.: 12-14 hours

Absorption: Oral: From intestines in presence of bile; SubQ: Variable

Metabolism: Rapidly hepatic

Excretion: Urine and feces

Dosage Note: According to the manufacturer, SubQ is the preferred parenteral route; I.M. route should be avoided due to the risk of hematoma formation; I.V. route should be restricted for emergency use only. The American College of Chest Physicians recommends the I.V. route in patients with serious or life-threatening bleeding secondary to use of vitamin K antagonists.

Adequate intake:

Children:

1-3 years: 30 mcg/day

4-8 years: 55 mcg/day

9-13 years: 60 mcg/day

14-18 years: 75 mcg/day

Adults: Males: 120 mcg/day; Females: 90 mcg/day

Hemorrhagic disease of the newborn:

Prophylaxis: I.M.: 0.5-1 mg within 1 hour of birth

Treatment: I.M., SubQ: 1 mg/dose/day; higher doses may be necessary if mother has been receiving oral anticoagulants

Hypoprothrombinemia due to drugs (other than coumarin derivatives) or factors limiting absorption or synthesis: Adults: Oral, SubQ, I.M., I.V.: Initial: 2.5-25 mg (rarely up to 50 mg)

Vitamin K deficiency (supratherapeutic INR) secondary to coumarin derivative (Ansell, 2008): Adults:

If INR above therapeutic range to <5 (no significant bleeding and rapid reversal unnecessary): Lower or hold next dose and monitor frequently; when INR approaches desired range, resume dosing with a lower dose.

If INR ≥5 and <9 (no significant bleeding): If no risk factors for bleeding exist, omit next 1 or 2 doses, monitor INR more frequently, and resume with an appropriately adjusted dose when INR in desired range.

Alternatively, if other risk factors for bleeding exist, omit next dose and administer vitamin K orally 1-2.5 mg; resume with an appropriately adjusted dose when INR in desired range.

If INR ≥5 and <9 (no significant bleeding and rapid reversal required for surgery): Administer vitamin K orally ≤5 mg and hold warfarin. Expect INR to be reduced within 24 hours; if INR still elevated, another 1-2 mg of vitamin K orally may be given.

If INR ≥9 (no significant bleeding): Hold warfarin, administer vitamin K orally 2.5-5 mg, expect INR to be reduced within 24-48 hours, monitor INR more frequently and give additional vitamin K at an appropriate dose if necessary. Resume warfarin at an appropriately adjusted dose when INR is in desired range.

If serious bleeding at any INR elevation: Hold warfarin, administer vitamin K 10 mg by slow I.V. infusion and supplement with FFP, PCC, or rFVIIa depending on the urgency of the situation; I.V. Vitamin K may be repeated every 12 hours.

If life-threatening bleeding: Hold warfarin, give FFP, PCC, or rFVIIa supplemented with vitamin K 10 mg slow I.V. infusion; repeat if necessary, depending on INR.

Notes:

If mild-moderate INR elevation without major bleeding occurs, administer vitamin K orally instead of subcutaneously.

Use of high doses of vitamin K (eg, 10-15 mg) may cause warfarin resistance for ≥1 week. During this period of resistance, heparin or low molecular weight heparin may be given until INR responds.

FFP=fresh frozen plasma; PCC=prothrombin complex concentrate; rFVIIa=recombinant factor VIIa

Administration

I.V. administration: Infuse slowly; rate of infusion should not exceed 1 mg/minute (3 mg/m²/minute in children and infants). The injectable route should be used only if the oral route is not feasible or there is a greater urgency to reverse anticoagulation.

Oral: The parenteral preparation has been administered orally to neonates.

Monitoring Parameters PT, INR

Dosage Forms Excipient information presented when available (limited, particularly for generics); consult specific product labeling.

Injection, aqueous colloidal: 2 mg/mL (0.5 mL); 10 mg/mL (1 mL) [contains benzyl alcohol]

Injection, aqueous colloidal [preservative free]: 2 mg/mL (0.5 mL) [contains polysorbate 80, propylene glycol 10.4 mg/0.5 mL]

Tablet: 100 mcg [OTC]

Mephyton®: 5 mg

Extemporaneous Preparations A 1 mg/mL oral suspension was stable for only 3 days when refrigerated when compounded as follows:

Triturate six 5 mg tablets in a mortar, reduce to a fine powder, then add 5 mL each of water and methylcellulose 1% while mixing; then transfer to a graduate and qs to 30 mL with sorbitol

Shake well before using and keep in refrigerator

Nahata MC and Hipple TF, *Pediatric Drug Formulations*, 3rd ed, Cincinnati, OH: Harvey Whitney Books Co, 1997.

References

Ansell J, Hirsh J, Hylek E, et al, "Pharmacology and Management of the Vitamin K Antagonists: American College of Chest Physicians Evidence-Based Clinical Practice Guidelines (8th Edition)," *Chest*, 2008, 133(6 Suppl):160-98.

Barash P, Kitahata LM, and Mandel S, "Acute Cardiovascular Collapse After Intravenous Phytonadione," *Anesth Analg*, 1976, 55(2):304-6.

Crowther MA, Douketis JD, Schnurr T, et al, "Oral Vitamin K Lowers the International Normalized Ratio More Rapidly Than Subcutaneous Vitamin K in the Treatment of Warfarin-Associated Coagulopathy. A Randomized, Controlled Trial," *Ann Intern Med*, 2002, 137(4):251-4.

"Dietary Reference Intakes for Vitamin A, Vitamin K, Arsenic, Boron, Chromium, Copper, Iodine, Iron, Manganese, Molybdenum, Nickel, Silicon, Vanadium, and Zinc," Food and Nutrition Board, Institute of Medicine. National Academy of Sciences, Washington, DC: National Academy Press, 2001, 162-84.

Fiore LD, Scola MA, Cantillon CE, et al, "Anaphylactoid Reactions to Vitamin K," *J Thromb Thrombolysis*, 2001, 11(2): 175-83.

Harrell CC and Kline SS, "Oral Vitamin K1: An Option to Reduce Warfarin's Activity," *Ann Pharmacother*, 1995, 29(12):1228-32.

Hopkins CS, "Adverse Reaction to a Cremophor-Containing Preparation of Intravenous Vitamin K," *Intensive Therapy Clin Monit*, 1988, 9:254-5.

Weibert RT, Le DT, Kayser SR, et al, "Correction of Excessive Anticoagulation With Low-Dose Oral Vitamin K1," *Ann Intern Med*, 1997, 126(12):959-62.

◆ **Pidorubicin** *see* Epirubicin *on page 408*

◆ **Pidorubicin Hydrochloride** *see* Epirubicin *on page 408*

Pilocarpine (pye loe KAR peen)

Medication Safety Issues

Sound-alike/look-alike issues:

Isopto® Carpine may be confused with Isopto® Carbachol

Salagen® may be confused with Salacid®, selegiline

International issues:

Salagen® may be confused with Poagen® which is a brand name for grass pollen extract in Portugal

Related Information

Oral Mucositis / Stomatitis *on page 1460*

U.S. Brand Names Isopto® Carpine; Pilopine HS®; Salagen®

Index Terms Pilocarpine Hydrochloride

Generic Available Yes: Hydrochloride solution, tablet

Canadian Brand Names Diocarpine; Isopto® Carpine; Pilopine HS®; Salagen®

Pharmacologic Category Cholinergic Agonist; Ophthalmic Agent, Anti-glaucoma; Ophthalmic Agent, Miotic

Use

Ophthalmic: Management of chronic simple glaucoma, chronic and acute angle-closure glaucoma

Oral: Symptomatic treatment of xerostomia caused by salivary gland hypofunction resulting from radiotherapy for cancer of the head and neck or Sjögren's syndrome

Unlabeled/Investigational Use Counter effects of cycloplegics

Pregnancy Risk Factor C

Lactation Excretion in breast milk unknown/not recommended

Labeled Contraindications Hypersensitivity to pilocarpine or any component of the formulation; acute inflammatory disease of the anterior chamber of the eye; in addition, tablets are also contraindicated in patients with uncontrolled asthma, angle-closure glaucoma, severe hepatic impairment

Warnings/Precautions Use caution with cardiovascular disease; patients may have difficulty compensating for transient changes in hemodynamics or rhythm induced by pilocarpine.

Ophthalmic products: May cause decreased visual acuity, especially at night or with reduced lighting.

Oral tablets: Use caution with controlled asthma, chronic bronchitis or COPD; may increase airway resistance, bronchial smooth muscle tone, and bronchial secretions. Use caution with cholelithiasis, biliary tract disease, nephrolithiasis; adjust dose with moderate hepatic impairment.

Adverse Reactions

Ophthalmic: Frequency not defined:

Cardiovascular: Hypertension, tachycardia

Gastrointestinal: Diarrhea, nausea, salivation, vomiting

Ocular: Burning, ciliary spasm, conjunctival vascular congestion, corneal granularity (gel 10%), lacrimation, lens opacity, myopia, retinal detachment, supraorbital or temporal headache, visual acuity decreased

Respiratory: Bronchial spasm, pulmonary edema

Miscellaneous: Diaphoresis

Oral (frequency varies by indication and dose):

>10%:

Cardiovascular: Flushing (8% to 13%)

Central nervous system: Chills (3% to 15%), dizziness (5% to 12%), headache (11%)

Gastrointestinal: Nausea (6% to 15%)

Genitourinary: Urinary frequency (9% to 12%)

Neuromuscular & skeletal: Weakness (2% to 12%)

Respiratory: Rhinitis (5% to 14%)

Miscellaneous: Diaphoresis (29% to 68%)

1% to 10%:

Cardiovascular: Edema (<1% to 5%), facial edema, hypertension (3%), palpitation, tachycardia

Central nervous system: Pain (4%), fever, somnolence

Dermatologic: Pruritus, rash

Gastrointestinal: Diarrhea (4% to 7%), dyspepsia (7%), vomiting (3% to 4%), constipation, flatulence, glossitis, salivation increased, stomatitis, taste perversion

Genitourinary: Vaginitis, urinary incontinence

Neuromuscular & skeletal: Myalgias, tremor

Ocular: Lacrimation (6%), amblyopia (4%), abnormal vision, blurred vision, conjunctivitis

Otic: Tinnitus

Respiratory: Cough increased, dysphagia, epistaxis, sinusitis

Miscellaneous: Allergic reaction, voice alteration

<1%: Abnormal dreams, abnormal thinking, alopecia, angina pectoris, anorexia, anxiety, aphasia, appetite increased, arrhythmia, arthralgia, arthritis, bilirubinemia, body odor, bone disorder, bradycardia, breast pain, bronchitis, cataract, cholelithiasis, colitis, confusion, contact dermatitis, cyst, deafness, depression, dry eyes, dry mouth, dry skin, dyspnea, dysuria, ear pain, ECG abnormality, eczema, emotional lability, eructation, erythema nodosum, esophagitis, exfoliative dermatitis, eye hemorrhage, eye pain, gastritis, gastroenteritis, gastrointestinal disorder, gingivitis, glaucoma, hematuria, hepatitis, herpes simplex, hiccup, hyperkinesias, hypoesthesia, hypoglycemia, hypotension, hypothermia, insomnia, intracranial hemorrhage, laryngismus, laryngitis, leg cramps, leukopenia, liver function test abnormal, lymphadenopathy, mastitis, melena, menorrhagia, metrorrhagia, migraine, moniliasis, myasthenia, MI, neck pain, photosensitivity reaction, nervousness, ovarian disorder, pancreatitis, paresthesia, parotid gland enlargement, peripheral edema, platelet abnormality, pneumonia, pyuria, salivary gland enlargement, salpingitis, seborrhea, skin ulcer, speech disorder, sputum increased, stridor, syncope, taste loss, tendon disorder, tenosynovitis, thrombocythemia, thrombocytopenia, thrombosis, tongue disorder, twitching, urethral pain, urinary impairment, urinary urgency, vaginal hemorrhage, vaginal moniliasis, vesiculobullous rash, WBC abnormality, yawning

Drug Interactions

Metabolism/Transport Effects Inhibits CYP2A6 (weak), 2E1 (weak), 3A4 (weak)

Avoid Concomitant Use There are no known interactions where it is recommended to avoid concomitant use.

Increased Effect/Toxicity

The levels/effects of Pilocarpine may be increased by: Acetylcholinesterase Inhibitors

Decreased Effect There are no known significant interactions involving a decrease in effect.

Ethanol/Nutrition/Herb Interactions Food: Avoid administering oral formulation with high-fat meal; fat decreases the rate of absorption, maximum concentration and increases the time it takes to reach maximum concentration.

Storage/Stability

Gel: Store at room temperature of 2°C to 27°C (36°F to 80°F); do not freeze. Avoid excessive heat.

Tablets: Store at controlled room temperature of 15°C to 30°C (59°F to 86°F).

Mechanism of Action Directly stimulates cholinergic receptors in the eye causing miosis (by contraction of the iris sphincter), loss of accommodation (by constriction of ciliary muscle), and lowering of intraocular pressure (with decreased resistance to aqueous humor outflow)

Pharmacodynamics/Kinetics

Onset of action:

Ophthalmic: Miosis: 10-30 minutes; Intraocular pressure reduction: 1 hour

Oral: 20 minutes

Duration:

Ophthalmic: Miosis: 4-8 hours; Intraocular pressure reduction: 4-12 hours

Oral: 3-5 hours

Half-life elimination: Oral: 0.76-1.35 hours; increased with hepatic impairment

Excretion: Urine

Dosage Adults:

Ophthalmic:

Glaucoma:

Solution: Instill 1-2 drops up to 6 times/day; adjust the concentration and frequency as required to control elevated intraocular pressure

Gel: Instill 0.5" ribbon into lower conjunctival sac once daily at bedtime

To counteract the mydriatic effects of sympathomimetic agents (unlabeled use): Solution: Instill 1 drop of a 1% solution in the affected eye

Oral: Xerostomia:

Following head and neck cancer: 5 mg 3 times/day, titration up to 10 mg 3 times/day may be considered for patients who have not responded adequately; do not exceed 2 tablets/dose

Sjögren's syndrome: 5 mg 4 times/day

Dosage adjustment in hepatic impairment: Oral: Patients with moderate impairment: 5 mg 2 times/day regardless of indication; adjust dose based on response and tolerability. Do not use with severe impairment (Child-Pugh score 10-15).

Administration

Oral: Avoid administering with high-fat meal. Fat decreases the rate of absorption, maximum concentration, and increases the time it takes to reach maximum concentration.

Ophthalmic: If both solution and gel are used, the solution should be applied first, then the gel at least 5 minutes later. Following administration of the solution, finger pressure should be applied on the lacrimal sac for 1-2 minutes.

Monitoring Parameters Intraocular pressure, funduscopic exam, visual field testing

Dosage Forms Excipient information presented when available (limited, particularly for generics); consult specific product labeling.

Gel, ophthalmic, as hydrochloride (Pilopine HS®): 4% (4 g) [contains benzalkonium chloride]

Solution, ophthalmic, as hydrochloride: 0.5% (15 mL); 1% (2 mL, 15 mL); 2% (2 mL, 15 mL); 3% (15 mL); 4% (2 mL, 15 mL); 6% (15 mL) [may contain benzalkonium chloride]

Isopto® Carpine: 1% (15 mL); 2% (15 mL); 4% (15 mL) [contains benzalkonium chloride]

Tablet, as hydrochloride: 5 mg, 7.5 mg

Salagen®: 5 mg, 7.5 mg

References

Hawthorne M and Sullivan K, "Pilocarpine for Radiation-Induced Xerostomia in Head and Neck Cancer," *Int J Palliat Nurs*, 2000, 6(5):228-32.

Jacobs CD and van der Pas M, "A Multicenter Maintenance Study of Oral Pilocarpine Tablets for Radiation-Induced Xerostomia," *Oncology*, 1996, 10(3 Suppl):16-20.

Johnson JT, Ferretti GA, Nethery WJ, et al, "Oral Pilocarpine for Postirradiation Xerostomia in Patients With Head and Neck Cancer," *N Engl J Med*, 1993, 329(6):390-5.

LeVeque FG, Montgomery M, Potter D, et al, "A Multicenter, Randomized, Double-Blind, Placebo-Controlled, Dose-Titration Study of Oral Pilocarpine for Treatment of Radiation-Induced Xerostomia in Head and Neck Cancer Patients," *J Clin Oncol*, 1993, 11(6):1124-31.

Rieke JW, Hafermann MD, Johnson JT, et al, "Oral Pilocarpine for Radiation-Induced Xerostomia: Integrated Efficacy and Safety Results From Two Prospective Randomized Clinical Trials," *Int J Radiat Oncol Biol Phys*, 1995, 31(3):661-9.

Schuller DE, Stevens P, Clausen KP, et al, "Treatment of Radiation Side Effects With Oral Pilocarpine," *J Surg Oncol*, 1989, 42(4):272-6.

Taylor SE, "Efficacy and Economic Evaluation of Pilocarpine in Treating Radiation-Induced Xerostomia," *Expert Opin Pharmacother*, 2003, 4(9):1489-97.

♦ **Pilocarpine Hydrochloride** *see* Pilocarpine *on page 956*

♦ **Pilopine HS®** *see* Pilocarpine *on page 956*

Piperacillin and Tazobactam Sodium
(pi PER a sil in & ta zoe BAK tam SOW dee um)

Medication Safety Issues
Sound-alike/look-alike issues:
Zosyn® may be confused with Zofran®, Zyvox®

U.S. Brand Names Zosyn®

Index Terms Piperacillin Sodium and Tazobactam Sodium; Tazobactam and Piperacillin

Generic Available No

Canadian Brand Names Tazocin®

Pharmacologic Category Antibiotic, Penicillin

Use Treatment of moderate-to-severe infections caused by susceptible organisms, including infections of the lower respiratory tract (community-acquired pneumonia, nosocomial pneumonia); urinary tract; uncomplicated and complicated skin and skin structures; gynecologic (endometritis, pelvic inflammatory disease); bone and joint infections; intra-abdominal infections (appendicitis with rupture/abscess, peritonitis); and septicemia. Tazobactam expands activity of piperacillin to include beta-lactamase producing strains of *S. aureus*, *H. influenzae*, *Bacteroides*, and other gram-negative bacteria.

Pregnancy Risk Factor B

Lactation Enters breast milk/use caution

Labeled Contraindications Hypersensitivity to penicillins, beta-lactamase inhibitors, or any component of the formulation

Warnings/Precautions Bleeding disorders have been observed, particularly in patients with renal impairment; discontinue if thrombocytopenia or bleeding occurs. Due to sodium load and to the adverse effects of high serum concentrations of penicillins, dosage modification is required in patients with impaired or underdeveloped renal function; use with caution in patients with seizures or in patients with history of beta-lactam allergy; associated with an increased incidence of rash and fever in cystic fibrosis patients. Prolonged use may result in fungal or bacterial superinfection, including *C. difficile*-associated diarrhea (CDAD) and pseudomembranous colitis; CDAD has been observed >2 months postantibiotic treatment. Safety and efficacy have not been established in children <2 months of age.

Adverse Reactions
>10%: Gastrointestinal: Diarrhea (7% to 11%)

>1% to 10%:
Cardiovascular: Hypertension (2%)
Central nervous system: Insomnia (7%), headache (8%), fever (2% to 5%), agitation (2%), pain (2%)
Dermatologic: Rash (4%), pruritus (3%)

Gastrointestinal: Constipation (1% to 8%), nausea (7%), vomiting (3% to 4%), dyspepsia (3%), stool changes (2%), abdominal pain (1% to 2%)

Hepatic: Transaminases increased

Local: Local reaction (3%), abscess (2%)

Respiratory: Pharyngitis (2%)

Miscellaneous: Moniliasis (2%), sepsis (2%), infection (2%)

≤1%, postmarketing, and/or case reports: Agranulocytosis, anaphylaxis/anaphylactoid reaction, anemia, anxiety, arrhythmia, arthralgia, atrial fibrillation, back pain, bradycardia, bronchospasm, candidiasis, cardiac arrest, cardiac failure, circulatory failure, chest pain, cholestatic jaundice, confusion, convulsions, coughing, depression, diaphoresis, dizziness, dyspnea, dysuria, edema, epistaxis, erythema multiforme, flatulence, flushing, gastritis, genital pruritus, hallucination, hematuria, hemolytic anemia, hemorrhage, hepatitis, hiccough, hypoglycemia, hypotension, ileus, incontinence, inflammation, injection site reaction, interstitial nephritis, leukorrhea, malaise, mesenteric embolism, myalgia, myocardial infarction, oliguria, pancytopenia, phlebitis, photophobia, pseudomembranous colitis, pulmonary edema, pulmonary embolism, purpura, renal failure, rhinitis, rigors, Stevens-Johnson syndrome, syncope, tachycardia (supraventricular and ventricular), taste perversion, thirst, thrombocytopenia, thrombocytosis, thrombophlebitis, tinnitus, toxic epidermal necrolysis, tremor, ulcerative stomatitis, urinary retention, vaginitis, ventricular fibrillation, vertigo

Drug Interactions

Avoid Concomitant Use There are no known interactions where it is recommended to avoid concomitant use.

Increased Effect/Toxicity

Piperacillin and Tazobactam Sodium may increase the levels/effects of: Methotrexate

The levels/effects of Piperacillin and Tazobactam Sodium may be increased by: Uricosuric Agents

Decreased Effect

Piperacillin and Tazobactam Sodium may decrease the levels/effects of: Aminoglycosides; Mycophenolate; Typhoid Vaccine

The levels/effects of Piperacillin and Tazobactam Sodium may be decreased by: Fusidic Acid; Tetracycline Derivatives

Storage/Stability

Vials: Store at controlled room temperature of 20°C to 25°C (68°F to 77°F). Use single-dose vials immediately after reconstitution (discard unused portions after 24 hours at room temperature and 48 hours if refrigerated). After reconstitution, vials or solution are stable in NS or D_5W for 24 hours at room temperature and 48 hours (vials) or 7 days (solution) when refrigerated.

Premixed solution: Store frozen at -20°C (-4°F). Thawed solution is stable for 24 hours at room temperature or 14 days under refrigeration; do not refreeze.

Reconstitution Reconstitute with 5 mL of diluent per 1 g of piperacillin and then further dilute.

Compatibility Stable in dextran 6% in NS, D_5W, NS, sterile water for injection; LR (EDTA-formulated product only); **variable stability (consult detailed reference)** in peritoneal dialysis solution.

Y-site administration: Compatible: Amikacin (EDTA formulated product only), aminophylline, aztreonam, bleomycin, bumetanide, buprenorphine, butorphanol, calcium gluconate, carboplatin, carmustine, cefepime, cimetidine, clindamycin, co-trimoxazole, cyclophosphamide, cytarabine, dexamethasone sodium phosphate, diphenhydramine, docetaxel, dopamine, ▶

enalaprilat, etoposide, etoposide phosphate, floxuridine, fluconazole, fludarabine, fluorouracil, furosemide, gentamicin (EDTA formulated product only), granisetron, heparin, hydrocortisone sodium phosphate, hydrocortisone sodium succinate, hydromorphone, ifosfamide, leucovorin, linezolid, lorazepam, magnesium sulfate, mannitol, meperidine, mesna, methotrexate, methylprednisolone sodium succinate, metoclopramide, metronidazole, morphine, ondansetron, plicamycin, potassium chloride, ranitidine, remifentanil, sargramostim, sodium bicarbonate, thiotepa, vinblastine, vincristine, zidovudine. **Incompatible:** Acyclovir, alatrofloxacin, amphotericin B, amphotericin B cholesteryl sulfate complex, chlorpromazine, cisplatin, dacarbazine, daunorubicin, dobutamine, doxorubicin, doxorubicin liposome, doxycycline, droperidol, famotidine, ganciclovir, gatifloxacin, gemcitabine, haloperidol, hydroxyzine, idarubicin, minocycline, mitomycin, mitoxantrone, nalbuphine, prochlorperazine edisylate, promethazine, streptozocin, tobramycin. **Variable (consult detailed reference):** Cisatracurium, vancomycin.

Compatibility when admixed: Compatible: Potassium chloride. **Incompatible:** Aminoglycosides.

Mechanism of Action Inhibits bacterial cell wall synthesis by binding to one or more of the penicillin binding proteins (PBPs); which in turn inhibits the final transpeptidation step of peptidoglycan synthesis in bacterial cell walls, thus inhibiting cell wall biosynthesis. Bacteria eventually lyse due to ongoing activity of cell wall autolytic enzymes (autolysins and murein hydrolases) while cell wall assembly is arrested. Tazobactam inhibits many beta-lactamases, including staphylococcal penicillinase and Richmond and Sykes types II, III, IV, and V, including extended spectrum enzymes; it has only limited activity against class I beta-lactamases other than class Ic types.

Pharmacodynamics/Kinetics Both AUC and peak concentrations are dose proportional; hepatic impairment does not affect kinetics

Distribution: Well into lungs, intestinal mucosa, skin, muscle, uterus, ovary, prostate, gallbladder, and bile; penetration into CSF is low in subject with noninflamed meninges

Protein binding: Piperacillin and tazobactam: ~30%

Metabolism:
Piperacillin: 6% to 9% to desethyl metabolite (weak activity)
Tazobactam: ~26% to inactive metabolite

Bioavailability:
Piperacillin: I.M.: 71%
Tazobactam: I.M.: 84%

Half-life elimination: Piperacillin and tazobactam: 0.7-1.2 hours

Time to peak, plasma: Immediately following infusion of 30 minutes

Excretion: Clearance of both piperacillin and tazobactam are directly proportional to renal function
Piperacillin: Urine (68% as unchanged drug); feces (10% to 20%)
Tazobactam: Urine (80% as unchanged drug; remainder as inactive metabolite)

Dosage

Usual dosage range:

Children: I.V.:
2-8 months: 80 mg of piperacillin component/kg every 8 hours
≥9 months and ≤40 kg: 100 mg of piperacillin component/kg every 8 hours
Adults: I.V.: 3.375 g every 6 hours **or** 4.5 g every 6-8 hours; maximum: 18 g/day

Indication-specific dosing: I.V.:

Children: **Note:** Dosing based on piperacillin component:

Appendicitis, peritonitis:

2-8 months: 80 mg/kg every 8 hours

≥9 months and ≤40 kg: 100 mg/kg every 8 hours

>40 kg: refer to Adult dosing

Cystic fibrosis, pseudomonal infections (unlabeled use): 350-450 mg/kg/day in divided doses

Adults:

Diverticulitis, intra-abdominal abscess, peritonitis: I.V.: 3.375 g every 6 hours; **Note:** Some clinicians use 4.5 g every 8 hours for empiric coverage since the %time>MIC is similar between the regimens for most pathogens; however, this regimen is NOT recommended for nosocomial pneumonia or *Pseudomonas* coverage.

Pneumonia (nosocomial): I.V.: 4.5 g every 6 hours for 7-14 days (when used empirically, combination with an aminoglycoside or antipseudomonal fluoroquinolone is recommended; consider discontinuation of additional agent if *P. aeruginosa* is not isolated)

Severe infections: I.V.: 3.375 g every 6 hours for 7-10 days; **Note:** Some clinicians use 4.5 g every 8 hours for empiric coverage since the %time>MIC is similar between the regimens for most pathogens; however, this regimen is NOT recommended for nosocomial pneumonia or *Pseudomonas* coverage.

Dosing interval in renal impairment:

Cl_{cr} 20-40 mL/minute: Administer 2.25 g every 6 hours (3.375 g every 6 hours for nosocomial pneumonia)

Cl_{cr} <20 mL/minute: Administer 2.25 g every 8 hours (2.25 g every 6 hours for nosocomial pneumonia)

Hemodialysis/CAPD: Administer 2.25 g every 12 hours (2.25 g every 8 hours for nosocomial pneumonia) with an additional dose of 0.75 g after each hemodialysis session

Continuous renal replacement therapy (CRRT): Drug clearance is highly dependent on the method of renal replacement, filter type, and flow rate. Appropriate dosing requires close monitoring of pharmacologic response, signs of adverse reactions due to drug accumulation, as well as drug levels in relation to target trough (if appropriate). The following are general recommendations only (based on dialysate flow/ultrafiltration rates of 1 L/hour) and should not supersede clinical judgment:

CVVH: 2.25 g every 6 hours

CVVHD/CVVHDF: 2.25-3.375 g every 6 hours

Note: Higher dose of 3.375 g should be considered when treating resistant pathogens (especially *Pseudomonas*); alternative recommendations suggest dosing of 4.5 g every 8 hours; regardless of regimen, there is some concern of tazobactam (TAZ) accumulation, given its lower clearance relative to piperacillin (PIP). Some clinicians advocate dosing with PIP to alternate with PIP/TAZ, particularly in CVVH-dependent patients, to lessen this concern.

Administration Administer by I.V. infusion over 30 minutes

Some penicillins (eg, carbenicillin, ticarcillin and piperacillin) have been shown to inactivate aminoglycosides *in vitro*. This has been observed to a greater extent with tobramycin and gentamicin, while amikacin has shown greater stability against inactivation. Concurrent use of these agents may pose a risk of reduced antibacterial efficacy *in vivo*, particularly in the setting of profound renal impairment. However, definitive clinical evidence is lacking. If combination penicillin/aminoglycoside therapy is desired in a patient with renal dysfunction, separation of doses (if feasible), and routine monitoring of aminoglycoside levels, CBC, and clinical response should be considered. **Note:** Reformulated Zosyn® containing EDTA has been shown to be compatible *in vitro* for Y-site infusion with amikacin and gentamicin, but not compatible with tobramycin.

Monitoring Parameters Creatinine, BUN, CBC with differential, PT, PTT; signs of bleeding; monitor for signs of anaphylaxis during first dose

Test Interactions Positive Coombs' [direct] test; false positive reaction for urine glucose using copper-reduction method (Clinitest®); may result in false positive results with the Platelia® *Aspergillus* enzyme immunoassay (EIA)

Some penicillin derivatives may accelerate the degradation of aminoglycosides *in vitro*, leading to a potential underestimation of aminoglycoside serum concentration. **Note:** Reformulated Zosyn® containing EDTA has been shown to be compatible *in vitro* for Y-site infusion with amikacin and gentamicin, but not compatible with tobramycin.

Dietary Considerations
Infusion, premixed: 2.25 g contains sodium 5.58 mEq (128 mg); 3.375 g contains sodium 8.38 mEq (192 mg); 4.5 g contains sodium 11.17 mEq (256 mg)

Injection, powder for reconstitution: 2.25 g contains sodium 5.58 mEq (128 mg); 3.375 g contains sodium 8.38 mEq (192 mg); 4.5 g contains sodium 11.17 mEq (256 mg); 40.5 g contains sodium 100.4 mEq (2304 mg, bulk pharmacy vial)

Dosage Forms Excipient information presented when available (limited, particularly for generics); consult specific product labeling.

Note: 8:1 ratio of piperacillin sodium/tazobactam sodium

Infusion [premixed iso-osmotic solution, frozen]:
2.25 g: Piperacillin 2 g and tazobactam 0.25 g (50 mL) [contains sodium 5.58 mEq (128 mg) and EDTA]

3.375 g: Piperacillin 3 g and tazobactam 0.375 g (50 mL) [contains sodium 8.38 mEq (192 mg) and EDTA]

4.5 g: Piperacillin 4 g and tazobactam 0.5 g (50 mL) [contains sodium 11.17 mEq (256 mg) and EDTA]

Injection, powder for reconstitution:
2.25 g: Piperacillin 2 g and tazobactam 0.25 g [contains sodium 5.58 mEq (128 mg) and EDTA]

3.375 g: Piperacillin 3 g and tazobactam 0.375 g [contains sodium 8.38 mEq (192 mg) and EDTA]

4.5 g: Piperacillin 4 g and tazobactam 0.5 g [contains sodium 11.17 mEq (256 mg) and EDTA]

40.5 g: Piperacillin 36 g and tazobactam 4.5 g [contains sodium 100.4 mEq (2304 mg) and EDTA; bulk pharmacy vial]

References
Kim M-K, Capitano B, Mattoes HM, et al, "Pharmacokinetic and Pharmacodynamic Evaluation of Two Dosing Regimens for Piperacillin-Tazobactam," *Pharmacother*, 2002, 22(5):569-77.

Lau A, Lee M, Flascha S, et al, "Effect of Piperacillin on Tobramycin Pharmacokinetics in Patients with Normal Renal Function,"*Antimicrob Agents Chemother*, 1983, 24(4):533-37.

Perez-Vazquez A, Pastor JM, and Riancho JA, "Immune Thrombocytopenia Caused by Piperacillin/Tazobactam," *Clin Infect Dis*, 1998, 27(3):650-1.

Reichardt P, Handrick W, Linke A, et al, "Leukocytopenia, Thrombocytopenia and Fever Related to Piperacillin/Tazobactam Treatment – a Retrospective Analysis in 38 Children With Cystic Fibrosis," *Infection*, 1999, 27(6):355-6.

◆ **Piperacillin Sodium and Tazobactam Sodium** *see* Piperacillin and Tazobactam Sodium *on page 960*

Plerixafor (pler IX a fore)

Related Information

Hematopoietic Stem Cell Transplantation *on page 1501*

U.S. Brand Names Mozobil™

Index Terms AMD3100; LM3100

Generic Available No

Pharmacologic Category Hematopoietic Stem Cell Mobilizer

Use Mobilization of hematopoietic stem cells (HSC) for collection and subsequent autologous transplantation (in combination with filgrastim) in patients with non-Hodgkin's lymphoma (NHL) and multiple myeloma (MM)

Pregnancy Risk Factor D

Lactation Excretion in breast milk unknown/not recommended

Labeled Contraindications There are no contraindications listed within the manufacturer's labeling.

Warnings/Precautions Increases circulating leukocytes when used in conjunction with filgrastim; monitor WBC; use with caution in patients with neutrophil count >50,000/mm^3. Thrombocytopenia has been observed with use; monitor platelet count. Not intended for mobilization in patients with leukemia; may contaminate apheresis product by mobilizing leukemic cells. When used in combination with filgrastim, tumor cells released from marrow could be collected in leukapheresis product; potential effect of tumor cell reinfusion is unknown. Splenomegaly and splenic rupture have been reported (rarely) with filgrastim use; instruct patients to report left upper quadrant pain or scapular/shoulder tip pain; promptly evaluate in any patient who report these.

Primary route of elimination is urinary; dosage reduction is recommended in patients with moderate-severe renal impairment (Cl$_{cr}$ ≤50 mL/minute). Medications that may reduce renal function or compete for active tubular secretion may increase serum concentrations of plerixafor. Use has not been studied in patients weighing >175% of ideal body weight. Safety and efficacy have not been established in children.

Adverse Reactions Adverse reactions reported with filgrastim combination therapy.

>10%:

Central nervous system: Fatigue (27%), headache (22%), dizziness (11%)

Gastrointestinal: Diarrhea (37%), nausea (34%)

Local: Injection site reactions (34%, including erythema, hematoma, hemorrhage, induration, inflammation, irritation, pain, paresthesia, pruritus, rash, swelling, urticaria)

Neuromuscular & skeletal: Arthralgia (13%)

5% to 10%:

Central nervous system: Insomnia (7%)

Gastrointestinal: Vomiting (10%), flatulence (7%)

<5%, postmarketing, and/or case reports: Abdominal discomfort, abdominal distension, abdominal pain, constipation, diaphoresis, dyspnea, erythema, hypesthesia (oral), hypoxia, leukocytes increased, malaise, musculoskeletal pain, orthostatic hypotension, periorbital swelling, syncope, thrombocytopenia, urticaria, vasovagal reaction, xerostomia

Drug Interactions

Avoid Concomitant Use There are no known interactions where it is recommended to avoid concomitant use.

Increased Effect/Toxicity There are no known significant interactions involving an increase in effect.

Decreased Effect There are no known significant interactions involving a decrease in effect.

Storage/Stability Store at 25°C (77°F); excursions permitted to 15°C to 30°C (59°F to 86°F). The manufacturer recommends discarding unused drug remaining in the vial after use.

Mechanism of Action Reversibly inhibits binding of stromal cell-derived factor-1-alpha (SDF-1α), expressed on bone marrow stromal cells, to the CXC chemokine receptor 4 (CXCR4), resulting in mobilization of hematopoietic stem and progenitor cells from bone marrow into peripheral blood. Plerixafor used in combination with filgrastim results in synergistic increase in CD34+ cell mobilization. Mobilized CD34+ cells are capable of engrafting with extended repopulating capacity.

Pharmacodynamics/Kinetics

Onset of action: Peak CD34+ mobilization: Plerixafor monotherapy: 6-9 hours after administration; Plerixafor + filgrastim: 10-14 hours

Duration: WBC counts return toward baseline at ~24 after administration

Absorption: SubQ: Rapid

Distribution: 0.3L/kg; primarily to extravascular fluid space

Protein binding: ≤58%

Metabolism: Not metabolized

Half-life elimination: Terminal: 3-6 hours

Time to peak, plasma: SubQ: 30-60 minutes

Excretion: Urine (~70%; as parent drug)

Dosage Note: Dosing is based on actual body weight. Begin plerixafor after patient has received filgrastim 10 mcg/kg once daily for 4 days; plerixafor, filgrastim and apheresis should be continued daily until sufficient cell collection up to a maximum of 4 days.

SubQ: Adults: HSC mobilization: 0.24 mg/kg once daily ~11 hours prior to apheresis for up to 4 consecutive days; maximum dose: 40 mg/day

Dosage adjustment in renal impairment:

Cl_{cr} >50 mL/minute: No adjustment required

Cl_{cr} ≤50 mL/minute: 0.16 mg/kg; maximum dose: 27 mg/day

Hemodialysis: Insufficient information for dosing recommendation

Administration Administer subcutaneously, ~11 hours prior to initiation of apheresis. In some clinical trials, plerixafor administration began in the evening prior to apheresis. (filgrastim was begun on day 1, plerixafor initiated in the evening on day 4 and apheresis in the morning on day 5; with filgrastim, plerixafor and apheresis then continued daily until sufficient cell collection for autologous transplant.)

Monitoring Parameters CBC with differential and platelets

Dosage Forms Excipient information presented when available (limited, particularly for generics); consult specific product labeling.

Injection, solution [preservative free]:

Mozobil™: 20 mg/mL (1.2 mL)

References

Calandra G, McCarty J, McGuirk J, et al, "AMD3100 Plus G-CSF Can Successfully Mobilize CD34 + Cells From Non-Hodgkin's Lymphoma, Hodgkin's Disease and Multiple Myeloma Patients Previously Failing Mobilization With Chemotherapy and/or Cytokine Treatment: Compassionate Use Data," *Bone Marrow Transplant,* 2008, 41(4):331-8.

Cashen A, Lopez S, Gao F, et al, "A Phase II Study of Plerixafor (AMD3100) Plus G-CSF for Autologous Hematopoietic Progenitor Cell Mobilization in Patients With Hodgkin Lymphoma," *Biol Blood Marrow Transplant,* 2008, 14(11):1253-61.

Devine SM, Flomenberg N, Vesole DH, et al, "Rapid Mobilization of CD34+ Cells Following Administration of the CXCR4 Antagonist AMD3100 to Patients With Multiple Myeloma and Non-Hodgkin's Lymphoma," *J Clin Oncol,* 2004, 22(6):1095-102.

Devine SM, Vij R, Rettig M, et al, "Rapid Mobilization of Functional Donor Hematopoietic Cells Without G-CSF Using AMD3100, an Antagonist of the CXCR4/SDF-1 Interaction," *Blood*, 2008, 112(4):990-8.

Flomenberg N, Devine SM, DiPersio JF, et al, "The Use of AMD3100 Plus G-CSF for Autologous Hematopoietic Progenitor Cell Mobilization is Superior to G-CSF Alone," *Blood*, 2005, 106 (5):1867-74.

Lack NA, Green B, Dale DC, et al, "A Pharmacokinetic-Pharmacodynamic Model for the Mobilization of CD34+ Hematopoietic Progenitor Cells by AMD3100," *Clin Pharmacol Ther*, 2005, 77(5):427-36.

Liles WC, Broxmeyer HE, Rodger E, et al, "Mobilization of Hematopoietic Progenitor Cells in Healthy Volunteers by AMD3100, a CXCR4 Antagonist," *Blood*, 2003, 102(8):2728-30.

- ◆ **PMS-Anagrelide (Can)** *see* Anagrelide *on page* 83
- ◆ **PMS-Benzydamine (Can)** *see* Benzydamine *on page* 136
- ◆ **PMS-Bicalutamide (Can)** *see* Bicalutamide *on page* 147
- ◆ **PMS-Ciprofloxacin (Can)** *see* Ciprofloxacin *on page* 228
- ◆ **PMS-Deferoxamine (Can)** *see* Deferoxamine *on page* 334
- ◆ **PMS-Desmopressin (Can)** *see* Desmopressin *on page* 344
- ◆ **PMS-Dexamethasone (Can)** *see* Dexamethasone *on page* 350
- ◆ **PMS-Famciclovir (Can)** *see* Famciclovir *on page* 455
- ◆ **PMS-Fluconazole (Can)** *see* Fluconazole *on page* 485
- ◆ **PMS-Haloperidol LA (Can)** *see* Haloperidol *on page* 556
- ◆ **PMS-Hydromorphone (Can)** *see* HYDROmorphone *on page* 584
- ◆ **PMS-Hydroxyzine (Can)** *see* HydrOXYzine *on page* 594
- ◆ **PMS-Levofloxacin (Can)** *see* Levofloxacin *on page* 707
- ◆ **PMS-Lorazepam (Can)** *see* LORazepam *on page* 731
- ◆ **PMS-Metoclopramide (Can)** *see* Metoclopramide *on page* 788
- ◆ **PMS-Morphine Sulfate SR (Can)** *see* Morphine Sulfate *on page* 816
- ◆ **PMS-Nystatin (Can)** *see* Nystatin *on page* 855
- ◆ **PMS-Ofloxacin (Can)** *see* Ofloxacin *on page* 863
- ◆ **PMS-Olanzapine (Can)** *see* OLANZapine *on page* 869
- ◆ **PMS-Ondansetron (Can)** *see* Ondansetron *on page* 874
- ◆ **PMS-Oxycodone (Can)** *see* OxyCODONE *on page* 889
- ◆ **PMS-Pamidronate (Can)** *see* Pamidronate *on page* 914
- ◆ **PMS-Promethazine (Can)** *see* Promethazine *on page* 997
- ◆ **PMS-Tamoxifen (Can)** *see* Tamoxifen *on page* 1072
- ◆ **PMS-Tobramycin (Can)** *see* Tobramycin *on page* 1110
- ◆ **PMS-Valacyclovir (Can)** *see* Valacyclovir *on page* 1154
- ◆ **PN401** *see* Vistonuridine *on page* 1186
- ◆ **Polyethylene Glycol-L-asparaginase** *see* Pegaspargase *on page* 925

Porfimer (POR fi mer)

Medication Safety Issues
High alert medication: The Institute for Safe Medication Practices (ISMP) includes this medication among its list of drug classes which have a heightened risk of causing significant patient harm when used in error.

Related Information
Safe Handling of Hazardous Drugs *on page* 1517

U.S. Brand Names Photofrin®

◄ **Index Terms** CL-184116; Dihematoporphyrin Ether; Porfimer Sodium

Generic Available No

Canadian Brand Names Photofrin®

Pharmacologic Category Antineoplastic Agent, Miscellaneous

Use Palliation in patients with obstructing (partial or complete) esophageal cancer; treatment of microinvasive endobronchial nonsmall cell lung cancer (NSCLC); reduction of obstruction and palliation in patients with obstructing (partial or complete) NSCLC; ablation of high-grade dysplasia in Barrett's esophagus

Unlabeled/Investigational Use Treatment of gastric cancer (obstruction); treatment of actinic keratoses and low-risk basal and squamous cell skin cancers

Pregnancy Risk Factor C

Lactation Excretion in breast milk unknown/not recommended

Labeled Contraindications Porphyria

Photodynamic therapy (PDT) is contraindicated in patients with tracheoesophageal or bronchoesophageal fistula; tumors eroding into a major blood vessel; severe acute respiratory distress when caused by endobronchial lesion; esophageal or gastric varices; esophageal ulcers >1 cm in diameter

Warnings/Precautions Hazardous agent - use appropriate precautions for handling and disposal. When treating endobronchial tumors, use caution if treatment-induced inflammation may obstruct airway. Assess patient for possibility of tumor erosion into a pulmonary blood vessel (contraindication); fatal massive pulmonary hemoptysis (FMH) may occur. Risk factors for FMH include large, centrally-located tumors, cavitating tumors, or extensive tumor extrinsic to the bronchus. Fistula formation may occur after resolution of endobronchial tumors with deep bronchial wall invasion. Generally not suited for treatment of patients with esophageal or gastric varices; if used in esophageal varices, extreme caution is warranted and light exposure to the varices should be avoided. In patients with Barrett's esophagus, conduct rigorous surveillance (endoscopic biopsy every 3 months until 4 consecutive negative results for high-grade dysplasia followed by further follow-up per physician judgement). Esophageal strictures are common adverse events associated with photodynamic therapy of Barrett's esophagus; esophageal dilation may be required. Porfimer treatment for esophageal tumors which erode into the trachea or bronchial tree are likely to cause fistula; use in not recommended; use is contraindicated in patients with existing tracheoesophageal or bronchoesophageal fistula.

Photosensitivity reactions are common is patients are exposed to direct sunlight or bright indoor light (eg fluorescent lights, unshaded light bulbs, examination/operating lights). Photosensitivity may last 30-90 days. Encourage ambient indoor light exposure (aids in gradually inactivating residual porfimer). Ocular discomfort has been reported; for at least 30 days, when outdoors, patients should wear dark sunglasses which have an average white light transmittance of <4%. Patients should be educated to test for residual photosensitivity before resuming exposure to direct sunlight. Conventional sunscreens are **not** protective. Allow 2-4 weeks to elapse after phototherapy prior to initiating radiation therapy; 4 weeks should elapse after radiation therapy prior to initiating phototherapy. Concurrent use with other photosensitizing agents may increase the risk for photosensitivity reactions. Avoid extravasation; if occurs, protect affected area from light. Elimination may be prolonged in hepatic and renal impairment; toxicities may be increased; photosensitivity may be increased beyond 90 days in patients mild-to-severe hepatic impairment and in patients with severe renal impairment. Safety and efficacy in children have not been established.

Adverse Reactions

>10%:

Cardiovascular: Chest pain (7% to 31%; substernal: 5%), edema (5% to 18%)

Central nervous system: Fever (8% to 31%), pain (1% to 22%), insomnia (5% to 14%)

Dermatologic: Photosensitivity reaction (19% to 22% in cancer patients; 37% to 69% in Barrett's esophagus patients; severe: 10%)

Gastrointestinal: Esophageal stricture/stenosis (6% in esophageal cancer patients; 30% to 36% in Barrett's esophagus patients), nausea (24% to 37%), vomiting (17% to 31%), constipation (5% to 24%), dysphagia (10% to 24%), mucositis (20% in superficial endobronchial cancer), abdominal pain (5% to 20%)

Hematologic: Anemia (32% in esophageal cancer patients)

Neuromuscular & skeletal: Back pain (3% to 11%)

Respiratory: Pleural effusion (32% in esophageal cancer patients; 12% in Barrett's esophagus patients; ≤5% in endobronchial cancer patients), dyspnea (7% to 30%), bronchial obstruction/mucus plug (21%), pneumonia (6% to 18%), hemoptysis (7% to 16%), cough (5% to 15%), bronchostenosis (11%), pharyngitis (11%)

5% to 10%:

Cardiovascular: Atrial fibrillation (10%), hypotension (7%), cardiac failure (7% in esophageal cancer), hypertension (6%), tachycardia (6%)

Central nervous system: Anxiety (3% to 7%), dysphonia (3% to 5%)

Endocrine & metabolic: Dehydration (7% to 10%)

Gastrointestinal: Weight loss (5% to 9%), anorexia (8%), esophageal edema (8%), hematemesis (8%), esophageal pain (7%), dyspepsia (1% to 6%), diarrhea (5%), eructation (5%), esophagitis (5%), melena (5%), odynophagia (5%)

Genitourinary: Urinary tract infection (7%)

Respiratory: Respiratory insufficiency (≤10%), bronchitis (10%), bronchial ulceration (9%), tracheoesophageal fistula (6%), fatal massive hemoptysis (≤5%)

Miscellaneous: Moniliasis (9%), tumor hemorrhage (8%), hiccups (5%), surgical complication (5% in esophageal cancer patients)

<5%, postmarketing, and/or case reports (limited to important or life-threatening): Abnormal vision, angina, bradycardia, bronchospasm, cataracts, diplopia, erythema, esophageal perforation, eye pain, fluid imbalance, gastric ulcer, hair growth increased, ileus, jaundice, laryngotracheal edema, lung abscess, MI, ocular sensitivity, peritonitis, photophobia, pneumonitis, pruritus, pseudoporphyria state, pulmonary edema, pulmonary embolism, pulmonary hemorrhage, pulmonary thrombosis, respiratory failure, sepsis, sick sinus syndrome, skin blistering, skin discoloration, skin fragility, skin nodules, skin wrinkles, stridor, supraventricular tachycardia

Drug Interactions

Avoid Concomitant Use There are no known interactions where it is recommended to avoid concomitant use.

Increased Effect/Toxicity There are no known significant interactions involving an increase in effect.

Decreased Effect There are no known significant interactions involving a decrease in effect.

◄ **Storage/Stability** Store intact vials at controlled room temperature of 20°C to 25°C (68°F to 77°F). Reconstituted solutions should be protected from light and used immediately after preparation.

Reconstitution Reconstitute each vial of porfimer with 31.8 mL of either D_5W or NS injection resulting in a final concentration of 2.5 mg/mL. Shake well until dissolved. Protect the reconstituted product from bright light and use immediately. Use appropriate precautions for handling and disposal.

Compatibility Do not mix porfimer with other drugs in the same solution.

Mechanism of Action Porfimer's cytotoxic activity is dependent on light and oxygen. Following administration, the drug is selectively retained in neoplastic tissues. Exposure of the drug to laser light at wavelengths >630 nm results in the production of oxygen free-radicals. Release of thromboxane A_2, leading to vascular occlusion and ischemic necrosis, may also occur.

Pharmacodynamics/Kinetics

Distribution: V_{dss}: 0.49 L/kg

Protein binding, plasma: ~90%

Half-life elimination: Mean: 17 days (range: 13-21 days)

Time to peak, serum: Adults: Females: ~90 minutes; Males: ~10 minutes

Excretion: Feces; Clearance: Plasma: Total: 0.051 mL/minute/kg

Dosage I.V.: Adults: 2 mg/kg, followed by exposure to the appropriate laser light; repeat courses must be separated by at least 30 days (esophageal or endobronchial cancer) or 90 days (Barrett's esophagus); delay subsequent treatment for insufficient healing) for a maximum of 3 courses

Administration Administer slow I.V. injection over 3-5 minutes. Avoid contact with skin during administration.

Dosage Forms Excipient information presented when available (limited, particularly for generics); consult specific product labeling.

Injection, powder for reconstitution, as sodium:

Photofrin®: 75 mg

References

National Comprehensive Cancer Network® (NCCN), "Clinical Practice Guidelines in Oncology™: Gastric Cancer," Version 2.2009. Available at http://www.nccn.org/professionals/physician_gls/PDF/gastric.pdf.

National Comprehensive Cancer Network® (NCCN), "Clinical Practice Guidelines in Oncology™: Basal Cell and Squamous Cell Skin Cancers," Version 1.2008. Available at http://www.nccn.org/professionals/physician_gls/PDF/nmsc.pdf.

Rosenthal DI and Glatstein E, "Clinical Applications of Photodynamic Therapy," *Ann Med*, 1994, 26 (6):405-9.

◆ **Porfimer Sodium** see Porfimer on page 967

Posaconazole (poe sa KON a zole)

Medication Safety Issues

Sound-alike/look-alike issues:

Noxafil® may be confused with minoxidil

International issues:

Noxafil® may be confused with Noxidil® which is a brand name for minoxidil in Thailand

U.S. Brand Names Noxafil®

Index Terms SCH 56592

Generic Available No

Canadian Brand Names Posanol™

Pharmacologic Category Antifungal Agent, Oral

Use Prophylaxis of invasive *Aspergillus* and *Candida* infections in severely-immunocompromised patients [eg, hematopoietic stem cell transplant (HSCT)

recipients with graft-versus-host disease (GVHD) or those with prolonged neutropenia secondary to chemotherapy for hematologic malignancies]; treatment of oropharyngeal candidiasis (including patients refractory to itraconazole and/or fluconazole)

Unlabeled/Investigational Use Salvage therapy of refractory invasive fungal infections; mucormycosis

Pregnancy Risk Factor C

Lactation Excretion in breast milk unknown/not recommended

Labeled Contraindications Hypersensitivity to posaconazole or any component of the formulation; coadministration of cisapride, ergot alkaloids, pimozide, quinidine, or sirolimus

Warnings/Precautions Hepatic dysfunction has occurred, ranging from reversible mild/moderate increases of ALT, AST, alkaline phosphatase, total bilirubin, and/or clinical hepatitis to severe reactions (cholestasis, hepatic failure including death). Consider discontinuation of therapy in patients who develop clinical evidence of liver disease that may be secondary to posaconazole. Use caution in patients with an increased risk of arrhythmia (long QT syndrome, concurrent QT$_c$-prolonging drugs, hypokalemia). Correct electrolyte abnormalities (eg, potassium, magnesium, and calcium) before initiating therapy. Concurrent use may significantly increase cyclosporine levels and may result in rare serious adverse events (eg, nephrotoxicity, leukoencephalopathy, and death); dose reduction and close monitoring are recommended with initiation of posaconazole therapy.

Use caution in hypersensitivity with other azole antifungal agents; cross-reaction may occur, but has not been established. Consider alternative therapy or closely monitor for breakthrough fungal infections in patients receiving drugs that decrease absorption or increase the metabolism of posaconazole or in any patient unable to eat or tolerate an oral liquid nutritional supplement. Use caution in severe renal impairment or GI disturbances; monitor for break-through fungal infections. Safety and efficacy have not been established in children <13 years of age.

Adverse Reactions Note: A higher frequency of adverse reactions was observed in studies with refractory oropharyngeal candidiasis patients and percentages are included below.

>10%: Gastrointestinal: Diarrhea (3% to 11%)

1% to 10%:

Cardiovascular: QT$_c$ prolongation (≤4%), hypertension (≤1%)

Central nervous system: Headache (1% to 8%), dizziness (1% to 3%), fatigue (1% to 3%), insomnia (1% to 3%), fever (≤3%), somnolence (≤1%)

Dermatologic: Rash (1% to 4%), pruritus (1% to 2%)

Endocrine & metabolic: Hypokalemia (≤3%)

Gastrointestinal: Nausea (5% to 8%), vomiting (4% to 7%), abdominal pain (1% to 5%), flatulence (1% to 5%), anorexia (1% to 3%), mucositis (≤2%), dyspepsia (1% to 2%), xerostomia (1% to 2%), constipation (≤1%), taste perversion (≤1%)

Hematologic: Neutropenia (2% to 8%), anemia (≤3%), thrombocytopenia (≤2%)

Hepatic: ALT increased (2% to 17%), AST increased (2% to 17%), alkaline phosphatase increased (1% to 13%), bilirubin increased (2% to 9%), GGT increased (2% to 3%), hepatocellular damage (≤1%)

Neuromuscular & skeletal: Weakness (1% to 3%), myalgia (≤2%), tremor (≤1%)

Ocular: Blurred vision (≤1%)

Renal: Serum creatinine increased (≤2%)

<1%, postmarketing, and/or case reports: Adrenal insufficiency, allergic/hypersensitivity reactions, atrial fibrillation, cholestasis, ejection fraction decreased, hemolytic uremic syndrome, hepatic failure, hepatitis, jaundice, pulmonary embolus, syncope, thrombotic thrombocytopenic purpura, torsade de pointes

Drug Interactions

Metabolism/Transport Effects Inhibits CYP3A4 (strong)

Avoid Concomitant Use

Avoid concomitant use of Posaconazole with any of the following: Alfuzosin; Cisapride; Conivaptan; Dofetilide; Dronedarone; Efavirenz; Eplerenone; Ergot Derivatives; Everolimus; Halofantrine; Nilotinib; Nisoldipine; Pimozide; Proton Pump Inhibitors; QuiNIDine; Ranolazine; Rivaroxaban; Salmeterol; Silodosin; Sirolimus; Tolvaptan

Increased Effect/Toxicity

Posaconazole may increase the levels/effects of: Alfentanil; Alfuzosin; Almotriptan; Alosetron; Antineoplastic Agents (Vinca Alkaloids); Aprepitant; Benzodiazepines (metabolized by oxidation); Bosentan; BusPIRone; Busulfan; Calcium Channel Blockers; CarBAMazepine; Cardiac Glycosides; Ciclesonide; Cilostazol; Cinacalcet; Cisapride; Colchicine; Conivaptan; Corticosteroids (Orally Inhaled); Corticosteroids (Systemic); CycloSPORINE; CYP3A4 Substrates; Docetaxel; Dofetilide; Dronedarone; Dutasteride; Eletriptan; Eplerenone; Ergot Derivatives; Erlotinib; Eszopiclone; Everolimus; FentaNYL; Fesoterodine; Fosaprepitant; Gefitinib; Halofantrine; HMG-CoA Reductase Inhibitors; Imatinib; Irinotecan; Ixabepilone; Losartan; Macrolide Antibiotics; Maraviroc; Methadone; Nilotinib; Nisoldipine; Paricalcitol; Phenytoin; Phosphodiesterase 5 Inhibitors; Pimecrolimus; Pimozide; Protease Inhibitors; QuiNIDine; Ramelteon; Ranolazine; Repaglinide; Rifamycin Derivatives; Rivaroxaban; Salmeterol; Saxagliptin; Silodosin; Sirolimus; Solifenacin; Sorafenib; Sunitinib; Tacrolimus; Tadalafil; Temsirolimus; Tolterodine; Tolvaptan; Trimetrexate; Vitamin K Antagonists; Ziprasidone; Zolpidem

The levels/effects of Posaconazole may be increased by: Grapefruit Juice; Macrolide Antibiotics; Protease Inhibitors

Decreased Effect

Posaconazole may decrease the levels/effects of: Amphotericin B; Prasugrel; Saccharomyces boulardii

The levels/effects of Posaconazole may be decreased by: Antacids; Didanosine; Efavirenz; H2-Antagonists; Metoclopramide; Phenytoin; Proton Pump Inhibitors; Rifamycin Derivatives; Sucralfate

Ethanol/Nutrition/Herb Interactions Food: Bioavailability increased ~3 times when posaconazole is administered with a nonfat meal or an oral liquid nutritional supplement; increased ~4 times when administered with a high-fat meal. Grapefruit juice may decrease the levels/effects of posaconazole; concurrent use should be avoided.

Storage/Stability Store at 25°C (77°F); excursions permitted to 15°C to 30°C (59°C to 86°C). Do not freeze.

Mechanism of Action Interferes with fungal cytochrome P450 (latosterol-14α-demethylase) activity, decreasing ergosterol synthesis (principal sterol in fungal cell membrane) and inhibiting fungal cell membrane formation.

Pharmacodynamics/Kinetics

Absorption: Coadministration with food, liquid nutritional supplements, and/or acidic carbonated beverages (eg, ginger ale) increases absorption; fasting states do not provide sufficient absorption to ensure adequate plasma concentrations.

Distribution: V_d: 465-1774 L

Protein binding: >98%; predominantly bound to albumin

Metabolism: Not significantly metabolized; ~15% to 17% undergoes non-CYP-mediated metabolism, primarily via hepatic glucuronidation into metabolites

Half-life elimination: 35 hours (range: 20-66 hours)

Time to peak, plasma: ~3-5 hours

Excretion: Feces 71% to 77% (~66% of the total dose as unchanged drug); urine 13% to 14% (<0.2% of the total dose as unchanged drug)

Dosage Oral:

Children ≥13 years and Adults:

Aspergillosis, invasive:

Prophylaxis: 200 mg 3 times/day

Salvage treatment of refractory infection (unlabeled use): 200 mg 4 times/day initially; after disease stabilization may decrease frequency to 400 mg twice daily (Walsh, 2007). **Note:** Duration of therapy should be a minimum of 6-12 weeks or throughout period of immunosuppression.

Candidal infections:

Prophylaxis: 200 mg 3 times/day

Treatment of oropharyngeal infection: Initial: 100 mg twice daily for 1 day; maintenance: 100 mg once daily for 13 days

Treatment of refractory oropharyngeal infection: 400 mg twice daily

Adults: **Mucormycosis (unlabeled use):** 800 mg/day in 2 or 4 divided doses (Greenburg, 2006)

Dosage adjustment in renal impairment:

Mild-to-moderate renal insufficiency (Cl_{cr} 20-80 mL/minute): No adjustment necessary

Severe renal insufficiency (Cl_{cr} <20 mL/minute): No adjustment necessary; however, monitor for breakthrough fungal infections due to variability in posaconazole exposure.

Dosage adjustment in hepatic impairment:

Mild-to-severe hepatic insufficiency (Child-Pugh classes A, B, and C): No adjustment necessary

Clinical signs and symptoms of liver disease due to posaconazole: Consider discontinuing therapy

Administration Oral: Shake well before use. Must be administered during or within 20 minutes following a full meal or an oral liquid nutritional supplement; alternatively, posaconazole may be administered with an acidic carbonated beverage (eg, ginger ale). In patients able to swallow, administer oral suspension using dosing spoon provided by the manufacturer; spoon should be rinsed clean with water after each use and before storage.

Monitoring Parameters Hepatic function (eg, AST/ALT, alkaline phosphatase and bilirubin) prior to initiation and during treatment; renal function; electrolyte disturbances (eg, calcium, magnesium, potassium); CBC

Dietary Considerations Give during or within 20 minutes following a full meal or liquid nutritional supplement; alternatively, posaconazole may be administered with an acidic carbonated beverage (eg, ginger ale). Consider alternative antifungal therapy in patients with inadequate oral intake or severe diarrhea/vomiting; if alternative therapy is not an option, closely monitoring for breakthrough fungal infections. Adequate posaconazole absorption from GI tract and subsequent plasma concentrations are dependent on food for efficacy. Lower average plasma concentrations have been associated with an increased risk of treatment failure.

◀ **Dosage Forms** Excipient information presented when available (limited, particularly for generics); consult specific product labeling.

Suspension, oral:

Noxafil®: 40 mg/mL (123 mL) [contains sodium benzoate; delivers 105 mL of suspension; cherry flavor; packaged with calibrated dosing spoon]

References

Cornely OA, Maertens J, Winston DJ, et al, "Posaconazole vs. Fluconazole or Itraconazole Prophylaxis in Patients With Neutropenia," *N Engl J Med*, 2007, 356(4):348-59.

Herbrecht R, "Posaconazole: A Potent, Extended-Spectrum Triazole Anti-Fungal for the Treatment of Serious Fungal Infections," *Int J Clin Pract*, 2004, 58(6): 612-24.

National Comprehensive Cancer Network® (NCCN), "Clinical Practice Guidelines in Oncology™: Prevention and Treatment of Cancer-Related Infections," Version 1.2008. Available at http://www.nccn.org/professionals/physician_gls/PDF/infections.pdf.

Raad II, Graybill JR, Bustamante AB, "Safety of Long-Term Oral Posaconazole Use in the Treatment of Refractory Invasive Fungal Infections," *Clin Infect Dis*, 2006, 42(12):1726-34.

Ullmann AJ, Lipton JH, Vesole DH, et al, "Posaconazole or Fluconazole for Prophylaxis in Severe Graft-Versus-Host Disease," *N Engl J Med*, 2007, 356(4):335-47.

Walsh TJ, Anaissie EJ, Denning DW, et al, "Treatment of Aspergillosis: Clinical Practice Guidelines of the Infectious Diseases Society of America," *Clin Infect Dis*, 2008, 46(3):327-60.

Walsh RJ, Raad I, Patterson TF, "Treatment of Invasive Aspergillosis With Posaconazole in Patients Who are Refractory to or Intolerant of Conventional Therapy: An Externally Controlled Trial," *Clin Infect Dis*, 2007, 44(1):2-12.

◆ **Posanol™ (Can)** *see* Posaconazole *on page 970*

◆ **Post Peel Healing Balm [OTC]** *see* Hydrocortisone *on page 575*

Pralatrexate (pral a TREX ate)

Medication Safety Issues

Sound-alike/look-alike issues:

Pralatrexate may be confused with methotrexate, pemetrexed

Folotyn™ may be confused with Focalin®

High alert medication: The Institute for Safe Medication Practices (ISMP) includes this medication among its list of drug classes which have a heightened risk of causing significant patient harm when used in error.

Related Information

Safe Handling of Hazardous Drugs *on page 1517*

U.S. Brand Names Folotyn™

Index Terms PDX

Generic Available No

Pharmacologic Category Antineoplastic Agent, Antimetabolite (Antifolate)

Use Treatment of relapsed or refractory peripheral T-cell lymphoma (PTCL)

Pregnancy Risk Factor D

Lactation Excretion in breast milk unknown/not recommended

Labeled Contraindications There are no contraindications listed within the manufacturer's labeling.

Warnings/Precautions Hazardous agent - use appropriate precautions for handling and disposal. May cause bone marrow suppression (thrombocytopenia, neutropenia and anemia); may require dosage modification. Mucositis, including stomatitis or mucosal inflammation of gastrointestinal and genitourinary tracts, may occur with treatment; may require dosage modification. Prophylactic folic acid and vitamin B_{12} supplements are necessary to reduce hematologic toxicity and treatment-related mucositis.

Use with caution in patients with moderate-to-severe renal impairment (has not been studied in patients with renal impairment); monitor renal function and for systemic toxicity due to increased exposure. Concurrent use with drugs with substantial renal clearance (eg, NSAIDs, sulfamethoxazole/trimethoprim) may result in delayed pralatrexate clearance. Liver function test abnormalities have been observed with use; monitor liver function; persistent abnormalities may indicate hepatotoxicity and may require dosage modification.

Adverse Reactions

>10%:

Cardiovascular: Edema (30%)

Central nervous system: Fatigue (36%), fever (32%)

Dermatologic: Rash (15%), pruritus (14%)

Endocrine & metabolic: Hypokalemia (15%)

Gastrointestinal: Mucositis (70%; grade 3: 17%; grade 4: 4%), nausea (40%), constipation (33%), vomiting (25%), diarrhea (21%), anorexia (15%), abdominal pain (12%)

Hematologic: Thrombocytopenia (41%; grade 3: 14%; grade 4: 19%), anemia (34%; grade 4: 2%), neutropenia (24%; grade 3: 13%; grade 4: 7%), leukopenia (11%; grade 4: 4%)

Hepatic: Transaminases increased (13%; grade 3: 5%; grade 4: 0%)

Neuromuscular & skeletal: Limb pain (12%), back pain (11%)

Respiratory: Cough (28%), epistaxis (26%), dyspnea (19%), pharyngolaryngeal pain (14%)

Miscellaneous: Night sweats (11%), infection

1% to 10%:

Cardiovascular: Tachycardia (10%)

Endocrine & metabolic: Dehydration (serious >3%)

Hematologic: Neutropenic fever (serious >3%)

Neuromuscular & skeletal: Weakness (10%)

Respiratory: Upper respiratory infection (10%)

Miscellaneous: Sepsis (serious >3%)

<1%, postmarketing, and/or case reports: Bowel obstruction, cardiopulmonary arrest, lymphopenia, odynophagia, pancytopenia

Drug Interactions

Avoid Concomitant Use

Avoid concomitant use of Pralatrexate with any of the following: Natalizumab; Vaccines (Live)

Increased Effect/Toxicity

Pralatrexate may increase the levels/effects of: Leflunomide; Natalizumab; Vaccines (Live); Vitamin K Antagonists

The levels/effects of Pralatrexate may be increased by: Nonsteroidal Anti-Inflammatory Agents; Penicillins; Salicylates; Sulfonamide Derivatives; Trastuzumab; Trimethoprim; Uricosuric Agents

Decreased Effect

Pralatrexate may decrease the levels/effects of: Cardiac Glycosides; Sapropterin; Vaccines (Inactivated); Vaccines (Live); Vitamin K Antagonists

The levels/effects of Pralatrexate may be decreased by: Echinacea

Storage/Stability Store intact vials refrigerated at 2°C to 8°C (36°F to 46°F). Store in original carton and protect from light until use. Unopened vials (stored in the original carton) are stable for up to 72 hours at room temperature (discard after 72 hours).

Reconstitution Use appropriate precautions for handling (hazardous agent). Withdraw into syringe for administration; do not dilute (manufacturer recommends immediate use after placing in syringe). Discard unused portion in the vial.

Compatibility Y-site administration: **Compatible:** Normal saline

Mechanism of Action Antifolate analog; inhibits DNA, RNA, and protein synthesis by selectively entering cells expressing reduced folate carrier (RFC-1), is polyglutamylated by folylpolyglutamate synthetase (FPGS) and then competes for the DHFR-folate binding site to inhibit dihydrofolate reductase (DHFR)

Pharmacodynamics/Kinetics

Distribution: *S*-diastereomer: 105 L; *R*-diastereomer: 37 L

Protein binding: ~67%

Half-life elimination: 12-18 hours

Excretion: Urine (~34% as unchanged drug)

Dosage Note: Start vitamin supplements 1 week before initial pemetrexed dose: Folic acid 1-1.25 mg/day orally beginning within 10 days prior to initiating pralatrexate (continue during treatment and for 30 days after last pralatrexate dose) and vitamin B_{12} 1000 mcg I.M. within 10 weeks prior to treatment and every 8-10 weeks thereafter (after initial dose, B_{12} may be administered on the same day as pralatrexate).

Prior to administering any dose, mucositis should be ≤grade 1, platelets should be ≥100,000/mm^3 for the first dose and ≥50,000/mm^3 for subsequent doses, and absolute neutrophil count (ANC) should be ≥1000/mm^3.

I.V.: Adults: PTCL: 30 mg/m^2 once weekly for 6 weeks of a 7-week treatment cycle (continue until disease progression or unacceptable toxicity)

Dosage adjustment for toxicity: Severe or intolerable adverse events may require dose omission, reduction or interruption. Do not make up omitted doses at the end of the cycle; do not re-escalate dose after a reduction due to toxicity.

Hematologic toxicity:

Platelets:

<50,000/mm^3 (for 1-week duration): Omit dose; continue at previous dose if platelets recover within 1 week

<50,000/mm^3 (for 2-week duration): Omit dose; decrease to 20 mg/m^2 if platelets recover within 2 weeks

<50,000/mm^3 (for 3-week duration): Discontinue treatment

ANC:

500-1000/mm^3 without fever (for 1-week duration): Omit dose; continue at previous dose if ANC recovers within 1 week

500-1000/mm^3 with fever **or** ANC <500/mm^3 (for 1-week duration): Omit dose, give filgrastim or sargramostim support; continue at previous dose (with growth factor support) if ANC recovers within 1 week

500-1000/mm^3 with fever **or** ANC <500/mm^3 (recurrent or for 2-week duration): Omit dose and give filgrastim or sargramostim support; decrease to 20 mg/m^2 (with growth factor support) if ANC recovers within 2 weeks

500-1000/mm^3 with fever **or** ANC <500/mm^3 (second recurrence or for 3-week duration): Discontinue treatment

Nonhematologic toxicity: Mucositis (on day of treatment):

Grade 2: Omit dose; continue at previous dose when recovers to ≤grade 1

Grade 3 or recurrent grade 2: Omit dose and decrease to 20 mg/m^2 when recovers to ≤grade 1

Grade 4: Discontinue treatment

Nonhematologic toxicity: Other than mucositis:

Grade 3: Omit dose; decrease to 20 mg/m^2 when recovers to ≤grade 2

Grade 4: Discontinue treatment

Dosage adjustment in renal impairment: Moderate-to-severe renal impairment: Use with caution (has not been studied in patients with renal impairment). Monitor for possible systemic toxicity due to increased exposure.

Dosage adjustment in hepatic impairment: Patients with total bilirubin >1.5 mg/dL, AST or ALT >2.5 times the upper limit of normal (ULN), and ALT or AST >5 times ULN if documented hepatic lymphoma involvement were excluded from clinical trials. Persistent abnormalities may indicate hepatotoxicity requiring dosage modification; refer to dosage adjustment for nonhematologic (other than mucositis) toxicity for adjustment recommendations.

Administration Administer I.V. push over 3-5 minutes into the line of a free-flowing normal saline I.V.

Monitoring Parameters CBC with differential (weekly), serum chemistries, including renal and liver function tests (prior to the first and fourth doses in each cycle); mucositis severity (weekly)

Dosage Forms Excipient information presented when available (limited, particularly for generics); consult specific product labeling.
Injection, solution [preservative free]:
Folotyn™: 20 mg/mL (1 mL, 2 mL)

References

Izbicka E, Diaz A, Streeper R, et al, "Distinct Mechanistic Activity Profile of Pralatrexate in Comparison to Other Antifolates in *in vitro* and *in vivo* Models of Human Cancers," *Cancer Chemother Pharmacol*, 2009, 64(5): 993-9.

O'Connor OA, Horwitz S, Hamlin P, et al, "Phase II-I-II Study of Two Different Doses and Schedules of Pralatrexate, a High-Affinity Substrate for the Reduced Folate Carrier, in Patients With Relapsed or Refractory Lymphoma Reveals Marked Activity in T-Cell Malignancies," *J Clin Oncol*, 2009, 27(26):4357-64.

O'Connor O, Pro B, Pinter-Brown L, et al, "PROPEL: Results of the Pivotal, Multicenter, Phase II Study of Pralatrexate in Patients With Relapsed or Refractory Peripheral T-Cell Lymphoma (PTCL)," *J Clin Oncol*, 2009, 27(15S) [abstract 8561 from 2009 ASCO Annual Meeting]

◆ **Pred Forte®** see PrednisoLONE *on page 977*

◆ **Pred Mild®** see PrednisoLONE *on page 977*

PrednisoLONE (pred NISS oh lone)

Medication Safety Issues

Sound-alike/look-alike issues:
PrednisoLONE may be confused with predniSONE
Pediapred® may be confused with Pediazole®
Prelone® may be confused with Prozac®

U.S. Brand Names Econopred® Plus [DSC]; Millipred™; Omnipred™; Orapred ODT®; Orapred®; Pediapred®; Pred Forte®; Pred Mild®; Prelone®; Veripred™ 20

Index Terms Deltahydrocortisone; Metacortandralone; Prednisolone Acetate; Prednisolone Acetate, Ophthalmic; Prednisolone Sodium Phosphate; Prednisolone Sodium Phosphate, Ophthalmic

Generic Available Yes

Canadian Brand Names Diopred®; Hydeltra T.B.A.®; Inflamase® Mild; Novo-Prednisolone; Ophtho-Tate®; Pediapred®; Pred Forte®; Pred Mild®; Sab-Prenase

Pharmacologic Category Corticosteroid, Ophthalmic; Corticosteroid, Systemic

Use Treatment of palpebral and bulbar conjunctivitis; corneal injury from chemical, radiation, thermal burns, or foreign body penetration; endocrine disorders, rheumatic disorders, collagen diseases, dermatologic diseases, allergic states, ophthalmic diseases, respiratory diseases, hematologic disorders, neoplastic diseases, edematous states, and gastrointestinal diseases; resolution of acute exacerbations of multiple sclerosis; management of fulminating or disseminated tuberculosis and trichinosis; acute or chronic solid organ rejection

Pregnancy Risk Factor C

Lactation Enters breast milk/use caution (AAP rates "compatible")

Labeled Contraindications Hypersensitivity to prednisolone or any component of the formulation; acute superficial herpes simplex keratitis; live or attenuated virus vaccines (with immunosuppressive doses of corticosteroids); systemic fungal infections; varicella

Warnings/Precautions May cause hypercorticism or suppression of hypothalamic-pituitary-adrenal (HPA) axis, particularly in younger children or in patients receiving high doses for prolonged periods. HPA axis suppression may lead to adrenal crisis. Withdrawal and discontinuation of a corticosteroid should be done slowly and carefully. Particular care is required when patients are transferred from systemic corticosteroids to inhaled products due to possible adrenal insufficiency or withdrawal from steroids, including an increase in allergic symptoms. Patients receiving >20 mg per day of prednisone (or equivalent) may be most susceptible. Fatalities have occurred due to adrenal insufficiency in asthmatic patients during and after transfer from systemic corticosteroids to aerosol steroids; aerosol steroids do **not** provide the systemic steroid needed to treat patients having trauma, surgery, or infections.

Acute myopathy has been reported with high dose corticosteroids, usually in patients with neuromuscular transmission disorders; may involve ocular and/or respiratory muscles; monitor creatine kinase; recovery may be delayed. Corticosteroid use may cause psychiatric disturbances, including depression, euphoria, insomnia, mood swings, and personality changes. Pre-existing psychiatric conditions may be exacerbated by corticosteroid use. Prolonged use of corticosteroids may also increase the incidence of secondary infection, mask acute infection (including fungal infections), prolong or exacerbate viral infections, or limit response to vaccines. Exposure to chickenpox should be avoided; corticosteroids should not be used to treat ocular herpes simplex. Corticosteroids should not be used for cerebral malaria or viral hepatitis. Close observation is required in patients with latent tuberculosis and/or TB reactivity; restrict use in active TB (only in conjunction with antituberculosis treatment). Prolonged use of corticosteroids may result in glaucoma; damage to the optic nerve (not indicated for treatment of optic neuritis), defects in visual acuity and fields of vision, and posterior subcapsular cataract formation may occur. Use following cataract surgery may delay healing or increase the incidence of bleb formation. Prolonged treatment with corticosteroids has been associated with the development of Kaposi's sarcoma (case reports); if noted, discontinuation of therapy should be considered.

Use with caution in patients with thyroid disease, hepatic impairment, renal impairment, cardiovascular disease, diabetes, glaucoma, cataracts, myasthenia gravis, patients at risk for osteoporosis, patients at risk for seizures, or GI diseases (diverticulitis, peptic ulcer, ulcerative colitis) due to perforation risk. Use caution following acute MI (corticosteroids have been associated with myocardial rupture). Because of the risk of adverse effects, systemic corticosteroids should be used cautiously in the elderly in the smallest possible effective dose for the shortest duration. Do not use occlusive dressings on weeping or exudative lesions and general caution with occlusive dressings should be observed; adverse effects may be increased. Discontinue if skin irritation or contact dermatitis should occur; do not use in patients with decreased skin circulation. Withdraw therapy with gradual tapering of dose. May affect growth velocity; growth should be routinely monitored in pediatric patients.

Adverse Reactions Frequency not defined.

Ophthalmic formulation:

Endocrine & metabolic: Hypercorticoidism (rare)

Ocular: Conjunctival hyperemia, conjunctivitis, corneal ulcers, delayed wound healing, glaucoma, intraocular pressure increased, keratitis, loss of accommodation, optic nerve damage, mydriasis, posterior subcapsular cataract formation, ptosis, secondary ocular infection

Oral formulation:

Cardiovascular: Cardiomyopathy, CHF, edema, facial edema, hypertension

Central nervous system: Convulsions, headache, insomnia, malaise, nervousness, pseudotumor cerebri, psychic disorders, vertigo

Dermatologic: Bruising, facial erythema, hirsutism, petechiae, skin test reaction suppression, thin fragile skin, urticaria

Endocrine & metabolic: Carbohydrate tolerance decreased, Cushing's syndrome, diabetes mellitus, growth suppression, hyperglycemia, hypernatremia, hypokalemia, hypokalemic alkalosis, menstrual irregularities, negative nitrogen balance, pituitary adrenal axis suppression

Gastrointestinal: Abdominal distention, increased appetite, indigestion, nausea, pancreatitis, peptic ulcer, ulcerative esophagitis, weight gain

Hepatic: LFTs increased (usually reversible)

Neuromuscular & skeletal: Arthralgia, aseptic necrosis (humeral/femoral heads), fractures, muscle mass decreased, muscle weakness, osteoporosis, steroid myopathy, tendon rupture, weakness

Ocular: Cataracts, exophthalmus, eyelid edema, glaucoma, intraocular pressure increased, irritation

Respiratory: Epistaxis

Miscellaneous: Diaphoresis increased, impaired wound healing

Drug Interactions

Metabolism/Transport Effects Substrate of CYP3A4 (minor); **Inhibits** CYP3A4 (weak)

Avoid Concomitant Use

Avoid concomitant use of PrednisoLONE with any of the following: Natalizumab; Vaccines (Live)

Increased Effect/Toxicity

PrednisoLONE may increase the levels/effects of: Acetylcholinesterase Inhibitors; Amphotericin B; CycloSPORINE; Leflunomide; Loop Diuretics; Natalizumab; NSAID (COX-2 Inhibitor); NSAID (Nonselective); Thiazide Diuretics; Vaccines (Live); Warfarin

The levels/effects of PrednisoLONE may be increased by: Antifungal Agents (Azole Derivatives, Systemic); Aprepitant; Calcium Channel Blockers (Nondihydropyridine); CycloSPORINE; Estrogen Derivatives; Fluconazole; Fosaprepitant; Macrolide Antibiotics; Neuromuscular-Blocking Agents (Nondepolarizing); Quinolone Antibiotics; Salicylates; Trastuzumab

Decreased Effect

PrednisoLONE may decrease the levels/effects of: Antidiabetic Agents; Calcitriol; Corticorelin; Isoniazid; Salicylates; Vaccines (Inactivated); Vaccines (Live)

The levels/effects of PrednisoLONE may be decreased by: Amino-glutethimide; Antacids; Barbiturates; Bile Acid Sequestrants; Echinacea; Mitotane; Primidone; Rifamycin Derivatives

Ethanol/Nutrition/Herb Interactions

Ethanol: Avoid ethanol (may increase gastric mucosal irritation).

Food: Prednisolone interferes with calcium absorption. Limit caffeine.

Herb/Nutraceutical: St John's wort may decrease prednisolone levels. Avoid cat's claw, echinacea (have immunostimulant properties).

Storage/Stability Store Orapred ODT® at 20°C to 25°C (68°F to 77°F) in blister pack. Protect from moisture.

Mechanism of Action Decreases inflammation by suppression of migration of polymorphonuclear leukocytes and reversal of increased capillary permeability; suppresses the immune system by reducing activity and volume of the lymphatic system

Pharmacodynamics/Kinetics

Duration: 18-36 hours

Protein binding (concentration dependent): 65% to 91%; decreased in elderly

Metabolism: Primarily hepatic, but also metabolized in most tissues, to inactive compounds

Half-life elimination: 3.6 hours; End-stage renal disease: 3-5 hours

Excretion: Primarily urine (as glucuronides, sulfates, and unconjugated metabolites)

Dosage Dose depends upon condition being treated and response of patient; dosage for infants and children should be based on severity of the disease and response of the patient rather than on strict adherence to dosage indicated by age, weight, or body surface area. Oral dosage expressed in terms of prednisolone base. Consider alternate day therapy for long-term therapy. Discontinuation of long-term therapy requires gradual withdrawal by tapering the dose. Patients undergoing unusual stress while receiving corticosteroids, should receive increased doses prior to, during, and after the stressful situation.

Children: Oral:

Acute asthma: 1-2 mg/kg/day in divided doses 1-2 times/day for 3-5 days

Anti-inflammatory or immunosuppressive dose: 0.1-2 mg/kg/day in divided doses 1-4 times/day

Nephrotic syndrome:

Initial (first 3 episodes): 2 mg/kg/day **or** 60 mg/m^2/day (maximum: 80 mg/day) in divided doses 3-4 times/day until urine is protein free for 3 consecutive days (maximum: 28 days); followed by 1-1.5 mg/kg/dose **or** 40 mg/m^2/dose given every other day for 4 weeks

Maintenance (long-term maintenance dose for frequent relapses): 0.5-1 mg/kg/dose given every other day for 3-6 months

Adults: Oral:

Usual range: 5-60 mg/day

Multiple sclerosis: 200 mg/day for 1 week followed by 80 mg every other day for 1 month

Rheumatoid arthritis: Initial: 5-7.5 mg/day; adjust dose as necessary

Ophthalmic suspension/solution: Conjunctivitis, corneal injury: Children and Adults: Instill 1-2 drops into conjunctival sac every hour during day, every 2 hours at night until favorable response is obtained, then use 1 drop every 4 hours.

Elderly: Use lowest effective dose

Dosing adjustment in hyperthyroidism: Prednisolone dose may need to be increased to achieve adequate therapeutic effects

Hemodialysis: Slightly dialyzable (5% to 20%); administer dose posthemodialysis

Peritoneal dialysis: Supplemental dose is not necessary

Combination Regimens

Lymphoma, Hodgkin's:

LOPP on page 1363

MOPP (Lymphoma, Hodgkin's Disease) on page 1372

Administration Administer oral formulation with food or milk to decrease GI effects.

Orapred ODT®: Do not break or use partial tablet. Remove tablet from blister pack just prior to use. May swallow whole or allow to dissolve on tongue.

Monitoring Parameters Blood pressure; blood glucose, electrolytes; intra-ocular pressure (use >6 weeks); bone mineral density

Test Interactions Response to skin tests

Dietary Considerations Should be taken after meals or with food or milk to decrease GI effects; increase dietary intake of pyridoxine, vitamin C, vitamin D, folate, calcium, and phosphorus.

Dosage Forms Excipient information presented when available (limited, particularly for generics); consult specific product labeling. [DSC] = Discontinued product

Solution, ophthalmic, as sodium phosphate: 1% (5 mL, 10 mL, 15 mL) [contains benzalkonium chloride]

Solution, oral, as base: 15 mg/5 mL (240 mL, 480 mL)

Solution, oral, as sodium phosphate: Prednisolone base 5 mg/5 mL (120 mL, 240 mL); prednisolone base 15 mg/5 mL (240 mL)

Millipred™: Prednisolone base 10 mg/5 mL (237 mL) [dye free; grape flavor]

Orapred®: Prednisolone base 15 mg/5 mL (20 mL, 240 mL) [dye free; contains ethanol 2%, sodium benzoate; grape flavor]

Pediapred®: Prednisolone base 5 mg/5 mL (120 mL) [dye free; raspberry flavor]

Veripred™ 20: Prednisolone base 20 mg/5 mL (237 mL) [dye free, ethanol free; grape flavor]

Suspension, ophthalmic, as acetate: 1% (5 mL, 10 mL, 15 mL)

Econopred® Plus [DSC], Omnipred™: 1% (5 mL, 10 mL) [contains benzalkonium chloride]

Pred Forte®: 1% (1 mL, 5 mL, 10 mL, 15 mL) [contains benzalkonium chloride and sodium bisulfite]

Pred Mild®: 0.12% (5 mL, 10 mL) [contains benzalkonium chloride and sodium bisulfite]

Syrup, as base: 5 mg/5 mL (120 mL); 15 mg/5 mL (5 mL [DSC], 240 mL, 480 mL)

Prelone®: 15 mg/5 mL (240 mL, 480 mL) [contains ethanol 5%, benzoic acid, propylene glycol; wild cherry flavor]

Tablet, as base: 5 mg

Tablet, orally disintegrating, as sodium phosphate [strength expressed as base]:

Orapred ODT®: 10 mg, 15 mg, 30 mg [grape flavor]

References

Annane D, Sebille V, Charpentier C, et al, "Effect of Treatment With Low Doses of Hydrocortisone and Fludrocortisone on Mortality in Patients With Septic Shock," *JAMA*, 2002, 288(7):862-71.

Cooper MS and Stewart PM, "Corticosteroid Insufficiency in Acutely Ill Patients," *N Engl J Med*, 2003, 348(8):727-34.

Coursin DB and Wood KE, "Corticosteroid Supplementation for Adrenal Insufficiency," *JAMA*, 2002, 287(2):236-40.

Frey BM and Frey FJ, "Clinical Pharmacokinetics of Prednisone and Prednisolone," *Clin Pharmacokinet*, 1990, 19(2):126-46.

Frey FJ, "Kinetics and Dynamics of Prednisolone," *Endocr Rev*, 1987, 8(4):453-73.

Gambertoglio JG, Amend WJ Jr and Benet LZ, "Pharmacokinetics and Bioavailability of Prednisone and Prednisolone in Healthy Volunteers and Patients: A Review," *J Pharmacokinet Biopharm*, 1980, 8(1):1-52.

Goedert JJ, Vitale F, Lauria C, et al, "Risk Factors for Classical Kaposi's Sarcoma," *J Natl Cancer Inst*, 2002, 94(22):1712-8.

Hotchkiss RS and Karl IE, "The Pathophysiology and Treatment of Sepsis," *N Engl J Med*, 2003, 348(2):138-50.

Report of a Workshop by the British Association for Paediatric Nephrology and Research Unit, Royal College of Physicians, "Consensus Statement on Management and Audit Potential for Steroid Responsive Nephrotic Syndrome," *Arch Dis Child*, 1994, 70(2):151-7.

Salem M, Tainsh RE Jr, Bromberg J, et al, "Perioperative Glucocorticoid Coverage. A Reassessment 42 Years After Emergence of a Problem," *Ann Surg*, 1994, 219(4):416-25.

◆ **Prednisolone Acetate** *see* PrednisoLONE *on page* 977

◆ **Prednisolone Acetate, Ophthalmic** *see* PrednisoLONE *on page* 977

◆ **Prednisolone Sodium Phosphate** *see* PrednisoLONE *on page* 977

◆ **Prednisolone Sodium Phosphate, Ophthalmic** *see* PrednisoLONE *on page* 977

PredniSONE (PRED ni sone)

Medication Safety Issues

Sound-alike/look-alike issues:

PredniSONE may be confused with methylPREDNISolone, Pramosone®, prazosin, prednisoLONE, Prilosec®, primidone, promethazine

U.S. Brand Names PredniSONE Intensol™; Sterapred®; Sterapred® DS

Index Terms Deltacortisone; Deltadehydrocortisone

Generic Available Yes

Canadian Brand Names Apo-Prednisone®; Novo-Prednisone; Winpred™

Pharmacologic Category Corticosteroid, Systemic

Use Treatment of a variety of diseases, including:

Allergic states (including adjunctive treatment of anaphylaxis)

Autoimmune disorders (including systemic lupus erythematosus [SLE])

Collagen diseases

Dermatologic conditions/diseases

Edematous states (including nephrotic syndrome)

Endocrine disorders

Gastrointestinal diseases

Hematologic disorders (including idiopathic thrombocytopenia purpura [ITP])

Multiple sclerosis exacerbations

Neoplastic diseases

Ophthalmic diseases

Respiratory diseases (including acute asthma exacerbation)

Rheumatic disorders (including rheumatoid arthritis)

Trichinosis with neurologic or myocardial involvement

Tuberculous meningitis

Unlabeled/Investigational Use Adjunctive therapy for *Pneumocystis jiroveci* (formerly *carinii*) pneumonia (PCP); autoimmune hepatitis; adjunctive therapy for pain management in immunocompetent patients with herpes zoster; tuberculosis (severe, paradoxical reactions)

Lactation Enters breast milk/AAP rates "compatible"

Labeled Contraindications Hypersensitivity to any component of the formulation; systemic fungal infections; administration of live or live attenuated vaccines with immunosuppressive doses of prednisone

Warnings/Precautions May cause hypercorticism or suppression of hypothalamic-pituitary-adrenal (HPA) axis, particularly in younger children or in patients receiving high doses for prolonged periods. HPA axis suppression may lead to adrenal crisis. Withdrawal and discontinuation of a corticosteroid should be done slowly and carefully. Particular care is required when patients are transferred from systemic corticosteroids to inhaled products due to possible adrenal insufficiency or withdrawal from steroids, including an increase in allergic symptoms. Patients receiving >20 mg per day of prednisone (or equivalent) may be most susceptible. Fatalities have occurred due to adrenal insufficiency in asthmatic patients during and after transfer from systemic corticosteroids to aerosol steroids; aerosol steroids do **not** provide the systemic steroid needed to treat patients having trauma, surgery, or infections.

Acute myopathy has been reported with high dose corticosteroids, usually in patients with neuromuscular transmission disorders; may involve ocular and/or respiratory muscles; monitor creatine kinase; recovery may be delayed. Prolonged use of corticosteroids may increase the incidence of secondary infection, mask acute infection (including fungal infections), prolong or exacerbate viral infections, or limit response to vaccines. Exposure to chickenpox should be avoided. Corticosteroids should not be used to treat ocular herpes simplex or cerebral malaria. Close observation is required in patients with latent tuberculosis and/or TB reactivity; restrict use in active TB (only in conjunction with antituberculosis treatment). Prolonged treatment with corticosteroids has been associated with the development of Kaposi's sarcoma (case reports); if noted, discontinuation of therapy should be considered. Prolonged use may cause posterior subcapsular cataracts, glaucoma (with possible nerve damage) and may increase the risk for ocular infections. Corticosteroid use may cause psychiatric disturbances, including depression, euphoria, insomnia, mood swings, and personality changes. Pre-existing psychiatric conditions may be exacerbated by corticosteroid use.

Use with caution in patients with HF, diabetes, GI diseases (diverticulitis, peptic ulcer, ulcerative colitis; due to risk of perforation), hepatic impairment, myasthenia gravis, MI, patients with or who are at risk for osteoporosis, seizure disorders or thyroid disease. May affect growth velocity; growth should be routinely monitored in pediatric patients.

Prior to use, the dose and duration of treatment should be based on the risk versus benefit for each individual patient. In general, use the smallest effective dose for the shortest duration of time to minimize adverse events. A gradual tapering of dose may be required prior to discontinuing therapy.

Adverse Reactions Frequency not defined.

Cardiovascular: Congestive heart failure (in susceptible patients), hypertension

Central nervous system: Emotional instability, headache, intracranial pressure increased (with papilledema), psychic derangements (including euphoria, insomnia, mood swings, personality changes, severe depression), seizure, vertigo

Dermatologic: Bruising, facial erythema, petechiae, thin fragile skin, urticaria, wound healing impaired

Endocrine & metabolic: Adrenocortical and pituitary unresponsiveness (in times of stress), carbohydrate intolerance, Cushing's syndrome, diabetes mellitus, fluid retention, growth suppression (in children), hypokalemic

◀

alkalosis, hypothyroidism enhanced, menstrual irregularities, negative nitrogen balance due to protein catabolism, potassium loss, sodium retention

Gastrointestinal: Abdominal distension, pancreatitis, peptic ulcer (with possible perforation and hemorrhage), ulcerative esophagitis

Hepatic: ALT increased, AST increased, alkaline phosphatase increased

Neuromuscular & skeletal: Aseptic necrosis of femoral and humeral heads, muscle mass loss, muscle weakness, osteoporosis, pathologic fracture of long bones, steroid myopathy, tendon rupture (particularly Achilles tendon), vertebral compression fractures

Ocular: Exophthalmos, glaucoma, intraocular pressure increased, posterior subcapsular cataracts

Miscellaneous: Allergic reactions, anaphylactic reactions, diaphoresis, hypersensitivity reactions, infections, Kaposi's sarcoma

Drug Interactions

Metabolism/Transport Effects Substrate of CYP3A4 (minor); **Induces** CYP2C19 (weak), 3A4 (weak)

Avoid Concomitant Use

Avoid concomitant use of PredniSONE with any of the following: Natalizumab; Vaccines (Live)

Increased Effect/Toxicity

PredniSONE may increase the levels/effects of: Acetylcholinesterase Inhibitors; Amphotericin B; CycloSPORINE; Leflunomide; Loop Diuretics; Natalizumab; NSAID (COX-2 Inhibitor); NSAID (Nonselective); Thiazide Diuretics; Vaccines (Live); Warfarin

The levels/effects of PredniSONE may be increased by: Antifungal Agents (Azole Derivatives, Systemic); Aprepitant; Calcium Channel Blockers (Nondihydropyridine); CycloSPORINE; Estrogen Derivatives; Fluconazole; Fosaprepitant; Macrolide Antibiotics; Neuromuscular-Blocking Agents (Nondepolarizing); Quinolone Antibiotics; Salicylates; Trastuzumab

Decreased Effect

PredniSONE may decrease the levels/effects of: Antidiabetic Agents; Calcitriol; Corticorelin; Isoniazid; Salicylates; Vaccines (Inactivated); Vaccines (Live)

The levels/effects of PredniSONE may be decreased by: Aminoglutethimide; Antacids; Barbiturates; Bile Acid Sequestrants; Echinacea; Mitotane; Primidone; Rifamycin Derivatives; Somatropin

Ethanol/Nutrition/Herb Interactions

Ethanol: Avoid ethanol (may increase gastric mucosal irritation)

Food: Prednisone interferes with calcium absorption. Limit caffeine.

Herb/Nutraceutical: St John's wort may decrease prednisone levels. Avoid cat's claw, echinacea (have immunostimulant properties).

Mechanism of Action Decreases inflammation by suppression of migration of polymorphonuclear leukocytes and reversal of increased capillary permeability; suppresses the immune system by reducing activity and volume of the lymphatic system; suppresses adrenal function at high doses. Antitumor effects may be related to inhibition of glucose transport, phosphorylation, or induction of cell death in immature lymphocytes. Antiemetic effects are thought to occur due to blockade of cerebral innervation of the emetic center via inhibition of prostaglandin synthesis.

Pharmacodynamics/Kinetics

Absorption: 50% to 90% (may be altered in IBS or hyperthyroidism)

Protein binding (concentration dependent): 65% to 91%

Metabolism: Hepatically converted from prednisone (inactive) to prednisolone (active); may be impaired with hepatic dysfunction

Half-life elimination: Normal renal function: ~3.5 hours

Excretion: Urine (small portion)

Dosage Oral:

General dosing range: Children and Adults: Initial: 5-60 mg/day: **Note:** Dose depends upon condition being treated and response of patient; dosage for infants and children should be based on severity of the disease and response of the patient rather than on strict adherence to dosage indicated by age, weight, or body surface area. Consider alternate day therapy for long-term therapy. Discontinuation of long-term therapy requires gradual withdrawal by tapering the dose.

Prednisone taper (other regimens also available):

Day 1: 30 mg divided as 10 mg before breakfast, 5 mg at lunch, 5 mg at dinner, 10 mg at bedtime

Day 2: 5 mg at breakfast, 5 mg at lunch, 5 mg at dinner, 10 mg at bedtime

Day 3: 5 mg 4 times/day (with meals and at bedtime)

Day 4: 5 mg 3 times/day (breakfast, lunch, bedtime)

Day 5: 5 mg 2 times/day (breakfast, bedtime)

Day 6: 5 mg before breakfast

Indication-specific dosing:

Children:

Acute asthma (NIH guidelines, 2007):
0-11 years 1-2 mg/kg/day for 3-10 days (maximum: 60 mg/day)
≥12 years: Refer to Adults dosing

Autoimmune hepatitis (unlabeled use; Czaja 2002): Initial treatment: 2 mg/kg/day for 2 weeks (maximum: 60 mg/day), followed by a taper over 6-8 weeks to a dose of 0.1-0.2 mg/kg/day or 5 mg/day

Nephrotic syndrome (Pediatric Nephrology Panel recommendations [Hogg, 2000]): Initial: 2 mg/kg/day or 60 mg/m^2/day given every day in 1-3 divided doses (maximum: 80 mg/day) until urine is protein free or for 4-6 weeks; followed by maintenance dose: 2 mg/kg/dose or 40 mg/m^2/dose given every other day in the morning; gradually taper and discontinue after 4-6 weeks. **Note:** No definitive treatment guidelines exist. Dosing is dependant on institution protocols and individual response.

PCP pneumonia (AIDSinfo guidelines, 2008): 1 mg/kg twice daily for 5 days, *followed by* 0.5-1 mg/kg twice daily for 5 days, *followed by* 0.5 mg/kg once daily for 11-21 days

Adolescents and Adults:

PCP pneumonia (AIDSinfo guidelines, 2008): Note: Begin within 72 hours of PCP therapy: 40 mg twice daily for 5 days, *followed by* 40 mg once daily for 5 days, *followed by* 20 mg once daily for 11 days or until antimicrobial regimen is completed

Adults:

Acute asthma (NIH guidelines, 2007): 40-60 mg per day for 3-10 days; administer as single or 2 divided doses

Anaphylaxis, adjunctive treatment (Lieberman 2005): 0.5 mg/kg

Antineoplastic: Usual range: 10 mg/day to 100 mg/m^2/day (depending on indication). **Note:** Details concerning dosing in combination regimens should also be consulted.

Autoimmune hepatitis (unlabeled use; Czaja 2002): Initial treatment: 60 mg/day for 1 week, *followed by* 40 mg/day for 1 week, *then* 30 mg/day for 2 weeks, *then* 20 mg/day. Half this dose should be given when used in combination with azathioprine

Herpes zoster (unlabeled use; Dworkin 2007): 60 mg/day for 7 days, *followed by* 30 mg/day for 7 days, *then* 15 mg/day for 7 days

Idiopathic thrombocytopenia purpura (American Society of Hematology 1997): 1-2 mg/kg/day

Rheumatoid arthritis (American College of Rheumatology 2002): ≤10 mg/day

Systemic lupus erythematosus (American College of Rheumatology 1999):

Mild SLE: ≤10 mg/day

Refractory or severe organ-threatening disease: 20-60 mg/day

Thyrotoxicosis (type II amiodarone induced; unlabeled use): 30-40 mg/day for 7-14 days, gradually taper over 3 months

Tuberculosis, severe, paradoxical reactions (unlabeled use, AIDSinfo guidelines 2008): 1 mg/kg/day, gradually reduce after 1-2 weeks

Elderly: Use the lowest effective dose

Dosing adjustment in hepatic impairment: Prednisone is inactive and must be metabolized by the liver to prednisolone. This conversion may be impaired in patients with liver disease, however, prednisolone levels are observed to be higher in patients with severe liver failure than in normal patients. Therefore, compensation for the inadequate conversion of prednisone to prednisolone occurs.

Dosing adjustment in hyperthyroidism: Prednisone dose may need to be increased to achieve adequate therapeutic effects

Hemodialysis: Supplemental dose is not necessary

Peritoneal dialysis: Supplemental dose is not necessary

Combination Regimens Note: In the U.S. prednisone is the preferred corticosteroid. However, in the British literature prednisolone is often used. The oral doses of these two agents are equivalent (ie, 1 mg prednisone = 1 mg prednisolone). Also, early clinical trials gave prednisone only with the first and fourth cycles. Some clinicians give prednisone with every cycle.

Brain tumors:
  MOPP (Medulloblastoma) on page 1373
  POC on page 1396
Breast cancer:
  CFP on page 1259
  CMFP on page 1276
  CMFVP (Cooper Regimen, VPCMF) on page 1276
Leukemia, acute lymphocytic:
  DVP on page 1298
  Hyper-CVAD + Imatinib on page 1348
  Hyper-CVAD (Leukemia, Acute Lymphocytic) on page 1349
  Larson Regimen on page 1361
  Linker Protocol on page 1362
  MTX/6-MP/VP (Maintenance) on page 1374
  POMP on page 1397
  PVA (POG 8602) on page 1398
  PVDA on page 1400
Leukemia, chronic lymphocytic:
  CHL + PRED on page 1262
  CP (Leukemia) on page 1281
  CVP (Leukemia) on page 1283
Lymphoma, Hodgkin's:
  BEACOPP on page 1229
  CAD/MOPP/ABV on page 1242

Chlorambucil-VPP (Hodgkin's Lymphoma) on page 1262
COMP on page 1280
LOPP on page 1363
MOPP (Lymphoma, Hodgkin's Disease) on page 1372
MOPP/ABV Hybrid on page 1372
MOPP/ABVD on page 1369
MVPP on page 1380
OPA on page 1382
OPPA on page 1383
Stanford V Regimen on page 1403
Lymphoma, non-Hodgkin's:
CEPP(B) on page 1254
CHOP on page 1262
CNOP on page 1277
COMP on page 1280
COP-BLAM on page 1280
COPP on page 1281
CVP (Lymphoma, non-Hodgkin's) on page 1284
EPOCH Dose-Adjusted (AIDS-Related Lymphoma) on page 1307
EPOCH Dose-Adjusted (NHL) on page 1307
EPOCH (Dose-Adjusted)-Rituximab (NHL) on page 1308
EPOCH (NHL) on page 1309
EPOCH-Rituximab (NHL) on page 1310
MACOP-B on page 1364
Pro-MACE-CytaBOM on page 1397
R-CVP on page 1401
Rituximab-CHOP on page 1402
Multiple myeloma:
Bortezomib-Melphalan-Prednisone on page 1240
Bortezomib-Melphalan-Prednisone-Thalidomide on page 1241
M-2 on page 1364
Melphalan-Prednisone-Thalidomide on page 1365
MP (Multiple Myeloma) on page 1374
VBAP on page 1418
VBMCP on page 1419
VCAP on page 1419
Prostate cancer:
Docetaxel-Prednisone on page 1292
Estramustine + Docetaxel + Prednisone on page 1314
Mitoxantrone-Prednisone (Prostate Cancer) on page 1368

Administration Administer with food to decrease gastrointestinal upset

Monitoring Parameters Blood pressure, blood glucose, electrolytes

Following prolonged use: Bone mass density, growth in children, signs and symptoms of infection, cataract formation

Test Interactions Decreased response to skin tests

Dietary Considerations Should be taken after meals or with food or milk; may require increased dietary intake of pyridoxine, vitamin C, vitamin D, folate, calcium, and phosphorus; may require decreased dietary intake of sodium

Additional Information Tapering of corticosteroids after a short course of therapy (<7-10 days) is generally not required unless the disease/inflammatory process is slow to respond. Tapering after prolonged exposure is dependent upon the individual patient, duration of corticosteroid treatments, and size of steroid dose. Recovery of the HPA axis may require several months. Subtle but important HPA axis suppression may be present for as long as several months ▶

after a course of as few as 10-14 days duration. Testing of HPA axis (cosyntropin) may be required, and signs/symptoms of adrenal insufficiency should be monitored in patients with a history of use.

Dosage Forms Excipient information presented when available (limited, particularly for generics); consult specific product labeling.

Solution, oral: 1 mg/mL (5 mL, 120 mL, 500 mL) [contains alcohol 5%, sodium benzoate; peppermint vanilla flavor]

Solution, oral [concentrate]:

PredniSONE Intensol™: 5 mg/mL (30 mL) [contains alcohol 30%]

Tablet: 1 mg, 2.5 mg, 5 mg, 10 mg, 20 mg, 50 mg

Sterapred®: 5 mg [supplied as 21 tablet 6-day unit-dose package or 48 tablet 12-day unit-dose package]

Sterapred® DS: 10 mg [supplied as 21 tablet 6-day unit-dose package or 48 tablet 12-day unit-dose package]

References

Coursin DB and Wood KE, "Corticosteroid Supplementation for Adrenal Insufficiency," *JAMA*, 2002, 287(2):236-40.

Dellinger RP, Levy MM, Carlet JM, et al, "Surviving Sepsis Campaign: International Guidelines for Management of Severe Sepsis and Septic Shock: 2008," *Intensive Care Med*, 2008, 34(1):17-60. Available at http://www.survivingsepsis.org/system/files/images/2008_20International_20SSC_20Guidelines_1_.pdf

"Diagnosis And Treatment of Idiopathic Thrombocytopenic Purpura: Recommendations of the American Society of Hematology. The American Society of Hematology ITP Practice Guideline Panel," *Ann Intern Med*, 1997, 126(4):319-26.

Dworkin RH, Johnson RW, Breuer J, et al, "Recommendations for the management of herpes zoster," *Clin Infect Dis*, 2007, 44(Suppl 1):1-26.

Frey BM and Frey FJ, "Clinical Pharmacokinetics of Prednisone and Prednisolone," *Clin Pharmacokinet*, 1990, 19(2):126-46.

Goedert JJ, Vitale F, Lauria C, et al, "Risk Factors for Classical Kaposi's Sarcoma," *J Natl Cancer Inst*, 2002, 94(22):1712-8.

"Guidelines for Referral and Management of Systemic Lupus Erythematosus in Adults. American College of Rheumatology Ad Hoc Committee on Systemic Lupus Erythematosus Guidelines," *Arthritis Rheum*, 1999, 42(9):1785-96.

Gutin PH, "Corticosteroid Therapy in Patients With Brain Tumors," *Natl Cancer Inst Monogr*, 1977, 46:151-6.

Hogg RJ, Portman RJ, Milliner D, et al, "Evaluation and Management of Proteinuria and Nephrotic Syndrome in Children: Recommendations From a Pediatric Nephrology Panel Established at the National Kidney Foundation Conference on Proteinuria, Albuminuria, Risk, Assessment, Detection, and Elimination (PARADE)," *Pediatrics*, 2000, 105(6):1242-9.

Report of a Workshop by the British Association for Paediatric Nephrology and Research Unit, Royal College of Physicians, "Consensus Statement on Management and Audit Potential for Steroid Responsive Nephrotic Syndrome," *Arch Dis Child*, 1994, 70(2):151-7.

Wallace DV, Dykewicz MS, Bernstein DI, et al, "The Diagnosis and Management of Anaphylaxis: An Updated Practice Parameter," *J Allergy Clin Immunol*, 2005, 115(3 Suppl 2):483-523.

Wolkowitz OM, "Long-Lasting Behavioral Changes Following Prednisone Withdrawal," *JAMA*, 1989, 261(12):1731-2.

♦ **Pro-Calcitonin (Can)** *see Calcitonin on page 165*

Procarbazine (proe KAR ba zeen)

Medication Safety Issues
Sound-alike/look-alike issues:
Procarbazine may be confused with dacarbazine
Matulane® may be confused with Materna®

High alert medication: The Institute for Safe Medication Practices (ISMP) includes this medication among its list of drugs which have a heightened risk of causing significant patient harm when used in error.

Related Information
Fertility and Cancer Therapy *on page 1430*
Management of Chemotherapy-Induced Nausea and Vomiting *on page 1434*
Safe Handling of Hazardous Drugs *on page 1517*

U.S. Brand Names Matulane®

Index Terms Benzmethyzin; N-Methylhydrazine; Procarbazine Hydrochloride

Generic Available No

Canadian Brand Names Matulane®; Natulan®

Pharmacologic Category Antineoplastic Agent, Alkylating Agent

Use Treatment of Hodgkin's disease

Unlabeled/Investigational Use Treatment of non-Hodgkin's lymphoma, brain tumors

Pregnancy Risk Factor D

Lactation Excretion in breast milk unknown/not recommended

Labeled Contraindications Hypersensitivity to procarbazine or any component of the formulation; pre-existing bone marrow aplasia; ethanol ingestion; pregnancy

Warnings/Precautions Hazardous agent - use appropriate precautions for handling and disposal. Use with caution in patients with pre-existing renal or hepatic impairment. Procarbazine possesses MAO inhibitor activity and has potential for severe drug and food interactions; follow MAO-I diet. Avoid ethanol consumption, may cause disulfiram-like reaction. May cause hemolysis and/or presence of Heinz inclusion bodies in erythrocytes. Bone marrow depression may occur 2-8 weeks after treatment initiation. Allow ≥1 month interval between radiation therapy or myelosuppressive chemotherapy and initiation of treatment. Withhold treatment for CNS toxicity, leukopenia (WBC <4000/mm^3), thrombocytopenia (platelets <100,000/mm^3), hypersensitivity, stomatitis, diarrhea or hemorrhage. Procarbazine is a carcinogen which may cause acute leukemia. May cause infertility. **[U.S. Boxed Warning]: Should be administered under the supervision of an experienced cancer chemotherapy physician.**

Adverse Reactions Most frequencies not defined.
Cardiovascular: Edema, flushing, hypotension, syncope, tachycardia
Central nervous system: Apprehension, ataxia, chills, coma, confusion, depression, dizziness, drowsiness, fatigue, fever, hallucination, headache, insomnia, lethargy, nervousness, nightmares, pain, seizure, slurred speech
Dermatologic: Alopecia, dermatitis, hyperpigmentation, petechiae, pruritus, purpura, rash, urticaria
Endocrine & metabolic: Gynecomastia (in prepubertal and early pubertal males)
Hematologic: Eosinophilia; hemolysis (in patients with G6PD deficiency); hemolytic anemia; myelosuppression (leukopenia, anemia, thrombocytopenia); pancytopenia

Gastrointestinal: Abdominal pain, anorexia, constipation, diarrhea, dysphagia, hematemesis, melena; nausea and vomiting ([60% to 90%], increasing the dose in a stepwise fashion over several days may minimize); stomatitis, xerostomia

Genitourinary: Azoospermia (reported with combination chemotherapy), hematuria, nocturia, polyuria, reproductive dysfunction (>10%)

Hepatic: Hepatic dysfunction, jaundice

Neuromuscular & skeletal: Arthralgia, falling, foot drop, myalgia, neuropathy, paresthesia, reflex diminished, tremor, unsteadiness, weakness

Ocular: Diplopia, inability to focus, nystagmus, papilledema, photophobia, retinal hemorrhage

Otic: Hearing loss

Respiratory: Cough, epistaxis, hemoptysis, hoarseness, pleural effusion, pneumonitis, pulmonary toxicity (<1%)

Miscellaneous: Allergic reaction, diaphoresis, herpes, infection, secondary malignancies (2% to 15%; reported with combination therapy)

Drug Interactions

Avoid Concomitant Use

Avoid concomitant use of Procarbazine with any of the following: Alpha-/Beta-Agonists (Indirect-Acting); Alpha1-Agonists; Alpha2-Agonists (Ophthalmic); Amphetamines; Anilidopiperidine Opioids; Atomoxetine; BuPROPion; BusPIRone; CarBAMazepine; Cyclobenzaprine; Dexmethylphenidate; Dextromethorphan; Linezolid; Maprotiline; Meperidine; Methyldopa; Methylphenidate; Mirtazapine; Natalizumab; Propoxyphene; Selective Serotonin Reuptake Inhibitors; Serotonin 5-HT1D Receptor Agonists; Serotonin/Norepinephrine Reuptake Inhibitors; Sibutramine; Tapentadol; Tetrabenazine; Tricyclic Antidepressants; Vaccines (Live)

Increased Effect/Toxicity

Procarbazine may increase the levels/effects of: Alpha-/Beta-Agonists (Direct-Acting); Alpha-/Beta-Agonists (Indirect-Acting); Alpha1-Agonists; Alpha2-Agonists (Ophthalmic); Amphetamines; Antihypertensives; Atomoxetine; Beta2-Agonists; BuPROPion; Dexmethylphenidate; Dextromethorphan; Leflunomide; Linezolid; Lithium; Meperidine; Methyldopa; Methylphenidate; Mirtazapine; Natalizumab; Orthostasis Producing Agents; Rauwolfia Alkaloids; Selective Serotonin Reuptake Inhibitors; Serotonin 5-HT1D Receptor Agonists; Serotonin Modulators; Serotonin/Norepinephrine Reuptake Inhibitors; Tricyclic Antidepressants; Vaccines (Live); Vitamin K Antagonists

The levels/effects of Procarbazine may be increased by: Altretamine; Anilidopiperidine Opioids; BusPIRone; CarBAMazepine; COMT Inhibitors; Cyclobenzaprine; Levodopa; MAO Inhibitors; Maprotiline; Propoxyphene; Sibutramine; Tapentadol; Tetrabenazine; TraMADol; Trastuzumab

Decreased Effect

Procarbazine may decrease the levels/effects of: Cardiac Glycosides; Vaccines (Inactivated); Vaccines (Live); Vitamin K Antagonists

The levels/effects of Procarbazine may be decreased by: Echinacea

Ethanol/Nutrition/Herb Interactions

Ethanol: May enhance the adverse/toxic effects of procarbazine; concurrent use not recommended.

Food: Concurrent ingestion of foods rich in tyramine may cause sudden and severe high blood pressure (hypertensive crisis). Avoid tyramine-containing foods with MAO-Is. Food's freshness is also an important concern; improperly stored or spoiled food can create an environment where tyramine concentrations may increase.

Herb/Nutraceuticals: Avoid supplements containing caffeine, tyrosine, tryptophan, or phenylalanine. Ingestion of large quantities may increase the risk of severe side effects (eg, hypertensive reactions, serotonin syndrome).

Storage/Stability Protect from light.

Mechanism of Action Mechanism of action is not clear, methylating of nucleic acids; inhibits DNA, RNA, and protein synthesis; may damage DNA directly and suppresses mitosis; metabolic activation required by host

Pharmacodynamics/Kinetics

Absorption: Rapid and complete

Distribution: Crosses blood-brain barrier; equilibrates between plasma and CSF

Metabolism: Hepatic and renal

Half-life elimination: 1 hour

Time to peak, plasma: 1 hour

Excretion: Urine and respiratory tract (<5% as unchanged drug, 70% as metabolites)

Dosage Refer to individual protocols. Manufacturer states that the dose is based on patient's ideal weight if the patient is obese or has abnormal fluid retention. Other studies suggest that ideal body weight may not be necessary. Oral (may be given as a single daily dose or in 2-3 divided doses):

Children:

BMT aplastic anemia conditioning regimen (unlabeled use): 12.5 mg/kg/day every other day for 4 doses

Hodgkin's disease: MOPP/IC-MOPP regimens: 100 mg/m^2/day for 14 days and repeated every 4 weeks

Neuroblastoma and medulloblastoma (unlabeled use): Doses as high as 100-200 mg/m^2/day once daily have been used

Adults: Initial: 2-4 mg/kg/day in single or divided doses for 7 days then increase dose to 4-6 mg/kg/day until response is obtained or leukocyte count decreased <4000/mm^3 or the platelet count decreased <100,000/mm^3; maintenance: 1-2 mg/kg/day

Dosing in renal impairment: The FDA-approved labeling does not contain dosing adjustment guidelines; use with caution; may result in increased toxicity.

Dosing in hepatic impairment: The FDA-approved labeling does not contain dosing adjustment guidelines; use with caution; may result in increased toxicity. The following guidelines have been used by some clinicians:

Floyd, 2006:

Transaminases 1.6-6 times ULN: Administer 75% of dose

Transaminases >6 times ULN: Use clinical judgment

Serum bilirubin >5 mg/dL or transaminases >3 times ULN: Avoid use

King, 2001: Serum bilirubin >5 mg/dL or transaminases >180 units/L: Avoid use

Combination Regimens

Brain tumors:

8 in 1 (Brain Tumors) on page 1221

MOP on page 1369

MOPP (Medulloblastoma) on page 1373

PCV (Brain Tumor Regimen) on page 1392

Lymphoma, Hodgkin's:

BEACOPP on page 1229

CAD/MOPP/ABV on page 1242

Administration May be given as a single daily dose or in 2-3 divided doses.

Monitoring Parameters CBC with differential, platelet and reticulocyte count, urinalysis, liver function test, renal function test.

Dietary Considerations Avoid tyramine-containing foods/beverages. Some examples include aged or matured cheese, air-dried or cured meats (including sausages and salamis), fava or broad bean pods, tap/draft beers, Marmite concentrate, sauerkraut, soy sauce and other soybean condiments.

Emetic Potential High (>90%)

Dosage Forms Excipient information presented when available (limited, particularly for generics); consult specific product labeling.

Capsule, as hydrochloride:
Matulane®: 50 mg

References

Floyd J, Mirza I, Sachs B, et al, "Hepatotoxicity of Chemotherapy," *Semin Oncol*, 2006, 33 (1):50-67.

King PD and Perry MC, "Hepatotoxicity of Chemotherapy," *Oncologist*, 2001, 6(2):162-76.

Longo DL, Young RC, Wesley M, et al, "Twenty Years of MOPP Therapy for Hodgkin's Disease," *J Clin Oncol*, 1986, 4(9):1295-306.

Rodriguez LA, Prados M, Silver P, et al, "Re-evaluation of Procarbazine for the Treatment of Recurrent Malignant Central Nervous System Tumors," *Cancer*, 1989, 64(12):2420-3.

Shulman KI and Walker SE, "A Reevaluation of Dietary Restrictions for Irreversible Monoamine Oxidase Inhibitors," *Psychiatr Ann*, 2001, 31(6):378-84.

Shulman KI and Walker SE, "Refining the MAOI Diet: Tyramine Content of Pizzas and Soy Products," *J Clin Psychiatry*, 1999, 60(3):191-3.

Walker SE, Shulman KI, Tailor SA, et al, "Tyramine Content of Previously Restricted Foods in Monoamine Oxidase Inhibitor Diets," *J Clin Psychopharmacol*, 1996, 16(5):383-8.

◆ **Procarbazine Hydrochloride** *see* Procarbazine *on page 989*

Prochlorperazine (proe klor PER a zeen)

Medication Safety Issues

Sound-alike/look-alike issues:
Prochlorperazine may be confused with chlorproMAZINE
Compazine® may be confused with Copaxone®, Coumadin®

CPZ (occasional abbreviation for Compazine®) is an error-prone abbreviation (mistaken as chlorpromazine)

Related Information

Management of Chemotherapy-Induced Nausea and Vomiting *on page 1434*

U.S. Brand Names Compro™

Index Terms Chlormeprazine; Compazine; Prochlorperazine Edisylate; Prochlorperazine Maleate

Generic Available Yes: Injection, tablet, suppository

Canadian Brand Names Apo-Prochlorperazine®; Nu-Prochlor; Stemetil®

Pharmacologic Category Antiemetic; Antipsychotic Agent, Typical, Phenothiazine

Use Management of nausea and vomiting; psychotic disorders, including schizophrenia and anxiety

Unlabeled/Investigational Use Behavioral syndromes in dementia; psychosis/agitation related to Alzheimer's dementia

Lactation Excretion in breast milk unknown/use caution

Labeled Contraindications Hypersensitivity to prochlorperazine or any component of the formulation (cross-reactivity between phenothiazines may occur); severe CNS depression; coma; pediatric surgery; Reye's syndrome; should not be used in children <2 years of age or <9 kg

Warnings/Precautions [U.S. Boxed Warning]: Elderly patients with dementia-related psychosis treated with antipsychotics are at an increased risk of death compared to placebo. Most deaths appeared to be either cardiovascular (eg, heart failure, sudden death) or infectious (eg, pneumonia) in nature. Prochlorperazine is not approved for the treatment of dementia-related psychosis.

May be sedating; use with caution in disorders where CNS depression is a feature. May obscure intestinal obstruction or brain tumor. May impair physical or mental abilities. Effects with other sedative drugs or ethanol may be potentiated. Use with caution in Parkinson's disease; hemodynamic instability; predisposition to seizures; subcortical brain damage; and in severe cardiac, hepatic, or renal disease. May alter temperature regulation or mask toxicity of other drugs. Use caution with exposure to heat. May alter cardiac conduction. May cause orthostatic hypotension. Hypotension may occur following administration, particularly when parenteral form is used or in high dosages. Antipsychotic use has been associated with esophageal dysmotility and aspiration; use with caution in patients at risk of pneumonia (ie, Alzheimer's disease). Blood dyscrasias have occurred; check blood counts periodically. May cause pigmentary retinopathy, and lenticular and corneal deposits, particularly with prolonged therapy. Use associated with increased prolactin levels; clinical significance of hyperprolactinemia in patients with breast cancer or other prolactin-dependent tumors is unknown.

Phenothiazines may cause anticholinergic effects; therefore, they should be used with caution in patients with decreased gastrointestinal motility, urinary retention, BPH, xerostomia, or visual problems. Conditions which also may be exacerbated by cholinergic blockade include narrow-angle glaucoma and worsening of myasthenia gravis. May cause extrapyramidal symptoms (EPS), including pseudoparkinsonism, acute dystonic reactions, akathisia, and tardive dyskinesia (risk of these reactions is high relative to other neuroleptics). Risk of dystonia (and possibly other EPS) may be greater with increased doses, use of conventional antipsychotics, males, and younger patients. Use caution in the elderly. Children with acute illness or dehydration are more susceptible to neuromuscular reactions; use cautiously. May be associated with neuroleptic malignant syndrome (NMS). Injection contains benzyl alcohol which has been associated with "gasping syndrome" in neonates.

Adverse Reactions Reported with prochlorperazine or other phenothiazines. Frequency not defined.

Cardiovascular: Cardiac arrest, hypotension, peripheral edema, Q-wave distortions, T-wave distortions

Central nervous system: Agitation, catatonia, cerebral edema, cough reflex suppressed, dizziness, drowsiness, fever (mild - I.M.), headache, hyperactivity, hyperpyrexia, impairment of temperature regulation, insomnia,

◀ neuroleptic malignant syndrome (NMS), paradoxical excitement, restlessness, seizure

Dermatologic: Angioedema, contact dermatitis, discoloration of skin (blue-gray), epithelial keratopathy, erythema, eczema, exfoliative dermatitis (injectable), itching, photosensitivity, rash, skin pigmentation, urticaria

Endocrine & metabolic: Amenorrhea, breast enlargement, galactorrhea, gynecomastia, glucosuria, hyperglycemia, hypoglycemia, lactation, libido (changes in), menstrual irregularity, SIADH

Gastrointestinal: Appetite increased, atonic colon, constipation, ileus, nausea, weight gain, xerostomia

Genitourinary: Ejaculating dysfunction, ejaculatory disturbances, impotence, incontinence, polyuria, priapism, urinary retention, urination difficulty

Hematologic: Agranulocytosis, aplastic anemia, eosinophilia, hemolytic anemia, leukopenia, pancytopenia, thrombocytopenic purpura

Hepatic: Biliary stasis, cholestatic jaundice, hepatotoxicity

Neuromuscular & skeletal: Dystonias (torticollis, opisthotonos, carpopedal spasm, trismus, oculogyric crisis, protusion of tongue); extrapyramidal symptoms (pseudoparkinsonism, akathisia, dystonias, tardive dyskinesia); SLE-like syndrome, tremor

Ocular: blurred vision, cornea and lens changes, lenticular/corneal deposits, miosis, mydriasis, pigmentary retinopathy

Respiratory: Asthma, laryngeal edema, nasal congestion

Miscellaneous: Allergic reactions, diaphoresis

Drug Interactions

Avoid Concomitant Use
Avoid concomitant use of Prochlorperazine with any of the following: Dofetilide

Increased Effect/Toxicity
Prochlorperazine may increase the levels/effects of: Alcohol (Ethyl); Analgesics (Opioid); Anticholinergics; Beta-Blockers; CNS Depressants; Dofetilide; Methotrimeprazine

The levels/effects of Prochlorperazine may be increased by: Acetylcholinesterase Inhibitors (Central); Antimalarial Agents; Beta-Blockers; Lithium formulations; Methotrimeprazine; Pramlintide; Tetrabenazine

Decreased Effect
Prochlorperazine may decrease the levels/effects of: Amphetamines; Anti-Parkinson's Agents (Dopamine Agonist)

The levels/effects of Prochlorperazine may be decreased by: Antacids; Lithium formulations

Ethanol/Nutrition/Herb Interactions
Ethanol: Avoid ethanol (may increase CNS depression).

Food: Limit caffeine.

Herb/Nutraceutical: Avoid dong quai, St John's wort (may also cause photosensitization). Avoid kava kava, gotu kola, valerian, St John's wort (may increase CNS depression).

Storage/Stability
Injection: Store at <30°C (<86°F); do not freeze. Protect from light. Clear or slightly yellow solutions may be used.

I.V. infusion: Injection may be diluted in 50-100 mL NS or D₅W.

Suppository, tablet: Store at 15°C to 30°C (59°F to 86°F). Protect from light.

Compatibility Stable in dextran 6% in dextrose, dextran 6% in NS, D₅W, D₁₀W, D₅LR, D₅¹/₄NS, D₅¹/₂NS, D₅NS, LR, ¹/₂NS, NS.

Y-site administration: Compatible: Amsacrine, calcium gluconate, cis-atracurium, cisplatin, cladribine, clarithromycin, cyclophosphamide, cytarabine, docetaxel, doxorubicin, doxorubicin liposome, fluconazole, gatifloxacin, granisetron, heparin, hydrocortisone sodium succinate, linezolid, melphalan, methotrexate, ondansetron, paclitaxel, potassium chloride, propofol, remifentanil, sargramostim, sufentanil, teniposide, thiotepa, topotecan, vinorelbine, vitamin B complex with C. **Incompatible:** Aldesleukin, allopurinol, amifostine, amphotericin B cholesteryl sulfate complex, aztreonam, cefepime, etoposide phosphate, fludarabine, foscarnet, filgrastim, gemcitabine, piperacillin/tazobactam.

Compatibility in syringe: Compatible: Atropine, butorphanol, chlorpromazine, cimetidine, diamorphine, diphenhydramine, droperidol, fentanyl, glycopyrrolate, hydroxyzine, meperidine, metoclopramide, nalbuphine, pentazocine, perphenazine, promazine, promethazine, ranitidine, scopolamine, sufentanil. **Incompatible:** Dimenhydrinate, ketorolac, midazolam, morphine tartrate, pentobarbital, thiopental. **Variable (consult detailed reference):** Hydromorphone, morphine sulfate.

Compatibility when admixed: Compatible: Amikacin, ascorbic acid injection, cephalothin, dexamethasone sodium phosphate, dimenhydrinate, erythromycin lactobionate, ethacrynate, lidocaine, nafcillin, sodium bicarbonate, vitamin B complex with C. **Incompatible:** Aminophylline, amphotericin B, ampicillin, chloramphenicol, chlorothiazide, floxacillin, furosemide, heparin, hydrocortisone sodium succinate, methohexital, penicillin G sodium, phenobarbital, phenytoin, thiopental. **Variable (consult detailed reference):** Calcium gluconate, penicillin G potassium.

Mechanism of Action Prochlorperazine is a piperazine phenothiazine antipsychotic which blocks postsynaptic mesolimbic dopaminergic D_1 and D_2 receptors in the brain, including the chemoreceptor trigger zone; exhibits a strong alpha-adrenergic and anticholinergic blocking effect and depresses the release of hypothalamic and hypophyseal hormones; believed to depress the reticular activating system, thus affecting basal metabolism, body temperature, wakefulness, vasomotor tone and emesis

Pharmacodynamics/Kinetics

Onset of action: Oral: 30-40 minutes; I.M.: 10-20 minutes; Rectal: ~60 minutes Peak antiemetic effect: I.V.: 30-60 minutes

Duration: Rectal: 12 hours; Oral: 3-4 hours; I.M., I.V.: Adults: 4-6 hours; I.M.: Children: 12 hours

Distribution: V_d: 1400-1548 L; crosses placenta; enters breast milk

Metabolism: Primarily hepatic; N-desmethyl prochlorperazine (major active metabolite)

Bioavailability: Oral: 12.5%

Half-life elimination: Oral: 6-10 hours (single dose), 14-22 hours (repeated dosing); I.V.: 6-10 hours

Dosage

Antiemetic: Children (therapy >1 day usually not required): **Note:** Not recommended for use in children <9 kg or <2 years:

Oral, rectal: >9 kg: 0.4 mg/kg/24 hours in 3-4 divided doses; **or**

9-13 kg: 2.5 mg every 12-24 hours as needed; maximum: 7.5 mg/day

13.1-17 kg: 2.5 mg every 8-12 hours as needed; maximum: 10 mg/day

17.1-37 kg: 2.5 mg every 8 hours or 5 mg every 12 hours as needed; maximum: 15 mg/day

I.M.: 0.13 mg/kg/dose; change to oral as soon as possible

Antiemetic: Adults:

Oral (tablet): 5-10 mg 3-4 times/day; usual maximum: 40 mg/day; larger doses may rarely be required

I.M. (deep): 5-10 mg every 3-4 hours; usual maximum: 40 mg/day

I.V.: 2.5-10 mg; maximum 10 mg/dose or 40 mg/day; may repeat dose every 3-4 hours as needed

Rectal: 25 mg twice daily

Surgical nausea/vomiting: Adults: **Note:** Should not exceed 40 mg/day

I.M.: 5-10 mg 1-2 hours before induction or to control symptoms during or after surgery; may repeat once if necessary

I.V. (administer slow IVP <5 mg/minute): 5-10 mg 15-30 minutes before induction or to control symptoms during or after surgery; may repeat once if necessary

Rectal (unlabeled use): 25 mg

Antipsychotic:

Children 2-12 years (not recommended in children <9 kg or <2 years):

Oral, rectal: 2.5 mg 2-3 times/day; do not give more than 10 mg the first day; increase dosage as needed to maximum daily dose of 20 mg for 2-5 years and 25 mg for 6-12 years

I.M.: 0.13 mg/kg/dose; change to oral as soon as possible

Adults:

Oral: 5-10 mg 3-4 times/day; titrate dose slowly every 2-3 days; doses up to 150 mg/day may be required in some patients for treatment of severe disturbances

I.M.: Initial: 10-20 mg; if necessary repeat initial dose every 1-4 hours to gain control; more than 3-4 doses are rarely needed. If parenteral administration is still required; give 10-20 mg every 4-6 hours; change to oral as soon as possible.

Nonpsychotic anxiety: Oral (tablet): Adults: Usual dose: 15-20 mg/day in divided doses; do not give doses >20 mg/day or for longer than 12 weeks

Elderly: Behavioral symptoms associated with dementia (unlabeled use): Initial: 2.5-5 mg 1-2 times/day; increase dose at 4- to 7-day intervals by 2.5-5 mg/day; increase dosing intervals (twice daily, 3 times/day, etc) as necessary to control response or side effects; maximum daily dose should probably not exceed 75 mg in elderly; gradual increases (titration) may prevent some side effects or decrease their severity

Administration May be administered orally, I.M., or I.V.

I.M.: Inject by deep IM into outer quadrant of buttocks.

I.V.: Doses should be given as a short (~30 minute) infusion to avoid orthostatic hypotension; administer at ≤5 mg/minute

Monitoring Parameters Vital signs; lipid profile, fasting blood glucose/Hgb A_{1c}; BMI; mental status, abnormal involuntary movement scale (AIMS); periodic ophthalmic exams (if chronically used); extrapyramidal symptoms (EPS)

Test Interactions False-positives for phenylketonuria, pregnancy, urinary amylase, uroporphyrins, urobilinogen

Dietary Considerations Increase dietary intake of riboflavin; should be administered with food or water. Rectal suppositories may contain coconut and palm oil.

Additional Information Not recommended as an antipsychotic due to inferior efficacy compared to other phenothiazines.

Dosage Forms Excipient information presented when available (limited, particularly for generics); consult specific product labeling.

Injection, solution, as edisylate: 5 mg/mL (2 mL, 10 mL) [contains benzyl alcohol]

Suppository, rectal: 25 mg (12s) [may contain coconut and palm oil]

Compro™: 25 mg (12s) [contains coconut and palm oils]

Tablet, as maleate: 5 mg, 10 mg [strength expressed as base]

References

Ernst AA, Weiss SJ, Park S, et al, "Prochlorperazine Versus Promethazine for Uncomplicated Nausea and Vomiting in the Emergency Department: A Randomized, Double-Blind Clinical Trial," *Ann Emerg Med*, 2000, 36(2):89-94.

Goldstein D, Levi JA, Woods RL, et al, "Double-Blind Randomized Cross-Over Trial of Dexamethasone and Prochlorperazine as Antiemetics for Cancer Chemotherapy," *Oncology*, 1989, 46(2):105-8.

Hesketh PJ, Gandara DR, Hesketh AM, et al, "Improved Control of High-Dose-Cisplatin-Induced Acute Emesis With the Addition of Prochlorperazine to Granisetron/Dexamethasone," *Cancer J Sci Am*, 1997, 3(3):180-3.

Olver IN, Webster LK, Bishop JF, et al, "A Dose Finding Study of Prochlorperazine as an Antiemetic for Cancer Chemotherapy," *Eur J Cancer Clin Oncol*, 1989, 25(10):1457-61.

Owens NH, Schauer AR, Nightingale CH, et al, "Antiemetic Efficacy of Prochlorperazine, Haloperidol, Droperidol in Cisplatin-Induced Emesis," *Clin Pharm*, 1984, 3(2):167-70.

◆ **Prochlorperazine Edisylate** see Prochlorperazine on page 992

◆ **Prochlorperazine Maleate** see Prochlorperazine on page 992

◆ **PRO-Ciprofloxacin (Can)** see Ciprofloxacin on page 228

◆ **Procrit®** see Epoetin Alfa on page 412

◆ **Proctocort®** see Hydrocortisone on page 575

◆ **ProctoCream® HC** see Hydrocortisone on page 575

◆ **Procto-Kit™** see Hydrocortisone on page 575

◆ **Procto-Pak™** see Hydrocortisone on page 575

◆ **Proctosert** see Hydrocortisone on page 575

◆ **Proctosol-HC®** see Hydrocortisone on page 575

◆ **Proctozone-HC™** see Hydrocortisone on page 575

◆ **Procytox® (Can)** see Cyclophosphamide on page 260

◆ **Profilnine® SD** see Factor IX Complex (Human) on page 452

◆ **Pro-Fluconazole (Can)** see Fluconazole on page 485

◆ **Prograf®** see Tacrolimus on page 1062

◆ **Proleukin®** see Aldesleukin on page 25

◆ **Promacta®** see Eltrombopag on page 398

Promethazine (proe METH a zeen)

Medication Safety Issues

Sound-alike/look-alike issues:

Promethazine may be confused with chlorproMAZINE, predniSONE, promazine

Phenergan® may be confused with Phenaphen®, PHENobarbital, Phrenilin®, Theragran®

High alert medication: The Institute for Safe Medication Practices (ISMP) includes this medication (I.V. formulation) among its list of drugs which have a heightened risk of causing significant patient harm when used in error.

Administration issues:

To prevent or minimize tissue damage during I.V. administration, the Institute for Safe Medication Practices (ISMP) has the following recommendations: Limit concentration available to the 25 mg/mL product

◄

   Consider limiting initial doses to 6.25-12.5 mg

   Further dilute the 25 mg/mL strength into 10-20 mL NS

   Administer through a large bore vein (not hand or wrist)

   Administer via running I.V. line at port farthest from patient's vein

   Consider administering over 10-15 minutes

   Instruct patients to report immediately signs of pain or burning

Related Information

  Management of Chemotherapy-Induced Nausea and Vomiting *on page 1434*

  Management of Drug Extravasations *on page 1447*

U.S. Brand Names Phenadoz™; Phenergan®; Promethegan™

Index Terms Promethazine Hydrochloride

Generic Available Yes

Canadian Brand Names Bioniche Promethazine; Histantil; Phenergan®; PMS-Promethazine

Pharmacologic Category Antiemetic; Histamine H$_1$ Antagonist; Histamine H$_1$ Antagonist, First Generation

Use Symptomatic treatment of various allergic conditions; antiemetic; motion sickness; sedative

Pregnancy Risk Factor C

Lactation Excretion in breast milk unknown/not recommended

Labeled Contraindications Hypersensitivity to promethazine or any component of the formulation (cross-reactivity between phenothiazines may occur); coma; treatment of lower respiratory tract symptoms, including asthma; children <2 years of age

Warnings/Precautions [U.S. Boxed Warning]: Respiratory fatalities have been reported in children <2 years of age. Contraindicated in children <2 years of age. In children ≥2 years, use the lowest possible dose; other drugs with respiratory depressant effects should be avoided. Not for SubQ or intra-arterial administration. Injection may contain sodium metabisulfite. I.M. is the preferred route of parenteral administration. I.V. use has been associated with severe tissue damage; follow specific administration techniques to minimize risk; discontinue immediately if burning or pain occurs with administration. May be sedating; use with caution in disorders where CNS depression is a feature. May impair physical or mental abilities; patients must be cautioned about performing tasks which require mental alertness. Use with caution in Parkinson's disease; hemodynamic instability; bone marrow suppression; subcortical brain damage; and in severe cardiac, hepatic or respiratory disease. Avoid use in Reye's syndrome. May lower seizure threshold; use caution in persons with seizure disorders or in persons using narcotics or local anesthetics which may also affect seizure threshold. May alter temperature regulation or mask toxicity of other drugs due to antiemetic effects. May alter cardiac conduction (life-threatening arrhythmias have occurred with therapeutic doses of phenothiazines). May cause orthostatic hypotension; use with caution in patients at risk of hypotension or where transient hypotensive episodes would be poorly tolerated (cardiovascular disease or cerebrovascular disease).

Phenothiazines may cause anticholinergic effects; therefore, they should be used with caution in patients with decreased gastrointestinal motility, GI or GU obstruction, urinary retention, BPH, xerostomia, or visual problems. Conditions which also may be exacerbated by cholinergic blockade include narrow-angle glaucoma (screening is recommended) and worsening of myasthenia gravis. May cause extrapyramidal symptoms, including pseudoparkinsonism, acute dystonic reactions, akathisia, and tardive dyskinesia. May be associated with neuroleptic malignant syndrome (NMS). Use cautiously in the elderly.

Adverse Reactions Frequency not defined.

Cardiovascular: Bradycardia, hypertension, postural hypotension, tachycardia, nonspecific QT changes

Central nervous system: Akathisia, catatonic states, confusion, delirium, disorientation, dizziness, drowsiness, dystonias, euphoria, excitation, extrapyramidal symptoms, fatigue, hallucinations, hysteria, insomnia, lassitude, pseudoparkinsonism, tardive dyskinesia, nervousness, neuroleptic malignant syndrome, nightmares, sedation, seizure, somnolence

Dermatologic: Angioneurotic edema, photosensitivity, dermatitis, skin pigmentation (slate gray), urticaria

Endocrine & metabolic: Lactation, breast engorgement, amenorrhea, gynecomastia, hyperglycemia

Gastrointestinal: Xerostomia, constipation, nausea, vomiting

Genitourinary: Urinary retention, ejaculatory disorder, impotence

Hematologic: Agranulocytosis, eosinophilia, leukopenia, hemolytic anemia, aplastic anemia, thrombocytopenia, thrombocytopenic purpura

Hepatic: Jaundice

Local: Venous thrombosis; injection site reactions (burning, erythema, pain, edema)

Neuromuscular & skeletal: Incoordination, tremor

Ocular: Blurred vision, corneal and lenticular changes, diplopia, epithelial keratopathy, pigmentary retinopathy

Otic: Tinnitus

Respiratory: Apnea, asthma, nasal congestion, respiratory depression

Drug Interactions

Metabolism/Transport Effects Substrate (major) of CYP2B6, 2D6; Inhibits CYP2D6 (weak)

Avoid Concomitant Use

Avoid concomitant use of Promethazine with any of the following: Sibutramine

Increased Effect/Toxicity

Promethazine may increase the levels/effects of: Anticholinergics; Serotonin Modulators

The levels/effects of Promethazine may be increased by: CYP2B6 Inhibitors (Moderate); CYP2B6 Inhibitors (Strong); CYP2D6 Inhibitors (Moderate); CYP2D6 Inhibitors (Strong); Darunavir; MAO Inhibitors; Pramlintide; Sibutramine

Decreased Effect

Promethazine may decrease the levels/effects of: Acetylcholinesterase Inhibitors (Central)

The levels/effects of Promethazine may be decreased by: Acetylcholinesterase Inhibitors (Central); CYP2B6 Inducers (Strong); Peginterferon Alfa-2b

Ethanol/Nutrition/Herb Interactions

Ethanol: Avoid ethanol (may increase CNS depression).

Herb/Nutraceutical: Avoid valerian, St John's wort, kava kava, gotu kola (may increase CNS depression).

Storage/Stability

Injection: Prior to dilution, store at room temperature. Protect from light. Solutions in NS or D_5W are stable for 24 hours at room temperature.

Suppositories: Store refrigerated at 2°C to 8°C (36°F to 46°F).

Tablets, oral solution: Store at room temperature. Protect from light.

◄ **Compatibility** Stable in dextran 6% in dextrose, dextran 6% in NS, D_5W, $D_{10}W$, D_5LR, $D_5{}^{1}/_4NS$, $D_5{}^{1}/_2NS$, D_5NS, LR, $^{1}/_2NS$, NS.

Y-site administration: Compatible: Amifostine, amsacrine, aztreonam, bivalirudin, ciprofloxacin, cisatracurium, cisplatin, cladribine, cyclophosphamide, cytarabine, dexmedetomidine, docetaxel, doxorubicin hydrochloride, etoposide phosphate, fenoldopam, filgrastim, fluconazole, fludarabine, gatifloxacin, gemcitabine, granisetron, linezolid, melphalan, ondansetron, oxaliplatin, palonosetron, pemetrexed, remifentanil, sargramostim, teniposide, thiotepa, vinorelbine. **Incompatible:** Aldesleukin, allopurinol, amphotericin B cholesteryl sulfate complex, cefazolin, cefepime, cefoperazone, cefotetan, doxorubicin liposome, foscarnet, furosemide, lansoprazole, methotrexate, piperacillin/tazobactam. **Variable (consult detailed reference):** Cefazolin, ceftizoxime, heparin, hydrocortisone sodium succinate, potassium chloride, vitamin B complex with C.

Compatibility in syringe: Compatible: Atropine, atropine with meperidine, butorphanol, chlorpromazine, cimetidine, dihydroergotamine, diphenhydramine, droperidol, fentanyl, glycopyrrolate, hydromorphone, hydroxyzine, meperidine, metoclopramide, midazolam, pentazocine, perphenazine, prochlorperazine edisylate, promazine, ranitidine, scopolamine. **Incompatible:** Cefotetan, ceftriaxone, chloroquine, dexamethasone, diatrizoate sodium 75%, diatrizoate meglumine 52% with diatrizoate sodium 8%, diatrizoate meglumine 34.3% with diatrizoate sodium 35%, dimenhydrinate, heparin, iodipamide meglumine 52%, iothalamate meglumine 60%, iothalamate sodium 80%, ketorolac, pentobarbital, thiopental. **Variable (consult detailed reference):** Morphine, nalbuphine.

Compatibility when admixed: Compatible: Amikacin, ascorbic acid injection, buprenorphine, butorphanol, chloroquine, cimetidine, dopamine, glycopyrrolate, hydromorphone, morphine, netilmicin, procainamide, prochlorperazine, vancomycin, vinorelbine, vitamin B complex with C. **Incompatible:** Aminophylline, ampicillin, cefazolin, cefotetan, ceftriaxone, chloramphenicol, chlordiazepoxide, chlorothiazide, codeine, floxacillin, furosemide, heparin, hydrocortisone sodium succinate, ketorolac, meperidine, methylprednisolone, methohexital, pentobarbital, phenobarbital, phenytoin, sodium bicarbonate, thiopental. **Variable (consult detailed reference):** Dimenhydrinate, penicillin G potassium.

Mechanism of Action Blocks postsynaptic mesolimbic dopaminergic receptors in the brain; exhibits a strong alpha-adrenergic blocking effect and depresses the release of hypothalamic and hypophyseal hormones; competes with histamine for the H_1-receptor; muscarinic-blocking effect may be responsible for antiemetic activity; reduces stimuli to the brainstem reticular system

Pharmacodynamics/Kinetics

Onset of action: Oral, I.M.: ~20 minutes; I.V.: 3-5 minutes

Peak effect: C_{max}: 9.04 ng/mL (suppository); 19.3 ng/mL (syrup)

Duration: Usually 4-6 hours (up to 12 hours)

Absorption:

I.M.: Bioavailability may be greater than with oral or rectal administration

Oral: Rapid and complete; large first pass effect limits systemic bioavailability

Distribution: V_d: 171 L

Protein binding: 93%

Metabolism: Hepatic; primarily oxidation; forms metabolites

Half-life elimination: 9-16 hours

Time to maximum serum concentration: 4.4 hours (syrup); 6.7-8.6 hours (suppositories)

Excretion: Primarily urine and feces (as inactive metabolites)

Dosage

Children ≥2 years:

Allergic conditions: Oral, rectal: 0.1 mg/kg/dose (maximum: 12.5 mg) every 6 hours during the day and 0.5 mg/kg/dose (maximum: 25 mg) at bedtime as needed

Antiemetic: Oral, I.M., I.V., rectal: 0.25-1 mg/kg 4-6 times/day as needed (maximum: 25 mg/dose)

Motion sickness: Oral, rectal: 0.5 mg/kg/dose 30 minutes to 1 hour before departure, then every 12 hours as needed (maximum dose: 25 mg twice daily)

Sedation: Oral, I.M., I.V., rectal: 0.5-1 mg/kg/dose every 6 hours as needed (maximum: 50 mg/dose)

Adults:

Allergic conditions (including allergic reactions to blood or plasma):

Oral, rectal: 25 mg at bedtime **or** 12.5 mg before meals and at bedtime (range: 6.25-12.5 mg 3 times/day)

I.M., I.V.: 25 mg, may repeat in 2 hours when necessary; switch to oral route as soon as feasible

Antiemetic: Oral, I.M., I.V., rectal: 12.5-25 mg every 4-6 hours as needed

Motion sickness: Oral, rectal: 25 mg 30-60 minutes before departure, then every 12 hours as needed

Sedation: Oral, I.M., I.V., rectal: 12.5-50 mg/dose

Administration Formulations available for oral, rectal, I.M./I.V.; not for SubQ or intra-arterial administration. Administer I.M. into deep muscle (preferred route of administration). I.V. administration is **not** the preferred route; severe tissue damage may occur. Solution for injection should be administered in a maximum concentration of 25 mg/mL (more dilute solutions are recommended). Administer via running I.V. line at port farthest from patient's vein, or through a large bore vein (not hand or wrist). Consider administering over 10-15 minutes (maximum: 25 mg/minute). Discontinue immediately if burning or pain occurs with administration.

Monitoring Parameters Relief of symptoms, mental status

Test Interactions Alters the flare response in intradermal allergen tests; hCG-based pregnancy tests may result in false-negatives or false-positives

Dietary Considerations Increase dietary intake of riboflavin.

Vesicant Yes; see Management of Drug Extravasations on page 1447.

Dosage Forms Excipient information presented when available (limited, particularly for generics); consult specific product labeling. [DSC] = Discontinued product

Injection, solution, as hydrochloride: 25 mg/mL (1 mL); 50 mg/mL (1 mL)

Phenergan®: 25 mg/mL (1 mL); 50 mg/mL (1 mL) [contains sodium metabisulfite]

Suppository, rectal, as hydrochloride: 12.5 mg, 25 mg, 50 mg

Phenadoz™: 12.5 mg, 25 mg

Phenergan®: 25 mg, 50 mg [DSC]

Promethegan™: 12.5 mg, 25 mg, 50 mg

Syrup, as hydrochloride: 6.25 mg/5 mL (120 mL, 480 mL) [contains ethanol, sodium benzoate]

Tablet, as hydrochloride: 12.5 mg, 25 mg, 50 mg

Phenergan®: 25 mg [DSC]

References
Grunberg SM and Hesketh PJ, "Control of Chemotherapy-Induced Emesis," *N Engl J Med*, 1993, 329(24):1790-6.
Institute for Safe Medication Practice, "Action Needed to Prevent Serious Tissue Injury With I.V. Promethazine." Available at http://www.ismp.org/Newsletters/acutecare/articles/20060810.asp

◆ **Promethazine Hydrochloride** *see* Promethazine *on page 997*

◆ **Promethegan™** *see* Promethazine *on page 997*

◆ **Propecia®** *see* Finasteride *on page 480*

◆ **Proquin® XR** *see* Ciprofloxacin *on page 228*

◆ **Proscar®** *see* Finasteride *on page 480*

◆ **Protein-Bound Paclitaxel** *see* Paclitaxel (Protein Bound) *on page 904*

◆ **Prothrombin Complex Concentrate** *see* Factor IX Complex (Human) *on page 452*

◆ **Protopic®** *see* Tacrolimus *on page 1062*

◆ **Provera®** *see* MedroxyPROGESTERone *on page 739*

◆ **Provera-Pak (Can)** *see* MedroxyPROGESTERone *on page 739*

◆ **PS-341** *see* Bortezomib *on page 155*

◆ **Purinethol®** *see* Mercaptopurine *on page 754*

◆ **Quadrivalent Human Papillomavirus Vaccine** *see* Papillomavirus (Types 6, 11, 16, 18) Vaccine (Human, Recombinant) *on page 922*

◆ **Quixin®** *see* Levofloxacin *on page 707*

◆ **RAD001** *see* Everolimus *on page 440*

◆ **rAHF** *see* Antihemophilic Factor (Recombinant) *on page 93*

◆ **Ralivia™ ER (Can)** *see* TraMADol *on page 1130*

Raloxifene (ral OKS i feen)

Medication Safety Issues
Sound-alike/look-alike issues:
Evista® may be confused with Avinza™, Eovist®

Related Information
Safe Handling of Hazardous Drugs *on page 1517*

U.S. Brand Names Evista®

Index Terms Keoxifene Hydrochloride; Raloxifene Hydrochloride

Generic Available No

Canadian Brand Names Apo-Raloxifene; Evista®; Novo-Raloxifene

Pharmacologic Category Selective Estrogen Receptor Modulator (SERM)

Use Prevention and treatment of osteoporosis in postmenopausal women; risk reduction for invasive breast cancer in postmenopausal women with osteoporosis and in postmenopausal women with high risk for invasive breast cancer

Pregnancy Risk Factor X

Lactation Excretion in breast milk unknown/contraindicated

Labeled Contraindications History of or current venous thromboembolic disorders (including DVT, PE, and retinal vein thrombosis); pregnancy or women who could become pregnant; breast-feeding

Warnings/Precautions Hazardous agent - use appropriate precautions for handling and disposal. **[U.S. Boxed Warning]: May increase the risk for DVT or PE; use contraindicated in patients with history of or current venous thromboembolic disorders.** Use with caution in patients at high risk for venous thromboembolism; the risk for DVT and PE are higher in the first 4 months of treatment. Discontinue at least 72 hours prior to and during prolonged immobilization (postoperative recovery or prolonged bedrest). **[U.S. Boxed Warning]: The risk of death due to stroke may be increased in women with coronary heart disease or in women at risk for coronary events;** use with caution in patients with cardiovascular disease. Not be used for the prevention of cardiovascular disease. Use caution with moderate-to-severe renal dysfunction, hepatic impairment, unexplained uterine bleeding, and in women with a history of elevated triglycerides in response to treatment with oral estrogens (or estrogen/progestin). Safety with concomitant estrogen therapy has not been established. Safety and efficacy in premenopausal women or men have not been established. Not indicated for treatment of invasive breast cancer, to reduce the risk of recurrence of invasive breast cancer or to reduce the risk of noninvasive breast cancer. The efficacy (for breast cancer risk reduction) in women with inherited BRCA1 and BRCA1 mutations has not been established.

Adverse Reactions Note: Raloxifene has been associated with increased risk of thromboembolism (DVT, PE) and superficial thrombophlebitis; risk is similar to reported risk of HRT

>10%:

Cardiovascular: Peripheral edema (3% to 14%)

Endocrine & metabolic: Hot flashes (8% to 29%)

Neuromuscular & skeletal: Arthralgia (11% to 16%), leg cramps/muscle spasm (6% to 12%)

Miscellaneous: Flu syndrome (14% to 15%), infection (11%)

1% to 10%:

Cardiovascular: Chest pain (3%), venous thromboembolism (1% to 2%)

Central nervous system: Insomnia (6%)

Dermatologic: Rash (6%)

Endocrine & metabolic: Breast pain (4%)

Gastrointestinal: Weight gain (9%), abdominal pain (7%), vomiting (5%), flatulence (2% to 3%), cholelithiasis (≤3%), gastroenteritis (≤3%)

Genitourinary: Vaginal bleeding (6%), leukorrhea (3%), urinary tract disorder (3%), uterine disorder (3%), vaginal hemorrhage (3%), endometrial disorder (≤3%)

Neuromuscular & skeletal: Myalgia (8%), tendon disorder (4%)

Respiratory: Bronchitis (10%), sinusitis (10%), pharyngitis (8%), pneumonia (3%), laryngitis (≤2%)

Miscellaneous: Diaphoresis (3%)

<1%, postmarketing, and/or case reports: Apolipoprotein A-1 increased, apolipoprotein B decreased, death related to VTE, fibrinogen decreased, hypertriglyceridemia (in women with a history of increased triglycerides in response to oral estrogens), intermittent claudication, LDL cholesterol decreased, lipoprotein decreased, retinal vein occlusion, stroke related to VTE, superficial thrombophlebitis, total serum cholesterol decreased

Drug Interactions

Avoid Concomitant Use There are no known interactions where it is recommended to avoid concomitant use.

Increased Effect/Toxicity There are no known significant interactions involving an increase in effect.

Decreased Effect

Raloxifene may decrease the levels/effects of: Levothyroxine

The levels/effects of Raloxifene may be decreased by: Bile Acid Sequestrants

◄ **Ethanol/Nutrition/Herb Interactions** Ethanol: Avoid ethanol (may increase risk of osteoporosis).

Storage/Stability Store at controlled room temperature of 20°C to 25°C (68°F to 77°F); excursions permitted to 15°C to 30°C (59°F to 86°F).

Mechanism of Action A selective estrogen receptor modulator (SERM), meaning that it affects some of the same receptors that estrogen does, but not all, and in some instances, it antagonizes or blocks estrogen; it acts like estrogen to prevent bone loss and has the potential to block some estrogen effects in the breast and uterine tissues. Raloxifene decreases bone resorption, increasing bone mineral density and decreasing fracture incidence.

Pharmacodynamics/Kinetics

Onset of action: 8 weeks

Absorption: Rapid; ~60%

Distribution: 2348 L/kg

Protein binding: >95% to albumin and α-glycoprotein; does not bind to sex-hormone-binding globulin

Metabolism: Hepatic, extensive first-pass effect; metabolized to glucuronide conjugates

Bioavailability: ~2%

Half-life elimination: 28-33 hours

Excretion: Primarily feces; urine (<0.2% as unchanged drug; <6% as glucuronide conjugates)

Dosage Adults: Females: Oral:

Osteoporosis: 60 mg once daily

Invasive breast cancer risk reduction: 60 mg once daily for 5 years per ASCO guidelines (Visvanathan, 2009)

Dosage adjustment in renal impairment: Moderate-to-severe impairment: Use caution; safety and efficacy have not been established.

Dosage adjustment in hepatic impairment: Mild impairment (Child-Pugh class A): Plasma concentrations were higher and correlated with total bilirubin. Safety and efficacy in hepatic insufficiency have not been established.

Administration May be administered any time of the day without regard to meals.

Monitoring Parameters Bone mineral density (BMD), lipid profile; adequate diagnostic measures, including endometrial sampling, if indicated, should be performed to rule out malignancy in all cases of undiagnosed abnormal vaginal bleeding

Dietary Considerations Osteoporosis prevention or treatment: Ensure adequate calcium and vitamin D intake; postmenopausal women should consume ~1500 mg/day of elemental calcium and 400-800 int. units/day of vitamin D.

Additional Information The decrease in estrogen-related adverse effects with the selective estrogen-receptor modulators in general and raloxifene in particular should improve compliance and decrease the incidence of cardiovascular events and fractures while not increasing breast cancer.

Oncology Comment: The American Society of Clinical Oncology (ASCO) guidelines for breast cancer risk reduction (Visvanathan, 2009) recommend raloxifene (for 5 years) as an option to reduce the risk of ER-positive invasive breast cancer in postmenopausal women with a 5-year projected risk (based on NCI trial model) of ≥1.66%, or with lobular carcinoma *in situ*. Raloxifene should not be used in premenopausal women. Women with osteoporosis may use raloxifene beyond 5 years of treatment. According to the NCCN breast cancer risk reduction guidelines (v.2.2009), raloxifene is only recommended for postmenopausal women (≥35 years of age), and is equivalent to tamoxifen although, raloxifene has a better adverse event profile; however, tamoxifen is superior in reducing the risk on noninvasive breast cancer.

Dosage Forms Excipient information presented when available (limited, particularly for generics); consult specific product labeling.

Tablet, as hydrochloride:

Evista®: 60 mg

References

Barrett-Connor E, Mosca L, Collins P, et al, "Raloxifene Use for The Heart (RUTH) Trial Investigators. Effects of Raloxifene on Cardiovascular Events and Breast Cancer in Postmenopausal Women," *N Engl J Med*, 2006, 355(2):125-37.

Chlebowski RT, Col N, Winer EP, et al, "American Society of Clinical Oncology Technology Assessment of Pharmacologic Interventions for Breast Cancer Risk Reduction Including Tamoxifen, Raloxifene, and Aromatase Inhibition," *J Clin Oncol*, 2002, 20(15):3328-43.

Cummings SR, Eckert S, Krueger KA, et al, "The Effect of Raloxifene on Risk of Breast Cancer in Postmenopausal Women: Results from the MORE Randomized Trial," *JAMA*, 1999, 281(23) 2189-97.

Delmas PD, Bjarnason NH, Mitlak BH, et al, "Effects of Raloxifene on Bone Mineral Density, Serum Cholesterol Concentrations, and Uterine Endometrium in Postmenopausal Women," *N Engl J Med*, 1997, 337(23):1641-7.

Land SR, Wickerham DL, Costantino JP, et al, "Patient-Reported Symptoms and Quality of Life During Treatment With Tamoxifen or Raloxifene for Breast Cancer Prevention: The NSABP Study of Tamoxifen and Raloxifene (STAR) P-2 Trial," *JAMA*, 2006, 295(23):2742-51.

Martino S, Cauley JA, Barrett-Connor E, et al, "Continuing Outcomes Relevant to Evista: Breast Cancer Incident in Postmenopausal Women in a Randomized Trial of Raloxifene," *J Natl Cancer Inst*, 2004, 96(23):1751-61.

National Comprehensive Cancer Network® (NCCN), "Clinical Practice Guidelines in Oncology™: Breast Cancer," Version 1.2009. Available at http://www.nccn.org/professionals/physician_gls/PDF/breast.pdf.

National Comprehensive Cancer Network (NCCN), "Clinical Practice Guidelines in Oncology™: Breast Cancer Risk Reduction," Version 2.2009. Available at http://www.nccn.org/professionals/physician_gls/PDF/breast_risk.pdf.

Siris ES, Harrris ST, Eastell R, et al, "Skeletal Effects of Raloxifene After 8 Years: Results From the Continuing Outcomes Relevant to Evista (CORE) Study," *J Bone Miner Res*, 2005, 20 (9):1514-24.

Visvanathan K, Chlebowski RT, Hurley P, et al, "American Society of Clinical Oncology Clinical Practice Guideline Update on the Use of Pharmacologic Interventions Including Tamoxifen, Raloxifene, and Aromatase Inhibition for Breast Cancer Risk Reduction," *J Clin Oncol*, 2009, 27 (19):3235-58.

Vogel VG, Costantino JP, Wickerham DL, "Effects of Tamoxifen vs Raloxifene on the Risk of Developing Invasive Breast Cancer and Other Disease Outcomes: The NSABP Study of Tamoxifen and Raloxifene (STAR) P-2 Trial," *JAMA*, 2006, 295(23):2727-41.

◆ **Raloxifene Hydrochloride** *see* Raloxifene *on page 1002*

Raltitrexed (ral ti TREX ed)

Medication Safety Issues

High alert medication: The Institute for Safe Medication Practices (ISMP) includes this medication among its list of drug classes which have a heightened risk of causing significant patient harm when used in error.

Related Information

Safe Handling of Hazardous Drugs *on page 1517*

Index Terms ICI-D1694; Raltitrexed Disodium; ZD1694

Generic Available No

Canadian Brand Names Tomudex®

Pharmacologic Category Antineoplastic Agent, Antimetabolite

Use Treatment of advanced colorectal neoplasms

Restrictions Not available in U.S./Investigational

Pregnancy Risk Factor X

Lactation Excretion in breast milk unknown/contraindicated

Labeled Contraindications Hypersensitivity to raltitrexed or any component of the formulation; uncontrolled diarrhea; severe renal or hepatic impairment; pregnancy or breast-feeding

Warnings/Precautions Hazardous agent - use appropriate precautions for handling and disposal. Use caution in patients heavily pretreated with chemotherapy or radiation, especially if myelosuppression, stomatitis, renal toxicity persist. Therapy interruption is required in patients with hepatotoxicity. Use caution in elderly, mild-to-moderate hepatic or renal dysfunction, or a history of gastrointestinal problems (particularly diarrhea). Folinic acid, folic acid, or folate-containing medications (eg, multivitamins) may interfere with raltitrexed; do not administer immediately prior to or concurrently with raltitrexed. May cause malaise/weakness (caution patients concerning operation of machinery/driving). Safety and efficacy in pediatric patients have not been established.

Adverse Reactions

>10%:

Central nervous system: Fever (2% to 23%), may be delayed until several days after administration

Dermatologic: Rashes (14%), usually pruritic papular lesions on head and thorax

Gastrointestinal: Nausea (58%; grade 3 or 4 in 12%), mucositis/stomatitis (12% to 48%; grade 3 or 4 in 2%), diarrhea (38%; grade 3 or 4 in 11%), vomiting (37%), anorexia (27%), abdominal pain (18%), constipation (13% to 15%; grade 3 or 4 in 2%)

Hematologic: Myelosuppression; leukopenia occurs in about 21% of patients (grade 3 or 4 in 12%), nadirs occur in ~8 days, but may be delayed to day 21, with recovery in ~10 days; thrombocytopenia (5% to 6%; grade 3 or 4 in 4%), anemia (15% to 18%; grade 3 or 4 in 7%)

Hepatic: Transaminases increased (14% to 18%; grade 3 or 4 in 10%)

Neuromuscular & skeletal: Weakness (46% to 48%; grade 3 or 4 in 9%)

1% to 10%:

Cardiovascular: Edema (9% to 10%), arrhythmias (3%), CHF (2%)

Central nervous system: Malaise, headache, pain, chills, insomnia, depression, paresthesia

Dermatologic: Alopecia, cellulitis, exfoliative eruptions

Endocrine & metabolic: Dehydration, hypokalemia

Gastrointestinal: Dyspepsia, flatulence, xerostomia, weight loss, taste perversion

Genitourinary: Urinary tract infection

Hepatic: Alkaline phosphatase increased, bilirubin increased

Neuromuscular & skeletal: Arthralgia, myalgia, hypotonia

Ocular: Conjunctivitis

Renal: Serum creatinine increased

Respiratory: Cough increased, dyspnea, pharyngitis

Miscellaneous: Flu-like syndrome (6% to 8%), diaphoresis, infection, sepsis

<1%: Hypersensitivity/allergic reaction (including stridor and wheezing following the first dose), desquamation

Drug Interactions

Avoid Concomitant Use

Avoid concomitant use of Raltitrexed with any of the following: Folic Acid; Leucovorin-Levoleucovorin; Methylfolate

Increased Effect/Toxicity There are no known significant interactions involving an increase in effect.

Decreased Effect

The levels/effects of Raltitrexed may be decreased by: Folic Acid; Leucovorin-Levoleucovorin; Methylfolate

Ethanol/Nutrition/Herb Interactions Herb/Nutraceutical: Avoid folic acid and multivitamins with folic acid close to and during administration.

Storage/Stability Intact vials should be refrigerated at 2°C to 25°C. Protect from light. Solutions reconstituted with saline or dextrose to a concentrate of 0.5 mg/mL are stable for up to 24 hours under refrigeration at 2°C to 8°C.

Reconstitution Reconstitute 2 mg vial with 4 mL SWFI; add to 50-250 mL NS or D_5W.

Compatibility Stable in D_5W, NS. Do not mix with other medications.

Mechanism of Action Raltitrexed is a folate analogue that inhibits thymidylate synthase, blocking purine synthesis. This results in an overall inhibition of DNA synthesis.

Pharmacodynamics/Kinetics

Distribution: V_{ss}: 548 L

Protein binding: 93%

Metabolism: Undergoes extensive intracellular metabolism to active poly-glutamate forms; appears to be little or no systemic metabolism of the drug

Half-life elimination: Triphasic; Beta: 2 hours; Terminal: Up to 198 hours

Excretion: Urine (50% as unchanged drug); feces (15%)

Dosage Refer to individual protocols.

I.V.: 3 mg/m² every 3 weeks

Dosage adjustment in renal impairment:

Cl_{cr} 55-65 mL/minute: Administer 75% of dose every 4 weeks

Cl_{cr} 25-54 mL/minute: Administer % of dose equivalent to Cl_{cr} every 4 weeks (ie, 25% of dose for Cl_{cr} of 25 mL/minute)

Cl_{cr} <25 mL/minute: Do not administer

Dosage adjustment for hepatic impairment: No adjustment required for mild-moderate hepatic insufficiency. Patients who develop hepatic toxicity should have treatment held until returns to grade 2.

Dosage adjustment for toxicity:

Grade 4 gastrointestinal toxicity or grade 3 gastrointestinal toxicity in combination with grade 4 hematologic toxicity: Discontinue therapy

Grade 3 hematologic toxicity or grade 2 gastrointestinal toxicity: Reduce dose by 25%

Grade 4 hematologic toxicity or grade 3 gastrointestinal toxicity: Reduce dose by 50%

Administration Infuse over 15 minutes.

Monitoring Parameters CBC with differential, hepatic function tests, serum lipids, serum creatinine

Dietary Considerations Avoid folic acid, folinic acid, and multivitamins with folic acid close to and during administration.

Additional Information Not available in U.S.

Dosage Forms Excipient information presented when available (limited, particularly for generics); consult specific product labeling.

Injection, powder for reconstitution, as disodium: 2 mg

References

Clarke SJ, Beale PJ, and Rivory LP, "Clinical and Preclinical Pharmacokinetics of Raltitrexed," *Clin Pharmacokinet*, 2000, 39(6):429-43.

Taylor SC, "Raltitrexed for Advanced Colorectal Cancer. The Story So Far," *Cancer Pract*, 2000, 8 (1):51-4.

Van Cutsem E, Cunningham D, Maroun J, et al, "Raltitrexed: Current Clinical Status and Future Directions," *Ann Oncol*, 2002, 13(4):513-22.

Rasburicase (ras BYOOR i kayse)

Related Information
Tumor Lysis Syndrome *on page 1468*

U.S. Brand Names Elitek®

Index Terms Recombinant Urate Oxidase; Urate Oxidase

Generic Available No

Canadian Brand Names Fasturtec®

Pharmacologic Category Enzyme; Enzyme, Urate-Oxidase (Recombinant)

Use Initial management of uric acid levels in pediatric patients with leukemia, lymphoma, and solid tumor malignancies receiving chemotherapy expected to result in tumor lysis and elevation of plasma uric acid

Unlabeled/Investigational Use Prevention and treatment of malignancy-associated hyperuricemia in adults

Pregnancy Risk Factor C

Lactation Excretion in breast milk unknown/not recommended

Labeled Contraindications Hypersensitivity, hemolytic or methemoglobinemia reactions to rasburicase or any component of the formulation; glucose-6-phosphatase dehydrogenase (G6PD) deficiency

Warnings/Precautions [U.S. Boxed Warning]: Severe hypersensitivity reactions (including anaphylaxis) have been reported; immediately and permanently discontinue in patients developing serious hypersensitivity reaction; reactions may occur at any time during treatment, including the initial dose. Signs and symptoms of hypersensitivity may include bronshospasm, chest pain/tightness, dyspnea, hypotension, hypoxia, shock, or urticaria. **[U.S. Boxed Warning]: Hemolysis may be associated with G6PD deficiency; discontinue immediately and permanently in any patient developing hemolysis. Patients at higher risk for G6PD deficiency (eg, African, Mediterranean, or Southeas Asian descent) should be screened prior to therapy;** use is contraindicated in patients with G6PD deficiency. [U.S. Boxed Warning]: Methemoglobinemia has been reported. Discontinue immediately and permanently in any patient developing methemoglobinemia.

[U.S. Boxed Warning]: Enzymatic degradation of uric acid in blood samples will occur if left at room temperature; specific guidelines for the collection of plasma uric acid samples must be followed, including collection in pre-chilled tubes with heparin anticoagulant, immediate ice water bath immersion and assay within 4 hours. Patients at risk for tumor lysis syndrome should receive appropriate I.V. hydration as part of uric acid management; however, alkalinization (with sodium bicarbonate) concurrently with rasburicase is not recommended (Coiffier, 2008). Rasburicase is immunogenic and can elicit an antibody response; administration of more than one course is not recommended.

Adverse Reactions

>10%:
Central nervous system: Fever (46%; serious: 5%), headache (26%)
Dermatologic: Rash (13%; serious: 1%)

Gastrointestinal: Vomiting (50%), nausea (27%), abdominal pain (20%), constipation (20%), diarrhea (20%), mucositis (15%; serious: 2%)

Miscellaneous: Antibody formation (healthy volunteers: 61% to 64%; patients with malignancies: 11%)

1% to 10%:

Hematologic: Neutropenic fever (serious: 4%), neutropenia (serious: 2%)

Respiratory: Respiratory distress (serious: 3%)

Miscellaneous: Sepsis (serious: 3%)

<1%, postmarketing, and/or case reports: Acute renal failure, anaphylaxis, arrhythmia, cardiac arrest, cardiac failure, cellulitis, cerebrovascular disorder, chest pain, cyanosis, dehydration, hemolysis, hemorrhage, hot flashes, ileus, infection, intestinal obstruction, liver enzymes increased, methemoglobinemia, MI, pancytopenia, paresthesia, pneumonia, pulmonary edema, pulmonary hypertension, retinal hemorrhage, rigors, seizure, thrombosis, thrombophlebitis

Drug Interactions

Avoid Concomitant Use There are no known interactions where it is recommended to avoid concomitant use.

Increased Effect/Toxicity There are no known significant interactions involving an increase in effect.

Decreased Effect There are no known significant interactions involving a decrease in effect.

Storage/Stability Prior to reconstitution, store with diluent at 2°C to 8°C (36°F to 46°F); do not freeze. Protect from light. Reconstituted and final solution may be stored up to 24 hours at 2°C to 8°C (36°F to 46°F). Discard unused product.

Reconstitution Reconstitute with provided diluent (use 1 mL diluent for the 1.5 mg vial and 5 mL diluent for the 7.5 mg vial). Mix by gently swirling; do **not** shake or vortex. Discard if discolored or containing particulate matter. Total dose should be further diluted in NS to a final volume of 50 mL.

Mechanism of Action Rasburicase is a recombinant urate-oxidase enzyme, which converts uric acid to allantoin (an inactive and soluble metabolite of uric acid); it does not inhibit the formation of uric acid.

Pharmacodynamics/Kinetics

Onset: Uric acid levels decrease within 4 hours of initial administration

Distribution: Children: 110-127 mL/kg

Half-life elimination: Children: 0.15 mg/kg: ~16 hours; 0.2 mg/kg: ~21 hours

Dosage I.V.: Hyperuricemia associated with malignancy:

Children: 0.15 mg/kg or 0.2 mg/kg once daily for 5 days (manufacturer-recommended dose and duration); begin chemotherapy 4-24 hours after the first dose **or**

Alternate dosing (unlabeled; Coiffier, 2008): 0.05-0.2 mg/kg once daily for 1-7 days (average of 2-3 days) with the duration of treatment dependant on plasma uric acid levels and clinical judgment (patients with significant tumor burden may require an increase to twice daily); the following dose levels are recommended based on risk of tumor lysis syndrome (TLS):

High risk: 0.2 mg/kg once daily (duration is based on plasma uric acid levels)

Intermediate risk: 0.15 mg/kg once daily (duration is based on plasma uric acid levels); may consider managing initially with a single dose

Low risk: 0.1 mg/kg once daily (duration is based on clinical judgment); a dose of 0.05 mg/kg was used (with good results) in one trial

Single-dose rasburicase (unlabeled use; based on limited data): 0.15 mg/kg; additional doses may be needed based on serum uric acid levels (Liu, 2005)

Adults (unlabeled use; Coiffier, 2008): 0.05-0.2 mg/kg once daily for 1-7 days (average of 2-3 days) with the duration of treatment dependant on plasma uric acid levels and clinical judgment (patients with significant tumor burden may require an increase to twice daily); the following dose levels are recommended based on risk of tumor lysis syndrome (TLS):

High risk: 0.2 mg/kg once daily (duration is based on plasma uric acid levels)

Intermediate risk: 0.15 mg/kg once daily (duration is based on plasma uric acid levels)

Low risk: 0.1 mg/kg once daily (duration is based on clinical judgment); a dose of 0.05 mg/kg was used (with good results) in one trial

Single-dose rasburicase (unlabeled use; based on limited data): 0.15 mg/kg (Campara, 2009; Liu, 2005) **or** 3-7.5 mg as a single dose (Hutcherson, 2006; McDonnell, 2006; Reeves, 2008; Trifilio, 2006); repeat doses (1.5-6 mg) may be needed based on serum uric acid levels

Administration I.V. infusion over 30 minutes; do **not** administer as a bolus infusion. Do **not** filter during infusion. If not possible to administer through a separate line, I.V. line should be flushed with at least 15 mL saline prior to and following rasburicase infusion.

Monitoring Parameters Plasma uric acid levels (4 hours after rasburicase administration, then every 6-8 hours until TLS resolution), CBC, G6PD deficiency screening (in patients at high risk for deficiency); monitor for hypersensitivity

Test Interactions Specific handling procedures must be followed to prevent the degradation of uric acid in plasma samples. Blood must be collected in prechilled tubes containing heparin anticoagulant. Samples must then be **immediately** immersed in an ice water bath. Prepare samples by centrifugation in a precooled centrifuge (4°C). Samples must be kept in ice water bath and analyzed within 4 hours of collection.

Additional Information

Specific handling procedures must be followed to prevent the degradation of uric acid in plasma samples. Blood must be collected in prechilled tubes containing heparin anticoagulant. Samples must then be **immediately** immersed in an ice water bath. Prepare samples by centrifugation in a precooled centrifuge (4°C). Samples must be kept in ice water bath and analyzed within 4 hours of collection.

Dosage Forms Excipient information presented when available (limited, particularly for generics); consult specific product labeling.

Injection, powder for reconstitution:

Elitek®: 1.5 mg [packaged with three 1 mL ampuls of diluent]; 7.5 mg [packaged with 5 mL of diluent]

References

Arnold TM, Reuter JP, Delman BS, et al, "Use of Single-Dose Rasburicase in an Obese Female," *Ann Pharmacother*, 2004, 38(9):1428-31.

Campara M, Shord SS, and Haaf CM, "Single-Dose Rasburicase for Tumour Lysis Syndrome in Adults: Weight-Based Approach," *J Clin Pharm Ther*, 2009, 34(2):207-13.

Coiffier B, Altman A, Pui CH, et al, "Guidelines for the Management of Pediatric and Adult Tumor Lysis Syndrome: An Evidence-Based Review," *J Clin Oncol*, 2008, 26(16):2767-78.

Coiffier B, Mounier N, Bologna S, et al, "Efficacy and Safety of Rasburicase (Recombinant Urate Oxidase) for the Prevention and Treatment of Hyperuricemia During Induction Chemotherapy of Aggressive Non-Hodgkin's Lymphoma: Results of GRAALI (Groupe d'Etude des Lymphomes de l'Adulte Trial on Rasburicase Activity in Adult Lymphoma) Study," *J Clin Oncol*, 2003, 21 (23):4402-6.

Hutcherson DA, Gammon DC, Bhatt MS, et al, "Reduced-Dose Rasburicase in the Treatment of Adults With Hyperuricemia Associated With Malignancy," *Pharmacother*, 2006, 26(2):242-7.

Jeha S, Kantarjian H, Irwin D, et al, "Efficacy and Safety of Rasburicase, a Recombinant Urate Oxidase (Elitek), in the Management of Malignancy-Associated Hyperuricemia in Pediatric and

Adult Patients: Final Results of a Multicenter Compassionate Use Trial," *Leukemia*, 2005, 19 (1):34-8.

Lee AC, Li CH, So KT, et al, "Treatment of Impending Tumor Lysis With Single-Dose Rasburicase," *Ann Pharmacother*, 2003, 37(11):1614-7.

Liu CY, Sims-McCallum RP, and Schiffer CA, "A Single Dose of Rasburicase is Sufficient for the Treatment of Hyperuricemia in Patients Receiving Chemotherapy," *Leuk Res*, 2005, 29(4):463-5.

McDonnell AM, Lenz KL, Frei-Lahr DA, et al, "Single-Dose Rasburicase 6 mg in the Management of Tumor Lysis Syndrome in Adults," *Pharmacother*, 2006, 26(6):806-12.

Reeves DJ and Bestul DJ, "Evaluation of a Single Fixed Dose of Rasburicase 7.5 mg for the Treatment of Hyperuricemia in Adults With Cancer," *Pharmacother*, 2008; 28(6):685–90.

Trifilio S, Gordon L, Singhall S, et al, "Reduced Dose Rasburicase (Recombinant Xanthine Oxidase) in Adult Cancer Patients With Hyperuricemia," *Bone Marrow Transplant*, 2006, 37 (11):997-1001.

Rh_o(D) Immune Globulin (ar aych oh (dee) i MYUN GLOB yoo lin)

U.S. Brand Names HyperRHO™ S/D Full Dose; HyperRHO™ S/D Mini Dose; MICRhoGAM®; RhoGAM®; Rhophylac®; WinRho® SDF

Index Terms RhIG; Rho(D) Immune Globulin (Human); RhoIGIV; RhoIVIM

Generic Available No

Canadian Brand Names WinRho® SDF

Pharmacologic Category Blood Product Derivative; Immune Globulin

Use

Suppression of Rh isoimmunization: Use in the following situations when an Rh₀(D)-negative individual is exposed to Rh₀(D)-positive blood: During delivery of an Rh₀(D)-positive infant; abortion; amniocentesis; chorionic villus sampling; ruptured tubal pregnancy; abdominal trauma; hydatidiform mole; transplacental hemorrhage. Used when the mother is Rh₀(D) negative, the father of the child is either Rh₀(D) positive or Rh₀(D) unknown, the baby is either Rh₀(D) positive or Rh₀(D) unknown.

Transfusion: Suppression of Rh isoimmunization in Rh₀(D)-negative individuals transfused with Rh₀(D) antigen-positive RBCs or blood components containing Rh₀(D) antigen-positive RBCs

Treatment of idiopathic thrombocytopenic purpura (ITP): Used in the following nonsplenectomized Rh₀(D) positive individuals: Children with acute or chronic ITP, adults with chronic ITP, children and adults with ITP secondary to HIV infection

Pregnancy Risk Factor C

Lactation Does not enter breast milk

Labeled Contraindications Hypersensitivity to immune globulins or any component of the formulation; prior sensitization to Rh₀(D)

Warnings/Precautions Rare but serious signs and symptoms (eg, back pain, shaking, chills, fever, discolored urine; onset within 4 hours of infusion) of intravascular hemolysis (IVH) have been reported in postmarketing experience in patients treated for ITP. Clinically-compromising anemia, acute renal insufficiency and disseminated intravascular coagulation (DIC) have also been reported. ITP patients should be advised of the signs and symptoms of IVH and instructed to report them immediately.

Product of human plasma; may potentially contain infectious agents which could transmit disease. Screening of donors, as well as testing and/or inactivation or removal of certain viruses, reduces the risk. Infections thought to be transmitted by this product should be reported to the manufacturer. Not for replacement therapy in immune globulin deficiency syndromes. Use caution with IgA deficiency, may contain trace amounts of IgA; patients who are IgA deficient may have the potential for developing IgA antibodies, anaphylactic reactions may occur. Administer I.M. injections with caution in patients with thrombocytopenia or coagulation disorders. Some products may contain maltose, which may result in falsely-elevated blood glucose readings. Use caution with renal dysfunction; may require an infusion rate reduction or discontinuation. Safety and efficacy have not been established for Rhophylac® in patients with anemia.

ITP: Do not administer I.M. or SubQ for the treatment of ITP; administer dose I.V. only. Safety and efficacy not established in Rh₀(D) negative, non-ITP thrombocytopenia, or splenectomized patients. When using WinRho® SDF, decrease dose with hemoglobin <10 g/dL; use with extreme caution if hemoglobin <8 g/dL. Safety and efficacy have not been established for Rhophylac® in patients with anemia.

Rh₀(D) suppression: For use in the mother; do not administer to the neonate.

Adverse Reactions Frequency not defined.

Cardiovascular: Hyper-/hypotension, pallor, tachycardia, vasodilation

Central nervous system: Chills, dizziness, fever, headache, malaise, somnolence

Dermatologic: Pruritus, rash

Gastrointestinal: Abdominal pain, diarrhea, nausea, vomiting

Hematologic: Haptoglobin decreased, hemoglobin decreased (patients with ITP), intravascular hemolysis (patients with ITP)

Hepatic: Bilirubin increased, LDH increased

Local: Injection site reaction: Discomfort, induration, mild pain, redness, swelling

Neuromuscular & skeletal: Arthralgia, back pain, hyperkinesia, myalgia, weakness

Renal: Acute renal insufficiency

Miscellaneous: Anaphylaxis, diaphoresis, infusion-related reactions, positive anti-C antibody test (transient), shivering

Postmarketing and/or case reports: Anemia (clinically-compromising), DIC, dyspnea, erythema, hemoglobinuria (transient in patients with ITP), injection site irritation, vertigo

Drug Interactions

Avoid Concomitant Use There are no known interactions where it is recommended to avoid concomitant use.

Increased Effect/Toxicity There are no known significant interactions involving an increase in effect.

Decreased Effect

Rho(D) Immune Globulin may decrease the levels/effects of: Vaccines (Live)

Storage/Stability Store at 2°C to 8°C (35°F to 46°F); do not freeze. Rhophylac®: Protect from light.

Mechanism of Action

Rh suppression: Prevents isoimmunization by suppressing the immune response and antibody formation by Rh₀(D) negative individuals to Rh₀(D) positive red blood cells.

ITP: Not completely characterized; Rh₀(D) immune globulin is thought to form anti-D-coated red blood cell complexes which bind to macrophage Fc receptors within the spleen; blocking or saturating the spleens ability to clear antibody-coated cells, including platelets. In this manner, platelets are spared from destruction.

Pharmacodynamics/Kinetics

Onset of platelet increase: ITP: Platelets should rise within 1-2 days

Peak effect: In 7-14 days

Duration: Suppression of Rh isoimmunization: ~12 weeks; Treatment of ITP: 30 days (variable)

Distribution: V_d: I.M.: 8.59 L

Bioavailability: I.M.: Rhophylac®: 69%

Half-life elimination: 12-30 days

Time to peak, plasma: I.M.: 5-10 days; I.V. (WinRho® SDF): ≤2 hours

Dosage

ITP: Children and Adults:

Rhophylac®: I.V.: 50 mcg/kg

WinRho® SDF: I.V.:

Initial: 50 mcg/kg as a single injection, or can be given as a divided dose on separate days. If hemoglobin is <10 g/dL: Dose should be reduced to 25-40 mcg/kg.

Subsequent dosing: 25-60 mcg/kg can be used if required to elevate platelet count

Maintenance dosing if patient **did respond** to initial dosing: 25-60 mcg/kg based on platelet and hemoglobin levels

Maintenance dosing if patient **did not respond** to initial dosing:

Hemoglobin 8-10 g/dL: Redose between 25-40 mcg/kg

Hemoglobin >10 g/dL: Redose between 50-60 mcg/kg

Hemoglobin <8 g/dL: Use with caution

Rh$_O$(D) suppression: Adults: **Note:** One "full dose" (300 mcg) provides enough antibody to prevent Rh sensitization if the volume of RBC entering the circulation is ≤15 mL. When >15 mL is suspected, a fetal red cell count should be performed to determine the appropriate dose.

Pregnancy:

Antepartum prophylaxis: In general, dose is given at 28 weeks. If given early in pregnancy, administer every 12 weeks to ensure adequate levels of passively acquired anti-Rh

HyperRHO™ S/D Full Dose, RhoGAM®: I.M.: 300 mcg

Rhophylac®, WinRho® SDF: I.M., I.V.: 300 mcg

Postpartum prophylaxis: In general, dose is administered as soon as possible after delivery, preferably within 72 hours. Can be given up to 28 days following delivery

HyperRHO™ S/D Full Dose, RhoGAM®: I.M.: 300 mcg

Rhophylac®: I.M., I.V.: 300 mcg

WinRho® SDF: I.M., I.V.: 120 mcg

Threatened abortion, any time during pregnancy (with continuation of pregnancy):

HyperRHO™ S/D Full Dose, RhoGAM®: I.M.: 300 mcg; administer as soon as possible

Rhophylac®, WinRho® SDF: I.M., I.V.: 300 mcg; administer as soon as possible

Abortion, miscarriage, termination of ectopic pregnancy:

RhoGAM®: I.M.: ≥13 weeks gestation: 300 mcg.

HyperRHO™ S/D Mini Dose, MICRhoGAM®: <13 weeks gestation: I.M.: 50 mcg

Rhophylac®: I.M., I.V.: 300 mcg

WinRho® SDF: I.M., I.V.: After 34 weeks gestation: 120 mcg; administer immediately or within 72 hours

Amniocentesis, chorionic villus sampling:

HyperRHO™ S/D Full Dose, RhoGAM®: I.M.: At 15-18 weeks gestation or during the 3rd trimester: 300 mcg. If dose is given between 13-18 weeks, repeat at 26-28 weeks and within 72 hours of delivery.

Rhophylac®: I.M., I.V.: 300 mcg

WinRho® SDF: I.M., I.V.: Before 34 weeks gestation: 300 mcg; administer immediately, repeat dose every 12 weeks during pregnancy; After 34 weeks gestation: 120 mcg, administered immediately or within 72 hours

Excessive fetomaternal hemorrhage (>15 mL): Rhophylac®: I.M., I.V.: 300 mcg within 72 hours plus 20 mcg/mL fetal RBCs in excess of 15 mL if excess transplacental bleeding is quantified **or** 300 mcg/dose if bleeding cannot be quantified

Abdominal trauma, manipulation:

HyperRHO™ S/D Full Dose, RhoGAM®: I.M.: 2nd or 3rd trimester: 300 mcg. If dose is given between 13-18 weeks, repeat at 26-28 weeks and within 72 hours of delivery

Rhophylac®: I.M., I.V.: 300 mcg within 72 hours

WinRho® SDF: I.M./I.V.: After 34 weeks gestation: 120 mcg; administer immediately or within 72 hours

Transfusion:

Children and Adults: WinRho® SDF: Administer within 72 hours after exposure of incompatible blood transfusions or massive fetal hemorrhage.

I.V.: Calculate dose as follows; administer 600 mcg every 8 hours until the total dose is administered:

Exposure to $Rh_o(D)$ positive whole blood: 9 mcg/mL blood

Exposure to $Rh_o(D)$ positive red blood cells: 18 mcg/mL cells

I.M.: Calculate dose as follows; administer 1200 mcg every 12 hours until the total dose is administered:

Exposure to $Rh_o(D)$ positive whole blood: 12 mcg/mL blood

Exposure to $Rh_o(D)$ positive red blood cells: 24 mcg/mL cells

Adults:

HyperRHO™ S/D Full Dose, RhoGAM®: I.M.: Multiply the volume of Rh positive whole blood administered by the hematocrit of the donor unit to equal the volume of RBCs transfused. The volume of RBCs is then divided by 15 mL, providing the number of 300 mcg doses (vials/syringes) to administer. If the dose calculated results in a fraction, round up to the next higher whole 300 mcg dose (vial/syringe).

Rhophylac®: I.M., I.V.: 20 mcg/2 mL transfused blood or 20 mcg/mL erythrocyte concentrate

Dosage adjustment in renal impairment: I.V. infusion: Use caution; may require infusion rate reduction or discontinuation.

Administration The total volume can be administered in divided doses at different sites at one time or may be divided and given at intervals, provided the total dosage is given within 72 hours of the fetomaternal hemorrhage or transfusion.

I.M.: Administer into the deltoid muscle of the upper arm or anterolateral aspect of the upper thigh; avoid gluteal region due to risk of sciatic nerve injury. If large doses (>5 mL) are needed, administration in divided doses at different sites is recommended. **Note:** Do not administer I.M. Rho(D) immune globulin for ITP.

I.V.:

WinRho® SDF: Infuse over at least 3-5 minutes; do not administer with other medications

Rhophylac®: ITP: Infuse at 2 mL per 15-60 seconds

Note: If preparing dose using liquid formulation, withdraw the entire contents of the vial to ensure accurate calculation of the dosage requirement.

Monitoring Parameters Signs and symptoms of intravascular hemolysis (IVH), anemia, and renal insufficiency; observe patient for side effects for at least 20 minutes following administration; patients with suspected IVH should have CBC, haptoglobin, plasma hemoglobin, urine dipstick, BUN, serum creatinine, liver function tests; DIC-specific tests (D-dimer, fibrin degradation products [FDP] or fibrin split products [FSP]) for differential diagnosis. Clinical response may be determined by monitoring platelets, red blood cell (RBC) counts, hemoglobin, and reticulocyte levels.

Test Interactions Some infants born to women given $Rh_o(D)$ antepartum have a weakly positive Coombs' test at birth. Fetal-maternal hemorrhage may cause false blood-typing result in the mother; when there is any doubt to the patients' Rh type, $Rh_o(D)$ immune globulin should be administered. WinRho® SDF liquid contains maltose; may result in falsely elevated blood glucose levels with dehydrogenase pyrroloquinolinequinone or glucose-dye-oxidoreductase testing methods. WinRho® SDF contains trace amounts of anti-A, B, C and E; may alter Coombs' tests following administration.

◀ **Additional Information** A "full dose" of Rh_o(D) immune globulin has previously been referred to as a 300 mcg dose. It is not the actual anti-D content. Although dosing has traditionally been expressed in mcg, potency is listed in int. units (1 mcg = 5 int. units). ITP patients requiring transfusions should be transfused with Rho-negative blood cells to avoid exacerbating hemolysis; platelet products may contain red blood cells; caution should be exercised if platelets are from Rh_o-positive donors.

Dosage Forms Excipient information presented when available (limited, particularly for generics); consult specific product labeling. [DSC] = Discontinued product

Injection, solution [preservative free]:

HyperRHO™ S/D Full Dose: 300 mcg [for I.M. use only]

HyperRHO™ S/D Mini Dose: 50 mcg [for I.M. use only]

MICRhoGAM®: 50 mcg [for I.M. use only; contains polysorbate 80]

RhoGAM®: 300 mcg [for I.M. use only; contains polysorbate 80]

Rhophylac®: 300 mcg/2 mL (2 mL) [1500 int. units; for I.M. or I.V. use; contains human albumin]

WinRho® SDF:

120 mcg/~0.5 mL (~0.5 mL) [600 int. units; contains maltose and polysorbate 80; for I.M. or I.V. use] [DSC]

300 mcg/~1.3 mL (~1.3 mL) [1500 int. units; contains maltose and polysorbate 80; for I.M. or I.V. use]

500 mcg/~2.2 mL (~2.2 mL) [2500 int. units; contains maltose and polysorbate 80; for I.M. or I.V. use]

1000 mcg/~4.4 mL (~4.4 mL) [5000 int. units; contains maltose and polysorbate 80; for I.M. or I.V. use]

3000 mcg/~13 mL (~13 mL) [15,000 int. units; contains maltose and polysorbate 80; for I.M. or I.V. use]

References

Gaines AR, "Acute Onset Hemoglobinemia and/or Hemoglobinuria and Sequelae Following Rho (D) Immune Globulin Intravenous Administration in Immune Thrombocytopenic Purpura Patients," *Blood*, 2000, 95(8):2523-9.

Gaines AR, "Disseminated Intravascular Coagulation Associated with Acute Hemoglobinemia or Hemoglobinuria Following Rho(D) Immune Globulin Intravenous Administration for Immune Thrombocytopenic Purpura," *Blood*, 2005, 106(5):1532-37.

George JN, Woolf SH, Raskob GE, et al, "Clinical Guideline: Diagnosis and Treatment of Idiopathic Thrombocytopenic Purpura: Recommendations of the American Society of Hematology," *Ann Intern Med*, 1997, 126(4):319-26.

"Rh_o(D) Immune Globulin I.V. for Prevention of Rh Isoimmunization and for Treatment of ITP," *Med Lett Drugs Ther*, 1996, 38(966):6-8.

Simpson KN, Coughlin CM, Eron J, et al, "Idiopathic Thrombocytopenia Purpura: Treatment Patterns and an Analysis of Cost Associated With Intravenous Immunoglobulin and Anti-D Therapy," *Semin Hematol*, 1998, 35(1 Suppl 1):58-64.

Scaradavou A, Bussel J. "Clinical Experience With Anti-D in the Treatment of Idiopathic Thrombocytopenic Purpura." *Semin Hematol*, 1998, 35(1 Suppl 1):52-7.

♦ **rhu Keratinocyte Growth Factor** *see* Palifermin *on page 908*

♦ **rHu-KGF** *see* Palifermin *on page 908*

♦ **rHuMAb-EGFr** *see* Panitumumab *on page 919*

♦ **rhuMAb-VEGF** *see* Bevacizumab *on page 137*

♦ **RiaSTAP™** *see* Fibrinogen Concentrate (Human) *on page 474*

♦ **rIL-11** *see* Oprelvekin *on page 880*

♦ **Rituxan®** *see* RiTUXimab *on page 1017*

RiTUXimab (ri TUK si mab)

Medication Safety Issues

Sound-alike/look-alike issues:

Rituxan® may be confused with Remicade®

RiTUXimab may be confused with bevacizumab, inFLIXimab

High alert medication: The Institute for Safe Medication Practices (ISMP) includes this medication among its list of drug classes which have a heightened risk of causing significant patient harm when used in error.

The rituximab dose for rheumatoid arthritis is a flat dose (1000 mg) and is not based on body surface area (BSA).

U.S. Brand Names Rituxan®

Index Terms Anti-CD20 Monoclonal Antibody; C2B8 Monoclonal Antibody; IDEC-C2B8

Generic Available No

Canadian Brand Names Rituxan®

Pharmacologic Category Antineoplastic Agent, Monoclonal Antibody; Monoclonal Antibody

Use Treatment of low-grade or follicular CD20-positive, B-cell non-Hodgkin's lymphoma (NHL); treatment of diffuse large B-cell CD20-positive NHL; treatment of moderately- to severely-active rheumatoid arthritis (RA) in combination with methotrexate

Canadian labeling: Additional uses (not in U.S. labeling): Treatment of B-cell chronic lymphocytic leukemia (B-CLL), stage B or C, in combination with cyclophosphamide and fludarabine

Unlabeled/Investigational Use Treatment of Burkitt's lymphoma, central nervous system lymphoma, Hodgkin's lymphoma (lymphocyte predominant); mucosal associated lymphoid tissue (MALT) lymphoma (gastric and non-gastric), splenic marginal zone lymphoma, chronic lymphocytic leukemia (CLL); small lymphocytic lymphoma (SLL); Waldenström's macroglobulinemia (WM); autoimmune hemolytic anemia (AIHA) in children; chronic immune thrombocytopenic purpura (ITP); refractory pemphigus vulgaris, treatment of systemic autoimmune diseases (other than rheumatoid arthritis); treatment of steroid-refractory chronic graft-versus-host disease (GVHD)

Pregnancy Risk Factor C

Lactation Excretion in breast milk unknown/not recommended

Labeled Contraindications There are no contraindications listed in the FDA-approved manufacturer's labeling.

Canadian labeling (not in U.S. labeling): Type 1 hypersensitivity or anaphylactic reaction to murine proteins, Chinese Hamster Ovary (CHO) cell proteins, or any component of the formulation

◄ **Warnings/Precautions [U.S. Boxed Warning]: Severe (occasionally fatal) infusion-related reactions have been reported, usually with the first infusion; fatalities have been reported within 24 hours of infusion; monitor closely and discontinue with grades 3 or 4 infusion reactions.** Reactions usually occur within 30-120 minutes and may include hypotension, angioedema, bronchospasm, hypoxia, urticaria, and in more severe cases pulmonary infiltrates, acute respiratory distress syndrome, myocardial infarction, ventricular fibrillation, cardiogenic shock and/or anaphylaxis. Risk factors associated with fatal outcomes include chronic lymphocytic leukemia, female gender, mantle cell lymphoma, or pulmonary infiltrates. Closely monitor patients with a history of prior cardiopulmonary reactions or with pre-existing cardiac or pulmonary conditions and patients with high numbers of circulating malignant cells (>25,000/mm^3). Prior to infusion, premedicate patients with acetaminophen and an antihistamine. Discontinue infusion for severe reactions; treatment is symptomatic. Medications for the treatment of hypersensitivity reactions (eg, bronchodilators, epinephrine, antihistamines, corticosteroids) should be available for immediate use. Discontinue infusion for serious or life-threatening cardiac arrhythmias; subsequent doses should include cardiac monitoring during and after the infusion. Mild-to-moderate infusion-related reactions (eg, chills, fever, rigors) occur frequently and are typically managed through slowing or interrupting the infusion. Infusion may be resumed at a 50% infusion rate reduction upon resolution of symptoms. Due to the potential for hypotension, consider withholding antihypertensives 12 hours prior to treatment.

[U.S. Boxed Warning]: Progressive multifocal leukoencephalopathy (PML) due to JC virus infection has been reported with rituximab use. Cases were reported in patients with hematologic malignancies receiving rituximab either with combination chemotherapy, or with hematopoietic stem cell transplant. Cases were also reported in patients receiving rituximab for autoimmune diseases who had received prior or concurrent immunosuppressant therapy. Onset may be delayed, although most cases were diagnosed within 12 months of the last rituximab dose. A retrospective analysis of patients (n=57) diagnosed with PML following rituximab therapy, found a median of 16 months (following rituximab initiation), 5.5 months (following last rituximab dose), and 6 rituximab doses preceded PML diagnosis. Clinical findings included confusion/disorientation, motor weakness/hemiparesis, altered vision/ speech, and poor motor coordination with symptoms progressing over weeks to months (Carson, 2009). Promptly evaluate any patient presenting with neurological changes; consider neurology consultation, brain MRI and lumbar puncture for suspected PML. Discontinue rituximab in patients who develop PML; consider reduction/discontinuation of concurrent chemotherapy or immunosuppressants. Avoid use if severe active infection is present. Serious and potentially fatal viral infections, either new or reactivated, associated with rituximab use include cytomegalovirus, herpes simplex virus, parvovirus B19, varicella zoster virus, West Nile virus, and hepatitis C. Viral infections may be delayed; occurring up to 1 year after discontinuation of rituximab. Rarely, reactivation of hepatitis B (with fulminant hepatitis and hepatic failure) has been reported in association with rituximab; median time to hepatitis diagnosis was ~4 months after initiation of therapy and 1 month following last dose; screen high-risk patients prior to therapy initiation.

[U.S. Boxed Warning]: Tumor lysis syndrome leading to acute renal failure requiring dialysis may occur 12-24 hours following the first dose. Hyperkalemia, hypocalcemia, hyperuricemia, and/or hyperphosphatemia may occur. Consider prophylaxis (allopurinol, hydration) in patients at high risk (high numbers of circulating malignant cells ≥25,000/mm³ or high tumor burden). May cause renal toxicity in patients with hematologic malignancies; correct electrolyte abnormalities; monitor renal function and hydration status; consider discontinuation with increasing serum creatinine or oliguria. **[U.S. Boxed Warning]: Severe and sometimes fatal mucocutaneous reactions (lichenoid dermatitis, paraneoplastic pemphigus, Stevens-Johnson syndrome, toxic epidermal necrolysis and vesiculobullous dermatitis) have been reported,** occurring from 1-13 weeks following exposure. Discontinue in patients experiencing severe mucocutaneous skin reactions; the safety of re-exposure following mucocutaneous reactions has not been evaluated. Use caution with pre-existing cardiac or pulmonary disease, or prior cardiopulmonary events. Rheumatoid arthritis patients are at increased risk for cardiovascular events; monitor closely during and after each infusion. Elderly patients are at higher risk for cardiac (supraventricular arrhythmia) and pulmonary adverse events (pneumonia, pneumonitis). Bowel obstruction and perforation (rarely fatal) have been reported with an average onset of symptoms of ~6 days; complaints of abdominal pain should be evaluated, especially if early in the treatment course. Live vaccines should not be given concurrently with rituximab; there is no data available concerning secondary transmission of live vaccines with or following rituximab treatment. RA patients should be brought up to date with nonlive immunizations (following current guidelines) before initiating therapy; evaluate risks of therapy delay versus benefit (of nonlive vaccines) for NHL patients. Safety and efficacy of rituximab in combination with biologic agents or disease-modifying antirheumatic drugs (DMARD) other than methotrexate have not been established. Safety and efficacy of retreatment for RA have not been established.

Adverse Reactions Note: Patients treated with rituximab for rheumatoid arthritis (RA) may experience fewer adverse reactions.

>10%:

Central nervous system: Fever (5% to 53%), chills (3% to 33%), headache (19%), pain (12%)

Dermatologic: Rash (15%; grades 3/4: 1%), pruritus (5% to 14%), angioedema (11%; grades 3/4: 1%)

Gastrointestinal: Nausea (8% to 23%), abdominal pain (2% to 14%)

Hematologic: Cytopenias (grades 3/4: ≤48%; may be prolonged); lymphopenia (48%; grades 3/4: 40%; median duration 14 days), leukopenia (14%; grades 3/4: 4%), neutropenia (14%; grades 3/4: 6%; median duration 13 days), thrombocytopenia (12%; grades 3/4: 2%)

Neuromuscular & skeletal: Weakness (2% to 26%)

Respiratory: Cough (13%), rhinitis (3% to 12%)

Miscellaneous: Infusion-related reactions (lymphoma: first dose 77%; decreases with subsequent infusions; may include angioedema, bronchospasm, chills, dizziness, fever, headache, hyper-/hypotension, myalgia, nausea, pruritus, rash, rigors, urticaria, and vomiting; reactions reported are lower [first infusion: 32%] in RA); infection (31%; grades 3/4: 4%; bacterial: 19%; viral 10%; fungal: 1%), night sweats (15%); human antichimeric antibody (HACA) positive (1% to 11%)

1% to 10%:

Cardiovascular: Hypotension (10%), peripheral edema (8%), hypertension (6% to 8%), flushing (5%), edema (<5%)

Central nervous system: Dizziness (10%), anxiety (2% to 5%), agitation (<5%), depression (<5%), hypoesthesia (<5%), insomnia (<5%), malaise (<5%), nervousness (<5%), neuritis (<5%), somnolence (<5%), vertigo (<5%), migraine (RA: 2%)

Dermatologic: Urticaria (2% to 8%)

Endocrine & metabolic: Hyperglycemia (9%), hypoglycemia (<5%), hyper-cholesterolemia (2%)

Gastrointestinal: Diarrhea (10%), vomiting (10%), dyspepsia (3%), anorexia (<5%), weight loss (<5%)

Hematologic: Anemia (8%; grades 3/4: 3%)

Local: Pain at the injection site (<5%)

Neuromuscular & skeletal: Back pain (10%), myalgia (10%), arthralgia (6% to 10%), paresthesia (2%), arthritis (<5%), hyperkinesia (<5%), hypertonia (<5%), neuropathy (<5%)

Ocular: Conjunctivitis (<5%), lacrimation disorder (<5%)

Respiratory: Throat irritation (2% to 9%), bronchospasm (8%), dyspnea (7%), upper respiratory tract infection (RA: 7%), sinusitis (6%)

Miscellaneous: LDH increased (7%)

Postmarketing and/or case reports: Acute renal failure, anaphylactoid reaction/anaphylaxis, angina, aplastic anemia, ARDS, arrhythmia, bowel obstruction/perforation, bronchiolitis obliterans, cardiac failure, cardiogenic shock, disease progression (Kaposi's sarcoma), encephalomyelitis, fatal infusion-related reactions, fulminant hepatitis, gastrointestinal perforation, hemolytic anemia, hepatic failure, hepatitis, hepatitis B reactivation, hyperviscosity syndrome (in Waldenström's macroglobulinemia), hypogammaglobulinemia, hypoxia, interstitial pneumonitis, laryngeal edema, lichenoid dermatitis, lupus-like syndrome, marrow hypoplasia, MI, mucositis, mucocutaneous reaction, neutropenia (late-onset occurring >40 days after last dose), optic neuritis, pancytopenia (prolonged), paraneoplastic pemphigus (uncommon), pleuritis, pneumonia, pneumonitis, polyarticular arthritis, polymyositis, progressive multifocal leukoencephalopathy (PML), pure red cell aplasia, renal toxicity, serum sickness, Stevens-Johnson syndrome, supraventricular arrhythmia, systemic vasculitis, toxic epidermal necrolysis, tuberculosis reactivation, tumor lysis syndrome, urticaria, uveitis, vasculitis with rash, ventricular fibrillation, ventricular tachycardia, vesiculobullous dermatitis, viral reactivation (includes JC virus, cytomegalovirus, herpes simplex virus, parvovirus B19, varicella zoster virus, West Nile virus, and hepatitis C), wheezing

Drug Interactions

Avoid Concomitant Use

Avoid concomitant use of RiTUXimab with any of the following: Certolizumab Pegol; Natalizumab; Vaccines (Live)

Increased Effect/Toxicity

RiTUXimab may increase the levels/effects of: Certolizumab Pegol; Hypoglycemic Agents; Leflunomide; Natalizumab; Vaccines (Live)

The levels/effects of RiTUXimab may be increased by: Abciximab; Antihypertensives; Herbs (Hypoglycemic Properties); Trastuzumab

Decreased Effect

RiTUXimab may decrease the levels/effects of: Vaccines (Inactivated); Vaccines (Live)

The levels/effects of RiTUXimab may be decreased by: Echinacea

Ethanol/Nutrition/Herb Interactions Herb/Nutraceutical: Avoid echinacea (may diminish the therapeutic effect of immunosuppressants). Avoid hypoglycemic herbs, including alfalfa, aloe, bilberry, bitter melon, burdock, celery, damiana, fenugreek, garcinia, garlic, ginger, ginseng (American), gymnema, marshmallow, and stinging nettle (may enhance the hypoglycemic effect of rituximab).

Storage/Stability Store vials under refrigeration at 2°C to 8°C (36°F to 46°F); do not freeze. Do not shake. Protect vials from direct sunlight. Solutions for infusion are stable at 2°C to 8°C (36°F to 46°F) for 24 hours and at room temperature for an additional 24 hours.

Reconstitution Withdraw necessary amount of rituximab and dilute to a final concentration of 1-4 mg/mL with 0.9% sodium chloride or 5% dextrose in water. Gently invert the bag to mix the solution. Do not shake.

Mechanism of Action Rituximab is a monoclonal antibody directed against the CD20 antigen on B-lymphocytes. CD20 regulates cell cycle initiation; and, possibly, functions as a calcium channel. Rituximab binds to the antigen on the cell surface, activating complement-dependent B-cell cytotoxicity; and to human Fc receptors, mediating cell killing through an antibody-dependent cellular toxicity. B-cells are believed to play a role in the development and progression of rheumatoid arthritis. Signs and symptoms of RA are reduced by targeting B-cells and the progression of structural damage is delayed.

Pharmacodynamics/Kinetics

Duration: Detectable in serum 3-6 months after completion of treatment; B-cell recovery begins ~6 months following completion of treatment; median B-cell levels return to normal by 12 months following completion of treatment

Absorption: I.V.: Immediate and results in a rapid and sustained depletion of circulating and tissue-based B cells

Distribution: 4.3 L (following two 1000 mg doses for rheumatoid arthritis)

Half-life elimination:

Cancer: Proportional to dose; wide ranges reflect variable tumor burden and changes in CD20 positive B-cell populations with repeated doses:

>100 mg/m^2: 4.4 days (range: 1.6-10.5 days)

375 mg/m^2:

Following first dose: Mean half-life: 3.2 days (range: 1.3-6.4 days)

Following fourth dose: Mean half-life: 8.6 days (range: 3.5-17 days)

RA: Mean terminal half-life: 19 days

Excretion: Uncertain; may undergo phagocytosis and catabolism in the reticuloendothelial system (RES)

Dosage Note: Pretreatment with acetaminophen and an antihistamine is recommended. Details concerning dosing in combination regimens should also be consulted.

Children: AIHA, chronic ITP (unlabeled uses): I.V.: 375 mg/m^2 once weekly for 2-4 doses

Adults: I.V. infusion:

NHL (relapsed/refractory, low-grade or follicular CD20-positive, B-cell): 375 mg/m^2 once weekly for 4 or 8 doses

Retreatment following disease progression: 375 mg/m^2 once weekly for 4 doses

NHL (diffuse large B-cell): 375 mg/m^2 given on day 1 of each chemotherapy cycle for up to 8 doses

NHL (follicular, CD20-positive, B-cell, previously untreated): 375 mg/m^2 given on day 1 of each chemotherapy cycle for up to 8 doses

NHL (nonprogressing, low-grade, CD20-positive, B-cell, after first line CVP): 375 mg/m^2 once weekly for 4 doses every 6 months for up to 4 cycles (initiate after 6-8 cycles of chemotherapy are completed)

NHL maintenance treatment for (low grade or follicular) responding to induction therapy: *Canadian labeling (not in U.S. labeling):* 375 mg/m^2 every 3 months until disease progression or up to 2 years

Rheumatoid arthritis: 1000 mg on days 1 and 15 in combination with methotrexate

◀ **Note:** Premedication with a corticosteroid (eg, methylprednisolone 100 mg I.V.) 30 minutes prior to each rituximab dose is recommended. In clinical trials, patients received oral corticosteroids on a tapering schedule from baseline through day 16.

CLL: *Canadian labeling (unlabeled use in U.S.):* 375 mg/m² day 1 (cycle one only), then 500 mg/m² on day 1 of each subsequent chemotherapy cycle for up to 6 cycles (Keating, 2005; Tam, 2008)

Note: To decrease risk of tumor lysis syndrome, administer uricostatic agent (eg, allopurinol) and maintain adequate hydration 48 hours prior to rituximab initiation. Premedication with a corticosteroid (eg, methylprednisolone 80 mg I.V.) prior to each rituximab dose is recommended in patients with lymphocytes >25,000/mm³.

Refractory pemphigus vulgaris (unlabeled use): 375 mg/m² once weekly of weeks 1, 2, and 3 of a 4-week cycle, repeat for 1 additional cycle, then 1 dose per month for 4 months (total of 10 doses in 6 months)

Refractory chronic GVHD, Waldenström's macroglobulinemia (unlabeled uses): 375 mg/m² once weekly for 4 weeks

Combination therapy with ibritumomab: 250 mg/m² I.V. day 1; repeat in 7-9 days with ibritumomab (also see Ibritumomab monograph):

Combination Regimens

Leukemia, chronic lymphocytic:
Lymphoma, non-Hodgkin's:
Lymphoma, non-Hodgkin's (Mantle cell):

Administration Do **not** administer I.V. push or bolus.

Initial infusion: Start rate of 50 mg/hour; if there is no reaction, increase the rate by 50 mg/hour increments every 30 minutes, to a maximum rate of 400 mg/hour.

Subsequent infusions: If patient did not tolerate initial infusion follow initial infusion guidelines. If patient tolerated initial infusion, start at 100 mg/hour; if there is no reaction, increase the rate by 100 mg/hour increments every 30 minutes, to a maximum rate of 400 mg/hour.

Note: If a reaction occurs, slow or stop the infusion. If the reaction abates, restart infusion at 50% of the previous rate.

In patients with NHL who are receiving a corticosteroid as part of their combination chemotherapy regimen and after tolerance has been established at the recommended infusion rate in cycle 1, a rapid infusion rate has been used beginning with cycle 2. The daily corticosteroid, acetaminophen, and diphenhydramine are administered prior to treatment, then the rituximab dose is administered over 90 minutes, with 20% of the dose administered in the first 30 minutes and the remaining 80% is given over 60 minutes (Sehn, 2007).

Monitoring Parameters CBC with differential and platelets, peripheral CD20⁺ cells; HAMA/HACA titers (high levels may increase the risk of allergic reactions); renal function, fluid balance; vital signs; monitor for infusion reactions, cardiac monitoring during and after infusion in rheumatoid arthritis patients and in patients with pre-existing cardiac disease or if arrhythmias develop during or after subsequent infusions

Screen for hepatitis B in high-risk patients prior to initiation of rituximab therapy (the NCCN NHL guidelines recommend screening **all** NHL patients prior to therapy). In addition, carriers and patients with evidence of recovery from prior hepatitis B infection should be monitored closely for clinical and laboratory signs of HBV infection during therapy and for up to a year following completion of treatment. High-risk patients should be screened for hepatitis C (per NCCN guidelines).

Complaints of abdominal pain, especially early in the course of treatment, should prompt a thorough diagnostic evaluation and appropriate treatment. Signs or symptoms of progressive multifocal leukoencephalopathy (focal neurologic deficits, which may present as hemiparesis, visual field deficits, cognitive impairment, aphasia, ataxia, and/or cranial nerve deficits). If PML is suspected, obtain brain MRI scan and lumbar puncture.

Emetic Potential Very low (<10%)

Dosage Forms Excipient information presented when available (limited, particularly for generics); consult specific product labeling.

Injection, solution [preservative free]:

Rituxan®: 10 mg/mL (10 mL, 50 mL) [contains polysorbate 80]

References

Ahmed AR, Spigelman Z, Cavacini LA, et al, "Treatment of Pemphigus Vulgaris With Rituximab and Intravenous Immune Globulin," *N Engl J Med*, 2006, 355(17):1772-9.

Byrd JC, Murphy T, Howard RS, et al, "Rituximab Using a Thrice Weekly Dosing Schedule in B-Cell Chronic Lymphocytic Leukemia and Small Lymphocytic Lymphoma Demonstrates Clinical Activity and Acceptable Toxicity," *J Clin Oncol*, 2001, 19(8):2153-64.

Coiffier B, "State-of-the-Art Therapeutics: Diffuse Large B-Cell Lymphoma," *J Clin Oncol*, 2005, 23 (26): 6387-93.

Coiffier B, Haioun C, Ketterer N, et al, "Rituximab (Anti-CD20 Monoclonal Antibody) for the Treatment of Patients With Relapsing or Refractory Aggressive Lymphoma: A Multicenter Phase II Study," *Blood*, 1998, 92(6):1927-32.

Coiffier B, Lepage E, Briere J, "CHOP Chemotherapy Plus Rituximab Compared With CHOP Alone in Elderly Patients With Diffuse Large-B-Cell Lymphoma," *N Engl J Med*, 2002, 346(4):235-42.

Cutler C, Miklos D, Kim HT, et al, "Rituximab for Steroid-Refractory Chronic Graft-Versus-Host Disease," *Blood*, 2006, 108(2):756-62.

Dimopoulos MA, Kyle RA, Anagnostopoulos A, et al, "Diagnosis and Management of Waldenstrom's Macroglobulinemia," *J Clin Oncol*, 2005, 23(7):1564-77.

Edwards JC, Szczepanski L, Szechinski J, et al, "Efficacy of B-Cell-Targeted Therapy With Rituximab in Patients With Rheumatoid Arthritis," *N Engl J Med*, 2004, 350(25):2572-81.

Garcia-Suarez J, de Miguel D, Krsnik I, et al, "Changes in the Natural History of Progressive Multifocal Leukoencephalopathy in HIV-Negative Lymphoproliferative Disorders: Impact of Novel Therapies," *Am J Hematol*, 2005, 80(4):271-81.

Goldberg SL, Pecora AL, Alter RS, et al, "Unusual Viral Infections (Progressive Multifocal Leukoencephalopathy and Cytomegalovirus Disease) After High-Dose Chemotherapy With Autologous Blood Stem Cell Rescue and Peritransplantation Rituximab," *Blood*, 2002, 99 (4):1486-8.

Gottenberg JE, Guillevin L, Lambotte O, et al, "Tolerance and Short Term Efficacy of Rituximab in 43 Patients With Systemic Autoimmune Diseases," *Ann Rheum Dis*, 2005, 64(6):913-20.

Higashida J, Wun T, Schmidt S, et al, "Safety and Efficacy of Rituximab in Patients With Rheumatoid Arthritis Refractory to Disease Modifying Antirheumatic Drugs and Anti-Tumor Necrosis Factor-Alpha Treatment," *J Rheumatol*, 2005, 32(11):2109-15.

Keating MJ, O'Brien S, Albitar M, et al, "Early Results of a Chemoimmunotherapy Regimen of Fludarabine, Cyclophosphamide, and Rituximab as Initial Therapy for Chronic Lymphocytic Leukemia," *J Clin Oncol*, 2005, 23(18):4079-88.

Marcus R, Imrie K, Belch A, et al, "CVP Chemotherapy Plus Rituximab Compared With CVP as First-Line Treatment for Advanced Follicular Lymphoma," *Blood*, 2005, 105(4):1417-23.

McLaughlin P, Grillo-Lopez AJ, Link BK, et al, "Rituximab Chimeric Anti-CD20 Monoclonal Antibody Therapy for Relapsed Indolent Lymphoma: Half of Patients Respond to a Four-Dose Treatment Program," *J Clin Oncol*, 1998, 16(8):2825-33.

Moore J, Ma D, Will R, et al, "A phase II Study of Rituximab in Rheumatoid Arthritis Patients With Recurrent Disease Following Haematopoietic Stem Cell Transplantation," *Bone Marrow Transplant*, 2004, 34(3):241-7

National Comprehensive Cancer Network® (NCCN), "Clinical Practice Guidelines in Oncology™: Central Nervous System Cancers," Version 2.2009. Available at http://www.nccn.org/profes-sionals/physician_gls/PDF/cns.pdf

National Comprehensive Cancer Network® (NCCN), "Clinical Practice Guidelines in Oncology™: Hodgkin Disease/Lymphoma," Version 2.2009. Available at http://www.nccn.org/professionals/physician_gls/PDF/hodgkins.pdf

National Comprehensive Cancer Network® (NCCN), "Clinical Practice Guidelines in Oncology™: Multiple Myeloma," Version 2.2010. Available at http://www.nccn.org/professionals/physician_gls/PDF/myeloma.pdf.

National Comprehensive Cancer Network® (NCCN), "Clinical Practice Guidelines in Oncology™: Non-Hodgkin's Lymphomas," V.2.2009. Available at http://www.nccn.org/professionals/phys-ician_gls/PDF/nhl.pdf

Ng CM, Bruno R, Combs D, et al, "Population Pharmacokinetics of Rituximab (Anti-CD20 Monoclonal Antibody) in Rheumatoid Arthritis Patients During a Phase II Clinical Trial," *J Clin Pharmacol*, 2005, 45(7):792-801

Sehn LH, Donaldson J, Filewich A, et al, "Rapid Infusion Rituximab in Combination With Corticosteroid-Containing Chemotherapy or as Maintenance Therapy is Well Tolerated and Can Safely be Delivered in the Community Setting," *Blood*, 2007, 109(10):4171-3.

Tam CS, O'Brien S, Wierda W, et al, "Long-Term Results of the Fludarabine, Cyclophosphamide, and Rituximab Regimen as Initial Therapy of Chronic Lymphocytic Leukemia," *Blood*, 2008, 112(4):975-80.

Wang J, Wiley JM, Luddy R, et al, "Chronic Immune Thrombocytopenic Purpura in Children: Assessment of Rituximab Treatment," *J Pediatr*, 2005, 146(2):217-21.

Zecca M, Nobili B, Ramenghi U, et al, "Rituximab in the Treatment of Refractory Autoimmune Hemolytic Anemia in Children," *Blood*, 2003, 101(10): 3857-61.

◆ **Riva-Ciprofloxacin (Can)** *see* Ciprofloxacin *on page* 228

◆ **Riva-Fluconazole (Can)** *see* Fluconazole *on page* 485

◆ **Riva-Lorazepam (Can)** *see* LORazepam *on page* 731

◆ **Riva-Valacyclovir (Can)** *see* Valacyclovir *on page* 1154

◆ **rLFN-α2** *see* Interferon Alfa-2b *on page* 642

◆ **Ro 5488** *see* Tretinoin, Systemic *on page* 1141

◆ **Rocaltrol®** *see* Calcitriol *on page* 168

◆ **Rocephin®** *see* CefTRIAXone *on page* 199

Romiplostim (roe mi PLOE stim)

U.S. Brand Names Nplate™

Index Terms AMG 531

Generic Available No

Canadian Brand Names Nplate™

Pharmacologic Category Colony Stimulating Factor; Thrombopoietic Agent

Use Treatment of thrombocytopenia in patients with chronic immune (idiopathic) thrombocytopenia purpura (ITP) who have had insufficient response to corticosteroids, immune globulin, or splenectomy

Restrictions Approved for use only under a risk management and restricted distribution program, Nplate™ NEXUS (Network of Experts Understanding and Supporting Nplate™ and Patients) program (1-877-675-2831 or www.nplate.com). Prescribers and patients must be registered with the program.

Pregnancy Risk Factor C

Lactation Excretion in breast milk unknown/ not recommended.

Labeled Contraindications There are no contraindications listed within the manufacturer's labeling.

Warnings/Precautions May increase the risk for bone marrow reticulin formation or progression. Collagen fibrosis with cytopenias was not observed in clinical trials, although patients receiving romiplostim may be at risk for marrow fibrosis with cytopenias. Onset of new or worsening cellular abnormalities or cytopenias may warrant therapy discontinuation and subsequent bone marrow biopsy. Thromboembolism may occur with treatment; use with caution in patients with a history of cerebrovascular disease. Stimulation of cell surface thrombopoietin (TPO) receptors may increase the risk for hematologic malignancies; may increase the risk for progression of underlying myelodysplastic syndrome (MDS).

Inadequate platelet response may be due to neutralizing antibodies (to romiplostim or TPO) or bone marrow fibrosis. Indicated only when the degree of thrombocytopenia and clinical conditions increase the risk for bleeding; use the lowest dose necessary to achieve and maintain platelet count platelet count ≥50,000/mm³. Do not use to normalize platelet counts. Discontinue if platelet count does not respond to a level to avoid clinically important bleeding after 4 weeks at the maximum recommended dose. May be used in combination with other therapies for ITP, including corticosteroids, danazol, azathioprine, immune globulin, or Rho(D) immune globulin. Reduce dose of or discontinue ITP medications when platelet count ≥50,000/mm³.

Upon discontinuation of therapy, thrombocytopenia may worsen. Severity may be greater than pretreatment level. Risk of bleeding is increased, particularly in patients receiving anticoagulants or antiplatelet agents; monitor closely. Rebound thrombocytopenia generally resolves within 14 days.

Use with caution in patients with hepatic and renal impairment (has not been studied). Safety and efficacy have not been established in children.

Adverse Reactions

>10%:

Central nervous system: Headache (35%), fatigue (33%), dizziness (17%), insomnia (16%)

Gastrointestinal: Diarrhea (17%), nausea (13%), abdominal pain (11%)

Neuromuscular & skeletal: Arthralgia (26%), myalgia (14%), back pain (13%), limb pain (13%)

Respiratory: Epistaxis (32%), upper respiratory tract infection (17%)

1% to 10%:

Gastrointestinal: Dyspepsia (7%)

Hematologic: Rebound thrombocytopenia (7%), bone marrow reticulin formation/deposition (4%)

Neuromuscular & skeletal: Shoulder pain (8%), paresthesia (6%)

Miscellaneous: Antibody formation (romiplostim 10%; TPO 5%)

<1%, postmarketing, and/or case reports: Thromboembolism

Drug Interactions

Avoid Concomitant Use There are no known interactions where it is recommended to avoid concomitant use.

Increased Effect/Toxicity There are no known significant interactions involving an increase in effect.

Decreased Effect There are no known significant interactions involving a decrease in effect.

◄ **Storage/Stability** Store intact vials refrigerated at 2°C to 8°C (36°F to 46°F); do not freeze. Protect from light. Reconstituted solution may be stored at room temperature of 25°C (77°F) or refrigerated at 2°C to 8°C (36°F to 46°F) for up to 24 hours. Protect reconstituted solution from light.

Reconstitution Reconstitute with preservative free SWFI to a final concentration of 500 mcg/mL. Gently invert vial and swirl; do not shake.

Mechanism of Action Thrombopoietin (TPO) peptide mimetic which increases platelet counts in ITP by binding to and activating the human TPO receptor.

Pharmacodynamics/Kinetics

Onset of action: Platelet count increase: SubQ: 4-9 days; Peak platelet count increase: Days 12-16

Duration: Platelet counts return to baseline by day 28

Absorption: SubQ: Slow

Half-life elimination: Median: 3.5 days (range: 1-34 days)

Time to peak, plasma: SubQ: Median: 14 hours (range: 7-50 hours)

Dosage Note: Initial dose is based on actual body weight. Discontinue if platelet count does not respond to a level that avoids clinically important bleeding after 4 weeks at the maximum recommended dose.

SubQ: Adults: ITP: Initial: 1 mcg/kg once weekly; adjust dose by 1 mcg/kg/ week to achieve platelet count ≥50,000/mm^3 and to reduce the risk of bleeding; Maximum: 10 mcg/kg (median dose needed to achieve response in clinical trials: 2 mcg/kg)

Dosage adjustment recommendations:

Platelet count <50,000/mm^3: Increase dose by 1 mcg/kg

Platelet count >200,000/mm^3 for 2 consecutive weeks: Reduce dose by 1 mcg/kg

Platelet count >400,000/mm^3: Withhold dose; assess platelet count weekly; when platelet count <200,000/mm^3, resume with the dose reduced by 1 mcg/kg

Administration Administer SubQ. Administration volume may be small; use appropriate syringe (with graduations to 0.01 mL) for administration.

Monitoring Parameters CBC with differential and platelets (baseline, during treatment [weekly until platelet response stable for 4 weeks then monthly] and weekly for at least 2 weeks following completion of treatment)

Evaluate for neutralizing antibodies in patients with inadequate response (blood samples may be submitted to Amgen for assay [1-800-772-6436]).

Dietary Considerations Nplate™ 250 mcg vial contains sucrose 15 mg and 500 mcg vial contains sucrose 25 mg.

Dosage Forms Excipient information presented when available (limited, particularly for generics); consult specific product labeling.

Injection, powder for reconstitution:

Nplate™: 250 mcg [contains sucrose 15 mg/vial]; 500 mcg [contains sucrose 25 mg/vial]

References

Bussel JB, Kuter DJ, George JN, et al, "AMG 531, a Thrombopoiesis-Stimulating Protein, for Chronic ITP," *N Engl J Med*, 2006, 355(16):1672-81.

Kuter DJ, "New Thrombopoietic Growth Factors," *Blood*, 2007, 109(11):4607-16.

Kuter DJ, Bussel JB, Lyons RM, et al, "Efficacy of Romiplostim in Patients With Chronic Immune Thrombocytopenic Purpura: A Double-Blind Randomised Controlled Trial," *Lancet*, 2008, 371 (9610):395-403.

Wang B, Nichol JL, and Sullivan JT, "Pharmacodynamics and Pharmacokinetics of AMG 531, a Novel Thrombopoietin Receptor Ligand," *Clin Pharmacol Ther*, 2004, 76(6):628-38.

◆ **Roxanol™** *see* Morphine Sulfate *on page 816*

- ◆ **Roxicodone®** *see* OxyCODONE *on page 889*
- ◆ **RP-6976** *see* Docetaxel *on page 361*
- ◆ **RS-25259** *see* Palonosetron *on page 911*
- ◆ **RS-25259-197** *see* Palonosetron *on page 911*
- ◆ **RU-486** *see* Mifepristone *on page 800*
- ◆ **RU-23908** *see* Nilutamide *on page 851*
- ◆ **RU-38486** *see* Mifepristone *on page 800*
- ◆ **Rubidomycin Hydrochloride** *see* DAUNOrubicin Hydrochloride *on page 323*
- ◆ **Ryzolt™** *see* TraMADol *on page 1130*
- ◆ **SAB-Gentamicin (Can)** *see* Gentamicin *on page 542*
- ◆ **Sab-Prenase (Can)** *see* PrednisoLONE *on page 977*
- ◆ **SAHA** *see* Vorinostat *on page 1193*
- ◆ **Salagen®** *see* Pilocarpine *on page 956*
- ◆ **Salivart® [OTC]** *see* Saliva Substitute *on page 1027*

Saliva Substitute (sa LYE va SUB stee tute)

U.S. Brand Names Aquoral™; Caphosol®; Entertainer's Secret® [OTC]; Moi-Stir® [OTC]; Mouthkote® [OTC]; Numoisyn™; Oasis®; Oral Balance® [OTC]; Saliva Substitute® [OTC] [DSC]; Salivart® [OTC]; SalivaSure™ [OTC]

Index Terms Artificial Saliva

Generic Available No

Pharmacologic Category Gastrointestinal Agent, Miscellaneous

Use Relief of dry mouth and throat in xerostomia or hyposalivation; adjunct to standard oral care in relief of symptoms associated with chemotherapy or radiation therapy-induced mucositis

Drug Interactions

Avoid Concomitant Use There are no known interactions where it is recommended to avoid concomitant use.

Increased Effect/Toxicity There are no known significant interactions involving an increase in effect.

Decreased Effect There are no known significant interactions involving a decrease in effect.

Storage/Stability

Caphosol®: Store at room temperature; do not refrigerate.

Numoisyn™ liquid: Store at room temperature; do not refrigerate. Use within 3 months after opening.

Numoisyn™ lozenges: Store at room temperature.

Reconstitution Caphosol®: Mix contents of 1 blue (A) and 1 clear (B) ampul in clean container; use immediately after mixing.

Mechanism of Action Protein or electrolyte mixtures which restore/replace saliva, lubricate, moisten, and provide a coating on oral mucosa

Dosage Adults: Use as needed or product-specific dosing:

Caphosol®:

Mucositis symptoms: Swish and spit 4-10 doses per day (begin at onset of chemo-or radiation therapy)

Xerostomia: Swish and spit 2-10 doses per day

Numoisyn™ liquid: Use 2 mL as needed

Numoisyn™ lozenges: Dissolve 1 slowly; maximum 16 lozenges/day

Oasis® mouthwash: Rinse mouth with ~30 mL twice daily or as needed; do not swallow

Oasis® spray: 1-2 sprays as needed; maximum 60 sprays/day

Oral Balance®: Use after meals, at bedtime and as needed

Administration Oral:

Caphosol®: Mix contents of 1 blue (A) and 1 clear (B) ampul in clean container, swish thoroughly with ½ of mixture (15 mL) for 1 minute and spit; repeat. Avoid eating or drinking for at least 15 minutes after use.

Numoisyn™ liquid: Rinse in mouth before swallowing.

Numoisyn™ lozenges: Dissolve slowly in mouth.

Oasis® mouthwash: Rinse for 30 seconds.

Oasis® spray: Spray into mouth holding bottle upright; do not rinse.

Dietary Considerations Caphosol®: Contains sodium 75 mg/30 mL dose

Dosage Forms Excipient information presented when available (limited, particularly for generics); consult specific product labeling. [DSC] = Discontinued product

Liquid:

Numoisyn™: Water, sorbitol, linseed extract, *Chondrus crispus*, methylparaben, sodium benzoate, potassium sorbate, dipotassium phosphate, propylparaben (300 mL)

Oral Balance®: Water, starch, sunflower oil, propylene glycol, xylitol, glycerine, purified milk extract (45 mL) [sugar-free]

Lozenge:

Numoisyn™: Sorbitol 0.3 g/lozenge, polyethylene glycol, malic acid, sodium citrate, calcium phosphate dibasic, hydrogenated cottonseed oil, citric acid, magnesium stearate, silicon dioxide (100s)

SalivaSure™: Xylitol, citric acid, apple acid, sodium citrate dihydrate, sodium carboxymethylcellulose, dibasic calcium phosphate, silica colloidal, magnesium stearate, stearic acid (90s)

Solution, oral:

Caphosol®: Dibasic sodium phosphate 0.032%, monobasic sodium phosphate 0.009%, calcium chloride 0.052%, sodium chloride 0.569%, purified water (30 mL) [packaged in two 15 mL ampuls when mixed together provide one 30 mL dose]

Entertainer's Secret®: Sodium carboxymethylcellulose, aloe vera gel, glycerin (60 mL) [alcohol-free; honey-apple flavor]

Saliva Substitute®: Sorbitol, sodium carboxymethylcellulose, methylparaben (120 mL) [alcohol free, dye free, sugar free; mild mint flavor] [DSC]

Solution, oral [mouthwash/gargle]:

Oasis®: Water, glycerin, sorbitol, poloxamer 338, PEG-60, hydrogenated castor oil, copovidone, sodium benzoate, carboxymethycellulose (473 mL) [alcohol free, sugar free; mild mint flavor]

Solution, oral [preservative free; spray]:

Salivart®: Water, sodium carboxymethylcellulose, sorbitol, sodium chloride, potassium chloride, calcium chloride, magnesium chloride, potassium phosphate (74 mL) [alcohol free]

Solution, oral [spray]:

Aquoral™: Oxidized glycerol triesters and silicon dioxide (40 mL) [contains aspartame; delivers 400 sprays, citrus flavor]

Moi-Stir®: Water, sorbitol, sodium carboxymethylcellulose, methylparaben, propylparaben, potassium chloride, dibasic sodium phosphate, calcium chloride, magnesium chloride, sodium chloride (120 mL)

Mouthkote®: Water, xylitol, sorbitol, yerba santa, citric acid, ascorbic acid, sodium saccharin, sodium benzoate (5 mL, 60 mL, 240 mL) [alcohol free, sugar free; lemon-lime flavor]

Oasis®: Glycerin, cetylpyridinium, copovidone (30 mL) [alcohol free, sugar free; contains sodium benzoate; delivers ~150 sprays, mild mint flavor]

References

Papas AS, Clark RE, Martuscelli G, et al, "A Prospective, Randomized Trial for the Prevention of Mucositis in Patients Undergoing Hematopoietic Stem Cell Transplantation," *Bone Marrow Transplant*, 2003, 31(8): 705-12.

Scully C and Epstein JB, " Oral Health Care for the Cancer Patient," *Oral Oncology*, 1996, 32(5): 281-92.

Sweeney MP and Bagg J, "The Mouth and Palliative Care," *Am J Palliat Care*, 2000, 17(2):118-24.

Sargramostim (sar GRAM oh stim)

Medication Safety Issues
Sound-alike/look-alike issues:
Leukine® may be confused with Leukeran®, leucovorin

Related Information
Hematopoietic Stem Cell Transplantation on page 1501
Oral Mucositis / Stomatitis on page 1460

U.S. Brand Names Leukine®

Index Terms GM-CSF; Granulocyte-Macrophage Colony Stimulating Factor; NSC-613795; rhuGM-CSF

Generic Available No

Canadian Brand Names Leukine®

Pharmacologic Category Colony Stimulating Factor

Use

Acute myelogenous leukemia (AML) following induction chemotherapy in older adults (≥55 years of age) to shorten time to neutrophil recovery and to reduce the incidence of severe and life-threatening infections and infections resulting in death

Bone marrow transplant (allogeneic or autologous) failure or engraftment delay

Myeloid reconstitution after allogeneic bone marrow transplantation

Myeloid reconstitution after autologous bone marrow transplantation: Non-Hodgkin's lymphoma (NHL), acute lymphoblastic leukemia (ALL), Hodgkin's lymphoma

Peripheral stem cell transplantation: Mobilization and myeloid reconstitution following autologous peripheral stem cell transplantation

Pregnancy Risk Factor C

Lactation Excretion in breast milk unknown/use caution

Labeled Contraindications Hypersensitivity to sargramostim, yeast-derived products, or any component of the formulation; concurrent (24 hours preceding/following) myelosuppressive chemotherapy or radiation therapy; patients with excessive (≥10%) leukemic myeloid blasts in bone marrow or peripheral blood

Warnings/Precautions Simultaneous administration, or administration 24 hours preceding/following cytotoxic chemotherapy or radiotherapy is not recommended. Use with caution in patients with pre-existing cardiac problems or HF; supraventricular arrhythmias have been reported in patients with history of arrhythmias. Edema, capillary leak syndrome, pleural and/or pericardial effusion have been reported; use with caution in patients with pre-existing fluid retention; may worsen. Use with caution in patients with hepatic or renal impairment; monitor hepatic and/or renal function in patients with history of hepatic or renal dysfunction. Elevations in bilirubin, transaminases, and serum creatinine have been observed with use. Dyspnea may occur; monitor respiratory symptoms during and following infusion; use with caution in patients with hypoxia or pulmonary infiltrates.

With rapid increase in blood counts (ANC >20,000/mm^3, WBC >50,000/mm^3, or platelets >500,000/mm^3); decrease dose by 50% or discontinue drug (counts will fall to normal within 3-7 days after discontinuing drug). May potentially act as a growth factor for any tumor type, particularly myeloid malignancies; caution should be exercised when using in any malignancy with myeloid characteristics; tumors of nonhematopoietic origin may have surface receptors for sargramostim. Discontinue use if disease progression occurs during treatment.

There is a "first-dose effect" (refer to Adverse Reactions for details) which is seen (rarely) with the first dose of a cycle and does not usually occur with subsequent doses within that cycle. Anaphylaxis or other serious allergic reactions have been reported; discontinue immediately if occur. Solution contains benzyl alcohol; do not use in premature infants or neonates.

Adverse Reactions

>10%:

Cardiovascular: Hypertension (34%), pericardial effusion (4% to 25%), edema (13% to 25%), chest pain (15%), peripheral edema (11%), tachycardia (11%)

Central nervous system: Fever (81%), malaise (57%), headache (26%), chills (25%), anxiety (11%), insomnia (11%)

Dermatologic: Rash (44%), pruritus (23%)

Endocrine & metabolic: Hyperglycemia (25%), hypercholesterolemia (17%), hypomagnesemia (15%)

Gastrointestinal: Diarrhea (≤89%), nausea (58% to 70%), vomiting (46% to 70%), abdominal pain (38%), weight loss (37%), anorexia (13%), hematemesis (13%), dysphagia (11%), gastrointestinal hemorrhage (11%)

Genitourinary: Urinary tract disorder (14%)

Hepatic: Hyperbilirubinemia (30%)

Neuromuscular & skeletal: Weakness (66%), bone pain (21%), arthralgia (11% to 21%) myalgia (18%)

Ocular: Eye hemorrhage (11%)

Renal: BUN increased (23%), serum creatinine increased (15%)

Respiratory: Pharyngitis (23%), epistaxis (17%), dyspnea (15%)

Miscellaneous: Antibody formation (2%)

1% to 10%: Respiratory: Pleural effusion (1%)

<1%, postmarketing, and/or case reports: Allergic reaction, anaphylaxis, arrhythmia, capillary leak syndrome, constipation, dizziness, eosinophilia; first-dose effect (syndrome with respiratory distress, hypoxia, flushing, hypotension, syncope, and/or tachycardia occurring with the first dose of a treatment cycle); injection site reaction, lethargy, leukocytosis, liver function abnormalities (transient), pain, pericarditis, prothrombin time prolonged, rigors, sore throat, supraventricular arrhythmia (transient), thrombocytosis, thrombophlebitis, thrombosis

Drug Interactions

Avoid Concomitant Use There are no known interactions where it is recommended to avoid concomitant use.

Increased Effect/Toxicity There are no known significant interactions involving an increase in effect.

Decreased Effect There are no known significant interactions involving a decrease in effect.

Storage/Stability Store at 2°C to 8°C (36°F to 46°F); do not freeze. Do not shake.

Solution for injection: May be stored for up to 20 days at 2°C to 8°C (36°F to 46°F) once the vial has been entered. Discard remaining solution after 20 days.

Powder for injection: Preparations made with SWFI should be administered as soon as possible, and discarded within 6 hours of reconstitution. Preparations made with bacteriostatic water may be stored for up to 20 days at 2°C to 8°C (36°F to 46°F).

I.V. infusion administration: Preparations diluted with NS are stable for 48 hours at room temperature and refrigeration.

Reconstitution

Powder for injection: May be reconstituted with preservative free SWFI or bacteriostatic water for injection (with benzyl alcohol 0.9%). Gently swirl to reconstitute; do not shake.

Sargramostim may also be further diluted in 25-50 mL NS to a concentration ≥10 mcg/mL for I.V. infusion administration.

If the final concentration of sargramostim is <10 mcg/mL, 1 mg of human albumin/1 mL of NS (eg, 1 mL of 5% human albumin/50 mL of NS) should be added.

Compatibility Stable in NS, sterile water for injection, bacteriostatic water; **incompatible** with dextrose-containing solutions.

Y-site administration: Compatible: Amikacin, aminophylline, aztreonam, bleomycin, butorphanol, calcium gluconate, carboplatin, carmustine, cefazolin, cefepime, cefotaxime, cefotetan, ceftizoxime, ceftriaxone, cefuroxime, cimetidine, cisplatin, clindamycin, co-trimoxazole, cyclophosphamide, cyclosporine, cytarabine, dacarbazine, dactinomycin, dexamethasone sodium phosphate, diphenhydramine, dopamine, doxorubicin, doxycycline, droperidol, etoposide, famotidine, fentanyl, floxuridine, fluconazole, fluorouracil, furosemide, gentamicin, granisetron, heparin, idarubicin, ifosfamide, immune globulin, magnesium sulfate, mannitol, mechlorethamine, meperidine, mesna, methotrexate, metoclopramide, metronidazole, minocycline, mitoxantrone, netilmicin, pentostatin, piperacillin/tazobactam, potassium chloride, prochlorperazine edisylate, promethazine, ranitidine, teniposide, ticarcillin, ticarcillin/clavulanate, vinblastine, vincristine, zidovudine. **Incompatible:** Acyclovir, ampicillin, ampicillin/sulbactam, cefoperazone, chlorpromazine, ganciclovir, haloperidol, hydrocortisone sodium phosphate, hydrocortisone sodium succinate, hydromorphone, hydroxyzine, imipenem/cilastatin,

◄ lorazepam, methylprednisolone sodium succinate, mitomycin, morphine, nalbuphine, ondansetron, piperacillin, sodium bicarbonate, tobramycin. **Variable (consult detailed reference):** Amphotericin B, amsacrine, ceftazidime, vancomycin.

Mechanism of Action Stimulates proliferation, differentiation and functional activity of neutrophils, eosinophils, monocytes, and macrophages, as indicated.

Pharmacodynamics/Kinetics

Onset of action: Increase in WBC: 7-14 days

Duration: WBCs return to baseline within 1 week of discontinuing drug

Half-life elimination: I.V.: 60 minutes; SubQ: 2.7 hours

Time to peak, serum: SubQ: 1-3 hours

Dosage

Children (unlabeled use) and Adults: I.V. infusion over ≥2 hours or SubQ: **Rounding the dose to the nearest vial size enhances patient convenience and reduces costs without clinical detriment**

Myeloid reconstitution after allogeneic or autologous bone marrow transplant: I.V.: 250 mcg/m²/day (over 2 hours), begin 2-4 hours after the marrow infusion and ≥24 hours after chemotherapy or radiotherapy, when the post marrow infusion ANC is <500 cells/mm³, and continue until ANC >1500 cells/mm³ for 3 consecutive days

If a severe adverse reaction occurs, reduce dose by 50% or temporarily discontinue the dose until the reaction abates

If blast cells appear or progression of the underlying disease occurs, discontinue treatment

If ANC >20,000 cells/mm³, interrupt treatment or reduce the dose by 50%

Neutrophil recovery following chemotherapy in AML: I.V.: 250 mcg/m²/day (over 4 hours) starting approximately on day 11 or 4 days following the completion of induction chemotherapy, if day 10 bone marrow is hypoplastic with <5% blasts

If a second cycle of chemotherapy is necessary, administer ~4 days after the completion of chemotherapy if the bone marrow is hypoplastic with <5% blasts

Continue sargramostim until ANC is >1500 cells/mm³ for 3 consecutive days or a maximum of 42 days

Discontinue sargramostim immediately if leukemic regrowth occurs

If a severe adverse reaction occurs, reduce the dose by 50% or temporarily discontinue the dose until the reaction abates

If ANC >20,000 cells/mm³, interrupt treatment or reduce the dose by 50%

Mobilization of peripheral blood progenitor cells: I.V., SubQ: 250 mcg/m²/day I.V. over 24 hours or SubQ once daily

Continue the same schedule through the period of PBPC collection

The optimal schedule for PBPC collection has not been established (usually begun by day 5 and performed daily until protocol specified targets are achieved)

If WBC >50,000 cells/mm³, reduce the dose by 50%

If adequate numbers of progenitor cells are not collected, consider other mobilization therapy

Postperipheral blood progenitor cell transplantation: I.V., SubQ: 250 mcg/m²/day I.V. over 24 hours or SubQ once daily beginning immediately following infusion of progenitor cells and continuing until ANC is >1500 cells/mm³ for 3 consecutive days is attained

BMT failure or engraftment delay: I.V.: 250 mcg/m²/day over 2 hours for 14 days

May be repeated after 7 days off therapy if engraftment has not occurred

If engraftment still has not occurred, a third course of 500 mcg/m²/day for 14 days may be tried after another 7 days off therapy; if there is still no improvement, it is unlikely that further dose escalation will be beneficial

If a severe adverse reaction occurs, reduce the dose by 50% or temporarily discontinue the dose until the reaction abates

If blast cells appear or disease progression occurs, discontinue treatment

If ANC >20,000 cells/mm³, interrupt treatment or reduce the dose by 50%

Combination Regimens

Lymphoma, non-Hodgkin's:
CODOX-M on page 1278
IVAC on page 1361

Administration Can premedicate with analgesics and antipyretics (eg, acetaminophen) to control adverse events (eg, fever, chills, myalgia, etc); control bone pain with non-narcotic analgesics. Sargramostim is administered as a subcutaneous injection or intravenous infusion; intravenous infusion should be over 2-24 hours; continuous infusions may be more effective than short infusion or bolus injection. An in-line membrane filter should **NOT** be used for intravenous administration. When administering GM-CSF subcutaneously, rotate injection sites.

Monitoring Parameters Vital signs, hydration status, weight, CBC with differential twice weekly during therapy, renal/liver function tests at least biweekly during therapy (in patients displaying renal or hepatic dysfunction prior to initiation of treatment), pulmonary function

Test Interactions May interfere with bone imaging studies; increased hematopoietic activity of the bone marrow may appear as transient positive bone imaging changes

Additional Information Reimbursement Hotline (Leukine®): 1-800-321-4669

Dosage Forms Excipient information presented when available (limited, particularly for generics); consult specific product labeling.

Injection, powder for reconstitution:

Leukine®: 250 mcg [contains sucrose 10 mg/mL]

Injection, solution:

Leukine®: 500 mcg/mL (1 mL) [contains benzyl alcohol and sucrose 10 mg/mL]

References

Lieschke GJ and Burgess AW, "Granulocyte Colony-Stimulating Factor and Granulocyte-Macrophage Colony-Stimulating Factor," (1) N Engl J Med, 1992, 327(1):28-35.

Lieschke GJ and Burgess AW, "Granulocyte Colony-Stimulating Factor and Granulocyte-Macrophage Colony-Stimulating Factor," (2) N Engl J Med, 1992, 327(2):99-106.

Mayer D and Bednarczyk EM, "Interaction of Colony-Stimulating Factors and Fluorodeoxyglucose F[18] Positron Emission Tomography," Ann Pharmacother, 2002, 36(11):1796-9.

Smith TJ, Khatcheressian J, Lyman GH, et al, "2006 Update of Recommendations for the Use of White Blood Cell Growth Factors: An Evidence-Based Clinical Practice Guideline," J Clin Oncol, 2006, 24(19):3187-205.

◆ **Sarna® HC (Can)** see Hydrocortisone on page 575

◆ **Sarnol®-HC [OTC]** see Hydrocortisone on page 575

◆ **Sativex® (Can)** see Tetrahydrocannabinol and Cannabidiol on page 1090

◆ **SB-497115** see Eltrombopag on page 398

◆ **SB-497115-GR** see Eltrombopag on page 398

◆ **SC 33428** see IDArubicin on page 605

- ◆ **SCH 13521** *see* Flutamide *on page* 506
- ◆ **SCH 56592** *see* Posaconazole *on page* 970
- ◆ **SCIG** *see* Immune Globulin (Subcutaneous) *on page* 633
- ◆ **Sclerosol®** *see* Talc (Sterile) *on page* 1071
- ◆ **SD/01** *see* Pegfilgrastim *on page* 929
- ◆ **SDX-105** *see* Bendamustine *on page* 132
- ◆ **Sensipar®** *see* Cinacalcet *on page* 225
- ◆ **Septra®** *see* Sulfamethoxazole and Trimethoprim *on page* 1051
- ◆ **Septra® DS** *see* Sulfamethoxazole and Trimethoprim *on page* 1051
- ◆ **Septra® Injection (Can)** *see* Sulfamethoxazole and Trimethoprim *on page* 1051
- ◆ **Simulect®** *see* Basiliximab *on page* 125

Sirolimus (sir OH li mus)

Medication Safety Issues
Sound-alike/look-alike issues:
Rapamune® may be confused with Rapaflo™
Sirolimus may be confused with everolimus, tacrolimus, temsirolimus

U.S. Brand Names Rapamune®

Generic Available No

Canadian Brand Names Rapamune®

Pharmacologic Category Immunosuppressant Agent; mTOR Kinase Inhibitor

Use Prophylaxis of organ rejection in patients receiving renal transplants

Unlabeled/Investigational Use Prophylaxis of organ rejection in heart transplant recipients; immunosuppression in peripheral stem cell/bone marrow transplantation

Pregnancy Risk Factor C

Lactation Excretion in breast milk unknown/not recommended

Labeled Contraindications Hypersensitivity to sirolimus or any component of the formulation

Warnings/Precautions [U.S. Boxed Warning]: Immunosuppressive agents, including sirolimus, increase the risk of infection and may be associated with the development of lymphoma. Immune suppression may also increase the risk of opportunistic infections, fatal infections, and sepsis. Prophylactic treatment for *Pneumocystis jirovec* pneumonia (PCP) should be administered for 1 year post-transplant; prophylaxis for cytomegalovirus (CMV) should be taken for 3 months post-transplant in patients at risk for CMV.

[U.S. Boxed Warning]: Sirolimus is not recommended for *de novo* use in liver or lung transplant patients. Bronchial anastomotic dehiscence cases have been reported in lung transplant patients when sirolimus was used as part of an immunosuppressive regimen; most of these reactions were fatal. Studies indicate an association with an increase risk of hepatic artery thrombosis (HAT), graft failure, and increased mortality (with evidence of infection) in liver transplant patients when sirolimus is used in combination with cyclosporine and/or tacrolimus. Most cases of HAT occurred within 30 days of transplant.

In renal transplant patients, *de novo* use without cyclosporine has been associated with higher rates of acute rejection. Sirolimus should be used in combination with cyclosporine (and corticosteroids) initially. Cyclosporine may be withdrawn in low-to-moderate immunologic risk patients after 2-4 months, in conjunction with an increase in sirolimus dosage. In high immunologic risk patients, use in combination with cyclosporine and corticosteroids is recommended for the first year. Safety and efficacy of combination therapy with cyclosporine in high-risk patients has not been studied beyond 12 months of treatment; adjustment of immunosuppressive therapy beyond 12 months should be considered based on clinical judgement. Monitor renal function closely when combined with cyclosporine; consider dosage adjustment or discontinue in patients with increasing serum creatinine. Separate dosing; sirolimus should be administered 4 hours after oral cyclosporine dose.

May increase serum creatinine and decrease GFR. Use caution when used concurrently with medications which may alter renal function. May delay recovery of renal function in patients with delayed allograft function. Increased urinary protein excretion has been observed when converting renal transplant patients from calcineurin inhibitors to sirolimus during maintenance therapy. A higher level of proteinuria prior to sirolimus conversion correlates with a higher degree of proteinuria after conversion. In some patients, proteinuria may reach nephrotic levels; nephrotic syndrome (new onset) has been reported.

Use caution with hepatic impairment; a reduction in the maintenance dose is recommended. Has been associated with an increased risk of fluid accumulation and lymphocele; peripheral edema, lymphedema, and pleural and pericardial effusions (including significant effusions and tamponade) were reported; use with caution in patients in whom fluid accumulation may be poorly tolerated, such as in cardiovascular disease (heart failure or hypertension) and pulmonary disease. Cases of interstitial lung disease (eg, pneumonitis, bronchiolitis obliterans organizing pneumonia [BOOP], pulmonary fibrosis) have been observed; risk may be increased with higher trough levels. Avoid concurrent use of strong CYP3A4 and/or P-glycoprotein (P-gp) inhibitors (eg, clarithromycin, erythromycin, telithromycin, itraconazole, ketoconazole, voriconazole) and strong inducers of CYP3A4 and/or P-gp (eg, rifampin, rifabutin). Concurrent use with a calcineurin inhibitor (cyclosporine, tacrolimus) may increase the risk of calcineurin inhibitor-induced hemolytic uremic syndrome/thrombotic thrombocytopenic purpura/thrombotic microangiopathy (HUS/TTP/TMA).

Hypersensitivity reactions, including anaphylactic/anaphylactoid reactions, angioedema, exfoliative dermatitis, and hypersensitivity vasculitis have been reported. Concurrent use with other drugs known to cause angioedema (eg, ACE inhibitors) may increase risk. Immunosuppressant therapy is associated with an increased risk of skin cancer; limit sun and ultraviolet light exposure; use appropriate sun protection. May increase serum lipids (cholesterol and triglycerides); use with caution in patients with hyperlipidemia. May be associated with wound dehiscence and impaired healing; use caution in the perioperative period. Patients with a body mass index (BMI) >30 kg/m^2 are at increased risk for abnormal wound healing. Not labeled for use in children <13 years of age, or in adolescent patients <18 years of age considered at high immunological risk.

Adverse Reactions Incidence of many adverse effects is dose related.
>20%:
  Cardiovascular: Peripheral edema (54% to 64%), hypertension (39% to 49%), edema (16% to 24%), chest pain (16% to 24%)
  Central nervous system: Fever (23% to 34%), headache (23% to 34%), pain (24% to 33%), insomnia (13% to 22%)
  Dermatologic: Acne (20% to 31%)

Endocrine & metabolic: Hypertriglyceridemia (38% to 57%), hypercholesterolemia (38% to 46%), hypophosphatemia (15% to 23%), hypokalemia (11% to 21%)

Gastrointestinal: Diarrhea (25% to 42%), constipation (28% to 38%), abdominal pain (28% to 36%), nausea (25% to 36%), vomiting (19% to 25%), dyspepsia (17% to 25%), weight gain (8% to 21%)

Genitourinary: Urinary tract infection (20% to 33%)

Hematologic: Anemia (23% to 37%), thrombocytopenia (13% to 30%)

Neuromuscular & skeletal: Weakness (22% to 40%), arthralgia (25% to 31%), tremor (21% to 31%), back pain (16% to 26%)

Renal: Serum creatinine increased (35% to 40%)

Respiratory: Dyspnea (22% to 30%), upper respiratory infection (20% to 26%), pharyngitis (16% to 21%)

3% to 20%:

Cardiovascular: Atrial fibrillation, CHF, DVT, facial edema, hypervolemia, hypotension, palpitation, peripheral vascular disorder, postural hypotension, syncope, tachycardia, thrombosis, vasodilation, venous thromboembolism

Central nervous system: Chills, malaise, anxiety, confusion, depression, dizziness, emotional lability, hypoesthesia, hypotonia, neuropathy, somnolence

Dermatologic: Rash (10% to 20%), dermatitis (fungal), hirsutism, pruritus, skin hypertrophy, dermal ulcer, ecchymosis, cellulitis, skin carcinoma (up to 3%; includes basal cell carcinoma, squamous cell carcinoma, melanoma), wound healing abnormal

Endocrine & metabolic: Hyperkalemia (12% to 17%), Cushing's syndrome, diabetes mellitus, glycosuria, acidosis, dehydration, hypercalcemia, hyperglycemia, hyperphosphatemia, hypocalcemia, hypoglycemia, hypomagnesemia, hyponatremia

Gastrointestinal: Enlarged abdomen, anorexia, dysphagia, eructation, esophagitis, flatulence, gastritis, gastroenteritis, gingivitis, gingival hyperplasia, ileus, mouth ulceration, oral moniliasis, stomatitis, weight loss

Genitourinary: Pelvic pain, scrotal edema, testis disorder, impotence

Hematologic: Leukopenia (9% to 15%), leukocytosis, polycythemia, TTP, hemolytic-uremic syndrome, hemorrhage

Hepatic: Abnormal liver function tests, alkaline phosphatase increased, ascites, LDH increased, transaminases increased

Local: Thrombophlebitis

Neuromuscular & skeletal: Arthrosis, bone necrosis, CPK increased, leg cramps, myalgia, osteoporosis, tetany, hypertonia, paresthesia

Ocular: Abnormal vision, cataract, conjunctivitis

Otic: Ear pain, otitis media, tinnitus

Renal: Albuminuria, bladder pain, BUN increased, dysuria, hematuria, hydronephrosis, kidney pain, tubular necrosis, nocturia, oliguria, pyelonephritis, pyuria, nephropathy (toxic), urinary frequency, urinary incontinence, urinary retention

Respiratory: Asthma, atelectasis, bronchitis, cough, epistaxis, hypoxia, lung edema, pleural effusion, pneumonia, pulmonary embolism, rhinitis, sinusitis

Miscellaneous: Abscess, diaphoresis, flu-like syndrome, herpesvirus infection, hernia, infection (including opportunistic), lymphadenopathy, lymphocele, lymphoproliferative disease/lymphoma (1% to 3%), peritonitis, sepsis

Infrequent, postmarketing, and/or case reports: Alveolar proteinosis, anaphylactoid reaction, anaphylaxis, anastomotic disruption, angioedema, azoospermia, cytomegalovirus, Epstein-Barr virus, exfoliative dermatitis, fascial dehiscence, focal segmental glomerulosclerosis, hepatic necrosis, hepatotoxicity, hypersensitivity reaction, hypersensitivity vasculitis; incisional hernia;

interstitial lung disease (dose-related; includes pneumonitis, pulmonary fibrosis, and bronchiolitis obliterans organizing pneumonia [BOOP] with no identified infectious etiology); joint disorders, lymphedema, nephrotic syndrome, neutropenia, pancreatitis, pancytopenia, pericardial effusion, *Pneumocystis* pneumonia, proteinuria, pulmonary hemorrhage, tamponade, tuberculosis, wound dehiscence

Note: Hepatic artery thrombosis (HAT) and graft failure have been reported in liver transplant patients (not an approved use); bronchial anastomotic dehiscence has been reported in lung transplant patients (not an approved use); and calcineurin inhibitor-induced hemolytic uremic syndrome/thrombotic thrombocytopenic purpura/thrombotic microangiopathy (HUS/TTP/TMA) has been reported with concurrent cyclosporine and/or tacrolimus.

Drug Interactions

Metabolism/Transport Effects Substrate of CYP3A4 (major), P-glycoprotein; **Inhibits** CYP3A4 (weak)

Avoid Concomitant Use

Avoid concomitant use of Sirolimus with any of the following: Natalizumab; Posaconazole; Tacrolimus; Vaccines (Live); Voriconazole

Increased Effect/Toxicity

Sirolimus may increase the levels/effects of: ACE Inhibitors; CycloSPORINE; Hypoglycemic Agents; Leflunomide; Natalizumab; Tacrolimus; Vaccines (Live)

The levels/effects of Sirolimus may be increased by: CycloSPORINE; CYP3A4 Inhibitors (Moderate); CYP3A4 Inhibitors (Strong); Dasatinib; Fluconazole; Herbs (Hypoglycemic Properties); Itraconazole; Ketoconazole; Macrolide Antibiotics; Miconazole; P-Glycoprotein Inhibitors; Posaconazole; Protease Inhibitors; Tacrolimus; Trastuzumab; Voriconazole

Decreased Effect

Sirolimus may decrease the levels/effects of: Vaccines (Inactivated); Vaccines (Live)

The levels/effects of Sirolimus may be decreased by: CYP3A4 Inducers (Strong); Deferasirox; Echinacea; Herbs (CYP3A4 Inducers); P-Glycoprotein Inducers; Phenytoin; Rifampin

Ethanol/Nutrition/Herb Interactions

Food: Avoid grapefruit juice; may decrease clearance of sirolimus. Ingestion with high-fat meals decreases peak concentrations but increases AUC by 23% to 35%. Sirolimus should be taken consistently (either with or without food) to minimize variability.

Herb/Nutraceutical: St John's wort may decrease sirolimus levels; avoid concurrent use. Avoid cat's claw, echinacea (have immunostimulant properties; consider therapy modifications). Herbs with hypoglycemic properties may increase the risk of sirolimus-induced hypoglycemia; includes alfalfa, aloe, bilberry, bitter melon, burdock, celery, damiana, fenugreek, garcinia, garlic, ginger, ginseng (American), gymnema, marshmallow, stinging nettle.

Storage/Stability

Oral solution: Store under refrigeration, 2°C to 8°C (36°F to 46°F). Protect from light. A slight haze may develop in refrigerated solutions, but the quality of the product is not affected. After opening, solution should be used in 1 month. If necessary, may be stored at temperatures up to 25°C (77°F) for ≤15 days after opening. Product may be stored in amber syringe for a maximum of 24 hours (at room temperature or refrigerated). Solution should be used immediately following dilution.

Tablet: Store at room temperature of 20°C to 25°C (68°F to 77°F). Protect from light.

Mechanism of Action Sirolimus inhibits T-lymphocyte activation and proliferation in response to antigenic and cytokine stimulation and inhibits antibody production. Its mechanism differs from other immunosuppressants. Sirolimus binds to FKBP-12, an intracellular protein, to form an immunosuppressive complex which inhibits the regulatory kinase, mTOR (mammalian target of rapamycin). This inhibition suppresses cytokine mediated T-cell proliferation, halting progression from the G1 to the S phase of the cell cycle. It inhibits acute rejection of allografts and prolongs graft survival.

Pharmacodynamics/Kinetics

Absorption: Rapid

Distribution: 12 L/kg (range: 4-20 L/kg)

Protein binding: ~92%, primarily to albumin

Metabolism: Extensive; in intestinal wall via P-gp and hepatic via CYP3A4; to 7 major metabolites

Bioavailability: Oral solution: 14%; Oral tablet: 18%

Half-life elimination: Mean: 62 hours (range: 46-78 hours); extended in hepatic impairment (Child-Pugh class A or B) to 113 hours

Time to peak: Oral solution: 1-3 hours; Tablet: 1-6 hours

Excretion: Feces (91% due to P-glycoprotein-mediated efflux into gut lumen); urine (2%)

Dosage Oral:

Combination therapy with cyclosporine: Doses should be taken 4 hours after cyclosporine, and should be taken consistently either with or without food.

Low-to-moderate immunologic risk renal transplant patients: Children ≥13 years and Adults: Dosing by body weight:

<40 kg: Loading dose: 3 mg/m^2 on day 1, followed by maintenance dosing of 1 mg/m^2 once daily

≥40 kg: Loading dose: 6 mg on day 1; maintenance: 2 mg once daily

High immunologic risk renal transplant patients: Adults: Loading dose: Up to 15 mg on day 1; maintenance: 5 mg/day; obtain trough concentration between days 5-7 and adjust accordingly. Continue concurrent cyclosporine/sirolimus therapy for 1 year following transplantation. Further adjustment of the regimen must be based on clinical status.

Dosage adjustment: Sirolimus dosages should be adjusted to maintain trough concentrations within desired range based on risk and concomitant therapy. Maximum daily dose: 40 mg. Dosage should be adjusted at intervals of 7-14 days to account for the long half-life of sirolimus. In general, dose proportionality may be assumed. New sirolimus dose **equals** current dose **multiplied by** (target concentration/current concentration). **Note:** If large dose increase is required, consider loading dose calculated as:

Loading dose **equals** (new maintenance dose **minus** current maintenance dose) **multiplied by** 3

Maximum dose in 1 day: 40 mg; if required dose is >40 mg (due to loading dose), divide over 2 days. Serum concentrations should not be used as the sole basis for dosage adjustment (monitor clinical signs/symptoms, tissue biopsy, and laboratory parameters).

Maintenance therapy after withdrawal of cyclosporine: Cyclosporine withdrawal is not recommended in high immunological risk patients. Following 2-4 months of combined therapy, withdrawal of cyclosporine may be considered in low-to-moderate immunologic risk patients. Cyclosporine should be discontinued over 4-8 weeks, and a necessary increase in the dosage of sirolimus (up to fourfold) should be anticipated due to removal of metabolic inhibition by cyclosporine and to maintain adequate immunosuppressive effects. Dose-adjusted trough target concentrations are typically 16-24 ng/mL for the first year post-transplant and 12-20 ng/mL thereafter (measured by chromatographic methodology).

Dosage adjustment in renal impairment: No dosage adjustment (in loading or maintenance dose) is necessary in renal impairment. However, adjustment of regimen (including discontinuation of therapy) should be considered when used concurrently with cyclosporine and elevated or increasing serum creatinine is noted.

Dosage adjustment in hepatic impairment:

Loading dose: No adjustment required

Maintenance dose:

Mild-to-moderate hepatic impairment: reduce maintenance dose by ~33%

Severe hepatic impairment: reduce maintenance dose by ~50%

Administration Initial dose should be administered as soon as possible after transplant. Sirolimus should be taken 4 hours after oral cyclosporine (Neoral® or Gengraf®).

Solution: Mix with at least 2 ounces of water or orange juice. No other liquids should be used for dilution. Patient should drink diluted solution immediately. The cup should then be refilled with an additional 4 ounces of water or orange juice, stirred vigorously, and the patient should drink the contents at once.

Tablet: Do not crush, split, or chew.

Monitoring Parameters Monitor LFTs and CBC during treatment. Monitor sirolimus levels in all patients (especially in pediatric patients, patients ≥13 years of age weighing <40 kg, patients with hepatic impairment, on concurrent potent inhibitors or inducers of CYP3A4 or P-gp, and/or if cyclosporine dosing is markedly reduced or discontinued), and when changing dosage forms of sirolimus. Also monitor serum cholesterol and triglycerides, blood pressure, serum creatinine, and urinary protein. Serum drug concentrations should be determined 3-4 days after loading doses and 7-14 days after dosage adjustments; however, these concentrations should not be used as the sole basis for dosage adjustment, especially during withdrawal of cyclosporine (monitor clinical signs/symptoms, tissue biopsy, and laboratory parameters). **Note:** Specific ranges will vary with assay methodology (chromatographic or immunoassay) and are not interchangeable.

Dietary Considerations Take consistently (with or without food) to minimize variability of absorption.

Additional Information Sirolimus tablets and oral solution are not bioequivalent, due to differences in absorption. Clinical equivalence was seen using 2 mg tablet and 2 mg solution. It is not known if higher doses are also clinically equivalent. Monitor sirolimus levels if changes in dosage forms are made.

Sirolimus solution may cause irritation if administered undiluted.

High-risk renal transplant patients are defined (per the manufacturer's labeling) as African-American transplant recipients and/or repeat renal transplant recipients who lost a previous allograft based on an immunologic process and/or patients with high PRA (panel-reactive antibodies; peak PRA level >80%). Individual transplant centers may have differences in their definitions. For example, some centers would consider a PRA >50% to be at higher risk of rejection.

◀ **Dosage Forms** Excipient information presented when available (limited, particularly for generics); consult specific product labeling.

Solution, oral:
Rapamune®: 1 mg/mL (60 mL) [contains ethanol 1.5% to 2.5%; packaged with oral syringes and a carrying case]

Tablet:
Rapamune®: 1 mg, 2 mg

References
Antin J, Kim H, Cutler C, et al, "Sirolimus, Tacrolimus, and Low-Dose Methotrexate for Graft-Versus-Host Disease Prophylaxis in Mismatched Related Donor or Unrelated Donor Transplantation," *Blood*, 2003, 102(5):1601-5.

Cutler C, Kim H, Hochberg E, et al, "Sirolimus and Tacrolimus Without Methotrexate as Graft-Versus-Host Disease Prophylaxis After Matched Related Donor Peripheral Blood Stem Cell Transplantation," *Biol Blood Marrow Transplant*, 2004, 10(5):328-36.

◆ **SKF 104864** see Topotecan on page 1116

◆ **SKF 104864-A** see Topotecan on page 1116

◆ **S-leucovorin** see LEVOleucovorin on page 714

◆ **6S-leucovorin** see LEVOleucovorin on page 714

◆ **SMZ-TMP** see Sulfamethoxazole and Trimethoprim on page 1051

◆ **Sodium 2-Mercaptoethane Sulfonate** see Mesna on page 758

◆ **Sodium Ferric Gluconate** see Ferric Gluconate on page 469

◆ **Sodium Hyposulfate** see Sodium Thiosulfate on page 1040

◆ **Sodium Nafcillin** see Nafcillin on page 840

Sodium Thiosulfate (SOW dee um thye oh SUL fate)

Related Information
Management of Drug Extravasations on page 1447

U.S. Brand Names Versiclear™

Index Terms Disodium Thiosulfate Pentahydrate; Pentahydrate; Sodium Hyposulfate; Sodium Thiosulphate; Thiosulfuric Acid Disodium Salt

Generic Available Yes: Injection

Pharmacologic Category Antidote

Use

Parenteral: Used alone or with sodium nitrite or amyl nitrite in cyanide poisoning; reduce the risk of nephrotoxicity associated with cisplatin therapy; treatment of cyanide poisoning due to nitroprusside

Topical: Treatment of tinea versicolor

Unlabeled/Investigational Use Management of I.V. extravasation

Pregnancy Risk Factor C

Labeled Contraindications Hypersensitivity to sodium thiosulfate or any component of the formulation

Warnings/Precautions Safety in pregnancy has not been established; discontinue topical use if irritation or sensitivity occurs; rapid I.V. infusion has caused transient hypotension and ECG changes in dogs; can increase risk of thiocyanate intoxication; use caution with renal impairment.

Fire victims may present with both cyanide and carbon monoxide poisoning. Collection of pretreatment blood cyanide concentrations does not preclude administration and should not delay administration in the emergency management of highly suspected or confirmed cyanide toxicity. Patients receiving treatment for acute cyanide toxicity must be monitored for return of symptoms for 24–48 hours.

Adverse Reactions Frequency not defined
Cardiovascular: Hypotension (infusion rate-dependent)
Dermatologic: Contact dermatitis, local irritation
Gastrointestinal: Nausea, vomiting
Miscellaneous: Hypersensitivity reactions

Drug Interactions

Avoid Concomitant Use There are no known interactions where it is recommended to avoid concomitant use.

Increased Effect/Toxicity There are no known significant interactions involving an increase in effect.

Decreased Effect There are no known significant interactions involving a decrease in effect.

Mechanism of Action

Cyanide toxicity: Accelerates the clearance of cyanide via the rhodanase-catalyzed detoxification of cyanide to thiocyanate (much less toxic than cyanide). The accelerated action of rhodanase is a result of the exogenous sulfur provided by sodium thiosulfate.

Cisplatin toxicity: Complexes with cisplatin to form a compound that is nontoxic to either normal or cancerous cells

Pharmacodynamics/Kinetics

Absorption: Oral: Poor
Distribution: Extracellular fluid
Half-life elimination: 0.65 hour
Excretion: Urine (28.5% as unchanged drug)

Dosage

Cyanide poisoning: I.V.: **Note:** Death from cyanide poisoning may occur rapidly, do not delay antidote administration in the event of highly suspected or confirmed cyanide poisoning; usually given in conjunction with amyl nitrite and sodium nitrite

Children: 7 g/m^2 (maximum dose: 12.5 g) given over 10 minutes; may repeat at ¹/₂ the original dose if symptoms return

Adults: 12.5 g given over 10 minutes; may repeat at ¹/₂ the original dose if symptoms return

Cisplatin rescue should be given before or during cisplatin administration: I.V. infusion (in sterile water): 12 g/m^2 over 6 hours or 9 g/m^2 I.V. push followed by 1.2 g/m^2 continuous infusion for 6 hours

Tinea versicolor: Children and Adults: Topical: 20% to 25% solution: Apply a thin layer to affected areas twice daily

Drug extravasation (unlabeled use): Children and Adults: SubQ: 1/6 M (~4%) solution: Inject into the affected area; various volumes have also been suggested for direct injection into existing I.V. line; however, the optimal volume and efficacy of such practices have not been thoroughly evaluated. **Note:** Use only for large cisplatin infiltrates (>20 mL) and cisplatin concentrations >0.5 mg/mL.

Administration

I.V.: Inject slowly, over at least 10 minutes; rapid administration may cause hypotension.

Topical: Do not apply to or near eyes.

Monitoring Parameters Monitor for signs of thiocyanate toxicity; monitor for hypotension and hypersensitivity reactions

Dosage Forms Excipient information presented when available (limited, particularly for generics); consult specific product labeling.

Injection, solution [preservative free]: 100 mg/mL (10 mL); 250 mg/mL (50 mL)

Lotion: Sodium thiosulfate 25% and salicylic acid 1% (120 mL) [contains isopropyl alcohol 10%]

References

Bertelli G, "Prevention and Management of Extravasation of Cytotoxic Drugs," *Drug Saf*, 1995, 12 (4):245-55.

Dorr RT, "Antidotes to Vesicant Chemotherapy Extravasations," *Blood Rev*, 1990, 4(1):41-60.

Ener RA, Meglathery SB, and Styler M, "Extravasation of Systemic Hemato-Oncological Therapies," *Ann Oncol*, 2004, 15(6):858-62.

Fuks JZ, Wadler S, and Wiernik PH, "Phase I and II Agents in Cancer Therapy: Two Cisplatin Analogues and High-Dose Cisplatin in Hypertonic Saline or With Thiosulfate Protection," *J Clin Pharmacol*, 1987, 27(5):357-65.

Gandara DR, Wiebe VJ, Perez EA, et al, "Cisplatin Rescue Therapy: Experience With Sodium Thiosulfate, WR2721, and Diethyldithiocarbamate," *Crit Rev Oncol Hematol*, 1990, 10(4):353-65.

Howell SB, Pfeifle CL, Wung WE, et al, "Intraperitoneal Cisplatin With Systemic Thiosulfate Protection," *Ann Intern Med*, 1982, 97(6):845-51.

MullinS, Beckwith MC, Tyler LS, "Prevention and Management of Antineoplastic Extravasation Injury," *Hospital Pharmacy*, 2000, 35(1):57-76.

Pfeifle CE, Howell SB, Felthouse RD, et al, "High-Dose Cisplatin With Sodium Thiosulfate Protection," *J Clin Oncol*, 1985, 3(2):237-44.

Skinner R, "Strategies to Prevent Nephrotoxicity of Anticancer Drugs," *Curr Opin Oncol*, 1995, 7 (4):310-5.

Tognella S, "Pharmacological Interventions to Reduce Platinum-Induced Toxicity," *Cancer Treat Rev*, 1990, 17(2-3):139-42.

Sorafenib (sor AF e nib)

Medication Safety Issues

Sound-alike/look-alike issues:
Nexavar® may be confused with Nexium®
Sorafenib may be confused with imatinib, sunitinib

High alert medication: The Institute for Safe Medication Practices (ISMP) includes this medication among its list of drug classes which have a heightened risk of causing significant patient harm when used in error.

Related Information

Safe Handling of Hazardous Drugs *on page* 1517

U.S. Brand Names Nexavar®

Index Terms BAY 43-9006; NSC-724772; Sorafenib Tosylate

Generic Available No

Canadian Brand Names Nexavar®

Pharmacologic Category Antineoplastic Agent, Tyrosine Kinase Inhibitor; Vascular Endothelial Growth Factor (VEGF) Inhibitor

Use Treatment of advanced renal cell cancer (RCC), unresectable hepatocellular cancer (HCC)

Unlabeled/Investigational Use Treatment of advanced thyroid cancer, recurrent or metastatic angiosarcoma, resistant gastrointestinal stromal tumor (GIST)

Pregnancy Risk Factor D

Lactation Excretion in breast milk unknown/not recommended

Labeled Contraindications Hypersensitivity to sorafenib or any component of the formulation

Warnings/Precautions Hazardous agent - use appropriate precautions for handling and disposal. May cause hypertension, especially in the first 6 weeks of treatment; monitor; use caution in patients with underlying or poorly-controlled hypertension. May cause cardiac ischemia or infarction; consider discontinuing (temporarily or permanently) in patients who develop these; use in patients with unstable coronary artery disease or recent myocardial infarction has not been studied. Use with caution in patients with cardiovascular disease. Serious bleeding events may occur; monitor PT/INR in patients on warfarin therapy. May complicate wound healing; temporarily withhold treatment for patients undergoing major surgical procedures. Gastrointestinal perforation has been reported (rare); monitor patients for signs/symptoms (abdominal pain, constipation, or vomiting); discontinue treatment if gastrointestinal perforation occurs. Avoid concurrent use (if possible) with strong CYP3A4 inducers (eg, carbamazepine, dexamethasone, phenobarbital, phenytoin, rifampin, St. John's wort); may decrease sorafenib levels/effects. Use caution when administering sorafenib with compounds that are metabolized predominantly via UGT1A1 (eg, irinotecan). Hand-foot skin reaction and rash are the most common adverse events; usually managed with topical treatment, treatment delays, and/or dose reductions. The risk for hand-foot syndrome increased with cumulative doses of sorafenib. The incidence of hand-foot syndrome is also increased in patients treated with sorafenib plus bevacizumab in comparison to those treated with sorafenib monotherapy. Sorafenib levels may be lower in HCC patients with mild-to-moderate hepatic impairment (Child-Pugh classes A and B); has not been studied in patients with severe hepatic impairment. Use with extreme caution in patients with HCC with elevated bilirubin levels. The optimal dose in non-HCC patients with hepatic impairment has not been established. In a small study of Asian patients with advanced HCC, sorafenib demonstrated efficacy with adequate tolerability in a hepatitis B-endemic area (Yau, 2009). Safety and efficacy have not been established in children.

Adverse Reactions

>10%:

Cardiovascular: Hypertension (9% to 17%; grade 3: 3% to 4%; grade 4: <1%; onset: ~3 weeks)

Central nervous system: Fatigue (37% to 46%), sensory neuropathy (≤13%), pain (11%)

Dermatologic: Rash/desquamation (19% to 40%; grade 3: ≤1%), hand-foot syndrome (21% to 30%; grade 3: 6% to 8%), alopecia (14% to 27%), pruritus (14% to 19%), dry skin (10% to 11%), erythema

Endocrine & metabolic: Hypoalbuminemia (≤59%), hypophosphatemia (35% to 45%; grade 3: 11% to 13%; grade 4: <1%)

Gastrointestinal: Diarrhea (43% to 55%; grade 3: 2% to 10%; grade 4: <1%), lipase increased (40% to 41% [usually transient]), amylase increased (30% to 34% [usually transient]), abdominal pain (11% to 31%), weight loss (10% to 30%), anorexia (16% to 29%), nausea (23% to 24%), vomiting (15% to 16%), constipation (14% to 15%)

Hematologic: Lymphopenia (23% to 47%; grades 3/4: ≤13%), thrombocytopenia (12% to 46%; grades 3/4: 1% to 4%), INR increased (≤42%), neutropenia (≤18%; grades 3/4: ≤5%), hemorrhage (15% to 18%; grade 3: 2% to 3%; grade 4: ≤2%), leukopenia

Hepatic: Liver dysfunction (≤11%; grade 3: 2%; grade 4: 1%)

Neuromuscular & skeletal: Muscle pain, weakness

Respiratory: Dyspnea (≤14%), cough (≤13%)

1% to 10%:

Cardiovascular: Cardiac ischemia/infarction (≤3%), flushing

Central nervous system: Headache (≤10%), depression, fever

Dermatologic: Acne, exfoliative dermatitis

Gastrointestinal: Appetite decreased, dyspepsia, dysphagia, esophageal varices bleeding (2%), glossodynia, mucositis, stomatitis, xerostomia

Genitourinary: Erectile dysfunction

Hematologic: Anemia

Hepatic: Transaminases increased (transient)

Neuromuscular & skeletal: Joint pain (≤10%), arthralgia, myalgia

Respiratory: Hoarseness

Miscellaneous: Flu-like syndrome

<1%, postmarketing, and/or case reports: Acute renal failure, alkaline phosphatase increased, arrhythmia, bilirubin increased, bone pain, cardiac failure, cerebral hemorrhage, CHF, dehydration, eczema, epistaxis, erythema multiforme, folliculitis, gastritis, gastrointestinal hemorrhage, gastrointestinal perforation, gastrointestinal reflux, gynecomastia, hypersensitivity (skin reaction, urticaria), hypertensive crisis, hyponatremia, hypothyroidism, infection, jaundice, MI, mouth pain, myocardial ischemia, pancreatitis, pleural effusion, preeclampsia-like syndrome (reversible hypertension and proteinuria), renal failure, respiratory hemorrhage, reversible posterior leukoencephalopathy syndrome (RPLS), rhinorrhea, skin cancer (squamous cell/keratoacanthomas), thromboembolism, tinnitus, transient ischemic attack, tumor lysis syndrome, tumor pain, voice alteration

Drug Interactions

Metabolism/Transport Effects Substrate of CYP3A4 (minor); **Inhibits** CYP2B6 (moderate), 2C8 (strong), 2C9 (moderate)

Avoid Concomitant Use

Avoid concomitant use of Sorafenib with any of the following: Natalizumab; Vaccines (Live)

Increased Effect/Toxicity

Sorafenib may increase the levels/effects of: Carvedilol; CYP2B6 Substrates; CYP2C8 Substrates (High risk); CYP2C9 Substrates (High risk); DOXOrubicin; Fluorouracil; Irinotecan; Leflunomide; Natalizumab; Treprostinil; Vaccines (Live); Vitamin K Antagonists; Warfarin

The levels/effects of Sorafenib may be increased by: Bevacizumab; CYP3A4 Inhibitors (Strong); Trastuzumab

Decreased Effect

Sorafenib may decrease the levels/effects of: Cardiac Glycosides; Dacarbazine; Fluorouracil; Vaccines (Inactivated); Vaccines (Live); Vitamin K Antagonists

The levels/effects of Sorafenib may be decreased by: CYP3A4 Inducers (Strong); Echinacea; Herbs (CYP3A4 Inducers)

Ethanol/Nutrition/Herb Interactions

Food: Bioavailability is decreased 29% with a high-fat meal (bioavailability is similar to fasting state when administered with a moderate-fat meal).

Herb/Nutraceutical: Avoid St John's wort (may decrease the levels/effects of sorafenib).

Storage/Stability Store at room temperature of 25°C (77°F); excursions permitted to 15°C and 30°C (59°F and 86°F). Protect from moisture.

Mechanism of Action Multikinase inhibitor; inhibits tumor growth and angiogenesis by inhibiting intracellular Raf kinases (CRAF, BRAF, and mutant BRAF), and cell surface kinase receptors (VEGFR-2, VEGFR-3, PDGFR-beta, cKIT, and FLT-3)

Pharmacodynamics/Kinetics

Protein binding: 99.5%

Metabolism: Hepatic, via CYP3A4 (primarily oxidated to the pyridine N-oxide; active, minor) and UGT1A9 (glucuronidation)

Bioavailability: 38% to 49%; reduced when administered with a high-fat meal

Half-life elimination: 25-48 hours

Time to peak, plasma: ~3 hours

Excretion: Feces (77%, 51% as unchanged drug); urine (19%, as metabolites)

Dosage Oral: Adults:

Advanced renal cell carcinoma: 400 mg twice daily

Hepatocellular cancer: 400 mg twice daily

Angiosarcoma (unlabeled use): 400 mg twice daily (Maki, 2009)

Thyroid cancer (unlabeled use): 400 mg twice daily (Gupta-Abramson, 2008)

Dosage adjustment for concomitant CYP3A4 inducers: Avoid the concomitant use of a strong CYP3A4 inducer (eg, carbamazepine, dexamethasone, phenobarbital, phenytoin, rifampin, St. John's wort) with sorafenib. If a strong CYP3A4 inducer is required, the sorafenib dose may need to be increased, with careful monitoring. When the strong CYP3A4 inducer is discontinued, reduce sorafenib to the indicated dose.

Dosage adjustment for toxicity: Temporary interruption and/or dosage reduction may be necessary for management of adverse drug reactions. The dose may be reduced to 400 mg once daily and then further reduced to 400 mg every other day.

Dose modification for severe/persistent hypertension (despite antihypertensive therapy) or cardiac ischemia/infarction: Consider temporarily or permanently discontinuing treatment.

Dose modification for hemorrhage requiring medical intervention or gastrointestinal perforation: Consider permanently discontinuing treatment.

Dose modification for skin toxicity:

Grade 1 (numbness, dysesthesia, paresthesia, tingling, painless swelling, erythema or discomfort of the hands or feet which do not disrupt normal activities): Continue sorafenib and consider symptomatic treatment with topical therapy.

Grade 2 (painful erythema and swelling of the hands or feet and/or discomfort affecting normal activities):

1st occurrence: Continue sorafenib and consider symptomatic treatment with topical therapy. **Note:** If no improvement within 7 days, see dosing for 2nd or 3rd occurrence.

2nd or 3rd occurrence: Hold treatment until resolves to grade 0-1; resume treatment with dose reduced by one dose level (400 mg daily or 400 mg every other day)

4th occurrence: Discontinue treatment

Grade 3 (moist desquamation, ulceration, blistering, or severe pain of the hands or feet or severe discomfort that prevents working or performing daily activities):

1st or 2nd occurrence: Hold treatment until resolves to grade 0-1; resume treatment with dose reduced by one dose level (400 mg daily or 400 mg every other day)

3rd occurrence: Discontinue treatment

Dosage adjustment in renal impairment:

FDA-approved labeling: No adjustment is required for mild, moderate, or severe renal impairment (not dependant on dialysis); has not been studied in dialysis patients.

Safety and pharmacokinetics were studied in varying degrees of renal dysfunction with the following empiric dose levels recommended based on patient tolerance (Miller, 2009):

Mild renal dysfunction (Cl_{cr} 40-59 mL/minute): 400 mg twice daily

Moderate renal dysfunction (Cl_{cr} 20-39 mL/minute): 200 mg twice daily

Severe renal dysfunction (Cl_{cr} <20 mL/minute): Data inadequate to define dose

Hemodialysis (any Cl_{cr}): 200 mg once daily

Dosage adjustment in hepatic impairment:

FDA-approved labeling: No adjustment is required for mild (Child-Pugh class A) to moderate (Child-Pugh class B) hepatic impairment; not studied in severe hepatic impairment (Child-Pugh class C). Use with extreme caution in patients with HCC with elevated bilirubin levels.

Safety and pharmacokinetics were studied in varying degrees of hepatic dysfunction with the following empiric dose levels recommended based on patient tolerance (Miller, 2009):

Mild hepatic dysfunction (bilirubin >1 to ≤1.5 times ULN and/or AST >ULN): 400 mg twice daily

Moderate hepatic dysfunction (bilirubin >1.5 to 3 times ULN; any AST): 200 mg twice daily

Severe hepatic dysfunction:

Bilirubin >3-10 x ULN (any AST): 200 mg every 3 days was **not** tolerated

Albumin <2.5 g/dL (any bilirubin and AST): 200 mg once daily

Administration Administer with water on an empty stomach (1 hour before or 2 hours after eating). Swallow tablet whole.

Monitoring Parameters CBC with differential, electrolytes, phosphorus, lipase and amylase levels; blood pressure (baseline, weekly for the first 6 weeks, then periodic); monitor for hand-foot syndrome

Dietary Considerations Take without food (1 hour before or 2 hours after eating).

Additional Information Hand-foot skin reaction (HFSR) management (Lacouture, 2008): The following treatments may be used in addition to the recommended dosage modifications. Prior to treatment initiation, a pedicure is recommended to remove hyperkeratotic areas/calluses, which may predispose to HFSR; avoid vigorous exercise/activities which may stress hands or feet. During therapy, patients should reduce exposure to hot water (may exacerbate hand-foot symptoms); avoid constrictive footwear and excessive skin friction. Grade 1 HFSR may be relieved with moisturizing creams, cotton gloves and socks (at night) and/or keratolytic creams such as urea or salicylic acid. Apply topical steroid (eg, clobetasol ointment) to erythematous areas of Grade 2 HFSR; topical anesthetics and then systemic analgesics (if appropriate) may be used for pain control. Resolution of acute erythema may result in keratotic areas which may be softened with keratolytic agents.

Emetic Potential Very low (<10%)

Dosage Forms Excipient information presented when available (limited, particularly for generics); consult specific product labeling.

Tablet, as tosylate:

Nexavar®: 200 mg

References

Abou-Alfa GK, Schwarts L, Ricci S, et al, "Phase II Study of Sorafenib in Patients With Advanced Hepatocellular Carcinoma," *J Clin Oncol*, 2006, 24(26):4293-300.

Escudier B, Eisen T, Stadler WM, et al, "Sorafenib in Advanced Clear-Cell Renal-Cell Carcinoma," *N Engl J Med*, 2007, 356(2):125-34.

Gupta-Abramson V, Troxel AB, Nellore A, et al, "Phase II Trial of Sorafenib in Advanced Thyroid Cancer," *J Clin Oncol*, 2008, 26(29):4714-9.

Llovet J Ricci S, Mazzaferro V, et al, "Sorafenib in Advanced Hepatocellular Carcinoma," *N Engl J Med*, 2008 Jul 24;359(4):378-90.

Miller AA, Murry DJ, Owzar K, et al, "Pharmacokinetic (PK) and Phase I Study of Sorafenib (S) for Solid Tumors and Hematologic Malignancies in Patients With Hepatic or Renal Dysfunction," *J Clin Oncol*, 2007, 25(18S):3538 [abstract from 2007 ASCO Annual Meeting Proceedings, Part I]

National Comprehensive Cancer Network®, "NCCN Clinical Practice Guidelines in Oncology™: Hepatobiliary Cancers," Version 2.2008. Accessible at http://www.nccn.org/professionals/physician_gls/PDF/hepatobiliary.pdf

Patel TV, Morgan JA, Demetri GD, et al, "A Preeclampsia-Like Syndrome Characterized by Reversible Hypertension and Proteinuria Induced by the Multitargeted Kinase Inhibitors Sunitinib and Sorafenib," *J Natl Cancer Inst*, 2008, 100(4):282-4.

Ratain, MJ, Eisen T, Stadler WM, et al, "Phase II Placebo-Controlled Randomized Discontinuation Trial of Sorafenib in Patients With Metastatic Renal Cell Carcinoma," *J Clin Oncol*, 2006, 24(16):2505-12.

Rini BI and Small EJ, "Biology and Clinical Development of Vascular Endothelial Growth Factor-Targeted Therapy in Renal Cell Carcinoma," *J Clin Oncol*, 2005, 23(5):1028-43.

Siu LL, Awada A, Takimoto CH, et al, "Phase I Trial of Sorafenib and Gemcitabine in Advanced Solid Tumors with an Expanded Cohort in Advanced Pancreatic Cancer," *Clin Cancer Res*, 2006, 12(1):144-51.

Strumberg D, Richly H, Hilger RA, et al, "Phase I Clinical and Pharmacokinetic Study of the Novel Raf Kinase and Vascular Endothelial Growth Factor Receptor Inhibitor BAY 43-9006 in Patients With Advanced Refractory Solid Tumors," *J Clin Oncol*, 2005, 23(5):965-72.

Veronese ML, Mosenkis A, Flaherty KT, et al, "Mechanisms of Hypertension Associated With BAY 43-9006," *J Clin Oncol*, 2006, 24(9):1363-9.

- ◆ **Sorafenib Tosylate** *see* Sorafenib *on page 1042*
- ◆ **Sporanox®** *see* Itraconazole *on page 667*
- ◆ **Sprycel®** *see* Dasatinib *on page 314*
- ◆ **Statex® (Can)** *see* Morphine Sulfate *on page 816*
- ◆ **Stemetil® (Can)** *see* Prochlorperazine *on page 992*
- ◆ **Sterapred®** *see* PredniSONE *on page 982*
- ◆ **Sterapred® DS** *see* PredniSONE *on page 982*
- ◆ **Sterile Talc** *see* Talc (Sterile) *on page 1071*
- ◆ **Sterile Talc Powder™** *see* Talc (Sterile) *on page 1071*
- ◆ **STI-571** *see* Imatinib *on page 613*
- ◆ **Stimate®** *see* Desmopressin *on page 344*

Streptozocin (strep toe ZOE sin)

Medication Safety Issues

Sound-alike/look-alike issues:

Streptozocin may be confused with streptomycin

High alert medication: The Institute for Safe Medication Practices (ISMP) includes this medication among its list of drugs which have a heightened risk of causing significant patient harm when used in error.

Related Information

Management of Chemotherapy-Induced Nausea and Vomiting *on page 1434*

Management of Drug Extravasations *on page 1447*

Safe Handling of Hazardous Drugs *on page 1517*

U.S. Brand Names Zanosar®

Generic Available No

Canadian Brand Names Zanosar®

Pharmacologic Category Antineoplastic Agent, Alkylating Agent

Use Treatment of metastatic islet cell carcinoma of the pancreas

Unlabeled/Investigational Use Treatment of adrenal tumors

Pregnancy Risk Factor D

Lactation Enters breast milk/contraindicated

Labeled Contraindications Pregnancy

Warnings/Precautions Hazardous agent - use appropriate precautions for handling and disposal. **[U.S. Boxed Warnings]: Renal toxicity is dose-related and cumulative and may be severe or fatal; other major toxicities include liver dysfunction, diarrhea, nausea, and vomiting. Should be administered under the supervision of an experienced cancer chemotherapy physician.** There may be an acute release of insulin during treatment. Keep syringe of $D_{50}W$ at bedside during administration. Local tissue irritation may occur; extravasation may cause local tissue lesions and necrosis.

Adverse Reactions

>10%:
  Gastrointestinal: Nausea and vomiting (100%)
  Hepatic: LFTs increased
  Miscellaneous: Hypoalbuminemia
  Renal: BUN increased, Cl_{cr} decreased, hypophosphatemia, nephrotoxicity (25% to 75%), proteinuria, renal dysfunction (65%), renal tubular acidosis

1% to 10%:
  Endocrine & metabolic: Hypoglycemia (6%)
  Gastrointestinal: Diarrhea (10%)
  Local: Pain at injection site

<1%: Confusion, lethargy, depression, leukopenia, thrombocytopenia, liver dysfunction, secondary malignancy

  Myelosuppressive:
    WBC: Mild
    Platelets: Mild
    Onset: 7 days
    Nadir: 14 days
    Recovery: 21 days

Drug Interactions

Avoid Concomitant Use
  Avoid concomitant use of Streptozocin with any of the following: Natalizumab; Vaccines (Live)

Increased Effect/Toxicity
  Streptozocin may increase the levels/effects of: Hypoglycemic Agents; Leflunomide; Natalizumab; Vaccines (Live)

  The levels/effects of Streptozocin may be increased by: Herbs (Hypoglycemic Properties); Trastuzumab

Decreased Effect
  Streptozocin may decrease the levels/effects of: Vaccines (Inactivated); Vaccines (Live)

  The levels/effects of Streptozocin may be decreased by: Echinacea

Storage/Stability Store intact vials under refrigeration. Vials are stable for 1 year at room temperature. Solution reconstituted with SWFI or NS is stable for 48 hours at room temperature and 96 hours under refrigeration. Further dilution in D_5W or NS is stable for 48 hours at room temperature and 96 hours under refrigeration when protected from light. Manufacturer recommends that reconstituted solution be used within 12 hours; vial does not contain a preservative

Reconstitution Dilute powder with 9.5 mL SWFI or NS to a concentration of 100 mg/mL.

Compatibility Stable in D_5W, NS.

Y-site administration: Compatible: Amifostine, etoposide phosphate, filgrastim, gemcitabine, granisetron, melphalan, ondansetron, teniposide, thiotepa, vinorelbine. **Incompatible:** Allopurinol, aztreonam, cefepime, piperacillin/tazobactam.

Mechanism of Action Interferes with the normal function of DNA by alkylation and cross-linking the strands of DNA, and by possible protein modification

Pharmacodynamics/Kinetics

Duration: Disappears from serum in 4 hours

Distribution: Concentrates in liver, intestine, pancreas, and kidney

Metabolism: Rapidly hepatic

Half-life elimination: 35-40 minutes

Excretion: Urine (60% to 70% as metabolites); exhaled gases (5%); feces (1%)

Dosage I.V. (refer to individual protocols):

Children and Adults:

Single-agent therapy: 1-1.5 g/m^2 weekly for 6 weeks followed by a 4-week rest period

Combination therapy: 0.5-1 g/m^2 for 5 consecutive days followed by a 4- to 6-week rest period

Dosing adjustment in renal impairment: The FDA-approved labeling does not contain dosing adjustments; however, it is recommended to use clinical judgment weighing benefit vs risk of renal toxicity in patients with pre-existing renal impairment. The following dosing adjustments have been used by some clinicians (Aronoff, 2007): Adults:

Cl_{cr} 10-50 mL/minute: Administer 75% of dose

Cl_{cr} <10 mL/minute: Administer 50% of dose

Dosing adjustment in hepatic impairment: There are no specific guidelines on dosage adjustment in patients with hepatic impairment. Streptozocin is rapidly hepatically metabolized; dose should be decreased in patients with severe liver disease.

Administration Administer as short (30-60 minutes) or 6-hour infusion; may be given by rapid I.V. push

Monitoring Parameters Monitor renal function closely

Emetic Potential Very high (>90%)

Vesicant Yes; see Management of Drug Extravasations on page 1447.

Dosage Forms Excipient information presented when available (limited, particularly for generics); consult specific product labeling.

Injection, powder for reconstitution: 1 g

References

Aronoff GR, Bennett WM, Berns JS, et al, *Drug Prescribing in Renal Failure: Dosing Guidelines for Adults and Children*, 5th ed. Philadelphia, PA: American College of Physicians; 2007, p 101.

Bolzan AD and Bianchi MS, "Genotoxicity of Streptozotocin," *Mutat Res*, 2002, 512(2-3):121-34.

◆ **Strontium-89 Chloride** *see* Strontium-89 *on page 1049*

Strontium-89 (STRON shee um atey nine)

U.S. Brand Names Metastron®

Index Terms Strontium-89 Chloride

Generic Available No

Canadian Brand Names Metastron®

◄ **Pharmacologic Category** Radiopharmaceutical

Use Relief of bone pain in patients with skeletal metastases

Pregnancy Risk Factor D

Labeled Contraindications Hypersensitivity to any strontium-containing compounds or any other component of the formulation; pregnancy; breast-feeding

Warnings/Precautions Use caution in patients with bone marrow compromise; incontinent patients may require urinary catheterization. Body fluids may remain radioactive up to one week after injection. Not indicated for use in patients with cancer not involving bone and should be used with caution in patients whose platelet counts fall <60,000/mm^3 or whose white blood cell counts fall <2400/mm^3. A small number of patients have experienced a transient increase in bone pain at 36-72 hours postdose; this reaction is generally mild and self-limiting. Use with caution in patients with renal impairment; renally eliminated. It should be handled cautiously, in a similar manner to other radioactive drugs. Appropriate safety measures to minimize radiation to personnel should be instituted. Safety and efficacy have not been established in children.

Adverse Reactions Most severe reactions of marrow toxicity can be managed by conventional means

Frequency not defined:

Cardiovascular: Flushing (most common after rapid injection)

Central nervous system: Fever and chills (rare)

Hematologic: Thrombocytopenia, leukopenia

Neuromuscular & skeletal: Increase in bone pain may occur (10% to 20% of patients)

Drug Interactions

Avoid Concomitant Use There are no known interactions where it is recommended to avoid concomitant use.

Increased Effect/Toxicity There are no known significant interactions involving an increase in effect.

Decreased Effect There are no known significant interactions involving a decrease in effect.

Storage/Stability Store vial and its contents inside its transportation container at room temperature.

Dosage Adults: I.V.: 148 megabecquerel (4 millicurie) administered by slow I.V. injection over 1-2 minutes or 1.5-2.2 megabecquerel (40-60 microcurie)/kg; repeated doses are generally not recommended at intervals <90 days; measure the patient dose by a suitable radioactivity calibration system immediately prior to administration

Monitoring Parameters Routine blood tests

Additional Information During the first week after injection, strontium-89 will be present in the blood and urine, therefore, the following common sense precautions should be instituted:

1. Where a normal toilet is available, use in preference to a urinal, flush the toilet twice
2. Wipe away any spilled urine with a tissue and flush it away
3. Have patient wash hands after using the toilet
4. Immediately wash any linen or clothes that become stained with blood or urine
5. Wash away any spilled blood if a cut occurs

Dosage Forms Excipient information presented when available (limited, particularly for generics); consult specific product labeling.

Injection, solution, as chloride [preservative free]:
Metastron®: 1 mCi/mL (4 mL) [37 megabecquerel per mL]

References

Brandi ML, "New Treatment Strategies: Ipriflavone Strontium, Vitamin D Metabolites and Analogs," *Am J Med*, 1993, 95(Suppl 5A):5A-69S-5A-74S.

Lincoln TA, "Importance of Initial Management of Persons Internally Contaminated With Radionuclides," *Am Ind Hyg Assoc J*, 1976, 37(1):16-21.

Robinson RG, Preston DF, Schiefelbein M, et al, "Strontium 89 Therapy for the Palliation of Pain Due to Osseous Metastases," *JAMA*, 1995, 274(5):420-4.

◆ **SU011248** *see* Sunitinib *on page 1057*

◆ **Suberoylanilide Hydroxamic Acid** *see* Vorinostat *on page 1193*

◆ **Sublimaze®** *see* FentaNYL *on page 458*

Sulfamethoxazole and Trimethoprim

(sul fa meth OKS a zole & trye METH oh prim)

Medication Safety Issues

Sound-alike/look-alike issues:

Bactrim™ may be confused with bacitracin, Bactine®, Bactroban®

Co-trimoxazole may be confused with clotrimazole

Septra® may be confused with Ceptaz®, Sectral®

Septra® DS may be confused with Semprex®-D

U.S. Brand Names Bactrim™; Bactrim™ DS; Septra®; Septra® DS; Sulfatrim®

Index Terms Co-Trimoxazole; SMZ-TMP; Sulfatrim; TMP-SMZ; Trimethoprim and Sulfamethoxazole

Generic Available Yes

Canadian Brand Names Apo-Sulfatrim®; Apo-Sulfatrim® DS; Apo-Sulfatrim® Pediatric; Novo-Trimel; Novo-Trimel D.S.; Nu-Cotrimox; Septra® Injection

Pharmacologic Category Antibiotic, Miscellaneous; Antibiotic, Sulfonamide Derivative

Use

Oral treatment of urinary tract infections due to *E. coli*, *Klebsiella* and *Enterobacter* sp, *M. morganii*, *P. mirabilis* and *P. vulgaris*; acute otitis media in children; acute exacerbations of chronic bronchitis in adults due to susceptible strains of *H. influenzae* or *S. pneumoniae*; treatment and prophylaxis of *Pneumocystis jiroveci* pneumonitis (PCP); traveler's diarrhea due to enterotoxigenic *E. coli*; treatment of enteritis caused by *Shigella flexneri* or *Shigella sonnei*

I.V. treatment or severe or complicated infections when oral therapy is not feasible, for documented PCP, empiric treatment of PCP in immune compromised patients; treatment of documented or suspected shigellosis, typhoid fever, *Nocardia asteroides* infection, or other infections caused by susceptible bacteria

Unlabeled/Investigational Use Cholera and *Salmonella*-type infections and nocardiosis; chronic prostatitis; as prophylaxis in neutropenic patients with *P. jiroveci* infections, in leukemia patients, and in patients following renal transplantation, to decrease incidence of PCP; treatment of *Cyclospora* infection, typhoid fever, *Nocardia asteroides* infection; prophylaxis against urinary tract infection; skin/soft tissue infections due to community-acquired MRSA

Pregnancy Risk Factor C

Lactation Enters breast milk/contraindicated (AAP rates "compatible")

Labeled Contraindications Hypersensitivity to any sulfa drug, trimethoprim, or any component of the formulation; megaloblastic anemia due to folate deficiency; infants <2 months of age; marked hepatic damage or severe renal disease (if patient not monitored); pregnancy (at term); breast-feeding

Warnings/Precautions Use with caution in patients with G6PD deficiency, impaired renal or hepatic function or potential folate deficiency (malnourished, chronic anticonvulsant therapy, or elderly); maintain adequate hydration to prevent crystalluria; adjust dosage in patients with renal impairment. Injection vehicle contains benzyl alcohol and sodium metabisulfite.

Chemical similarities are present among sulfonamides, sulfonylureas, carbonic anhydrase inhibitors, thiazides, and loop diuretics (except ethacrynic acid). Use in patients with sulfonamide allergy is specifically contraindicated in product labeling, however, a risk of cross-reaction exists in patients with allergy to any of these compounds; avoid use when previous reaction has been severe.

Fatalities associated with severe reactions including Stevens-Johnson syndrome, toxic epidermal necrolysis, hepatic necrosis, agranulocytosis, aplastic anemia and other blood dyscrasias; discontinue use at first sign of rash or serious adverse reactions. Elderly patients appear at greater risk for more severe adverse reactions. May cause hypoglycemia, particularly in malnourished, or patients with renal or hepatic impairment. Use with caution in patients with porphyria or thyroid dysfunction. Slow acetylators may be more prone to adverse reactions. Caution in patients with allergies or asthma. May cause hyperkalemia (associated with high doses of trimethoprim). Incidence of adverse effects appears to be increased in patients with AIDS. Prolonged use may result in fungal or bacterial superinfection, including *C. difficile*-associated diarrhea (CDAD) and pseudomembranous colitis; CDAD has been observed >2 months postantibiotic treatment.

Adverse Reactions The most common adverse reactions include gastrointestinal upset (nausea, vomiting, anorexia) and dermatologic reactions (rash or urticaria). Rare, life-threatening reactions have been associated with cotrimoxazole, including severe dermatologic reactions, blood dyscrasias, and hepatotoxic reactions. Most other reactions listed are rare, however, frequency cannot be accurately estimated.

Cardiovascular: Allergic myocarditis

Central nervous system: Apathy, aseptic meningitis, ataxia, chills, depression, fatigue, fever, hallucinations, headache, insomnia, kernicterus (in neonates), nervousness, peripheral neuritis, seizure, vertigo

Dermatologic: Photosensitivity, pruritus, rash, skin eruptions, urticaria; rare reactions include erythema multiforme, exfoliative dermatitis, Henoch-Schönlein purpura, Stevens-Johnson syndrome, and toxic epidermal necrolysis

Endocrine & metabolic: Hyperkalemia (generally at high dosages), hypoglycemia (rare), hyponatremia

Gastrointestinal: Abdominal pain, anorexia, diarrhea, glottis, nausea, pancreatitis, pseudomembranous colitis, stomatitis, vomiting

Hematologic: Agranulocytosis, aplastic anemia, eosinophilia, hemolysis (with G6PD deficiency), hemolytic anemia, hypoprothrombinemia, leukopenia, megaloblastic anemia, methemoglobinemia, neutropenia, thrombocytopenia

Hepatic: Hepatotoxicity (including hepatitis, cholestasis, and hepatic necrosis), hyperbilirubinemia, transaminases increased

Neuromuscular & skeletal: Arthralgia, myalgia, rhabdomyolysis, weakness

Otic: Tinnitus

Renal: BUN increased, crystalluria, diuresis (rare), interstitial nephritis, nephrotoxicity (in association with cyclosporine), renal failure, serum creatinine increased, toxic nephrosis (with anuria and oliguria)

Respiratory: Cough, dyspnea, pulmonary infiltrates

Miscellaneous: Allergic reaction, anaphylaxis, angioedema, periarteritis nodosa (rare), serum sickness, systemic lupus erythematosus (rare)

Drug Interactions

Metabolism/Transport Effects

Sulfamethoxazole: **Substrate** of CYP2C9 (major), 3A4 (minor); **Inhibits** CYP2C9 (moderate)

Trimethoprim: **Substrate** (major) of CYP2C9, 3A4; **Inhibits** CYP2C8 (moderate), 2C9 (moderate)

Avoid Concomitant Use

Avoid concomitant use of Sulfamethoxazole and Trimethoprim with any of the following: Dofetilide; Procaine

Increased Effect/Toxicity

Sulfamethoxazole and Trimethoprim may increase the levels/effects of: ACE Inhibitors; Amantadine; Angiotensin II Receptor Blockers; Antidiabetic Agents (Thiazolidinedione); AzaTHIOprine; Carvedilol; CycloSPORINE; CYP2C8 Substrates (High risk); CYP2C9 Substrates (High risk); Dapsone; Dofetilide; LamiVUDine; Memantine; Methotrexate; Phenytoin; Procainamide; Repaglinide; Sulfonylureas; Vitamin K Antagonists

The levels/effects of Sulfamethoxazole and Trimethoprim may be increased by: Amantadine; CYP2C9 Inhibitors (Moderate); CYP2C9 Inhibitors (Strong); Dapsone; Memantine

Decreased Effect

Sulfamethoxazole and Trimethoprim may decrease the levels/effects of: CycloSPORINE; Typhoid Vaccine

The levels/effects of Sulfamethoxazole and Trimethoprim may be decreased by: CYP2C9 Inducers (Highly Effective); CYP3A4 Inducers (Strong); Deferasirox; Herbs (CYP3A4 Inducers); Leucovorin-Levoleucovorin; Peginterferon Alfa-2b; Procaine

Ethanol/Nutrition/Herb Interactions Herb/Nutraceutical: Avoid dong quai; St John's wort (may diminish effects and also cause photosensitization).

Storage/Stability

Injection: Store at room temperature; do not refrigerate. Less soluble in more alkaline pH. Protect from light. Solution must be diluted prior to administration. Following dilution, store at room temperature; do not refrigerate. Manufacturer recommended dilutions and stability of parenteral admixture at room temperature (25°C):

5 mL/125 mL D_5W; stable for 6 hours.

5 mL/100 mL D_5W; stable for 4 hours.

5 mL/75 mL D_5W; stable for 2 hours.

Studies have also confirmed limited stability in NS; detailed references should be consulted.

Suspension, tablet: Store at controlled room temperature of 15°C to 25°C (59°F to 77°F). Protect from light.

Compatibility Stable in D_5½NS, LR, ½NS; **variable stability (consult detailed reference)** in D_5W, NS.

Y-site administration: Compatible: Acyclovir, aldesleukin, allopurinol, amifostine, amphotericin B cholesteryl sulfate complex, atracurium, aztreonam, bivalirudin, cefepime, cyclophosphamide, dexmedetomidine, diltiazem, docetaxel, doxorubicin liposome, enalaprilat, esmolol, etoposide phosphate, fenoldopam, filgrastim, fludarabine, gallium nitrate, gatifloxacin, gemcitabine, granisetron, hydromorphone, labetalol, linezolid, lorazepam, magnesium sulfate, melphalan, meperidine, morphine, nicardipine, pancuronium, pemetrexed, perphenazine, piperacillin/tazobactam, remifentanil, sargramostim, tacrolimus, teniposide, thiotepa, vecuronium, zidovudine. **Incompatible:** Fluconazole, midazolam, vinorelbine. **Variable (consult detailed reference):** Cisatracurium, foscarnet.

Compatibility in syringe: Compatible: Dimenhydramine, heparin. **Incompatible:** Pantoprazole.

Compatibility when admixed: Incompatible: Fluconazole, linezolid, verapamil.

Mechanism of Action Sulfamethoxazole interferes with bacterial folic acid synthesis and growth via inhibition of dihydrofolic acid formation from paraaminobenzoic acid; trimethoprim inhibits dihydrofolic acid reduction to tetrahydrofolate resulting in sequential inhibition of enzymes of the folic acid pathway

Pharmacodynamics/Kinetics

Absorption: Oral: Almost completely, 90% to 100%

Protein binding: SMX: 68%, TMP: 45%

Metabolism: SMX: N-acetylated and glucuronidated; TMP: Metabolized to oxide and hydroxylated metabolites

Half-life elimination: SMX: 9 hours, TMP: 6-17 hours; both are prolonged in renal failure

Time to peak, serum: Within 1-4 hours

Excretion: Both are excreted in urine as metabolites and unchanged drug

Effects of aging on the pharmacokinetics of both agents has been variable; increase in half-life and decreases in clearance have been associated with reduced creatinine clearance

Dosage Dosage recommendations are based on the trimethoprim component. double strength tablets are equivalent to sulfamethoxazole 800 mg and trimethoprim 160 mg.

Usual dosage ranges:

Children >2 months:

Mild-to-moderate infections: Oral: 8-12 mg TMP/kg/day in divided doses every 12 hours

Serious infection:

Oral: 20 mg TMP/kg/day in divided doses every 6 hours

I.V.: 8-12 mg TMP/kg/day in divided doses every 6 hours

Adults:

Oral: One double strength tablet (sulfamethoxazole 800 mg; trimethoprim 160 mg) every 12-24 hours

I.V.: 8-20 mg TMP/kg/day divided every 6-12 hours

Indication-specific dosing:

Children >2 months:

Acute otitis media: Oral: 8 mg TMP/kg/day in divided doses every 12 hours for 10 days. **Note:** Recommended by the American Academy of Pediatrics as an alternative agent in penicillin-allergic patients at a dose of 6-10 mg TMP/kg/day (AOM guidelines, 2004).

Cyclospora **(unlabeled use):** Oral, I.V.: 5 mg TMP/kg twice daily for 7-10 days

Pneumocystis jiroveci:

Treatment: Oral, I.V.: 15-20 mg TMP/kg/day in divided doses every 6-8 hours

Prophylaxis: Oral, 150 mg TMP/m^2/day in divided doses every 12 hours for 3 days/week; dose should not exceed trimethoprim 320 mg and sulfamethoxazole 1600 mg daily

Alternative prophylaxis dosing schedules include:

150 mg TMP/m^2/day as a single daily dose 3 times/week on consecutive days

or

150 mg TMP/m^2/day in divided doses every 12 hours administered 7 days/week

or

150 mg TMP/m^2/day in divided doses every 12 hours administered 3 times/week on alternate days

Shigellosis:

Oral: 8 mg TMP/kg/day in divided doses every 12 hours for 5 days

I.V.: 8-10 mg TMP/kg/day in divided doses every 6, 8, or 12 hours for up to 5 days

Urinary tract infection:

Treatment:

Oral: 6-12 mg TMP/kg/day in divided doses every 12 hours

I.V.: 8-10 mg TMP/kg/day in divided doses every 6, 8, or 12 hours for up to 14 days with serious infections

Prophylaxis: Oral: 2 mg TMP/kg/dose daily or 5 mg TMP/kg/dose twice weekly

Adults:

Chronic bronchitis (acute): Oral: One double strength tablet every 12 hours for 10-14 days

Cyclospora (unlabeled use): Oral, I.V.: 160 mg TMP twice daily for 7-10 days. **Note:** AIDS patients: Oral: One double strength tablet 2-4 times/day for 10 days, then 1 double strength tablet 3 times/week for 10 weeks (Pape, 1994; Verdier, 2000).

Meningitis (bacterial): I.V.: 10-20 mg TMP/kg/day in divided doses every 6-12 hours

Nocardia (unlabeled use): Oral, I.V.:

Cutaneous infections: 5-10 mg TMP/kg/day in 2-4 divided doses

Severe infections (pulmonary/cerebral): 15 mg TMP/kg/day in 2-4 divided doses for 3-4 weeks, then 10 mg TMP/kg/day in 2-4 divided doses. Treatment duration is controversial; an average of 7 months has been reported.

Note: Therapy for severe infection may be initiated I.V. and converted to oral therapy (frequently converted to approximate dosages of oral solid dosage forms: 2 DS tablets every 8-12 hours). Although not widely available, sulfonamide levels should be considered in patients with questionable absorption, at risk for dose-related toxicity, or those with poor therapeutic response.

Pneumocystis jiroveci:

Prophylaxis: Oral: One double strength tablet daily or 3 times/week

Treatment: Oral, I.V.: 15-20 mg TMP/kg/day in 3-4 divided doses

Sepsis: I.V.: 20 TMP/kg/day divided every 6 hours

Shigellosis:

Oral: One double strength tablet every 12 hours for 5 days

I.V.: 8-10 mg TMP/kg/day in divided doses every 6, 8, or 12 hours for up to 5 days

Skin/soft tissue infection due to community-acquired MRSA (unlabeled use): Oral: 1-2 double strength tablets every 12 hours (Stevens, 2005)

Travelers' diarrhea: Oral: One double strength tablet every 12 hours for 5 days

Urinary tract infection:
Oral: One double strength tablet every 12 hours
Duration of therapy: Uncomplicated: 3-5 days; Complicated: 7-10 days
Pyelonephritis: 14 days
Prostatitis: Acute: 2 weeks; Chronic: 2-3 months
I.V.: 8-10 mg TMP/kg/day in divided doses every 6, 8, or 12 hours for up to 14 days with severe infections

Dosing adjustment in renal impairment: Oral, I.V.:
Cl_{cr} 15-30 mL/minute: Administer 50% of recommended dose
Cl_{cr} <15 mL/minute: Use is not recommended

Administration
I.V.: Infuse over 60-90 minutes, must dilute well before giving; may be given less diluted in a central line; not for I.M. injection
Oral: May be taken with or without food. Administer with at least 8 ounces of water.

Monitoring Parameters Perform culture and sensitivity testing prior to initiating therapy; CBC, serum potassium, creatinine, BUN

Test Interactions Increased creatinine (Jaffé alkaline picrate reaction); increased serum methotrexate by dihydrofolate reductase method

Dietary Considerations Should be taken with 8 oz of water.

Dosage Forms Excipient information presented when available (limited, particularly for generics); consult specific product labeling. **Note:** The 5:1 ratio (SMX:TMP) remains constant in all dosage forms.
Injection, solution: Sulfamethoxazole 80 mg and trimethoprim 16 mg per mL (5 mL, 10 mL, 30 mL) [contains benzyl alcohol, ethanol 12.2%, propylene glycol 400 mg/mL, sodium metabisulfite]
Suspension, oral: Sulfamethoxazole 200 mg and trimethoprim 40 mg per 5 mL (480 mL)
Sulfatrim®: Sulfamethoxazole 200 mg and trimethoprim 40 mg per 5 mL (100 mL, 480 mL) [contains alcohol ≤0.5% propylene glycol; cherry flavor]
Tablet: Sulfamethoxazole 400 mg and trimethoprim 80 mg
Bactrim™: Sulfamethoxazole 400 mg and trimethoprim 80 mg
Septra®: Sulfamethoxazole 400 mg and trimethoprim 80 mg
Tablet, double strength: Sulfamethoxazole 800 mg and trimethoprim 160 mg
Bactrim™ DS: Sulfamethoxazole 800 mg and trimethoprim 160 mg
Septra® DS: Sulfamethoxazole 800 mg and trimethoprim 160 mg

References
Bissuel F, Cotte L, Crapanne JB, et al, "Trimethoprim-Sulphamethoxazole Rechallenge in 20 Previously Allergic HIV-Infected Patients After Homeopathic," *AIDS*, 1995, 9(4):407-8.
Masur H, "Prevention and Treatment of *Pneumocystis* Pneumonia," *N Engl J Med*, 1992, 327 (26):1853-60.
Singh N, Gayowski T, Yu VL, et al, "Trimethoprim-Sulfamethoxazole for the Prevention of Spontaneous Bacterial Peritonitis in Cirrhosis: A Randomized Trial," *Ann Intern Med*, 1995, 122 (8):595-8.
Stevens DL, Bisno AL, Chambers HF, et al, "Practice Guidelines for the Diagnosis and Management of Skin and Soft-Tissue Infections," *Clin Infect Dis*, 2005; 41(10):1373–406.

Sunitinib (su NIT e nib)

Medication Safety Issues

Sound-alike/look-alike issues:

Sunitinib may be confused with imatinib, sorafenib

High alert medication: The Institute for Safe Medication Practices (ISMP) includes this medication among its list of drug classes which have a heightened risk of causing significant patient harm when used in error.

Related Information

Safe Handling of Hazardous Drugs on page 1517

U.S. Brand Names Sutent®

Index Terms SU011248; SU11248; Sunitinib Malate

Generic Available No

Canadian Brand Names Sutent®

Pharmacologic Category Antineoplastic Agent, Tyrosine Kinase Inhibitor; Vascular Endothelial Growth Factor (VEGF) Inhibitor

Use Treatment of gastrointestinal stromal tumor (GIST) intolerance to or disease progression on imatinib; treatment of advanced renal cell cancer (RCC)

Unlabeled/Investigational Use Treatment of advanced thyroid cancer

Pregnancy Risk Factor D

Lactation Excretion in breast milk unknown/not recommended

Labeled Contraindications There are no contraindications listed within the FDA-approved manufacturer's labeling.

Canadian labeling: Hypersensitivity to sunitinib or any component of the formulation; pregnancy

Warnings/Precautions May cause a decrease in left ventricular ejection fraction (LVEF), including grade 3 reductions; monitor with baseline and periodic LVEF evaluations. Mean onset of symptomatic HF is 22 days from treatment initiation. Interrupt therapy or decrease dose with LVEF <50% or >20% reduction from baseline. Discontinue with clinical signs and symptoms of heart failure (HF). QT_c prolongation and torsade de pointes have been observed; a baseline and periodic ECG should be obtained; correct electrolyte abnormalities prior to treatment and monitor and correct potassium, calcium and magnesium levels during therapy; use caution in patients with a history of QT_c prolongation, with medications known to prolong the QT_c interval, or patients with pre-existing (relevant) cardiac disease, bradycardia, or electrolyte imbalance. Use caution with cardiac dysfunction; patients with MI, bypass grafts, HF, vascular diseases (including CVA and TIA), and PE were excluded from clinical trials. May cause hypertension; monitor and control with antihypertensives if needed; interrupt therapy until hypertension is controlled for severe hypertension. Use caution and closely monitor in patients with underlying or poorly-controlled hypertension. Use with caution in patients concurrently taking strong CYP3A4 inhibitors (may increase sunitinib levels; eg, ketoconazole) or inducers (may decrease sunitinib levels; eg, rifampin); dosage adjustments of sunitinib may be required.

Hemorrhagic events have been reported including epistaxis, rectal, gingival, upper GI, genital, wound bleeding, tumor-related, and hemoptysis/pulmonary hemorrhage. Microangiopathic hemolytic anemia (MAHA) and dose-limiting hypertension have been reported when sunitinib has been used in combination with bevacizumab. Serious and fatal gastrointestinal complications, including gastrointestinal perforation, have occurred (rarely). Hypothyroidism may occur; the risk for hypothyroidism appears to increase with therapy duration; ▶

hyperthyroidism, sometimes followed by hypothyroidism has also been reported; monitor thyroid function at baseline and if symptomatic. Adrenal function abnormalities have been reported; monitor for adrenal insufficiency for patients with trauma, severe infection, or undergoing surgery. May cause skin and/or hair depigmentation or discoloration. Reversible posterior leukoence-phalopathy syndrome (RPLS) has been reported (rarely); symptoms include confusion, headache, hypertension, lethargy, seizure, blindness and/or other vision, or neurologic disturbances; interrupt treatment and begin hypertension management. Has not been studied in patients with severe hepatic impairment (Child-Pugh class C). Safety and effectiveness in children have not been established.

Adverse Reactions

>10%:

Cardiovascular: Hypertension (15% to 30%; grades 3/4: 4% to 10%), LVEF decreased (11% to 21%; grades 3/4: 1%), heart failure (≤15%), peripheral edema (11%)

Central nervous system: Fatigue (42% to 58%), fever (17% to 18%), headache (13% to 18%), chills (11%), insomnia (11%)

Dermatologic: Hyperpigmentation (19% to 33%), skin discoloration (19% to 30%), rash (14% to 27%), hand-foot syndrome (12% to 21%), dry skin (17% to 18%), hair color changes (7% to 16%)

Endocrine & metabolic: Hyperuricemia (15% to 41%), hypophosphatemia (9% to 36%), hypocalcemia (35%), hypoglycemia (19%), hypoalbuminemia (18%), hyperglycemia (15%), hyponatremia (6% to 14%), hypokalemia (12%), hyperkalemia (6% to 11%), hypernatremia (10% to 11%)

Gastrointestinal: Diarrhea (40% to 58%), lipase increased (25% to 52%), nausea (31% to 49%), taste perversion (21% to 44%), mucositis/stomatitis (29% to 43%), anorexia (31% to 38%), constipation (16% to 34%), abdominal pain (22% to 33%), dyspepsia (28%), vomiting (24% to 28%), amylase increased (5% to 17%), weight loss (12%), xerostomia (12%), GERD/reflux (11%)

Hematologic: Leukopenia (up to 78%; grades 3/4: 5%), neutropenia (53% to 72%; grades 3/4: 10% to 12%), anemia (26% to 72%; grades 3/4: 3% to 7%), thrombocytopenia (38% to 65%; grades 3/4: 5% to 8%), lymphopenia (38% to 59%; grades 3/4: up to 59%), hemorrhage/bleeding (18% to 30%)

Hepatic: AST increased (39% to 52%), ALT increased (39% to 46%), alkaline phosphatase increased (24% to 42%), hyperbilirubinemia (10% to 19%)

Neuromuscular & skeletal: Creatine kinase increased (41%), weakness (21% to 22%), back pain (11% to 19%), arthralgia (12% to 18%), limb pain (14% to 17%), myalgia (14%)

Renal: Creatinine increased (12% to 66%)

Respiratory: Dyspnea (10% to 28%), cough (8% to 17%)

1% to 10%:

Cardiovascular: Venous thrombotic events (2% to 3%), DVT (1% to 3%), myocardial ischemia (1%)

Central nervous system: Depression (8%), dizziness (7%)

Dermatologic: Skin blistering (7%), alopecia (5%)

Endocrine & metabolic: Dehydration (8%), hypothyroidism (3% to 7%)

Gastrointestinal: Flatulence (10%), glossodynia (10%), oral pain (6% to 10%), appetite disturbance (9%), pancreatitis (1%)

Neuromuscular & skeletal: Peripheral neuropathy (10%)

Ocular: Periorbital edema (7%), lacrimation increased (6%)

Respiratory: Pulmonary embolism (1%)

<1%, postmarketing, and/or case reports: Acute renal failure, adrenal dysfunction, atrial flutter, coma, febrile neutropenia, gastrointestinal

perforation, hepatic failure, hyperthyroidism, infection, macrocytosis, micro-angiopathic hemolytic anemia (when used in combination with bevacizumab), MI, myopathy, nephrotic syndrome, neutropenic infection, preeclampsia-like syndrome (proteinuria and reversible hypertension), proteinuria, pulmonary hemorrhage, QT_c prolongation, reversible posterior leukoencephalopathy syndrome (RPLS), rhabdomyolysis, seizure, thrombotic microangiopathy, torsade de pointes, ventricular arrhythmia

Drug Interactions

Metabolism/Transport Effects Substrate of CYP3A4 (major)

Avoid Concomitant Use

Avoid concomitant use of Sunitinib with any of the following: Artemether; Bevacizumab; Dabigatran Etexilate; Dronedarone; Lumefantrine; Natalizumab; Nilotinib; Pimozide; QuiNINE; Silodosin; Tetrabenazine; Thioridazine; Vaccines (Live); Ziprasidone

Increased Effect/Toxicity

Sunitinib may increase the levels/effects of: Bevacizumab; Colchicine; Dabigatran Etexilate; Dronedarone; Leflunomide; Natalizumab; P-Glycoprotein Substrates; Pimozide; QTc-Prolonging Agents; QuiNINE; Rivaroxaban; Silodosin; Tetrabenazine; Thioridazine; Topotecan; Vaccines (Live); Vitamin K Antagonists; Ziprasidone

The levels/effects of Sunitinib may be increased by: Alfuzosin; Antifungal Agents (Azole Derivatives, Systemic); Artemether; Bevacizumab; Chloroquine; Ciprofloxacin; CYP3A4 Inhibitors (Moderate); CYP3A4 Inhibitors (Strong); Gadobutrol; Lumefantrine; Nilotinib; QuiNINE; Trastuzumab

Decreased Effect

Sunitinib may decrease the levels/effects of: Cardiac Glycosides; Vaccines (Inactivated); Vaccines (Live); Vitamin K Antagonists

The levels/effects of Sunitinib may be decreased by: CYP3A4 Inducers (Strong); Deferasirox; Echinacea; Herbs (CYP3A4 Inducers); Rifamycin Derivatives

Ethanol/Nutrition/Herb Interactions

Food: Grapefruit juice may increase the levels/effects of sunitinib. Food has no effect on the bioavailability of sunitinib.

Herb/Nutraceutical: Avoid St John's wort (may increase metabolism and decrease sunitinib concentrations).

Storage/Stability Store at room temperature of 25°C (77°F); excursions permitted to 15°C to 30°C (59°F to 86°F).

Mechanism of Action Exhibits antitumor and antiangiogenic properties by inhibiting multiple receptor tyrosine kinases, including platelet-derived growth factors (PDGFRα and PDGFRβ), vascular endothelial growth factors (VEGFR1, VEGFR2, and VEGFR3), FMS-like tyrosine kinase-3 (FLT3), colony-stimulating factor type 1 (CSF-1R), and glial cell-line-derived neurotrophic factor receptor (RET).

Pharmacodynamics/Kinetics

Distribution: V_d/F: 2230 L

Protein binding: Sunitinib: 95%; SU12662: 90%

Metabolism: Hepatic; primarily metabolized by CYP3A4 to the N-desethyl metabolite SU12662 (active)

Half-life elimination: Sunitinib: 40-60 hours; SU12662: 80-110 hours

Time to peak, plasma: 6-12 hours

Excretion: Feces (61%); urine (16%)

Dosage Oral: Adults:

Gastrointestinal stromal tumor, renal cell cancer: 50 mg once daily for 4 weeks of a 6-week treatment cycle (4 weeks on, 2 weeks off). **Note:** Dosage modifications should be done in increments of 12.5 mg; individualize based on safety and tolerability.

Thyroid cancer (unlabeled use): 50 mg once daily for 4 weeks of a 6-week treatment cycle (Cohen, 2008; Ravaud, 2008)

Dosage adjustment with concurrent CYP3A4 inhibitor: Dose reductions are more likely to be needed when sunitinib is administered concomitantly with strong CYP3A4 inhibitors (eg, clarithromycin, erythromycin, itraconazole, ketoconazole, nefazodone, protease inhibitors, telithromycin, voriconazole); dose reductions to a minimum of 37.5 mg/day should be considered with strong CYP3A4 inhibitors.

Dosage adjustment with concurrent CYP3A4 inducer: May require increased doses; dosage increases to a maximum of 87.5 mg/day with careful monitoring should be considered with strong CYP3A4 inducers (eg, carbamazepine, dexamethasone, phenobarbital, phenytoin, rifampin, St. John's wort).

Dosage adjustment for toxicity:

Cardiac toxicity:

Ejection fraction <50% and >20% below baseline without evidence of CHF: Interrupt treatment and/or reduce dose

LV dysfunction with CHF clinical manifestations: Discontinue treatment

Severe hypertension: Temporarily interrupt treatment until hypertension is controlled

Hepatic failure, nephrotic syndrome, or pancreatitis: Discontinue treatment

RPLS or thrombotic microangiopathy: Temporarily withhold treatment; after resolution, may resume with discretion.

Dosage adjustment in renal impairment: Most studies excluded patients with a serum creatinine >2 x ULN; pharmacokinetics were unaltered in patients with Cl_{cr} ≥42 mL/minute. Limited case reports of sunitinib use in patients with renal cell cancer requiring hemodialysis suggest efficacy; doses were initiated at 25 mg once daily (for 4 weeks of a 6-week cycle) and increased to 37.5 or 50 mg/day in later cycles (Zastrow, 2009).

Dosage adjustment in hepatic impairment: No adjustment is necessary with mild-to-moderate (Child-Pugh Class A or B) hepatic impairment; not studied in patients with severe (Child-Pugh Class C) hepatic impairment. Studies excluded patients with ALT/AST >2.5 x ULN, or if due to liver metastases, ALT/AST >5 x ULN.

Administration May be administered with or without food.

Monitoring Parameters LVEF, baseline (and periodic with cardiac risk factors), ECG (12-lead; baseline and periodic), blood pressure, adrenal function, CBC with differential and platelets (prior to each treatment cycle), serum chemistries including magnesium, phosphate, and potassium (prior to each treatment cycle), thyroid function (baseline; then if symptomatic), urinalysis (for proteinuria development or worsening)

Dietary Considerations May be taken with or without food. Avoid grapefruit juice.

Additional Information Hand-foot skin reaction (HFSR) management (Lacouture, 2008): The following treatments may be used in addition to the recommended dosage modifications. Prior to treatment initiation, a pedicure is recommended to remove hyperkeratotic areas/calluses, which may predispose to HFSR; avoid vigorous exercise/activities which may stress hands or feet.

During therapy, patients should reduce exposure to hot water (may exacerbate hand-foot symptoms); avoid constrictive footwear and excessive skin friction. Grade 1 HFSR may be relieved with moisturizing creams, cotton gloves and socks (at night) and/or keratolytic creams such as urea or salicylic acid. Apply topical steroid (eg, clobetasol ointment) to erythematous areas of Grade 2 HFSR; topical anesthetics and then systemic analgesics (if appropriate) may be used for pain control. Resolution of acute erythema may result in keratotic areas which may be softened with keratolytic agents.

Emetic Potential Very low (<10%)

Dosage Forms Excipient information presented when available (limited, particularly for generics); consult specific product labeling.
Capsule:
Sutent®: 12.5 mg, 25 mg, 50 mg

Extemporaneous Preparations

Sunitinib 10 mg/mL oral suspension: In a mortar, mix the contents of three 50-mg sunitinib capsules with a 1:1 mixture of Ora-Sweet® and Ora-Plus® to a final volume of 15 mL, yielding a final sunitinib concentration of 10 mg/mL; transfer to amber plastic bottle. This suspension maintains an average concentration of 96% to 106% (of the original concentration) at room temperature or refrigerated for up to 60 days in plastic amber prescription bottles. Note: Shake well before use.

Navid F, Christensen R, Minkin P, et al, "Stability of Sunitinib in Oral Suspension," *Ann Pharmacother*, 2008, 42(7):962-6.

References

Chu TF, Rupnick MA, Kerkela R, et al, "Cardiotoxicity Associated With Tyrosine Kinase Inhibitor Sunitinib," *Lancet*, 2007, 370(9604):2011-9.

Cohen EE, Needles BM, Cullen KJ, et al, "Phase 2 Study of Sunitinib in Refractory Thyroid Cancer," *J Clin Oncol*, 2008, 26(Supp): [abstract 6025 from 2008 ASCO Annual Meeting]

Demetri GD, van Oosterom AT, Garret CR, et al, "Efficacy and Safety of Sunitinib in Patients With Advanced Gastrointestinal Stromal Tumour After Failure of Imatinib: A Randomised Controlled Trial," *Lancet*, 2006, 368(9544):1329-38.

Desai J, Yassa L, Marqusee E, et al, "Hypothyroidism After Sunitinib Treatment for Patients With Gastrointestinal Stromal Tumors," *Ann Intern Med*, 2006, 145(9):660-4.

Faivre S, Delbaldo C, and Vera K, "Safety, Pharmacokinetic, and Antitumor Activity of SU11248, a Novel Oral Multitarget Tyrosine Kinase Inhibitor, in Patients With Cancer," *J Clin Oncol*, 2006, 24 (1):25-35.

Feldman DR, Baum MS, Ginsberg MS, et al, "Phase I Trial of Bevacizumab Plus Escalated Doses of Sunitinib in Patients With Metastatic Renal Cell Carcinoma," *J Clin Oncol*, 2009, 27(9):1432-9.

Feldman DR, Ginsberg MS, Baum M, et al, "Phase I Trial of Bevacizumab Plus Sunitinib in Patients With Metastatic Renal Cell Carcinoma," *J Clin Oncol*, 2008, 26(Supp): [abstract 5100 from 2008 ASCO Annual Meeting]

Feldman DR, Martorella AJ, Robbins RJ, et al, "Re: Hypothyroidism in Patients With Metastatic Renal Cell Carcinoma Treated With Sunitinib," *J Natl Cancer Inst*, 2007, 99(12):974-5.

Khakoo AY, Kassiotis CM, Tannir N, et al, "Heart Failure Associated with Sunitinib Malate," *Cancer*, 2008, 112(11):2500-8.

Motzer RJ, Hutson TE, Tomczak P, et al, "Sunitinib Versus Interferon Alfa in Metastatic Renal-Cell Cancer," *N Engl J Med*, 2007, 356(2):115-24.

Motzer RJ, Michaelson MD, and Redman BG, "Activity of SU11248, a Multitargeted Inhibitor of Vascular Endothelial Growth Factor Receptor, in Patients With Metastatic Renal Cell Cancer," *J Clin Oncol*, 2006, 24(1):16-24.

Ravaud A, de la Fouchardiere C, Courbon F, et al, "Sunitinib in Patients With Refractory Advanced Thyroid Cancer: The THYSU Phase II Trial," *J Clin Oncol*, 2008, 26(Supp): [abstract 6058 from 2008 ASCO Annual Meeting]

Rini BI, Choueiri TK, Elson P, et al, "Sunitinib-Induced Macrocytosis in Patients With Metastatic Renal Cell Carcinoma," *Cancer*, 2008, 113(6):1309-14.

Rini BI, Tamaskar I, Shaheen P, et al, "Hypothyroidism in Patients With Metastatic Renal Cell Carcinoma Treated With Sunitinib," *J Natl Cancer Inst*, 2007, 99(1):81-3.

Telli ML, Witteles RM, Fisher GA, et al, "Cardiotoxicity Associated With the Cancer Therapeutic Agent Sunitinib Malate," *Ann Oncol*, 2008, 19(9):1613-8.

Zastrow S, Froehner M, Platzek I, et al, "Treatment of Metastatic Renal Cell Cancer With Sunitinib During Chronic Hemodialysis," *Urology*, 2009, 73(4):868-70.

Tacrolimus (ta KROE li mus)

Medication Safety Issues

Sound-alike/look-alike issues:

Prograf® may be confused with Gengraf®, Prozac®

Tacrolimus may be confused with everolimus, pimecrolimus, sirolimus, temsirolimus

Related Information

Hematopoietic Stem Cell Transplantation *on page* 1501

Safe Handling of Hazardous Drugs *on page* 1517

U.S. Brand Names Prograf®; Protopic®

Index Terms FK506

Generic Available Yes: Capsule

Canadian Brand Names Advagraf™; Prograf®; Protopic®

Pharmacologic Category Calcineurin Inhibitor; Immunosuppressant Agent; Topical Skin Product

Use

Oral/injection: Prevention of organ rejection in heart, kidney, or liver transplant recipients

Topical: Moderate-to-severe atopic dermatitis in patients not responsive to conventional therapy or when conventional therapy is not appropriate

Unlabeled/Investigational Use Prevention of organ rejection in lung, small bowel transplant recipients; prevention and treatment of graft-versus-host disease (GVHD) in allogenic hematopoietic stem cell transplantation

Pregnancy Risk Factor C

Lactation Enters breast milk/not recommended

Labeled Contraindications Hypersensitivity to tacrolimus or any component of the formulation

Warnings/Precautions

Oral/injection: **[U.S. Boxed Warning]: Increased susceptibility to infection and the possible development of lymphoma may result from immunosuppression with tacrolimus.** The risk of developing other malignancies may also be increased. Insulin-dependent post-transplant diabetes mellitus (PTDM) has been reported including in patients without pretransplant history of diabetes mellitus; risk increases in African-American and Hispanic kidney transplant patients. Posterior reversible encephalopathy syndrome (PRES) may occur with therapy; symptoms are reversible with dose reduction or discontinuation of immunosuppressant therapy; stabilize blood pressure and reduce dose with suspected or confirmed diagnosis. Nephrotoxicity has has been reported, especially with higher doses; to avoid excess nephrotoxicity do not administer simultaneously with other nephrotoxic drugs (eg sirolimus, cyclosporine). Neurotoxicity may occur especially when used in high doses; tremor headache, coma and delirium have been reported and are associated with serum concentrations. Seizures may also occur. Monitoring of serum concentrations (trough for oral therapy) is essential to prevent organ rejection and reduce drug-related toxicity. Variable absorption is seen in bone marrow transplantation relative to total body radiation and/or methotrexate use. A period of ≥24 hours should elapse between discontinuation of cyclosporine and the initiation of tacrolimus. Delay initiation further with persistently elevated tacrolimus/cyclosporine levels. Use caution in renal or hepatic dysfunction, dosing adjustments may be required. Delay initiation if postoperative oliguria occurs. Use may be associated with the development of hypertension (common); hyperkalemia has been reported; avoid use of potassium-sparing diuretics. Myocardial hypertrophy has been reported (rare). Each mL of injection contains polyoxyl 60 hydrogenated castor oil (HCO-60) (200 mg) and dehydrated alcohol USP 80% v/v. Anaphylaxis has been reported with the injection, use should be reserved for those patients not able to take oral medications. **[U.S. Boxed Warning]: Should be administered under the supervision of a physician experienced in immunosuppressive therapy and organ transplantation in a facility appropriate for monitoring and managing therapy.**

Topical: **[U.S. Boxed Warning]: Topical calcineurin inhibitors have been associated with rare cases of malignancy (including skin and lymphoma), therefore it should be limited to short-term and intermittent treatment using the minimum amount necessary for the control of symptoms and only on involved areas. Use in children <2 years of age is not recommended, children ages 2-15 should only use the 0.03% ointment.** Avoid use on malignant or premalignant skin conditions (eg cutaneous T-cell lymphoma). Should not be used in immunocompromised patients. Do not apply to areas of active bacterial or viral infection; infections at the treatment site should be cleared prior to therapy. Topical calcineurin agents are considered second-line therapies in the treatment of atopic dermatitis/eczema, and should be limited to use in patients who have failed treatment with other therapies. Patients with atopic dermatitis are predisposed to skin infections, and tacrolimus therapy has been associated with risk of developing eczema herpeticum, varicella zoster, and herpes simplex. If atopic dermatitis is not improved in <6 weeks, re-evaluate to confirm diagnosis. May be associated with development of lymphadenopathy; possible infectious causes should be investigated. Discontinue use in patients with unknown cause of lymphadenopathy or acute infectious mononucleosis. Acute renal failure has been observed (rarely) with topical use. Not recommended for use in patients with skin disease which may increase systemic absorption (eg, Netherton's syndrome). Minimize sunlight exposure during treatment. Safety not established in patients with generalized erythroderma. Safety of intermittent use for >1 year has not been established, particularly since the effect on immune system development is unknown.

Adverse Reactions As reported for kidney, liver, and heart transplantation:

Oral, I.V.:

≥15%:

Cardiovascular: Hypertension (13% to 62%), edema (peripheral 11% to 36%), chest pain (19%), edema (18%), pericardial effusion (heart transplant 15%)

Central nervous system: Headache (25% to 64%), insomnia (30% to 64%), pain (24% to 63%), fever (19% to 48%), postprocedural pain (kidney transplant 29%), dizziness (19%)

Dermatologic: Pruritus (15% to 36%), rash (10% to 24%)

Endocrine & metabolic: Hypophosphatemia (28% to 49%), hypomagnesemia (16% to 48%), hyperglycemia (21% to 47%), hyperkalemia (8% to 45%), hyperlipemia (10% to 31%), hypokalemia (13% to 29%), diabetes mellitus (24% to 26%)

Gastrointestinal: Diarrhea (24% to 72%), abdominal pain (29% to 59%), nausea (32% to 46%), constipation (23% to 36%), anorexia (7% to 34%), vomiting (14% to 29%), dyspepsia (18% to 28%)

Genitourinary: Urinary tract infection (16% to 34%)

Hematologic: Anemia (5% to 50%), leukopenia (13% to 48%), leukocytosis (8% to 32%), thrombocytopenia (14% to 24%)

Hepatic: Liver function tests abnormal (6% to 36%), ascites (7% to 27%)

Local: Incision site complication (kidney transplant 28%)

Neuromuscular & skeletal: Tremor (34% to 56%; heart transplant 15%), weakness (11% to 52%), paresthesia (17% to 40%), back pain (17% to 30%), arthralgia (25%)

Renal: Abnormal kidney function (36% to 56%), creatinine increased (23% to 45%), BUN increased (12% to 30%), oliguria (18% to 19%)

Respiratory: Atelectasis (5% to 28%), pleural effusion (30% to 36%), dyspnea (5% to 29%), cough increased (18%), bronchitis (17%)

Miscellaneous: Infection (24% to 45%), CMV infection (32%), graft dysfunction (kidney transplant 24%)

<15%:

Cardiovascular: Abnormal ECG (QRS or ST segment abnormal), arrhythmia, atrial fibrillation, atrial flutter, bradycardia, cardiopulmonary failure, deep thrombophlebitis, heart failure, heart rate decreased, hemorrhage, hemorrhagic stroke, hypervolemia, hypotension, peripheral vascular disorder, phlebitis, postural hypotension, syncope, tachycardia, thrombosis, vasodilation, ventricular fibrillation

Central nervous system: Abnormal dreams, abnormal thinking, agitation, amnesia, anxiety, chills, confusion, depression, emotional lability, encephalopathy, flaccid paralysis, hallucinations, mood elevated, nervousness, psychosis, quadriparesis, seizure, somnolence

Dermatologic: Acne, alopecia, bruising, cellulitis, exfoliative dermatitis, fungal dermatitis, hirsutism, photosensitivity reaction, skin discoloration, skin disorder, skin neoplasm, skin ulcer, wound healing impaired

Endocrine & metabolic: Acidosis, alkalosis, bicarbonate decreased, Cushing's syndrome, dehydration, gout, hypercholesterolemia, hyper-/hypocalcemia, hyperphosphatemia, hyperuricemia, hypoproteinemia, serum iron decreased

Gastrointestinal: Appetite increased, cramps, duodenitis, dysphagia, enlarged abdomen, esophagitis (including ulcerative), flatulence, gastritis, gastroesophagitis, GI perforation/hemorrhage, ileus, oral moniliasis, pancreatic pseudocyst, rectal disorder, stomatitis, weight gain

Genitourinary: Bladder spasm, cystitis, dysuria, nocturia, urge incontinence, urinary frequency, urinary incontinence, urinary retention, vaginitis

Hematologic: Coagulation disorder, decreased prothrombin, hypochromic anemia, polycythemia

Hepatic: Alkaline phosphatase increased, bilirubinemia, cholangitis, cholestatic jaundice, GGT increased, hepatitis (including granulomatous), jaundice, LDH increased, liver damage

Local: Phlebitis

Neuromuscular & skeletal: Hypertonia, incoordination, joint disorder, leg cramps, myalgia, myasthenia, myoclonus, nerve compression, neuropathy, osteoporosis

Ocular: Abnormal vision, amblyopia

Otic: Ear pain, otitis media, tinnitus

Renal: Acute renal failure, albuminuria, BK nephropathy, hematuria, hydronephrosis, renal tubular necrosis, toxic nephropathy

Respiratory: Asthma, lung disorder, pharyngitis, pneumonia, pneumothorax, pulmonary edema, respiratory disorder, rhinitis, sinusitis, voice alteration

Miscellaneous: Abscess, abnormal healing, allergic reaction, crying, diaphoresis, flu-like syndrome, generalized spasm, hernia, herpes simplex, peritonitis, sepsis, writing impaired

Topical (as reported in children and adults, unless otherwise noted):
>10%:
Central nervous system: Headache (5% to 20%), fever (1% to 21%)
Dermatologic: Skin burning (43% to 58%; tends to improve as lesions resolve), pruritus (41% to 46%), erythema (12% to 28%)
Respiratory: Increased cough (children 18%)
Miscellaneous: Flu-like syndrome (23% to 31%), allergic reaction (4% to 12%)

1% to 10%:
Cardiovascular: Peripheral edema (adults 3% to 4%)
Central nervous system: Hyperesthesia (adults 3% to 7%), pain (1% to 2%)
Dermatologic: Skin tingling (2% to 8%), acne (adults 4% to 7%), localized flushing (following ethanol consumption; adults 3% to 7%), folliculitis (3% to 6%), urticaria (1% to 6%), rash (2% to 5%), pustular rash (2% to 4%), vesiculobullous rash (children 4%), contact dermatitis (3% to 4%), cyst (adults 1% to 3%), eczema herpeticum (1% to 2%), fungal dermatitis (adults 1% to 2%), sunburn (adults 1% to 2%), alopecia (adults 1%), dry skin (children 1%)
Endocrine & metabolic: Dysmenorrhea (adult females 4%)
Gastrointestinal: Diarrhea (3% to 5%), dyspepsia (adults 1% to 4%), abdominal pain (children 3%), vomiting (adults 1%), gastroenteritis (adults 2%), nausea (children 1%), tooth disorder (adults 1%)
Neuromuscular & skeletal: Paresthesia (adults 3%), myalgia (adults 2% to 3%), weakness (adults 2% to 3%), arthralgia (adults 1% to 3%), back pain (adults 2%)
Ocular: Conjunctivitis (2% adults)
Otic: Otitis media (12% children)
Respiratory: Rhinitis (6% children), sinusitis (2% to 4% adults), bronchitis (2% adults), pneumonia (1% adults)
Miscellaneous: Varicella/herpes zoster (1% to 5%), lymphadenopathy (3% children)

Oral, I.V., topical: Postmarketing and/or case reports (limited to important or life-threatening): Acute renal failure, anaphylaxis, anaphylactoid reaction, angioedema, ARDS, arrhythmia, atrial fibrillation, atrial flutter, basal cell carcinoma, bile duct stenosis, blindness, cardiac arrest, cerebral infarction, cerebrovascular accident, deafness, delirium, DIC, hemiparesis, hemolytic-uremic syndrome, hemorrhagic cystitis, hepatic necrosis, hepatotoxicity, interstitial lung disease, leukoencephalopathy, lymphoproliferative disorder (related to EBV), malignant melanoma, myocardial hypertrophy (associated with ventricular dysfunction; reversible upon discontinuation), MI, neutropenia, osteomyelitis, pancreatitis (hemorrhagic and necrotizing), pancytopenia, paresthesia, photosensitivity reaction (topical), posterior reversible encephalopathy syndrome (PRES), progressive multifocal leukoencephalopathy (PML), quadriplegia, QT_c prolongation, respiratory failure, seizure, septicemia, skin discoloration (topical), squamous cell carcinoma, Stevens-Johnson syndrome, syncope, toxic epidermal necrolysis, thrombocytopenic purpura, torsade de pointes, TTP, veno-occlusive hepatic disease, venous thrombosis, ventricular fibrillation

Note: Calcineurin inhibitor-induced hemolytic uremic syndrome/thrombotic thrombocytopenic purpura/thrombotic microangiopathy (HUS/TTP/TMA) have been reported (with concurrent sirolimus).

Drug Interactions

Metabolism/Transport Effects Substrate of CYP3A4 (major); **Inhibits** CYP3A4 (weak)

Avoid Concomitant Use

Avoid concomitant use of Tacrolimus with any of the following: Artemether; CycloSPORINE; Dabigatran Etexilate; Dronedarone; Grapefruit Juice; Lumefantrine; Natalizumab; Nilotinib; Pimozide; QuiNINE; Silodosin; Sirolimus; Tetrabenazine; Thioridazine; Topotecan; Vaccines (Live); Ziprasidone

Increased Effect/Toxicity

Tacrolimus may increase the levels/effects of: Alcohol (Ethyl); Colchicine; CycloSPORINE; Dabigatran Etexilate; Dronedarone; Leflunomide; Natalizumab; P-Glycoprotein Substrates; Phenytoin; Pimozide; QTc-Prolonging Agents; QuiNINE; Rivaroxaban; Silodosin; Sirolimus; Tetrabenazine; Thioridazine; Topotecan; Vaccines (Live); Ziprasidone

The levels/effects of Tacrolimus may be increased by: Alfuzosin; Antidepressants (Serotonin Reuptake Inhibitor/Antagonist); Antifungal Agents (Azole Derivatives, Systemic); Artemether; Calcium Channel Blockers (Dihydropyridine); Calcium Channel Blockers (Nondihydropyridine); Chloroquine; Ciprofloxacin; CycloSPORINE; CYP3A4 Inhibitors (Moderate); CYP3A4 Inhibitors (Strong); Fluconazole; Gadobutrol; Grapefruit Juice; Lumefantrine; Macrolide Antibiotics; MetroNIDAZOLE; Nilotinib; P-Glycoprotein Inhibitors; Protease Inhibitors; Proton Pump Inhibitors; QuiNINE; Sirolimus; Temsirolimus; Trastuzumab

Decreased Effect

Tacrolimus may decrease the levels/effects of: Vaccines (Inactivated); Vaccines (Live)

The levels/effects of Tacrolimus may be decreased by: Caspofungin; Cinacalcet; CYP3A4 Inducers (Strong); Deferasirox; Echinacea; P-Glycoprotein Inducers; Phenytoin; Rifamycin Derivatives; St Johns Wort

Ethanol/Nutrition/Herb Interactions

Ethanol: Localized flushing (redness, warm sensation) may occur at application site of topical tacrolimus following ethanol consumption.

Food: Decreases rate and extent of absorption. High-fat meals have most pronounced effect (37% decrease in AUC, 77% decrease in C_{max}). Grapefruit juice, CYP3A4 inhibitor, may increase serum level and/or toxicity of tacrolimus; avoid concurrent use.

Herb/Nutraceutical: St John's wort: May reduce tacrolimus serum concentrations (avoid concurrent use).

Storage/Stability

Injection: Prior to dilution, store at 5°C to 25°C (41°F to 77°F). Following dilution, stable for 24 hours in D_5W or NS in glass or polyethylene containers.

Capsules and ointment: Store at room temperature of 25°C (77°F); excursions permitted to 15°C to 30°C (59°F to 86°F).

Reconstitution Dilute with 5% dextrose injection or 0.9% sodium chloride injection to a final concentration between 0.004 mg/mL and 0.02 mg/mL.

Compatibility Variable stability (consult detailed reference) in D_5W, NS (only in glass or polyethylene containers).

Y-site administration: Compatible: Aminophylline, amphotericin B, ampicillin, ampicillin/sulbactam, anidulafungin, benztropine, calcium gluconate, cefazolin, cefotetan, ceftazidime, ceftriaxone, cefuroxime, chloramphenicol,

cimetidine, ciprofloxacin, clindamycin, co-trimoxazole, dexamethasone sodium phosphate, digoxin, diphenhydramine, dobutamine, dopamine, doxycycline, erythromycin lactobionate, esmolol, fluconazole, furosemide, gentamicin, haloperidol, heparin, hydrocortisone sodium succinate, hydromorphone, imipenem/cilastatin, insulin (regular), isoproterenol, leucovorin, lorazepam, methylprednisolone sodium succinate, metoclopramide, metronidazole, micafungin, morphine, multivitamins, nitroglycerin, oxacillin, penicillin G potassium, phenytoin, piperacillin, potassium chloride, propranolol, ranitidine, sodium bicarbonate, sodium nitroprusside, sodium tetradecyl sulfate, tobramycin, vancomycin. **Incompatible:** Acyclovir, ganciclovir.
Compatibility when admixed: Compatible: Cimetidine.

Mechanism of Action Suppresses cellular immunity (inhibits T-lymphocyte activation), by binding to an intracellular protein, FKBP-12 and complexes with calcineurin dependant proteins to inhibit calcineurin phosphatase activity

Pharmacodynamics/Kinetics

Absorption: Better in resected patients with a closed stoma; unlike cyclosporine, clamping of the T-tube in liver transplant patients does not alter trough concentrations or AUC

Oral: Incomplete and variable; the rate and extent of absorption is affected by food and may be most pronounced with a high-fat meal

Topical: Minimally absorbed; serum concentrations range from undetectable to 20 ng/mL (~2 ng/mL in majority of adult patients studied)

Distribution: V_d: Children: 0.5-4.7 L/kg; Adults: 0.55-2.47 L/kg

Protein binding: 99% primarily to albumin and alpha$_1$-acid glycoprotein glycoprotein

Metabolism: Extensively hepatic via CYP3A4 to eight possible metabolites (major metabolite, 31-demethyl tacrolimus, shows same activity as tacrolimus *in vitro*)

Bioavailability: Oral: Children: 7% to 55%, Adults: 7% to 32%; Topical: <0.5%; Absolute: Unknown

Half-life elimination: Variable, 23-46 hours in healthy volunteers; 2.1-36 hours in transplant patients

Time to peak: 0.5-6 hours

Excretion: Feces (~93%); urine (<2% as unchanged drug)

Dosage

Oral:

Prevention of organ rejection in transplant recipients: The initial dose of tacrolimus should begin no sooner than 6 hours post-transplant; adjunctive therapy with corticosteroids is recommended early post-transplant. I.V. route should only be used in patients not able to take oral medications and continued only until oral medication can be tolerated; anaphylaxis has been reported with I.V. administration. If switching from I.V. to oral, the oral dose should be started 8-12 hours after stopping the infusion.

Children: Patients without pre-existing renal or hepatic dysfunction have required (and tolerated) higher doses than adults to achieve similar blood concentrations. It is recommended that therapy be initiated at *high end* of the recommended adult I.V. and oral dosing ranges; dosage adjustments may be required.

Liver transplant: Initial dose: 0.15-0.20 mg/kg/day in 2 divided doses, given every 12 hours

Adults:

Heart transplant: Initial dose: 0.075 mg/kg/day in 2 divided doses, given every 12 hours. Use in combination with azathioprine or mycophenolate mofetil is recommended.

Kidney transplant: Initial dose: 0.2 mg/kg/day in combination with azathioprine **or** 0.1 mg/kg/day in combination with mycophenolate mofetil. Administer in 2 divided doses, given every 12 hours; initial dose may be given within 24 hours of transplant, but should be delayed until renal function has recovered; African-American patients may require larger doses to maintain trough concentration.

Liver transplant: Initial dose: 0.1-0.15 mg/kg/day in 2 divided doses, given every 12 hours

Prevention of graft-versus-host disease (unlabeled use): Children and Adults: Convert from I.V. to oral dose (1:4 ratio): Multiply total daily I.V. dose times 4 and administer in 2 divided oral doses per day, every 12 hours (Uberti 1999; Yanik, 2000).

Treatment of graft-versus-host disease (unlabeled use): Adults: 0.06 mg/kg twice daily (Furlong, 2000; Przepiorka, 1999)

I.V.:

Prevention of organ rejection in transplant recipients: The initial dose of tacrolimus should begin no sooner than 6 hours post-transplant; adjunctive therapy with corticosteroids is recommended early post-transplant. I.V. route should only be used in patients not able to take oral medications and continued only until oral medication can be tolerated; anaphylaxis has been reported with I.V. administration. If switching from I.V. to oral, the oral dose should be started 8-12 hours after stopping the infusion.

Children: It is recommended that therapy be initiated at the ***high end*** of the dosing range.

Liver transplant: Initial dose: 0.03-0.05 mg/kg/day as a continuous infusion

Adults: It is recommended that therapy be initiated at the ***lower end*** of the dosing range.

Heart transplant: Initial dose: 0.01 mg/kg/day as a continuous infusion. Use in combination with azathioprine or mycophenolate mofetil is recommended.

Kidney transplant: Initial dose: 0.03-0.05 mg/kg/day as a continuous infusion. Use in combination with azathioprine or mycophenolate mofetil is recommended.

Liver transplant: Initial dose: 0.03-0.05 mg/kg/day as a continuous infusion.

Prevention of graft-versus-host disease (unlabeled use): Children and Adults: Initial: 0.03 mg/kg/day (based on lean body weight) as continuous infusion. Treatment should begin at least 24 hours prior to stem cell infusion and continued only until oral medication can be tolerated (Przepiorka, 1999; Yanik, 2000).

Treatment of graft-versus-host disease (unlabeled use): Adults: Initial: 0.03 mg/kg/day (based on lean body weight) as continuous infusion (Furlong 2000, Przepiorka 1999)

Topical:

Atopic dermatitis (moderate-to-severe):

Children ≥2 years: Apply minimum amount of 0.03% ointment to affected area twice daily; rub in gently and completely. Discontinue use when symptoms have cleared. If no improvement within 6 weeks, patients should be re-examined to confirm diagnosis.

Adults: Apply minimum amount of 0.03% or 0.1% ointment to affected area twice daily; rub in gently and completely. Discontinue use when symptoms have cleared. If no improvement within 6 weeks, patients should be re-examined to confirm diagnosis.

Dosing adjustment in renal impairment: Systemic therapy: Evidence suggests that lower doses should be used; patients should receive doses at the lowest value of the recommended I.V. and oral dosing ranges; further reductions in dose below these ranges may be required.

Tacrolimus therapy should usually be delayed up to 48 hours or longer in patients with postoperative oliguria.

Hemodialysis: Not removed by hemodialysis; supplemental dose is not necessary.

Peritoneal dialysis: Significant drug removal is unlikely based on physiochemical characteristics.

Dosing adjustment in hepatic impairment: Systemic therapy: Use of tacrolimus in liver transplant recipients experiencing post-transplant hepatic impairment may be associated with increased risk of developing renal insufficiency related to high whole blood levels of tacrolimus. The presence of moderate-to-severe hepatic dysfunction (serum bilirubin >2 mg/dL; Child-Pugh score ≥10) appears to affect the metabolism of tacrolimus. The half-life of the drug was prolonged and the clearance reduced after I.V. administration. The bioavailability of tacrolimus was also increased after oral administration. The higher plasma concentrations as determined by ELISA, in patients with severe hepatic dysfunction are probably due to the accumulation of metabolites of lower activity. These patients should be monitored closely and dosage adjustments should be considered. Some evidence indicates that lower doses could be used in these patients.

Administration

I.V.: If I.V. administration is necessary, administer by continuous infusion only. Do not use PVC tubing when administering diluted solutions. Tacrolimus is usually intended to be administered as a continuous infusion over 24 hours. Do not mix with solutions with a pH ≥9 (eg, acyclovir or ganciclovir) due to chemical degradation of tacrolimus (use different ports in multilumen lines). Do not alter dose with concurrent T-tube clamping. Adsorption of the drug to PVC tubing may become clinically significant with low concentrations.

Oral: Administer on an empty stomach; be consistent with timing and composition of meals if GI intolerance occurs and administration with food becomes necessary (per manufacturer). If dosed once daily (not common), administer in the morning. If dosed twice daily, doses should be 12 hours apart. If the morning and evening doses differ, the larger dose (differences are never >0.5-1 mg) should be given in the morning. If dosed 3 times/day, separate doses by 8 hours.

Topical: Do not use with occlusive dressings. Burning at the application site is most common in first few days; improves as atopic dermatitis improves. Limit application to involved areas. Continue as long as signs and symptoms persist; discontinue if resolution occurs; re-evaluate if symptoms persist >6 weeks.

Monitoring Parameters Renal function, hepatic function, serum electrolytes (especially potassium), glucose and blood pressure, measure 3 times/week for first few weeks, then gradually decrease frequency as patient stabilizes. Whole blood concentrations should be used for monitoring (trough for oral therapy). Signs/symptoms of anaphylactic reactions during infusion should also be monitored. Patients should be monitored during the first 30 minutes of the infusion, and frequently thereafter.

Dietary Considerations Capsule: Take on an empty stomach; be consistent with timing and composition of meals if GI intolerance occurs and administration with food becomes necessary (per manufacturer). Avoid grapefruit juice.

Additional Information Additional dosing considerations:

Switch from I.V. to oral therapy: Threefold increase in dose; initiate oral therapy 8-12 hours after discontinuation of I.V.

Pediatric patients: Dose requirements are about 2 times higher compared to adults

Dosage Forms Excipient information presented when available (limited, particularly for generics); consult specific product labeling.

Capsule: 0.5 mg, 1 mg, 5 mg

Prograf®: 0.5 mg, 1 mg, 5 mg

Injection, solution:

Prograf®: 5 mg/mL (1 mL) [contains dehydrated alcohol 80% and polyoxyl 60 hydrogenated castor oil]

Ointment, topical:

Protopic®: 0.03% (30 g, 60 g, 100 g); 0.1% (30 g, 60 g, 100 g)

Extemporaneous Preparations Tacrolimus 0.5 mg/mL oral suspension: Mix the contents of six 5-mg tacrolimus capsules with equal amounts of Ora-Plus® and Simple Syrup, N.F., to make a final volume of 60 mL. The suspension is stable for 56 days at room temperature in glass or plastic amber prescription bottles.

Esquivel C, So S, McDiarmid S, Andrews W, and Colombani PM, "Suggested Guidelines for the Use of Tacrolimus in Pediatric Liver Transplant Patients," *Transplantation*, 1996, 61(5):847-8.

Foster JA, Jacobson PA, Johnson CE, et al, "Stability of Tacrolimus in an Extemporaneously Compounded Oral Liquid (Abstract of Meeting Presentation)," *American Society of Health-System Pharmacists Annual Meeting*, 1996, 53:P-52(E).

Tacrolimus 1 mg/mL oral suspension: Mix the contents of six 5-mg capsules in approximately 5 mL of sterile water; add capsule contents to an empty amber bottle first, then add sterile water and agitate bottle until drug disperses and a slurry is formed. Add equal parts of Ora-Plus® (suspending agent) and Ora-Sweet® (sweetening agent) to a total volume of 30 mL. The suspension is stable for 4 months at room temperature in plastic amber prescription bottles.

Elefante A, Muindi J, West K, et al, "Long-Term Stability of a Patient-Convenient 1 mg/mL Suspension of Tacrolimus for Accurate Maintenance of Stable Therapeutic Levels," *Bone Marrow Transplant*, 2006, 37(8):781-4.

References

French AE, Soldin SJ, Soldin OP, et al, "Milk Transfer and Neonatal Safety of Tacrolimus," *Ann Pharmacother*, 2003, 37(6):815-8.

Furlong T, Storb R, Anasetti C, et al, "Clinical Outcome After Conversion to FK 506 (Tacrolimus) Therapy for Acute Graft-Versus-Host Disease Resistant to Cyclosporine or for Cyclosporine-Associated Toxicities," *Bone Marrow Transplant*, 2000, 26(9):985-91.

Gardiner SJ and Begg EJ, "Breastfeeding During Tacrolimus Therapy," *Obstet Gynecol*, 2006, 107 (2 Pt 2):453-5.

Grimer M and Caring for Australians with Renal Impairment (CARI), "The CARI Guidelines. Calcineurin Inhibitors in Renal Transplantation: Pregnancy, Lactation and Calcineurin Inhibitors," *Nephrology (Carlton)*, 2007, 12(Suppl 1):98-105.

Jain A, Venkataramanan R, Fung JJ, et al, "Pregnancy After Liver Transplantation Under Tacrolimus," *Transplantation*, 1997, 64(4):559-65.

Kainz A, Harabacz I, Cowlrick IS, et al, "Analysis of 100 Pregnancy Outcomes in Women Treated Systemically With Tacrolimus," *Transpl Int*, 2000, 13(Suppl 1):299-300.

Kelly PA, Burckart GJ, and Venkataramanan R, "Tacrolimus: A New Immunosuppressive Agent," *Am J Health Syst Pharm*, 1995, 52(14):1521-35.

Messina M, Faraci M, de Fazio V, et al, "Paediatric Working Party. Prevention and Treatment of Acute GvHD," *Bone Marrow Transplant*, 2008, 41(Suppl 2):65-70.

Natazuka T, Ogawa R, Kizaki T, et al, "Immunosuppressive Drugs and Hypertrophic Cardiomyopathy," *Lancet*, 1995, 345(8965):1641.

Przepiorka D, Devine S, Fay J, et al, "Practical Considerations in the Use of Tacrolimus for Allogeneic Marrow Transplantation," *Bone Marrow Transplant*, 1999, 24(10):1053-6.

Przepiorka D, Suzuki J, Ippoliti C, et al, "Blood Tacrolimus Concentration Unchanged by Plasmapheresis," *Am J Hosp Pharm*, 1994, 51(13):1708.

Uberti JP, Cronin S, and Ratanatharathorn V, "Optimum Use of Tacrolimus in the Prophylaxis of Graft Versus Host Disease," *BioDrugs*, 1999, 11(5):343-58.

Yanik G, Levine JE, Ratanatharathorn V, et al, "Tacrolimus (FK506) and Methotrexate as Prophylaxis for Acute Graft-Versus-Host Disease in Pediatric Allogeneic Stem Cell Transplantation," *Bone Marrow Transplant*, 2000, 26(2):161-7.

♦ **Talc** *see* Talc (Sterile) *on page 1071*

♦ **Talc for Pleurodesis** *see* Talc (Sterile) *on page 1071*

Talc (Sterile) (talk STARE il)

U.S. Brand Names Sclerosol®; Sterile Talc Powder™

Index Terms Intrapleural Talc; Sterile Talc; Talc; Talc for Pleurodesis

Pharmacologic Category Sclerosing Agent

Use Prevention of recurrence of malignant pleural effusion in symptomatic patients

Pregnancy Risk Factor B

Labeled Contraindications There are no contraindications listed within the manufacturer's labeling.

Warnings/Precautions Acute pneumonitis and acute respiratory distress syndrome (including one death) have rarely been reported with higher doses (10 g). Should not be used to treat malignancies; does not have antineoplastic activity. Clinicians should evaluate need for future diagnostic procedures before use; sclerosis of pleural space may preclude subsequent procedures (eg, pneumonectomy for transplantation). Sclerosol® contents under pressure and should be kept away from any heat source.

Adverse Reactions Frequency not defined.

Cardiovascular: Asystolic arrest, chest pain, hypotension (transient), hypovolemia, MI, tachycardia

Central nervous system: Fever (generally lasting <24 hours)

Local: Bleeding (localized), infection at administration site, pain

Respiratory: ARDS, bronchopleural fistula, dyspnea, empyema, hemoptysis, hypoxemia, pneumonia, pulmonary edema, pulmonary embolism, subcutaneous emphysema

Storage/Stability

Sclerosol® Intrapleural Aerosol: Store at room temperature 15°C to 30°C (59°F to 86°F); do not freeze. Protect from heat and light.

Sterile Talc Powder™: Store at controlled room temperature of 18°C to 25°C (64°F to 77°F). Protect from light. Use within 12 hours of slurry preparation.

Reconstitution Sterile Talc Powder™: Vent bottle with needle; slowly add 50 mL of NS to bottle using aseptic technique. For doses >5 g, use a second bottle. Swirl the bottle to disperse talc and avoid settling. Divide the contents of each bottle into two 60 mL irrigation syringes (25 mL of talc slurry in each). Add an additional 25 mL of NS to each syringe for a total of 50 mL (2.5 g/50 mL). If not used immediately, label "For IntraPleural Use Only."

Mechanism of Action Induces an inflammatory reaction that promotes adherence of the visceral to the parietal pleura, therefore, preventing reaccumulation of pleural fluid.

Dosage Adults: Pleural effusion:

Intrapleural aerosol: 4-8 g (1-2 cans) as a single dose

Intrapleural instillation: 5 g

Administration Administer after adequate drainage of the effusion.

Sclerosol® Intrapleural Aerosol: Shake well and attach delivery tube. Insert delivery tube through pleural trocar, manually press on actuator button of canister to release; point in several different directions to distribute to all pleural surfaces. Keep canister in an upright position. Rate of delivery is 0.4 g per second.

Sterile Talc Powder™: Administer as a slurry. Shake well before instillation. Empty contents of each syringe into chest cavity through the chest tube by gently applying pressure to syringe plunger. After administration, flush with 10-25 mL of NS. Clamp chest tube and have patient rotate from supine to alternating decubitus positions at 20-30 minute intervals for 2 hours. For intrapleural use only; **not for I.V. administration.**

Dosage Forms Excipient information presented when available (limited, particularly for generics); consult specific product labeling.

Aerosol, intrapleural [powder]:

Sclerosol®: 4 g [contains chlorofluorocarbon]

Powder, intrapleural:

Sterile Talc Powder™: Talc USP (5 g)

References

Dresler CM, Olak J, Herndon JE, et al, "Phase III Intergroup Study of Talc Poudrage vs Talc Slurry Sclerosis for Malignant Pleural Effusion," *Chest*, 2005, 127(3):909-15.

Kvale PA, Seleecky PA, and Prakash UB, "Palliative Care in Lung Cancer: ACCP Evidence-Based Clinical Guidelines (2nd Edition)," *Chest*, 2007, 132(3 Suppl):368-403.

◆ **Tamofen® (Can)** *see* Tamoxifen *on page 1072*

Tamoxifen (ta MOKS i fen)

Medication Safety Issues

Sound-alike/look-alike issues:

Tamoxifen may be confused with pentoxifylline, Tambocor™, tamsulosin, temazepam

Related Information

Safe Handling of Hazardous Drugs *on page 1517*

Index Terms ICI-46474; Nolvadex; Tamoxifen Citras; Tamoxifen Citrate

Generic Available Yes

Canadian Brand Names Apo-Tamox®; Mylan-Tamoxifen; Nolvadex®-D; Novo-Tamoxifen; PMS-Tamoxifen; Tamofen®

Pharmacologic Category Antineoplastic Agent, Estrogen Receptor Antagonist; Selective Estrogen Receptor Modulator (SERM)

Use Treatment of metastatic (female and male) breast cancer; adjuvant treatment of breast cancer; reduce risk of invasive breast cancer in women with ductal carcinoma *in situ* (DCIS); reduce the incidence of breast cancer in women at high risk

Unlabeled/Investigational Use Treatment of mastalgia, gynecomastia, ovarian cancer, endometrial cancer, uterine sarcoma, and desmoid tumors; risk reduction in women with Paget's disease of the breast (with DCIS or without associated cancer); induction of ovulation; treatment of precocious puberty in females, secondary to McCune-Albright syndrome

Pregnancy Risk Factor D

Lactation Excretion in breast milk unknown/not recommended

Labeled Contraindications Hypersensitivity to tamoxifen or any component of the formulation; concurrent warfarin therapy or history of deep vein thrombosis or pulmonary embolism (when tamoxifen is used for cancer risk reduction)

Warnings/Precautions Hazardous agent - use appropriate precautions for handling and disposal. **[U.S. Boxed Warning]: Serious and life-threatening events (including stroke, pulmonary emboli, and uterine malignancy) have occurred at an incidence greater than placebo during use for breast**

cancer risk reduction; these events are rare, but require consideration in risk:benefit evaluation. An increased incidence of thromboembolic events, including DVT and pulmonary embolism, has been associated with use for breast cancer; risk is increased with concomitant chemotherapy; use with caution in individuals with a history of thromboembolic events. Thrombocytopenia and/or leukopenia may occur; neutropenia and pancytopenia have been reported rarely. Although the relationship to tamoxifen therapy is uncertain, rare hemorrhagic episodes have occurred in patients with significant thrombocytopenia. Use with caution in patients with hyperlipidemias; infrequent postmarketing cases of hyperlipidemias have been reported. Decreased visual acuity, retinal vein thrombosis, retinopathy, corneal changes, color perception changes, and increased incidence of cataracts (and the need for cataract surgery), have been reported. Hypercalcemia has occurred in patients with bone metastasis, usually within a few weeks of therapy initiation; institute appropriate hypercalcemia management; discontinue if severe. Local disease flare and increased bone and tumor pain may occur in patients with metastatic breast cancer; may be associated with (good) tumor response.

Tamoxifen is associated with a high potential for drug interactions, including CYP-and Pgp-mediated interactions. Decreased efficacy and an increased risk of breast cancer recurrence has been reported with concurrent moderate or strong CYP2D6 inhibitors (Aubert, 2009; Dezentje, 2009). Concomitant use with select SSRIs may result in decreased tamoxifen efficacy. Strong CYP2D6 inhibitors (eg, fluoxetine, paroxetine) and moderate CYP2D6 inhibitors (eg, sertraline) are reported to interfere with transformation to the active metabolite endoxifen. Weak CYP2D6 inhibitors (eg, venlafaxine, citalopram) have minimal effect on the conversion to endoxifen (Jin, 2005; NCCN Breast Cancer Risk Reduction Guidelines v.1.2009); escitalopram is also a weak CYP2D6 inhibitor. Lower plasma concentrations of endoxifen (active metabolite) have been observed in patients associated with reduced CYP2D6 activity (Jin, 2005) and may be associated with reduced efficacy.

Tamoxifen use may be associated with changes in bone mineral density (BMD) and the effects may be dependant upon menstrual status. In postmenopausal women, tamoxifen use is associated with a protective effect on bone mineral density (BMD), preventing loss of BMD which lasts over the 5 year treatment period. In premenopausal women, a decline (from baseline) in BMD mineral density has been observed in women who continued to menstruate; may be associated with an increased risk of fractures. Liver abnormalities such as cholestasis, fatty liver, hepatitis, and hepatic necrosis have occurred. Hepatocellular carcinomas have been reported in some studies; relationship to treatment is unclear. Tamoxifen is associated with an increased incidence of uterine or endometrial cancers. Endometrial hyperplasia, polyps, endometriosis, uterine fibroids, and ovarian cysts have occurred. Monitor and promptly evaluate any report of abnormal vaginal bleeding. Amenorrhea and menstrual irregularities have been reported with tamoxifen use.

Adverse Reactions

>10%:

Cardiovascular: Flushing (33% to 41%), hypertension (11%), peripheral edema (11%)

Central nervous system: Mood changes (12% to 18%), pain (3% to 16%), depression (2% to 12%)

Dermatologic: Skin changes (6% to 19%), rash (13%)

Endocrine & metabolic: Hot flashes (3% to 80%), fluid retention (32%), altered menses (13% to 25%), amenorrhea (16%)

◀ Gastrointestinal: Nausea (5% to 26%), weight loss (23%)
Genitourinary: Vaginal discharge (13% to 55%), vaginal bleeding (2% to 23%)
Neuromuscular & skeletal: Weakness (19%), arthritis (14%), arthralgia (11%)
Respiratory: Pharyngitis (14%)

1% to 10%:
Cardiovascular: Chest pain (5%), venous thrombotic events (5%), edema (4%), cardiovascular ischemia (3%), cerebrovascular ischemia (3%), angina (2%), deep venous thrombus (≤2%), MI (1%)
Central nervous system: Insomnia (9%), dizziness (8%), headache (8%), anxiety (6%), fatigue (4%)
Dermatologic: Alopecia (<1% to 5%)
Endocrine & metabolic: Oligomenorrhea (9%), breast pain (6%), menstrual disorder (6%), breast neoplasm (5%), hypercholesterolemia (4%)
Gastrointestinal: Abdominal pain (9%), weight gain (9%), constipation (4% to 8%), diarrhea (7%), dyspepsia (6%), throat irritation (oral solution 5%), abdominal cramps (1%), anorexia (1%)
Genitourinary: Urinary tract infection (10%), leukorrhea (9%), vaginal hemorrhage (6%), vaginitis (5%), ovarian cyst (3%)
Hematologic: Thrombocytopenia (≤10%), anemia (5%)
Hepatic: AST increased (5%), serum bilirubin increased (2%)
Neuromuscular & skeletal: Back pain (10%), bone pain (6% to 10%), osteoporosis (7%), fracture (7%), arthrosis (5%), myalgia (5%), paresthesia (5%), musculoskeletal pain (3%)
Ocular: Cataract (7%)
Renal: Serum creatinine increased (≤2%)
Respiratory: Cough (4% to 9%), dyspnea (8%), bronchitis (5%), sinusitis (5%)
Miscellaneous: Infection/sepsis (≤9%), diaphoresis (6%), flu-like syndrome (6%), allergic reaction (3%)

<1%, infrequent, or frequency not defined: Cholestasis, corneal changes, endometriosis, endometrial cancer, endometrial hyperplasia, endometrial polyps, fatty liver, hepatic necrosis, hepatitis, hypercalcemia, hyperlipidemia, lightheadedness, phlebitis, pruritus vulvae, pulmonary embolism, retinal vein thrombosis, retinopathy, second primary tumors, stroke, superficial phlebitis, taste disturbances, tumor pain and local disease flare (including increase in lesion size and erythema) during treatment of metastatic breast cancer (generally resolves with continuation), uterine fibroids, vaginal dryness

Postmarketing and/or case reports: Angioedema, bullous pemphigoid, erythema multiforme, hypersensitivity reactions, hypertriglyceridemia, impotence (males), interstitial pneumonitis, loss of libido (males), pancreatitis, Stevens-Johnson syndrome, visual color perception changes

Drug Interactions

Metabolism/Transport Effects Substrate of CYP2A6 (minor), 2B6 (minor), 2C9 (major), 2D6 (major), 2E1 (minor), 3A4 (major); **Inhibits** CYP2B6 (weak), 2C8 (moderate), 2C9 (weak), 3A4 (weak), p-glycoprotein

Avoid Concomitant Use
Avoid concomitant use of Tamoxifen with any of the following: CYP2D6 Inhibitors (Strong); Dabigatran Etexilate; Silodosin; Topotecan; Vitamin K Antagonists

Increased Effect/Toxicity
Tamoxifen may increase the levels/effects of: Colchicine; CYP2C8 Substrates (High risk); Dabigatran Etexilate; P-Glycoprotein Substrates; Rivaroxaban; Silodosin; Topotecan; Vitamin K Antagonists

The levels/effects of Tamoxifen may be increased by: CYP2C9 Inhibitors (Moderate); CYP2C9 Inhibitors (Strong); CYP2D6 Inhibitors (Moderate);

CYP2D6 Inhibitors (Strong); CYP3A4 Inhibitors (Moderate); CYP3A4 Inhibitors (Strong); Darunavir; Dasatinib

Decreased Effect

Tamoxifen may decrease the levels/effects of: Anastrozole; Letrozole

The levels/effects of Tamoxifen may be decreased by: Aminoglutethimide; CYP2C9 Inducers (Highly Effective); CYP3A4 Inducers (Strong); Deferasirox; Herbs (CYP3A4 Inducers); Peginterferon Alfa-2b; Rifamycin Derivatives

Ethanol/Nutrition/Herb Interactions

Food: Avoid grapefruit juice (may decrease the metabolism of tamoxifen).

Herb/Nutraceutical: Avoid black cohosh, dong quai in estrogen-dependent tumors. Avoid St John's wort (may decrease levels/effects of tamoxifen).

Storage/Stability Store at room temperature of 20°C to 25°C (68°F to 77°F). Protect from light.

Mechanism of Action Competitively binds to estrogen receptors on tumors and other tissue targets, producing a nuclear complex that decreases DNA synthesis and inhibits estrogen effects; nonsteroidal agent with potent antiestrogenic properties which compete with estrogen for binding sites in breast and other tissues; cells accumulate in the G_0 and G_1 phases; therefore, tamoxifen is cytostatic rather than cytocidal.

Pharmacodynamics/Kinetics

Absorption: Well absorbed

Distribution: High concentrations found in uterus, endometrial and breast tissue

Protein binding: 99%

Metabolism: Hepatic; via CYP2D6 to 4-hydroxytamoxifen and via CYP3A4/5 to N-desmethyl-tamoxifen. Each is then further metabolized into endoxifen (4-hydroxy-tamoxifen via CYP3A4/5 and N-desmethyl-tamoxifen via CYP2D6); both 4-hydroxy-tamoxifen and endoxifen are 30- to 100-fold more potent than tamoxifen

Half-life elimination: Tamoxifen: ~5-7 days; N-desmethyl tamoxifen: ~14 days

Time to peak, serum: ~5 hours

Excretion: Feces (26% to 51%); urine (9% to 13%)

Dosage Oral: **Note:** For the treatment of breast cancer, patients receiving both tamoxifen and chemotherapy, should receive treatment sequentially, with tamoxifen following completion of chemotherapy.

Children: Females: Precocious puberty and McCune-Albright syndrome (unlabeled use): A dose of 20 mg/day has been reported in patients 2-10 years of age; safety and efficacy have not been established for treatment of longer than 1 year duration

Adults:

Breast cancer treatment:

Adjuvant therapy (females): 20 mg once daily for 5 years

Metastatic (males and females): 20-40 mg/day; daily doses >20 mg should be given in 2 divided doses (morning and evening)

DCIS (females): 20 mg once daily for 5 years

Breast cancer risk reduction (pre- and postmenopausal high-risk females): 20 mg once daily for 5 years

Induction of ovulation (unlabeled use): 20 mg once daily (range: 20-80 mg once daily) for 5 days (Steiner, 2005)

Paget's disease of the breast (risk reduction; with DCIS or without associated cancer): 20 mg once daily for 5 years (NCCN Breast Cancer Guidelines, v.1.2009)

Dosage adjustment for DVT, pulmonary embolism, cerebrovascular accident, or prolonged immobilization: Discontinue tamoxifen (NCCN Breast Cancer Risk Reduction Guidelines, v.1.2009)

Combination Regimens

Breast cancer: Tamoxifen-Epirubicin on page 1405

Melanoma:

CCDT (Melanoma) on page 1253

Dartmouth Regimen on page 1286

Administration Administer orally once or twice daily with or without food. Doses >20 mg/day should be given in divided doses.

Monitoring Parameters CBC with platelets, serum calcium, LFTs; triglycerides and cholesterol (in patients with pre-existing hyperlipidemias); abnormal vaginal bleeding; breast and gynecologic exams (baseline and routine), mammogram (baseline and routine); signs/symptoms of DVT (leg swelling, tenderness) or PE (shortness of breath); ophthalmic exam (if vision problem or cataracts); bone mineral density (premenopausal women)

Test Interactions T_4 elevations (which may be explained by increases in thyroid-binding globulin) have been reported; not accompanied by clinical hyperthyroidism

Dietary Considerations May be taken with or without food. Avoid grapefruit and grapefruit juice.

Additional Information Oral clonidine is being studied for the treatment of tamoxifen-induced "hot flashes." The tumor flare reaction may indicate a good therapeutic response, and is often considered a good prognostic factor.

Estrogen receptor status may predict if adjuvant treatment with tamoxifen is of benefit. In metastatic breast cancer, patients with estrogen receptor positive tumors are more likely to benefit from tamoxifen treatment. With tamoxifen use to reduce the incidence of breast cancer in high risk-women, high risk is defined as women ≥35 years of age with a 5 year NCI Gail model predicted risk of breast cancer ≥1.67%.

Dosage Forms Excipient information presented when available (limited, particularly for generics); consult specific product labeling.

Tablet: 10 mg, 20 mg

References

Aubert RE, Stanek EJ, Yao J, et al, "Risk of Breast Cancer Recurrence in Women Initiating Tamoxifen With CYP2D6 Inhibitors," *J Clin Oncol*, 2009, 27(18S):CRA508 [abstract from 2009 ASCO Annual Meeting].

Dezentje V, Van Blijderveen NJ, Gelderblom H, et al, "Concomitant CYP2D6 Inhibitor Use and Tamoxifen Adherence in Early-Stage Breast Cancer: A Pharmacoepidemiologic Study," *J Clin Oncol*, 2009, 27(18S):CRA509 [abstract from 2009 ASCO Annual Meeting].

Early Breast Cancer Trialists' Collaborative Group (EBCTCG), "Effects of Chemotherapy and Hormonal Therapy for Early Breast Cancer on Recurrence and 15-Year Survival: An Overview of the Randomised Trials," *Lancet*, 2005, 365(9472):1687-717.

Eastell R, Adams JE, Coleman RE, et al, "Effect of Anastrozole on Bone Mineral Density: 5-Year Results From the Anastrozole, Tamoxifen, Alone or in Combination Trial 18233230," *J Clin Oncol*, 2008, 26(7):1051-7.

Goetz MP, Kamal A, and Ames MM, "Tamoxifen Pharmacogenomics: The Role of CYP2D6 as a Predictor of Drug Response," *Clin Pharmacol Ther*, 2008, 83(1):160-6.

Jin Y, Desta Z, Stearns V, et al, "CYP2D6 Genotype, Antidepressant Use, and Tamoxifen Metabolism During Adjuvant Breast Cancer Treatment," *J Natl Cancer Inst*, 2005, 97(1):30-9.

Khatcheressian JL, Wolff AC, Smith TJ, et al, "American Society of Clinical Oncology 2006 Update of the Breast Cancer Follow-Up and Management Guidelines in the Adjuvant Setting," *J Clin Oncol*, 2006, 24(31):5091-7.

LiVolsi VA, Salhany KE, and Dowdy YG, "Endocervical Adenocarcinoma in Tamoxifen-Treated Patient," *Am J Obstet Gynecol*, 1995, 172(3):1065.

National Comprehensive Cancer Network (NCCN)®, "Clinical Practice Guidelines in Oncology™: Breast Cancer," Version 1.2009. Available at http://www.nccn.org/professionals/physician_gls/PDF/breast.pdf.

National Comprehensive Cancer Network (NCCN)®, "Clinical Practice Guidelines in Oncology™: Breast Cancer Risk Reduction, Version 1.2009." Accessible at http://www.nccn.org/professionals/physician_gls/PDF/breast_risk.pdf

National Comprehensive Cancer Network (NCCN)®, "Clinical Practice Guidelines in Oncology™: Ovarian Cancer," Version 1.2009. Available at http://www.nccn.org/professionals/physician_gls/PDF/ovarian.pdf

National Comprehensive Cancer Network (NCCN)®, "Clinical Practice Guidelines in Oncology™: Uterine Neoplasms," Version 2.2009. Available at http://www.nccn.org/professionals/physician_gls/PDF/uterine.pdf

Rutqvist LE, Johansson H, Signomklao T, et al, "Adjuvant Tamoxifen Therapy for Early Stage Breast Cancer and Second Primary Malignancies. Stockholm Breast Cancer Study Group," *J Natl Cancer Inst*, 1995, 87(9):645-51.

Steiner AZ, Terplan M, and Paulson RJ, "Comparison of Tamoxifen and Clomifene Citrate for Ovulation Induction: A Meta-Analysis," *Hum Reprod*, 2005, 20(6):1511-5.

Thessaloniki ESHRE/ASRM-Sponsored PCOS Consensus Workshop Group, "Consensus on Infertility Treatment Related to Polycystic Ovary Syndrome," *Fertil Steril*, 2008, 89(3):505-22.

Vehmanen L, Elomaa I, Blomqvist C, et al, "Tamoxifen Treatment After Adjuvant Chemotherapy Has Opposite Effects on Bone Mineral Density in Premenopausal Patients Depending on Menstrual Status," *J Clin Oncol*, 2006, 24(4):675-80.

Visvanathan K, Chlebowski RT, Hurley P, et al, "American Society of Clinical Oncology Clinical Practice Guideline Update on the Use of Pharmacologic Interventions Including Tamoxifen, Raloxifene, and Aromatase Inhibition for Breast Cancer Risk Reduction," *J Clin Oncol*, 2009, 27 (19):3235-58.

Winer EP, Hudis C, Burstein HJ, et al, "American Society of Clinical Oncology Technology Assessment on the Use of Aromatase Inhibitors as Adjuvant Therapy for Postmenopausal Women With Hormone Receptor-Positive Breast Cancer: Status Report 2004," *J Clin Oncol*, 2005, 23(3):619-29.

Temozolomide (te moe ZOE loe mide)

Medication Safety Issues

Sound-alike/look-alike issues:

Temodar® may be confused with Tambocor®

◀ **High alert medication:** The Institute for Safe Medication Practices (ISMP) includes this medication among its list of drug classes which have a heightened risk of causing significant patient harm when used in error.

Related Information

Safe Handling of Hazardous Drugs *on page 1517*

U.S. Brand Names Temodar®

Index Terms TMZ

Generic Available No

Canadian Brand Names Temodal®

Pharmacologic Category Antineoplastic Agent, Alkylating Agent (Triazene)

Use Treatment of newly-diagnosed glioblastoma multiforme (initially in combination with radiotherapy, then as maintenance treatment); treatment of refractory anaplastic astrocytoma

Note: The following use is approved in Canada (not an approved indication in the U.S.): Treatment of recurrent glioblastoma multiforme

Unlabeled/Investigational Use Treatment of recurrent glioblastoma multiforme, advanced or metastatic melanoma, anaplastic oligodendroglioma, ependymoma, metastatic CNS lesions, cutaneous T-cell lymphomas (mycosis fungoides [MF] and Sézary syndrome [SS]), carcinoid tumors

Pregnancy Risk Factor D

Lactation Excretion in breast milk unknown/not recommended

Labeled Contraindications Hypersensitivity (eg, allergic reaction, anaphylaxis, urticaria, Stevens-Johnson syndrome, toxic epidermal necrolysis) to temozolomide or any component of the formulation; hypersensitivity to dacarbazine (both drugs are metabolized to MTIC)

Canadian labeling: Additional contraindications (not in U.S. labeling): Not recommended in patients with severe myelossuppression

Warnings/Precautions Hazardous agent - use appropriate precautions for handling and disposal. Pneumocystis *jiroveci* pneumonia (PCP) may occur; risk is increased in those receiving steroids or longer dosing regimens; PCP prophylaxis is required in patients receiving radiotherapy in combination with the 42-day temozolomide regimen. Myelosuppression may occur; an increased incidence has been reported in geriatric and female patients. Prolonged pancytopenia resulting in aplastic anemia has been reported; concurrent use of temozolomide with medications associated with aplastic anemia may obscure assessment for development of aplastic anemia (eg, carbamazepine, cotrimoxazole, phenytoin) may obscure assessment for development of aplastic anemia. Rare cases of myelodysplastic syndrome and secondary malignancies, including acute myeloid leukemia have been reported. Use caution in patients with severe hepatic or renal impairment; has not been studied in dialysis patients.

Increased MGMT (O-6-methylguanine-DNA methyltransferase) activity/levels within tumor tissue is associated with temozolomide resistance. Glioblastoma patients with decreased levels (due to methylated MGMT promoter) may be more likely to benefit from the combination of radiation therapy and temozolomide (Hegi, 2008; Stupp, 2009). Determination of MGMT status may be predictive for response to alkylating agents.

Adverse Reactions Note: With CNS malignancies, it may be difficult to distinguish between CNS adverse events caused by temozolomide versus the effects of progressive disease.

>10%:

Cardiovascular: Peripheral edema (11%)

Central nervous system: Fatigue (34% to 61%), headache (23% to 41%), seizure (6% to 23%), hemiparesis (18%), fever (13%), dizziness (5% to 12%), coordination abnormality (11%)

Dermatologic: Alopecia (55%), rash (8% to 13%)

Gastrointestinal: Nausea (49% to 53%; grades 3/4: 1% to 10%), vomiting (29% to 42%; grades 3/4: 2% to 6%), constipation (22% to 33%), anorexia (9% to 27%), diarrhea (10% to 16%)

Hematologic: Lymphopenia (grades 3/4: 55%), thrombocytopenia (grades 3/4: adults: 4% to 19%; children: 25%), neutropenia (grades 3/4: adults: 8% to 14%; children: 20%), leukopenia (grades 3/4: 11%)

Neuromuscular & skeletal: Weakness (7% to 13%)

Miscellaneous: Viral infection (11%)

1% to 10%:

Central nervous system: Amnesia (10%), insomnia (4% to 10%), somnolence (9%), ataxia (8%), paresis (8%), anxiety (7%), memory impairment (7%), depression (6%), confusion (5%)

Dermatologic: Pruritus (5% to 8%), dry skin (5%), radiation injury (2% maintenance phase after radiotherapy), erythema (1%)

Endocrine & metabolic: Hypercorticism (8%), breast pain (females 6%)

Gastrointestinal: Stomatitis (9%), abdominal pain (5% to 9%), dysphagia (7%), taste perversion (5%), weight gain (5%)

Genitourinary: Incontinence (8%), urinary tract infection (8%), urinary frequency (6%)

Hematologic: Anemia (grades 3/4: 4%)

Neuromuscular & skeletal: Paresthesia (9%), back pain (8%), abnormal gait (6%), arthralgia (6%), myalgia (5%)

Ocular: Blurred vision (5% to 8%), diplopia (5%), vision abnormality (visual deficit/vision changes 5%)

Respiratory: Pharyngitis (8%), upper respiratory tract infection (8%), cough (5% to 8%), sinusitis (6%), dyspnea (5%)

Miscellaneous: Allergic reaction (≤3%)

<1%, postmarketing, and/or case reports (limited to important or life-threatening): Agitation, alkaline phosphatase increased, anaphylaxis, apathy, aplastic anemia, emotional lability, erythema multiforme, febrile neutropenia, flu-like syndrome, hallucination, hematoma, hemorrhage, herpes simplex, herpes zoster, hyperglycemia, hypokalemia, injection site reactions (erythema, irritation, pain, pruritus, swelling, warmth), interstitial pneumonitis, myelodysplastic syndrome, neuropathy, opportunistic infection (eg, PCP), oral candidiasis, pancytopenia (may be prolonged), peripheral neuropathy, petechiae, pneumonitis, secondary malignancies (including myeloid leukemia), Stevens-Johnson syndrome, toxic epidermal necrolysis, weight loss

Drug Interactions

Avoid Concomitant Use

Avoid concomitant use of Temozolomide with any of the following: Natalizumab; Vaccines (Live)

Increased Effect/Toxicity

Temozolomide may increase the levels/effects of: Leflunomide; Natalizumab; Vaccines (Live)

The levels/effects of Temozolomide may be increased by: Trastuzumab; Valproic Acid

Decreased Effect

Temozolomide may decrease the levels/effects of: Vaccines (Inactivated); Vaccines (Live)

The levels/effects of Temozolomide may be decreased by: Echinacea

◄ **Ethanol/Nutrition/Herb Interactions** Food: Food reduces rate and extent of absorption.

Storage/Stability

Injection: Store intact vials refrigerated at 2°C to 8°C (36°F to 46°F). Reconstituted vials may be stored for up to 14 hours at room temperature of 25°C (77°F); infusion must be completed within 14 hours of reconstitution. Capsule: Store at room temperature of 25°C (77°F); excursions permitted to 15°C to 30°C (59°F to 86°F).

Reconstitution

Bring to room temperature prior to reconstitution. Reconstitute each 100 mg vial with 41 mL sterile water for injection to a final concentration of 2.5 mg/mL. Swirl gently; do not shake. Place dose without further dilution into a 250 mL empty sterile PVC infusion bag. Infusion must be completed within 14 hours of reconstitution. Use appropriate precautions for handling and disposal.

Mechanism of Action Like dacarbazine, temozolomide (a prodrug) is rapidly and nonenzymatically converted to the active alkylating metabolite MTIC [(methyl-triazene-1-yl)-imidazole-4-carboxamide]. Unlike dacarbazine, however, this conversion is spontaneous, nonenzymatic, and occurs under physiologic conditions in all tissues to which the drug distributes. The cytotoxic effects of MTIC are manifested through alkylation of DNA at the O^6, N^7 guanine positions.

Pharmacodynamics/Kinetics

Absorption: Oral: Rapid and complete

Distribution: V_d: Parent drug: 0.4 L/kg; penetrates blood brain barrier; CSF levels are ~35% to 39% of plasma levels

Protein binding: 15%

Metabolism: Prodrug, hydrolyzed to the active form, MTIC; MTIC is eventually eliminated as CO_2 and 5-aminoimidazole-4-carboxamide (AIC), a natural constituent in urine; CYP isoenzymes play only a minor role in metabolism (of temozolomide and MTIC)

Bioavailability: Oral: 100% (on a mg-per-mg basis, I.V. temozolomide, infused over 90 minutes, is bioequivalent to an oral dose)

Half-life elimination: Mean: Parent drug: 1.8 hours

Time to peak: Oral: Empty stomach: 1 hour; with food (high-fat meal): 2.25 hours

Excretion: Urine (~38%; parent drug 6%); feces <1%

Dosage Oral, I.V.: Adults:

Anaplastic astrocytoma (refractory): Initial dose: 150 mg/m^2/day for 5 days; repeat every 28 days. Subsequent doses of 100-200 mg/m^2/day for 5 days per treatment cycle; based upon hematologic tolerance.

Dosage modification for toxicity:

ANC <1000/mm^3 or platelets <50,000/mm^3 on day 22 or day 29 (day 1 of next cycle): Postpone therapy until ANC >1500/mm^3 and platelets >100,000/mm^3; reduce dose by 50 mg/m^2/day for subsequent cycle

ANC 1000-1500/mm^3 or platelets 50,000-100,000/mm^3 on day 22 or day 29 (day 1 of next cycle): Postpone therapy until ANC >1500/mm^3 and platelets >100,000/mm^3; maintain initial dose

ANC >1500/mm^3 and platelets >100,000/mm^3 on day 22 or day 29 (day 1 of next cycle): Increase dose to or maintain dose at 200 mg/m^2/day for 5 days for subsequent cycle

Glioblastoma multiforme (newly diagnosed, high-grade glioma):

Concomitant phase: 75 mg/m^2/day for 42 days with focal radiotherapy (60Gy administered in 30 fractions). **Note:** PCP prophylaxis is required during concomitant phase and should continue in patients who develop lymphocytopenia until lymphocyte recovery to ≤ grade 1. Obtain weekly CBC.

ANC ≥1500/mm^3, platelet count ≥100,000/mm^3, and nonhematologic toxicity ≤ grade 1 (excludes alopecia, nausea/vomiting): Temodar® 75 mg/m^2/day may be continued throughout the 42-day concomitant period up to 49 days

Dosage modification for toxicity:

ANC ≥500/mm^3 but <1500/mm^3 **or** platelet count ≥10,000/mm^3 but <100,000/mm^3 **or** grade 2 nonhematologic toxicity (excludes alopecia, nausea/vomiting): Interrupt therapy

ANC <500/mm^3 **or** platelet count <10,000/mm^3 **or** grade 3/4 non-hematologic toxicity (excludes alopecia, nausea/vomiting): Discontinue therapy

Maintenance phase (consists of 6 treatment cycles): Begin 4 weeks after concomitant phase completion. **Note:** Each subsequent cycle is 28 days (consisting of 5 days of drug treatment followed by 23 days without treatment). Draw CBC within 48 hours of day 22; hold next cycle and do weekly CBC until ANC >1500/mm^3 and platelet count >100,000/mm^3; dosing modification should be based on lowest blood counts and worst non-hematologic toxicity during the previous cycle.

Cycle 1: 150 mg/m^2/day for 5 days; repeat every 28 days

Cycles 2-6: May increase to 200 mg/m^2/day for 5 days every 28 days (if ANC >1500/mm^3, platelets >100,000/mm^3 and nonhematologic toxicities for cycle 1 are ≤ grade 2; if dose was not escalated at the onset of cycle 2, do not increase for cycles 3-6)

Dosage modification (during maintenance phase) for toxicity:

ANC <1000/mm^3, platelet count <50,000/mm^3, or grade 3 nonhematologic toxicity (excludes alopecia, nausea/vomiting) during previous cycle: Decrease dose by 1 dose level (by 50 mg/m^2/day for 5 days), unless dose has already been lowered to 100 mg/m^2/day, then discontinue therapy.

If dose reduction <100 mg/m^2/day is required or grade 4 nonhematologic toxicity (excludes alopecia, nausea/vomiting), or if the same grade 3 nonhematologic toxicity occurs after dose reduction: Discontinue therapy

Glioblastoma multiforme (recurrent glioma): *Canadian labeling (not an approved use in the U.S.):* 200 mg/m^2/day for 5 days every 28 days; if previously treated with chemotherapy, initiate at 150 mg/m^2/day for 5 days every 28 days and increase to 200 mg/m^2/day for 5 days every 28 days with cycle 2 if no hematologic toxicity

Metastatic melanoma (unlabeled use): Oral: 200 mg/m^2/day for 5 days every 28 days (for up to 12 cycles). For subsequent cycles reduce dose to 75% of the original dose for grade 3/4 hematologic toxicity and reduce the dose to 50% of the original dose for grade 3/4 nonhematologic toxicity (Middletown, 2000).

Elderly: Refer to adult dosing. **Note:** Patients ≥70 years of age had a higher incidence of grade 4 neutropenia and thrombocytopenia in the first cycle of therapy than patients <70 years of age.

Dosage adjustment in renal impairment: Oral:

Cl$_{cr}$ ≥36 mL/minute: No effect on temozolomide clearance was demonstrated

Severe renal impairment (Cl$_{cr}$ <36 mL/minute): Use with caution

Dialysis patients: Use has not been studied

Dosage adjustment in hepatic impairment: Severe hepatic impairment: Use with caution

◀ **Administration** Standard antiemetics may be administered if needed.

Oral: Swallow capsules whole with a glass of water. Absorption is affected by food. Administer consistently either with food or without food (was administered in studies under fasting and non-fasting conditions). May administer on an empty stomach or at bedtime to reduce nausea and vomiting. Do not repeat if vomiting occurs after dose is administered, wait until the next scheduled dose. Do not open or chew capsules; avoid contact with skin if capsules are accidentally opened or damaged.

I.V.: Infuse over 90 minutes. Flush line before and after administration. Do not administer other medications through the same I.V. line.

Monitoring Parameters CBC with differential and platelets (prior to each cycle; weekly during glioma concomitant phase treatment; at or within 48 hours of day 22 and weekly until ANC >1500/mm^3 for glioma maintenance and astrocytoma treatment)

Dietary Considerations The incidence of nausea/vomiting is decreased when the drug is taken on an empty stomach. Take capsules consistently either with food or without food (absorption is affected by food).

Emetic Potential Moderate (30% to 90%)

Dosage Forms Excipient information presented when available (limited, particularly for generics); consult specific product labeling.

Capsule:

Temodar®: 5 mg, 20 mg, 100 mg, 140 mg, 180 mg, 250 mg

Injection, powder for reconstitution:

Temodar®: 100 mg [contains polysorbate 80]

Extemporaneous Preparations Temozolomide 10 mg/mL oral suspension: In a glass mortar, mix the contents of ten 100-mg capsules and 500 mg of povidine K-30 powder; add 25 mg anhydrous citric acid dissolved in 1.5 mL purified water; mix to form a paste; add 50 mL Ora-Plus® (add a small amount at first, mix, add balance); mix; transfer to amber plastic bottle; add enough Ora-Sweet® or Ora-Sweet® SF to bring a total volume of 100 mL by rinsing the mortar with small amounts of Ora-Sweet®; repeat rinsing 3 more times. The suspension is stable for 7 days at room temperature or 60 days refrigerated in plastic amber prescription bottles. **Note:** Use appropriate handling precautions during preparation.

Trissel LA, Yanping Z, and Koontz SE. "Temozolomide Stability in Extemporaneously Compounded Oral Suspension," *Int J Pharm Compounding*, 2006, 10(5):396-9.

References

Agarwala SS, Kirkwood JM, Gore M, et al, " Temozolomide for the Treatment of Brain metastases Associated With Metastatic Melanoma: A Phase II Study," *J Clin Oncol*, 2004, 22(11):2101-7.

Hegi ME, Diserens AC, Gorlia T, et al, "MGMT Gene Silencing and Benefit From Temozolomide in Glioblastoma," *N Engl J Med*, 2005, 352(10):997-1003.

Hegi ME, Liu L, Herman JG, et al, "Correlation of O6-Methylguanine Methyltransferase (MGMT) Promoter Methylation With Clinical Outcomes in Glioblastoma and Clinical Strategies to Modulate MGMT Activity," *J Clin Oncol*, 2008, 26(25):4189-99.

Middleton MR, Grob JJ, Aaronson N, et al, "Randomized Phase III Study of Temozolomide Versus Dacarbazine in the Treatment of Patients With Advanced Metastatic Malignant Melanoma," *J Clin Oncol*, 2000, 18(1):158-66.

National Comprehensive Cancer Network® (NCCN), "Clinical Practice Guidelines in Oncology™: Central Nervous System Cancers," Version 1.2009. Available at http://www.nccn.org/profession als/physician_gls/PDF/cns.pdf

National Comprehensive Cancer Network® (NCCN), "Clinical Practice Guidelines in Oncology™: Non-Hodgkin's Lymphomas," Version 1.2009. Available at http://www.nccn.org/professionals/ physician_gls/PDF/nhl.pdf

Stupp R, Dietrich PY, Ostermann Kraljevic S, et al, "Promising Survival for Patients With Newly Diagnosed Glioblastoma Multiforme Treated With Concomitant Radiation Plus Temozolomide Followed by Adjuvant Temozolomide," *J Clin Oncol*, 2002, 20(5):1375-82.

Stupp R, Gander M, Leyvraz S, et al, "Current and Future Developments in the Use of Temozolomide for the Treatment of Brain Tumours," *Lancet Oncol*, 2001, 2(9):552-60.

Stupp R, Hegi ME, Mason WP, et al, "Effects of Radiotherapy With Concomitant and Adjuvant Temozolomide Versus Radiotherapy Alone on Survival in Glioblastoma in a Randomised Phase III Study: 5-year Analysis of the EORTC-NCIC Trial," *Lancet Oncol*, 2009 [epub ahead of print]

Stupp R, Mason WP, van den Bent MJ, et al, "Radiotherapy Plus Concomitant and Adjuvant Temozolomide for Glioblastoma," *N Engl J Med*, 2005, 352(10):987-96.

Villano JL, Collins CA, Manasanch EE, et al, "Aplastic Anaemia in Patient With Glioblastoma Multiforme Treated With Temozolomide," *Lancet Oncol*, 2006, 7(5):436-8.

Yung WK, Prados MD, Yaya-Tur R, et al, "Multicenter Phase II Trial of Temozolomide in Patients With Anaplastic Astrocytoma or Anaplastic Oligoastrocytoma at First Relapse," *J Clin Oncol*, 1999, 17(9):2762-71.

Temsirolimus (tem sir OH li mus)

Medication Safety Issues

Sound-alike/look-alike issues:

Temsirolimus may be confused with everolimus, sirolimus, tacrolimus

High alert medication: The Institute for Safe Medication Practices (ISMP) includes this medication among its list of drug classes which have a heightened risk of causing significant patient harm when used in error.

Temsirolimus, for the treatment of advanced renal cell cancer, is a flat dose (25 mg) and is not based on body surface area (BSA).

Related Information

Management of Chemotherapy-Induced Nausea and Vomiting *on page 1434*

Safe Handling of Hazardous Drugs *on page 1517*

U.S. Brand Names Torisel®

Index Terms CCI-779; NSC-683864

Generic Available No

Canadian Brand Names Torisel®

Pharmacologic Category Antineoplastic Agent, mTOR Kinase Inhibitor

Use Treatment of advanced renal cell cancer (RCC)

Pregnancy Risk Factor D

Lactation Excretion in breast milk unknown/not recommended

Labeled Contraindications There are no contraindications listed within the FDA-approved manufacturer's labeling.

Canadian labeling: Additional contraindications (not in U.S. labeling): History of anaphylaxis after exposure to temsirolimus, sirolimus, or any component of the formulation

Warnings/Precautions Hazardous agent - use appropriate precautions for handling and disposal.

Hypersensitivity/infusion reactions (eg, anaphylaxis, apnea, dyspnea, flushing, loss of consciousness, hypotension, and/or chest pain) have been reported. Infusion reaction may occur with initial or subsequent infusions. Premedicate with an antihistamine (H$_1$ antagonist) prior to infusion; monitor during infusion; interrupt infusion for severe reaction. With discretion, treatment may be resumed at a slower infusion rate; administer an H$_1$ antagonist (if not given as premedication) and/or an H$_2$ antagonist 30 minutes prior to resuming infusion. Use with caution in patients with hypersensitivity to polysorbate 80. Angioneurotic edema has been reported; concurrent use with other drugs known to cause angioedema (eg, ACE inhibitors) may increase risk.

Use with caution in patients taking strong CYP3A4 inhibitors and moderate or strong CYP3A4 inducers (see Drug Interactions); consider alternative agents that avoid or lessen the potential for CYP-mediated interactions. Patients should not be immunized with live, viral vaccines during or shortly after treatment and should avoid close contact with recently vaccinated (live vaccine) individuals. Patients who are receiving anticoagulant therapy or those with CNS tumors/metastases may be at increased risk for developing intracerebral bleeding.

Increases in serum glucose are common; may alter insulin and/or oral hypoglycemic therapy requirements in patients with diabetes; monitor. Serum cholesterol and triglyceride elevations are also common; may require initiation or dose increases of antihyperlipidemic agents. Treatment may result in immunosuppression, may increase risk of opportunistic infections and/or sepsis. Interstitial lung disease (ILD), sometimes fatal, has been reported; symptoms include dyspnea, cough, hypoxia, and/or fever, although asymptomatic cases may present; promptly evaluate worsening respiratory symptoms. Cases of bowel perforation (fatal) have occurred; promptly evaluate any new or worsening abdominal pain or bloody stools. Temsirolimus may be associated with impaired wound healing; use caution in the perioperative period. Cases of acute renal failure with rapid progression have been reported, including cases unresponsive to dialysis.

Has not been studied in patients with hepatic impairment; use caution; temsirolimus is predominantly cleared by the liver. Safety and efficacy in children have not been established.

Adverse Reactions

>10%:
Cardiovascular: Edema (35%), peripheral edema (27%), chest pain (16%)
Central nervous system: Pain (28%), fever (24%), headache (15%), insomnia (12%)
Dermatologic: Rash (47%), pruritus (19%), nail disorder/thinning (14%), dry skin (11%)
Endocrine & metabolic: Hyperglycemia (26% to 89%; grades 3/4: 16%), hypercholesterolemia (24% to 87%; grades 3/4: 2%), hyperlipidemia (27% to 83%; grades 3/4: 44%), hypophosphatemia (49%; grades 3/4: 18%), hypokalemia (21%; grades 3/4: 5%)
Gastrointestinal: Mucositis (41%), nausea (37%), anorexia (32%), diarrhea (27%), abdominal pain (21%), constipation (20%), stomatitis (20%), taste disturbance (20%), vomiting (19%), weight loss (19%)
Genitourinary: Urinary tract infection (15%)
Hematologic: Anemia (45% to 94%; grades 3/4: 20%), lymphopenia (53%; grades 3/4: 16%), thrombocytopenia (14% to 40%; grades 3/4: 1%; dose-limiting toxicity), leukopenia (6% to 32%; grades 3/4: 1%), neutropenia (7% to 19%; grades 3/4: 3% to 5%)
Hepatic: Alkaline phosphatase increased (68%; grades 3/4: 3%), AST increased (8% to 38%; grades 3/4: 1% to 2%)
Neuromuscular & skeletal: Weakness (51%), back pain (20%), arthralgia (18%)
Renal: Creatinine increased (14% to 57%; grades 3/4: 3%)
Respiratory: Dyspnea (28%), cough (26%), epistaxis (12%), pharyngitis (12%)
Miscellaneous: Infection (20% to 27%; includes abscess, bronchitis, cellulitis, herpes simplex, herpes zoster)
1% to 10%:
Cardiovascular: Hypertension (7%), venous thromboembolism (2%, includes DVT and PE), thrombophlebitis (1%)
Central nervous system: Chills (8%), depression (4%)
Dermatologic: Acne (10%), wound healing impaired (1%)

Gastrointestinal: Bowel perforation (fatal: 1%)

Hepatic: Hyperbilirubinemia (8%)

Neuromuscular & skeletal: Myalgia (8%)

Ocular: Conjunctivitis (7%)

Respiratory: Rhinitis (10%), pneumonia (8%), upper respiratory tract infection (7%), interstitial lung disease (2%)

Miscellaneous: Allergic/hypersensitivity/infusion reaction (9%; includes anaphylaxis, apnea, chest pain, dyspnea, flushing, hypotension, loss of consciousness)

<1%, postmarketing, and/or case reports: Acute renal failure, angioneurotic edema, pneumonitis

Drug Interactions

Metabolism/Transport Effects Substrate of CYP3A4 (major); **Inhibits** CYP3A4 (weak), 2D6 (weak)

Avoid Concomitant Use

Avoid concomitant use of Temsirolimus with any of the following: Natalizumab; Vaccines (Live)

Increased Effect/Toxicity

Temsirolimus may increase the levels/effects of: ACE Inhibitors; Cyclo-SPORINE; Hypoglycemic Agents; Leflunomide; Natalizumab; Tacrolimus; Vaccines (Live)

The levels/effects of Temsirolimus may be increased by: Antifungal Agents (Azole Derivatives, Systemic); CYP3A4 Inhibitors (Moderate); CYP3A4 Inhibitors (Strong); Dasatinib; Herbs (Hypoglycemic Properties); Macrolide Antibiotics; P-Glycoprotein Inhibitors; Protease Inhibitors; Trastuzumab

Decreased Effect

Temsirolimus may decrease the levels/effects of: Vaccines (Inactivated); Vaccines (Live)

The levels/effects of Temsirolimus may be decreased by: CarBAMazepine; CYP3A4 Inducers (Strong); Deferasirox; Echinacea; Herbs (CYP3A4 Inducers); P-Glycoprotein Inducers; Phenytoin; Rifamycin Derivatives

Ethanol/Nutrition/Herb Interactions Herb/Nutraceutical: St John's wort may decrease sirolimus (the active metabolite of temsirolimus) levels; avoid concurrent use. Herbs with hypoglycemic properties may increase the risk of temsirolimus-induced hypoglycemia; includes alfalfa, aloe, bilberry, bitter melon, burdock, celery, damiana, fenugreek, garcinia, garlic, ginger, ginseng (American), gymnema, marshmallow, stinging nettle. Avoid grapefruit and grapefruit juice (may increase the levels/effects of sirolimus).

Storage/Stability Store intact vials under refrigeration at 2°C to 8°C (36°F to 46°F). Diluted solution in the vial (10 mg/mL) is stable for 24 hours at room temperature. Solutions diluted for infusion (in normal saline) must be infused within 6 hours of preparation. Protect from light during storage, preparation, and handling.

Reconstitution Vials should be diluted with 1.8 mL of provided diluent to a concentration of 10 mg/mL (vial contains overfill). Mix by inverting vial. After allowing air bubbles to subside, further dilute in 250 mL of NS in a non-DEHP/non-PVC container (glass, polyolefin or polypropylene). Avoid excessive shaking (may result in foaming). Use appropriate precautions for handling and disposal.

Compatibility Compatible with normal saline; do not mix with other solutions or medications. Temsirolimus is degraded by acids and bases.

Mechanism of Action Temsirolimus and its active metabolite, sirolimus, are targeted inhibitors of mTOR (mammalian target of rapamycin) kinase activity. ▶

Temsirolimus (and sirolimus) bind to FKBP-12, an intracellular protein, to form a complex which inhibits mTOR signaling, halting the cell cycle at the G1 phase in tumor cells. In renal cell carcinoma, mTOR inhibition also exhibits anti-angiogenesis activity by reducing levels of HIF-1 and HIF-2 alpha (hypoxia inducible factors) and vascular endothelial growth factor (VEGF).

Pharmacodynamics/Kinetics

Distribution: V_{dss}: 172 L

Metabolism: Hepatic; via CYP3A4 to sirolimus (primary active metabolite) and 4 minor metabolites

Half-life elimination: Temsirolimus: ~17 hours; Sirolimus: ~55 hours

Time to peak, plasma: Temsirolimus: At end of infusion; Sirolimus: 0.5-2 hours after temsirolimus infusion

Excretion: Feces (78%); urine (<5%)

Dosage Note: For infusion reaction prophylaxis, premedicate with an H_1 antagonist (eg, diphenhydramine 25-50 mg I.V.) 30 minutes prior to infusion.

I.V.: Adults: RCC: 25 mg weekly

Dosage adjustment for concomitant CYP3A4 inhibitors/inducers:

CYP3A4 inhibitors: Dose reductions are likely to be needed when temsirolimus is administered concomitantly with a strong CYP3A4 inhibitor (an alternate medication for CYP3A4 enzyme inhibitors should be investigated first); in the event that temsirolimus must be administered concomitantly with a potent enzyme inhibitor, consider reducing temsirolimus to 12.5 mg/week with careful monitoring. (When a strong CYP3A4 inhibitor is discontinued; allow ~1 week to elapse prior to adjusting the temsirolimus upward to the dose used prior to initiation of the CYP3A4 inhibitor.)

CYP3A4 inducers: Concomitant administration with CYP3A4 inducers may require increased temsirolimus doses (alternatives to the enzyme-inducing agent should be utilized first); consider adjusting temsirolimus dose to 50 mg/week, with careful monitoring. (If the strong CYP3A4 enzyme inducer is discontinued, reduce the temsirolimus to the dose used prior to initiation of the CYP3A4 inducer.)

Dosage adjustment for toxicity:

Hematologic toxicity: ANC <1000/mm^3 or platelets <75,000/mm^3: Withhold treatment until resolves and reinitiate treatment with a 5 mg/week dose reduction; minimum dose: 15 mg/week if adjustment for toxicity is needed.

Nonhematologic toxicity: Any toxicity ≥grade 3: Withhold treatment until resolves to ≤grade 2; reinitiate treatment with a 5 mg/week dose reduction; minimum dose: 15 mg/week if adjustment for toxicity is needed.

Dosage adjustment in renal impairment: Not studied in renal dysfunction; however, due to the minimal renal elimination (<5%), dosage adjustment for renal dysfunction is not recommended.

Hemodialysis: Has not been studied in hemodialysis patients.

Dosage adjustment in hepatic impairment (DOH) The FDA-approved labeling does not contain hepatic dosing adjustment guidelines. Patients with AST >3 times ULN (>5 times ULN in the presence of liver metastases) and total bilirubin >1.5 times ULN were excluded from clinical trials. Temsirolimus is primarily cleared hepatically.

Administration Infuse over 30-60 minute via an infusion pump (preferred). Use non-DEHP containing administration tubing. Administer through an inline polyethersulfone filter ≤5 micron. Premedicate with an H_1 antagonist (eg, diphenhydramine 25-50 mg I.V.) 30 minutes prior to infusion. Monitor during infusion; interrupt infusion for hypersensitivity/infusion reaction; monitor for

30-60 minutes; may reinitiate at a reduced infusion rate (over 60 minutes) with discretion, 30 minutes after administration of a histamine H_1 antagonist and/or a histamine H_2 antagonist (eg, famotidine or ranitidine).

Monitoring Parameters CBC with differential and platelets (weekly), serum chemistries including glucose (baseline and every other week), serum cholesterol and triglycerides (baseline and periodic), liver and renal function tests

Monitor for infusion reactions; infection; symptoms of ILD (or radiographic changes)

Emetic Potential Very low (<10%)

Dosage Forms Excipient information presented when available (limited, particularly for generics); consult specific product labeling.

Injection, solution [concentrate]:

Torisel®: 25 mg/mL [contains dehydrated ethanol, propylene glycol; diluent contains dehydrated ethanol, polyethylene glycol, polysorbate 80]

References

Atkins MB, Hidalgo M, Stadler WM, et al, "Randomized Phase II Study of Multiple Dose Levels of CCI-779, a Novel Mammalian Target of Rapamycin Kinase Inhibitor, in Patients With Advanced Refractory Renal Cell Carcinoma," *J Clin Oncol*, 2004, 22(5): 909-18.

Bellmunt J, Szczylik C, Feingold J, et al, "Temsirolimus Safety Profile and Management of Toxic Effects in Patients With Advanced Renal Cell Carcinoma and Poor Prognostic Features," *Ann Oncol*, 2008, 19(8):1387-92.

Hidalgo M, Buckner JC, Erlichman C, et al, "A Phase I and Pharmacokinetics Study of Temsirolimus (CCI-779) Administered Intravenously Daily for 5 Days Every 2 Weeks to Patients With Advanced Cancer," *Clin Cancer Res*, 2006, 12(19):5755-63.

Hudes G, Carducci M, Tomczak P, et al, "Temsirolimus, Interferon Alfa, or Both for Advanced Renal-Cell Carcinoma," *N Engl J Med*, 2007, 356(22):2271-81.

Raymond E, Alexandre J, Faivre S, et al, "Safety and Pharmacokinetics of Escalated Doses of Weekly Intravenous Infusion of CCI-779, a Novel mTOR Inhibitor, in Patients With Cancer," *J Clin Oncol*, 2004, 22(12): 2336-47.

Witzig TE, Geyer SM, Ghobrial I, et al, "Phase II Trial of Single-Agent Temsirolimus (CCI-779) for Relapsed Mantle Cell Lymphoma," *J Clin Oncol*, 2005, 23(23):5347-56.

Teniposide (ten i POE side)

Medication Safety Issues

Sound-alike/look-alike issues:

Teniposide may be confused with etoposide

High alert medication: The Institute for Safe Medication Practices (ISMP) includes this medication among its list of drugs which have a heightened risk of causing significant patient harm when used in error.

Related Information

Management of Drug Extravasations *on page 1447*
Safe Handling of Hazardous Drugs *on page 1517*

U.S. Brand Names Vumon®

Index Terms EPT; VM-26

Generic Available No

Canadian Brand Names Vumon®

Pharmacologic Category Antineoplastic Agent, Miscellaneous

Use Treatment of acute lymphocytic leukemia (ALL)

Pregnancy Risk Factor D

Lactation Not recommended

Labeled Contraindications Hypersensitivity to teniposide, Cremophor® EL (polyoxyethylated castor oil), or any component of the formulation; pregnancy

Warnings/Precautions Hazardous agent - use appropriate precautions for handling and disposal. **[U.S. Boxed Warning]: Severe myelosuppression**

may occur; monitor for infection and bleeding. **[U.S. Boxed Warning]: Hypersensitivity reactions, including anaphylaxis-like reactions, have been reported;** monitor during infusion; immediate treatment for anaphylactic reaction should be available during administration. Teniposide injection contains benzyl alcohol and should be avoided in neonates. The injection contains about 43% alcohol. For I.V. use only; may cause local tissue necrosis or thrombophlebitis if extravasation occurs. **[U.S. Boxed Warning]: Should be administered under the supervision of an experienced cancer chemotherapy physician.**

Adverse Reactions

>10%:
  Gastrointestinal: Mucositis (75%); diarrhea, nausea, vomiting (20% to 30%); anorexia
  Hematologic: Myelosuppression, leukopenia, neutropenia (95%), thrombocytopenia (65% to 80%), anemia
  Onset: 5-7 days
  Nadir: 7-10 days
  Recovery: 21-28 days
1% to 10%:
  Cardiovascular: Hypotension (2%), associated with rapid (<30 minutes) infusions
  Dermatologic: Alopecia (9%), rash (3%)
  Miscellaneous: Anaphylactoid reactions (5%; fever, rash, hyper-/hypotension, dyspnea, bronchospasm), usually seen with rapid (<30 minutes) infusions
<1%: Lethargy, peripheral neuropathy, somnolence

Drug Interactions

Metabolism/Transport Effects Substrate of CYP3A4 (major); **Inhibits** CYP2C9 (weak), 3A4 (weak)

Avoid Concomitant Use
  Avoid concomitant use of Teniposide with any of the following: Natalizumab; Vaccines (Live)

Increased Effect/Toxicity
  Teniposide may increase the levels/effects of: Leflunomide; Natalizumab; Vaccines (Live)

  The levels/effects of Teniposide may be increased by: CYP3A4 Inhibitors (Moderate); CYP3A4 Inhibitors (Strong); Dasatinib; P-Glycoprotein Inhibitors; Trastuzumab

Decreased Effect
  Teniposide may decrease the levels/effects of: Vaccines (Inactivated); Vaccines (Live)

  The levels/effects of Teniposide may be decreased by: Barbiturates; CYP3A4 Inducers (Strong); Deferasirox; Echinacea; Herbs (CYP3A4 Inducers); P-Glycoprotein Inducers; Phenytoin

Ethanol/Nutrition/Herb Interactions Herb/Nutraceutical: St John's wort may decrease teniposide levels.

Storage/Stability Store ampuls in refrigerator at 2°C to 8°C (36°F to 46°F). Reconstituted solutions are stable at room temperature for up to 24 hours after preparation.

Reconstitution Teniposide must be diluted with either D_5W or 0.9% sodium chloride solutions to a final concentration of 0.1, 0.2, 0.4, or 1 mg/mL. However, precipitation may occur at any concentration. **Solutions should be prepared in non-DEHP-containing containers such as glass or polyolefin containers.** The use of polyvinyl chloride (PVC) containers is not recommended. Administer 1 mg/mL solutions within 4 hours of preparation to reduce the potential for precipitation.

Compatibility Stable in D_5W, LR, NS.

Y-site administration: Compatible: Acyclovir, allopurinol, amifostine, amikacin, aminophylline, amphotericin B, ampicillin, ampicillin/sulbactam, aztreonam, bleomycin, bumetanide, buprenorphine, butorphanol, calcium gluconate, carboplatin, carmustine, cefazolin, cefoperazone, cefotaxime, cefotetan, cefoxitin, ceftazidime, ceftizoxime, ceftriaxone, cefuroxime, chlorpromazine, cimetidine, ciprofloxacin, cisplatin, cladribine, clindamycin, co-trimoxazole, cyclophosphamide, cytarabine, dacarbazine, dactinomycin, daunorubicin, dexamethasone sodium phosphate, diphenhydramine, doxorubicin, doxycycline, droperidol, enalaprilat, etoposide, etoposide phosphate, famotidine, floxuridine, fluconazole, fludarabine, fluorouracil, furosemide, ganciclovir, gemcitabine, gentamicin, granisetron, haloperidol, hydrocortisone sodium phosphate, hydrocortisone sodium succinate, hydromorphone, hydroxyzine, ifosfamide, imipenem/cilastatin, leucovorin, lorazepam, mannitol, mechlorethamine, melphalan, meperidine, mesna, methotrexate, methylprednisolone sodium succinate, metoclopramide, metronidazole, minocycline, mitomycin, mitoxantrone, morphine, nalbuphine, netilmicin, ondansetron, piperacillin, plicamycin, potassium chloride, prochlorperazine edisylate, promethazine, ranitidine, sargramostim, sodium bicarbonate, streptozocin, thiotepa, ticarcillin, ticarcillin/clavulanate, tobramycin, vancomycin, vinblastine, vincristine, vinorelbine, zidovudine. **Incompatible:** Idarubicin, heparin.

Mechanism of Action Teniposide does not inhibit microtubular assembly; it has been shown to delay transit of cells through the S phase and arrest cells in late S or early G_2 phase. Teniposide is a topoisomerase II inhibitor, and appears to cause DNA strand breaks by inhibition of strand-passing and DNA ligase action.

Pharmacodynamics/Kinetics

Distribution: V_d: 0.28 L/kg; Adults: 8-44 L; Children: 3-11 L; mainly into liver, kidneys, small intestine, and adrenals; crosses blood-brain barrier to a limited extent

Protein binding: 99.4%

Metabolism: Extensively hepatic

Half-life elimination: 5 hours

Excretion: Urine (44%, 21% as unchanged drug); feces (≤10%)

Dosage I.V.:

Children: 130 mg/m^2/week, increasing to 150 mg/m^2 after 3 weeks and up to 180 mg/m^2 after 6 weeks

Acute lymphoblastic leukemia (ALL): 165 mg/m^2 twice weekly for 8-9 doses **or** 250 mg/m^2 weekly for 4-8 weeks

Adults: 50-180 mg/m^2 once or twice weekly for 4-6 weeks or 20-60 mg/m^2/day for 5 days

Dosage adjustment in Down syndrome patients: Reduce initial dosing; administer the first course at half the usual dose. Patients with both Down syndrome and leukemia may be especially sensitive to myelosuppressive chemotherapy.

Dosage adjustment in renal/hepatic impairment: Data is insufficient, but dose adjustments may be necessary in patient with significant renal or hepatic impairment

Combination Regimens

Leukemia, acute lymphocytic: Linker Protocol on page 1362

◀ Neuroblastoma:

CCDDT (Neuroblastoma) on page 1252
CCT (Neuroblastoma) on page 1253
OPEC on page 1382
OPEC-D on page 1382
PE-CAdO on page 1393

Administration Must be administered slowly (over at least 30-60 minutes).

Vesicant No; may be an irritant

High Dose Considerations

High Dose I.V.: 750-1000 mg/m^2

Dosage Forms Excipient information presented when available (limited, particularly for generics); consult specific product labeling.

Injection, solution: 10 mg/mL (5 mL) [contains benzyl alcohol, dehydrated ethanol 42.7%, and polyoxyethylated castor oil]

References

Clark PI and Slevin ML, "The Clinical Pharmacology of Etoposide and Teniposide," *Clin Pharmacokinet*, 1987, 12(4):223-52.

Muggia FM, "Teniposide: Overview of Its Therapeutic Potential in Adult Cancers," *Cancer Chemother Pharmacol*, 1994, 34(Suppl):127-33.

O'Dwyer PJ, Alonso MT, Leyland-Jones B, et al, "Teniposide: A Review of 12 Years of Experience," *Cancer Treat Rep*, 1984, 68(12):1455-66.

Rivera GK and Evans WE, "Clinical Trials of Teniposide (VM-26) in Childhood Acute Lymphocytic Leukemia," *Semin Oncol*, 1992, 19(2 Suppl 6):51-8.

Sonneveld P, "Teniposide in Lymphomas and Leukemias," *Semin Oncol*, 1992, 19(2 Suppl 6):59-64.

◆ **TESPA** see Thiotepa on page 1100

◆ **Tetrahydrocannabinol** see Dronabinol on page 387

Tetrahydrocannabinol and Cannabidiol

(TET ra hye droe can NAB i nol & can nab e DYE ol)

Index Terms Cannabidiol and Tetrahydrocannabinol; Delta-9-Tetrahydrocannabinol and Cannabinol; GW-1000-02; THC and CBD

Generic Available No

Canadian Brand Names Sativex®

Pharmacologic Category Analgesic, Miscellaneous

Use Adjunctive treatment of neuropathic pain in multiple sclerosis; adjunctive treatment of moderate-to-severe pain in advanced cancer

Restrictions Not available in U.S.; CDSA-II

Lactation Enters breast milk/contraindicated

Labeled Contraindications Hypersensitivity to cannabinoids or any component of the formulation; serious cardiovascular disease (including arrhythmias, severe heart failure, poorly controlled hypertension, and ischemic heart disease); history of psychotic disorders (including schizophrenia); women of childbearing potential who are not using a reliable form of contraception; males intending to start a family; children <18 years of age; pregnancy; breast-feeding

Warnings/Precautions [Canadian Boxed Warnings]: May cause physical and psychological dependence in long-term use; avoid use in patients with a history or risk of drug or alcohol dependency. Prescriptions should be written for the minimal amount needed between clinic visits. Use may be associated with changes in mood, cognitive performance, memory, impulsivity, and coordination, as well as an altered perception of reality, particularly with respect to an awareness/sensation of time. May impair physical or mental abilities; patients must be cautioned about performing tasks which require mental alertness (eg, operating machinery or driving). **[Canadian Boxed Warnings]: Use with caution in patients with a history of seizures. Concurrent use of ethanol or other CNS active drugs may be additive.** Dosage must be carefully titrated and monitored, with downward adjustment in patients with unacceptable adverse events. Drug discontinuation is recommended, and a period of close observation should be instituted, in patients experiencing a psychotic reaction.

[Canadian Boxed Warning]: May be associated with adverse cardiovascular effects, including tachycardia and alterations in blood pressure (including orthostatic changes).

Use with caution in severe hepatic and renal dysfunction. Use with caution in elderly patients. May be irritating to the buccal mucosa; avoid administration in an area of soreness or inflammation. Use in cancer patients associated with increased risk of urinary retention and infection. Formulation contains ethanol; use may be harmful in patients with alcoholism. Due to accumulation in body fat, cannabinoids may be detectable in the urine and serum for several weeks following drug discontinuation.

Adverse Reactions

>10%:

Central nervous system: Dizziness (up to 32%), somnolence (9% to 15%), fatigue (14%)

Gastrointestinal: Oral application site events (≤20%), nausea (12%)

1% to 10%:

Cardiovascular: Hypotension (2% to 5%), hypertension (2%), flushing (1%), syncope (1%),

Central nervous system: Confusion (1% to 7%), disorientation (5%), vertigo (4% to 5%), attention disturbance (3% to 5%), impaired balance (3% to 5%), dissociation (3%), euphoria (3%), headache (3%), insomnia (3%), panic attack (3%), hallucination (up to 3%), amnesia (2%), anxiety (2%), lethargy (2%), malaise (2%), depression (1% to 2%), memory impairment (1%), paranoia (1%)

Endocrine & metabolic: Thirst (1%)

Gastrointestinal: Xerostomia (8%), vomiting (4% to 8%), oral discomfort/pain (up to 8%), diarrhea (5% to 7%), constipation (4% to 5%), abnormal taste (4%), tooth discoloration (4%), dysgeusia (3% to 5%), oral candidiasis (3%), anorexia (2%), appetite increased (2%), abdominal pain (1%), appetite decreased (1%)

Genitourinary: Urinary retention (5%)

Hepatic: ALT increased, AST increased (2.6%)

Neuromuscular & skeletal: Weakness (5% to 6%), muscle spasticity (3%), dysarthria (2%), fall (2%), paresthesia (2%)

Ocular: Vision blurred (2%)

Renal: Hematuria (3%)

Respiratory: Pharyngitis (2%), cough (1%), respiratory tract infection (1%), throat irritation (1%)

Miscellaneous: Drunken feeling (5%), sensation of heaviness (1%)

<1% and/or frequency not defined: Auditory hallucination, delusions, suicidal ideation, tachycardia, urinary infection

Drug Interactions

Metabolism/Transport Effects Substrate (minor) of CYP2C9, 2C19, 2D6, 3A4; **Inhibits** (weak) CYP1A2, 2C19, 2D6, 3A4

Avoid Concomitant Use There are no known interactions where it is recommended to avoid concomitant use.

Increased Effect/Toxicity

Tetrahydrocannabinol and Cannabidiol may increase the levels/effects of: Alcohol (Ethyl); CNS Depressants; Methotrimeprazine; Sympathomimetics

The levels/effects of Tetrahydrocannabinol and Cannabidiol may be increased by: Anticholinergic Agents; Cocaine; Methotrimeprazine

Decreased Effect There are no known significant interactions involving a decrease in effect.

Ethanol/Nutrition/Herb Interactions

Ethanol: Avoid ethanol (may increase CNS depression).

Food: Administration with high-lipid meals may increase absorption.

Storage/Stability Prior to first use, store unopened at 2°C to 8°C (36°F to 46°F); do not freeze. After opening, may be stored at room temperature of 15°C to 25°C (59°F to 77°F) for up to 28 days. Avoid heat and direct sunlight.

Mechanism of Action Stimulates cannabinoid receptors CB1 and CB2 in the CNS and dorsal root ganglia as well as other sites in the body. Cannabinoid receptors in the pain pathways of the brain and spinal cord mediate cannabinoid-induced analgesia. Peripheral CB2 receptors modulate immune function through cytokine release.

Pharmacodynamics/Kinetics

Absorption: Rapidly absorbed from the buccal mucosa

Distribution: Widely distributed, particularly to fatty tissues

Protein binding: Extensive

Metabolism: Hepatic, via CYP isoenzymes (2C9, 2C19, 2D6 and 3A4) to THC metabolite 11-hydroxy-tetrahydrocannabinol (11-OH-THC, psycho-active) and CBD metabolite 7-hydroxy-cannabidiol.

Half-life elimination: Initial: 1-2 hours; terminal half-life may require 24-36 hours (or longer) due to redistribution from fatty tissue

Time to peak, plasma: 2-4 hours

Excretion: As metabolites, urine and feces

Dosage Buccal spray: Adults: Neuropathic pain (MS), cancer pain: Initial: One spray every 4 hours to a maximum of 4 sprays on first day

Titration and individualization: Dosage is self-titrated by the patient. In the treatment of MS, the mean daily dosage after titration in clinical trials was 5 sprays per day. The usual maximum dose is 12 sprays per day although some patients may require and tolerate a higher number of sprays per day. In the treatment of cancer pain, the mean daily dosage after titration was 8 sprays per day. Dosage should be adjusted as necessary, based on effect and tolerance. Sprays should be evenly distributed over the course of the day during initial titration. If adverse reactions, including intoxication-type symptoms, are noted the dosage should be suspended until resolution of the symptoms; a dosage reduction or extension of the interval between doses may be used to avoid a recurrence of symptoms. Retitration may be required in the event of adverse reactions and/or worsening of symptoms.

Elderly: Refer to adult dosing. Use with caution and monitor closely.

Dosage adjustment in renal impairment: Use with caution; has not been studied in patients with significant renal dysfunction.

Dosage adjustment in hepatic impairment: Use with caution; has not been studied in patients with significant hepatic dysfunction.

Administration Note: For buccal use only; spray should be directed below the tongue or on the inside of the cheeks (the site should be varied); avoid direction to the pharynx.

Shake vial before use and remove protective cap; replace protective cap following use. Do not apply spray to sore or inflamed mucosa.

Priming: Vial should be held in an upright position and primed prior to the initial use by depression of the actuator 2-3 times until a fine spray appears. Priming should not be required for subsequent uses. Do not spray near an open flame.

Normal use: Hold vial in upright position and spray into mouth; spray should be directed below the tongue or on the inside of the cheeks, avoiding direction to the pharynx. The site should be varied.

Monitoring Parameters Mental status, response to pain; mucosal integrity and inflammation

Dosage Forms Excipient information presented when available (limited, particularly for generics); consult specific product labeling. [CAN] = Canadian brand name

Solution, buccal [spray]:

Sativex® [CAN]: Delta-9 tetrahydrocannabinol 27 mg/mL and cannabidiol 25 mg/mL (5.5 mL) [delivers 100 microliters/spray; 51 metered sprays; contains ethanol 50%, peppermint oil, and propylene glycol] [not available in U.S.]

References

Berman JS, Symonds C, and Birch R, "Efficacy of Two Cannabis Based Medicinal Extracts for Relief of Central Neuropathic Pain From Brachial Plexus Avulsion: Results of a Randomised Controlled Trial," *Pain*, 2004, 112(3):299-306.

♦ **Texacort®** see Hydrocortisone on page 575

♦ **TG** see Thioguanine on page 1098

♦ **6-TG (error-prone abbreviation)** see Thioguanine on page 1098

Thalidomide (tha LI doe mide)

Medication Safety Issues

Sound-alike/look-alike issues:

Thalidomide may be confused with flutamide, lenalidomide

Thalomid® may be confused with thiamine

High alert medication: The Institute for Safe Medication Practices (ISMP) includes this medication among its list of drugs which have a heightened risk of causing significant patient harm when used in error.

International issues:

Thalomid® may be confused with Thilomide® which is a brand name for Iodoxamide in Greece and Turkey

Related Information

Safe Handling of Hazardous Drugs on page 1517

U.S. Brand Names Thalomid®

Generic Available No

Canadian Brand Names Thalomid®

Pharmacologic Category Angiogenesis Inhibitor; Immunomodulator, Systemic; Tumor Necrosis Factor (TNF) Blocking Agent

Use Treatment of multiple myeloma; treatment and maintenance of cutaneous manifestations of erythema nodosum leprosum (ENL)

Unlabeled/Investigational Use Treatment of Crohn's disease; graft-versus-host reactions after bone marrow transplantation; AIDS-related aphthous stomatitis; Behçet's syndrome; Waldenström's macroglobulinemia; Langerhans cell histiocytosis

Restrictions Thalidomide is approved for marketing only under a special distribution program. This program, called the "System for Thalidomide Education and Prescribing Safety" (STEPS® 1-888-423-5436), has been approved by the FDA. Prescribers and pharmacists must be registered with the program. No more than a 4-week supply should be dispensed. Blister packs should be dispensed intact (do not repackage capsules). Prescriptions must be filled within 7 days. Subsequent prescriptions may be filled only if fewer than 7 days of therapy remain on the previous prescription. A new prescription is required for further dispensing (a telephone prescription may not be accepted.)

Pregnancy Risk Factor X

Lactation Excretion in breast milk unknown/not recommended

Labeled Contraindications Hypersensitivity to thalidomide or any component of the formulation; neuropathy (peripheral); patient unable to comply with STEPS® program (including males); women of childbearing potential unless alternative therapies are inappropriate and adequate precautions are taken to avoid pregnancy; pregnancy

Warnings/Precautions Hazardous agent - use appropriate precautions for handling and disposal. **[U.S. Boxed Warning]: Thalidomide is a known teratogen; effective contraception must be used for at least 4 weeks before initiating therapy, during therapy, and for 4 weeks following discontinuation of thalidomide for women of childbearing potential.** Use caution with drugs which may decrease the efficacy of hormonal contraceptives.

[U.S. Boxed Warning]: Thrombotic events have been reported, generally in patients with other risk factors for thrombosis (neoplastic disease, inflammatory disease, or concurrent therapy with combination chemotherapy. Use in combination with dexamethasone is associated with increased risk for deep vein thrombosis (DVT) and pulmonary embolism (PE), monitor for signs and symptoms of thromboembolism; patients at risk may benefit from prophylactic anticoagulation or aspirin.

May cause sedation; patients must be warned to use caution when performing tasks which require alertness. Use caution in patients with renal or hepatic impairment, neurological disorders, or constipation. Thalidomide has been associated with the development of peripheral neuropathy, which may be irreversible; use caution with other medications which may cause peripheral neuropathy. Consider immediate discontinuation (if clinically appropriate) in patients who develop neuropathy. May cause seizures; use caution in patients with a history of seizures, concurrent therapy with drugs which alter seizure threshold, or conditions which predispose to seizures. May cause neutropenia; discontinue therapy if absolute neutrophil count decreases to <750/mm^3. Use caution in patients with HIV infection; has been associated with increased viral loads. May cause orthostasis and/or bradycardia; use with caution in patients with cardiovascular disease or in patients who would not tolerate transient hypotensive episodes. Hypersensitivity, Stevens-Johnson syndrome (SJS) and toxic epidermal necrolysis (TEN) have been reported; withhold therapy and evaluate with skin rashes; permanently discontinue if rash is exfoliative, purpuric, bullous or if SJS or TEN is suspected. Safety and efficacy have not been established in children <12 years of age.

Adverse Reactions

>10%:

  Cardiovascular: Edema (57%), thrombosis/embolism (23%; grade 3: 13%, grade 4: 9%), hypotension (16%)

  Central nervous system: Fatigue (79%; grade 3: 3%, grade 4: 1%), somnolence (36% to 38%), dizziness (4% to 20%), sensory neuropathy (54%), confusion (28%), anxiety/agitation (9% to 26%), fever (19% to 23%), motor neuropathy (22%), headache (13% to 19%)

Dermatologic: Rash (21% to 31%), rash/desquamation (30%; grade 3: 4%), dry skin (21%), maculopapular rash (4% to 19%), acne (3% to 11%)

Endocrine & metabolic: Hypocalcemia (72%)

Gastrointestinal: Constipation (3% to 55%), anorexia (3% to 28%), nausea (4% to 24%), weight loss (23%), weight gain (22%), diarrhea (4% to 19%), oral moniliasis (4% to 11%)

Hematologic: Leukopenia (17% to 35%), neutropenia (31%), anemia (6% to 13%), lymphadenopathy (6% to 13%)

Hepatic: AST increased (3% to 25%), bilirubin increased (14%)

Neuromuscular & skeletal: Muscle weakness (40%), tremor (4% to 26%), weakness (6% to 22%), myalgia (17%), paresthesia (6% to 16%), arthralgia (13%)

Renal: Hematuria (11%)

Respiratory: Dyspnea (42%)

Miscellaneous: Diaphoresis (13%)

1% to 10%:

Cardiovascular: Facial edema (4%), peripheral edema (3% to 8%)

Central nervous system: Insomnia (9%), nervousness (3% to 9%), malaise (8%), vertigo (8%), pain (3% to 8%)

Dermatologic: Dermatitis (fungal 4% to 9%), pruritus (3% to 8%), nail disorder (3% to 4%)

Endocrine & metabolic: Hyperlipemia (6% to 9%)

Gastrointestinal: Xerostomia (8% to 9%), flatulence (8%), tooth pain (4%)

Genitourinary: Impotence (3% to 8%)

Hepatic: LFTs abnormal (9%)

Neuromuscular & skeletal: Neuropathy (8%), back pain (4% to 6%), neck pain (4%), neck rigidity (4%)

Renal: Albuminuria (3% to 8%)

Respiratory: Pharyngitis (4% to 8%), rhinitis (4%), sinusitis (4% to 8%)

Miscellaneous: Infection (6% to 8%)

Postmarketing and/or case reports (limited to important or life-threatening): Acute renal failure, alkaline phosphatase increased, ALT increased, amenorrhea, aphthous stomatitis, arrhythmia, atrial fibrillation, bile duct obstruction, bradycardia, BUN increased, carpal tunnel, CML, creatinine clearance decreased, creatinine increased, deafness, depression, diplopia, dysesthesia, ECG abnormalities, electrolyte imbalances, enuresis, eosinophilia, epistaxis, erythema multiforme, erythema nodosum, erythroleukemia, exfoliative dermatitis, febrile neutropenia, foot drop, galactorrhea, granulocytopenia, gynecomastia, hepatomegaly, Hodgkin's disease, hypercalcemia, hyper-/hypokalemia, hypersensitivity, hypertension, hyper-/hypothyroidism, hyperuricemia, hypomagnesemia, hyponatremia, hypoproteinemia, intestinal obstruction, intestinal perforation, interstitial pneumonitis, LDH increased, lethargy, leukocytosis, lymphedema, lymphopenia, mental status changes, metrorrhagia, migraine, myxedema, nystagmus, oliguria, orthostatic hypotension, pancytopenia, paresthesia, petechiae, peripheral neuritis, photosensitivity, pleural effusion, prothrombin time changes, psychosis, pulmonary embolus, pulmonary hypertension, purpura, Raynaud's syndrome, seizure, status epilepticus, Stevens-Johnson syndrome, stomach ulcer, stupor, suicide attempt, syncope, tachycardia, thrombocytopenia, toxic epidermal necrolysis, tumor lysis syndrome

Drug Interactions

Avoid Concomitant Use

Avoid concomitant use of Thalidomide with any of the following: Abatacept; Anakinra; Canakinumab; Certolizumab Pegol; Natalizumab; Rilonacept; Vaccines (Live)

◀ **Increased Effect/Toxicity**

Thalidomide may increase the levels/effects of: Abatacept; Alcohol (Ethyl); Anakinra; Canakinumab; Certolizumab Pegol; CNS Depressants; Leflunomide; Methotrimeprazine; Natalizumab; Pamidronate; Rilonacept; Vaccines (Live); Zoledronic Acid

The levels/effects of Thalidomide may be increased by: Dexamethasone; Methotrimeprazine; Trastuzumab

Decreased Effect

Thalidomide may decrease the levels/effects of: Vaccines (Inactivated); Vaccines (Live)

The levels/effects of Thalidomide may be decreased by: Echinacea

Ethanol/Nutrition/Herb Interactions

Ethanol: Avoid ethanol (may increase sedation).

Herb/Nutraceutical: Avoid cat's claw and echinacea (have immunostimulant properties; consider therapy modifications).

Storage/Stability Store at 15°C to 30°C (50°F to 86°F). Protect from light. Keep in original package.

Mechanism of Action Has immunomodulatory and antiangiogenic characteristics. Immunologic effects may vary based on conditions; may suppress excessive tumor necrosis factor-alpha production in patients with ENL, yet may increase plasma tumor necrosis factor-alpha levels in HIV-positive patients. In multiple myeloma, thalidomide is associated with an increase in natural killer cells and increased levels of interleukin-2 and interferon gamma. Other proposed mechanisms of action include suppression of angiogenesis, prevention of free-radical-mediated DNA damage, increased cell mediated cytotoxic effects, and altered expression of cellular adhesion molecules.

Pharmacodynamics/Kinetics

Distribution: V_d: 120 L

Protein binding: 55% to 66%

Metabolism: Nonenzymatic hydrolysis in plasma; forms multiple metabolites

Half-life elimination: 5-7 hours

Time to peak, plasma: 3-6 hours

Excretion: Urine (<1% as unchanged drug)

Dosage Oral:

Multiple myeloma: 200 mg once daily (with dexamethasone 40 mg daily on days 1-4, 9-12, and 17-20 of a 28-day treatment cycle)

Cutaneous ENL:

Initial: 100-300 mg/day taken once daily at bedtime with water (at least 1 hour after evening meal)

Patients weighing <50 kg: Initiate at lower end of the dosing range

Severe cutaneous reaction or patients previously requiring high dose may be initiated at 400 mg/day; doses may be divided, but taken 1 hour after meals

Maintenance: Dosing should continue until active reaction subsides (usually at least 2 weeks), then tapered in 50 mg decrements every 2-4 weeks

Patients who flare during tapering or with a history or requiring prolonged maintenance should be maintained on the minimum dosage necessary to control the reaction. Efforts to taper should be repeated every 3-6 months, in increments of 50 mg every 2-4 weeks

Behçet's syndrome (unlabeled use): 100-400 mg/day

Graft-vs-host reactions (unlabeled use): 100-1600 mg/day; usual initial dose: 200 mg 4 times/day for use up to 700 days

AIDS-related aphthous stomatitis (unlabeled use): 200 mg twice daily for 5 days, then 200 mg/day for up to 8 weeks

Combination Regimens
Multiple myeloma:
  Bortezomib-Melphalan-Prednisone-Thalidomide on page 1241
  DTPACE on page 1297
  Melphalan-Prednisone-Thalidomide on page 1365
  Thalidomide-Dexamethasone on page 1405
Prostate cancer: Docetaxel-Thalidomide on page 1292

Administration Oral: Administer with water, preferably at bedtime once daily on an empty stomach, at least 1 hour after the evening meal. Doses >400 mg/day may be given in 2-3 divided doses. Avoid extensive handling of capsules; capsules should remain in blister pack until ingestion. If exposed to the powder content from broken capsules or body fluids from patients receiving thalidomide, the exposed area should be washed with soap and water.

Monitoring Parameters CBC with differential, platelets; signs of neuropathy monthly for the first 3 months, then periodically during treatment; consider monitoring of sensory nerve application potential amplitudes (at baseline and every 6 months) to detect asymptomatic neuropathy. In HIV-seropositive patients: viral load after 1 and 3 months, then every 3 months. Pregnancy testing (sensitivity of at least 50 mIU/mL) is required within 24 hours prior to initiation of therapy, weekly during the first 4 weeks, then every 4 weeks in women with regular menstrual cycles or every 2 weeks in women with irregular menstrual cycles.

Dietary Considerations Should be taken at least 1 hour after the evening meal.

Emetic Potential Very low (<10%)

Dosage Forms Excipient information presented when available (limited, particularly for generics); consult specific product labeling.
Capsule:
  Thalomid®: 50 mg, 100 mg, 150 mg, 200 mg

References
Eriksson T, Bjorkman S, and Hoglund P, "Clinical Pharmacology of Thalidomide," *Eur J Clin Pharmacol*, 2001, 57(5):365-76.

Franks ME, Macpherson GR, and Figg WD, "Thalidomide," *Lancet*, 2004, 363(9423):1802-11.

Hamuryudan V, Mat C, Saip S, et al, "Thalidomide in the Treatment of the Mucocutaneous Lesions of the Behçet Syndrome. A Randomized, Double-Blind, Placebo-Controlled Trial," *Ann Intern Med*, 1998, 128(6):443-50.

Jacobson JM, Greenspan JS, Spritzler J, et al, "Thalidomide for the Treatment of Oral Aphthous Ulcers in Patients With Human Immunodeficiency Virus Infection. National Institute of Allergy and Infectious Diseases AIDS Clinical Trials Group," *N Engl J Med*, 1997, 336(21):1487-93.

Kyle RA and Rajkumar SV, "Multiple Myeloma," *N Engl J Med*, 2004, 351(18): 1860-73.

Rajkumar SV, Blood E, Vesole D, et al, "Phase III Clinical Trial of Thalidomide Plus Dexamethasone Compared With Dexamethasone Alone in Newly Diagnosed Multiple Myeloma: A Clinical Trial Coordinated by the Eastern Cooperative Oncology Group," *J Clin Oncol*, 2006, 24 (3):431-6.

Teo SK, Colburn WA, Tracewell WG, et al, "Clinical Pharmacokinetics of Thalidomide," *Clin Pharmacokinet*, 2004, 43(5):311-27.

Uhl K, Cox E, Rogan R, et al, "Thalidomide Use in the US: Experience With Pregnancy Testing in the S.T.E.P.S.® Programme," *Drug Saf*, 2006, 29(4):231-9.

Thioguanine (thye oh GWAH neen)

Medication Safety Issues

High alert medication: The Institute for Safe Medication Practices (ISMP) includes this medication among its list of drugs which have a heightened risk of causing significant patient harm when used in error.

6-thioguanine and 6-TG are error-prone abbreviations (associated with six-fold overdoses of thioguanine)

Related Information

Management of Chemotherapy-Induced Nausea and Vomiting *on page 1434*
Safe Handling of Hazardous Drugs *on page 1517*

U.S. Brand Names Tabloid®

Index Terms 2-Amino-6-Mercaptopurine; 6-TG (error-prone abbreviation); 6-Thioguanine (error-prone abbreviation); TG; Tioguanine

Generic Available No

Canadian Brand Names Lanvis®

Pharmacologic Category Antineoplastic Agent, Antimetabolite (Purine Antagonist)

Use Treatment of acute myelogenous (nonlymphocytic) leukemia (AML)

Restrictions The I.V. formulation is not available in U.S.

Pregnancy Risk Factor D

Lactation Excretion in breast milk unknown

Labeled Contraindications Hypersensitivity to thioguanine or any component of the formulation; pregnancy

Warnings/Precautions Hazardous agent - use appropriate precautions for handling and disposal. Use with caution and reduce dose in patients with renal or hepatic impairment. Not recommended for long-term continuous therapy due to potential for hepatotoxicity (hepatic veno-occlusive disease). Discontinue in patients with evidence of hepatotoxicity. Thioguanine is potentially carcinogenic and teratogenic; myelosuppression may be delayed. Caution with history of previous therapy resistance with either thioguanine or mercaptopurine (there is usually complete cross resistance between these two). Patients with genetic deficiency of thiopurine methyltransferase (TPMT) or who are receiving drugs which inhibit this enzyme (mesalazine, olsalazine, sulfasalazine) may be highly sensitive to myelosuppressive effects.

Adverse Reactions

>10%: Hematologic: Myelosuppressive:
  WBC: Moderate
  Platelets: Moderate
  Onset: 7-10 days
  Nadir: 14 days
  Recovery: 21 days
1% to 10%:
  Dermatologic: Skin rash
  Endocrine & metabolic: Hyperuricemia
  Gastrointestinal: Mild nausea or vomiting, anorexia, stomatitis, diarrhea
  Neuromuscular & skeletal: Unsteady gait
<1%: Ascites, esophageal varices, hepatic necrosis, hepatitis, jaundice, LFTs increased, neurotoxicity, photosensitivity, portal hypertension, splenomegaly, thrombocytopenia, veno-occlusive hepatic disease

Drug Interactions

Avoid Concomitant Use

Avoid concomitant use of Thioguanine with any of the following: Natalizumab; Vaccines (Live)

Increased Effect/Toxicity

Thioguanine may increase the levels/effects of: Leflunomide; Natalizumab; Vaccines (Live)

The levels/effects of Thioguanine may be increased by: 5-ASA Derivatives; Trastuzumab

Decreased Effect

Thioguanine may decrease the levels/effects of: Vaccines (Inactivated); Vaccines (Live)

The levels/effects of Thioguanine may be decreased by: Echinacea

Ethanol/Nutrition/Herb Interactions Food: Enhanced absorption if administered between meals.

Storage/Stability Store tablet at room temperature.

Mechanism of Action Purine analog that is incorporated into DNA and RNA resulting in the blockage of synthesis and metabolism of purine nucleotides

Pharmacodynamics/Kinetics

Absorption: 30% (highly variable)

Distribution: Crosses placenta

Metabolism: Hepatic; rapidly and extensively via TPMT to 2-amino-6-methylthioguanine (active) and inactive compounds

Half-life elimination: Terminal: 11 hours

Time to peak, serum: Within 8 hours

Excretion: Urine

Dosage Total daily dose can be given at one time.

Oral (refer to individual protocols):

Infants and Children <3 years: Combination drug therapy for acute nonlymphocytic leukemia: 3.3 mg/kg/day in divided doses twice daily for 4 days

Children and Adults: 2-3 mg/kg/day calculated to nearest 20 mg or 75-200 mg/m²/day in 1-2 divided doses for 5-7 days or until remission is attained

Dosing comments in renal or hepatic impairment: Reduce dose

Combination Regimens

Leukemia, acute myeloid:

DAT on page 1288

TAD on page 1405

V-TAD on page 1427

Monitoring Parameters CBC with differential and platelet count; liver function tests (weekly when beginning therapy then monthly, more frequently in patients with liver disease or concurrent hepatotoxic drugs); hemoglobin, hematocrit, serum uric acid; some laboratories offer testing for TPMT deficiency

Hepatotoxicity may present with signs of portal hypertension (splenomegaly, esophageal varices, thrombocytopenia) or veno-occlusive disease (fluid retention, ascites, hepatomegaly with tenderness, or hyperbilirubinemia)

Emetic Potential Very low (<10%)

Dosage Forms Excipient information presented when available (limited, particularly for generics); consult specific product labeling.

Tablet [scored]:

Tabloid®: 40 mg

Extemporaneous Preparations A 20 mg/mL oral suspension can be prepared by crushing fifteen 40 mg tablets in a mortar, and then adding 10 mL of methylcellulose 1% (in small amounts). Transfer to a graduate, then add a sufficient quantity of syrup to make 30 mL of suspension. Label "shake well."

Room temperature stability is 60 days.

Dressman JB and Poust RI, "Stability of Allopurinol and Five Antineoplastics in Suspension," *Am J Hosp Pharm*, 1983, 40:616-8.

Nahata MC, Morosco RS, and Hipple TF, 4th ed, *Pediatric Drug Formulations*, Cincinnati, OH: Harvey Whitney Books Co, 2000.

References

Broxson EH, Dole M, Wong R, et al, "Portal Hypertension Develops in a Subset of Children With Standard Risk Acute Lymphoblastic Leukemia Treated With Oral 6-Thioguanine During Maintenance Therapy," *Pediatr Blood Cancer*, 2005, 44(3):226-31

Elgemeie GH, "Thioguanine, Mercaptopurine: Their Analogs and Nucleosides as Antimetabolites," *Curr Pharm Des*, 2003, 9(31):2627-42.

Estlin EJ, "Continuing Therapy for Childhood Acute Lymphoblastic Leukaemia: Clinical and Cellular Pharmacology of Methotrexate, 6-Mercaptopurine and 6-Thioguanine," *Cancer Treat Rev*, 2001, 27(6):351-63.

◆ **6-Thioguanine (error-prone abbreviation)** see Thioguanine *on page 1098*

◆ **Thiophosphoramide** see Thiotepa *on page 1100*

◆ **Thiosulfuric Acid Disodium Salt** see Sodium Thiosulfate *on page 1040*

Thiotepa (thye oh TEP a)

Medication Safety Issues

High alert medication: The Institute for Safe Medication Practices (ISMP) includes this medication among its list of drugs which have a heightened risk of causing significant patient harm when used in error.

Related Information

Management of Drug Extravasations *on page 1447*

Safe Handling of Hazardous Drugs *on page 1517*

Index Terms TESPA; Thiophosphoramide; Triethylenethiophosphoramide; TSPA

Generic Available Yes

Pharmacologic Category Antineoplastic Agent, Alkylating Agent

Use Treatment of superficial tumors of the bladder; palliative treatment of adenocarcinoma of breast or ovary; controlling intracavitary effusions caused by metastatic tumors

Unlabeled/Investigational Use Intrathecal treatment of neoplastic meningitis

Pregnancy Risk Factor D

Lactation Enters breast milk/not recommended

Labeled Contraindications Hypersensitivity to thiotepa or any component of the formulation; pregnancy

Warnings/Precautions Hazardous agent - use appropriate precautions for handling and disposal. Myelosuppression is common. Potentially mutagenic, carcinogenic, and teratogenic. Reduce dosage and use extreme caution in patients with hepatic, renal, or bone marrow damage. Use should be limited to cases where benefit outweighs risk.

Adverse Reactions

>10%:

Hematopoietic: Dose-limiting toxicity which is dose related and cumulative; moderate-to-severe leukopenia and severe thrombocytopenia have occurred. Anemia and pancytopenia may become fatal, so careful hematologic monitoring is required; intravesical administration may cause bone marrow suppression as well.

Hematologic: Myelosuppression (WBC: moderate; platelets: severe; onset: 7-10 days, nadir: 14 days, recovery: 28 days)

Local: Injection site pain

1% to 10%:

Central nervous system: Dizziness, fatigue, fever, headache

Dermatologic: Alopecia, depigmentation (with topical treatment), hyper-pigmentation (with high-dose therapy), pruritus, rash, urticaria

Endocrine & metabolic: Amenorrhea, hyperuricemia

Gastrointestinal: Anorexia, nausea and vomiting rarely occur

Emetic potential: Low (<10%)

Genitourinary: Dysuria, hemorrhagic cystitis (intravesicular administration: rare), urinary retention

Neuromuscular & skeletal: Weakness

Ocular: Conjunctivitis

Renal: Hematuria

Miscellaneous: Tightness of the throat, allergic reactions

<1%: Stomatitis, anaphylaxis; like other alkylating agents, this drug is carcinogenic

Drug Interactions

Metabolism/Transport Effects Inhibits CYP2B6 (strong)

Avoid Concomitant Use

Avoid concomitant use of Thiotepa with any of the following: Natalizumab; Vaccines (Live)

Increased Effect/Toxicity

Thiotepa may increase the levels/effects of: CYP2B6 Substrates; Lefluno-mide; Natalizumab; Vaccines (Live)

The levels/effects of Thiotepa may be increased by: Trastuzumab

Decreased Effect

Thiotepa may decrease the levels/effects of: Vaccines (Inactivated); Vaccines (Live)

The levels/effects of Thiotepa may be decreased by: Echinacea

Ethanol/Nutrition/Herb Interactions

Ethanol: Avoid ethanol (due to GI irritation).

Herb/Nutraceutical: Avoid black cohosh, dong quai in estrogen-dependent tumors.

Storage/Stability Store intact vials under refrigeration (2°C to 8°C). Protect from light. Reconstituted solutions (10 mg/mL) are stable for up to 28 days under refrigeration (4°C to 8°C) or 7 days at room temperature (25°C).

Solutions for infusion in D_5W (≥5 mg/mL) are stable for 14 days under refrigeration (4°C) or 3 days at room temperature (23°C).

Solutions for infusion in NS (1, 3, or 5 mg/mL) are stable for 48 hours under refrigeration (4°C to 8°C) or 24 hours at room temperature (25°C). Solutions in NS at a concentration ≤0.5 mg/mL are stable for <1 hour.

Reconstitution Reconstitute each vial to 10 mg/mL. Solutions for infusion should be diluted to a concentration ≥5 mg/mL in 5% dextrose or 1, 3, or 5 mg/mL in 0.9% sodium chloride injection. Solutions for intravesicular admin-istration should be diluted in 30-60 mL SWFI or NS. Solutions for intrathecal administration should be diluted in 1-5 mL NS or Elliott's B solution. Filter through a 0.22 micron filter prior to administration.

Compatibility Variable stability (consult detailed reference) in D_5W, NS.

Y-site administration: Compatible: Acyclovir, allopurinol, amifostine, amikacin, aminophylline, amphotericin B, ampicillin, ampicillin/sulbactam, aztreonam, bleomycin, bumetanide, buprenorphine, butorphanol, calcium gluconate, carboplatin, carmustine, cefazolin, cefepime, cefoperazone, cefotaxime, cefotetan, cefoxitin, ceftazidime, ceftizoxime, ceftriaxone, cefuroxime, chlorpromazine, cimetidine, ciprofloxacin, clindamycin, co-trimoxazole, cyclophosphamide, cytarabine, dacarbazine, dactinomycin, daunorubicin, dexamethasone sodium phosphate, diphenhydramine, dobutamine, dopamine, doxorubicin, doxycycline, droperidol, enalaprilat, etoposide, etoposide phosphate, famotidine, floxuridine, fluconazole, fludarabine, fluorouracil, furosemide, ganciclovir, gemcitabine, gentamicin, granisetron, haloperidol, heparin, hydrocortisone sodium phosphate, hydrocortisone sodium succinate, hydromorphone, hydroxyzine, idarubicin, ifosfamide, imipenem/cilastatin, leucovorin, lorazepam, magnesium sulfate, mannitol, melphalan, meperidine, mesna, methotrexate, methylprednisolone sodium succinate, metoclopramide, metronidazole, mitomycin, mitoxantrone, morphine, nalbuphine, netilmicin, ofloxacin, ondansetron, paclitaxel, piperacillin, piperacillin/tazobactam, plicamycin, potassium chloride, prochlorperazine edisylate, promethazine, ranitidine, sodium bicarbonate, streptozocin, teniposide, ticarcillin, ticarcillin/clavulanate, tobramycin, vancomycin, vinblastine, vincristine, zidovudine. **Incompatible:** Cisplatin, filgrastim, minocycline, vinorelbine. **Variable (consult detailed reference):** TPN.

Compatibility when admixed: Compatible: Epinephrine, lidocaine. **Incompatible:** Cisplatin.

Mechanism of Action Alkylating agent that reacts with DNA phosphate groups to produce cross-linking of DNA strands leading to inhibition of DNA, RNA, and protein synthesis; mechanism of action has not been explored as thoroughly as the other alkylating agents, it is presumed that the aziridine rings open and react as nitrogen mustard; reactivity is enhanced at a lower pH

Pharmacodynamics/Kinetics

Absorption: Intracavitary instillation: Unreliable (10% to 100%) through bladder mucosa; I.M.: variable

Metabolism: Extensively hepatic; major metabolite (active): TEPA

Half-life elimination: Terminal (dose-dependent clearance): 109 minutes

Excretion: Urine (as metabolites and unchanged drug)

Dosage Adults:

Bladder cancer: Intravesical: 60 mg in 30-60 mL NS retained for 2 hours once weekly for 4 weeks

Ovarian, breast cancer: I.V.: 0.3-0.4 mg/kg by rapid I.V. administration every 1-4 weeks

Effusions: Intracavitary: 0.6-0.8 mg/kg

Neoplastic meningitis (unlabeled use): Intrathecal: 10 mg twice a week for 4 weeks, then weekly for 4 weeks then monthly for 4 doses (NCCN CNS cancer guidelines v.2.2009)

Dosing comments/adjustment in renal impairment: Use with extreme caution, reduced dose may be warranted.

Combination Regimens

Breast cancer: VATH on page 1418

Leukemia, acute lymphocytic: TVTG on page 1416

Leukemia, acute myeloid: TVTG on page 1416

Administration

I.V.: Administer either as a short (10-60 minute) infusion or 1-2 minute push; a 1 mg/mL solution is considered isotonic; not a vesicant

Intravesical lavage: Instill directly into the bladder and retain for at least 2 hours; patient should be repositioned every 15-30 minutes for maximal exposure

Monitoring Parameters CBC with differential and platelet count (monitor for at least 3 weeks after treatment); uric acid, urinalysis

Additional Information A 1 mg/mL solution is considered isotonic.

Vesicant May be an irritant

High Dose Considerations

Comments Administration of thiotepa over 30 minutes, 1 hour before infusion of cyclophosphamide over 60 minutes, reduced bioactivation of cyclophosphamide to 4-hydroxycyclophosphamide in 20 patients. This effect did not occur with administration of thiotepa 1 hour following infusion of cyclophosphamide.

High Dose I.V.: 360-1125 mg/m^2 as a single dose or divided into 2 daily doses; generally combined with other high-dose chemotherapeutic drugs.

Unique Toxicities

Central nervous system: Effect increased with doses >1000 mg/m^2: Confusion, inappropriate behavior, somnolence

Dermatologic: Hyperpigmentation (most common on occluded areas of skin)

Gastrointestinal: Mucositis, mild nausea and vomiting

Hepatic: Serum transaminitis, hyperbilirubinemia

Dosage Forms Excipient information presented when available (limited, particularly for generics); consult specific product labeling.

Injection, powder for reconstitution: 15 mg, 30 mg

References

Antman K, Eder JP, Elias A, et al, "High-Dose Thiotepa Alone and in Combination Regimens With Bone Marrow Support," *Semin Oncol*, 1990, 17(1 Suppl 3):33-8.

Badalament RA and Farah RN, "Treatment of Superficial Bladder Cancer With Intravesicle Chemotherapy," *Semin Surg Oncol*, 1997, 13(5):335-41.

deJonge ME, Huitema AD, vanDam SM, et al, "Significant Induction of Cyclophosphamide and Thiotepa Metabolism by Phenytoin," *Cancer Chemother Pharmacol*, 2005, 55(5):507-10.

Dimopoulos MA, Alexanian R, Przepiorka D, et al, "Thiotepa, Busulfan, and Cyclophosphamide: A New Preparative Regimen for Autologous Marrow or Blood Stem Cell Transplantation in High-Risk Multiple Myeloma," *Blood*, 1993, 82(8):2324-8.

Gutin PH, Weiss HD, Wiernik PH, et al, "Intrathecal N,N',N''-triethylenethiophosphoramide [thio-TEPA (NSC-6396)] in the Treatment of Malignant Meningeal Disease: Phase I-II Study," *Cancer*, 1976, 38(4):1471-5.

Heideman RL, Cole D, Balis F, et al, "Phase I and Pharmacokinetic Evaluation of Thiotepa in the Cerebrospinal Fluid and Plasma of Pediatric Patients: Evidence for Dose-Dependent Plasma Clearance of Thiotepa," *Cancer Res*, 1989, 49(3):736-41.

Herzig GP, "Phase I-II Studies of High-Dose Thiotepa and Autologous BMT in Patients With Refractory Malignancies," *Adv Cancer Chemotherapy*, 1987, 17-29 (proceedings of a symposium, Oct 1986)

Maanen MJ, Smeets CJ, and Beijnen JH, "Chemistry, Pharmacology and Pharmacokinetics of N, N',N'', -Triethylenethiophosphoramide (ThioTEPA)," *Cancer Treat Rev*, 2000, 26(4):257-68.

National Comprehensive Cancer Network® (NCCN), "Clinical Practice Guidelines in Oncology™: Central Nervous System Cancers," Version 2.2009. Available at http://www.nccn.org/professionals/physician_gls/PDF/cns.pdf

Saarinen UM, Hovi L, and Makipern CA, "High Dose Thiotepa With Autologous Bone Marrow Rescue in Pediatric Solid Tumors," *Proc Am Soc Clin Oncol*, 1989, 8:303.

◆ **Thorazine** see ChlorproMAZINE *on page 220*

◆ **Thrombate III®** see Antithrombin III *on page 96*

◆ **Thymocyte Stimulating Factor** see Aldesleukin *on page 25*

◆ **Thymoglobulin®** see Antithymocyte Globulin (Rabbit) *on page 101*

◆ **Thyrogen®** see Thyrotropin Alfa *on page 1103*

Thyrotropin Alfa (thye roe TROH pin AL fa)

Medication Safety Issues

Sound-alike/look-alike issues:

Thyrogen® may be confused with Thyrolar®

U.S. Brand Names Thyrogen®

Index Terms Human Thyroid Stimulating Hormone; Recombinant Human Thyrotropin; Rh-TSH; Thyrotropin Alpha; TSH

Generic Available No

Canadian Brand Names Thyrogen®

Pharmacologic Category Diagnostic Agent

Use As an adjunctive diagnostic tool for serum thyroglobulin (Tg) testing; adjunctive treatment for radioiodine ablation of thyroid tissue remnants after total or near-total thyroidectomy in patients with well-differentiated thyroid cancer without evidence of metastatic disease

Potential clinical uses include: Patients with an undetectable Tg on thyroid hormone suppressive therapy to exclude the diagnosis of residual or recurrent thyroid cancer, patients requiring serum Tg testing and radioiodine imaging who are unwilling to undergo thyroid hormone withdrawal testing and whose treating physician believes that use of a less sensitive test is justified, patients who are either unable to mount an adequate endogenous TSH response to thyroid hormone withdrawal or in whom withdrawal is medically contraindicated, and patients without evidence of metastatic disease to ablate thyroid remnants (in combination with radioiodine [I^{131}]) following near-total thyroidectomy.

Pregnancy Risk Factor C

Lactation

Excretion in breast milk unknown/use caution

Labeled Contraindications There are no contraindications listed within the manufacturer's labeling.

Warnings/Precautions For I.M. use only. Caution should be exercised when administered to patients who have been previously treated with bovine TSH and, in particular, to those patients who have experienced hypersensitivity reactions to bovine TSH. In patients with significant residual thyroid tissue, thyrotropin will cause significant increases in thyroid hormone levels; use caution in patients with known history of heart disease or serious underlying illness; may lead to serious complications. Use caution with extensive metastatic disease; may cause edema and/or hemorrhage at metastatic sites, leading to impingement of vital anatomic structures. Pretreatment with corticosteroids may be considered. Thyrotropin elimination is significantly reduced in dialysis-dependent end-stage renal impairment, leading to prolonged elevation of thyroid-stimulating hormone (TSH) levels. Thyrotropin use in elderly (with functioning thyroid tumors) may result in palpitations or cardiac rhythm disorders; arrhythmia has been reported in elderly patients with pre-existing cardiac disease; carefully evaluate risk versus benefit. Safety and efficacy in children <16 years of age have not been established.

Considerations in the use of thyrotropin alfa:

1. There remains a meaningful risk of missing the diagnosis of thyroid cancer or of underestimating the extent of disease when thyrotropin-stimulated Tg testing is performed even in combination with radioiodine imaging.
2. Thyrotropin Tg levels are generally lower than, and do not correlate with, Tg levels after thyroid hormone withdrawal.
3. Newly detectable Tg level or a Tg level rising over time after thyrotropin or a high index of suspicion of metastatic disease, even in the setting of a negative or low-stage thyrotropin radioiodine scan, should prompt further evaluation such as thyroid hormone withdrawal to definitively establish the location and extent of thyroid cancer.
4. Decision to perform a thyrotropin radioiodine scan in conjunction with a thyrotropin serum Tg test and whether or when to withdraw a patient from thyroid hormones are complex. Pertinent factors in this decision include the sensitivity of the Tg assay used, the thyrotropin Tg level obtained, and the index of suspicion of recurrent or persistent local or metastatic disease.

5. The signs and symptoms of hypothyroidism which accompany thyroid hormone withdrawal are avoided with thyrotropin use.

6. Clinical experience in thyroid remnant ablation with thyrotropin is limited; long-term outcome data have not been established compared to withholding thyroid hormone.

7. Thyrotropin studies for thyroid remnant ablation used I^{131} activity of 100 mCi ± 10%; activity of I^{131} used in clinical practice may vary; lower radioiodine doses may not be as effective.

Adverse Reactions

>10%: Gastrointestinal: Nausea (3% to 12%)

1% to 10%:

Central nervous system: Headache (1% to 7%), dizziness (≤3%), fatigue (1% to 3%), insomnia (≤2%)

Endocrine & metabolic: Hypercholesterolemia (≤3%), cholesterol abnormal (≤1%)

Gastrointestinal: Vomiting (1% to 3%), diarrhea (≤1%)

Neuromuscular & skeletal: Paresthesia (≤2%), weakness (≤2%)

Respiratory: Nasopharyngitis (≤1%)

Adverse reactions which may be related to local edema or hemorrhage at metastatic sites: Acute visual loss; enlargement of locally-recurring papillary carcinoma (accompanied by dyspnea, stridor, or dysphonia); hemiplegia, hemiparesis, laryngeal edema with respiratory distress, pain

<1%, postmarketing, and/or case reports: Atrial arrhythmia; flu-like syndrome (arthralgia, chills, fever, myalgia, shivering); hypersensitivity reactions (eg, flushing, pruritus, rash, respiratory difficulty, urticaria); hyperthyroidism, MI, taste loss, thyrotropin alfa antibody formation

Drug Interactions

Avoid Concomitant Use There are no known interactions where it is recommended to avoid concomitant use.

Increased Effect/Toxicity There are no known significant interactions involving an increase in effect.

Decreased Effect There are no known significant interactions involving a decrease in effect.

Storage/Stability Store intact vials at 2°C to 8°C (36°F to 46°F). If necessary, the reconstituted solution can be stored for up to 24 hours at 2°C to 8°C (36°F to 46°F). Protect from light.

Reconstitution Reconstitute each vial with 1.2 mL of sterile water for injection to a final concentration of 0.9 mg/mL. Each vial should be reconstituted immediately prior to use with diluent provided.

Mechanism of Action Thyrotropin alfa, derived from a recombinant DNA source, has the identical amino acid sequence as endogenous human thyroid stimulating hormone (TSH). As a diagnostic tool in conjunction with serum thyroglobulin (Tg) testing, thyrotropin alfa stimulates the secretion of Tg from any remaining thyroid tissues (remnants). Under conditions of successful thyroidectomy and complete ablation, very little serum Tg should be detected under TSH stimulatory conditions; conversely, elevated Tg levels suggest the presence of remnant thyroid tissues. Since the source of TSH is exogenous, stimulation of Tg synthesis can be achieved in euthyroid patients, avoiding the need for thyroid hormone withdrawal.

As an adjunctive agent for radioiodine ablation treatment of thyroid cancer tissue remnants, thyrotropin alfa binds to TSH receptors on these tissues, stimulating the uptake and organification of iodine, including radiolabeled iodine (I^{131}). Cancerous tissue is destroyed via gamma emission from the radioiodine concentrated in these tissues.

Pharmacodynamics/Kinetics

Half-life elimination: 25 ± 10 hours

Time to peak: Median: 10 hours (range: 3-24 hours)

Dosage I.M.: Children >16 years and Adults: Radioiodine imaging or ablation: 0.9 mg, followed 24 hours later by a second 0.9 mg dose

For radioiodine imaging or remnant ablation, radioiodine administration should be given 24 hours following the second thyrotropin injection. Diagnostic scanning should be performed 48 hours after radioiodine administration (72 hours after the second thyrotropin injection). Post-therapy scanning may be delayed (additional days) to allow decline of background activity.

For serum Tg testing, serum Tg should be obtained 72 hours after final injection of thyrotropin.

Administration After reconstitution with 1.2 mL sterile water for injection, 1 mL of the resulting solution (0.9 mg/mL) should be administered I.M. into the buttock.

Test Interactions Thyroglobulin assay may be confounded by thyroglobulin antibodies, possibly leading to misinterpreted or difficult to interpret thyroglobulin levels.

Dosage Forms Excipient information presented when available (limited, particularly for generics); consult specific product labeling.

Injection, powder for reconstitution:

Thyrogen®: 1.1 mg

References

Haugen BR, Pacini F, Reiners C, et al, "A Comparison of Recombinant Human Thyrotropin and Thyroid Hormone Withdrawal for the Detection of Thyroid Remnant or Cancer," *J Clin Endocrinol Metab*, 1999, 94(11):3877-85.

Pacini F, Ladenson PW, Schlumberger M, et al, "Radioiodine Ablation of Thyroid Remnants After Preparation With Recombinant Human Thyrotropin in Differentiated Thyroid Carcinoma: Results of an International, Randomized, Controlled Study," *J Clin Endocrinol Metab*, 2006, 91(3):926-32.

Schroeder PR, Haugen BR, Pacini F, et al, "A Comparison of Short-Term Changes in Health-Related Quality of Life in Thyroid Carcinoma Patients Undergoing Diagnostic Evaluation With Recombinant Human Thyrotropin Compared With Thyroid Hormone Withdrawal," *J Clin Endocrinol Metab*, 2006, 91(3):878-84.

◆ **Thyrotropin Alpha** *see* Thyrotropin Alfa *on page* 1103

Ticarcillin and Clavulanate Potassium

(tye kar SIL in & klav yoo LAN ate poe TASS ee um)

U.S. Brand Names Timentin®

Index Terms Ticarcillin and Clavulanic Acid

Generic Available No

Canadian Brand Names Timentin®

Pharmacologic Category Antibiotic, Penicillin

Use Treatment of lower respiratory tract, urinary tract, skin and skin structures, bone and joint, gynecologic (endometritis) and intra-abdominal (peritonitis) infections, and septicemia caused by susceptible organisms. Clavulanate expands activity of ticarcillin to include beta-lactamase producing strains of *S. aureus*, *H. influenzae*, *Bacteroides* species, and some other gram-negative bacilli

Pregnancy Risk Factor B

Lactation Enters breast milk/use caution

Labeled Contraindications Hypersensitivity to ticarcillin, clavulanate, any penicillin, or any component of the formulation

Warnings/Precautions Use with caution and modify dosage in patients with renal impairment; serious and occasionally severe or fatal hypersensitivity (anaphylactoid) reactions have been reported in patients on penicillin therapy (especially with a history of beta-lactam hypersensitivity and/or a history of sensitivity to multiple allergens); use with caution in patients with seizures and in patients with HF due to high sodium load. Particularly in patients with renal impairment, bleeding disorders have been observed; discontinue if thrombocytopenia or bleeding occurs. Prolonged use may result in fungal or bacterial superinfection, including *C. difficile*-associated diarrhea (CDAD) and pseudomembranous colitis; CDAD has been observed >2 months postantibiotic treatment. Safety and efficacy have not been established in children <3 months of age.

Adverse Reactions Frequency not defined.

Central nervous system: Confusion, drowsiness, fever, headache, Jarisch-Herxheimer reaction, seizure

Dermatologic: Erythema multiforme, pruritus, rash, Stevens-Johnson syndrome, toxic epidermal necrolysis, urticaria

Endocrine & metabolic: Electrolyte imbalance

Gastrointestinal: *Clostridium difficile* colitis, diarrhea, nausea, vomiting

Hematologic: Bleeding, eosinophilia, hemolytic anemia, leukopenia, neutropenia, positive Coombs' reaction, prothrombin time prolonged, thrombocytopenia

Hepatic: Hepatotoxicity, jaundice

Local: Injection site reaction (pain, burning, induration); thrombophlebitis

Neuromuscular & skeletal: Myoclonus

Renal: BUN increased, interstitial nephritis (acute), serum creatinine increased

Miscellaneous: Anaphylaxis, hypersensitivity reactions

Drug Interactions

Avoid Concomitant Use There are no known interactions where it is recommended to avoid concomitant use.

Increased Effect/Toxicity

Ticarcillin and Clavulanate Potassium may increase the levels/effects of: Methotrexate

The levels/effects of Ticarcillin and Clavulanate Potassium may be increased by: Uricosuric Agents

Decreased Effect

Ticarcillin and Clavulanate Potassium may decrease the levels/effects of: Aminoglycosides; Mycophenolate; Typhoid Vaccine

The levels/effects of Ticarcillin and Clavulanate Potassium may be decreased by: Fusidic Acid; Tetracycline Derivatives

Storage/Stability

Vials: Store intact vials at <24°C (<75°F). Reconstituted solution is stable for 6 hours at room temperature and 72 hours when refrigerated. I.V. infusion in NS or LR is stable for 24 hours at room temperature, 7 days when refrigerated, or 30 days when frozen. I.V. infusion in D_5W solution is stable for 24 hours at room temperature, 3 days when refrigerated, or 7 days when frozen. After freezing, thawed solution is stable for 8 hours at room temperature. Darkening of drug indicates loss of potency of clavulanate potassium.

Premixed solution: Store frozen at ≤-20°C (-4°F). Thawed solution is stable for 24 hours at room temperature or 7 days under refrigeration; do not refreeze.

Compatibility Stable in D_5W, LR, NS, sterile water for injection.

Y-site administration: Compatible: Allopurinol, amifostine, aztreonam, cefepime, clarithromycin, cyclophosphamide, diltiazem, docetaxel, doxorubicin liposome, etoposide, famotidine, filgrastim, fluconazole, fludarabine, foscarnet, gatifloxacin, gemcitabine, granisetron, heparin, insulin (regular), melphalan, meperidine, morphine, ondansetron, perphenazine, propofol, ▶

remifentanil, sargramostim, teniposide, theophylline, thiotepa, vinorelbine.
Incompatible: Alatrofloxacin, amphotericin B cholesteryl sulfate complex.
Variable (consult detailed reference): Cisatracurium, topotecan, vancomycin.

Compatibility when admixed: Incompatible: Sodium bicarbonate, aminoglycosides.

Mechanism of Action Inhibits bacterial cell wall synthesis by binding to one or more of the penicillin binding proteins (PBPs); which in turn inhibits the final transpeptidation step of peptidoglycan synthesis in bacterial cell walls, thus inhibiting cell wall biosynthesis. Bacteria eventually lyse due to ongoing activity of cell wall autolytic enzymes (autolysins and murein hydrolases) while cell wall assembly is arrested.

Pharmacodynamics/Kinetics

Absorption: Ticarcillin: Not absorbed orally

Protein binding: Ticarcillin: ~45%; Clavulanic acid: ~25%

Metabolism: Clavulanic acid: Hepatic

Half-life elimination: Ticarcillin: 1.1 hours; Clavulanic acid: 1.1 hours

Excretion: Ticarcillin: Urine (60% to 70%); Clavulanic acid: Urine (35% to 45% as unchanged drug)

Clearance: Clavulanic acid does not affect clearance of ticarcillin

Dosage Note: Timentin® (ticarcillin/clavulanate) is a combination product; each 3.1 g dosage form contains 3 g ticarcillin disodium and 0.1 g clavulanic acid.

Usual dosage range:

Children and Adults <60 kg: I.V.: 200-300 mg of ticarcillin component/kg/day in divided doses every 4-6 hours

Children ≥60 kg and Adults: I.V.: 3.1 g (ticarcillin 3 g plus clavulanic acid 0.1 g) every 4-6 hours (maximum: 24 g of ticarcillin component/day)

Indication-specific dosing:

Children: I.V.:

Bite wounds (animal): 200 mg of ticarcillin component/kg/day in divided doses

Neutropenic fever: 75 mg of ticarcillin component/kg every 6 hours (maximum: 3.1 g/dose)

Pneumonia (nosocomial): 300 mg of ticarcillin component/kg/day in 4 divided doses (maximum: 18-24 g of ticarcillin component/day)

Children ≥60 kg and Adults: I.V.:

Amnionitis, cholangitis, diverticulitis, endometritis, epididymo-orchitis, mastoiditis, orbital cellulitis, peritonitis, pneumonia (aspiration): 3.1 g every 6 hours

Liver abscess, parafascial space infections, septic thrombophlebitis: 3.1 g every 4 hours

***Pseudomonas* infections:** 3.1 g every 4 hours

Urinary tract infections: 3.1 g every 6-8 hours

Dosing adjustment in renal impairment: Loading dose: I.V.: 3.1 g one dose, followed by maintenance dose based on creatinine clearance:

Cl_{cr} 30-60 mL/minute: Administer 2 g of ticarcillin component every 4 hours or 3.1 g every 8 hours

Cl_{cr} 10-30 mL/minute: Administer 2 g of ticarcillin component every 8 hours or 3.1 g every 12 hours

Cl_{cr} <10 mL/minute: Administer 2 g of ticarcillin component every 12 hours

Cl_{cr} <10 mL/minute with concomitant hepatic dysfunction: 2 g of ticarcillin component every 24 hours

Moderately dialyzable (20% to 50%)

Continuous ambulatory peritoneal dialysis: 3.1 g every 12 hours

Hemodialysis: 2 g of ticarcillin component every 12 hours; supplemented with 3.1 g after each dialysis

Continuous renal replacement therapy (CRRT): Drug clearance is highly dependent on the method of renal replacement, filter type, and flow rate. Appropriate dosing requires close monitoring of pharmacologic response, signs of adverse reactions due to drug accumulation, as well as drug levels in relation to target trough (if appropriate). The following are general recommendations only (based on dialysate flow/ultrafiltration rates of 1 L/hour) and should not supersede clinical judgment:

CVVH: 2 g every 6-8 hours

CVVHD/CVVHDF: 3.1 g every 6 hours

Note: Do not administer in intervals exceeding every 8 hours. Clavulanate component is hepatically eliminated; extending the dosing interval beyond 8 hours may result in loss of beta-lactamase inhibition.

Dosing adjustment in hepatic dysfunction: With concomitant renal dysfunction (Cl_{cr} <10 mL/minute): 2 g of ticarcillin component every 24 hours

Administration Infuse over 30 minutes.

Some penicillins (eg, carbenicillin, ticarcillin, and piperacillin) have been shown to inactivate aminoglycosides *in vitro*. This has been observed to a greater extent with tobramycin and gentamicin, while amikacin has shown greater stability against inactivation. Concurrent use of these agents may pose a risk of reduced antibacterial efficacy *in vivo*, particularly in the setting of profound renal impairment. However, definitive clinical evidence is lacking. If combination penicillin/aminoglycoside therapy is desired in a patient with renal dysfunction, separation of doses (if feasible), and routine monitoring of aminoglycoside levels, CBC, and clinical response should be considered.

Monitoring Parameters Observe for signs and symptoms of anaphylaxis during first dose.

Test Interactions Positive Coombs' test, false-positive urinary proteins

Some penicillin derivatives may accelerate the degradation of aminoglycosides *in vitro*, leading to a potential underestimation of aminoglycoside serum concentration.

Dietary Considerations Sodium content of 1 g: 4.51 mEq; potassium content of 1 g: 0.15 mEq

Dosage Forms Excipient information presented when available (limited, particularly for generics); consult specific product labeling.

Infusion [premixed, frozen]: Ticarcillin 3 g and clavulanic acid 0.1 g (100 mL) [contains sodium 4.51 mEq and potassium 0.15 mEq per g]

Injection, powder for reconstitution: Ticarcillin 3 g and clavulanic acid 0.1 g (3.1 g, 31 g) [contains sodium 4.51 mEq and potassium 0.15 mEq per g]

References

Donowitz GR and Mandell GL, "Beta-Lactam Antibiotics," *N Engl J Med*, 1988, 318(7):419-26 and 318(8):490-500.

Stutman HR and Marks MI, "Review of Pediatric Antimicrobial Therapies," *Semin Pediatr Infect Dis*, 1991, 2:3-17.

Wright AJ, "The Penicillins," *Mayo Clin Proc*, 1999, 74(3):290-307.

◆ **Ticarcillin and Clavulanic Acid** *see* Ticarcillin and Clavulanate Potassium *on page 1106*

◆ **TICE® BCG** *see* BCG Vaccine *on page 128*

◆ **Tigan®** *see* Trimethobenzamide *on page 1147*

◆ **Timentin®** *see* Ticarcillin and Clavulanate Potassium *on page 1106*

◆ **Tioguanine** *see* Thioguanine *on page 1098*

Tobramycin (toe bra MYE sin)

Medication Safety Issues

Sound-alike/look-alike issues:

Tobramycin may be confused with Trobicin®, vancomycin

AKTob® may be confused with AK-Trol®

Nebcin® may be confused with Inapsine®, Naprosyn®, Nubain®

Tobrex® may be confused with TobraDex®

High alert medication: The Institute for Safe Medication Practices (ISMP) includes this medication (intrathecal administration) among its list of drug classes which have a heightened risk of causing significant patient harm when used in error.

U.S. Brand Names AKTob®; TOBI®; Tobrex®

Index Terms Tobramycin Sulfate

Generic Available Yes: Excludes ophthalmic ointment, solution for nebulization

Canadian Brand Names PMS-Tobramycin; Sandoz-Tobramycin; TOBI®; Tobramycin Injection, USP; Tobrex®

Pharmacologic Category Antibiotic, Aminoglycoside; Antibiotic, Ophthalmic

Use Treatment of documented or suspected infections caused by susceptible gram-negative bacilli including *Pseudomonas aeruginosa*; topically used to treat superficial ophthalmic infections caused by susceptible bacteria. Tobramycin solution for inhalation is indicated for the management of cystic fibrosis patients (>6 years of age) with *Pseudomonas aeruginosa*.

Pregnancy Risk Factor D (injection, inhalation); B (ophthalmic)

Lactation Enters breast milk/not recommended

Labeled Contraindications Hypersensitivity to tobramycin, other aminoglycosides, or any component of the formulation; pregnancy (injection/inhalation)

Warnings/Precautions [U.S. Boxed Warning]: Aminoglycosides may cause neurotoxicity and/or nephrotoxicity; usual risk factors include preexisting renal impairment, concomitant neuro-/nephrotoxic medications, advanced age and dehydration. Ototoxicity may be directly proportional to the amount of drug given and the duration of treatment; tinnitus or vertigo are indications of vestibular injury and impending hearing loss; renal damage is usually reversible. May cause neuromuscular blockade and respiratory paralysis; especially when given soon after anesthesia or muscle relaxants.

Not intended for long-term therapy due to toxic hazards associated with extended administration; use caution in pre-existing renal insufficiency, vestibular or cochlear impairment, myasthenia gravis, hypocalcemia, conditions which depress neuromuscular transmission. Dosage modification required in patients with impaired renal function. Prolonged use may result in fungal or bacterial superinfection, including *C. difficile*-associated diarrhea (CDAD) and pseudomembranous colitis; CDAD has been observed >2 months postantibiotic treatment. Solution may contain sodium metabisulfate; use caution in patients with sulfite allergy.

Adverse Reactions

Injection: Frequency not defined:

Central nervous system: Confusion, disorientation, dizziness, fever, headache, lethargy, vertigo

Dermatologic: Exfoliative dermatitis, itching, rash, urticaria

Endocrine & metabolic: Serum calcium, magnesium, potassium, and/or sodium decreased

Gastrointestinal: Diarrhea, nausea, vomiting

Hematologic: Anemia, eosinophilia, granulocytopenia, leukocytosis, leukopenia, thrombocytopenia

Hepatic: ALT increased, AST increased, bilirubin increased, LDH increased

Local: Pain at the injection site

Otic: Hearing loss, tinnitus, ototoxicity (auditory), ototoxicity (vestibular), roaring in the ears

Renal: BUN increased, cylindruria, serum creatinine increased, oliguria, proteinuria

Inhalation:

>10%:

Gastrointestinal: Sputum discoloration (21%)

Respiratory: Voice alteration (13%)

1% to 10%:

Central nervous system: Malaise (6%)

Otic: Tinnitus (3%)

Postmarketing and/or case reports: Hearing loss

Ophthalmic: <1%: Ocular: Conjunctival erythema, lid itching, lid swelling

Drug Interactions

Avoid Concomitant Use

Avoid concomitant use of Tobramycin with any of the following: Gallium Nitrate

Increased Effect/Toxicity

Tobramycin may increase the levels/effects of: AbobotulinumtoxinA; Bisphosphonate Derivatives; CARBOplatin; Colistimethate; CycloSPORINE; Gallium Nitrate; Neuromuscular-Blocking Agents; OnabotulinumtoxinA; RimabotulinumtoxinB

The levels/effects of Tobramycin may be increased by: Amphotericin B; Capreomycin; CISplatin; Loop Diuretics; Nonsteroidal Anti-Inflammatory Agents; Vancomycin

Decreased Effect

Tobramycin may decrease the levels/effects of: Typhoid Vaccine

The levels/effects of Tobramycin may be decreased by: Penicillins

Storage/Stability

Injection: Stable at room temperature both as the clear, colorless solution and as the dry powder. Reconstituted solutions remain stable for 24 hours at room temperature and 96 hours when refrigerated.

Ophthalmic solution: Store at 8°C to 27°C (46°F to 80°F).

Solution, for inhalation (TOBI®): Store under refrigeration at 2°C to 8°C (36°F to 46°F). May be stored in foil pouch at room temperature of 25°C (77°F) for up to 28 days. Avoid intense light. Solution may darken over time; however, do not use if cloudy or contains particles.

Reconstitution Dilute in 50-100 mL NS, D$_5$W for I.V. infusion.

Compatibility Stable in dextran 40 10% in dextrose, D$_5$NS, D$_5$W, D$_{10}$W, mannitol 20%, LR, NS; **variable stability (consult detailed reference)** in peritoneal dialysis solutions.

◄ **Y-site administration: Compatible:** Acyclovir, alatrofloxacin, amifostine, amiodarone, amsacrine, aztreonam, ciprofloxacin, cisatracurium, cyclophosphamide, diltiazem, docetaxel, doxorubicin liposome, enalaprilat, esmolol, etoposide phosphate, filgrastim, fluconazole, fludarabine, foscarnet, furosemide, gatifloxacin, gemcitabine, granisetron, hydromorphone, IL-2, insulin (regular), labetalol, linezolid, magnesium sulfate, melphalan, meperidine, midazolam, morphine, perphenazine, remifentanil, tacrolimus, teniposide, theophylline, thiotepa, tolazoline, vinorelbine, zidovudine. **Incompatible:** Allopurinol, amphotericin B cholesteryl sulfate complex, cefoperazone, heparin, hetastarch, indomethacin, propofol, sargramostim.

Compatibility in syringe: Compatible: Doxapram. **Incompatible:** Cefamandole, clindamycin, heparin.

Compatibility when admixed: Compatible: Aztreonam, bleomycin, calcium gluconate, cefoxitin, ciprofloxacin, clindamycin, furosemide, metronidazole, metronidazole with sodium bicarbonate, ofloxacin, ranitidine, verapamil. **Incompatible:** Cefamandole, cefepime, cefotaxime, cefotetan, floxacillin, heparin.

Mechanism of Action Interferes with bacterial protein synthesis by binding to 30S and 50S ribosomal subunits resulting in a defective bacterial cell membrane

Pharmacodynamics/Kinetics

Absorption:
Oral: Poorly absorbed
I.M.: Rapid and complete
Inhalation: Peak serum concentrations are ~1 mcg/mL following a 300 mg dose

Distribution: V_d: 0.2-0.3 L/kg; Pediatrics: 0.2-0.7 L/kg; to extracellular fluid including serum, abscesses, ascitic, pericardial, pleural, synovial, lymphatic, and peritoneal fluids; poor penetration into CSF, eye, bone, prostate
Inhalation: Tobramycin remains concentrated primarily in the airways

Protein binding: <30%

Half-life elimination:
Neonates: ≤1200 g: 11 hours; >1200 g: 2-9 hours
Adults: 2-3 hours; directly dependent upon glomerular filtration rate
Adults with impaired renal function: 5-70 hours

Time to peak, serum: I.M.: 30-60 minutes; I.V.: ~30 minutes

Excretion: Normal renal function: Urine (~90% to 95%) within 24 hours

Dosage Note: Dosage individualization is **critical** because of the low therapeutic index.

Use of ideal body weight (IBW) for determining the mg/kg/dose appears to be more accurate than dosing on the basis of total body weight (TBW). In morbid obesity, dosage requirement may best be estimated using a dosing weight of IBW + 0.4 (TBW - IBW).

Initial and periodic plasma drug levels (eg, peak and trough with conventional dosing) should be determined, particularly in critically-ill patients with serious infections or in disease states known to significantly alter aminoglycoside pharmacokinetics (eg, cystic fibrosis, burns, or major surgery).

Usual dosage range:
Infants and Children <5 years: I.M., I.V.: 2.5 mg/kg/dose every 8 hours
Children ≥5 years: I.M., I.V.: 2-2.5 mg/kg/dose every 8 hours
Note: Higher individual doses and/or more frequent intervals (eg, every 6 hours) may be required in selected clinical situations (cystic fibrosis) or serum levels document the need.

Children and Adults:

Inhalation:

Aerosolized tobramycin injection (unlabeled use): 80 mg 2 times/day. **Note:** Injectable formulation may contain preservatives, which may increase risk of bronchospasm.

TOBI®: Children ≥6 years and Adults: 300 mg every 12 hours (do not administer doses <6 hours apart); administer in repeated cycles of 28 days on drug followed by 28 days off drug.

Intrathecal: 4-8 mg/day

Ophthalmic: Children ≥2 months and Adults:

Ointment: Instill ½" (1.25 cm) 2-3 times/day every 3-4 hours

Solution: Instill 1-2 drops every 2-4 hours, up to 2 drops every hour for severe infections

Topical: Apply 3-4 times/day to affected area

Adults: I.M., I.V.:

Conventional: 1-2.5 mg/kg/dose every 8-12 hours; to ensure adequate peak concentrations early in therapy, higher initial dosage may be considered in selected patients when extracellular water is increased (edema, septic shock, postsurgical, and/or trauma)

Once-daily: 4-7 mg/kg/dose once daily; some clinicians recommend this approach for all patients with normal renal function; this dose is at least as efficacious with similar, if not less, toxicity than conventional dosing.

Indication-specific dosing:

Neonates:

Meningitis: I.M., I.V.:

0-7 days: <2000 g: 2.5 mg/kg every 18-24 hours; >2000 g: 2.5 mg/kg every 12 hours

8-28 days: <2000 g: 2.5 mg/kg every 8-12 hours; >2000 g: 2.5 mg/kg every 8 hours

Children:

Cystic fibrosis:

I.M., I.V.: 2.5-3.3 mg/kg every 6-8 hours; **Note:** Some patients may require larger or more frequent doses if serum levels document the need (eg, cystic fibrosis or febrile granulocytopenic patients).

Inhalation: See adult dosing.

Adults:

I.M., I.V.:

Brucellosis: 240 mg (I.M.) daily or 5 mg/kg (I.V.) daily for 7 days; either regimen recommended in combination with doxycycline

Cholangitis: 4-6 mg/kg once daily with ampicillin

Diverticulitis, complicated: 1.5-2 mg/kg every 8 hours (with ampicillin and metronidazole)

Infective endocarditis or synergy (for gram-positive infections): I.M., I.V.: 1 mg/kg every 8 hours (with ampicillin)

Meningitis *(Enterococcus or Pseudomonas aeruginosa):* I.V.: Loading dose: 2 mg/kg, then 1.7 mg/kg/dose every 8 hours (administered with another bactericidal drug)

Pelvic inflammatory disease: Loading dose: 2 mg/kg, then 1.5 mg/kg every 8 hours **or** 4.5 mg/kg once daily

Plague *(Yersinia pestis):* Treatment: 5 mg/kg/day, followed by postexposure prophylaxis with doxycycline

Pneumonia, hospital- or ventilator-associated: 7 mg/kg/day (with antipseudomonal beta-lactam or carbapenem)

Prophylaxis against endocarditis (dental, oral, upper respiratory procedures, GI/GU procedures): 1.5 mg/kg with ampicillin (50 mg/kg) 30 minutes prior to procedure. **Note:** AHA guidelines now recommend prophylaxis only in patients undergoing invasive procedures and in whom underlying cardiac conditions may predispose to a higher risk of adverse outcomes should infection occur. As of April 2007, routine prophylaxis no longer recommended by the AHA.

Tularemia: 5 mg/kg/day divided every 8 hours for 1-2 weeks

Urinary tract infection: 1.5 mg/kg/dose every 8 hours

Inhalation:

Cystic fibrosis:

Aerosolized tobramycin injection (unlabeled use): 80 mg 2 times/day; **Note:** Injectable formulation may contain preservatives, which may increase risk of bronchospasm.

TOBI®: 300 mg every 12 hours (do not administer doses <6 hours apart); administer in repeated cycles of 28 days on drug followed by 28 days off drug.

Dosing interval in renal impairment: I.M., I.V.:

Conventional dosing:

Cl_{cr} ≥60 mL/minute: Administer every 8 hours

Cl_{cr} 40-60 mL/minute: Administer every 12 hours

Cl_{cr} 20-40 mL/minute: Administer every 24 hours

Cl_{cr} 10-20 mL/minute: Administer every 48 hours

Cl_{cr} <10 mL/minute: Administer every 72 hours

High-dose therapy: Interval may be extended (eg, every 48 hours) in patients with moderate renal impairment (Cl_{cr} 30-59 mL/minute) and/or adjusted based on serum level determinations.

Hemodialysis: Dialyzable; 30% removal of aminoglycosides occurs during 4 hours of HD - administer dose after dialysis and follow levels

Continuous arteriovenous or venovenous hemofiltration: Dose as for Cl_{cr} of 10-40 mL/minute and follow levels

Administration in CAPD fluid:

Gram-negative infection: 4-8 mg/L (4-8 mcg/mL) of CAPD fluid

Gram-positive infection (ie, synergy): 3-4 mg/L (3-4 mcg/mL) of CAPD fluid

Administration IVPB/I.M.: Dose as for Cl_{cr} <10 mL/minute and follow levels

Dosing adjustment/comments in hepatic disease: Monitor plasma concentrations

Administration

I.V.: Infuse over 30-60 minutes. Flush with saline before and after administration.

Inhalation (TOBI®): To be inhaled over ~15 minutes using a handheld nebulizer (PARI-LC PLUS™). If multiple different nebulizer treatments are required, administer bronchodilator first, followed by chest physiotherapy, any other nebulized medications, and then TOBI® last. Do not mix with other nebulizer medications.

Ophthalmic: Contact lenses should not be worn during treatment of ophthalmic infections.

Ointment: Do not touch tip of tube to eye. Instill ointment into pocket between eyeball and lower lid; patient should look downward before closing eye.

Solution: Allow 5 minutes between application of "multiple-drop" therapy.

Suspension: Shake well before using; tilt head back, instill suspension in conjunctival sac and close eye(s). Do not touch dropper to eye. Apply light finger pressure on lacrimal sac for 1 minute following instillation.

Some penicillins (eg, carbenicillin, ticarcillin and piperacillin) have been shown to inactivate aminoglycosides *in vitro*. This has been observed to a greater extent with tobramycin and gentamicin, while amikacin has shown greater stability against inactivation. Concurrent use of these agents may pose a risk of reduced antibacterial efficacy *in vivo*, particularly in the setting of profound renal impairment. However, definitive clinical evidence is lacking. If combination penicillin/aminoglycoside therapy is desired in a patient with renal dysfunction, separation of doses (if feasible), and routine monitoring of aminoglycoside levels, CBC, and clinical response should be considered.

Monitoring Parameters Urinalysis, urine output, BUN, serum creatinine, peak and trough plasma tobramycin levels; be alert to ototoxicity; hearing should be tested before and during treatment

Some penicillin derivatives may accelerate the degradation of aminoglycosides *in vitro*. This may be clinically-significant for certain penicillin (ticarcillin, piperacillin, carbenicillin) and aminoglycoside (gentamicin, tobramycin) combination therapy in patients with significant renal impairment. Close monitoring of aminoglycoside levels is warranted.

Test Interactions Some penicillin derivatives may accelerate the degradation of aminoglycosides *in vitro*, leading to a potential underestimation of aminoglycoside serum concentration.

Dietary Considerations May require supplementation of calcium, magnesium, potassium.

Additional Information Once-daily dosing: Higher peak serum drug concentration to MIC ratios, demonstrated aminoglycoside postantibiotic effect, decreased renal cortex drug uptake, and improved cost-time efficiency are supportive reasons for the use of once daily dosing regimens for aminoglycosides. Current research indicates these regimens to be as effective for non-life-threatening infections, with no higher incidence of nephrotoxicity, than those requiring multiple daily doses. Doses are determined by calculating the entire day's dose via usual multiple dose calculation techniques and administering this quantity as a single dose. Doses are then adjusted to maintain mean serum concentrations above the MIC(s) of the causative organism(s). (Example: 2.5-5 mg/kg as a single dose; expected Cp_{max}: 10-20 mcg/mL and Cp_{min}: <1 mcg/mL). Further research is needed for universal recommendation in all patient populations and gram-negative disease; exceptions may include those with known high clearance (eg, children, patients with cystic fibrosis, or burns who may require shorter dosage intervals) and patients with renal function impairment for whom longer than conventional dosage intervals are usually required.

Dosage Forms Excipient information presented when available (limited, particularly for generics); consult specific product labeling.

Infusion [premixed in NS]: 60 mg (50 mL); 80 mg (100 mL)

Injection, powder for reconstitution: 1.2 g

Injection, solution: 10 mg/mL (2 mL, 8 mL); 40 mg/mL (2 mL, 30 mL, 50 mL) [may contain sodium metabisulfite]

Ointment, ophthalmic (Tobrex®): 0.3% (3.5 g)

Solution for nebulization [preservative free] (TOBI®): 60 mg/mL (5 mL)

Solution, ophthalmic (AKTob®, Tobrex®): 0.3% (5 mL) [contains benzalkonium chloride]

References

American Thoracic Society and Infectious Diseases Society of America, "Guidelines for the Management of Adults With Hospital-Acquired, Ventilator-Associated, and Healthcare-Associated Pneumonia," *Am J Respir Crit Care Med*, 2005, 171(4):388-416.

Bauer LA and Blouin RA, "Influence of Age on Tobramycin. Pharmacokinetics in Patients With Normal Renal Function," *Antimicrob Agents Chemother*, 1981, 20:587-9.

Gilbert DN, "Once-Daily Aminoglycoside Therapy," *Antimicrob Agents Chemother*, 1991, 35 (3):399-405.

Hustinx WN and Hoepelman IM, "Aminoglycoside Dosage Regimens. Is Once a Day Enough?" *Clin Pharmacokinet*, 1993, 25(6):427-32.

Lortholary O, Tod M, Cohen Y, et al, "Aminoglycosides," *Med Clin North Am*, 1995, 79(4):761-87.

Mayer PR, Brown CH, Carter RA, et al, "Intramuscular Tobramycin Pharmacokinetics in Geriatric Patients," *Drug Intell Clin Pharm*, 1986, 20:611-5.

McCormack JP and Jewesson PJ, "A Critical Re-evaluation of the "Therapeutic Range" of Aminoglycosides," *Clin Infect Dis*, 1992, 14(1):320-39.

Nicolau DP, Freeman CD, Belliveau PP, et al, "Experience With a Once-Daily Aminoglycoside Program Administered to 2184 Adult Patients," *Antimicrob Agents Chemother*, 1995, 39(3):650-5.

Preston SL and Briceland LL, "Single Daily Dosing of Aminoglycosides," *Pharmacotherapy*, 1995, 15(3):297-316.

◆ **Tobramycin Injection, USP (Can)** *see* Tobramycin *on page* 1110

◆ **Tobramycin Sulfate** *see* Tobramycin *on page* 1110

◆ **Tobrex®** *see* Tobramycin *on page* 1110

◆ **Tomudex® (Can)** *see* Raltitrexed *on page* 1005

◆ **Toposar™** *see* Etoposide *on page* 429

Topotecan (toe poe TEE kan)

Medication Safety Issues

Sound-alike/look-alike issues:

Hycamtin® may be confused with Hycomine®, Mycamine®

High alert medication: The Institute for Safe Medication Practices (ISMP) includes this medication among its list of drugs which have a heightened risk of causing significant patient harm when used in error.

Related Information

Management of Chemotherapy-Induced Nausea and Vomiting *on page* 1434

Management of Drug Extravasations *on page* 1447

Safe Handling of Hazardous Drugs *on page* 1517

U.S. Brand Names Hycamtin®

Index Terms Hycamptamine; SKF 104864; SKF 104864-A; Topotecan Hydrochloride

Generic Available No

Canadian Brand Names Hycamtin®

Pharmacologic Category Antineoplastic Agent, Camptothecin; Antineoplastic Agent, Natural Source (Plant) Derivative

Use Treatment of ovarian cancer and small cell lung cancer; cervical cancer (in combination with cisplatin)

Unlabeled/Investigational Use Investigational: Treatment of nonsmall cell lung cancer, myelodysplastic syndrome, sarcoma (pediatrics), neuroblastoma (pediatrics), refractory solid tumors (pediatrics)

Pregnancy Risk Factor D

Lactation Excretion in breast milk unknown/contraindicated

Labeled Contraindications Hypersensitivity to topotecan or any component of the formulation; severe bone marrow depression; pregnancy; breast-feeding

Warnings/Precautions Hazardous agent - use appropriate precautions for handling and disposal. The dose-limiting toxicity is bone marrow suppression (primarily neutropenia; may also cause thrombocytopenia and anemia); monitor bone marrow function. Neutropenia is not cumulative overtime. [U.S. **Boxed Warning]: Should only administer to patients with adequate bone marrow reserves, baseline neutrophils at least 1500 cells/mm³** and platelet counts at least 100,000/mm³. In a clinical study comparing I.V. to oral topotecan, G-CSF support was administered in a higher percentage of patients receiving oral topotecan. Topotecan-induced neutropenia may lead to neutropenic colitis; should be considered in patients presenting with neutropenia, fever and abdominal pain. Diarrhea has been reported with oral topotecan; may be severe; incidence may be higher in the elderly; educate patients on proper management. Use caution in renal impairment; may require dose adjustment. **[U.S. Boxed Warning]: Should be administered under the supervision of an experienced cancer chemotherapy physician.** Safety and efficacy in children have not been established.

Adverse Reactions

>10%:

Central nervous system: Fatigue (11% to 29%), fever (5% to 28%), pain (23%), headache (18%)

Dermatologic: Alopecia (10% to 49%), rash (16%)

Gastrointestinal: Nausea (27% to 64%), vomiting (19% to 45%), diarrhea (14% to 32%; Oral: grade 3: 4%; grade 4: ≤1%; onset: 9 days), constipation (29%), abdominal pain (22%), anorexia (7% to 19%), stomatitis (18%)

Hematologic: Neutropenia (83% to 97%; grade 4: 32% to 80%; nadir 8-11 days; duration: 7 days; recovery <21 days), leukopenia (86% to 97%; grade 4: 15% to 32%), anemia (89% to 98%; grade 4: 7% to 10%), thrombocytopenia (69% to 81%; grade 4: 6% to 29%; duration: 3 days), neutropenic fever/sepsis (2% to 28%)

Neuromuscular & skeletal: Weakness (3% to 25%)

Respiratory: Dyspnea (22%), cough (15%)

1% to 10%:

Hepatic: Liver enzymes increased (transient; 8%)

Neuromuscular & skeletal: Paresthesia (7%)

Miscellaneous: Sepsis (grades 3/4: 5%)

<1%, postmarketing, and/or case reports: Abdominal pain, allergic reactions, anaphylactoid reactions, angioedema, bleeding (severe, associated with thrombocytopenia), dermatitis (severe), injection site reactions (mild erythema, bruising), neutropenic colitis, pancytopenia, pruritus (severe)

Drug Interactions

Avoid Concomitant Use

Avoid concomitant use of Topotecan with any of the following: Natalizumab; P-Glycoprotein Inhibitors; Vaccines (Live)

Increased Effect/Toxicity

Topotecan may increase the levels/effects of: Leflunomide; Natalizumab; Vaccines (Live)

The levels/effects of Topotecan may be increased by: BCRP/ABCG2 Inhibitors; Filgrastim; P-Glycoprotein Inhibitors; Platinum Derivatives; Trastuzumab

Decreased Effect

Topotecan may decrease the levels/effects of: Vaccines (Inactivated); Vaccines (Live)

The levels/effects of Topotecan may be decreased by: Echinacea

Ethanol/Nutrition/Herb Interactions Ethanol: Avoid ethanol (due to GI irritation).

Storage/Stability

I.V.: Store intact vials of lyophilized powder for injection at room temperature of 20°C to 25°C (68°F to 77°F); protect from light. Reconstituted solution is stable for up to 28 days at room temperature of 20°C to 25°C (68°F to 77°F). When further diluted in 50-100 mL D_5W or NS, solution is stable for 24 hours at room temperature or up to 7 days under refrigeration.

Oral: Store at 2°C to 8°C (36°F to 46°F). Protect from light.

◀ **Reconstitution** Reconstitute vials with 4 mL SWFI. May be further diluted in 50-100 mL D_5W or NS for infusion.

Compatibility Stable in D_5W, NS.

Y-site administration: Compatible: Carboplatin, cimetidine, cisplatin, cyclophosphamide, doxorubicin, etoposide, gemcitabine, granisetron, ifosfamide, methylprednisolone sodium succinate, metoclopramide, ondansetron, paclitaxel, prochlorperazine edisylate, vincristine. **Incompatible:** Dexamethasone sodium phosphate, fluorouracil, mitomycin. **Variable (consult detailed reference):** Ticarcillin/clavulanate.

Mechanism of Action Binds to topoisomerase I and stabilizes the cleavable complex so that religation of the cleaved DNA strand cannot occur. This results in the accumulation of cleavable complexes and single-strand DNA breaks. Topotecan acts in S phase of the cell cycle.

Pharmacodynamics/Kinetics

Absorption: Oral: Rapid

Distribution: V_{dss} of the lactone is high (mean: 87.3 L/mm^2; range: 25.6-186 L/mm^2), suggesting wide distribution and/or tissue sequestering

Protein binding: ~35%

Metabolism: Undergoes a rapid, pH-dependent hydrolysis of the lactone ring to yield a relatively inactive hydroxy acid in plasma; metabolized in the liver to N-demethylated metabolite

Bioavailability: Oral: ~40%

Half-life elimination: I.V.: 2-3 hours; renal impairment: 5 hours; Oral: 3-6 hours

Time to peak, plasma: Oral 1-2 hours; delayed with high-fat meal (1.5-4 hours)

Excretion:

I.V.: Urine (51%; 3% as N-desmethyl topotecan); feces (18%; 2% as N-desmethyl topotecan)

Oral: Urine (20%; 2% as N-desmethyl topotecan); feces (33%; <2% as N-desmethyl topotecan)

Dosage Adults (refer to individual protocols): **Note:** Baseline neutrophil count should be >1500/mm^3; retreatment neutrophil count should be >1000/mm^3; baseline and retreatment platelet count should be >100,000/mm^3; (also, for oral topotecan, retreatment hemoglobin should be ≥9 g/dL):

Small cell lung cancer:

IVPB: 1.5 mg/m^2/day for 5 days; repeated every 21 days

Oral: 2.3 mg/m^2/day for 5 days; repeated every 21 days (round dose to the nearest 0.25 mg); if patient vomits after dose is administered, do not give a replacement dose.

Metastatic ovarian cancer:

IVPB: 1.5 mg/m^2/day for 5 days; repeated every 21 days

I.V. continuous infusion (unlabeled dose) 0.2-0.7 mg/m^2/day for 7-21 days

Cervical cancer: IVPB: 0.75 mg/m^2/day for 3 days (followed by cisplatin 50 mg/m^2 on day 1 only, [with hydration]); repeated every 21 days

Dosage adjustment for toxicity:

I.V.:

Ovarian and small cell lung cancer: Dosage adjustment for hematological effects: Severe neutropenia or platelet count <25,000/mm^3: Reduce dose to 1.25 mg/m^2/day for subsequent cycles (may consider G-CSF support [beginning on day 6] prior to instituting dose reduction for neutropenia)

Cervical cancer: Severe febrile neutropenia (ANC <1000/mm^3 with temperature of 38°C) or platelet count <10,000/mm^3: Reduce topotecan to 0.6 mg/m^2/day for subsequent cycles (may consider C-CSF support [beginning on day 4] prior to instituting dose reduction for neutropenic fever.

For neutropenic fever despite G-CSF use, reduce dose to 0.45 mg/m^2/day for subsequent cycles). **Note:** Cisplatin may also require dose adjustment.

Oral:

Small cell lung cancer: Severe neutropenia (neutrophils <500/mm^3 associated with fever or infection or lasting >7 days) or prolonged neutropenia (neutrophils ≥500/mm^3 to ≤1000/mm^3 lasting beyond day 21) or platelets <25,000/mm^3 or grades 3/4 diarrhea: Reduce dose to 1.9 mg/m^2/day for subsequent cycles (may consider same dosage reduction for grade 2 diarrhea if clinically indicated).

Dosing adjustment in renal impairment:

The FDA-approved labeling recommends the following dosage adjustment:

I.V.:

Cl$_{cr}$ 20-39 mL/minute: Reduce to 0.75 mg/m^2/dose

Cl$_{cr}$ <20 mL/minute: Insufficient data available for dosing recommendation

Note: For topotecan in combination with cisplatin for cervical cancer, do not initiate treatment in patients with serum creatinine >1.5 mg/dL; consider discontinuing treatment in patients with serum creatinine >1.5 mg/dL in subsequent cycles.

Oral:

Cl$_{cr}$ 30-49 mL/minute: Reduce dose to 1.8 mg/m^2/day

Cl$_{cr}$ <30 mL/minute: Insufficient data available for dosing recommendation

The following guidelines have been used by some clinicians:

Aronoff, 2007: *I.V.:*

Children:

Cl$_{cr}$ 30-50 mL/minute: Administer 75% of dose

Cl$_{cr}$ 10-29 mL/minute: Administer 50% of dose or reduce by 0.75 mg/m^2/dose

Cl$_{cr}$ <10 mL/minute: Administer 25% of dose

Hemodialysis: 0.75 mg/m^2

Continuous renal replacement therapy (CRRT): Administer 50% of dose or reduce by 0.75 mg/m^2/dose

Adults:

Cl$_{cr}$ >50 mL/minute: Administer 75% of dose

Cl$_{cr}$ 10-50 mL/minute: Administer 50% of dose

Cl$_{cr}$ <10 mL/minute: Administer 25% of dose

Hemodialysis: Avoid use

Continuous ambulatory peritoneal dialysis (CAPD): Avoid use

Continuous renal replacement therapy (CRRT): 0.75 mg/m^2

Kintzel, 1995:

Cl$_{cr}$ 46-60 mL/minute: Administer 80% of dose

Cl$_{cr}$ 31-45 mL/minute: Administer 75% of dose

Cl$_{cr}$ <30 mL/minute: Administer 70% of dose

Dosing adjustment in hepatic impairment:

The FDA-approved labeling recommends the following:

I.V.: Bilirubin 1.5-10 mg/dL: No adjustment necessary

Oral: Bilirubin >1.5 mg/dL: No adjustment necessary

Combination Regimens

Cervical cancer: Topotecan-Cisplatin on page 1407
Leukemia, acute lymphocytic: TVTG on page 1416
Leukemia, acute myeloid: TVTG on page 1416
Lung cancer, nonsmall cell: Topotecan (Oral Regimen) on page 1407
Lung cancer, small cell:
Topotecan (Oral Regimen) on page 1407

Administration

I.V.: Administer IVPB over 30 minutes or by 24-hour continuous infusion. For combination chemotherapy with cisplatin, administer pretreatment hydration.
Oral: Administer with or without food. Swallow whole; do not crush, chew, or divide capsule. If vomiting occurs after dose, do not take replacement dose.

Monitoring Parameters CBC with differential and platelet count, renal function tests, bilirubin

Test Interactions None known

Dietary Considerations May be taken with or without food.

Emetic Potential Moderate (30% to 90%)

Vesicant May be an irritant; inadvertent extravasation may result in mild erythema and bruising.

Dosage Forms Excipient information presented when available (limited, particularly for generics); consult specific product labeling.

Capsule:
Hycamtin®: 0.25 mg, 1 mg
Injection, powder for reconstitution:
Hycamtin®: 4 mg

References

Aronoff GR, Bennett WM, Berns JS, et al, *Drug Prescribing in Renal Failure: Dosing Guidelines for Adults and Children*, 5th ed. Philadelphia, PA: American College of Physicians; 2007, p 102, 174.

Craig SB, Bhatt UH, and Patel K, "Stability and Compatibility of Topotecan Hydrochloride for Injection With Common Infusion Solutions and Containers," *J Pharm Biomed Anal*, 1997, 16 (2):199-205.

Eckardt JR, von Pawel J, Pujol JL, et al, "Phase III Study of Oral Compared With Intravenous Topotecan as Second-Line Therapy in Small-Cell Lung Cancer," *J Clin Oncol*, 2007, 25 (15):2086-92.

Kintzel PE and Dorr RT, "Anticancer Drug Renal Toxicity and Elimination: Dosing Guidelines for Altered Renal Function," *Cancer Treat Rev*, 1995, 21(1):33-64.

Kruijtzer CMF, Beijnen JH, Rosing H, et al, "Increased Oral Bioavailability of Topotecan in Combination With the Breast Cancer Resistance Protein and P-Glycoprotein Inhibitor GF120918," *J Clin Oncol*, 2002, 20(13):2943-50.

Long HJ 3rd, Bundy BN, Grendys EC Jr, et al, "Randomized Phase III Trial of Cisplatin With or Without Topotecan in Carcinoma of the Uterine Cervix: a Gynecologic Oncology Group Study," *J Clin Oncol*, 2005, 23(21):4626-33.

O'Brien ME, Ciuleanu TE, Tsekov H, et al, "Phase III Trial Comparing Supportive Care Alone With Supportive Care With Oral Topotecan in Patients With Relapsed Small-Cell Lung Cancer," *J Clin Oncol*, 2006, 24(34):5441-7.

O'Reilly S, Rowinsky EK, Slichenmyer W, et al, "Phase I and Pharmacologic Study of Topotecan in Patients With Impaired Hepatic Function," *J Natl Cancer Inst*, 1996, 88(12):817-24.

O'Reilly S, Rowinsky EK, Slichenmyer W, et al, "Phase I and Pharmacologic Study of Topotecan in Patients With Impaired Renal Function," *J Clin Oncol*, 1996, 14(12):3062-73.

Patel K, Craig SB, McBride MG, et al, "Microbial Inhibitory Properties and Stability of Topotecan Hydrochloride Injection," *Am J Health Syst Pharm*, 1998, 55(15):1584-7.

◆ **Topotecan Hydrochloride** *see* Topotecan *on page 1116*

Toremifene (tore EM i feen)

Related Information
Safe Handling of Hazardous Drugs *on page 1517*

U.S. Brand Names Fareston®

Index Terms FC1157a; Toremifene Citrate

Generic Available No

Canadian Brand Names Fareston®

Pharmacologic Category Antineoplastic Agent, Estrogen Receptor Antagonist; Selective Estrogen Receptor Modulator (SERM)

Use Treatment of postmenopausal metastatic breast cancer (estrogen receptor positive or estrogen receptor status unknown)

Unlabeled/Investigational Use Treatment of soft tissue sarcoma (desmoid tumors)

Pregnancy Risk Factor D

Lactation Excretion in breast milk unknown/not recommended

Labeled Contraindications Hypersensitivity to toremifene or any component of the formulation

Warnings/Precautions Hazardous agent - use appropriate precautions for handling and disposal. Hypercalcemia and tumor flare have been reported during the first weeks of treatment in some breast cancer patients with bone metastases. Tumor flare is a syndrome of diffuse musculoskeletal pain and erythema with increased size of tumor lesions that later regress. It is often accompanied by hypercalcemia. Tumor flare does not imply treatment failure or represent tumor progression. Institute appropriate measures if hypercalcemia occurs, and if severe, discontinue treatment. Drugs that decrease renal calcium excretion (eg, thiazide diuretics) may increase the risk of hypercalcemia in patients receiving toremifene. Leukopenia and thrombocytopenia have been reported rarely. Endometrial hyperplasia has been reported; endometrial cancer has been reported, although a role of toremifene in endometrial cancer development has not been established. Use with caution in patients with hepatic failure. Avoid use in patients with thromboembolic disease.

Adverse Reactions

>10%:

Endocrine & metabolic: Hot flashes (35%)

Gastrointestinal: Nausea (14%)

Genitourinary: Vaginal discharge (13%)

Hepatic: Alkaline phosphatase increased (8% to 19%), AST increased (5% to 19%)

Miscellaneous: Diaphoresis (20%)

1% to 10%:

Cardiovascular: Edema (5%), arrhythmia (≤2%), CVA/TIA (≤2%), thrombosis (≤2%), cardiac failure (≤1%), MI (≤1%)

Central nervous system: Dizziness (9%)

Endocrine & metabolic: Hypercalcemia (≤3%)

Gastrointestinal: Vomiting (4%)

Genitourinary: Vaginal bleeding (2%)

Hepatic: Bilirubin increased (1% to 2%)

Local: Thrombophlebitis (≤2%)

Ocular: Cataracts (≤10%), xerophthalmia (≤9%), visual field abnormal (≤4%), corneal keratopathy (≤2%), glaucoma (≤2%), vision abnormal/diplopia (≤2%)

Respiratory: Pulmonary embolism (≤2%)

<1%, postmarketing, and/or case reports: Alopecia, angina, anorexia, arthritis, ataxia, constipation, corneal opacity (reversible), corneal verticulata, deep vein thrombosis, depression, dermatitis, dyspnea, endometrial cancer, endometrial hyperplasia, fatigue, hepatitis (toxic), incoordination, ischemic attack, jaundice, lethargy, leukopenia, paresis, pruritus, QT prolongation, retinopathy, rigors, skin discoloration, thrombocytopenia, thrombophlebitis, tremor, tumor flare, vaginal dryness, vertigo, weakness

Drug Interactions

Metabolism/Transport Effects Substrate of CYP1A2 (minor), 3A4 (major)

Avoid Concomitant Use

Avoid concomitant use of Toremifene with any of the following: Artemether; Dronedarone; Lumefantrine; Nilotinib; Pimozide; QuiNINE; Tetrabenazine; Thioridazine; Ziprasidone

Increased Effect/Toxicity

Toremifene may increase the levels/effects of: Dronedarone; Pimozide; QTc-Prolonging Agents; QuiNINE; Tetrabenazine; Thioridazine; Ziprasidone

The levels/effects of Toremifene may be increased by: Alfuzosin; Artemether; Chloroquine; Ciprofloxacin; Gadobutrol; Lumefantrine; Nilotinib; QuiNINE

Decreased Effect

The levels/effects of Toremifene may be decreased by: CYP3A4 Inducers (Strong); Deferasirox; Herbs (CYP3A4 Inducers)

Ethanol/Nutrition/Herb Interactions Herb/Nutraceutical: Avoid St John's wort (may decrease toremifene levels).

Storage/Stability Store at 25°C (77°F); excursions permitted to 15°C to 30°C (59°F to 86°F); protect from heat. Protect from light.

Mechanism of Action Nonsteroidal, triphenylethylene derivative with potent antiestrogenic properties (also has estrogenic effects). Competitively binds to estrogen receptors on tumors and other tissue targets, producing a nuclear complex that decreases DNA synthesis and inhibits estrogen effects. Competes with estrogen for binding sites in breast and other tissues; cells accumulate in the G_0 and G_1 phases; therefore, toremifene is cytostatic rather than cytocidal.

Pharmacodynamics/Kinetics

Absorption: Well absorbed

Distribution: V_d: 580 L (range: 457-958 L)

Protein binding, plasma: >99.5%, primarily to albumin

Metabolism: Extensively hepatic, principally by CYP3A4 to N-demethyltoremifene, which is also antiestrogenic but with weak *in vivo* antitumor potency

Half-life elimination: ~5 days

Time to peak, serum: ~3 hours (range: 2-6 hours)

Excretion: Primarily feces; urine (10%) during a 1-week period

Dosage Adults: Oral: 60 mg once daily, generally continued until disease progression is observed

Dosage adjustment in renal impairment: No dosage adjustment necessary

Dosage adjustment in hepatic impairment: Toremifene is extensively metabolized in the liver and dosage adjustments may be indicated in patients with liver disease; however, no specific guidelines have been developed

Administration Administer orally, as a single daily dose.

Monitoring Parameters Obtain periodic complete blood counts, calcium levels, and liver function tests. Closely monitor patients with bone metastases for hypercalcemia during the first few weeks of treatment. Leukopenia and thrombocytopenia have been reported rarely; monitor leukocyte and platelet counts during treatment.

Dosage Forms Excipient information presented when available (limited, particularly for generics); consult specific product labeling.

Tablet:

Fareston®: 60 mg

References

National Comprehensive Cancer Network (NCCN), "Clinical Practice Guidelines in Oncology™: Breast Cancer, Version 2.2008." Available at http://www.nccn.org/professionals/physician_gls/PDF/breast.pdf

National Comprehensive Cancer Network® (NCCN), "Clinical Practice Guidelines in Oncology™: Soft Tissue Sarcoma," Version 2.2009. Available at http://www.nccn.org/professionals/physician_gls/PDF/sarcoma.pdf

Osborne CK, Zhao H, and Fuqua SA, "Selective Estrogen Receptor Modulators: Structure, Function, and Clinical Use," *J Clin Oncol*, 2000, 18(17):3172-86.

Pagani O, Gelber S, Price K, et al, "Toremifene and Tamoxifen are Equally Effective for Early-Stage Breast Cancer: First Results of International Breast Cancer Study Group Trials 12-93 and 14-93," *Ann Oncol*, 2004, 15(12):1749-59.

Pyrhönen S, Valavaara R, Modig H, et al, "Comparison of Toremifene and Tamoxifen in Postmenopausal Patients With Advanced Breast Cancer: A Randomized Double-Blind, the "Nordic" Phase III Study," *Br J Cancer*, 1997, 76(2):270-7.

Taras TL, Wurz GT, Linares GR, et al, "Clinical Pharmacokinetics of Toremifene," *Clin Pharmacokinet*, 2000, 39(5):327-34.

◆ **Toremifene Citrate** see Toremifene *on page 1120*

◆ **Torisel®** see Temsirolimus *on page 1083*

◆ **Tositumomab I-131** see Tositumomab and Iodine I 131 Tositumomab *on page 1123*

Tositumomab and Iodine I 131 Tositumomab

(toe si TYOO mo mab & EYE oh dyne eye one THUR tee one toe si TYOO mo mab)

Medication Safety Issues

High alert medication: The Institute for Safe Medication Practices (ISMP) includes this medication among its list of drug classes which have a heightened risk of causing significant patient harm when used in error.

Related Information

Safe Handling of Hazardous Drugs *on page 1517*

U.S. Brand Names Bexxar®

Index Terms 131 I Anti-B1 Antibody; 131 I-Anti-B1 Monoclonal Antibody; Anti-CD20-Murine Monoclonal Antibody I-131; Iodine I 131 Tositumomab and Tositumomab; Tositumomab I-131

Generic Available No

Pharmacologic Category Antineoplastic Agent, Monoclonal Antibody; Radiopharmaceutical

Use Treatment of relapsed or refractory CD20 positive, low-grade, follicular, or transformed non-Hodgkin's lymphoma (NHL)

Unlabeled/Investigational Use First-line treatment of follicular NHL

Pregnancy Risk Factor X

Lactation Enters breast milk/not recommended

Labeled Contraindications Hypersensitivity to murine proteins or any component of the formulation; pregnancy

Warnings/Precautions Hazardous agent - use appropriate precautions for handling and disposal. **[U.S. Boxed Warning]: Hypersensitivity reactions (including anaphylaxis) have been reported; discontinue for severe reaction; medications for the treatment of reactions should be readily available in the event of severe reactions.** Patients should be screened for human antimouse antibodies (HAMA); patients positive for HAMA may be at increased risk of allergic or serious hypersensitivity reactions. **[U.S. Boxed Warning]: Severe neutropenia and thrombocytopenia are common; do not administer in patients with >25% lymphoma marrow involvement and/or impaired bone marrow reserve.** Hematologic toxicity is reported to be the most common adverse effect with 27% patients requiring supportive care; cytopenias may be prolonged and severe. The duration of severe hematologic toxicity may be prolonged in the elderly. Safety has not been established in patients with >25% lymphoma marrow involvement, platelet count <100,000 cells/mm^3, or neutrophil count <1500 cells/mm^3. Secondary malignancies have been reported following use.

[U.S. Boxed Warning]: Treatment involves radioactive isotopes and should only be administered by trained physicians and staff; appropriate precautions for handling and administration must be followed. Patients must be instructed in measures to minimize exposure of others. **[U.S. Boxed Warning]: May cause fetal harm if administered during pregnancy;** women of childbearing potential should be advised of potential fetal risk; effective contraceptive measures should be used during and for 12 months following treatment (males and females). Treatment may lead to hypothyroidism; patients should receive thyroid-blocking medications beginning at least 24 hours prior to the dosimetric dose and continued for 2 weeks after the therapeutic dose; evaluate for signs and symptoms of hypothyroidism; screen annually. Patients should be premedicated to prevent infusion-related reactions.

Safety has not been established in patients with renal impairment; excretion is primarily renal; impaired renal function may increase exposure. Safety and efficacy have not been established in children. The safety and efficacy of live vaccines in patients who have received therapy with tositumomab have not been established.

Adverse Reactions

>10%:

Central nervous system: Fever (37%), pain (19%), chills (18%), headache (16%)

Dermatologic: Rash (17%; grades 3/4: <1%)

Endocrine & metabolic: Hypothyroidism (7% to 19%)

Gastrointestinal: Nausea (36%), abdominal pain (15%), vomiting (15%), anorexia (14%), diarrhea (12%)

Hematologic: Myelosuppression (grades 3/4: 71%; nadir: 4-7 weeks; duration: 30 days [>90 days in 5% to 7% of patients]), neutropenia (grades 3/4: 63%; median duration: 31 days; grade 4: 25%), thrombocytopenia (grades 3/4: 53%; median duration: 32 days; grade 4: 21%), lymphocytopenia (recovery: ~12 weeks after treatment), anemia (grades 3/4: 29%; median duration: 23 days; grade 4: 5%), hemorrhage (12%)

Neuromuscular & skeletal: Weakness (46%), myalgia (13%)

Respiratory: Cough (21%), pharyngitis (12%), dyspnea (11%)

Miscellaneous: Infusion-related reactions (29%, occurred within 14 days of infusion, included bronchospasm, chills, dyspnea, fever, hypotension, nausea, rigors, diaphoresis), infection (21% to 45%; serious: 9%), HAMA-positive seroconversion (11% to 21%)

1% to 10%:

Cardiovascular: Hypotension (7%), peripheral edema (9%), chest pain (7%), vasodilation (5%)

Central nervous system: Dizziness (5%), somnolence (5%)

Dermatologic: Pruritus (10%)

Gastrointestinal: Constipation (6%), dyspepsia (6%), weight loss (6%)

Local: Injection site hypersensitivity

Neuromuscular & skeletal: Arthralgia (10%), back pain (8%), neck pain (6%)

Respiratory: Rhinitis (10%), pneumonia (6%)

Miscellaneous: Diaphoresis (8%), hypersensitivity reaction (6%), secondary leukemia/myelodysplastic syndrome (overall: 4% at 29-month median follow up; 6% to 15% with 5-year follow up), secondary malignancies

<1%, postmarketing, and/or case reports: Anaphylactic reaction, angioedema, bacteremia, bronchitis, dehydration, flu-like syndrome, herpes virus infection, laryngismus, pleural effusion, septicemia, serum sickness, skin infections

Drug Interactions

Avoid Concomitant Use

Avoid concomitant use of Tositumomab and Iodine I 131 Tositumomab with any of the following: Natalizumab; Vaccines (Live)

Increased Effect/Toxicity

Tositumomab and Iodine I 131 Tositumomab may increase the levels/effects of: Leflunomide; Natalizumab; Vaccines (Live); Vitamin K Antagonists

The levels/effects of Tositumomab and Iodine I 131 Tositumomab may be increased by: Anticoagulants; Antiplatelet Agents; Trastuzumab

Decreased Effect

Tositumomab and Iodine I 131 Tositumomab may decrease the levels/effects of: Cardiac Glycosides; Vaccines (Inactivated); Vaccines (Live); Vitamin K Antagonists

The levels/effects of Tositumomab and Iodine I 131 Tositumomab may be decreased by: Echinacea

Storage/Stability

Tositumomab: Store under refrigeration at 2°C to 8°C (36°F to 46°F); do not freeze. Protect from strong light. Following dilution, tositumomab is stable for 24 hour when refrigerated or 8 hours at room temperature.

Iodine I 131 tositumomab: Store frozen at less than or equal to -20°C in the original lead pots. Allow 60 minutes for thawing at ambient temperature. Thawed doses are stable for up to 8 hours at 2°C to 8°C (36°F to 46°F) or room temperature. Solutions diluted for infusion should be refrigerated prior to administration; do not freeze.

Reconstitution

Tositumomab: Withdraw and discard 32 mL of saline from a 50 mL bag of NS. Add contents of both 225 mg vials of tositumomab (total 32 mL) to remaining NS to make a final volume of 50 mL. Gently mix by inverting bag; do not shake.

Iodine I 131 tositumomab: Calculate volume required for an iodine I 131 tositumomab activity of 5 mCi (specification sheet provided with product). If the amount of tositumomab contained in the iodine I 131 tositumomab solution contains <35 mg of tositumomab, use the 35 mg vial of tositumomab to prepare a final concentration of tositumomab 35 mg. Using NS, the final volume should equal 30 mL.

Mechanism of Action Tositumomab is a murine IgG_{2a} lambda monoclonal antibody which binds to the CD20 antigen, expressed on B-lymphocytes and on >90% of B-cell non-Hodgkin's lymphomas. Iodine I 131 tositumomab is a radio-iodinated derivative of tositumomab covalently linked to iodine 131. The possible actions of the regimen include apoptosis, complement-dependent cytotoxicity, antibody-dependent cellular cytotoxicity, and radiation-induced cell death. Administration results in depletion of CD20 positive cells.

Pharmacodynamics/Kinetics Note: Iodine-131 elimination occurs by decay and urinary excretion; after 5 days total body clearance is 67% of a dose.

Distribution: Tositumomab: V_d increased with high tumor burden, splenomegaly, or bone marrow involvement

◄

Half-life elimination: Tositumomab: 67 hours (range: 28-115 hours); decreased with high tumor burden, splenomegaly, or bone marrow involvement

Dosage I.V.: Adults: NHL: Dosing consists of four components administered in 2 steps. Refer to manufacturer's labeling for additional details. Thyroid protective agents (SSKI, Lugol's solution or potassium iodide) should be administered beginning at least 24 hours prior to step 1 (Refer to Additional Information). Premedicate with acetaminophen 650 mg and diphenhydramine 50 mg orally prior to step 1 and step 2.

Step 1: Dosimetric step (Day 0):
Tositumomab 450 mg in NS 50 mL administered over 60 minutes
Iodine I 131 tositumomab (containing I-131 5 mCi and tositumomab 35 mg) in NS 30 mL administered over 20 minutes

Note: Whole body dosimetry and biodistribution should be determined on Day 0; days 2, 3, or 4; and day 6 or 7 prior to administration of Step 2. If biodistribution is not acceptable, do not administer the therapeutic step. On day 6 or 7, calculate the patient specific activity of iodine I 131 tositumomab to deliver 75 cGy TBD or 65 cGy TBD (in mCi).

Step 2: Therapeutic step (one dose administered 7-14 days after step 1):
Tositumomab 450 mg in NS 50 mL administered over 60 minutes
Iodine I 131 tositumomab:
Platelets ≥150,000/mm^3: Iodine I 131 calculated to deliver 75 cGy total body irradiation and tositumomab 35 mg over 20 minutes
Platelets ≥100,000/mm^3 and <150,000/mm^3: Iodine I 131 calculated to deliver 65 cGy total body irradiation and tositumomab 35 mg over 20 minutes

Dosage adjustment for toxicity: Infusion-related toxicity (with tositumomab or iodine I-131 tositumomab):
Mild-to-moderate: Reduce infusion rate by 50%
Severe: Interrupt infusion; after complete resolution, resume with infusion rate reduced by 50%

Administration I.V.: Refer to manufacturer's labeling for additional details.
Tositumomab: Infuse over 60 minutes
Iodine I 131 tositumomab: Infuse over 20 minutes
Administer via an I.V. tubing set with an in-line 0.22 micron filter; pre-prime tubing and wet 0.22 micron filter with NS; do not change primary infusion set or filter at any time during the dosimetric or therapeutic step; changing the filter may result in up to a 7% loss of the iodine I 131 tositumomab dose (use the same infusion set and filter for tositumomab and iodine I 131 tositumomab; flush with NS in between).
Reduce the rate of tositumomab or iodine 131 tositumomab infusion by 50% for mild-to-moderate infusion-related toxicities; interrupt for severe toxicity. Once severe toxicity has resolved, infusion may be restarted at half the previous rate. Prior to infusion, patients should be premedicated (with acetaminophen and an antihistamine) and a thyroid-protective agent should be started.

Monitoring Parameters CBC with differential (baseline and weekly for 10-12 weeks, or longer for persistent severe cytopenia); signs and symptoms of hypothyroidism, TSH (prior to therapy and yearly); serum creatinine (immediately prior to administration)
Following infusion of the iodine I 131 tositumomab dosimetric dose, the total body gamma camera counts and whole body images should be taken within 1 hour of the infusion and prior to urination, and 2-4 days after the infusion and following urination, and 6-7 days after the infusion and following urination.

Test Interactions May interfere with tests using murine antibody technology.

Additional Information Thyroid protective agent: One of the following agents should be used starting at least 24 hours prior to the dosimetric dose and continued for 2 weeks after the therapeutic dose. Therapy should not begin without using one of the following agents 24 hours prior to Step 1:

SSKI: 4 drops 3 times/day

Lugol's solution: 20 drops 3 times/day

Potassium iodide: 130 mg once daily

Oncology Comment: Tositumomab and iodine I 131 tositumomab radioimmunotherapy has been studied for use as initial therapy in the treatment of follicular lymphoma and demonstrated a high overall survival rate; patients with complete responses have a 5-year progression free survival rate of 77% (Kaminski, 2005 [NEJM]). Tositumomab and iodine I 131 tositumomab has also been studied as front-line therapy following 6 cycles of CHOP chemotherapy for follicular lymphoma; high overall response and survival rates were demonstrated in this trial (Press, 2006). In a small study of patients with NHL who had previously responded (partial, clinical or complete response) to tositumomab and iodine I 131 tositumomab, 18 of 28 patients completing the therapeutic regimen responded to retreatment with tositumomab and iodine I 131 tositumomab (Kaminski, 2005 [JCO]).

Dosage Forms Excipient information presented when available (limited, particularly for generics); consult specific product labeling.

Note: Not all components are shipped from the same facility. When ordering, ensure that all will arrive on the same day.

Kit [dosimetric package]: Tositumomab 225 mg/16.1 mL [2 vials], tositumomab 35 mg/2.5 mL [1 vial], and iodine I 131 tositumomab 0.1 mg/mL and 0.61mCi/mL (20 mL) [1 vial]

Kit [therapeutic package]: Tositumomab 225 mg/16.1 mL [2 vials], tositumomab 35 mg/2.5 mL [1 vial], and iodine I 131 tositumomab 1.1 mg/mL and 5.6 mCi/mL (20 mL) [1 or 2 vials]

References

Kaminski MS, Radford JA, Gregory S, et al, "Re-Treatment With I-131 Tositumomab in Patients With Non-Hodgkin's Lymphoma Who Had Previously Responded to I-131 Tositumomab," *J Clin Oncol,* 2005, 23(31):7985-93.

Kaminski MS, Tuck M, Estes J, et al, "131I-Tositumomab Therapy as Initial Treatment for Follicular Lymphoma," *N Engl J Med,* 2005, 352(5):441-9.

Kaminski MS, Zelenetz AD, Press OW, et al, "Pivotal Study of Iodine I 131 Tositumomab for Chemotherapy-Refractory Low-Grade or Transformed Low-Grade B-Cell Non-Hodgkin's Lymphomas," *J Clin Oncol,* 2001, 19(19):3918-28.

National Comprehensive Cancer Network (NCCN®), "Clinical Practice Guidelines in Oncology™: Non-Hodgkin's Lymphomas," Version 2.2009. Available at http://www.nccn.org/professionals/physician_gls/PDF/nhl.pdf

Press OW, Eary JF, Appelbaum FR, et al, "Phase I Trial of 131I-B1 (Anti-CD20) Antibody Therapy With Autologous Stem Cell Transplantation for Relapsed B Cell Lymphomas," *Lancet,* 1995, 346 (8971):336-40.

Press OW, Unger JM, Braziel RM, et al, "Phase II Trial of CHOP Chemotherapy Followed by Tositumomab/Iodine I-131 Tositumomab for Previously Untreated Follicular Non-Hodgkin's Lymphoma: Five-Year Follow-up of Southwest Oncology Group Protocol S9911," *J Clin Oncol,* 2006, 24(25):4143-9.

◆ **Totect™** *see* Dexrazoxane *on page* 357

◆ **tPA** *see* Alteplase *on page* 41

◆ **tRA** *see* Tretinoin, Systemic *on page* 1141

Trabectedin (tra BEK te din)

Medication Safety Issues

High alert medication: The Institute for Safe Medication Practices (ISMP) ▶

includes this class of medications among its list of medications which have a heightened risk of causing significant patient harm when used in error.

Index Terms Ecteinascidin; Ecteinascidin 743; ET-743; Yondelis

Pharmacologic Category Antineoplastic Agent, Miscellaneous

Use Not approved for use in the U.S.; used investigationally and approved internationally for the treatment of refractory soft tissue sarcoma

Restrictions Not available in U.S.

Labeled Contraindications Hypersensitivity to trabectedin or any component of the formulation. Avoid use with concurrent serious or uncontrolled infection, breast-feeding, or with concurrent administration of yellow fever vaccine

Warnings/Precautions Hazardous agent - use appropriate precautions for handling and disposal. Use is not recommended in patients with elevated bilirubin. Systemic exposure and the risk for hepatotoxicity is increased in patients with hepatic impairment. Patient with active chronic hepatitis or other clinically significant liver disease should be monitored closely. Reversible increases in transaminases may occur; may require dosage modification.

Neutropenia and thrombocytopenia are common; may be severe and/or dose-limiting. Rhabdomyolysis has been reported with use rarely, usually in association with myelosuppression, severe liver impairment, or renal failure (not recommended for use if CPK >2.5 times upper limit of normal [ULN]). Use is not recommended in patients with Cl_{cr} <30 mL/minute.

HMG-CoA reductase inhibitors may increase the risk for rhabdomyolysis when used in combination with trabectedin. Concurrent use of trabectedin with phenytoin is not recommended; may reduce phenytoin absorption and increase the risk for seizure. Concurrent use of trabectedin with antiemetic regimens containing dexamethasone have been reported to increase the trabectedin AUC; concurrent use is recommended however, due to the hepatoprotective and antiemetic effect of dexamethasone. Patients should not be immunized with live viral vaccines during or shortly after treatment; concurrent administration of yellow fever vaccine is contraindicated. Central line administration is recommended; peripheral administration may cause severe injection site reactions.

Adverse Reactions Note: Toxicities associated with trabectedin are generally reversible and not cumulative.

Frequency not defined:

Cardiovascular: Edema, flushing, hypotension, peripheral edema

Central nervous system: Dizziness, fatigue, fever, headache, insomnia

Dermatologic: Alopecia

Endocrine & metabolic: Albumin decreased, dehydration, hypokalemia

Gastrointestinal: Abdominal pain, anorexia, appetite decreased, constipation, diarrhea, dyspepsia, nausea, stomatitis, taste alteration, vomiting, weight loss

Hematologic: Anemia, leukopenia, neutropenia, neutropenic fever, thrombocytopenia

Hepatic: Alkaline phosphatase increased, ALT increased, AST increased, bilirubin increased, GGT increased, hepatomegaly, jaundice, liver pain

Local: Injection pain, injection site reaction, phlebitis

Neuromuscular & skeletal: Arthralgia, back pain, creatine phosphokinase increased, myalgia, paresthesia, peripheral neuropathy, rhabdomyolysis, weakness

Renal: Acute renal failure, creatinine increased

Respiratory: Cough, dyspnea

Miscellaneous: Allergy, infection, septic shock

Storage/Stability Store intact vials under refrigeration.

Mechanism of Action A marine-derived compound which blocks the cell cycle at the G_2/M phase by covalently binding to the minor DNA groove, bending the helix toward the major groove and altering DNA transcription. Also alters DNA repair mechanism.

Dosage Note: Neutrophils should be ≥1500/mm^3 and platelets should be ≥100,000/mm^3 prior to initiating treatment (delay treatment for up to 2 weeks to allow for recovery). Premedication with dexamethasone is recommended for hepatoprotective and antiemetic effects; antiemetic regimens also usually included a 5HT$_3$ receptor antagonist.

I.V.: Adults: Soft tissue sarcoma (unlabeled/investigational use): 1.5 mg/m^2 over 24 hours every 3 weeks (Yovine, 2004)

Dosage adjustment for toxicity: The following dosage adjustments for toxicity were used in clinical trials (Yovine, 2004; Garcia-Carbonero, 2005):

Febrile neutropenia, infection, grade 4 neutropenia lasting ≥5 days or grade 4 thrombocytopenia: Reduce dose to 1.2 mg/m^2 over 24 hours every 3 weeks

Cardiac or neurologic toxicity grade 2, or other nonhematologic toxicity ≥ grade 3 lasting >21 days: Reduce dose to 1.2 mg/m^2 over 24 hours every 3 weeks

Recurrent severe toxicity: Further reduce dose to 1 mg/m^2 over 24 hours every 3 weeks

Cardiac or neurologic toxicity ≥ grade 3 lasting >35 days: Discontinue treatment

Dosage adjustment in renal impairment: Cl$_{cr}$ <30 mL/minute: Use is not recommended

Dosage adjustment in hepatic impairment:

AST, AST, alkaline phophatase >2.5 x ULN or bilirubin >ULN: Use is not recommended; **Note:**Some studies excluded patients for alkaline phosphatase >ULN.

The following dosage adjustments for hepatotoxicity were used in clinical trials (Yovine, 2004; Garcia-Carbonero, 2005):

Bilirubin or alkaline phosphatase elevation ≥ grade 1: Reduce dose to 1.2 mg/m^2 over 24 hours every 3 weeks

ALT or AST elevation of any grade lasting 21-35 days: Reduce dose to 1.2 mg/m^2 over 24 hours every 3 weeks

ALT or AST elevation of any grade lasting ≥35 days: Discontinue treatment

Administration Infuse as a continuous infusion through a central line over 24 hours. Antiemetic prophylaxis was utilized in clinical trials.

Monitoring Parameters CBC with differential, liver function, renal function, creatine kinase

References

Garcia-Carbonero R, Supko JG, Maki RG, et al, "Ecteinascidin-743 (ET-743) for Chemotherapy-Naive Patients With Advanced Soft Tissue Sarcomas: Multicenter Phase II and Pharmacokinetic Study," *J Clin Oncol*, 2005, 23(24):5484-92.

Le Cesne A, Blay JY, Judson I, et al, "Phase II Study of ET-743 in Advanced Soft Tissue Sarcomas: A European Organisation for the Research and Treatment of Cancer (EORTC) Soft Tissue and Bone Sarcoma Group Trial," *J Clin Oncol*, 2005, 23(3):576-84.

National Comprehensive Cancer Network® (NCCN), "Clinical Practice Guidelines in Oncology™: Soft Tissue Sarcoma," Version 1.2009. Available at http://www.nccn.org/professionals/physician_gls/PDF/sarcoma.pdf

Yovine A, Riofrio M, Blay JY, et al, "Phase II Study of Ecteinascidin-743 in Advanced Pretreated Soft Tissue Sarcoma Patients," *J Clin Oncol*, 2004, 22(5):890-9.

TraMADol (TRA ma dole)

Medication Safety Issues

Sound-alike/look-alike issues:

TraMADol may be confused with tapentadol, Toradol®, Trandate®, traZODone, Voltaren®

Ultram® may be confused with Ultane®, Ultracet®, Voltaren®

International issues:

Theradol® [Netherlands] may be confused with Foradil® which is a brand name for formoterol in the U.S.

Theradol® [Netherlands] may be confused with Terazol® which is a brand name for terconazole in the U.S.

Theradol® [Netherlands] may be confused with Toradol® which is a brand name for ketorolac in the U.S.

U.S. Brand Names Ryzolt™; Ultram®; Ultram® ER

Index Terms Tramadol Hydrochloride

Generic Available Yes: Excludes extended release tablet

Canadian Brand Names Ralivia™ ER; Tridural™; Zytram® XL

Pharmacologic Category Analgesic, Opioid

Use Relief of moderate to moderately-severe pain

Extended release formulations are indicated for patients requiring around-the-clock management of moderate to moderately-severe pain for an extended period of time

Pregnancy Risk Factor C

Lactation Enters breast milk/not recommended

Labeled Contraindications Hypersensitivity to tramadol, opioids, or any component of the formulation; opioid-dependent patients; acute intoxication with alcohol, hypnotics, centrally-acting analgesics, opioids, or psychotropic drugs

Additional contraindications for Ryzolt™: Severe/acute bronchial asthma, hypercapnia, or significant respiratory depression in the absence of appropriately monitored setting and/or resuscitative equipment

Note: Based on Canadian product labeling:

Tramadol is contraindicated during or within 14 days following MAO inhibitor therapy

Extended release formulations (Ralivia™ ER [CAN], Tridural™[CAN], and Zytram® XL [CAN]): Additional contraindications: Severe (Cl_{cr} <30 mL/minute) renal dysfunction, severe (Child-Pugh class C) hepatic dysfunction

Warnings/Precautions Rare but serious anaphylactoid reactions (including fatalities) often following initial dosing have been reported. Pruritus, hives, bronchospasm, angioedema, toxic epidermal necrolysis (TEN) and Stevens-Johnson syndrome also have been reported with use. Previous anaphylactoid reactions to opioids may increase risks for similar reactions to tramadol. Caution patients to swallow extended release tablets whole. Rapid release and absorption of tramadol from extended release tablets that are broken, crushed, or chewed may lead to a potentially lethal overdose. May cause CNS depression, which may impair physical or mental abilities; patients must be cautioned about performing tasks which require mental alertness (eg, operating machinery or driving). May cause CNS depression and/or respiratory depression, particularly when combined with other CNS depressants. Use with caution and reduce dosage when administered to patients receiving other CNS depressants. An increased risk of seizures may occur in patients receiving serotonin reuptake inhibitors (SSRIs or anorectics), tricyclic antidepressants, other cyclic compounds (including cyclobenzaprine, promethazine), neuro-leptics, or drugs which may lower seizure threshold. Patients with a history of seizures, or with a risk of seizures (head trauma, metabolic disorders, CNS infection, or malignancy, or during ethanol/drug withdrawal) are also at increased risk. Avoid use with serotonergic agents such as TCAs, MAO inhibitors (contraindicated in Canadian product labeling), triptans, venlafaxine, trazodone, lithium, sibutramine, meperidine, dextromethorphan, St John's wort, SNRIs and SSRIs; concomitant use has been associated with the development of serotonin syndrome.

Elderly (particularly >75 years of age), debilitated patients and patients with chronic respiratory disorders may be at greater risk of adverse events. Use with caution in patients with increased intracranial pressure or head injury. Avoid use in patients who are suicidal or addiction prone. Healthcare provider should be alert to problems of abuse, misuse, and diversion. Use caution in heavy alcohol users. Use caution in treatment of acute abdominal conditions; may mask pain. Use tramadol with caution and reduce dosage in patients with liver disease or renal dysfunction. Avoid using extended release tablets in severe hepatic impairment. Do not use Ryzolt™ in any degree of hepatic impairment. Tolerance or drug dependence may result from extended use (withdrawal symptoms have been reported); abrupt discontinuation should be avoided. Tapering of dose at the time of discontinuation limits the risk of withdrawal symptoms. Safety and efficacy in pediatric patients have not been established.

Adverse Reactions

>10%:
Cardiovascular: Flushing (8% to 16%)
Central nervous system: Dizziness (10% to 33%), headache (4% to 32%), somnolence (7% to 25%), insomnia (2% to 11%)
Dermatologic: Pruritus (5% to 12%)
Gastrointestinal: Constipation (10% to 46%), nausea (15% to 40%), vomiting (5% to 17%), dyspepsia (1% to 13%)
Neuromuscular & skeletal: Weakness (4% to 12%)

1% to 10%:
Cardiovascular: Postural hypotension (2% to 5%), chest pain (1% to <5%), vasodilation (1% to <5%)
Central nervous system: Anxiety (1% to <5%), confusion (1% to <5%), coordination impaired (1% to <5%), depression (1% to <5%), euphoria (1% to <5%), hypoesthesia (1% to <5%), lethargy (1% to <5%), nervousness (1% to <5%), pain (1% to <5%), pyrexia (1% to <5%), restlessness (1% to <5%), malaise (<1% to <5%), fatigue (2%), vertigo (2%)
Dermatologic: Dermatitis (1% to <5%), rash (1% to <5%)
Endocrine & metabolic: Hot flashes (2% to 9%), menopausal symptoms (1% to <5%)
Gastrointestinal: Diarrhea (5% to 10%), xerostomia (3% to 10%), anorexia (1% to <6%), abdominal pain (1% to <5%), appetite decreased (1% to <5%), weight loss (1% to <5%), flatulence (<1% to <5%)
Genitourinary: Urinary tract infection (1% to <5%), urinary frequency (<1% to <5%), urinary retention (<1% to <5%)
Neuromuscular & skeletal: Arthralgia (1% to <5%), back pain (1% to <5%), hypertonia (1% to <5%), rigors (1% to <5%), paresthesia (1% to <5%), tremor (1% to <5%), creatine phosphokinase increased (1% to <5%)
Ocular: Blurred vision (1% to <5%), miosis (1% to <5%)
Respiratory: Bronchitis (1% to <5%), congestion (nasal/sinus) (1% to <5%), cough (1% to <5%), dyspnea (1% to <5%), nasopharyngitis (1% to <5%),

rhinorrhea (1% to <5%), sinusitis (1% to <5%), sneezing (1% to <5%), sore throat (1% to <5%), upper respiratory infection (1% to <5%)

Miscellaneous: Diaphoresis (2% to 9%), flu-like syndrome (1% to < 5%), shivering (<1% to <5%)

<1% (Limited to important or life-threatening): Abnormal ECG, abnormal gait, agitation, allergic reaction, amnesia, anaphylactoid reactions, anaphylaxis, anemia, angioedema, appendicitis, ALT increased/decreased, AST increased/decreased, bradycardia, bronchospasm, cataracts, cellulitis, cholecystitis, cholelithiasis, clamminess, cognitive dysfunction, concentration difficulty, creatinine increased, deafness, disorientation, diverticulitis, dreams abnormal, dysphagia, dysuria, ear infection, edema, fecal impaction, gastroenteritis, gastrointestinal bleeding, hallucination, hematuria, hemoglobin decreased, hepatitis, hyperglycemia, hyper-/hypotension, hypersensitivity, irritability, joint stiffness, libido decreased, liver enzymes increased, liver failure, menstrual disorder, MI, migraine, muscle cramps, muscle spasms, muscle twitching, myalgia, myocardial ischemia, night sweats, orthostatic hypotension, palpitation, pancreatitis, peripheral edema, peripheral ischemia, pneumonia, proteinuria, pulmonary edema, pulmonary embolism, sedation, seizure, serotonin syndrome, sleep disorder, speech disorder, Stevens-Johnson syndrome, stomatitis, suicidal tendency, syncope, taste perversion, tachycardia, thrombocytopenia, tinnitus, toxic epidermal necrolysis, urticaria, vesicles, visual disturbance

A withdrawal syndrome may occur with abrupt discontinuation; includes anxiety, diarrhea, hallucinations (rare), nausea, pain, piloerection, rigors, sweating, and tremor. Uncommon discontinuation symptoms may include severe anxiety, panic attacks, or paresthesia.

Drug Interactions

Metabolism/Transport Effects Substrate of CYP2D6 (major), 3A4 (major)

Avoid Concomitant Use

Avoid concomitant use of TraMADol with any of the following: Sibutramine

Increased Effect/Toxicity

TraMADol may increase the levels/effects of: Alcohol (Ethyl); CNS Depressants; MAO Inhibitors; Methotrimeprazine; Selective Serotonin Reuptake Inhibitors; Serotonin Modulators

The levels/effects of TraMADol may be increased by: CYP3A4 Inhibitors (Moderate); CYP3A4 Inhibitors (Strong); Dasatinib; Methotrimeprazine; Selective Serotonin Reuptake Inhibitors; Sibutramine; Tricyclic Antidepressants

Decreased Effect

The levels/effects of TraMADol may be decreased by: CYP2D6 Inhibitors (Moderate); CYP2D6 Inhibitors (Strong); CYP3A4 Inducers (Strong); Deferasirox

Ethanol/Nutrition/Herb Interactions

Ethanol: Avoid ethanol (may increase CNS depression).

Food:

Immediate release: Does not affect the rate or extent of absorption.

Extended release: Reduced C_{max} and AUC and T_{max} occurred 3 hours earlier when taken with a high-fat meal.

Ryzolt™: Increased C_{max}; no effect on AUC.

Herb/Nutraceutical: Avoid valerian, St John's wort, kava kava, gotu kola (may increase CNS depression).

Storage/Stability Store at controlled room temperature of 25°C (77°F).

Mechanism of Action Tramadol and its active metabolite (M1) binds to μ-opiate receptors in the CNS causing inhibition of ascending pain pathways, altering the perception of and response to pain; also inhibits the reuptake of norepinephrine and serotonin, which also modifies the ascending pain pathway

Pharmacodynamics/Kinetics

Onset of action: Immediate release: ~1 hour

Duration: 9 hours

Absorption: Immediate release formulation: Rapid and complete; Extended release formulation: Delayed

Distribution: V_d: 2.5-3 L/kg

Protein binding, plasma: 20%

Metabolism: Extensively hepatic via demethylation (mediated by CYP3A4 and CYP2B6), glucuronidation, and sulfation; has pharmacologically active metabolite formed by CYP2D6 (M1; O-desmethyl tramadol)

Bioavailability: Immediate release: 75%; Extended release: Ultram® ER: 85% to 90% (as compared to immediate release), Zytram® XL, Tridural™: 70%, Ryzolt™: ~95% (as compared to immediate release)

Half-life elimination: Tramadol: ~6-8 hours; Active metabolite: 7-9 hours; prolonged in elderly, hepatic or renal impairment; Zytram® XL: ~16 hours; Ralivia™ ER, Ryzolt™, Tridural™: ~5-9 hours

Time to peak: Immediate release: ~2 hours; Extended release: Ultram® ER: ~12 hours, Ryzolt™, Tridural™: ~4 hours

Excretion: Urine (30% as unchanged drug; 60% as metabolites)

Dosage Oral: Moderate-to-severe pain:

Children ≥17 years and Adults: Immediate release formulation: 50-100 mg every 4-6 hours (not to exceed 400 mg/day)

For patients not requiring rapid onset of effect, tolerability may be improved by starting dose at 25 mg/day and titrating dose by 25 mg every 3 days, until reaching 25 mg 4 times/day. The total daily dose may then be increased by 50 mg every 3 days as tolerated, to reach dose of 50 mg 4 times/day. After titration, 50-100 mg may be given every 4-6 hours as needed up to a maximum 400 mg/day.

Adults: Extended release formulations:

Ultram® ER:

Patients not currently on immediate-release: 100 mg once daily; titrate every 5 days (maximum: 300 mg/day)

Patients currently on immediate-release: Calculate 24-hour immediate release total dose and initiate total extended release daily dose (round dose to the next lowest 100 mg increment); titrate (maximum: 300 mg/day)

Ralivia™ ER (Canadian labeling, not available in U.S.): 100 mg once daily; titrate every 5 days as needed based on clinical response and severity of pain (maximum: 300 mg/day)

Ryzolt™:

Patients not currently on immediate-release: 100 mg once daily; titrate every 2-3 days by 100 mg/day increments; usual daily dose: 200-300 mg/day (maximum: 300 mg/day)

Patients currently on immediate-release: Calculate 24 hour immediate release total dose and initiate total extended release daily dose (round dose to the next lowest 100 mg increment); titrate (maximum: 300 mg/day)

Tridural™ (Canadian labeling, not available in U.S.): 100 mg once daily; titrate by 100 mg/day every 2 days as needed based on clinical response and severity of pain (maximum: 300 mg/day)

◄ Zytram® XL (Canadian labeling, not available in U.S.): 150 mg once daily; if pain relief is not achieved may titrate by increasing dosage incrementally, with sufficient time to evaluate effect of increased dosage; generally not more often than every 7 days (maximum: 400 mg/day)

Elderly >65 years: Use caution and initiate at the lower end of the dosing range

Immediate release: Elderly >75 years: Do not exceed 300 mg/day; see dosing adjustments for renal and hepatic impairment.

Extended release formulation: Elderly >75 years: Use with great caution. See adult, renal, and hepatic dosing.

Dosing adjustment in renal impairment:

Immediate release: Cl_{cr} <30 mL/minute: Administer 50-100 mg dose every 12 hours (maximum: 200 mg/day)

Extended release: Should not be used in patients with Cl_{cr} <30 mL/minute

Dosing adjustment in hepatic impairment:

Immediate release: Cirrhosis: Recommended dose: 50 mg every 12 hours

Extended release: Should not be used in patients with severe (Child-Pugh class C) hepatic dysfunction; Ryzolt™ should not be used in any degree of hepatic impairment

Administration Extended release tablet: Swallow whole; do not crush, chew, or split

Monitoring Parameters Pain relief, respiratory rate, blood pressure, and pulse; signs of tolerance or abuse

Dietary Considerations May be taken with or without food. Ultram® ER: Be consistent; always give with food or always give on an empty stomach.

Dosage Forms Excipient information presented when available (limited, particularly for generics); consult specific product labeling. [CAN] = Canadian brand name

Tablet, as hydrochloride: 50 mg

Ultram®: 50 mg

Tablet, extended release, as hydrochloride:

Ultram® ER: 100 mg, 200 mg, 300 mg

Ralivia™ ER [CAN]: 100 mg, 200 mg, 300 mg [not available in the U.S.]

Ryzolt™: 100 mg, 200 mg, 300 mg

Tridural™ [CAN]: 100 mg, 200 mg, 300 mg [not available in the U.S.]

Zytram® XL [CAN]: 150 mg, 200 mg, 300 mg, 400 mg [not available in the U.S.]

References

"Drugs for Pain," *Treat Guidel Med Lett*, 2004, 2(23):47-54.

Kahn LH, Alderfer RJ, and Graham DJ, "Seizures Reported With Tramadol," *JAMA*, 1997, 278 (20):1661.

Rauck RL, Ruoff GE, and McGillen, "Comparison of Tramadol and Acetaminophen With Codeine for Long-Term Pain Management in Elderly Patients," *Curr Ther Res*, 1994, 556:1417-31.

Ruoff GE, "Slowing the Initial Titration Rate of Tramadol Improves Tolerability," *Pharmacotherapy*, 1999, 19(1):88-93.

◆ **Tramadol Hydrochloride** see TraMADol on page 1130

Tranexamic Acid (tran eks AM ik AS id)

Medication Safety Issues

Sound-alike/look-alike issues:

Cyklokapron® may be confused with cycloSPORINE

U.S. Brand Names Cyklokapron®

Generic Available No

Canadian Brand Names Cyklokapron®; Tranexamic Acid Injection BP

Pharmacologic Category Antifibrinolytic Agent; Antihemophilic Agent; Hemostatic Agent; Lysine Analog

Use Short-term use (2-8 days) in hemophilia patients to reduce or prevent hemorrhage and reduce need for replacement therapy during and following tooth extraction

Pregnancy Risk Factor B

Lactation Enters breast milk/use caution

Labeled Contraindications Acquired defective color vision; active intravascular clotting; subarachnoid hemorrhage

Warnings/Precautions Venous and arterial thrombosis or thromboembolism, including central retinal artery/vein obstruction, has been reported. Use with caution in patients with thromboembolic disease. Use with caution in patients with upper urinary tract bleeding, ureteral obstruction due to clot formation has been reported. Use with extreme caution in patients with DIC requiring antifibrinolytic therapy; patients should be under strict supervision of a physician experienced in treating this disorder. Use with caution in patients with uncorrected cardiovascular or cerebrovascular disease due to complications of thrombosis. Concurrent use with anti-inhibitor coagulant complex/factor IX complex concentrates is not recommended due to the increased risk of thrombosis.

Visual defects (eg, color vision change, visual loss) have been reported; in patients being treated for longer than several days, ophthalmic examination recommended at baseline and regular intervals during the course of therapy; discontinue treatment if changes in ophthalmic examination occur. Use is contraindicated in patients with acquired defective color vision since this would prohibit monitoring one endpoint as a measure of ophthalmic toxicity. Use with caution in patients with renal impairment; dosage modification may be required.

Adverse Reactions

Frequency not defined:

Cardiovascular: Hypotension (with rapid I.V. injection)

Endocrine & metabolic: Unusual menstrual discomfort

Gastrointestinal: Diarrhea, nausea, vomiting

Ocular: Blurred vision

Postmarketing and/or case reports: Cerebral thrombosis, deep venous thrombosis (DVT), postoperative visual loss, pulmonary embolus (PE), renal cortical necrosis, retinal artery obstruction, retinal vein obstruction, ureteral obstruction, visual disturbances (defective color vision)

Drug Interactions

Avoid Concomitant Use

Avoid concomitant use of Tranexamic Acid with any of the following: Anti-inhibitor Coagulant Complex

Increased Effect/Toxicity

Tranexamic Acid may increase the levels/effects of: Anti-inhibitor Coagulant Complex; Fibrinogen Concentrate (Human)

The levels/effects of Tranexamic Acid may be increased by: Fibrinogen Concentrate (Human); Tretinoin (Oral)

Decreased Effect There are no known significant interactions involving a decrease in effect.

Storage/Stability Store at 25°C (77°F); excursions permitted to 15°C to 30°C (59°F to 86°F).

Reconstitution For intravenous infusion, tranexamic acid may be further diluted with dextrose, saline, or other compatible solutions. The mixture should be used on the same day as prepared.

◀ **Compatibility** Compatible with dextrose, saline, electrolyte, amino acid, or dextran solutions, heparin; **incompatible** with solutions containing penicillin.

Mechanism of Action Forms a reversible complex that displaces plasminogen from fibrin resulting in inhibition of fibrinolysis; it also inhibits the proteolytic activity of plasmin

Pharmacodynamics/Kinetics

Distribution: V_d: 9-12 L

Protein binding: ~3%, primarily to plasminogen

Half-life elimination: ~2 hours

Excretion: Urine (>95% as unchanged drug)

Dosage I.V.: Children and Adults: Tooth extraction in patients with hemophilia (in combination with replacement therapy): 10 mg/kg immediately before surgery, then 10 mg/kg/dose 3-4 times/day; may be used for 2-8 days

Dosing adjustment/interval in renal impairment:

Cl_{cr} 50-80 mL/minute: Administer 50% of normal maintenance dose

Cl_{cr} 10-50 mL/minute: Administer 25% of normal maintenance dose

Cl_{cr} <10 mL/minute: Administer 10% of normal maintenance dose

OR

Serum creatinine 1.36-2.83 mg/dL: Maintenance dose of 10 mg/kg/dose twice daily

Serum creatinine 2.83-5.66 mg/dL: Maintenance dose of 10 mg/kg/dose once daily

Serum creatinine >5.66 mg/dL: Maintenance dose of 10 mg/kg/dose every 48 hours **or** 5 mg/kg/dose once daily

Administration May be administered by direct I.V. injection at a maximum rate of 100 mg/minute; use plastic syringe only for I.V. push

Monitoring Parameters

Ophthalmic examination (visual acuity, color vision, eye-ground and visual fields) at baseline and regular intervals during the course of therapy in patients being treated for longer than several days

Additional Information Tranexamic acid is 6-10 times more potent in plasminogen/plasmin binding compared to epsilon-aminocaproic acid.

Dosage Forms Excipient information presented when available (limited, particularly for generics); consult specific product labeling.

Injection, solution:

Cyklokapron®: 100 mg/mL (10 mL)

References

Nilsson IM, "Clinical Pharmacology of Aminocaproic and Tranexamic Acids," *J Clin Pathol Suppl* (Royal College of Pathologists), 1980, 14:41-7.

Seto AH and Dunlap DS, "Tranexamic Acid in Oncology," *Ann Pharmacother*, 1996, 30 (7-8):868-70.

♦ **Tranexamic Acid Injection BP (Can)** *see* Tranexamic Acid *on page 1134*

♦ ***trans*-Retinoic Acid** *see* Tretinoin, Systemic *on page 1141*

♦ ***trans* Vitamin A Acid** *see* Tretinoin, Systemic *on page 1141*

Trastuzumab (tras TU zoo mab)

Medication Safety Issues

High alert medication: The Institute for Safe Medication Practices (ISMP) includes this medication among its list of drug classes which have a heightened risk of causing significant patient harm when used in error.

Related Information

Safe Handling of Hazardous Drugs *on page 1517*

U.S. Brand Names Herceptin®

Index Terms NSC-688097

Generic Available No

Canadian Brand Names Herceptin®

Pharmacologic Category Antineoplastic Agent, Monoclonal Antibody; Monoclonal Antibody

Use Adjuvant treatment of HER-2 overexpressing breast cancer; treatment of HER-2 overexpressing metastatic breast cancer

Pregnancy Risk Factor D

Lactation Excretion in breast milk unknown/not recommended

Labeled Contraindications There are no contraindications listed within the manufacturer's labeling.

Warnings/Precautions Hazardous agent - use appropriate precautions for handling and disposal. **[U.S. Boxed Warning]: Trastuzumab is associated with symptomatic and asymptomatic reductions in left ventricular ejection fraction (LVEF) and severe heart failure (HF) and may result in mural thrombus formation and stroke, and even cardiac death; discontinue for cardiomyopathy.** Evaluate LVEF in all patients prior to and during treatments. Extreme caution should be used in patients with pre-existing cardiac disease or dysfunction. Concomitant administration of anthracyclines and prior exposure to anthracyclines or radiation therapy significantly increases the risk of cardiomyopathy; other potential risk factors include advanced age, high or low body mass index, smoking, diabetes, and hyper/hypothyroidism. Discontinuation should be strongly considered in patients who develop a clinically significant reduction in LVEF during therapy; treatment with HF medications (eg, ACE inhibitors, beta-blockers) should be initiated. Cardiomyopathy due to trastuzumab is generally reversible over a period of 1-3 months after discontinuation. (When LVEF returns to baseline, reinitiation may be considered if indicated.) Trastuzumab is also associated with arrhythmias and hypertension.

[U.S. Boxed Warning]: Serious adverse events, including hypersensitivity reaction (anaphylaxis), infusion reactions (including fatalities), and pulmonary events (including acute respiratory distress syndrome [ARDS]) have been associated with trastuzumab. Discontinue for anaphylaxis, angioedema, ARDS or interstitial pneumonitis. Most of these events occur with the first infusion; pulmonary events may occur during or within 24 hours of the first infusion; delayed reactions have occurred. Interrupt infusion for dyspnea or significant hypotension. Retreatment of patients who experienced severe hypersensitivity reactions has been attempted (with premedication). Some patients tolerated retreatment, while others experienced a second severe reaction. When used in combination with myelosuppressive chemotherapy, trastuzumab may increase the incidence of neutropenia (moderate-to-severe) and febrile neutropenia. May cause serious pulmonary toxicity (dyspnea, hypoxia, interstitial pneumonitis, pulmonary infiltrates, pleural effusion, noncardiogenic pulmonary edema, pulmonary insufficiency, acute respiratory distress syndrome, and/or pulmonary fibrosis); use caution in patients with pre-existing pulmonary disease or patients with extensive pulmonary tumor involvement. Safety and efficacy in children have not been established.

Adverse Reactions Note: Percentages reported with single-agent therapy.

>10%:

Cardiovascular: LVEF decreased (4% to 22%)

Central nervous system: Pain (47%), fever (6% to 36%), chills (5% to 32%), headache (10% to 26%), insomnia (14%), dizziness (4% to 13%)

◀ Dermatologic: Rash (4% to 18%)
Gastrointestinal: Nausea (6% to 33%), diarrhea (7% to 25%), vomiting (4% to 23%), abdominal pain (2% to 22%), anorexia (14%)
Neuromuscular & skeletal: Weakness (4% to 42%), back pain (5% to 22%)
Respiratory: Cough (5% to 26%), dyspnea (3% to 22%), rhinitis (2% to 14%), pharyngitis (12%)
Miscellaneous: Infusion reaction (21% to 40%, chills and fever most common; severe: 1%), infection (20%)
1% to 10%:
Cardiovascular: Peripheral edema (5% to 10%), edema (8%), CHF (2% to 7%; severe: <1%), tachycardia (5%), hypertension (4%), arrhythmia (3%), palpitation (3%)
Central nervous system: Depression (6%)
Dermatologic: Acne (2%), nail disorder (2%), pruritus (2%)
Gastrointestinal: Constipation (2%), dyspepsia (2%)
Genitourinary: Urinary tract infection (3% to 5%)
Hematologic: Anemia (4%), leukopenia (3%)
Neuromuscular & skeletal: Paresthesia (2% to 9%), bone pain (3% to 7%), arthralgia (6% to 8%), myalgia (4%), muscle spasm (3%), peripheral neuritis (2%), neuropathy (1%)
Respiratory: Sinusitis (2% to 9%), nasopharyngitis (8%), upper respiratory infection (3%), epistaxis (2%), pharyngolaryngeal pain (2%)
Miscellaneous: Flu-like syndrome (2% to 10%), accidental injury (6%), influenza (4%), allergic reaction (2%), herpes simplex (2%)
<1%, postmarketing, and/or case reports: Acute respiratory distress syndrome (ARDS), amblyopia, anaphylaxis, anaphylactoid reaction, angioedema, apnea, ascites, asthma, ataxia, bone necrosis, bronchospasm, cardiac arrest, cardiomyopathy, cellulitis, coagulopathy, colitis, confusion, deafness, esophageal ulcer, gastroenteritis, glomerulonephritis (membraneous, focal and fibrillary), glomerulopathy, glomerulosclerosis, hematemesis, hemorrhage, hemorrhagic cystitis, hepatic failure, hepatitis, herpes zoster, hydrocephalus, hydronephrosis, hypercalcemia, hypersensitivity, hypotension, hypothyroidism, hypoxia, ileus, intestinal obstruction, interstitial pneumonitis, laryngitis, leukemia (acute), lymphangitis, mania, mural thrombosis, myopathy, nephrotic syndrome, neutropenia, oligohydramnios, pancreatitis, pancytopenia, paroxysmal nocturnal dyspnea, pathological fracture, pericardial effusion, pleural effusion, pneumonitis, pneumothorax, pulmonary edema (noncardiogenic), pulmonary fibrosis, pulmonary hypertension, pulmonary infiltrate, pyelonephritis, radiation injury, renal failure, respiratory distress, respiratory failure, seizure, sepsis, shock, skin ulcers, stroke, syncope, stomatitis, thyroiditis (autoimmune), vascular thrombosis, ventricular dysfunction, volume overload

Drug Interactions

Avoid Concomitant Use There are no known interactions where it is recommended to avoid concomitant use.

Increased Effect/Toxicity

Trastuzumab may increase the levels/effects of: Antineoplastic Agents (Anthracycline); Immunosuppressants

The levels/effects of Trastuzumab may be increased by: Abciximab; Paclitaxel

Decreased Effect

Trastuzumab may decrease the levels/effects of: Paclitaxel

Storage/Stability Prior to reconstitution, store intact vials under refrigeration at 2°C to 8°C (36°F to 46°F). Following reconstitution with bacteriostatic SWFI, the solution in the vial is stable refrigerated for 28 days from the date of reconstitution; do not freeze. Solutions reconstituted with sterile water for injection without preservatives must be used immediately. The solution diluted in 250 mL NS for infusion is stable for 24 hours refrigerated; do not freeze.

Reconstitution Reconstitute each vial with 20 mL of bacteriostatic sterile water for injection to a concentration of 21 mg/mL. Swirl gently; do not shake. Allow vial to rest for ~5 minutes. If the patient has a known hypersensitivity to benzyl alcohol, trastuzumab may be reconstituted with sterile water for injection without preservatives, which must be used immediately. Determine the appropriate volume for the trastuzumab dose and further dilute in 250 mL NS prior to administration. Avoid rapid expulsion from syringe; gently invert bag to mix

Compatibility Stable in NS; **incompatible** with D_5W.

Mechanism of Action Trastuzumab is a monoclonal antibody which binds to the extracellular domain of the human epidermal growth factor receptor 2 protein (HER-2); it mediates antibody-dependent cellular cytotoxicity by inhibiting proliferation of cells which overexpress HER-2 protein.

Pharmacodynamics/Kinetics

Distribution: V_d: 44 mL/kg; not likely to cross the (intact) blood brain barrier (due to the large molecule size)

Half-life elimination: Weekly dosing: Mean: 6 days (range: 1-32 days); every 3 week regimen: Mean: 16 days (range: 11-23 days)

Dosage Details concerning dosing in combination regimens should also be consulted. Adults: I.V. infusion:

Adjuvant treatment of breast cancer:

With concurrent paclitaxel or docetaxel:

Initial loading dose: 4 mg/kg infused over 90 minutes

Maintenance dose: 2 mg/kg infused over 30 minutes weekly for total of 12 weeks, followed 1 week later (when concurrent chemotherapy completed) by 6 mg/kg infused over 30-60 minutes every 3 weeks for total therapy duration of 52 weeks

With concurrent docetaxel/carboplatin:

Initial loading dose: 4 mg/kg infused over 90 minutes

Maintenance dose: 2 mg/kg infused over 30 minutes weekly for total of 18 weeks, followed 1 week later (when concurrent chemotherapy completed) by 6 mg/kg infused over 30-60 minutes every 3 weeks for total therapy duration of 52 weeks

Following completion of anthracycline-based chemotherapy:

Initial loading dose: 8 mg/kg infused over 90 minutes

Maintenance dose: 6 mg/kg infused over 30 minutes every 3 weeks for total therapy duration of 52 weeks

Metastatic breast cancer (either as a single agent or in combination with paclitaxel):

Initial loading dose: 4 mg/kg infused over 90 minutes

Maintenance dose: 2 mg/kg infused over 30 minutes weekly until disease progression

Dosage adjustment for toxicity:

Cardiotoxicity: LVEF ≥16% decrease from baseline within normal limits or LVEF below normal limits and ≥10% decrease from baseline: Withhold treatment for 4 weeks and repeat LVEF every 4 weeks. May resume trastuzumab treatment if LVEF returns to normal limits within 4-8 weeks and remains at ≤15% decrease from baseline value. Discontinue permanently for persistent (>8 weeks) LVEF decline or for >3 incidents of treatment interruptions for cardiomyopathy.

Infusion-related events:
Mild-moderate infusion reactions: Decrease infusion rate
Dyspnea, clinically significant hypotension: Interrupt infusion
Severe or life-threatening infusion reactions: Consider permanent discontinuation

Dosing adjustment in renal impairment: Data suggest that the disposition of trastuzumab is not altered based on age or serum creatinine (up to 2 mg/dL); however, no formal interaction studies have been performed

Dosing adjustment in hepatic impairment: No data is currently available

Combination Regimens
Breast cancer:
AC-Paclitaxel-Trastuzumab on page 1224
Capecitabine-Trastuzumab on page 1245
Docetaxel-Trastuzumab on page 1293
Docetaxel-Trastuzumab-Carboplatin on page 1293
Docetaxel-Trastuzumab-Cisplatin on page 1294
Docetaxel-Trastuzumab-FEC on page 1294
Docetaxel (Weekly)-Trastuzumab on page 1295
Trastuzumab-Paclitaxel on page 1408
Trastuzumab-Paclitaxel-Carboplatin on page 1409
Trastuzumab-Paclitaxel (Weekly) on page 1410
Vinorelbine-Trastuzumab on page 1423
Vinorelbine-Trastuzumab-FEC on page 1424

Administration Administered by I.V. infusion; loading doses are infused over 90 minutes; maintenance doses may be infused over 30 minutes if tolerated. Do not administer with D_5W. Do not administer I.V. push or by rapid bolus. Treatment with acetaminophen, diphenhydramine, and/or meperidine is usually effective for managing infusion-related events.

Monitoring Parameters HER2 expression assessment (pretherapy); monitor vital signs during infusion; signs and symptoms of cardiac dysfunction; LVEF (baseline, every 3 months during treatment, upon therapy completion and every 6 months for at least 2 years; if treatment is withheld for significant LVEF dysfunction, monitor LVEF at 4-week intervals)

Emetic Potential Low (10% to 30%)

Dosage Forms Excipient information presented when available (limited, particularly for generics); consult specific product labeling.
Injection, powder for reconstitution:
Herceptin®: 440 mg [packaged with bacteriostatic water for injection; diluent contains benzyl alcohol]

References
Bader AA, Schlembach D, Tamussino KF, et al, "Anhydramnios Associated With Administration of Trastuzumab and Paclitaxel for Metastatic Breast Cancer During Pregnancy," *Lancet Oncol*, 2007, 8(1):79-81.

Baselga J, Albanell J, Molina MA, et al, "Mechanism of Action of Trastuzumab and Scientific Update," *Semin Oncol*, 2001, 28(5 Suppl 16):4-11.

Ewer MS, Vooletich MT, Durand JB, et al, "Reversibility of Trastuzumab-Related Cardiotoxicity: New Insights Based on Clinical Course and Response to Medical Treatment," *J Clin Oncol*, 2005, 23(31):7820-6.

Feldman AM, Lorell BH, and Reis SE, "Trastuzumab in the Treatment of Metastatic Breast cancer: Anticancer Therapy Versus Cardiotoxicity," *Circulation*, 2000, 102(3):272-4.

Floyd JD, Nguyen DT, Lobins RL, et al, "Cardiotoxicity of Cancer Therapy," *J Clin Oncol*, 2005, 23 (30):7685-96.

Hudis CA, "Trastuzumab - Mechanism of Action and Use in Clinical Practice," *N Engl J Med*, 2007, 357(1): 39-51.

Leyland-Jones B, Gelmon K, Ayoub JP, et al, "Pharmacokinetics, Safety, and Efficacy of Trastuzumab Administered Every Three Weeks in Combination With Paclitaxel," *J Clin Oncol*, 2003, 21(21):3965-71.

National Comprehensive Cancer Network (NCCN), "Clinical Practice Guidelines in Oncology™: Breast Cancer," Version 2.2008. Available at http://www.nccn.org/professionals/physician_gls/PDF/breast.pdf.

Romond EH, Perez EA, Bryant J, et al, "Trastuzumab Plus Adjuvant Chemotherapy for Operable HER2-Positive Breast Cancer," *N Engl J Med*, 2005, 353(16):1673-84.

Sekar R and Stone PR, "Trastuzumab Use for Metastatic Breast Cancer in Pregnancy," *Obstet Gynecol*, 2007, 110(2 Pt 2):507-10.

Suter TM, Procter M, van Veldhuisen DJ, et al, "Trastuzumab Associated Cardiac Adverse Effects int eh Herceptin Adjuvant Trial," J Clin Oncol, 2007, 25(25):3859-65.

Watson WJ, "Herceptin (Trastuzumab) Therapy During Pregnancy: Association With Reversible Anhydramnios," *Obstet Gynecol*, 2005, 105(3):642-3.

◆ **Treanda®** see Bendamustine *on page 132*

◆ **Trelstar® (Can)** see Triptorelin *on page 1150*

◆ **Trelstar® Depot** see Triptorelin *on page 1150*

◆ **Trelstar® LA** see Triptorelin *on page 1150*

Tretinoin, Systemic (TRET i noyn, sis TEM ik)

Related Information
Safe Handling of Hazardous Drugs *on page 1517*

U.S. Brand Names Vesanoid®

Index Terms *trans* Vitamin A Acid ; *trans*-Retinoic Acid; All-*trans* Retinoic Acid; All-*trans* Vitamin A Acid; ATRA; Ro 5488; tRA; Tretinoinum

Generic Available Yes

Canadian Brand Names Vesanoid®

Pharmacologic Category Antineoplastic Agent, Miscellaneous; Retinoic Acid Derivative

Use Induction of remission in patients with acute promyelocytic leukemia (APL), French American British (FAB) classification M3 (including the M3 variant) characterized by t(15;17) translocation and/or PML/RARα gene presence

Unlabeled/Investigational Use Post consolidation and maintenance therapy in APL; combination therapy (with arsenic trioxide) for remission induction in APL

Pregnancy Risk Factor D

Lactation Excretion in breast milk unknown/not recommended

Labeled Contraindications Hypersensitivity to tretinoin, other retinoids, parabens, or any component of the formulation

Warnings/Precautions Hazardous agent - use appropriate precautions for handling and disposal.

[U.S. Boxed Warning]: About 25% of patients with APL treated with tretinoin have experienced APL differentiation syndrome (DS; formerly called retinoic acid-APL [RA-APL] syndrome), which is characterized by fever, dyspnea, acute respiratory distress, weight gain, radiographic pulmonary infiltrates and pleural or pericardial effusions, edema, and hepatic, renal, and/or multiorgan failure. DS usually occurs during the first month of treatment, with some cases reported following the first dose. DS has been observed with or without concomitant leukocytosis and has occasionally been accompanied by impaired myocardial contractility and episodic hypotension; endotracheal intubation and mechanical ventilation have been required in some cases due to progressive hypoxemia, and several patients have expired with multiorgan failure. About one-half of DS cases are severe, which is associated with increased mortality. Management has not been defined, although high-dose steroids given at the first suspicion appear to reduce morbidity and mortality. Regardless of the leukocyte count, at the first signs suggestive of DS, immediately initiate steroid therapy with ▶

dexamethasone 10 mg I.V. every 12 hours for 3-5 days; taper off over 2 weeks. Most patients do not require termination of tretinoin therapy during treatment of DS.

[U.S. Boxed Warning]: During treatment, ~40% of patients will develop rapidly evolving leukocytosis. A high WBC at diagnosis increases the risk for further leukocytosis and may be associated with a higher risk of life-threatening complications. If signs and symptoms of the APL-DS syndrome are present together with leukocytosis, initiate treatment with high-dose steroids immediately. Consider adding full-dose chemotherapy (including an anthracycline, if not contraindicated) to the tretinoin therapy on day 1 or 2 for patients presenting with a WBC count of >5 x 10^9/L or immediately, for patients presenting with a WBC count of <5 x 10^9/L, if the WBC count reaches ≥6 x 10^9/L by day 5, or ≥10 x 10^9/L by day 10 or ≥15 x 10^9/L by day 28.

[U.S. Boxed Warning]: High risk of teratogenicity; if treatment with tretinoin is required in women of childbearing potential, two reliable forms of contraception should be used during and for 1 month after treatment. Repeat pregnancy testing and contraception counseling monthly throughout the period of treatment. If possible, initiation of treatment with tretinoin should be delayed until negative pregnancy test result is confirmed.

Retinoids have been associated with pseudotumor cerebri (benign intracranial hypertension), especially in children. Concurrent use of other drugs associated with this effect (eg, tetracyclines) may increase risk. Early signs and symptoms include papilledema, headache, nausea, vomiting, visual disturbances, intracranial noises, or pulsate tinnitus.

Up to 60% of patients experienced hypercholesterolemia or hypertriglyceridemia, which were reversible upon completion of treatment. Venous thrombosis and MI have been reported in patient without risk factors for thrombosis or MI; the risk for thrombosis (arterial and venous) is increased during the first month of treatment. Use with caution with antifibrinolytic agents; thrombotic complications have been reported (rarely) with concomitant use. Elevated liver function test results occur in 50% to 60% of patients during treatment. Carefully monitor liver function test results during treatment and give consideration to a temporary withdrawal of tretinoin if test results reach >5 times the upper limit of normal. Most liver function test abnormalities will resolve without interruption of treatment or after therapy completion. May cause headache, malaise, and/or dizziness; caution patients about performing tasks which require mental alertness (eg, operating machinery or driving). Patients with APL are at high risk and can have severe adverse reactions to tretinoin. **[U.S. Boxed Warning]: Should be administered under the supervision of an experienced cancer chemotherapy physician.** Tretinoin treatment for APL should be initiated early, discontinue if pending cytogenetic analysis does not confirm APL by t(15;17) translocation or the presence of the PML/RARα fusion protein (caused by translocation of the promyelocytic [PML] gene on chromosome 15 and retinoic acid receptor [RAR] alpha gene on chromosome 17).

Adverse Reactions Most patients will experience drug-related toxicity, especially headache, fever, weakness and fatigue. These are seldom permanent or irreversible and do not typically require therapy interruption.

>10%:

Cardiovascular: Peripheral edema (52%), chest discomfort (32%), edema (29%), arrhythmias (23%), flushing (23%), hypotension (14%), hypertension (11%)

Central nervous system: Headache (86%), fever (83%), malaise (66%), pain (37%), dizziness (20%), anxiety (17%), depression (14%), insomnia (14%), confusion (11%)

Dermatologic: Skin/mucous membrane dryness (77%), rash (54%), pruritus (20%), alopecia (14%), skin changes (14%)

Endocrine & metabolic: Hypercholesterolemia and/or hypertriglyceridemia (≤60%)

Gastrointestinal: Nausea/vomiting (57%), GI hemorrhage (34%), abdominal pain (31%), mucositis (26%), diarrhea (23%), weight gain (23%), anorexia (17%), constipation (17%), weight loss (17%), dyspepsia (14%), abdominal distention (11%)

Hematologic: Hemorrhage (60%), leukocytosis (40%), disseminated intravascular coagulation (DIC) (26%)

Hepatic: Liver function tests increased (50% to 60%)

Local: Phlebitis (11%)

Neuromuscular & skeletal: Bone pain (77%), paresthesia (17%), myalgia (14%)

Ocular: Ocular disorder (17%), visual disturbances (17%)

Otic: Earache/ear fullness (23%)

Renal: Renal insufficiency (11%)

Respiratory: Upper respiratory tract disorders (63%), dyspnea (60%), respiratory insufficiency (26%), pleural effusion (20%), expiratory wheezing (14%), pneumonia (14%), rales (14%)

Miscellaneous: Shivering (63%), infections (58%), retinoic acid-acute promyelocytic leukemia syndrome differentiation syndrome (≤25%), diaphoresis (20%)

1% to 10%:

Cardiovascular: Cerebral hemorrhage (9%), cardiac failure (6%), facial edema (6%), pallor (6%), cardiac arrest (3%), cardiomyopathy (3%), heart enlarged (3%), heart murmur (3%), ischemia (3%), MI (3%), myocarditis (3%), pericarditis (3%), stroke (3%)

Central nervous system: Agitation (9%), intracranial hypertension (9%), hallucination (6%), aphasia (3%), cerebellar edema (3%), CNS depression (3%), coma (3%), dementia (3%), encephalopathy (3%), facial paralysis (3%), forgetfulness (3%), hypotaxia (3%), hypothermia (3%), light reflex absent (3%), seizure (3%), slow speech (3%), somnolence (3%), spinal cord disorder (3%), unconsciousness (3%)

Dermatologic: Cellulitis (8%)

Endocrine & metabolic: Fluid imbalance (6%), acidosis (3%)

Gastrointestinal: Hepatosplenomegaly (9%), ulcer (3%)

Genitourinary: Dysuria (9%), micturition frequency (3%), prostate enlarged (3%)

Hepatic: Ascites (3%), hepatitis (3%)

Neuromuscular & skeletal: Flank pain (9%), abnormal gait (3%), asterixis (3%), bone inflammation (3%), dysarthria (3%), hemiplegia (3%), hyporeflexia (3%), leg weakness (3%), tremor (3%)

Ocular: Visual acuity change (6%), agnosia (3%), visual field deficit (3%)

Otic: Hearing loss (6%)

Renal: Acute renal failure (3%), renal tubular necrosis (3%)

Respiratory: Lower respiratory tract disorders (9%), pulmonary infiltration (6%), bronchial asthma (3%), larynx edema (3%), pulmonary hypertension (3%)

Miscellaneous: Lymph disorder (6%)

<1%, postmarketing, and/or case reports: Arterial thrombosis, basophilia, erythema nodosum, genital ulceration, hypercalcemia, hyperhistaminemia,

irreversible hearing loss, myositis, organomegaly, pancreatitis, pseudotumor cerebri, renal infarct, Sweet's syndrome, thrombocytosis, vasculitis (skin), venous thrombosis

Drug Interactions

Metabolism/Transport Effects Substrate (minor) of CYP2A6 (minor), 2B6 (minor), 2C8 (major), 2C9 (minor); **Inhibits** CYP2C9 (weak); **Induces** CYP2E1 (weak)

Avoid Concomitant Use

Avoid concomitant use of Tretinoin (Oral) with any of the following: Natalizumab; Tetracycline Derivatives; Vaccines (Live); Vitamin A

Increased Effect/Toxicity

Tretinoin (Oral) may increase the levels/effects of: Antifibrinolytic Agents; Leflunomide; Natalizumab; Vaccines (Live); Vitamin A

The levels/effects of Tretinoin (Oral) may be increased by: CYP2C8 Inhibitors (Moderate); CYP2C8 Inhibitors (Strong); Deferasirox; Tetracycline Derivatives; Trastuzumab

Decreased Effect

Tretinoin (Oral) may decrease the levels/effects of: Oral Contraceptive (Estrogens); Oral Contraceptive (Progestins); Vaccines (Inactivated); Vaccines (Live)

The levels/effects of Tretinoin (Oral) may be decreased by: CYP2C8 Inducers (Highly Effective); Echinacea

Ethanol/Nutrition/Herb Interactions

Ethanol: Avoid ethanol (may increase CNS depression).

Food: Absorption of retinoids has been shown to be enhanced when taken with food.

Herb/Nutraceutical: St John's wort may decrease tretinoin levels. Avoid dong quai, St John's wort (may also cause photosensitization). Avoid additional vitamin A supplementation; may lead to vitamin A toxicity.

Storage/Stability Store capsule at 15°C to 30°C (59°F to 86°F). Protect from light.

Mechanism of Action Tretinoin appears to bind one or more nuclear receptors and decreases proliferation and induces differentiation of APL cells; initially produces maturation of primitive promyelocytes and repopulates the marrow and peripheral blood with normal hematopoietic cells to achieve complete remission

Pharmacodynamics/Kinetics

Absorption: Well absorbed

Protein binding: >95%, predominantly to albumin

Metabolism: Hepatic via CYP; primary metabolite: 4-oxo-all-*trans*-retinoic acid; displays autometabolism

Half-life elimination: Terminal: Parent drug: 0.5-2 hours

Time to peak, serum: 1-2 hours

Excretion: Urine (63%); feces (30%)

Dosage Details concerning dosing in combination regimens should also be consulted. **Note:** Induction treatment of APL with tretinoin should be initiated early; discontinue if pending cytogenetic analysis does not confirm t(15;17) translocation or the presence of the PML/RARα fusion protein.Oral: Children and Adults: APL:

Remission induction: 45 mg/m^2/day in 2 equally divided doses until documentation of complete remission (CR); discontinue 30 days after CR or after 90 days of treatment, whichever occurs first

Remission induction (in combination with an anthracycline; unlabeled use):
Children: 25 mg/m²/day in 2 equally divided doses until complete remission or 90 days (Ortega, 2005)
Adults: 45 mg/m²/day in 2 equally divided doses until complete remission or 90 days (Sanz, 2004; Sanz, 2008)

Consolidation therapy, intermediate- and high-risk patients (unlabeled use):
Children: 25 mg/m²/day in 2 equally divided doses for 15 days each month for 3 months (Ortega, 2005)
Adults: 45 mg/m²/day in 2 equally divided doses for 15 days each month for 3 months (Sanz, 2004)

Maintenance therapy, intermediate- and high-risk patients (unlabeled use):
Children: 25 mg/m²/day in 2 equally divided doses for 15 days every 3 months for 2 years (Ortega, 2005)
Adults: 45 mg/m²/day in 2 equally divided doses for 15 days every 3 months for 2 years (Sanz, 2004)

Dosage adjustment for toxicity:
APL differentiation syndrome: Initiate dexamethasone 10 mg I.V. every 12 hours for 3-5 days; consider interrupting tretinoin until resolution of hypoxia
Liver function tests >5 times the upper limit of normal: Consider temporarily withholding treatment

Combination Regimens
Leukemia, acute promyelocytic:
Tretinoin-Arsenic Trioxide (APL) on page 1410
Tretinoin-Arsenic Trioxide-Gemtuzumab (APL) on page 1411
Tretinoin-Daunorubicin (APL) on page 1411
Tretinoin-Daunorubicin-Cytarabine (APL) on page 1412
Tretinoin-Idarubicin (APL) on page 1414

Administration Administer orally with a meal; do not crush capsules.
Although the manufacturer does not recommend the use of the capsule contents to extemporaneously prepare tretinoin suspension, there are limited case reports of use in patients who are unable to swallow the capsules whole. In a patient with a nasogastric (NG) tube, tretinoin capsules were cut open, with partial aspiration of the contents into a glass syringe, the residual capsule contents were mixed with soy bean oil and aspirated into the same syringe and administered (Shaw, 1995). Tretinoin capsules have also been mixed with sterile water (~20 mL) and heated in a water bath (37°C) to melt the capsules and create an oily suspension for NG tube administration (Bargetzi, 1996). Tretinoin has also been administered sublingually by squeezing the capsule contents beneath the tongue (Kueh, 1999). Low plasma levels have been reported when tretinoin has been administered through a feeding tube, although patient-specific impaired absorption may have been a contributing factor (Takitani, 2004).

Monitoring Parameters Bone marrow cytology to confirm t(15;17) translocation or the presence of the PML/RARα fusion protein (do not withhold treatment initiation for results); monitor CBC with differential, coagulation profile, liver function test results, and triglyceride and cholesterol levels frequently; monitor closely for signs of APL differentiation syndrome (eg, monitor volume status, pulmonary status, temperature, respiration)

Dietary Considerations The absorption of retinoids (as a class) is enhanced when taken with food. Capsule contains soybean oil.

Emetic Potential Low (10% to 30%)

Dosage Forms Excipient information presented when available (limited, particularly for generics); consult specific product labeling.
Capsule: 10 mg
Vesanoid®: 10 mg [contains soybean oil and parabens]

Extemporaneous Preparations Although the manufacturer does not recommend the use of the capsule contents (data on file) to extemporaneously prepare a suspension of tretinoin (due to reports of low plasma levels), there are limited case reports of use in patients who are unable to swallow the capsules whole. In a patient with a nasogastric (NG) tube, tretinoin capsules were cut open, with partial aspiration of the contents aspirated into a glass syringe, the residual capsule contents were mixed with soy bean oil and aspirated into the syringe and administered (Shaw, 1995). Tretinoin capsules have also been mixed with sterile water (~20 mL) and heated in a water bath to melt the capsules and create an oily suspension for NG tube administration (Bargetzi, 1996). Tretinoin has also been administered sublingually by squeezing the capsule contents beneath the tongue (Kueh, 1999).

Bargetzi MJ, Tichelli A, Gratwohl A, et al, "Oral All-Transretinoic Acid Administration in Intubated Patients With Acute Promyelocytic Leukemia," *Schweiz Med Wochenschr*, 1996, 126 (45):1944-5.

Kueh YK, Liew PP, Ho PC, et al, "Sublingual Administration of All-*Trans*-Retinoic Acid to a Comatose Patient With Acute Promyelocytic Leukemia," *Ann Pharmacother*, 1999, 33(4):503-5.

Shaw PJ, Atkins MC, Nath CE, et al, "ATRA Administration in the Critically Ill Patient," *Leukemia*, 1995, 9(7):1288.

Vesanoid® data on file, Roche Pharmaceuticals

References

Bargetzi MJ, Tichelli A, Gratwohl A, et al, "Oral All-Transretinoic Acid Administration in Intubated Patients With Acute Promyelocytic Leukemia," *Schweiz Med Wochenschr*, 1996, 126 (45):1944-5.

Chen GQ, Shen ZX, Wu F, et al, "Pharmacokinetics and Efficacy of Low-Dose All-*trans* Retinoic Acid in the Treatment of Acute Promyelocytic Leukemia," *Leukemia*, 1996, 10(5):825-8.

Kueh YK, Liew PP, Ho PC, et al, "Sublingual Administration of All-*Trans*-Retinoic Acid to a Comatose Patient With Acute Promyelocytic Leukemia," *Ann Pharmacother*, 1999, 33(4):503-5.

Kurzrock R, Estey E, and Talpaz M, "All-*trans* Retinoic Acid: Tolerance and Biologic Effects in Myelodysplastic Syndrome," *J Clin Oncol*, 1993, 11(8):1489-95.

Lazzarino M, Regazzi MB, and Corso A, "Clinical Relevance of All-*trans* Retinoic Acid Pharmacokinetics and Its Modulation in Acute Promyelocytic Leukemia," *Leuk Lymphoma*, 1996, 23(5-6):539-43.

Montesinos P, Bergua JM, Vellenga E, et al, "Differentiation Syndrome in Patients With Acute Promyelocytic Leukemia Treated with All-*Trans* Retinoic Acid and Anthracycline Chemotherapy: Characteristics, Outcomes, and Prognostic Factors," *Blood*, 2009, 113(4):775-83.

Muindi JR, Frankel SR, Huselton C, et al, "Clinical Pharmacology of Oral All-*trans* Retinoic Acid in Patients With Acute Promyelocytic Leukemia," *Cancer Res*, 1992, 52(8):2138-42.

National Comprehensive Cancer Network® (NCCN), "Practice Guidelines in Oncology™: Acute Myeloid Leukemia," Version 1, 2009. Accessible at http://www.nccn.org/professionals/physician_gls/PDF/aml.pdf

Ortega JJ, Madero L, Martin G, et al, "Treatment With All-*Trans* Retinoic Acid and Anthracycline Monochemotherapy for Children With Acute Promyelocytic Leukemia: A Multicenter Study by the PETHEMA Group," *J Clin Oncol*, 2005, 23(30):7632-40.

Sanz MA, Grimwade D, Tallman MS, et al, "Management of Acute Promyelocytic Leukemia: Recommendations From an Expert Panel on Behalf of the European LeukemiaNet," *Blood*, 2009, 113(9):1875-91.

Sanz MA, Martin G, Gonzalez M, et al, "Risk-Adapted Treatment of Acute Promyelocytic Leukemia With All-*Trans*-Retinoic Acid and Anthracycline Monochemotherapy: A Multicenter Study by the PETHEMA Group," *Blood*, 2004, 103(4):1237-43.

Sanz MA, Montesinos P, Vellenga E, et al, "Risk-Adapted Treatment of Acute Promyelocytic Leukemia With All-*Trans*-Retinoic Acid and Anthracycline Monochemotherapy: Long-Term Outcome of the LPA 99 Multicenter Study by the PETHEMA Group," *Blood*, 2008, 112(8):3130-4.

Shaw PJ, Atkins MC, Nath CE, et al, "ATRA Administration in the Critically Ill Patient," *Leukemia*, 1995, 9(7):1288.

Smith MA, Adamson PC, Balis FM, et al, "Phase I and Pharmacokinetic Evaluation of All-*trans*-Retinoic Acid in Pediatric Patients With Cancer," *J Clin Oncol*, 1992, 10(11):1666-73.

Takitani K, Nakao Y, Kosada Y, et al, "Low Plasma Levels of All-*Trans* Retinoic Acid After Feeding Tube Administration for Acute Promyelocytic Leukemia," *Am J Hematol*, 2004, 71(1):97-8.

Testi AM, Biondi A, Lo Coco F, et al, "GIMEMA_AIEOPAIDA Protocol for the Treatment of Newly Diagnosed Acute Promyelocutic Leukemia (APL) in Children," *Blood*, 2005, 106(2): 447-53.

◆ **Tretinoinum** *see Tretinoin, Systemic on page 1141*

◆ **Trexall™** *see Methotrexate on page 768*

◆ **Tridural™ (Can)** *see TraMADol on page 1130*

◆ **Triethylenethiophosphoramide** *see Thiotepa on page 1100*

◆ **Trikacide (Can)** *see MetroNIDAZOLE on page 793*

Trimethobenzamide (trye meth oh BEN za mide)

Medication Safety Issues
Sound-alike/look-alike issues:
Tigan® may be confused with Tiazac®, Ticar®, Ticlid®
Trimethobenzamide may be confused with metoclopramide, trimethoprim

Related Information
Management of Chemotherapy-Induced Nausea and Vomiting *on page 1434*

U.S. Brand Names Tigan®

Index Terms Trimethobenzamide Hydrochloride

Generic Available Yes

Canadian Brand Names Tigan®

Pharmacologic Category Anticholinergic Agent; Antiemetic

Use Treatment of postoperative nausea and vomiting; treatment of nausea associated with gastroenteritis

Lactation Excretion in breast milk unknown

Labeled Contraindications Hypersensitivity to trimethobenzamide or any component of the formulation; injection contraindicated in children

Warnings/Precautions May mask emesis due to Reye's syndrome or mimic CNS effects of Reye's syndrome in patients with emesis of other etiologies. Antiemetic effects may mask toxicity of other drugs or conditions (eg, intestinal obstruction). May cause drowsiness; patient should avoid tasks requiring alertness (eg, driving, operating machinery). May cause extrapyramidal symptoms (EPS) which may be confused with CNS symptoms of primary disease responsible for emesis. Risk of CNS adverse effects (eg, coma, EPS, seizure) may be increased in patients with acute febrile illness, dehydration, electrolyte imbalance, encephalitis, or gastroenteritis; use caution. Allergic-type skin reactions have been reported with use; discontinue with signs of sensitization. Trimethobenzamide clearance is predominantly renal; dosage reductions may be recommended in patient with renal impairment. Use capsule formulation with caution in children; antiemetics are not recommended for uncomplicated vomiting in children, limit antiemetic use to prolonged vomiting of known etiology. Use of injection is contraindicated in children.

Adverse Reactions Frequency not defined.
Cardiovascular: Hypotension (I.V. administration)
Central nervous system: Coma, depression, disorientation, dizziness, drowsiness, EPS, headache, Parkinson-like symptoms, seizure
Dermatologic: Allergic-type skin reactions
Gastrointestinal: Diarrhea
Hematologic: Blood dyscrasias
Hepatic: Jaundice
Local: Injection site burning, pain, redness, stinging, or swelling
Neuromuscular & skeletal: Muscle cramps, opisthotonos
Ocular: Blurred vision
Miscellaneous: Hypersensitivity reactions

Drug Interactions
Avoid Concomitant Use There are no known interactions where it is recommended to avoid concomitant use.

Increased Effect/Toxicity
Trimethobenzamide may increase the levels/effects of: Anticholinergics; Cannabinoids; Potassium Chloride

The levels/effects of Trimethobenzamide may be increased by: Pramlintide

Decreased Effect
Trimethobenzamide may decrease the levels/effects of: Acetylcholinesterase Inhibitors (Central); Secretin

The levels/effects of Trimethobenzamide may be decreased by: Acetylcholinesterase Inhibitors (Central)

Ethanol/Nutrition/Herb Interactions Ethanol: Concomitant use should be avoided (sedative effects may be additive).

Storage/Stability Store capsules and injection solution at room temperature of 25°C (77°F); excursions permitted to 15°C to 30°C (59°F to 86°F).

Compatibility
Compatibility in syringe: Compatible: Glycopyrrolate, hydromorphone, midazolam, nalbuphine.

Mechanism of Action Acts centrally to inhibit the medullary chemoreceptor trigger zone by blocking emetic impulses to the vomiting center

Pharmacodynamics/Kinetics
Onset of action: Antiemetic: Oral: 10-40 minutes; I.M.: 15-35 minutes

Duration: 3-4 hours

Metabolism: Via oxidation, forms metabolite trimethobenzamide N-oxide

Bioavailability: Oral: 60% to 100%

Half-life elimination: 7-9 hours

Time to peak: Oral: ~45 minutes; I.M.: ~30 minutes

Excretion: Urine (30% to 50%, as unchanged drug)

Dosage
Children >40 kg: Oral: 300 mg 3-4 times/day

Adults:

Oral: 300 mg 3-4 times/day

I.M.: 200 mg 3-4 times/day

Postoperative nausea and vomiting (PONV): I.M.: 200 mg, followed 1 hour later by a second 200 mg dose

Elderly: Refer to adult dosing. Consider dosage reduction or increasing dosing interval in elderly patients with renal impairment (specific adjustment guidelines are not provided in the manufacturer's labeling).

Dosage adjustment in renal impairment: Cl_{cr} ≤70 mL/minute: Consider dosage reduction or increasing dosing interval (specific adjustment guidelines are not provided in the manufacturer's labeling)

Administration
Injection: Administer I.M. only; not for I.V. administration. Inject deep into upper outer quadrant of gluteal muscle. Capsule: Administer capsule orally without regard to meals.

Monitoring Parameters Renal function (at baseline)

Dosage Forms Excipient information presented when available (limited, particularly for generics); consult specific product labeling.

Capsule, as hydrochloride: 300 mg

Tigan®: 300 mg

Injection, solution, as hydrochloride: 100 mg/mL (2 mL)

Tigan®: 100 mg/mL (20 mL)

Injection, solution, as hydrochloride [preservative free]:

Tigan®: 100 mg/mL (2 mL)

References

Ginsburg CM and Clahsen J, "Evaluation of Trimethobenzamide Hydrochloride (Tigan®) Suppositories for Treatment of Nausea and Vomiting in Children," *J Pediatr*, 1980, 96(4):767-9.

◆ **Trimethobenzamide Hydrochloride** *see* Trimethobenzamide *on page 1147*

Trimethoprim (trye METH oh prim)

Medication Safety Issues
Sound-alike/look-alike issues:
Trimethoprim may be confused with trimethaphan

U.S. Brand Names Primsol®

Index Terms TMP

Generic Available Yes: Tablet

Canadian Brand Names Apo-Trimethoprim®

Pharmacologic Category Antibiotic, Miscellaneous

Use Treatment of urinary tract infections due to susceptible strains of *E. coli, P. mirabilis, K. pneumoniae, Enterobacter* sp and coagulase-negative *Staphylococcus* including *S. saprophyticus*; acute otitis media in children; acute exacerbations of chronic bronchitis in adults; in combination with other agents for treatment of toxoplasmosis, *Pneumocystis carinii*; treatment of superficial ocular infections involving the conjunctiva and cornea

Pregnancy Risk Factor C

Lactation Enters breast milk/use caution

Labeled Contraindications Hypersensitivity to trimethoprim or any component of the formulation; megaloblastic anemia due to folate deficiency

Warnings/Precautions Use with caution in patients with impaired renal or hepatic function or with possible folate deficiency. Prolonged use may result in fungal or bacterial superinfection, including *C. difficile*-associated diarrhea (CDAD) and pseudomembranous colitis; CDAD has been observed >2 months postantibiotic treatment.

Adverse Reactions Frequency not defined.
Central nervous system: Aseptic meningitis (rare), fever
Dermatologic: Maculopapular rash (3% to 7% at 200 mg/day; incidence higher with larger daily doses), erythema multiforme (rare), exfoliative dermatitis (rare), pruritus (common), phototoxic skin eruptions, Stevens-Johnson syndrome (rare), toxic epidermal necrolysis (rare)
Endocrine & metabolic: Hyperkalemia, hyponatremia
Gastrointestinal: Epigastric distress, glossitis, nausea, vomiting
Hematologic: Leukopenia, megaloblastic anemia, methemoglobinemia, neutropenia, thrombocytopenia
Hepatic: Cholestatic jaundice (rare), liver enzymes increased
Renal: BUN and creatinine increased
Miscellaneous: Anaphylaxis, hypersensitivity reactions

Drug Interactions

Metabolism/Transport Effects Substrate (major) of CYP2C9, 3A4; **Inhibits** CYP2C8 (moderate), 2C9 (moderate)

Avoid Concomitant Use
Avoid concomitant use of Trimethoprim with any of the following: Dofetilide

Increased Effect/Toxicity
Trimethoprim may increase the levels/effects of: ACE Inhibitors; Amantadine; Angiotensin II Receptor Blockers; Antidiabetic Agents (Thiazolidinedione); AzaTHIOprine; Carvedilol; CYP2C8 Substrates (High risk); CYP2C9 Substrates (High risk); Dapsone; Dofetilide; LamiVUDine; Memantine; Methotrexate; Phenytoin; Procainamide; Repaglinide

◄

The levels/effects of Trimethoprim may be increased by: Amantadine; CYP2C9 Inhibitors (Moderate); CYP2C9 Inhibitors (Strong); Dapsone; Memantine

Decreased Effect

Trimethoprim may decrease the levels/effects of: Typhoid Vaccine

The levels/effects of Trimethoprim may be decreased by: CYP2C9 Inducers (Highly Effective); CYP3A4 Inducers (Strong); Deferasirox; Herbs (CYP3A4 Inducers); Leucovorin-Levoleucovorin; Peginterferon Alfa-2b

Storage/Stability Protect the 200 mg tablet from light.

Mechanism of Action Inhibits folic acid reduction to tetrahydrofolate, and thereby inhibits microbial growth

Pharmacodynamics/Kinetics

Absorption: Readily and extensive

Distribution: Widely into body tissues and fluids (middle ear, prostate, bile, aqueous humor, CSF)

Protein binding: 42% to 46%

Metabolism: Partially hepatic

Half-life elimination: 8-14 hours; prolonged with renal impairment

Time to peak, serum: 1-4 hours

Excretion: Urine (60% to 80%) as unchanged drug

Dosage Oral:

Children: 4 mg/kg/day in divided doses every 12 hours

Adults: 100 mg every 12 hours or 200 mg every 24 hours for 10 days; longer treatment periods may be necessary for prostatitis (ie, 4-16 weeks); in the treatment of *Pneumocystis carinii* pneumonia; dose may be as high as 15-20 mg/kg/day in 3-4 divided doses

Dosing interval in renal impairment:

Cl_{cr} 15-30 mL/minute: Administer 100 mg every 18 hours or 50 mg every 12 hours

Cl_{cr} <15 mL/minute: Administer 100 mg every 24 hours or avoid use

Hemodialysis: Moderately dialyzable (20% to 50%)

Administration Administer with milk or food.

Dietary Considerations May cause folic acid deficiency, supplements may be needed. Should be taken with milk or food.

Dosage Forms Excipient information presented when available (limited, particularly for generics); consult specific product labeling.

Solution, oral:

Primsol®: 50 mg (base)/5 mL (473 mL) [dye free, ethanol free; contains propylene glycol, sodium benzoate; bubble gum flavor]

Tablet: 100 mg

References

Varoquaux O, Lajoie D, Gobert C, et al, "Pharmacokinetics of the Trimethoprim-Sulfamethoxazole Combination in the Elderly," *Br J Clin Pharmacol*, 1985, 20:575-81.

♦ **Trimethoprim and Sulfamethoxazole** *see* Sulfamethoxazole and Trimethoprim *on page 1051*

♦ **Triptoraline** *see* Triptorelin *on page 1150*

Triptorelin (trip toe REL in)

Related Information

Safe Handling of Hazardous Drugs *on page 1517*

U.S. Brand Names Trelstar® Depot; Trelstar® LA

Index Terms AY-25650; CL-118,532; D-Trp(6)-LHRH; Triptoraline; Triptorelin Pamoate; Tryptoreline

Generic Available No

Canadian Brand Names Trelstar®; Trelstar® Depot; Trelstar® LA

Pharmacologic Category Gonadotropin Releasing Hormone Agonist

Use Palliative treatment of advanced prostate cancer as an alternative to orchiectomy or estrogen administration

Unlabeled/Investigational Use Treatment of endometriosis, growth hormone deficiency, hyperandrogenism, *in vitro* fertilization, precocious puberty, uterine sarcoma

Pregnancy Risk Factor X

Lactation Excretion in breast milk unknown/contraindicated

Labeled Contraindications Hypersensitivity to triptorelin or any component of the formulation, other LHRH agonists or LHRH; pregnancy

Warnings/Precautions Hazardous agent - use appropriate precautions for handling and disposal. Transient increases in testosterone can lead to worsening symptoms (bone pain, hematuria, bladder outlet obstruction) of prostate cancer during the first few weeks of therapy. Cases of spinal cord compression have been reported with LHRH agonists. Closely observe patients with metastatic vertebral lesions or lower urinary tract obstruction. Hypersensitivity reactions including angioedema and anaphylaxis have rarely occurred. Rare cases of pituitary apoplexy (frequently secondary to pituitary adenoma) have been observed with leuprolide administration (onset from 1 hour to usually <2 weeks); may present as sudden headache, vomiting, visual or mental status changes, and infrequently cardiovascular collapse; immediate medical attention required. Safety and efficacy has not established in pediatric population.

Adverse Reactions As reported with Trelstar® Depot and Trelstar® LA; frequency of effect may vary by product:

>10%:

Central nervous system: Headache (30% to 60%)

Endocrine & metabolic: Hot flashes (95% to 100%), glucose increased

Hematologic: Hemoglobin decreased, RBC count decreased

Hepatic: Alkaline phosphatase increased, ALT increased, AST increased

Neuromuscular & skeletal: Skeletal pain (12% to 13%)

Renal: BUN increased

1% to 10%:

Cardiovascular: Leg edema (6%), hypertension (4%), chest pain (2%), peripheral edema (1%)

Central nervous system: Dizziness (1% to 3%), pain (2% to 3%), fatigue (2%), insomnia (2%), emotional lability (1%)

Dermatologic: Rash (2%), pruritus (1%)

Endocrine & metabolic: Tumor flare (8%), alkaline phosphatase increased (2%), breast pain (2%), gynecomastia (2%), libido decreased (2%)

Gastrointestinal: Nausea (3%), anorexia (2%), constipation (2%), dyspepsia (2%), vomiting (2%), abdominal pain (1%), diarrhea (1%)

Genitourinary: Impotence (2% to 7%), dysuria (5%), urinary retention (1%), urinary tract infection (1%)

Hematologic: Anemia (1%)

Local: Injection site pain (4%)

Neuromuscular & skeletal: Leg pain (2% to 5%), back pain (3%), arthralgia (2%), leg cramps (2%), myalgia (1%), weakness (1%)

Ocular: Conjunctivitis (1%), eye pain (1%)

Respiratory: Cough (2%), dyspnea (1%), pharyngitis (1%)

Postmarketing and/or case reports: Anaphylaxis, angioedema, hypersensitivity reactions, pituitary apoplexy, spinal cord compression, renal dysfunction

◄ **Drug Interactions**
Avoid Concomitant Use There are no known interactions where it is recommended to avoid concomitant use.
Increased Effect/Toxicity There are no known significant interactions involving an increase in effect.
Decreased Effect
Triptorelin may decrease the levels/effects of: Antidiabetic Agents
Storage/Stability
Trelstar® Depot: Store at 15°C to 30°C (59°F to 86°F).
Trelstar® LA: Store at 20°C to 25°C (68°F to 77°F).
Reconstitution Reconstitute with 2 mL sterile water for injection. Shake well to obtain a uniform suspension.
Debioclip™: Follow manufacturer's instructions for mixing prior to use.
Mechanism of Action Causes suppression of ovarian and testicular steroidogenesis due to decreased levels of LH and FSH with subsequent decrease in testosterone (male) and estrogen (female) levels. After chronic and continuous administration, usually 2-4 weeks after initiation, a sustained decrease in LH and FSH secretion occurs.
Pharmacodynamics/Kinetics
Absorption: Oral: Not active
Distribution: V_d: 30-33 L
Protein binding: None
Metabolism: Unknown; unlikely to involve CYP; no known metabolites
Half-life elimination: 2.8 ± 1.2 hours
Moderate-to-severe renal impairment: 6.5-7.7 hours
Hepatic impairment: 7.6 hours
Time to peak: 1-3 hours
Excretion: Urine (42% as intact peptide); hepatic
Dosage I.M.: Adults: Prostate cancer:
Trelstar® Depot: 3.75 mg once every 28 days
Trelstar® LA: 11.25 mg once every 84 days
Dosage adjustment in renal/hepatic impairment: Although this drug is excreted renally, no guidelines for adjustments are available.
Administration Administer by I.M. injection into the buttock; alternate injection sites.
Monitoring Parameters Serum testosterone levels, prostate-specific antigen
Test Interactions Pituitary-gonadal function may be suppressed with chronic administration and for up to 8 weeks after triptorelin therapy has been discontinued.
Dosage Forms Excipient information presented when available (limited, particularly for generics); consult specific product labeling.
Injection, powder for reconstitution:
Trelstar® Depot: 3.75 mg [contains polylactide-co-glycolide; polysorbate 80]
Trelstar® LA: 11.25 mg [contains polylactide-co-glycolide; polysorbate 80]
References
Filicor M, "Gonadotrophin-Releasing Hormone Agonists. A Guide to Use and Selection," *Drugs*, 1994, 48(1):41-58.
Swanson LJ, Seely JH, and Garnick MB, "Gonadotropin-Releasing Hormone Analogs and Prostatic Cancer," *Crit Rev Oncol Hematol*, 1988, 8(1):1-26.

◆ **Triptorelin Pamoate** *see* Triptorelin *on page* 1150
◆ **Trisenox®** *see* Arsenic Trioxide *on page* 107
◆ **Trivagizole-3® (Can)** *see* Clotrimazole *on page* 253
◆ **Tryptoreline** *see* Triptorelin *on page* 1150

- **TSH** *see* Thyrotropin Alfa *on page 1103*
- **TSPA** *see* Thiotepa *on page 1100*
- **Tucks® Anti-Itch [OTC]** *see* Hydrocortisone *on page 575*
- **Tykerb®** *see* Lapatinib *on page 684*
- **506U78** *see* Nelarabine *on page 843*

UFT

U.S. Brand Names Orzel® [DSC]

Index Terms Uracil and Ftorafur; Uracil and Tegafur; Uracil and Tetrahydrofuranyl-5-Fluorouracil

Generic Available No

Pharmacologic Category Antineoplastic Agent, Antimetabolite (Pyrimidine Antagonist)

Unlabeled/Investigational Use Investigational: Treatment of unresectable or metastatic colorectal cancer

Warnings/Precautions

Hazardous agent - use appropriate precautions for handling and disposal.

Adverse Reactions Frequency not defined.

Central nervous system: Fatigue, cerebellar toxicity (rare)

Dermatologic: Rash, skin pigmentation, photosensitivity, hand-foot syndrome (rare)

Gastrointestinal: Nausea, vomiting, anorexia, diarrhea (may be dose limiting)

Hematologic: Neutropenia (may be dose limiting)

Neuromuscular & skeletal: Neurotoxicity (peripheral neuropathy)

Ocular: Lacrimation

Mechanism of Action Tegafur is a prodrug of fluorouracil. It is converted *in vivo* to fluorouracil through hepatic microsomal cytochrome P450, and also via thymidine phosphorylase and spontaneous anabolic conversion. Uracil is a competitive inhibitor of dihydropyrimidine dehydrogenase (DPD), the enzyme responsible for catabolism of approximately 85% of fluorouracil to fluoro-β alanine.

Pharmacodynamics/Kinetics

Plasma levels: Tegafur > uracil > fluorouracil

Time to C_{pmax}: Tegafur: 0.6-2.1 hours; uracil: 0.6-4.1 hours; fluorouracil: 0.7-2.0 hours; the relationship between UFT dose and fluorouracil C_{pmax} is not linear

Dosage Refer to individual protocols.

Oral: Adults: 300 mg/m^2/day (expressed as tegafur) in combination with oral leucovorin

Emetic Potential Moderate (30% to 90%)

Dosage Forms Excipient information presented when available (limited, particularly for generics); consult specific product labeling. [DSC] = Discontinued product

Capsule:

Orzel® [DSC]: Tegafur 100 mg and uracil 224 mg

References

Ho DH, Covington WP, Pazdur R, et al, "Clinical Pharmacology of Combined Oral Uracil and Ftorafur," *Drug Metab Disp*, 1992, 20(6):936-40.

Kohne CH and Peters GJ, "UFT: Mechanism of Drug Action," *Oncology (Huntingt)*, 2000, 14(10 Suppl 9):13-8.

Sun W and Haller D, "UFT in the Treatment of Colorectal and Breast Cancer," *Oncology (Huntingt)*, 2001, 15(1 Suppl 2):49-56.

- **UK109496** *see* Voriconazole *on page 1187*
- **Ultram®** *see* TraMADol *on page 1130*

Valacyclovir (val ay SYE kloe veer)

Medication Safety Issues
Sound-alike/look-alike issues:
Valtrex® may be confused with Valcyte™, Zovirax®
ValACYclovir may be confused with acyclovir, valGANCIclovir, vancomycin

U.S. Brand Names Valtrex®

Index Terms Valacyclovir Hydrochloride

Generic Available No

Canadian Brand Names Apo-Valacyclovir®; PMS-Valacyclovir; Riva-Valacyclovir; Valtrex®

Pharmacologic Category Antiviral Agent; Antiviral Agent, Oral

Use Treatment of herpes zoster (shingles) in immunocompetent patients; treatment of first-episode and recurrent genital herpes; suppression of recurrent genital herpes and reduction of heterosexual transmission of genital herpes in immunocompetent patients; suppression of genital herpes in HIV-infected individuals; treatment of herpes labialis (cold sores); chickenpox in immunocompetent children

Unlabeled/Investigational Use Prophylaxis of cancer-related HSV, VZV, and CMV infections; treatment of cancer-related HSV, VZV infection

Pregnancy Risk Factor B

Lactation Enters breast milk/use caution

Labeled Contraindications Hypersensitivity to valacyclovir, acyclovir, or any component of the formulation

Warnings/Precautions Thrombotic thrombocytopenic purpura/hemolytic uremic syndrome has occurred in immunocompromised patients (at doses of 8 g/day). Safety and efficacy have not been established for treatment/suppression of recurrent genital herpes or disseminated herpes in patients with profound immunosuppression (eg, advanced HIV with CD4 <100 cells/mm^3). Use caution in patients with renal impairment, the elderly, and/or those receiving nephrotoxic agents. Acute renal failure and CNS effects have been observed in patients with renal dysfunction; dose adjustment may be required. Decreased precipitation in renal tubules may occur leading to urinary precipitation; adequately hydrate patient. For cold sores, treatment should begin at with earliest symptom (tingling, itching, burning). For genital herpes, treatment should begin as soon as possible after the first signs and symptoms (within 72 hours of onset of first diagnosis or within 24 hours of onset of recurrent episodes). For herpes zoster, treatment should begin within 72 hours of onset of rash. For chickenpox, treatment should begin with earliest sign or symptom. Use with caution in the elderly; CNS effects have been reported. Safety and efficacy have not been established in patients <2 years of age.

Adverse Reactions
>10%:
Central nervous system: Headache (13% to 38%)
Gastrointestinal: Nausea (5% to 15%), abdominal pain (1% to 11%)

Hematologic: Neutropenia (≤18%)
Hepatic: ALT increased (≤14%), AST increased (2% to 16%)
Respiratory: Nasopharyngitis (≤16%)
1% to 10%:
Central nervous system: Fatigue (≤8%), depression (≤7%), fever (children 4%), dizziness (2% to 4%)
Dermatologic: Rash (≤8%)
Endocrine: Dysmenorrhea (≤1% to 8%), dehydration (children 2%)
Gastrointestinal: Vomiting (<1% to 6%), diarrhea (children 5%; adults <1%)
Hematologic: Thrombocytopenia (≤3%)
Hepatic: Alkaline phosphatase increased (≤4%)
Neuromuscular & skeletal: Arthralgia (<1 to 6%)
Respiratory: Rhinorrhea (children 2%)
Miscellaneous: Herpes simplex (children 2%)
<1%, postmarketing, and/or case reports: Acute hypersensitivity reactions (angioedema, anaphylaxis, dyspnea, pruritus, rash, urticaria); aggression, agitation, alopecia, anemia, aplastic anemia, ataxia, creatinine increased, coma, confusion, consciousness decreased, dysarthria, encephalopathy, erythema multiforme, facial edema, hallucinations (auditory and visual), hemolytic uremic syndrome (HUS), hepatitis, hypertension, leukocytoclastic vasculitis, leukopenia, mania, photosensitivity reaction, psychosis, renal failure, renal pain, seizure, tachycardia, thrombotic thrombocytopenic purpura (TTP), tremor, urinary precipitation, visual disturbances

Drug Interactions

Avoid Concomitant Use
Avoid concomitant use of ValACYclovir with any of the following: Zoster Vaccine

Increased Effect/Toxicity
ValACYclovir may increase the levels/effects of: Mycophenolate; Tenofovir; Zidovudine

The levels/effects of ValACYclovir may be increased by: Mycophenolate

Decreased Effect
ValACYclovir may decrease the levels/effects of: Zoster Vaccine

Storage/Stability Store at 15°C to 25°C (59°F to 77°F).

Mechanism of Action Valacyclovir is rapidly and nearly completely converted to acyclovir by intestinal and hepatic metabolism. Acyclovir is converted to acyclovir monophosphate by virus-specific thymidine kinase then further converted to acyclovir triphosphate by other cellular enzymes. Acyclovir triphosphate inhibits DNA synthesis and viral replication by competing with deoxyguanosine triphosphate for viral DNA polymerase and being incorporated into viral DNA.

Pharmacodynamics/Kinetics
Absorption: Rapid
Distribution: Acyclovir is widely distributed throughout the body including brain, kidney, lungs, liver, spleen, muscle, uterus, vagina, and CSF
Protein binding: ~14% to 18%
Metabolism: Hepatic; valacyclovir is rapidly and nearly completely converted to acyclovir and L-valine by first-pass effect; acyclovir is hepatically metabolized to a very small extent by aldehyde oxidase and by alcohol and aldehyde dehydrogenase (inactive metabolites)
Bioavailability: ~55% once converted to acyclovir
Half-life elimination: Normal renal function: Adults: Acyclovir: 2.5-3.3 hours, Valacyclovir: ~30 minutes; End-stage renal disease: Acyclovir: 14-20 hours; During hemodialysis: 4 hours

◄ Excretion: Urine, primarily as acyclovir (89%); **Note:** Following oral administration of radiolabeled valacyclovir, 46% of the label is eliminated in the feces (corresponding to nonabsorbed drug), while 47% of the radiolabel is eliminated in the urine.

Dosage Oral:

Children 2 to <18 years: Chickenpox: 20 mg/kg/dose 3 times/day for 5 days (maximum: 1 g 3 times/day)

Children ≥12 and Adults: Herpes labialis (cold sores): 2 g twice daily for 1 day (separate doses by ~12 hours)

Adults:

CMV prophylaxis in allogeneic HSCT recipients (unlabeled use): 2 g 4 times/ day

Herpes zoster (shingles): 1 g 3 times/day for 7 days

HSV, VZV in cancer patients (unlabeled use): Prophylaxis: 500 mg 2-3 times/ day; Treatment: 1 g 3 times/day

Genital herpes:

Initial episode: 1 g twice daily for 10 days

Recurrent episode: 500 mg twice daily for 3 days

Reduction of transmission: 500 mg once daily (source partner)

Suppressive therapy:

Immunocompetent patients: 1000 mg once daily (500 mg once daily in patients with <9 recurrences per year)

HIV-infected patients (CD4 ≥100 cells/mm^3): 500 mg twice daily

Dosing adjustment in renal impairment:

Herpes zoster: Adults:

Cl_{cr} 30-49 mL/minute: 1 g every 12 hours

Cl_{cr} 10-29 mL/minute: 1 g every 24 hours

Cl_{cr} <10 mL/minute: 500 mg every 24 hours

Genital herpes: Adults:

Initial episode:

Cl_{cr} 10-29 mL/minute: 1 g every 24 hours

Cl_{cr} <10 mL/minute: 500 mg every 24 hours

Recurrent episode: Cl_{cr} <29 mL/minute: 500 mg every 24 hours

Suppressive therapy: Cl_{cr} <29 mL/minute:

For usual dose of 1 g every 24 hours, decrease dose to 500 mg every 24 hours

For usual dose of 500 mg every 24 hours, decrease dose to 500 mg every 48 hours

HIV-infected patients: 500 mg every 24 hours

Herpes labialis: Adolescents and Adults:

Cl_{cr} 30-49 mL/minute: 1 g every 12 hours for 2 doses

Cl_{cr} 10-29 mL/minute: 500 mg every 12 hours for 2 doses

Cl_{cr} <10 mL/minute: 500 mg as a single dose

Hemodialysis: Dialyzable (~33% removed during 4-hour session); administer dose postdialysis

Chronic ambulatory peritoneal dialysis/continuous arteriovenous hemofiltration dialysis: Pharmacokinetic parameters are similar to those in patients with ESRD; supplemental dose not needed following dialysis

Dosing adjustment in hepatic impairment: No adjustment required.

Administration If GI upset occurs, administer with meals.

Monitoring Parameters Urinalysis, BUN, serum creatinine, liver enzymes, and CBC

Dietary Considerations May be taken with or without food.

Dosage Forms Excipient information presented when available (limited, particularly for generics); consult specific product labeling.
Caplet:

Valtrex®: 500 mg, 1000 mg

Extemporaneous Preparations

To prepare a valacyclovir 25 mg/mL oral suspension, crush five valacyclovir 500 mg caplets (10 caplets for 50 mg/mL suspension) into a fine powder in a mortar. Gradually add 5 mL aliquots of Suspension Structured Vehicle USP-NF (SSV) to powder and triturate until a paste is formed. Continue adding 5 mL aliquots of SSV to the mortar until a suspension is formed (minimum 20 mL SSV and maximum 40 mL SSV). Transfer to 100 mL bottle. Add the cherry flavor (amount recommended on package) to the mortar and dissolve in ~5 mL of SSV. Add to bottle once dissolved. Rinse the mortar at least 3 times with ~5 mL of SSV, transferring contents between additions of SSV. Continue to add the SSV to bring final volume to 100 mL. The preparation is stable for 28 days under refrigeration; shake well before using. (Refer to manufacturer's current labeling.)

References

Acosta EP and Fletcher CV, "Valacyclovir," *Ann Pharmacother*, 1997, 31(2):185-91.

Alrabiah FA and Sacks SL, "New Antiherpesvirus Agents. Their Targets and Therapeutic Potential," *Drugs*, 1996, 52(1):17-32.

Beutner KR, Friedman DJ, Forszpaniak C, et al, "Valacyclovir Compared With Acyclovir for Improved Therapy for Herpes Zoster in Immunocompetent Adults," *Antimicrob Agents Chemother*, 1995, 39(7):1546-53.

Bodsworth NJ, Crooks RJ, Borelli S, et al, "Valaciclovir Versus Aciclovir in Patients Initiated Treatment of Recurrent Genital Herpes: A Randomized, Double-Blind Clinical Trial. International Valaciclovir HSV Study Group," *Genitourin Med*, 1997, 73(2):110-6.

Grant DM, Mauskopf JA, Bell L, et al, "Comparison of Valaciclovir and Acyclovir for the Treatment of Herpes Zoster in Immunocompetent Patients Over 50 Years of Age: A Cost-Consequence Model," *Pharmacotherapy*, 1997, 17(2):333-41.

National Comprehensive Cancer Network (NCCN), "Clinical Practice Guidelines in Oncology™: Prevention and Treatment of Cancer-Related Infections," Version 1.2008. Available at http://www.nccn.org/professionals/physician_gls/PDF/infections.pdf.

Patel R, Bodsworth NJ, Woolley P, et al, "Valaciclovir for the Suppression of Recurrent Genital HSV Infection: A Placebo Controlled Study of Once Daily Therapy. International Valaciclovir HSV Study Group," *Genitourin Med*, 1997, 73(2):105-9.

Reitano M, Tyring S, Lang W, et al, "Valaciclovir for the Suppression of Recurrent Genital Herpes Simplex Virus Infection: A Large-Scale Dose Range-Finding Study. International Valaciclovir HSV Study Group," *J Infect Dis*, 1998, 178(3):603-10.

Tyring SK, Douglas JM Jr, Corey L, et al, "A Randomized, Placebo-Controlled Comparison of Oral Valacyclovir and Acyclovir in Immunocompetent Patients With Recurrent Genital Herpes Infections. The Valaciclovir International Study Group," *Arch Dermatol*, 1998, 134(2):185-91.

◆ **Valacyclovir Hydrochloride** *see* Valacyclovir *on page 1154*

◆ **Valcyte®** *see* Valganciclovir *on page 1157*

Valganciclovir (val gan SYE kloh veer)

Medication Safety Issues

Sound-alike/look-alike issues:

Valcyte™ may be confused with Valium®, Valtrex®

ValGANCIclovir may be confused with valACYclovir

Related Information

Safe Handling of Hazardous Drugs *on page 1517*

U.S. Brand Names Valcyte®

Index Terms Valganciclovir Hydrochloride

Generic Available No

Canadian Brand Names Valcyte®

Pharmacologic Category Antiviral Agent

◄ **Use** Treatment of cytomegalovirus (CMV) retinitis in patients with acquired immunodeficiency syndrome (AIDS); prevention of CMV disease in high-risk patients (donor CMV positive/recipient CMV negative) undergoing kidney, heart, or kidney/pancreas transplantation

Pregnancy Risk Factor C

Lactation Excretion in breast milk unknown/contraindicated

Labeled Contraindications Hypersensitivity to valganciclovir, ganciclovir, acyclovir, or any component of the formulation; absolute neutrophil count <500/mm³; platelet count <25,000/mm³; hemoglobin <8 g/dL

Warnings/Precautions Hazardous agent - use appropriate precautions for handling and disposal. **[U.S. Boxed Warning]: May cause dose- or therapy-limiting granulocytopenia, anemia, and/or thrombocytopenia;** use caution in patients with impaired renal function (dose adjustment required). **[U.S. Boxed Warning]: Ganciclovir may adversely affect spermatogenesis and fertility;** due to its mutagenic potential, contraceptive precautions for female and male patients need to be followed during and for at least 90 days after therapy with the drug. Due to differences in bioavailability, valganciclovir tablets cannot be substituted for ganciclovir capsules on a one-to-one basis. Not indicated for use in liver transplant patients (higher incidence of tissue-invasive CMV relative to oral ganciclovir was observed in trials).

Adverse Reactions

>10%:

  Central nervous system: Fever (31%), headache (9% to 22%), insomnia (16%)

  Gastrointestinal: Diarrhea (16% to 41%), nausea (8% to 30%), vomiting (21%), abdominal pain (15%)

  Hematologic: Granulocytopenia (11% to 27%), anemia (8% to 26%)

  Ocular: Retinal detachment (15%)

1% to 10%:

  Central nervous system: Peripheral neuropathy (9%), paresthesia (8%), seizure (<5%), psychosis, hallucinations (<5%), confusion (<5%), agitation (<5%)

  Hematologic: Thrombocytopenia (8%), pancytopenia (<5%), bone marrow depression (<5%), aplastic anemia (<5%), bleeding (potentially life-threatening due to thrombocytopenia <5%)

  Renal: Renal function decreased (<5%)

  Miscellaneous: Local and systemic infection, including sepsis (<5%); allergic reaction (<5%)

<1%: Valganciclovir is expected to share the toxicities which may occur at a low incidence or due to idiosyncratic reactions which have been associated with ganciclovir

Drug Interactions

Avoid Concomitant Use There are no known interactions where it is recommended to avoid concomitant use.

Increased Effect/Toxicity

ValGANCIclovir may increase the levels/effects of: Mycophenolate; Reverse Transcriptase Inhibitors (Nucleoside); Tenofovir

The levels/effects of ValGANCIclovir may be increased by: Mycophenolate

Decreased Effect There are no known significant interactions involving a decrease in effect.

Ethanol/Nutrition/Herb Interactions Food: Coadministration with a high-fat meal increased AUC by 30%.

Storage/Stability Store at 25°C (77°F); excursions permitted to 15°C to 30°C (59°F to 86°F).

Mechanism of Action Valganciclovir is rapidly converted to ganciclovir in the body. The bioavailability of ganciclovir from valganciclovir is increased 10-fold compared to oral ganciclovir. A dose of 900 mg achieved systemic exposure of ganciclovir comparable to that achieved with the recommended doses of intravenous ganciclovir of 5 mg/kg. Ganciclovir is phosphorylated to a substrate which competitively inhibits the binding of deoxyguanosine triphosphate to DNA polymerase resulting in inhibition of viral DNA synthesis.

Pharmacodynamics/Kinetics

Absorption: Well absorbed; high-fat meal increases AUC by 30%

Distribution: Ganciclovir: V_d: 15.26 L/1.73 m^2; widely to all tissue including CSF and ocular tissue

Protein binding: 1% to 2%

Metabolism: Converted to ganciclovir by intestinal mucosal cells and hepatocytes

Bioavailability: With food: 60%

Half-life elimination: Ganciclovir: 4.08 hours; prolonged with renal impairment; Severe renal impairment: Up to 68 hours

Excretion: Urine (primarily as ganciclovir)

Dosage Oral: Adults:

CMV retinitis:

Induction: 900 mg twice daily for 21 days (with food)

Maintenance: Following induction treatment, or for patients with inactive CMV retinitis who require maintenance therapy: Recommended dose: 900 mg once daily (with food)

Prevention of CMV disease following transplantation: 900 mg once daily (with food) beginning within 10 days of transplantation; continue therapy until 100 days post-transplantation

Dosage adjustment in renal impairment:

Induction dose:

Cl_{cr} 40-59 mL/minute: 450 mg twice daily

Cl_{cr} 25-39 mL/minute: 450 mg once daily

Cl_{cr} 10-24 mL/minute: 450 mg every 2 days

Maintenance dose:

Cl_{cr} 40-59 mL/minute: 450 mg once daily

Cl_{cr} 25-39 mL/minute: 450 mg every 2 days

Cl_{cr} 10-24 mL/minute: 450 mg twice weekly

Note: Valganciclovir is not recommended in patients receiving hemodialysis. For patients on hemodialysis (Cl_{cr} <10 mL/minute), it is recommended that ganciclovir be used (dose adjusted as specified for ganciclovir).

Administration Avoid direct contact with broken or crushed tablets. Consideration should be given to handling and disposal according to guidelines issued for antineoplastic drugs. However, there is no consensus on the need for these precautions.

Monitoring Parameters Retinal exam (at least every 4-6 weeks), CBC, platelet counts, serum creatinine

Dietary Considerations Should be taken with meals.

Product Availability

Valcyte® oral solution: FDA approved August 2009; availability expected January 2010

Dosage Forms Excipient information presented when available (limited, particularly for generics); consult specific product labeling.

Tablet, oral: 450 mg

References

Ljungman P, de La Camara R, Milpied N, et al, "Randomized Study of Valacyclovir as Prophylaxis Against Cytomegalovirus Reactivation in Recipients of Allogeneic Bone Marrow Transplants," *Blood*, 2002, 99(8):3050-6.

◆ **Valganciclovir Hydrochloride** *see* Valganciclovir *on page 1157*

Valrubicin (val ROO bi sin)

Medication Safety Issues

Sound-alike/look-alike issues:

Valrubicin may be confused with DAUNOrubicin, DOXOrubicin, epirubicin, IDArubicin

Valstar® may be confused with valsartan

High alert medication: The Institute for Safe Medication Practices (ISMP) includes this medication among its list of drug classes which have a heightened risk of causing significant patient harm when used in error.

Related Information

Management of Drug Extravasations *on page 1447*

Safe Handling of Hazardous Drugs *on page 1517*

U.S. Brand Names Valstar®

Index Terms *N*-trifluoroacetyladriamycin-14-valerate; AD32

Generic Available No

Canadian Brand Names Valtaxin®

Pharmacologic Category Antineoplastic Agent, Anthracycline

Use Intravesical therapy of BCG-refractory bladder carcinoma *in situ*

Pregnancy Risk Factor C

Lactation Excretion in breast milk unknown/not recommended

Labeled Contraindications Hypersensitivity to anthracyclines, polyoxyl castor oil (Cremophor® EL), or any component of the formulation; concurrent urinary tract infection; small bladder capacity (unable to tolerate a 75 mL instillation)

Warnings/Precautions Hazardous agent - use appropriate precautions for handling and disposal. Delay valrubicin therapy for at least 2 weeks after transurethral resection and/or fulguration. Do not administer if mucosal integrity of bladder has been compromised or bladder perforation is present; evaluate bladder status prior to instillation. Use aseptic technique to prevent urinary tract infection or traumatizing urinary mucosa. Although clamping of the urinary catheter after administration is not recommended, use caution and appropriate medical supervision if performed. Irritable bladder symptoms may occur during instillation and retention, and for a brief time after voiding. Use caution in patients with severe irritable bladder symptoms. Red-tinged urine is typical for the first 24 hours after instillation. Prolonged symptoms or discoloration should prompt contact with the physician.

Contains polyoxyl castor oil (Cremophor® EL) which is associated with hypersensitivity reactions; use is contraindicated in patients with hypersensitivity to polyoxyl castor oil. Delaying cystectomy during treatment may lead to metastatic bladder cancer; reconsider cystectomy if complete response to treatment does not occur within 3 months.

Adverse Reactions Note: In general, local adverse reactions occur during or shortly after instillation and resolve within 1-7 days.

>10%: Genitourinary: Bladder irritation (88%), urinary frequency (61%), urinary urgency (57%), dysuria (56%), bladder spasm (31%), hematuria (29%; gross:

1%), bladder pain (28%), urinary incontinence (22%), cystitis (15%), urinary tract infection (15%), urine red-tinged

1% to 10%:

Cardiovascular: Chest pain (3%), vasodilation (2%), peripheral edema (1%)

Central nervous system: Headache (4%), malaise (4%), dizziness (3%), fever (2%)

Dermatologic: Rash (3%)

Endocrine & metabolic: Hyperglycemia (1%)

Gastrointestinal: Abdominal pain (5%), nausea (5%), diarrhea (3%), vomiting (2%), flatulence (1%)

Genitourinary: Nocturia (7%), burning symptoms (5%), urinary retention (4%), urethral pain (3%), pelvic pain (1%), hematuria (microscopic) (3%)

Hematologic: Anemia (2%)

Neuromuscular & skeletal: Weakness (4%), back pain (3%), myalgia (1%)

Respiratory: Pneumonia (1%)

<1%, postmarketing, and/or case reports: Hematologic toxicity (following instillation with perforated bladder), nonprotein nitrogen increased, pruritus, skin irritation (local), taste loss, urine flow decreased, urethritis, tenesmus

Drug Interactions

Avoid Concomitant Use

Avoid concomitant use of Valrubicin with any of the following: Natalizumab; Vaccines (Live)

Increased Effect/Toxicity

Valrubicin may increase the levels/effects of: Leflunomide; Natalizumab; Vaccines (Live)

The levels/effects of Valrubicin may be increased by: Bevacizumab; Taxane Derivatives; Trastuzumab

Decreased Effect

Valrubicin may decrease the levels/effects of: Cardiac Glycosides; Vaccines (Inactivated); Vaccines (Live)

The levels/effects of Valrubicin may be decreased by: Cardiac Glycosides; Echinacea

Storage/Stability Store unopened vials under refrigeration at 2°C to 8°C (36°F to 48°F). Stable for 12 hours at room temperature when diluted in 0.9% sodium chloride.

Reconstitution Allow vials to warm to room temperature (without heating) prior to use. A waxy precipitate (due to polyoxyl castor oil) may form at temperatures <4°C, warm vial in the hand until solution is clear (do not use vial if particulate still present). Use appropriate precautions for handling and disposal. Dilute 800 mg (20 mL) with 55 mL NS (total volume of 75 mL). Use non-PVC containers (glass, polyolefin or polypropylene) and administration sets to avoid leaching of DEHP plasticizers. Stable for 12 hours at room temperature when diluted in 0.9% sodium chloride. Do not mix with other drugs.

Mechanism of Action Blocks function of DNA topoisomerase II; inhibits DNA synthesis, causes extensive chromosomal damage, and arrests cell development; unlike other anthracyclines, does not appear to intercalate DNA; readily penetrates cells.

Pharmacodynamics/Kinetics

Absorption: Intravesical: Penetrates into bladder wall; negligible systemic absorption (dependant on bladder wall condition; trauma to mucosa may increase absorption, bladder wall perforation may significantly increase absorption and systemic myelotoxicity).

Metabolism: Negligible after intravesical instillation and 2-hour retention

Excretion: Urine (post 2-hour retention): 98.6% as intact drug; 0.4% as *N*-trifluoroacetyladriamycin)

Dosage Adults: Intravesical: Bladder cancer: 800 mg once weekly (retain for 2 hours) for 6 weeks

Dosage adjustment for toxicity: In clinical trials (Steinberg, 2000), treatment was delayed for 1 week for the following adverse events: Grade 3 dysuria (not controlled with phenazopyridine), frequency/urgency lasting >24 hours, grade 2 gross hematuria (without clots) lasting >48 hours, grade 3 hematuria (with clots) lasting >48 hours. For local toxicities <grade 4 (eg, dysuria [not controlled with phenazopyridine] or severe bladder spasm), anticholinergic therapy (systemic or topical) or topical anesthesia was administered prior to subsequent instillations.

Administration Intravesicular bladder instillation: Insert urinary catheter, empty bladder prior to instillation, slowly by gravity flow, instill 800 mg/75 mL (in 0.9% sodium chloride injection), remove catheter. Retain in the bladder for 2 hours, then void. Administer through non-PVC tubing due to the polyoxyl castor oil (Cremophor® EL) diluent. Maintain adequate hydration following treatment.

Monitoring Parameters Cystoscopy, biopsy, and urine cytology every 3 months for recurrence or progression

Dosage Forms Excipient information presented when available (limited, particularly for generics); consult specific product labeling.

Injection, solution [preservative free]:

Valstar®: 40 mg/mL (5 mL) [contains polyoxyl castor oil and dehydrated ethanol 50%]

References

Newling DW, Hetherington J, Sundaram SK, et al, "The Use of Valrubicin for the Chemoresection of Superficial Bladder Cancer – A Marker Lesion Study," *Eur Urol*, 2001, 39(6):643-7.

Steinberg G, Bahnson R, Brosman S, et al, "Efficacy and Safety of Valrubicin for the Treatment of Bacillus Calmette-Guerin Refractory Carcinoma *in situ* of the Bladder: The Valrubicin Study Group," *J Urol*, 2000, 163(3):761-7.

◆ **Valstar®** *see* Valrubicin *on page 1160*

◆ **Valtaxin® (Can)** *see* Valrubicin *on page 1160*

◆ **Valtrex®** *see* Valacyclovir *on page 1154*

◆ **Vancocin®** *see* Vancomycin *on page 1162*

Vancomycin (van koe MYE sin)

Medication Safety Issues

Sound-alike/look-alike issues:

I.V. vancomycin may be confused with Invanz®

Vancomycin may be confused with clindamycin, gentamicin, tobramycin, valACYclovir, vecuronium, Vibramycin®

High alert medication: The Institute for Safe Medication Practices (ISMP) includes this medication (intrathecal administration) among its list of drug classes which have a heightened risk of causing significant patient harm when used in error.

U.S. Brand Names Vancocin®

Index Terms Vancomycin Hydrochloride

Generic Available Yes: Injection

Canadian Brand Names Vancocin®

Pharmacologic Category Antibiotic, Miscellaneous

Use Treatment of patients with infections caused by staphylococcal species and streptococcal species; used orally for staphylococcal enterocolitis or for antibiotic-associated pseudomembranous colitis produced by *C. difficile*

Unlabeled/Investigational Use Bacterial endophthalmitis; treatment of infections caused by gram-positive organisms in patients who have serious allergies to beta-lactam agents; treatment of beta-lactam resistant gram-positive infections

Pregnancy Risk Factor B (oral); C (injection)

Lactation Enters breast milk/not recommended

Labeled Contraindications Hypersensitivity to vancomycin or any component of the formulation; avoid in patients with previous severe hearing loss

Warnings/Precautions May cause nephrotoxicity although limited data suggest direct causal relationship; usual risk factors include pre-existing renal impairment, concomitant nephrotoxic medications, advanced age, and dehydration. If multiple sequential (≥2) serum creatinine concentrations demonstrate an increase of 0.5 mg/dL or ≥50% increase from baseline (whichever is greater) in the absence of an alternative explanation, the patient should be identified as having vancomycin-induced nephrotoxicity (Rybak, 2009). Discontinue treatment if signs of nephrotoxicity occur; renal damage is usually reversible. May cause neurotoxicity; usual risk factors include pre-existing renal impairment, concomitant neuro-/nephrotoxic medications, advanced age, and dehydration. Ototoxicity, although rarely associated with monotherapy, is proportional to the amount of drug given and the duration of treatment. Tinnitus or vertigo may be indications of vestibular injury and impending bilateral irreversible damage. Discontinue treatment if signs of ototoxicity occur. Prolonged therapy (>1 week) or total doses exceeding 25 g may increase the risk of neutropenia; prompt reversal of neutropenia is expected after discontinuation of therapy. Prolonged use may result in fungal or bacterial superinfection, including *C. difficile*-associated diarrhea (CDAD) and pseudomembranous colitis; CDAD has been observed >2 months postantibiotic treatment. Use with caution in patients with renal impairment or those receiving other nephrotoxic or ototoxic drugs; dosage modification required in patients with impaired renal function (especially elderly). Rapid I.V. administration may result in hypotension, flushing, erythema, urticaria, and/or pruritus. Oral vancomycin is only indicated for the treatment of pseudomembranous colitis due to *C. difficile* and enterocolitis due to *S. aureus* and is not effective for systemic infections; parenteral vancomycin is not effective for the treatment of colitis due to *C. difficile* and enterocolitis due to *S. aureus*.

Adverse Reactions

Oral:
>10%: Gastrointestinal: Bitter taste, nausea, vomiting
1% to 10%:
  Central nervous system: Chills, drug fever
  Hematologic: Eosinophilia
<1%: Interstitial nephritis, ototoxicity, renal failure, thrombocytopenia, vasculitis

Parenteral:
>10%:
  Cardiovascular: Hypotension accompanied by flushing
  Dermatologic: Erythematous rash on face and upper body (red neck or red man syndrome - infusion rate related)
1% to 10%:
  Central nervous system: Chills, drug fever
  Dermatologic: Rash

Hematologic: Eosinophilia, reversible neutropenia

Local: Phlebitis

<1%, postmarketing, and/or case reports: Drug rash with eosinophilia and systemic symptoms (DRESS), ototoxicity (rare; use of other ototoxic agents may increase risk), renal failure (limited data suggesting direct relationship), Stevens-Johnson syndrome, thrombocytopenia, vasculitis

Drug Interactions

Avoid Concomitant Use

Avoid concomitant use of Vancomycin with any of the following: Gallium Nitrate

Increased Effect/Toxicity

Vancomycin may increase the levels/effects of: Aminoglycosides; Colistimethate; Gallium Nitrate; Neuromuscular-Blocking Agents

The levels/effects of Vancomycin may be increased by: Nonsteroidal Anti-Inflammatory Agents

Decreased Effect

Vancomycin may decrease the levels/effects of: Typhoid Vaccine

Storage/Stability Reconstituted 500 mg and 1 g vials are stable for at either room temperature or under refrigeration for 14 days. **Note:** Vials contain no bacteriostatic agent. Solutions diluted for administration in either D_5W or NS are stable under refrigeration for 14 days or at room temperature for 7 days.

Reconstitution Reconstitute vials with 20 mL of SWFI for each 1 g of vancomycin (10 mL/500 mg vial; 20 mL/1 g vial; 100 mL/5 g vial; 200 mL/10 g vial). The reconstituted solution must be further diluted with at least 100 mL of a compatible diluent per 500 mg of vancomycin prior to parenteral administration.

Intrathecal: Vancomycin is available as a powder for injection and may be diluted to 1-5 mg/mL concentration in preservative free 0.9% sodium chloride for administration into the CSF.

Compatibility Stable in dextran 6% in NS, D_5NS, D_5W, $D_{10}W$, LR, NS; **variable stability (consult detailed reference)** in peritoneal dialysis solutions, TPN.

Y-site administration: Compatible: Acyclovir, aldesleukin, allopurinol, amifostine, amiodarone, amsacrine, anidulafungin, atracurium, cisatracurium, clarithromycin, cyclophosphamide, dexmedetomidine, diltiazem, docetaxel, doxapram, doxorubicin liposome, enalaprilat, esmolol, etoposide phosphate, fenoldopam, filgrastim, fluconazole, fludarabine, gallium nitrate, gemcitabine, granisetron, hetastarch, hydromorphone, insulin (regular), labetalol, levofloxacin, linezolid, lorazepam, magnesium sulfate, melphalan, meperidine, meropenem, midazolam, milrinone, morphine, nicardipine, ondansetron, paclitaxel, pancuronium, pemetrexed, perphenazine, remifentanil, sodium bicarbonate, tacrolimus, teniposide, theophylline, thiotepa, tigecycline, tolazoline, vecuronium, vinorelbine, zidovudine. **Incompatible:** Albumin, amphotericin B cholesteryl sulfate complex, bivalirudin, drotrecogin alfa, idarubicin, omeprazole. **Variable (consult detailed reference):** Ampicillin, ampicillin/sulbactam, aztreonam, cefazolin, cefepime, cefotaxime, cefotetan, cefoxitin, ceftazidime, ceftizoxime, ceftriaxone, cefuroxime, foscarnet, heparin, methotrexate, nafcillin, piperacillin, piperacillin/tazobactam, propofol, sargramostim, ticarcillin/clavulanate, TPN, warfarin.

Compatibility in syringe: Compatible: Caffeine citrate, pantoprazole. **Incompatible:** Dimenhydrinate, heparin.

Compatibility when admixed: Compatible: Amikacin, atracurium, calcium gluconate, cefepime, cimetidine, corticotropin, dimenhydrinate, famotidine, fusidate sodium, hydrocortisone sodium succinate, meropenem, ofloxacin, potassium chloride, ranitidine, verapamil, vitamin B complex with C. **Incompatible:** Amobarbital, chloramphenicol, chlorothiazide, dexamethasone sodium phosphate, penicillin G potassium, pentobarbital, phenobarbital. **Variable (consult detailed reference):** Aminophylline, aztreonam, heparin, sodium bicarbonate.

Mechanism of Action Inhibits bacterial cell wall synthesis by blocking glycopeptide polymerization through binding tightly to D-alanyl-D-alanine portion of cell wall precursor

Pharmacodynamics/Kinetics

Absorption: Oral: Poor; I.M.: Erratic; Intraperitoneal: ~38%

Distribution: V_d: 0.4-1 L/kg; Distributes widely in body tissue and fluids, except for CSF

Relative diffusion from blood into CSF: Good only with inflammation (exceeds usual MICs)

Uninflamed meninges: 0-4 mcg/mL; serum concentration dependent

Inflamed meninges: 6-11 mcg/mL; serum concentration dependent

CSF:blood level ratio: Normal meninges: Nil; Inflamed meninges: 20% to 30%

Protein binding: ~50%

Half-life elimination: Biphasic: Terminal:

Newborns: 6-10 hours

Infants and Children 3 months to 4 years: 4 hours

Children >3 years: 2.2-3 hours

Adults: 5-11 hours; significantly prolonged with renal impairment

End-stage renal disease: 200-250 hours

Time to peak, serum: I.V.: Immediately after completion of infusion

Excretion: I.V.: Urine (80% to 90% as unchanged drug); Oral: Primarily feces

Dosage

Usual dosage range:

Infants >1 month and Children: I.V.: 10-15 mg/kg every 6 hours

Adults:

I.V.: 2-3 g/day (or 30-60 mg/kg/day) in divided doses every 8-12 hours (Rybak, 2009); **Note:** Dose requires adjustment in renal impairment

Oral: 500-1000 mg/day in divided doses every 6 hours

Indication-specific dosing:

Infants >1 month and Children:

Colitis *(C. difficile)*, enterocolitis *(S. aureus)*: Oral: 40 mg/kg/day in 3-4 divided doses added to fluids for 7-10 days (maximum: 2000 mg/day)

Meningitis/CNS infection:

I.V.: 15 mg/kg every 6 hours

Intrathecal: 5-20 mg/day

Prophylaxis against infective endocarditis: I.V.:

Dental, oral, or upper respiratory tract surgery: 20 mg/kg 1 hour prior to the procedure. **Note:** American Heart Association (AHA) guidelines now recommend prophylaxis only in patients undergoing invasive procedures and in whom underlying cardiac conditions may predispose to a higher risk of adverse outcomes should infection occur.

GI/GU procedure: 20 mg/kg plus gentamicin 2 mg/kg 1 hour prior to surgery. **Note:** As of April 2007, routine prophylaxis no longer recommended by the AHA.

Susceptible gram-positive infections: I.V.: 10 mg/kg every 6 hours

Adults: Initial intravenous dosing should be based on actual body weight; subsequent dosing adjusted based on serum trough vancomycin concentrations.

Complicated infections in seriously-ill patients (Rybak, 2009): I.V.: Loading dose: 25-30 mg/kg (based on actual body weight) may be used to rapidly achieve target concentration; then 15-20 mg/kg/dose every 8-12 hours.

Catheter-related infections: Antibiotic lock technique (Mermel, 2009): 2 mg/mL ± 10 units heparin/mL **or** 2.5 mg/mL ± 2500 **or** 5000 units heparin/mL **or** 5 mg/mL ± 5000 units heparin/mL (preferred regimen); instill into catheter port with a volume sufficient to fill the catheter (2-5 mL). **Note:** May use SWFI/NS or D$_5$W as diluents. Do not mix with any other solutions. Dwell times generally should not exceed 48 hours before renewal of lock solution. Remove lock solution prior to catheter use then replace.

Colitis *(C. difficile)*, enterocolitis *(S. aureus)*: Oral: 500-2000 mg/day in 3-4 divided doses for 7-10 days (usual dose: 125-250 mg every 6 hours)

Endophthalmitis (unlabeled use): Intravitreal: Usual dose: 1 mg/0.1 mL NS instilled into vitreum; may repeat administration if necessary in 3-4 days, usually in combination with ceftazidime or an aminoglycoside **Note:** Some clinicians have recommended using a lower dose of 0.2 mg/0.1 mL, based on concerns for retinotoxicity.

Hospital-acquired pneumonia (HAP): I.V.: 15 mg/kg/dose every 12 hours (American Thoracic Society [ATS] 2005 guidelines)

Meningitis *(Pneumococcus* or *Staphylococcus)*:
I.V.: 30-60 mg/kg/day in divided doses every 8-12 hours (Rybak, 2009) **or** 500-750 mg every 6 hours (with third-generation cephalosporin for PCN-resistant *Streptococcus pneumoniae*)
Intrathecal: 5-20 mg/day

Prophylaxis against infective endocarditis: I.V.:
Dental, oral, or upper respiratory tract surgery: 1 g 1 hour before surgery. **Note:** AHA guidelines now recommend prophylaxis only in patients undergoing invasive procedures and in whom underlying cardiac conditions may predispose to a higher risk of adverse outcomes should infection occur
GI/GU procedure: 1 g plus 1.5 mg/kg gentamicin 1 hour prior to surgery. **Note:** As of April 2007, routine prophylaxis no longer recommended by the AHA.

Susceptible (MIC ≤1 mcg/mL; Rybak, 2009) gram-positive infections:
I.V.: 15-20 mg/kg/dose (usual: 750-1500 mg) every 8-12 hours
Note: If MIC ≥2 mcg/mL, the targeted AUC:MIC >400 is not achievable with conventional dosing methods in patients with normal renal function and alternative therapies are recommended.

Dosing interval in renal impairment (vancomycin levels should be monitored in patients with any renal impairment):
Cl$_{cr}$ >50 mL/minute: Start with 15-20 mg/kg/dose (usual: 750-1500 mg) every 8-12 hours
Cl$_{cr}$ 20-49 mL/minute: Start with 15-20 mg/kg/dose (usual: 750-1500 mg) every 24 hours
Cl$_{cr}$ <20 mL/minute: Will need longer intervals; determine by serum concentration monitoring
Note: In the critically-ill patient with renal insufficiency, the initial loading dose (25-30 mg/kg) should not be reduced. However, subsequent dosage adjustments should be made based on renal function and trough serum concentrations.

Dialysis: Variable, depending on method; poorly dialyzable by conventional hemodialysis (0% to 5%). Use of high-flux membranes and continuous renal replacement therapy (CRRT) increases vancomycin clearance, and generally requires replacement dosing.

Hemodialysis (HD): Following loading dose of 15-20 mg/kg, give 500 mg to 1 g after each dialysis session, depending on factors such as HD membrane type and flow rate; monitor levels closely.

Continuous ambulatory peritoneal dialysis (CAPD):

Administration via CAPD fluid: 15-30 mg/L (15-30 mcg/mL) of CAPD fluid

Systemic: 1 g loading dose, followed by 500 mg to 1 g every 48-72 hours with close monitoring of levels

Continuous renal replacement therapy (CRRT): Removal of vancomycin is highly dependent on the method of replacement, filter type, and flow rate. Appropriate dosing requires close monitoring of levels in relation to target trough. The following are general recommendations only (Trotman, 2005), and require consideration of the aforementioned parameters.

CVVH: Following loading dose of 15-20 mg/kg, give 1 g every 48 hours

CVVHD or CVVHDF: Following loading dose of 15-20 mg/kg, give 1 g every 24 hours

Trotman RL, Williamson JC, Shoemaker DM, et al, "Antibiotic Dosing in Critically Ill Adult Patients Receiving Continuous Renal Replacement Therapy," *Clin Infect Dis*, 2005, 41:1159-66.

Administration

Intravenous: Administer vancomycin with a final concentration not to exceed 5 mg/mL by I.V. intermittent infusion over at least 60 minutes (recommended infusion period of ≥30 minutes for every 500 mg administered).

If a maculopapular rash appears on the face, neck, trunk, and/or upper extremities (red man syndrome), slow the infusion rate to over 1½ to 2 hours and increase the dilution volume. Hypotension, shock, and cardiac arrest (rare) have also been reported with too rapid of infusion. Reactions are often treated with antihistamines and steroids.

Intrathecal: Vancomycin is available as a powder for injection and may be diluted to 1-5 mg/mL concentration in preservative free 0.9% sodium chloride for intrathecal administration.

Intravitreal: May be administered by intravitreal injection (unlabeled use).

Oral: May be administered with food. If patient cannot swallow capsules, the powder for injection may be reconstituted and diluted for oral administration. Not for I.M. administration.

Extravasation treatment: Monitor I.V. site closely; extravasation will cause serious injury with possible necrosis and tissue sloughing. Rotate infusion site frequently.

Monitoring Parameters Periodic renal function tests, urinalysis, WBC; serum trough vancomycin concentrations in select patients (eg, aggressive dosing, unstable renal function, concurrent nephrotoxins, prolonged courses)

Frequency of trough vancomycin concentration monitoring (Rybak, 2009):

Hemodynamically stable patients: Draw trough concentrations at least once-weekly.

Hemodynamically unstable patients: Draw trough concentrations more frequently or in some instances daily.

Prolonged courses (>3-5 days): Draw at least one steady-state trough concentration; repeat as clinically appropriate.

Note: Drawing >1 trough concentration prior to the fourth dose for short course (<3 days) or lower intensity dosing (target trough concentrations <15 mcg/mL) is not recommended.

Dietary Considerations May be taken with food.

Additional Information Because of its long half-life, vancomycin should be dosed on an every 8- to 12-hour basis. Monitoring of trough serum concentrations is advisable in certain situations. "Red man syndrome", characterized by skin rash and hypotension, is not an allergic reaction but rather is associated with too rapid infusion of the drug. To alleviate or prevent the reaction, infuse vancomycin at a rate of ≥30 minutes for each 500 mg of drug being administered (eg, 1 g over ≥60 minutes); 1.5 g over ≥90 minutes.

Dosage Forms Excipient information presented when available (limited, particularly for generics); consult specific product labeling.

Capsule (Vancocin®): 125 mg, 250 mg

Infusion [premixed in iso-osmotic dextrose] (Vancocin®): 500 mg (100 mL); 1 g (200 mL)

Injection, powder for reconstitution: 500 mg, 1 g, 5 g, 10 g

References

American Thoracic Society and Infectious Diseases Society of America, "Guidelines for the Management of Adults With Hospital-Acquired, Ventilator-Associated, and Healthcare-Associated Pneumonia," *Am J Respir Crit Care Med*, 2005, 171(4):388-416.

Centers for Disease Control and Prevention, "Recommendations for Preventing the Spread of Vancomycin Resistance - Recommendations of the Hospital Infection Control Practice Advisory Committee (HICPAC)," *MMWR Recomm Rep*, 1995, 44(RR-12):1-9.

Chang D, Liem L, and Malogolowkin M, "A Prospective Study of Vancomycin Pharmacokinetics and Dosage Requirements in Pediatric Cancer Patients," *Pediatr Infect Dis J*, 1994, 13 (11):969-74.

Chang D, "Influence of Malignancy on the Pharmacokinetics of Vancomycin in Infants and Children," *Pediatr Infect Dis J*, 1995, 14(8):667-73.

DeVries E, van Rossum MAJ, Garritsen EJA, et al, "No Difference in Frequency of Adverse Reactions to Either Vancomycin or Teicoplanin in 70 Pediatric Bone Marrow Transplant Patients," *Bone Marrow Transplant*, 1995, 15(Suppl 2):124.

Frimat L, Hestin D, Hanesse B, et al, "Acute Renal Failure Due to Vancomycin Alone," *Nephrol Dial Transplant*, 1995, 10(4):550-1.

Kelly CP, Pothoulakis C, and LaMont JT, "Clostridium difficile colitis," *N Engl J Med*, 1994, 330 (4):257-62.

Leader WG, Chandler MH, and Castiglia M, "Pharmacokinetic Optimization of Vancomycin Therapy," *Clin Pharmacokinet*, 1995, 28(4):327-42.

Luer MS and Hatton J, "Vancomycin Administration Into the Cerebrospinal Fluid: A Review," *Ann Pharmacother*, 1993, 27(7-8):912-21.

Lyon GD and Bruce DL, "Diphenhydramine Reversal of Vancomycin-Induced Hypotension," *Anesth Analg*, 1988, 67(11):1109-10.

Matzke GR, Zhanel GG, and Guay DRP, "Clinical Pharmacokinetics of Vancomycin," *Clin Pharmacokinet*, 1986, 11(4):257-82.

Murray BE, "Vancomycin-Resistant Enterococcal Infections," *N Engl J Med*, 2000, 342(10):710-21.

Rodvold KA, Blum RA, Fischer JH, et al, "Vancomycin Pharmacokinetics in Patients With Various Degrees of Renal Function," *Antimicrob Agents Chemother*, 1988, 32(6):848-52.

Rybak MJ, Albrecht LM, Boike SC, et al, "Nephrotoxicity of Vancomycin, Alone and With an Aminoglycoside," *J Antimicrob Chemother*, 1990, 25(4):679-87.

Rybak M, Lomaestro B, Rotschafer JC, et al, "Therapeutic Monitoring of Vancomycin in Adult Patients: A Consensus Review of the American Society of Health-System Pharmacists, the Infectious Diseases Society of America, and the Society of Infectious Diseases Pharmacists," *Am J Health-Syst Pharm*, 2009, 66(1):82-98

◆ **Versiclear™** *see* Sodium Thiosulfate *on page 1040*

◆ **Vesanoid®** *see* Tretinoin, Systemic *on page 1141*

◆ **VFEND®** *see* Voriconazole *on page 1187*

◆ **Vidaza®** *see* AzaCITIDine *on page 117*

VinBLAStine (vin BLAS teen)

Medication Safety Issues

Sound-alike/look-alike issues:

VinBLAStine may be confused with vinCRIStine, vinorelbine

High alert medication: The Institute for Safe Medication Practices (ISMP) includes this medication among its list of drug classes which have a heightened risk of causing significant patient harm when used in error.

Note: Must be dispensed in overwrap which bears the statement **"Do not remove covering until the moment of injection. Fatal if given intrathecally. For I.V. use only."** Syringes should be labeled: **"Fatal if given intrathecally. For I.V. use only."**

Related Information

Management of Chemotherapy-Induced Nausea and Vomiting *on page 1434*
Management of Drug Extravasations *on page 1447*
Safe Handling of Hazardous Drugs *on page 1517*

Index Terms Velban; Vinblastine Sulfate; Vincaleukoblastine; VLB

Generic Available Yes

Pharmacologic Category Antineoplastic Agent, Natural Source (Plant) Derivative; Antineoplastic Agent, Vinca Alkaloid

Use Treatment of Hodgkin's and non-Hodgkin's lymphoma; testicular cancer; breast cancer; mycosis fungoides; Kaposi's sarcoma; histiocytosis (Letterer-Siwe disease); choriocarcinoma

Unlabeled/Investigational Use Treatment of bladder cancer, melanoma, nonsmall cell lung cancer (NSCLC), ovarian cancer, soft tissue sarcoma (desmoid tumors)

Pregnancy Risk Factor D

Lactation Excretion in breast milk unknown/not recommended

Labeled Contraindications Significant granulocytopenia; presence of bacterial infection; I.T. administration is contraindicated (may result in death)

Warnings/Precautions Hazardous agent - use appropriate precautions for handling and disposal. **[U.S. Boxed Warning]: For I.V. use only. Intrathecal administration may result in death.** Must be dispensed in overwrap which bears the statement **"Do not remove covering until the moment of injection. Fatal if given intrathecally. For I.V. use only." [U.S. Boxed Warning]: Vinblastine is a moderate vesicant; avoid extravasation. Individuals administering should be experienced in vinblastine administration;** assure proper needle or catheter placement prior to administration. Leukopenia is common; granulocytopenia may be severe with higher doses. Leukopenia may be more pronounced in cachectic patients and patients with skin ulceration. Thrombocytopenia and anemia may occur rarely.

Use with caution in patients with hepatic impairment; toxicity may be increased; may require dosage modification. Neurotoxicity is rare at clinical doses; may occur with high doses (symptoms are similar to vincristine toxicity, including peripheral neuropathy, loss of deep tendon reflexes, headache, weakness, urinary retention, and GI symptoms). May rarely cause disabling neurotoxicity (usually reversible). Itraconazole may decrease the metabolism of vinblastine via CYP3A4 inhibition and may increase the effects of vinblastine via P-glycoprotein effects; severe myelosuppression and neurotoxicity may occur. Acute shortness of breath and severe bronchospasm have been reported, most often in association with concurrent administration of mitomycin; may occur within minutes to several hours following vinblastine administration or up to 14 days following mitomycin administration; use caution in patients with pre-existing pulmonary disease. Use with caution in patients with ischemic heart disease. **[U.S. Boxed Warning]: Should be administered under the supervision of an experienced cancer chemotherapy physician.** Some dosage forms may contain benzyl alcohol which has been associated with "gasping syndrome" in neonates.

Adverse Reactions Frequency not defined.

Common:
Cardiovascular: Hypertension
Central nervous system: Malaise
Dermatologic: Alopecia
Gastrointestinal: Constipation
Hematologic: Myelosuppression, leukopenia/granulocytopenia (nadir: 5-10 days; recovery: 7-14 days; dose-limiting toxicity)
Neuromuscular & skeletal: Bone pain, jaw pain, tumor pain

Less common:
Cardiovascular: Angina, cerebrovascular accident, coronary ischemia, ECG abnormalities, MI, Raynaud's phenomenon
Central nervous system: Depression, dizziness, headache, neurotoxicity (duration: >24 hours), seizure, vertigo
Dermatologic: Dermatitis, photosensitivity (rare), rash, skin blistering
Endocrine & metabolic: Aspermia, hyperuricemia, SIADH
Gastrointestinal: Abdominal pain, anorexia, diarrhea, gastrointestinal bleeding, hemorrhagic enterocolitis, ileus, metallic taste, nausea (mild), paralytic ileus, rectal bleeding, stomatitis, vomiting (mild)
Genitourinary: Urinary retention
Hematologic: Anemia, thrombocytopenia (recovery within a few days)
Local: Cellulitis (with extravasation), irritation, phlebitis (with extravasation), radiation recall
Neuromuscular & skeletal: Deep tendon reflex loss, myalgia, paresthesia, peripheral neuritis, weakness
Ocular: Nystagmus
Otic: Auditory damage, deafness, vestibular damage
Respiratory: Bronchospasm, dyspnea, pharyngitis

Drug Interactions

Metabolism/Transport Effects Substrate of CYP2D6 (minor), 3A4 (major); **Inhibits** CYP2D6 (weak), 3A4 (weak)

Avoid Concomitant Use

Avoid concomitant use of VinBLAStine with any of the following: Natalizumab; Vaccines (Live)

Increased Effect/Toxicity

VinBLAStine may increase the levels/effects of: Leflunomide; Mitomycin; Natalizumab; Tolterodine; Vaccines (Live)

The levels/effects of VinBLAStine may be increased by: CYP3A4 Inhibitors (Moderate); CYP3A4 Inhibitors (Strong); Dasatinib; Itraconazole; Lopinavir; Macrolide Antibiotics; MAO Inhibitors; P-Glycoprotein Inhibitors; Posaconazole; Ritonavir; Trastuzumab; Voriconazole

Decreased Effect

VinBLAStine may decrease the levels/effects of: Dabigatran Etexilate; P-Glycoprotein Substrates; Vaccines (Inactivated); Vaccines (Live)

The levels/effects of VinBLAStine may be decreased by: CYP3A4 Inducers (Strong); Deferasirox; Echinacea; Herbs (CYP3A4 Inducers); Peginterferon Alfa-2b; P-Glycoprotein Inducers

Ethanol/Nutrition/Herb Interactions Herb/Nutraceutical: Avoid St John's wort (may decrease vinblastine levels). Avoid black cohosh, dong quai in estrogen-dependent tumors.

Storage/Stability Note: Must be dispensed in overwrap which bears the statement "Do not remove covering until the moment of injection. Fatal if given intrathecally. For I.V. use only." Syringes should be labeled: "Fatal if given intrathecally. For I.V. use only."

Store intact vials under refrigeration at 2°C to 8°C (36°F to 46°F). Protect from light. Solutions reconstituted in bacteriostatic NS are stable for 28 days under refrigeration.

Reconstitution Reconstitute lyophilized powder to a concentration of 1 mg/mL with NS or bacteriostatic NS. For infusion, may dilute in 50 mL NS or D_5W; dilution in larger volumes (≥100 mL) of I.V. fluids is not recommended. Use appropriate precautions for handling and disposal.

Compatibility Stable in D_5W, LR, NS

Y-site administration: Compatible: Allopurinol, amifostine, amphotericin B cholesteryl sulfate complex, aztreonam, bleomycin, cisplatin, cyclophosphamide, doxorubicin, doxorubicin liposome, droperidol, etoposide phosphate, filgrastim, fludarabine, fluorouracil, gatifloxacin, gemcitabine, granisetron, heparin, leucovorin calcium, melphalan, methotrexate, metoclopramide, mitomycin, ondansetron, paclitaxel, piperacillin/tazobactam, sargramostim, teniposide, thiotepa, vincristine, vinorelbine. **Incompatible:** Cefepime, furosemide, lansoprazole.

Compatibility in syringe: Compatible: Bleomycin, cisplatin, cyclophosphamide, droperidol, fluorouracil, leucovorin calcium, methotrexate, metoclopramide, mitomycin, vincristine. **Incompatible:** Furosemide. **Variable (consult detailed reference):** Doxorubicin, heparin.

Compatibility when admixed: Compatible: Bleomycin, dacarbazine. **Variable (consult detailed reference):** Doxorubicin.

Mechanism of Action Vinblastine binds to tubulin and inhibits microtubule formation, therefore, arresting the cell at metaphase by disrupting the formation of the mitotic spindle; it is specific for the M and S phases. Vinblastine may also interfere with nucleic acid and protein synthesis by blocking glutamic acid utilization.

Pharmacodynamics/Kinetics

Distribution: V_d: 27.3 L/kg; binds extensively to tissues; does not penetrate CNS or other fatty tissues; distributes to liver

Protein binding: 99%

Metabolism: Hepatic to active metabolite

Half-life elimination: Biphasic: Initial: 4 minutes; Terminal: 25 hours

Excretion: Feces (95%); urine (<1% as unchanged drug)

Dosage Details concerning dosing in combination regimens should also be consulted. **Note:** Frequency and duration of therapy may vary by indication, concomitant combination chemotherapy and hematologic response. **For I.V. use only.**

◀ Children: I.V.:
   Hodgkin's disease: Initial dose: 6 mg/m^2; do not administer more frequently than every 7 days
   Letterer-Siwe disease: Initial dose: 6.5 mg/m^2; do not administer more frequently than every 7 days
   Testicular cancer: Initial dose: 3 mg/m^2; do not administer more frequently than every 7 days
Adults: I.V.: Initial: 3.7 mg/m^2; adjust dose every 7 days (based on white blood cell response) up to 5.5 mg/m^2 (second dose); 7.4 mg/m^2 (third dose); 9.25 mg/m^2 (fourth dose); and 11.1 mg/m^2 (fifth dose); do not administer more frequently than every 7 days.
   Usual range: 5.5-7.4 mg/m^2 every 7 days; Maximum dose: 18.5 mg/m^2; dosage adjustment goal is to reduce white blood cell count to ~3000/mm^3
Indication-specific dosing:
Hodgkin's disease: Usual dose: 6 mg/m^2 every 2 weeks (as part of a combination chemotherapy regimen) (Bartlett, 1995; Horning, 2002)
Testicular cancer: Usual dose: 0.11 mg/kg daily for 2 days every 3 weeks (as part of a combination chemotherapy regimen) (Loehrer, 1998) **or** 6 mg/m^2/day for 2 days every 3-4 weeks (as part of a combination chemotherapy regimen) (Clemm, 1986)
Bladder cancer (unlabeled use): Usual dose: 3 mg/m^2 every 7 days for 3 out of 4 weeks (as part of combination chemotherapy) (Sternberg, 2001) **or** 3 mg/m^2 days 2, 15, and 22 of a 28-day treatment cycle (as part of a combination chemotherapy regimen) (von der Maase, 2000)
Melanoma (unlabeled used): 2 mg/m^2 days 1-4 and 22-25 of a 6-week treatment cycle (as part of a combination chemotherapy regimen) (Eton, 2002)
Nonsmall cell lung cancer (unlabeled use): 4 mg/m^2 days 1, 8, 15, 22, and 29, then every 2 weeks (as part of combination chemotherapy) (Arriagada, 2004)
Ovarian cancer (unlabeled use): 0.11 mg/kg daily for 2 days every 3 weeks (as part of a combination chemotherapy regimen) (Loehrer, 1998)

Dosing adjustment in renal impairment: According to FDA-approved labeling, no adjustment is necessary in patients with renal impairment.
Dosing adjustment in hepatic impairment:
The FDA-approved labeling recommends the following guidelines: Serum bilirubin >3 mg/dL: Administer 50% of dose
The following guidelines have been used by some clinicians:
   Serum bilirubin >3.1 or transaminases >3 times ULN: Avoid use (Floyd, 2006)
      or
   Serum bilirubin 1.5-3 mg/dL or AST 60-180 units: Administer 50% of dose
   Serum bilirubin 3-5 mg/dL: Administer 25% of dose
   Serum bilirubin >5 mg/dL or AST >180 units: Avoid use
Combination Regimens

Administration FATAL IF GIVEN INTRATHECALLY. For I.V. administration only, usually as a slow (2-3 minutes) push, or a bolus (5-15 minutes) infusion; the manufacturer recommends an undiluted 1-minute infusion to prevent venous irritation/extravasation. Prolonged administration times and/or increased administration volumes may the risk of vein irritation and extravasation. Assure proper needle or catheter placement prior to administration.

Monitoring Parameters CBC with differential and platelet count, serum uric acid, hepatic function tests

Emetic Potential Very low (<10%)

Vesicant Yes; see Management of Drug Extravasations on page 1447.

Dosage Forms Excipient information presented when available (limited, particularly for generics); consult specific product labeling.

Injection, powder for reconstitution, as sulfate: 10 mg

Injection, solution, as sulfate: 1 mg/mL (10 mL) [contains benzyl alcohol]

References

Arriagada R, Bergman B, Dunant A, et al, "Cisplatin-Based Adjuvant Chemotherapy in Patients With Completely Resected Non-Small-Cell Lung Cancer," *N Engl J Med*, 2004, 350(4):351-60.

Bartlett NL, Rosenberg SA, Hoppe RT, et al, "Brief Chemotherapy, Stanford V, and Adjuvant Radiotherapy for Bulky or Advanced-Stage Hodgkin's Disease: A Preliminary Report," *J Clin Oncol*, 1995, 13(5):1080-8.

Bashir H, Motl S, Metzger ML, et al, "Itraconazole-Enhanced Chemotherapy Toxicity in a Patient With Hodgkin Lymphoma," *J Pediatr Hematol Oncol*, 2006, 28(1):33-5.

Bonadonna G, Valagussa P, and Santoro A, "Alternating Non-Cross-Resistant Combination Chemotherapy or MOPP in Stage IV Hodgkin's Disease: A Report of 8-Year Results," *Ann Intern Med*, 1986, 104(6):739-46.

Chong CD, Logothetis CJ, Savaraj N, et al, "The Correlation of Vinblastine Pharmacokinetics to Toxicity in Testicular Cancer Patients," *J Clin Pharmacol*, 1998, 28(8):714-8.

Clemm C, Hartenstein R, Willich N, et al, "Vinblastine-Ifosfamide-Cisplatin Treatment of Bulky Seminoma," *Cancer*, 1986, 58(10):2203-7.

Eton O, Legha SS, Bedikian AY, et al, "Sequential Biochemotherapy Versus Chemotherapy for Metastatic Melanoma: Results From a Phase III Randomized Trial," *J Clin Oncol*, 2002, 20 (8):2045-52.

Floyd J, Mirza I, Sachs B, et al, "Hepatotoxicity of Chemotherapy," *Semin Oncol*, 2006, 33 (1):50-67.

Friedman M, Venkatesan TK, and Caldarelli DD, "Intralesional Vinblastine for Treating AIDS-Associated Kaposi's Sarcoma of the Oropharynx and Larynx," *Ann Otol Rhinol Laryngol*, 1996, 105(4):272-4.

Horning SJ, Hoppe RT, Breslin S, et al, "Stanford V and Radiotherapy for Locally Extensive and Advanced Hodgkin's Disease: Mature Results of a Prospective Clinical Trial," *J Clin Oncol*, 2002, 20(3):630-7.

Loehrer PJ Sr, Gonin R, Nichols CR, et al, "Vinblastine Plus Ifosfamide Plus Cisplatin as Initial Salvage Therapy in Recurrent Germ Cell Tumor," *J Clin Oncol*, 1998, 16(7):2500-4.

Pronzato P, Queirolo P, Vidili MG, et al, "Continuous Venous Infusion of Vinblastine in Metastatic Breast Cancer," *Chemotherapy*, 1991, 37(2):146-9.

Sternberg CN, de Mulder PH, Schornagel JH, et al, "Randomized Phase III Trial of High-Dose-Intensity Methotrexate, Vinblastine, Doxorubicin, and Cisplatin (M-VAC) Chemotherapy and Recombinant Human Granulocyte Colony-Stimulating Factor Versus Classic M-VAC in Advanced Urothelial Tract Tumors: European Organization for Research and Treatment of Cancer Protocol No. 30924," *J Clin Oncol*, 2001, 19(10):2638-46.

van der Maase H, Hansen SW, Roberts JT, et al, "Gemcitabine and Cisplatin Versus Methotrexate, Vinblastine, Doxorubicin, and Cisplatin in Advanced or Metastatic Bladder Cancer: Results of a Large, Randomized, Multinational, Multicenter, Phase III Study," *J Clin Oncol*, 2000, 18 (17):3068-77.

Williams SD, Birch R, Einhorn LH, et al, "Treatment of Disseminated Germ-Cell Tumors With Cisplatin, Bleomycin, and Either Vinblastine or Etoposide," *N Engl J Med*, 1987, 316 (23):1435-40.

♦ **Vinblastine Sulfate** *see* VinBLAStine *on page* 1169

♦ **Vincaleukoblastine** *see* VinBLAStine *on page* 1169

♦ **Vincasar PFS®** *see* VinCRIStine *on page* 1174

♦ **Vincasar® PFS® (Can)** *see* VinCRIStine *on page* 1174

VinCRIStine (vin KRIS teen)

Medication Safety Issues

Sound-alike/look-alike issues:

VinCRIStine may be confused with vinBLAStine

Oncovin® may be confused with Ancobon®

High alert medication: The Institute for Safe Medication Practices (ISMP) includes this medication among its list of drugs which have a heightened risk of causing significant patient harm when used in error.

To prevent fatal inadvertent intrathecal injection, it is recommended that all doses be dispensed in a small minibag. If dispensing vincristine in a syringe, vincristine must be packaged in the manufacturer-provided overwrap which bears the statement **"Do not remove covering until the moment of injection. For intravenous use only. Fatal if given intrathecally."**

Related Information

Management of Drug Extravasations *on page* 1447

Safe Handling of Hazardous Drugs *on page* 1517

U.S. Brand Names Vincasar PFS®

Index Terms Leurocristine Sulfate; Oncovin; Vincristine Sulfate

Generic Available Yes

Canadian Brand Names Vincasar® PFS®

Pharmacologic Category Antineoplastic Agent, Natural Source (Plant) Derivative; Antineoplastic Agent, Vinca Alkaloid

Use Treatment of acute lymphocytic leukemia (ALL), Hodgkin's disease, non-Hodgkin's lymphomas, Wilms' tumor, neuroblastoma, rhabdomyosarcoma

Unlabeled/Investigational Use Treatment of multiple myeloma, chronic lymphocytic leukemia (CLL), brain tumors, small cell lung cancer, ovarian germ cell tumors

Pregnancy Risk Factor D

Lactation Enters breast milk/not recommended

Labeled Contraindications Hypersensitivity to vincristine or any component of the formulation; **for I.V. use only, fatal if given intrathecally;** patients with demyelinating form of Charcot-Marie-Tooth syndrome; pregnancy

Warnings/Precautions Hazardous agent - use appropriate precautions for handling and disposal. **[U.S. Boxed Warning]: Vincristine is a vesicant; avoid extravasation. (Individuals administering should be experienced in vincristine administration.)**

Dosage modification required in patients with impaired hepatic function or who have pre-existing neuromuscular disease. Use with caution in the elderly. Avoid eye contamination. Observe closely for shortness of breath, bronchospasm, especially in patients treated with mitomycin C. Alterations in mental status such as depression, confusion, or insomnia; constipation, paralytic ileus, and urinary tract disturbances may occur. All patients should be on a prophylactic bowel management regimen.

[U.S. Boxed Warning]: Intrathecal administration of vincristine has uniformly caused severe neurologic damage and/or death; vincristine should never be administered by this route. For I.V. use only. Neurologic effects of vincristine may be additive with those of other neurotoxic agents and spinal cord irradiation.

Adverse Reactions

>10%: Dermatologic: Alopecia (20% to 70%)

1% to 10%:

Cardiovascular: Orthostatic hypotension or hypertension, hyper-/hypotension

Central nervous system: CNS depression, confusion, cranial nerve paralysis, fever, headache, insomnia, motor difficulties, seizure

Intrathecal administration of vincristine has uniformly caused death; vincristine should never be administered by this route. Neurologic effects of vincristine may be additive with those of other neurotoxic agents and spinal cord irradiation.

Dermatologic: Rash

Endocrine & metabolic: Hyperuricemia

Gastrointestinal: Abdominal cramps, anorexia, bloating, constipation (and possible paralytic ileus secondary to neurologic toxicity), diarrhea, metallic taste, nausea (mild), oral ulceration, vomiting, weight loss

Genitourinary: Bladder atony (related to neurotoxicity), dysuria, polyuria, urinary retention

Hematologic: Leukopenia (mild), thrombocytopenia, myelosuppression (onset: 7 days; nadir: 10 days; recovery: 21 days)

Local: Phlebitis, tissue irritation and necrosis if infiltrated

Neuromuscular & skeletal: Cramping, jaw pain, leg pain, myalgia, numbness, weakness

Peripheral neuropathy: Frequently the dose-limiting toxicity of vincristine. Most frequent in patients >40 years of age; occurs usually after an average of 3 weekly doses, but may occur after just one dose. Manifested as loss of the deep tendon reflexes in the lower extremities, numbness, tingling, pain, paresthesia of the fingers and toes (stocking glove sensation), and "foot drop" or "wrist drop."

Ocular: Optic atrophy, photophobia

<1%: SIADH (rare), stomatitis

Drug Interactions

Metabolism/Transport Effects Substrate of CYP3A4 (major); **Inhibits** CYP3A4 (weak)

◀ **Avoid Concomitant Use**
Avoid concomitant use of VinCRIStine with any of the following: Natalizumab; Vaccines (Live)

Increased Effect/Toxicity
VinCRIStine may increase the levels/effects of: Leflunomide; Mitomycin; Natalizumab; Vaccines (Live); Vitamin K Antagonists

The levels/effects of VinCRIStine may be increased by: CYP3A4 Inhibitors (Moderate); CYP3A4 Inhibitors (Strong); Dasatinib; Itraconazole; Lopinavir; Macrolide Antibiotics; MAO Inhibitors; NIFEdipine; P-Glycoprotein Inhibitors; Posaconazole; Ritonavir; Trastuzumab; Voriconazole

Decreased Effect
VinCRIStine may decrease the levels/effects of: Cardiac Glycosides; Vaccines (Inactivated); Vaccines (Live); Vitamin K Antagonists

The levels/effects of VinCRIStine may be decreased by: CYP3A4 Inducers (Strong); Deferasirox; Echinacea; Herbs (CYP3A4 Inducers); P-Glycoprotein Inducers

Ethanol/Nutrition/Herb Interactions Herb/Nutraceutical: St John's wort may decrease vincristine levels.

Storage/Stability
Undiluted vials: Store under refrigeration. May be stable for up to 30 days at room temperature.
I.V. solution: Diluted in 20-50 mL NS or D_5W, stable for 7 days under refrigeration, or 2 days at room temperature. In ambulatory pumps, solution is stable for 7-10 days at room temperature.

Reconstitution Solutions for I.V. infusion may be mixed in NS or D_5W. **Note:** The World Health Organization (WHO) recommends dispensing vincristine in a minibag, rather than a syringe.

Compatibility Stable in D_5W, LR, NS.
Y-site administration: Compatible: Allopurinol, amifostine, amphotericin B cholesteryl sulfate complex, aztreonam, bleomycin, cisplatin, cladribine, cyclophosphamide, doxorubicin, doxorubicin liposome, droperidol, etoposide phosphate, filgrastim, fludarabine, fluorouracil, gatifloxacin, gemcitabine, granisetron, heparin, leucovorin, linezolid, melphalan, methotrexate, metoclopramide, mitomycin, ondansetron, paclitaxel, piperacillin/tazobactam, sargramostim, teniposide, thiotepa, topotecan, vinblastine, vinorelbine. **Incompatible:** Cefepime, furosemide, idarubicin, sodium bicarbonate.
Compatibility in syringe: Compatible: Bleomycin, cisplatin, cyclophosphamide, doxapram, doxorubicin, droperidol, fluorouracil, heparin, leucovorin, methotrexate, metoclopramide, mitomycin, vinblastine. **Incompatible:** Furosemide.
Compatibility when admixed: Compatible: Bleomycin, cytarabine, doxorubicin with ondansetron, fluorouracil, methotrexate. **Variable (consult detailed reference):** Doxorubicin with etoposide.

Mechanism of Action Binds to tubulin and inhibits microtubule formation, therefore, arresting the cell at metaphase by disrupting the formation of the mitotic spindle; it is specific for the M and S phases. Vincristine may also interfere with nucleic acid and protein synthesis by blocking glutamic acid utilization.

Pharmacodynamics/Kinetics
Absorption: Oral: Poor
Distribution: V_d: 163-165 L/m²; poor penetration into CSF; rapidly removed from bloodstream and tightly bound to tissues; penetrates blood-brain barrier poorly

Protein binding: 75%

Metabolism: Extensively hepatic

Half-life elimination: Terminal: 24 hours

Excretion: Feces (~80%); urine (<1% as unchanged drug)

Dosage Note: Doses are often capped at 2 mg; however, this may reduce the efficacy of the therapy and may not be advisable. Refer to individual protocols; orders for single doses >2.5 mg or >5 mg/treatment cycle should be verified with the specific treatment regimen and/or an experienced oncologist prior to dispensing. I.V.:

Children ≤10 kg or BSA <1 m^2: Initial therapy: 0.05 mg/kg once weekly then titrate dose

Children >10 kg or BSA ≥1 m^2: 1-2 mg/m^2, may repeat once weekly for 3-6 weeks; maximum single dose: 2 mg

Neuroblastoma: I.V. continuous infusion with doxorubicin: 1 mg/m^2/day for 72 hours

Adults: 0.4-1.4 mg/m^2, may repeat every week **or**

0.4-0.5 mg/day continuous infusion for 4 days every 4 weeks **or**

0.25-0.5 mg/m^2/day for 5 days every 4 weeks

Dosing adjustment in renal impairment: No adjustment is necessary in patients with renal impairment.

Dosing adjustment in hepatic impairment:

The FDA-approved labeling recommends the following guidelines: Serum bilirubin >3 mg/dL: Administer 50% of normal dose

The following guidelines have been used by some clinicians:

Serum bilirubin 1.5-3 mg/dL or AST 60-180 units: Administer 50% of dose

Serum bilirubin 3-5 mg/dL: Administer 25% of dose

Serum bilirubin >5 mg/dL or AST >180 units: Avoid use

Floyd, 2006: Serum bilirubin 1.5-3 mg/dL or transaminases 2-3 times ULN or alkaline phosphatase elevated: Administer 50% of dose

Combination Regimens

Brain tumors:

Breast cancer:

Gestational trophoblastic tumor:

Head and neck cancer:

Leukemia, acute lymphocytic:

Administration FATAL IF GIVEN INTRATHECALLY.

I.V.: Usually administered as short (10-15 minutes) infusion (preferred) or as slow (1-2 minutes) push; 24-hour continuous infusions are occasionally used
Intralesional injection has been reported for Kaposi's sarcoma.

Monitoring Parameters Serum electrolytes (sodium), hepatic function tests, neurologic examination, CBC, serum uric acid

Emetic Potential Very low (<10%)

Vesicant Yes; moderate. See Management of Drug Extravasations on page 1447.

Dosage Forms Excipient information presented when available (limited, particularly for generics); consult specific product labeling.

Injection, solution, as sulfate [preservative free]:
  Vincasar PFS® 1 mg/mL (1 mL, 2 mL)

References

Aronoff GR, Bennett WM, Berns JS, et al, *Drug Prescribing in Renal Failure: Dosing Guidelines for Adults and Children*, 5th ed. Philadelphia, PA: American College of Physicians; 2007, p 102, 174.

Bermudez M, Fuster JL, Llinares E, et al, "Itraconazole-Related Increased Vincristine Neurotoxicity: Case Report and Review of Literature," *J Pediatr Hematol Oncol*, 2005, 27(7):389-92.

Bohme A, Ganser A, and Hoelzer D, "Aggravation of Vincristine-Induced Neurotoxicity by Itraconazole in the Treatment of Adult ALL," *Ann Hematol*, 1995, 71(6):311-2.

Floyd J, Mirza I, Sachs B, et al, "Hepatotoxicity of Chemotherapy," *Semin Oncol*, 2006, 33 (1):50-67.

Legha SS, "Vincristine Neurotoxicity. Pathophysiology and Management," *Med Toxicol*, 1986, 1 (6):421-7.

McCune JS and Lindley C, "Appropriateness of Maximum-Dose Guidelines for Vincristine," *Am J Health Syst Pharm*, 1997, 54(15):1755-8.

◆ **Vincristine Sulfate** *see* VinCRIStine *on page 1174*

Vindesine (VIN de seen)

Medication Safety Issues

High alert medication: The Institute for Safe Medication Practices (ISMP) includes this medication among its list of drugs which have a heightened risk of causing significant patient harm when used in error.

To prevent fatal inadvertent intrathecal injection, it is recommended by ISMP that all doses be dispensed in a small minibag. **Fatal if given intrathecally.**

Related Information

Management of Drug Extravasations *on page 1447*
Safe Handling of Hazardous Drugs *on page 1517*

Index Terms DAVA; Deacetyl Vinblastine Carboxamide; Desacetyl Vinblastine Amide Sulfate; DVA; Eldisine Lilly 99094; Lilly CT-3231; NSC-245467; Vindesine Sulfate

Generic Available No

Pharmacologic Category Antineoplastic Agent, Vinca Alkaloid

Unlabeled/Investigational Use Investigational: Management of acute lymphocytic leukemia, chronic myelogenous leukemia; breast, head, neck, and lung cancers; lymphomas (Hodgkin's and non-Hodgkin's)

Restrictions Not available in U.S./Investigational

Lactation Breast-feeding is not recommended.

Labeled Contraindications Hypersensitivity to vindesine, vinca alkaloids, or any component of the formulation

Warnings/Precautions Hazardous agent - use appropriate precautions for handling and disposal. Vindesine should be used cautiously, if at all, in patients with impaired hepatic function or neurologic problems. **Intrathecal administration may be fatal.** Vindesine has been reported to be cross-resistance with vincristine.

Adverse Reactions

>10%:

Central nervous system: Pyrexia, malaise (up to 60%)

Dermatologic: Alopecia (6% to 92%)

Gastrointestinal: Mild nausea and vomiting (7% to 27%), constipation (10% to 17%) - related to the neurotoxicity

Hematologic: Leukopenia (50%) and thrombocytopenia (14% to 26%), may be dose limiting; thrombocytosis (20% to 28%)

Nadir: 6-12 days

Recovery: Days 14-18

Neuromuscular & skeletal: Paresthesia (40% to 70%); loss of deep tendon reflexes (35% to 60%, may be dose limiting); myalgia (up to 60%)

1% to 10%:

Dermatologic: Rashes

Gastrointestinal: Loss of taste

Hematologic: Anemia

Local: Phlebitis

Neuromuscular & skeletal: Facial paralysis

<1%: Acute chest pain, ECG changes, paralytic ileus, jaw pain, photophobia

Storage/Stability Reconstituted solutions are stable for 30 days under refrigeration (2°C to 8°C/36°F to 46°F). Solutions diluted in dextrose or saline for I.V. infusion are stable for 24 hours at room temperature (15°C to 30°C/59°F to 86°F). **The drug will precipitate at pH >6.**

Reconstitution The powder is reconstituted to a concentration of 1 mg/mL.

Mechanism of Action Vindesine is a semisynthetic vinca alkaloid, having a mechanism of action similar to the other vinca derivatives. It arrests cell division in metaphase through inhibition of microtubular formation of the mitotic spindle. The drug is cell-cycle specific for the S phase.

Pharmacodynamics/Kinetics

Distribution: V_d: 8 L/kg; minimal distribution to adipose tissue or CNS

Metabolism: Hepatic

Half-life elimination:

Triphasic; Alpha: 2 minutes; Beta: 1 hour

Terminal: 24 hours

Excretion: Feces; urine (~3% to 25% of dose as unchanged drug)

Dosage Refer to individual protocols. I.V.: Adults:

3-4 mg/m^2/week **or**

1-2 mg/m^2 days 1 and 2 every 2 weeks **or**

1-2 mg/m^2 days 1-5 (continuous infusion) every 2-4 weeks **or**

1-2 mg/m^2 days 1-5 every 3-4 weeks

Dosage adjustment in hepatic impairment: Dosage reductions of 50% to 75% have been suggested for "severe" hepatic dysfunction; however, specific guidelines have not been published.

Combination Regimens

Breast cancer: VM on page 1426

Lymphoma, Hodgkin's disease: CAD/MOPP/ABV on page 1242

Administration Usually administered as a rapid I.V. push (2-3 minutes) or short (15-20 minutes) infusion; 24-hour continuous infusions are occasionally used.

Vesicant Yes; see Management of Drug Extravasations on page 1447.

Dosage Forms Excipient information presented when available (limited, particularly for generics); consult specific product labeling.

Injection, powder for reconstitution: 5 mg

References

Dancey J and Steward WP, "The Role of Vindesine in Oncology - Recommendations After 10 Years' Experience," *Anticancer Drugs*, 1995, 6(5):625-36.

Rhomberg W, Eiter H, Soltesz E, et al, "Long-Term Application of Vindesine: Toxicity and Tolerance," *J Cancer Res Clin Oncol*, 1990, 116(6):651-3.

Sorenson JB and Hansen HH, "Is There a Role for Vindesine in the Treatment of Nonsmall Cell Lung Cancer?" *Invest New Drugs*, 1993, 11(2-3):103-33.

◆ **Vindesine Sulfate** *see* Vindesine on page 1180

Vinorelbine (vi NOR el been)

Medication Safety Issues

Sound-alike/look-alike issues:

Vinorelbine may be confused with vinBLAStine

High alert medication: The Institute for Safe Medication Practices (ISMP) includes this medication among its list of drug classes which have a heightened risk of causing significant patient harm when used in error.

Vinorelbine is intended **for I. V. use only**: Inadvertent intrathecal administration of other vinca alkaloids has resulted in death. Syringes containing vinorelbine should be labeled **"For I.V. use only. Fatal if given intrathecally."**

Related Information

Management of Drug Extravasations on page 1447

Safe Handling of Hazardous Drugs on page 1517

U.S. Brand Names Navelbine®

Index Terms Dihydroxydeoxynorvinkaleukoblastine; Vinorelbine Tartrate

Generic Available Yes

◀ **Canadian Brand Names** Navelbine®; Vinorelbine Injection, USP; Vinorelbine Tartrate for Injection

Pharmacologic Category Antineoplastic Agent, Natural Source (Plant) Derivative; Antineoplastic Agent, Vinca Alkaloid

Use Treatment of nonsmall cell lung cancer (NSCLC)

Unlabeled/Investigational Use Treatment of breast cancer, cervical cancer, and ovarian cancer

Pregnancy Risk Factor D

Lactation Excretion in breast milk unknown/not recommended

Labeled Contraindications Pretreatment granulocyte counts <1000/mm^3

Warnings/Precautions Hazardous agent - use appropriate precautions for handling and disposal. **[U.S. Boxed Warning]: For I.V. use only; do not administer intrathecally;** intrathecal administration may result in death. **[U.S. Boxed Warning]: Avoid extravasation;** infiltration may cause irritation, thrombophlebitis and/or local tissue necrosis. **[U.S. Boxed Warning]: Severe granulocytopenia may occur with treatment;** granulocytopenia is a dose-limiting toxicity; granulocyte counts should be ≥1000/mm^3 prior to treatment initiation; monitor closely for infections and/or fever; may require dosage adjustment. The incidence of granulocytopenia is significantly higher when given in combination with cisplatin when compared to single-agent vinorelbine. Use with caution in patients with compromised marrow reserve due to prior chemotherapy therapy or prior radiation therapy.

Fatal cases of interstitial pulmonary changes and ARDS have been reported (with single-agent therapy); promptly evaluate changes in baseline pulmonary symptoms or any new onset pulmonary symptoms. Acute shortness of breath and severe bronchospasm have been reported rarely; usually associated with the concurrent administration of mitomycin.

Dosage modification required in patients with impaired hepatic function and neurotoxicity; use with caution. May cause new onset or worsening of pre-existing neuropathy; use with caution in patients with neuropathy. May cause severe constipation (grade 3-4), paralytic ileus, intestinal obstruction, necrosis, and/or perforation. May have radiosensitizing effects with prior or concurrent radiation therapy; radiation recall reactions may occur in patients who have received prior radiation therapy. Avoid eye contamination (exposure may cause severe irritation). **[U.S. Boxed Warning]: Should be administered under the supervision of an experienced cancer chemotherapy physician.**

Adverse Reactions Note: Reported with single-agent therapy.

>10%:

Central nervous system: Fatigue (27%)

Dermatologic: Alopecia (12% to 30%)

Gastrointestinal: Nausea (31% to 44%; grade 3: 1% to 2%), constipation (35%; grade 3: 3%), vomiting (20% to 31%; grade 3: 1% to 2%), diarrhea (12% to 17%)

Hematologic: Leukopenia (83% to 92%; grade 4: 6% to 15%), granulocytopenia (90%; grade 4: 36%; nadir: 7-10 days; recovery 14-21 days; dose-limiting), neutropenia (85%; grade 4: 28%), anemia (83%; grades 3/4: 9%)

Hepatic: AST increased (67%; grade 3: 5%; grade 4: 1%), total bilirubin increased (5% to 13%; grade 3: 4%; grade 4: 3%)

Local: Injection site reaction (22% to 28%; includes erythema, vein discoloration), injection site pain (16%)

Neuromuscular & skeletal: Weakness (36%), peripheral neuropathy (25%; grade 3: 1%; grade 4: <1%)

Renal: Creatinine increased (13%)
1% to 10%:
Cardiovascular: Chest pain (5%)
Dermatologic: Rash (<5%)
Gastrointestinal: Paralytic ileus (1%)
Hematologic: Neutropenic fever/sepsis (8%; grade 4: 4%), thrombocytopenia (3% to 5%; grades 3/4: 1%)
Local: Phlebitis (7% to 10%)
Neuromuscular & skeletal: Loss of deep tendon reflexes (<5%), myalgia (<5%), arthralgia (<5%), jaw pain (<5%)
Otic: Ototoxicity (≤1%)
Respiratory: Dyspnea (7%)
<1%, postmarketing, and/or case reports: Abdominal pain, allergic reactions, anaphylaxis, angioedema, back pain, DVT, dysphagia, esophagitis, flushing, gait instability, headache, hemorrhagic cystitis, hyper-/hypotension, hyponatremia, intestinal necrosis, intestinal obstruction, intestinal perforation, interstitial pulmonary changes, local rash, local urticaria, MI (rare), mucositis, muscle weakness, pancreatitis, paralytic ileus, pneumonia, pruritus, pulmonary edema, pulmonary embolus, radiation recall (dermatitis, esophagitis), skin blistering, syndrome of inappropriate ADH secretion, tachycardia, thromboembolic events, tumor pain, urticaria, vasodilation

Drug Interactions

Metabolism/Transport Effects Substrate of CYP2D6 (minor), 3A4 (major); **Inhibits** CYP2D6 (weak), 3A4 (weak)

Avoid Concomitant Use

Avoid concomitant use of Vinorelbine with any of the following: Natalizumab; Vaccines (Live)

Increased Effect/Toxicity

Vinorelbine may increase the levels/effects of: Leflunomide; Mitomycin; Natalizumab; Vaccines (Live)

The levels/effects of Vinorelbine may be increased by: CISplatin; CYP3A4 Inhibitors (Moderate); CYP3A4 Inhibitors (Strong); Dasatinib; Macrolide Antibiotics; Paclitaxel; Paclitaxel (Protein Bound); Posaconazole; Trastuzumab; Voriconazole

Decreased Effect

Vinorelbine may decrease the levels/effects of: Vaccines (Inactivated); Vaccines (Live)

The levels/effects of Vinorelbine may be decreased by: CYP3A4 Inducers (Strong); Deferasirox; Echinacea; Herbs (CYP3A4 Inducers); Peginterferon Alfa-2b

Ethanol/Nutrition/Herb Interactions Herb/Nutraceutical: Avoid St John's wort (may decrease vinorelbine levels).

Storage/Stability Store intact vials under refrigeration at 2°C to 8°C (36°F to 46°F); do not freeze. Protect from light. Intact vials are stable at room temperature of 25°C (77°F) for up to 72 hours. Dilutions in D₅W or NS are stable for 24 hours at room temperature.

Reconstitution Dilute in D₅W or NS to a final concentration of 1.5-3 mg/mL (for syringe) or 0.5-2 mg/mL (for I.V. bag).

Compatibility Stable in D₅¹/₂NS, D₅W, LR, NS, ¹/₂NS.

Y-site administration: Compatible: Amikacin, aztreonam, bleomycin, bumetanide, buprenorphine, butorphanol, calcium gluconate, carboplatin, carmustine, cefotaxime, ceftazidime, ceftizoxime, chlorpromazine, cimetidine, cisplatin, clindamycin, cyclophosphamide, cytarabine, dacarbazine, ▶

dactinomycin, daunorubicin, dexamethasone sodium phosphate, diphenhydramine, doxorubicin, doxorubicin liposome, doxycycline, droperidol, enalaprilat, etoposide, famotidine, filgrastim, floxuridine, fluconazole, fludarabine, gatifloxacin, gemcitabine, gentamicin, granisetron, haloperidol, hydrocortisone sodium phosphate, hydrocortisone sodium succinate, hydromorphone, hydroxyzine, idarubicin, ifosfamide, imipenem/cilastatin, lorazepam, mannitol, mechlorethamine, melphalan, meperidine, mesna, methotrexate, metoclopramide, metronidazole, minocycline, mitoxantrone, morphine, nalbuphine, netilmicin, ondansetron, plicamycin, streptozocin, teniposide, ticarcillin, ticarcillin/clavulanate, tobramycin, vancomycin, vinblastine, vincristine, zidovudine. **Incompatible:** Acyclovir, allopurinol, aminophylline, amphotericin B, amphotericin B cholesteryl sulfate complex, ampicillin, cefazolin, cefoperazone, cefotetan, ceftriaxone, cefuroxime, co-trimoxazole, fluorouracil, furosemide, ganciclovir, methylprednisolone sodium succinate, mitomycin, piperacillin, sodium bicarbonate, thiotepa. **Variable (consult detailed reference):** Heparin.

Mechanism of Action Semisynthetic vinca alkaloid which binds to tubulin and inhibits microtubule formation, therefore, arresting the cell at metaphase by disrupting the formation of the mitotic spindle; it is specific for the M and S phases. Vinorelbine may also interfere with nucleic acid and protein synthesis by blocking glutamic acid utilization.

Pharmacodynamics/Kinetics

Absorption: Unreliable; must be given I.V.

Distribution: V_d: 25-40 L/kg; binds extensively to human platelets and lymphocytes (80% to 91%)

Protein binding: 80% to 91%

Metabolism: Extensively hepatic, via CYP3A4, to two metabolites, deacetylvinorelbine (active) and vinorelbine N-oxide

Bioavailability: Oral (not approved in the U. S.): 26% to 45%

Half-life elimination: Triphasic: Terminal: 28-44 hours

Excretion: Feces (46%); urine (18%, 10% to 12% as unchanged drug)

Clearance: Plasma: Mean: 0.97-1.26 L/hour/kg

Dosage Details concerning dosing in combination regimens should also be consulted.

I.V.: Adults:

NSCLC:

Single-agent therapy: 30 mg/m²/dose every 7 days

Combination therapy with cisplatin: 25-30 mg/m²/dose every 7 days (in combination with cisplatin)

Breast cancer (unlabeled use): 25 mg/m²/dose every 7 days

Cervical cancer (unlabeled use): 30 mg/m²/dose days 1 and 8 of a 21-day treatment cycle

Ovarian cancer (unlabeled use): 25 mg/m²/dose every 7 days **or** 30 mg/m²/dose days 1 and 8 of a 21-day treatment cycle

Dosage adjustment in hematological toxicity: Granulocyte counts should be ≥1000 cells/mm³ prior to the administration of vinorelbine. Adjustments in the dosage of vinorelbine should be based on granulocyte counts obtained on the day of treatment as follows:

Granulocytes ≥1500 cells/mm³ on day of treatment: Administer 100% of starting dose

Granulocytes 1000-1499 cells/mm³ on day of treatment: Administer 50% of starting dose

Granulocytes <1000 cells/mm^3 on day of treatment: Do not administer. Repeat granulocyte count in one week; if 3 consecutive doses are held because granulocyte count is <1000 cells/mm^3, discontinue vinorelbine.

For patients who, during treatment, have experienced fever and/or sepsis while granulocytopenic or had 2 consecutive weekly doses held due to granulocytopenia, subsequent doses of vinorelbine should be:

75% of starting dose for granulocytes ≥1500 cells/mm^3

37.5% of starting dose for granulocytes 1000-1499 cells/mm^3

Dosage adjustment for neurotoxicity: Neurotoxicity ≥grade 2: Discontinue treatment

Dosage adjustment in renal impairment: No adjustment is necessary.

Dosing adjustment in hepatic impairment: The FDA-approved labeling guidelines are as follows: Vinorelbine should be administered with caution in patients with hepatic insufficiency. In patients who develop hyperbilirubinemia during treatment with vinorelbine, the dose should be adjusted for total bilirubin as follows:

Serum bilirubin ≤2 mg/dL: Administer 100% of dose

Serum bilirubin 2.1-3 mg/dL: Administer 50% of dose

Serum bilirubin >3 mg/dL: Administer 25% of dose

Dosing adjustment in patients with concurrent hematologic toxicity and hepatic impairment: Administer the lower of the doses determined from the adjustment recommendations.

Combination Regimens

Breast cancer:

Paclitaxel-Vinorelbine on page 1389

VD on page 1420

Vinorelbine-FEC on page 1423

Vinorelbine-Trastuzumab on page 1423

Vinorelbine-Trastuzumab-FEC on page 1424

Cervical cancer: Cisplatin-Vinorelbine on page 1275

Leukemia, acute lymphocytic: TVTG on page 1416

Leukemia, acute myeloid: TVTG on page 1416

Lung cancer (nonsmall cell):

Cetuximab-Cisplatin-Vinorelbine on page 1256

Gemcitabine-Vinorelbine on page 1346

Vinorelbine-Cisplatin on page 1422

Vinorelbine-Gemcitabine on page 1423

Lymphoma, Hodgkin's disease: Gemcitabine-Vinorelbine-Doxorubicin (Liposomal) on page 1346

Prostate cancer: Estramustine + Vinorelbine on page 1317

Administration FATAL IF GIVEN INTRATHECALLY. Administer as a direct intravenous push or rapid bolus, over 6-10 minutes (up to 30 minutes). Longer infusions may increase the risk of pain and phlebitis. Intravenous doses should be followed by at least 75-125 mL of saline or D$_5$W to reduce the incidence of phlebitis and inflammation. Assure proper needle or catheter position prior to administration.

Monitoring Parameters CBC with differential and platelet count, hepatic function tests; monitor for new-onset pulmonary symptoms (or worsening from baseline); monitor for neuropathy

Emetic Potential

Oral: Moderate (30% to 90%)

I.V.: Very low (<10%)

Vesicant Yes; moderate. See Management of Drug Extravasations on page 1447.

Dosage Forms Excipient information presented when available (limited, particularly for generics); consult specific product labeling.
Injection, solution [preservative free]: 10 mg/mL (1 mL, 5 mL)
   Navelbine®: 10 mg/mL (1 mL, 5 mL)

References

Bajetta E, Di Leo A, Biganzoli L, et al, "Phase II Study of Vinorelbine in Patients With Pretreated Advanced Ovarian Cancer: Activity in Platinum-Resistant Disease," *J Clin Oncol*, 1996, 14 (9):2546-51.

Muggia FM, Blessing JA, Method M, et al, "Evaluation of Vinorelbine in Persistent or Recurrent Squamous Cell Carcinoma of the Cervix: A Gynecologic Oncology Group Study," *Gynecol Oncol*, 2004, 92(2):639-43.

Muggia FM, Blessing JA, Waggoner S, et al, "Evaluation of Vinorelbine in Persistent or Recurrent Nonsquamous Carcinoma of the Cervix: A Gynecologic Oncology Group Study," *Gynecol Oncol*, 2005, 96(1):108-11.

Rothenberg ML, Liu PY, Wilczynski s, et al, "Phase II Trial of Vinorelbine for Relapsed Ovarian Cancer: A Southwest Oncology Group Study," *Gynecol Oncol*, 2004, 95(3):506-12.

Zelek L, Barthier S, Riofrio M, et al, "Weekly Vinorelbine is an Effective Palliative Regimen After Failure With Anthracyclines and Taxanes in Metastatic Breast Carcinoma," *Cancer*, 2001, 92 (9):2267-72.

◆ **Vinorelbine Injection, USP (Can)** *see* Vinorelbine *on page 1181*

◆ **Vinorelbine Tartrate** *see* Vinorelbine *on page 1181*

◆ **Vinorelbine Tartrate for Injection (Can)** *see* Vinorelbine *on page 1181*

◆ **Vistaril®** *see* HydrOXYzine *on page 594*

Vistonuridine (VIST oh nur i deen)

Index Terms PN401

Pharmacologic Category Antidote

Unlabeled/Investigational Use Antidote for fluorouracil overdose or overexposure

Restrictions Investigational agent - not approved for use in the U.S.

Vistonuridine is supplied for emergency use under a single-patient Investigational New Drug (IND) provision. Procurement information is available from Wellstat Therapeutics at 1-443-831-5626.

Drug Interactions

Avoid Concomitant Use There are no known interactions where it is recommended to avoid concomitant use.

Increased Effect/Toxicity There are no known significant interactions involving an increase in effect.

Decreased Effect There are no known significant interactions involving a decrease in effect.

Mechanism of Action Vistonuridine is a prodrug of uridine, is converted to uridine triphosphate (UTP) which competes with FUTP for incorporation into RNA and therefore preventing cell death and dose-limiting toxicity.

Pharmacodynamics/Kinetics Metabolism: Deacetylated (by esterases) to uridine

Dosage Oral: Adults: Fluorouracil overdose (unlabeled use): 10 g every 6 hours for 20 doses beginning as soon as possible (8 hours to 4 days) after fluorouracil overdose (von Borstel, 2009)

Administration Administer orally (tablets); begin as soon as possible following of fluorouracil overdose (within 8-96 hours).

Monitoring Parameters CBC with differential; gastrointestinal toxicity

Additional Information Oncology Comment: Vistonuridine has been studied in a limited number of cases of fluorouracil overdose. Of 17 patients receiving vistonuridine beginning within 8-96 hours after fluorouracil overdose, all patients fully recovered (von Borstel, 2009).

References

Hidalgo M, Villalona-Calero MA, Eckhardt SG, et al, "Phase I and Pharmacologic Study of PN401 and Fluorouracil in Patients With Advanced Solid Malignancies," *J Clin Oncol*, 2000, 18 (1):167-77.

Kelson DP, Martin D, O'Neil J, et al, "Phase I Trial of PN401, an Oral Prodrug of Uridine, to Prevent Toxicity From Fluorouracil in Patients With Advanced Cancer," *J Clin Oncol*, 1997, 15(4):1511-7.

von Borstel R, O'Neil J, and Bamat M, "Vistonuridine: An Orally Administered, Life-Saving Antidote for 5-Fluorouracil (5FU) Overdose," *J Clin Oncol*, 2009, 27(15S):9616 [abstract from 2009 ASCO Annual Meeting].

♦ **Vitamin K₁** *see* Phytonadione *on page 953*

♦ **Vitrase®** *see* Hyaluronidase *on page 573*

♦ **Vitrasert®** *see* Ganciclovir *on page 525*

♦ **Vivaglobin®** *see* Immune Globulin (Subcutaneous) *on page 633*

♦ **VLB** *see* VinBLAStine *on page 1169*

♦ **VM-26** *see* Teniposide *on page 1087*

♦ **Voraxaze** *see* Glucarpidase *on page 547*

Voriconazole (vor i KOE na zole)

Related Information
Safe Handling of Hazardous Drugs *on page 1517*

U.S. Brand Names VFEND®

Index Terms UK109496

Generic Available No

Canadian Brand Names VFEND®

Pharmacologic Category Antifungal Agent, Oral; Antifungal Agent, Parenteral

Use Treatment of invasive aspergillosis; treatment of esophageal candidiasis; treatment of candidemia (in non-neutropenic patients); treatment of disseminated *Candida* infections of the skin and viscera; treatment of serious fungal infections caused by *Scedosporium apiospermum* and *Fusarium* spp (including *Fusarium solani*) in patients intolerant of, or refractory to, other therapy

Unlabeled/Investigational Use
Fungal infection prophylaxis in intermediate or high risk neutropenic cancer patients with myelodysplastic syndrome (MDS) or acute myelogenous leukemia (AML), neutropenic allogeneic hematopoietic stem cell recipients, and patients with significant graft-versus-host disease; empiric antifungal therapy (second-line) for persistent neutropenic fever

Pregnancy Risk Factor D

Lactation Excretion in breast milk unknown/not recommended

Labeled Contraindications Hypersensitivity to voriconazole or any component of the formulation (cross-reaction with other azole antifungal agents may occur but has not been established, use caution); coadministration of CYP3A4 substrates which may lead to QT_c prolongation (cisapride, pimozide, or quinidine); coadministration with barbiturates (long acting), carbamazepine, efavirenz (with standard [eg, not adjusted] voriconazole and efavirenz doses), ergot derivatives, rifampin, rifabutin, ritonavir (≥800 mg/day), sirolimus, St John's wort

Warnings/Precautions Visual changes, including blurred vision, changes in visual acuity, color perception, and photophobia, are commonly associated with treatment. Patients should be warned to avoid tasks which depend on vision, including operating machinery or driving. Changes are reversible on discontinuation following brief exposure/treatment regimens (≤28 days). ▶

Serious hepatic reactions (including hepatitis, cholestasis, and fulminant hepatic failure) have occurred during treatment, primarily in patients with serious concomitant medical conditions. However, hepatotoxicity has occurred in patients with no identifiable risk factors. Use caution in patients with pre-existing hepatic impairment (dose adjustment or discontinuation may be required).

Voriconazole tablets contain lactose; avoid administration in hereditary galactose intolerance, Lapp lactase deficiency, or glucose-galactose malabsorption. Suspension contains sucrose; use caution with fructose intolerance, sucrose-isomaltase deficiency, or glucose-galactose malabsorption. Avoid/limit use of intravenous formulation in patients with renal impairment; intravenous formulation contains excipient cyclodextrin (sulfobutyl ether beta-cyclodextrin), which may accumulate in renal insufficiency. Acute renal failure has been observed in severely ill patients; use with caution in patients receiving concomitant nephrotoxic medications. Anaphylactoid-type infusion-related reactions may occur with intravenous dosing. Consider discontinuation of infusion if reaction is severe.

Use caution in patients taking strong cytochrome P450 inducers, CYP2C9 inhibitors, and major 3A4 substrates (see Drug Interactions); consider alternative agents that avoid or lessen the potential for CYP-mediated interactions. QT interval prolongation has been associated with voriconazole use; rare cases of arrhythmia (including torsade de pointes), cardiac arrest, and sudden death have been reported, usually in seriously ill patients with comorbidities and/or risk factors (eg, prior cardiotoxic chemotherapy, cardiomyopathy, electrolyte imbalance, or concomitant QT_c-prolonging drugs). Use with caution in these patient populations; correct electrolyte abnormalities (eg, hypokalemia, hypomagnesemia, hypocalcemia) prior to initiating therapy. Do not infuse concomitantly with blood products or short-term concentrated electrolyte solutions, even if the two infusions are running in separate intravenous lines (or cannulas). Rarely, serious cutaneous reactions (including Stevens-Johnson syndrome) have been reported with treatment. Consider discontinuing in patients developing a rash. Avoid strong, direct exposure to sunlight; may cause photosensitivity, especially with long-term use. Monitor pancreatic function in patients (children and adults) at risk for acute pancreatitis (eg, recent chemotherapy or hematopoietic stem cell transplantation); there have been postmarketing reports of pancreatitis in children. Safety and efficacy have not been established in children <12 years of age.

Adverse Reactions
>10%:
  Central nervous system: Hallucinations (4% to 12%; auditory and/or visual and likely serum concentration-dependent)
  Ocular: Visual changes (dose related; photophobia, color changes, increased or decreased visual acuity, or blurred vision occur in ~21%)
  Renal: Creatinine increased (1% to 21%)
2% to 10%:
  Cardiovascular: Tachycardia (≤2%)
  Central nervous system: Fever (≤6%), chills (≤4%), headache (≤3%)
  Dermatologic: Rash (≤7%)
  Endocrine & metabolic: Hypokalemia (≤2%)
  Gastrointestinal: Nausea (1% to 5%), vomiting (1% to 4%)
  Hepatic: Alkaline phosphatase increased (4% to 5%), AST increased (2% to 4%), ALT increased (2% to 3%), cholestatic jaundice (1% to 2%)
  Ocular: Photophobia (2% to 3%)

<2% (Limited to important or life-threatening): Acute tubular necrosis, adrenal cortical insufficiency, agranulocytosis, allergic reaction, alopecia, anaphylactoid reaction, anemia (aplastic, hemolytic, macrocytic, megaloblastic, or microcytic), angioedema, anuria, ascites, ataxia, atrial arrhythmia, atrial fibrillation, AV block, bigeminy, bleeding time increased, bone marrow depression, bone necrosis, bradycardia, brain edema, bundle branch block, BUN increased, cardiac arrest, cardiomegaly, cardiomyopathy, cerebral hemorrhage, cerebral ischemia, cerebrovascular accident, chest pain, CHF, cholecystitis, cholelithiasis, chromatopsia, color blindness, coma, confusion, cyanosis, delirium, dementia, depersonalization, depression, diabetes insipidus, diarrhea, DIC, discoid lupus erythematosus, duodenal ulcer perforation, DVT, dyspnea, edema, encephalopathy, endocarditis, eosinophilia, erythema multiforme, exfoliative dermatitis, extrapyramidal symptoms, fixed drug eruption, fulminant hepatic failure, gastrointestinal hemorrhage, GGT/LDH increased, glucose tolerance decreased, grand mal seizure, Guillain-Barré syndrome, hematemesis, hepatic coma, hepatic failure, hepatitis, hepatomegaly, hydronephrosis, hyperbilirubinemia, hypercholesterolemia, hyper-/hypocalcemia, hyper-/hypoglycemia, hyper-/hypomagnesemia, hyper-/hyponatremia, hyper-/hypotension, hyper-/hypothyroidism, hyperkalemia, hyperuricemia, hypophosphatemia, hypoxia, intestinal perforation, intracranial hypertension, jaundice, leukopenia, liver enlarged, lung edema, lymphadenopathy, lymphangitis, maculopapular rash, MI, multiorgan failure, myasthenia, myopathy, nephritis, nephrosis, neuropathy, night blindness, nodal arrhythmia, oculogyric crisis, optic atrophy, optic neuritis, osteomalacia, osteoporosis, palpitation, pancreatitis, pancytopenia, papilledema, paresthesia, peripheral edema, peritonitis, petechia, photosensitivity, pleural effusion, postural hypotension, pruritus, pseudomembranous colitis, psychosis, pulmonary embolus, purpura, QT interval prolongation, renal dysfunction, renal failure (acute), respiratory distress syndrome, retinal hemorrhage, seizure, sepsis, somnolence, spleen enlarged, Stevens-Johnson syndrome, substernal chest pain, suicidal ideation, supraventricular extrasystoles, supraventricular tachycardia, syncope, thrombocytopenia, thrombophlebitis, thrombotic thrombocytopenic purpura, tongue edema, torsade de pointes, toxic epidermal necrolysis, uremia, urinary retention, urticaria, uveitis, vasodilation, ventricular arrhythmia, ventricular fibrillation, ventricular tachycardia, visual field defect

Drug Interactions

Metabolism/Transport Effects Substrate of CYP2C9 (major), 2C19 (major), 3A4 (minor); **Inhibits** CYP2C9 (weak), 2C19 (weak), 3A4 (moderate)

Avoid Concomitant Use

Avoid concomitant use of Voriconazole with any of the following: Alfuzosin; Artemether; Barbiturates; CarBAMazepine; Cisapride; Conivaptan; Darunavir; Dofetilide; Dronedarone; Eplerenone; Ergot Derivatives; Everolimus; Halofantrine; Lopinavir; Lumefantrine; Nilotinib; Nisoldipine; Pimozide; QuiNIDine; QuiNINE; Ranolazine; Rifamycin Derivatives; Ritonavir; Rivaroxaban; Salmeterol; Silodosin; Sirolimus; St Johns Wort; Tetrabenazine; Thioridazine; Tolvaptan; Ziprasidone

Increased Effect/Toxicity

Voriconazole may increase the levels/effects of: Alfentanil; Alfuzosin; Almotriptan; Alosetron; Antineoplastic Agents (Vinca Alkaloids); Aprepitant; Benzodiazepines (metabolized by oxidation); Bosentan; BusPIRone; Busulfan; Calcium Channel Blockers; CarBAMazepine; Cardiac Glycosides; Ciclesonide; Cilostazol; Cinacalcet; Cisapride; Colchicine; Conivaptan; Corticosteroids (Orally Inhaled); Corticosteroids (Systemic); CycloSPORINE;

CYP3A4 Substrates; Diclofenac; Docetaxel; Dofetilide; Dronedarone; Dutasteride; Eletriptan; Eplerenone; Ergot Derivatives; Erlotinib; Eszopiclone; Everolimus; FentaNYL; Fesoterodine; Fosaprepitant; Gefitinib; Halofantrine; HMG-CoA Reductase Inhibitors; Imatinib; Irinotecan; Ixabepilone; Losartan; Macrolide Antibiotics; Maraviroc; Methadone; Nilotinib; Nisoldipine; Oral Contraceptive (Estrogens); Oral Contraceptive (Progestins); Paricalcitol; Phenytoin; Phosphodiesterase 5 Inhibitors; Pimecrolimus; Pimozide; Protease Inhibitors; QTc-Prolonging Agents; QuiNIDine; QuiNINE; Ramelteon; Ranolazine; Repaglinide; Reverse Transcriptase Inhibitors (Non-Nucleoside); Rifamycin Derivatives; Rivaroxaban; Salmeterol; Saxagliptin; Silodosin; Sirolimus; Solifenacin; Sorafenib; Sunitinib; Tacrolimus; Tadalafil; Temsirolimus; Tetrabenazine; Thioridazine; Tolterodine; Tolvaptan; Trimetrexate; Venlafaxine; Vitamin K Antagonists; Ziprasidone; Zolpidem

The levels/effects of Voriconazole may be increased by: Alfuzosin; Artemether; Chloroquine; Ciprofloxacin; CYP2C9 Inhibitors (Moderate); CYP2C9 Inhibitors (Strong); Gadobutrol; Grapefruit Juice; Lumefantrine; Macrolide Antibiotics; Nilotinib; Oral Contraceptive (Estrogens); Oral Contraceptive (Progestins); Protease Inhibitors; Proton Pump Inhibitors; QuiNINE

Decreased Effect

Voriconazole may decrease the levels/effects of: Amphotericin B; Prasugrel; Saccharomyces boulardii

The levels/effects of Voriconazole may be decreased by: Barbiturates; CarBAMazepine; CYP2C19 Inducers (Strong); CYP2C9 Inducers (Highly Effective); Darunavir; Didanosine; Lopinavir; Peginterferon Alfa-2b; Phenytoin; Reverse Transcriptase Inhibitors (Non-Nucleoside); Rifamycin Derivatives; Ritonavir; St Johns Wort; Sucralfate

Ethanol/Nutrition/Herb Interactions

Food: May decrease voriconazole absorption. Voriconazole should be taken 1 hour before or 1 hour after a meal. Avoid grapefruit juice (may decrease voriconazole levels).

Herb/Nutraceutical: St John's wort may decrease voriconazole levels; concurrent use with voriconazole is contraindicated.

Storage/Stability

Powder for injection: Store at 15°C to 30°C (59°F to 86°F). Reconstituted solutions are stable for up to 24 hours under refrigeration at 2°C to 8°C (36°F to 46°F).

Powder for oral suspension: Store at 2°C to 8°C (36°F to 46°F). Reconstituted oral suspension may be stored at 15°C to 30°C (59°F to 86°F).

Tablets: Store at 15°C to 30°C (59°F to 86°F).

Reconstitution

Powder for injection: Reconstitute 200 mg vial with 19 mL of sterile water for injection (use of automated syringe is not recommended). Resultant solution (20 mL) has a concentration of 10 mg/mL. Prior to infusion, must dilute to 0.5-5 mg/mL with NS, LR, D_5WLR, $D_5W^1/_2NS$, D_5W, D_5W with KCl 20 mEq, $^1/_2NS$, or D_5WNS. Do not dilute with 4.2% sodium bicarbonate infusion.

Powder for oral suspension: Add 46 mL of water to the bottle to make 40 mg/mL suspension. Discard unused portion after 14 days.

Compatibility Stable in NS, LR, D_5WLR, $D_5W^1/_2NS$, D_5W, D_5W with KCl 20 mEq, $^1/_2NS$, or D_5WNS. Do not infuse **concomitantly** into same line or cannula with other drug infusions, including TPN. May be infused simultaneously with TPN through a separate I.V. line.

Incompatible: Do not infuse simultaneously with blood products.

Mechanism of Action Interferes with fungal cytochrome P450 activity (selectively inhibits 14-alpha-lanosterol demethylation), decreasing ergosterol synthesis (principal sterol in fungal cell membrane) and inhibiting fungal cell membrane formation.

Pharmacodynamics/Kinetics

Absorption: Well absorbed after oral administration; administration of crushed tablets is considered bioequivalent to whole tablets

Distribution: V_d: 4.6 L/kg

Protein binding: 58%

Metabolism: Hepatic, via CYP2C19 (major pathway) and CYP2C9 and CYP3A4 (less significant); saturable (may demonstrate nonlinearity)

Bioavailability: 96%

Half-life elimination: Variable, dose-dependent

Time to peak: Oral: 1-2 hours; 0.5 hours (crushed tablet)

Excretion: Urine (as inactive metabolites; <2% as unchanged drug)

Dosage

Usual dosage ranges:

Children <12 years: Dosage not established

Children ≥12 years and Adults:

Oral: 100-300 mg every 12 hours

I.V.: 6 mg/kg every 12 hours for 2 doses; followed by maintenance dose of 4 mg/kg every 12 hours

Indication-specific dosing: Children ≥12 years and Adults:

Aspergillosis, invasive, including disseminated and extrapulmonary infection: Duration of therapy should be a minimum of 6-12 weeks or throughout period of immunosuppression:

I.V.: Initial: Loading dose: 6 mg/kg every 12 hours for 2 doses; followed by maintenance dose of 4 mg/kg every 12 hours

Oral: May consider oral therapy in place of I.V. with dosing of 4 mg/kg (rounded up to convenient tablet dosage form) every 12 hours; however, I.V. administration is preferred in serious infections since comparative efficacy with the oral formulation has not been established.

Scedosporiosis, fusariosis: I.V.: Initial: Loading dose: 6 mg/kg every 12 hours for 2 doses; followed by maintenance dose of 4 mg/kg every 12 hours

Candidemia and other deep tissue *Candida* infections: I.V.: Initial: Loading dose 6 mg/kg every 12 hours for 2 doses; followed by maintenance dose of 3-4 mg/kg every 12 hours

Endophthalmitis, fungal (unlabeled use, Pappas, 2009): I.V.: 6 mg/kg every 12 hours for 2 doses, then 3-4 mg/kg every 12 hours

Esophageal candidiasis: Oral:

Patients <40 kg: 100 mg every 12 hours; maximum: 300 mg/day

Patients ≥40 kg: 200 mg every 12 hours; maximum: 600 mg/day

Note: Treatment should continue for a minimum of 14 days, and for at least 7 days following resolution of symptoms.

Conversion to oral dosing:

Patients <40 kg: 100 mg every 12 hours; increase to 150 mg every 12 hours in patients who fail to respond adequately

Patients ≥40 kg: 200 mg every 12 hours; increase to 300 mg every 12 hours in patients who fail to respond adequately

Dosage adjustment in patients unable to tolerate treatment:

I.V.: Dose may be reduced to 3 mg/kg every 12 hours

Oral: Dose may be reduced in 50 mg decrements to a minimum dosage of 200 mg every 12 hours in patients weighing ≥40 kg (100 mg every 12 hours in patients <40 kg)

Dosage adjustment in patients receiving concomitant CYP450 enzyme inducers or substrates:
Cyclosporine: Reduce cyclosporine dose by 1/2 and monitor closely.
Efavirenz: Oral: Increase maintenance dose of voriconazole to 400 mg every 12 hours and reduce efavirenz dose to 300 mg once daily
Phenytoin:
I.V.: Increase maintenance dosage to 5 mg/kg every 12 hours
Oral: Increase dose to 400 mg every 12 hours in patients ≥40 kg (200 mg every 12 hours in patients <40 kg)

Dosage adjustment in renal impairment: In patients with Cl_{cr} <50 mL/minute, accumulation of the intravenous vehicle (cyclodextrin) occurs. After initial I.V. loading dose, oral voriconazole should be administered to these patients, unless an assessment of the benefit:risk to the patient justifies the use of I.V. voriconazole. Monitor serum creatinine and change to oral voriconazole therapy when possible.
Hemodialysis: Oral dosage adjustment not required; I.V. dosing not recommended since cyclodextrin vehicle is cleared at half the rate of voriconazole and may accumulate

Dosage adjustment in hepatic impairment:
Mild-to-moderate hepatic dysfunction (Child-Pugh class A and B): Following standard loading dose, reduce maintenance dosage by 50%
Severe hepatic impairment: Should only be used if benefit outweighs risk; monitor closely for toxicity

Administration
Oral: Administer 1 hour before or 1 hour after a meal.
I.V.: Infuse over 1-2 hours (rate not to exceed 3 mg/kg/hour). Do not infuse concomitantly into same line or cannula with other drug infusions, including TPN.

Monitoring Parameters Hepatic function at initiation and during course of treatment; renal function; serum electrolytes (particularly calcium, magnesium and potassium) prior to therapy initiation; visual function (visual acuity, visual field and color perception) if treatment course continues >28 days; may consider obtaining voriconazole trough level in patients failing therapy or exhibiting signs of toxicity; pancreatic function (in patients at risk for acute pancreatitis)

Dietary Considerations Oral: Should be taken 1 hour before or 1 hour after a meal. Voriconazole tablets contain lactose; avoid administration in hereditary galactose intolerance, Lapp lactase deficiency, or glucose-galactose malabsorption. Suspension contains sucrose; use caution with fructose intolerance, sucrose-isomaltase deficiency, or glucose-galactose malabsorption.

Dosage Forms Excipient information presented when available (limited, particularly for generics); consult specific product labeling.
Injection, powder for reconstitution:
VFEND®: 200 mg 200 mg [contains cyclodextrin]
Powder for oral suspension:
VFEND®: 200 mg/5 mL (70 mL) [contains sodium benzoate and sucrose; orange flavor]
Tablet:
VFEND®: 50 mg, 200 mg

References
Dodds-Ashley ES, Zaas AK, Fang AF, et al, "Comparative Pharmacokinetics of Voriconazole Administered Orally as Either Crushed or Whole Tablets," *Antimicrob Agents Chemother*, 2007, 51(3):877-80.

Herbrecht R, Denning DW, Patterson TF, et al, "Voriconazole Versus Amphotericin B for Primary Therapy of Invasive Aspergillosis," *N Engl J Med*, 2002, 347(6):408-15.

Kullberg BJ, Sobel JD, Ruhnke M, et al, "Voriconazole Versus a Regimen of Amphotericin B Followed by Fluconazole for Candidaemia in Non-Neutropenic Patients: A Randomised Non-Inferiority Trial," *Lancet*, 2005, 366(9495):1435-42.

National Comprehensive Cancer Network (NCCN), "Clinical Practice Guidelines in Oncology™: Prevention and Treatment of Cancer-Related Infections," Version 1.2008. Available at http://www.nccn.org/professionals/physician_gls/PDF/infections.pdf.

Pappas PG, Kauffman CA, Andes D, et al, "Clinical Practice Guidelines for the Management of Candidiasis: 2009 Update by the Infectious Diseases Society of America," *Clin Infect Dis*, 2009, 48(5):503-35.

Walsh TJ, Anaissie EJ, Denning DW, et al, "Treatment of Aspergillosis: Clinical Practice Guidelines of the Infectious Diseases Society of America," *Clin Infect Dis*, 2008, 46(3):327-60.

Walsh TJ, Pappas P, Winston DJ et al, "Voriconazole Compared with Liposomal Amphotericin B for Empirical Antifungal Therapy in Patients with Neutropenia and Persistent Fever," *N Engl J Med*, 2002, 346(4):225-34.

Vorinostat (vor IN oh stat)

Medication Safety Issues
High alert medication: The Institute for Safe Medication Practices (ISMP) includes this medication among its list of drug classes which have a heightened risk of causing significant patient harm when used in error.

Related Information
Safe Handling of Hazardous Drugs *on page 1517*

U.S. Brand Names Zolinza™

Index Terms NSC-701852; SAHA; Suberoylanilide Hydroxamic Acid

Generic Available No

Canadian Brand Names Zolinza™

Pharmacologic Category Antineoplastic Agent, Histone Deacetylase Inhibitor

Use Treatment of progressive, persistent, or recurrent cutaneous T-cell lymphoma (CTCL)

Pregnancy Risk Factor D

Lactation Excretion in breast milk unknown/not recommended

Labeled Contraindications There are no contraindications listed within the manufacturer's labeling.

Warnings/Precautions Hazardous agent - use appropriate precautions for handling and disposal. Pulmonary embolism and deep vein thrombosis (DVT) have been reported; monitor. Use caution in patients with a history of thrombotic events. Dose-related thrombocytopenia and/or anemia may occur; may require dosage adjustments or discontinuation. QT_c prolongation has been observed; a baseline and periodic 12-lead ECG should be obtained. Correct electrolyte abnormalities prior to treatment and monitor and correct potassium, calcium, and magnesium levels during therapy. Use caution in patients with a history of QT_c prolongation or with medications known to prolong the QT interval. May cause hyperglycemia; monitor and use with caution in diabetics; may require diet and/or therapy modifications. Nausea, vomiting, and diarrhea may occur; antiemetics and antidiarrheals may be required; replace fluids and electrolytes to avoid dehydration. Safety and efficacy in children have not been established.

Adverse Reactions
>10%:
Cardiovascular: Peripheral edema (13%)
Central nervous system: Fatigue (46% to 73%), chills (12% to 16%), dizziness (15%), headache (12%), fever (11%)
Dermatologic: Alopecia (18% to 19%), pruritus (12%)

◄

Endocrine & metabolic: Hyperglycemia (8% to 69%; grade 3: 5%), dehydration (16%)

Gastrointestinal: Diarrhea (49% to 52%), nausea (41% to 49%), taste perversion (24% to 46%), xerostomia (11% to 35%), weight loss (20% to 27%), anorexia (22% to 24%), vomiting (12% to 24%), appetite decreased (14% to 22%), constipation (11% to 15%)

Hematologic: Thrombocytopenia (22% to 54%; grades 3/4: 5% to 19%), anemia (2% to 14%; grades 3/4: 1% to 3%)

Neuromuscular & skeletal: Muscle spasm (16% to 20%)

Renal: Proteinuria (51%), creatinine increased (15% to 47%)

Respiratory: Dyspnea (34%), cough (11%), upper respiratory infection (11%)

1% to 10%:

Cardiovascular: QT_c prolongation (3% to 6%)

Dermatologic: Squamous cell carcinoma (4%)

Respiratory: Pulmonary embolism (5%)

<1%, postmarketing, and/or case reports: Angioneurotic edema, blurred vision, chest pain, cholecystitis, creatine phosphokinase (CPK) increased, DVT, enterococcal infection, exfoliative dermatitis, gastrointestinal hemorrhage, hemoptysis, hypertension, hypocalcemia, hypokalemia, hyponatremia, hypophosphatemia, infection, lethargy, leukopenia, MI, neutropenia, pneumonia, renal failure, sepsis, spinal cord injury, streptococcal bacteremia, stroke (ischemic), syncope, T-cell lymphoma, transaminases increased, tumor hemorrhage, ureteric obstruction, ureteropelvic junction obstruction, urinary retention, vasculitis, weakness

Drug Interactions

Avoid Concomitant Use

Avoid concomitant use of Vorinostat with any of the following: Artemether; Dronedarone; Lumefantrine; Nilotinib; Pimozide; QuiNINE; Tetrabenazine; Thioridazine; Ziprasidone

Increased Effect/Toxicity

Vorinostat may increase the levels/effects of: Dronedarone; Pimozide; QTc-Prolonging Agents; QuiNINE; Tetrabenazine; Thioridazine; Vitamin K Antagonists; Ziprasidone

The levels/effects of Vorinostat may be increased by: Alfuzosin; Artemether; Chloroquine; Ciprofloxacin; Gadobutrol; Lumefantrine; Nilotinib; QuiNINE; Valproic Acid

Decreased Effect There are no known significant interactions involving a decrease in effect.

Storage/Stability Store at 20°C to 25°C (68°F to 77°F); excursions permitted to 15°C to 30°C (59°F to 86°F).

Mechanism of Action Inhibition of histone deacetylase enzymes, HDAC1, HDAC2, HDAC3, and HDAC6, which catalyze acetyl group removal from protein lysine residues (including histones and transcription factors). Inhibition of histone deacetylase results in accumulation of acetyl groups, leading to alterations in chromatin structure and transcription factor activation causing termination of cell growth leading to cell death.

Pharmacodynamics/Kinetics

Protein binding: ~71%

Metabolism: Glucuronidated and hydrolyzed (followed by beta-oxidation) to inactive metabolites

Bioavailability: Fasting: ~43%

Half-life elimination: ~2 hours

Time to peak, plasma: With high-fat meal: ~4 hours (range: 2-10 hours)

Excretion: Urine: 52% (<1% as unchanged drug, ~52% as inactive metabolites)

Dosage Oral: Adults: Cutaneous T-cell lymphoma: 400 mg once daily

Dosage adjustment for intolerance: Reduce dose to 300 mg once daily; may further reduce to 300 mg daily for 5 consecutive days per week

In clinical trials, treatment was withheld for grade 4 anemia or thrombocytopenia or other grade 3 or 4 drug related toxicity, until resolved to ≤ grade 1. Therapy was reinitiated with dose modification (Olsen, 2007).

Dosage adjustment in renal impairment: Not studied, however, based on the minimal renal elimination, adjustment may not be required.

Dosage adjustment in hepatic impairment: Not studied; use caution based on predominant hepatic metabolism.

Administration Administer with food. Do not open, crush, or chew capsules.

Monitoring Parameters Baseline, then periodic 12-lead ECG; baseline, then every other week serum electrolytes (including calcium, magnesium and potassium), CBC with differential and platelets, serum creatinine and blood glucose for 2 months, then monthly

Dietary Considerations Take with food.

Emetic Potential Low (10% to 30%)

Dosage Forms Excipient information presented when available (limited, particularly for generics); consult specific product labeling.

Capsule:

Zolinza™: 100 mg

References

Duvic M, Talpur R, Ni X, et al, "Phase II Trial of Oral Vorinostat (Suberoylanilide Hydroxamic Acid, SAHA) for Refractory Cutaneous T-Cell Lymphoma (CTCL)," *Blood*, 2007, 109(1):31-9.

Kelly WK, O'Connor OA, Krug LM, et al, "Phase I Study of an Oral Histone Deacetylase Inhibitor, Suberoylanilide Hydroxamic Acid, in Patients With Advanced Cancer," *J Clin Oncol*, 2005, 23 (17):3923-31.

O'Connor OA, Heaney ML, Schwartz L, et al, "Clinical Experience With Intravenous and Oral Formulations of the Novel Histone Deacetylase Inhibitor Suberoylanilide Hydroxamic Acid in Patients With Advanced Hematologic Malignancies," *J Clin Oncol*, 2006, 24(1):166-73.

Olsen EA, Kim YH, Kuzel TM, et al, "Phase IIb Multicenter Trial of Vorinostat in Patients With Persistent, Progressive, or Treatment Refractory Cutaneous T-Cell Lymphoma," *J Clin Oncol*, 2007, 25(21):3109-15.

Ziconotide (zi KOE no tide)

Medication Safety Issues
High alert medication: The Institute for Safe Medication Practices (ISMP) includes this medication among its list of drugs which have a heightened risk of causing significant patient harm when used in error.

U.S. Brand Names Prialt®

Generic Available No

Pharmacologic Category Analgesic, Nonopioid; Calcium Channel Blocker, N-Type

Use Management of severe chronic pain in patients requiring intrathecal (I.T.) therapy and who are intolerant or refractory to other therapies

Pregnancy Risk Factor C

Lactation Excretion in breast milk unknown/not recommended

Labeled Contraindications Hypersensitivity to ziconotide or any component of the formulation; history of psychosis; I.V. administration

I.T. administration is contraindicated in patients with infection at the injection site, uncontrolled bleeding, or spinal canal obstruction that impairs CSF circulation

Warnings/Precautions [U.S Boxed Warning]: Severe psychiatric symptoms and neurological impairment have been reported; interrupt or discontinue therapy if cognitive impairment, hallucinations, mood changes, or changes in consciousness occur. May cause or worsen depression and/or risk of suicide. Cognitive impairment may appear gradually during treatment and is generally reversible after discontinuation (may take up to 2 weeks for cognitive effects to reverse). Use caution in the elderly; may experience a higher incidence of confusion. Patients should be instructed to use caution in performing tasks which require alertness (eg, operating machinery or driving). May have additive effects with opiates or other CNS-depressant medications; may potentiate opioid-induced decreased GI motility; does not interact with opioid receptors or potentiate opiate-induced respiratory depression. Will not prevent or relieve symptoms associated with opiate withdrawal and opiates should not be abruptly discontinued. Unlike opioids, ziconotide therapy can be interrupted abruptly or discontinued without evidence of withdrawal.

Meningitis may occur with use of I.T. pumps; monitor for signs and symptoms of meningitis; treatment of meningitis may require removal of system and discontinuation of intrathecal therapy. Elevated serum creatine kinase can occur, particularly during the first 2 months of therapy; consider dose reduction or discontinuing if combined with new neuromuscular symptoms (myalgias, myasthenia, muscle cramps, weakness) or reduction in physical activity. Safety and efficacy have not been established with renal or hepatic dysfunction, or in pediatric patients. Should not be used in combination with intrathecal opiates.

Adverse Reactions

>10%:

Central nervous system: Dizziness (46%), confusion (15% to 33%), memory impairment (7% to 22%), somnolence (17%), ataxia (14%), speech disorder (14%), headache (13%), aphasia (12%), hallucination (12%; including auditory and visual)

Gastrointestinal: Nausea (40%), diarrhea (18%), vomiting (16%)

Neuromuscular & skeletal: Creatine kinase increased (40%; ≥3 times ULN: 11%), weakness (18%), gait disturbances (14%)

Ocular: Blurred vision (12%)

2% to 10%:

Cardiovascular: Hypotension, peripheral edema, postural hypotension

Central nervous system: Abnormal thinking (8%), amnesia (8%), anxiety (8%), vertigo (7%), insomnia (6%), fever (5%), paranoid reaction (3%), delirium (2%), hostility (2%), stupor (2%), agitation, attention disturbance, balance impaired, burning sensation, coordination abnormal, depression, disorientation, fatigue, fever, hypoesthesia, irritability, lethargy, mental impairment, mood disorder, nervousness, pain, sedation

Dermatologic: Pruritus (7%)

Gastrointestinal: Anorexia (6%), taste perversion (5%), abdominal pain, appetite decreased, constipation, xerostomia

Genitourinary: Urinary retention (9%), dysuria, urinary hesitance

Neuromuscular & skeletal: Dysarthria (7%), paresthesia (7%), rigors (7%), tremor (7%), muscle spasm (6%), limb pain (5%), areflexia, muscle cramp, muscle weakness, myalgia

Ocular: Nystagmus (8%), diplopia, visual disturbance

Respiratory: Sinusitis (5%)

Miscellaneous: Diaphoresis (5%)

<2%, postmarketing, and/or case reports: Acute renal failure, aspiration pneumonia (<1%), atrial fibrillation, cerebral vascular accident, ECG abnormalities, incoherence, loss of consciousness, mania, meningitis, myoclonus, psychosis (1%), psychotic disorder, respiratory distress, rhabdomyolysis, seizure (clonic and grand mal), sepsis, suicidal ideation, suicide attempt (<1%)

Drug Interactions

Avoid Concomitant Use There are no known interactions where it is recommended to avoid concomitant use.

Increased Effect/Toxicity

Ziconotide may increase the levels/effects of: Alcohol (Ethyl); CNS Depressants; Methotrimeprazine

The levels/effects of Ziconotide may be increased by: Methotrimeprazine

Decreased Effect There are no known significant interactions involving a decrease in effect.

Ethanol/Nutrition/Herb Interactions Ethanol: Avoid ethanol (may increase CNS adverse effects).

Storage/Stability Prior to use, store vials at 2°C to 8°C (36°F to 46°F). Once diluted, may be stored at 2°C to 8°C (36°F to 46°F) for 24 hours; refrigerate during transit. Do not freeze. Protect from light.

When using the Medtronic SynchroMed® EL or SynchroMed® II Infusion System, solutions expire as follows:

25 mcg/mL: Undiluted:

Initial fill: Use within 14 days.

Refill: Use within 84 days.

100 mcg/mL:
  Undiluted: Refill: Use within 84 days.
  Diluted: Refill: Use within 40 days.

Reconstitution Preservative free NS should be used when dilution is needed.
  CADD-Micro® ambulatory infusion pump: Initial fill: Dilute to final concentration of 5 mcg/mL.
  Medtronic SynchroMed® EL or SynchroMed® II infusion system: Prior to initial fill, rinse internal pump surfaces with 2 mL ziconotide (25 mcg/mL), repeat twice. Only the 25 mcg/mL concentration (undiluted) should be used for initial pump fill.

Mechanism of Action Ziconotide selectively binds to N-type voltage-sensitive calcium channels located on the nociceptive afferent nerves of the dorsal horn in the spinal cord. This binding is thought to block N-type calcium channels, leading to a blockade of excitatory neurotransmitter release and reducing sensitivity to painful stimuli.

Pharmacodynamics/Kinetics
Distribution: I.T.: V_d: ~140 mL
Protein binding: ~50%
Metabolism: Metabolized via endopeptidases and exopeptidases present on multiple organs including kidney, liver, lung; degraded to peptide fragments and free amino acids
Half-life elimination: I.V.: 1-1.6 hours (plasma); I.T.: 2.9-6.5 hours (CSF)
Excretion: I.V.: Urine (<1%)

Dosage I.T.:
Adults: Chronic pain: Initial dose: ≤2.4 mcg/day (0.1 mcg/hour)
  Dose may be titrated by ≤2.4 mcg/day (0.1 mcg/hour) at intervals ≤2-3 times/week to a maximum dose of 19.2 mcg/day (0.8 mcg/hour) by day 21; average dose at day 21: 6.9 mcg/day (0.29 mcg/hour). A faster titration should be used only if the urgent need for analgesia outweighs the possible risk to patient safety.
Dosage adjustment for toxicity:
  Cognitive impairment: Reduce dose or discontinue. Effects are generally reversible within 3-15 days of discontinuation.
  Reduced level of consciousness: Discontinue until event resolves.
  CK elevation with neuromuscular symptoms: Consider dose reduction or discontinuation.
Elderly: Refer to adult dosing; use with caution.

Administration Not for I.V. administration. For I.T. administration only using Medtronic SynchroMed® EL, SynchroMed® II Infusion System, or CADD-Micro® ambulatory infusion pump.
  Medtronic SynchroMed® EL or SynchroMed® II Infusion Systems:
    Naive pump priming (first time use with ziconotide): Use 2 mL of undiluted ziconotide 25 mcg/mL solution to rinse the internal surfaces of the pump; repeat twice for a total of 3 rinses
    Initial pump fill: Use only undiluted 25 mcg/mL solution and fill pump after priming. Following the initial fill only, adsorption on internal device surfaces will occur, requiring the use of the undiluted solution and refill within 14 days.
    Pump refills: Contents should be emptied prior to refill. Subsequent pump refills should occur at least every 40 days if using diluted solution or at least every 84 days if using undiluted solution.
  CADD-Micro® ambulatory infusion pump: Refer to manufacturers' manual for initial fill and refill instructions

Monitoring Parameters Monitor for psychiatric or neurological impairment; signs and symptoms of meningitis or other infection; serum CPK (every other week for first month then monthly); pain relief

Dosage Forms Excipient information presented when available (limited, particularly for generics); consult specific product labeling.
Injection, solution, as acetate [preservative free]:
Prialt®: 25 mcg/mL (20 mL); 100 mcg/mL (1 mL, 5 mL)

References

Jain KK, "An Evaluation of Intrathecal Ziconotide for the Treatment of Chronic Pain," *Expert Opin Investig Drugs*, 2000, 9(10):2403-10.

Miljanich GP, "Ziconotide: Neuronal Calcium Channel Blocker for Treating Severe Chronic Pain," *Curr Med Chem*, 2004, 11(23):3029-40.

Staats PS, Yearwood T, Charapata SG, et al, "Intrathecal Ziconotide in the Treatment of Refractory Pain in Patients With Cancer or AIDS: A Randomized Controlled Trial," *JAMA*, 2004, 291 (1):63-70.

Wermeling D, Drass M, Ellis D, et al, "Pharmacokinetics and Pharmacodynamics of Intrathecal Ziconotide in Chronic Pain Patients," *J Clin Pharmacol*, 2003, 43(6):624-36.

Zoledronic Acid (zoe le DRON ik AS id)

Medication Safety Issues

Sound-alike/look-alike issues:
Zometa® may be confused with Zofran®, Zoladex®

Duplicate therapy issues:
Reclast® and Aclasta® contain zoledronic acid, which is the same ingredient contained in Zometa®; patients receiving Zometa® should not be treated with Reclast® or Aclasta®

Related Information

Safe Handling of Hazardous Drugs *on page 1517*

U.S. Brand Names Reclast®; Zometa®

Index Terms CGP-42446; Zol 446; Zoledronate

Generic Available No

Canadian Brand Names Aclasta®; Zometa®

Pharmacologic Category Antidote; Bisphosphonate Derivative

Use

Oncology-related uses: Treatment of hypercalcemia of malignancy (albumin-corrected serum calcium >12 mg/dL); treatment of multiple myeloma; treatment of bone metastases of solid tumors

Nononcology uses: Treatment of Paget's disease of bone; treatment of osteoporosis in postmenopausal women (to reduce the incidence of fractures or to reduce the incidence of new clinical fractures in patients with low-trauma hip fracture); prevention of osteoporosis in postmenopausal women, treatment of osteoporosis in men (to increase bone mass); treatment and prevention of glucocorticoid-induced osteoporosis (in patients initiating or continuing prednisone ≥7.5 mg/day [or equivalent] and expected to remain on glucocorticoids for at least 12 months)

Unlabeled/Investigational Use Prevention of bone loss associated with aromatase inhibitor therapy in postmenopausal women with breast cancer; prevention of bone loss associated with androgen deprivation therapy in prostate cancer

Pregnancy Risk Factor D

Lactation Excretion in breast milk unknown/not recommended

Labeled Contraindications Hypersensitivity to zoledronic acid, other bisphosphonates, or any component of the formulation; hypocalcemia (Reclast®)

Note: In Canada, Aclasta® is also contraindicated with uncorrected hypocalcemia at the time of infusion and in pregnancy and breast-feeding.

Warnings/Precautions Bisphosphonate therapy has been associated with osteonecrosis, primarily of the jaw; this has been observed mostly in cancer patients, but also in patients with postmenopausal osteoporosis and other diagnoses. Most reported cases occurred after I.V. bisphosphonate therapy; however, cases have been reported following oral therapy. Literature suggests ONJ is found more frequently in certain tumor types, such as multiple myeloma and advanced breast cancer. Dental exams and preventive dentistry should be performed prior to placing patients with risk factors on chronic bisphosphonate therapy. Good oral hygiene should be maintained and invasive dental procedures should be avoided during treatment.

Infrequently, severe (and occasionally debilitating) musculoskeletal (bone, joint, and/or muscle) pain have been reported during bisphosphonate treatment. The onset of pain ranged from a single day to several months. Consider discontinuing therapy in patients who experience severe symptoms; symptoms usually resolve upon discontinuation. Some patients experienced recurrence when rechallenged with same drug or another bisphosphonate; avoid use in patients with a history of these symptoms in association with bisphosphonate therapy.

May cause hypocalcemia in patients with Paget's disease, in whom the pretreatment rate of bone turnover may be greatly elevated. Hypocalcemia must be corrected before initiation of therapy in patients with Paget's disease and osteoporosis. Ensure adequate calcium and vitamin D intake during therapy. Use caution in patients with disturbances of calcium and mineral metabolism (eg, hypoparathyroidism, thyroid surgery, malabsorption syndromes).

Reclast®: Use is not recommended in patients with Cl_{cr} <35 mL/minute.

Zometa®: Use caution in mild-to-moderate renal dysfunction; dosage adjustment required. In cancer patients, renal toxicity has been reported with doses >4 mg or infusions administered over 15 minutes. Risk factors for renal deterioration include pre-existing renal insufficiency and repeated doses of zoledronic acid and other bisphosphonates. Dehydration and the use of other nephrotoxic drugs which may contribute to renal deterioration should be identified and managed. Use is not recommended in patients with severe renal impairment (serum creatinine >3 mg/dL) and bone metastases (limited data); use in patients with hypercalcemia of malignancy and severe renal impairment should only be done if the benefits outweigh the risks. Renal function should be assessed prior to treatment; if decreased after treatment, additional treatments should be withheld until renal function returns to within 10% of baseline. Diuretics should not be used before correcting hypovolemia. Renal deterioration, resulting in renal failure and dialysis has occurred in patients treated with zoledronic acid after single and multiple infusions at recommended doses of 4 mg over 15 minutes.

Aclasta® [CAN; not available in U.S.]: Use is not recommended in patients with Cl_{cr} <30 mL/minute.

According to the American Society of Clinical Oncology (ASCO) guidelines for bisphosphonates in multiple myeloma, treatment with zoledronic acid is not recommended for asymptomatic (smoldering) or indolent myeloma or with solitary plasmacytoma (Kyle, 2007). The National Comprehensive Cancer Network® (NCCN) multiple myeloma guidelines (v.2.2009) also do not recommend zoledronic acid use in stage 1 or smoldering disease, unless part of a clinical trial.

Adequate hydration is required during treatment (urine output ~2 L/day); avoid overhydration, especially in patients with heart failure. Pre-existing renal compromise, severe dehydration, and concurrent use with diuretics or other nephrotoxic drugs may increase the risk for renal impairment. Single and multiple infusions in patients with both normal and impaired renal function have been associated with renal deterioration, resulting in renal failure and dialysis (rare). Use caution in patients with aspirin-sensitive asthma (may cause bronchoconstriction) and the elderly. Women of childbearing age should be advised against becoming pregnant. Not approved for use in children.

Adverse Reactions Note: An acute reaction (eg, arthralgia, fever, flu-like symptoms, myalgia) may occur within the first 3 days following infusion in up to 44% of patients; usually resolves within 3-4 days of onset, although may take up to 14 days to resolve. The incidence may be decreased with acetaminophen (prior to infusion and for 72 hours postinfusion).

Zometa®:

>10%:

Cardiovascular: Leg edema (5% to 21%), hypotension (11%)

Central nervous system: Fatigue (39%), fever (32% to 44%), headache (5% to 19%), dizziness (18%), insomnia (15% to 16%), anxiety (11% to 14%), depression (14%), agitation (13%), confusion (7% to 13%), hypoesthesia (12%)

Dermatologic: Alopecia (12%), dermatitis (11%)

Endocrine & metabolic: Dehydration (5% to 14%), hypophosphatemia (12% to 13%), hypokalemia (12%), hypomagnesemia (11%)

Gastrointestinal: Nausea (29% to 46%), constipation (27% to 31%), vomiting (14% to 32%), diarrhea (17% to 24%), anorexia (9% to 22%), abdominal pain (14% to 16%), weight loss (16%), appetite decreased (13%)

Genitourinary: Urinary tract infection (12% to 14%)

Hematologic: Anemia (22% to 33%), neutropenia (12%)

Neuromuscular & skeletal: Bone pain (55%), weakness (5% to 24%), myalgia (23%), arthralgia (5% to 21%), back pain (15%), paresthesia (15%), limb pain (14%), skeletal pain (12%), rigors (11%)

Renal: Renal deterioration (8% to 17%; up to 40% in patients with abnormal baseline creatinine)

Respiratory: Dyspnea (22% to 27%), cough (12% to 22%)

Miscellaneous: Cancer progression (16%), moniliasis (12%)

1% to 10%:

Cardiovascular: Chest pain (5% to 10%)

Central nervous system: Somnolence (5% to 10%)

Endocrine & metabolic: Hypocalcemia (5% to 10%; grades 3/4: ≤1%), hypermagnesemia (2%)

Gastrointestinal: Dysphagia (5% to 10%), dyspepsia (10%), mucositis (5% to 10%), stomatitis (8%), sore throat (8%)

Hematologic: Thrombocytopenia (5% to 10%), pancytopenia (5% to 10%), granulocytopenia (5% to 10%)

Renal: Serum creatinine increased (grades 3/4: 2%)

Respiratory: Pleural effusion, upper respiratory tract infection (10%)

Miscellaneous: Metastases (5% to 10%), nonspecific infection (5% to 10%)

Reclast®:

>10%:

Cardiovascular: Hypertension (5% to 13%)

Central nervous system: Pain (2% to 24%), fever (9% to 22%), headache (4% to 20%), chills (2% to 18%), fatigue (2% to 18%)

Endocrine & metabolic: Hypocalcemia (≤3%; Paget's disease 21%)

Gastrointestinal: Nausea (5% to 18%)

Neuromuscular & skeletal: Arthralgia (9% to 27%), myalgia (5% to 23%), back pain (4% to 18%), limb pain (3% to 16%), musculoskeletal pain (≤12%)

Miscellaneous: Acute phase reaction (4% to 25%), flu-like syndrome (1% to 11%)

1% to 10%:

Cardiovascular: Chest pain (1% to 8%), peripheral edema (3% to 6%), atrial fibrillation (1% to 3%), palpitation (≤3%)

Central nervous system: Dizziness (2% to 9%), malaise (1% to 7%), hypoesthesia (≤6%), lethargy (3% to 5%), vertigo (1% to 4%), hyperthermia (≤2%)

Dermatologic: Rash (2% to 3%), hyperhidrosis (≤3%)

Gastrointestinal: Abdominal pain (1% to 9%), diarrhea (5% to 8%), vomiting (2% to 8%), constipation (6% to 7%), dyspepsia (2% to 7%), abdominal discomfort/distension (1% to 2%), anorexia (1% to 2%)

Neuromuscular & skeletal: Bone pain (3% to 9%), arthritis (2% to 9%), rigors (8%), shoulder pain (≤7%), neck pain (1% to 7%), weakness (2% to 6%), muscle spasm (2% to 6%), stiffness (1% to 5%), jaw pain (2% to 4%), joint swelling (≤3%), paresthesia (2%)

Ocular: Eye pain (≤2%)

Renal: Serum creatinine increased (2%)

Respiratory: Dyspnea (5% to 7%)

Miscellaneous: C-reactive protein increased (≤5%)

Zometa® and/or Reclast®: <1%, postmarketing, and/or case reports: Acute renal failure (requiring hospitalization/dialysis), allergic reaction, anaphylactic reaction/shock, angioedema, arrhythmia, blurred vision, bradycardia, bronchoconstriction, conjunctivitis, diaphoresis, episcleritis; flu-like syndrome (fever, chills, flushing, bone pain, arthralgia, myalgia); hematuria, hyperesthesia, hyperkalemia, hypernatremia, hypersensitivity, hypertension; injection site reaction (eg, itching, pain, redness); iritis, joint and/or muscle pain (sometimes severe and/or incapacitating), muscle cramps, osteonecrosis (primarily of the jaws), proteinuria, pruritus, rash, renal failure, renal impairment, taste perversion, toxic acute renal tubular necrosis, tremor, urticaria, uveitis, weight gain, xerostomia

Drug Interactions

Avoid Concomitant Use There are no known interactions where it is recommended to avoid concomitant use.

Increased Effect/Toxicity

Zoledronic Acid may increase the levels/effects of: Phosphate Supplements

The levels/effects of Zoledronic Acid may be increased by: Aminoglycosides; Nonsteroidal Anti-Inflammatory Agents; Thalidomide

Decreased Effect There are no known significant interactions involving a decrease in effect.

Storage/Stability

Aclasta® [CAN]: Store at room temperature of 15°C to 30°C (59°F to 86°F).

Reclast®: Store at room temperature of 25°C (77°F); excursions permitted to 15°C to 30°C (59°F to 86°F). After opening, stable for 24 hours at 2°C to 8°C (36°F to 46°F).

Zometa®: Store vials at 25°C (77°F); excursions permitted to 15°C to 30°C (59°F to 86°F). Solutions for infusion may be stored for 24 hours at 15°C to 30°C (59°F to 86°F). Infusion of solution must be completed within 24 hours.

Reconstitution Zometa®: Dilute solution for injection in 100 mL NS or D_5W prior to administration.

Compatibility Incompatible with calcium-containing solutions (eg, LR).

Mechanism of Action A bisphosphonate which inhibits bone resorption via actions on osteoclasts or on osteoclast precursors; inhibits osteoclastic activity and skeletal calcium release induced by tumors. Decreases serum calcium and phosphorus, and increases their elimination. In osteoporosis, zoledronic acid inhibits osteoclast-mediated resorption, therefore reducing bone turnover.

Pharmacodynamics/Kinetics

Distribution: Binds to bone

Protein binding: 28% to 53%

Half-life elimination: Triphasic; Terminal: 146 hours

Excretion: Urine (39% ± 16% as unchanged drug) within 24 hours; feces (<3%)

Dosage I.V.: Adults: **Note:** Acetaminophen administration after the infusion may reduce symptoms of acute-phase reactions. Patients treated for multiple myeloma, osteoporosis, and Paget's disease should receive a daily calcium supplement and multivitamin containing vitamin D (if dietary intake is inadequate).

Hypercalcemia of malignancy (albumin-corrected serum calcium ≥12 mg/dL) (Zometa®): 4 mg (maximum) given as a single dose. Wait at least 7 days before considering retreatment. Dosage adjustment may be needed in patients with decreased renal function following treatment.

Multiple myeloma or metastatic bone lesions from solid tumors (Zometa®): 4 mg every 3-4 weeks

Osteoporosis, glucocorticoid-induced, treatment and prevention (Reclast®, Aclasta® [CAN]): 5 mg infused over at least 15 minutes once a year

Osteoporosis, prevention (Reclast®): 5 mg infused over at least 15 minutes every 2 years

Osteoporosis, treatment (Reclast®, Aclasta® [CAN]): 5 mg infused over at least 15 minutes once a year

Paget's disease: 5 mg infused over at least 15 minutes. **Note:** Data concerning retreatment is not available; retreatment may be considered for relapse if appropriate, for inadequate response, or in patients who are symptomatic.

Prevention of aromatase inhibitor-induced bone loss in breast cancer (unlabeled use): 4 mg every 6 months

Prevention of androgen deprivation-induced bone loss in nonmetastatic prostate cancer (unlabeled use): 4 mg every 3-12 months

Dosage adjustment in renal impairment (at treatment initiation):
Reclast®:
Cl$_{cr}$ ≥35 mL/minute: No adjustment required
Cl$_{cr}$ <35 mL/minute: Use is not recommended
Zometa®: Multiple myeloma and bone metastases:
Cl$_{cr}$ >60 mL/minute: 4 mg
Cl$_{cr}$ 50-60 mL/minute: 3.5 mg
Cl$_{cr}$ 40-49 mL/minute: 3.3 mg
Cl$_{cr}$ 30-39 mL/minute: 3 mg
Cl$_{cr}$ <30 mL/minute: Not recommended
Zometa®: Hypercalcemia of malignancy:
Mild-to-moderate impairment: No adjustment necessary
Severe impairment (serum creatinine >4.5 mg/dL): Evaluate risk versus benefit
Aclasta® [CAN]:
Cl$_{cr}$ ≥30 mL/minute: No adjustment required
Cl$_{cr}$ <30 mL/minute: Use is not recommended

Dosage adjustment for renal toxicity (during treatment):
Hypercalcemia of malignancy: Evidence of renal deterioration: Evaluate risk versus benefit.
Multiple myeloma and bone metastases: Evidence of renal deterioration: Withhold dose until renal function returns to within 10% of baseline: renal deterioration defined as follows:
Normal baseline creatinine: Increase of 0.5 mg/dL
Abnormal baseline creatinine: Increase of 1 mg/dL
Reinitiate dose at the same dose administered prior to treatment interruption.
Multiple myeloma: Albuminuria >500 mg/24 hours (unexplained): Withhold dose until return to baseline, then reevaluate every 3-4 weeks; consider reinitiating with a longer infusion time of at least 30 minutes (Kyle, 2007).

Dosage adjustment in hepatic impairment: Specific guidelines are not available.

Administration Infuse over 15-30 minutes; do not infuse over <15 minutes. Infuse in a line separate from other medications. Patients should be appropriately hydrated prior to treatment.
Reclast®: If refrigerated, allow to reach room temperature prior to administration. Acetaminophen or ibuprofen after administration may reduce the incidence of acute reaction (eg, arthralgia, fever, flu-like symptoms, myalgia).

Monitoring Parameters Prior to initiation of therapy, dental exam and preventative dentistry for patients at risk for osteonecrosis, including all cancer patients
Aclasta® [CAN]: Serum creatinine, calcium and vitamin D levels
Reclast®: Alkaline phosphatase, serum creatinine (prior to each dose; high-risk patients may require interim monitoring), calcium and mineral (phosphorus and magnesium) levels
Zometa®: Serum creatinine prior to each dose; serum electrolytes, phosphate, magnesium, and hemoglobin/hematocrit should be evaluated regularly. Monitor serum calcium to assess response and avoid overtreatment. In patients with multiple myeloma, monitor urine every 3-6 months for albuminuria.

Test Interactions Bisphosphonates may interfere with diagnostic imaging agents such as technetium-99m-diphosphonate in bone scans.

Dietary Considerations
Multiple myeloma or metastatic bone lesions from solid tumors: Take daily

calcium supplement (500 mg) and daily multivitamin (with 400 int. units vitamin D).

Osteoporosis: Ensure adequate calcium and vitamin D supplementation; general requirements are calcium 1200 mg/day and vitamin D 800-1000 int. units/day.

Paget's disease: Take calcium 1500 mg/day and vitamin D 800 units/day, particularly during the first 2 weeks after administration.

Dosage Forms Excipient information presented when available (limited, particularly for generics); consult specific product labeling. [CAN] = Canadian brand name

Infusion, solution [premixed]:

Aclasta® [CAN]: 5 mg (100 mL) [not available in U.S.]

Reclast®: 5 mg (100 mL)

Injection, solution:

Zometa®: 4 mg/5 mL (5 mL) [as monohydrate 4.264 mg]

References

Black DM, Delmas PD, Eastell R, et al, "Once-Yearly Zoledronic Acid for Treatment of Postmenopausal Osteoporosis," *New Engl J Med*, 2007, 356(18):1809-22.

Boonen S, Sellmeyer DE, Lippuner K, et al, "Renal Safety of Annual Zoledronic Acid Infusions in Osteoporotic Postmenopausal Women," *Kidney Int*, 2008, 74(5):641-8.

Brufsky A, Harker WG, Beck JT, et al, "Zoledronic Acid Inhibits Adjuvant Letrozole-Induced Bone Loss in Postmenopausal Women With Early Breast Cancer," *J Clin Oncol* 2007, 25(7):829-36.

Coleman RE and Seaman JJ, "The Role of Zoledronic Acid in Cancer: Clinical Studies in the Treatment and Prevention of Bone Metastases," *Semin Oncol*, 2001, 28(2 Suppl 6):11-6.

Durie BG, Katz M, and Crowley J, "Osteonecrosis of the Jaw and Bisphosphonates," *N Engl J Med*, 2005, 353(1):99-102.

Hillner BE, Ingle JN, Chlebowski RT, et al, "American Society of Clinical Oncology 2003 Update on the Role of Bisphosphonates and Bone Health Issues in Women With Breast Cancer," *J Clin Oncol*, 2003, 21(21):4042-57.

Kyle RA, Yee GC, Somerfield MR, et al, "American Society of Clinical Oncology 2007 Clinical Practice Guideline Update on the Role of Bisphosphonates in Multiple Myeloma," *J Clin Oncol*, 2007, 25(17):2464-72.

Lyles KW, Colon-Emeric CS, Magaziner JS, et al, "Zoledronic Acid and Clinical Fractures and Mortality After Hip Fracture," *N Engl J Med*, 2007, 357(18):1799-809.

Maerevoet M, Martin C, and Duck L, "Osteonecrosis of the Jaw and Bisphosphonates," *N Engl J Med*, 2005, 353(1):99-102.

Michaelson MD, Kaufman DS, Lee H, et al, "Randomized Controlled Trial of Annual Zoledronic Acid to Prevent Gonadotropin-Releasing Hormone Agonist-Induced Bone Loss in Men With Prostate Cancer," *J Clin Oncol*, 2007, 25(9):1038-42.

National Comprehensive Cancer Network® (NCCN), "Clinical Practice Guidelines in Oncology™: Multiple Myeloma," Version 2.2009. Available at http://www.nccn.org/professionals/physician_gls/PDF/myeloma.pdf.

Reid DM, Devogelaer JP, Saag K, et al, "Zoledronic Acid and Risedronate in the Prevention and Treatment of Glucocorticoid-Induced Osteoporosis (HORIZON): A Multicentre, Double-Blind, Double-Dummy, Randomised Controlled Trial," *Lancet*, 2009, 373(9671):1253-63.

Reid IR, Miller P, Lyles K, et al, "Comparison of a Single Infusion of Zoledronic Acid With Risedronate for Paget's Disease," *N Engl J Med*, 2005, 353(9):898-908.

Smith MR, Eastham J, Gleason DM, et al, "Randomized Controlled Trial of Zoledronic Acid to Prevent Bone Loss in Men Receiving Androgen Deprivation Therapy for Nonmetastatic Prostate Cancer," *J Urol*, 2003, 169(6):2008-12.

CHEMOTHERAPY REGIMEN INDEX

CHEMOTHERAPY REGIMEN INDEX

GASTROINTESTINAL

Anal Cancer

Biliary Adenocarcinoma

Colorectal Cancer

HEMATOLOGIC/LEUKEMIA

ALPHABETICAL LISTING OF CHEMOTHERAPY REGIMENS

5 + 2

Index Terms Cytarabine-Daunorubicin (5 + 2); Daunorubicin-Cytarabine (5 + 2)

Use Leukemia, acute myeloid (induction)

Regimen

Cytarabine: I.V.: 100-200 mg/m^2/day continuous infusion days 1 to 5
  [total dose/cycle = 500-1000 mg/m^2]

with

Daunorubicin: I.V.: 45 mg/m^2/day days 1 and 2
  [total dose/cycle = 90 mg/m^2]

References

Rai KR, Holland JF, Glidewell OJ, et al, "Treatment of Acute Myelocytic Leukemia: A Study by Cancer and Leukemia Group B," *Blood*, 1981, 58(6):1203-12.

7 + 3 + 7

Index Terms Cytarabine-Daunorubicin-Etoposide (7 + 3 + 7)

Use Leukemia, acute myeloid

Regimen

Cytarabine: I.V.: 100 mg/m^2/day continuous infusion days 1 to 7
  [total dose/cycle = 700 mg/m^2]
Daunorubicin: I.V.: 50 mg/m^2/day days 1, 2, and 3
  [total dose/cycle = 150 mg/m^2]
Etoposide: I.V.: 75 mg/m^2/day days 1 to 7
  [total dose/cycle = 525 mg/m^2]
Repeat cycle every 21 days; up to 3 cycles may be given based on individual response

References

Bishop JF, Lowenthal RM, Joshua D, et al, "Etoposide in Acute Nonlymphocytic Leukemia, Australian Leukemia Study Group," *Blood*, 1990, 75(1):27-32.

7 + 3 (Daunorubicin)

Index Terms Cytarabine-Daunorubicin (7 + 3)

Use Leukemia, acute myeloid (induction)

Regimen

Cytarabine: I.V.: 100 mg/m^2/day continuous infusion days 1 to 7
  [total dose/cycle = 700 mg/m^2]
Daunorubicin: I.V.: 45 mg/m^2/day days 1, 2, and 3
  [total dose/cycle = 135 mg/m^2]
Administer one cycle only

References

Dilman RO, Davis RB, Green MR, et al, "A Comparative Study of Two Different Doses of Cytarabine for Acute Myeloid Leukemia: A Phase III Trial of Cancer and Leukemia Group B," *Blood*, 1991, 78(10):2520-6.

Preisler H, Davis RB, Kirschner J, et al, "Comparison of Three Remission Induction Regimens and Two Postinduction Strategies for the Treatment of Acute Nonlymphocytic Leukemia: A Cancer and Leukemia Group B Study," *Blood*, 1987, 69(5):1441-9.

Rai KR, Holland JF, Glidewell OJ, et al, "Treatment of Acute Myelocytic Leukemia: A Study by Cancer and Leukemia Group B," *Blood*, 1981, 58(6):1203-12.

Vogler WR, Velez-Garcia E, Weiner RS, et al, "A Phase III Trial Comparing Idarubicin and Daunorubicin in Combination With Cytarabine in Acute Myelogenous Leukemia: A Southeastern Cancer Study Group Study," *J Clin Oncol*, 1992, 10(7):1103-11.

Yates J, Glidewell O, Wiernik P, et al, "Cytosine Arabinoside With Daunorubicin or Adriamycin® for Therapy of Acute Myelocytic Leukemia: A CALGB Study," *Blood*, 1982, 60(2):454-62.

Yates JW, Wallace HJ Jr, Ellison RR, et al, "Cytosine Arabinoside (NSC-63878) and Daunorubicin (NSC-83142) Therapy in Acute Nonlymphocytic Leukemia," *Cancer Chemother Rep*, 1973, 57 (4):485-8.

7 + 3 (Idarubicin)

Index Terms Cytarabine-Idarubicin (7 + 3)

Use Leukemia, acute myeloid (induction)

Regimen

Cytarabine: I.V.: 100-200 mg/m^2/day continuous infusion days 1 to 7
[total dose/cycle = 700-1400 mg/m^2]
Idarubicin: I.V.: 12 mg/m^2/day days 1, 2, and 3
[total dose/cycle = 36 mg/m^2]
Administer one cycle only

References

Vogler WR, Velez-Garcia E, Weiner RS, et al, "A Phase III Trial Comparing Idarubicin and Daunorubicin in Combination With Cytarabine in Acute Myelogenous Leukemia: A Southeastern Cancer Study Group Study," *J Clin Oncol*, 1992, 10(7):1103-11.

7 + 3 (Mitoxantrone)

Index Terms Cytarabine-Mitoxantrone (7 + 3)

Use Leukemia, acute myeloid (induction)

Regimen

Cytarabine: I.V.: 100-200 mg/m^2/day continuous infusion days 1 to 7
[total dose/cycle = 700-1400 mg/m^2]
Mitoxantrone: I.V.: 12 mg/m^2/day days 1, 2, and 3
[total dose/cycle = 36 mg/m^2]
Administer one cycle only

References

Arlin Z, Case DC Jr, Moore J, et al, "Randomized Multicenter Trial of Cytosine Arabinoside With Mitoxantrone or Daunorubicin in Previously Untreated Adult Patients With Acute Nonlymphocytic Leukemia (ANLL)," Lederle Cooperative Group," *Leukemia*, 1990, 4(3):177-83.

8 in 1 (Brain Tumors)

Use Brain tumors

Regimen NOTE: Multiple variations are listed.

Variation 1:

Methylprednisolone: I.V.: 300 mg/m^2 every 6 hours day 1 (3 doses)
[total dose/cycle = 900 mg/m^2]
Vincristine: I.V.: 1.5 mg/m^2 (maximum dose: 2 mg) day 1
Lomustine: Oral: 75 mg/m^2 day 1
Procarbazine: Oral: 75 mg/m^2 day 1; 1 hour after methylprednisolone and vincristine
Hydroxyurea: Oral: 3000 mg/m^2 day 1; 2 hours after methylprednisolone and vincristine
Cisplatin: I.V.: 90 mg/m^2 day 1; 3 hours after methylprednisolone and vincristine
Cytarabine: I.V.: 300 mg/m^2 day 1; 9 hours after methylprednisolone and vincristine
Dacarbazine: I.V.: 150 mg/m^2 day 1; 12 hours after methylprednisolone and vincristine
Repeat cycle every 14 days

Variation 2:

Methylprednisolone: I.V.: 300 mg/m^2 every 6 hours day 1 (3 doses)
[total dose/cycle = 900 mg/m^2]
Vincristine: I.V.: 1.5 mg/m^2 (maximum dose: 2 mg) day 1
Lomustine: Oral: 75 mg/m^2 day 1
Procarbazine: Oral: 75 mg/m^2 day 1; 1 hour after methylprednisolone and vincristine

◄

Hydroxyurea: Oral: 3000 mg/m² day 1; 2 hours after methylprednisolone and vincristine

Cisplatin: I.V.: 60 mg/m² day 1; 3 hours after methylprednisolone and vincristine

Cytarabine: I.V.: 300 mg/m² day 1; 9 hours after methylprednisolone and vincristine

Cyclophosphamide: I.V.: 300 mg/m² day 1; 12 hours after methylprednisolone and vincristine

Repeat cycle every 14 days

References

Pendergrass TW, Milstein JM, Geyer JR, et al, "Eight Drugs in One Day Chemotherapy for Brain Tumors: Experience in 107 Children and Rationale for Preradiation Chemotherapy," *J Clin Oncol*, 1987, 5(8):1221-31.

8 in 1 (Retinoblastoma)

Use Retinoblastoma

Regimen

Vincristine: I.V.: 1.5 mg/m² day 1
Methylprednisolone: I.V.: 300 mg/m² day 1
Lomustine: Oral: 75 mg/m² day 1
Procarbazine: Oral: 75 mg/m² day 1
Hydroxyurea: Oral: 1500 mg/m² day 1
Cisplatin: I.V.: 60 mg/m² day 1
Cytarabine: I.V.: 300 mg/m² day 1
Repeat cycle every 28 days

References

Doz F, Khelfaoui F, Mosseri V, et al, "The Role of Chemotherapy in Orbital Involvement of Retinoblastoma. The Experience of a Single Institution With 33 Patients," *Cancer*, 1994, 74 (2):722-32.

AAV (DD)

Use Wilms' tumor

Regimen

Dactinomycin: I.V.: 15 mcg/kg/day days 1 to 5 of weeks 0, 13, 26, 39, 52, and 65
  [total dose/cycle = 450 mcg/kg]
Doxorubicin: I.V.: 20 mg/m²/day days 1, 2, and 3 of weeks 6, 19, 32, 45, and 58
  [total dose/cycle = 300 mg/m²]
Vincristine: I.V.: 1.5 mg/m² day 1 of weeks 0-10, 13, 14, 26, 27, 39, 40, 52, 53, 65, and 66
  [total dose/cycle = 31.5 mg/m²]

References

D'Angio GJ, Breslow N, Beckwith JB, et al, "Treatment of Wilms' Tumor. Results of the Third National Wilms' Tumor Study," *Cancer*, 1989, 64(2):349-60.

ABVD

Use Lymphoma, Hodgkin's disease

Regimen

Doxorubicin: I.V.: 25 mg/m²/day days 1 and 15
  [total dose/cycle = 50 mg/m²]
Bleomycin: I.V.: 10 units/m²/day days 1 and 15
  [total dose/cycle = 20 units/m²]
Vinblastine: I.V.: 6 mg/m²/day days 1 and 15
  [total dose/cycle = 12 mg/m²]

Dacarbazine: I.V.: 375 mg/m^2/day days 1 and 15
[total dose/cycle = 750 mg/m^2]
Repeat cycle every 28 days

References

Bonadonna G, Zucali R, DeLena M, et al, "Combined Chemotherapy (MOPP or ABVD) - Radiotherapy Approach in Advanced Hodgkin's Disease," *Cancer Treat Rep*, 1977, 61(5):769-77.

Canellos GP, Anderson JR, Propert KJ, et al, "Chemotherapy of Advanced Hodgkin's Disease With MOPP, ABVD, or MOPP Alternating With ABVD," *N Engl J Med*, 1992, 327(21):1478-84.

AC

Use Breast cancer

Regimen NOTE: Multiple variations are listed.

Variation 1: AC (conventional):
Doxorubicin: I.V.: 60 mg/m^2 day 1
[total dose/cycle = 60 mg/m^2]
Cyclophosphamide: I.V.: 600 mg/m^2 day 1
[total dose/cycle = 600 mg/m^2]
Repeat cycle every 21 days

Variation 2:
Cyclophosphamide: Oral: 200 mg/m^2/day days 3 to 6
[total dose/cycle = 800 mg/m^2]
Doxorubicin: I.V.: 40 mg/m^2 day 1
[total dose/cycle = 40 mg/m^2]
Repeat cycle every 3 weeks for 3 cycles, then every 4 weeks

References

Variation 1:

Fisher B, Brown AM, Dimitrov NV, et al, "Two Months of Doxorubicin-Cyclophosphamide With and Without Interval Reinduction Therapy Compared With 6 Months of Cyclophosphamide, Methotrexate, and Fluorouracil in Positive-Node Breast Cancer Patients With Tamoxifen-Nonresponsive Tumors: Results From the National Surgical Adjuvant Breast and Bowel Project B-15," *J Clin Oncol*, 1990, 8(9):1483-96.

Variation 2:

Jones SE, Durie BG, and Salmon SE, "Combination Chemotherapy With Adriamycin and Cyclophosphamide for Advanced Breast Cancer," *Cancer*, 1975, 36(1):90-7.

AC/Paclitaxel (Sequential)

Use Breast cancer

Regimen

Variation 1: AC + Paclitaxel (conventional):
Doxorubicin: I.V.: 60 mg/m^2 day 1
[total dose/cycle = 60 mg/m^2]
Cyclophosphamide: I.V.: 600 mg/m^2 day 1
[total dose/cycle = 600 mg/m^2]
Repeat cycle every 21 days for 4 cycles
followed by
Paclitaxel: I.V.: 175 mg/m^2 day 1
[total dose/cycle = 175 mg/m^2]
Repeat cycle every 21 days for 4 cycles

Variation 2: AC + Paclitaxel (dose dense):
Doxorubicin: I.V.: 60 mg/m^2 day 1
[total dose/cycle = 60 mg/m^2]
Cyclophosphamide: I.V.: 600 mg/m^2 day 1
[total dose/cycle = 600 mg/m^2]
Filgrastim: SubQ: 5 mcg/kg/day days 3 to 10
[total dose/cycle = 40 mcg/kg]
Repeat cycle every 14 days for 4 cycles

followed by
Paclitaxel: I.V.: 175 mg/m² day 1
[total dose/cycle = 175 mg/m²]
Filgrastim: SubQ: 5 mcg/kg/day days 3 to 10
[total dose/cycle = 40 mcg/kg]
Repeat cycle every 14 days for 4 cycles

References

Variation 1:
Henderson IC, Berry DA, Demetri GD, et al, "Improved Outcomes From Adding Sequential Paclitaxel but Not From Escalating Doxorubicin Dose in an Adjuvant Chemotherapy Regimen for Patients With Node-Positive Primary Breast Cancer," *J Clin Oncol*, 2003, 21(6):976-83.
Variation 2:
Citron ML, Berry DA, Cirrincione C, et al, "Randomized Trial of Dose-Dense Versus Conventionally Scheduled Versus Concurrent Combination Chemotherapy as Postoperative Adjuvant Treatment of Node-Positive Primary Breast Cancer: First Report of Intergroup Trial C9741/Cancer Leukemia Group B Trial 9741," *J Clin Oncol*, 2003, 21(8):1431-9.

AC-Paclitaxel-Trastuzumab

Use Breast cancer

Regimen NOTE: Multiple variations are listed.

Variation 1:
Doxorubicin: I.V.: 60 mg/m² day 1
[total dose/cycle = 60 mg/m²]
Cyclophosphamide: I.V.: 600 mg/m² day 1
[total dose/cycle = 600 mg/m²]
Repeat cycle every 21 days for 4 cycles
followed by
Paclitaxel: I.V.: 175 mg/m² day 1
[total dose/cycle = 175 mg/m²]
Trastuzumab: I.V.: 4 mg/kg (loading dose) day 1 (cycle 1 only)
[total dose/cycle = 4 mg/kg]
   followed by I.V.: 2 mg/kg/day days 8 and 15 (cycle 1)
   [total dose/cycle = 4 mg/kg]
      then I.V.: 2 mg/kg/day days 1, 8, and 15 (cycles 2, 3, and 4)
      [total dose/cycle = 6 mg/kg]
Repeat cycle every 21 days for 4 cycles
followed by
Trastuzumab: I.V.: 2 mg/kg weekly for 40 weeks

Variation 2:
Doxorubicin: I.V.: 60 mg/m² day 1
[total dose/cycle = 60 mg/m²]
Cyclophosphamide: I.V.: 600 mg/m² day 1
[total dose/cycle = 600 mg/m²]
Repeat cycle every 21 days for 4 cycles
followed by
Paclitaxel: I.V.: 80 mg/m²day 1 week 13
[total dose/cycle = 80 mg/m²]
Trastuzumab: I.V.: 4 mg/kg (loading dose) day 1 week 13 only
[total dose/cycle = 4 mg/kg]
followed by
Paclitaxel: I.V.: 80 mg/m² weekly
[total dose/cycle = 80 mg/m²]
Trastuzumab: I.V.: 2 mg/kg /weekly
[total dose/cycle = 2 mg/kg]
Repeat cycle every week for 11 cycles

followed by
Trastuzumab: I.V.: 2 mg/kg/weekly for 40 weeks
References
Romond EH, Perez EA, Bryant J, et al, "Trastuzumab Plus Adjuvant Chemotherapy for Operable HER2-Positive Breast Cancer," *N Engl J Med*, 2005, 353(16):1673-84.

AD

Use Soft tissue sarcoma
Regimen
Doxorubicin: I.V.: 60 mg/m^2 day 1
[total dose/cycle = 60 mg/m^2]
Dacarbazine: I.V.: 250 mg/m^2/day days 1 to 5
[total dose/cycle = 1250 mg/m^2]
Repeat cycle every 21 days
References
Borden EC, Amato DA, Rosenbaum C, et al, "Randomized Comparison of Three Adriamycin Regimens for Metastatic Soft Tissue Sarcomas," *J Clin Oncol*, 1987, 5(6):840-50.

AI

Use Soft tissue sarcoma
Regimen NOTE: Multiple variations are listed.
Variation 1:
Doxorubicin: I.V.: 25 mg/m^2/day continuous infusion days 1, 2, and 3
[total dose/cycle = 75 mg/m^2]
Ifosfamide: I.V.: 2 g/m^2/day days 1 to 5
[total dose/cycle = 10 g/m^2]
Mesna: I.V.: 400 mg/m^2 day 1
followed by I.V.: 1200 mg/m^2/day continuous infusion days 1 to 5
[total dose/cycle = 6400 mg/m^2]
Repeat cycle every 3 weeks
Variation 2:
Doxorubicin: I.V.: 30 mg/m^2/day continuous infusion days 1, 2, and 3
[total dose/cycle = 90 mg/m^2]
Ifosfamide: I.V.: 2.5 g/m^2/day days 1 to 4
[total dose/cycle = 10 g/m^2]
Mesna: I.V.: 500 mg/m^2 day 1
followed by I.V.: 1500 mg/m^2/day continuous infusion days 1 to 4
[total dose/cycle = 6500 mg/m^2]
Filgrastim: SubQ: 5 mcg/kg/day days 5 through ANC recovery
Repeat cycle every 3 weeks
References
Patel SR, Vadhan-Raj S, Burgess MA, et al, "Results of Two Consecutive Trials of Dose-Intensive Chemotherapy With Doxorubicin and Ifosfamide in Patients With Sarcomas," *Am J Clin Oncol*, 1998, 21(3):317-21.

◆ **Aldesleukin (Low Dose)-Interferon Alfa 2b** see Interleukin 2 (Low Dose)-Interferon Alfa 2b on page 1359

◆ **AlinC 14** see PVA (POG 8602) on page 1398

AP

Use Endometrial cancer
Regimen
Doxorubicin: I.V.: 60 mg/m^2 day 1
[total dose/cycle = 60 mg/m^2]

Cisplatin: I.V.: 60 mg/m^2 day 1
[total dose/cycle = 60 mg/m^2]
Repeat cycle every 21-28 days

References

Barrett RJ, Blessing JA, Homesley HD, et al, "Circadian-Timed Combination Doxorubicin-Cisplatin Chemotherapy for Advanced Endometrial Carcinoma. A Phase II Study of the Gynecologic Oncology Group," *Am J Clin Oncol*, 1993, 16(6):494-6.

♦ **Arsenic Trioxide-ATRA (APL)** *see* Tretinoin-Arsenic Trioxide (APL) *on page 1410*

AT

Use Breast cancer

Regimen NOTE: Multiple variations are listed.

Variation 1:
Doxorubicin: I.V.: 50 mg/m^2 day 1
[total dose/cycle = 50 mg/m^2]
Docetaxel: I.V.: 75 mg/m^2 day 1
[total dose/cycle = 75 mg/m^2]
Repeat cycle every 3 weeks

Variation 2:
Doxorubicin: I.V.: 60 mg/m^2 day 1
[total dose/cycle = 60 mg/m^2]
Docetaxel: I.V.: 60 mg/m^2 day 1
[total dose/cycle = 60 mg/m^2]
Repeat cycle every 3 weeks

Variation 3:
Doxorubicin: I.V.: 50 mg/m^2 day 1
[total dose/cycle = 50 mg/m^2]
Docetaxel: I.V.: 75 mg/m^2 day 1
[total dose/cycle = 75 mg/m^2]
Repeat cycle every 14 days

Variation 4:
Doxorubicin: I.V.: 50 mg/m^2 day 1
[total dose/cycle = 50 mg/m^2]
Docetaxel: I.V.: 60 mg/m^2 day 1
[total dose/cycle = 60 mg/m^2]
Repeat cycle every 3 weeks

Variation 5:
Doxorubicin: I.V.: 50 mg/m^2 day 1
[total dose/cycle = 50 mg/m^2]
Docetaxel: I.V.: 60 mg/m^2 day 1
[total dose/cycle = 60 mg/m^2]
Repeat cycle every 3-4 weeks

Variation 6:
Doxorubicin: I.V.: 56 mg/m^2 day 1
[total dose/cycle = 56 mg/m^2]
Docetaxel: I.V.: 75 mg/m^2 day 1
[total dose/cycle = 75 mg/m^2]
Repeat cycle every 3 weeks

Variation 7:
Doxorubicin: I.V.: 50 mg/m^2 day 1
[total dose/cycle = 50 mg/m^2]

Docetaxel: I.V.: 75 mg/m² day 2

[total dose/cycle = 75 mg/m²]

Repeat cycle every 4 weeks

References

Variation 1:

von Minckwitz G, Costa SD, Eiermann W, et al, "Maximized Reduction of Primary Breast Tumor Size Using Preoperative Chemotherapy With Doxorubicin and Docetaxel," *J Clin Oncol*, 1999, 17 (7):1999-2005.

Variation 2:

Dieras V, "Docetaxel in Combination With Doxorubicin: A Phase I Dose-Finding Study," *Oncology (Williston Park)*, 1997, 11(6 Suppl 6):17-20.

Variation 3:

von Minckwitz G, Costa SD, Raab G, et al, "Dose-Dense Doxorubicin, Docetaxel, and Granulocyte Colony-Stimulating Factor Support With or Without Tamoxifen as Preoperative Therapy in Patients With Operable Carcinoma of the Breast: A Randomized, Controlled, Open Phase IIB Study," *J Clin Oncol*, 2001, 19(15):3506-15.

Variation 4:

Muthalib A, Darwis I, Prayogo N, et al, "Preliminary Results of Multicenter Phase II Trial of Docetaxel (Taxotere) in Combination With Doxorubicin as First-Line Chemotherapy in Indonesian Patients With Advanced or Metastatic Breast Cancer," *Gan To Kagaku Ryoho*, 2000, 27(Suppl 2):498-504.

Variation 5:

Aihara T, Takatsuka Y, Itoh K, et al, "Phase II Study of Concurrent Administration of Doxorubicin and Docetaxel as First-Line Chemotherapy for Metastatic Breast Cancer," *Oncology*, 2003, 64 (2):124-30.

Variation 6:

Miller KD, McCaskill-Stevens W, Sisk J, et al, "Combination Versus Sequential Doxorubicin and Docetaxel as Primary Chemotherapy for Breast Cancer: A Randomized Pilot Trial of the Hoosier Oncology Group," *J Clin Oncol*, 1999, 17(10):3033-7.

Variation 7:

Palmeri S, Leonardi V, Tamburo De Bella M, et al, "Doxorubicin-Docetaxel Sequential Schedule: Results of Front-Line Treatment in Advanced Breast Cancer," *Oncology*, 2002, 63(3):205-12.

- **ATC** *see* TAC *on page 1404*

- **ATRA-Arsenic Trioxide-Gemtuzumab (APL)** *see* Tretinoin-Arsenic Trioxide-Gemtuzumab (APL) *on page 1411*

- **ATRA-Arsenic Trixoide (APL)** *see* Tretinoin-Arsenic Trioxide (APL) *on page 1410*

- **ATRA-Daunorubicin (APL)** *see* Tretinoin-Daunorubicin (APL) *on page 1411*

- **ATRA-Daunorubicin-Cytarabine (APL)** *see* Tretinoin-Daunorubicin-Cytarabine (APL) *on page 1412*

- **ATRA-Idarubicin (APL)** *see* Tretinoin-Idarubicin (APL) *on page 1414*

AVD

Use Wilms' tumor

Regimen

Dactinomycin: I.V.: 15 mcg/kg/day days 1 to 5 of weeks 0, 13, 26, 39, 52, and 65

[total dose/cycle = 450 mcg/kg]

Doxorubicin: I.V.: 60 mg/m² day 1 of weeks 6, 19, 32, 45, and 58

[total dose/cycle = 300 mg/m²]

Vincristine: I.V.: 1.5 mg/m² day 1 of weeks 1 to 8, 13, 14, 26, 27, 39, 40, 52, 53, 65, and 66

[total dose/cycle = 27 mg/m²]

References

Green DM, Breslow NE, Evans I, et al, "Treatment of Children With Stage IV Favorable Histology Wilms Tumor: A Report From the National Wilms' Tumor Study Group," *Med Pediatr Oncol*, 1996, 26(3):147-52.

AV (EE)

Use Wilms' tumor

Regimen

Dactinomycin: I.V.: 15 mcg/kg/day days 1 to 5 of weeks 0, 5, 13, and 26
[total dose/cycle = 300 mcg/kg]

Vincristine: I.V.: 1.5 mg/m^2/dose day 1 of weeks 1 to 10, and days 1 and 5 of
weeks 13 and 26
[total dose/cycle = 21 mg/m^2]

References

D'Angio GJ, Breslow N, Beckwith JB, et al, "Treatment of Wilms' Tumor. Results of the Third
National Wilms' Tumor Study," *Cancer*, 1989, 64(2):349-60.

AV (K)

Use Wilms' tumor

Regimen

Dactinomycin: I.V.: 15 mcg/kg/day days 1 to 5 of weeks 0, 5, 13, 22, 31, 40, 49,
and 58
[total dose/cycle = 600 mcg/kg]

Vincristine: I.V.: 1.5 mg/m^2/dose day 1 of weeks 0-10, 15-20, 24-29, 33-38,
42-47, 51-56, and 60-65
[total dose/cycle = 70.5 mg/m^2]

References

D'Angio GJ, Breslow N, Beckwith JB, et al, "Treatment of Wilms' Tumor. Results of the Third
National Wilms' Tumor Study," *Cancer*, 1989, 64(2):349-60.

AV (L)

Use Wilms' tumor

Regimen

Dactinomycin: I.V.: 15 mcg/kg/day days 1 to 5 of weeks 0 and 5
[total dose/cycle = 150 mcg/kg]

Vincristine: I.V.: 1.5 mg/m^2 day 1 of weeks 0-10
[total dose/cycle = 16.5 mg/m^2]

References

D'Angio GJ, Breslow N, Beckwith JB, et al, "Treatment of Wilms' Tumor. Results of the Third
National Wilms' Tumor Study," *Cancer*, 1989, 64(2):349-60.

AV (Wilms' Tumor)

Use Wilms' tumor

Regimen

Dactinomycin: I.V.: 15 mcg/kg/day days 1 to 5 of weeks 0, 13, 26, 39, 52, and
65
[total dose/cycle = 450 mcg/kg]

Vincristine: I.V.: 1.5 mg/m^2/dose day 1 of weeks 1 to 8, 13, 14, 26, 27, 39, 40,
52, 53, 65, and 66
[total dose/cycle = 27 mg/m^2]

References

Green DM, Breslow NE, Evans I, et al, "Treatment of Children With Stage IV Favorable Histology
Wilms' Tumor: A Report From the National Wilms Tumor Study Group," *Med Pediatr Oncol*, 1996,
26(3):147-52.

◆ **Baby Brain I** *see* COPE *on page* 1280

BEACOPP

Use Lymphoma, Hodgkin's disease
Regimen
Bleomycin: I.V.: 10 units/m² day 8
  [total dose/cycle = 10 units/m²]
Etoposide: I.V.: 100 mg/m²/day days 1, 2, and 3
  [total dose/cycle = 300 mg/m²]
Doxorubicin: I.V.: 25 mg/m² day 1
  [total dose/cycle = 25 mg/m²]
Cyclophosphamide: I.V.: 650 mg/m² day 1
  [total dose/cycle = 650 mg/m²]
Vincristine: I.V.: 1.4 mg/m² (maximum dose: 2 mg) day 8
  [total dose/cycle = 1.4 mg/m²; maximum: 2 mg]
Procarbazine: Oral: 100 mg/m²/day days 1 to 7
  [total dose/cycle = 700 mg/m²]
Prednisone: Oral: 40 mg/m²/day days 1 to 14
  [total dose/cycle = 560 mg/m²]
Repeat cycle every 21 days

References
Diehl V, Franklin J, Hasenclever D, et al, "BEACOPP, a New Dose-Escalated and Accelerated Regimen, Is at Least as Effective as COPP/ABVD in Patients With Advanced-Stage Hodgkin's Lymphoma: Interim Report From a Trial of the German Hodgkin's Lymphoma Study Group," *J Clin Oncol*, 1998, 16(12):3810-21.

Bendamustine-Rituximab

Index Terms Rituximab-Bendamustine
Use Lymphoma, non-Hodgkin's (Mantle cell or low-grade NHL)
Regimen NOTE: Multiple variations are listed.
Variation 1:
  Pretreatment:
    Rituximab: I.V.: 375 mg/m² 1 week before the start of cycle 1
      [total dose/pretreatment = 375 mg/m²]
  Cycles:
    Rituximab: I.V.: 375 mg/m² day 1
      [total dose/cycle = 375 mg/m²]
    Bendamustine: I.V.: 90 mg/m² days 2 and 3
      [total dose/cycle = 180 mg/m²]
    Repeat cycle every 4 weeks for up to 4 cycles
  Post-Treatment:
    Rituximab: I.V.: 375 mg/m² 4 weeks after the last cycle
      [total dose/post-treatment = 375 mg/m²]
Variation 2:
  Pretreatment:
    Rituximab: I.V.: 375 mg/m² 1 week before the start of cycle 1
      [total dose/pretreatment = 375 mg/m²]
  Cycles:
    Rituximab: I.V.: 375 mg/m² day 1
      [total dose/cycle = 375 mg/m²]
    Bendamustine: I.V.: 90 mg/m² days 2 and 3
      [total dose/cycle = 180 mg/m²]
    Repeat cycle every 4 weeks for 4-6 cycles
  Post-Treatment:
    Rituximab: I.V.: 375 mg/m² 4 weeks after the last cycle
      [total dose/post-treatment = 375 mg/m²]

References

Variation 1:
Rummel MJ, Al-Batran SE, Kim SZ, et al, "Bendamustine Plus Rituximab Is Effective and Has a Favorable Toxicity Profile in the Treatment of Mantle Cell and Low-Grade Non-Hodgkin's Lymphoma," *J Clin Oncol*, 2005, 23(15):3383-9.

Variation 2:
Robinson KS, Williams ME, van der Jagt RH, et al, "Phase II Multicenter Study of Bendamustine Plus Rituximab in Patients With Relapsed Indolent B-Cell and Mantle Cell Non-Hodgkin's Lymphoma," *J Clin Oncol*, 2008, 26(27):4473-9.

BEP (Ovarian Cancer)

Use Ovarian cancer

Regimen

Bleomycin: I.V.: 20 units/m^2 (maximum dose: 30 units) day 1
[total dose/cycle = 20 units/m^2]

Etoposide: I.V.: 75 mg/m^2/day days 1 to 5
[total dose/cycle = 375 mg/m^2]
or I.V.: 75 mg/m^2/day days 1 to 4 (if received prior radiation therapy)
[total dose/cycle = 300 mg/m^2]

Cisplatin: I.V.: 20 mg/m^2/day days 1 to 5
[total dose/cycle = 100 mg/m^2]

Repeat cycle every 3 weeks for 4 cycles

References

Homesley HD, Bundy BN, Hurteau JA, et al, "Bleomycin, Etoposide, and Cisplatin Combination Therapy of Ovarian Granulosa Cell Tumors and Other Stromal Malignancies: A Gynecologic Oncology Group Study," *Gynecol Oncol*, 1999, 72(2):131-7.

BEP (Ovarian Cancer, Testicular Cancer)

Use Ovarian cancer; Testicular cancer

Regimen

Bleomycin: I.V.: 30 units/day days 2, 9, and 16
[total dose/cycle = 90 units]

Etoposide: I.V.: 100 mg/m^2/day days 1 to 5
[total dose/cycle = 500 mg/m^2]
or I.V.: 120 mg/m^2/day days 1, 2, and 3
[total dose/cycle = 360 mg/m^2]

Cisplatin: I.V.: 20 mg/m^2/day days 1 to 5
[total dose/cycle = 100 mg/m^2]

Repeat cycle every 21 days

References

Horwich A, Sleijfer DT, Fossa SD, et al, "Randomized Trial of Bleomycin, Etoposide, and Cisplatin Compared With Bleomycin, Etoposide, and Carboplatin in Good-Prognosis Metastatic Non-seminomatous Germ Cell Cancer: A Multiinstitutional Medical Research Council/European Organization for Research and Treatment of Cancer Trial," *J Clin Oncol*, 1997, 15(5):1844-52.

Nichols CR, Catalano PJ, Crawford ED, et al, "Randomized Comparison of Cisplatin and Etoposide and Either Bleomycin or Ifosfamide in Treatment of Advanced Disseminated Germ Cell Tumors: An Eastern Cooperative Oncology Group, Southwest Oncology Group, and Cancer and Leukemia Group B Study," *J Clin Oncol*, 1998, 16(4):1287-93.

Williams S, Blessing JA, Liao SY, et al, "Adjuvant Therapy of Ovarian Germ Cell Tumors With Cisplatin, Etoposide, and Bleomycin: A Trial of the Gynecologic Oncology Group," *J Clin Oncol*, 1994, 12(4):701-6.

BEP (Testicular Cancer)

Index Terms Bleomycin–Etoposide–Cisplatin (Testicular Cancer)

Use Testicular cancer

Regimen NOTE: Multiple variations are listed.

Variation 1:

Bleomycin: I.V.: 30 units/day days 1, 8, and 15
[total dose/cycle = 90 units]

Etoposide: I.V.: 100 mg/m^2/day days 1 to 5
  [total dose/cycle = 500 mg/m^2]
Cisplatin: I.V.: 20 mg/m^2/day days 1 to 5
  [total dose/cycle = 100 mg/m^2]
Repeat cycle every 21 days for 3-4 cycles
Variation 2:
Bleomycin: I.V.: 30 units/day days 2, 9, and 16
  [total dose/cycle = 90 units]
Etoposide: I.V.: 100 mg/m^2/day days 1 to 5
  [total dose/cycle = 500 mg/m^2]
Cisplatin: I.V.: 20 mg/m^2/day days 1 to 5
  [total dose/cycle = 100 mg/m^2]
Repeat cycle every 21 days
Variation 3:
Bleomycin: I.V.: 30 units once weekly
  [total dose/cycle = 90 units]
Etoposide: I.V.: 120 mg/m^2/day days 1, 3, and 5
  [total dose/cycle = 360 mg/m^2]
Cisplatin: I.V.: 20 mg/m^2/day days 1 to 5
  [total dose/cycle = 100 mg/m^2]
Repeat cycle every 21 days
Variation 4:
Bleomycin: I.V.: 30 units/day days 1, 8, and 15
  [total dose/cycle = 90 units]
Etoposide: I.V.: 165 mg/m^2/day days 1, 2, and 3
  [total dose/cycle = 495 mg/m^2]
Cisplatin: I.V.: 50 mg/m^2/day days 1 and 2
  [total dose/cycle = 100 mg/m^2]
Repeat cycle every 21 days

References

Variation 1:
Saxman SB, Finch D, Gonin R, et al, "Long-Term Follow-Up of a Phase III Study of Three Versus Four Cycles of Bleomycin, Etoposide, and Cisplatin in Favorable-Prognosis Germ-Cell Tumors: The Indian University Experience," *J Clin Oncol*, 1998, 16(2):702-6.
Variation 2:
Williams SD, Birch R, Einhorn LH, et al, "Treatment of Disseminated Germ-Cell Tumors With Cisplatin, Bleomycin, and Either Vinblastine or Etoposide," *N Engl J Med*, 1987, 316 (23):1435-40.
Variation 3:
de Wit R, Stoter G, Sleijfer DT, et al, "Four Cycles of BEP Vs Four Cycles of VIP in Patients With Intermediate-Prognosis Metastatic Testicular Nonseminoma: A Randomized Study of the EORTC Genitourinary Tract Cancer Cooperative Group. European Organization for Research and Treatment of Cancer," *Br J Cancer*, 1998, 78(6):828-32.
Variation 4:
de Wit R, Roberts JT, Wilkinson PM, et al, "Equivalence of Three or Four Cycles of Bleomycin, Etoposide, and Cisplatin Chemotherapy and of a 3- or 5-Day Schedule in Good-Prognosis Germ Cell Cancer: A Randomized Study of the European Organization for Research and Treatment of Cancer Genitourinary Tract Cancer Cooperative Group and the Medical Research Council," *J Clin Oncol*, 2001, 19(6):1629-40.

Bevacizumab-Capecitabine
Index Terms Capecitabine-Bevacizumab
Use Breast cancer
Regimen
Capecitabine: Oral: 1250 mg/m^2 twice daily days 1 to 14
  [total dose/cycle = 35,000 mg/m^2]

Bevacizumab: I.V.: 15 mg/kg day 1
[total dose/cycle = 15 mg/kg]
Repeat cycle every 21 days for up to 35 cycles

References
Miller KD, Chap LI, Holmes FA, et al, "Randomized Phase III Trial of Capecitabine Compared With Bevacizumab Plus Capecitabine in Patients With Previously Treated Metastatic Breast Cancer," *J Clin Oncol*, 2005, 23(4):792-9.

Bevacizumab-Cisplatin-Gemcitabine (NSCLC)

Index Terms Cisplatin-Gemcitabine-Bevacizumab (NSCLC)

Use Lung cancer, nonsmall cell

Regimen
Bevacizumab: I.V.: 7.5 or 15 mg/kg/dose day 1
[total dose/cycle = 7.5 or 15 mg/kg]
Cisplatin: I.V.: 80 mg/m^2/dose day 1
[total dose/cycle = 80 mg/m^2]
Gemcitabine: I.V.: 1250 mg/m^2/dose days 1 and 8
[total dose/cycle = 2500 mg/m^2]
Repeat cycle every 21 days for up to 6 cycles (bevacizumab monotherapy may be continued thereafter until disease progression)

References
Manegold C, von Pawel J, Zatloukal P, et al, "Randomised, Double-Blind Multicentre Phase III Study of Bevacizumab in Combination With Cisplatin and Gemcitabine in Chemotherapy-Naïve Patients With Advanced or Recurrent Non-Squamous Non-Small Cell Lung Cancer (NSCLC): BO17704," *J Clin Oncol*, 2007, 25(18S) [abstract LBA7514 from 2007 ASCO Annual Meeting].

◆ **Bevacizumab-Docetaxel** see Docetaxel-Bevacizumab on page 1289

Bevacizumab-Fluorouracil-Leucovorin

Index Terms Fluorouracil-Leucovorin-Bevacizumab

Use Colorectal cancer

Regimen
Bevacizumab: I.V.: 5 mg/kg/day days 1, 15, 29, and 43
[total dose/cycle = 20 mg/kg]
Leucovorin: I.V.: 500 mg/m^2/day days 1, 8, 15, 22, 29, and 36
[total dose/cycle = 3000 mg/m^2]
Fluorouracil: I.V.: 500 mg/m^2/day days 1, 8, 15, 22, 29, and 36
[total dose/cycle = 3000 mg/m^2]
Repeat cycle every 56 days

References
Kabbinavar FF, Schulz J, McCleod M, et al, "Addition of Bevacizumab to Bolus Fluorouracil and Leucovorin in First-Line Metastatic Colorectal Cancer: Results of a Randomized Phase II Trial," *J Clin Oncol*, 2005, 23(16):3697-705.

Bevacizumab-Interferon Alfa (RCC)

Index Terms Interferon Alfa-Bevacizumab (RCC)

Use Renal cell cancer

Regimen NOTE: Multiple variations are listed.
Variation 1:
Interferon Alfa-2a: SubQ: 9 million units 3 times/week
[total dose/cycle = 54 million units]
Bevacizumab: I.V.: 10 mg/kg day 1
[total dose/cycle = 10 mg/kg]
Repeat cycle every 14 days for up to 1 year or until disease progression

Variation 2:
Interferon Alfa-2b: SubQ: 9 million units 3 times/week
[total dose/cycle = 108 million units]
Bevacizumab: I.V.: 10 mg/kg day 1 and 15
[total dose/cycle = 20 mg/kg]
Repeat cycle every 28 days until disease progression or unacceptable toxicity

References

Variation 1:

Escudier B, Koralewski P, Pluzanska A, et al, "A Randomized, Controlled, Double-Blind Phase III Study (AVOREN) of Bevacizumab/Interferon-α2a vs Placebo/Interferon-α2a as First-Line Therapy in Metastatic Renal Cell Carcinoma," *J Clin Oncol*, 2007, 25(18S):3 [abstract from 2007 ASCO Annual Meeting Proceedings, Part I].

Escudier B, Pluzanska A, Koralewski P, et al, "Bevacizumab Plus Interferon Alfa-2a for Treatment of Metastatic Renal Cell Carcinoma: A Randomised, Double-Blind Phase III Trial," *Lancet*, 2007, 370(9605):2103-11.

Variation 2:

Rini BI, Halabi S, Rosenberg JE, et al, "Bevacizumab Plus Interferon Alfa Compared With Interferon Alfa Monotherapy in Patients With Metastatic Renal Cell Carcinoma: CALGB 90206," *J Clin Oncol*, 2008, 26(33):5422-8.

Bevacizumab-Irinotecan-Fluorouracil-Leucovorin

Index Terms Irinotecan-Fluorouracil-Leucovorin-Bevacizumab

Use Colorectal cancer

Regimen

Bevacizumab: I.V.: 5 mg/kg/day days 1, 15, and 29
[total dose/cycle = 15 mg/kg]
Irinotecan: I.V.: 125 mg/m^2/day days 1, 8, 15, and 22
[total dose/cycle = 500 mg/m^2]
Fluorouracil: I.V.: 500 mg/m^2/day days 1, 8, 15, and 22
[total dose/cycle = 2000 mg/m^2]
Leucovorin: I.V.: 20 mg/m^2/day days 1, 8, 15, and 22
[total dose/cycle = 80 mg/m^2]
Repeat cycle every 42 days

References

Hurwitz H, Fehrenbacher L, Novotny W, et al, "Bevacizumab Plus Irinotecan, Fluorouracil, and Leucovorin for Metastatic Colorectal Cancer," *N Engl J Med*, 2004, 350(23):2335-42.

Bevacizumab-Irinotecan (Glioblastoma)

Index Terms Irinotecan-Bevacizumab (Glioblastoma)

Use Brain tumors

Regimen Note: Patients receiving concurrent antiepileptic enzyme-inducing drugs received an increased dose of irinotecan (340 mg/m^2/dose).
Bevacizumab: I.V.: 10 mg/kg day 1
[total dose/cycle = 10 mg/kg]
Irinotecan: I.V.: 125 mg/m^2 day 1
[total dose/cycle = 125 mg/m^2]
Repeat cycle every 14 days

References

Vredenburgh JJ, Desjardins A, Herndon JE 2nd, et al, "Bevacizumab Plus Irinotecan in Recurrent Glioblastoma Multiforme," *J Clin Oncol*, 2007, 25(30):4722-9.

Bevacizumab-Oxaliplatin-Fluorouracil-Leucovorin

Index Terms Bevacizumab-Oxaliplatin-Leucovorin-Fluorouracil; Oxaliplatin-Fluorouracil-Leucovorin-Bevacizumab

Use Colorectal cancer

Regimen

Bevacizumab: I.V.: 10 mg/kg day 1
[total dose/cycle = 10 mg/kg]
Oxaliplatin: I.V.: 85 mg/m^2 day 1
[total dose/cycle = 85 mg/m^2]
Leucovorin: I.V.: 200 mg/m^2/day days 1 and 2
[total dose/cycle = 400 mg/m^2]
Fluorouracil: I.V. bolus: 400 mg/m^2/day days 1 and 2
followed by I.V.: 600 mg/m^2 continuous infusion over 22 hours days 1 and 2
[total dose/cycle = 2000 mg/m^2]
Repeat cycle every 14 days

References

Giantonio BJ, Catalano PJ, Meropol NJ, et al, "Bevacizumab in Combination With Oxaliplatin, Fluorouracil, and Leucovorin (FOLFOX4) for Previously Treated Metastatic Colorectal Cancer: Results From the Eastern Cooperative Oncology Group Study E3200," *J Clin Oncol*, 2007, 25 (12):1539-44.

- ◆ **Bevacizumab-Oxaliplatin-Leucovorin-Fluorouracil** *see* Bevacizumab-Oxaliplatin-Fluorouracil-Leucovorin *on page 1233*

- ◆ **Bevacizumab-Paclitaxel** *see* Paclitaxel-Bevacizumab *on page 1385*

- ◆ **Bevacizumab-Paclitaxel-Carboplatin** *see* Paclitaxel-Carboplatin-Bevacizumab *on page 1385*

Bicalutamide-Goserelin

Index Terms Goserelin-Bicalutamide

Use Prostate cancer

Regimen

Bicalutamide: Oral: 50 mg/day
[total dose/cycle = 1400 mg]
Goserelin acetate: SubQ: 3.6 mg day 1
[total dose/cycle = 3.6 mg]
Repeat cycle every 28 days

References

Schellhammer PF, Scharifi R, Block NL, et al, "A Controlled Trial of Bicalutamide Versus Flutamide, Each in Combination With Luteinizing Hormone-Releasing Hormone Analogue Therapy, in Patients With Advanced Prostate Cancer. Casodex Combination Study Group," *Urology*, 1995, 45(5):745-52.

Schellhammer PF, Sharifi R, Block NL, et al, "Clinical Benefits of Bicalutamide Compared With Flutamide in Combined Androgen Blockade for Patients With Advanced Prostatic Carcinoma: Final Report of a Double-Blind, Randomized, Multicenter Trial. Casodex Combination Study Group," *Urology*, 1997, 50(3):330-6.

Bicalutamide-Leuprolide

Index Terms Leuprolide-Bicalutamide

Use Prostate cancer

Regimen

Bicalutamide: Oral: 50 mg/day
[total dose/cycle = 1400 mg]
Leuprolide depot: I.M.: 7.5 mg day 1
[total dose/cycle = 7.5 mg]
Repeat cycle every 28 days

References

Schellhammer PF, Scharifi R, Block NL, et al, "A Controlled Trial of Bicalutamide Versus Flutamide, Each in Combination With Luteinizing Hormone-Releasing Hormone Analogue Therapy, in Patients With Advanced Prostate Cancer. Casodex Combination Study Group," *Urology*, 1995, 45(5):745-52.

Schellhammer PF, Sharifi R, Block NL, et al, "Clinical Benefits of Bicalutamide Compared With Flutamide in Combined Androgen Blockade for Patients With Advanced Prostatic Carcinoma: Final Report of a Double-Blind, Randomized, Multicenter Trial. Casodex Combination Study Group," *Urology*, 1997, 50(3):330-6.

BIP

Use Cervical cancer

Regimen

Bleomycin: I.V.: 30 units continuous infusion day 1
[total dose/cycle = 30 units]

Cisplatin: I.V.: 50 mg/m^2 day 2
[total dose/cycle = 50 mg/m^2]

Ifosfamide: I.V.: 5 g/m^2 continuous infusion day 2
[total dose/cycle = 5 g/m^2]

Mesna: I.V.: 6 g/m^2 continuous infusion over 36 hours day 2 (start with ifosfamide)
[total dose/cycle = 6 g/m^2]

Repeat cycle every 21 days

References

Buxton EJ, Meanwell CA, Hilton C, et al, "Combination Bleomycin, Ifosfamide, and Cisplatin Chemotherapy in Cervical Cancer," *J Natl Cancer Inst*, 1989, 81(5):359-61.

♦ **Bleomycin–Etoposide–Cisplatin (Testicular Cancer)** *see* BEP (Testicular Cancer) *on page 1230*

BOLD

Use Melanoma

Regimen

Dacarbazine: I.V.: 200 mg/m^2/day days 1 to 5
[total dose/cycle = 1000 mg/m^2]

Vincristine: I.V.: 1 mg/m^2/day days 1 and 4
[total dose/cycle = 2 mg/m^2]

Bleomycin: I.V.: 15 units/day days 2 and 5
[total dose/cycle = 30 units]

Lomustine: Oral: 80 mg day 1
[total dose/cycle = 80 mg]

Repeat cycle every 4 weeks

References

Nathan FE, Berd D, Sato T, et al, "BOLD + Interferon in the Treatment of Metastatic Uveal Melanoma: First Report of Active Systemic Therapy," *J Exp Clin Cancer Res*, 1997, 16(2):201-8.

Punt CJ, van Herpen CM, Janasen RL, et al, "Chemoimmunotherapy With Bleomycin, Vincristine, Lomustine, Dacarbazine (BOLD) Plus Interferon Alpha for Metastatic Melanoma: A Multicentre Phase II Study," *Br J Cancer*, 1997, 76(2):266-9.

BOLD + Interferon

Use Melanoma

Regimen NOTE: Multiple variations are listed.

Variation 1:

Bleomycin: I.V.: 15 units/day days 2 and 5
[total dose/cycle = 30 units]

Vincristine: I.V.: 1 mg/m^2/day days 1 and 4
[total dose/cycle = 2 mg/m^2]

Lomustine: Oral: 80 mg day 1
[total dose/cycle = 80 mg]

Dacarbazine: I.V.: 200 mg/m^2/day days 1 to 5
[total dose/cycle = 1000 mg/m^2]

◀

Interferon Alfa-2b: SubQ: 3 million units/day days 8 to 49 (cycles 1 and 2)
[total dose through day 49 = 126 million units]
followed by SubQ: 6 million units 3 times/week (beginning day 50 and subsequent cycles)
[total dose/cycle = 72 million units]
Repeat cycle every 4 weeks

Variation 2:
Bleomycin: I.V.: 30 units day 1
[total dose/cycle = 30 units]
Vincristine: I.V.: 2 mg day 1
[total dose/cycle = 2 mg]
Lomustine: Oral: 80 mg day 1
[total dose/cycle = 80 mg]
Dacarbazine: I.V.: 700 mg/m^2 day 1
[total dose/cycle = 700 mg/m^2]
Interferon Alfa-2b: SubQ: 3 million units 3 times/week
[total dose/cycle = 36 million units]
Repeat cycle every 4 weeks

Variation 3:
Bleomycin: I.V.: 15 units/day days 2 and 5
[total dose/cycle = 30 units]
Vincristine: I.V.: 1-2 mg/day days 1 and 4
[total dose/cycle = 2-4 mg]
Lomustine: Oral: 80 mg day 1
[total dose/cycle = 80 mg]
Dacarbazine: I.V.: 200 mg/m^2/day days 1 to 5
[total dose/cycle = 1000 mg/m^2]
Interferon Alfa-2b: SubQ: 6 million units 3 times/week, for 6 doses, starting day 8
[total dose/cycle = 36 million units]
Repeat cycle every 4 weeks

Variation 4:
Bleomycin: I.V.: 15 units/day days 2 and 5
[total dose/cycle = 30 units]
Vincristine: I.V.: 1 mg/m^2/day (maximum dose: 2 mg) days 1 and 4
[total dose/cycle = 2 mg/m^2]
Lomustine: Oral: 80 mg day 1
[total dose/cycle = 80 mg]
Dacarbazine: I.V.: 200 mg/m^2/day days 1 to 5
[total dose/cycle = 1000 mg/m^2]
Interferon Alfa-2b: SubQ: 3 million units/day days 8, 10, 12, 15, 17, and 19
[total dose/cycle = 18 million units]
Repeat cycle every 4 weeks

References

Variation 1:
Pyrhonen S, Hahka-Kemppinen M, and Muhonen T, "A Promising Interferon Plus Four-Drug Chemotherapy Regimen for Metastatic Melanoma," *J Clin Oncol*, 1992, 10(12):1919-26.
Variation 2:
Vuoristo MS, Grohn P, Kumpulainen E, et al, "Treatment of Patients With Metastatic Melanoma With a One Day Regimen of Dacarbazine, Vincristine, Bleomycin, and Lomustine Plus Interferon Alfa," *Eur J Cancer*, 1994, 30A(3):420.
Variation 3:
Vuoristo M, Grohn P, Kellokumpu-Lehtinen P, et al, "Intermittent Interferon and Polychemotherapy in Metastatic Melanoma," *J Cancer Res Clin Oncol*, 1995, 121(3):175-80.
Variation 4:
Nathan FE, Berd D, Sato T, et al, "BOLD + Interferon in the Treatment of Metastatic Uveal Melanoma: First Report of Active Systemic Therapy," *J Exp Clin Cancer Res*, 1997, 16(2):201-8.

BOLD (Melanoma)

Use Melanoma

Regimen NOTE: Multiple variations are listed.

Variation 1:

Bleomycin: SubQ: 7.5 units/day days 1 and 4 (cycle 1 only)
   followed by SubQ: 15 units/day days 1 and 4 (subsequent cycles)
   [total dose/cycle = 45 units; maximum total dose (all cycles): 400 units]
Vincristine: I.V.: 1 mg/m^2/day days 1 and 5
   [total dose/cycle = 2 mg/m^2]
Lomustine: Oral: 80 mg/m^2 (maximum dose: 150 mg) day 1
   [total dose/cycle = 80 mg/m^2]
Dacarbazine: I.V.: 200 mg/m^2/day (maximum dose: 400 mg) days 1 to 5
   [total dose/cycle = 1000 mg/m^2; maximum: 2000 mg]
Repeat cycle every 4-6 weeks

Variation 2:

Bleomycin: I.V.: 15 units/day days 1 and 4
   [total dose/cycle = 30 units]
Vincristine: I.V.: 1 mg/m^2/day days 1 and 5
   [total dose/cycle = 2 mg/m^2]
Lomustine: Oral: 80 mg/m^2 (maximum dose: 150 mg) day 1
   [total dose/cycle = 80 mg/m^2]
Dacarbazine: I.V.: 200 mg/m^2/day days 1 to 5
   [total dose/cycle = 1000 mg/m^2]
Repeat cycle every 4 weeks

Variation 3:

Bleomycin: I.V.: 15 units/day days 1 and 4
   [total dose/cycle = 30 units]
Vincristine: I.V.: 1 mg/m^2 day 1
   [total dose/cycle = 1 mg/m^2]
Lomustine: Oral: 80 mg/m^2 day 3 (odd numbered cycles)
   [total dose/cycle = 80 mg/m^2; every other cycle]
Dacarbazine: I.V.: 200 mg/m^2/day days 1 to 5
   [total dose/cycle = 1000 mg/m^2]
Repeat cycle every 4 weeks

References

Variation 1:
Seigler HF, Lucas VS, Pickett NJ, et al, "DTIC, CCNU, Bleomycin and Vincristine (BOLD) in Metastatic Melanoma," *Cancer*, 1980, 46(11):2346-8.
Variation 2:
York RM and Foltz AT, "Bleomycin, Vincristine, Lomustine, and DTIC Chemotherapy for Metastatic Melanoma," *Cancer*, 1988, 61(11):2183-6.
Variation 3:
Lakhani S, Selby P, Bliss JM, et al, "Chemotherapy for Malignant Melanoma: Combinations and High Doses Produce More Responses Without Survival Benefit," *Br J Cancer*, 1990, 61(2):330-4.

Bortezomib-Dexamethasone

Index Terms Dexamethasone-Bortezomib

Use Multiple myeloma

Regimen NOTE: Multiple variations are listed.

Variation 1:

Cycles 1 and 2:

Bortezomib: I.V.: 1.3 mg/m^2/day days 1, 4, 8, and 11
   [total dose/cycle = 5.2 mg/m^2]

Dexamethasone: Oral: 40 mg/day days 1 to 4 and days 9 to 12
  [total dose/cycle = 320 mg]
Treatment cycle is 21 days
Cycles 3 and 4:
  Bortezomib: I.V.: 1.3 mg/m^2/day days 1, 4, 8, and 11
    [total dose/cycle = 5.2 mg/m^2]
  Dexamethasone: Oral: 40 mg/day days 1 to 4
    [total dose/cycle = 160 mg]
  Treatment cycle is 21 days
Variation 2:
Cycles 1 and 2:
  Bortezomib: I.V.: 1.3 mg/m^2/day days 1, 4, 8, and 11
    [total dose/cycle = 5.2 mg/m^2]
  Treatment cycle is 21 days
Cycles 3 through 6 (begin dexamethasone after cycle 2 if partial response not achieved or after cycle 4 if complete response not achieved):
  Bortezomib: I.V.: 1.3 mg/m^2/day days 1, 4, 8, and 11
    [total dose/cycle = 5.2 mg/m^2]
  Dexamethasone: Oral: 40 mg/day days 1 and 2
    [total dose/cycle = 80 mg]
  Treatment cycle is 21 days (for up to a total of 6 cycles)

References

Variation 1:
Harousseau JL, Attal M, Leleu X, et al, "Bortezomib Plus Dexamethasone as Induction Treatment Prior to Autologous Stem Cell Transplantation in Patients With Newly Diagnosed Multiple Myeloma: Results of an IFM Phase II Study," *Haematologica*, 2006, 91(11):1498-505.

Harousseau JL, Mathiot C, Attal M, et al, "VELCADE/Dexamethasone (Vel/D) Versus VAD as Induction Treatment Prior to Autologous Stem Cell Transplantation (ASCT) in Newly Diagnosed Multiple Myeloma (MM): Updated Results of the IFM 2005/01 Trial," *Blood*, 2007, 110(11): 450, ASH 2007 Annual Meeting Abstract 450.

Variation 2:
Jagannath S, Durie BG, Wolf J, et al, "Bortezomib Therapy Alone and in Combination With Dexamethasone for Previously Untreated Symptomatic Multiple Myeloma," *Br J Haematol*, 2005, 129(6):776-83.

Bortezomib-Doxorubicin-Dexamethasone

Index Terms Dexamethasone-Bortezomib-Doxorubicin; Doxorubicin-Dexamethasone-Bortezomib; PAD

Use Multiple myeloma

Regimen NOTE: Multiple variations are listed.

Variation 1:
Cycle 1:
  Bortezomib: I.V.: 1.3 mg/m^2/day days 1, 4, 8, and 11
    [total dose/cycle = 5.2 mg/m^2]
  Dexamethasone: Oral: 40 mg/day days 1 to 4, 8 to 11, and 15 to 18
    [total dose/cycle = 480 mg]
  Doxorubicin: I.V.: 4.5 or 9 mg/m^2/day days 1 to 4
    [total dose/cycle = 18 or 36 mg/m^2]
  Treatment cycle is 21 days
Cycles 2-4:
  Bortezomib: I.V.: 1.3 mg/m^2/day days 1, 4, 8, and 11
    [total dose/cycle = 5.2 mg/m^2]
  Dexamethasone: Oral: 40 mg/day days 1 to 4
    [total dose/cycle = 160 mg]

Doxorubicin: I.V.: 4.5 or 9 mg/m^2/day days 1 to 4
[total dose/cycle = 18 or 36 mg/m^2]
Treatment cycle is 21 days
Variation 2:
Cycle 1:
Bortezomib: I.V.: 1 mg/m^2/day days 1, 4, 8, and 11
[total dose/cycle = 4 mg/m^2]
Dexamethasone: Oral: 40 mg/day days 1 to 4, 8 to 11, and 15 to 18
[total dose/cycle = 480 mg]
Doxorubicin: I.V.: 9 mg/m^2/day days 1 to 4
[total dose/cycle = 36 mg/m^2]
Treatment cycle is 21 days
Cycles 2-4:
Bortezomib: I.V.: 1 mg/m^2/day days 1, 4, 8, and 11
[total dose/cycle = 4 mg/m^2]
Dexamethasone: Oral: 40 mg/day days 1 to 4
[total dose/cycle = 160 mg]
Doxorubicin: I.V.: 9 mg/m^2/day days 1 to 4
[total dose/cycle = 36 mg/m^2]
Treatment cycle is 21 days
Variation 3:
Bortezomib: I.V.: 1.3 mg/m^2/day days 1, 4, 8, and 11
[total dose/cycle = 5.2 mg/m^2]
Dexamethasone: Oral: 40 mg/day days 1 to 4
[total dose/cycle = 160 mg]
Doxorubicin: I.V.: 20 mg/m^2/day days 1 and 4
[total dose/cycle = 40 mg/m^2]
Repeat cycle every 28 days for up to 6 cycles

References

Variation 1:

Oakervee HE, Popat R, Curry N, et al, "PAD Combination Therapy (PS-341/Bortezomib, Doxorubicin and Dexamethasone) for Previously Untreated Patients With Multiple Myeloma," Br J Haematol, 2005, 129(6):755-62.

Popat R, Oakervee HE, Hallam S, et al, "Bortezomib, Doxorubicin and Dexamethasone (PAD) Front-Line Treatment of Multiple Myeloma: Updated Results After Long-Term Follow-Up," Br J Haematol, 2008, 41(4):512-6.

Variation 2:

Popat R, Oakervee HE, Hallam S, et al, "Bortezomib, Doxorubicin and Dexamethasone (PAD) Front-Line Treatment of Multiple Myeloma: Updated Results After Long-Term Follow-Up," Br J Haematol, 2008, 41(4):512-6.

Variation 3:

Palumbo A, Gay F, Bringhen S, et al, "Bortezomib, Doxorubicin and Dexamethasone in Advanced Multiple Myeloma," Ann Oncol, 2008, 19(6):1160-5.

Bortezomib-Doxorubicin (Liposomal)

Index Terms Doxorubicin (Liposomal)-Bortezomib

Use Multiple myeloma

Regimen

Bortezomib: I.V.: 1.3 mg/m^2/day days 1, 4, 8, and 11
[total dose/cycle = 5.2 mg/m^2]
Doxorubicin (liposomal): I.V.: 30 mg/m^2 day 4
[total dose/cycle = 30 mg/m^2]
Repeat cycle every 21 days for up to 8 cycles

References

Biehn SE, Moore DT, Voorhees PM, et al, "Extended Follow-Up of Outcome Measures in Multiple Myeloma Patients Treated on a Phase I Study With Bortezomib and Pegylated Liposomal Doxorubicin," Ann Hematol, 2007, 86(3):211-6.

Orlowski RZ, Nagler A, Sonneveld P, et al, "Randomized Phase III Study of Pegylated Liposomal Doxorubicin Plus Bortezomib Compared With Bortezomib Alone in Relapsed or Refractory Multiple Myeloma: Combination Therapy Improves Time to Progression," *J Clin Oncol*, 2007, 25 (25):3892-901.

Orlowski RZ, Voorhees PM, Garcia RA, et al, "Phase 1 Trial of the Proteasome Inhibitor Bortezomib and Pegylated Liposomal Doxorubicin in Patients With Advanced Hematologic Malignancies," *Blood*, 2005, 105(8):3058-65.

Bortezomib-Doxorubicin (Liposomal)-Dexamethasone

Index Terms Dexamethasone-Bortezomib-Doxorubicin (Liposomal); Doxorubicin (Liposomal)-Dexamethasone-Bortezomib

Use Multiple myeloma

Regimen
Bortezomib: I.V.: 1.3 mg/m^2/day days 1, 4, 8, and 11
  [total dose/cycle = 5.2 mg/m^2]
Doxorubicin (Liposomal): I.V.: 30 mg/m^2 day 1
  [total dose/cycle = 30 mg/m^2]
Dexamethasone: Oral: 40 mg/day days 1 to 4
  [total dose/cycle = 160 mg]
Repeat cycle every 28 days for up to 6 cycles

References
Palumbo A, Gay F, Bringhen S, et al, "Bortezomib, Doxorubicin and Dexamethasone in Advanced Multiple Myeloma," *Ann Oncol*, 2008, 19(6):1160-5.

Bortezomib-Melphalan-Prednisone

Index Terms Melphalan-Prednisone-Bortezomib; VMP

Use Multiple myeloma

Regimen NOTE: Multiple variations are listed.
Variation 1:
  Bortezomib: I.V.: 1.3 mg/m^2/day days 1, 4, 8, 11, 22, 25, 29, and 32
    [total dose/cycle = 10.4 mg/m^2]
  Melphalan: Oral: 9 mg/m^2/day days 1 to 4
    [total dose/cycle = 36 mg/m^2]
  Prednisone: Oral: 60 mg/m^2/day days 1 to 4
    [total dose/cycle = 240 mg/m^2]
  Repeat cycle every 42 days for 4 cycles
  followed by
  Bortezomib: I.V.: 1.3 mg/m^2/day days 1, 8, 22, and 29
    [total dose/cycle = 5.2 mg/m^2]
  Melphalan: Oral: 9 mg/m^2/day days 1 to 4
    [total dose/cycle = 36 mg/m^2]
  Prednisone: Oral: 60 mg/m^2/day days 1 to 4
    [total dose/cycle = 240 mg/m^2]
  Repeat cycle every 42 days for 5 cycles
Variation 2:
  Bortezomib: I.V.: 1-1.3 mg/m^2/day days 1, 4, 8, 11, 22, 25, 29, and 32
    [total dose/cycle = 8-10.4 mg/m^2]
  Melphalan: Oral: 9 mg/m^2/day days 1 to 4
    [total dose/cycle = 36 mg/m^2]
  Prednisone: Oral: 60 mg/m^2/day days 1 to 4
    [total dose/cycle = 240 mg/m^2]
  Repeat cycle every 42 days for 4 cycles
  followed by
  Bortezomib: I.V.: 1-1.3 mg/m^2/day days 1, 8, 15, and 22
    [total dose/cycle = 4-5.2 mg/m^2]

Melphalan: Oral: 9 mg/m^2/day days 1 to 4
[total dose/cycle = 36 mg/m^2]
Prednisone: Oral: 60 mg/m^2/day days 1 to 4
[total dose/cycle = 240 mg/m^2]
Repeat cycle every 35 days for 5 cycles

References

Variation 1:

San Miguel JF, Schlag R, Khuageva NK, et al, "Bortezomib Plus Melphalan and Prednisone for Initial Treatment of Multiple Myeloma," *N Engl J Med*, 2008, 359(9):906-17.

Variation 2:

Mateos MV, Hernández JM, Hernández MT, et al, "Bortezomib Plus Melphalan and Prednisone in Elderly Untreated Patients With Multiple Myeloma: Results of a Multicenter Phase 1/2 Study," *Blood*, 2006, 108(7):2165-72.

Mateos MV, Hernández JM, Hernández MT, et al, "Bortezomib Plus Melphalan and Prednisone in Elderly Untreated Patients With Multiple Myeloma: Updated Time-to-Events Results and Prognostic Factors for Time to Progression," *Haematologica*, 2008, 93(4):560-5.

Bortezomib-Melphalan-Prednisone-Thalidomide

Index Terms Melphalan-Prednisone-Bortezomib-Thalidomide; VMPT

Use Multiple myeloma

Regimen

Bortezomib: I.V.: 1-1.3 mg/m^2/day days 1, 4, 15, and 22
[total dose/cycle = 4-5.2 mg/m^2]
Melphalan: Oral: 6 mg/m^2/day days 1 to 5
[total dose/cycle = 30 mg/m^2]
Prednisone: Oral: 60 mg/m^2/day days 1 to 5
[total dose/cycle = 300 mg/m^2]
Thalidomide: Oral: 50 mg/day days 1 to 35
[total dose/cycle = 1750 mg]
Repeat cycle every 35 days for 6 cycles

References

Palumbo A, Ambrosini MT, Benevolo G, et al, "Bortezomib, Melphalan, Prednisone, and Thalidomide for Relapsed Multiple Myeloma," *Blood*, 2007, 109(7):2767-72.

CA

Use Leukemia, acute myeloid

Regimen

Cytarabine: I.V.: 3000 mg/m^2 every 12 hours days 1 and 2 (4 doses)
[total dose/cycle = 12,000 mg/m^2]
Asparaginase: I.M.: 6000 units/m^2 at hour 42
[total dose/cycle = 6000 units/m^2]
Repeat cycle every 7 days for 2 or 3 cycles

References

Capizzi RL, Davis R, Powell B, et al, "Synergy Between High-Dose Cytarabine and Asparaginase in the Treatment of Adults With Refractory and Relapsed Acute Myelogenous Leukemia: A Cancer and Leukemia Group B Study," *J Clin Oncol*, 1988, 6(3):499-508.

CABO

Use Head and neck cancer

Regimen

Cisplatin: I.V.: 50 mg/m^2 day 4
[total dose/cycle = 50 mg/m^2]
Methotrexate: I.V.: 40 mg/m^2 days 1 and 15
[total dose/cycle = 80 mg/m^2]
Bleomycin: I.V.: 10 units/day days 1, 8, and 15
[total dose/cycle = 30 units]

◀ Vincristine: I.V.: 2 mg/day days 1, 8, and 15
[total dose/cycle = 6 mg]
Repeat cycle every 21 days

References
Clavel M, Vermorken JB, Cognetti F, et al, "Randomized Comparison of Cisplatin, Methotrexate, Bleomycin, and Vincristine (CABO) Versus Cisplatin and 5-Fluorouracil (CF) Versus Cisplatin in Recurrent or Metastatic Squamous Cell Carcinoma of the Head and Neck. A Phase III Study of the EORTC Head and Neck Cancer Cooperative Group," *Ann Oncol*, 1994, 5(6):521-6.

CAD/MOPP/ABV

Use Lymphoma, Hodgkin's disease

Regimen

CAD:
Lomustine: Oral: 100 mg/m^2 day 1
[total dose/cycle = 100 mg/m^2]
Melphalan: Oral: 6 mg/m^2/day days 1 to 4
[total dose/cycle = 24 mg/m^2]
Vindesine: I.V.: 3 mg/m^2/day days 1 and 8
[total dose/cycle = 6 mg/m^2]

MOPP:
Mechlorethamine: I.V.: 6 mg/m^2/day days 1 and 8
[total dose/cycle = 12 mg/m^2]
Vincristine: I.V.: 1.4 mg/m^2/day days 1 and 8
[total dose/cycle = 2.8 mg/m^2]
Procarbazine: Oral: 100 mg/m^2/day days 1 to 14
[total dose/cycle = 1400 mg/m^2]
Prednisone: Oral: 40 mg/m^2/day days 1 to 14
[total dose/cycle = 560 mg/m^2]

ABV:
Doxorubicin: I.V.: 25 mg/m^2/day days 1 and 14
[total dose/cycle = 50 mg/m^2]
Bleomycin: SubQ: 6 units/m^2/day days 1 and 14
[total dose/cycle = 12 units/m^2]
Vinblastine: I.V.: 2 mg/m^2 continuous infusion days 4 to 12 and 18 to 26
[total dose/cycle = 36 mg/m^2]

CAD is administered first, then MOPP begins on day 29 or day 37 following CAD. ABV is administered on day 29 following MOPP; CAD recycles on day 29 following ABV.

References
Straus DJ, Myers J, Koziner B, et al, "Combination Chemotherapy for the Treatment of Hodgkin's Disease in Relapse. Results With Lomustine (CCNU), Melphalan (Alkeran), and Vindesine (DVA) Alone (CAD) and in Alternation With MOPP and Doxorubicin (Adriamycin), Bleomycin, and Vinblastine (ABV)," *Cancer Chemother Pharmacol*, 1983, 11(2):80-5.

CAF

Use Breast cancer

Regimen NOTE: Multiple variations are listed.

Variation 1:
Cyclophosphamide: Oral: 100 mg/m^2/day days 1 to 14
[total dose/cycle = 1400 mg/m^2]
Doxorubicin: I.V.: 30 mg/m^2/day days 1 and 8
[total dose/cycle = 60 mg/m^2]
Fluorouracil: I.V.: 500 mg/m^2/day days 1 and 8
[total dose/cycle = 1000 mg/m^2]
Repeat cycle every 28 days

Variation 2:
  Cyclophosphamide: Oral: 100 mg/m^2/day days 1 to 14
    [total dose/cycle = 1400 mg/m^2]
  Doxorubicin: I.V.: 25 mg/m^2/day days 1 and 8
    [total dose/cycle = 50 mg/m^2]
  Fluorouracil: I.V.: 500 mg/m^2/day days 1 and 8
    [total dose/cycle = 1000 mg/m^2]
  Repeat cycle every 28 days

References

Variation 1:
Bull JM, Tormey DC, Li SH, et al, "A Randomized Comparative Trial of Adriamycin® Versus Methotrexate in Combination Drug Therapy," *Cancer*, 1978, 41(5):1649-57.
Variation 2:
Aisner J, Weinberg V, Perloff M, et al, "Chemotherapy Versus Chemoimmunotherapy (CAF v CAFVP v CMF each +/- MER) for Metastatic Carcinoma of the Breast," *J Clin Oncol*, 1987, 5 (10):1523-33.

◆ **CAF-IV** see FAC on page 1318

CAP

Use Bladder cancer
Regimen
  Cyclophosphamide: I.V.: 400 mg/m^2 day 1
    [total dose = 400 mg/m^2]
  Doxorubicin: I.V.: 40 mg/m^2 day 1
    [total dose = 40 mg/m^2]
  Cisplatin: I.V.: 60 mg/m^2 day 1
    [total dose = 60 mg/m^2]
  Repeat cycle every 21 days

References

Eagan RT, Frytak S, Creagan ET, et al, "Phase II Study of Cyclophosphamide, Adriamycin, and Cis-Dichlorodiammineplatinum (II) by Infusion in Patients With Adenocarcinoma and Large Cell Carcinoma of the Lung," *Cancer Treat Rep*, 1979, 63(9-10):1589-91.

◆ **Capecitabine-Bevacizumab** see Bevacizumab-Capecitabine on page 1231

Capecitabine + Docetaxel (Breast Cancer)

Use Breast cancer
Regimen NOTE: Multiple variations are listed.
  Variation 1:
  Capecitabine: Oral: 1250 mg/m^2 twice daily days 1 to 14
    [total dose/cycle = 35,000 mg/m^2]
  Docetaxel: I.V.: 75 mg/m^2 day 1
    [total dose/cycle = 75 mg/m^2]
  Repeat cycle every 3 weeks
  Variation 2:
  Capecitabine: Oral: 1000 mg/m^2 twice daily days 2 to 15
    [total dose/cycle = 28,000 mg/m^2]
  Docetaxel: I.V.: 75 mg/m^2 day 1
    [total dose/cycle = 75 mg/m^2]
  Repeat cycle every 3 weeks
  Variation 3:
  Capecitabine: Oral: 937.5 mg/m^2 twice daily days 2 to 15
    [total dose/cycle = 26,250 mg/m^2]
  Docetaxel: I.V.: 60 mg/m^2 day 1
    [total dose/cycle = 60 mg/m^2]
  Repeat cycle every 3 weeks

References
Variation 1:
O'Shaughnessy J, Miles D, Vukelja S, et al, "Superior Survival With Capecitabine Plus Docetaxel Combination Therapy in Anthracycline-Pretreated Patients With Advanced Breast Cancer: Phase III Trial Results," *J Clin Oncol*, 2002, 20(12):2812-23.

Variations 2 and 3:
Lebowitz PF, Eng-Wong J, Swain SM, et al, "A Phase II Trial of Neoadjuvant Docetaxel and Capecitabine for Locally Advanced Breast Cancer," *Clin Cancer Res*, 2004, 10(20):6764-9.

Capecitabine + Docetaxel (Gastric Cancer)

Use Gastric cancer

Regimen NOTE: Multiple variations are listed.

Variation 1:
Capecitabine: Oral: 1000 mg/m^2 twice daily days 1 to 14
[total dose/cycle = 28,000 mg/m^2]
Docetaxel: I.V.: 75 mg/m^2 day 1
[total dose/cycle = 75 mg/m^2]
Repeat cycle every 3 weeks

Variation 2:
Capecitabine: Oral: 1000 mg/m^2 twice daily days 1 to 14
[total dose/cycle = 28,000 mg/m^2]
Docetaxel: I.V.: 36 mg/m^2 days 1 and 8
[total dose/cycle = 72 mg/m^2]
Repeat cycle every 3 weeks

References
Variation 1:
Kim JG, Sohn SK, Kim DH, et al, "Phase II Study of Docetaxel and Capecitabine in Patients With Metastatic or Recurrent Gastric Cancer," *Oncology*, 2005, 68(2-3):190-5.

Variation 2:
Chun JH, Kim HK, Lee JS, et al, "Weekly Docetaxel in Combination With Capecitabine in Patients With Metastatic Gastric Cancer," *Am J Clin Oncol*, 2005, 28(2):188-94.

Capecitabine-Docetaxel (NSCLC)

Use Lung cancer, nonsmall cell

Regimen NOTE: Multiple variations are listed.

Variation 1:
Capecitabine: Oral: 1000 mg/m^2 twice daily days 1 to 14
[total dose/cycle = 28,000 mg/m^2]
Docetaxel: I.V.: 36 mg/m^2 days 1 and 8
[total dose/cycle = 72 mg/m^2]
Repeat cycle every 3 weeks

Variation 2:
Capecitabine: Oral: 625 mg/m^2 twice daily days 5 to 18
[total dose/cycle = 17,500 mg/m^2]
Docetaxel: I.V.: 36 mg/m^2 days 1, 8, and 15
[total dose/cycle = 108 mg/m^2]
Repeat cycle every 4 weeks

References
Variation 1:
Han JY, Lee DH, Kim HY, et al, "A Phase II Study of Weekly Docetaxel Plus Capecitabine for Patients With Advanced Nonsmall Cell Lung Carcinoma," *Cancer*, 2003, 98(9):1918-24.

Variation 2:
Kindwall-Keller T, Otterson GA, Young D, et al, "Phase II Evaluation of Docetaxel-Modulated Capecitabine in Previously Treated Patients With Non-Small Cell Lung Cancer," *Clin Cancer Res*, 2005, 11(5):1870-6.

◆ **Capecitabine-Ixabepilone** see Ixabepilone-Capecitabine *on page 1361*

Capecitabine + Lapatinib
Index Terms Lapatinib-Capecitabine
Use Breast cancer
Regimen
Capecitabine: Oral: 1000 mg/m^2 twice daily days 1 to 14
[total dose/cycle = 28,000 mg/m^2]
Lapatinib: Oral: 1250 mg/day days 1 to 21
[total dose/cycle = 26,250 mg]
Repeat cycle every 3 weeks
References
Geyer CE, Forster J, Lindquist D, et al, "Lapatinib Plus Capecitabine for HER2-Positive Advanced Breast Cancer," *N Engl J Med*, 2006, 355(26):2733-43.

◆ **Capecitabine-Oxaliplatin (Biliary Cancer)** *see* CAPOX (Biliary Cancer) *on page 1246*

◆ **Capecitabine-Oxaliplatin (Colorectal Cancer)** *see* CAPOX (Colorectal Cancer) *on page 1246*

◆ **Capecitabine-Oxaliplatin-Epirubicin** *see* Epirubicin-Oxaliplatin-Capecitabine *on page 1306*

◆ **Capecitabine-Oxaliplatin (Pancreatic Cancer)** *see* CAPOX (Pancreatic Cancer) *on page 1247*

Capecitabine-Trastuzumab
Index Terms Trastuzumab-Capecitabine
Use Breast cancer
Regimen NOTE: Multiple variations are listed.
Variation 1:
Cycle 1:
Capecitabine: Oral: 1250 mg/m^2 twice daily days 1 to 14
[total dose/cycle 1 = 35,000 mg/m^2]
Trastuzumab: I.V.: 4 mg/kg (loading dose) day 1 cycle 1
followed by I.V.: 2 mg/kg/day days 8 and 15 cycle 1
[total dose/cycle 1 = 8 mg/kg]
Treatment cycle is 21 days
Subsequent cycles:
Capecitabine: Oral: 1250 mg/m^2 twice daily days 1 to 14
[total dose/cycle = 35,000 mg/m^2]
Trastuzumab: I.V.: 2 mg/kg/day days 1, 8, and 15
[total dose/cycle = 6 mg/kg]
Repeat cycle every 21 days
Variation 2:
Cycle 1:
Capecitabine: Oral: 1250 mg/m^2 twice daily days 1 to 14
[total dose/cycle 1 = 35,000 mg/m^2]
Trastuzumab: I.V.: 8 mg/kg (loading dose) day 1 cycle 1
[total dose/cycle 1 = 8 mg/kg]
Treatment cycle is 21 days
Subsequent cycles:
Capecitabine: Oral: 1250 mg/m^2 twice daily days 1 to 14
[total dose/cycle = 35,000 mg/m^2]
Trastuzumab: I.V.: 6 mg/kg day 1
[total dose/cycle = 6 mg/kg]
Repeat cycle every 21 days

References

Variation 1:
Schaller G, Fuchs I, Gonsch T, et al, "Phase II Study of Capecitabine Plus Trastuzumab in Human Epidermal Growth Factor Receptor 2 Overexpressing Metastatic Breast Cancer Pretreated With Anthracyclines or Taxanes," *J Clin Oncol*, 2007, 25(22):3246-50.

Variation 2:
Bartsch R, Wenzel C, Altorjai G, et al, "Capecitabine and Trastuzumab in Heavily Pretreated Metastatic Breast Cancer," *J Clin Oncol*, 2007, 25(25):3853-8.

CAPOX (Biliary Cancer)

Index Terms Capecitabine-Oxaliplatin (Biliary Cancer); Oxaliplatin-Capecitabine (Biliary Cancer)

Use Biliary adenocarcinoma

Regimen
Capecitabine: Oral: 1000 mg/m^2/dose twice daily days 1 to 14
  [total dose/cycle = 28,000 mg/m^2]
Oxaliplatin: I.V.: 130 mg/m^2 over 2 hours day 1
  [total dose/cycle = 130 mg/m^2]
Repeat cycle every 3 weeks

References

Nehls O, Oettle H, Hartmann JT, et al, "Capecitabine Plus Oxaliplatin as First-Line Treatment in Patients With Advanced Biliary System Adenocarcinoma: A Prospective Multicentre Phase II Trial," *Br J Cancer*, 2008, 98(2):309-15.

CAPOX (Colorectal Cancer)

Index Terms Capecitabine-Oxaliplatin (Colorectal Cancer); Oxaliplatin-Capecitabine (Colorectal Cancer); Xelox (Colorectal Cancer)

Use Colorectal cancer

Regimen Note: Multiple variations are listed.
Variation 1:
  Oxaliplatin: I.V.: 130 mg/m^2 day 1
    [total dose/cycle = 130 mg/m^2]
  Capecitabine: Oral: 2500 mg/m^2/day days 1 to 14
    [total dose/cycle = 35,000 mg/m^2]
  Repeat cycle every 21 days
Variation 2:
  Oxaliplatin: I.V.: 85 mg/m^2 day 1
    [total dose/cycle = 85 mg/m^2]
  Capecitabine: Oral: 3500 mg/m^2/day days 1 to 7
    [total dose/cycle = 24,500 mg/m^2]
  Repeat cycle every 14 days
Variation 3:
  Oxaliplatin: I.V.: 50-80 mg/m^2/day days 1, 8, 22, and 29
    [total dose/cycle = 200-320 mg/m^2]
  Capecitabine: Oral: 1650 mg/m^2/day days 1 to 14 and 22 to 35
    [total dose/cycle = 46,200 mg/m^2]
Variation 4:
  Oxaliplatin: I.V.: 70 mg/m^2/day days 1 and 8
    [total dose/cycle = 140 mg/m^2]
  Capecitabine: Oral: 2000 mg/m^2/day days 1 to 14
    [total dose/cycle = 28,000 mg/m^2]
  Repeat cycle every 21 days
Variation 5:
  Oxaliplatin: I.V.: 120 mg/m^2 day 1
    [total dose/cycle = 120 mg/m^2]

Capecitabine: Oral: 2500 mg/m^2/day days 1 to 14
  [total dose/cycle = 35,000 mg/m^2]
Repeat cycle every 21 days
Variation 6:
  Oxaliplatin: I.V.: 85 mg/m^2 day 1
    [total dose/cycle = 85 mg/m^2]
  Capecitabine: Oral: 2500 mg/m^2/day days 1 to 7
    [total dose/cycle = 17,500 mg/m^2]
  or Capecitabine: Oral: 3000 mg/m^2/day days 1 to 7
    [total dose/cycle = 21,000 mg/m^2]
  or Capecitabine: Oral: 3500 mg/m^2/day days 1 to 7
    [total dose/cycle = 24,500 mg/m^2]
  or Capecitabine: Oral: 4000 mg/m^2/day days 1 to 7
    [total dose/cycle = 28,000 mg/m^2]
  Repeat cycle every 14 days
Variation 7:
  Oxaliplatin: I.V.: 130 mg/m^2 day 1
    [total dose/cycle = 130 mg/m^2]
  Capecitabine: Oral: 1000 mg/m^2 twice daily days 1 (beginning with evening
    dose) to 15 (ending with morning dose)
    [total dose/cycle = 28,000 mg/m^2]
  Repeat cycle every 21 days

References

Variation 1:
Borner MM, Dietrich D, Stupp R, et al, "Phase I Study of Capecitabine and Oxaliplatin in First- and Second-Line Treatment of Advanced or Metastatic Colorectal Cancer," *J Clin Oncol*, 2002, 20 (7):1759-66.
Variation 2:
Scheithauer W, Kornek GV, Raderer M, et al, "Randomized Multicenter Phase II Trial of Two Different Schedules of Capecitabine Plus Oxaliplatin as First-Line Treatment in Advanced Colorectal Cancer," *J Clin Oncol*, 2003, 21(7):1307-12.
Variation 3:
Rodel C, Grabenbauer GG, Papadopoulos T, et al, "Phase I/II Trial of Capecitabine, Oxaliplatin, and Radiation for Rectal Cancer," *J Clin Oncol*, 2003, 21(16):3098-104.
Variation 4:
Jordan K, Grothey A, Kellner O, et al, "Randomized Phase II Trial of Capecitabine Plus Irinotecan vs Capecitabine Plus Oxaliplatin as First-Line Therapy in Advanced Colorectal Cancer (ACRC): Results of an Interim Analysis," *Proc Annu Meet Am Soc Clin Oncol*, 2002, 21:2225.
Variation 5:
Zeuli M, Nardoni C, Pino MS, et al, "Phase II Study of Capecitabine and Oxaliplatin as First-Line Treatment in Advanced Colorectal Cancer," *Ann Oncol*, 2003, 14(9):1378-82.
Variation 6:
Scheithauer W, Kornek GV, Raderer M, et al, "Intermittent Weekly High-Dose Capecitabine in Combination With Oxaliplatin: A Phase I/II Study in First-Line Treatment of Patients With Advanced Colorectal Cancer," *Ann Oncol*, 2002, 13(10):1583-9.
Variation 7:
Cassidy J, Tabernero J, Twelves C, et al, "XELOX (Capecitabine Plus Oxaliplatin): Active First-Line Therapy for Patients With Metastatic Colorectal Cancer," *J Clin Oncol*, 2004, 22(11):2084-91.

CAPOX (Pancreatic Cancer)

Index Terms Capecitabine-Oxaliplatin (Pancreatic Cancer); Oxaliplatin-Capecitabine (Pancreatic Cancer)

Use Pancreatic cancer

Regimen NOTE: Multiple variations are listed.

Variation 1 (patients ≤65 years of age or ECOG PS <2):
  Capecitabine: Oral: 1000 mg/m^2/dose twice daily days 1 to 14
    [total dose/cycle = 28,000 mg/m^2]
  Oxaliplatin: I.V.: 130 mg/m^2/dose over 2 hours day 1
    [total dose/cycle = 130 mg/m^2]

Repeat cycle every 21 days until disease progression or unacceptable toxicity

Variation 2 (patients >65 years of age or ECOG PS of 2):

Capecitabine: Oral: 750 mg/m^2/dose twice daily days 1 to 14

[total dose/cycle = 21,000 mg/m^2]

Oxaliplatin: I.V.: 110 mg/m^2/dose over 2 hours day 1

[total dose/cycle = 110 mg/m^2]

Repeat cycle every 21 days until disease progression or unacceptable toxicity

References

Variations 1 and 2:

Xiong HQ, Varadhachary GR, Blais JC, et al, "Phase 2 Trial of Oxaliplatin Plus Capecitabine (XELOX) as Second-Line Therapy for Patients With Advanced Pancreatic Cancer," *Cancer*, 2008, 113(8):2046-52.

Carboplatin-Cetuximab

Index Terms Cetuximab-Carboplatin

Use Head and neck cancer

Regimen

Cycle 1:

Cetuximab: I.V.: 400 mg/m^2 (loading dose) day 1 (week 1, cycle 1 only)

[total loading dose = 400 mg/m^2]

followed by I.V.: 250 mg/m^2/day days 8 and 15

[total dose/cycle 1 = 900 mg/m^2]

Carboplatin: I.V.: AUC 5 day 1

[total dose/cycle = AUC = 5]

Treatment cycle is 3 weeks

Subsequent cycles:

Cetuximab: I.V.: 250 mg/m^2/day days 1, 8, and 15

[total dose/cycle = 750 mg/m^2]

Carboplatin: I.V.: AUC 5 day 1

[total dose/cycle = AUC = 5]

Repeat cycle every 3 weeks

References

Chan AT, Hsu MM, Goh BC, et al, "Multicenter, Phase II Study of Cetuximab in Combination With Carboplatin in Patients With Recurrent or Metastatic Nasopharyngeal Carcinoma," *J Clin Oncol*, 2005, 23(15):3568-76.

Carboplatin-Paclitaxel (Ovarian Cancer)

Index Terms Carbo-Tax (Ovarian Cancer); Paclitaxel-Carboplatin (Ovarian Cancer)

Use Ovarian cancer

Regimen NOTE: Multiple variations are listed.

Variation 1:

Carboplatin: I.V.: AUC 7.5 day 1

[total dose/cycle = AUC = 7.5]

Paclitaxel: I.V.: 175 mg/m² over 3 hours day 1

[total dose/cycle = 175 mg/m²]

Repeat cycle every 3 weeks for a total for 6 cycles

Variation 2:

Carboplatin: I.V.: AUC 5-6 day 1

[total dose/cycle = AUC = 5-6]

Paclitaxel: I.V.: 175 mg/m² over 3 hours day 1

[total dose/cycle = 175 mg/m²]

Repeat cycle every 3 weeks for a total of 6-8 cycles

Variation 3:

Carboplatin: I.V.: AUC 5 day 1

[total dose/cycle = AUC = 5]

Paclitaxel: I.V.: 175 mg/m² over 3 hours day 1

[total dose/cycle = 175 mg/m²]

Repeat cycle every 3 weeks for 6 cycles

Variation 4:

Carboplatin: I.V.: AUC 6 (maximum dose: 880 mg) day 1

[total dose/cycle = AUC = 6; maximum dose: 880 mg]

Paclitaxel: I.V.: 185 mg/m² (maximum dose: 400 mg) over 3 hours day 1

[total dose/cycle = 185 mg/m²; maximum dose: 400 mg]

Repeat cycle every 3 weeks

Variation 5:

Carboplatin: I.V.: AUC 7.5 day 1

[total dose/cycle = AUC = 7.5]

Paclitaxel: I.V.: 175 mg/m² over 3 hours day 1

[total dose/cycle = 175 mg/m²]

Repeat cycle every 3 weeks for 3-6 cycles

References

Variation 1:

Ozols RF, Bundy BN, Greer BE, et al, "Phase III Trial of Carboplatin and Paclitaxel Compared With Cisplatin and Paclitaxel in Patients With Optimally Resected Stage III Ovarian Cancer: A Gynecologic Oncology Group Study," *J Clin Oncol*, 2003, 21(17):3194-200.

Variation 2:

Parmar MK, Ledermann JA, Colombo N, et al, "Paclitaxel Plus Platinum-Based Chemotherapy Versus Conventional Platinum-Based Chemotherapy in Women With Relapsed Ovarian Cancer: The ICON4/AGO-OVAR-2.2 Trial," *Lancet*, 2003, 361(9375):2099-106.

Variation 3:

Neijt JP, Engelholm SA, Tuxen MK, et al, "Exploratory Phase III Study of Paclitaxel and Cisplatin Versus Paclitaxel and Carboplatin in Advanced Ovarian Cancer," *J Clin Oncol*, 2000, 18 (17):3084-92.

Vasey PA, Jayson GC, Gordon A, et al, "Phase III Randomized Trial of Docetaxel-Carboplatin Versus Paclitaxel-Carboplatin as First-Line Chemotherapy for Ovarian Carcinoma," *J Natl Cancer Inst*, 2004, 96(22):1682-91.

Variation 4:

du Bois A, Lück HJ, Meier W, et al, "A Randomized Clinical Trial of Cisplatin/Paclitaxel Versus Carboplatin/Paclitaxel as First-Line Treatment of Ovarian Cancer," *J Natl Cancer Inst*, 2003, 95 (17):1320-9.

Variation 5:

Bell J, Brady MF, Young RC, et al, "Randomized Phase III Trial of Three Versus Six Cycles of Adjuvant Carboplatin and Paclitaxel in Early Stage Epithelial Ovarian Carcinoma: A Gynecologic Oncology Group Study," *Gynecol Oncol*, 2006, 102(3):432-9.

◆ **Carboplatin-Pemetrexed (Mesothelioma)** *see* Pemetrexed-Carboplatin (Mesothelioma) *on page 1394*

♦ **Carboplatin–Etoposide (Ovarian Cancer)** *see* Etoposide-Carboplatin (Ovarian Cancer) *on page 1317*

Carbo-Tax (Adenocarcinoma)
Index Terms Paclitaxel-Carboplatin (Adenocarcinoma)
Use Adenocarcinoma, unknown primary
Regimen
  Paclitaxel: I.V.: 135 mg/m^2 infused over 24 hours day 1
    [total dose = 135 mg/m^2]
    followed by
  Carboplatin: I.V.: Target AUC 7.5
    [total dose = AUC = 7.5]
  Repeat cycle every 21 days
References
  Sulkes A, Uziely B, Isacson R, et al, "Combination Chemotherapy in Metastatic Tumors of Unknown Origin. 5-Fluorouracil, Adriamycin®, and Mitomycin C for Adenocarcinomas and Adriamycin®, Vinblastine and Mitomycin C for Anaplastic Carcinomas," *Isr J Med Sci*, 1988, 24 (9-10):604-10.

Carbo-Tax (NSCLC)
Index Terms Paclitaxel-Carboplatin (Nonsmall Cell Lung Cancer)
Use Lung cancer, nonsmall cell
Regimen
  Paclitaxel: I.V.: 135-215 mg/m^2 infused over 24 hours day 1
    [total dose/cycle = 135-215 mg/m^2]
    or I.V.: 175 mg/m^2 infused over 3 hours day 1
      [total dose/cycle = 175 mg/m^2]
    followed by
  Carboplatin: I.V.: Target AUC 7.5
    [total dose/cycle = AUC = 7.5]
  Repeat cycle every 21 days
References
  Langer CJ, Leighton JC, Comis RL, et al, "Paclitaxel By 24- or 1-Hour Infusion in Combination With Carboplatin in Advanced Nonsmall-Cell Lung Cancer: The Fox Chase Cancer Center Experience," *Semin Oncol*, 1995, 22(4 Suppl 9):18-29.

♦ **Carbo-Tax (Ovarian Cancer)** *see* Carboplatin-Paclitaxel (Ovarian Cancer) *on page 1248*
♦ **Carmustine-Cisplatin-Dacarbazine** *see* Cisplatin-Dacarbazine-Carmustine (Melanoma) *on page 1265*
♦ **Carmustine-Cisplatin-Dacarbazine-Tamoxifen** *see* Dartmouth Regimen *on page 1286*

CaT (NSCLC)
Use Lung cancer, nonsmall cell
Regimen NOTE: Multiple variations are listed.
  Variation 1:
    Paclitaxel: I.V.: 175 mg/m^2 day 1
      [total dose/cycle = 175 mg/m^2]
      or I.V.: 135 mg/m^2 continuous infusion day 1
        [total dose/cycle = 135 mg/m^2]
    Carboplatin: I.V.: AUC 7.5 day 1 or 2
      [total dose/cycle = AUC = 7.5]
    Repeat cycle every 21 days

Variation 2:
    Paclitaxel: I.V.: 225 mg/m^2 day 1
        [total dose/cycle = 225 mg/m^2]
    Carboplatin: I.V.: AUC 6 day 1
        [total dose/cycle = AUC = 6]
    Repeat cycle every 21 days

References

Variation 1:
Langer CJ, Leighton JC, Comis RL, et al, "Paclitaxel by 24- or 1-Hour Infusion in Combination With Carboplatin in Advanced Nonsmall-Cell Lung Cancer: The Fox Chase Cancer Center Experience," *Semin Oncol*, 1995, 22(4 Suppl 9):18-29.
Variation 2:
Schiller JH, Harrington D, Belani CP, et al, "Comparison of Four Chemotherapy Regimens for Advanced Nonsmall-Cell Lung Cancer," *N Engl J Med*, 2002, 346(2):92-8.

CAVE

Use Lung cancer, small cell
Regimen
Cyclophosphamide: I.V.: 750 mg/m^2 day 1
    [total dose/cycle = 750 mg/m^2]
Doxorubicin: I.V.: 50 mg/m^2 day 1
    [total dose/cycle = 50 mg/m^2]
Vincristine: I.V.: 1.4 mg/m^2 (maximum dose: 2 mg) day 1
    [total dose/cycle = 1.4 mg/m^2]
Etoposide: I.V.: 60-100 mg/m^2/day days 1, 2, and 3
    [total dose/cycle = 180-300 mg/m^2]
Repeat cycle every 21 days

References

Jett JR, Everson L, Therneau TM, et al, "Treatment of Limited-Stage Small-Cell Lung Cancer With Cyclophosphamide, Doxorubicin, and Vincristine With Or Without Etoposide: A Randomized Trial of the North Central Cancer Treatment Group," *J Clin Oncol*, 1990, 8(1):33-8.
Sufarlan AW and Zainudin BM, "Combination Chemotherapy for Small Cell Lung Cancer," *Med J Malaysia*, 1993, 48(2):166-70.

CAV-P/VP

Use Neuroblastoma
Regimen
Course 1, 2, 4, and 6:
    Cyclophosphamide: I.V.: 70 mg/kg/day days 1 and 2
        [total dose/cycle = 140 mg/kg]
    Doxorubicin: I.V.: 25 mg/m^2/day continuous infusion days 1, 2, and 3
        [total dose/cycle = 75 mg/m^2]
    Vincristine: I.V.: 0.033 mg/kg/day continuous infusion days 1, 2, and 3
        [total dose/cycle = 0.099 mg/kg]
    Vincristine: I.V.: 1.5 mg/m^2 day 9
        [total dose/cycle = 1.5 mg/m^2]
Course 3, 5, and 7:
    Etoposide: I.V.: 200 mg/m^2/day days 1, 2, and 3
        [total dose/cycle = 600 mg/m^2]
    Cisplatin: I.V.: 50 mg/m^2/day days 1 to 4
        [total dose/cycle = 200 mg/m^2]

References

Kushner BH, LaQuaglia MP, Bonilla MA, et al, "Highly Effective Induction Therapy for Stage 4 Neuroblastoma in Children Over 1 Year of Age," *J Clin Oncol*, 1994, 12(12):2607-13.

CC

Use

Ovarian cancer

Regimen

Carboplatin: I.V.: Target AUC 5-7.5 day 1
[total dose/cycle = AUC = 5-7.5]
Cyclophosphamide: I.V.: 600 mg/m^2 day 1
[total dose/cycle = 600 mg/m^2]
Repeat cycle every 28 days

References

Alberts DS, Green S, Hannigan EV, et al, "Improved Therapeutic Index of Carboplatin Plus Cyclophosphamide Versus Cisplatin Plus Cyclophosphamide: Final Report by the Southwest Oncology Group of a Phase III Randomized Trial in Stages III and IV Ovarian Cancer," *J Clin Oncol*, 1992, 10(5):706-17.

Swenerton K, Jeffrey J, Stuart G, et al, "Cisplatin-Cyclophosphamide Versus Carboplatin-Cyclophosphamide in Advanced Ovarian Cancer: A Randomized Phase III Study of the National Cancer Institute of Canada Clinical Trials Group," *J Clin Oncol*, 1992, 10(5):718-26.

CCCDE (Retinoblastoma)

Use Retinoblastoma

Regimen

Cyclophosphamide: I.V.: 150 mg/m^2/day days 1 to 7
[total dose/cycle = 1050 mg/m^2]
Cyclophosphamide: Oral: 150 mg/m^2/day days 22 to 28 and 43 to 49
[total dose/cycle = 2100 mg/m^2]
Doxorubicin: I.V.: 35 mg/m^2/day days 10 and 52
[total dose/cycle = 70 mg/m^2]
Cisplatin: I.V.: 90 mg/m^2/day days 8, 50, and 71
[total dose/cycle = 270 mg/m^2]
Etoposide: I.V.: 150 mg/m^2/day continuous infusion days 29, 30, and 31 and 73, 74, and 75
[total dose/cycle = 900 mg/m^2]

References

Advani SH, Rao SR, Iyer RS, et al, "Pilot Study of Sequential Combination Chemotherapy in Advanced and Recurrent Retinoblastoma," *Med Pediatr Oncol*, 1994, 22(2):125-8.

CCDDT (Neuroblastoma)

Use Neuroblastoma

Regimen

Cyclophosphamide: I.V.: 40 mg/kg/day days 1 and 2
[total dose/cycle = 80 mg/kg]
Cisplatin: I.V.: 20 mg/m^2/day days 1 to 5
[total dose/cycle = 100 mg/m^2]
Teniposide: I.V.: 100 mg/m^2 day 7
[total dose/cycle = 100 mg/m^2]
Doxorubicin: I.V.: 60 mg/m^2 day 1
[total dose/cycle = 60 mg/m^2]
Dacarbazine: I.V.: 250 mg/m^2/day days 1 to 5
[total dose/cycle = 1250 mg/m^2]
Repeat cycle every 21-28 days

References

Ikeda K, Nakagawara A, Yano H, et al, "Improved Survival Rates in Children Over 1 Year of Age With Stage III or IV Neuroblastoma Following an Intensive Chemotherapeutic Regimen," *J Pediatr Surg*, 1989, 24(2):189-93.

CCDT (Melanoma)

Use Melanoma

Regimen

Dacarbazine: I.V.: 220 mg/m^2/day days 1, 2, and 3, every 21 to 28 days
  [total dose/cycle = 660 mg/m^2]
Carmustine: I.V.: 150 mg/m^2 day 1, every 42 to 56 days
  [total dose/cycle = 150 mg/m^2]
Cisplatin: I.V.: 25 mg/m^2/day days 1, 2, and 3, every 21 to 28 days
  [total dose/cycle = 75 mg/m^2]
Tamoxifen: Oral: 20 mg/day (use of tamoxifen is optional)

References

Del Prete SA, Maurer LH, O'Donnell J, et al, "Combination Chemotherapy With Cisplatin, Carmustine, Dacarbazine, and Tamoxifen in Metastatic Melanoma," *Cancer Treat Rep*, 1984, 68 (11):1403-5.

Rusthoven JJ, Quirt IC, Iscoe NA, et al, "Randomized, Double-Blind, Placebo-Controlled Trial Comparing the Response Rates of Carmustine, Dacarbazine, and Cisplatin With and Without Tamoxifen in Patients With Metastatic Melanoma. National Cancer Institute of Canada Clinical Trials Group," *J Clin Oncol*, 1996, 14(7):2083-90.

CCT (Neuroblastoma)

Use Neuroblastoma

Regimen

Cyclophosphamide: I.V.: 40 mg/kg/day days 1 and 2
  [total dose/cycle = 80 mg/kg]
Cisplatin: I.V.: 20 mg/m^2/day days 22 to 26
  [total dose/cycle = 100 mg/m^2]
Teniposide: I.V.: 100 mg/m^2 day 28
  [total dose/cycle = 100 mg/m^2]
Repeat every 42 days for 3 cycles

References

Ikeda K, Nakagawara A, Yano H, et al, "Improved Survival Rates in Children Over 1 Year of Age With Stage III or IV Neuroblastoma Following an Intensive Chemotherapeutic Regimen," *J Pediatr Surg*, 1989, 24(2):189-93.

CDDP/VP-16

Use Brain tumors

Regimen

Cisplatin: I.V.: 90 mg/m^2 day 1
  [total dose/cycle = 90 mg/m^2]
Etoposide: I.V.: 150 mg/m^2/day days 3 and 4
  [total dose/cycle = 300 mg/m^2]
Repeat cycle every 21 days

References

Kovnar EH, Kellie SJ, Horowitz ME, et al, "Preirradiation Cisplatin and Etoposide in the Treatment of High-Risk Medulloblastoma and Other Malignant Embryonal Tumors of the Central Nervous System: A Phase II Study," *J Clin Oncol*, 1990, 8(2):330-6.

CE-CAdO

Use Neuroblastoma

Regimen

Carboplatin: I.V.: 160 mg/m^2/day days 1 to 5
  [total dose/cycle = 800 mg/m^2]
Etoposide: I.V.: 100 mg/m^2/day days 1 to 5
  [total dose/cycle = 500 mg/m^2]

◄ or
Carboplatin: I.V.: 200 mg/m^2/day days 1, 2, and 3
 [total dose/cycle = 600 mg/m^2]
Etoposide: I.V.: 150 mg/m^2/day days 1, 2, and 3
 [total dose/cycle = 450 mg/m^2]
and
Cyclophosphamide: I.V.: 300 mg/m^2/day days 1 to 5
 [total dose/cycle = 1500 mg/m^2]
Doxorubicin: I.V.: 60 mg/m^2 day 5
 [total dose/cycle = 60 mg/m^2]
Vincristine: I.V.: 1.5 mg/m^2/day days 1 and 5
 [total dose/cycle = 3 mg/m^2]
Repeat cycle every 21 days

References

Rubie H, Michon J, Plantaz D, et al, "Unresectable Localized Neuroblastoma: Improved Survival After Primary Chemotherapy Including Carboplatin-Etoposide. Neuroblastoma Study Group of the Societe Francaise d'Oncologie Pediatrique (SFOP)," *Br J Cancer*, 1998, 77(12):2310-7.

CEF

Use Breast cancer

Regimen
Cyclophosphamide: Oral: 75 mg/m^2/day days 1 to 14
 [total dose/cycle = 1050 mg/m^2]
Epirubicin: I.V.: 60 mg/m^2/day days 1 and 8
 [total dose/cycle = 120 mg/m^2]
Fluorouracil: I.V.: 500 mg/m^2/day days 1 and 8
 [total dose/cycle = 1000 mg/m^2]
Repeat cycle every 28 days

References

Levine MN, Bramwell VH, Pritchard KI, et al, "Randomized Trial of Intensive Cyclophosphamide, Epirubicin, and Fluorouracil Chemotherapy Compared With Cyclophosphamide, Methotrexate, and Fluorouracil in Premenopausal Women With Node-Positive Breast Cancer, National Cancer Institute of Canada Clinical Trials Group," *J Clin Oncol*, 1998, 16(8):2651-8.

CE (Neuroblastoma)

Use Neuroblastoma

Regimen
Carboplatin: I.V.: 500 mg/m^2/day days 1 and 2
 [total dose/cycle = 1000 mg/m^2]
Etoposide: I.V.: 100 mg/m^2/day days 1, 2, and 3
 [total dose/cycle = 300 mg/m^2]
Repeat cycle every 21-28 days

References

Alvarado CS, Kretschmar C, Joshi VV, et al, "Chemotherapy for Patients With Recurrent or Refractory Neuroblastoma: A POG Phase II Study," *J Pediatr Hematol Oncol*, 1997, 19(1):62-7.

CEPP(B)

Use Lymphoma, non-Hodgkin's

Regimen
Cyclophosphamide: I.V.: 600-650 mg/m^2/day days 1 and 8
 [total dose/cycle = 1200-1300 mg/m^2]
Etoposide: I.V.: 70-85 mg/m^2/day days 1, 2, and 3
 [total dose/cycle = 210-255 mg/m^2]
Procarbazine: Oral: 60 mg/m^2/day days 1 to 10
 [total dose/cycle = 600 mg/m^2]

Prednisone: Oral: 60 mg/m^2/day days 1 to 10
[total dose/cycle = 600 mg/m^2]
Bleomycin: I.V.: 15 units/m^2/day days 1 and 15 (Bleomycin is sometimes omitted)
[total dose/cycle = 30 units/m^2]
Repeat cycle every 28 days

References

Chao NJ, Rosenberg SA, and Horning SJ, "CEPP(B): An Effective and Well-Tolerated Regimen in Poor-Risk, Aggressive Non-Hodgkin's Lymphoma," *Blood*, 1990, 76(7):1293-8.

CE (Retinoblastoma)

Use Retinoblastoma

Regimen

Etoposide: I.V.: 100 mg/m^2/day days 1 to 5
[total dose/cycle = 500 mg/m^2]
Carboplatin: I.V.: 160 mg/m^2/day days 1 to 5
[total dose/cycle = 800 mg/m^2]
Repeat cycle every 21 days

References

Doz F, Neuenschwander S, Plantaz D, et al, "Etoposide and Carboplatin in Extraocular Retinoblastoma: A Study by the Societe Francaise d'Oncologie Pediatrique," *J Clin Oncol*, 1995, 13(4):902-9.

Cetuximab (Biweekly)-Irinotecan

Index Terms Irinotecan-Biweekly Cetuximab

Use Colorectal cancer

Regimen

Cycle 1:
Cetuximab: I.V.: 500 mg/m^2 over 120 minutes day 1 (cycle 1 only)
[total dose/cycle = 500 mg/m^2]
Irinotecan: I.V.: 180 mg/m^2 day 1
[total dose/cycle = 180 mg/m^2]
Subsequent cycles:
Cetuximab: I.V.: 500 mg/m^2 over 60 minutes day 1
[total dose/cycle = 500 mg/m^2]
Irinotecan: I.V.: 180 mg/m^2 day 1
[total dose/cycle = 180 mg/m^2]
Repeat cycle every 14 days

References

Pfeiffer P, Nielsen D, Bjerregaard J, et al, "Biweekly Cetuximab and Irinotecan as Third-Line Therapy in Patients With Advanced Colorectal Cancer After Failure to Irinotecan, Oxaliplatin and 5-Fluorouracil," *Ann Oncol*, 2008, 19(6):1141-5.

◆ **Cetuximab-Carboplatin** *see* Carboplatin-Cetuximab *on page 1248*

Cetuximab-Carboplatin-Fluorouracil

Index Terms Carboplatin-Fluorouracil-Cetuximab

Use Head and neck cancer

Regimen

Cycle 1:
Cetuximab: I.V.: 400 mg/m^2 (loading dose) day 1 (week 1, cycle 1 only)
[total loading dose = 400 mg/m^2]
followed by I.V.: 250 mg/m^2/day days 8 and 15
[total dose/cycle 1 = 900 mg/m^2]
Carboplatin: I.V.: AUC 5 day 1
[total dose/cycle = AUC = 5]

◄ Fluorouracil: I.V.: 1000 mg/m^2/day continuous infusion days 1 to 4
  [total dose/cycle = 4000 mg/m^2]
Treatment cycle is 3 weeks
Subsequent cycles:
  Cetuximab: I.V.: 250 mg/m^2/day days 1, 8, and 15
    [total dose/cycle = 750 mg/m^2]
  Carboplatin: I.V.: AUC 5 day 1
    [total dose/cycle = AUC = 5]
  Fluorouracil: I.V.: 1000 mg/m^2/day continuous infusion days 1 to 4
    [total dose/cycle = 4000 mg/m^2]
  Repeat cycle every 3 weeks for a total of up to 6 cycles (cetuximab monotherapy may be continued thereafter until disease progression or unacceptable toxicity)

References
Vermorken JB, Mesia R, Rivera F, et al, "Platinum-Based Chemotherapy Plus Cetuximab in Head and Neck Cancer," *N Engl J Med*, 2008, 359(11):1116-27.

◆ **Cetuximab-Cisplatin** *see* Cisplatin-Cetuximab *on page 1264*

Cetuximab-Cisplatin-Fluorouracil

Index Terms Cisplatin-Fluorouracil-Cetuximab
Use Head and neck cancer
Regimen
  Cycle 1:
    Cetuximab: I.V.: 400 mg/m^2 (loading dose) day 1 (week 1, cycle 1 only)
      [total loading dose = 400 mg/m^2]
      followed by I.V.: 250 mg/m^2/day days 8 and 15
        [total dose/cycle 1 = 900 mg/m^2]
    Cisplatin: I.V.: 100 mg/m^2 day 1
      [total dose/cycle = 100 mg/m^2]
    Fluorouracil: I.V.: 1000 mg/m^2/day continuous infusion days 1 to 4
      [total dose/cycle = 4000 mg/m^2]
    Treatment cycle is 3 weeks
  Subsequent cycles:
    Cetuximab: I.V.: 250 mg/m^2/day days 1, 8, and 15
      [total dose/cycle = 750 mg/m^2]
    Cisplatin: I.V.: 100 mg/m^2 day 1
      [total dose/cycle = 100 mg/m^2]
    Fluorouracil: I.V.: 1000 mg/m^2/day continuous infusion days 1 to 4
      [total dose/cycle = 4000 mg/m^2]
    Repeat cycle every 3 weeks for a total of up to 6 cycles (cetuximab monotherapy may be continued thereafter until disease progression or unacceptable toxicity)

References
Vermorken JB, Mesia R, Rivera F, et al, "Platinum-Based Chemotherapy Plus Cetuximab in Head and Neck Cancer," *N Engl J Med*, 2008, 359(11):1116-27.

Cetuximab-Cisplatin-Vinorelbine

Index Terms Cisplatin-Vinorelbine-Cetuximab
Use Lung cancer, nonsmall cell
Regimen
  Cycle 1:
    Cetuximab: I.V.: 400 mg/m^2 (loading dose) day 1 (week 1, cycle 1 only)
      [total loading dose = 400 mg/m^2]

followed by I.V.: 250 mg/m² /dose days 8 and 15
  [total dose/cycle 1 = 900 mg/m²]
Cisplatin: I.V.: 80 mg/m² /dose day 1
  [total dose/cycle = 80 mg/m²]
Vinorelbine: I.V.: 25 mg/m² /dose days 1 and 8
  [total dose/cycle = 50 mg/m²]
Treatment cycle is 3 weeks
Subsequent cycles:
Cetuximab: I.V.: 250 mg/m² /day days 1, 8, and 15
  [total dose/cycle = 750 mg/m²]
Cisplatin: I.V.: 80 mg/m² day 1
  [total dose/cycle = 80 mg/m²]
Vinorelbine: I.V.: 25 mg/m² /dose days 1 and 8
  [total dose/cycle = 50 mg/m²]
Repeat cycle every 3 weeks

References
Pirker R, Szczesna A, von Pawel J, et al, "FLEX: A Randomized, Multicenter, Phase III Study of Cetuximab in Combination With Cisplatin/Vinorelbine (CV) Versus CV Alone in the First-Line Treatment of Patients With Advanced Non-Small Cell Lung Cancer (NSCLC)," *J Clin Oncol*, 2008, 26(Supp) [abstract 3 from 2008 ASCO Annual Meeting].

Rosell R, Robinet G, Szczesna A, et al, "Randomized Phase II Study of Cetuximab Plus Cisplatin/Vinorelbine Compared With Cisplatin/Vinorelbine Alone as First-Line Therapy in EGFR-Expressing Advanced Non-Small-Cell Lung Cancer," *Ann Oncol*, 2008, 19(2):362-9.

Cetuximab-FOLFOX4
Index Terms FOLFOX4-Cetuximab
Use Colorectal cancer
Regimen
Cycle 1:
Cetuximab: I.V.: 400 mg/m² (loading dose) day 1 (week 1, cycle 1 only)
  followed by I.V.: 250 mg/m² /day day 8
  [total dose/cycle 1 = 650 mg/m²]
Oxaliplatin: I.V.: 85 mg/m² (over 2 hours) day 1
  [total dose/cycle = 85 mg/m²]
Leucovorin: I.V.: 200 mg/m² /day (over 2 hours) days 1 and 2
  [total dose/cycle = 400 mg/m²]
Fluorouracil: I.V. bolus: 400 mg/m² /day days 1 and 2
  followed by I.V.: 600 mg/m² continuous infusion (over 22 hours) days 1 and 2
  [total dose/cycle = 2000 mg/m²]
Note: Bolus fluorouracil and continuous infusion are both given on each day.
Treatment cycle is 14 days
Subsequent cycles:
Cetuximab: I.V.: 250 mg/m² /day days 1 and 8
  [total dose/cycle = 500 mg/m²]
Oxaliplatin: I.V.: 85 mg/m² day 1
  [total dose/cycle = 85 mg/m²]
Leucovorin: I.V.: 200 mg/m² /day (over 2 hours) days 1 and 2
  [total dose/cycle = 400 mg/m²]
Fluorouracil: I.V. bolus: 400 mg/m² /day days 1 and 2
  followed by I.V.: 600 mg/m² continuous infusion (over 22 hours) days 1 and 2
  [total dose/cycle = 2000 mg/m²]
Note: Bolus fluorouracil and continuous infusion are both given on each day.
Repeat cycle every 14 days

References

Tabernero J, Van Cutsem E, Díaz-Rubio E, et al, "Phase II Trial of Cetuximab in Combination With Fluorouracil, Leucovorin, and Oxaliplatin in the First-Line Treatment of Metastatic Colorectal Cancer," *J Clin Oncol*, 2007, 25(33):5225-32.

Cetuximab-Irinotecan

Index Terms Irinotecan-Cetuximab

Use Colorectal cancer

Regimen NOTE: Multiple variations are listed.

Variation 1:

Cycle 1:

Cetuximab: I.V.: 400 mg/m^2 (loading dose) day 1 (week 1, cycle 1 only)
[total loading dose = 400 mg/m^2]
followed by I.V.: 250 mg/m^2/day days 8, 15, 22, 29, and 36
[total dose/cycle 1 = 1650 mg/m^2]
Irinotecan: I.V.: 125 mg/m^2/day days 1, 8, 15, and 22
[total dose/cycle = 500 mg/m^2]

Subsequent cycles:

Cetuximab: I.V.: 250 mg/m^2/day days 1, 8, 15, 22, 29, and 36
[total dose/cycle = 1500 mg/m^2]
Irinotecan: I.V.: 125 mg/m^2/day days 1, 8, 15, and 22
[total dose/cycle = 500 mg/m^2]

Repeat cycle every 42 days

Variation 2:

Cycle 1:

Cetuximab: I.V.: 400 mg/m^2 (loading dose) day 1 (week 1, cycle 1 only)
[total loading dose = 400 mg/m^2]
followed by I.V.: 250 mg/m^2 day 8
[total dose/cycle 1 = 650 mg/m^2]
Irinotecan: I.V.: 180 mg/m^2 day 1
[total dose/cycle = 180 mg/m^2]

Subsequent cycles:

Cetuximab: I.V.: 250 mg/m^2/day days 1 and 8
[total dose/cycle = 500 mg/m^2]
Irinotecan: I.V.: 180 mg/m^2 day 1
[total dose/cycle = 180 mg/m^2]

Repeat cycle every 14 days

Variation 3:

Cycle 1:

Cetuximab: I.V.: 400 mg/m^2 (loading dose) day 1 (week 1, cycle 1 only)
[total loading dose = 400 mg/m^2]
followed by I.V.: 250 mg/m^2/day days 8 and 15 (cycle 1)
[total dose/cycle 1 = 900 mg/m^2]
Irinotecan: I.V.: 350 mg/m^2 day 1
[total dose/cycle = 350 mg/m^2]

Subsequent cycles:

Cetuximab: I.V.: 250 mg/m^2/day days 1, 8, and 15
[total dose/cycle = 750 mg/m^2]
Irinotecan: I.V.: 350 mg/m^2 day 1
[total dose/cycle = 350 mg/m^2]

Repeat cycle every 21 days

References

Cunningham D, Humblet Y, Siena S, et al, "Cetuximab Monotherapy and Cetuximab Plus Irinotecan in Irinotecan-Refractory Metastatic Colorectal Cancer," *N Engl J Med*, 2004, 351 (4):337-45.

◆ **Cetuximab-Paclitaxel** see Paclitaxel-Cetuximab on page 1387

CEV

Use Rhabdomyosarcoma
Regimen
Carboplatin: I.V.: 500 mg/m² day 1
  [total dose/cycle = 500 mg/m²]
Epirubicin: I.V.: 150 mg/m² day 1
  [total dose/cycle = 150 mg/m²]
Vincristine: I.V.: 1.5 mg/m²/day days 1 and 7
  [total dose/cycle = 3 mg/m²]
Repeat cycle every 21 days
References

Frascella E, Pritchard-Jones K, Modak S, et al, "Response of Previously Untreated Metastatic Rhabdomyosarcoma to Combination Chemotherapy With Carboplatin, Epirubicin and Vincristine," *Eur J Cancer*, 1996, 32A(5):821-5.

◆ **CF (Esophageal Cancer)** see Cisplatin-Fluorouracil (Esophageal Cancer) on page 1268

◆ **CF (Head and Neck Cancer)** see Cisplatin-Fluorouracil (Head and Neck Cancer) on page 1270

◆ **CFM** see CNF on page 1277

◆ **CF (NHL-Mantle Cell)** see Fludarabine-Cyclophosphamide (NHL-Mantle Cell) on page 1327

CFP

Use Breast cancer
Regimen
Cyclophosphamide: I.V.: 150 mg/m²/day days 1 to 5
  [total dose/cycle = 750 mg/m²]
Fluorouracil: I.V.: 300 mg/m²/day days 1 to 5
  [total dose/cycle = 1500 mg/m²]
Prednisone: Oral: 30 mg/day days 1 to 14 (cycle 1 only)
  followed by Oral: 20 mg/day days 15 to 21 (cycle 1 only)
    followed by Oral: 10 mg daily thereafter as maintenance
      [total dose/cycle = 700 mg in cycle 1; 350 mg in subsequent cycles]
Repeat cycle every 35 days
References

Marschke RF Jr, Ingle JN, Schaid DJ, et al, "Randomized Clinical Trial of CFP Versus CMFP in Women With Metastatic Breast Cancer," *Cancer*, 1989, 63(10):1931-7.

CHAMOCA (Modified Bagshawe Regimen)

Use Gestational trophoblastic tumor
Regimen NOTE: Multiple variations are listed.
Variation 1:
Hydroxyurea: Oral: 500 mg every 6 hours, for 4 doses, day 1 (start at 6 AM)
  [total dose/cycle = 2000 mg]
Dactinomycin: I.V.: 0.2 mg/day days 1, 2, and 3 (give at 7 PM)
  followed by I.V.: 0.5 mg/day days 4 and 5 (give at 7 PM)
    [total dose/cycle = 1.6 mg]
Cyclophosphamide: I.V.: 500 mg/m²/day days 3 and 8 (give at 7 PM)
  [total dose/cycle = 1000 mg/m²]
Vincristine: I.V.: 1 mg/m² (maximum dose: 2 mg) day 2 (give at 7 AM)
  [total dose/cycle = 1 mg/m²; maximum: 2 mg]

Methotrexate: I.V. bolus: 100 mg/m^2 day 2 (give at 7 PM)
  followed by I.V.: 200 mg/m^2 continuous infusion over 12 hours day 2
   [total dose/cycle = 300 mg/m^2]
Leucovorin: I.M.: 14 mg every 6 hours, for 6 doses, days 3, 4, and 5 (begin at
 7 PM on day 3; start 24 hours after the start of methotrexate)
   [total dose/cycle = 84 mg]
Doxorubicin: I.V.: 30 mg/m^2 day 8 (give at 7 PM)
   [total dose/cycle = 30 mg/m^2]
Repeat cycle every 18 days or as toxicity permits (cycle may be repeated 10
 days after last treatment)
Variation 2:
 Hydroxyurea: Oral: 500 mg every 12 hours, for 4 doses, days 1 and 2
  (usually started in early morning)
   [total dose/cycle = 2000 mg]
 Dactinomycin: I.V.: 10 mcg/kg/day days 5, 6, and 7
   [total dose/cycle = 30 mcg/kg]
 Vincristine: I.V.: 1 mg/m^2 day 3
   [total dose/cycle = 1 mg/m^2]
 Methotrexate: I.V. bolus: 100 mg/m^2 day 3
  followed by I.V.: 200 mg/m^2 continuous infusion over 12 hours day 3
   [total dose/cycle = 300 mg/m^2]
 Leucovorin: I.M.: 10 mg/m^2 every 12 hours, for 4 doses, days 4 and 5 (start
  24 hours after the start of methotrexate)
   [total dose/cycle = 40 mg/m^2]
 Cyclophosphamide: I.V.: 600 mg/m^2 day 5
   [total dose/cycle = 600 mg/m^2]
 Doxorubicin: I.V.: 30 mg/m^2 day 10
   [total dose/cycle = 30 mg/m^2]
 Repeat cycle every 3 weeks
Variation 3:
 Hydroxyurea: Oral: 500 mg every 12 hours, for 4 doses, days 1 and 2
  (usually started in early morning)
   [total dose/cycle = 2000 mg/m^2]
 Vincristine: I.V.: 1 mg/m^2 day 3
   [total dose/cycle = 1 mg/m^2]
 Methotrexate: I.V. bolus: 100 mg/m^2 day 3
  followed by I.V.: 200 mg/m^2 continuous infusion over 12 hours day 3
   [total dose/cycle = 300 mg/m^2]
 Leucovorin: I.M.: 14 mg every 6 hours, for 6 doses, days 4, 5, and 6 (start 24
  hours after start of methotrexate)
   [total dose/cycle = 84 mg]
 Dactinomycin: I.V.: 0.2 mg/day days 2, 3, and 4
  followed by I.V.: 0.5 mg/day days 5 and 6
   [total dose/cycle = 1.6 mg]
 Cyclophosphamide: I.V.: 500 mg/m^2 day 4
   [total dose/cycle = 500 mg/m^2]
 Doxorubicin: I.V.: 30 mg/m^2 day 9
   [total dose/cycle = 30 mg/m^2]
 Melphalan: I.V.: 6 mg/m^2 day 9
   [total dose/cycle = 6 mg/m^2]
 Repeat cycle approximately every 3 weeks
Variation 4:
 Hydroxyurea: Oral: 500 mg 4 times/day, for 4 doses, day 1
   [total dose/cycle = 2000 mg/m^2]

Vincristine: I.V.: 1 mg/m^2 day 2
[total dose/cycle = 1 mg/m^2]
Methotrexate: I.V. bolus: 100 mg/m^2 day 2
followed by I.V.: 200 mg/m^2 continuous infusion over 12 hours day 2
[total dose/cycle = 300 mg/m^2]
Leucovorin: I.M.: 14 mg every 6 hours, for 6 doses, days 3, 4, and 5 (start 24 hours after the start of methotrexate)
[total dose/cycle = 84 mg]
Dactinomycin: I.V.: 0.2 mg days 1, 2, and 3
followed by I.V.: 0.5 mg days 4 and 5
[total dose/cycle = 1.6 mg]
Cyclophosphamide: I.V.: 500 mg/m^2 day 3
[total dose/cycle = 500 mg/m^2]
Cyclophosphamide: I.V.: 300 mg/m^2 on day 8
[total dose/cycle = 300 mg/m^2]
Doxorubicin: I.V.: 30 mg/m^2 day 8
[total dose/cycle = 30 mg/m^2]
Repeat cycle approximately every 3 weeks

References

Variation 1:
Weed JC Jr, Barnard DE, Currie JL, et al, "Chemotherapy With the Modified Bagshawe Protocol for Poor Prognosis Metastatic Trophoblastic Disease," *Obstet Gynecol*, 1982, 59(3):377-80.
Variation 2:
Wong LC, Choo YC, and Ma HK, "Modified Bagshawe's Regimen in High-Risk Gestational Trophoblastic Disease," *Gynecol Oncol*, 1986, 23(1):87-93.
Variation 3:
Surwit EA, Suciu TN, Schmidt HJ, et al, "A New Combination Chemotherapy for Resistant Trophoblastic Disease," *Gynecol Oncol*, 1979, 8(1):110-8.
Variation 4:
Surwit EA and Hammond CB, "Treatment of Metastatic Trophoblastic Disease With Poor Prognosis," *Obstet Gynecol*, 1980, 55(5):565-70.

CHAMOMA (Bagshawe Regimen)

Use Gestational trophoblastic tumor

Regimen

Hydroxyurea: Oral: 500 mg every 12 hours, for 4 doses, days 1 and 2
[total dose/cycle = 2000 mg]
Vincristine: I.V.: 1 mg/m^2 day 3
[total dose/cycle = 1 mg/m^2]
Methotrexate: I.V. bolus: 100 mg/m^2 day 3
followed by I.V.: 200 mg/m^2 continuous infusion over 12 hours day 3
[total dose/cycle = 300 mg/m^2]
Leucovorin: I.M.: 12 mg/m^2 every 12 hours, for 4 doses, days 4 and 5 (start 12 hours after the end of methotrexate infusion)
[total dose/cycle = 48 mg/m^2]
Dactinomycin: I.V.: 10 mcg/kg/day days 5, 6, and 7
[total dose/cycle = 30 mcg/kg]
Cyclophosphamide: I.V.: 600 mg/m^2 day 5
[total dose/cycle = 600 mg/m^2]
Doxorubicin: I.V.: 30 mg/m^2 day 10
[total dose/cycle = 30 mg/m^2]
Melphalan: I.V.: 6 mg/m^2 day 10
[total dose/cycle = 6 mg/m^2]
Repeat cycle approximately every 3 weeks

References

Bagshawe KD, "Treatment of Trophoblastic Tumors," *Ann Acad Med Singapore*, 1976, 5:273-9.

Chlorambucil-VPP (Hodgkin's Lymphoma)

Use Lymphoma, Hodgkin's disease

Regimen

Chlorambucil: Oral: 6 mg/m^2/day (maximum dose: 10 mg) days 1 to 14
[total dose/cycle = 84 mg/m^2]
Vinblastine: I.V.: 6 mg/m^2/day (maximum dose: 10 mg) days 1 and 8
[total dose/cycle = 12 mg/m^2]
Procarbazine: Oral: 100 mg/m^2/day (maximum dose: 150 mg) days 1 to 14
[total dose/cycle = 1400 mg/m^2]
Prednisone: Oral: 40-50 mg/day days 1 to 14
[total dose/cycle = 560-700 mg]
Repeat cycle every 28 days

References

Selby P, Patel P, Milan S, et al, "ChlVPP Combination Chemotherapy for Hodgkin's Disease: Long-Term Results," *Br J Cancer*, 1990, 62(2):279-85.

CHL + PRED

Use Leukemia, chronic lymphocytic

Regimen

Chlorambucil: Oral: 0.4 mg/kg/day for 1 day every other week; increase initial dose of 0.4 mg/kg by 0.1 mg/kg every 2 weeks until toxicity or disease control is achieved
Prednisone: Oral: 100 mg/day for 2 days every other week

References

Han T, Ezdinli EZ, Shimaoka K, et al, "Chlorambucil Vs Combined Chlorambucil-Corticosteroid Therapy in Chronic Lymphocytic Leukemia," *Cancer*, 1973,31(3):502-8.

CHOP

Use Lymphoma, non-Hodgkin's

Regimen NOTE: Multiple variations are listed.

Variation 1:
Cyclophosphamide: I.V.: 750 mg/m^2 day 1
[total dose/cycle = 750 mg/m^2]
Doxorubicin: I.V.: 50 mg/m^2 day 1
[total dose/cycle = 50 mg/m^2]
Vincristine: I.V.: 1.4 mg/m^2 (maximum dose: 2 mg) day 1
[total dose/cycle = 1.4 mg/m^2]
Prednisone: Oral: 100 mg/day days 1 to 5
[total dose/cycle = 500 mg]
or Oral: 50 mg/m^2/day days 1 to 5
[total dose/cycle = 250 mg/m^2]
or Oral: 100 mg/m^2/day days 1 to 5
[total dose/cycle = 500 mg/m^2]
Repeat cycle every 21 days

Variation 2:
Cyclophosphamide: I.V.: 750 mg/m^2 day 1
[total dose/cycle = 750 mg/m^2]
Doxorubicin: I.V.: 50 mg/m^2 day 1
[total dose/cycle = 50 mg/m^2]
Vincristine: I.V.: 2 mg day 1
[total dose/cycle = 2 mg]
Prednisone: Oral: 75 mg/day days 1 to 5
[total dose/cycle = 375 mg]
Repeat cycle every 21 days

Variation 3:

Cyclophosphamide: I.V.: 750 mg/m^2/day days 1 and 8
[total dose/cycle = 1500 mg/m^2]

Doxorubicin: I.V.: 25 mg/m^2/day days 1 and 8
[total dose/cycle = 50 mg/m^2]

Vincristine: I.V.: 1.4 mg/m^2/day (maximum dose: 2 mg) days 1 and 8
[total dose/cycle = 2.8 mg/m^2]

Prednisone: Oral: 50 mg/m^2/day days 1 to 8
[total dose/cycle = 400 mg/m^2]

Repeat cycle every 28 days

Variation 4 - "mini-CHOP":

Cyclophosphamide: I.V.: 250 mg/m^2/day days 1, 8, and 15
[total dose/cycle = 750 mg/m^2]

Doxorubicin: I.V.: 16.7 mg/m^2/day days 1, 8, and 15
[total dose/cycle = 50.1 mg/m^2]

Vincristine: I.V.: 0.67 mg/day days 1, 8, and 15
[total dose/cycle = 2.01 mg]

Prednisone: Oral: 75 mg/day days 1 to 5
[total dose/cycle = 375 mg]

Repeat cycle every 21 days

References

Variation 1:

Bezwoda W, Rastogi RB, Erazo Valla A, et al, "Long-Term Results of a Multicentre Randomised, Comparative Phase III Trial of CHOP Versus CNOP Regimens in Patients With Intermediate- and High-Grade Non-Hodgkin's Lymphomas, Novantrone International Study Group," *Eur J Cancer*, 1995, 31A(6):903-11.

McKelvey EM, Gottlieb JA, Wilson HE, et al, "Hydroxyldaunomycin (Adriamycin®) Combination Chemotherapy in Malignant Lymphoma," *Cancer*, 1976, 38(4):1484-93.

Miller TP, Dahlberg S, Cassady JR, et al, "Chemotherapy Alone Compared With Chemotherapy Plus Radiotherapy for Localized Intermediate- and High-Grade Non-Hodgkin's Lymphoma," *N Engl J Med*, 1998, 339(1):21-6.

Variation 2 and 4:

Meyer RM, Browman GP, Samosh ML, et al, "Randomized Phase II Comparison of Standard CHOP With Weekly CHOP in Elderly Patients With Non-Hodgkin's Lymphoma," *J Clin Oncol*, 1995, 13(9):2386-93.

Variation 3:

Linch DC, Vaughan Hudson B, Hancock BW, et al, "A Randomised Comparison of a Third-Generation Regimen (PACEBOM) With a Standard Regimen (CHOP) in Patients With Histologically Aggressive Non-Hodgkin's Lymphoma: A British National Lymphoma Investigation Report," *Br J Cancer*, 1996, 74(2):318-22.

♦ **CHOP-Rituximab** *see* Rituximab-CHOP *on page 1402*

CI (Neuroblastoma)

Use Neuroblastoma

Regimen

Ifosfamide: I.V.: 1500 mg/m^2/day days 1, 2, and 3
[total dose/cycle = 4500 mg/m^2]

Mesna: I.V.: 500 mg/m^2 every 3 hours, for 3 doses each day, days 1, 2, and 3
[total dose/cycle = 4500 mg/m^2]

Carboplatin: I.V.: 400 mg/m^2 day 4
[total dose/cycle = 400 mg/m^2]

Repeat cycle every 21-28 days

References

Alvarado CS, Kretschmar C, Joshi VV, et al, "Chemotherapy for Patients With Recurrent or Refractory Neuroblastoma: A POG Phase II Study," *J Pediatr Hematol Oncol*, 1997, 19(1):62-7.

CISCA

Use Bladder cancer

Regimen

Cyclophosphamide: I.V.: 650 mg/m^2 day 1
 [total dose = 650 mg/m^2]
Doxorubicin: I.V.: 50 mg/m^2 day 1
 [total dose = 50 mg/m^2]
Cisplatin: I.V.: 100 mg/m^2 day 2
 [total dose = 100 mg/m^2]
Repeat cycle every 21-28 days

References

Sternberg JJ, Bracken RB, Handel PB, et al, "Combination Chemotherapy (CISCA) for Advanced Urinary Tract Carcinoma. A Preliminary Report," *JAMA*, 1977, 238(21):2282-7.

Cisplatin-Cetuximab

Index Terms Cetuximab-Cisplatin

Use Head and neck cancer

Regimen NOTE: Multiple variations are listed.

Variation 1:

Cycle 1:

Cetuximab: I.V.: 400 mg/m^2 (loading dose) day 1 (week 1, cycle 1 only)
 [total loading dose = 400 mg/m^2]
 followed by I.V.: 250 mg/m^2/day days 8, 15, and 22
 [total dose/cycle 1 = 1150 mg/m^2]
Cisplatin: I.V.: 100 mg/m^2 day 1
 [total dose/cycle = 100 mg/m^2]
Treatment cycle is 4 weeks

Subsequent cycles:

Cetuximab: I.V.: 250 mg/m^2/day days 1, 8, 15, and 22
 [total dose/cycle = 1000 mg/m^2]
Cisplatin: I.V.: 100 mg/m^2 day 1
 [total dose/cycle = 100 mg/m^2]
Repeat cycle every 4 weeks

Variation 2:

Cycle 1:

Cetuximab: I.V.: 400 mg/m^2 (loading dose) day 1 (week 1, cycle 1 only)
 [total loading dose = 400 mg/m^2]
 followed by I.V.: 250 mg/m^2/day days 8 and 15
 [total dose/cycle 1 = 900 mg/m^2]
Cisplatin: I.V.: 75-100 mg/m^2 day 1
 [total dose/cycle = 75-100 mg/m^2]
Treatment cycle is 3 weeks

Subsequent cycles:

Cetuximab: I.V.: 250 mg/m^2/day days 1, 8, and 15
 [total dose/cycle = 750 mg/m^2]
Cisplatin: I.V.: 75-100 mg/m^2 day 1
 [total dose/cycle = 75-100 mg/m^2]
Repeat cycle every 3 weeks

References

Variation 1:
Burtness B, Goldwasser MA, Flood W, et al, "Phase III Randomized Trial of Cisplatin Plus Placebo Compared With Cisplatin Plus Cetuximab in Metastatic/Recurrent Head and Neck Cancer: An Eastern Cooperative Oncology Group Study," *J Clin Oncol*, 2005, 23(34):8646-54.

Variation 2:

Herbst RS, Arquette M, Shin DM, et al, "Phase II Multicenter Study of the Epidermal Growth Factor Receptor Antibody Cetuximab and Cisplatin for Recurrent and Refractory Aquamous Cell Carcinoma of the Head and Neck," *J Clin Oncol*, 2005, 23(24):5578-87.

Cisplatin-Cytarabine-Dexamethasone (NHL Regimen)

Index Terms DHAP (NHL Regimen)

Use Lymphoma, non-Hodgkin's

Regimen NOTE: Multiple variations are listed.

Variation 1:

Dexamethasone: I.V. or Oral: 40 mg/day days 1 to 4
  [total dose/cycle = 160 mg]
Cisplatin: I.V.: 100 mg/m^2 over 24 hours day 1
  [total dose/cycle = 100 mg/m^2]
Cytarabine: I.V.: 2000 mg/m^2 every 12 hours for 2 doses day 2 (begins at the
  end of the cisplatin infusion)
  [total dose/cycle = 4000 mg/m^2]
Repeat cycle every 3-4 weeks for 6-10 cycles

Variation 2 (patients >70 years of age):

Dexamethasone: I.V. or Oral: 40 mg/day days 1 to 4
  [total dose/cycle = 160 mg]
Cisplatin: I.V.: 100 mg/m^2 over 24 hours day 1
  [total dose/cycle = 100 mg/m^2]
Cytarabine: I.V.: 1000 mg/m^2 every 12 hours for 2 doses day 2 (begins at the
  end of the cisplatin infusion)
  [total dose/cycle = 2000 mg/m^2]
Repeat cycle every 3-4 weeks for 6-10 cycles

References

Variation 1 and 2:

Velasquez WS, Cabanillas F, Salvador P, et al, "Effective Salvage Therapy for Lymphoma With Cisplatin in Combination With High-Dose Ara-C and Dexamethasone (DHAP)," *Blood*, 1988, 71 (1):117-22.

Cisplatin-Dacarbazine-Carmustine (Melanoma)

Index Terms Carmustine-Cisplatin-Dacarbazine; Dacarbazine-Carmustine-Cisplatin

Use Melanoma

Regimen NOTE: Multiple variations are listed.

Variation 1:

Cisplatin: I.V.: 25 mg/m^2/day days 1, 2, and 3
  [total dose/cycle = 75 mg/m^2]
Dacarbazine: I.V.: 220 mg/m^2/day days 1, 2, and 3
  [total dose/cycle = 660 mg/m^2]
Carmustine: I.V.: 150 mg/m^2 day 1 (every other cycle **[odd cycles]**)
  [total dose/**odd** cycles = 150 mg/m^2]
Repeat cycle every 21 days

Variation 2:

Carmustine: I.V.: 150 mg/m^2 day 1
  [total dose/cycle = 150 mg/m^2]
Cisplatin: I.V.: 25 mg/m^2/day days 1, 2, 3, 22, 23, and 24
  [total dose/cycle = 150 mg/m^2]
Dacarbazine: I.V.: 220 mg/m^2/day days 1, 2, 3, 22, 23, and 24
  [total dose/cycle = 1320 mg/m^2]
Repeat cycle every 42 days

References

Variation 1:
Creagan ET, Suman VJ, Dalton RJ, et al, "Phase III Clinical Trial of the Combination of Cisplatin, Dacarbazine, and Carmustine With or Without Tamoxifen in Patients With Advanced Malignant Melanoma," *J Clin Oncol*, 1999, 17(6):1884-90.

Variation 2:
Rusthoven JJ, Quirt IC, Iscoe NA, et al, "Randomized, Double-Blind, Placebo-Controlled Trial Comparing the Response Rates of Carmustine, Dacarbazine, and Cisplatin With and Without Tamoxifen in Patients With Metastatic Melanoma. National Cancer Institute of Canada Clinical Trials Group," *J Clin Oncol*, 1996, 14(7):2083-90.

♦ Cisplatin-Dacarbazine-Carmustine-Tamoxifen *see* Dartmouth Regimen on page 1286

Cisplatin-Dacarbazine-Interferon Alfa-2b-Aldesleukin

Index Terms Dacarbazine-Cisplatin-Interferon Alfa-2b-Aldesleukin

Use Melanoma

Regimen

Cisplatin: I.V.: 25 mg/m^2/day days 1, 2, and 3
[total dose/cycle = 75 mg/m^2]
Dacarbazine: 250 mg/m^2/day days 1, 2, and 3
[total dose/cycle = 750 mg/m^2]
Interferon Alfa-2b: SubQ: 5 million units/m^2/day days 6, 8, 10, 13, and 15
[total dose/cycle = 25 million units/m^2]
Aldesleukin: I.V.: 18 million units/m^2/day days 6 to 10, 13, 14, and 15
[total dose/cycle = 144 million units/m^2]
Repeat cycle every 28 days

References

Flaherty LE, Atkins M, Sosman J, et al, "Outpatient Biochemotherapy With Interleukin-2 and Interferon Alfa-2b in Patients With Metastatic Malignant Melanoma: Results of Two Phase II Cytokine Working Group Trials," *J Clin Oncol*, 2001, 19(13):3194-202.

Cisplatin-Docetaxel

Use Bladder cancer

Regimen

Cisplatin: I.V.: 30 mg/m^2 day 1
[total dose/cycle = 30 mg/m^2]
Docetaxel: I.V.: 40 mg/m^2 day 4
[total dose/cycle = 40 mg/m^2]
Repeat cycle weekly for 8 weeks

References

Varveris H, Delakas D, Anezinis P, et al, "Concurrent Platinum and Docetaxel Chemotherapy and External Radical Radiotherapy in Patients With Invasive Transitional Cell Bladder Carcinoma. A Preliminary Report of Tolerance and Local Control," *Anticancer Res*, 1997, 17(6D):4771-80.

Cisplatin-Etoposide (NSCLC)

Index Terms Etoposide-Cisplatin

Use Lung cancer, nonsmall cell

Regimen NOTE: Multiple variations are listed.

Variation 1:
Cisplatin: I.V.: 80 mg/m^2 day 1
[total dose/cycle = 80 mg/m^2]
Etoposide: I.V.: 100 mg/m^2/day days 1, 2, and 3
[total dose/cycle = 300 mg/m^2]
Repeat cycle every 21 days for a total of 4 cycles

Variation 2:
Cisplatin: I.V.: 100 mg/m^2 day 1
[total dose/cycle = 100 mg/m^2]
Etoposide: I.V.: 100 mg/m^2/day days 1, 2, and 3
[total dose/cycle = 300 mg/m^2]
Repeat cycle every 28 days for a total of 3 cycles
Variation 3:
Cisplatin: I.V.: 100 mg/m^2 day 1
[total dose/cycle = 100 mg/m^2]
Etoposide: I.V.: 100 mg/m^2/day days 1, 2, and 3
[total dose/cycle = 300 mg/m^2]
Repeat cycle every 28 days for a total of 4 cycles
Variation 4:
Cisplatin: I.V.: 120 mg/m^2/day days 1, 29, and 71
[total dose/treatment = 360 mg/m^2]
Etoposide: I.V.: 100 mg/m^2/day days 1, 2, 3, 29, 30, 31, 71, 72, and 73
[total dose/treatment = 900 mg/m^2]
Variation 5:
Cisplatin: I.V.: 75 mg/m^2 day 1
[total dose/cycle = 75 mg/m^2]
Etoposide: I.V.: 100 mg/m^2/day days 1, 2, and 3
[total dose/cycle = 300 mg/m^2]
Repeat cycle every 21 days for up to 10 cycles

References

Variations 1-4:
Arriagada R, Bergman B, Dunant A, et al, "Cisplatin-Based Adjuvant Chemotherapy in Patients With Completely Resected Non-Small-Cell Lung Cancer," *N Engl J Med*, 2004, 350(4):351-60.
Variation 5:
Belani CP, Lee JS, Socinski MA, et al, "Randomized Phase III Trial Comparing Cisplatin-Etoposide to Carboplatin-Paclitaxel in Advanced or Metastatic Non-Small Cell Lung Cancer," *Ann Oncol*, 2005, 16(7):1069-75.

Cisplatin-Fluorouracil (Bladder Cancer)

Index Terms Fluorouracil-Cisplatin (Bladder Cancer)

Use Bladder cancer

Regimen In combination with radiation therapy

Note: Begin infusion(s) 2 hours before radiation therapy on days 1, 3, 15, and 17:
Cisplatin: I.V.: 15 mg/m^2/day over 2 hours days 1, 2, 3, 15, 16, and 17
[total dose/cycle = 90 mg/m^2]
Fluorouracil: I.V.: 400 mg/m^2/day over 2 hours days 1, 2, 3, 15, 16, and 17
[total dose/cycle = 2400 mg/m^2]

References

Housset M, Maulard C, Chretien Y, et al, "Combined Radiation and Chemotherapy for Invasive Transitional-Cell Carcinoma of the Bladder: A Prospective Study," *J Clin Oncol*, 1993, 11 (11):2150-7.

Cisplatin-Fluorouracil (Cervical Cancer)

Index Terms Fluorouracil-Cisplatin (Cervical Cancer)

Use Cervical cancer

Regimen NOTE: Multiple variations are listed.
Variation 1:
Cisplatin: I.V.: 75 mg/m^2 day 1
[total dose/cycle = 75 mg/m^2]
Fluorouracil: I.V.: 1000 mg/m^2/day continuous infusion days 1 to 4 (96 hours)
[total dose/cycle = 4000 mg/m^2]
Repeat cycle every 21 days

◀ Variation 2:
Cisplatin: I.V.: 50 mg/m^2 day 1 starting 4 hours before radiotherapy
[total dose/cycle = 50 mg/m^2]
Fluorouracil: I.V.: 1000 mg/m^2/day continuous infusion days 2 to 5 (96 hours)
[total dose/cycle = 4000 mg/m^2]
Repeat cycle every 28 days
Variation 3:
Cisplatin: I.V.: 70 mg/m^2 day 1
[total dose/cycle = 70 mg/m^2]
Fluorouracil: I.V.: 1000 mg/m^2/day continuous infusion days 1 to 4 (96 hours)
[total dose/cycle = 4000 mg/m^2]
Repeat cycle every 21 days

References

Variation 1:
Morris M, Eifel PJ, Lu J, et al, "Pelvic Radiation With Concurrent Chemotherapy Compared With Pelvic and Para-aortic Radiation for High-Risk Cervical Cancer," *N Engl J Med*, 1999, 340 (15):1137-43.
Variation 2:
Whitney CW, Sause W, Bundy BN, et al, "Randomized Comparison of Fluorouracil Plus Cisplatin Versus Hydroxyurea as an Adjunct to Radiation Therapy in Stage IIB-IVA Carcinoma of the Cervix With Negative Para-aortic Lymph Nodes: A Gynecologic Oncology Group and Southwest Oncology Group Study," *J Clin Oncol*, 1999, 17(5):1339-48.
Variation 3:
Peters WA 3rd, Liu PY, Barrett RJ 2nd, et al, "Concurrent Chemotherapy and Pelvic Radiation Therapy Compared With Pelvic Radiation Therapy Alone as Adjuvant Therapy After Radical Surgery in High-Risk Early-Stage Cancer of the Cervix," *J Clin Oncol*, 2000, 18(8):1606-13.

◆ **Cisplatin-Fluorouracil-Cetuximab** *see* Cetuximab-Cisplatin-Fluorouracil
on page 1256

Cisplatin-Fluorouracil (Esophageal Cancer)

Index Terms CF (Esophageal Cancer); Fluorouracil-Cisplatin (Esophageal Cancer)

Use Esophageal cancer

Regimen NOTE: Multiple variations are listed.
Variation 1:
Cisplatin: I.V.: 100 mg/m^2/dose day 1
[total dose/cycle = 100 mg/m^2]
Fluorouracil: I.V.: 1000 mg/m^2/day continuous infusion days 1 to 5
[total dose/cycle = 5000 mg/m^2]
Repeat cycle every 28 days
Variation 2:
Cycles 1 to 3 (prior to surgery):
Cisplatin: I.V.: 100 mg/m^2/dose day 1
[total dose/cycle = 100 mg/m^2]
Fluorouracil: I.V.: 1000 mg/m^2/day continuous infusion days 1 to 5
[total dose/cycle = 5000 mg/m^2]
Treatment cycles 1-3 are 28 days each
Cycles 4 and 5 (postoperative):
Cisplatin: I.V.: 75 mg/m^2/dose day 1
[total dose/cycle = 75 mg/m^2]
Fluorouracil: I.V.: 1000 mg/m^2/day continuous infusion days 1 to 5
[total dose/cycle = 5000 mg/m^2]
Treatment cycles 4 and 5 are 28 days each

Variation 3 (in combination with radiation therapy):
Cycle 1:
Cisplatin: I.V.: 75 mg/m^2/dose day 1
[total dose/cycle = 75 mg/m^2]
Fluorouracil: I.V.: 1000 mg/m^2/day continuous infusion days 1 to 4
[total dose/cycle = 4000 mg/m^2]
Treatment cycle is 28 days
Cycles 2 to 4:
Cisplatin: I.V.: 75 mg/m^2/dose day 1
[total dose/cycle = 75 mg/m^2]
Fluorouracil: I.V.: 1000 mg/m^2/day continuous infusion days 1 to 4
[total dose/cycle = 4000 mg/m^2]
Repeat cycle every 21 days for 3 more cycles (total of 4 cycles)
Variation 4 (in combination with radiation therapy):
Cisplatin: I.V.: 100 mg/m^2/dose day 1
[total dose/cycle = 100 mg/m^2]
Fluorouracil: I.V.: 1000 mg/m^2/day continuous infusion days 1 to 4
[total dose/cycle = 4000 mg/m^2]
Repeat cycle every 28 days for total of 2 cycles
Variation 5 (in combination with radiation therapy):
Cisplatin: I.V.: 75 mg/m^2/dose day 1
[total dose/cycle = 75 mg/m^2]
Fluorouracil: I.V.: 1000 mg/m^2/day continuous infusion days 1 to 4
[total dose/cycle = 4000 mg/m^2]
Repeat cycle every 28 days for 4 cycles
Variation 6 (in combination with radiation therapy):
Cycles 1 and 2:
Cisplatin: I.V.: 75 mg/m^2/dose day 1
[total dose/cycle = 75 mg/m^2]
Fluorouracil: I.V.: 1000 mg/m^2/day continuous infusion days 1 to 4
[total dose/cycle = 4000 mg/m^2]
Treatment cycles 1 and 2 are 28 days each; cycle 2 is followed by a 2-week rest
Cycles 3 and 4 (begin cycle 3 at week 11):
Cisplatin: I.V.: 75 mg/m^2/dose day 1
[total dose/cycle = 75 mg/m^2]
Fluorouracil: I.V.: 1000 mg/m^2/day continuous infusion days 1 to 4
[total dose/cycle = 4000 mg/m^2]
Treatment cycles 3 and 4 are 28 days each
Variation 7 (in combination with radiation therapy):
Cycles 1 to 4:
Cisplatin: I.V.: 15 mg/m^2/day days 1 to 5
[total dose/cycle = 75 mg/m^2]
Fluorouracil: I.V.: 800 mg/m^2/day continuous infusion days 1 to 5
[total dose/cycle = 4000 mg/m^2]
Repeat cycles 1-4 every 21 days; cycle 4 is followed by a 1-week rest
Cycles 5 (begin cycle 5 at week 14):
Cisplatin: I.V.: 15 mg/m^2/day days 1 to 5
[total dose/cycle = 75 mg/m^2]
Fluorouracil: I.V.: 800 mg/m^2/day continuous infusion days 1 to 5
[total dose/cycle = 4000 mg/m^2]

References

Variation 1:
Ajani JA, Moiseyenko VM, Tjulandin S, et al, "Quality of Life With Docetaxel Plus Cisplatin and Fluorouracil Compared With Cisplatin and Fluorouracil From a Phase III Trial for Advanced

Gastric or Gastroesophageal Adenocarcinoma: The V-325 Study Group," *J Clin Oncol*, 2007, 25 (22):3210-6.

Variation 2:

Kelsen DP, Ginsberg R, Pajak TF, et al, "Chemotherapy Followed by Surgery Compared With Surgery Alone for Localized Esophageal Cancer," *N Engl J Med*, 1998, 339(27):1979-84.

Variation 3:

Cooper JS, Guo MD, Herskovic A, et al, "Chemoradiotherapy of Locally Advanced Esophageal Cancer: Long-Term Follow-Up of a Prospective Randomized Trial (RTOG 85-01). Radiation Therapy Oncology Group," *JAMA*, 1999, 281(17):1623-7.

Variation 4:

Tepper J, Krasna MJ, Niedzwiecki D, et al, "Phase III Trial of Trimodality Therapy With Cisplatin, Fluorouracil, Radiotherapy, and Surgery Compared With Surgery Alone for Esophageal Cancer: CALGB 9781," *J Clin Oncol*, 2008, 26(7):1086-92.

Variation 5 and 6:

Minsky BD, Pajak TF, Ginsberg RJ, et al, "INT 0123 (Radiation Therapy Oncology Group 94-05) Phase III Trial of Combined-Modality Therapy for Esophageal Cancer: High-Dose Versus Standard-Dose Radiation Therapy," *J Clin Oncol*, 2002, 20(5):1167-74.

Variation 7:

Bedenne L, Michel P, Bouché O, et al, "Chemoradiation Followed by Surgery Compared With Chemoradiation Alone in Squamous Cancer of the Esophagus: FFCD 9102," *J Clin Oncol*, 2007, 25(10):1160-8.

Cisplatin-Fluorouracil (Head and Neck Cancer)

Index Terms CF (Head and Neck Cancer); Fluorouracil-Cisplatin (Head and Neck Cancer)

Use Head and neck cancer

Regimen NOTE: Multiple variations are listed.

Variation 1:

Cisplatin: I.V.: 100 mg/m^2 day 1

[total dose/cycle = 100 mg/m^2]

Fluorouracil: I.V.: 1000 mg/m^2/day continuous infusion days 1 to 4

[total dose/cycle = 4000 mg/m^2]

Repeat cycle every 3 or 4 weeks

Variation 2:

Cisplatin: I.V.: 100 mg/m^2 day 1

[total dose/cycle = 100 mg/m^2]

Fluorouracil: I.V.: 1000 mg/m^2/day continuous infusion days 1 to 5

[total dose/cycle = 5000 mg/m^2]

Repeat cycle every 3 or 4 weeks

Variation 3:

Cisplatin: I.V.: 60 mg/m^2 day 1

[total dose/cycle = 60 mg/m^2]

Fluorouracil: I.V.: 800 mg/m^2/day continuous infusion days 1 to 5

[total dose/cycle = 4000 mg/m^2]

Repeat cycle every 14 days

Variation 4:

Cisplatin: I.V.: 20 mg/m^2/day days 1 to 5

[total dose/cycle = 100 mg/m^2]

Fluorouracil: I.V.: 200 mg/m^2/day days 1 to 5

[total dose/cycle = 1000 mg/m^2]

Repeat cycle every 3 weeks

Variation 5:

Cisplatin: I.V.: 80 mg/m^2 continuous infusion day 1

[total dose/cycle = 80 mg/m^2]

Fluorouracil: I.V.: 800 mg/m^2/day continuous infusion days 2 to 6

[total dose/cycle = 4000 mg/m^2]

Repeat cycle every 3 weeks

Variation 6:
  Cisplatin: I.V.: 75 mg/m² day 1
    [total dose/cycle = 75 mg/m²]
  Fluorouracil: I.V.: 1000 mg/m²/day continuous infusion days 1 to 4
    [total dose/cycle = 4000 mg/m²]
  Repeat cycle every 4 weeks
Variation 7:
  Cisplatin: I.V.: 120 mg/m² day 1
    [total dose/cycle = 120 mg/m²]
  Fluorouracil: I.V.: 1000 mg/m²/day continuous infusion days 1 to 5
    [total dose/cycle = 5000 mg/m²]
  Repeat cycle every 3 weeks
Variation 8:
  Cisplatin: I.V.: 25 mg/m²/day continuous infusion days 1 to 4
    [total dose/cycle = 100 mg/m²]
  Fluorouracil: I.V.: 1000 mg/m²/day days 1 to 4
    [total dose/cycle = 4000 mg/m²]
  Repeat cycle every 3 weeks
Variation 9:
  Fluorouracil: I.V.: 350 mg/m²/day days 1 to 5
    [total dose/cycle = 1750 mg/m²]
  Cisplatin: I.V.: 50 mg/m² day 6
    [total dose/cycle = 50 mg/m²]
  Repeat cycle every 3 weeks
Variation 10:
  Cisplatin: I.V.: 5 mg/m²/day continuous infusion days 1 to 14
    [total dose/cycle = 70 mg/m²]
  Fluorouracil: I.V.: 200 mg/m²/day continuous infusion days 1 to 14
    [total dose/cycle = 2800 mg/m²]
  With concurrent radiation therapy, cycle does not repeat

References

Variation 1:
Kish J, Drelichman A, Jacobs J, et al, "Clinical Trial of Cisplatin and 5-FU Infusion as Initial Treatment for Advanced Squamous Cell Carcinoma of the Head and Neck," *Cancer Treat Rep*, 1982, 66(3):471-4.

Mercier RJ, Neal GD, Mattox DE, et al, "Cisplatin and 5-Fluorouracil Chemotherapy in Advanced or Recurrent Squamous Cell Carcinoma of the Head and Neck," *Cancer*, 1987, 60(11):2609-12.
Variation 2:
Rooney M, Kish J, Jacobs J, et al, "Improved Complete Response Rate and Survival in Advanced Head and Neck Cancer After Three-Course Induction Therapy With 120-Hour 5-FU Infusion and Cisplatin," *Cancer*, 1985, 55(5):1123-8.

Dasmahapatra KS, Citrin P, Hill GJ, et al, "A Prospective Evaluation of 5-Fluorouracil Plus Cisplatin in Advanced Squamous-Cell Cancer of the Head and Neck," *J Clin Oncol*, 1985, 3(11):1486-9.
Variation 3:
Taylor SG 4th, Murthy AK, Showel JL, et al, "Improved Control in Advanced Head and Neck Cancer With Simultaneous Radiation and Cisplatin/5-FU Chemotherapy," *Cancer Treat Rep*, 1985, 69 (9):933-9.
Variation 4:
Merlano M, Tatarek R, Grimaldi A, et al, "Phase I-II Trial With Cisplatin and 5-FU in Recurrent Head and Neck Cancer: An Effective Outpatient Schedule," *Cancer Treat Rep*, 1985, 69(9):961-4.
Variation 5:
Amrein PC and Weitzman SA, "Treatment of Squamous-Cell Carcinoma of the Head and Neck With Cisplatin and 5-Fluorouracil," *J Clin Oncol*, 1985, 3(12):1632-9.
Variation 6:
Adelstein DJ, Li Y, Adams GL, et al, "An Intergroup Phase III Comparison of Standard Radiation and Two Schedules of Concurrent Chemoradiotherapy in Patients With Unresectable Squamous Cell Head and Neck Cancer," *J Clin Oncol*, 2003, 21(1):92-8.

Adelstein DJ, Sharan VM, Earle AS, et al, "Chemoradiotherapy as Initial Management in Patients With Squamous Cell Carcinoma of the Head and Neck," *Cancer Treat Rep*, 1986, 70(6):761-7.

Variation 7:
Paredes J, Hong WK, Felder TB, et al, "Prospective Randomized Trial of High-Dose Cisplatin and Fluorouracil Infusion With or Without Sodium Diethyldithiocarbamate in Recurrent and/or Metastatic Squamous Cell Carcinoma of the Head and Neck," *J Clin Oncol*, 1988, 6(6):955-62.

Variation 8:
Bernal AG, Cruz JJ, Sanchez P, et al, "Four-Day Continuous Infusion of Cisplatin and 5-Fluorouracil in Head and Neck Cancer," *Cancer*, 1989, 63(10):1927-30.

Variation 9:
Denham JW and Abbott RL, "Concurrent Cisplatin, Infusional Fluorouracil, and Conventionally Fractionated Radiation Therapy in Head and Neck Cancer: Dose-Limiting Mucosal Toxicity," *J Clin Oncol*, 1991, 9(3):458-63.

Variation 10:
Arcangeli G, Saracino B, Danesi DT, et al, "Accelerated Hyperfractionated Radiotherapy and Concurrent Protracted Venous Infusion Chemotherapy in Locally-Advanced Head and Neck Cancer," *Am J Clin Oncol*, 2002, 25(5):431-7.

Cisplatin-Irinotecan (Small Cell Lung Cancer)

Index Terms Irinotecan-Cisplatin (Small Cell Lung Cancer)

Use Lung cancer, small cell

Regimen
Cisplatin: I.V.: 60 mg/m^2 day 1
[total dose/cycle = 60 mg/m^2]
Irinotecan: I.V.: 60 mg/m^2/dose days 1, 8, and 15
[total dose/cycle = 180 mg/m^2]
Repeat cycle every 28 days for 4 cycles

References
Noda K, Nishiwaki Y, Kawahara M, et al, "Irinotecan Plus Cisplatin Compared With Etoposide Plus Cisplatin for Extensive Small-Cell Lung Cancer," *N Engl J Med*, 2002, 346(2):85-91.

Cisplatin-Paclitaxel (Intraperitoneal Regimen)

Index Terms Paclitaxel-Cisplatin (Intraperitoneal Regimen)

Use Ovarian cancer

Regimen Note: I.P. therapies administered in 2 liters warmed saline
Paclitaxel: I.V.: 135 mg/m^2 continuous infusion (over 24 hours) day 1
[total dose/cycle = 135 mg/m^2]
Cisplatin: I.P.: 100 mg/m^2 day 2
[total dose/cycle = 100 mg/m^2]
Paclitaxel: I.P.: 60 mg/m^2 day 8
[total dose/cycle = 60 mg/m^2]
Repeat cycle every 21 days for 6 cycles

References

Armstrong DK, Bundy B, Wenzel L, et al, "Intraperitoneal Cisplatin and Paclitaxel in Ovarian Cancer," *N Engl J Med*, 2006, 354(1):34-43.

Cisplatin-Paclitaxel (Ovarian Cancer)

Index Terms Paclitaxel-Cisplatin (Ovarian Cancer)

Use Ovarian cancer

Regimen NOTE: Multiple variations are listed.

Variation 1:

Paclitaxel: I.V.: 135 mg/m^2 continuous infusion over 24 hours day 1

[total dose/cycle = 135 mg/m^2]

Cisplatin: I.V.: 75 mg/m^2 day 2

[total dose/cycle = 75 mg/m^2]

Repeat cycle every 21 days for a total of 6 cycles

Variation 2:

Paclitaxel: I.V.: 175 mg/m^2 over 3 hours day 1

[total dose/cycle = 175 mg/m^2]

Cisplatin: I.V.: 75 mg/m^2 day 1

[total dose/cycle = 75 mg/m^2]

Repeat cycle every 21 days for a total of at least 6 cycles

Variation 3:

Paclitaxel: I.V.: 185 mg/m^2 (maximum dose: 400 mg) over 3 hours day 1

[total dose/cycle = 185 mg/m^2; maximum: 400 mg]

Cisplatin: I.V.: 75 mg/m^2 (maximum dose: 165 mg) day 1

[total dose/cycle = 75 mg/m^2; maximum: 165 mg]

Repeat cycle every 21 days

References

Variation 1:

McGuire WP, Hoskins WJ, Brady MF, et al, "Cyclophosphamide and Cisplatin Compared With Paclitaxel and Cisplatin in Patients With Stage III and Stage IV Ovarian Cancer," *N Engl J Med*, 1996, 334(1):1-6.

Muggia FM, Braly PS, Brady MF, et al, "Phase III Randomized Study of Cisplatin Versus Paclitaxel Versus Cisplatin and Paclitaxel in Patients With Suboptimal Stage III or IV Ovarian Cancer: A Gynecologic Oncology Group Study," *J Clin Oncol*, 2000, 18(1):106-15.

Variation 2:

Neijt JP, Engelholm SA, Tuxen MK, et al, "Exploratory Phase III Study of Paclitaxel and Cisplatin Versus Paclitaxel and Carboplatin in Advanced Ovarian Cancer," *J Clin Oncol*, 2000, 18 (17):3084-92.

Variation 3:

du Bois A, Lück HJ, Meier W, et al, "A Randomized Clinical Trial of Cisplatin/Paclitaxel Versus Carboplatin/Paclitaxel as First-Line Treatment of Ovarian Cancer," *J Natl Cancer Inst*, 2003, 95 (17):1320-9.

Cisplatin-Pemetrexed (Mesothelioma)

Index Terms Pemetrexed-Cisplatin (Mesothelioma)

Use Malignant pleural mesothelioma

Regimen

Pemetrexed: I.V.: 500 mg/m^2 infused over 10 minutes day 1

[total dose/cycle = 500 mg/m^2]

Cisplatin: I.V.: 75 mg/m^2 infused over 2 hours day 1 (start 30 minutes after pemetrexed)

[total dose/cycle = 75 mg/m^2]

Repeat cycle every 21 days

References

Vogelzang NJ, Rusthoven JJ, Symanowski J, et al, "Phase III Study of Pemetrexed in Combination With Cisplatin Versus Cisplatin Alone in Patients With Malignant Pleural Mesothelioma," *J Clin Oncol*, 2003, 21(14):2636-44.

◆ **Cisplatin-Pemetrexed (NSCLC)** *see* Pemetrexed-Cisplatin (NSCLC) *on page 1394*

◆ **Cisplatin-Topotecan (Oral)** *see* Topotecan (Oral)-Cisplatin *on page 1407*

Cisplatin-Vinblastine-Dacarbazine (Melanoma)

Index Terms CVD; Dacarbazine-Cisplatin-Vinblastine; Vinblastine-Cisplatin-Dacarbazine

Use Melanoma

Regimen NOTE: Multiple variations are listed.

Variation 1:
Cisplatin: I.V.: 20 mg/m^2/day days 2 to 5
[total dose/cycle = 80 mg/m^2]
Vinblastine: I.V.: 1.6 mg/m^2/day days 1 to 5
[total dose/cycle = 8 mg/m^2]
Dacarbazine: I.V.: 800 mg/m^2 day 1
[total dose/cycle = 800 mg/m^2]
Repeat cycle every 21 days

Variation 2:
Cisplatin: I.V.: 20 mg/m^2/day days 1 to 4
[total dose/cycle = 80 mg/m^2]
Vinblastine: I.V.: 2 mg/m^2/day days 1 to 4
[total dose/cycle = 8 mg/m^2]
Dacarbazine: I.V.: 800 mg/m^2 day 1
[total dose/cycle = 800 mg/m^2]
Repeat cycle every 21 days

References

Variation 1:
Legha SS, Ring S, Papadopoulos N, et al, "A Prospective Evaluation of a Triple-Drug Regimen Containing Cisplatin, Vinblastine, and Dacarbazine (CVD) for Metastatic Melanoma," *Cancer*, 1989, 64(10):2024-9.

Variation 2:
Eton O, Legha SS, Bedikian AY, et al, "Sequential Biochemotherapy Versus Chemotherapy for Metastatic Melanoma: Results From a Phase III Randomized Trial," *J Clin Oncol*, 2002, 20 (8):2045-52.

Cisplatin-Vinblastine (NSCLC)

Index Terms Vinblastine-Cisplatin

Use Lung cancer, nonsmall cell

Regimen NOTE: Multiple variations are listed.

Variation 1:
Cisplatin: I.V.: 80 mg/m^2/day days 1, 22, 43, and 64
[total dose/treatment = 320 mg/m^2]
Vinblastine: I.V.: 4 mg/m^2/day days 1, 8, 15, 22, 29, 43, and 57
[total dose/treatment = 28 mg/m^2]

Variation 2:
Cisplatin: I.V.: 100 mg/m^2/day days 1, 29, and 57
[total dose/treatment = 300 mg/m^2]
Vinblastine: I.V.: 4 mg/m^2/day days 1, 8, 15, 22, 29, 43, and 57
[total dose/treatment = 28 mg/m^2]

Variation 3:
Cisplatin: I.V.: 100 mg/m^2/day days 1, 29, 57, and 85
[total dose/treatment = 400 mg/m^2]
Vinblastine: I.V.: 4 mg/m^2/day days 1, 8, 15, 22, 29, 43, 57, 71, and 85
[total dose/treatment = 36 mg/m^2]

Variation 4:
Cisplatin: I.V.: 120 mg/m^2/day days 1, 29, and 71
[total dose/treatment = 360 mg/m^2]
Vinblastine: I.V.: 4 mg/m^2/day days 1, 8, 15, 22, 29, 43, 57, and 71
[total dose/treatment = 32 mg/m^2]

References

Arriagada R, Bergman B, Dunant A, et al, "Cisplatin-Based Adjuvant Chemotherapy in Patients With Completely Resected Non-Small-Cell Lung Cancer," *N Engl J Med*, 2004, 350(4):351-60.

Cisplatin-Vinorelbine

Use Cervical cancer
Regimen
Cisplatin: I.V.: 80 mg/m^2 day 1
[total dose/cycle = 80 mg/m^2]
Vinorelbine: I.V.: 25 mg/m^2/day days 1 and 8
[total dose/cycle = 50 mg/m^2]
Repeat cycle every 21 days

References

Pignata S, Silvestro G, Ferrari E, et al, "Phase II Study of Cisplatin and Vinorelbine as First-Line Chemotherapy in Patients With Carcinoma of the Uterine Cervix," *J Clin Oncol*, 1999, 17 (3):756-60.

♦ **Cisplatin-Vinorelbine** see Vinorelbine-Cisplatin *on page 1422*

♦ **Cisplatin-Vinorelbine-Cetuximab** see Cetuximab-Cisplatin-Vinorelbine *on page 1256*

♦ **Cisplatin-Vinblastine-Dacarbazine-Interleukin-Interferon (Melanoma)** see CVD-Interleukin-Interferon (Melanoma) *on page 1282*

CMF

Use Breast cancer
Regimen NOTE: Multiple variations are listed.
Variation 1:
Methotrexate: I.V.: 40 mg/m^2/day days 1 and 8
[total dose/cycle = 80 mg/m^2]
Fluorouracil: I.V.: 600 mg/m^2/day days 1 and 8
[total dose/cycle = 1200 mg/m^2]
Cyclophosphamide: Oral: 100 mg/m^2/day days 1 to 14
[total dose/cycle = 1400 mg/m^2]
Repeat cycle every 28 days
Variation 2 (>60 years of age):
Methotrexate: I.V.: 30 mg/m^2/day days 1 and 8
[total dose/cycle = 60 mg/m^2]
Fluorouracil: I.V.: 400 mg/m^2/day days 1 and 8
[total dose/cycle = 800 mg/m^2]
Cyclophosphamide: Oral: 100 mg/m^2/day days 1 to 14
[total dose/cycle = 1400 mg/m^2]
Repeat cycle every 28 days

References

Variations 1 and 2:
Bonadonna G, Brusamolino E, Valagussa P, et al, "Combination Chemotherapy as an Adjuvant Treatment in Operable Breast Cancer," *N Engl J Med*, 1976, 294(8):405-10.
Canellos GP, Pocock SJ, Taylor SG III, et al, "Combination Chemotherapy for Metastatic Breast Carcinoma, Prospective Comparison of Multiple Drug Therapy With L-Phenylalanine Mustard," *Cancer*, 1976, 38(5):1882-6.

CMF-IV

Use Breast cancer

Regimen

Cyclophosphamide: I.V.: 600 mg/m^2 day 1
  [total dose/cycle = 600 mg/m^2]
Methotrexate: I.V.: 40 mg/m^2 day 1
  [total dose/cycle = 40 mg/m^2]
Fluorouracil: I.V.: 600 mg/m^2 day 1
  [total dose/cycle = 600 mg/m^2]
Repeat cycle every 21 or 28 days

References

Bonadonna G, Veronesi U, Brambilla C, et al, "Primary Chemotherapy to Avoid Mastectomy in Tumors With Diameters of Three Centimeters or More," *J Natl Cancer Inst*, 1990, 82 (19):1539-45.

Tannock IF, Boyd NF, DeBoer G, et al, "A Randomized Trial of Two Dose Levels of Cyclophosphamide, Methotrexate, and Fluorouracil Chemotherapy for Patients With Metastatic Breast Cancer," *J Clin Oncol*, 1988, 6(9):1377-87.

CMFP

Use Breast cancer

Regimen

Cyclophosphamide: Oral: 100 mg/m^2/day days 1 to 14
  [total dose = 1400 mg/m^2]
Methotrexate: I.V.: 30 or 40 mg/m^2/day days 1 and 8
  [total dose = 60 or 80 mg/m^2]
Fluorouracil: I.V.: 400 or 600 mg/m^2/day days 1 and 8
  [total dose = 800 or 1200 mg/m^2]
Prednisone: Oral: 40 mg/m^2/day days 1 to 14
  [total dose = 560 mg/m^2]
Repeat cycle every 28 days

References

Marschke RF Jr, Ingle JN, Schaid DJ, et al, "Randomized Clinical Trial of CFP Versus CMFP in Women With Metastatic Breast Cancer," *Cancer*, 1989, 63(10):1931-7.

CMFVP (Cooper Regimen, VPCMF)

Use Breast cancer

Regimen

Cyclophosphamide: Oral: 2 mg/kg/day days 1 to 252
  [total dose/cycle = 504 mg/kg]
Methotrexate: I.V.: 0.7 mg/kg day 1, weeks 1 to 8, 10, 12, 14, 16, 18, 20, 22, 24, 26, 28, 30, 32, 34, and 36
  [total dose/cycle = 15.4 mg/kg]
Fluorouracil: I.V.: 12 mg/kg day 1, weeks 1 to 8, 10, 12, 14, 16, 18, 20, 22, 24, 26, 28, 30, 32, 34, and 36
  [total dose/cycle = 264 mg/kg]
Vincristine: I.V.: 0.035 mg/kg (maximum dose: 2 mg) day 1, weeks 1 to 5, 8, 12, 16, 20, 24, 28, 32, and 36
  [total dose/cycle = 0.455 mg/kg]
Prednisone: Oral: 0.75 mg/kg/day days 1 to 10, taper off over next 40 days
Administer one cycle only

References

Cooper RG, Holland JF, and Glidewell O, "Adjuvant Chemotherapy of Breast Cancer," *Cancer*, 1979, 44(3):793-8.

◆ **C MOPP** *see* COPP *on page* 1281

CMV

Use Bladder cancer

Regimen

Cisplatin: I.V.: 100 mg/m² infused over 4 hours (start at least 12 hours after methotrexate) day 2
[total dose = 100 mg/m²]
Methotrexate: I.V.: 30 mg/m²/day days 1 and 8
[total dose = 60 mg/m²]
Vinblastine: I.V.: 4 mg/m²/day days 1 and 8
[total dose = 8 mg/m²]
Repeat cycle every 21 days

References

Harker WG, Meyers FJ, Freiha FS, et al, "Cisplatin, Methotrexate, and Vinblastine (CMV): An Effective Chemotherapy Regimen for Metastatic Transitional Cell Carcinoma of the Urinary Tract. A Northern California Oncology Group Study," *J Clin Oncol*, 1985, 3(11):1463-70.

CNF

Index Terms CFM; FNC

Use Breast cancer

Regimen NOTE: Multiple variations are listed.

Variation 1:
Cyclophosphamide: I.V.: 500 mg/m² day 1
[total dose/cycle = 500 mg/m²]
Mitoxantrone: I.V.: 10 mg/m² day 1
[total dose/cycle = 10 mg/m²]
Fluorouracil: I.V.: 500 mg/m² day 1
[total dose/cycle = 500 mg/m²]
Repeat cycle every 21 days

Variation 2:
Cyclophosphamide: I.V.: 500-600 mg/m² day 1
[total dose/cycle = 500-600 mg/m²]
Fluorouracil: I.V.: 500-600 mg/m² day 1
[total dose/cycle = 500-600 mg/m²]
Mitoxantrone: I.V.: 10-12 mg/m² day 1
[total dose/cycle = 10-12 mg/m²]
Repeat cycle every 21 days

References

Variation 1:
Bennett JM, Muss HB, Doroshow JH, et al, "A Randomized Multicenter Trial Comparing Mitixantrone, Cyclophosphamide, and Fluorouracil With Doxorubicin, Cyclophosphamide, and Fluorouracil in the Therapy of Metastatic Breast Carcinoma," *J Clin Oncol*, 1988, 6(10):1611-20.

Variation 2:
Alonso MC, Tabernero JM, Ojeda B, "A Phase III Randomized Trial of Cyclophosphamide, Mitoxantrone, and 5-Fluorouracil (CNF) Versus Cyclophosphamide, Adriamycin®, and 5-Fluorouracil (CAF) in Patients With Metastatic Breast Cancer," *Breast Cancer Res Treat*, 1995, 34(1):15-24.

Casciato DA and Lowitz BB, eds, *Manual of Clinical Oncology*, 3rd ed, Boston, MA: Little, Brown, 1995, 596.

CNOP

Use Lymphoma, non-Hodgkin's

Regimen

Cyclophosphamide: I.V.: 750 mg/m² day 1
[total dose/cycle = 750 mg/m²]
Mitoxantrone: I.V.: 10 mg/m² day 1
[total dose/cycle = 10 mg/m²]

Vincristine: I.V.: 1.4 mg/m^2 day 1
[total dose/cycle = 1.4 mg/m^2]
Prednisone: Oral: 50 mg/m^2/day days 1 to 5
[total dose/cycle = 250 mg/m^2]
Repeat cycle every 21 days

References
Pavlovsky S, Santarelli MT, Erazo A, et al, "Results of a Randomized Study of Previously Untreated Intermediate and High Grade Lymphoma Using CHOP Versus CNOP," *Ann Oncol*, 1992, 3(3):205-9.

CO

Use Retinoblastoma
Regimen
Cyclophosphamide: I.V.: 10 mg/kg/day days 1, 2, and 3
[total dose/cycle = 30 mg/kg]
Vincristine: I.V.: 1.5 mg/m^2 day 1
[total dose/cycle = 1.5 mg/m^2]
Repeat cycle every 21 days

References
Doz F, Khelfaoui F, Mosseri V, et al, "The Role of Chemotherapy in Orbital Involvement of Retinoblastoma. The Experience of a Single Institution With 33 Patients," *Cancer*, 1994, 74 (2):722-32.

CODOX-M

Use Lymphoma, non-Hodgkin's
Regimen
Cytarabine: I.T.: 70 mg/day days 1 and 3
[total dose/cycle = 140 mg]
Cyclophosphamide: I.V.: 800 mg/m^2 day 1
followed by I.V.: 200 mg/m^2/day days 2 to 5
[total dose/cycle = 1600 mg/m^2]
Vincristine: I.V.: 1.5 mg/m^2/day days 1 and 8 (cycle 1); days 1, 8, and 15 (cycle 3)
[total dose/cycle = 3-4.5 mg/m^2]
Doxorubicin: I.V.: 40 mg/m^2 day 1
[total dose/cycle = 40 mg/m^2]
Methotrexate:
I.T.: 12 mg day 15
[total dose/cycle = 12 mg]
I.V.: 1200 mg/m^2 loading dose
followed by I.V.: 240 mg/m^2/hour for 23 hours day 10
[total dose/cycle = 6720 mg/m^2]
Leucovorin: I.V.: 192 mg/m^2 day 11
followed by I.V.: 12 mg/m^2 every 6 hours until methotrexate level <5 X 10^{-8}M
(begin 36 hours after the start of methotrexate infusion)
Sargramostim: SubQ: 7.5 mcg/kg/day day 13 until ANC >1000 cells/mm^3
Repeat cycle when ANC >1000 cells/mm^3

References
Magrath I, Adde M, Shad A, et al, "Adults and Children With Small Non-Cleaved-Cell Lymphoma Have a Similar Excellent Outcome When Treated With the Same Chemotherapy Regimen," *J Clin Oncol*, 1996, 14(3):925-34.

CODOX-M/IVAC

Use Lymphoma, non-Hodgkin's (Burkitt's)
Regimen
CODOX-M

Cyclophosphamide: I.V.: 800 mg/m^2/day days 1 and 2
[total dose/cycle = 1600 mg/m^2]
Vincristine: I.V.: 1.4 mg/m^2/day (maximum dose: 2 mg) days 1 and 10
[total dose/cycle = 2.8 mg/m^2; maximum: 4 mg/cycle]
Doxorubicin: I.V.: 50 mg/m^2 day 1
[total dose/cycle = 50 mg/m^2]
Methotrexate: I.V.: 3 g/m^2 day 10
[total dose/cycle = 3 g/m^2]
Leucovorin: I.V.: 200 mg/m^2 day 11
followed by Oral, I.V.: 15 mg/m^2 every 6 hours until methotrexate level <0.1 Mmol/L
Cytarabine: I.T.: 50 mg/day days 1 and 3
[total dose/cycle = 100 mg]
Methotrexate: I.T.: 12 mg day 1
[total dose/cycle = 12 mg]
Filgrastim: SubQ: Dose not specified, days 3 to 8 and day 12 until ANC >1000 cells/mm^3
Cycle alternates with IVAC (cycles begin when ANC >1000 cells/mm^3)
Note: Hydrocortisone 50 mg may be added to intrathecal therapy to reduce the incidence of side effects/chemical arachnoiditis.

IVAC
Ifosfamide: I.V.: 1500 mg/m^2/day days 1 to 5
[total dose/cycle = 7500 mg/m^2]
Mesna: I.V.: 1500 mg/m^2/day (in divided doses) days 1 to 5
[total dose/cycle = 7500 mg/m^2]
Etoposide: I.V.: 60 mg/m^2/day days 1 to 5
[total dose/cycle = 300 mg/m^2]
Cytarabine: I.V.: 2 g/m^2 every 12 hours, for 4 doses, days 1 and 2
[total dose/cycle = 8 g/m^2]
Methotrexate: I.T.: 12 mg day 5
[total dose/cycle = 12 mg]
Filgrastim: SubQ: Dose not specified, day 6 until ANC >1000 cells/mm^3
Cycle alternates with CODOX-M (cycles begin when ANC >1000 cells/mm^3)
Note: Hydrocortisone 50 mg may be added to intrathecal therapy to reduce the incidence of side effects/chemical arachnoiditis.

References
Lacasce A, Howard O, Lib S, et al, "Modified Magrath Regimens for Adults With Burkitt and Burkitt-Like Lymphomas: Preserved Efficacy With Decreased Toxicity," *Leuk Lymphoma*, 2004, 45 (4):761-7.

COMLA

Use Lymphoma, non-Hodgkin's
Regimen
Cyclophosphamide: I.V.: 1500 mg/m^2 day 1
[total dose/cycle = 1500 mg/m^2]
Vincristine: I.V.: 1.4 mg/m^2/day (maximum dose: 2 mg) days 1, 8, and 15
[total dose/cycle = 4.2 mg/m^2]
Methotrexate: I.V.: 120 mg/m^2/day days 22, 29, 36, 43, 50, 57, 64, and 71
[total dose/cycle = 960 mg/m^2]
Leucovorin: Oral: 25 mg/m^2 every 6 hours for 4 doses (beginning 24 hours after each methotrexate dose)
[total dose/cycle = 800 mg/m^2]
Cytarabine: I.V.: 300 mg/m^2/day days 22, 29, 36, 43, 50, 57, 64, and 71
[total dose/cycle = 2400 mg/m^2]
Repeat cycle every 85 days

References

Sweet DL, Golomb HM, Ultmann JE, et al, "Cyclophosphamide, Vincristine, Methotrexate With Leucovorin Rescue, and Cytarabine (COMLA) Combination Sequential Chemotherapy for Advanced Diffuse Histiocytic Lymphoma," *Ann Intern Med*, 1980, 92(6):785-90.

COMP

Use Lymphoma, Hodgkin's disease; Lymphoma, non-Hodgkin's disease

Regimen

Cyclophosphamide: I.V.: 1200 mg/m² day 1, cycle 1
[total dose/cycle = 1200 mg/m²]
  followed by I.V.: 1000 mg/m² day 1 on subsequent cycles
  [total dose/cycle = 1000 mg/m²]

Vincristine: I.V.: 2 mg/m²/day (maximum dose: 2 mg) days 3, 10, 17, 24, cycle 1
[total dose/cycle = 8 mg/m²]
  followed by I.V.: 1.5 mg/m²/day days 1 and 4, on subsequent cycles
  [total dose/cycle = 3 mg/m²]

Methotrexate: I.V.: 300 mg/m² day 12
[total dose/cycle = 300 mg/m²]

Prednisone: Oral: 60 mg/m²/day (maximum dose: 60 mg) days 3 to 30 then taper over next 7 days, cycle 1
[total dose/cycle = 1680 mg/m² then taper over next 7 days]
  followed by Oral: 60 mg/m² (maximum dose: 60 mg) days 1 to 5, on subsequent cycles
  [total dose/cycle = 300 mg/m²]

Maintenance cycles repeat every 28 days

References

Anderson JR, Wilson JF, Jenkin DT, et al, "Childhood Non-Hodgkin's Lymphoma. The Results of a Randomized Therapeutic Trial Comparing a 4-Drug Regimen (COMP) With a 10-Drug Regimen (LSA2-L2)." *N Engl J Med*, 1983, 308(10):559-65.

COP-BLAM

Use Lymphoma, non-Hodgkin's

Regimen

Cyclophosphamide: I.V.: 400 mg/m² day 1
[total dose/cycle = 400 mg/m²]

Vincristine: I.V.: 1 mg/m² day 1
[total dose/cycle = 1 mg/m²]

Prednisone: Oral: 40 mg/m²/day days 1 to 10
[total dose/cycle = 400 mg/m²]

Bleomycin: I.V.: 15 mg day 14
[total dose/cycle = 15 mg]

Doxorubicin: I.V.: 40 mg/m² day 1
[total dose/cycle = 40 mg/m²]

Procarbazine: Oral: 100 mg/m²/day days 1 to 10
[total dose/cycle = 1000 mg/m²]

References

Salles G, Shipp MA, and Coiffier B, "Chemotherapy of Non-Hodgkin's Aggressive Lymphomas," *Semin Hematol*, 1994, 31(1):46-69.

Urba WJ, Duffey PL, and Longo DL, "Treatment of Patients With Aggressive Lymphomas: An Overview," *J Natl Cancer Inst Monogr*, 1990, (10):29-37.

COPE

Index Terms Baby Brain I

Use Brain tumors

Regimen
Cycle A:
Vincristine: I.V.: 0.065 mg/kg/day (maximum dose: 1.5 mg) days 1 and 8
[total dose/cycle = 0.13 mg/kg]
Cyclophosphamide: I.V.: 65 mg/kg day 1
[total dose/cycle = 65 mg/kg]
Cycle B:
Cisplatin: I.V.: 4 mg/kg day 1
[total dose/cycle = 4 mg/kg]
Etoposide: I.V.: 6.5 mg/kg/day days 3 and 4
[total dose/cycle = 13 mg/kg]
Repeat cycle every 28 days in the following sequence: AABAAB

References
Duffner PK, Horowitz ME, Krischer JP, et al "Postoperative Chemotherapy and Delayed Radiation in Children Less Than Three Years of Age With Malignant Brain Tumors," *N Engl J Med*, 1993, 328(24):1725-31.

COPP

Index Terms C MOPP

Use Lymphoma, non-Hodgkin's

Regimen
Cyclophosphamide: I.V.: 450-650 mg/m^2/day days 1 and 8
[total dose/cycle = 900-1300 mg/m^2]
Vincristine: I.V.: 1.4-2 mg/m^2/day (maximum dose: 2 mg) days 1 and 8
[total dose/cycle = 2.8-4 mg/m^2]
Procarbazine: Oral: 100 mg/m^2/day days 1 to 14
[total dose/cycle = 1400 mg/m^2]
Prednisone: Oral: 40 mg/m^2/day days 1 to 14
[total dose/cycle = 560 mg/m^2]
Repeat cycle every 3-4 weeks

References
Brereton HD, Young RC, Longo DL, et al, "A Comparison Between Combination Chemotherapy and Total Body Irradiation Plus Combination Chemotherapy in Non-Hodgkin's Lymphoma," *Cancer*, 1979, 43(6):2227-31.

CP (Leukemia)

Use Leukemia, chronic lymphocytic

Regimen
Chlorambucil: Oral: 30 mg/m^2 day 1
[total dose/cycle = 30 mg/m^2]
Prednisone: Oral: 80 mg/day days 1 to 5
[total dose/cycle = 400 mg]
Repeat cycle every 14 days

References
Raphael B, Anderson JW, Silber R, et al, "Comparison of Chlorambucil and Prednisone Versus Cyclophosphamide, Vincristine, and Prednisone as Initial Treatment for Chronic Lymphocytic Leukemia: Long-Term Follow-up of an Eastern Cooperative Oncology Group Randomized Clinical Trial," *J Clin Oncol*, 1991, 9(5):770-6.

CP (Ovarian Cancer)

Use Ovarian cancer

Regimen
Cyclophosphamide: I.V.: 750 mg/m^2 day 1
[total dose/cycle = 750 mg/m^2]
Cisplatin: I.V.: 75 mg/m^2 day 1
[total dose/cycle = 75 mg/m^2]
Repeat cycle every 21 days

References

Hainsworth JD, Grosh WW, Burnett LS, et al, "Advanced Ovarian Cancer: Long-Term Results of Treatment With Intensive Cisplatin-Based Chemotherapy of Brief Duration," *Ann Intern Med*, 1988, 108(2):165-70.

Neijt JP, ten Bokkel Huinink WW, van der Burg ME, et al, "Randomized Trial Comparing Two Combination Chemotherapy Regimens (CHAP-5 v CP) in Advanced Ovarian Carcinoma," *J Clin Oncol*, 1987, 5(8):1157-68.

Omura GA, Brady MF, Homesley HD, et al, "Long-Term Follow-up and Prognostic Factor Analysis in Advanced Ovarian Carcinoma: The Gynecologic Oncology Group Experience," *J Clin Oncol*, 1991, 9(7):1138-50.

CV

Use Retinoblastoma

Regimen

Cyclophosphamide: I.V.: 300 mg/m^2
 [total dose/cycle = 300 mg/m^2]
Vincristine: I.V.: 1.5 mg/m^2
 [total dose/cycle = 1.5 mg/m^2]
Repeat weekly for 6 weeks

followed by

Cyclophosphamide: I.V.: 200 mg/m^2
 [total dose/cycle = 200 mg/m^2]
Vincristine: I.V.: 1.5 mg/m^2
 [total dose/cycle = 1.5 mg/m^2]
Repeat weekly for 42 weeks

References

Zelter M, Damel A, Gonzalez G, et al, "A Prospective Study on the Treatment of Retinoblastoma in 72 Patients," *Cancer*, 1991, 68(8):1685-90.

◆ **CVD** see Cisplatin-Vinblastine-Dacarbazine (Melanoma) *on page 1274*

◆ **CVD-IL-2-IFN (Melanoma)** see CVD-Interleukin-Interferon (Melanoma) *on page 1282*

CVD-Interleukin-Interferon (Melanoma)

Index Terms Cisplatin-Vinblastine-Dacarbazine-Interleukin-Interferon (Melanoma); CVD-IL-2-IFN (Melanoma)

Use Melanoma

Regimen NOTE: Multiple variations are listed.

Variation 1:

Cisplatin: I.V.: 20 mg/m^2/day days 1 to 4 and 22 to 25
 [total dose/cycle = 160 mg/m^2]
Vinblastine: I.V.: 1.5 mg/m^2/day days 1 to 4 and 22 to 25
 [total dose/cycle = 12 mg/m^2]
Dacarbazine: I.V.: 800 mg/m^2/day days 1 and 22
 [total dose/cycle = 1600 mg/m^2]
Aldesleukin: I.V.: 9 million units/m^2/day continuous infusion days 5 to 8, 17 to 20, and 26 to 29
 [total dose/cycle = 108 million units/m^2]
Interferon alfa-2b: SubQ: 5 million units/m^2/day days 5 to 9, 17 to 21, and 26 to 30
 [total dose/cycle = 75 million units/m^2]
Repeat every 42 days (maximum of five 21-day cycles for cytokine [interleukin and interferon] component)

Variation 2:
Cisplatin: I.V.: 20 mg/m^2/day days 1 to 4
  [total dose/cycle = 80 mg/m^2]
Vinblastine: I.V.: 1.6 mg/m^2/day days 1 to 4
  [total dose/cycle = 6.4 mg/m^2]
Dacarbazine: I.V.: 800 mg/m^2 day 1
  [total dose/cycle = 800 mg/m^2]
Aldesleukin: I.V.: 9 million units/m^2/day continuous infusion days 1 to 4
  [total dose/cycle = 36 million units/m^2]
Interferon alfa-2a: SubQ: 5 million units/m^2/day days 1 to 5, 7, 9, 11, and 13
  [total dose/cycle = 45 million units/m^2]
Repeat cycle every 21 days for a total of 6 cycles
Variation 3:
Cisplatin: I.V.: 20 mg/m^2/day days 1 to 4
  [total dose/cycle = 80 mg/m^2]
Vinblastine: I.V.: 1.2 mg/m^2/day days 1 to 4
  [total dose/cycle = 4.8 mg/m^2]
Dacarbazine: I.V.: 800 mg/m^2 day 1
  [total dose/cycle = 800 mg/m^2]
Aldesleukin: I.V.: 9 million units/m^2/day continuous infusion days 1 to 4
  [total dose/cycle = 36 million units/m^2]
Interferon alfa-2b: SubQ: 5 million units/m^2/day days 1 to 5, 8, 10, and 12
  [total dose/cycle = 40 million units/m^2]
Repeat cycle every 21 days (maximum: 4 cycles)

References

Variation 1:
Eton O, Legha SS, Bedikian AY, et al, "Sequential Biochemotherapy Versus Chemotherapy for Metastatic Melanoma: Results From a Phase III Randomized Trial," *J Clin Oncol*, 2002, 20 (8):2045-52.
Variation 2:
Legha SS, Ring S, Eton O, et al, "Development of a Biochemotherapy Regimen With Concurrent Administration of Cisplatin, Vinblastine, Dacarbazine, Interferon Alfa, and Interleukin-2 for Patients With Metastatic Melanoma," *J Clin Oncol*, 1998, 16(5):1752-9.
Variation 3:
McDermott DF, Mier JW, Lawrence DP, et al, "A Phase II Pilot Trial of Concurrent Biochemotherapy With Cisplatin, Vinblastine, Dacarbazine, Interleukin 2, and Interferon Alpha-2B in Patients With Metastatic Melanoma," *Clin Cancer Res*, 2000, 6(6):2201-8.

CVP (Leukemia)

Use Leukemia, chronic lymphocytic

Regimen NOTE: Multiple variations are listed.
Variation 1:
Cyclophosphamide: Oral: 300 or 400 mg/m^2/day days 1 to 5
  [total dose/cycle = 1500 or 2000 mg/m^2]
Vincristine: I.V.: 1.4 mg/m^2 (maximum dose: 2 mg) day 1
  [total dose/cycle = 1.4 mg/m^2]
Prednisone: Oral: 100 mg/m^2/day days 1 to 5
  [total dose/cycle = 500 mg/m^2]
Repeat cycle every 21 days
Variation 2:
Cyclophosphamide: I.V.: 800 mg/m^2 day 1
  [total dose/cycle = 800 mg/m^2]
Vincristine: I.V.: 1.4 mg/m^2 (maximum dose: 2 mg) day 1
  [total dose/cycle = 1.4 mg/m^2]
Prednisone: Oral: 100 mg/m^2/day days 1 to 5
  [total dose/cycle = 500 mg/m^2]
Repeat cycle every 21 days

References
Variation 1:
Bagley CM, DeVita VT, Berard CW, et al, "Advanced Lymphosarcoma: Intensive Cyclical Combination Chemotherapy With Cyclophosphamide, Vincristine, and Prednisone," *Ann Int Med*, 1972, 76(2):227-34.
Raphael B, Anderson JW, Silber R, et al, "Comparison of Chlorambucil and Prednisone Versus Cyclophosphamide, Vincristine, and Prednisone as Initial Treatment for Chronic Lymphocytic Leukemia: Long-Term Follow-up of an Eastern Cooperative Oncology Group Randomized Clinical Trial," *J Clin Oncol*, 1991, 9(5):770-6.
Variation 2:
Oken MM and Kaplan ME, "Combination Chemotherapy With Cyclophosphamide, Vincristine, and Prednisone in the Treatment of Refractory Chronic Lymphocytic Leukemia," *Cancer Treat Rep*, 1979, 63(3):441-7.

CVP (Lymphoma, non-Hodgkin's)

Index Terms Cyclophosphamide-Vincristine-Prednisone (NHL)

Use Lymphoma, non-Hodgkin's

Regimen NOTE: Multiple variations are listed.

Variation 1:
Cyclophosphamide: I.V.: 750 mg/m² day 1
[total dose/cycle = 750 mg/m²]
Vincristine: I.V.: 1.2 mg/m² day 1
[total dose/cycle = 1.2 mg/m²]
Prednisone: Oral: 40 mg/m²/day days 1 to 5
[total dose/cycle = 200 mg/m²]
Repeat cycle every 21 days for up to 10 cycles

Variation 2:
Cyclophosphamide: I.V.: 750 mg/m² day 1
[total dose/cycle = 750 mg/m²]
Vincristine: I.V.: 1.2 mg/m² day 1 (maximum dose: 2 mg)
[total dose/cycle = 1.2 mg/m² (maximum: 2 mg)]
Prednisone: Oral: 40 mg/m²/day days 1 to 5
[total dose/cycle = 200 mg/m²]
Repeat cycle every 28 days for up to 8 cycles

Variation 3:
Cyclophosphamide: I.V.: 750 mg/m² day 1
[total dose/cycle = 750 mg/m²]
Vincristine: I.V.: 1.4 mg/m² day 1 (maximum dose: 2 mg)
[total dose/cycle = 1.4 mg/m² (maximum: 2 mg)]
Prednisone: Oral: 40 mg/m²/day days 1 to 5
[total dose/cycle = 200 mg/m²]
Repeat cycle every 21 days for up to 8 cycles

Variation 4:
Cyclophosphamide: Oral: 400 mg/m²/day days 1 to 5
[total dose/cycle = 2000 mg/m²]
Vincristine: I.V.: 1.4 mg/m² day 1 (maximum dose: 2 mg)
[total dose/cycle = 1.4 mg/m² (maximum: 2 mg)]
Prednisone: Oral: 100 mg/m²/day days 1 to 5
[total dose/cycle = 500 mg/m²]
Repeat cycle every 21 days

References
Variation 1:
Klasa RJ, Meyer RM, Shustik C, et al, "Randomized Phase III Study of Fludarabine Phosphate Versus Cyclophosphamide, Vincristine, and Prednisone in Patients With Recurrent Low-Grade Non-Hodgkin's Lymphoma Previously Treated With an Alkylating Agent or Alkylator-Containing Regimen," *J Clin Oncol*, 2002, 20(24):4649-54.

Variation 2:
Hagenbeek A, Eghbali H, Monfardini S, et al, "Phase III Intergroup Study of Fludarabine Phosphate Compared With Cyclophosphamide, Vincristine, and Prednisone Chemotherapy in Newly Diagnosed Patients With Stage III and IV Low-Grade Malignant Non-Hodgkin's Lymphoma," *J Clin Oncol*, 2006, 24(10):1590-6.

Variation 3:
Marcus R, Imrie K, Belch A, et al, "CVP Chemotherapy Plus Rituximab Compared With CVP as First-Line Treatment for Advanced Follicular Lymphoma," *Blood*, 2005, 105(4):1417-23.

Variation 4:
Bagley CM Jr, Devita VT Jr, Berard CW, et al, "Advanced Lymphosarcoma: Intensive Cyclical Combination Chemotherapy With Cyclophosphamide, Vincristine, and Prednisone," *Ann Intern Med*, 1972, 76(2):227-34.

Portlock CS, Rosenberg SA, Glatstein E, et al, "Treatment of Advanced Non-Hodgkin's Lymphomas With Favorable Histologies: Preliminary Results of a Prospective Trial," *Blood*, 1976, 47(5):747-56.

- ◆ **CVP-R** *see* R-CVP *on page 1401*

- ◆ **Cyclophosphamide-Fludarabine (CLL)** *see* Fludarabine-Cyclophosphamide (CLL) *on page 1325*

- ◆ **Cyclophosphamide-Fludarabine (NHL-Mantle Cell)** *see* Fludarabine-Cyclophosphamide (NHL-Mantle Cell) *on page 1327*

- ◆ **Cyclophosphamide-Vincristine-Prednisone (NHL)** *see* CVP (Lymphoma, non-Hodgkin's) *on page 1284*

- ◆ **Cytarabine-Daunorubicin (5 + 2)** *see* 5 + 2 *on page 1220*

- ◆ **Cytarabine-Daunorubicin (7 + 3)** *see* 7 + 3 (Daunorubicin) *on page 1220*

- ◆ **Cytarabine-Daunorubicin-Etoposide (7 + 3 + 7)** *see* 7 + 3 + 7 *on page 1220*

- ◆ **Cytarabine-Idarubicin (7 + 3)** *see* 7 + 3 (Idarubicin) *on page 1221*

- ◆ **Cytarabine-Mitoxantrone (7 + 3)** *see* 7 + 3 (Mitoxantrone) *on page 1221*

CYVADIC

Use Sarcoma

Regimen
Cyclophosphamide: I.V.: 500 mg/m² day 1
  [total dose/cycle = 500 mg/m²]
Vincristine: I.V.: 1.4 mg/m²/day days 1 and 5
  [total dose/cycle = 2.8 mg/m²]
Doxorubicin: I.V.: 50 mg/m² day 1
  [total dose/cycle = 50 mg/m²]
Dacarbazine: I.V.: 250 mg/m²/day days 1 to 5
  [total dose/cycle = 1250 mg/m²]
Repeat cycle every 21 days

References
Pinedo HM, Bramwell VH, Mouridsen HT, et al, "Cyvadic in Advanced Soft Tissue Sarcoma: A Randomized Study Comparing Two Schedules. A Study of the EORTC Soft Tissue and Bone Sarcoma Group," *Cancer*, 1984, 53(9):1825-32.

DA

Use Leukemia, acute myeloid (induction)

Regimen Induction:
Daunorubicin: I.V.: 45 mg/m²/day days 1, 2, and 3
  [total dose/cycle = 135 mg/m²]
Cytarabine: I.V.: 100 mg/m²/day continuous infusion days 1 to 7
  [total dose/cycle = 700 mg/m²]

References
Rai KR, Holland JF, Glidewell OJ, et al, "Treatment of Acute Myelocytic Leukemia: A Study by Cancer and Leukemia Group B," *Blood*, 1981, 58(6):1203-12.

Yates J, Glidewell O, Wiernik P, et al, "Cytosine Arabinoside With Daunorubicin or Adriamycin for Therapy of Acute Myelocytic Leukemia: A CALGB Study," *Blood*, 1982, 60(2):454-62.

Dacarbazine-Carboplatin-Aldesleukin-Interferon

Use Melanoma

Regimen

Dacarbazine: I.V.: 750 mg/m^2/day days 1 and 22
[total dose/cycle = 1500 mg/m^2]

Carboplatin: I.V.: 400 mg/m^2/day days 1 and 22
[total dose/cycle = 800 mg/m^2]

Aldesleukin: SubQ: 4,800,000 units every 8 hours days 36 and 57
[total dose/cycle = 28,800,000 units]

then 4,800,000 units every 12 hours days 37 and 58
[total dose/cycle = 19,200,000 units]

then 4,800,000 units/day days 38 to 40, 43 to 47, 50 to 54, 59 to 61, 65 to 68, 71 to 75
[total dose/cycle = 120,000,000 units]

Interferon alpha-2a: SubQ: 6,000,000 units days 38, 40, 43, 45, 47, 50, 52, 54, 59, 61, 64, 66, 68, 71, 73, and 75
[total dose/cycle = 96,000,000 units]

Repeat cycle every 78 days for 3 cycles

References

Ron IG, Mordish Y, Eisenthal A, et al, "A Phase II Study of Combined Administration of Dacarbazine and Carboplatin With Home Therapy of Recombinant Interleukin-2 and Interferon-Alpha 2a in Patients With Advanced Malignant Melanoma," *Cancer Immunol Immunother*, 1994, 38(6):379-84.

- **Dacarbazine-Carmustine-Cisplatin** see Cisplatin-Dacarbazine-Carmustine (Melanoma) on page 1265

- **Dacarbazine-Carmustine-Cisplatin-Tamoxifen** see Dartmouth Regimen on page 1286

- **Dacarbazine-Cisplatin-Interferon Alfa-2b-Aldesleukin** see Cisplatin-Dacarbazine-Interferon Alfa-2b-Aldesleukin on page 1266

- **Dacarbazine-Cisplatin-Vinblastine** see Cisplatin-Vinblastine-Dacarbazine (Melanoma) on page 1274

Dartmouth Regimen

Index Terms Carmustine-Cisplatin-Dacarbazine-Tamoxifen; Cisplatin-Dacarbazine-Carmustine-Tamoxifen; Dacarbazine-Carmustine-Cisplatin-Tamoxifen

Use Melanoma

Regimen NOTE: Multiple variations are listed.

Variation 1:

Cisplatin: I.V.: 25 mg/m^2/day days 1, 2, and 3
[total dose/cycle = 75 mg/m^2]

Dacarbazine: I.V.: 220 mg/m^2/day days 1, 2, and 3
[total dose/cycle = 660 mg/m^2]

Carmustine: I.V.: 150 mg/m^2 day 1 (every other cycle)
[total dose/cycle = 150 mg/m^2; every other cycle]

Tamoxifen: Oral: 10 mg twice daily (begin 1 week before chemotherapy)
[total dose/cycle = 420 mg]

Repeat cycle every 21 days

Variation 2:
  Carmustine: I.V.: 150 mg/m^2 day 1
    [total dose/cycle = 150 mg/m^2]
  Cisplatin: I.V.: 25 mg/m^2/day days 1, 2, 3, 22, 23, and 24
    [total dose/cycle = 150 mg/m^2]
  Dacarbazine: I.V.: 220 mg/m^2/day days 1, 2, 3, 22, 23, and 24
    [total dose/cycle = 1320 mg/m^2]
  Tamoxifen: Oral: 10 mg twice daily days 1 to 42
    [total dose/cycle = 840 mg]
  Repeat cycle every 42 days
Variation 3:
  Carmustine: I.V.: 150 mg/m^2 day 1
    [total dose/cycle = 150 mg/m^2]
  Cisplatin: I.V.: 25 mg/m^2/day days 1, 2, 3, 22, 23, and 24
    [total dose/cycle = 150 mg/m^2]
  Dacarbazine: I.V.: 220 mg/m^2/day days 1, 2, 3, 22, 23, and 24
    [total dose/cycle = 1320 mg/m^2]
  Tamoxifen: Oral: 160 mg/day days -6 to 0 (cycle 1 only)
    [total dose/cycle = 1120 mg]
    followed by Oral: 40 mg/day days 1 to 42
      [total dose/cycle = 1680 mg]
  Repeat cycle every 42 days
Variation 4:
  Carmustine: I.V.: 150 mg/m^2 day 1
    [total dose/cycle = 150 mg/m^2]
  Cisplatin: I.V.: 25 mg/m^2/day days 1, 2, 3, 29, 30, and 31
    [total dose/cycle = 150 mg/m^2]
  Dacarbazine: I.V.: 220 mg/m^2/day days 1, 2, 3, 29, 30, and 31
    [total dose/cycle = 1320 mg/m^2]
  Tamoxifen: Oral: 10-20 mg twice daily days 1 to 56
    [total dose/cycle = 1120-2240 mg]
  Repeat cycle every 56 days
Variation 5:
  Cisplatin: I.V.: 25 mg/m^2/day days 1, 2, and 3
    [total dose/cycle = 75 mg/m^2]
  Dacarbazine: I.V.: 220 mg/m^2/day days 1, 2, and 3
    [total dose/cycle = 660 mg/m^2]
  Carmustine: I.V.: 100 mg/m^2 day 1 (give in cycles 1, 3, and 6 **only**)
    [total dose/cycles 1, 3, and 6 = 100 mg/m^2]
  Tamoxifen: Oral: 160 mg loading dose immediately before cycle 1
    [total dose/loading dose + cycle 1 = 580 mg]
    followed by Oral: 20 mg daily days 1 to 21
      [total dose/subsequent cycles = 420 mg]
  Repeat cycle every 21 days
Note: Tamoxifen is continued until 3 weeks after last cycle.

References

Variation 1:

Chapman PB, Einhorn LH, Meyers ML, et al, "Phase III Multicenter Randomized Trial of the Dartmouth Regimen Versus Dacarbazine in Patients With Metastatic Melanoma," *J Clin Oncol*, 1999, 17(9):2745-51.

Gause BL, Sharfman WH, Janik JE, et al, "A Phase II Study of Carboplatin, Interferon-Alpha, and Tamoxifen for Patients With Metastatic Melanoma," *Cancer Invest*, 1998, 16(6):374-80.

McClay EF, Berd D, and Mastrangelo MJ, "The Dartmouth Regimen: Gone or Going Strong? " *Cancer Invest*, 1998, 16(6):421-3.

◄ Variation 2

Del Prete SA, Maurer LH, O'Donnell J, et al, "Combination Chemotherapy With Cisplatin, Carmustine, Dacarbazine, and Tamoxifen in Metastatic Melanoma," *Cancer Treat Rep*, 1984, 68 (11):1403-5.

Variation 3:

Rusthoven JJ, Quirt IC, Iscoe NA, et al, "Randomized, Double-Blind, Placebo-Controlled Trial Comparing the Response Rates of Carmustine, Dacarbazine, and Cisplatin With and Without Tamoxifen in Patients With Metastatic Melanoma," *J Clin Oncol*, 1996, 14(7):2083-90.

Variation 4:

McClay EF, Mastrangelo MJ, Berd D, et al, "Effective Combination Chemo/Hormonal Therapy for Malignant Melanoma: Experience With Three Consecutive Trials," *Int J Cancer*, 1992, 50 (4):553-6.

Variation 5:

Propper DJ, Braybrooke JP, Levitt NC, et al, "Phase II Study of Second-Line Therapy With DTIC, BCNU, Cisplatin and Tamoxifen (Dartmouth Regimen) Chemotherapy in Patients With Malignant Melanoma Previously Treated With Dacarbazine," *Br J Cancer*, 2000, 82(11):1759-63.

DAT

Use Leukemia, acute myeloid (induction)

Regimen Induction:

Daunorubicin: I.V. bolus: 45 mg/m^2/day days 1, 2, and 3
[total dose/cycle = 135 mg/m^2]
Cytarabine: I.V. bolus: 200 mg/m^2
[total dose/cycle = 200 mg/m^2]
Thioguanine: Oral: 100 mg/m^2/day days 1 to 7
[total dose/cycle = 700 mg/m^2]

References

Gale RP and Cline MJ, "High Remission-Induction Rate in Acute Myeloid Leukaemia," *Lancet*, 1977, 1(8010):497-9.

◆ **Daunorubicin-ATRA (APL)** *see* Tretinoin-Daunorubicin (APL) *on page* 1411
◆ **Daunorubicin-Cytarabine (5 + 2)** *see* 5 + 2 *on page* 1220
◆ **Daunorubicin-Tretinoin (APL)** *see* Tretinoin-Daunorubicin (APL) *on page* 1411

DAV

Use Leukemia, acute myeloid

Regimen

Daunorubicin: I.V.: 60 mg/m^2/day days 3, 4, and 5
[total dose/cycle = 180 mg/m^2]
Cytarabine I.V.: 100 mg/m^2/day continuous infusion days 1 and 2
[total dose/cycle = 200 mg/m^2]
followed by I.V.: 100 mg/m^2 over 30 minutes every 12 hours days 3 to 8
(12 doses)
[total dose/cycle = 1200 mg/m^2]
Etoposide: I.V.: 150 mg/m^2/day days 6, 7, and 8
[total dose/cycle = 450 mg/m^2]
Administer one cycle only

References

Creutzig U, Ritter J, and Schellong G, "Identification of Two Risk Groups in Childhood Acute Myelogenous Leukemia After Therapy Intensification in Study AML-BFM-83 as Compared With Study AML-BFM-78, AML-BFM Study Group," *Blood*, 1990, 75(10):1932-40.

◆ **DCF (Gastric/Esophageal Cancer)** *see* Docetaxel-Cisplatin-Fluorouracil (Gastric/Esophageal Cancer) *on page* 1290

Decitabine (Low Dose Regimen)

Use Leukemia, chronic myelogenous; Myelodysplastic syndrome

Regimen
Decitabine: I.V.: 20 mg/m^2/day days 1 to 5
[total dose/cycle = 100 mg/m^2]
Repeat cycle every 28 days for at least 3 cycles

References

Kantarjian H, Oki Y, Garcia-Manero G, et al, "Results of a Randomized Study of 3 Schedules of Low-Dose Decitabine in Higher-Risk Myelodysplastic Syndrome and Chronic Myelomonocytic Leukemia," *Blood*, 2007, 109(1):52-7.

- ◆ **Dexamethasone-Bortezomib** *see* Bortezomib-Dexamethasone *on page 1237*

- ◆ **Dexamethasone-Bortezomib-Doxorubicin** *see* Bortezomib-Doxorubicin-Dexamethasone *on page 1238*

- ◆ **Dexamethasone-Bortezomib-Doxorubicin (Liposomal)** *see* Bortezomib-Doxorubicin (Liposomal)-Dexamethasone *on page 1240*

- ◆ **Dexamethasone-Lenalidomide** *see* Lenalidomide-Dexamethasone *on page 1362*

- ◆ **Dexamethasone (Low Dose)-Lenalidomide** *see* Lenalidomide-Dexamethasone (Low Dose) *on page 1362*

- ◆ **Dexamethasone-Thalidomide** *see* Thalidomide-Dexamethasone *on page 1405*

- ◆ **DHAP (NHL Regimen)** *see* Cisplatin-Cytarabine-Dexamethasone (NHL Regimen) *on page 1265*

- ◆ **DHAX (NHL Regimen)** *see* Oxaliplatin-Cytarabine-Dexamethasone (NHL Regimen) *on page 1383*

Docetaxel-Bevacizumab

Index Terms Bevacizumab-Docetaxel

Use Breast cancer

Regimen NOTE: Multiple variations are listed.
Variation 1:
Docetaxel: I.V.: 100 mg/m^2 day 1
[total dose/cycle = 100 mg/m^2]
Bevacizumab: I.V.: 7.5 mg/kg day 1
[total dose/cycle = 7.5 mg/kg]
Repeat cycle every 21 days (administer docetaxel for up to 9 cycles, bevacizumab until disease progression or unacceptable toxicity)
Variation 2:
Docetaxel: I.V.: 100 mg/m^2 day 1
[total dose/cycle = 100 mg/m^2]
Bevacizumab: I.V.: 15 mg/kg day 1
[total dose/cycle = 15 mg/kg]
Repeat cycle every 21 days (administer docetaxel for up to 9 cycles, bevacizumab until disease progression or unacceptable toxicity)

References

Miles D, Chan A, Romieu G, et al, "Randomized, Double-Blind, Placebo-Controlled, Phase III Study of Bevacizumab With Docetaxel or Docetaxel With Placebo as First-Line Therapy for Patients With Locally Recurrent or Metastatic Breast Cancer (mBC): AVADO," [LBA1011abstract from 2008 ASCO Annual Meeting]

Docetaxel-Carboplatin (Ovarian Cancer)

Index Terms Carboplatin-Docetaxel (Ovarian Cancer)

Use Ovarian cancer

Regimen NOTE: Multiple variations are listed.

Variation 1:
Docetaxel: I.V.: 60 mg/m² day 1
[total dose/cycle = 60 mg/m²]
Carboplatin: I.V.: Target AUC 6
[total dose/cycle = AUC = 6]
Repeat cycle every 21 days for 6 cycles
Variation 2:
Docetaxel: I.V.: 75 mg/m² day 1
[total dose/cycle = 75 mg/m²]
Carboplatin: I.V.: AUC 5 day 1
[total dose/cycle = AUC = 5]
Repeat cycle every 21 days for 6 cycles

References

Variation 1:
Markman M, Kennedy A, Webster K, et al, "Combination Chemotherapy With Carboplatin and Docetaxel in the Treatment of Cancers of the Ovary and Fallopian Tube and Primary Carcinoma of the Peritoneum," *J Clin Oncol*, 2001, 19(7):1901-5.

Variation 2:
Vasey PA, Jayson GC, Gordon A, et al, "Phase III Randomized Trial of Docetaxel-Carboplatin Versus Paclitaxel-Carboplatin as First-line Chemotherapy for Ovarian Carcinoma," *J Natl Cancer Inst*, 2004, 96(22):1682-91.

Docetaxel-Cisplatin

Use Lung cancer, nonsmall cell

Regimen
Docetaxel: I.V.: 75 mg/m² day 1
[total dose/cycle = 75 mg/m²]
Cisplatin: I.V.: 75 mg/m² day 1
[total dose/cycle = 75 mg/m²]
Repeat cycle every 21 days

References

Zalcberg J, Millward M, Bishop J, et al, "Phase II Study of Docetaxel and Cisplatin in Advanced Nonsmall-Cell Lung Cancer," *J Clin Oncol*, 1998, 16(5):1948-53.

Docetaxel-Cisplatin-Fluorouracil (Gastric/Esophageal Cancer)

Index Terms DCF (Gastric/Esophageal Cancer)

Use Esophageal cancer; Gastric cancer

Regimen
Docetaxel: I.V.: 75 mg/m² day 1
[total dose/cycle = 75 mg/m²]
Cisplatin: I.V.: 75 mg/m² day 1
[total dose/cycle = 75 mg/m²]
Fluorouracil: I.V.: 750 mg/m²/day continuous infusion days 1 to 5
[total dose/cycle = 3750 mg/m²]
Repeat cycle every 21 days

References

Ajani JA, Fodor MB, Tjulandin SA, et al, "Phase II Multi-Institutional Randomized Trial of Docetaxel Plus Cisplatin With or Without Fluorouracil in Patients With Untreated, Advanced Gastric, or Gastroesophageal Adenocarcinoma," *J Clin Oncol*, 2005, 23(24):5660-7.

Ajani JA, Moiseyenko VM, Tjulandin S, et al, "Quality of Life With Docetaxel Plus Cisplatin and Fluorouracil Compared With Cisplatin and Fluorouracil From a Phase III Trial for Advanced Gastric or Gastroesophageal Adenocarcinoma: The V-325 Study Group," *J Clin Oncol*, 2007, 25 (22):3210-6.

Van Cutsem E, Moiseyenko VM, Tjulandin S, et al, "Phase III Study of Docetaxel and Cisplatin Plus Fluorouracil Compared With Cisplatin and Fluorouracil as First-Line Therapy for Advanced Gastric Cancer: A Report of the V325 Study Group," *J Clin Oncol*, 2006, 24(31):4991-7.

Docetaxel-Cisplatin-Fluorouracil (Head and Neck Cancer)

Index Terms TPF

Use Head and neck cancer

Regimen NOTE: Multiple variations are listed.

Variation 1:

Docetaxel: I.V.: 75 mg/m^2 day 1
[total dose/cycle = 75 mg/m^2]
Cisplatin: I.V.: 75 mg/m^2 day 1
[total dose/cycle = 75 mg/m^2]
Fluorouracil: I.V.: 750 mg/m^2/day continuous infusion days 1 to 5
[total dose/cycle = 3750 mg/m^2]
Repeat cycle every 21 days for 4 cycles

Variation 2:

Docetaxel: I.V.: 75 mg/m^2 day 1
[total dose/cycle = 75 mg/m^2]
Cisplatin: I.V.: 75-100 mg/m^2 day 1
[total dose/cycle = 75-100 mg/m^2]
Fluorouracil: I.V.: 1000 mg/m^2/day continuous infusion days 1 to 4
[total dose/cycle = 4000 mg/m^2]
Repeat cycle every 21 days for total of 3 cycles

References

Variation 1:

Schrijvers D, van Herpen C, Kerger J, et al, "Docetaxel, Cisplatin and 5-Fluorouracil in Patients With Locally Advanced Unresectable Head and Neck Cancer: A Phase I-II Feasibility Study," *Ann Oncol*, 2004, 15(4):638-45.

Vermorken JB, Remenar E, van Herpen C, et al, "Cisplatin, Fluorouracil, and Docetaxel in Unresectable Head and Neck Cancer," *N Engl J Med*, 2007, 357(17):1695-1704.

Variation 2:

Posner MR, Glisson B, Frenette G, et al, "Multicenter Phase I-II Trial of Docetaxel, Cisplatin, and Fluorouracil Induction Chemotherapy for Patients With Locally Advanced Squamous Cell Cancer of the Head and Neck," *J Clin Oncol*, 2001, 19(4):1096-104.

Posner MR, Hershock DM, Blajman CR, et al, "Cisplatin and Fluorouracil Alone or With Docetaxel in Head and Neck Cancer," *N Engl J Med*, 2007, 357(17):1705-15.

Docetaxel-Cyclophosphamide (TC)

Index Terms TC

Use Breast cancer

Regimen

Docetaxel: I.V.: 75 mg/m^2 day 1
[total dose/cycle = 75 mg/m^2]
Cyclophosphamide: I.V.: 600 mg/m^2 day 1
[total dose/cycle = 600 mg/m^2]
Repeat cycle every 21 days for 4 cycles

References

Jones SE, Savin MA, Holmes FA, et al, "Phase III Trial Comparing Doxorubicin Plus Cyclophosphamide With Docetaxel Plus Cyclophosphamide as Adjuvant Therapy for Operable Breast Cancer," *J Clin Oncol*, 2006, 24(34):5381-7.

◆ **Docetaxel-Doxorubicin Liposomal (Breast Cancer)** *see* Doxorubicin (Liposomal)-Docetaxel (Breast Cancer) *on page 1296*

Docetaxel-FEC

Index Terms FEC-Docetaxel

Use Breast cancer

Regimen

Cycles 1, 2, and 3:
  Docetaxel: I.V.: 80-100 mg/m² day 1
    [total dose/cycle = 80-100 mg/m²]
  Repeat cycle every 21 days for 3 cycles
Cycles 4, 5, and 6 (FEC):
  Fluorouracil: I.V.: 600 mg/m² day 1
    [total dose/cycle = 600 mg/m²]
  Epirubicin: I.V.: 60 mg/m² day 1
    [total dose/cycle = 60 mg/m²]
  Cyclophosphamide: I.V.: 600 mg/m² day 1
    [total dose/cycle = 600 mg/m²]
  Repeat FEC cycle every 21 days for total of 3 cycles

References

Joensuu H, Kellokumpu-Lehtinen PL, Bono P, et al, "Adjuvant Docetaxel or Vinorelbine With or Without Trastuzumab for Breast Cancer," *N Engl J Med*, 2006, 354(8):809-20.

Docetaxel-Oxaliplatin (Ovarian Cancer)

Index Terms Oxaliplatin-Docetaxel (Ovarian Cancer)

Use Ovarian cancer

Regimen

Docetaxel: I.V.: 75 mg/m²/dose over 60 minutes day 1
  [total dose/cycle = 75 mg/m²]
Oxaliplatin: I.V.: 100 mg/m²/dose over 2 hours day 1
  [total dose/cycle = 100 mg/m²]
Repeat cycle every 21 days

References

Ferrandina G, Ludovisi M, De Vincenzo R, et al, "Docetaxel and Oxaliplatin in the Second-Line Treatment of Platinum-Sensitive Recurrent Ovarian Cancer: A Phase II Study," *Ann Oncol*, 2007, 18(8):1348-53.

Docetaxel-Prednisone

Use Prostate cancer

Regimen

Docetaxel: I.V.: 75 mg/m² day 1
  [total dose/cycle = 75 mg/m²]
Prednisone: Oral: 5 mg twice daily
  [total dose/cycle = 210 mg]
Repeat cycle every 21 days for up to 10 cycles

References

Dagher R, Li N, Abraham S, et al, "Approval Summary: Docetaxel in Combination With Prednisone for the Treatment of Androgen-Independent Hormone-Refractory Prostate Cancer," *Clin Cancer Res*, 2004, 10(24):8147-51.

Tannock IF, de Wit R, Berry WR, et al, "Docetaxel Plus Prednisone or Mitoxantrone Plus Prednisone for Advanced Prostate Cancer," *N Engl J Med*, 2004, 351(15):1502-12

Docetaxel-Thalidomide

Use Prostate cancer

Regimen

Docetaxel: I.V.: 30 mg/m²/day days 1, 8, and 15
  [total dose/cycle = 90 mg/m²]

Thalidomide: Oral: 200 mg daily (at bedtime)
[total dose/cycle = 5600 mg]
Repeat cycle every 28 days

References

Dahut WL, Gulley JL, Arlen PM, et al, "Randomized Phase II Trial of Docetaxel Plus Thalidomide in Androgen-Independent Prostate Cancer," *J Clin Oncol*, 2004, 22(13):2532-9.

Docetaxel-Trastuzumab

Index Terms Trastuzumab-Docetaxel
Use Breast cancer
Regimen
Cycle 1:
Docetaxel: I.V.: 100 mg/m^2 day 1
[total dose/cycle 1 = 100 mg/m^2]
Trastuzumab: I.V.: 4 mg/kg (loading dose) day 1 cycle 1
followed by I.V.: 2 mg/kg/day days 8 and 15 cycle 1
[total dose/cycle 1 = 8 mg/kg]
Treatment cycle is 21 days
Subsequent cycles:
Docetaxel: I.V.: 100 mg/m^2 day 1
[total dose/cycle = 100 mg/m^2]
Trastuzumab: I.V.: 2 mg/kg/day days 1, 8, and 15
[total dose/cycle = 6 mg/kg]
Repeat cycle every 21 days for a total of at least 6 cycles (continue weekly trastuzumab until disease progression)

References

Marty M, Cognetti F, Maraninchi D, et al, "Randomized Phase II Trial of the Efficacy and Safety of Trastuzumab Combined With Docetaxel in Patients With Human Epidermal Growth Factor Receptor 2-Positive Metastatic Breast Cancer Administered as First-Line Treatment: The M77001 Study Group," *J Clin Oncol*, 2005, 23(19):4265-74.

Docetaxel-Trastuzumab-Carboplatin

Index Terms Trastuzumab-Docetaxel-Carboplatin
Use Breast cancer
Regimen
Cycle 1:
Trastuzumab: I.V.: 4 mg/kg (loading dose) day 1 cycle 1
followed by I.V.: 2 mg/kg/day days 8 and 15 cycle 1
[total dose/cycle 1 = 8 mg/kg]
Docetaxel: I.V.: 75 mg/m^2 day 2
[total dose/cycle 1 = 75 mg/m^2]
Carboplatin: I.V.: AUC 6 day 2
[total dose/cycle 1 = AUC = 6]
Treatment cycle is 21 days
Subsequent cycles:
Trastuzumab: I.V.: 2 mg/kg/day days 1, 8, and 15
[total dose/cycle = 6 mg/kg]
Docetaxel: I.V.: 75 mg/m^2 day 1
[total dose/cycle = 75 mg/m^2]
Carboplatin: I.V.: AUC 6 day 1
[total dose/cycle = AUC = 6]
Repeat cycle every 21 days for a total of ~6 cycles (continue weekly trastuzumab for 1 year after chemotherapy, or until disease progression or unacceptable toxicity)

◄ **References**
Pegram MD, Pienkowski T, Northfelt DW, et al, "Results of Two Open-Label, Multicenter Phase II Studies of Docetaxel, Platinum Salts, and Trastuzumab in HER2-Positive Advanced Breast Cancer," *J Natl Cancer Inst*, 2004, 96(10):759-69.

Docetaxel-Trastuzumab-Cisplatin

Index Terms Trastuzumab-Docetaxel-Cisplatin

Use Breast cancer

Regimen

Cycle 1:
Trastuzumab: I.V.: 4 mg/kg (loading dose) day 1 cycle 1
followed by I.V.: 2 mg/kg/day days 8 and 15 cycle 1
[total dose/cycle 1 = 8 mg/kg]
Docetaxel: I.V.: 75 mg/m² day 2
[total dose/cycle 1 = 75 mg/m²]
Cisplatin: I.V.: 75 mg/m² day 2
[total dose/cycle 1 = 75 mg/m²]
Treatment cycle is 21 days

Subsequent cycles:
Trastuzumab: I.V.: 2 mg/kg/day days 1, 8, and 15
[total dose/cycle = 6 mg/kg]
Docetaxel: I.V.: 75 mg/m² day 1
[total dose/cycle = 75 mg/m²]
Cisplatin: I.V.: 75 mg/m² day 1
[total dose/cycle = 75 mg/m²]
Repeat cycle every 21 days for a total of ~6 cycles (continue weekly trastuzumab for 1 year after chemotherapy, or until disease progression or unacceptable toxicity)

References
Pegram MD, Pienkowski T, Northfelt DW, et al, "Results of Two Open-Label, Multicenter Phase II Studies of Docetaxel, Platinum Salts, and Trastuzumab in HER2-Positive Advanced Breast Cancer," *J Natl Cancer Inst*, 2004, 96(10):759-69.

Docetaxel-Trastuzumab-FEC

Index Terms Trastuzumab-Docetaxel-FEC

Use Breast cancer

Regimen

Cycle 1:
Trastuzumab: I.V.: 4 mg/kg (loading dose) day 1 cycle 1
followed by I.V.: 2 mg/kg/day days 8 and 15 cycle 1
[total dose/cycle 1 = 8 mg/kg]
Docetaxel: I.V.: 80-100 mg/m² day 1
[total dose/cycle 1 = 80-100 mg/m²]
Treatment cycle is 21 days

Cycles 2 and 3:
Trastuzumab: I.V.: 2 mg/kg/day days 1, 8, and 15
[total dose/cycle = 6 mg/kg]
Docetaxel: I.V.: 80-100 mg/m² day 1
[total dose/cycle = 80-100 mg/m²]
Treatment cycle is 21 days

Cycles 4, 5, and 6 (FEC):
Fluorouracil: I.V.: 600 mg/m² day 1
[total dose/cycle = 600 mg/m²]
Epirubicin: I.V.: 60 mg/m² day 1
[total dose/cycle = 60 mg/m²]

References

Sparano JA, Makhson AN, Semiglazov VF, et al, "Pegylated Liposomal Doxorubicin Plus Docetaxel Significantly Improves Time to Progression Without Additive Cardiotoxicity Compared With Docetaxel Monotherapy in Patients With Advanced Breast Cancer Previously Treated With Neoadjuvant-Adjuvant Anthracycline Therapy: Results From a Randomized Phase III Study," *J Clin Oncol*, 2009 [epub ahead of print].

Doxorubicin (Liposomal)-Vincristine-Dexamethasone

Index Terms DVd; DVD

Use Multiple myeloma

Regimen NOTE: Multiple variations are listed.

Variation 1:

Doxorubicin, liposomal: I.V.: 40 mg/m^2 day 1
[total dose/cycle = 40 mg/m^2]

Vincristine: I.V.: 2 mg day 1
[total dose/cycle = 2 mg]

Dexamethasone: Oral or I.V.: 40 mg/day days 1 to 4
[total dose/cycle = 160 mg]

Repeat cycle every 4 weeks

Variation 2:

Doxorubicin, liposomal: I.V.: 40 mg/m^2 day 1
[total dose/cycle = 40 mg/m^2]

Vincristine: I.V.: 1.4 mg/m^2 (maximum dose: 2 mg) day 1
[total dose/cycle = 1.4 mg/m^2; maximum: 2 mg]

Dexamethasone: Oral: 40 mg/day days 1 to 4
[total dose/cycle = 160 mg]

Repeat cycle every 4 weeks

References

Variation 1:

Hussein MA, Wood L, Hsi E, et al, "A Phase II Trial of Pegylated Liposomal Doxorubicin, Vincristine, and Reduced-Dose Dexamethasone Combination Therapy in Newly Diagnosed Multiple Myeloma Patients," *Cancer*, 2002, 95(10):2160-8.

Variation 2:

Rifkin RM, Gregory SA, Mohrbacher A, et al, "Pegylated Liposomal Doxorubicin, Vincristine, and Dexamethasone Provide Significant Reduction in Toxicity Compared With Doxorubicin, Vincristine, and Dexamethasone in Patients With Newly Diagnosed Multiple Myeloma: A Phase III Multicenter Randomized Trial," *Cancer*, 2006, 106(4):848-58.

DTPACE

Use Multiple myeloma

Regimen

Dexamethasone: Oral: 40 mg/day days 1 to 4
[total dose/cycle = 160 mg]

Thalidomide: Oral: 400 mg/day
[total dose/cycle = 11,200 - 16,800 mg]

Cisplatin: I.V.: 10 mg/m^2/day continuous infusion days 1 to 4
[total dose/cycle = 40 mg/m^2]

Doxorubicin: I.V.: 10 mg/m^2/day continuous infusion days 1 to 4
[total dose/cycle = 40 mg/m^2]

Cyclophosphamide: I.V.: 400 mg/m^2 continuous infusion days 1 to 4
[total dose/cycle = 1600 mg/m^2]

Etoposide: I.V.: 40 mg/m^2 continuous infusion days 1 to 4
[total dose/cycle = 160 mg/m^2]

Repeat cycle every 4-6 weeks

References

Lee CK, Barlogie B, Munshi N, et al, "DTPACE: An Effective, Novel Combination Chemotherapy With Thalidomide for Previously Treated Patients With Myeloma," *J Clin Oncol*, 2003, 21 (14):2732-9.

◆ **DVd** *see* Doxorubicin (Liposomal)-Vincristine-Dexamethasone *on page 1297*

DVP

Use Leukemia, acute lymphocytic

Regimen Induction:

Daunorubicin: I.V.: 25 mg/m^2/day days 1, 8, and 15
[total dose/cycle = 75 mg/m^2]

Vincristine: I.V.: 1.5 mg/m^2/day (maximum dose: 2 mg) days 1, 8, 15, and 22
[total dose/cycle = 6 mg/m^2]

Prednisone: Oral: 60 mg/m^2/day days 1 to 28 then taper over next 14 days
[total dose/cycle = 1680 mg/m^2 + taper over next 14 days]

Administer single cycle; used in conjunction with intrathecal chemotherapy

References

Belasco JB, Luery N, and Scher C, "Multiagent Chemotherapy in Relapsed Acute Lymphoblastic Leukemia in Children," *Cancer*, 1990, 66(12):2492-7.

EAP

Use Gastric cancer

Regimen

Etoposide: I.V.: 120 mg/m^2/day days 4, 5, and 6
[total dose/cycle = 360 mg/m^2]

Doxorubicin: I.V.: 20 mg/m^2/day days 1 and 7
[total dose/cycle = 40 mg/m^2]

Cisplatin: I.V.: 40 mg/m^2/day days 2 and 8
[total dose/cycle = 80 mg/m^2]

Repeat cycle every 22-28 days

References

Preusser P, Wilke H, Achterrath W, et al, "Phase II Study With the Combination Etoposide, Doxorubicin, and Cisplatin in Advanced Measurable Gastric Cancer," *J Clin Oncol*, 1989, 7 (9):1310-17.

Wilke H, Preusser P, Fink U, et al, "New Developments in the Treatment of Gastric Carcinoma," *Semin Oncol*, 1990, 17(1 Suppl 2):61-70.

Wilke H, Preusser P, Fink U, et al, "Preoperative Chemotherapy in Locally Advanced and Nonresectable Gastric Cancer: A Phase II Study With Etoposide, Doxorubicin, and Cisplatin," *J Clin Oncol*, 1989, 7(9):1318-26.

◆ **ECF (Gastric/Esophageal Cancer)** *see* Epirubicin-Cisplatin-Fluorouracil (Gastric/Esophageal Cancer) *on page 1305*

EC (NSCLC)

Use Lung cancer, nonsmall cell

Regimen

Etoposide: I.V.: 120 mg/m^2/day days 1, 2, and 3
[total dose/cycle = 360 mg/m^2]

Carboplatin: I.V.: AUC 6 day 1
[total dose/cycle = AUC = 6]

Repeat cycle every 21-28 days

References

Birch R, Weaver CH, Hainsworth JD, et al, "A Randomized Study of Etoposide and Carboplatin With or Without Paclitaxel in the Treatment of Small Cell Lung Cancer," *Semin Oncol*, 1997, 24(4 Suppl 12):S12-135, 137.

EC (Small Cell Lung Cancer)

Use Lung cancer, small cell

Regimen NOTE: Multiple variations are listed.

Variation 1:

Etoposide: I.V.: 100-120 mg/m²/day days 1, 2, and 3
[total dose/cycle = 300-360 mg/m²]

Carboplatin: I.V.: 325-400 mg/m² day 1
[total dose/cycle = 325-400 mg/m²]

Repeat cycle every 28 days

Variation 2:

Etoposide: I.V.: 120 mg/m²/day days 1, 2, and 3
[total dose/cycle = 360 mg/m²]

Carboplatin: I.V.: AUC 6 day 1
[total dose/cycle = AUC = 6]

Repeat cycle every 21-28 days

References

Variation 1:

Kosmidis PA, Samantas E, Fountzilas G, et al, "Cisplatin/Etoposide Versus Carboplatin/Etoposide Chemotherapy and Irradiation in Small Cell Lung Cancer: A Randomized Phase III Study. Hellenic Cooperative Oncology Group for Lung Cancer Trials," *Semin Oncol*, 1994, 1(3 Suppl 6):23-30.

Variation 2:

Birch R, Weaver CH, Hainsworth JD, et al, "A Randomized Study of Etoposide and Carboplatin With or Without Paclitaxel in the Treatment of Small Cell Lung Cancer," *Semin Oncol*, 1997, 24(4 Suppl 12):135, 137.

♦ **ECX (Esophageal Cancer)** *see* Epirubicin-Cisplatin-Capecitabine (Esophageal Cancer) *on page 1305*

EE

Use Wilms' tumor

Regimen

Dactinomycin: I.V.: 15 mcg/kg/day days 1 to 5 of weeks 0, 5, 13, and 24
[total dose/cycle = 300 mcg/kg]

Vincristine: I.V.: 1.5 mg/m² day 1 of weeks 1-10, 13, 14, 24, and 25
[total dose/cycle = 21 mg/m²]

References

Green DM, Breslow NE, Beckwith JB, et al, "Effect of Duration of Treatment on Treatment Outcome and Cost of Treatment for Wilms' Tumor: A Report From the National Wilms' Tumor Study Group," *J Clin Oncol*, 1998, 16(12):3744-51.

EE-4A

Use Wilms' tumor

Regimen

Dactinomycin: I.V.: 45 mcg/kg day 1 of weeks 0, 3, 6, 9, 12, 15, and 18
[total dose/cycle = 315 mcg/kg]

Vincristine: I.V.: 2 mg/m² day 1 of weeks 1-10, 12, 15, and 18
[total dose/cycle = 26 mg/m²]

References

Green DM, Breslow NE, Beckwith JB, et al, "Effect of Duration of Treatment on Treatment Outcome and Cost of Treatment for Wilms' Tumor: A Report From the National Wilms' Tumor Study Group," *J Clin Oncol*, 16(12):3744-51.

EFP

Use Gastric cancer

Regimen NOTE: Multiple variations are listed.

Variation 1:

Etoposide: I.V.: 90 mg/m^2/day days 1, 3, and 5
[total dose/cycle = 270 mg/m^2]

Fluorouracil: I.V.: 900 mg/m^2/day (20-hour infusion) days 1 to 5
[total dose/cycle = 4500 mg/m^2]

Cisplatin: I.V.: 20 mg/m^2/day days 1 to 5
[total dose/cycle = 100 mg/m^2]

Repeat cycle every 24-28 days

Variation 2:

Etoposide: I.V.: 100 mg/m^2/day days 1, 3, and 5
[total dose/cycle = 300 mg/m^2]

Fluorouracil: I.V.: 800 mg/m^2/day (12-hour infusion) days 1 to 5
[total dose/cycle = 4000 mg/m^2]

Cisplatin: I.V.: 20 mg/m^2/day days 1 to 5
[total dose/cycle = 100 mg/m^2]

Repeat cycle every 3 weeks

References

Variation 1:
Ajani JA, Roth JA, Ryan B, et al, "Evaluation of Pre- and Postoperative Chemotherapy for Resectable Adenocarcinoma of the Esophagus or Gastroesophageal Junction," *J Clin Oncol*, 1990, 8(7):1231-8.

Variation 2:
Ryoo BY, Kang YK, Im YH, et al, "Adjuvant (Cisplatin, Etoposide, and 5-Fluorouracil) Chemotherapy After Curative Resection of Gastric Adenocarcinomas Involving the Esophagogastric Junction," *Am J Clin Oncol*, 1999, 22(3):253-7.

ELF

Use Gastric cancer

Regimen

Leucovorin calcium: I.V.: 300 mg/m^2/day days 1, 2, and 3
[total dose/cycle = 900 mg/m^2]

followed by

Etoposide: I.V.: 120 mg/m^2/day days 1, 2, and 3
[total dose/cycle = 360 mg/m^2]

followed by

Fluorouracil: I.V.: 500 mg/m^2/day days 1, 2, and 3
[total dose/cycle = 1500 mg/m^2]

Repeat cycle every 21-28 days

References

Wilke H, Preusser P, Fink U, et al, "New Developments in the Treatment of Gastric Carcinoma," *Semin Oncol*, 1990, 17(1 Suppl 2):61-70.

EMA 86

Use Leukemia, acute myeloid

Regimen

Mitoxantrone: I.V.: 12 mg/m^2/day days 1, 2, and 3
[total dose/cycle = 36 mg/m^2]

Etoposide: I.V.: 200 mg/m^2/day continuous infusion days 8, 9, and 10
[total dose/cycle = 600 mg/m^2]

Cytarabine: I.V.: 500 mg/m^2/day continuous infusion days 1, 2, and 3 and days 8, 9, and 10
[total dose/cycle = 3000 mg/m^2]

Administer one cycle only

References
Archimbaud E, Fenaux P, Reiffers J, et al, "Granulocyte-Macrophage Colony-Stimulating Factor in Association to Timed-Sequential Chemotherapy With Mitoxantrone, Etoposide, and Cytarabine for Refractory Acute Myelogenous Leukemia," *Leukemia*, 1993, 7(3):372-7.

EMA/CO

Use Gestational trophoblastic tumor

Regimen NOTE: Multiple variations are listed.

Variation 1:

Etoposide: I.V.: 100 mg/m^2/day days 1 and 2
[total dose/cycle = 200 mg/m^2]

Methotrexate: I.V.: 300 mg/m^2 continuous infusion over 12 hours day 1
[total dose/cycle = 300 mg/m^2]

Dactinomycin: I.V. push: 0.5 mg/day days 1 and 2
[total dose/cycle = 1 mg]

Leucovorin: Oral, I.M.: 15 mg twice daily for 2 days (start 24 hours after the start of methotrexate) days 2 and 3
[total dose/cycle = 60 mg]

Alternate weekly with:

Cyclophosphamide: I.V.: 600 mg/m^2 day 1
[total dose/cycle = 600 mg/m^2]

Vincristine: I.V. push: 0.8 mg/m^2 (maximum dose: 2 mg) day 1
[total dose/cycle = 0.8 mg/m^2]

Repeat cycle every 2 weeks

Variation 2:

Dactinomycin: I.V.: 0.5 mg/day days 1 and 2
[total dose/cycle = 1 mg]

Etoposide: I.V.: 100 mg/m^2/day days 1 and 2
[total dose/cycle = 200 mg/m^2]

Methotrexate: I.V. bolus: 100 mg/m^2 then 200 mg/m^2 continuous infusion over 12 hours day 1
[total dose/cycle = 300 mg/m^2]

Leucovorin: Oral, I.M.: 15 mg every 12 hours for 4 doses (start 24 hours after methotrexate) days 2 and 3
[total dose/cycle = 60 mg]

Vincristine: I.V.: 1 mg/m^2 day 8
[total dose/cycle = 1 mg/m^2]

Cyclophosphamide: I.V.: 600 mg/m^2 day 8
[total dose/cycle = 600 mg/m^2]

Repeat cycle every 2 weeks

Variation 3:

Dactinomycin: I.V.: 0.5 mg/day days 1 and 2
[total dose/cycle = 1 mg]

Etoposide: I.V.: 100 mg/m^2/day days 1 and 2
[total dose/cycle = 200 mg/m^2]

Methotrexate: I.V.: 300 mg/m^2 continuous infusion over 12 hours day 1
[total dose/cycle = 300 mg/m^2]

Leucovorin: Oral, I.M.: 15 mg every 12 hours for 4 doses (start 24 hours after start of methotrexate) days 2 and 3
[total dose/cycle = 60 mg]

Vincristine: I.V.: 1 mg/m^2 day 8
[total dose/cycle = 1 mg/m^2]

◀ Cyclophosphamide: I.V.: 600 mg/m² day 8
[total dose/cycle = 600 mg/m²]
Repeat cycle every 2 weeks
Variation 4:
Dactinomycin: I.V.: 0.35 mg/m²/day days 1 and 2
[total dose/cycle = 0.7 mg/m²]
Etoposide: I.V.: 100 mg/m²/day days 1 and 2
[total dose/cycle = 200 mg/m²]
Methotrexate: I.V. bolus: 100 mg/m² then 200 mg/m² continuous infusion over 12 hours day 1
[total dose/cycle = 300 mg/m²]
Leucovorin: Oral, I.M.: 15 mg every 12 hours for 4 doses (start 24 hours after start of methotrexate) days 2 and 3
[total dose/cycle = 60 mg]
Vincristine: I.V.: 1 mg/m² day 8
[total dose/cycle = 1 mg/m²]
Cyclophosphamide: I.V.: 600 mg/m² day 8
[total dose/cycle = 600 mg/m²]
Repeat cycle every 2 weeks
Variation 5 (patients with brain metastases):
Dactinomycin: I.V.: 0.5 mg/day days 1 and 2
[total dose/cycle = 1 mg]
Etoposide:I.V.: 100 mg/m²/day days 1 and 2
[total dose/cycle = 200 mg/m²]
Methotrexate: I.V.: 1 g/m² continuous infusion over 12 hours day 1
[total dose/cycle = 1 g/m²]
Leucovorin: I.M.: 20 mg/m² every 6 hours for 12 doses (start 24 hours after start of methotrexate) days 2, 3, and 4
[total dose/cycle = 240 mg/m²]
Vincristine: I.V.: 1 mg/m² day 8
[total dose/cycle = 1 mg/m²]
Cyclophosphamide: I.V.: 600 mg/m² day 8
[total dose/cycle = 600 mg/m²]
Repeat cycle every 2 weeks
Variation 6 (patients with brain metastases):
Dactinomycin: I.V.: 0.5 mg/day days 1 and 2
[total dose/cycle = 1 mg]
Etoposide: I.V.: 100 mg/m²/day days 1 and 2
[total dose/cycle = 200 mg/m²]
Methotrexate: I.V.: 1 g/m² continuous infusion over 12 hours day 1
[total dose/cycle = 1 g/m²]
Leucovorin: Oral, I.M.: 30 mg/m² every 12 hours for 6 doses (start 32 hours after start of methotrexate) days 2, 3, and 4
[total dose/cycle = 180 mg/m²]
Vincristine: I.V.: 1 mg/m² day 8
[total dose/cycle = 1 mg/m²]
Cyclophosphamide: I.V.: 600 mg/m² day 8
[total dose/cycle = 600 mg/m²]
Repeat cycle every 2 weeks
Variation 7:
Dactinomycin: I.V.: 0.5 mg/day days 1 and 2
[total dose/cycle = 1 mg]
Etoposide: I.V.: 100 mg/m²/day days 1 and 2
[total dose/cycle = 200 mg/m²]

Methotrexate: I.V.: 1 g/m^2 continuous infusion over 24 hours day 1
  [total dose/cycle = 1 g/m^2]
Leucovorin: Oral, I.M.: 15 mg every 8 hours for 9 doses (start 32 hours after start of methotrexate) days 2, 3, and 4
  [total dose/cycle = 135 mg/m^2]
Vincristine: I.V.: 1 mg/m^2 day 8
  [total dose/cycle = 1 mg/m^2]
Cyclophosphamide: I.V.: 600 mg/m^2 day 8
  [total dose/cycle = 600 mg/m^2]
Repeat cycle every 2 weeks

Variation 8 (patients with lung metastases):
Dactinomycin: I.V.: 0.5 mg/day days 1 and 2
  [total dose/cycle = 1 mg]
Etoposide: I.V.: 100 mg/m^2/day days 1 and 2
  [total dose/cycle = 200 mg/m^2]
Methotrexate: I.V. bolus: 100 mg/m^2 then 200 mg/m^2 continuous infusion over 12 hours day 1
  [total dose/cycle = 300 mg/m^2]
Leucovorin: Oral, I.M.: 15 mg every 12 hours for 4 doses (start 24 hours after start of methotrexate) days 2 and 3
  [total dose/cycle = 60 mg]
Vincristine: I.V.: 1 mg/m^2 day 8
  [total dose/cycle = 1 mg/m^2]
Cyclophosphamide: I.V.: 600 mg/m^2 day 8
  [total dose/cycle = 600 mg/m^2]
Methotrexate: I.T.: 10 mg day 1 (every other cycle)
  [total dose/cycle = 10 mg, every other cycle]
Repeat cycle every 2 weeks

Variation 9 (patients with lung metastases):
Dactinomycin: I.V.: 0.5 mg/day days 1 and 2
  [total dose/cycle = 1 mg]
Etoposide: I.V.: 100 mg/m^2/day days 1 and 2
  [total dose/cycle = 200 mg/m^2]
Methotrexate: I.V. bolus: 100 mg/m^2 then 200 mg/m^2 continuous infusion over 12 hours day 1
  [total dose/cycle = 300 mg/m^2]
Leucovorin: Oral, I.M.: 15 mg every 12 hours for 4 doses (start 24 hours after start of methotrexate) days 2 and 3
  [total dose/cycle = 60 mg]
Vincristine: I.V.: 1 mg/m^2 day 8
  [total dose/cycle = 1 mg/m^2]
Cyclophosphamide: I.V.: 600 mg/m^2 day 8
  [total dose/cycle = 600 mg/m^2]
Methotrexate: I.T.: 12.5 mg day 8
  [total dose/cycle = 12.5 mg]
Repeat cycle every 2 weeks

References

Variation 1:
Bagshawe KD, "High-Risk Metastatic Trophoblastic Disease," *Obstet Gynecol Clin North Am,* 1988, 15(3):531-43.
Variation 2:
Newlands ES, Bagshawe KD, Begent RH, et al, "Developments in Chemotherapy for Medium- and High-Risk Patients With Gestational Trophoblastic Tumours (1979-1984)," *Br J Obstet Gynaecol,* 1986, 93(1):63-9.

Variation 3:
Newlands ES, Bagshawe KD, Begent RH, et al, "Results With the EMA/CO (Etoposide, Methotrexate, Actinomycin D, Cyclophosphamide, Vincristine) Regimen in High-Risk Gestational Trophoblastic Tumours, 1979 to 1989," *J Obstet Gynecol*, 1991, 98(6):550-7.

Variation 4:
Soper JT, Evans AC, Clarke-Pearson DL, et al, "Alternating Weekly Chemotherapy With Etoposide-Methotrexate-Dactinomycin/Cyclophosphamide-Vincristine for High-Risk Gestational Trophoblastic Disease," *Obstet Gynecol*, 1994, 83(1):113-7.

Variation 5:
Bolis G, Bonazzi C, Landoni F, et al, "EMA/CO Regimen in High-Risk Gestational Trophoblastic Tumor (GTT)," *Gynecol Oncol*, 1988, 31(3):439-44.

Variation 6:
Schink JC, Singh Dk, Rademaker AW, et al, "Etoposide, Methotrexate, Actinomycin-D, Cyclophosphamide, and Vincristine for the Treatment of Metastatic, High-Risk Gestational Trophoblastic Disease," *Obstet Gynecol*, 1992, 80(5):817-20.

Variation 7:
Newlands ES, Bagshawe KD, Begent RH, et al, "Results With the EMA/CO (Etoposide, Methotrexate, Actinomycin D, Cyclophosphamide, Vincristine) Regimen in High-Risk Gestational Trophoblastic Tumours, 1979 to 1989," *Br J Obstet Gynaecol*, 1991, 98(6):550-7.

Variation 8:
Bolis G, Bonazzi C, Landoni F, et al, "EMA/CO Regimen in High-Risk Gestational Trophoblastic Tumor (GTT)," *Gynecol Oncol*, 1988, 31(3):439-44.

Variation 9:
Newlands ES, Bagshawe KD, Begent RH, et al, "Developments in Chemotherapy for Medium- and High-Risk Patients With Gestational Trophoblastic Tumours (1979-1984)," *Br J Obstet Gynaecol*, 1986, 93(1):63-9.

◆ **EMA/EP** see EP/EMA on page 1304

◆ **EOF (Esophageal Cancer)** see Epirubicin-Oxaliplatin-Fluorouracil (Esophageal Cancer) on page 1306

◆ **EOX** see Epirubicin-Oxaliplatin-Capecitabine on page 1306

EP (Adenocarcinoma)

Use Adenocarcinoma, unknown primary

Regimen

Cisplatin: I.V.: 60-100 mg/m² day 1
 [total dose = 60-100 mg/m²]
Etoposide: I.V.: 80-100 mg/m²/day days 1, 2, and 3
 [total dose = 240-300 mg/m²]
Repeat cycle every 21 days

References

Sulkes A, Uziely B, Isacson R, et al, "Combination Chemotherapy in Metastatic Tumors of Unknown Origin. 5-Fluorouracil, Adriamycin® and Mitomycin C for Adenocarcinomas and Adriamycin®, Vinblastine, and Mitomycin C for Anaplastic Carcinomas," *Isr J Med Sci*, 1988, 24 (9-10):604-10.

EP/EMA

Index Terms EMA/EP

Use Gestational trophoblastic tumor

Regimen NOTE: Multiple variations are listed.

Variation 1:

Etoposide: I.V.: 150 mg/m² day 1
 [total dose/cycle = 150 mg/m²]
Cisplatin: I.V.: 25 mg/m² infused over 4 hours for 3 consecutive doses, day 1
 [total dose/cycle = 75 mg/m²]

Alternate weekly with:

Etoposide: I.V.: 100 mg/m² day 1
 [total dose/cycle = 100 mg/m²]

Methotrexate: I.V.: 300 mg/m^2 infused over 12 hours day 1
[total dose/cycle = 300 mg/m^2]
Dactinomycin: I.V. push: 0.5 mg day 1
[total dose/cycle = 0.5 mg]
Leucovorin: Oral, I.M.: 15 mg twice daily for 2 days (start 24 hours after the start of methotrexate) days 2 and 3
[total dose/cycle = 60 mg]
Variation 2:
Dactinomycin: I.V.: 0.5 mg/day days 1 and 2
[total dose/cycle = 1 mg]
Etoposide: I.V.: 100 mg/m^2/day days 1 and 2
[total dose/cycle = 200 mg/m^2]
Methotrexate: I.V.: 300 mg/m^2 continuous infusion over 12 hours day 1
[total dose/cycle = 300 mg/m^2]
Leucovorin: Oral, I.M.: 15 mg every 12 hours for 4 doses (start 24 hours after start of methotrexate) days 2 and 3
[total dose/cycle = 60 mg]
Etoposide: I.V.: 150 mg/m^2 day 8
[total dose/cycle = 150 mg/m^2]
Cisplatin: I.V.: 75 mg/m^2 day 8
[total dose/cycle = 75 mg/m^2]
Repeat cycle every 2 weeks

References

Variation 1:
Newlands ES, Bower M, Holden L, et al, "Management of Resistant Gestational Trophoblastic Tumors," *J Reprod Med*, 1998, 43(2):111-8.
Variation 2:
Newlands ES, Bagshawe KD, Begent RH, et al, "Results With the EMA/CO (Etoposide, Methotrexate, Actinomycin D, Cyclophosphamide, Vincristine) Regimen in High Risk Gestational Trophoblastic Tumours, 1979 to 1989," *J Obstet Gynaecol*, 1991, 98(6):550-7.

Epirubicin-Cisplatin-Capecitabine (Esophageal Cancer)

Index Terms ECX (Esophageal Cancer)
Use Esophageal cancer
Regimen
Epirubicin: I.V.: 50 mg/m^2 day 1
[total dose/cycle = 50 mg/m^2]
Cisplatin: I.V.: 60 mg/m^2 day 1
[total dose/cycle = 60 mg/m^2]
Capecitabine: Oral: 625 mg/m^2 twice daily days 1 to 21
[total dose/cycle = 26,250 mg/m^2]
Repeat cycle every 21 days for up to 8 cycles

References

Cunningham D, Starling N, Rao S, et al, "Capecitabine and Oxaliplatin for Advanced Esophagogastric Cancer," *N Engl J Med*, 2008, 358(1):36-46.

Epirubicin-Cisplatin-Fluorouracil (Gastric/Esophageal Cancer)

Index Terms ECF (Gastric/Esophageal Cancer)
Use Esophageal cancer; Gastric cancer
Regimen NOTE: Multiple variations are listed.
Variation 1:
Epirubicin: I.V.: 50 mg/m^2 day 1
[total dose/cycle = 50 mg/m^2]

Cisplatin: I.V.: 60 mg/m^2 day 1
  [total dose/cycle = 60 mg/m^2]
Fluorouracil: I.V.: 200 mg/m^2/day continuous infusion days 1 to 21
  [total dose/cycle = 4200 mg/m^2]
Repeat cycle every 3 weeks for up to 8 cycles
Variation 2:
Epirubicin: I.V.: 50 mg/m^2 day 1
  [total dose/cycle = 50 mg/m^2]
Cisplatin: I.V.: 60 mg/m^2 day 1
  [total dose/cycle = 60 mg/m^2]
Fluorouracil: I.V.: 200 mg/m^2/day continuous infusion days 1 to 21
  [total dose/cycle = 4200 mg/m^2]
Repeat cycle every 3 weeks for up to 6 cycles (3 cycles before surgery and 3
cycles postoperatively)

References

Variation 1:
Cunningham D, Starling N, Rao S, et al, "Capecitabine and Oxaliplatin for Advanced Esophagogastric Cancer," *N Engl J Med*, 2008, 358(1):36-46.

Ross P, Nicolson M, Cunningham D, et al, "Prospective Randomized Trial Comparing Mitomycin, Cisplatin, and Protracted Venous-Infusion Fluorouracil (PVI 5-FU) With Epirubicin, Cisplatin, and PVI 5-FU in Advanced Esophagogastric Cancer," *J Clin Oncol*, 2002, 20(8):1996-2004.

Webb A, Cunningham D, Scarffe JH, et al, "Randomized Trial Comparing Epirubicin, Cisplatin, and Fluorouracil Versus Fluorouracil, Doxorubicin, and Methotrexate in Advanced Esophagogastric Cancer," *J Clin Oncol*, 1997, 15(1):261-7.

Variation 2:
Cunningham D, Allum WH, Stenning SP, et al, "Perioperative Chemotherapy Versus Surgery Alone for Resectable Gastroesophageal Cancer," *N Engl J Med*, 2006, 355(1):11-20.

Epirubicin-Oxaliplatin-Capecitabine

Index Terms Capecitabine-Oxaliplatin-Epirubicin; EOX; Oxaliplatin-Capecitabine-Epirubicin

Use Esophageal cancer; Gastric cancer

Regimen

Epirubicin: I.V.: 50 mg/m^2 day 1
  [total dose/cycle = 50 mg/m^2]
Oxaliplatin: I.V.: 130 mg/m^2 day 1
  [total dose/cycle = 130 mg/m^2]
Capecitabine: Oral: 625 mg/m^2 twice daily days 1 to 21
  [total dose/cycle = 26,250 mg/m^2]
Repeat cycle every 21 days for up to 8 cycles

References

Cunningham D, Starling N, Rao S, et al, "Capecitabine and Oxaliplatin for Advanced Esophagogastric Cancer," *N Engl J Med*, 2008, 358(1):36-46.

Epirubicin-Oxaliplatin-Fluorouracil (Esophageal Cancer)

Index Terms EOF (Esophageal Cancer)

Use Esophageal cancer

Regimen

Epirubicin: I.V.: 50 mg/m^2 day 1
  [total dose/cycle = 50 mg/m^2]
Oxaliplatin: I.V.: 130 mg/m^2 day 1
  [total dose/cycle = 130 mg/m^2]
Fluorouracil: I.V.: 200 mg/m^2/day continuous infusion days 1 to 21
  [total dose/cycle = 4200 mg/m^2]
Repeat cycle every 21 days for up to 8 cycles

References

Cunningham D, Starling N, Rao S, et al, "Capecitabine and Oxaliplatin for Advanced Esophagogastric Cancer," *N Engl J Med*, 2008, 358(1):36-46.

EP (NSCLC)

Use Lung cancer, nonsmall cell

Regimen

Etoposide: I.V.: 80-120 mg/m^2/day days 1, 2, and 3
[total dose/cycle = 240-360 mg/m^2]
Cisplatin: I.V.: 80-100 mg/m^2 day 1
[total dose/cycle = 80-100 mg/m^2]
Repeat cycle every 21-28 days

References

Goldhirsch A, Joss RA, Cavalli F, et al, "Cis-Dichlorodiammineplatinum (II) and VP 16-213 Combination Chemotherapy for Nonsmall-Cell Lung Cancer," *Med Pediatr Oncol*, 1981, 9 (3):205-8.

EPOCH Dose-Adjusted (AIDS-Related Lymphoma)

Index Terms Dose-Adjusted EPOCH (AIDS-Related Lymphoma)

Use Lymphoma, AIDS-related

Regimen

Etoposide: I.V.: 50 mg/m^2/day continuous infusion days 1 to 4
[total dose/cycle = 200 mg/m^2]
Vincristine: I.V.: 0.4 mg/m^2/day continuous infusion days 1 to 4
[total dose/cycle = 1.6 mg/m^2]
Doxorubicin: I.V.: 10 mg/m^2/day continuous infusion days 1 to 4
[total dose/cycle = 40 mg/m^2]
Cyclophosphamide: I.V.: 375 mg/m^2 day 5 for CD4+ cells ≥100/mm^3 **or** 187 mg/m^2 day 5 for CD4+ cells <100/mm^3
[total dose/cycle = 187-375 mg/m^2]
Prednisone: Oral: 60 mg/m^2/day days 1 to 5
[total dose/cycle = 300 mg/m^2]
Filgrastim: SubQ: 5 mcg/kg/day beginning day 6; continue until ANC >5000/mm^3 (past nadir)
Repeat cycle every 21 days for 6 cycles with cyclophosphamide dose adjusted based on previous cycle nadir according to the following schedule:
Nadir ANC >500/mm^3: Increase cyclophosphamide dose by 187 mg/m^2 above previous cycle dose (maximum dose: 750 mg/m^2)
Nadir ANC <500/mm^3 or platelet <25,000/mm^3: Decrease cyclophosphamide dose by 187 mg/m^2 below previous cycle dose

References

Little RF, Pittaluga S, Grant N, et al, "Highly Effective Treatment of Acquired Immunodeficiency Syndrome-Related Lymphoma With Dose-Adjusted EPOCH: Impact of Antiretroviral Therapy Suspension and Tumor Biology," *Blood*, 2003, 101(12):4653-9.

EPOCH Dose-Adjusted (NHL)

Index Terms Dose-Adjusted EPOCH (NHL)

Use Lymphoma, non-Hodgkin's

Regimen

Etoposide: I.V.: 50 mg/m^2/day continuous infusion days 1 to 4
[total dose/cycle = 200 mg/m^2]
Vincristine: I.V.: 0.4 mg/m^2/day continuous infusion days 1 to 4
[total dose/cycle = 1.6 mg/m^2]
Doxorubicin: I.V.: 10 mg/m^2/day continuous infusion days 1 to 4
[total dose/cycle = 40 mg/m^2]

Cyclophosphamide: I.V.: 750 mg/m^2 day 5
[total dose/cycle = 750 mg/m^2]

Prednisone: Oral: 60 mg/m^2 twice daily days 1 to 5
total dose/cycle = 600 mg/m^2]

Filgrastim: SubQ: 5 mcg/kg/day beginning day 6; continue until ANC >5000/mm^3

Repeat cycle every 21 days with etoposide, doxorubicin, and cyclophosphamide dose adjustments (based on CBC 2 times/week) according to the following schedule:

Nadir ANC ≥500/mm^3: 20% increase (above previous cycle) for etoposide, doxorubicin, and cyclophosphamide

Nadir ANC <500/mm^3 (on 1 or 2 measurements): Same doses as previous cycle

Nadir ANC <500/mm^3 (on ≥3 measurements) or nadir platelet <25,000/mm^3 (on 1 measurement): 20% decrease below previous cycle for etoposide, doxorubicin, and cyclophosphamide (dosing adjustments below starting dose levels only apply to cyclophosphamide)

References

Wilson WH, Grossbard ML, Pittaluga S, et al, "Dose-Adjusted EPOCH Chemotherapy for Untreated Large B-Cell Lymphomas: A Pharmacodynamic Approach With High Efficacy," *Blood*, 2002, 99(8):2685-93.

EPOCH (Dose-Adjusted)-Rituximab (NHL)

Index Terms EPOCH (Dose-Adjusted)-R (NHL); R-EPOCH Dose Adjusted (NHL); Rituximab-EPOCH Dose Adjusted (NHL)

Use Lymphoma, non-Hodgkin's

Regimen NOTE: Multiple variations are listed.

Variation 1:

Rituximab: I.V.: 375 mg/m^2 day 1
[total dose/cycle = 375 mg/m^2]

Etoposide: I.V.: 50 mg/m^2/day continuous infusion days 1 to 4
[total dose/cycle = 200 mg/m^2]

Vincristine: I.V.: 0.4 mg/m^2/day continuous infusion days 1 to 4
[total dose/cycle = 1.6 mg/m^2]

Doxorubicin: I.V.: 10 mg/m^2/day continuous infusion days 1 to 4
[total dose/cycle = 40 mg/m^2]

Cyclophosphamide: I.V.: 750 mg/m^2 day 5
[total dose/cycle = 750 mg/m^2]

Prednisone: Oral: 60 mg/m^2 twice daily days 1 to 5
[total dose/cycle = 600 mg/m^2]

Filgrastim: SubQ: 5 mcg/kg/day beginning day 6; continue until ANC >5000/mm^3

Repeat cycle every 21 days (for at least 2 cycles beyond best response; minimum of 6 cycles) with etoposide, doxorubicin, and cyclophosphamide dose adjustments (based on CBC 2 times/week) according to the following schedule:

Nadir ANC ≥500/mm^3: 20% increase (above previous cycle) for etoposide, doxorubicin, and cyclophosphamide

Nadir ANC <500/mm^3 (on 1 or 2 measurements): Same doses as previous cycle

Nadir ANC <500/mm^3 (on ≥3 measurements): 20% decrease below previous cycle for etoposide, doxorubicin, and cyclophosphamide (dosing adjustments below starting dose levels only apply to cyclophosphamide)

Variation 2:
  Rituximab: I.V.: 375 mg/m² day 1
    [total dose/cycle = 375 mg/m²]
  Etoposide: I.V.: 50 mg/m²/day continuous infusion days 1 to 4
    [total dose/cycle = 200 mg/m²]
  Vincristine: I.V.: 0.4 mg/m²/day continuous infusion days 1 to 4
    [total dose/cycle = 1.6 mg/m²]
  Doxorubicin: I.V.: 10 mg/m²/day continuous infusion days 1 to 4
    [total dose/cycle = 40 mg/m²]
  Cyclophosphamide: I.V.: 750 mg/m² day 5
    [total dose/cycle = 750 mg/m²]
  Prednisone: Oral: 60 mg/m²/day days 1 to 5
    [total dose/cycle = 300 mg/m²]
  Filgrastim: SubQ: 5 mcg/kg/day beginning day 6; continue until ANC >500/mm³
  Repeat cycle every 21 days (for 6-8 cycles); refer to variation 1 for dose adjustments

References

Variation 1:
Wilson WH, Gutierrez M, O'Connor P, et al, "The Role of Rituximab and Chemotherapy in Aggressive B-Cell Lymphoma: A Preliminary Report of Dose-Adjusted EPOCH-R," *Semin Oncol,* 2002, 29(1 Suppl 2):41-7.
Variation 2:
García-Suárez J, Bañas H, Arribas I, et al, "Dose-Adjusted EPOCH Plus Rituximab is an Effective Regimen in Patients With Poor-Prognostic Untreated Diffuse Large B-Cell Lymphoma: Results From a Prospective Observational Study," *Br J Haematol,* 2007, 136(2):276-85.

◆ **EPOCH (Dose-Adjusted)-R (NHL)** *see* EPOCH (Dose-Adjusted)-Rituximab (NHL) *on page 1308*

EPOCH (NHL)

Use Lymphoma, non-Hodgkin's

Regimen NOTE: Multiple variations are listed.
Variation 1:
  Etoposide: I.V.: 50 mg/m²/day continuous infusion days 1 to 4
    [total dose/cycle = 200 mg/m²]
  Vincristine: I.V.: 0.4 mg/m²/day continuous infusion days 1 to 4
    [total dose/cycle = 1.6 mg/m²]
  Doxorubicin: I.V.: 10 mg/m²/day continuous infusion days 1 to 4
    [total dose/cycle = 40 mg/m²]
  Cyclophosphamide: I.V.: 750 mg/m² day 5
    [total dose/cycle = 750 mg/m²]
  Prednisone: Oral: 60 mg/m²/day days 1 to 5
    [total dose/cycle = 300 mg/m²]
  Repeat cycle (with cyclophosphamide dose adjustments if needed based on ANC) every 21 days (best response seen in a median of 4 cycles)
Variation 2:
  Etoposide: I.V.: 50 mg/m²/day continuous infusion days 1 to 4
    [total dose/cycle = 200 mg/m²]
  Vincristine: I.V.: 0.4 mg/m²/day continuous infusion days 1 to 4
    [total dose/cycle = 1.6 mg/m²]
  Doxorubicin: I.V.: 10 mg/m²/day continuous infusion days 1 to 4
    [total dose/cycle = 40 mg/m²]
  Cyclophosphamide: I.V.: 750 mg/m² day 6
    [total dose/cycle = 750 mg/m²]

Prednisone: Oral: 60 mg/m^2/day days 1 to 6
[total dose/cycle = 360 mg/m^2]
Repeat cycle (with cyclophosphamide dose adjustments if needed based on ANC) every 21 days (best response seen in a median of 4 cycles)

References

Variation 1:
Gutierrez M, Chabner BA, Pearson D, et al, "Role of a Doxorubicin-Containing Regimen in Relapsed and Resistant Lymphomas: An 8-Year Follow-Up Study of EPOCH," *J Clin Oncol*, 2000, 18(21):3633-42.
Variation 2:
Wilson WH, Bryant G, Bates S, et al, "EPOCH Chemotherapy: Toxicity and Efficacy in Relapsed and Refractory Non-Hodgkin's Lymphoma," *J Clin Oncol*, 1993, 11(8):1573-82.

EPOCH-Rituximab (NHL)

Index Terms EPOCH-R (NHL); R-EPOCH (NHL); Rituximab-EPOCH (NHL)
Use Lymphoma, non-Hodgkin's
Regimen
Rituximab: I.V.: 375 mg/m^2 day 1
[total dose/cycle = 375 mg/m^2]
Etoposide: I.V.: 65 mg/m^2/day continuous infusion days 2, 3, and 4
[total dose/cycle = 195 mg/m^2]
Vincristine: I.V.: 0.5 mg/m^2/day continuous infusion days 2, 3, and 4
[total dose/cycle = 1.5 mg/m^2]
Doxorubicin: I.V.: 15 mg/m^2/day continuous infusion days 2, 3, and 4
[total dose/cycle = 45 mg/m^2]
Cyclophosphamide: I.V.: 750 mg/m^2 day 5
[total dose/cycle = 750 mg/m^2]
Prednisone: Oral: 60 mg/m^2/day days 1 to 14
[total dose/cycle = 840 mg/m^2]
Repeat cycle every 21 days for 4-6 cycles

References

Jermann M, Jost LM, Taverna Ch, et al, "Rituximab-EPOCH, An Effective Salvage Therapy for Relapsed, Refractory or Transformed B-Cell Lymphomas: Results of a Phase II Study," *Ann Oncol*, 2004, 15(3):511-6.

◆ **EPOCH-R (NHL)** *see* EPOCH-Rituximab (NHL) *on page 1310*

EP/PE

Use Lung cancer, nonsmall cell
Regimen
Etoposide: I.V.: 120 mg/m^2/day days 1, 2, and 3
[total dose/cycle = 360 mg/m^2]
Cisplatin: I.V.: 60-120 mg/m^2 day 1
[total dose/cycle = 60-120 mg/m^2]
Repeat cycle every 21-28 days

References

Weick JK, Crowley J, Natale RB, et al, "A Randomized Trial of Five Cisplatin-Containing Treatments in Patients With Metastatic Nonsmall-Cell Lung Cancer: A Southwest Oncology Group Study," *J Clin Oncol*, 1991, 9(7):1157-62.

EP (Small Cell Lung Cancer)

Use Lung cancer, small cell
Regimen NOTE: Multiple variations are listed.
Variation 1:
Etoposide: I.V.: 100 mg/m^2/day days 1, 2, and 3
[total dose/cycle = 300 mg/m^2]

Cisplatin: I.V.: 100 mg/m² day 1
[total dose/cycle = 100 mg/m²]
Repeat cycle every 21 days
Variation 2:
Etoposide: I.V.: 80 mg/m²/day days 1, 2, and 3
[total dose/cycle = 240 mg/m²]
Cisplatin: I.V.: 80 mg/m² day 1
[total dose/cycle = 80 mg/m²]
Repeat cycle every 21-28 days

References

Variation 1:
Goodman GE, Crowley JJ, Blasko JC, et al, "Treatment of Limited Small-Cell Lung Cancer With Etoposide and Cisplatin Alternating With Vincristine, Doxorubicin, and Cyclophosphamide Versus Concurrent Etoposide, Vincristine, Doxorubicin, and Cyclophosphamide and Chest Radiotherapy: A Southwest Oncology Group Study," *J Clin Oncol*, 1990, 8(1):39-47.
Variation 2:
Perng RP, Chen YM, Ming-Liu J, et al, "Gemcitabine Versus the Combination of Cisplatin and Etoposide in Patients With Inoperable Nonsmall Cell Lung Cancer in a Phase II Randomized Study," *J Clin Oncol*, 1997, 15(5):2097-102.

EP (Testicular Cancer)

Use Testicular cancer

Regimen NOTE: Multiple variations are listed.
Variation 1:
Etoposide: I.V.: 100 mg/m²/day days 1 to 5
[total dose/cycle = 500 mg/m²]
Cisplatin: I.V.: 20 mg/m²/day days 1 to 5
[total dose/cycle = 100 mg/m²]
Repeat cycle every 21 days
Variation 2:
Etoposide: I.V.: 120 mg/m²/day days 1, 2, and 3
[total dose/cycle = 360 mg/m²]
Cisplatin: I.V.: 20 mg/m²/day days 1 to 5
[total dose/cycle = 100 mg/m²]
Repeat cycle every 3 or 4 weeks
Variation 3:
Etoposide: I.V.: 120 mg/m²/day days 1, 3, and 5
[total dose/cycle = 360 mg/m²]
Cisplatin: I.V.: 20 mg/m²/day days 1 to 5
[total dose/cycle = 100 mg/m²]
Repeat cycle every 3 weeks

References

Variation 1:
Hainsworth JD, Williams SD, Einhorn LH, et al, "Successful Treatment of Resistant Germinal Neoplasms With VP-16 and Cisplatin: Results of a Southeastern Cancer Study Group Trial," *J Clin Oncol*, 1985, 3(5):666-71.
Variation 2:
Peckham MJ, Horwich A, Blackmore C, et al, "Etoposide and Cisplatin With or Without Bleomycin as First-Line Chemotherapy for Patients With Small-Volume Metastases of Testicular Non-seminoma," *Cancer Treat Rep*, 1985, 69(5):483-8.
Variation 3:
de Wit R, Stoter G, Kaye SB, et al, "Importance of Bleomycin in Combination Chemotherapy for Good-Prognosis Testicular Nonseminoma: A Randomized Study of the European Organization for Research and Treatment of Cancer Genitourinary Tract Cancer Cooperative Group," *J Clin Oncol*, 1997, 15(5):1837-43.

◆ **Erlotinib-Gemcitabine** *see* Gemcitabine-Erlotinib *on page 1344*

Erlotinib-Paclitaxel-Carboplatin (NSCLC)

Index Terms Carboplatin-Paclitaxel-Erlotinib (NSCLC); Paclitaxel-Carboplatin-Erlotinib (NSCLC)

Use Lung cancer, nonsmall cell (in never smokers)

Regimen

Erlotinib: Oral: 150 mg once daily days 1 to 21
[total dose/cycle = 3150 mg]
Paclitaxel: I.V.: 200 mg/m^2/dose day 1
[total dose/cycle = 200 mg/m^2]
Carboplatin: I.V.: AUC 6 day 1
[total dose/cycle = AUC = 6]
Repeat cycle every 21 days (maximum: 6 cycles)

References

Herbst RS, Prager D, Hermann R, et al, "TRIBUTE: A Phase III Trial of Erlotinib Hydrochloride (OSI-774) Combined With Carboplatin and Paclitaxel Chemotherapy in Advanced Non-Small-Cell Lung Cancer," *Clin Oncol*, 2005, 23(25):5892-9.

ESHAP

Use Lymphoma, non-Hodgkin's

Regimen NOTE: Multiple variations are listed.

Variation 1:
Etoposide: I.V.: 40 mg/m^2/day days 1 to 4
[total dose/cycle = 160 mg/m^2]
Methylprednisolone: I.V.: 250-500 mg/day days 1 to 5
[total dose/cycle = 1250-2500 mg]
Cytarabine: I.V.: 2000 mg/m^2 day 5
[total dose/cycle = 2000 mg/m^2]
Cisplatin: I.V.: 25 mg/m^2/day continuous infusion days 1 to 4
[total dose/cycle = 100 mg/m^2]
Repeat cycle every 21-28 days

Variation 2:
Etoposide: I.V.: 40 mg/m^2/day days 1 to 4
[total dose/cycle = 160 mg/m^2]
Methylprednisolone: I.V.: 500 mg/day days 1 to 5
[total dose/cycle = 2500 mg]
Cytarabine: I.V.: 2000 mg/m^2 day 5
[total dose/cycle = 2000 mg/m^2]
Cisplatin: I.V.: 25 mg/m^2/day continuous infusion days 1 to 4
[total dose/cycle = 100 mg/m^2]
Repeat cycle every 21-28 days

Variation 3:
Etoposide: I.V.: 60 mg/m^2/day days 1 to 4
[total dose/cycle = 240 mg/m^2]
Methylprednisolone: I.V.: 500 mg/day days 1 to 4
[total dose/cycle = 2000 mg]
Cytarabine: I.V.: 2000 mg/m^2 day 5
[total dose/cycle = 2000 mg/m^2]
Cisplatin: I.V.: 25 mg/m^2/day continuous infusion days 1 to 4
[total dose/cycle = 100 mg/m^2]
Repeat cycle every 21 days

References

Variation 1:
Velasquez WF, McLaughlin P, Tucker S, et al, "ESHAP - An Effective Chemotherapy Regimen in Refractory and Relapsing Lymphoma: A 4-Year Follow-up Study," *J Clin Oncol*, 1994, 12 (6):1169-76.

Variation 2:

Wang WS, Chiou TJ, Liu JH, et al, "ESHAP as Salvage Therapy for Refractory Non-Hodgkin's Lymphoma: Taiwan Experience," *Jpn J Clin Oncol*, 1999, 29(1):33-7.

Variation 3:

Rodriguez MA, Cabanillas FC, Velasquez W, et al, "Results of a Salvage Treatment Program for Relapsing Lymphoma: MINE Consolidated With ESHAP," *J Clin Oncol*, 1995, 13(7):1734-41.

Estramustine + Docetaxel

Use Prostate cancer

Regimen NOTE: Multiple variations are listed.

Variation 1:

Docetaxel: I.V.: 20-80 mg/m^2 day 2

[total dose/cycle = 20-80 mg/m^2]

Estramustine: Oral: 280 mg 3 times/day days 1 to 5

[total dose/cycle = 4200 mg]

Repeat cycle every 21 days

Variation 2:

Docetaxel: I.V.: 20-80 mg/m^2 day 2

[total dose/cycle = 20-80 mg/m^2]

Estramustine: Oral: 14 mg/kg/day days 1 to 21

[total dose/cycle = 294 mg/kg]

Repeat cycle every 21 days

Variation 3:

Docetaxel: I.V.: 35 mg/m^2/day days 2 and 9

[total dose/cycle = 70 mg/m^2]

Estramustine: Oral: 420 mg 3 times/day for 4 doses, then 280 mg 3 times/day for 5 doses days 1, 2, 3, 8, 9, and 10

[total dose/cycle = 6160 mg]

Repeat cycle every 21 days

Variation 4:

Docetaxel: I.V.: 60 mg/m^2 day 2 cycle 1

[total dose/cycle = 60 mg/m^2]

followed by I.V.: 60-70 mg/m^2 day 2 (subsequent cycles)

[total dose/cycle = 60-70 mg/m^2]

Estramustine: Oral: 280 mg 3 times/day days 1 to 5

[total dose/cycle = 4200 mg]

Repeat cycle every 21 days for up to 12 cycles

References

Variation 1:

Petrylak DP, Macarthur RB, O'Connor J, et al, "Phase I Trial of Docetaxel With Estramustine in Androgen-Independent Prostate Cancer," *J Clin Oncol*, 1999, 17(3):958-67.

Variation 2:

Kreis W, Budman DR, Fetten J, et al, "Phase I Trial of The Combination of Daily Estramustine Phosphate and Intermittent Docetaxel in Patients With Metastatic Hormone Refractory Prostate Carcinoma," *Ann Oncol*, 1999, 10(1):33-8.

Variation 3:

Sitka Copur M, Ledakis P, Lynch J, et al, "Weekly Docetaxel and Estramustine in Patients With Hormone-Refractory Prostate Cancer," *Semin Oncol*, 2001, 28(4 Suppl 15):16-21.

Variation 4:

Petrylak DP, Tangen CM, Hussain MH, et al, "Docetaxel and Estramustine Compared With Mitoxantrone and Prednisone for Advanced Refractory Prostate Cancer," *N Engl J Med*, 2004, 351(15):1513-20.

Estramustine + Docetaxel + Calcitriol

Use Prostate cancer

Regimen

Cycle 1:

Calcitriol: Oral: 60 mcg (in divided doses) day 1

[total dose/cycle = 60 mcg]

Estramustine: Oral: 280 mg 3 times/day days 1 to 5
  [total dose/cycle = 4200 mg]
Docetaxel: I.V.: 60 mg/m^2 day 2
  [total dose/cycle = 60 mg/m^2]
Treatment cycle is 21 days
Subsequent cycles:
  Calcitriol: Oral: 60 mcg (in divided doses) day 1
    [total dose/cycle = 60 mcg]
  Estramustine: Oral: 280 mg 3 times/day days 1 to 5
    [total dose/cycle = 4200 mg]
  Docetaxel: I.V.: 70 mg/m^2 day 2
    [total dose/cycle = 70 mg/m^2]
  Repeat cycle every 21 days for up to 12 cycles

References
Tiffany NM, Ryan CW, Garzotto M, et al, "High Dose Pulse Calcitriol, Docetaxel and Estramustine for Androgen Independent Prostate Cancer: A Phase I/II Study," *J Urol*, 2005, 174(3):888-92.

Estramustine + Docetaxel + Carboplatin

Use Prostate cancer
Regimen
Docetaxel: I.V.: 70 mg/m^2 day 2
  [total dose/cycle = 70 mg/m^2]
Estramustine: Oral: 280 mg 3 times/day days 1 to 5
  [total dose/cycle = 4200 mg]
Carboplatin: I.V.: Target AUC 5 day 2
  [total dose/cycle = AUC = 5]
Repeat cycle every 3 weeks

References
Oh WK, Halabi S, Kelly WK, et al, "A Phase II Study of Estramustine, Docetaxel, and Carboplatin (EDC) with G-CSF Support in Men With Hormone Refractory Prostate Cancer: CALGB 99813," *Proc Am Soc Clin Oncol*, 2002, 21:195a.

Oh WK, Halabi S, Kelly WK, et al, "A Phase II Study of Estramustine, Docetaxel, and Carboplatin With Granulocyte-Colony-Stimulating Factor Support in Patients With Hormone-Refractory Prostate Carcinoma: Cancer and Leukemia Group B 99813," *Cancer*, 2003, 98(12):2592-8.

Estramustine + Docetaxel + Hydrocortisone

Use Prostate cancer
Regimen
Docetaxel: I.V.: 70 mg/m^2 day 2
  [total dose/cycle = 70 mg/m^2]
Estramustine: Oral: 10 mg/kg/day days 1 to 5
  [total dose/cycle = 50 mg/kg]
Hydrocortisone: Oral: 40 mg daily
  [total dose/cycle = 840 mg]
Repeat cycle every 3 weeks

References
Savarese DM, Halabi S, Hars V, et al, "Phase II Study of Docetaxel, Estramustine, and Low-Dose Hydrocortisone in Men With Hormone-Refractory Prostate Cancer: A Final Report of CALGB 9780. Cancer and Leukemia Group B," *J Clin Oncol*, 2001, 19(9):2509-16.

Estramustine + Docetaxel + Prednisone

Use Prostate cancer

Regimen
Estramustine: Oral: 280 mg 3 times/day days 1 to 5 and days 7 to 11
  [total dose/cycle = 8400 mg]
Docetaxel: I.V.: 70 mg/m^2 day 2
  [total dose/cycle = 70 mg/m^2]
Prednisone: Oral: 10 mg daily
  [total dose/cycle = 210 mg]
Repeat cycle every 21 days for up to 6 cycles

References
Boehmer A, Anastasiadis AG, Feyerabend S, et al, "Docetaxel, Estramustine and Prednisone for Hormone-Refractory Prostate Cancer: A Single-Center Experience," *Anticancer Res*, 2005, 25 (6C):4481-6.

Estramustine + Etoposide

Use Prostate cancer

Regimen NOTE: Multiple variations are listed.
Variation 1:
  Estramustine: Oral: 15 mg/kg/day days 1 to 21
    [total dose/cycle = 315 mg/kg]
  Etoposide: Oral: 50 mg/m^2/day days 1 to 21
    [total dose/cycle = 1050 mg/m^2]
  Repeat cycle every 4 weeks
Variation 2:
  Estramustine: Oral: 10 mg/kg/day days 1 to 21
    [total dose/cycle = 210 mg/kg]
  Etoposide: Oral: 50 mg/m^2/day days 1 to 21
    [total dose/cycle = 1050 mg/m^2]
  Repeat cycle every 4 weeks
Variation 3:
  Estramustine: Oral: 140 mg 3 times/day days 1 to 21
    [total dose/cycle = 8820 mg]
  Etoposide: Oral: 50 mg/m^2/day days 1 to 21
    [total dose/cycle = 1050 mg/m^2]
  Repeat cycle every 4 weeks

References
Variation 1:
Pienta KJ, Redman B, Hussain M, et al, "Phase II Evaluation of Oral Estramustine and Oral Etoposide in Hormone-Refractory Adenocarcinoma of the Prostate," *J Clin Oncol*, 1994, 12 (10):2005-12.
Variation 2:
Pienta KJ, Redman BG, Bandekar R, et al, "A Phase II Trial of Oral Estramustine and Oral Etoposide in Hormone Refractory Prostate Cancer," *Urology*, 1997, 50(3):401-6; discussion 406-7.
Variation 3:
Dimopoulos MA, Panopoulos C, Bamia C, et al, "Oral Estramustine and Oral Etoposide for Hormone-Refractory Prostate Cancer," *Urology*, 1997, 50(5):754-8.

Estramustine-Paclitaxel

Index Terms Paclitaxel-Estramustine; PE (Prostate Cancer)

Use Prostate cancer

Regimen NOTE: Multiple variations are listed.
Variation 1:
  Paclitaxel: I.V.: 30-35 mg/m^2/day continuous infusion (given in 2-3 divided doses daily) either days 1 to 4 or days 2 to 5
    [total dose/cycle = 120-140 mg/m^2]

◄ Estramustine: Oral: 600 mg/m²/day days 1 to 21
[total dose/cycle = 12,600 mg/m²]
Repeat cycle every 21 days

Variation 2:
Paclitaxel: I.V. 60-107 mg/m² infused over 3 hours weekly for 6 weeks
[total dose/cycle = 360-642 mg/m²]
Estramustine: Oral: 280 mg twice daily 3 days/week for 6 weeks
[total dose/cycle = 3360 mg]
Repeat cycle every 8 weeks

Variation 3:
Paclitaxel: I.V. 150 mg/m²/day days 2, 9, and 16
[total dose/cycle = 450 mg/m²]
Estramustine: Oral: 280 mg 3 times/day days 1, 2, 3, 8, 9, 10, 15, 16, and 17
[total dose/week = 7560 mg/m²]
Repeat cycle every 4 weeks

Variation 4:
Paclitaxel: I.V.: 100 mg/m²/day days 2, 9, and 16
[total dose/cycle = 300 mg/m²]
Estramustine: Oral: 280 mg 3 times/day days 1, 2, 3, 8, 9, 10, 15, 16, and 17
[total dose/cycle = 7560 mg]
Repeat cycle every 4 weeks

References

Variation 1:
Hudes GR, Nathan FE, Khater C, et al, "Paclitaxel Plus Estramustine in Metastatic Hormone-Refractory Prostate Cancer," *Semin Oncol*, 1995, 22(5 Suppl 12):41-5.
Hudes GR, Nathan F, Khater C, et al, "Phase II Trial of 96-Hour Paclitaxel Plus Oral Estramustine Phosphate in Metastatic Hormone-Refractory Prostate Cancer," *J Clin Oncol*, 1997, 15 (9):3156-63.
Variation 2:
Haas N, Roth B, Garay C, et al, "Phase I Trial of Weekly Paclitaxel Plus Oral Estramustine Phosphate in Patients With Hormone-Refractory Prostate Cancer," *Urology*, 2001, 58(1):59-64
Variation 3:
Vaishampayan U, Fontana J, Du W, et al, "An Active Regimen of Weekly Paclitaxel and Estramustine in Metastatic Androgen-Independent Prostate Cancer," *Urology*, 2002, 60 (6):1050-4.
Variation 4:
Berry W, Gregurich M, Dakhil S, et al, "Phase II Randomized Trial of Weekly Paclitaxel With or Without Estramustine Phosphate in Patients With Symptomatic, Hormone-Refractory Metastatic Carcinoma of the Prostate." *Proc Am Soc Clin Oncol*, 2001, 20:175a.

Estramustine-Vinblastine

Index Terms EV

Use Prostate cancer

Regimen NOTE: Multiple variations are listed.

Variation 1:
Estramustine: Oral: 10 mg/kg/day days 1 to 42
[total dose/cycle = 420 mg/kg]
Vinblastine: I.V.: 4 mg/m²/day days 1, 8, 15, 22, 29, and 36
[total dose/cycle = 24 mg/m²]
Repeat cycle every 8 weeks

Variation 2:
Estramustine: Oral: 600 mg/m²/day days 1 to 42
[total dose/cycle = 25,200 mg/m²]
Vinblastine: I.V.: 4 mg/m²/day days 1, 8, 15, 22, 29, and 36
[total dose/cycle = 24 mg/m²]
Repeat cycle every 8 weeks

References
Variation 1:

Seidman AD, Scher HI, Petrylak D, et al, "Estramustine and Vinblastine: Use of Prostate Specific Antigen as a Clinical Trial Endpoint for Hormone Refractory Prostatic Cancer," *J Urol*, 1992, 147 (3 Pt 2):931-4.

Variation 2:

Hudes GR, Greenberg R, Krigel RL, et al, "Phase II Study of Estramustine and Vinblastine, Two Microtubule Inhibitors, in Hormone-Refractory Prostate Cancer," *J Clin Oncol*, 1992, 10 (11):1754-61.

Estramustine + Vinorelbine

Use Prostate cancer

Regimen NOTE: Multiple variations are listed.

Variation 1:

Estramustine: Oral: 140 mg 3 times/day days 1 to 14

[total dose/cycle = 5880 mg]

Vinorelbine: I.V.: 25 mg/m^2/day days 1 and 8

[total dose/cycle = 50 mg/m^2]

Repeat cycle every 21 days

Variation 2:

Estramustine: Oral: 280 mg 3 times/day days 1, 2, and 3

[total dose/cycle = 2520 mg/m^2]

Vinorelbine: I.V.: 15 or 20 mg/m^2 day 2

[total dose/cycle = 15 or 20 mg/m^2]

Repeat cycle weekly for 8 weeks, then every other week

References
Variation 1:

Smith MR, Kaufman D, Oh W, et al, "Vinorelbine and Estramustine in Androgen-Independent Metastatic Prostate Cancer: A Phase II Study," *Cancer*, 2000, 89(8):1824-8.

Variation 2:

Sweeney CJ, Monaco FJ, Jung SH, et al, "A Phase II Hoosier Oncology Group Study of Vinorelbine and Estramustine Phosphate in Hormone-Refractory Prostate Cancer," *Ann Oncol*, 2002, 13(3):435-40.

Etoposide-Carboplatin (Ovarian Cancer)

Index Terms Carboplatin–Etoposide (Ovarian Cancer)

Use Ovarian cancer

Regimen

Etoposide: I.V.: 120 mg/m^2/day days 1, 2, and 3

[total dose/cycle = 360 mg/m^2]

Carboplatin: I.V.: 400 mg/m^2 day 1

[total dose/cycle = 400 mg/m^2]

Repeat cycle every 28 days for a total of 3 cycles

References
Williams SD, Kauderer J, Burnett AF, et al, "Adjuvant Therapy of Completely Resected Dysgerminoma With Carboplatin and Etoposide: A Trial of the Gynecologic Oncology Group," *Gynecol Oncol*, 2004, 95(3):496-9.

♦ **Etoposide-Cisplatin** see Cisplatin-Etoposide (NSCLC) *on page 1266*

♦ **Etoposide-Ifosfamide-Mitoxantrone-Dexamethasone** see VIM-D (Hodgkin's Lymphoma) *on page 1420*

Etoposide-Vinblastine-Doxorubicin (Hodgkin's)

Index Terms EVA (Hodgkin's)

Use Lymphoma, Hodgkin's disease

Regimen

Etoposide: I.V.: 100 mg/m^2/day days 1, 2, and 3
  [total dose/cycle = 300 mg/m^2]
Vinblastine: I.V.: 6 mg/m^2 day 1
  [total dose/cycle = 6 mg/m^2]
Doxorubicin: I.V.: 50 mg/m^2 day 1
  [total dose/cycle = 50 mg/m^2]
Repeat cycle every 28 days

References

Canellos GP, Petroni GR, Barcos M, et al, "Etoposide, Vinblastine, and Doxorubicin: An Active Regimen for the Treatment of Hodgkin's Disease in Relapse Following MOPP. Cancer and Leukemia Group B," *J Clin Oncol*, 1995, 13(8):2005-11.

◆ **EV** *see* Estramustine-Vinblastine *on page 1316*

◆ **EVA (Hodgkin's)** *see* Etoposide-Vinblastine-Doxorubicin (Hodgkin's) *on page 1317*

◆ **F-CL** *see* Fluorouracil-Leucovorin *on page 1331*

FAC

Index Terms CAF-IV; IVCAF

Use Breast cancer

Regimen NOTE: Multiple variations are listed.

Variation 1:
  Fluorouracil: I.V.: 500 mg/m^2/day days 1 and 8
    [total dose/cycle = 1000 mg/m^2]
    or 500 mg/m^2 day 1
    [total dose/cycle = 500 mg/m^2]
  Doxorubicin: I.V.: 50 mg/m^2 day 1
    [total dose/cycle = 50 mg/m^2]
  Cyclophosphamide: I.V.: 500 mg/m^2 day 1
    [total dose/cycle = 500 mg/m^2]
  Repeat cycle every 21-28 days

Variation 2:
  Fluorouracil: I.V.: 200 mg/m^2/day days 1, 2, and 3
    [total dose/cycle = 600 mg/m^2]
  Doxorubicin: I.V.: 40 mg/m^2 day 1
    [total dose/cycle = 40 mg/m^2]
  Cyclophosphamide: I.V.: 400 mg/m^2 day 1
    [total dose/cycle = 400 mg/m^2]
  Repeat cycle every 28 days

Variation 3:
  Fluorouracil: I.V.: 400 mg/m^2/day days 1 and 8
    [total dose/cycle = 800 mg/m^2]
  Doxorubicin: I.V.: 40 mg/m^2 day 1
    [total dose/cycle = 40 mg/m^2]
  Cyclophosphamide: I.V.: 400 mg/m^2 day 1
    [total dose/cycle = 400 mg/m^2]
  Repeat cycle every 28 days

Variation 4:
  Fluorouracil: I.V.: 600 mg/m^2/day days 1 and 8
    [total dose/cycle = 1200 mg/m^2]
  Doxorubicin: I.V.: 60 mg/m^2 day 1
    [total dose/cycle = 60 mg/m^2]

Cyclophosphamide: I.V.: 600 mg/m² day 1
[total dose/cycle = 600 mg/m²]
Repeat cycle every 28 days
Variation 5:
Fluorouracil: I.V.: 300 mg/m²/day days 1 and 8
[total dose/cycle = 600 mg/m²]
Doxorubicin: I.V.: 30 mg/m² day 1
[total dose/cycle = 30 mg/m²]
Cyclophosphamide: I.V.: 300 mg/m² day 1
[total dose/cycle = 300 mg/m²]
Repeat cycle every 28 days

References

Variation 1:

Smalley RV, Carpenter J, Bartolucci A, et al, "A Comparison of Cyclophosphamide, Adriamycin®, 5-Fluorouracil (CAF), and Cyclophosphamide, Methotrexate, 5-Fluorouracil, Vincristine, Prednisone (CMFVP) in Patients With Metastatic Breast Cancer: A Southeastern Cancer Study Group Project," *Cancer*, 1977, 40(2):625-32.

Swenerton KD, Legha SS, Smith T, et al, "Prognostic Factors in Metastatic Breast Cancer Treated With Combination Chemotherapy," *Cancer Res*, 1979, 39(5):1552-62.

Variation 2:

Nemoto T, Horton J, Simon R, et al, "Comparison of Four-Combination Chemotherapy Programs in Metastatic Breast Cancer: Comparison of Multiple Drug Therapy With Cytoxan, 5-FU, and Prednisone, Versus Cytoxan and Adriamycin, Versus Cytoxan, 5-FU, and Adriamycin, Versus Cytoxan, 5-FU, and Prednisone Alternation With Cytoxan and Adriamycin," *Cancer*, 1982, 49 (10):1988-93.

Variation 3-5:

Wood WC, Budman DR, Korzun AH, et al, "Dose and Dose Intensity of Adjuvant Chemotherapy for State II, Node-Positive Breast Carcinoma," *N Engl J Med*, 1994, 330(18):1253-9.

FAM

Use Gastric cancer; Pancreatic cancer

Regimen NOTE: Multiple variations are listed.
Variation 1:
Fluorouracil: I.V.: 600 mg/m²/day days 1, 8, 29, and 36
[total dose/cycle = 2400 mg/m²]
Doxorubicin: I.V.: 30 mg/m²/day days 1 and 29
[total dose/cycle = 60 mg/m²]
Mitomycin: I.V.: 10 mg/m² day 1
[total dose/cycle = 10 mg/m²]
Repeat cycle every 8 weeks
Variation 2:
Fluorouracil: I.V.: 600 mg/m²/day days 29 to 32
[total dose/cycle = 2400 mg/m²]
Doxorubicin: I.V.: 50 mg/m² day 1
[total dose/cycle = 50 mg/m²]
Mitomycin: I.V.: 10 mg/m² day 3
[total dose/cycle = 10 mg/m²]
Repeat cycle every 8 weeks
Variation 3:
Fluorouracil: I.V.: 500 mg/m²/day days 1, 8, 21, and 28
[total dose/cycle = 2000 mg/m²]
Doxorubicin: I.V.: 30 mg/m²/day days 1 and 21
[total dose/cycle = 60 mg/m²]
Mitomycin: I.V.: 10 mg/m² day 1
[total dose/cycle = 10 mg/m²]
Repeat cycle every 6 weeks

Variation 4:
Fluorouracil: I.V.: 275 mg/m^2/day days 1 to 5 and 36 to 40
[total dose/cycle = 2750 mg/m^2]
Doxorubicin: I.V.: 30 mg/m^2/day days 1 and 36
[total dose/cycle = 60 mg/m^2]
Mitomycin: I.V.: 10 mg/m^2 day 1
[total dose/cycle = 10 mg/m^2]
Repeat cycle every 10 weeks
Variation 5:
Fluorouracil: I.V.: 600 mg/m^2/day days 1, 8, 22, and 29
[total dose/cycle = 2400 mg/m^2]
Doxorubicin: I.V.: 30 mg/m^2/day days 1 and 22
[total dose/cycle = 60 mg/m^2]
Mitomycin: I.V.: 10 mg/m^2 day 1
[total dose/cycle = 10 mg/m^2]
Repeat cycle every 6 weeks

References

Variation 1:
Cullinan SA, Moertel CG, Fleming TR, et al, "A Comparison of Three Chemotherapeutic Regimens in the Treatment of Advanced Pancreatic and Gastric Carcinoma. Fluorouracil vs Fluorouracil and Doxorubicin vs Fluorouracil, Doxorubicin, and Mitomycin," *JAMA*, 1985, 253(14):2061-7.

Preusser P, Achterrath W, Wilke H, et al, "Chemotherapy of Gastric Cancer," *Cancer Treat Rev*, 1988, 15(4):257-77.

Variation 2:
Panettiere FJ, Haas C, McDonald B, et al, "Drug Combinations in the Treatment of Gastric Adenocarcinoma: A Randomized Southwest Oncology Group Study," *J Clin Oncol*, 1984, 2 (5):420-4.

Variation 3:
Bitran JD, Desser RK, Kozloff MF, et al, "Treatment of Metastatic Pancreatic and Gastric Adenocarcinomas With 5-Fluorouracil, Adriamycin, and Mitomycin C (FAM)," *Cancer Treat Rep*, 1979, 63(11-12):2049-51.

Variation 4:
"A Comparative Clinical Assessment of Combination Chemotherapy in the Management of Advanced Gastric Carcinoma: The Gastrointestinal Tumor Study Group," *Cancer*, 1982, 49 (7):1362-6.

Variation 5:
Haim N, Epelbaum R, Cohen Y, et al, "Further Studies on the Treatment of Advanced Gastric Cancer by 5-Fluorouracil, Adriamycin (Doxorubicin), and Mitomycin C (Modified FAM)," *Cancer*, 1984, 54(9):1999-2002.

FAMe

Use Gastric cancer

Regimen
Fluorouracil: I.V.: 325 mg/m^2/day days 1 to 5 and days 36 to 40
[total dose/cycle = 3250 mg/m^2]
Doxorubicin: I.V.: 40 mg/m^2 days 1 and 36
[total dose/cycle = 80 mg/m^2]
Lomustine: Oral: 110 mg/m^2 day 1
[total dose/cycle = 110 mg/m^2]
Repeat cycle every 10 weeks

References

Cullinan SA, Moertel CG, Wieand HS, et al, "Controlled Evaluation of Three Drug Combination Regimens Versus Fluorouracil Alone for the Therapy of Advanced Gastric Cancer. North Central Cancer Treatment Group," *J Clin Oncol*, 1994, 12(2):412-6.

FAMTX

Use Gastric cancer

Regimen NOTE: Multiple variations are listed.

Variation 1:

Methotrexate: I.V.: 1500 mg/m^2 day 1
[total dose/cycle = 1500 mg/m^2]

Fluorouracil: I.V.: 1500 mg/m^2 (1 hour after methotrexate) day 1
[total dose/cycle = 1500 mg/m^2]

Leucovorin: Oral: 15 mg/m^2 every 6 hours for 48 hours (start 24 hours after methotrexate) day 2
[total dose/cycle = 120 mg/m^2]

Doxorubicin: I.V.: 30 mg/m^2 day 15
[total dose/cycle = 30 mg/m^2]

Repeat cycle every 28 days

Variation 2:

Methotrexate: I.V.: 1500 mg/m^2 day 1
[total dose/cycle = 1500 mg/m^2]

Fluorouracil: I.V.: 1500 mg/m^2 (1 hour after methotrexate) day 1
[total dose/cycle = 1500 mg/m^2]

Leucovorin: Oral: 30 mg/m^2 every 6 hours for 8 doses (start 24 hours after methotrexate)
[total dose/cycle = 240 mg/m^2]
followed by Oral: 30 mg/m^2 every 6 hours for 8 more doses if 24-hour methotrexate level ≥2.5 mol/L
[total cumulative dose/cycle = 480 mg/m^2]

Doxorubicin: I.V.: 30 mg/m^2 day 15
[total dose/cycle = 30 mg/m^2]

Repeat cycle every 28 days

Variation 3:

Methotrexate: I.V.: 1000 mg/m^2 day 1
[total dose/cycle = 1000 mg/m^2]

Fluorouracil: I.V.: 1500 mg/m^2 (1 hour after methotrexate) day 1
[total dose/cycle = 1500 mg/m^2]

Leucovorin: Oral: 15 mg every 6 hours for 8 doses (start 24 hours after methotrexate)
[total dose/cycle = 120 mg/m^2]

Doxorubicin: I.V.: 30 mg/m^2 day 15
[total dose/cycle = 30 mg/m^2]

Repeat cycle every 28 days

References

Variation 1:

Kelsen D, Atiq O, Salz L, et al, "FAMTX (Fluorouracil, Methotrexate, Adriamycin®) Is as Effective and Less Toxic Than EAP (Etoposide, Adriamycin®, Cisplatin): A Random Assignment Trial in Gastric Cancer," *Proc Am Soc Clin Oncol*, 1991, 10:137.

Variation 2:

Wils J, Bleiberg H, Dalesio O, et al, "An EORTC Gastrointestinal Group Evaluation of the Combination of Sequential Methotrexate and 5-Fluorouracil, Combined With Adriamycin in Advanced Measurable Gastric Cancer," *J Clin Oncol*, 1986, 4(12):1799-803.

Variation 3:

Murad AM, Santiago FF, Petroianu A, et al, "Modified Therapy With 5-Fluorouracil, Doxorubicin, and Methotrexate in Advanced Gastric Cancer," *Cancer*, 1993, 72(1):37-41.

FAP

Use Gastric cancer

Regimen

Fluorouracil: I.V.: 300 mg/m^2/day days 1 to 5
[total dose/cycle = 1500 mg/m^2]
Doxorubicin: I.V.: 40 mg/m^2 day 1
[total dose/cycle = 40 mg/m^2]
Cisplatin: I.V.: 60 mg/m^2 day 1
[total dose/cycle = 60 mg/m^2]
Repeat cycle every 5 weeks

References

Cullinan SA, Moertel CG, Wieand HS, et al, "Controlled Evaluation of Three Drug Combination Regimens Versus Fluorouracil Alone for the Therapy of Advanced Gastric Cancer. North Central Cancer Treatment Group," *J Clin Oncol*, 1994, 12(2):412-6.

◆ **FC (CLL)** see Fludarabine-Cyclophosphamide (CLL) *on page 1325*

◆ **FCMR (NHL)** see Fludarabine-Cyclophosphamide-Mitoxantrone-Rituximab *on page 1326*

◆ **FC (NHL-Mantle Cell)** see Fludarabine-Cyclophosphamide (NHL-Mantle Cell) *on page 1327*

◆ **FCR (CLL)** see Fludarabine-Cyclophosphamide-Rituximab (CLL) *on page 1327*

◆ **FCR (NHL-Follicular)** see Fludarabine-Cyclophosphamide-Rituximab (NHL-Follicular) *on page 1328*

FEC

Use Breast cancer

Regimen

Fluorouracil: I.V.: 500 mg/m^2 day 1
[total dose/cycle = 500 mg/m^2]
Cyclophosphamide: I.V.: 500 mg/m^2 day 1
[total dose/cycle = 500 mg/m^2]
Epirubicin: I.V.: 100 mg/m^2 day 1
[total dose/cycle = 100 mg/m^2]
Repeat cycle every 21 days

References

Bonneterre J, Roché H, Bremond A, et al, "Results of a Randomized Trial of Adjuvant Chemotherapy With FEC 50 vs FEC 100 in High Risk Node-Positive Breast Cancer Patients," *Proc Am Soc Clin Oncol*, 1998, 17:124a (abstract 473).

◆ **FEC-Docetaxel** see Docetaxel-FEC *on page 1292*

◆ **FEC-Vinorelbine** see Vinorelbine-FEC *on page 1423*

FIS-HAM

Use Leukemia, acute lymphocytic; Leukemia, acute myeloid

Regimen

Fludarabine: I.V.: 15 mg/m^2/day every 12 hours days 1, 2, 8, and 9
[total dose/cycle = 120 mg/m^2]
Cytarabine: I.V.: 750 mg/m^2/day every 3 hours days 1, 2, 8, and 9
[total dose/cycle = 24,000 mg/m^2]
Mitoxantrone: I.V.: 10 mg/m^2/day days 3, 4, 10, and 11
[total dose/cycle = 40 mg/m^2]

References

Kern W, Schleyer E, Braess J, et al, "Efficacy of Fludarabine, Intermittent Sequential High-Dose Cytosine Arabinoside, and Mitoxantrone (FIS-HAM) Salvage Therapy in Highly Resistant Acute Leukemias," *Ann Hematol*, 2001, 80(6):334-9.

FL

Index Terms Flutamide + Leuprolide

Use Prostate cancer

Regimen NOTE: Multiple variations are listed.

Variation 1:

Flutamide: Oral: 250 mg every 8 hours
[total dose/cycle = 21,000 mg]

Leuprolide acetate: SubQ: 1 mg/day
[total dose/cycle = 28 mg]

Repeat cycle every 28 days

Variation 2:

Flutamide: Oral: 250 mg every 8 hours
[total dose/cycle = 67,500 mg]

Leuprolide acetate depot: I.M.: 22.5 mg day 1
[total dose/cycle = 22.5 mg]

Repeat cycle every 3 months

References

Variation 1: Crawford ED, Eisenberger MA, McLeod DG, et al, "A Controlled Trial of Leuprolide With and Without Flutamide in Prostatic Carcinoma," *N Engl J Med*, 1989, 17:321(7):419-24.

Variation 2: McLeod DG, Schellhammer PF, Vogelzang NJ, et al, "Exploratory Analysis on the Effect of Race on Clinical Outcome in Patients With Advanced Prostate Cancer Receiving Bicalutamide or Flutamide, Each in Combination With LHRH Analogues. The Casodex Combination Study Group." *Prostate*, 1999, 1:40(4):218-24.

FLAG (AML)

Index Terms Fludarabine-ARAC-GCSF (AML); Fludarabine-Cytarabine-Filgrastim (AML)

Use Leukemia, acute myeloid

Regimen NOTE: Multiple variations are listed.

Variation 1:

Fludarabine: I.V.: 30 mg/m^2/day over 30 minutes days 1 to 5
[total dose/cycle = 150 mg/m^2]

Cytarabine: I.V.: 2 g/m^2/day over 4 hours days 1 to 5 (begin 4 hours after fludarabine infusion)
[total dose/cycle = 10 g/m^2]

Filgrastim: SubQ: 300 mcg 12 hours prior to start of fludarabine then 300 mcg/day days 2 through 5
[total dose/cycle = 1500 mcg]

followed by Filgrastim: SubQ: 300 mcg/day beginning one week after the end of treatment and continuing until complete neutrophil recovery

Variation 2:

Fludarabine: I.V.: 30 mg/m^2/day over 30 minutes days 1 to 5
[total dose/cycle = 150 mg/m^2]

Cytarabine: I.V.: 2 g/m^2/day over 4 hours days 1 to 5 (begin 3.5 hours after end of fludarabine infusion)
[total dose/cycle = 10 g/m^2]

Filgrastim: SubQ: 5 mcg/kg/day beginning 24 hours prior to start of fludarabine and continuing until ANC >500 cells/mm^3

May repeat cycle one time for partial remission

Variation 3:

Fludarabine: I.V.: 30 mg/m^2/day over 30 minutes days 1 to 5
[total dose/cycle = 150 mg/m^2]

Cytarabine: I.V.: 2 g/m^2/day over 2 hours days 1 to 5 (begin 4 hours after the start of fludarabine infusion)
[total dose/cycle = 10 g/m^2]

◀ Filgrastim: SubQ or I.V.: 300 mcg/day beginning the day prior to start of chemotherapy and continuing during chemotherapy and until ANC >1000 cells/mm³

May receive a second cycle

Variation 4:

Fludarabine: I.V.: 25 mg/m²/day over 30 minutes days 1 to 5
  [total dose/cycle = 125 mg/m²]

Cytarabine: I.V.: 2 g/m²/day over 4 hours days 1 to 5 (begin 4 hours after start of fludarabine infusion)
  [total dose/cycle = 10 g/m²]

Filgrastim: SubQ: 5 mcg/kg/day beginning 24 hours prior to start of cytarabine and continuing until ANC >500 cells/mm³

References

Variation 1:
Clavio M, Carrara P, Miglino M, et al, "High Efficacy of Fludarabine-Containing Therapy (FLAG-FLANG) in Poor Risk Acute Myeloid Leukemia," *Haematologica*, 1996, 81(6):513-20.

Variation 2:
Montillo M, Mirto S, Petti MC, et al, "Fludarabine, Cytarabine, and G-CSF (FLAG) for the Treatment of Poor Risk Acute Myeloid Leukemia," *Am J Hematol*, 1998, 58(2):105-9.

Variation 3:
Virchis A, Koh M, Rankin P, et al, "Fludarabine, Cytosine Arabinoside, Granulocyte-Colony Stimulating Factor With or Without Idarubicin in the Treatment of High Risk Acute Leukaemia or Myelodysplastic Syndromes," *Br J Haematol*, 2004, 124(1):26-32.

Variation 4:
Ossenkoppele GJ, Graveland WJ, Sonneveld P, et al, "The Value of Fludarabine in Addition to ARA-C and G-CSF in the Treatment of Patients With High-Risk Myelodysplastic Syndromes and AML in Elderly Patients," *Blood*, 2004, 103(8):2908-13.

FLAG-IDA

Use Leukemia, acute myeloid

Regimen

Fludarabine: I.V.: 30 mg/m²/day days 1 to 5
  [total dose/cycle = 150 mg/m²]

Cytarabine: I.V.: 2 g/m²/day days 1 to 5
  [total dose/cycle = 10 g/m²]

Idarubicin: I.V.: 10 mg/m²/day days 1, 2, and 3
  [total dose/cycle = 30 mg/m²]

Filgrastim: 5 mcg/kg from day 6 until neutrophil recovery

Administer one cycle only

References

Pastore D, Specchia G, Carluccio P, et al, "FLAG-IDA in the Treatment of Refractory/Relapsed Acute Myeloid Leukemia: Single-Center Experience," *Ann Hematol*, 2003, 82(4):231-5.

◆ **FLO (Gastric Cancer)** *see* Fluorouracil-Leucovorin-Oxaliplatin (Gastric Cancer) *on page 1334*

◆ **FLO (Gastric/Esophageal Cancer)** *see* Fluorouracil-Leucovorin-Oxaliplatin (Gastric/Esophageal Cancer) *on page 1334*

◆ **Flox** *see* FLOX (Nordic FLOX) *on page 1324*

FLOX (Nordic FLOX)

Index Terms Flox

Use Colorectal cancer

Regimen

Oxaliplatin: I.V.: 85 mg/m² day 1
  [total dose/cycle = 85 mg/m²]

Fluorouracil: I.V.: 500 mg/m²/day days 1 and 2
  [total dose/cycle = 1000 mg/m²]

Leucovorin: I.V.: 60 mg/m²/day days 1 and 2
[total dose/cycle = 120 mg/m²]
Repeat cycle every 2 weeks

References

Sorbye H and Dahl O, "Nordic 5-Fluorouracil/Leucovorin Bolus Schedule Combined With Oxaliplatin (Nordic FLOX) as First-Line Treatment of Metastatic Colorectal Cancer," *Acta Oncol*, 2003, 42(8):827-31.

◆ **Fludarabine-ARAC-GCSF (AML)** see FLAG (AML) on page 1323

Fludarabine-Cyclophosphamide (CLL)

Index Terms Cyclophosphamide-Fludarabine (CLL); FC (CLL)
Use Leukemia, chronic lymphocytic
Regimen NOTE: Multiple variations are listed.
Variation 1:
Fludarabine: I.V.: 25 mg/m²/day days 1, 2, and 3
[total dose/cycle = 75 mg/m²]
Cyclophosphamide: I.V.: 250 mg/m²/day days 1, 2, and 3
[total dose/cycle = 750 mg/m²]
Repeat cycle every 4 weeks for up to 6 cycles
Variation 2:
Fludarabine: I.V.: 30 mg/m²/day days 1, 2, and 3
[total dose/cycle = 90 mg/m²]
Cyclophosphamide: I.V.: 250 mg/m²/day days 1, 2, and 3
[total dose/cycle = 750 mg/m²]
Repeat cycle every 4 weeks for up to 6 cycles
Variation 3:
Cyclophosphamide: I.V.: 600 mg/m² day 1
[total dose/cycle = 600 mg/m²]
Fludarabine: I.V.: 20 mg/m²/day days 1 to 5
[total dose/cycle = 100 mg/m²]
Repeat cycle every 4 weeks for up to 6 cycles
Variation 4:
Fludarabine: I.V.: 30 mg/m²/day days 1, 2, and 3
[total dose/cycle = 90 mg/m²]
Cyclophosphamide: I.V.: 300 mg/m²/day days 1, 2, and 3
[total dose/cycle = 900 mg/m²]
Repeat cycle every 4 weeks for up to 6 cycles
Variation 5:
Fludarabine: I.V.: 30 mg/m²/day days 1, 2, and 3
[total dose/cycle = 90 mg/m²]
Cyclophosphamide: I.V.: 300 mg/m²/day days 1, 2, and 3
[total dose/cycle = 900 mg/m²]
Repeat cycle every 4-6 weeks for up to 6 cycles

References

Variation 1:
Catovsky D, Richards S, Matutes E, et al, "Assessment of Fludarabine Plus Cyclophosphamide for Patients With Chronic Lymphocytic Leukaemia (The LRF CLL4 Trial): A Randomised Controlled Trial," *Lancet*, 2007, 370(9583):230-9.
O'Brien S, Moore JO, Boyd TE, et al, "Randomized Phase III Trial of Fludarabine Plus Cyclophosphamide With or Without Oblimersen Sodium (Bcl-2 Antisense) in Patients With Relapsed or Refractory Chronic Lymphocytic Leukemia," *J Clin Oncol*, 2007, 25(9):1114-20.
Variation 2:
Eichhorst BF, Busch R, Obwandner T, et al, "Health-Related Quality of Life in Younger Patients With Chronic Lymphocytic Leukemia Treated With Fludarabine Plus Cyclophosphamide or Fludarabine Alone for First-Line Therapy: A Study by the German CLL Study Group," *J Clin Oncol*, 2007, 25(13):1722-31.

◄ Variation 3:

Flinn IW, Neuberg DS, Grever MR, et al, "Phase III Trial of Fludarabine Plus Cyclophosphamide Compared With Fludarabine for Patients With Previously Untreated Chronic Lymphocytic Leukemia: US Intergroup Trial E2997," *J Clin Oncol*, 2007, 25(7):793-8.

Variation 4:

Wierda W, O'Brien S, Faderl S, et al, "A Retrospective Comparison of Three Sequential Groups of Patients With Recurrent/Refractory Chronic Lymphocytic Leukemia Treated With Fludarabine-Based Regimens," *Cancer*, 2006, 106(2):337-45.

Variation 5:

O'Brien SM, Kantarjian HM, Cortes J, et al, "Results of the Fludarabine and Cyclophosphamide Combination Regimen in Chronic Lymphocytic Leukemia," *J Clin Oncol*, 2001, 19(5):1414-20.

Fludarabine-Cyclophosphamide-Mitoxantrone-Rituximab

Index Terms FCMR (NHL); R-FCM (NHL); Rituximab-Fludarabine-Cyclophosphamide-Mitoxantrone

Use Lymphoma, non-Hodgkin's

Regimen NOTE: Multiple variations are listed.

Consider pretherapy cytoreduction with cyclophosphamide 200 mg/m²/ day for 3-5 days for patients with high tumor burden and/or lymphocytes >20,000/mm³

Variation 1:

Rituximab: I.V.: 375 mg/m²/dose day 1

[total dose/cycle = 375 mg/m²]

Fludarabine: I.V.: 25 mg/m²/day days 2, 3, and 4

[total dose/cycle = 75 mg/m²]

Cyclophosphamide: I.V.: 200 mg/m²/day days 2, 3, and 4

[total dose/cycle = 600 mg/m²]

Mitoxantrone: I.V.: 8 mg/m²/dose day 2

[total dose/cycle = 8 mg/m²]

Repeat cycle every 28 days for total of 4 cycles

Variation 2 (with maintenance rituximab):

Rituximab: I.V.: 375 mg/m²/dose day 1

[total dose/cycle = 375 mg/m²]

Fludarabine: I.V.: 25 mg/m²/day days 2, 3, and 4

[total dose/cycle = 75 mg/m²]

Cyclophosphamide: I.V.: 200 mg/m²/day days 2, 3, and 4

[total dose/cycle = 600 mg/m²]

Mitoxantrone: I.V.: 8 mg/m²/dose day 2

[total dose/cycle = 8 mg/m²]

Repeat cycle every 28 days for total of 4 cycles

followed by:

Maintenance rituximab (begin 3 months after completion of cycle 4):

Rituximab: I.V.: 375 mg/m²/dose day 1, 8, 15, and 22

[total dose/cycle = 1500 mg/m²]

Repeat maintenance cycle (once) in 6 months

References

Variation 1:

Forstpointner R, Dreyling M, Repp R, et al, "The Addition of Rituximab to a Combination of Fludarabine, Cyclophosphamide, Mitoxantrone (FCM) Significantly Increases the Response Rate and Prolongs Survival as Compared With FCM Alone in Patients With Relapsed and Refractory Follicular and Mantle Cell Lymphomas: Results of a Prospective Randomized Study of the German Low-Grade Lymphoma Study Group," *Blood*, 2004, 104(10):3064-71.

Variation 2:

Forstpointner R, Unterhalt M, Dreyling M, et al, "Maintenance Therapy With Rituximab Leads to a Significant Prolongation of Response Duration After Salvage Therapy With a Combination of Rituximab, Fludarabine, Cyclophosphamide, and Mitoxantrone (R-FCM) in Patients With Recurring and Refractory Follicular and Mantle Cell Lymphomas: Results of a Prospective Randomized Study of the German Low Grade Lymphoma Study Group (GLSG)," *Blood*, 2006, 108(13):4003-8.

Fludarabine-Cyclophosphamide (NHL-Mantle Cell)

Index Terms CF (NHL-Mantle Cell); Cyclophosphamide-Fludarabine (NHL-Mantle Cell); FC (NHL-Mantle Cell)

Use Lymphoma, non-Hodgkin's (Mantle cell)

Regimen NOTE: Multiple variations are listed.

Variation 1:

Fludarabine: I.V.: 20 mg/m^2/day days 1 to 5
[total dose/cycle = 100 mg/m^2]
Cyclophosphamide: I.V.: 800 mg/m^2/dose day 1
[total dose/cycle = 800 mg/m^2]
Repeat cycle every 3-4 weeks for up to a total of 5 cycles

Variation 2:

Fludarabine: I.V.: 20 mg/m^2/day days 1 to 5
[total dose/cycle = 100 mg/m^2]
Cyclophosphamide: I.V.: 1000 mg/m^2/dose day 1
[total dose/cycle = 1000 mg/m^2]
Repeat cycle every 3-4 weeks for up to a total of 5 cycles

Variation 3:

Fludarabine: I.V.: 25 mg/m^2/day days 1 to 4
[total dose/cycle = 100 mg/m^2]
Cyclophosphamide: I.V.: 1000 mg/m^2/dose day 1
[total dose/cycle = 1000 mg/m^2]
Repeat cycle every 3-4 weeks for up to a total of 5 cycles

References

Variations 1-3:

Cohen BJ, Moskowitz C, Straus D, et al, "Cyclophosphamide/Fludarabine (CF) is Active in the Treatment of Mantle Cell Lymphoma," *Leuk Lymphoma*, 2001, 42(5):1015-22.

Fludarabine-Cyclophosphamide-Rituximab (CLL)

Index Terms FCR (CLL); Rituximab-Fludarabine-Cyclophosphamide (CLL)

Use Leukemia, chronic lymphocytic

Regimen

Cycle 1:

Rituximab: I.V.: 375 mg/m^2 day 1
[total dose/cycle = 375 mg/m^2]
Fludarabine: I.V.: 25 mg/m^2/day days 2, 3, and 4
[total dose/cycle = 75 mg/m^2]
Cyclophosphamide: I.V.: 250 mg/m^2/day days 2, 3, and 4
[total dose/cycle = 750 mg/m^2]
Treatment cycle is 4 weeks

Cycles 2-6:

Rituximab: I.V.: 500 mg/m^2 day 1
[total dose/cycle = 500 mg/m^2]
Fludarabine: I.V.: 25 mg/m^2/day days 1, 2, and 3
[total dose/cycle = 75 mg/m^2]
Cyclophosphamide: I.V.: 250 mg/m^2/day days 1, 2, and 3
[total dose/cycle = 750 mg/m^2]
Repeat cycle every 4 weeks

References

Keating MJ, O'Brien S, Albitar M, et al, "Early Results of a Chemoimmunotherapy Regimen of Fludarabine, Cyclophosphamide, and Rituximab as Initial Therapy for Chronic Lymphocytic Leukemia," *J Clin Oncol*, 2005, 23(18):4079-88.

Wierda W, O'Brien S, Wen S, et al, "Chemoimmunotherapy With Fludarabine, Cyclophosphamide, and Rituximab for Relapsed and Refractory Chronic Lymphocytic Leukemia," *J Clin Oncol*, 2005, 23(18):4070-8.

Fludarabine-Cyclophosphamide-Rituximab (NHL-Follicular)

Index Terms FCR (NHL-Follicular); Rituximab-Fludarabine-Cyclophosphamide (NHL-Follicular)

Use Lymphoma, non-Hodgkin's (Follicular lymphoma)

Regimen

Cycle 1:
Rituximab: I.V.: 375 mg/m^2 day 15
  [total dose/cycle = 375 mg/m^2]
Fludarabine: I.V.: 25 mg/m^2/day days 1, 2, and 3
  [total dose/cycle = 75 mg/m^2]
Cyclophosphamide: I.V.: 300 mg/m^2/day days 1, 2, and 3
  [total dose/cycle = 900 mg/m^2]
Treatment cycle is 3 weeks

Cycles 2-4:
Rituximab: I.V.: 375 mg/m^2 day 1
  [total dose/cycle = 375 mg/m^2]
Fludarabine: I.V.: 25 mg/m^2/day days 1, 2, and 3
  [total dose/cycle = 75 mg/m^2]
Cyclophosphamide: I.V.: 300 mg/m^2/day days 1, 2, and 3
  [total dose/cycle = 900 mg/m^2]
Each treatment cycle is 3 weeks

References

Sacchi S, Pozzi S, Marcheselli R, et al, "Rituximab in Combination With Fludarabine and Cyclophosphamide in the Treatment of Patients With Recurrent Follicular Lymphoma," *Cancer*, 2007, 110(1):121-8.

◆ **Fludarabine-Cytarabine-Filgrastim (AML)** *see* FLAG (AML) *on page 1323*

Fludarabine-Mitoxantrone

Index Terms FM (NHL)

Use Lymphoma, non-Hodgkin's

Regimen

Fludarabine: I.V.: 25 mg/m^2/day days 1, 2, and 3
  [total dose/cycle = 75 mg/m^2]
Mitoxantrone: I.V.: 10 mg/m^2/dose day 1
  [total dose/cycle = 10 mg/m^2]
Repeat cycle every 21 days for total of 6 cycles

References

Zinzani PL, Pulsoni A, Perrotti A, et al, "Fludarabine Plus Mitoxantrone With and Without Rituximab Versus CHOP With and Without Rituximab as Front-Line Treatment for Patients With Follicular Lymphoma," *J Clin Oncol*, 2004, 22(13):2654-61.

Fludarabine-Mitoxantrone-Dexamethasone (NHL)

Index Terms FND (NHL)

Use Lymphoma, non-Hodgkin's

Regimen
Fludarabine: I.V.: 25 mg/m^2/day days 1, 2, and 3
[total dose/cycle = 75 mg/m^2]
Mitoxantrone: I.V.: 10 mg/m^2/dose day 1
[total dose/cycle = 10 mg/m^2]
Dexamethasone: I.V. or Oral: 20 mg/day days 1 to 5
[total dose/cycle = 100 mg]
Repeat cycle every 28 days for up to a total of 8 cycles

References
McLaughlin P, Hagemeister FB, Romaguera JE, et al, "Fludarabine, Mitoxantrone, and Dexamethasone: An Effective New Regimen for Indolent Lymphoma," *J Clin Oncol*, 1996, 14 (4):1262-8.

Tsimberidou AM, McLaughlin P, Younes A, et al, "Fludarabine, Mitoxantrone, Dexamethasone (FND) Compared With an Alternating Triple Therapy (ATT) Regimen in Patients With Stage IV Indolent Lymphoma," *Blood*, 2002, 100(13):4351-7.

Fludarabine-Mitoxantrone-Dexamethasone-Rituximab
Index Terms FNDR (NHL); Rituximab-Fludarabine-Mitoxantrone-Dexamethasone

Use Lymphoma, non-Hodgkin's

Regimen
Cycle 1:
Rituximab: I.V.: 375 mg/m^2/day days 1 and 8
[total dose/cycle = 750 mg/m^2]
Fludarabine: I.V.: 25 mg/m^2/day days 1, 2, and 3
[total dose/cycle = 75 mg/m^2]
Mitoxantrone: I.V.: 10 mg/m^2/dose day 1
[total dose/cycle = 10 mg/m^2]
Dexamethasone: I.V. or Oral: 20 mg/m^2/day days 1 to 5
[total dose/cycle = 100 mg/m^2]
Treatment cycle is 28 days

Cycles 2-5:
Rituximab: I.V.: 375 mg/m^2 day 1
[total dose/cycle = 375 mg/m^2]
Fludarabine: I.V.: 25 mg/m^2/day days 2, 3, and 4
[total dose/cycle = 75 mg/m^2]
Mitoxantrone: I.V.: 10 mg/m^2/dose day 2
[total dose/cycle = 10 mg/m^2]
Dexamethasone: I.V. or Oral: 20 mg/m^2/day days 1 to 5
[total dose/cycle = 100 mg/m^2]
Repeat cycle every 28 days

Cycles 6-8:
Fludarabine: I.V.: 25 mg/m^2/day days 1, 2, and 3
[total dose/cycle = 75 mg/m^2]
Mitoxantrone: I.V.: 10 mg/m^2/dose day 1
[total dose/cycle = 10 mg/m^2]
Dexamethasone: I.V. or Oral: 20 mg/m^2/day days 1 to 5
[total dose/cycle = 100 mg/m^2]
Repeat cycle every 28 days

followed by:
Interferon maintenance:
Interferon alfa-2b: SubQ: 3 million units/m^2 days 1 to 14
[total dose/cycle = 42 million units/m^2]
Dexamethasone: Oral: 8 mg/day days 1, 2, and 3
[total dose/cycle = 24 mg]
Repeat cycle every month for 1 year

References

McLaughlin P, Hagemeister FB, Rodriguez MA, et al, "Safety of Fludarabine, Mitoxantrone, and Dexamethasone Combined With Rituximab in the Treatment of Stage IV Indolent Lymphoma," *Semin Oncol*, 2000, 27(6 Suppl 12):37-41.

Fludarabine-Mitoxantrone-Rituximab

Index Terms FMR (NHL); RFM (NHL); Rituximab-Fludarabine-Mitoxantrone

Use Lymphoma, non-Hodgkin's

Regimen

Fludarabine: I.V.: 25 mg/m^2/day days 1, 2, and 3
[total dose/cycle = 75 mg/m^2]
Mitoxantrone: I.V.: 10 mg/m^2/dose day 1
[total dose/cycle = 10 mg/m^2]
Repeat cycle every 21 days for total of 6 cycles

followed by:

Sequential rituximab (after completion of cycle 6):
Rituximab: I.V.: 375 mg/m^2/dose weekly for 4 doses
[total dose/4 weeks = 1500 mg/m^2]

References

Zinzani PL, Pulsoni A, Perrotti A, et al, "Fludarabine Plus Mitoxantrone With and Without Rituximab Versus CHOP With and Without Rituximab as Front-Line Treatment for Patients With Follicular Lymphoma," *J Clin Oncol*, 2004, 22(13):2654-61.

Fludarabine-Rituximab (CLL)

Use Leukemia, chronic lymphocytic

Regimen

Rituximab: I.V.: 375 mg/m^2/day days 1 and 4 (cycle 1); day 1 (cycles 2 to 6)
Fludarabine: I.V.: 25 mg/m^2/day days 1 to 5
Repeat cycle every 4 weeks

References

Byrd JC, Peterson BL, Morrison VA, et al, "Randomized Phase 2 Study of Fludarabine With Concurrent vs Sequential Treatment With Rituximab in Symptomatic, Untreated Patients With B-Cell Chronic Lymphocytic Leukemia: Results From Cancer and Leukemia Group B 9712 (CALGB 9712)," *Blood*, 2003, 101(1):6-14.

Fluorouracil + Carboplatin

Use Head and neck cancer

Regimen NOTE: Multiple variations are listed.

Variation 1:
Fluorouracil: I.V.: 600 mg/m^2/day continuous infusion days 1 to 4
[total dose/cycle = 2400 mg/m^2]
Carboplatin: I.V.: 70 mg/m^2/day days 1 to 4
[total dose/cycle = 280 mg/m^2]
Repeat cycle every 3 weeks for 3 cycles

Variation 2:
Carboplatin: I.V.: 400 mg/m^2 day 1
[total dose/cycle = 400 mg/m^2]
Fluorouracil: I.V.: 1000 mg/m^2/day continuous infusion days 1 to 4
[total dose/cycle = 4000 mg/m^2]
Repeat cycle every 28 days

References

Variation 1:
Denis F, Garaud P, Bardet E, et al, "Final Results of the 94-01 French Head and Neck Oncology and Radiotherapy Group Randomized Trial Comparing Radiotherapy Alone With Concomitant

Radiochemotherapy in Advanced-Stage Oropharynx Carcinoma," *J Clin Oncol*, 2004, 22 (1):69-76.

Variation 2:

Gregoire V, Beauduin M, Humblet Y, et al, "A Phase I-II Trial of Induction Chemotherapy With Carboplatin and Fluorouracil in Locally Advanced Head and Neck Squamous Cell Carcinoma: A Report From the UCL-Oncology Group, Belgium," *J Clin Oncol*, 1991, 9(8):1385-92.

◆ **Fluorouracil-Cisplatin (Bladder Cancer)** *see* Cisplatin-Fluorouracil (Bladder Cancer) *on page 1267*

◆ **Fluorouracil-Cisplatin (Cervical Cancer)** *see* Cisplatin-Fluorouracil (Cervical Cancer) *on page 1267*

◆ **Fluorouracil-Cisplatin (Esophageal Cancer)** *see* Cisplatin-Fluorouracil (Esophageal Cancer) *on page 1268*

◆ **Fluorouracil-Cisplatin (Head and Neck Cancer)** *see* Cisplatin-Fluorouracil (Head and Neck Cancer) *on page 1270*

Fluorouracil-Leucovorin

Index Terms F-CL; FU-LV; FU/Leucovorin

Use Colorectal cancer

Regimen NOTE: Multiple variations are listed.

Variation 1 (Mayo Regimen):

Fluorouracil: I.V.: 370-425 mg/m^2/day days 1 to 5
[total dose/cycle = 1850-2125 mg/m^2]

Leucovorin: I.V.: 20 mg/m^2/day days 1 to 5
[total dose/cycle = 100 mg/m^2]

Repeat cycle at 4 weeks, 8 weeks, and every 5 weeks thereafter

Variation 2:

Fluorouracil: I.V.: 400 mg/m^2/day days 1 to 5
[total dose/cycle = 2000 mg/m^2]

Leucovorin: I.V.: 20 mg/m^2/day days 1 to 5
[total dose/cycle = 100 mg/m^2]

Repeat cycle every 28 days

Variation 3:

Fluorouracil: I.V.: 500 mg/m^2 day 1
[total dose/cycle = 500 mg/m^2]

Leucovorin: I.V.: 20 mg/m^2 (2-hour infusion) day 1
[total dose/cycle = 20 mg/m^2]

Repeat cycle weekly

Variation 4:

Fluorouracil: I.V.: 600 mg/m^2 weekly for 6 weeks
[total dose/cycle = 3600 mg/m^2]

Leucovorin: I.V.: 500 mg/m^2 (3-hour infusion) weekly for 6 weeks
[total dose/cycle = 3000 mg/m^2]

Repeat cycle every 8 weeks

Variation 5:

Fluorouracil: I.V.: 600 mg/m^2 weekly for 6 weeks
[total dose/cycle = 3600 mg/m^2]

Leucovorin: I.V.: 500 mg/m^2 (2-hour infusion) weekly for 6 weeks
[total dose/cycle = 3000 mg/m^2]

Repeat cycle every 8 weeks

Variation 6:

Fluorouracil: I.V.: 600 mg/m^2 weekly
[total dose/cycle = 600 mg/m^2]

◄ Leucovorin: I.V.: 500 mg/m^2 (2-hour infusion) weekly
   [total dose/cycle = 500 mg/m^2]
Repeat cycle weekly

Variation 7:
   Fluorouracil: I.V.: 2600 mg/m^2 continuous infusion over 24 hours day 1
      [total dose/cycle = 2600 mg/m^2]
   Leucovorin: I.V.: 500 mg/m^2 continuous infusion over 24 hours day 1
      [total dose/cycle = 500 mg/m^2]
   Repeat cycle weekly

Variation 8:
   Fluorouracil: I.V.: 2600 mg/m^2 continuous infusion over 24 hours day 1
      [total dose/cycle = 2600 mg/m^2]
   Leucovorin: I.V.: 300 mg/m^2 (maximum dose: 500 mg) continuous infusion
      over 24 hours day 1
      [total dose/cycle = 300 mg/m^2; maximum: 500 mg]
   Repeat cycle weekly

Variation 9:
   Fluorouracil: I.V.: 2600 mg/m^2 continuous infusion over 24 hours once weekly
      for 6 weeks
      [total dose/cycle = 15,600 mg/m^2]
   Leucovorin: I.V.: 500 mg/m^2 over 2 hours once weekly for 6 weeks
      [total dose/cycle = 3000 mg/m^2]
   Repeat cycle every 8 weeks

Variation 10:
   Fluorouracil: I.V.: 2300 mg/m^2 continuous infusion over 24 hours day 1
      [total dose/cycle = 2300 mg/m^2]
   Leucovorin: I.V.: 50 mg/m^2 continuous infusion over 24 hours day 1
      [total dose/cycle = 50 mg/m^2]
   Repeat cycle weekly

Variation 11:
   Fluorouracil: I.V.: 200 mg/m^2/day continuous infusion days 1 to 14
      [total dose/cycle = 2800 mg/m^2]
   Leucovorin: I.V.: 5 mg/m^2/day continuous infusion days 1 to 14
      [total dose/cycle = 70 mg/m^2]
   Repeat cycle every 28 days

Variation 12:
   Cycle 1:
      Fluorouracil: I.V.: 200 mg/m^2/day continuous infusion for 4 weeks
         [total dose/cycle = 5600 mg/m^2]
      Leucovorin: I.V.: 20 mg/m^2/day days 1, 8, 15, 22
         [total dose/cycle = 80 mg/m^2]
      Treatment cycle is 6 weeks
   Subsequent cycles (starting week 7):
      Fluorouracil: 200 mg/m^2 continuous infusion days 1 to 21
         [total dose/cycle = 4200 mg/m^2]
      Leucovorin: I.V.: 20 mg/m^2/day days 1, 8, and 15
         [total dose/cycle = 60 mg/m^2]
      Repeat cycle every 4 weeks

References

Variation 1:
Poon MA, O'Connell MJ, Moertel CG, et al, "Biochemical Modulation of Fluorouracil: Evidence of Significant Improvement of Survival and Quality of Life in Patients With Advanced Colorectal Carcinoma," *J Clin Oncol*, 1989, 7(10):1407-18.

Variation 2:

Borner MM, Castiglione M, Bacchi M, et al "The Impact of Adding Low-Dose Leucovorin to Monthly 5-Fluorouracil in Advanced Colorectal Carcinoma: Results of a Phase III Trial. Swiss Group for Clinical Cancer Research (SAKK)," *Ann Oncol*, 1998, 9(5):535-41.

Variation 3:

Jager E, Heike M, Bernhard H, et al, "Weekly High-Dose Leucovorin Versus Low-Dose Leucovorin Combined With Fluorouracil in Advanced Colorectal Cancer: Results of a Randomized Multicenter Trial. Study Group for Palliative Treatment of Metastatic Colorectal Cancer Study Protocol 1," *J Clin Oncol*, 1996, 14(8):2274-9.

Variation 4:

Leichman CG, Fleming TR, Muggia FM, et al, "Phase II Study of Fluorouracil and Its Modulation in Advanced Colorectal Cancer: A Southwest Oncology Group Study," *J Clin Oncol*, 1995, 13 (6):1303-11.

Variation 5:

Buroker TR, O'Connell MJ, Wieand HS, et al, "Randomized Comparison of Two Schedules of Fluorouracil and Leucovorin in the Treatment of Advanced Colorectal Cancer," *J Clin Oncol*, 1994, 12(1):14-20.

Variation 6:

Nobile MT, Rosso R, Sertoli MR, et al, "Randomised Comparison of Weekly Bolus 5-Fluorouracil With or Without Leucovorin in Metastatic Colorectal Carcinoma," *Eur J Cancer*, 1992, 28A (11):1823-7.

Variation 7:

Ardalan B, Chua L, Tian EM, et al, "A Phase II Study of Weekly 24-Hour Infusion With High-Dose Fluorouracil With Leucovorin in Colorectal Carcinoma," *J Clin Oncol*, 1991, 9(4):625-30.

Variation 8:

Yeh KH, Cheng AL, Lin MT, et al, "A Phase II Study of Weekly 24-Hour Infusion of High-Dose 5-Fluorouracil and Leucovorin (HDFL) in the Treatment of Recurrent or Metastatic Colorectal Cancers," *Anticancer Res*, 1997, 17(5B):3867-72.

Variation 9:

Kohne CH, Schoffski P, Wilke H, et al, "Effective Biomodulation by Leucovorin of High-Dose Infusion Fluorouracil Given as a Weekly 24-Hour Infusion: Results of a Randomized Trial in Patients With Advanced Colorectal Cancer," *J Clin Oncol*, 1998, 16(2):418-26.

Variation 10:

Haas NB, Schilder RJ, Nash S, et al, "A Phase II Trial of Weekly Infusional 5-Fluorouracil in Combination With Low-Dose Leucovorin in Patients With Advanced Colorectal Cancer," *Invest New Drugs*, 1995, 13(3):229-33.

Variation 11:

Falcone A, Allegrini G, Lencioni M, et al, "Protracted Continuous Infusion of 5-Fluorouracil and Low-Dose Leucovorin in Patients With Metastatic Colorectal Cancer Resistant to 5-Fluorouracil Bolus-Based Chemotherapy: A Phase II Study," *Cancer Chemother Pharmacol*, 1999, 44 (2):159-63.

Variation 12:

Leichman CG, Leichman L, Spears CP, et al, "Prolonged Continuous Infusion of Fluorouracil With Weekly Bolus Leucovorin: A Phase II Study in Patients With Disseminated Colorectal Cancer," *J Natl Cancer Inst*, 1993, 85(1):41-4.

◆ **Fluorouracil-Leucovorin-Bevacizumab** *see* Bevacizumab-Fluorouracil-Leucovorin *on page 1232*

◆ **Fluorouracil-Leucovorin-Irinotecan** *see* FU-LV-CPT-11 *on page 1338*

Fluorouracil-Leucovorin-Irinotecan (Saltz Regimen)

Index Terms FU-LV-CPT-11 (Saltz Regimen); Irinotecan-Fluorouracil-Leucovorin (Saltz Regimen); Saltz Regimen

Use Colorectal cancer

Regimen

Fluorouracil: I.V.: 500 mg/m^2/day days 1, 8, 15, and 22
[total dose/cycle = 2000 mg/m^2]
Leucovorin: I.V.: 20 mg/m^2/day days 1, 8, 15, and 22
[total dose/cycle = 80 mg/m^2]
Irinotecan: I.V.: 125 mg/m^2/day days 1, 8, 15, and 22
[total dose/cycle = 500 mg/m^2]
Repeat cycle every 42 days

References
Saltz LB, Cox JV, Blanke C, et al, "Irinotecan Plus Fluorouracil and Leucovorin for Metastatic Colorectal Cancer, Irinotecan Study Group," *N Engl J Med*, 2000, 343(13):905-14.

Fluorouracil-Leucovorin-Oxaliplatin (Gastric Cancer)

Index Terms FLO (Gastric Cancer); Oxaliplatin-Leucovorin-Fluorouracil (Gastric Cancer)

Use Gastric cancer

Regimen
Oxaliplatin: I.V.: 100 mg/m^2/dose over 2 hours day 1
[total dose/cycle = 100 mg/m^2]
Leucovorin: I.V.: 400 mg/m^2/dose over 2 hours day 1
[total dose/cycle = 400 mg/m^2]
Fluorouracil: I.V. bolus: 400 mg/m^2/dose over 10 minutes day 1
followed by I.V.: 3000 mg/m^2 continuous infusion over 46 hours day 1
[total dose/cycle = 3400 mg/m^2]
Note: Bolus fluorouracil and continuous infusion are both given on day 1.
Repeat cycle every 2 weeks for at least 6 cycles

References
Louvet C, André T, Tigaud JM, et al, "Phase II Study of Oxaliplatin, Fluorouracil, and Folinic Acid in Locally Advanced or Metastatic Gastric Cancer Patients," *J Clin Oncol*, 2002, 20(23):4543-8.

Fluorouracil-Leucovorin-Oxaliplatin (Gastric/Esophageal Cancer)

Index Terms FLO (Gastric/Esophageal Cancer); Oxaliplatin-Leucovorin-Fluorouracil (Gastric/Esophageal Cancer)

Use Esophageal Cancer; Gastric Cancer

Regimen NOTE: Multiple variations are listed.
Variation 1:
Oxaliplatin: I.V.: 85 mg/m^2/dose over 2 hours day 1
[total dose/cycle = 85 mg/m^2]
Leucovorin: I.V.: 200 mg/m^2/dose over 2 hours day 1
[total dose/cycle = 200 mg/m^2]
Fluorouracil: I.V.: 2600 mg/m^2/dose continuous infusion over 24 hours day 1
[total dose/cycle = 2600 mg/m^2]
Repeat cycle every 2 weeks
Variation 2:
Oxaliplatin: I.V.: 85 mg/m^2/dose over 2 hours day 1
[total dose/cycle = 85 mg/m^2]
Leucovorin: I.V.: 500 mg/m^2/day over 2 hours days 1 and 2
[total dose/cycle = 1000 mg/m^2]
Fluorouracil: I.V. bolus: 400 mg/m^2/day days 1 and 2
followed by I.V.: 600 mg/m^2/day continuous infusion over 22 hours days 1 and 2
[total dose/cycle = 2000 mg/m^2]
Note: Bolus fluorouracil and continuous infusion are both given on days 1 and 2.
Repeat cycle every 2 weeks

References
Variation 1:
Al-Batran SE, Hartmann JT, Probst S, et al, "Phase III Trial in Metastatic Gastroesophageal Adenocarcinoma With Fluorouracil, Leucovorin Plus Either Oxaliplatin or Cisplatin: A Study of the Arbeitsgemeinschaft Internistische Onkologie," *J Clin Oncol*, 2008, 26(9):1435-42.
Variation 2:
Mauer AM, Kraut EH, Krauss SA, et al, "Phase II Trial of Oxaliplatin, Leucovorin and Fluorouracil in Patients With Advanced Carcinoma of the Esophagus," *Ann Oncol*, 2005, 16(8):1320-5.

Fluorouracil-Mitomycin (Anal Cancer)

Index Terms Mitomycin–Fluorouracil (Anal Cancer)

Use Anal cancer

Regimen NOTE: Multiple variations are listed.

Variation 1 (in combination with radiotherapy):

Fluorouracil: I.V.: 1000 mg/m^2/day continuous infusion days 1 to 4 and days 29 to 32
[total dose/cycle = 8000 mg/m^2]

Mitomycin: I.V.: 10 mg/m^2/day (maximum dose: 20 mg) days 1 and 29
[total dose/cycle = 20 mg/m^2; maximum: 40 mg]

Variation 2 (in combination with radiotherapy):

Fluorouracil: I.V.: 1000 mg/m^2/day continuous infusion days 1 to 4
[total dose/cycle = 4000 mg/m^2]

Mitomycin: I.V.: 10 mg/m^2/dose (maximum dose: 20 mg) day 1
[total dose/cycle = 10 mg/m^2; maximum: 20 mg]

Repeat cycle in 28 days (total of 2 cycles)

References

Variation 1:

Ajani JA, Winter KA, Gunderson LL, et al, "Fluorouracil, Mitomycin, and Radiotherapy vs Fluorouracil, Cisplatin, and Radiotherapy for Carcinoma of the Anal Canal: A Randomized Controlled Trial," *JAMA*, 2008, 299(16):1914-21.

Variation 2:

Flam M, John M, Pajak TF, et al, "Role of Mitomycin in Combination With Fluorouracil and Radiotherapy, and of Salvage Chemoradiation in the Definitive Nonsurgical Treatment of Epidermoid Carcinoma of the Anal Canal: Results of a Phase III Randomized Intergroup Study," *J Clin Oncol*, 1996, 14(9):2527-39.

♦ **Fluorouracil-Oxaliplatin (Esophageal Cancer)** *see* Oxaliplatin-Fluorouracil (Esophageal Cancer) *on page 1384*

♦ **Flutamide + Goserelin** *see* FZ *on page 1340*

♦ **Flutamide + Leuprolide** *see* FL *on page 1323*

♦ **FM (NHL)** *see* Fludarabine-Mitoxantrone *on page 1328*

♦ **FMR (NHL)** *see* Fludarabine-Mitoxantrone-Rituximab *on page 1330*

♦ **FNC** *see* CNF *on page 1277*

♦ **FND (NHL)** *see* Fludarabine-Mitoxantrone-Dexamethasone (NHL) *on page 1328*

♦ **FNDR (NHL)** *see* Fludarabine-Mitoxantrone-Dexamethasone-Rituximab *on page 1329*

FOIL (Colorectal Cancer)

Use Colorectal cancer

Regimen

Irinotecan: I.V.: 175 mg/m^2 day 1
[total dose/cycle = 175 mg/m^2]

Oxaliplatin: I.V.: 100 mg/m^2 day 1
[total dose/cycle = 100 mg/m^2]

Leucovorin: I.V.: 200 mg/m^2 day 1
[total dose/cycle = 200 mg/m^2]

Fluorouracil: I.V.: 3800 mg/m^2/day continuous infusion days 1 and 2
[total dose/cycle = 7600 mg/m^2]

Repeat cycle every 14 days

References

Falcone A, Masi G, Allegrini G, et al, "Biweekly Chemotherapy With Oxaliplatin, Irinotecan, Infusional Fluorouracil, and Leucovorin: A Pilot Study in Patients With Metastatic Colorectal Cancer," *J Clin Oncol*, 2002, 20(19):4006-14.

FOLFIRINOX (Pancreatic Cancer)

Index Terms Irinotecan-Oxaliplatin-Fluorouracil-Leucovorin (Pancreatic Cancer) ; Oxaliplatin-Irinotecan-Fluorouracil-Leucovorin (Pancreatic Cancer)

Use Pancreatic cancer

Regimen

Oxaliplatin: I.V.: 85 mg/m^2/dose over 2 hours day 1
[total dose/cycle = 85 mg/m^2]
Irinotecan: I.V.: 180 mg/m^2/dose over 90 minutes day 1
[total dose/cycle = 180 mg/m^2]
Leucovorin: I.V.: 400 mg/m^2/dose over 2 hours day 1
[total dose/cycle = 400 mg/m^2]
Fluorouracil: I.V. bolus: 400 mg/m^2/dose day 1
followed by I.V.: 2400 mg/m^2 continuous infusion over 46 hours beginning day 1
[total dose/cycle = 2800 mg/m^2]
Note: Bolus fluorouracil and continuous infusion are both given on day 1.
Repeat cycle every 14 days for 12 cycles or until disease progression or unacceptable toxicity

References

Conroy T, Paillot B, François E, et al, "Irinotecan Plus Oxaliplatin and Leucovorin-Modulated Fluorouracil in Advanced Pancreatic Cancer–A Groupe Tumeurs Digestives of the Federation Nationale des Centres de Lutte Contre le Cancer Study," *J Clin Oncol*, 2005, 23(6):1228-36.

◆ **FOLFOX4-Cetuximab** *see* Cetuximab-FOLFOX4 *on page 1257*

FOLFOX 1

Use Colorectal cancer

Regimen

Oxaliplatin: I.V.: 130 mg/m^2 day 1 (every other cycle)
[total dose/cycle = 130 mg/m^2]
Leucovorin: I.V.: 500 mg/m^2/day days 1 and 2
[total dose/cycle = 1000 mg/m^2]
Fluorouracil: I.V.: 1.5-2 g/m^2/day continuous infusion days 1 and 2
[total dose/cycle = 3-4 g/m^2]
Repeat cycle every 14 days

References

de Gramont A, Tournigand C, Louvet C, et al, "Oxaliplatin, Folinic Acid, and 5-Fluorouracil (FOLFOX) in Pretreated Patients With Metastatic Advanced Cancer, The GERCOD," *Rev Med Interne*, 1997, 18(10):769-75.

FOLFOX 2

Use Colorectal cancer

Regimen

Oxaliplatin: I.V.: 100 mg/m^2 day 1
[total dose/cycle = 100 mg/m^2]
Leucovorin: I.V.: 500 mg/m^2/day days 1 and 2
[total dose/cycle = 1000 mg/m^2]
Fluorouracil: I.V.: 1.5-2 g/m^2/day continuous infusion days 1 and 2
[total dose/cycle = 3-4 g/m^2]
Repeat cycle every 14 days

References

de Gramont A, Vignoud J, Tournigand C, et al, "Oxaliplatin With High-Dose Leucovorin and 5-Fluorouracil 48-Hour Continuous Infusion in Pretreated Metastatic Colorectal Cancer," *Eur J Cancer*, 1997, 33(2):214-9.

FOLFOX 3

Use Colorectal cancer

Regimen

Oxaliplatin: I.V.: 85 mg/m^2 day 1
[total dose/cycle = 85 mg/m^2]

Leucovorin: I.V.: 500 mg/m^2/day days 1 and 2
[total dose/cycle = 1000 mg/m^2]

Fluorouracil: I.V.: 1.5-2 g/m^2/day continuous infusion days 1 and 2
[total dose/cycle = 3-4 g/m^2]

Repeat cycle every 14 days

References

de Gramont A, Tournigand C, Louvet C, et al, "Oxaliplatin, Folinic Acid, and 5-Fluorouracil (FOLFOX) in Pretreated Patients With Metastatic Advanced Cancer, The GERCOD," *Rev Med Interne*, 1997, 18(10):769-75.

FOLFOX 4

Use Colorectal cancer

Regimen

Oxaliplatin: I.V.: 85 mg/m^2 day 1
[total dose/cycle = 85 mg/m^2]

Leucovorin: I.V.: 200 mg/m^2/day days 1 and 2
[total dose/cycle = 400 mg/m^2]

Fluorouracil: I.V. bolus: 400 mg/m^2/day days 1 and 2
[total dose/cycle = 800 mg/m^2]

   followed by I.V.: 600 mg/m^2 continuous infusion (over 22 hours) days 1 and 2
   [total dose/cycle = 1200 mg/m^2]

Note: Bolus fluorouracil and continuous infusion are both given on each day.

Repeat cycle every 14 days

References

André T, Bensmaine MA, Louvet C, et al, "Multicenter Phase II Study of Bimonthly High-Dose Leucovorin, Fluorouracil Infusion, and Oxaliplatin for Metastatic Colorectal Cancer Resistant to the Same Leucovorin and Fluorouracil Regimen," *J Clin Oncol*, 1999, 17(11):3560-8.

FOLFOX 6

Use Colorectal cancer

Regimen

Oxaliplatin: I.V.: 100 mg/m^2 day 1
[total dose/cycle = 100 mg/m^2]

Leucovorin: I.V.: 400 mg/m^2 day 1
[total dose/cycle = 400 mg/m^2]

Fluorouracil: I.V. bolus: 400 mg/m^2 day 1
[total dose/cycle = 400 mg/m^2]

   followed by I.V.: 2.4-3 g/m^2 continuous infusion (46 hours) extending over days 1 and 2
   [total dose/cycle = 2.4-3 g/m^2]

Repeat cycle every 14 days

References

Maindrault-Goebel F, Louvet C, Andre T, et al, "Oxaliplatin Added to the Simplified Bimonthly Leucovorin and 5-Fluorouracil Regimen as Second-Line Therapy for Metastatic Colorectal Cancer (FOLFOX6), GERCOR," *Eur J Cancer*, 1999, 35(9):1338-42.

FOLFOX 7

Use Colorectal cancer
Regimen
Oxaliplatin: I.V.: 130 mg/m^2 day 1
[total dose/cycle = 130 mg/m^2]
Leucovorin: I.V.: 400 mg/m^2 day 1
[total dose/cycle = 400 mg/m^2]
Fluorouracil: I.V. bolus: 400 mg/m^2 day 1
[total dose/cycle = 400 mg/m^2]
  followed by I.V.: 2.4 g/m^2 continuous infusion (46 hours) extending over
  days 1 and 2
  [total dose/cycle = 2.4 g/m^2]
Repeat cycle every 14 days
References
Maindrault-Goebel F, de Gramont A, Louvet C, et al, "High-Dose Intensity Oxaliplatin Added to the Simplified Bimonthly Leucovorin and 5-Fluorouracil Regimen as Second-Line Therapy for Metastatic Colorectal Cancer (FOLFOX 7)," *Eur J Cancer*, 2001, 37(8):1000-5.

FOLFOXIRI (Colorectal Cancer)

Use Colorectal cancer
Regimen
Irinotecan: I.V.: 165 mg/m^2 over 1 hour day 1
[total dose/cycle = 165 mg/m^2]
Oxaliplatin: I.V.: 85 mg/m^2 over 2 hours day 1
[total dose/cycle = 85 mg/m^2]
Leucovorin: I.V.: 200 mg/m^2 over 2 hours day 1
[total dose/cycle = 200 mg/m^2]
Fluorouracil: I.V.: 3200 mg/m^2/day continuous infusion over 48 hours
beginning day 1
[total dose/cycle = 6400 mg/m^2]
Repeat cycle every 14 days (maximum: 12 cycles)
References
Falcone A, Ricci S, Brunetti I, et al, "Phase III Trial of Infusional Fluorouracil, Leucovorin, Oxaliplatin, and Irinotecan (FOLFOXIRI) Compared With Infusional Fluorouracil, Leucovorin, and Irinotecan (FOLFIRI) as First-Line Treatment for Metastatic Colorectal Cancer: The Gruppo Oncologico Nord Ovest," *J Clin Oncol*, 2007, 25(13):1670-6.

◆ **FU-LV** see Fluorouracil-Leucovorin on page 1331
◆ **FU-LV-CPT-11 (Saltz Regimen)** see Fluorouracil-Leucovorin-Irinotecan (Saltz Regimen) on page 1333
◆ **FU/Leucovorin** see Fluorouracil-Leucovorin on page 1331

FU-LV-CPT-11

Index Terms Fluorouracil-Leucovorin-Irinotecan; Irinotecan-Fluorouracil-Leucovorin
Use Colorectal cancer
Regimen NOTE: Multiple variations are listed.
Variation 1:
Irinotecan: I.V.: 350 mg/m^2 day 1
[total dose/cycle = 350 mg/m^2]
Leucovorin: I.V.: 20 mg/m^2/day days 22 to 26
[total dose/cycle = 100 mg/m^2]
Fluorouracil: I.V.: 425 mg/m^2/day days 22 to 26
[total dose/cycle = 2125 mg/m^2]
Repeat cycle every 6 weeks

Variation 2:

Irinotecan: I.V.: 80 mg/m^2 day 1
 [total dose/cycle = 80 mg/m^2]
Fluorouracil: I.V.: 2300 mg/m^2 continuous infusion day 1
 [total dose/cycle = 2300 mg/m^2]
Leucovorin: I.V.: 500 mg/m^2 day 1
 [total dose/cycle = 500 mg/m^2]
Repeat cycle weekly

or

Irinotecan: I.V.: 180 mg/m^2 day 1
 [total dose/cycle = 180 mg/m^2]
Leucovorin: I.V.: 200 mg/m^2/day days 1 and 2
 [total dose/cycle = 400 mg/m^2]
Fluorouracil: I.V.: 400 mg/m^2/day days 1 and 2
 [total dose/cycle = 800 mg/m^2]
  followed by I.V.: 600 mg/m^2/day continuous infusion days 1 and 2
   [total dose/cycle = 1200 mg/m^2]
Repeat cycle every 2 weeks

Variation 3:

Irinotecan: I.V.: 175 mg/m^2 day 1
 [total dose/cycle = 175 mg/m^2]
Leucovorin: I.V.: 250 mg/m^2 day 2
 [total dose/cycle = 250 mg/m^2]
Fluorouracil: I.V.: 950 mg/m^2 day 2
 [total dose/cycle = 950 mg/m^2]

or

Irinotecan: I.V.: 200 mg/m^2 day 1
 [total dose/cycle = 200 mg/m^2]
Leucovorin: I.V.: 250 mg/m^2 day 2
 [total dose/cycle = 250 mg/m^2]
Fluorouracil: I.V.: 850 mg/m^2 day 2
 [total dose/cycle = 850 mg/m^2]
Repeat cycle every other week

References

Variation 1:

Van Cutsem E, Pozzo C, Starkhammar H, et al, "A Phase II Study of Irinotecan Alternated With Five Days Bolus of 5-Fluorouracil and Leucovorin in First-Line Chemotherapy of Metastatic Colorectal Cancer," *Ann Oncol*, 1998, 9(11):1199-204.

Variation 2:

Douillard JY, Cunningham D, Roth AD, et al, "Irinotecan Combined With Fluorouracil Compared With Fluorouracil Alone as First-Line Treatment for Metastatic Colorectal Cancer: A Multicentre Randomised Trial," *Lancet*, 2000, 355(9209):1041-7.

Variation 3:

Comella P, Casaretti F, De Vita F, et al, "Concurrent Irinotecan and 5-Fluorouracil Plus Levo-Folinic Acid Given Every Other Week in the First-Line Management of Advanced Colorectal Carcinoma: A Phase I Study of the Southern Italy Cooperative Oncology Group," *Ann Oncol*, 1999, 10 (8):915-21.

FUP

Use Gastric cancer

Regimen

Fluorouracil: I.V.: 1000 mg/m^2/day continuous infusion days 1 to 5
 [total dose/cycle = 5000 mg/m^2]
Cisplatin: I.V.: 100 mg/m^2 day 2
 [total dose/cycle = 100 mg/m^2]
Repeat cycle every 28 days

References

Vanhoefer U, Rougier P, Wilke H, et al, "Final Results of a Randomized Phase III Trial of Sequential High-Dose Methotrexate, Fluorouracil, and Doxorubicin Versus Etoposide, Leucovorin, and Fluorouracil Versus Infusional Fluorouracil and Cisplatin in Advanced Gastric Cancer: A Trial of the European Organization for Research and Treatment of Cancer Gastrointestinal Tract Cancer Cooperative Group," *J Clin Oncol*, 2000, 18(14):2648-57.

FZ

Index Terms Flutamide + Goserelin

Use Prostate cancer

Regimen NOTE: Multiple variations are listed.

Variation 1:

Flutamide: Oral: 250 mg every 8 hours

[total dose/cycle = 21,000 mg]

Goserelin acetate: SubQ: 3.6 mg day 1

[total dose/cycle = 3.6 mg]

Repeat cycle every 28 days

Variation 2:

Flutamide: Oral: 250 mg every 8 hours

[total dose/cycle = 67,500 mg]

Goserelin acetate: SubQ: 10.8 mg day 1

[total dose/cycle = 10.8 mg]

Repeat cycle every 3 months

References

McLeod DG, Schellhammer PF, Vogelzang NJ, et al, "Exploratory Analysis on the Effect of Race on Clinical Outcome in Patients With Advanced Prostate Cancer Receiving Bicalutamide or Flutamide, Each in Combination With LHRH Analogues. The Casodex Combination Study Group," *Prostate*, 1999, 40(4):218-24.

Gemcitabine-Capecitabine

Use Biliary adenocarcinoma; Pancreatic cancer

Regimen

Gemcitabine: I.V.: 1000 mg/m^2/day days 1 and 8

[total dose/cycle = 2000 mg/m^2]

Capecitabine: Oral: 650 mg/m^2 twice daily days 1 to 14

[total dose/cycle = 18,200 mg/m^2]

Repeat cycle every 21 days

References

Hess V, Salzberg M, Borner M, et al, "Combining Capecitabine and Gemcitabine in Patients With Advanced Pancreatic Carcinoma: A Phase I/II Trial," *J Clin Oncol*, 2003, 21(1):66-8.

Knox JJ, Hedley D, Oza A, et al, "Combining Gemcitabine and Capecitabine in Patients With Advanced Biliary Cancer: A Phase II Trial," *J Clin Oncol*, 2005, 23(10):2332-8.

Gemcitabine-Carboplatin (Bladder Cancer)

Use Bladder cancer

Regimen

Gemcitabine: I.V.: 1000 mg/m^2/day days 1 and 8

[total dose/cycle = 2000 mg/m^2]

Carboplatin: I.V.: AUC 5 day 1

[total dose/cycle = AUC = 5]

Repeat cycle every 21 days for up to 6 cycles

References

Bamias A, Moulopoulos LA, Koutras A, et al, "The Combination of Gemcitabine and Carboplatin as First-Line Treatment in Patients With Advanced Urothelial Carcinoma. A Phase II Study of the Hellenic Cooperative Oncology Group," *Cancer*, 2006, 106(2):297-303.

Gemcitabine-Carboplatin (NSCLC)

Index Terms Carboplatin-Gemcitabine (NSCLC)
Use Lung cancer, nonsmall cell
Regimen NOTE: Multiple variations are listed.
Variation 1:
Gemcitabine: I.V.: 1000 mg/m^2/dose days 1, 8, and 15
[total dose/cycle = 3000 mg/m^2]
Carboplatin: I.V.: AUC 5 day 1
[total dose/cycle = AUC = 5]
Repeat cycle every 28 days for up to 4 cycles
Variation 2:
Gemcitabine: I.V.: 1000 or 1100 mg/m^2/day days 1 and 8
[total dose/cycle = 2000 or 2200 mg/m^2]
Carboplatin: I.V.: AUC 5 day 8
[total dose/cycle = AUC = 5]
Repeat cycle every 28 days

References

Variation 1:
Danson S, Middleton MR, O'Byrne KJ, et al, "Phase III Trial of Gemcitabine and Carboplatin Versus Mitomycin, Ifosfamide, and Cisplatin or Mitomycin, Vinblastine, and Cisplatin in Patients With Advanced Nonsmall Cell Lung Carcinoma," *Cancer*, 2003, 98(3):542-53.
Variation 2:
Iaffaioli RV, Tortoriello A, Facchini G, et al, "Phase I-II Study of Gemcitabine and Carboplatin in Stage IIIB-IV Nonsmall-Cell Lung Cancer," *J Clin Oncol*, 1999, 17(3):921-6.

Gemcitabine-Carboplatin (Ovarian Cancer)

Use Ovarian cancer
Regimen
Gemcitabine: I.V.: 1000 mg/m^2/day days 1 and 8
[total dose/cycle = 2000 mg/m^2]
Carboplatin: I.V.: AUC 4 day 1
[total dose/cycle = AUC = 4]
Repeat cycle every 21 days for 6-10 cycles

References

Pfisterer J, Plante M, Vergote I, et al, "Gemcitabine Plus Carboplatin Compared With Carboplatin in Patients With Platinum-Sensitive Recurrent Ovarian Cancer: An Intergroup Trial of the AGO-OVAR, the NCIC CTG, and the EORTC GCG," *J Clin Oncol*, 2006, 24(29):4699-707.

Gemcitabine-Cisplatin (Biliary Cancer)

Index Terms Cisplatin-Gemcitabine (Biliary Cancer)
Use Biliary adenocarcinoma
Regimen NOTE: Multiple variations are listed.
Variation 1:
Gemcitabine: I.V.: 1250 mg/m^2/dose days 1 and 8
[total dose/cycle = 2500 mg/m^2]
Cisplatin: I.V.: 75 mg/m^2/dose day 1
[total dose/cycle = 75 mg/m^2]
Repeat cycle every 3 weeks
Variation 2:
Gemcitabine: I.V.: 1000 mg/m^2/dose days 1 and 8
[total dose/cycle = 2000 mg/m^2]
Cisplatin: I.V.: 70 mg/m^2/dose day 1
[total dose/cycle = 70 mg/m^2]
Repeat cycle every 3 weeks (maximum: 6 cycles)

◀ **References**

Variation 1:
Thongprasert S, Napapan S, Charoentum C, et al, "Phase II Study of Gemcitabine and Cisplatin as First-Line Chemotherapy in Inoperable Biliary Tract Carcinoma," *Ann Oncol*, 2005, 16(2):279-81.

Variation 2:
Doval DC, Sekhon JS, Gupta SK, et al, "A Phase II Study of Gemcitabine and Cisplatin in Chemotherapy-Naive, Unresectable Gall Bladder Cancer," *Br J Cancer*, 2004, 90(8):1516-20.

Gemcitabine-Cisplatin (Bladder Cancer)

Use Bladder cancer

Regimen

Gemcitabine: I.V.: 1000 mg/m^2/day days 1, 8, and 15

[total dose/cycle = 3000 mg/m^2]

Cisplatin: I.V.: 70 mg/m^2 day 2

[total dose/cycle = 70 mg/m^2]

Repeat cycle every 28 days for 6 cycles

References

von der Maase H, Hansen SW, Roberts JT, et al, "Gemcitabine and Cisplatin Versus Methotrexate, Vinblastine, Doxorubicin, and Cisplatin in Advanced or Metastatic Bladder Cancer: Results of a Large, Randomized, Multinational, Multicenter, Phase III Study," *J Clin Oncol*, 2000, 18 (17):3068-77.

Gemcitabine-Cisplatin (Cervical Cancer)

Index Terms Cisplatin-Gemcitabine (Cervical Cancer)

Use Cervical cancer

Regimen

Gemcitabine: I.V.: 1250 mg/m^2/day days 1 and 8

[total dose/cycle = 2500 mg/m^2]

Cisplatin: I.V.: 50 mg/m^2 day 1

[total dose/cycle = 50 mg/m^2]

Repeat cycle every 21 days

References

Burnett AF, Roman LD, Garcia AA, "A Phase II Study of Gemcitabine and Cisplatin in Patients With Advanced, Persistent, or Recurrent Squamous Cell Carcinoma of the Cervix," *Gynecol Oncol*, 2000, 76(1):63-6.

Gemcitabine-Cisplatin (NSCLC)

Index Terms Cisplatin-Gemcitabine (NSCLC)

Use Lung cancer, nonsmall cell

Regimen NOTE: Multiple variations are listed.

Variation 1:

Gemcitabine: I.V.: 1000 mg/m^2/day days 1, 8, and 15

[total dose/cycle = 3000 mg/m^2]

Cisplatin: I.V.: 100 mg/m^2 day 1

[total dose/cycle = 100 mg/m^2]

Repeat cycle every 28 days

Variation 2:

Gemcitabine: I.V.: 1250 mg/m^2/day days 1 and 8

[total dose/cycle = 2500 mg/m^2]

Cisplatin: I.V.: 100 mg/m^2 day 1

[total dose/cycle = 100 mg/m^2]

Repeat cycle every 21 days

Variation 3:

Gemcitabine: I.V.: 1000 mg/m^2/day days 1 and 8

[total dose/cycle = 2000 mg/m^2]

Cisplatin: I.V.: 80 mg/m^2 day 1
[total dose/cycle = 80 mg/m^2]
Repeat cycle every 21 days
Variation 4:
Gemcitabine: I.V.: 1250 mg/m^2/day days 1 and 8
[total dose/cycle = 2500 mg/m^2]
Cisplatin: I.V.: 75 mg/m^2 day 1
[total dose/cycle = 75 mg/m^2]
Repeat cycle every 21 days for up to 6 cycles
Variation 5:
Gemcitabine: I.V.: 1000 mg/m^2/day days 1, 8, and 15
[total dose/cycle = 3000 mg/m^2]
Cisplatin: I.V.: 100 mg/m^2 day 15
[total dose/cycle = 100 mg/m^2]
Repeat cycle every 28 days
Variation 6:
Gemcitabine: I.V.: 1000 mg/m^2/day days 1, 8, and 15
[total dose/cycle = 3000 mg/m^2]
Cisplatin: I.V.: 100 mg/m^2 day 2
[total dose/cycle = 100 mg/m^2]
Repeat cycle every 28 days for 5 cycles
Variation 7:
Gemcitabine: I.V.: 1200 mg/m^2/day days 1, 8, and 15
[total dose/cycle = 3600 mg/m^2]
Cisplatin: I.V.: 100 mg/m^2 day 15
[total dose/cycle = 100 mg/m^2]
Repeat cycle every 28 days for up to 6 cycles
Variation 8 (patients ≥70 years of age):
Gemcitabine: I.V.: 1000 mg/m^2/day days 1 and 8
[total dose/cycle = 2000 mg/m^2]
Cisplatin: I.V.: 60 mg/m^2 day 1
[total dose/cycle = 60 mg/m^2]
Repeat cycle every 21 days for up to 6 cycles

References

Variation 1:

Comella P, Frasci G, Panza N, et al, "Randomized Trial Comparing Cisplatin, Gemcitabine, and Vinorelbine With Either Cisplatin and Gemcitabine or Cisplatin and Vinorelbine in Advanced Non-Small-Cell Lung Cancer: Interim Analysis of a Phase III Trial of the Southern Italy Cooperative Oncology Group," *J Clin Oncol*, 2000, 18(7):1451-7.

Sandler AB, Nemunaitis J, Denham C, et al, "Phase III Trial of Gemcitabine Plus Cisplatin Versus Cisplatin Alone in Patients With Locally Advanced or Metastatic Nonsmall-Cell Lung Cancer," *J Clin Oncol*, 2000, 18(1):122-30.

Schiller JH, Harrington D, Belani CP, et al, "Comparison of Four Chemotherapy Regimens for Advanced Non-Small-Cell Lung Cancer," *N Engl J Med*, 2002, 346(2):92-8.

Variation 2:

Cardenal F, López-Cabrerizo MP, Antón A, et al, "Randomized Phase III Study of Gemcitabine-Cisplatin Versus Etoposide-Cisplatin in the Treatment of Locally Advanced or Metastatic Non-Small-Cell Lung Cancer," *J Clin Oncol*, 1999, 17(1):12-8.

Variation 3:

Ohe Y, Ohashi Y, Kubota K, et al, "Randomized Phase III Study of Cisplatin Plus Irinotecan Versus Carboplatin Plus Paclitaxel, Cisplatin Plus Gemcitabine, and Cisplatin Plus Vinorelbine for Advanced Non-Small-Cell Lung Cancer: Four-Arm Cooperative Study in Japan," *Ann Oncol*, 2007, 18(2):317-23.

Variation 4:

Scagliotti GV, Parikh P, von Pawel J, et al, "Phase III Study Comparing Cisplatin Plus Gemcitabine With Cisplatin Plus Pemetrexed in Chemotherapy-Naive Patients With Advanced-Stage Non-Small-Cell Lung Cancer," *J Clin Oncol*, 2008, 26(21):3543-51.

Variation 5:
Abratt RP, Bezwoda WR, Goedhals L, et al, "Weekly Gemcitabine With Monthly Cisplatin: Effective Chemotherapy for Advanced Nonsmall-Cell Lung Cancer," *J Clin Oncol*, 1997, 15(2):744-9.

Variation 6:
Crino L, Scagliotti G, Marangolo M, et al, "Cisplatin-Gemcitabine Combination in Advanced Nonsmall-Cell Lung Cancer: A Phase II Study," *J Clin Oncol*, 1997, 15(1):297-303.

Variation 7:
Anton A, Diaz-Fernandez N, Gonzalez Larriba JL, et al, "Phase II Trial Assessing the Combination of Gemcitabine and Cisplatin in Advanced Non-Small Cell Lung Cancer (NSCLC)," *Lung Cancer*, 1998, 22(2):139-48.

Variation 8:
Gridelli C, Maione P, Illiano A, et al, "Cisplatin Plus Gemcitabine or Vinorelbine for Elderly Patients With Advanced Non Small-Cell Lung Cancer: The MILES-2P Studies," *J Clin Oncol*, 2007, 25 (29):4663-9.

Gemcitabine-Docetaxel (Bladder Cancer)

Use Bladder cancer

Regimen

Docetaxel: I.V.: 40 mg/m^2/day days 1 and 8
[total dose/cycle = 80 mg/m^2]
Gemcitabine: 800 mg/m^2/day days 1 and 8
[total dose/cycle = 1600 mg/m^2]
Repeat cycle every 21 days for up to 6 cycles

References

Dreicer R, Manola J, Schneider DJ, et al, "Phase II Trial of Gemcitabine and Docetaxel in Patients With Advanced Carcinoma of the Urothelium: A Trial of the Eastern Cooperative Oncology Group," *Cancer*, 2003, 97(11):2743-7.

Gemcitabine-Docetaxel (Sarcoma)

Use Osteosarcoma; Soft tissue sarcoma

Regimen

Gemcitabine: I.V.: 675 mg/m^2/day days 1 and 8
[total dose/cycle = 1350 mg/m^2]
Docetaxel: I.V.: 100 mg/m^2 day 8
[total dose/cycle = 100 mg/m^2]
Repeat cycle every 21 days

References

Leu KM, Ostruszka LJ, Shewach D, et al, "Laboratory and Clinical Evidence of Synergistic Cytotoxicity of Sequential Treatment With Gemcitabine Followed by Docetaxel in the Treatment of Sarcoma," *J Clin Oncol*, 2004, 22(9):1706-12.

Gemcitabine-Erlotinib

Index Terms Erlotinib-Gemcitabine

Use Pancreatic cancer

Regimen

Cycle 1:
Gemcitabine: I.V.: 1000 mg/m^2/day days 1, 8, 15, 22, 29, 36, and 43 (cycle 1 only)
[total dose/cycle 1 = 7000 mg/m^2]
Erlotinib: Oral: 100 mg once daily days 1 to 56
[total dose/cycle 1 = 5600 mg]
Treatment cycle is 56 days

Subsequent cycles:
Gemcitabine: I.V.: 1000 mg/m^2/day days 1, 8, and 15
[total dose/cycle = 3000 mg/m^2]
Erlotinib: Oral: 100 mg once daily days 1 to 28
[total dose/cycle = 2800 mg]
Repeat cycle every 28 days

References

Moore MJ, Goldstein D, Hamm J, et al, "Erlotinib Plus Gemcitabine Compared With Gemcitabine Alone in Patients With Advanced Pancreatic Cancer: A Phase III Trial of the National Cancer Institute of Canada Clinical Trials Group," *J Clin Oncol*, 2007, 25(15):1960-6.

Gemcitabine-Irinotecan

Index Terms Irinotecan-Gemcitabine

Use Pancreatic cancer

Regimen

Gemcitabine: I.V.: 1000 mg/m^2/day days 1 and 8
  [total dose/cycle = 2000 mg/m^2]
Irinotecan: I.V.: 100 mg/m^2/day days 1 and 8
  [total dose/cycle = 200 mg/m^2]
Repeat cycle 21 days

References

Rocha Lima CM, Savarese D, Bruckner H, et al, "Irinotecan Plus Gemcitabine Induces Both Radiographic and CA 19-9 Tumor Marker Responses in Patients With Previously Untreated Advanced Pancreatic Cancer," *J Clin Oncol*, 2002, 20(5):1182-91.

Gemcitabine-Oxaliplatin (Pancreatic Cancer)

Index Terms Oxaliplatin-Gemcitabine (Pancreatic Cancer)

Use Pancreatic cancer

Regimen

Gemcitabine: I.V.: 1000 mg/m^2/day (infused at 10 mg/m^2/minute) day 1
  [total dose/cycle = 1000 mg/m^2]
Oxaliplatin: I.V.: 100 mg/m^2/day (over 2 hours) day 2
  [total dose/cycle = 100 mg/m^2]
Repeat cycle every 14 days

References

Louvet C, Labianca R, Hammel P, et al, "Gemcitabine in Combination With Oxaliplatin Compared With Gemcitabine Alone in Locally Advanced or Metastatic Pancreatic Cancer: Results of a GERCOR and GISCAD Phase III Trial," *J Clin Oncol*, 2005, 23(15):3509-16.

Gemcitabine-Oxaliplatin-Rituximab (NHL)

Index Terms GEMOX-R (NHL); Oxaliplatin-Gemcitabine-Rituximab (NHL)

Use Lymphoma, non-Hodgkins

Regimen

Oxaliplatin: I.V.: 100 mg/m^2/dose day 1
  [total dose/cycle = 100 mg/m^2]
Gemcitabine: I.V.: 1000 mg/m^2/dose day 1
  [total dose/cycle = 1000 mg/m^2]
Rituximab: I.V.: 375 mg/m^2/dose day 1
  [total dose/cycle = 375 mg/m^2]
Repeat cycle every 3 weeks (for a total of 6-8 cycles)

References

López A, Gutiérrez A, Palacios A, et al, "GEMOX-R Regimen is a Highly Effective Salvage Regimen in Patients With Refractory/Relapsing Diffuse Large-Cell Lymphoma: A Phase II Study," *Eur J Haematol*, 2008, 80(2):127-32.

Rodríguez J, Gutierrez A, Palacios A, et al, "Rituximab, Gemcitabine and Oxaliplatin: An Effective Regimen in Patients With Refractory and Relapsing Mantle Cell Lymphoma," *Leuk Lymphoma*, 2007, 48(11):2172-8.

◆ **Gemcitabine-Oxaliplatin (Testicular Cancer)** *see* GEMOX (Testicular Cancer) on page 1347

Gemcitabine-Paclitaxel

Use Ovarian cancer

Regimen

Paclitaxel: I.V.: 80 mg/m² (infused over 60 minutes) days 1, 8, and 15

[total dose/cycle = 240 mg/m²]

Gemcitabine: I.V.: 1000 mg/m²/day (start at end of paclitaxel infusion) days 1, 8, and 15

[total dose/cycle = 3000 mg/m²]

Repeat cycle every 4 weeks

References

Garcia AA, O'Meara A, Bahador A, et al, "Phase II Study of Gemcitabine and Weekly Paclitaxel in Recurrent Platinum-Resistant Ovarian Cancer," *Gynecol Oncol*, 2004, 93(2):493-8.

◆ **Gemcitabine-Paclitaxel** *see* Paclitaxel-Gemcitabine *on page* 1389

Gemcitabine-Vinorelbine

Use Lung cancer, nonsmall cell

Regimen NOTE: Multiple variations are listed.

Variation 1:

Gemcitabine: I.V.: 1200 mg/m²/day days 1 and 8

[total dose/cycle = 2400 mg/m²]

Vinorelbine: I.V.: 30 mg/m²/day days 1 and 8

[total dose/cycle = 60 mg/m²]

Repeat cycle every 21 days for 6 cycles

Variation 2:

Gemcitabine: I.V.: 1000 mg/m²/day days 1, 8, and 15

[total dose/cycle = 3000 mg/m²]

Vinorelbine: I.V.: 20 mg/m²/day days 1, 8, and 15

[total dose/cycle = 60 mg/m²]

Repeat cycle every 28 days for 6 cycles

References

Variation 1 and 2:

Frasci G, Lorusso V, Panza N, et al, "Gemcitabine Plus Vinorelbine Vs Vinorelbine Alone in Elderly Patients With Advanced Nonsmall Cell Lung Cancer," *J Clin Oncol*, 2000, 18(13):2529-36.

Hainsworth JD, Burris HA 3rd, Litchy S, et al, "Gemcitabine and Vinorelbine in the Second-Line Treatment of Nonsmall Cell Lung Carcinoma Patients: A Minnie Pearl Cancer Research Network Phase II Trial," *Cancer*, 2000, 88(6):1353-8.

Gemcitabine-Vinorelbine-Doxorubicin (Liposomal)

Index Terms GVD; Vinorelbine-Gemcitabine-Doxorubicin (Liposomal)

Use Lymphoma, Hodgkin's disease

Regimen NOTE: Multiple variations are listed.

Variation 1 (for transplant-naive patients):

Vinorelbine: I.V.: 20 mg/m²/day days 1 and 8

[total dose/cycle = 40 mg/m²]

Gemcitabine: I.V.: 1000 mg/m²/day days 1 and 8

[total dose/cycle = 2000 mg/m²]

Doxorubicin liposomal: I.V.: 15 mg/m²/day days 1 and 8

[total dose/cycle = 30 mg/m²]

Repeat cycle every 21 days for 2-6 cycles

Variation 2 (for patients with prior transplant):

Vinorelbine: I.V.: 15 mg/m²/day days 1 and 8

[total dose/cycle = 30 mg/m²]

Gemcitabine: I.V.: 800 mg/m²/day days 1 and 8

[total dose/cycle = 1600 mg/m²]

Doxorubicin liposomal: I.V.: 10 mg/m^2/day days 1 and 8
[total dose/cycle = 20 mg/m^2]
Repeat cycle every 21 days for 2-6 cycles

References

Variations 1 and 2:
Bartlett NL, Niedzwiecki D, Johnson JL, et al, "Gemcitabine, Vinorelbine, and Pegylated Liposomal Doxorubicin (GVD), a Salvage Regimen in Relapsed Hodgkin's Lymphoma: CALGB 59804," *Ann Oncol*, 2007, 18(6):1071-9.

GEMOX (Biliary Cancer)

Use Biliary adenocarcinoma
Regimen
Gemcitabine: I.V.: 1000 mg/m^2 day 1
[total dose/cycle = 1000 mg/m^2]
Oxaliplatin: I.V.: 100 mg/m^2 day 2
[total dose/cycle = 100 mg/m^2]
Repeat cycle every 2 weeks

References

Andre T, Tournigand C, Rosmorduc O, et al, "Gemcitabine Combined With Oxaliplatin (GEMOX) in Advanced Biliary Tract Adenocarcinoma: A GERCOR Study," *Ann Oncol*, 2004, 15(9):1339-43.

◆ **GEMOX-R (NHL)** *see* Gemcitabine-Oxaliplatin-Rituximab (NHL) *on page 1345*

GEMOX (Testicular Cancer)

Index Terms Gemcitabine-Oxaliplatin (Testicular Cancer); Oxaliplatin-Gemcitabine (Testicular Cancer)
Use Testicular cancer
Regimen NOTE: Multiple variations are listed.
Variation 1:
Gemcitabine: I.V.: 1000 mg/m^2/dose over 30 minutes days 1 and 8
[total dose/cycle = 2000 mg/m^2]
Oxaliplatin: I.V.: 130 mg/m^2/dose over 2 hours day 1
[total dose/cycle = 130 mg/m^2]
Repeat cycle every 21 days for a total of at least 2 cycles (maximum: 6 cycles)
Variation 2:
Gemcitabine: I.V.: 1250 mg/m^2/dose over 30 minutes days 1 and 8
[total dose/cycle = 2500 mg/m^2]
Oxaliplatin: I.V.: 130 mg/m^2/dose over 2 hours day 1
[total dose/cycle = 130 mg/m^2]
Repeat cycle every 21 days

References

Variation 1:
Kollmannsberger C, Beyer J, Liersch R, et al, "Combination Chemotherapy With Gemcitabine Plus Oxaliplatin in Patients With Intensively Pretreated or Refractory Germ Cell Cancer: A Study of the German Testicular Cancer Study Group," *J Clin Oncol*, 2004, 22(1):108-14.
Pectasides D, Pectasides M, Farmakis D, et al, "Gemcitabine and Oxaliplatin (GEMOX) in Patients With Cisplatin-Refractory Germ Cell Tumors: A Phase II Study," *Ann Oncol*, 2004, 15(3):493-7.
Variation 2:
De Giorgi U, Rosti G, Aieta M, et al, "Phase II Study of Oxaliplatin and Gemcitabine Salvage Chemotherapy in Patients With Cisplatin-Refractory Nonseminomatous Germ Cell Tumor," *Eur Urol*, 2006, 50(5):1032-8.

◆ **Goserelin-Bicalutamide** *see* Bicalutamide-Goserelin *on page 1234*

◆ **GVD** *see* Gemcitabine-Vinorelbine-Doxorubicin (Liposomal) *on page 1346*

HDMTX

Use Osteosarcoma

Regimen

Methotrexate: I.V.: 12 g/m²/week for 2-12 weeks

[total dose/cycle = 24-144 g/m²]

Leucovorin calcium rescue: Oral, I.V.: 15 mg/m² every 6 hours (beginning 30 hours after the beginning of the 4-hour methotrexate infusion) for 10 doses; **serum methotrexate levels must be monitored**

[total dose/cycle = 150 mg/m²]

References

Camitta BM and Holcenberg JS, "Safety of Delayed Leucovorin 'Rescue' Following High-Dose Methotrexate in Children," *Med Pediatr Oncol*, 1978, 5(1):55-9.

HIPE-IVAD

Use Neuroblastoma

Regimen

Cisplatin: I.V.: 40 mg/m²/day days 1 to 5

[total dose/cycle = 200 mg/m²]

Etoposide: I.V.: 100 mg/m²/day days 1 to 5

[total dose/cycle = 500 mg/m²]

Ifosfamide: I.V.: 3 g/m²/day days 21 to 23

[total dose/cycle = 9 g/m²]

Mesna: I.V.: 3 g/m²/day continuous infusion days 21, 22, and 23

[total dose/cycle = 9 g/m²]

Vincristine: I.V.: 1.5 mg/m² day 21

[total dose/cycle = 1.5 mg/m²]

Doxorubicin: I.V.: 60 mg/m² day 23

[total dose/cycle = 60 mg/m²]

Repeat cycle every 28 days

References

Pinkerton CR, Zucker JM, Hartmann O, et al, "Short Duration, High Dose, Alternating Chemotherapy in Metastatic Neuroblastoma. (ENSG 3C Induction Regimen). The European Neuroblastoma Study Group," *Br J Cancer*, 1990, 62(2):319-23.

Hyper-CVAD + Imatinib

Use Leukemia, acute lymphocytic

Regimen

Cycle A: (Cycles 1, 3, 5, and 7)

Imatinib: Oral: 400 mg/day days 1 to 14

[total dose/cycle = 5600 mg]

Cyclophosphamide: I.V.: 300 mg/m² every 12 hours, for 6 doses, days 1, 2, and 3

[total dose/cycle = 1800 mg/m²]

Mesna: I.V.: 600 mg/m²/day continuous infusion days 1, 2, and 3

[total dose/cycle = 1800 mg/m²]

Vincristine: I.V.: 2 mg/day days 4 and 11

[total dose/cycle = 4 mg]

Doxorubicin: I.V.: 50 mg/m²/day continuous infusion day 4

[total dose/cycle = 50 mg/m²]

Dexamethasone: Oral, I.V.: 40 mg/day days 1 to 4 and 11 to 14

[total dose/cycle = 320 mg]

Cycle B: (Cycles 2, 4, 6, and 8)

Imatinib: Oral: 400 mg/day days 1 to 14

[total dose/cycle = 5600 mg]

Methotrexate: I.V.: 1 g/m²/day continuous infusion day 1
[total dose/cycle = 1 g/m²]
Leucovorin: I.V.: 50 mg then 15 mg every 6 hours, for 8 doses (start 12 hours after the end of the methotrexate infusion)
[total dose/cycle = 170 mg]
Cytarabine: I.V.: 3 g/m² every 12 hours for 4 doses, days 2 and 3
[total dose/cycle = 12 g/m²]
Repeat every 6 weeks in the following sequence: ABABABAB

CNS Prophylaxis
Methotrexate: I.T.: 12 mg/day day 2
[total dose/cycle = 12 mg/day]
or 6 mg into Ommaya day 2
[total dose/cycle = 6 mg/day]
Cytarabine: I.T.: 100 mg/day day 7 or 8
[total dose/cycle = 100 mg/day]
Repeat cycle every 3 weeks for 3 or 4 cycles

Maintenance (POMP)
Imatinib: Oral: 600 mg/day
[total dose/cycle = 18,000 mg]
Vincristine: I.V.: 2 mg/day day 1
[total dose/cycle = 2 mg]
Prednisone: Oral: 200 mg/day days 1 to 5
[total dose/cycle = 1000 mg/m²]
Repeat cycle every month (except months 6 and 13) for 13 months

Intensification
Imatinib: Oral: 400 mg/day days 1 to 14
[total dose/cycle = 5600 mg]
Cyclophosphamide: I.V.: 300 mg/m² every 12 hours, for 6 doses, days 1, 2, and 3
[total dose/cycle = 1800 mg/m²]
Mesna: I.V.: 600 mg/m²/day continuous infusion days 1, 2, and 3
[total dose/cycle = 1800 mg/m²]
Vincristine: I.V.: 2 mg/day days 4 and 11
[total dose/cycle = 4 mg]
Doxorubicin: 50 mg/m²/day continuous infusion day 4
[total dose/cycle = 50 mg/m²]
Dexamethasone: I.V. or Oral: 40 mg/day days 1 to 4 and 11 to 14
[total dose/cycle = 320 mg]
Cycle is given in months 6 and 13 during maintenance

References
Thomas DA, Faderl S, Cortes J, et al, "Treatment of Philadelphia Chromosome-Positive Acute Lymphocytic Leukemia With Hyper-CVAD and Imatinib Mesylate," *Blood*, 2004, 103 (12):4396-407.

Hyper-CVAD (Leukemia, Acute Lymphocytic)

Use Leukemia, acute lymphocytic
Regimen NOTE: Multiple variations are listed.
Variation 1:
Cycle A: (Cycles 1, 3, 5, and 7)
Cyclophosphamide: I.V.: 300 mg/m² every 12 hours, for 6 doses, days 1, 2, and 3
[total dose/cycle = 1800 mg/m²]
Mesna: I.V.: 1200 mg/m²/day continuous infusion days 1, 2, and 3
[total dose/cycle = 3600 mg/m²]

Vincristine: I.V.: 2 mg/day days 4 and 11
[total dose/cycle = 4 mg]
Doxorubicin: I.V.: 50 mg/m^2 day 4
[total dose/cycle = 50 mg/m^2]
Dexamethasone: (route not specified): 40 mg/day days 1 to 4 and 11 to 14
[total dose/cycle = 320 mg]
Cycle B: (Cycles 2, 4, 6, and 8)
Methotrexate: I.V.: 1 g/m^2 continuous infusion day 1
[total dose/cycle = 1g/m^2]
Leucovorin: (route not specified): 15 mg every 6 hours, for 8 doses (start 12 hours after end of methotrexate infusion)
[total dose/cycle = 120 mg]
Cytarabine: I.V.: 3 g/m^2 every 12 hours, for 4 doses, days 2 and 3
[total dose/cycle = 12 g/m^2]
Methylprednisolone: I.V.: 50 mg twice daily, for 6 doses, days 1, 2, and 3
[total dose/cycle = 300 mg/m^2]
Repeat every 6 weeks in the following sequence: ABABABAB

CNS Prophylaxis
Methotrexate: I.T.: 12 mg/day day 2
[total dose/cycle = 12 mg]
or 6 mg/day into Ommaya day 2
[total dose/cycle = 6 mg]
Cytarabine: I.T: 100 mg day 8
[total dose/cycle = 100 mg]
Repeat cycle every 3 weeks

Maintenance (POMP)
Mercaptopurine: Oral: 50 mg 3 times/day
[total dose/cycle = 4200-4650 mg]
Vincristine: I.V.: 2 mg day 1
[total dose/cycle = 2 mg]
Methotrexate: Oral: 20 mg/m^2/day days 1, 8, 15, and 22
[total dose/cycle = 80 mg/m^2]
Prednisone: Oral: 200 mg/day days 1 to 5
[total dose/cycle = 1000 mg/m^2]
or
Mercaptopurine: I.V.: 1 g/m^2/day days 1 to 5
[total dose/cycle = 5 g/m^2]
Vincristine: I.V.: 2 mg day 1
[total dose/cycle = 2 mg]
Methotrexate: I.V.: 10 mg/m^2/day days 1 to 5
[total dose/cycle = 50 mg/m^2]
Prednisone: Oral: 200 mg/day days 1 to 5
[total dose/cycle = 1000 mg/m^2]
Repeat cycles every month for 2 years
Variation 2:
Cycle A: (Cycles 1, 3, 5, and 7)
Cyclophosphamide: I.V.: 300 mg/m^2 every 12 hours, for 6 doses, days 1, 2, and 3
[total dose/cycle = 1800 mg/m^2]
Mesna: I.V.: 600 mg/m^2/day continuous infusion days 1, 2, and 3
[total dose/cycle = 1800 mg/m^2]
Vincristine: I.V.: 2 mg/day days 4 and 11
[total dose/cycle = 4 mg]
Doxorubicin: I.V.: 50 mg/m^2 day 4
[total dose/cycle = 50 mg/m^2]

Dexamethasone: Oral, I.V.: 40 mg/day days 1 to 4 and 11 to 14
  [total dose/cycle = 320 mg]
Cycle B: (Cycles 2, 4, 6, and 8)
  Methotrexate: I.V.: 1 g/m^2 continuous infusion day 1
    [total dose/cycle = 1 g/m^2]
  Leucovorin: 50 mg (start 12 hours after end of methotrexate infusion)
    followed by I.V.: 15 mg every 6 hours, for 8 doses
      [total dose/cycle = 170 mg]
  Cytarabine: I.V.: 3 g/m^2 every 12 hours, for 4 doses, days 2 and 3
    [total dose/cycle = 12 g/m^2]
  Repeat every 6 weeks in the following sequence: ABABABAB
CNS Prophylaxis
  Methotrexate: I.T.: 12 mg day 2
    [total dose/cycle = 12 mg]
  or 6 mg into Ommaya day 2
    [total dose/cycle = 6 mg]
  Cytarabine: I.T.: 100 mg day 7
    [total dose/cycle = 100 mg]
  Repeat cycle every 3 weeks
Variation 3:
  Cycle A: (Cycles 1, 3, 5, and 7)
    Cyclophosphamide: I.V.: 300 mg/m^2 every 12 hours, for 6 doses, days 1, 2, and 3
      [total dose/cycle = 1800 mg/m^2]
    Mesna: I.V.: 600 mg/m^2/day continuous infusion days 1, 2, and 3
      [total dose/cycle = 1800 mg/m^2]
    Vincristine: I.V.: 2 mg/day days 4 and 11
      [total dose/cycle = 4 mg]
    Doxorubicin: I.V.: 50 mg/m^2 continuous infusion day 4
      [total dose/cycle = 50 mg/m^2]
    Dexamethasone: Oral, I.V.: 40 mg/day days 1 to 4 and 11 to 14
      [total dose/cycle = 320 mg]
  Cycle B: (Cycles 2, 4, 6, and 8)
    Methotrexate: I.V.: 200 mg/m^2 day 1
    followed by I.V.: 800 mg/m^2 continuous infusion day 1
      [total dose/cycle = 1 g/m^2]
    Leucovorin: I.V.: 50 mg (start 12 hours after end of methotrexate infusion)
    followed by I.V.: 15 mg every 6 hours, for 8 doses
      [total dose/cycle = 170 mg/m^2]
    Cytarabine: I.V.: 3 g/m^2 every 12 hours, for 4 doses, days 2 and 3
      [total dose/cycle = 12 g/m^2]
  Repeat every 6 weeks in the following sequence: ABABABAB
CNS Prophylaxis
  Methotrexate: I.T.: 12 mg day 2
    [total dose/cycle = 12 mg]
  or 6 mg into Ommaya day 2
    [total dose/cycle = 6 mg]
  Cytarabine: I.T.: 100 mg day 7 **or** 8
    [total dose/cycle = 100 mg]
  Repeat cycles every 3 weeks for 6 or 8 cycles
Maintenance (POMP)
  Mercaptopurine: Oral: 50 mg 3 times/day
    [total dose/cycle = 4200-4650 mg]
  Vincristine: I.V.: 2 mg day 1
    [total dose/cycle = 2 mg]

◄

Methotrexate: Oral, I V: 20 mg/m^2/ day days 1, 8, 15, and 22
[total dose/cycle = 80 mg/m^2]
Prednisone: Oral: 200 mg/day days 1 to 5
[total dose/cycle = 1000 mg/m^2]

or

Mercaptopurine: I.V.: 1 g/m^2/day days 1 to 5
[total dose/cycle = 5 g/m^2]
Vincristine: I.V.: 2 mg day 1
[total dose/cycle = 2 mg]
Methotrexate: I.V.: 10 mg/m^2/day days 1 to 5
[total dose/cycle = 50 mg/m^2]
Prednisone: Oral: 200 mg/day days 1 to 5
[total dose/cycle = 1000 mg]
Repeat cycles every month (except months 7 and 11 or 9 and 12) for 2 years

Intensification

Etoposide: I.V.: 100 mg/m^2/day days 1 to 5
[total dose/cycle = 500 mg/m^2]
Pegaspargase: I.V.: 2500 units/m^2 day 1
[total dose/cycle = 2500 units/m^2]
Given during months 9 and 12 of maintenance

or

Methotrexate: I.V.: 100 mg/m^2/day days 1, 8, 15, and 22
[total dose/cycle = 400 mg/m^2]
Asparaginase: I.V.: 20,000 units/day days 2, 9, 16, and 23
[total dose/cycle = 80,000 units]
Given during months 7 and 11 of maintenance

Variation 4:

Cycle A: (Cycles 1, 3, 5, and 7)
Cyclophosphamide: I.V.: 300 mg/m^2 every 12 hours, for 6 doses, days 1, 2, and 3
[total dose/cycle = 1800 mg/m^2]
Mesna: I.V.: 600 mg/m^2/day continuous infusion days 1, 2, and 3
[total dose/cycle = 1800 mg/m^2]
Vincristine: I.V.: 2 mg/day days 4 and 11
[total dose/cycle = 4 mg]
Doxorubicin: I.V.: 50 mg/m^{2}day 4
[total dose/cycle = 50 mg/m^2]
Dexamethasone: (route not specified): 40 mg/day days 1 to 4 and 11 to 14
[total dose/cycle = 320 mg]

Cycle B: (Cycles 2, 4, 6, and 8)
Methotrexate: I.V.: 200 mg/m^2 day 1
followed by I.V.: 800 mg/m^2 continuous infusion day 1
[total dose/cycle = 1 g/m^2]
Leucovorin: (route not specified): 15 mg every 6 hours, for 8 doses (start 24 hours after end of methotrexate infusion)
[total dose/cycle = 120 mg]
Cytarabine: I.V.: 3 g/m^2 every 12 hours, for 4 doses, days 2 and 3
[total dose/cycle = 12 g/m^2]
Repeat every 6 weeks in the following sequence: ABABABAB

CNS Prophylaxis

Methotrexate: I.T.: 12 mg day 2
[total dose/cycle = 12 mg]

Cytarabine: I.T.: 100 mg day 8
[total dose/cycle = 100 mg]
Repeat cycle every 3 weeks for 4 or 8 cycles

Maintenance (POMP)
Mercaptopurine: Oral: 50 mg 3 times/day
[total dose/cycle = 4200-4650 mg]
Vincristine: I.V.: 2 mg day 1
[total dose/cycle = 2 mg]
Methotrexate: Oral: 20 mg/m^2/day days 1, 8, 15, and 22
[total dose/cycle = 80 mg/m^2]
Prednisone: Oral: 200 mg/day days 1 to 5
[total dose/cycle = 1000 mg/m^2]
or
Mercaptopurine: I.V.: 1 g/m^2/day days 1 to 5
[total dose/cycle = 5 g/m^2]
Vincristine: I.V.: 2 mg day 1
[total dose/cycle = 2 mg]
Methotrexate: I.V.: 10 mg/m^2/day days 1 to 5
[total dose/cycle = 50 mg/m^2]
Prednisone: Oral: 200 mg/day days 1 to 5
[total dose/cycle = 1000 mg/m^2]
or
Interferon alfa: SubQ: 5 million units/m^2 daily
[total dose/cycle = 140-155 million units/m^2]
Cytarabine: SubQ: 10 mg daily
[total dose/cycle = 280-310 mg]
Repeat cycles every month for 2 years

Variation 5:
Cycle A: (Cycles 1, 4, 6, and 8)
Cyclophosphamide: I.V.: 300 mg/m^2 every 12 hours, for 6 doses, days 1, 2, and 3
[total dose/cycle = 1800 mg/m^2]
Mesna: I.V.: 600 mg/m^2/day continuous infusion days 1, 2, and 3
[total dose/cycle = 1800 mg/m^2]
Vincristine: I.V.: 2 mg/day days 4 and 11
[total dose/cycle = 4 mg]
Doxorubicin: I.V.: 50 mg/m^2 continuous infusion day 4
[total dose/cycle = 50 mg/m^2]
Dexamethasone: Oral, I.V.: 40 mg/day days 1 to 4 and 11 to 14
[total dose/cycle = 320 mg]
Cycle B: (Cycles 3, 5, 7, and 9)
Methotrexate: I.V.: 200 mg/m^2 day 1
followed by I.V.: 800 mg/m^2 continuous infusion day 1
[total dose/cycle = 1 g/m^2]
Leucovorin: I.V.: 50 mg (start 12 hours after end of methotrexate infusion)
followed by I.V.: 15 mg every 6 hours, for 8 doses
[total dose/cycle = 170 mg]
Cytarabine: I.V.: 3 g/m^2 every 12 hours, for 4 doses, days 2 and 3
[total dose/cycle = 12 g/m^2]
Cycle C: Liposomal Daunorubicin/Cytarabine (Cycle 2):
Daunorubicin, liposomal: I.V.: 150 mg/m^2/day days 1 and 2
[total dose/cycle = 300 mg/m^2]
Cytarabine: I.V.: 1.5 g/m^2/day continuous infusion days 1 and 2
[total dose/cycle = 3 g/m^2]

◀ Prednisone: Oral: 200 mg/day days 1 to 5
[total dose/cycle = 1000 mg]
Administer in the following sequence: ACBABABA (Cycle C does not repeat)

CNS Prophylaxis

Methotrexate: I.T.: 12 mg day 2
[total dose/cycle = 12 mg]
or 6 mg into Ommaya day 2
[total dose/cycle = 6 mg]
Cytarabine: I.T.: 100 mg day 7 **or** 8
[total dose/cycle = 100 mg]
Repeat cycle every 3 weeks for 6 or 8 cycles

Maintenance (POMP)

Mercaptopurine: I.V.: 1 g/m^2/day days 1 to 5
[total dose/cycle = 5 g/m^2]
Vincristine: I.V.: 2 mg day 1
[total dose/cycle = 2 mg]
Methotrexate: I.V.: 10 mg/m^2/day days 1 to 5
[total dose/cycle = 50 mg/m^2]
Prednisone: Oral: 200 mg/day days 1 to 5
[total dose/cycle = 1000 mg]
Repeat cycles monthly, except months 6, 7, 18, and 19 for 3 years

Intensification

Methotrexate: I.V.: 100 mg/m^2/day days 1, 8, 15, and 22
[total dose/cycle = 400 mg/m^2]
Asparaginase: I.V.: 20,000 units/day days 2, 9, 16, and 23
[total dose/cycle = 80,000 units]
Given during months 6 and 18 of maintenance
Cyclophosphamide: I.V.: 300 mg/m^2 every 12 hours, for 6 doses, days 1, 2, and 3
[total dose/cycle = 1800 mg/m^2]
Mesna: I.V.: 600 mg/m^2/day continuous infusion days 1, 2, and 3
[total dose/cycle = 1800 mg/m^2]
Vincristine: I.V.: 2 mg/day days 4 and 11
[total dose/cycle = 4 mg]
Doxorubicin: I.V.: 50 mg/m^2/day continuous infusion day 4
[total dose/cycle = 50 mg/m^2]
Dexamethasone: Oral, I.V.: 40 mg/day days 1 to 4 and 11 to 14
[total dose/cycle = 320 mg]
Given during months 7 and 19 of maintenance

References

Variation 1:
Kantarjian H, Thomas D, O'Brien S, et al, "Long-Term Follow-Up Results of Hyperfractionated Cyclophosphamide, Vincristine, Doxorubicin, and Dexamethasone (Hyper-CVAD), A Dose-Intensive Regimen, in Adult Acute Lymphocytic Leukemia," *Cancer*, 2004, 101(12):2788-2801.
Variation 2:
Thomas DA, Cortes J, O'Brien S, et al, "Hyper-CVAD Program in Burkitt's-Type Adult Acute Lymphoblastic Leukemia," *J Clin Oncol*, 1999, 17(8):2461-70.
Variation 3:
Thomas DA, O'Brien S, Cortes J, et al, "Outcome With the Hyper-CVAD Regimens in Lymphoblastic Lymphoma," *Blood*, 2004, 104(6):1624-30.
Variation 4:
Kantarjian HM, O'Brien S, Smith TL, et al, "Results of Treatment With Hyper-CVAD, A Dose-Intensive Regimen, in Adult Acute Lymphocytic Leukemia," *J Clin Oncol*, 2000, 18(3): 547-61.
Variation 5:
Thomas DA, O'Brien S, Cortes J, et al, "Outcome With the Hyper-CVAD Regimens in Lymphoblastic Lymphoma," *Blood*, 2004, 104(6):1624-30.

Hyper-CVAD (Lymphoma, non-Hodgkin's)

Use Lymphoma, non-Hodgkin's

Regimen

Cycle A: (Cycles 1, 3, 5, and 7)

Cyclophosphamide: I.V.: 300 mg/m^2 every 12 hours, for 6 doses, days 1, 2, and 3

[total dose/cycle = 1800 mg/m^2]

Vincristine: I.V.: 2 mg/day days 4 and 11

[total dose/cycle = 4 mg]

Doxorubicin: I.V.: 25 mg/m^2/day continuous infusion days 4 and 5

[total dose/cycle = 50 mg/m^2]

Dexamethasone: Oral, I.V.: 40 mg/day days 1 to 4 and 11 to 14

[total dose/cycle = 320 mg]

Cycle B: (Cycles 2, 4, 6, and 8)

Methotrexate: I.V.: 200 mg/m^2 day 1

followed by I.V.: 800 mg/m^2 continuous infusion day 1

[total dose/cycle = 1 g/m^2]

Leucovorin: Oral: 50 mg

followed by Oral: 15 mg every 6 hours, for 8 doses (start 24 hours after end of methotrexate infusion)

[total dose/cycle = 170 mg]

Cytarabine: I.V.: 3 g/m^2 every 12 hours, for 4 doses, days 2 and 3

[total dose/cycle = 12 g/m^2]

Repeat every 6 weeks in the following sequence: ABABABAB

References

Khouri IF, Romaguera J, Kantarjian H, et al, "Hyper-CVAD and High-Dose Methotrexate/Cytarabine Followed by Stem-Cell Transplantation: An Active Regimen for Aggressive Mantle-Cell Lymphoma," *J Clin Oncol*, 1998, 16(12):3803-9.

Hyper-CVAD (Multiple Myeloma)

Use Multiple myeloma

Regimen

Cyclophosphamide: I.V.: 300 mg/m^2 every 12 hours, for 6 doses, days 1, 2, and 3

[total dose/cycle = 1800 mg/m^2]

Mesna: I.V.: 600 mg/m^2/day continuous infusion days 1, 2, and 3

[total dose/cycle = 1800 mg/m^2]

Doxorubicin: I.V.: 25 mg/m^2/day continuous infusion days 4 and 5

[total dose/cycle = 50 mg/m^2]

Vincristine: I.V.: 1 mg/day continuous infusion days 4 and 5

followed by I.V.: 2 mg day 11

[total dose/cycle = 4 mg]

Dexamethasone: Oral, I.V.: 20 mg/m^2/day days 1 to 5 and 11 to 14

[total dose/cycle = 180 mg/m^2]

Repeat cycle once if ≥50% reduction in myeloma protein

Maintenance

Cyclophosphamide: Oral: 125 mg/m^2 every 12 hours, for 10 doses, days 1 to 5

[total dose/cycle = 1250 mg/m^2]

Dexamethasone: Oral: 20 mg/m^2/day days 1 to 5

[total dose/cycle = 100 mg/m^2]

Repeat maintenance cycle every 5 weeks

References

Dimopoulos MA, Weber D, Kantarjian H, et al, "HyperCVAD for VAD-Resistant Multiple Myeloma," *Am J Hematol*, 1996, 52(2):77-81.

Hyper-CVAD + Rituximab

Use Lymphoma, non-Hodgkin's (Mantle cell)

Regimen

Cycle A: (Cycles 1, 3, 5 [and 7, if needed])

Rituximab: I.V.: 375 mg/m^2 day 1
[total dose/cycle = 375 mg/m^2]

Cyclophosphamide: I.V.: 300 mg/m^2 every 12 hours, for 6 doses, days 2, 3, and 4
[total dose/cycle = 1800 mg/m^2]

Mesna: I.V.: 600 mg/m^2 continuous infusion days 2, 3, and 4
[total dose/cycle = 1800 mg/m^2]

Vincristine: I.V.: 1.4 mg/m^2 (maximum dose: 2 mg) days 5 and 12
[total dose/cycle = 2.8 mg/m^2; maximum: 4 mg]

Doxorubicin: I.V.: 16.7 mg/m^2 continuous infusion days 5, 6, and 7
[total dose/cycle = 50.1 mg/m^2]

Dexamethasone: Oral, I.V.: 40 mg/day days 2 to 5 and 12 to 15
[total dose/cycle = 320 mg]

Cycle B: (Cycles 2, 4, 6 [and 8, if needed])

Rituximab: I.V.: 375 mg/m^2 day 1
[total dose/cycle = 375 mg/m^2]

Methotrexate: I.V.: 200 mg/m^2 day 2
followed by I.V.: 800 mg/m^2 continuous infusion day 2
[total dose/cycle = 1000 mg/m^2]

Leucovorin: Oral: 50 mg (start 12 hours after the end of the methotrexate infusion)
followed by Oral: 15 mg every 6 hours, for 8 doses
[total dose/cycle = 170 mg]

Cytarabine: I.V.: 3 g/m^2 every 12 hours, for 4 doses, day 3 and 4
[total dose/cycle = 12 g/m^2]

Repeat every 6 weeks in the following sequence: ABABABAB

References

Romaguera JE, Fayad L, Rodriguez MA, et al, "High Rate of Durable Remissions After Treatment of Newly Diagnosed Aggressive Mantle-Cell Lymphoma With Rituximab Plus Hyper-CVAD Alternating With Rituximab Plus High-Dose Methotrexate and Cytarabine," *J Clin Oncol*, 2005, 23 (28):7013-23.

◆ **ICE (Leukemia)** *see* Idarubicin, Cytarabine, Etoposide (ICE Protocol) on page 1357

ICE (Lymphoma, non-Hodgkin's)

Use Lymphoma, non-Hodgkin's

Regimen

Etoposide: I.V.: 100 mg/m^2/day days 1, 2, and 3
[total dose/cycle = 300 mg/m^2]

Carboplatin: I.V.: AUC 5 (maximum dose: 800 mg) day 2
[total dose/cycle = AUC = 5]

Ifosfamide: I.V.: 5000 mg/m^2 continuous infusion day 2
[total dose/cycle = 5000 mg/m^2]

Mesna: I.V.: 5000 mg/m^2 continuous infusion day 2
[total dose/cycle = 5000 mg/m^2]

Filgrastim: SubQ: 5 mcg/kg/day days 5-12 (cycles 1 and 2 only)
[total dose/cycle = 40 mcg/kg]
followed by SubQ: 10 mcg/kg/day day 5 through completion of leukaphoresis (cycle 3 only)

Repeat cycle every 2 weeks for 3 cycles

References

Moskowitz CH, Bertino JR, Glassman JR, et al, "Ifosfamide, Carboplatin, and Etoposide: A Highly Effective Cytoreduction and Peripheral-Blood Progenitor-Cell Mobilization Regimen for Transplant-Eligible Patients With Non-Hodgkin's Lymphoma," *J Clin Oncol*, 1999, 17(12):3776-85.

ICE (Sarcoma)

Use Osteosarcoma; Soft tissue sarcoma

Regimen

Ifosfamide: I.V.: 1500 mg/m^2/day days 1, 2, and 3
  [total dose/cycle = 4500 mg/m^2]
Carboplatin: I.V.: 300-635 mg/m^2 day 3
  [total dose/cycle = 300-635 mg/m^2]
Etoposide: I.V.: 100 mg/m^2/day days 1, 2, and 3
  [total dose/cycle = 300 mg/m^2]
Mesna: I.V.: 500 mg/m^2 prior to each ifosfamide, and every 3 hours for 2 more doses/day days 1, 2, and 3
  [total dose/cycle = 4500 mg/m^2]
Repeat cycle every 21-28 days

References

Kung FH, Desai SJ, Dickerman JD, et al, "Ifosfamide/Carboplatin/Etoposide (ICE) for Recurrent Malignant Solid Tumors of Childhood: A Pediatric Oncology Group Phase I/II Study," *J Pediatr Hematol Oncol*, 1995, 17(3):265-9.

ICE-T

Use Breast cancer; Soft tissue sarcoma

Regimen

Ifosfamide: I.V.: 1250 mg/m^2/day days 1, 2, and 3
  [total dose/cycle = 3750 mg/m^2]
Carboplatin: I.V.: 300 mg/m^2 day 1
  [total dose/cycle = 300 mg/m^2]
Etoposide: I.V.: 80 mg/m^2/day days 1, 2, and 3
  [total dose/cycle = 240 mg/m^2]
Paclitaxel: I.V.: 175 mg/m^2 day 4
  [total dose/cycle = 175 mg/m^2]
Mesna: I.V.: 250 mg prior to ifosfamide days 1, 2, and 3
  followed by: Oral: 500 mg at 4 and 8 hours after ifosfamide days 1, 2, and 3
  [total dose/cycle = I.V. 750 mg; Oral: 3000 mg]
or
Mesna: I.V.: 1250 mg/m^2/day over 6 hours, days 1, 2, and 3
  [total dose/cycle = 3750 mg/m^2]
Repeat cycle every 28 days

References

Chang AY, Boros L, Garrow GC, et al, "Ifosfamide, Carboplatin, Etoposide, and Paclitaxel Chemotherapy: A Dose-Escalation Study," *Semin Oncol*, 1996, 23(3 Suppl 6):74-7.

♦ **Idarubicin-ATRA (APL)** *see* Tretinoin-Idarubicin (APL) *on page 1414*

♦ **Idarubicin-Cytarabine-Etoposide (BF12; AML)** *see* Idarubicin-Cytarabine (High Dose)-Etoposide (AML) *on page 1358*

Idarubicin, Cytarabine, Etoposide (ICE Protocol)

Index Terms ICE (Leukemia)

Use Leukemia, acute myeloid

Regimen

Idarubicin: I.V.: 6 mg/m^2/day days 1 to 5
  [total dose/cycle = 30 mg/m^2]

Cytarabine: I.V.: 600 mg/m²/day days 1 to 5
[total dose/cycle = 3000 mg/m²]
Etoposide: I.V.: 150 mg/m²/day days 1, 2, and 3
[total dose/cycle = 450 mg/m²]
Administer one cycle only

References
Carella AM, Carlier P, Pungolino E, et al, "Idarubicin in Combination With Intermediate-Dose Cytarabine and VP-16 in the Treatment of Refractory or Rapidly Relapsed Patients With Acute Myeloid Leukemia," *Leukemia*, 1993, 7(2):196-9.

Idarubicin-Cytarabine (High Dose)-Etoposide (AML)

Index Terms Idarubicin-Cytarabine-Etoposide (BF12; AML)
Use Leukemia, acute myeloid
Regimen Induction:
Idarubicin: I.V.: 5 mg/m²/day days 1 to 5
[total dose/cycle = 25 mg/m²]
Cytarabine: I.V.: 2000 mg/m² every 12 hours for 10 doses days 1 to 5
[total dose/cycle = 20,000 mg/m²]
Etoposide: I.V.: 100 mg/m²/day days 1 to 5
[total dose/cycle = 500 mg/m²]

References
Mehta J, Powles R, Singhal S, et al, "Idarubicin, High-Dose Cytarabine, and Etoposide for Induction of Remission in Acute Leukemia," *Semin Hematol*, 1996, 33(4 Suppl 3):18-23.

◆ **Idarubicin-Tretinoin (APL)** *see* Tretinoin-Idarubicin (APL) *on page 1414*

IE

Use Soft tissue sarcoma
Regimen
Etoposide: I.V.: 100 mg/m²/day days 1, 2, and 3
[total dose/cycle = 300 mg/m²]
Ifosfamide: I.V.: 2500 mg/m²/day days 1, 2, and 3
[total dose/cycle = 7500 mg/m²]
Mesna: I.V.: 500 mg/m² prior to ifosfamide, after ifosfamide, and every 4 hours for 3 more doses (total of 5 doses/day) days 1, 2, and 3
[total dose/cycle = 7500 mg/m²]
Repeat cycle every 28 days

References
Edmonson JH, Buckner JC, Long HJ, et al, "Phase II Study of Ifosfamide-Etoposide-Mesna in Adults With Advanced Nonosseous Sarcomas," *J Natl Cancer Inst*, 1989, 81(11):863-6.

◆ **IL-2-Interferon Alfa 2** *see* Interleukin 2-Interferon Alfa-2 *on page 1359*

◆ **IL-2 (Low Dose)-Interferon Alfa 2b** *see* Interleukin 2 (Low Dose)-Interferon Alfa 2b *on page 1359*

IMVP-16

Use Lymphoma, non-Hodgkin's
Regimen
Ifosfamide: I.V.: 4 g/m² continuous infusion over 24 hours day 1
[total dose/cycle = 4 g/m²]
Mesna: I.V.: 800 mg/m² bolus prior to ifosfamide, then 4 g/m² continuous infusion over 12 hours concurrent with ifosfamide, then 2.4 g/m² continuous infusion over 12 hours after ifosfamide infusion day 1
[total dose/cycle = 7.2 g/m²]
Methotrexate: I.V.: 30 mg/m²/day days 3 and 10
[total dose/cycle = 60 mg/m²]

Etoposide: I.V.: 100 mg/m^2/day days 1, 2, and 3
[total dose/cycle = 300 mg/m^2]
Repeat cycle every 21-28 days

References

Cabanillas F, Hagemeister FB, Bodey GP, et al, "IMVP-16: An Effective Regimen for Patients With Lymphoma Who Have Relapsed After Initial Combination Chemotherapy," *Blood*, 1982, 60 (3):693-7.

♦ **Interferon Alfa 2-Interleukin** *see* Interleukin 2-Interferon Alfa-2 *on page 1359*

♦ **Interferon Alfa-Bevacizumab (RCC)** *see* Bevacizumab-Interferon Alfa (RCC) *on page 1232*

Interleukin 2-Interferon Alfa-2

Index Terms IL-2-Interferon Alfa 2; Interferon Alfa 2-Interleukin
Use Renal cell cancer
Regimen
Weeks 1 and 4:
  Aldesleukin: SubQ: 20 million units/m^2 3 times weekly
  [total dose/cycle = 120 million units/m^2]
  Interferon Alfa-2: SubQ: 6 million units/m^2 once weekly
  [total dose/cycle = 12 million units/m^2]
Weeks 2, 3, 5, and 6:
  Aldesleukin: SubQ: 5 million units/m^2 3 times weekly
  [total dose/cycle = 60 million units/m^2]
  Interferon Alfa-2: SubQ: 6 million units/m^2 3 times weekly
  [total dose/cycle = 72 million units/m^2]
Repeat cycle every 56 days

References

Atzpodien J, Kirchner H, Hanninen EL, et al, "European Studies of Interleukin-2 in Metastatic Renal Cell Carcinoma," *Semin Oncol*, 1993, 20(6 Suppl 9):22-6.

Interleukin 2 (Low Dose)-Interferon Alfa 2b

Index Terms Aldesleukin (Low Dose)-Interferon Alfa 2b; IL-2 (Low Dose)-Interferon Alfa 2b
Use Renal cell cancer
Regimen
Cycle 1:
  Week 1:
    Aldesleukin: SubQ: 5 million units/m^2 every 8 hours for 3 doses day 1
    followed by SubQ: 5 million units/m^2/day days 2 to 5
      [total dose/week 1 = 35 million units/m^2]
    Interferon alfa-2b: SubQ: 5 million units/m^2 3 times/week
    [total dose/week 1 = 15 million units/m^2]
  Weeks 2-4:
    Aldesleukin: SubQ: 5 million units/m^2/day days 1 to 5
    [total dose/weeks 2-4 = 75 million units/m^2]
    Interferon alfa-2b: SubQ: 5 million units/m^2 3 times/week
    [total dose/weeks 2-4 = 45 million units/m^2]
  Treatment cycle is 6 weeks
Cycles 2-6:
  Weeks 1-4:
    Aldesleukin: SubQ: 5 million units/m^2/day days 1 to 5
    [total dose/cycle = 100 million units/m^2]
    Interferon alfa-2b: SubQ: 5 million units/m^2 3 times/week
    [total dose/cycle = 60 million units/m^2]
  Repeat cycle every 6 weeks for up to a total of 6 cycles

References

McDermott DF, Regan MM, Clark JI, et al, "Randomized Phase III Trial of High-Dose Interleukin-2 Versus Subcutaneous Interleukin-2 and Interferon in Patients With Metastatic Renal Cell Carcinoma," *J Clin Oncol*, 2005, 23(1):133-41.

IPA

Use Hepatoblastoma

Regimen

Ifosfamide: I.V.: 500 mg/m² day 1
[total dose/cycle = 500 mg/m²]
followed by I.V.: 1000 mg/m²/day continuous infusion days 1 to 3
[total dose/cycle = 3000 mg/m²]
Cisplatin: I.V.: 20 mg/m²/day days 4 to 8
[total dose/cycle = 100 mg/m²]
Doxorubicin: I.V.: 30 mg/m²/day continuous infusion days 9 and 10
[total dose/cycle = 60 mg/m²]
Repeat cycle every 21 days

References

von Schweinitz D, Byrd DJ, Hecker H, et al, "Efficiency and Toxicity of Ifosfamide, Cisplatin, and Doxorubicin in the Treatment of Childhood Hepatoblastoma. Study Committee of the Cooperative Paediatric Liver Tumour Study HB89 of the German Society for Paediatric Oncology and Haematology," *Eur J Cancer*, 1997, 33(8):1243-9.

♦ **Irinotecan-Bevacizumab (Glioblastoma)** *see* Bevacizumab-Irinotecan (Glioblastoma) *on page 1233*

♦ **Irinotecan-Biweekly Cetuximab** *see* Cetuximab (Biweekly)-Irinotecan *on page 1255*

♦ **Irinotecan-Cetuximab** *see* Cetuximab-Irinotecan *on page 1258*

Irinotecan-Cisplatin (Esophageal Cancer)

Index Terms Cisplatin-Irinotecan (Esophageal Cancer)

Use Esophageal cancer

Regimen

Cisplatin: I.V.: 30 mg/m²/day days 1, 8, 15, and 22
[total dose/cycle = 120 mg/m²]
Irinotecan: I.V.: 65 mg/m²/day days 1, 8, 15, and 22
[total dose/cycle = 260 mg/m²]
Repeat cycle every 6 weeks

References

Ilson DH, Saltz L, Enzinger P, et al, "Phase II Trial of Weekly Irinotecan Plus Cisplatin in Advanced Esophageal Cancer," *J Clin Oncol*, 1999, 17(10):3270-5.

♦ **Irinotecan-Cisplatin (Small Cell Lung Cancer)** *see* Cisplatin-Irinotecan (Small Cell Lung Cancer) *on page 1272*

♦ **Irinotecan-Fluorouracil-Leucovorin** *see* FU-LV-CPT-11 *on page 1338*

♦ **Irinotecan-Fluorouracil-Leucovorin-Bevacizumab** *see* Bevacizumab-Irinotecan-Fluorouracil-Leucovorin *on page 1233*

♦ **Irinotecan-Fluorouracil-Leucovorin (Saltz Regimen)** *see* Fluorouracil-Leucovorin-Irinotecan (Saltz Regimen) *on page 1333*

♦ **Irinotecan-Gemcitabine** *see* Gemcitabine-Irinotecan *on page 1345*

♦ **Irinotecan-Oxaliplatin-Fluorouracil-Leucovorin (Pancreatic Cancer)** *see* FOLFIRINOX (Pancreatic Cancer) *on page 1336*

IVAC

Use Lymphoma, non-Hodgkin's

Regimen

Ifosfamide: I.V.: 1500 mg/m^2/day days 1 to 5
[total dose/cycle = 7500 mg/m^2]
Etoposide: I.V.: 60 mg/m^2/day days 1 to 5
[total dose/cycle = 300 mg/m^2]
Cytarabine: I.V.: 2 g/m^2 every 12 hours days 1 and 2
[total dose/cycle = 8 g/m^2]
Mesna: I.V.: 360 mg/m^2 every 3 hours days 1 to 5
[total dose/cycle = 14,400 mg/m^2]
Methotrexate: I.T.: 12 mg day 5
Sargramostim: SubQ: 7.5 mcg/kg day 7 until ANC >1000 cells/mm^3
Repeat when ANC >1000 cells/mm^3

References

Magrath I, Adde M, Shad A, et al, "Adults and Children With Small Non-Cleaved-Cell Lymphoma Have a Similar Excellent Outcome When Treated With the Same Chemotherapy Regimen," *J Clin Oncol*, 1996, 14(3):925-34.

◆ **IVCAF** see FAC on page *1318*

Ixabepilone-Capecitabine

Index Terms Capecitabine-Ixabepilone

Use Breast cancer

Regimen

Capecitabine: Oral: 1000 mg/m^2 twice daily days 1 to 14
[total dose/cycle = 28,000 mg/m^2]
Ixabepilone: I.V.: 40 mg/m^2 day 1
[total dose/cycle = 40 mg/m^2]
Repeat cycle every 3 weeks

References

Thomas ES, Gomez HL, Li RK, et al, "Ixabepilone Plus Capecitabine for Metastatic Breast Cancer Progressing After Anthracycline and Taxane Treatment," *J Clin Oncol*, 2007, 25(33):5210-7.

Vahdat LT, Thomas E, Li R, et al, "Phase III Trial of Ixabepilone Plus Capecitabine Compared to Capecitabine Alone in Patients With Metastatic Breast Cancer (MBC) Previously Treated or Resistant to an Anthracycline and Resistant to Taxanes," *J Clin Onc*, 2007, 25(18S):1006 [abstract from 2007 Proceedings of ASCO Annual Meeting].

◆ **Lapatinib-Capecitabine** see Capecitabine + Lapatinib on page *1245*

Larson Regimen

Use Leukemia, acute lymphocytic

Regimen

Cyclophosphamide: I.V.: 1200 mg/m^2 day 1
[total dose/cycle = 1200 mg/m^2]
Daunorubicin: I.V.: 45 mg/m^2/day days 1, 2, and 3
[total dose/cycle = 135 mg/m^2]
Vincristine: I.V.: 2 mg/day days 1, 8, 15, and 22
[total dose/cycle = 8 mg]
Prednisone: Oral or I.V.: 60 mg/m^2/day days 1 to 21
[total dose/cycle = 1260 mg/m^2]
Asparaginase: SubQ: 6000 units/m^2/day days 5, 8, 11, 15, 18, and 22
[total dose/cycle = 36,000 units/m^2]
Administer one cycle only

◀ **References**
Larson RA, Dodge RK, Burns CP, et al, "A Five-Drug Remission Induction Regimen With Intensive Consolidation for Adults With Acute Lymphoblastic Leukemia: Cancer and Leukemia Group B Study 8811," *Blood*, 1995, 85(8):2025-37.

Lenalidomide-Dexamethasone

Index Terms Dexamethasone-Lenalidomide

Use Multiple myeloma

Regimen
Lenalidomide: Oral: 25 mg/day days 1 to 21
[total dose/cycle = 525 mg]
Dexamethasone: Oral: 40 mg/day days 1 to 4, 9 to 12, and 17 to 20 (cycles 1 to 4)
[total dose/cycle = 480 mg]
Dexamethasone: Oral 40 mg/day days 1 to 4 (cycle 5 and beyond)
[total dose/cycle = 160 mg]
Repeat cycle every 28 days

References
Dimopoulos M, Spencer A, Attal M, et al, "Lenalidomide Plus Dexamethasone for Relapsed or Refractory Multiple Myeloma," *N Engl J Med*, 2007, 357(21):2123-32.
Rajkumar SV, Hayman SR, Lacy MQ, et al, "Combination Therapy With Lenalidomide Plus Dexamethasone (Rev/Dex) for Newly Diagnosed Myeloma," *Blood*, 2005, 106(13):4050-3.
Weber DM, Chen C, Niesvizky R, et al, "Lenalidomide Plus Dexamethasone for Relapsed Multiple Myeloma in North America," *N Engl J Med*, 2007, 357(21):2133-42.

Lenalidomide-Dexamethasone (Low Dose)

Index Terms Dexamethasone (Low Dose)-Lenalidomide

Use Multiple myeloma

Regimen
Lenalidomide: Oral: 25 mg/day days 1 to 21
[total dose/cycle = 525 mg]
Dexamethasone: Oral: 40 mg/day days 1, 8, 15, and 22
[total dose/cycle = 160 mg]
Repeat cycle every 28 days

References
Rajkumar SV, Jacobus S, Callander N, et al, "A Randomized Phase III Trial of Lenalidomide Plus High-Dose Dexamethasone Versus Lenalidomide Plus Low-Dose Dexamethasone in Newly Diagnosed Multiple Myeloma (E4A03): A Trial Coordinated by the Eastern Cooperative Oncology Group," *Blood*, 2006, 108(11), ASH Abstract 799.
Rajkumar SV, Jacobus S, Callander N, et al, "Phase III Trial of Lenalidomide Plus High-Dose Dexamethasone Versus Lenalidomide Plus Low-Dose Dexamethasone in Newly Diagnosed Multiple Myeloma (E4A03): A Trial Coordinated by the Eastern Cooperative Oncology Group, *J Clin Onc*, 2007, 25(18S), ASCO Abstract LBA8025.

◆ **Leuprolide-Bicalutamide** *see* Bicalutamide-Leuprolide *on page 1234*

Linker Protocol

Use Leukemia, acute lymphocytic

Regimen
Remission induction:
Daunorubicin: I.V.: 50 mg/m^2/day days 1, 2, and 3
[total dose/cycle = 150 mg/m^2]
Vincristine: I.V.: 2 mg/day days 1, 8, 15, and 22
[total dose/cycle = 8 mg]
Prednisone: Oral: 60 mg/m^2/day days 1 to 28
[total dose/cycle = 1680 mg/m^2]

Asparaginase: I.M.: 6000 units/m²/day days 17 to 28
   [total dose/cycle = 72,000 units/m²]
If residual leukemia in bone marrow on day 14:
Daunorubicin: I.V.: 50 mg/m² day 15
   [total dose/cycle = 50 mg/m²]
If residual leukemia in bone marrow on day 28:
Daunorubicin: I.V.: 50 mg/m²/day days 29 and 30
   [total dose/cycle = 100 mg/m²]
Vincristine: I.V.: 2 mg/day days 29 and 36
   [total dose/cycle = 4 mg]
Prednisone: Oral: 60 mg/m²/day days 29 to 42
   [total dose/cycle = 840 mg/m²]
Asparaginase: I.M.: 6000 units/m²/day days 29 to 35
   [total dose/cycle = 42,000 units/m²]

Consolidation therapy:
Treatment A (cycles 1, 3, 5, and 7)
Daunorubicin: I.V.: 50 mg/m²/day days 1 and 2
   [total dose/cycle = 100 mg/m²]
Vincristine: I.V.: 2 mg/day days 1 and 8
   [total dose/cycle = 4 mg]
Prednisone: Oral: 60 mg/m²/day days 1 to 14
   [total dose/cycle = 840 mg/m²]
Asparaginase: I.M.: 12,000 units/m²/day days 2, 4, 7, 9, 11, and 14
   [total dose/cycle = 72,000 units/m²]
Treatment B (cycles 2, 4, 6, and 8)
Teniposide: I.V.: 165 mg/m²/day days 1, 4, 8, and 11
   [total dose/cycle = 660 mg/m²]
Cytarabine: I.V.: 300 mg/m²/day days 1, 4, 8, and 11
   [total dose/cycle = 1200 mg/m²]
Treatment C (cycle 9)
Methotrexate: I.V.: 690 mg/m² continuous infusion over 42 hours day 1
   [total dose/cycle = 690 mg/m²]
Leucovorin: I.V.: 15 mg/m² every 6 hours for 12 doses (start at end of
   methotrexate infusion)
   [total dose/cycle = 180 mg/m²]
Administer remission induction regimen for one cycle only. Repeat
consolidation cycle every 28 days.
References

Linker CA, Levitt LJ, O'Donnell M, et al, "Treatment of Adult Acute Lymphoblastic Leukemia With Intensive Cyclical Chemotherapy: A Follow-up Report," *Blood*, 1991 78(11):2814-22.

LOPP

Use Lymphoma, Hodgkin's disease
Regimen
Chlorambucil: Oral: 10 mg/day days 1 to 10
   [total dose/cycle = 100 mg/m²]
Vincristine: I.V.: 1.4 mg/m²/day (maximum dose: 2 mg) days 1 and 8
   [total dose/cycle = 2.8 mg/m²]
Procarbazine: Oral: 100 mg/m²/day days 1 to 10
   [total dose/cycle = 1000 mg/m²]

◀ Prednisone: Oral: 25 mg/m²/day (maximum dose: 60 mg) days 1 to 14
[total dose/cycle = 350 mg/m²]
or
Prednisolone: Oral: 25 mg/m²/day (maximum dose: 60 mg) days 1 to 14
[total dose/cycle = 350 mg/m²]
Repeat cycle every 28 days

References

Hancock BW, "Randomised Study of MOPP (Mustine, Oncovin, Procarbazine, Prednisone) Against LOPP (Leukeran Substituted for Mustine) in Advanced Hodgkin's Disease. British National Lymphoma Investigation," *Radiother Oncol*, 1986, 7(3):215-21.

M-2

Use Multiple myeloma

Regimen

Vincristine: I.V.: 0.03 mg/kg (maximum dose: 2 mg) day 1
[total dose/cycle = 0.03 mg/kg]
Carmustine: I.V.: 0.5-1 mg/kg day 1
[total dose/cycle = 0.5-1 mg/kg]
Cyclophosphamide: I.V.: 10 mg/kg day 1
[total dose/cycle = 10 mg/kg]
Melphalan: Oral: 0.25 mg/kg/day days 1 to 4
[total dose/cycle = 1 mg/kg]
   or 0.1 mg/kg/day days 1 to 7 or 1 to 10
   [total dose/cycle = 0.7 or 1 mg/kg]
Prednisone: Oral: 1 mg/kg/day days 1 to 7
[total dose/cycle = 7 mg/kg]
Repeat cycle every 35-42 days

References

Case DC Jr, Lee DJ 3rd, and Clarkson BD, "Improved Survival Times in Multiple Myeloma Treated With Melphalan, Prednisone, Cyclophosphamide, Vincristine, and BCNU: M-2 Protocol," *Am J Med*, 1977, 63(6):897-903.

MACOP-B

Use Lymphoma, non-Hodgkin's

Regimen

Methotrexate: I.V. bolus: 100 mg/m² weeks 2, 6, 10
   followed by I.V.: 300 mg/m² over 4 hours weeks 2, 6, and 10
   [total dose/cycle = 1200 mg/m²]
Doxorubicin: I.V.: 50 mg/m² weeks 1, 3, 5, 7, 9, and 11
[total dose/cycle = 300 mg/m²]
Cyclophosphamide: I.V.: 350 mg/m² weeks 1, 3, 5, 7, 9, and 11
[total dose/cycle = 2100 mg/m²]
Vincristine: I.V.: 1.4 mg/m² (maximum dose: 2 mg) weeks 2, 4, 6, 8, 10, and 12
[total dose/cycle = 8.4 mg/m²; maximum: 12 mg]
Bleomycin: I.V.: 10 units/m² weeks 4, 8, and 12
[total dose/cycle = 30 units/m²]
Prednisone: Oral: 75 mg/day for 12 weeks, then taper over 2 weeks
Leucovorin calcium: Oral: 15 mg/m² every 6 hours, for 6 doses (beginning 24 hours after methotrexate) weeks 2, 6, and 10
[total dose/cycle = 270 mg/m²]
Administer one cycle

References

Klimo P and Conors JM, "MACOP-B Chemotherapy for the Treatment of Diffuse Large-Cell Lymphoma," *Ann Intern Med*, 1985, 102(5):596-602.

MAID

Use Soft tissue sarcoma

Regimen

Mesna: I.V.: 2500 mg/m^2/day continuous infusion days 1 to 4
[total dose/cycle = 10,000 mg/m^2]

Doxorubicin: I.V.: 20 mg/m^2/day continuous infusion days 1, 2, and 3
[total dose/cycle = 60 mg/m^2]

Ifosfamide: I.V.: 2500 mg/m^2/day continuous infusion days 1, 2, and 3
[total dose/cycle = 7500 mg/m^2]

Dacarbazine: I.V.: 300 mg/m^2/day continuous infusion days 1, 2, and 3
[total dose/cycle = 900 mg/m^2]

Repeat cycle every 21-28 days

References

Elias A, Ryan L, Sulkes A, et al, "Response to Mesna, Doxorubicin, Ifosfamide, and Dacarbazine in 108 Patients With Metastatic or Unresectable Sarcoma and No Prior Chemotherapy," *J Clin Oncol*, 1989, 7(9):1208-16.

m-BACOD

Use Lymphoma, non-Hodgkin's

Regimen

Methotrexate: I.V.: 200 mg/m^2/day days 8 and 15
[total dose/cycle = 400 mg/m^2]

Leucovorin calcium: Oral: 10 mg/m^2 every 6 hours for 8 doses (beginning 24 hours after each methotrexate dose) days 9 and 16
[total dose/cycle = 160 mg/m^2]

Bleomycin: I.V.: 4 units/m^2 day 1
[total dose/cycle = 4 units/m^2]

Doxorubicin: I.V.: 45 mg/m^2 day 1
[total dose/cycle = 45 mg/m^2]

Cyclophosphamide: I.V.: 600 mg/m^2 day 1
[total dose/cycle = 600 mg/m^2]

Vincristine: I.V.: 1 mg/m^2 day 1
[total dose/cycle = 1 mg/m^2]

Dexamethasone: Oral: 6 mg/m^2/day days 1 to 5
[total dose/cycle = 30 mg/m^2]

Repeat cycle every 21 days

References

Salles G, Shipp MA, and Coiffier B, "Chemotherapy of Non-Hodgkin's Aggressive Lymphomas," *Semin Hematol*, 1994, 31(1):46-69.

Urba WJ, Duffey PL, and Longo DL, "Treatment of Patients With Aggressive Lymphomas: An Overview," *J Natl Cancer Inst Monogr*, 1990, (10):29-37.

◆ **Melphalan-Prednisone-Bortezomib** *see* Bortezomib-Melphalan-Prednisone *on page 1240*

◆ **Melphalan-Prednisone-Bortezomib-Thalidomide** *see* Bortezomib-Melphalan-Prednisone-Thalidomide *on page 1241*

Melphalan-Prednisone-Thalidomide

Use Multiple myeloma

Regimen

Melphalan: Oral: 4 mg/m^2/day days 1 to 7
[total dose/cycle = 28 mg/m^2]

Prednisone: Oral: 40 mg/m^2/day days 1 to 7
[total dose/cycle = 280 mg/m^2]

Thalidomide: Oral: 100 mg/day days 1 to 28
  [total dose/cycle = 2800 mg]
Repeat cycle every 28 days for 6 cycles
followed by
Thalidomide: Oral: 100 mg daily (as maintenance)

References
Palumbo A, Bertola A, Musto P, et al, "Oral Melphalan, Prednisone, and Thalidomide for Newly Diagnosed Patients With Myeloma," *Cancer* , 2005, 104(7):1428-33.

Palumbo A, Bringhen S, Caravita T, et al, "Oral Melphalan and Prednisone Chemotherapy Plus Thalidomide Compared With Melphalan and Prednisone Alone in Elderly Patients With Multiple Myeloma: Randomised Controlled Trial," *Lancet*, 2006, 367(9513):825-31.

Methotrexate-Vinblastine (Desmoid Tumor)
Index Terms Vinblastine-Methotrexate (Desmoid Tumor)
Use Soft tissue sarcoma (Desmoid tumor)
Regimen
Methotrexate: I.V.: 30 mg/m^2 every 7-10 days
  [total dose/treatment = 30 mg/m^2]
Vinblastine: I.V.: 6 mg/m^2 every 7-10 days
  [total dose/treatment = 6 mg/m^2]
Continue treatment for 1 year (52 treatments)

References
Azzarelli A, Gronchi A, Bertulli R, et al, "Low-Dose Chemotherapy With Methotrexate and Vinblastine for Patients With Advanced Aggressive Fibromatosis," *Cancer*, 2001, 92(5):1259-64.

MF
Use Breast cancer
Regimen
Methotrexate: I.V. 100 mg/m^2/day days 1 and 8
  [total dose/cycle = 200 mg/m^2]
Fluorouracil: I.V.: 600 mg/m^2/day (start 1 hour after methotrexate) days 1 and 8
  [total dose/cycle = 1200 mg/m^2]
Leucovorin: Oral, I.V.: 10 mg/m^2 every 6 hours for 6 doses (start 24 hours after methotrexate)
  [total dose/cycle = 60 mg/m^2]
Repeat cycle every 28 days for 12 cycles

References
Fisher B, Dignam J, Mamounas EP, et al, "Sequential Methotrexate and Fluorouracil for the Treatment of Node-Negative Breast Cancer Patients With Estrogen Receptor-Negative Tumors: Eight-Year Results from National Surgical Adjuvant Breast and Bowel Project (NSABP) B-13 and First Report of Findings from NSABP B-19 Comparing Methotrexate and Fluorouracil With Conventional Cyclophosphamide, Methotrexate, and Fluorouracil," *J Clin Oncol*, 1996, 14 (7):1982-92.

MINE
Use Lymphoma, non-Hodgkin's
Regimen
Mesna: I.V.: 1.33 g/m^2/day concurrent with ifosfamide dose, then 500 mg orally (4 hours after each ifosfamide infusion) days 1, 2, and 3
  [total dose/cycle = 3.99 g/m^2/1500 mg]
Ifosfamide: I.V.: 1.33 g/m^2/day days 1, 2, and 3
  [total dose/cycle = 3.99 g/m^2]
Mitoxantrone: I.V.: 8 mg/m^2 day 1
  [total dose/cycle = 8 mg/m^2]
Etoposide: I.V.: 65 mg/m^2/day days 1, 2, and 3
  [total dose/cycle = 195 mg/m^2]
Repeat cycle every 28 days

References
Rodriguez-Monge EJ and Cabanillas F, "Long-Term Follow-up of Platinum-Based Lymphoma Salvage Regimens. The M.D. Anderson Cancer Center Experience," *Hematol Oncol Clin North Am*, 1997, 11(5):937-47.

MINE-ESHAP

Use Lymphoma, non-Hodgkin's
Regimen
Mesna: I.V.: 1.33 g/m^2 concurrent with ifosfamide dose, then 500 mg orally (4 hours after ifosfamide) days 1, 2, and 3
[total dose/cycle = 4 g/m^2/1500 mg]
Ifosfamide: I.V.: 1.33 g/m^2/day days 1, 2, and 3
[total dose/cycle = 4 g/m^2]
Mitoxantrone: I.V.: 8 mg/m^2 day 1
[total dose/cycle = 8 mg/m^2]
Etoposide: I.V.: 65 mg/m^2/day days 1, 2, and 3
[total dose/cycle = 195 mg/m^2]
Repeat cycle every 21 days for 6 cycles, followed by 3-6 cycles of ESHAP

References
Rodriguez MA, Cabanillas FC, Velasquez W, et al, "Results of a Salvage Treatment Program for Relapsing Lymphoma: MINE Consolidated With ESHAP," *J Clin Oncol*, 1995, 13(7):1734-41.

mini-BEAM

Use Lymphoma, Hodgkin's disease
Regimen
Carmustine: I.V.: 60 mg/m^2 day 1
[total dose/cycle = 60 mg/m^2]
Etoposide: I.V.: 75 mg/m^2/day days 2 to 5
[total dose/cycle = 300 mg/m^2]
Cytarabine: I.V.: 100 mg/m^2 every 12 hours for 8 doses days 2 to 5
[total dose/cycle = 800 mg/m^2]
Melphalan: I.V.: 30 mg/m^2 day 6
[total dose/cycle = 30 mg/m^2]
Repeat cycle every 4-6 weeks

References
Colwill R, Crump M, Couture F, et al, "Mini-BEAM as Salvage Therapy for Relapsed or Refractory Hodgkin's Disease Before Intensive Therapy and Autologous Bone Marrow Transplantation," *J Clin Oncol*, 1995, 13(2):396-402.

Mitomycin-Vinblastine

Index Terms MV
Use Breast cancer
Regimen
Mitomycin: I.V.: 20 mg/m^2 day 1
[total dose/cycle = 20 mg/m^2]
Vinblastine: I.V.: 0.15 mg/kg/day days 1 and 21
[total dose/cycle = 0.3 mg/kg]
Repeat cycle every 6-8 weeks

References
Konits PH, Aisner J, van Echo DA, et al, "Mitomycin C and Vinblastine Chemotherapy for Advanced Breast Cancer," *Cancer*, 1981, 48(6):1295-8.

◆ **Mitomycin–Fluorouracil (Anal Cancer)** *see* Fluorouracil-Mitomycin (Anal Cancer) *on page 1335*

Mitoxantrone + Hydrocortisone

Use Prostate cancer

Regimen

Mitoxantrone: I.V.: 14 mg/m² day 1

[total dose/cycle = 14 mg/m²]

Hydrocortisone: Oral: 40 mg daily

[total dose/cycle = 840 mg]

Repeat cycle every 3 weeks

References

Kantoff PW, Halabi S, Conaway M, et al, "Hydrocortisone With or Without Mitoxantrone in Men With Hormone-Refractory Prostate Cancer: Results of the Cancer and Leukemia Group B 9182 Study," *J Clin Oncol*, 1999, 17(8):2506-13.

Mitoxantrone-Prednisone (Prostate Cancer)

Index Terms MP (Prostate Cancer); Prednisone-Mitoxantrone (Prostate Cancer)

Use Prostate cancer

Regimen NOTE: Multiple variations are listed.

Variation 1:

Mitoxantrone: I.V.: 12 mg/m² day 1

[total dose/cycle = 12 mg/m²]

Prednisone: Oral: 5 mg twice daily

[total dose/cycle = 210 mg]

Repeat cycle every 21 days for up to a total of 10 cycles

Variation 2:

Cycle 1:

Mitoxantrone: I.V.: 12 mg/m² day 1

[total dose/cycle = 12 mg/m²]

Prednisone: Oral: 5 mg twice daily

[total dose/cycle = 210 mg]

Treatment cycle is 21 days

Cycle 2 and beyond:

Mitoxantrone: I.V.: 12-14 mg/m² day 1 (increase to 14 mg/m² if no grade 3/4 adverse events)

[total dose/cycle = 12-14 mg/m²]

Prednisone: Oral: 5 mg twice daily

[total dose/cycle = 210 mg]

Repeat cycle every 21 days for up to a maximum cumulative mitoxantrone dose of 144 mg/m²

Variation 3:

Cycle 1:

Mitoxantrone: I.V.: 12 mg/m² day 1

[total dose/cycle = 12 mg/m²]

Prednisone: Oral: 5 mg twice daily

[total dose/cycle = 210 mg]

Treatment cycle is 21 days

Cycles 2-8:

Mitoxantrone: I.V.: 12-14 mg/m² day 1 (increase to 14 mg/m² if granulocyte nadir is >1000/mm³ and platelet nadir >50,000/ mm³)

[total dose/cycle = 12-14 mg/m²]

Prednisone: Oral: 5 mg twice daily

[total dose/cycle = 210 mg]

Treatment cycle is 21 days for up to a total of 8 cycles

References

Variation 1:

Tannock IF, de Wit R, Berry WR, et al, "Docetaxel Plus Prednisone or Mitoxantrone Plus Prednisone for Advanced Prostate Cancer," *N Engl J Med*, 2004, 351(15):1502-12.

Variation 2:

Petrylak DP, Tangen CM, Hussain MH, et al, "Docetaxel and Estramustine Compared With Mitoxantrone and Prednisone for Advanced Refractory Prostate Cancer," *N Engl J Med*, 2004, 351(15):1513-20.

Variation 3:

Moore MJ, Osoba D, Murphy K, et al, "Use of Palliative Endpoints to Evaluate the Effects of Mitoxantrone and Low-Dose Prednisone in Patients With Hormonally Resistant Prostate Cancer," *J Clin Oncol*, 1994, 12(4):689-94.

MOP

Use Brain tumors

Regimen

Mechlorethamine: I.V.: 6 mg/m^2/day days 1 and 8
  [total dose/cycle = 12 mg/m^2]
Vincristine: I.V.: 1.5 mg/m^2/day (maximum dose: 2 mg) days 1 and 8
  [total dose/cycle = 3 mg/m^2]
Procarbazine: Oral: 100 mg/m^2/day days 1 to 14
  [total dose/cycle = 1400 mg/m^2]
Repeat cycle every 28 days

References

Kretschmar CS, Tarbell NJ, Kupsky W, et al, "Preirradiation Chemotherapy for Infants and Children With Medulloblastoma: A Preliminary Report," *J Neurosurg*, 1989, 71(6):820-5.

MOPP/ABVD

Use Lymphoma, Hodgkin's disease

Regimen NOTE: Multiple variations are listed.

Variation 1:

Mechlorethamine: I.V.: 6 mg/m^2/day days 1 and 8
  [total dose/cycle = 12 mg/m^2]
Vincristine: I.V.: 1.4 mg/m^2/day (maximum dose: 2 mg) days 1 and 8
  [total dose/cycle = 2.8 mg/m^2]
Procarbazine: I.V.: 100 mg/m^2/day days 1 to 14
  [total dose/cycle = 1400 mg/m^2]
Prednisone: Oral: 40 mg/m^2/day days 1 to 14 (during cycles 1, 4, 7, and 10 only)
  [total dose/cycle = 560 mg/m^2]
Doxorubicin: I.V.: 25 mg/m^2/day days 29 and 43
  [total dose/cycle = 50 mg/m^2]
Bleomycin: I.V.: 10 units/m^2/day days 29 and 43
  [total dose/cycle = 20 units/m^2]
Vinblastine: I.V.: 6 mg/m^2/day days 29 and 43
  [total dose/cycle = 12 mg/m^2]
Dacarbazine: I.V.: 375 mg/m^2/day days 29 and 43
  [total dose/cycle = 750 mg/m^2]
Repeat cycle every 56 days

Variation 2:

Mechlorethamine: I.V.: 6 mg/m^2/day days 1 and 8
  [total dose/cycle = 12 mg/m^2]
Vincristine: I.V.: 1.4 mg/m^2/day (maximum dose: 2 mg) days 1 and 8
  [total dose/cycle = 2.8 mg/m^2]
Procarbazine: I.V.: 100 mg/m^2/day days 1 to 14
  [total dose/cycle = 1400 mg/m^2]

◄ Prednisone: Oral: 40 mg/m^2/day days 1 to 14 (during cycles 1 and 7 only)
  [total dose/cycle = 560 mg/m^2]
Doxorubicin: I.V.: 25 mg/m^2/day days 29 and 43
  [total dose/cycle = 50 mg/m^2]
Bleomycin: I.V.: 10 units/m^2/day days 29 and 43
  [total dose/cycle = 20 units/m^2]
Vinblastine: I.V.: 6 mg/m^2/day days 29 and 43
  [total dose/cycle = 12 mg/m^2]
Dacarbazine: I.V.: 375 mg/m^2/day days 29 and 43
  [total dose/cycle = 750 mg/m^2]
Repeat cycle every 56 days
Variation 3:
 Mechlorethamine: I.V.: 6 mg/m^2/day days 1 and 8
  [total dose/cycle = 12 mg/m^2]
 Vincristine: I.V.: 1.4 mg/m^2/day (maximum dose: 2 mg) days 1 and 8
  [total dose/cycle = 2.8 mg/m^2]
 Procarbazine: I.V.: 100 mg/m^2/day days 1 to 14
  [total dose/cycle = 1400 mg/m^2]
 Prednisone: Oral: 40 mg/m^2/day days 1 to 14 (every cycle)
  [total dose/cycle = 560 mg/m^2]
 Doxorubicin: I.V.: 25 mg/m^2/day days 29 and 43
  [total dose/cycle = 50 mg/m^2]
 Bleomycin: I.V.: 10 units/m^2/day days 29 and 43
  [total dose/cycle = 20 units/m^2]
 Vinblastine: I.V.: 6 mg/m^2/day days 29 and 43
  [total dose/cycle = 12 mg/m^2]
 Dacarbazine: I.V.: 375 mg/m^2/day days 29 and 43
  [total dose/cycle = 750 mg/m^2]
 Repeat cycle every 56 days
Variation 4:
 MOPP Regimen:
 Mechlorethamine: I.V.: 6 mg/m^2/day days 1 and 8
  [total dose/cycle = 12 mg/m^2]
 Vincristine: I.V.: 1.4 mg/m^2/day (maximum dose: 2 mg) days 1 and 8
  [total dose/cycle = 2.8 mg/m^2]
 Procarbazine: I.V.: 100 mg/m^2/day days 1 to 14
  [total dose/cycle = 1400 mg/m^2]
 Prednisone: Oral: 25 mg/m^2/day days 1 to 14
  [total dose/cycle = 350 mg/m^2]
 ABVD Regimen:
 Doxorubicin: I.V.: 25 mg/m^2/day days 1 and 15
  [total dose/cycle = 50 mg/m^2]
 Bleomycin: I.V.: 6 units/m^2/day days 1 and 15
  [total dose/cycle = 12 units/m^2]
 Vinblastine: I.V.: 6 mg/m^2/day days 1 and 15
  [total dose/cycle = 12 mg/m^2]
 Dacarbazine: I.V.: 250 mg/m^2/day days 1 and 15
  [total dose/cycle = 500 mg/m^2]
 Each regimen cycle is 28 days. Administer regimens in alternating fashion as
  follows: 2 cycles of MOPP alternating with 2 cycles of ABVD for a total of 8
  cycles
Variation 5 (pediatrics):
 Mechlorethamine: I.V.: 6 mg/m^2/day days 1 and 8
  [total dose/cycle = 12 mg/m^2]

Vincristine: I.V.: 1.4 mg/m^2/day days 1 and 8
  [total dose/cycle = 2.8 mg/m^2]
Procarbazine: Oral: 100 mg/m^2/day days 1 to 14
  [total dose/cycle = 1400 mg/m^2]
Prednisone: Oral: 40 mg/m^2/day days 1 to 14
  [total dose/cycle = 560 mg/m^2]
Doxorubicin: I.V.: 25 mg/m^2/day days 29 and 42
  [total dose/cycle = 50 mg/m^2]
Bleomycin: I.V.: 10 units/m^2/day days 29 and 42
  [total dose/cycle = 20 units/m^2]
Vinblastine: I.V.: 6 mg/m^2/day days 29 and 42
  [total dose/cycle = 12 mg/m^2]
Dacarbazine: I.V.: 150 mg/m^2/day days 29 to 33
  [total dose/cycle = 750 mg/m^2]
Repeat cycle every 56 days for 4 cycles
Variation 6 (pediatrics):
  Mechlorethamine: I.V.: 6 mg/m^2/day days 1 and 8
  [total dose/cycle = 12 mg/m^2]
Vincristine: I.V.: 1.4 mg/m^2/day days 1 and 8
  [total dose/cycle = 2.8 mg/m^2]
Procarbazine: Oral: 100 mg/m^2/day days 1 to 14
  [total dose/cycle = 1400 mg/m^2]
Prednisone: Oral: 40 mg/m^2/day days 1 to 14
  [total dose/cycle = 560 mg/m^2]
Doxorubicin: I.V.: 25 mg/m^2/day days 29 and 42
  [total dose/cycle = 50 mg/m^2]
Bleomycin: I.V.: 10 units/m^2/day days 29 and 42
  [total dose/cycle = 20 units/m^2]
Vinblastine: I.V.: 6 mg/m^2/day days 29 and 42
  [total dose/cycle = 12 mg/m^2]
Dacarbazine: I.V.: 375 mg/m^2/day days 29 and 43
  [total dose/cycle = 750 mg/m^2]
Repeat cycle every 56 days for 4 cycles

References

Variation 1:

Bonadonna G, Valagussa P, and Santoro A, "Alternating Noncross-Resistant Combination Chemotherapy or MOPP in State IV Hodgkin's Disease. A Report of 8-Year Results," *Ann Int Med*, 1986, 104(6):739-46.

Variation 2:

Canellos, GP, Anderson JR, Propert KJ, et al, "Chemotherapy of Advanced Hodgkin's Disease With MOPP, ABVD, or MOPP Alternating With ABVD," *N Engl J Med*, 1992, 327(21):1478-84.

Variation 3:

Glick JH, Young ML, Harrington D, et al, "MOPP/ABV Hybrid Chemotherapy for Advanced Hodgkin's Disease Significantly Improves Failure-Free and Overall Survival. The 8-Year Results of the Intergroup Trial," *J Clin Oncol* 1998, 16(1):19-26.

Variation 4:

Somers R, Carde P, Henry-Amar M, et al, "A Randomized Study in State IIIB and IV Hodgkin's Disease Comparing Eight Courses of MOPP Versus an Alternation of MOPP With ABVD. A European Organization for Research and Treatment of Cancer Lymphoma Cooperative Group and Groupe Pierre-et-Marie-Curie Controlled Clinical Trial," *J Clin Oncol*, 1994, 12(2):279-87.

Variation 5 (pediatrics):

Weiner MA, Leventhal BG, Marcus R, et al, "Intensive Chemotherapy and Low-Dose Radiotherapy for the Treatment of Advanced-Stage Hodgkin's Disease in Pediatric Patients. A Pediatric Oncology Group Study," *J Clin Oncol*, 1991, 9(9):1591-8.

Variation 6 (pediatrics):

Weiner MA, Leventhal B, Brecher ML, et al, "Randomized Study of Intensive MOPP-ABVD With or Without Low-Dose Total-Nodal Radiation Therapy in the Treatment of Stages IIB, IIIA2, IIIB, and IV Hodgkin's Disease in Pediatric Patients. A Pediatric Oncology Group Study," *J Clin Oncol*, 1997, 15(8):2769-79.

MOPP/ABV Hybrid

Use Lymphoma, Hodgkin's disease

Regimen

Mechlorethamine: I.V.: 6 mg/m^2 day 1
  [total dose/cycle = 6 mg/m^2]
Vincristine: I.V.: 1.4 mg/m^2 (maximum dose: 2 mg) day 1
  [total dose/cycle = 1.4 mg/m^2]
Procarbazine: Oral: 100 mg/m^2/day days 1 to 7
  [total dose/cycle = 700 mg/m^2]
Prednisone: Oral: 40 mg/m^2/day days 1 to 14
  [total dose/cycle = 560 mg/m^2]
Doxorubicin: I.V.: 35 mg/m^2 day 8
  [total dose/cycle = 35 mg/m^2]
Bleomycin: I.V.: 10 units/m^2 day 8
  [total dose/cycle = 10 units/m^2]
Vinblastine: I.V.: 6 mg/m^2 day 8
  [total dose/cycle = 6 mg/m^2]
Repeat cycle every 28 days

References

Klimo P and Connors JM, "MOPP/ABV Hybrid Program: Combination Chemotherapy Based on Early Introduction of Seven Effective Drugs for Advanced Hodgkin's Disease," *J Clin Oncol*, 1985, 3(9):1174-82.

MOPP (Lymphoma, Hodgkin's Disease)

Use Lymphoma, Hodgkin's disease

Regimen NOTE: Multiple variations are listed.

Variation 1:

Mechlorethamine: I.V.: 6 mg/m^2/day days 1 and 8
  [total dose/cycle = 12 mg/m^2]
Vincristine: I.V.: 1.4 mg/m^2/day days 1 and 8
  [total dose/cycle = 2.8 mg/m^2]
Procarbazine: Oral: 100 mg/m^2/day days 1 to 14
  [total dose/cycle = 1400 mg/m^2]
Prednisone: Oral: 40 mg/m^2/day days 1 to 14 (cycles 1 and 4)
  [total dose/cycle = 560 mg/m^2]
Repeat cycle every 28 days for 6-8 cycles

Variation 2:

Mechlorethamine: I.V.: 6 mg/m^2/day (maximum dose: 15 mg) days 1 and 8
  [total dose/cycle = 12 mg/m^2]
Vincristine: I.V.: 1.4 mg/m^2/day (maximum dose: 2 mg) days 1 and 8
  [total dose/cycle = 2.8 mg/m^2]
Procarbazine: Oral: 100 mg/m^2/day days 1 to 10
  [total dose/cycle = 1000 mg/m^2]
Prednisone: Oral: 25 mg/m^2/day (maximum dose: 60 mg) days 1 to 14
  [total dose/cycle = 350 mg/m^2]

or

Prednisolone: Oral: 25 mg/m^2/day (maximum dose: 60 mg) days 1 to 14
  [total dose/cycle = 350 mg/m^2]
Repeat cycle every 28 days

Variation 3:

Mechlorethamine: I.V.: 6 mg/m^2/day days 1 and 8
  [total dose/cycle = 12 mg/m^2]
Vincristine: I.V.: 1.4 mg/m^2/day days 1 and 8
  [total dose/cycle = 2.8 mg/m^2]

Procarbazine: Oral: 50 mg day 1, 100 mg day 2, 100 mg/m^2/day days 3 to 14
[total dose/cycle = 150 mg / 1200 mg/m^2]
Prednisone: Oral: 40 mg/m^2/day days 1 to 14
[total dose/cycle = 560 mg/m^2]
Repeat cycle every 28 days
Variation 4:
Mechlorethamine: I.V.: 6 mg/m^2/day days 1 and 8
[total dose/cycle = 12 mg/m^2]
Vincristine: I.V.: 1.4 mg/m^2/day days 1 and 8
[total dose/cycle = 2.8 mg/m^2]
Procarbazine: Oral: 50 mg day 1, 100 mg day 2, 100 mg/m^2/day days 3 to 10
[total dose/cycle = 150 mg / 800 mg/m^2]
Prednisone: Oral: 40 mg/m^2/day days 1 to 14
[total dose/cycle = 560 mg/m^2]
Repeat cycle every 28 days
Variation 5:
Mechlorethamine: I.V.: 6 mg/m^2/day days 1 and 8
[total dose/cycle = 12 mg/m^2]
Vincristine: I.V.: 1.4 mg/m^2/day days 1 and 8
[total dose/cycle = 2.8 mg/m^2]
Procarbazine: Oral: 50 mg/m^2 day 1, then 100 mg/m^2/day days 2 to 14
[total dose/cycle = 1350 mg/m^2]
Prednisone: Oral: 40 mg/m^2/day days 1 to 14
[total dose/cycle = 560 mg/m^2]
Repeat cycle every 28 days

References

Variation 1:
Devita VT Jr, Serpick AA, and Carbone PP, "Combination Chemotherapy in the Treatment of Advanced Hodgkin's Disease," *Ann Intern Med*, 1970, 73(6):881-95.
Variation 2:
Hancock BW, "Randomised Study Of MOPP (Mustine, Oncovin, Procarbazine, Prednisone) Against LOPP (Leukeran Substituted for Mustine) in Advanced Hodgkin's Disease. British National Lymphoma Investigation," *Radiother Oncol*, 1986, 7(3):215-21.
Variation 3:
Nissen NI, Pajak TF, Glidewell O, et al, "A Comparative Study of a BCNU Containing 4-Drug Program Versus MOPP 3-Drug Combinations in Advanced Hodgkin's Disease: A Cooperative Study by the Cancer and Leukemia Group B," *Cancer*, 1979, 43(1):31-40.
Variation 4:
Huguley CM Jr, Durant JR, Moores RR, et al, "A Comparison of Nitrogen Mustard, Vincristine, Procarbazine, and Prednisone (MOPP) Vs Nitrogen Mustard In Advanced Hodgkin's Disease," *Cancer*, 1975, 36(4):1227-40.
Variation 5:
Bakemeier RF, Anderson JR, Costello W, et al, "BCVPP Chemotherapy for Advanced Hodgkin's Disease: Evidence for Greater Duration of Complete Remission, Greater Survival, and Less Toxicity Than With a MOPP Regimen. Results of the Eastern Cooperative Oncology Group Study," *Ann Intern Med*, 1984, 101(4):447-56.

MOPP (Medulloblastoma)

Use Brain tumors

Regimen

Mechlorethamine: I.V.: 3 mg/m^2/day days 1 and 8
[total dose/cycle = 6 mg/m^2]
Vincristine: I.V.: 1.4 mg/m^2/day (maximum dose: 2 mg) days 1 and 8
[total dose/cycle = 2.8 mg/m^2]
Prednisone: Oral: 40 mg/m^2/day days 1 to 10
[total dose/cycle = 400 mg/m^2]
Procarbazine: Oral: 50 mg day 1
[total dose/cycle = 50 mg]

◄ **followed by** Oral: 100 mg day 2
[total dose/cycle = 100 mg]
followed by Oral: 100 mg/m^2/day days 3 to 10
[total dose/cycle = 800 mg/m^2]
Repeat cycle every 28 days

References

Krischer JP, Ragab AH, Kun L, et al, "Nitrogen Mustard, Vincristine, Procarbazine, and Prednisone as Adjuvant Chemotherapy in the Treatment of Medulloblastoma. A Pediatric Oncology Group Study," *J Neurosurg*, 1991, 74(6):905-9.

MP (Multiple Myeloma)

Use Multiple myeloma

Regimen

Melphalan: Oral: 8-10 mg/m^2/day days 1 to 4
[total dose/cycle = 32-40 mg/m^2]
Prednisone: Oral: 40-60 mg/m^2/day days 1 to 4
[total dose/cycle = 160-240 mg/m^2]
Repeat cycle every 28-42 days

References

Belch A, Shelley W, Bergsagel D, et al, "A Randomized Trial of Maintenance Versus No Maintenance Melphalan and Prednisone in Responding Multiple Myeloma Patients," *Br J Cancer*, 1988, 57(1):94-9.

◆ **MP (Prostate Cancer)** *see* Mitoxantrone-Prednisone (Prostate Cancer) *on page 1368*

MTX/6-MP/VP (Maintenance)

Use Leukemia, acute lymphocytic

Regimen

Methotrexate: Oral: 20 mg/m^2 weekly
[total dose/cycle = 80 mg/m^2]
Mercaptopurine: Oral: 75 mg/m^2/day
[total dose/cycle = 2250 mg/m^2]
Vincristine: I.V.: 1.5 mg/m^2 day 1
[total dose/cycle = 1.5 mg/m^2]
Prednisone: Oral: 40 mg/m^2/day days 1 to 5
[total dose/cycle = 200 mg/m^2]
Repeat monthly for 2-3 years

References

Bleyer WA, Sather HN, Nickerson HJ, et al, "Monthly Pulses of Vincristine and Prednisone Prevent Bone Marrow and Testicular Relapse in Low-Risk Childhood Acute Lymphoblastic Leukemia: A Report of the CCG-161 Study by the Childrens Cancer Study Group," *J Clin Oncol*, 1991, 9 (6):1012-21.

MTX-CDDPAdr

Use Osteosarcoma

Regimen

Cisplatin: I.V.: 75 mg/m^2 day 1 of cycles 1-7, then 120 mg/m^2 for cycles 8, 9, and 10
Doxorubicin: I.V.: 25 mg/m^2/day days 1, 2, and 3 of cycles 1 to 7
Methotrexate: I.V.: 12 g/m^2/day days 21 and 28
Leucovorin calcium rescue: I.V.: 20 mg/m^2 every 3 hours (beginning 16 hours after completion of methotrexate) for 8 doses, then orally every 6 hours for 8 doses

References

Meyers PA, Heller G, Healey J, et al, "Chemotherapy for Nonmetastatic Osteogenic Sarcoma: The Memorial Sloan-Kettering Experience," *J Clin Oncol*, 1992, 10(1):5-15.

MV

Use Leukemia, acute myeloid

Regimen Induction:

Mitoxantrone: I.V.: 10 mg/m^2/day days 1 to 5

[total dose/cycle = 50 mg/m^2]

Etoposide: I.V.: 100 mg/m^2/day days 1 to 5

[total dose/cycle = 500 mg/m^2]

Second cycle may be given based on individual response; time between cycles not specified

References

Ho AD, Lipp T, Ehninger G, et al, "Combination of Mitoxantrone and Etoposide in Refractory Acute Myelogenous Leukemia an Active and Well-Tolerated Regimen," *J Clin Oncol*, 1988, 6(2):213-17.

◆ **MV** see Mitomycin-Vinblastine *on page 1367*

M-VAC (Bladder Cancer)

Use Bladder cancer

Regimen NOTE: Multiple variations are listed.

Variation 1:

Methotrexate: I.V.: 30 mg/m^2/day days 1, 15, and 22

[total dose/cycle = 90 mg/m^2]

Vinblastine: I.V.: 3 mg/m^2/day days 2, 15, and 22

[total dose/cycle = 9 mg/m^2]

Doxorubicin: I.V.: 30 mg/m^2 day 2

[total dose/cycle = 30 mg/m^2]

Cisplatin: I.V.: 70 mg/m^2 day 2

[total dose/cycle = 70 mg/m^2]

Repeat cycle every 4 weeks

Variation 2:

Methotrexate: I.V.: 40 or 50 mg/m^2/day days 1, 15, and 22

[total dose/cycle = 120 or 150 mg/m^2]

Vinblastine: I.V.: 4 or 5 mg/m^2/day days 2, 15, and 22

[total dose/cycle = 12 or 15 mg/m^2]

Doxorubicin: I.V.: 40 or 50 mg/m^2 day 2

[total dose/cycle = 40 or 50 mg/m^2]

Cisplatin: I.V.: 100 mg/m^2 day 2

[total dose/cycle = 100 mg/m^2]

Repeat cycle every 4 weeks

Variation 3:

Methotrexate: I.V.: 30 mg/m^2/day days 1, 15, and 22

[total dose/cycle = 90 mg/m^2]

Vinblastine: I.V.: 3 mg/m^2 day 2

[total dose/cycle = 3 mg/m^2]

Doxorubicin: I.V.: 30 mg/m^2 day 2

[total dose/cycle = 30 mg/m^2]

Cisplatin: I.V.: 70 mg/m^2 day 2

[total dose/cycle = 70 mg/m^2]

Repeat cycle every 4 weeks

Variation 4:
 Methotrexate: I.V.: 60 mg/m^2 day 1
  [total dose/cycle = 60 mg/m^2]
  followed by I.V.: 30 mg/m^2 day 16
   [total dose/cycle = 30 mg/m^2]
 Vinblastine: I.V.: 4 mg/m^2/day days 2 and 16
  [total dose/cycle = 8 mg/m^2]
 Doxorubicin: I.V.: 60 mg/m^2 day 2
  [total dose/cycle = 60 mg/m^2]
 Cisplatin: I.V.: 100 mg/m^2 day 2
  [total dose/cycle = 100 mg/m^2]
 Repeat cycle every 23 days
Variation 5:
 Methotrexate: I.V.: 30 mg/m^2/day days 1, 16, and 23
  [total dose/cycle = 90 mg/m^2]
 Vinblastine: I.V.: 4 mg/m^2/day days 1, 16, and 23
  [total dose/cycle = 12 mg/m^2]
 Doxorubicin: I.V.: 60 mg/m^2 day 2
  [total dose/cycle = 60 mg/m^2]
 Cisplatin: I.V.: 100 mg/m^2 day 2
  [total dose/cycle = 100 mg/m^2]
 Repeat cycle every 23 days
Variation 6:
 Methotrexate: I.V.: 30 or 35 mg/m^2 day 1
  [total dose/cycle = 30 or 35 mg/m^2]
 Vinblastine: I.V.: 3 or 3.5 mg/m^2 day 2
  [total dose/cycle = 3 or 3.5 mg/m^2]
 Doxorubicin: I.V.: 30 or 35 mg/m^2 day 2
  [total dose/cycle = 30 or 35 mg/m^2]
 Cisplatin: I.V.: 70 or 80 mg/m^2 day 2
  [total dose/cycle = 70 or 80 mg/m^2]
 Repeat cycle every 2 weeks
Variation 7:
 Methotrexate: I.V.: 30 mg/m^2 day 1
  [total dose/cycle = 30 mg/m^2]
 Vinblastine: I.V.: 3 mg/m^2 day 2
  [total dose/cycle = 3 mg/m^2]
 Doxorubicin: I.V.: 30 mg/m^2 day 2
  [total dose/cycle = 30 mg/m^2]
 Cisplatin: I.V.: 70 mg/m^2 day 2
  [total dose/cycle = 70 mg/m^2]
 Repeat cycle every 14 days
Variation 8:
 Methotrexate: I.V.: 30 mg/m^2/day days 1, 15, and 22
  [total dose/cycle = 90 mg/m^2]
 Vinblastine: I.V.: 3 mg/m^2/day days 1, 15, and 22
  [total dose/cycle = 9 mg/m^2]
 Doxorubicin: I.V.: 45 mg/m^2 day 2
  [total dose/cycle = 45 mg/m^2]
 Cisplatin: I.V.: 70 mg/m^2 day 2
  [total dose/cycle = 70 mg/m^2]
 Repeat cycle every 4 weeks

Variation 9:
 Methotrexate: I.V.: 40 mg/m^2/day days 1 and 15
  [total dose/cycle = 80 mg/m^2]
 Vinblastine: I.V.: 4 mg/m^2/day days 1, 16, and 23
  [total dose/cycle = 12 mg/m^2]
 Doxorubicin: I.V.: 60 mg/m^2 day 2
  [total dose/cycle = 60 mg/m^2]
 Cisplatin: I.V.: 100 mg/m^2 day 2
  [total dose/cycle = 100 mg/m^2]
 Repeat cycle every 23 days
Variation 10:
 Methotrexate: I.V.: 30 mg/m^2/day days 1, 15, and 22
  [total dose/cycle = 90 mg/m^2]
 Vinblastine: I.V.: 3 mg/m^2/day days 1, 16, and 22
  [total dose/cycle = 9 mg/m^2]
 Doxorubicin: I.V.: 30 mg/m^2 day 1
  [total dose/cycle = 30 mg/m^2]
 Cisplatin: I.V.: 70 mg/m^2 day 1
  [total dose/cycle = 70 mg/m^2]
 Repeat cycle every 4 weeks
Variation 11:
 Methotrexate: I.V.: 30 mg/m^2/day days 1, 15, and 22
  [total dose/cycle = 90 mg/m^2]
 Vinblastine: I.V.: 3 mg/m^2/day days 2, 15, and 22
  [total dose/cycle = 9 mg/m^2]
 Doxorubicin: I.V.: 30 mg/m^2 day 2
  [total dose/cycle = 30 mg/m^2]
 Cisplatin: I.V.: 70 mg/m^2 day 2
  [total dose/cycle = 70 mg/m^2]
 Leucovorin: Oral: 15 mg every 6 hours for 4 doses days 2, 16, and 23
  [total dose/cycle = 180 mg]
 Repeat cycle every 4 weeks
Variation 12:
 Methotrexate: I.V.: 30 mg/m^2/day days 1 and 15
  [total dose/cycle = 60 mg/m^2]
 Vinblastine: I.V.: 3 mg/m^2/day days 2 and 15
  [total dose/cycle = 6 mg/m^2]
 Doxorubicin: I.V.: 30 or 40 mg/m^2 day 3
  [total dose/cycle = 30 or 40 mg/m^2]
 Cisplatin: I.V.: 70 mg/m^2 day 2
  [total dose/cycle = 70 mg/m^2]
 Repeat cycle every 4 weeks
Variation 13:
 Methotrexate: I.V.: 30 mg/m^2/day days 1 and 15
  [total dose/cycle = 60 mg/m^2]
 Vinblastine: I.V.: 3 mg/m^2/day days 2 and 15
  [total dose/cycle = 6 mg/m^2]
 Doxorubicin: I.V.: 30 or 40 mg/m^2 day 2
  [total dose/cycle = 30 or 40 mg/m^2]
 Cisplatin: I.V.: 70 mg/m^2 day 2
  [total dose/cycle = 70 mg/m^2]
 Repeat cycle every 4 weeks

References

Variation 1:

Sternberg CN, de Mulder PH, Schornagel JH, et al, "Randomized Phase III Trial of High-Dose-Intensity Methotrexate, Vinblastine, Doxorubicin, and Cisplatin (MVAC) Chemotherapy and Recombinant Human Granulocyte Colony-Stimulating Factor Versus Classic MVAC in Advanced Urothelial Tract Tumors: European Organization for Research and Treatment of Cancer Protocol No. 30924," *J Clin Oncol*, 2001, 19(10):2638-46.

Sternberg CN, Yagoda A, Scher HI, et al, "Preliminary Results of M-VAC (Methotrexate, Vinblastine, Doxorubicin, and Cisplatin) for Transitional Cell Carcinoma of the Urothelium," *J Urol*, 1985, 133(3):403-7.

Variation 2:

Loehrer PJ Sr, Elson P, Dreicer R, et al, "Escalated Dosages of Methotrexate, Vinblastine, Doxorubicin, and Cisplatin Plus Recombinant Human Granulocyte Colony-Stimulating Factor in Advanced Urothelial Carcinoma: An Eastern Cooperative Oncology Group Trial," *J Clin Oncol*, 1994, 12(3):483-8.

Variation 3:

Loehrer PJ Sr, Einhorn LH, Elson PJ, et al, "A Randomized Comparison of Cisplatin Alone or in Combination With Methotrexate, Vinblastine, and Doxorubicin in Patients With Metastatic Urothelial Carcinoma: A Cooperative Group Study," *J Clin Oncol*, 1992, 10(7):1066-73.

Variation 4:

Logothetis CJ, Finn LD, Smith T, et al, "Escalated MVAC With or Without Recombinant Human Granulocyte-Macrophage Colony-Stimulating Factor for the Initial Treatment of Advanced Malignant Urothelial Tumors: Results of a Randomized Trial," *J Clin Oncol*, 1995, 13(9):2272-7.

Variation 5:

Logothetis CJ, Dexeus FH, Sella A, et al, "Escalated Therapy for Refractory Urothelial Tumors: Methotrexate-Vinblastine-Doxorubicin-Cisplatin Plus Unglycosylated Recombinant Human Granulocyte-Macrophage Colony-Stimulating Factor," *J Natl Cancer Inst*, 1990, 82(8):667-72.

Variation 6:

Sternberg CN, de Mulder PH, van Oosterom AT, et al, "Escalated M-VAC Chemotherapy and Recombinant Human Granulocyte-Macrophage Colony Stimulating Factor (rhGM-CSF) in Patients With Advanced Urothelial Tract Tumors," *Ann Oncol*, 1993, 4(5):403-7.

Variation 7:

Sternberg CN, de Mulder PH, Schornagel JH, et al, "Randomized Phase III Trial of High-Dose-Intensity Methotrexate, Vinblastine, Doxorubicin, and Cisplatin (M-VAC) Chemotherapy and Recombinant Human Granulocyte Colony-Stimulating Factor Versus Classic M-VAC in Advanced Urothelial Tract Tumors: European Organization for Research and Treatment of Cancer Protocol No. 30924," *J Clin Oncol*, 2001, 19(10):2638-46.

Variation 8 and 9:

Seidman AD, Scher HI, Gabrilove JL, et al, "Dose-Intensification of MVAC With Recombinant Granulocyte Colony-Stimulating Factor as Initial Therapy in Advanced Urothelial Cancer," *J Clin Oncol*, 1993, 11(3):408-14.

Variation 10:

Bamias A, Aravantinos G, Deliveliotis C, et al, "Docetaxel and Cisplatin With Granulocyte Colony-Stimulating Factor (G-CSF) Versus M-VAC With G-CSF in Advanced Urothelial Carcinoma: A Multicenter, Randomized, Phase III Study From the Hellenic Cooperative Oncology Group," *J Clin Oncol*, 2004, 22(2):220-8.

Variation 11:

Simon SD and Srougi M, "Neoadjuvant M-VAC Chemotherapy and Partial Cystectomy for Treatment of Locally Invasive Transitional Cell Carcinoma of the Bladder," *Prog Clin Biol Res*, 1990, 353:169-74.

Variation 12:

Farah R, Chodak GW, Vogelzang NJ, et al, "Curative Radiotherapy Following Chemotherapy for Invasive Bladder Carcinoma (A Preliminary Report)," *Int J Radiat Oncol Biol Phys*, 1991, 20 (3):413-7.

Variation 13:

Vogelzang NJ, Moormeier JA, Awan AM, et al, "Methotrexate, Vinblastine, Doxorubicin, and Cisplatin Followed by Radiotherapy or Surgery for Muscle Invasive Bladder Cancer: The University of Chicago Experience," *J Urol*, 1993, 149(4):753-7.

M-VAC (Breast Cancer)

Use Breast cancer

Regimen

Methotrexate: I.V.: 30 mg/m^2/day days 1, 15, and 22

[total dose/cycle = 90 mg/m^2]

Vinblastine: I.V.: 3 mg/m^2/day days 2, 15, and 22
  [total dose/cycle = 9 mg/m^2]
Doxorubicin: I.V.: 30 mg/m^2 day 2
  [total dose/cycle = 30 mg/m^2]
Cisplatin: I.V.: 70 mg/m^2 day 2
  [total dose/cycle = 70 mg/m^2]
Leucovorin: Oral: 10 mg every 6 hours for 6 doses days 2, 16, and 23
  [total dose/cycle = 180 mg]
Repeat cycle every 4 weeks

References

Morrell LE, Lee YJ, Hurley J, et al, "A Phase II Trial of Neoadjuvant Methotrexate, Vinblastine, Doxorubicin, and Cisplatin in the Treatment of Patients With Locally Advanced Breast Carcinoma," *Cancer*, 1998, 82(3):503-11.

M-VAC (Cervical Cancer)

Use Cervical cancer

Regimen

Methotrexate: I.V.: 30 mg/m^2/day days 1, 15, and 22
  [total dose/cycle = 90 mg/m^2]
Vinblastine: I.V.: 3 mg/m^2/day days 2, 15, and 22
  [total dose/cycle = 9 mg/m^2]
Doxorubicin: I.V.: 30 mg/m^2 day 2
  [total dose/cycle = 30 mg/m^2]
Cisplatin: I.V.: 70 mg/m^2 day 2
  [total dose/cycle = 70 mg/m^2]
Repeat cycle every 4 weeks

References

Wilson TO, "Neoadjuvant MVAC (Methotrexate, Vinblastine, Doxorubicin, Cisplatin) Chemotherapy for Locally Advanced or Metastatic Cervical and Vaginal Cancer," *Adjuvant Therapy of Cancer VII*, Salmon SE, ed, Philadelphia, PA: J B Lipincott Co, 1997, 366-71.

M-VAC (Endometrial Cancer)

Use Endometrial cancer

Regimen

Methotrexate: I.V.: 30 mg/m^2/day days 1, 15, and 22
  [total dose/cycle = 90 mg/m^2]
Vinblastine: I.V.: 3 mg/m^2/day days 2, 15, and 22
  [total dose/cycle = 9 mg/m^2]
Doxorubicin: I.V.: 30 mg/m^2/day day 2
  [total dose/cycle = 30 mg/m^2]
Cisplatin: I.V.: 70 mg/m^2/day day 2
  [total dose/cycle = 70 mg/m^2]
Repeat cycle every 4 weeks

References

Long HJ 3rd, Langdon RM Jr, Cha SS, et al, "Phase II Trial of Methotrexate, Vinblastine, Doxorubicin, and Cisplatin in Advanced/Recurrent Endometrial Carcinoma," *Gynecol Oncol*, 1995, 58(2):240-3.

M-VAC (Head and Neck Cancer)

Use Head and neck cancer

Regimen

Methotrexate: I.V.: 30 mg/m^2/day days 1, 15, and 22
  [total dose/cycle = 90 mg/m^2]
Vinblastine: I.V.: 3 mg/m^2/day days 2, 15, and 22
  [total dose/cycle = 9 mg/m^2]

Doxorubicin: I.V.: 30 mg/m^2 day 2
[total dose/cycle = 30 mg/m^2]
Cisplatin: I.V.: 70 mg/m^2 day 2
[total dose/cycle = 70 mg/m^2]
Repeat cycle every 4 weeks

References

Okuno SH, Mailliard JA, Suman VJ, et al, "Phase II Study of Methotrexate, Vinblastine, Doxorubicin, and Cisplatin in Patients With Squamous Cell Carcinoma of the Upper Respiratory or Alimentary Passages of the Head and Neck," *Cancer*, 2002, 94(8):2224-31.

MVPP

Use Lymphoma, Hodgkin's disease

Regimen

Mechlorethamine: I.V.: 6 mg/m^2/day days 1 and 8
[total dose/cycle = 12 mg/m^2]
Vinblastine: I.V.: 4 mg/m^2/day days 1 and 8
[total dose/cycle = 8 mg/m^2]
Procarbazine: Oral: 100 mg/m^2/day days 1 to 14
[total dose/cycle = 1400 mg/m^2]
Prednisone: Oral: 40 mg/m^2/day days 1 to 14
[total dose/cycle = 560 mg/m^2]
Repeat cycle every 4-6 weeks

References

Cooper MR, Pajak TF, Nissen NI, et al, "A New Effective Four-Drug Combination of CCNU (1-[2-Chloroethyl]-3-Cyclohexyl-1-Nitrosourea) (NSC-79038), Vinblastine, Prednisone, and Procarbazine for the Treatment of Advanced Hodgkin's Disease," *Cancer*, 1980, 46(4):654-62.

N4SE Protocol

Use Neuroblastoma

Regimen

Vincristine: I.V.: 0.05 mg/kg/day days 1 and 2
[total dose/cycle = 0.1 mg/kg]
Doxorubicin: I.V.: 15 mg/m^2/day days 1 and 2
[total dose/cycle = 30 mg/m^2]
Cyclophosphamide: I.V.: 30 mg/kg/day days 1 and 2
[total dose/cycle = 60 mg/kg]
Fluorouracil: I.V.: 1 mg/kg/day days 3, 8, and 9
[total dose/cycle = 3 mg/kg]
Cytarabine: I.V.: 3 mg/kg/day days 3, 8, and 9
[total dose/cycle = 9 mg/kg]
Hydroxyurea: Oral: 40 mg/kg/day days 3, 8, and 9
[total dose/cycle = 120 mg/kg]
Repeat cycle every 21-28 days

References

Kushner BH and Helson L, "Coordinated Use of Sequentially Escalated Cyclophosphamide and Cell-Cycle-Specific Chemotherapy (N4SE Protocol) for Advanced Neuroblastoma: Experience With 100 Patients," *J Clin Oncol*, 1987, 5(11):1746-51.

N6 Protocol

Use Neuroblastoma

Regimen

Course 1, 2, 4, and 6:
Cyclophosphamide: I.V.: 70 mg/kg/day days 1 and 2
[total dose/cycle = 140 mg/kg]
Doxorubicin: I.V.: 25 mg/m^2/day continuous infusion days 1, 2, and 3
[total dose/cycle = 75 mg/m^2]

Vincristine: I.V.: 0.033 mg/kg/day continuous infusion days 1, 2, and 3
[total dose/cycle = 0.099 mg/kg]
Vincristine: I.V.: 1.5 mg/m² day 9
[total dose/cycle = 1.5 mg/m²]
Course 3, 5, and 7:
Etoposide: I.V.: 200 mg/m²/day days 1, 2, and 3
[total dose/cycle = 600 mg/m²]
Cisplatin: I.V.: 50 mg/m²/day days 1 to 4
[total dose/cycle = 200 mg/m²]

References

Kushner BH, LaQuaglia MP, Bonilla MA, et al, "Highly Effective Induction Therapy for Stage 4 Neuroblastoma in Children Over 1 Year of Age," *J Clin Oncol*, 1994, 12(12):2607-13.

NFL

Use Breast cancer

Regimen NOTE: Multiple variations are listed.
Variation 1:
Mitoxantrone: I.V.: 12 mg/m² day 1
[total dose/cycle = 12 mg/m²]
Fluorouracil: I.V.: 350 mg/m²/day days 1, 2, and 3
[total dose/cycle = 1050 mg/m²]
Leucovorin: I.V.: 300 mg/m²/day days 1, 2, and 3
[total dose/cycle = 900 mg/m²]
Repeat cycle every 21 days
Variation 2:
Mitoxantrone: I.V.: 10 mg/m² day 1
[total dose/cycle = 10 mg/m²]
Fluorouracil: I.V.: 1000 mg/m²/day continuous infusion days 1, 2, and 3
[total dose/cycle = 3000 mg/m²]
Leucovorin: I.V.: 100 mg/m²/day days 1, 2, and 3
[total dose/cycle = 300 mg/m²]
Repeat cycle every 21 days

References

Variation 1:
Hainsworth JD, Andrews MB, Johnson DH, et al, "Mitoxantrone, Fluorouracil, and High-Dose Leucovorin: An Effective, Well-Tolerated Regimen for Metastatic Breast Cancer," *J Clin Oncol*, 1991, 9(10):1731-5.
Variation 2:
Jones SE, Mennel RG, Brooks B, et al, "Phase II Study of Mitoxantrone, Leucovorin, and Infusional Fluorouracil for Treatment of Metastatic Breast Cancer," *J Clin Oncol*, 1991, 9(10):1736-9.

OFAR (CLL)

Index Terms Oxaliplatin-Fludarabine-Cytarabine-Rituximab (CLL)

Use Leukemia, chronic lymphocytic

Regimen
Cycle 1:
Oxaliplatin: I.V.: 25 mg/m²/dose day 1 to 4
[total dose/cycle = 100 mg/m²]
Fludarabine: I.V.: 30 mg/m²/dose days 2 and 3
[total dose/cycle = 60 mg/m²]
Cytarabine: I.V.: 1000 mg/m²/dose over 2 hours days 2 and 3
[total dose/cycle = 2000 mg/m²]
Rituximab: I.V.: 375 mg/m² day 3
[total dose/cycle = 375 mg/m²]
Treatment cycle is 4 weeks

Cycles 2-6:
Oxaliplatin: I.V.: 25 mg/m^2/dose day 1 to 4
[total dose/cycle = 100 mg/m^2]
Fludarabine: I.V.: 30 mg/m^2/dose days 2 and 3
[total dose/cycle = 60 mg/m^2]
Cytarabine: I.V.: 1000 mg/m^2/dose over 2 hours days 2 and 3
[total dose/cycle = 2000 mg/m^2]
Rituximab: I.V.: 375 mg/m^2 day 1
[total dose/cycle = 375 mg/m^2]
Repeat cycle every 4 weeks (maximum: 6 cycles)

References
Tsimberidou AM, Wierda WG, Plunkett W, et al, "Phase I-II Study of Oxaliplatin, Fludarabine, Cytarabine, and Rituximab Combination Therapy in Patients With Richter's Syndrome or Fludarabine-Refractory Chronic Lymphocytic Leukemia," *J Clin Oncol*, 2008, 26(2):196-203.

OPA

Use Lymphoma, Hodgkin's disease
Regimen
Vincristine: I.V.: 1.5 mg/m^2/day (maximum dose: 2 mg) days 1, 8, and 15
[total dose/cycle = 4.5 mg/m^2]
Prednisone: Oral: 60 mg/m^2/day in 3 divided doses days 1 to 15
[total dose/cycle = 900 mg/m^2]
Doxorubicin: I.V.: 40 mg/m^2/day days 1 and 15
[total dose/cycle = 80 mg/m^2]
Second cycle may be given based on individual response; time between cycles not specified

References
Schellong G, Riepenhausen M, Creutzig U, et al, "Low Risk of Secondary Leukemias After Chemotherapy Without Mechlorethamine in Childhood Hodgkin's Disease. German-Austrian Pediatric Hodgkin's Disease Group," *J Clin Oncol*, 1997, 15(6):2247-53.

OPEC

Use Neuroblastoma
Regimen
Vincristine: I.V.: 1.5 mg/m^2 day 1
[total dose/cycle = 1.5 mg/m^2]
Cyclophosphamide: I.V.: 600 mg/m^2 day 1
[total dose/cycle = 600 mg/m^2]
Cisplatin: I.V.: 100 mg/m^2 day 2
[total dose/cycle = 100 mg/m^2]
Teniposide: I.V.: 150 mg/m^2 day 4
[total dose/cycle = 150 mg/m^2]
Repeat cycle every 21 days

References
Shafford EA, Rogers DW, Pritchard J, et al, "Advanced Neuroblastoma: Improved Response Rate Using a Multiagent Regimen (OPEC) Including Sequential Cisplatin and VM-26," *J Clin Oncol*, 1984, 2(7):742-7.

OPEC-D

Use Neuroblastoma
Regimen
Vincristine: I.V.: 1.5 mg/m^2 day 1
[total dose/cycle = 1.5 mg/m^2]
Cyclophosphamide: I.V.: 600 mg/m^2 day 1
[total dose/cycle = 600 mg/m^2]

Doxorubicin: I.V.: 40 mg/m^2 day 1
[total dose/cycle = 40 mg/m^2]
Cisplatin: I.V.: 100 mg/m^2 day 2
[total dose/cycle = 100 mg/m^2]
Teniposide: I.V.: 150 mg/m^2 day 4
[total dose/cycle = 150 mg/m^2]
Repeat cycle every 21 days

References

Shafford EA, Rogers DW, Pritchard J, et al, "Advanced Neuroblastoma: Improved Response Rate Using a Multiagent Regimen (OPEC) Including Sequential Cisplatin and VM-26," *J Clin Oncol*, 1984, 2(7):742-7.

OPPA

Use Lymphoma, Hodgkin's disease

Regimen

Vincristine: I.V.: 1.5 mg/m^2/day (maximum dose: 2 mg) days 1, 8, and 15
[total dose/cycle = 4.5 mg/m^2]
Prednisone: Oral: 60 mg/m^2/day in 3 divided doses days 1 to 15
[total dose/cycle = 900 mg/m^2]
Doxorubicin: I.V.: 40 mg/m^2/day days 1 and 15
[total dose/cycle = 80 mg/m^2]
Procarbazine: Oral: 100 mg/m^2/day in 2 or 3 divided doses days 1 to 15
[total dose/cycle = 1500 mg/m^2]
Second cycle may be given based on individual response; time between cycles not specified

References

Schellong G, Riepenhausen M, Creutzig U, et al, "Low Risk of Secondary Leukemias After Chemotherapy Without Mechlorethamine in Childhood Hodgkin's Disease. German-Austrian Pediatric Hodgkin's Disease Group," *J Clin Oncol*, 1997, 15(6):2247-53.

♦ **Oxaliplatin-Capecitabine (Biliary Cancer)** *see* CAPOX (Biliary Cancer) *on page 1246*

♦ **Oxaliplatin-Capecitabine (Colorectal Cancer)** *see* CAPOX (Colorectal Cancer) *on page 1246*

♦ **Oxaliplatin-Capecitabine-Epirubicin** *see* Epirubicin-Oxaliplatin-Capecitabine *on page 1306*

♦ **Oxaliplatin-Capecitabine (Pancreatic Cancer)** *see* CAPOX (Pancreatic Cancer) *on page 1247*

Oxaliplatin-Cytarabine-Dexamethasone (NHL Regimen)

Index Terms DHAX (NHL Regimen)

Use Lymphoma, non-Hodgkin's

Regimen

Dexamethasone: I.V. or Oral: 40 mg/day days 1 to 4
[total dose/cycle = 160 mg]
Oxaliplatin: I.V.: 130 mg/m^2 over 2 hours day 1
[total dose/cycle = 130 mg/m^2]
Cytarabine: I.V.: 2000 mg/m^2 over 3 hours every 12 hours for 2 doses day 2
[total dose/cycle = 4000 mg/m^2]
Repeat cycle every 3 weeks

References

Chau I, Webb A, Cunningham D, et al, "An Oxaliplatin-Based Chemotherapy in Patients With Relapsed or Refractory Intermediate and High-Grade Non-Hodgkin's Lymphoma," *Br J Haematol*, 2001, 115(4):786-92.

- **Oxaliplatin-Docetaxel (Ovarian Cancer)** *see* Docetaxel-Oxaliplatin (Ovarian Cancer) *on page 1292*
- **Oxaliplatin-Fludarabine-Cytarabine-Rituximab (CLL)** *see* OFAR (CLL) *on page 1381*

Oxaliplatin-Fluorouracil (Esophageal Cancer)

Index Terms Fluorouracil-Oxaliplatin (Esophageal Cancer)

Use Esophageal cancer

Regimen In combination with radiation therapy:
Oxaliplatin: I.V.: 85 mg/m^2/day over 2 hours days 1, 15, and 29
[total dose/cycle = 255 mg/m^2]
Fluorouracil: I.V.: 180 mg/m^2/day continuous infusion days 8 to 42
[total dose/cycle = 6300 mg/m^2]

References
Khushalani NI, Leichman CG, Proulx G, et al, "Oxaliplatin in Combination With Protracted-Infusion Fluorouracil and Radiation: Report of a Clinical Trial for Patients With Esophageal Cancer," *J Clin Oncol*, 2002, 20(12):2844-50.

- **Oxaliplatin-Fluorouracil-Leucovorin-Bevacizumab** *see* Bevacizumab-Oxaliplatin-Fluorouracil-Leucovorin *on page 1233*
- **Oxaliplatin-Gemcitabine (Pancreatic Cancer)** *see* Gemcitabine-Oxaliplatin (Pancreatic Cancer) *on page 1345*
- **Oxaliplatin-Gemcitabine-Rituximab (NHL)** *see* Gemcitabine-Oxaliplatin-Rituximab (NHL) *on page 1345*
- **Oxaliplatin-Gemcitabine (Testicular Cancer)** *see* GEMOX (Testicular Cancer) *on page 1347*
- **Oxaliplatin-Irinotecan-Fluorouracil-Leucovorin (Pancreatic Cancer)** *see* FOLFIRINOX (Pancreatic Cancer) *on page 1336*
- **Oxaliplatin-Leucovorin-Fluorouracil (Gastric/Esophageal Cancer)** *see* Fluorouracil-Leucovorin-Oxaliplatin (Gastric/Esophageal Cancer) *on page 1334*
- **Oxaliplatin-Leucovorin-Fluorouracil (Gastric Cancer)** *see* Fluorouracil-Leucovorin-Oxaliplatin (Gastric Cancer) *on page 1334*

PAC (CAP)

Use Ovarian cancer

Regimen
Cisplatin: I.V.: 50 mg/m^2 day 1
[total dose/cycle = 50 mg/m^2]
Doxorubicin: I.V.: 50 mg/m^2 day 1
[total dose/cycle = 50 mg/m^2]
Cyclophosphamide: I.V.: 1000 mg/m^2 day 1
[total dose/cycle = 1000 mg/m^2]
Repeat cycle every 21 days for 8 cycles

References
Omura GA, Bundy BN, Berek JS, et al, "Randomized Trial of Cyclophosphamide Plus Cisplatin With or Without Doxorubicin in Ovarian Carcinoma: A Gynecologic Oncology Group Study," *J Clin Oncol*, 1989, 7(4):457-65.

PA-CI

Use Hepatoblastoma

Regimen NOTE: Multiple variations are listed.
Variation 1:
Cisplatin: I.V.: 90 mg/m^2 day 1
[total dose/cycle = 90 mg/m^2]

Doxorubicin: I.V.: 20 mg/m^2/day continuous infusion days 2 to 5
[total dose/cycle = 80 mg/m^2]
Repeat cycle every 21 days
Variation 2:
Cisplatin: I.V.: 20 mg/m^2/day days 1 to 4
[total dose/cycle = 80 mg/m^2]
Doxorubicin: I.V.: 100 mg/m^2 continuous infusion day 1
[total dose/cycle = 100 mg/m^2]
Repeat cycle every 21-28 days

References

Variation 1:
Ortega JA, Douglass EC, Feusner JH, et al, "Randomized Comparison of Cisplatin/Vincristine/ Fluorouracil and Cisplatin/Continuous Infusion Doxorubicin for Treatment of Pediatric Hepatoblastoma: A Report From the Children's Cancer Group and the Pediatric Oncology Group," *J Clin Oncol*, 2000, 18(14):2665-75.

Variation 2:
Ortega JA, Krailo MD, Haas JE, et al, "Effective Treatment of Unresectable or Metastatic Hepatoblastoma With Cisplatin and Continuous Infusion Doxorubicin Chemotherapy: A Report From the Childrens Cancer Study Group," *J Clin Oncol*, 1991, 9(12):2167-76.

Paclitaxel-Bevacizumab

Index Terms Bevacizumab-Paclitaxel

Use Breast cancer

Regimen

Paclitaxel: I.V.: 90 mg/m^2/day days 1, 8, and 15
[total dose/cycle = 270 mg/m^2]
Bevacizumab: I.V.: 10 mg/kg/day days 1 and 15
[total dose/cycle = 20 mg/kg]
Repeat cycle every 28 days

References

Miller KD, "E2100: A Phase III Trial of Paclitaxel Versus Paclitaxel/Bevacizumab for Metastatic Breast Cancer," *Clin Breast Cancer*, 2003, 3(6):421-2.

Miller K, Wang M, Gralow J, et al, "Paclitaxel Plus Bevacizumab Versus Paclitaxel Alone for Metastatic Breast Cancer," *N Engl J Med*, 2007, 357(26):2666-76.

◆ **Paclitaxel-Carboplatin (Adenocarcinoma)** *see* Carbo-Tax (Adenocarcinoma) *on page 1250*

Paclitaxel-Carboplatin-Bevacizumab

Index Terms Bevacizumab-Paclitaxel-Carboplatin

Use Lung cancer, nonsquamous, nonsmall cell

Regimen

Paclitaxel: I.V.: 200 mg/m^2 infused over 3 hours day 1
[total dose/cycle = 200 mg/m^2]
followed by
Carboplatin: I.V.: Target AUC 6 day 1
[total dose/cycle = AUC = 6]
followed by
Bevacizumab: I.V.: 15 mg/kg day 1
[total dose/cycle = 15 mg/kg]
Repeat cycle every 21 days for 6 cycles

References

Johnson DH, Fehrenbacher L, Novotny WF, "Randomized Phase II Trial Comparing Bevacizumab Plus Carboplatin and Paclitaxel With Carboplatin and Paclitaxel Alone in Previously Untreated Locally Advanced or Metastatic Nonsmall-Cell Lung Cancer," *J Clin Oncol*, 2004, 22(11):2184-91.

Sandler A, Gray R, Perry MC, et al, "Paclitaxel-Carboplatin Alone or With Bevacizumab for Nonsmall-Cell Lung Cancer," *N Engl J Med*, 2006, 355(24):2542-50.

Paclitaxel-Carboplatin (Bladder Cancer)

Index Terms Carboplatin-Paclitaxel (Bladder Cancer); PC (Bladder Cancer)

Use Bladder cancer

Regimen

Paclitaxel: I.V.: 200 mg/m^2 or 225 mg/m^2 day 1

[total dose/cycle = 200 or 225 mg/m^2]

Carboplatin: I.V.: AUC 5-6 day 1

[total dose/cycle = AUC = 5-6]

Repeat cycle every 21 days

References

Vaughn DJ, Malkowicz SB, Zoltick B, et al, "Paclitaxel Plus Carboplatin in Advanced Carcinoma of the Urothelium: An Active and Tolerable Outpatient Regimen," *J Clin Oncol*, 1998, 16(1):255-60.

Paclitaxel-Carboplatin (Cervical Cancer)

Index Terms Carboplatin-Paclitaxel (Cervical Cancer)

Use Cervical cancer

Regimen NOTE: Multiple variations are listed.

Variation 1:

Paclitaxel: I.V.: 175 mg/m^2 over 3 hours day 1

[total dose/cycle = 175 mg/m^2]

Carboplatin: I.V.: AUC 5 or 6 day 1

[total dose/cycle = AUC = 5 or 6]

Repeat cycle every 28 days for 6-9 cycles

Variation 2 (if patient has received prior pelvic radiation):

Paclitaxel: I.V.: 155 mg/m^2 over 3 hours day 1

[total dose/cycle = 155 mg/m^2]

Carboplatin: I.V.: AUC 5 or 6 day 1

[total dose/cycle = AUC = 5 or 6]

Repeat cycle every 28 days for 6-9 cycles

References

Tinker AV, Bhagat K, Swenerton KD, et al, "Carboplatin and Paclitaxel for Advanced and Recurrent Cervical Carcinoma: The British Columbia Cancer Agency Experience," *Gynecol Oncol*, 2005, 98 (1):54-8.

♦ **Paclitaxel-Carboplatin-Erlotinib (NSCLC)** *see* Erlotinib-Paclitaxel-Carboplatin (NSCLC) *on page 1312*

Paclitaxel-Carboplatin-Etoposide

Use Adenocarcinoma, unknown primary

Regimen

Paclitaxel: I.V.: 200 mg/m^2 infused over 1 hour day 1

[total dose/cycle = 200 mg/m^2]

followed by

Carboplatin: I.V.: Target AUC 6

[total dose = AUC = 6]

Etoposide: Oral: 50 mg/day days 1, 3, 5, 7, and 9

and Oral: 100 mg/day days 2, 4, 6, 8, and 10

[total dose/cycle = 750 mg]

Repeat cycle every 21 days

References

Hainsworth JD, Erland JB, Kalman LA, et al, "Carcinoma of Unknown Primary Site: Treatment With 1-Hour Paclitaxel, Carboplatin, and Extended-Schedule Etoposide," *J Clin Oncol*, 1997, 15 (6):2385-93.

Paclitaxel-Carboplatin-Gemcitabine

Use Bladder cancer

Regimen

Paclitaxel: I.V.: 200 mg/m^2 day 1
  [total dose/cycle = 200 mg/m^2]
Gemcitabine: I.V.: 1000 mg/m^2/day days 1 and 8
  [total dose/cycle = 2000 mg/m^2]
Carboplatin: I.V.: AUC 5 day 1
  [total dose/cycle = AUC = 5]
Repeat cycle every 21 days

References

Hainsworth JD, Meluch AA, Litchy S, et al, "Paclitaxel, Carboplatin, and Gemcitabine in the Treatment of Patients With Advanced Transitional Cell Carcinoma of the Urothelium," *Cancer*, 2005, 103(11):2298-303

♦ **Paclitaxel-Carboplatin (Nonsmall Cell Lung Cancer)** *see* Carbo-Tax (NSCLC) *on page 1250*

♦ **Paclitaxel-Carboplatin (Ovarian Cancer)** *see* Carboplatin-Paclitaxel (Ovarian Cancer) *on page 1248*

♦ **Paclitaxel-Carboplatin-Trastuzumab** *see* Trastuzumab-Paclitaxel-Carboplatin *on page 1409*

Paclitaxel-Cetuximab

Index Terms Cetuximab-Paclitaxel

Use Head and neck cancer

Regimen

Week 1:
Paclitaxel: I.V.: 80 mg/m^2 day 1
  [total dose/week 1 = 80 mg/m^2]
Cetuximab: I.V.: 400 mg/m^2 (loading dose) day 1 (week 1 only)
  [total loading dose (week 1) = 400 mg/m^2]
Subsequent weeks:
Paclitaxel: I.V.: 80 mg/m^2 day 1
  [total dose/week = 80 mg/m^2]
Cetuximab: I.V.: 250 mg/m^2 day 1
  [total dose/week = 250 mg/m^2]

References

Hitt R, Irigoyen H, Nunez J, et al, "Phase II Study of Combination Cetuximab and Weekly Paclitaxel in Patients With Metastatic/Recurrent Squamous Cell Carcinama of Head and Neck (SCCHN): Spanish Head and Neck Cancer Group (TTCC)," *J Clin Oncol*, 2007, 25(18S) [abstract 6012 from 2007 ASCO Annual Meeting].

Paclitaxel-Cisplatin (Cervical Cancer)

Index Terms Cisplatin-Paclitaxel (Cervical Cancer)

Use Cervical cancer

Regimen

Paclitaxel: I.V.: 135 mg/m^2 continuous infusion over 24 hours day 1
  [total dose/cycle = 135 mg/m^2]
Cisplatin: I.V.: 50 mg/m^2 day 1
  [total dose/cycle = 50 mg/m^2]
Repeat cycle every 21 days for 6 cycles

References

Moore DH, Blessing JA, McQuellon RP, et al, "Phase III Study of Cisplatin With or Without Paclitaxel in Stage IVB, Recurrent, or Persistent Squamous Cell Carcinoma of the Cervix: A Gynecologic Oncology Group Study," *J Clin Oncol*, 2004, 22(15):3113-9.

Paclitaxel-Cisplatin-Fluorouracil (Esophageal Cancer)

Index Terms Paclitaxel-Fluorouracil-Cisplatin (Esophageal Cancer); TCF (Esophageal Cancer)

Use Esophageal cancer

Regimen

Paclitaxel: I.V.: 175 mg/m^2 over 3 hours day 1
  [total dose/cycle = 175 mg/m^2]
Cisplatin: I.V.: 20 mg/m^2/day days 1 to 5 for cycles 1, 2, and 3
  [total dose/cycle = 100 mg/m^2]
    then 15 mg/m^2/day days 1 to 5
    [total dose/cycle = 75 mg/m^2]
Fluorouracil: I.V.: 750 mg/m^2/day continuous infusion days 1 to 5
  [total dose/cycle = 3750 mg/m^2]
Repeat cycle every 28 days

References

Ilson DH, Ajani J, Bhalla K, et al, "Phase II Trial of Paclitaxel, Fluorouracil, and Cisplatin in Patients With Advanced Carcinoma of the Esophagus," *J Clin Oncol*, 1998, 16(5):1826-34.

♦ **Paclitaxel-Cisplatin (Intraperitoneal Regimen)** see Cisplatin-Paclitaxel (Intra-peritoneal Regimen) *on page 1272*

♦ **Paclitaxel-Cisplatin (Ovarian Cancer)** see Cisplatin-Paclitaxel (Ovarian Cancer) *on page 1273*

♦ **Paclitaxel-Estramustine** see Estramustine-Paclitaxel *on page 1315*

Paclitaxel + Estramustine + Carboplatin

Use Prostate cancer

Regimen

Paclitaxel: I.V.: 100 mg/m^2 day 3 each week
  [total dose/cycle = 400 mg/m^2]
Estramustine: Oral: 10 mg/kg/day days 1 to 5 each week
  [total dose/cycle = 200 mg/kg]
Carboplatin: I.V.: Target AUC 6 day 3
  [total dose/cycle = AUC = 6]
Repeat cycle every 28 days

References

Kelly WK, Curley T, Slovin S, et al, "Paclitaxel, Estramustine Phosphate, and Carboplatin in Patients With Advanced Prostate Cancer," *J Clin Oncol*, 2001, 19(1):44-53.

Paclitaxel + Estramustine + Etoposide

Use Prostate cancer

Regimen

Paclitaxel: I.V.: 135 mg/m^2 day 2
  [total dose/cycle = 135 mg/m^2]
Estramustine: Oral: 280 mg 3 times/day days 1 to 14
  [total dose/cycle = 11,760 mg]
Etoposide: Oral: 100 mg/day days 1 to 14
  [total dose/cycle = 1400 mg]
Repeat cycle every 21 days

References

Smith DC, Esper P, Strawderman M, et al, "Phase II Trial of Oral Estramustine, Oral Etoposide, and Intravenous Paclitaxel in Hormone-Refractory Prostate Cancer," *J Clin Oncol*, 1999, 17 (6):1664-71.

♦ **Paclitaxel-Fluorouracil-Cisplatin (Esophageal Cancer)** see Paclitaxel-Cis-platin-Fluorouracil (Esophageal Cancer) *on page 1388*

Paclitaxel-Gemcitabine

Index Terms Gemcitabine-Paclitaxel

Use Bladder cancer

Regimen
Paclitaxel: I.V.: 200 mg/m² day 1
[total dose/cycle = 200 mg/m²]
Gemcitabine: I.V.: 1000 mg/m²/day days 1, 8, and 15
[total dose/cycle = 3000 mg/m²]
Repeat cycle every 21 days for a maximum of 6 cycles

References
Meluch AA, Greco FA, Burris HA 3rd, et al, "Paclitaxel and Gemcitabine Chemotherapy for Advanced Transitional-Cell Carcinoma of the Urothelial Tract: A Phase II Trial of the Minnie Pearl Cancer Research Network," *J Clin Oncol*, 2001, 19(12):3018-24.

Paclitaxel-Ifosfamide-Cisplatin

Index Terms Cisplatin-Ifosfamide-Paclitaxel

Use Testicular cancer

Regimen
Paclitaxel: I.V.: 250 mg/m² continuous infusion day 1
[total dose/cycle = 250 mg/m²]
Ifosfamide: I.V.: 1500 mg/m²/day days 2 to 5
[total dose/cycle = 6000 mg/m²]
Cisplatin: I.V.: 25 mg/m²/day days 2 to 5
[total dose/cycle = 100 mg/m²]
Mesna: I.V.: 500 mg/m² prior to ifosfamide and every 4 hours for 2 doses, days 2 to 5
[total dose/cycle = 6000 mg/m²]
Repeat cycle every 21 days for 4 cycles

References
Kondagunta GV, Bacik J, Donadio A, et al, "Combination of Paclitaxel, Ifosfamide, and Cisplatin is an Effective Second-Line Therapy for Patients With Relapsed Testicular Germ Cell Tumors," *J Clin Oncol*, 2005, 23(27):6549-55.

◆ **Paclitaxel-Trastuzumab** *see* Trastuzumab-Paclitaxel *on page 1408*

Paclitaxel-Vinorelbine

Use Breast cancer

Regimen NOTE: Multiple variations are listed.
Variation 1:
Paclitaxel: I.V.: 135 mg/m² day 1
[total dose/cycle = 135 mg/m²]
Vinorelbine: I.V.: 30 mg/m² day 1
[total dose/cycle = 30 mg/m²]
Repeat cycle every 21 days
Variation 2:
Paclitaxel: I.V.: 150 mg/m² day 1
[total dose/cycle = 150 mg/m²]
Vinorelbine: I.V.: 25 mg/m² day 1
[total dose/cycle = 25 mg/m²]
Repeat cycle every 21 days
Variation 3:
Paclitaxel: I.V.: 135 mg/m² day 1
[total dose/cycle = 135 mg/m²]
Vinorelbine: I.V.: 30 mg/m²/day days 1 and 8
[total dose/cycle = 60 mg/m²]
Repeat cycle every 28 days

References

Variation 1:
Martin M, Lluch A, Casado A, et al, "Paclitaxel Plus Vinorelbine: An Active Regimen in Metastatic Breast Cancer Patients With Prior Anthracycline Exposure," *Ann Oncol*, 2000, 11(1):85-9.

Variation 2:
Vici P, Amodio A, Di Lauro L, et al, "First-Line Chemotherapy With Vinorelbine and Paclitaxel As Simultaneous Infusion in Advanced Breast Cancer," *Oncology*, 2000, 58(1):3-7.

Variation 3:
Romero Acuna LR, Langhi M, Perez J, et al, "Vinorelbine and Paclitaxel as First-Line Chemotherapy in Metastatic Breast Cancer," *J Clin Oncol*, 1999, 17(1):74-81.

♦ **Paclitaxel (Weekly)-Trastuzumab** *see* Trastuzumab-Paclitaxel (Weekly) on page 1410

♦ **PAD** *see* Bortezomib-Doxorubicin-Dexamethasone *on page 1238*

♦ **PC (Bladder Cancer)** *see* Paclitaxel-Carboplatin (Bladder Cancer) *on page 1386*

PCE

Use Adenocarcinoma, unknown primary

Regimen

Paclitaxel: I.V.: 200 mg/m^2 day 1
[total dose/cycle = 200 mg/m^2]
Carboplatin: I.V.: AUC = 6 day 1
[total dose/cycle = AUC = 6]
Etoposide: Oral: 50 mg/day days 1, 3, 5, 7, and 9
and Oral: 100 mg/day days 2, 4, 6, 8, and 10
[total dose/cycle = 750 mg]
Repeat cycle every 3 weeks

References

Greco FA, Burris HA 3rd, Erland JB, et al, "Carcinoma of Unknown Primary Site," *Cancer*, 2000, 89 (12):2655-60.

PC (NSCLC)

Use Lung cancer, nonsmall cell

Regimen NOTE: Multiple variations are listed.

Variation 1:
Paclitaxel: I.V.: 175-225 mg/m^2 day 1
[total dose/cycle = 175-225 mg/m^2]
Carboplatin: I.V.: Target AUC 5-7 day 1
[total dose/cycle = AUC = 5-7]
Repeat cycle every 21 days for 2-8 cycles

Variation 2:
Paclitaxel: I.V.: 175 mg/m^2 day 1
[total dose/cycle = 175 mg/m^2]
Cisplatin: I.V.: 80 mg/m^2 day 1
[total dose/cycle = 80 mg/m^2]
Repeat cycle every 21 days

Variation 3:
Paclitaxel: I.V.: 135 mg/m^2 continuous infusion day 1
[total dose/cycle = 135 mg/m^2]
Carboplatin: I.V.: AUC 7.5 day 2
[total dose/cycle = AUC = 7.5]
Repeat cycle every 21 days

Variation 4:
Paclitaxel: I.V.: 135 mg/m^2 continuous infusion day 1
[total dose/cycle = 135 mg/m^2]

Cisplatin: I.V.: 75 mg/m² day 2
[total dose/cycle = 75 mg/m²]
Repeat cycle every 21 days

References

Variation 1:

Hainsworth JD, Urba WJ, Hon JK, et al, "One-Hour Paclitaxel Plus Carboplatin in the Treatment of Advanced Nonsmall-Cell Lung Cancer: Results of a Multicentre, Phase II Trial," *Eur J Cancer*, 1998, 34(5):654-8.

Helsing M, Thaning L, Sederholm C, et al, "Treatment With Paclitaxel 1-H Infusion and Carboplatin of Patients With Advanced Nonsmall-Cell Lung Cancer: A Phase II Multicentre Trial. Joint Lung Cancer Study Group," *Lung Cancer*, 1999, 24(2):107-13.

Kosmidis PA, Mylonakis N, Fountzilas G, et al, "Paclitaxel and Carboplatin in Inoperable Nonsmall-Cell Lung Cancer: A Phase II Study," *Ann Oncol*, 1997, 8(7):697-9.

Laohavinij S, Maoleekoonpairoj S, Cheirsilpa A, et al, "Phase II Study of Paclitaxel and Carboplatin for Advanced Nonsmall-Cell Lung Cancer," *Lung Cancer*, 1999, 26(3):175-85.

Variation 2:

Giaccone G, Splinter TA, Debruyne C, et al, "Randomized Study of Paclitaxel-Cisplatin Versus Cisplatin-Teniposide in Patients With Advanced Nonsmall-Cell Lung Cancer. The European Organization for Research and Treatment of Cancer Lung Cancer Cooperative Group," *J Clin Oncol*, 1998, 16(6):2133-41.

Variation 3:

Langer CJ, Leighton JC, Comis RL, et al, "Paclitaxel by 24- or 1-Hour Infusion in Combination With Carboplatin in Advanced Nonsmall Cell Lung Cancer: The Fox Chase Cancer Center Experience," *Semin Oncol*, 1995, 22(4 Suppl 9):18-29.

Variation 4:

Schiller JH, Harrington D, Belani CP, et al, "Comparison of Four Chemotherapy Regimens for Advanced Nonsmall-Cell Lung Cancer," *N Engl J Med*, 2002, 346(2):92-8.

PCR

Index Terms Pentostatin-Cyclophosphamide-Rituximab

Use Leukemia, chronic lymphocytic

Regimen NOTE: Multiple variations are listed.

Variation 1:

Cycle 1:

Cyclophosphamide: I.V.: 600 mg/m² day 1
[total dose/cycle = 600 mg/m²]
Pentostatin: I.V.: 4 mg/m² day 1
[total dose/cycle = 4 mg/m²]
Treatment cycle is 3 weeks

Cycles 2-6:

Cyclophosphamide: I.V.: 600 mg/m² day 1
[total dose/cycle = 600 mg/m²]
Pentostatin: I.V.: 4 mg/m² day 1
[total dose/cycle = 4 mg/m²]
Rituximab: I.V.: 375 mg/m² day 1
[total dose/cycle = 375 mg/m²]
Repeat cycle every 3 weeks

Variation 2:

Cycle 1:

Pentostatin: I.V.: 2 mg/m² day 1
[total dose/cycle = 2 mg/m²]
Cyclophosphamide: I.V.: 600 mg/m² day 1
[total dose/cycle = 600 mg/m²]
Rituximab: I.V.: 100 mg/m² day 1 only
followed by I.V.: 375 mg/m²/day days 3 and 5 only
[total dose/cycle 1 = 850 mg/m²]
Treatment cycle is 3 weeks

◀ Cycles 2-6:

Pentostatin: I.V.: 2 mg/m² day 1

[total dose/cycle = 2 mg/m²]

Cyclophosphamide: I.V.: 600 mg/m² day 1

[total dose/cycle = 600 mg/m²]

Rituximab: I.V.: 375 mg/m² day 1

[total dose/cycle = 375 mg/m²]

Repeat cycle every 3 weeks

References

Variation 1:

Lamanna N, Kalaycio M, Maslak P, et al, "Pentostatin, Cyclophosphamide, and Rituximab Is an Active, Well-Tolerated Regimen for Patients With Previously Treated Chronic Lymphocytic Leukemia," *J Clin Oncol*, 2006, 24(10):1575-81.

Variation 2:

Kay NE, Geyer SM, Call TG, et al, "Combination Chemoimmunotherapy With Pentostatin, Cyclophosphamide, and Rituximab Shows Significant Clinical Activity With Low Accompanying Toxicity in Previously Untreated B Chronic Lymphocytic Leukemia," *Blood*, 2007, 109(2):405-11.

PCV (Brain Tumor Regimen)

Index Terms Procarbazine-CCNU-Vincristine; Procarbazine-Lomustine-Vincristine

Use Brain tumors

Regimen NOTE: Multiple variations are listed.

Variation 1:

Lomustine: Oral: 110 mg/m² day 1

[total dose/cycle = 110 mg/m²]

Procarbazine: Oral: 60 mg/m²/day days 8 to 21

[total dose/cycle = 840 mg/m²]

Vincristine: I.V.: 1.4 mg/m²/day (maximum dose: 2 mg) days 8 and 29

[total dose/cycle = 2.8 mg/m²; maximum: 4 mg]

Repeat cycle every 6 weeks for a total of 6 cycles

Variation 2:

Lomustine: Oral: 110 mg/m² day 1

[total dose/cycle = 110 mg/m²]

Procarbazine: Oral: 60 mg/m²/day days 8 to 21

[total dose/cycle = 840 mg/m²]

Vincristine: I.V.: 1.4 mg/m²/day (maximum dose: 2 mg) days 8 and 29

[total dose/cycle = 2.8 mg/m²; maximum: 4 mg]

Repeat cycle every 6 weeks for a total of 7 cycles

Variation 3:

Procarbazine: Oral: 75 mg/m²/day days 8 to 21

[total dose/cycle = 1050 mg/m²]

Lomustine: Oral: 130 mg/m² day 1

[total dose/cycle = 130 mg/m²]

Vincristine: I.V.: 1.4 mg/m²/day (no maximum) days 8 and 29

[total dose/cycle = 2.8 mg/m²; no maximum]

Repeat cycle every 6 weeks for a total of 6 cycles

Variation 4:

Procarbazine: Oral: 75 mg/m²/day days 8 to 21

[total dose/cycle = 1050 mg/m²]

Lomustine: Oral: 130 mg/m² day 1

[total dose/cycle = 130 mg/m²]

Vincristine: I.V.: 1.4 mg/m²/day (no maximum) days 8 and 29

[total dose/cycle = 2.8 mg/m²; no maximum]

Repeat cycle every 6 weeks for up to a total of 4 cycles

Variation 5:
  Lomustine: Oral: 110 mg/m^2 day 1
    [total dose/cycle = 110 mg/m^2]
  Procarbazine: Oral: 60 mg/m^2/day days 8 to 21
    [total dose/cycle = 840 mg/m^2]
  Vincristine: I.V.: 1.4 mg/m^2/day days 8 and 29
    [total dose/cycle = 2.8 mg/m^2]
  Repeat cycle every 6-8 weeks for 1 year

References

Variation 1:
van den Bent MJ, Carpentier AF, Brandes AA, et al, "Adjuvant Procarbazine, Lomustine, and Vincristine Improves Progression-Free Survival But Not Overall Survival in Newly Diagnosed Anaplastic Oligodendrogliomas and Oligoastrocytomas: A Randomized European Organisation for Research and Treatment of Cancer Phase III Trial," *J Clin Oncol*, 2006, 24(18):2715-22.

Variation 2:
Levin VA, Uhm JH, Jaeckle KA, et al, "Phase III Randomized Study of Postradiotherapy Chemotherapy With Alpha-Difluoromethylornithine-Procarbazine, N-(2-Chloroethyl)-N'-Cyclohexyl-N-Nitrosurea, Vincristine (DFMO-PCV) Versus PCV for Glioblastoma Multiforme," *Clin Cancer Res*, 2000, 6(10):3878-84.

Variation 3:
Cairncross G, Macdonald D, Ludwin S, et al, "Chemotherapy for Anaplastic Oligodendroglioma. National Cancer Institute of Canada Clinical Trials Group," *J Clin Oncol*, 1994, 12(10):2013-21.

Variation 4:
Intergroup Radiation Therapy Oncology Group Trial 9402, Cairncross G, Berkey B, et al, "Phase III Trial of Chemotherapy Plus Radiotherapy Compared With Radiotherapy Alone for Pure and Mixed Anaplastic Oligodendroglioma: Intergroup Radiation Therapy Oncology Group Trial 9402," *J Clin Oncol*, 2006, 24(18):2707-14.

Variation 5:
Levin VA, Silver P, Hannigan J, et al, "Superiority of Post-Radiotherapy Adjuvant Chemotherapy With CCNU, Procarbazine, and Vincristine (PCV) Over BCNU for Anaplastic Gliomas: NCOG 6G61 Final Report," *Int J Radiat Oncol Biol Phys*, 1990, 18(2):321-4.

PE-CAdO

Use Neuroblastoma
Regimen
  Cisplatin: I.V.: 100 mg/m^2 day 1
    [total dose/cycle = 100 mg/m^2]
  Teniposide: I.V.: 160 mg/m^2 day 3
    [total dose/cycle = 160 mg/m^2]
alternating with
  Cyclophosphamide: I.V.: 300 mg/m^2/day days 1 to 5
    [total dose/cycle = 1500 mg/m^2]
  Doxorubicin: I.V.: 60 mg/m^2 day 5
    [total dose/cycle = 60 mg/m^2]
  Vincristine: I.V.: 1.5 mg/m^2/day days 1 and 5
    [total dose/cycle = 3 mg/m^2]
  Repeat cycle every 21 days

References

Bernard JL, Philip T, Zucker JM, et al, "Sequential Cisplatin/VM-26 and Vincristine/Cyclophosphamide/Doxorubicin in Metastatic Neuroblastoma: An Effective Alternating Non-Cross-Resistant Regimen?" *J Clin Oncol*, 1987, 5(12):1952-9.

Pemetrexed (Bladder Cancer Regimen)

Use Bladder cancer
Regimen
  Pemetrexed: I.V.: 500 mg/m^2 infused over 10 minutes day 1
    [total dose/cycle = 500 mg/m^2]
  Repeat cycle every 21 days

References

Sweeney CJ, Roth BJ, Kabbinavar FF, et al, "Phase II Study of Pemetrexed for Second-Line Treatment of Transitional Cell Cancer of the Urothelium," *J Clin Oncol*, 2006, 24(21):3451-7.

Pemetrexed-Carboplatin (Mesothelioma)

Index Terms Carboplatin-Pemetrexed (Mesothelioma)

Use Malignant pleural mesothelioma

Regimen

Pemetrexed: I.V.: 500 mg/m^2 infused over 10 minutes day 1
[total dose/cycle = 500 mg/m^2]
Carboplatin: I.V.: AUC 5 infused over 30 minutes day 1 (start 30 minutes after pemetrexed)
[total dose/cycle = AUC = 5]
Repeat cycle every 21 days

References

Ceresoli GL, Zucali PA, Favaretto AG, et al, "Phase II Study of Pemetrexed Plus Carboplatin in Malignant Pleural Mesothelioma," *J Clin Oncol*, 2006, 24(9):1443-8.

◆ **Pemetrexed-Cisplatin (Mesothelioma)** *see* Cisplatin-Pemetrexed (Mesothelioma) *on page 1273*

Pemetrexed-Cisplatin (NSCLC)

Index Terms Cisplatin-Pemetrexed (NSCLC)

Use Lung cancer, nonsmall cell

Regimen

Pemetrexed: I.V.: 500 mg/m^2/dose day 1
[total dose/cycle = 500 mg/m^2]
Cisplatin: I.V.: 75 mg/m^2/dose day 1
[total dose/cycle = 75 mg/m^2]
Repeat cycle every 21 days for up to 6 cycles

References

Scagliotti GV, Parikh P, von Pawel J, et al, "Phase III Study Comparing Cisplatin Plus Gemcitabine With Cisplatin Plus Pemetrexed in Chemotherapy-Naive Patients With Advanced-Stage Non-Small-Cell Lung Cancer," *J Clin Oncol*, 2008, 26(21):3543-51.

Pentostatin-Cyclophosphamide

Use Leukemia, chronic lymphocytic

Regimen

Cyclophosphamide: I.V.: 600 mg/m^2 day 1
[total dose/cycle = 600 mg/m^2]
Pentostatin: I.V.: 4 mg/m^2 day 1
[total dose/cycle = 4 mg/m^2]
Repeat cycle every 3 weeks for up to 6 cycles

References

Weiss MA, Maslak PG, Jurcic JG, et al, "Pentostatin and Cyclophosphamide: An Effective New Regimen in Previously Treated Patients With Chronic Lymphocytic Leukemia," *J Clin Oncol*, 2003, 21(7):1278-84.

◆ **Pentostatin-Cyclophosphamide-Rituximab** *see* PCR *on page 1391*

◆ **PE (Prostate Cancer)** *see* Estramustine-Paclitaxel *on page 1315*

PFL (Colorectal Cancer)

Use Colorectal cancer

Regimen

Cisplatin: I.V.: 25 mg/m^2/day continuous infusion days 1 to 5
[total dose/cycle = 125 mg/m^2]

Fluorouracil: I.V.: 800 mg/m^2/day continuous infusion days 2 to 5
[total dose/cycle = 3200 mg/m^2]
Leucovorin calcium: I.V.: 500 mg/m^2/day continuous infusion days 1 to 5
[total dose/cycle = 2500 mg/m^2]
Repeat cycle every 28 days

References

Dreyfuss AI, Clark JR, Wright JE, et al, "Continuous Infusion High-Dose Leucovorin With 5-Fluorouracil and Cisplatin for Untreated Stage IV Carcinoma of the Head and Neck," *Ann Intern Med*, 1990, 112(3):167-72.

PFL (Head and Neck Cancer)

Use Head and neck cancer

Regimen NOTE: Multiple variations are listed.

Variation 1:

Cisplatin: I.V.: 25 mg/m^2/day continuous infusion days 1 to 5
[total dose/cycle = 125 mg/m^2]
Fluorouracil: I.V.: 800 mg/m^2/day continuous infusion days 2 to 6
[total dose/cycle = 4000 mg/m^2]
Leucovorin: I.V.: 500 mg/m^2/day continuous infusion days 1 to 6
[total dose/cycle = 3000 mg/m^2]
Repeat cycle every 28 days

Variation 2:

Cisplatin: I.V.: 100 mg/m^2 day 1
[total dose/cycle = 100 mg/m^2]
Fluorouracil: I.V.: 600-1000 mg/m^2/day continuous infusion days 1 to 5
[total dose/cycle = 3000-5000 mg/m^2]
Leucovorin: Oral: 50 mg/m^2 every 4-6 hours days 1 to 6
[total dose/cycle = 1200-1800 mg/m^2]
Repeat cycle every 21 days

References

Variation 1:
Dreyfuss AI, Clark JR, Wright JE, et al, "Continuous Infusion High-Dose Leucovorin With 5-Fluorouracil and Cisplatin for Untreated Stage IV Carcinoma of the Head and Neck," *Ann Intern Med*, 1990, 112(3):167-72.
Variation 2:
Vokes EE, Schilsky RL, Weichselbaum RR, et al, "Cisplatin, 5-Fluorouracil, and High-Dose Oral Leucovorin for Advanced Head and Neck Cancer," *Cancer*, 1989, 63(6 Suppl):1048-53.

PFL + IFN

Use Head and neck cancer

Regimen

Cisplatin: I.V.: 100 mg/m^2 day 1
[total dose/cycle = 100 mg/m^2]
Fluorouracil: I.V.: 640 mg/m^2/day continuous infusion days 1 to 5
[total dose/cycle = 3200 mg/m^2]
Leucovorin calcium: Oral: 100 mg every 4 hours days 1 to 5
[total dose/cycle = 3000 mg/m^2]
Interferon alfa-2b: SubQ: 2 x 10^6 units/m^2 days 1 to 6
[total dose/cycle = 12 x 10^6 units/m^2]

References

Brockstein BE, Weichselbaum RW, and Vokes EE, "Concomitant and Rapidly Alternating Chemoradiotherapy for Head and Neck Cancer," *Advances in Oncology*, 1998, 14:8-15.
Kies MS, Haraf DJ, Athanasiadis I, et al, "Induction Chemotherapy Followed by Concurrent Chemoradiation for Advanced Head and Neck Cancer: Improved Disease Control And Survival," *J Clin Oncol*, 1998, 16(8):2715-21.

POC

Use Brain tumors

Regimen

Prednisone: Oral: 40 mg/m^2/day days 1 to 14
[total dose/cycle = 560 mg/m^2]
Vincristine: I.V.: 1.5 mg/m^2/day (maximum dose: 2 mg) days 1, 8, and 15
[total dose/cycle = 4.5 mg/m^2]
Lomustine: Oral: 100 mg/m^2 day 1
[total dose/cycle = 100 mg/m^2]
Repeat cycle every 6 weeks

References

Finlay JL, Boyett JM, Yates AJ, et al, "Randomized Phase III Trial in Childhood High-Grade Astrocytoma Comparing Vincristine, Lomustine, and Prednisone With the Eight-Drugs-In-1-Day Regimen. Childrens Cancer Group," *J Clin Oncol*, 1995, 13(1):112-23.

POG-8651

Use Osteosarcoma

Regimen

(Surgery at week 10)

Methotrexate: I.V.: 12 g/m^2 weeks 0, 1, 5, 6, 13, 14, 18, 19, 23, 24, 37, and 38
[total dose/cycle = 144 g/m^2]
Leucovorin: (route not specified): 15 mg every 6 hours for 10 doses, weeks 0, 1, 5, 6, 13, 14, 18, 19, 23, 24, 37, and 38
[total dose/cycle = 1800 mg]
Doxorubicin: I.V.: 37.5 mg/m^2/dose days 1 and 2 of weeks 2, 7, 25, and 28
followed by I.V.: 30 mg/m^2/dose days 1, 2, and 3 of week 20
[total dose/cycle = 390 mg/m^2]
Cisplatin: I.V.: 60 mg/m^2/day days 1 and 2, weeks 2, 7, 25, and 28
[total dose/cycle = 480 mg/m^2]
Cyclophosphamide: I.V.: 600 mg/m^2/day days 1, 2, and 3, weeks 15, 31, 34, 39, and 42
[total dose/cycle = 9000 mg/m^2]
Bleomycin: I.V.: 15 units/m^2/day days 1, 2, and 3, weeks 15, 31, 34, 39, and 42
[total dose/cycle = 225 units/m^2]
Dactinomycin: I.V.: 0.6 mg/m^2/day days 1, 2, and 3, weeks 15, 31, 34, 39, and 42
[total dose/cycle = 9 mg/m^2]

or

(Surgery at week 0)

Methotrexate: 12 g/m^2 weeks 3, 4, 8, 9, 13, 14, 18, 19, 23, 24, 37, and 38
[total dose/cycle = 144 g/m^2]
Leucovorin: (route not specified): 15 mg every 6 hours for 10 doses, weeks 3, 4, 8, 9, 13, 14, 18, 19, 23, 24, 37, and 38
[total dose/cycle = 1800 mg]
Doxorubicin: I.V.: 37.5 mg/m^2/day days 1 and 2, weeks 5, 10, 25, and 28 and 30 mg/m^2 days 1, 2, and 3, week 20
[total dose/cycle = 390 mg/m^2]
Cisplatin: I.V.: 60 mg/m^2/day days 1 and 2, weeks 5, 10, 25, and 28
[total dose/cycle = 480 mg/m^2]
Cyclophosphamide: I.V.: 600 mg/m^2/day days 1, 2, and 3, weeks 15, 31, 34, 39, and 42
[total dose/cycle = 9000 mg/m^2]
Bleomycin: I.V.: 15 units/m^2/day days 1, 2, and 3, weeks 15, 31, 34, 39, and 42
[total dose/cycle = 225 units/m^2]

Dactinomycin: I.V.: 0.6 mg/m^2/day days 1, 2, and 3, weeks 15, 31, 34, 39, and 42

[total dose/cycle = 9 mg/m^2]

References

Goorin AM, Schwartzentruber DJ, Devidas M, et al, "Presurgical Chemotherapy Compared With Immediate Surgery and Adjuvant Chemotherapy for Nonmetastatic Osteosarcoma: Pediatric Oncology Group Study POG-8651," *J Clin Oncol*, 2003, 21(8):1574-80.

POMP

Use Leukemia, acute lymphocytic

Regimen Maintenance:

Mercaptopurine: Oral: 50 mg 3 times/day

[total dose/cycle = 4200-4650 mg]

Methotrexate: Oral: 20 mg/m^2 once weekly

[total dose/cycle = 80 mg/m^2]

Vincristine: I.V.: 2 mg day 1

[total dose/cycle = 2 mg]

Prednisone: Oral: 200 mg/day days 1 to 5

[total dose/cycle = 1000 mg]

Repeat cycle monthly for 2 years

References

Kantarjian HM, O'Brien S, Smith TL, et al, "Results of Treatment With Hyper-CVAD, a Dose-Intensive Regimen, in Adult Acute Lymphocytic Leukemia," *J Clin Oncol*, 2000, 18(3):547-61.

◆ **Prednisone-Mitoxantrone (Prostate Cancer)** see Mitoxantrone-Prednisone (Prostate Cancer) *on page 1368*

◆ **Procarbazine-CCNU-Vincristine** see PCV (Brain Tumor Regimen) *on page 1392*

◆ **Procarbazine-Lomustine-Vincristine** see PCV (Brain Tumor Regimen) *on page 1392*

Pro-MACE-CytaBOM

Use Lymphoma, non-Hodgkin's

Regimen

Prednisone: Oral: 60 mg/m^2/day days 1 to 14

[total dose/cycle = 840 mg/m^2]

Doxorubicin: I.V.: 25 mg/m^2 day 1

[total dose/cycle = 25 mg/m^2]

Cyclophosphamide: I.V.: 650 mg/m^2 day 1

[total dose/cycle = 650 mg/m^2]

Etoposide: I.V.: 120 mg/m^2 day 1

[total dose/cycle = 120 mg/m^2]

Cytarabine: I.V.: 300 mg/m^2 day 8

[total dose/cycle = 300 mg/m^2]

Bleomycin: I.V.: 5 units/m^2 day 8

[total dose/cycle = 5 units/m^2]

Vincristine: I.V.: 1.4 mg/m^2 (maximum dose: 2 mg) day 8

[total dose/cycle = 1.4 mg/m^2]

Methotrexate: I.V.: 120 mg/m^2 day 8

[total dose/cycle = 120 mg/m^2]

Leucovorin: Oral: 25 mg/m^2 every 6 hours for 4 doses (start 24 hours after methotrexate dose) day 9

[total dose/cycle = 100 mg/m^2]

Repeat cycle every 21 days

References
Longo DL, DeVita VT Jr, Duffey PL, et al, "Superiority of ProMACE-CytaBOM Over ProMACE-MOPP in the Treatment of Advanced Diffuse Aggressive Lymphoma: Results of a Prospective Randomized Trial," *J Clin Oncol*, 1991, 9(1):25-38.

PVA (POG 8602)

Index Terms AlinC 14

Use Leukemia, acute lymphocytic

Regimen

Induction:

Prednisone: Oral: 40 mg/m^2/day (maximum dose: 60 mg) given in 3 divided doses days 0 to 28
   [total dose/cycle = 1160 mg/m^2]

Vincristine: I.V.: 1.5 mg/m^2/day (maximum dose: 2 mg) days 0, 7, 14, and 21
   [total dose/cycle = 6 mg/m^2; maximum = 8 mg]

Asparaginase: I.M.: 6000 units/m^2 3 times per week for 2 weeks
   [total dose/cycle = 36,000 units/m^2]

Intrathecal therapy (triple): Days 0 and 22

Leucovorin: Route and dose not specified: Single dose 24 hours after every intrathecal treatment days 1 and 23

Administer one cycle only

CNS consolidation:

Mercaptopurine: Oral: 75 mg/m^2/day days 29 to 43
   [total dose/cycle = 1125 mg/m^2]

Intrathecal therapy (triple): Days 29 and 36

Leucovorin: Route and dose not specified: Single dose 24 hours after every intrathecal treatment days 30 and 37

Administer one cycle only

Intensification:

Regimen A:

Methotrexate: I.V.: 1000 mg/m^2 continuous infusion over 24 hours day 1
   [total dose/cycle = 1000 mg/m^2]

Cytarabine: I.V.: 1000 mg/m^2 continuous infusion over 24 hours day 1 (start 12 hours after start of methotrexate)
   [total dose/cycle = 1000 mg/m^2]

Leucovorin: I.M., I.V., or Oral: 30 mg/m^2 at 24 and 36 hours after the start of methotrexate
   [total dose/cycle = 60 mg/m^2]
   followed by I.M., I.V., or Oral: 3 mg/m^2 at 48, 60, and 72 hours after the start of methotrexate
   [total dose/cycle = 9 mg/m^2]

Repeat cycle every 3 weeks for 6 cycles (administered weeks 7, 10, 13, 16, 19, and 22)

Intrathecal therapy (triple): Weeks 9, 12, 15, and 18

Leucovorin: Route and dose not specified: Single dose 24 hours after every intrathecal treatment weeks 9, 12, 15, and 18

or

Regimen B:

Methotrexate: I.V.: 1000 mg/m^2 continuous infusion over 24 hours day 1
   [total dose/cycle = 1000 mg/m^2]

Cytarabine: I.V.: 1000 mg/m^2 continuous infusion over 24 hours day 1 (start 12 hours after methotrexate)
   [total dose/cycle = 1000 mg/m^2]

Leucovorin: I.M., I.V., or Oral: 30 mg/m² at 24 and 36 hours after the start of methotrexate

[total dose/cycle = 60 mg/m²]

followed by I.M., I.V., or Oral: 3 mg/m² at 48, 60, and 72 hours after the start of methotrexate

[total dose/cycle = 9 mg/m²]

Repeat cycle every 12 weeks for 6 cycles (administer weeks 7, 19, 31, 43, 55, and 67)

Intrathecal therapy (triple): Weeks 9, 12, 15, and 18

Leucovorin: Route and dose not specified: Single dose 24 hours after every intrathecal treatment weeks 9, 12, 15, and 18

Maintenance:
Regimen A:

Methotrexate: I.M.: 20 mg/m² weekly, weeks 25 to 156

[total dose/cycle = 2640 mg/m²]

Mercaptopurine: Oral: 75 mg/m² daily, weeks 25 to 156

[total dose/cycle = 69,300 mg/m²]

Intrathecal therapy (triple): Every 8 weeks, weeks 26 through 105

Leucovorin: Route and dose not specified: Single dose 24 hours after every intrathecal treatment weeks 26 through 105

Prednisone: Oral: 40 mg/m²/day (maximum dose: 60 mg) days 1 to 7 (given in 3 divided doses), weeks 8, 17, 25, 41, 57, 73, 89, and 105

[total dose/cycle = 2240 mg/m²; maximum: 3360 mg]

Vincristine: I.V.: 1.5 mg/m²/day (maximum dose: 2 mg) day 1, weeks 8, 9, 17, 18, 25, 26, 41, 42, 57, 58, 73, 74, 89, 90, 105, and 106

[total dose/cycle = 24 mg/m²; maximum: 32 mg]

or
Regimen B:

Methotrexate: I.M.: 20 mg/m² weekly, weeks 22-28, 34-40, 46-52, and 58-64

[total dose/cycle = 560 mg/m²]

Mercaptopurine: Oral: 75 mg/m² daily for 7 weeks, weeks 22-28, 34-40, 46-52, and 58-64

[total dose/cycle = 14700 mg/m²]

followed by

Methotrexate: I.M.: 20 mg/m² weekly, weeks 70 to 156

[total dose/cycle = 1720 mg/m²]

Mercaptopurine: Oral: 75 mg/m² daily, weeks 70 to 156

[total dose/cycle = 45,150 mg/m²]

Intrathecal therapy (triple): Every 8 weeks, weeks 26 through 105

Leucovorin: Route and dose not specified: Single dose 24 hours after every intrathecal treatment weeks 26 through 105

Prednisone: Oral: 40 mg/m²/day (maximum dose: 60 mg) days 1 to 7 (given in 3 divided doses), weeks 8, 17, 25, 41, 57, 73, 89, and 105

[total dose/cycle = 2240 mg/m²]

Vincristine: I.V.: 1.5 mg/m²/day (maximum dose: 2 mg) day 1, weeks 8, 9, 17, 18, 25, 26, 41, 42, 57, 58, 73, 74, 89, 90, 105, and 106

[total dose/cycle = 24 mg/m²; maximum dose: 32 mg]

References

Land VJ, Shuster JJ, Crist WM, et al, "Comparison of Two Schedules of Intermediate-Dose Methotrexate and Cytarabine Consolidation Therapy for Childhood B-Precursor Cell Acute Lymphoblastic Leukemia: A Pediatric Oncology Group Study," *J Clin Oncol*, 1994, 12(9):1939-45.

PVB

Use Testicular cancer

Regimen NOTE: Multiple variations are listed.

Variation 1:

Cisplatin: I.V.: 20 mg/m²/day days 1 to 5

[total dose/cycle = 100 mg/m²]

Vinblastine: I.V.: 0.2 mg/kg/day days 1 and 2

[total dose/cycle = 0.4 mg/kg]

Bleomycin: I.V.: 30 units/day days 2, 9, and 16

[total dose/cycle = 90 units]

Repeat cycle every 3 weeks

Variation 2:

Cisplatin: I.V.: 20 mg/m²/day days 1 to 5

[total dose/cycle = 100 mg/m²]

Vinblastine: I.V.: 0.15 mg/kg/day days 1 and 2

[total dose/cycle = 0.3 mg/kg]

Bleomycin: I.V.: 30 units/day days 2, 9, and 16

[total dose/cycle = 90 units]

Repeat cycle every 3 weeks

Variation 3:

Cisplatin: I.V.: 20 mg/m²/day days 1 to 5

[total dose/cycle = 100 mg/m²]

Vinblastine: I.V.: 6 mg/m²/day days 1 and 2

[total dose/cycle = 12 mg/m²]

Bleomycin: I.M.: 30 units/day days 2, 9, and 16

[total dose/cycle = 90 units]

Repeat cycle every 3 weeks

References

Variation 1:

Einhorn LH and Donohue J, "Cis-Diamminedichloroplatinum, Vinblastine, and Bleomycin Combination Chemotherapy in Disseminated Testicular Cancer," *Ann Intern Med*, 1977, 87 (3):293-8.

Variation 2:

Williams SD, Birch R, Einhorn LH, et al, "Treatment of Disseminated Germ-Cell Tumors With Cisplatin, Bleomycin, and Either Vinblastine or Etoposide," *N Engl J Med*, 1987, 316 (23):1435-40.

Variation 3:

Bodrogi I, Baki M, Horti J, et al, "Vinblastine, Cisplatin, and Bleomycin Treatment of Advanced Nonseminomatous Testicular Tumors," *Neoplasma*, 1990, 37(4):445-50.

◆ **PVB** see VBP on page 1419

PVDA

Use Leukemia, acute lymphocytic

Regimen Induction:

Prednisone: Oral: 60 mg/m²/day days 1 to 28

[total dose/cycle = 1680 mg/m²]

Vincristine: I.V.: 1.5 mg/m²/day days 1, 8, 15, and 22

[total dose/cycle = 6 mg/m²]

Daunorubicin: I.V.: 25 mg/m²/day days 1, 8, 15, and 22

[total dose/cycle = 100 mg/m²]

Asparaginase: I.M., SubQ, or I.V.: 5000 units/m²/day days 1 to 14

[total dose/cycle = 70,000 units/m²]

Administer one cycle only; used in conjunction with intrathecal chemotherapy

References

Hoelzer D, Thiel E, Loffler H, et al, "Intensified Therapy in Acute Lymphoblastic and Acute Undifferentiated Leukemia in Adults," *Blood*, 1984, 64(1):38-47.

◆ **R-CHOP** *see* Rituximab-CHOP *on page 1402*

R-CVP

Index Terms CVP-R; Rituximab-CVP; Rituximab-Cyclophosphamide-Vincristine-Prednisone

Use Lymphoma, non-Hodgkin's

Regimen

Rituximab: I.V.: 375 mg/m^2 day 1
[total dose/cycle = 375 mg/m^2]
Cyclophosphamide: I.V.: 750 mg/m^2 day 1
[total dose/cycle = 750 mg/m^2]
Vincristine: I.V.: 1.4 mg/m^2 day 1
[total dose/cycle = 1.4 mg/m^2]
Prednisone: Oral: 40 mg/m^2/day days 1 to 5
[total dose/cycle = 200 mg/m^2]
Repeat cycle every 21 days

References

Marcus R, Imrie K, Belch A, et al, "CVP Chemotherapy Plus Rituximab Compared With CVP as First-Line Treatment for Advanced Follicular Lymphoma," *Blood*, 2005, 105(4):1417-23.

Regimen A1

Use Neuroblastoma

Regimen

Cyclophosphamide: I.V.: 1.2 g/m^2 day 1
[total dose/cycle = 1.2 g/m^2]
Vincristine: I.V.: 1.5 mg/m^2 day 1
[total dose/cycle = 1.5 mg/m^2]
Doxorubicin: I.V.: 40 mg/m^2 day 3
[total dose/cycle = 40 mg/m^2]
Cisplatin: I.V.: 90 mg/m^2 day 5
[total dose/cycle = 90 mg/m^2]
Repeat cycle every 28 days

References

Kaneko M, Nishihira H, Mugishima H, et al, "Stratification of Treatment of Stage 4 Neuroblastoma Patients Based on N-myc Amplification Status. Study Group of Japan for Treatment of Advanced Neuroblastoma, Tokyo, Japan," *Med Pediatr Oncol*, 1998, 31(1):1-7.

Regimen A2

Index Terms Regimen new A1

Use Neuroblastoma

Regimen

Cyclophosphamide: I.V.: 1.2 g/m^2 day 1
[total dose/cycle = 1.2 g/m^2]
Etoposide: I.V.: 100 mg/m^2/day days 1 to 5
[total dose/cycle = 500 mg/m^2]
Doxorubicin: I.V.: 40 mg/m^2 day 3
[total dose/cycle = 40 mg/m^2]
Cisplatin: I.V.: 90 mg/m^2 day 5
[total dose/cycle = 90 mg/m^2]
Repeat cycle every 28 days

References
Kaneko M, Nishihira H, Mugishima H, et al, "Stratification of Treatment of Stage 4 Neuroblastoma Patients Based on N-myc Amplification Status. Study Group of Japan for Treatment of Advanced Neuroblastoma, Tokyo, Japan," *Med Pediatr Oncol*, 1998, 31(1):1-7.

◆ **Regimen new A1** *see* Regimen A2 *on page* 1401

◆ **R-EPOCH Dose Adjusted (NHL)** *see* EPOCH (Dose-Adjusted)-Rituximab (NHL) *on page* 1308

◆ **R-EPOCH (NHL)** *see* EPOCH-Rituximab (NHL) *on page* 1310

◆ **R-FCM (NHL)** *see* Fludarabine-Cyclophosphamide-Mitoxantrone-Rituximab *on page* 1326

◆ **RFM (NHL)** *see* Fludarabine-Mitoxantrone-Rituximab *on page* 1330

RICE

Index Terms R-ICE; Rituximab-ICE

Use Lymphoma, non-Hodgkin's

Regimen

Rituximab: I.V.: 375 mg/m^2/day days -2 and 1 (cycle 1)
  [total dose/cycle = 750 mg/m^2]
Rituximab: I.V.: 375 mg/m^2 day 1 (cycles 2 and 3)
  [total dose/cycle = 375 mg/m^2]
Etoposide: I.V.: 100 mg/m^2/days days 3, 4, and 5
  [total dose/cycle = 300 mg/m^2]
Carboplatin: I.V.: AUC = 5 (maximum dose: 800 mg) day 4
  [total dose/cycle = AUC = 5]
Ifosfamide: I.V.: 5000 mg/m^2 continuous infusion day 4
  [total dose/cycle = 5000 mg/m^2]
Mesna: I.V.: 5000 mg/m^2 continuous infusion day 4
  [total dose/cycle = 5000 mg/m^2]
Filgrastim: SubQ: 5 mcg/kg/day days 7 to 14 (cycles 1 and 2)
  [total dose/cycle = 40 mcg/kg]
Filgrastim: SubQ: 10 mcg/kg/day days 7 to 14 (cycle 3)
  [total dose/cycle = 80 mcg/kg]
Repeat cycle every 2 weeks

References
Kewalramani T, Zelenetz AD, Nimer SD, et al, "Rituximab and ICE as Second-Line Therapy before Autologous Stem Cell Transplantation for Relapsed or Primary Refractory Diffuse Large B-Cell Lymphoma," *Blood*, 2004, 103(10):3684-8.

◆ **R-ICE** *see* RICE *on page* 1402

◆ **Rituximab-Bendamustine** *see* Bendamustine-Rituximab *on page* 1229

Rituximab-CHOP

Index Terms CHOP-Rituximab; R-CHOP

Use Lymphoma, non-Hodgkin's

Regimen

Rituximab: I.V.: 375 mg/m^2 day 1
  [total dose/cycle = 375 mg/m^2]
Cyclophosphamide: I.V.: 750 mg/m^2 day 1
  [total dose/cycle = 750 mg/m^2]
Doxorubicin: I.V.: 50 mg/m^2 day 1
  [total dose/cycle = 50 mg/m^2]
Vincristine: I.V.: 1.4 mg/m^2 (maximum dose: 2 mg) day 1
  [total dose/cycle = 1.4 mg/m^2; maximum: 2 mg]

Prednisone: Oral: 40 mg/m^2/day days 1 to 5
[total dose/cycle = 200 mg/m^2]
Repeat cycle every 21 days

References

Coiffier B, Lepage E, Briere J, et al, "CHOP Chemotherapy Plus Rituximab Compared With CHOP Alone in Elderly Patients With Diffuse Large-B-Cell Lymphoma," *N Engl J Med*, 2002, 346 (4):235-42.

- ◆ **Rituximab-CVP** *see* R-CVP *on page 1401*

- ◆ **Rituximab-Cyclophosphamide-Vincristine-Prednisone** *see* R-CVP *on page 1401*

- ◆ **Rituximab-EPOCH Dose Adjusted (NHL)** *see* EPOCH (Dose-Adjusted)-Rituximab (NHL) *on page 1308*

- ◆ **Rituximab-EPOCH (NHL)** *see* EPOCH-Rituximab (NHL) *on page 1310*

- ◆ **Rituximab-Fludarabine-Cyclophosphamide (CLL)** *see* Fludarabine-Cyclophosphamide-Rituximab (CLL) *on page 1327*

- ◆ **Rituximab-Fludarabine-Cyclophosphamide-Mitoxantrone** *see* Fludarabine-Cyclophosphamide-Mitoxantrone-Rituximab *on page 1326*

- ◆ **Rituximab-Fludarabine-Cyclophosphamide (NHL-Follicular)** *see* Fludarabine-Cyclophosphamide-Rituximab (NHL-Follicular) *on page 1328*

- ◆ **Rituximab-Fludarabine-Mitoxantrone** *see* Fludarabine-Mitoxantrone-Rituximab *on page 1330*

- ◆ **Rituximab-Fludarabine-Mitoxantrone-Dexamethasone** *see* Fludarabine-Mitoxantrone-Dexamethasone-Rituximab *on page 1329*

- ◆ **Rituximab-ICE** *see* RICE *on page 1402*

- ◆ **Saltz Regimen** *see* Fluorouracil-Leucovorin-Irinotecan (Saltz Regimen) *on page 1333*

Stanford V Regimen

Use Lymphoma, Hodgkin's disease

Regimen NOTE: Multiple variations are listed.
Variation 1:
Mechlorethamine: I.V.: 6 mg/m^2 day 1
[total dose/cycle = 6 mg/m^2]
Doxorubicin: I.V.: 25 mg/m^2/day days 1 and 15
[total dose/cycle = 50 mg/m^2]
Vinblastine: I.V.: 6 mg/m^2/day days 1 and 15
[total dose/cycle = 12 mg/m^2]
Vincristine: I.V.: 1.4 mg/m^2/day (maximum dose: 2 mg) days 8 and 22
[total dose/cycle = 2.8 mg/m^2; maximum: 4 mg]
Bleomycin: I.V.: 5 units/m^2/day days 8 and 22
[total dose/cycle = 10 units/m^2]
Etoposide: I.V.: 60 mg/m^2/day days 15 and 16
[total dose/cycle = 120 mg/m^2]
Prednisone: Oral: 40 mg/m^2 every other day for 9 weeks
followed by tapering of dose by 10 mg every other day, beginning at week 10
Repeat cycle every 28 days for 3 cycles; **Note:** In cycle 3, for patients ≥50 years of age, decrease vinblastine dose to 4 mg/m^2/dose and decrease vincristine dose to 1 mg/m^2/dose
Variation 2:
Mechlorethamine: I.V.: 6 mg/m^2/dose weeks 1, 5, and 9
[total dose/cycle = 18 mg/m^2]

◄ Doxorubicin: I.V.: 25 mg/m^2/dose weeks 1, 3, 5, 7, 9, and 11
    [total dose/cycle = 150 mg/m^2]
Vinblastine: I.V.: 6 mg/m^2/dose weeks 1, 3, 5, 7, 9, and 11
    [total dose/cycle = 36 mg/m^2]
Vincristine: I.V.: 1.4 mg/m^2/dose (maximum dose: 2 mg) weeks 2, 4, 6, 8, 10, and 12
    [total dose/cycle = 8.4 mg/m^2; maximum: 12 mg]
Bleomycin: I.V.: 5 units/m^2/dose weeks 2, 4, 6, 8, 10, and 12
    [total dose/cycle = 30 units/m^2]
Etoposide: I.V.: 60 mg/m^2/day for 2 consecutive days, weeks 3, 7, and 11
    [total dose/cycle = 360 mg/m^2]
Prednisone: Oral: 40 mg/m^2 every other day for 10 weeks
    [total dose prior to taper = 1400 mg/m^2]
    followed by tapering of prednisone dose during weeks 11 and 12
Treatment cycle is 12 weeks

References

Variation 1:
Bartlett NL, Rosenberg SA, Hoppe RT, et al, "Brief Chemotherapy, Stanford V, and Adjuvant Radiotherapy for Bulky or Advanced-Stage Hodgkin's Disease: A Preliminary Report," *J Clin Oncol*, 1995, 13(5):1080-8.

Variation 2:
Horning SJ, Hoppe RT, Breslin S, et al, "Stanford V and Radiotherapy for Locally Extensive and Advanced Hodgkin's Disease: Mature Results of a Prospective Clinical Trial," *J Clin Oncol*, 2002, 20(3):630-7.

TAC

Index Terms ATC

Use Breast cancer

Regimen NOTE: Multiple variations are listed.

Variation 1:
Docetaxel: I.V.: 75 mg/m^2 day 1
    [total dose/cycle = 75 mg/m^2]
Doxorubicin: I.V.: 50 mg/m^2 day 1
    [total dose/cycle = 50 mg/m^2]
Cyclophosphamide: I.V.: 500 mg/m^2 day 1
    [total dose/cycle = 500 mg/m^2]
Repeat cycle every 3 weeks
Variation 2:
Docetaxel: I.V.: 60 mg/m^2 day 1
    [total dose/cycle = 60 mg/m^2]
Doxorubicin: I.V.: 60 mg/m^2 day 1
    [total dose/cycle = 60 mg/m^2]
Cyclophosphamide: I.V.: 600 mg/m^2 day 1
    [total dose/cycle = 600 mg/m^2]
Repeat cycle every 3 weeks

References

Variation 1:
Martin M, Pienkowski T, Mackey J, et al, "Adjuvant Docetaxel for Node-Positive Breast Cancer," *N Engl J Med*, 2005, 352(22):2302-13.
Nabholtz JM, Smylie M, Mackey JR, et al, "Docetaxel/Doxorubicin/Cyclophosphamide in the Treatment of Metastatic Breast Cancer," *Oncology (Williston Park)*, 1997, 11(6 Suppl 6):25-7.

Variation 2:
Smith RE, Anderson SJ, Brown A, et al,"Phase II Trial of Doxorubicin/Docetaxel/Cyclophosphamide for Locally Advanced and Metastatic Breast Cancer: Results From NSABP Trial BP-58," *Clin Breast Cancer*, 2002, 3(5):333-40.

TAD
Use Leukemia, acute myeloid
Regimen
Daunorubicin: I.V.: 60 mg/m²/day days 3, 4, and 5
  [total dose/cycle = 180 mg/m²]
Cytarabine: I.V.: 100 mg/m²/day continuous infusion days 1 and 2
  [total dose/cycle = 200 mg/m²]
    followed by I.V.: 100 mg/m²/day over 30 minutes every 12 hours days 3 to 8
    [total dose/cycle = 1200 mg/m²]
Thioguanine: Oral: 100 mg/m²/day every 12 hours days 3 to 9
  [total dose/cycle = 1400 mg/m²]
Administer one cycle only
References
Buchner T, Hiddemann W, Wormann B, et al, "Double Inductions Strategy for Acute Myeloid Leukemia: The Effect of High-Dose Cytarabine With Mitoxantrone Instead of Standard-Dose Cytarabine With Daunorubicin and 6-Thioguanine: A Randomized Trial by the German AML Cooperative Group," *Blood*, 1999, 93(12):4116-24.

Tamoxifen-Epirubicin
Use Breast cancer
Regimen
Tamoxifen: Oral: 20 mg daily
  [total dose/cycle = 560 mg]
Epirubicin: I.V.: 50 mg/m²/day days 1 and 8
  [total dose/cycle = 100 mg/m²]
Repeat epirubicin cycle every 28 days for 6 cycles; continue tamoxifen for 4 years
References
Wils JA, Bliss JM, Marty M, et al, "Epirubicin Plus Tamoxifen Versus Tamoxifen Alone in Node-Positive Postmenopausal Patients With Breast Cancer: A Randomized Trial of the International Collaborative Cancer Group." *J Clin Oncol*, 1999, 17(7):1988-98.

◆ **TC** *see* Docetaxel-Cyclophosphamide (TC) *on page 1291*

◆ **TCF (Esophageal Cancer)** *see* Paclitaxel-Cisplatin-Fluorouracil (Esophageal Cancer) *on page 1388*

TEX (Capecitabine + Docetaxel + Epirubicin)
Use Breast cancer
Regimen
Capecitabine: Oral: 1000 mg/m² twice daily days 1 to 14
  [total dose/cycle = 28,000 mg/m²]
Docetaxel: I.V.: 75 mg/m² day 1
  [total dose/cycle = 75 mg/m²]
Epirubicin: I.V.: 75 mg/m² day 1
  [total dose/cycle = 75 mg/m²]
Repeat cycle every 3 weeks
References
Venturini M, Durando A, Garrone O, et al, "Capecitabine in Combination With Docetaxel and Epirubicin in Patients With Previously Untreated, Advanced Breast Carcinoma," *Cancer*, 2003, 97 (5):1174-80.

Thalidomide-Dexamethasone
Index Terms Dexamethasone-Thalidomide
Use Multiple myeloma

◄ **Regimen** Note: Multiple variations are listed.

Variation 1:

Thalidomide: Oral: 100 mg/day days 1 to 28

[total dose/cycle = 2800 mg]

Dexamethasone: Oral: 40 mg/day days 1 to 4

[total dose/cycle = 160 mg]

Repeat cycle every 28 days

Variation 2:

Thalidomide: Oral: 200 mg/day days 1 to 14 cycle 1

followed by Oral: 400 mg/day days 15 to 28 cycle 1

[total dose/cycle = 8400 mg]

Thalidomide: Oral: 400 mg/day days 1 to 28 (subsequent cycles)

[total dose/cycle = 11,200 mg]

Dexamethasone: Oral: 20 mg/m^2/day days 1 to 4, 9 to 12, and 17 to 20 cycle 1 (subsequent cycles)

[total dose/cycle = 240 mg/m^2]

followed by Oral: 20 mg/m^2/day days 1 to 4 (subsequent cycles)

[total dose/cycle = 80 mg/m^2]

Repeat cycle every 28 days

Variation 3:

Thalidomide: Oral: 100 mg/day days 1 to 7, 150 mg/day days 8 to 14, 200 mg/day days 15 to 21, 250 mg/day days 22 to 28, and 300 mg/day days 29 to 35 (cycle 1)

[total dose/cycle = 7000 mg]

Thalidomide: Oral: 300 mg/day days 1 to 35 (subsequent cycles)

[total dose/cycle = 10,500 mg]

Dexamethasone: Oral: 20 mg/m^2/day days 1 to 4, 9 to 12, and 17 to 20

[total dose/cycle = 240 mg/m^2]

Repeat cycle every 35 days

Variation 4:

Thalidomide: Oral: 200 mg/day days 1 to 28

[total dose/cycle = 5600 mg]

Dexamethasone: Oral: 40 mg/day days 1 to 4, 9 to 12, and 17 to 20 (odd cycles)

[total dose/cycle = 480 mg]

Dexamethasone: Oral: 40 mg/day days 1 to 4 (even cycles)

[total dose/cycle = 160 mg]

Repeat cycle every 28 days

References

Variation 1:

Palumbo A, Giaccone L, Bertola A, et al, "Low-Dose Thalidomide Plus Dexamethasone Is an Effective Salvage Therapy for Advanced Myeloma," *Haematologica*, 2001, 86(4):399-403.

Variation 2:

Dimopoulos MA, Zervas K, Kouvatseas G, et al, "Thalidomide and Dexamethasone Combination for Refractory Multiple Myeloma," *Ann Oncol*, 2001, 12(7):991-5.

Variation 3:

Alexanian R, Weber D, Giralt S, et al, "Consolidation Therapy of Multiple Myeloma With Thalidomide-Dexamethasone After Intensive Chemotherapy," *Ann Oncol*, 2002, 13(7):1116-9.

Variation 4:

Rajkumar SV, Hayman S, Gertz MA, et al, "Combination Therapy With Thalidomide Plus Dexamethasone for Newly Diagnosed Myeloma," *J Clin Oncol*, 2002, 20(21):4319-23.

TIP

Use Esophageal cancer; Head and neck cancer

Regimen

Paclitaxel: I.V.: 175 mg/m^2 day 1
  [total dose/cycle = 175 mg/m^2]
Ifosfamide: I.V.: 1000 mg/m^2/day days 1, 2, and 3
  [total dose/cycle = 3000 mg/m^2]
Mesna: I.V.: 400 mg/m^2/day before ifosfamide days 1, 2, and 3
  plus I.V.: 200 mg/m^2 4 hours after ifosfamide days 1, 2, and 3
    [total dose/cycle = 1800 mg/m^2]
Cisplatin: I.V.: 60 mg/m^2 day 1
  [total dose/cycle = 60 mg/m^2]
Repeat cycle every 21-28 days

References

Shin DM, Glisson BS, Khuri FR, et al, "Phase II Trial of Paclitaxel, Ifosfamide, and Cisplatin in Patients With Recurrent Head and Neck Squamous Cell Carcinoma," *J Clin Oncol*, 1998, 16 (4):1325-30.

Topotecan-Cisplatin

Use Cervical cancer

Regimen Note: Body surface area capped at 2 m^2 maximum
Topotecan: I.V.: 0.75 mg/m^2/day days 1, 2, and 3
  [total dose/cycle = 2.25 mg/m^2]
Cisplatin: I.V.: 50 mg/m^2 day 1 only
  [total dose/cycle = 50 mg/m^2]
Repeat cycle every 21 days

References

Long HJ 3rd, Bundy BN, Grendys EC Jr, et al, "Randomized Phase III Trial of Cisplatin With or Without Topotecan in Carcinoma of the Uterine Cervix: A Gynecologic Oncology Group Study," *J Clin Oncol*, 2005, 23(21):4626-33.

Topotecan (Oral)-Cisplatin

Index Terms Cisplatin-Topotecan (Oral)

Use Lung cancer, small cell

Regimen

Topotecan: Oral: 1.7 mg/m^2/day days 1 to 5
  [total dose/cycle = 8.5 mg/m^2]
Cisplatin: I.V.: 60 mg/m^2 day 5 only
  [total dose/cycle = 60 mg/m^2]
Repeat cycle every 21 days for 4 cycles (or for 2 cycles beyond best response)

References

Eckardt JR, von Pawel J, Papai Z, et al, "Open-Label, Multicenter, Randomized, Phase III Study Comparing Oral Topotecan/Cisplatin Versus Etoposide/Cisplatin as Treatment for Chemotherapy-Naive Patients With Extensive-Disease Small-Cell Lung Cancer," *J Clin Oncol*, 2006, 24 (13):2044-51.

Topotecan (Oral Regimen)

Use Lung cancer, nonsmall cell; Lung cancer, small cell; Ovarian cancer

Regimen

Topotecan: Oral: 2.3 mg/m^2/day days 1 to 5
  [total dose/cycle = 11.5 mg/m^2]
Repeat cycle every 21 days

References
Clarke-Pearson DL, Van Le L, Iveson T, et al, "Oral Topotecan as Single-Agent Second-Line Chemotherapy in Patients With Advanced Ovarian Cancer," *J Clin Oncol*, 2001, 19(19):3967-75.

Eckardt JR, von Pawel J, Pujol JL, et al, "Phase III Study of Oral Compared With Intravenous Topotecan as Second-Line Therapy in Small-Cell Lung Cancer," *J Clin Oncol*, 2007, 25 (15):2086-92.

O'Brien ME, Ciuleanu TE, Tsekov H, et al, "Phase III Trial Comparing Supportive Care Alone With Supportive Care With Oral Topotecan in Patients With Relapsed Small-Cell Lung Cancer," *J Clin Oncol*, 2006, 24(34):5441-7.

Ramlau R, Gervais R, Krzakowski M, et al, "Phase III Study Comparing Oral Topotecan to Intravenous Docetaxel in Patients With Pretreated Advanced Non-Small-Cell Lung Cancer," *J Clin Oncol*, 2006, 24(18):2800-7.

White SC, Cheeseman S, Thatcher N, et al, "Phase II Study of Oral Topotecan in Advanced Non-Small Cell Lung Cancer," *Clin Cancer Res*, 2000, 6(3):868-73.

Topotecan (Weekly)

Use Lung cancer, small cell; Ovarian cancer

Regimen

Topotecan: I.V.: 4 mg/m^2/day days 1, 8, and 15
[total dose/cycle = 12 mg/m^2]
Repeat cycle every 28 days

References
Homesley HD, Hall DJ, Martin DA, et al, "A Dose-Escalating Study of Weekly Bolus Topotecan in Previously Treated Ovarian Cancer Patients," *Gynecol Oncol*, 2001, 83(2):394-9.

Levy T, Inbar M, Menczer J, et al, "Phase II Study of Weekly Topotecan in Patients With Recurrent or Persistent Epithelial Ovarian Cancer," *Gynecol Oncol*, 2004, 95(3):686-90.

Shah C, Ready N, Perry M, et al, "A Multi-Center Phase II Study of Weekly Topotecan as Second-Line Therapy for Small Cell Lung Cancer," *Lung Cancer*, 2007, 57(1):84-8.

♦ **TPF** see Docetaxel-Cisplatin-Fluorouracil (Head and Neck Cancer) *on page 1291*

♦ **Trastuzumab-Capecitabine** see Capecitabine-Trastuzumab *on page 1245*

♦ **Trastuzumab-Docetaxel** see Docetaxel-Trastuzumab *on page 1293*

♦ **Trastuzumab-Docetaxel-Carboplatin** see Docetaxel-Trastuzumab-Carboplatin *on page 1293*

♦ **Trastuzumab-Docetaxel-Cisplatin** see Docetaxel-Trastuzumab-Cisplatin *on page 1294*

♦ **Trastuzumab-Docetaxel-FEC** see Docetaxel-Trastuzumab-FEC *on page 1294*

♦ **Trastuzumab-Docetaxel (Weekly)** see Docetaxel (Weekly)-Trastuzumab *on page 1295*

Trastuzumab-Paclitaxel

Index Terms Paclitaxel-Trastuzumab

Use Breast cancer

Regimen NOTE: Multiple variations are listed.

Variation 1:
Cycle 1:
Paclitaxel: I.V.: 175 mg/m^2 day 1
[total dose/cycle = 175 mg/m^2]
Trastuzumab: I.V.: 4 mg/kg (loading dose) day 1
followed by I.V.: 2 mg/kg/day days 8 and 15
[total dose/cycle 1 = 8 mg/kg]
Treatment cycle is 21 days
Subsequent cycles:
Paclitaxel: I.V.: 175 mg/m^2 day 1
[total dose/cycle = 175 mg/m^2]

Trastuzumab: I.V.: 2 mg/kg/day days 1, 8, and 15
[total dose/cycle = 6 mg/kg]
Repeat cycle every 21 days for a total of at least 6 cycles
Variation 2:
Cycle 1:
Trastuzumab: I.V.: 4 mg/kg (loading dose) day 1
followed by I.V.: 2 mg/kg/day days 8 and 15
[total dose/cycle 1 = 8 mg/kg]
Paclitaxel: I.V.: 175 mg/m^2 day 2
[total dose/cycle = 175 mg/m^2]
Treatment cycle is 21 days
Subsequent cycles:
Trastuzumab: I.V.: 2 mg/kg/day days 1, 8, and 15
[total dose/cycle = 6 mg/kg]
Paclitaxel: I.V.: 175 mg/m^2 day 2
[total dose/cycle = 175 mg/m^2]
Repeat cycle every 21 days for a total of at least 6 cycles (continue weekly
trastuzumab after chemotherapy until disease progression or unacceptable toxicity)

References

Variation 1:
Slamon DJ, Leyland-Jones B, Shak S, et al, "Use of Chemotherapy Plus a Monoclonal Antibody Against HER2 for Metastatic Breast Cancer That Overexpresses HER2," *N Engl J Med*, 2001, 344(11):783-92.
Variation 2:
Robert N, Leyland-Jones B, Asmar L, et al, "Randomized Phase III Study of Trastuzumab, Paclitaxel, and Carboplatin Compared With Trastuzumab and Paclitaxel in Women With HER-2-Overexpressing Metastatic Breast Cancer," *J Clin Oncol*, 2006, 24(18):2786-92.

Trastuzumab-Paclitaxel-Carboplatin

Index Terms Paclitaxel-Carboplatin-Trastuzumab
Use Breast cancer
Regimen
Cycle 1:
Trastuzumab: I.V.: 4 mg/kg (loading dose) day 1
followed by I.V.: 2 mg/kg/day days 8 and 15
[total dose/cycle 1 = 8 mg/kg]
Paclitaxel: I.V.: 175 mg/m^2 day 2
[total dose/cycle = 175 mg/m^2]
Carboplatin: I.V.: AUC 6 day 2
[total dose/cycle = AUC = 6]
Treatment cycle is 21 days
Subsequent cycles:
Trastuzumab: I.V.: 2 mg/kg/day days 1, 8, and 15
[total dose/cycle = 6 mg/kg]
Paclitaxel: I.V.: 175 mg/m^2 day 2
[total dose/cycle = 175 mg/m^2]
Carboplatin: I.V.: AUC 6 day 2
[total dose/cycle = AUC = 6]
Repeat cycle every 21 days for a total of at least 6 cycles (continue weekly
trastuzumab after chemotherapy until disease progression or unacceptable toxicity)

References

Robert N, Leyland-Jones B, Asmar L, et al, "Randomized Phase III Study of Trastuzumab, Paclitaxel, and Carboplatin Compared With Trastuzumab and Paclitaxel in Women With HER-2-Overexpressing Metastatic Breast Cancer," *J Clin Oncol*, 2006, 24(18):2786-92.

Trastuzumab-Paclitaxel (Weekly)

Index Terms Paclitaxel (Weekly)-Trastuzumab

Use Breast cancer

Regimen NOTE: Multiple variations are listed.

Variation 1:

Week 1:

Trastuzumab: I.V.: 4 mg/kg (loading dose) day 1

[total dose/week 1 = 4 mg/kg]

Paclitaxel: I.V.: 90 mg/m^2 day 2

[total dose/week 1 = 90 mg/m^2]

Subsequent weeks:

Paclitaxel: I.V.: 90 mg/m^2 day 1

[total dose/week = 90 mg/m^2]

Trastuzumab: I.V.: 2 mg/kg day 1

[total dose/week = 2 mg/kg]

Repeat weekly

Variation 2:

Week 1:

Trastuzumab: I.V.: 4 mg/kg (loading dose) day 1

[total dose/week 1 = 4 mg/kg]

Paclitaxel: I.V.: 80 mg/m^2 day 1

[total dose/week 1 = 80 mg/m^2]

Subsequent weeks:

Trastuzumab: I.V.: 2 mg/kg day 1

[total dose/week = 2 mg/kg]

Paclitaxel: I.V.: 80 mg/m^2 day 1

[total dose/week = 80 mg/m^2]

Repeat weekly

References

Variation 1:

Seidman AD, Fornier MN, Esteva FJ, et al, "Weekly Trastuzumab and Paclitaxel Therapy for Metastatic Breast Cancer With Analysis of Efficacy by HER2 Immunophenotype and Gene Amplification," *J Clin Oncol*, 2001, 19(10):2587-95.

Variation 2:

Seidman AD, Berry D, Cirrincione C, et al, "Randomized Phase III Trial of Weekly Compared With Every-3-Weeks Paclitaxel for Metastatic Breast Cancer, With Trastuzumab for all HER-2 Overexpressors and Random Assignment to Trastuzumab or Not in HER-2 Nonoverexpressors: Final Results of Cancer and Leukemia Group B Protocol 9840," *J Clin Oncol*, 2008, 26 (10):1642-9.

◆ **Trastuzumab-Vinorelbine** see Vinorelbine-Trastuzumab on page 1423

Tretinoin-Arsenic Trioxide (APL)

Index Terms Arsenic Trioxide-ATRA (APL); ATRA-Arsenic Trioxide (APL)

Use Leukemia, acute promyelocytic

Regimen

Induction (continue until <5% blasts in marrow and no abnormal promyelocytes):

Tretinoin: Oral: 45 mg/m^2/day (in 2 divided doses) day 1 up to day 85

[total induction dose = up to 3825 mg/m^2]

Arsenic Trioxide: I.V.: 0.15 mg/kg/day over 1 hour beginning day 10 up to day 85

[total induction dose = up to 11.25 mg/kg]

Postremission therapy (beginning with complete remission):
Tretinoin: Oral: 45 mg/m^2/day weeks 1, 2, 5, 6, 9, 10, 13, 14, 17, 18, 21, 22, 25, 26
[total postremission dose = 4410 mg/m^2]
Arsenic Trioxide: I.V.: 0.15 mg/kg/day Monday through Friday weeks 1 to 4, 9 to 12, 17 to 20, and 25 to 28
[total postremission dose = 12 mg/kg]

References

Estey E, Garcia-Manero G, Ferrajoli A, et al, "Use of All-*Trans* Retinoic Acid Plus Arsenic Trioxide as an Alternative to Chemotherapy in Untreated Acute Promyelocytic Leukemia," *Blood*, 2006, 107(9):3469-73.

Ravandi F, Estey E, Jones D, et al, "Effective Treatment of Acute Promyelocytic Leukemia With All-*Trans*-Retinoic Acid, Arsenic Trioxide, and Gemtuzumab Ozogamicin," *J Clin Oncol*, 2009, 27 (4):504-10.

Tretinoin-Arsenic Trioxide-Gemtuzumab (APL)

Index Terms ATRA-Arsenic Trioxide-Gemtuzumab (APL)
Use Leukemia, acute promyelocytic
Regimen
Induction (continue until <5% blasts in marrow and no abnormal promyelocytes):
Tretinoin: Oral: 45 mg/m^2/day (in 2 divided doses) day 1 up to day 85
[total induction dose = up to 3825 mg/m^2]
Arsenic Trioxide: I.V.: 0.15 mg/kg/day over 1 hour beginning day 10 up to day 85
[total induction dose = up to 11.25 mg/kg]
Gemtuzumab: I.V.: 9 mg/m^2/dose day 1
[total induction dose = 9 mg/m^2]
Postremission therapy (beginning with complete remission):
Tretinoin: Oral: 45 mg/m^2/day weeks 1, 2, 5, 6, 9, 10, 13, 14, 17, 18, 21, 22, 25, 26
[total postremission dose = 4410 mg/m^2]
Arsenic Trioxide: I.V.: 0.15 mg/kg/day Monday through Friday weeks 1 to 4, 9 to 12, 17 to 20, and 25 to 28
[total postremission dose = 12 mg/kg]
Gemtuzumab: I.V.: 9 mg/m^2/dose once every 4-5 weeks until 28 weeks after complete remission (if tretinoin or arsenic trioxide are discontinued due to toxicity)

References

Ravandi F, Estey E, Jones D, et al, "Effective Treatment of Acute Promyelocytic Leukemia With All-*Trans*-Retinoic Acid, Arsenic Trioxide, and Gemtuzumab Ozogamicin," *J Clin Oncol*, 2009, 27 (4):504-10.

Tretinoin-Daunorubicin (APL)

Index Terms ATRA-Daunorubicin (APL); Daunorubicin-ATRA (APL); Daunorubicin-Tretinoin (APL)
Use Leukemia, acute promyelocytic
Regimen
Induction:
Tretinoin: Oral: 45 mg/m^2/day (in 2 divided doses) day 1 until hematologic complete remission
Daunorubicin: I.V.: 60 mg/m^2/day days 1, 2, and 3
[total dose/cycle = 180 mg/m^2]
Consolidation:
Course 1:
Daunorubicin: I.V.: 60 mg/m^2/day days 1, 2, and 3
[total dose/cycle = 180 mg/m^2]

Course 2:
  Daunorubicin: I.V.: 45 mg/m²/day days 1, 2, and 3
  [total dose/cycle = 135 mg/m²]
Maintenance:
  Mercaptopurine: Oral: 90 mg/m² daily
  [total dose/cycle = 8100 mg/m² (90 days)]
  Methotrexate: Oral: 15 mg/m² weekly
  [total dose/cycle = 180 mg/m²]
  Tretinoin: Oral: 45 mg/m²/day (in 2 divided doses) days 1 to 15
  [total dose/cycle = 675 mg/m²]
  Repeat cycle every 3 months for 2 years

References

Adès L, Chevret S, Raffoux E, et al, "Is Cytarabine Useful in the Treatment of Acute Promyelocytic Leukemia? Results of a Randomized Trial From the European Acute Promyelocytic Leukemia Group," *J Clin Oncol*, 2006, 24(36):5703-10.

Tretinoin-Daunorubicin-Cytarabine (APL)

Index Terms ATRA-Daunorubicin-Cytarabine (APL)

Use Leukemia, acute promyelocytic

Regimen NOTE: Multiple variations are listed.

Variation 1 (patients ≤60 years of age and WBC <10,000/mm³):
  Induction:
    Tretinoin: Oral: 45 mg/m²/day (in 2 divided doses) day 1 until hematologic complete remission
    Daunorubicin: I.V.: 60 mg/m²/day days 1, 2, and 3
    [total dose/cycle = 180 mg/m²]
    Cytarabine: I.V.: 200 mg/m²/day days 3 to 10
    [total dose/cycle = 1400 mg/m²]
  Consolidation:
    Course 1:
      Daunorubicin: I.V.: 60 mg/m²/day days 1, 2, and 3
      [total dose/cycle = 180 mg/m²]
      Cytarabine: I.V.: 200 mg/m²/day days 1 to 7
      [total dose/cycle = 1400 mg/m²]
    Course 2:
      Daunorubicin: I.V.: 45 mg/m²/day days 1, 2, and 3
      [total dose/cycle = 135 mg/m²]
      Cytarabine: I.V.: 1000 mg/m²/dose every 12 hours for 8 doses
      [total dose/cycle = 8000 mg/m²]
  Maintenance:
    Mercaptopurine: Oral: 90 mg/m² daily
    [total dose/cycle = 8100 mg/m² (90 days)]
    Methotrexate: Oral: 15 mg/m² weekly
    [total dose/cycle = 180 mg/m²]
    Tretinoin: Oral: 45 mg/m²/day (in 2 divided doses) days 1 to 15
    [total dose/cycle = 675 mg/m²]
    Repeat cycle every 3 months for 2 years
Variation 2 (patients ≤60 years of age and WBC ≥10,000/mm³):
  Induction:
    Tretinoin: Oral: 45 mg/m²/day (in 2 divided doses) day 1 until hematologic complete remission
    Daunorubicin: I.V.: 60 mg/m²/day days 1, 2, and 3
    [total dose/cycle = 180 mg/m²]

Cytarabine: I.V.: 200 mg/m²/day days 3 to 10
[total dose/cycle = 1400 mg/m²]
Consolidation:
Course 1:
Daunorubicin: I.V.: 60 mg/m²/day days 1, 2, and 3
[total dose/cycle = 180 mg/m²]
Cytarabine: I.V.: 200 mg/m²/day days 1 to 7
[total dose/cycle = 1400 mg/m²]
Course 2:
Daunorubicin: I.V.: 45 mg/m²/day days 1, 2, and 3
[total dose/cycle = 135 mg/m²]
Cytarabine: I.V.: 2000 mg/m²/dose every 12 hours for 10 doses
[total dose/cycle = 20,000 mg/m²]
Intrathecal prophylaxis: Five intrathecal injections: First dose in between induction and consolidation and 2 doses during each consolidation phase:
Methotrexate (preservative free): I.T.: 15 mg
Cytarabine (preservative free): I.T.: 50 mg
Corticosteroids (preservative free): I.T.: Dose unspecified
Maintenance:
Mercaptopurine: Oral: 90 mg/m² daily
[total dose/cycle = 8100 mg/m² (90 days)]
Methotrexate: Oral: 15 mg/m² weekly
[total dose/cycle = 180 mg/m²]
Tretinoin: Oral: 45 mg/m²/day (in 2 divided doses) days 1 to 15
[total dose/cycle = 675 mg/m²]
Repeat cycle every 3 months for 2 years
Variation 3 (patients >60 years of age and WBC >10,000/mm³):
Induction:
Tretinoin: Oral: 45 mg/m²/day (in 2 divided doses) day 1 until hematologic complete remission
Daunorubicin: I.V.: 60 mg/m²/day days 1, 2, and 3
[total dose/cycle = 180 mg/m²]
Cytarabine: I.V.: 200 mg/m²/day days 3 to 10
[total dose/cycle = 1400 mg/m²]
Consolidation:
Course 1:
Daunorubicin: I.V.: 60 mg/m²/day days 1, 2, and 3
[total dose/cycle = 180 mg/m²]
Cytarabine: I.V.: 200 mg/m²/day days 1 to 7
[total dose/cycle = 1400 mg/m²]
Course 2:
Daunorubicin: I.V.: 45 mg/m²/day days 1, 2, and 3
[total dose/cycle = 135 mg/m²]
Cytarabine: I.V.: 1000 mg/m²/dose every 12 hours for 8 doses
[total dose/cycle = 8,000 mg/m²]
Intrathecal prophylaxis: Five intrathecal injections: First dose in between induction and consolidation and 2 doses during each consolidation phase:
Methotrexate (preservative free): I.T.: 15 mg
Cytarabine (preservative free): I.T.: 50 mg
Corticosteroids (preservative free): I.T.: Dose unspecified
Maintenance:
Mercaptopurine: Oral: 90 mg/m² daily
[total dose/cycle = 8100 mg/m² (90 days)]
Methotrexate: Oral: 15 mg/m² weekly
[total dose/cycle = 180 mg/m²]

◀ Tretinoin: Oral: 45 mg/m²/day (in 2 divided doses) days 1 to 15
[total dose/cycle = 675 mg/m²]
Repeat cycle every 3 months for 2 years

References

Variations 1, 2, and 3:
Adès L, Chevret S, Raffoux E, et al, "Is Cytarabine Useful in the Treatment of Acute Promyelocytic Leukemia? Results of a Randomized Trial From the European Acute Promyelocytic Leukemia Group," *J Clin Oncol*, 2006, 24(36):5703-10.

Tretinoin-Idarubicin (APL)

Index Terms ATRA-Idarubicin (APL); Idarubicin-ATRA (APL); Idarubicin-Tretinoin (APL)

Use Leukemia, acute promyelocytic

Regimen NOTE: Multiple variations are listed.

Variation 1:

Induction:

Tretinoin: Oral: 45 mg/m²/day (in 2 divided doses) day 1 up to 90 days
[total dose/cycle = up to 4050 mg/m²]
≤20 years: Oral: 25 mg/m²/day (in 2 divided doses) day 1 up to 90 days
[total dose/cycle = up to 2250 mg/m²]
Idarubicin: I.V.: 12 mg/m²/day days 2, 4, 6, and 8 (omit day 8 for patients >70 years of age)
[total dose/cycle = 36-48 mg/m²]

Consolidation (administer courses sequentially at 1-month intervals for 3 months):

Course 1:
Idarubicin: I.V.: 5 mg/m²/day days 1 to 4
[total dose/cycle = 20 mg/m²]
or
Idarubicin: I.V.: 7 mg/m²/day days 1 to 4
[total dose/cycle = 28 mg/m²]
Tretinoin: Oral: 45 mg/m²/day (in 2 divided doses) days 1 to 15
[total dose/cycle = 675 mg/m²]

Course 2:
Mitoxantrone: I.V.: 10 mg/m²/day days 1 to 5
[total dose/cycle = 50 mg/m²]
or
Mitoxantrone: I.V.: 10 mg/m²/day days 1 to 5
[total dose/cycle = 50 mg/m²]
Tretinoin: Oral: 45 mg/m²/day (in 2 divided doses) days 1 to 15
[total dose/cycle = 675 mg/m²]

Course 3:
Idarubicin: I.V.: 12 mg/m² day 1
[total dose/cycle = 12 mg/m²]
or
Idarubicin: I.V.: 12 mg/m²/day days 1 and 2
[total dose/cycle = 24 mg/m²]
Tretinoin: Oral: 45 mg/m²/day (in 2 divided doses) days 1 to 15
[total dose/cycle = 675 mg/m²]

Maintenance:

Mercaptopurine: Oral: 50 mg/m² daily
[total dose/cycle = 4500 mg/m² (90 days)]
Methotrexate: I.M.: 15 mg/m² weekly
[total dose/cycle = 180 mg/m²]

Tretinoin: Oral: 45 mg/m^2/day (in 2 divided doses) days 1 to 15
  [total dose/cycle = 675 mg/m^2]
Repeat cycle every 3 months for 2 years
Variation 2:
Induction:
  Tretinoin: Oral: 45 mg/m^2/day (in 2 divided doses) day 1 up to 90 days
    [total dose/cycle = up to 4050 mg/m^2]
      <15 years: Oral: 25 mg/m^2/day (in 2 divided doses) day 1 up to 90 days
        [total dose/cycle = up to 2250 mg/m^2]
  Idarubicin: I.V.: 12 mg/m^2/day days 2, 4, 6, and 8
    [total dose/cycle = 48 mg/m^2]
Consolidation (administer courses sequentially at 1-month intervals for 3 months):
Course 1:
  Idarubicin: I.V.: 5 mg/m^2/day days 1 to 4
    [total dose/cycle = 20 mg/m^2]
Course 2:
  Mitoxantrone: I.V.: 10 mg/m^2/day days 1 to 5
    [total dose/cycle = 50 mg/m^2]
Course 3:
  Idarubicin: I.V.: 12 mg/m^2 day 1
    [total dose/cycle = 12 mg/m^2]
Maintenance:
  Mercaptopurine: Oral: 90 mg/m^2 daily
    [total dose/cycle = 8100 mg/m^2(90 days)]
  Methotrexate: I.M.: 15 mg/m^2 weekly
    [total dose/cycle = 180 mg/m^2]
  Tretinoin: Oral: 45 mg/m^2/day (in 2 divided doses) days 1 to 15
    [total dose/cycle = 675 mg/m^2]
  Repeat cycle every 3 months for 2 years
Variation 3 (patients ≥60 years of age):
Induction:
  Tretinoin: Oral: 45 mg/m^2/day (in 2 divided doses) day 1 up to 90 days
    [total dose/cycle = up to 4050 mg/m^2]
  Idarubicin: I.V.: 12 mg/m^2/day days 2, 4, 6, and 8 (omit day 8 for patients ≥70 years of age)
    [total dose/cycle = 36-48 mg/m^2]
Consolidation (administer courses sequentially at 1-month intervals for 3 months):
Course 1:
  Idarubicin: I.V.: 5 mg/m^2/day days 1 to 4
    [total dose/cycle = 20 mg/m^2]
  Tretinoin: Oral: 45 mg/m^2/day (in 2 divided doses) days 1 to 15 (if intermediate or high risk)
    [total dose/cycle = 675 mg/m^2]
Course 2:
  Mitoxantrone: I.V.: 10 mg/m^2/day days 1 to 5
    [total dose/cycle = 50 mg/m^2]
  Tretinoin: Oral: 45 mg/m^2/day (in 2 divided doses) days 1 to 15 (if intermediate or high risk)
    [total dose/cycle = 675 mg/m^2]
Course 3:
  Idarubicin: I.V.: 12 mg/m^2 day 1
    [total dose/cycle = 12 mg/m^2]

Tretinoin: Oral: 45 mg/m^2/day (in 2 divided doses) days 1 to 15 (if intermediate or high risk)
[total dose/cycle = 675 mg/m^2]

Maintenance:
Mercaptopurine: Oral: 50 mg/m^2 daily
[total dose/cycle = 4500 mg/m^2 (90 days)]
Methotrexate: I.M.: 15 mg/m^2 weekly
[total dose/cycle = 180 mg/m^2]
Tretinoin: Oral: 45 mg/m^2/day (in 2 divided doses) days 1 to 15
[total dose/cycle = 675 mg/m^2]
Repeat cycle every 3 months for 2 years

References

Variation 1:
Sanz MA, Martin G, Gonzalez M, et al, "Risk-Adapted Treatment of Acute Promyelocytic Leukemia With All-*Trans*-Retinoic Acid and Anthracycline Monochemotherapy: A Multicenter Study by the PETHEMA Group," *Blood*, 2004, 103(4):1237-43.

Variation 2:
Sanz MA, Martin G, Rayon C, et al, "A Modified AIDA Protocol With Anthracycline-Based Consolidation Results in High Antileukemic Efficacy and Reduced Toxicity in Newly Diagnosed PML/RARalpha-Positive Acute Promyelocytic Leukemia," *Blood*, 1999, 94(9):3015-21.

Variation 3:
Sanz MA, Vellenga E, Rayón C, et al, "All-*Trans* Retinoic Acid and Anthracycline Monochemotherapy for the Treatment of Elderly Patients With Acute Promyelocytic Leukemia," *Blood*, 2004, 104(12):3490-3.

TVTG

Use Leukemia, acute lymphocytic; Leukemia, acute myeloid

Regimen
Topotecan: I.V.: 1 mg/m^2/day continuous infusion days 1 to 5
[total dose/cycle = 5 mg/m^2]
Vinorelbine: I.V.: 20 mg/m^2/day days 0, 7, 14, and 21
[total dose/cycle = 80 mg/m^2]
Thiotepa: I.V.: 15 mg/m^2 day 2
Gemcitabine: I.V.: 3600 mg/m^2 day 7
Dexamethasone: Oral or I.V.: 45 mg/m^2/day days 7 to 14 (given in 3 divided doses)
[total dose/cycle = 315 mg/m^2]
Repeat cycle when ANC >500 cells/mm^3 and platelet count >75,000 cells/mm^3

References

Kolb EA and Steinherz PG, "A New Multidrug Reinduction Protocol With Topotecan, Vinorelbine, Thiotepa, Dexamethasone, and Gemcitabine for Relapsed or Refractory Acute Leukemia," *Leukemia*, 2003, 17(10):1967-72.

VAC Alternating With IE (Ewing's Sarcoma)

Use Ewing's sarcoma

Regimen
Cycle A: (Odd numbered cycles)
Cyclophosphamide: I.V.: 1200 mg/m^2 day 1 (followed by mesna; dose not specified)
[total dose/cycle = 1200 mg/m^2]
Vincristine: I.V.: 2 mg/m^2 (maximum dose: 2 mg) day 1
[total dose/cycle = 2 mg/m^2; maximum: 2 mg]
Doxorubicin: I.V.: 75 mg/m^2 day 1, for 5 cycles (maximum cumulative dose: 375 mg/m^2)
[total dose/cycle = 75 mg/m^2; maximum cumulative dose: 375 mg/m^2]

Dactinomycin: I.V.: 1.25 mg/m^2 day 1, begin cycle 11 (after reaching maximum cumulative doxorubicin dose)
[total dose/cycle = 1.25 mg/m^2]
Cycle B: (Even numbered cycles)
Ifosfamide: I.V.: 1800 mg/m^2/day days 1 to 5 (given with mesna)
[total dose/cycle = 9000 mg/m^2]
Etoposide: I.V.: 100 mg/m^2/day days 1 to 5
[total dose/cycle = 500 mg/m^2]
Alternate Cycles A and B, administering a cycle every 3 weeks (alternating in the following sequence: ABABAB) for 17 cycles

References

Grier HE, Krailo MD, Tarbell NJ, et al, "Addition of Ifosfamide and Etoposide to Standard Chemotherapy for Ewing's Sarcoma and Primitive Neuroectodermal Tumor of Bone," *N Engl J Med*, 2003, 348(8):694-701.

♦ **VAC (Ovarian Cancer)** *see* Vincristine-Dactinomycin-Cyclophosphamide (Ovarian Cancer) *on page 1421*

VAC Pulse

Use Rhabdomyosarcoma

Regimen

Vincristine: I.V.: 2 mg/m^2/dose (maximum dose: 2 mg/dose) every 7 days, for 12 weeks
Dactinomycin: I.V.: 0.015 mg/kg/day (maximum dose: 0.5 mg/day) days 1 to 5, every 3 months for 5 courses
Cyclophosphamide: Oral, I.V.: 10 mg/kg/day for 7 days, repeat every 6 weeks

References

Wilbur JR, Sutow WW, Sullivan MP, et al, "Chemotherapy of Sarcomas," *Cancer*, 1975, 36 (2):765-9.

VAC (Rhabdomyosarcoma)

Use Rhabdomyosarcoma

Regimen

Induction (weeks 1 to 17):
Vincristine: I.V. push: 1.5 mg/m^2 (maximum dose: 2 mg) day 1 of weeks 1 to 13, then one dose at week 17
Dactinomycin: I.V. push: 0.015 mg/kg/day (maximum dose: 0.5 mg) days 1 to 5 of weeks 1, 4, 7, and 17
Cyclophosphamide: I.V.: 2.2 g/m^2 day 1 of weeks 1, 4, 7, 10, 13, and 17
Continuation (weeks 21 to 44):
Vincristine: I.V. push: 1.5 mg/m^2 (maximum dose: 2 mg) day 1 of weeks 21 to 26, 30 to 35, and 39 to 44
Dactinomycin: I.V. push: 0.015 mg/kg/day (maximum dose: 0.5 mg) days 1 to 5 of weeks 21, 24, 30, 33, 39, and 42
Cyclophosphamide: I.V.: 2.2 g/m^2 day 1 of weeks 21, 24, 30, 33, 39, and 42

References

Baker KS, Anderson JR, Link MP, et al, "Benefit of Intensified Therapy for Patients With Local or Regional Embryonal Rhabdomyosarcoma: Results From the Intergroup Rhabdomyosarcoma Study IV," *J Clin Oncol*, 2000, 18(12):2427-34.

VAD

Use Multiple myeloma

Regimen

Vincristine: I.V.: 0.4 mg/day continuous infusion days 1 to 4
[total dose/cycle = 1.6 mg]

Doxorubicin: I.V.: 9 mg/m^2/day continuous infusion days 1 to 4
[total dose/cycle = 36 mg/m^2]
Dexamethasone: Oral: 40 mg/day days 1 to 4, 9 to 12, and 17 to 20
[total dose/cycle = 480 mg]
Repeat cycle every 28-35 days

References

Barlogie B, Smith L, and Alexanian R, "Effective Treatment of Advanced Multiple Myeloma Refractory to Alkylating Agents," *N Engl J Med*, 1984, 310(21):1353-6.

◆ **VAD-C (Wilms' Tumor)** *see* VDA-C (Wilms' Tumor) *on page 1420*

VAD/CVAD

Use Leukemia, acute lymphocytic

Regimen Induction cycle:
Vincristine: I.V.: 0.4 mg/day continuous infusion days 1 to 4 and 24 to 27
[total dose/cycle = 3.2 mg]
Doxorubicin: I.V.: 12 mg/m^2/day continuous infusion days 1 to 4 and 24 to 27
[total dose/cycle = 96 mg/m^2]
Dexamethasone: Oral: 40 mg/day days 1 to 4, 9 to 12, 17 to 20, 24 to 27, 32 to 35, and 40 to 43
[total dose/cycle = 960 mg]
Cyclophosphamide: I.V.: 1 g/m^2 day 24
[total dose/cycle = 1 g/m^2]
Administer one cycle only

References

Kantarjian H, Walters RS, Keating MJ, et al, "Results of the Vincristine, Doxorubicin, and Dexamethasone Regimen in Adults With Standard and High-Risk Acute Lymphocytic Leukemia," *J Clin Oncol*, 1990, 8(6):994-1004.

VATH

Use Breast cancer

Regimen
Vinblastine: I.V.: 4.5 mg/m^2 day 1
[total dose/cycle = 4.5 mg/m^2]
Doxorubicin: I.V.: 45 mg/m^2 day 1
[total dose/cycle = 45 mg/m^2]
Thiotepa: I.V.: 12 mg/m^2 day 1
[total dose/cycle = 12 mg/m^2]
Fluoxymesterone: Oral: 10 mg 3 times/day days 1 to 21
[total dose/cycle = 630 mg]
Repeat cycle every 21 days

References

Hart RD, Perloff M, and Holland JF, "One-Day VATH (Vinblastine, Adriamycin®, Thiotepa, and Halotestin®) Therapy for Advanced Breast Cancer Refractory to Chemotherapy," *Cancer*, 1981, 48(7):1522-7.

VBAP

Use Multiple myeloma

Regimen
Vincristine: I.V.: 1 mg day 1
[total dose/cycle = 1 mg]
Carmustine: I.V.: 30 mg/m^2 day 1
[total dose/cycle = 30 mg/m^2]
Doxorubicin: I.V.: 30 mg/m^2 day 1
[total dose/cycle = 30 mg/m^2]

Prednisone: Oral: 100 mg/day days 1 to 4
  [total dose/cycle = 400 mg]
Repeat cycle every 21 days

References

Bonnet J, Alexanian R, Salmon S, et al, "Vincristine, BCNU, Doxorubicin, and Prednisone (VBAP) Combination in the Treatment of Relapsing or Resistant Multiple Myeloma: A Southwest Oncology Group Study," *Cancer Treat Rep*, 1982, 66(6):1267-71.

VBMCP

Use Multiple myeloma

Regimen

Vincristine: I.V.: 1.2 mg/m^2 (maximum dose: 2 mg) day 1
  [total dose/cycle = 1.2 mg/m^2; maximum: 2 mg]
Carmustine: I.V.: 20 mg/m^2 day 1
  [total dose/cycle = 20 mg/m^2]
Melphalan: Oral: 8 mg/m^2/day days 1 to 4
  [total dose/cycle = 32 mg/m^2]
Cyclophosphamide: I.V.: 400 mg/m^2 day 1
  [total dose/cycle = 400 mg/m^2]
Prednisone: Oral: 40 mg/m^2/day days 1 to 7 (all cycles)
  [total dose/cycle = 280 mg/m^2]
    followed by Oral: 20 mg/m^2/day days 8 to 14 (first 3 cycles only)
      [total dose/cycle = 140 mg/m^2]
Repeat cycle every 35 days

References

Oken MM, Harrington DP, Abramson N, et al, "Comparison of Melphalan and Prednisone With Vincristine, Carmustine, Melphalan, Cyclophosphamide, and Prednisone in the Treatment of Multiple Myeloma: Results of Eastern Cooperative Oncology Group Study E2479," *Cancer*, 1997, 79(8):1561-7.

VBP

Index Terms PVB

Use Testicular cancer

Regimen

Vinblastine: I.V.: 0.15 mg/kg/day days 1 and 2
  [total dose/cycle = 0.3 mg/kg]
Bleomycin: I.V.: 30 units/day days 2, 9, and 16
  [total dose/cycle = 90 units]
Cisplatin: I.V.: 20 mg/m^2/day days 1 to 5
  [total dose/cycle = 100 mg/m^2]
Repeat cycle every 21 days for 4 cycles

References

Williams SD, Birch R, Einhorn LH, et al, "Treatment of Disseminated Germ-Cell Tumors With Cisplatin, Bleomycin, and Either Vinblastine or Etoposide," *N Engl J Med*, 1987, 316 (23):1435-40.

♦ **VC** see Vinorelbine-Cisplatin *on page 1422*

VCAP

Use Multiple myeloma

Regimen

Vincristine: I.V.: 1 mg/m^2 (maximum dose: 1.5 mg) day 1
  [total dose/cycle = 1 mg/m^2]
Cyclophosphamide: Oral: 125 mg/m^2/day days 1 to 4
  [total dose/cycle = 500 mg/m^2]

Doxorubicin: I.V.: 30 mg/m^2 day 1
[total dose/cycle = 30 mg/m^2]
Prednisone: Oral: 60 mg/m^2/day days 1 to 4
[total dose/cycle = 240 mg/m^2]
Repeat cycle every 21 days for 6-12 months

References
Salmon SE, Haut A, Bonnet JD, et al, "Alternating Combination Chemotherapy and Levamisole Improves Survival in Multiple Myeloma: A Southwest Oncology Group Study," *J Clin Oncol*, 1983, 1(8):453-61.

VD

Use Breast cancer
Regimen
Vinorelbine: I.V.: 25 mg/m^2/day days 1 and 8
[total dose/cycle = 50 mg/m^2]
Doxorubicin: I.V.: 50 mg/m^2 day 1
[total dose/cycle = 50 mg/m^2]
Repeat cycle every 3 weeks

References
Spielmann M, Dorval T, Turpin F, et al, "Phase II Trial of Vinorelbine/Doxorubicin as First-Line Therapy of Advanced Breast Cancer," *J Clin Oncol*, 1994 12(9):1764-70.

VDA-C (Wilms' Tumor)

Index Terms VAD-C (Wilms' Tumor)
Use Wilms' tumor
Regimen
Dactinomycin: I.V.: 15 mcg/kg/day days 1 to 5 of weeks 0, 13, 26, 39, 52, and 65
[total dose/cycle = 450 mcg/kg]
Cyclophosphamide: I.V.: 10 mg/kg/day days 1, 2, and 3 of weeks 6, 13, 19, 26, 32, 39, 45, 52, 58, and 65
[total dose/cycle = 300 mg/kg]
Doxorubicin: I.V.: 20 mg/m^2/day days 1, 2, and 3 of weeks 6, 19, 32, 45, and 58
[total dose/cycle = 300 mg/m^2]
Vincristine: I.V.: 1.5 mg/m^2 day 1 of weeks 1-10, 13, 14, 19, 20, 26, 27, 32, 33, 39, 40, 45, 46, 52, 53, 58, 59, 65, and 66
[total dose/cycle = 42 mg/m^2]

References
D'Angio GJ, Breslow N, Beckwith JB, et al, "Treatment of Wilms' Tumor. Results of the Third National Wilms' Tumor Study," *Cancer*, 1989, 64(2):349-60.

VIM-D (Hodgkin's Lymphoma)

Index Terms Etoposide-Ifosfamide-Mitoxantrone-Dexamethasone
Use Lymphoma, Hodgkin's disease
Regimen
Cycle 1:
Etoposide: I.V.: 100 mg/m^2 day 1
[total dose/cycle = 100 mg/m^2]
Ifosfamide: I.V.: 4 g/m^2 continuous infusion over 24 hours day 1
[total dose/cycle = 4 g/m^2]
Mesna: I.V.: 1 g/m^2 bolus day 1, followed by 6 g/m^2 continuous infusion over 36 hours
[total dose/cycle = 7 g/m^2]
Mitoxantrone: I.V.: 10 mg/m^2 day 1
[total dose/cycle = 10 mg/m^2]

Dexamethasone: Oral: 40 mg/day days 1 to 5
  [total dose/cycle = 200 mg]
Treatment cycle is 28 days
Cycle 2 and subsequent cycles (if mid-cycle neutrophil count >1500/mm^3; if not, continue with cycle 1 regimen):
Etoposide: I.V.: 100 mg/m^2/day days 1 and 2
  [total dose/cycle = 200 mg/m^2]
Ifosfamide: I.V.: 4 g/m^2 continuous infusion over 24 hours day 1
  [total dose/cycle = 4 g/m^2]
Mesna: I.V.: 1 g/m^2 bolus day 1, followed by 6 g/m^2 continuous infusion over 36 hours
  [total dose/cycle = 7 g/m^2]
Mitoxantrone: I.V.: 10 mg/m^2 day 1
  [total dose/cycle = 10 mg/m^2]
Dexamethasone: Oral: 40 mg/day days 1 to 5
  [total dose/cycle = 200 mg]
Repeat cycle every 28 days for up to 6 cycles

References

Phillips JK, Spearing RL, Davies JM, et al, "VIM-D Salvage Chemotherapy in Hodgkin's Disease," *Cancer Chemother Pharmacol*, 1990, 27(2):161-3.

♦ **Vinblastine-Cisplatin** *see* Cisplatin-Vinblastine (NSCLC) *on page 1274*

♦ **Vinblastine-Cisplatin-Dacarbazine** *see* Cisplatin-Vinblastine-Dacarbazine (Melanoma) *on page 1274*

♦ **Vinblastine-Methotrexate (Desmoid Tumor)** *see* Methotrexate-Vinblastine (Desmoid Tumor) *on page 1366*

Vincristine-Dactinomycin-Cyclophosphamide (Ovarian Cancer)

Index Terms VAC (Ovarian Cancer)

Use Ovarian cancer (germ cell tumor)

Regimen NOTE: Multiple variations are listed.
Variation 1:
Vincristine: I.V.: 1.5 mg/m^2 (maximum dose: 2 mg) days 1, 8, 15, and 22 for 2-3 cycles
  [total dose/cycle = 6 mg/m^2 (maximum: 8 mg)] for 2-3 cycles
Dactinomycin: I.V.: 300 mcg/m^2/day days 1 to 5
  [total dose/cycle = 1500 mcg/m^2]
Cyclophosphamide: I.V.: 150 mg/m^2/day days 1 to 5
  [total dose/cycle = 750 mg/m^2]
Repeat cycle every 4 weeks for at least 10 cycles; vincristine is only administered for 8-12 weeks
Variation 2:
Vincristine: I.V.: 1-1.5 mg/m^2 day 1
  [total dose/cycle = 1-1.5 mg/m^2]
Dactinomycin: I.V.: 500 mcg/day days 1 to 5
  [total dose/cycle = 2500 mcg]
Cyclophosphamide: I.V.: 5-7 mg/kg/day days 1 to 5
  [total dose/cycle = 25-35 mg/kg]
Repeat cycle every 4 weeks for up to 12 cycles

References

Variation 1:
Slayton RE, Park RC, Silverberg SG, et al, "Vincristine, Dactinomycin, and Cyclophosphamide in the Treatment of Malignant Germ Cell Tumors of the Ovary. A Gynecologic Oncology Group Study (A Final Report)," *Cancer*, 1985, 56(2):243-8.

Variation 2:
Gershenson DM, Copeland LJ, Kavanagh JJ, et al, "Treatment of Malignant Nondysgerminomatous Germ Cell Tumors of the Ovary With Vincristine, Dactinomycin, and Cyclophosphamide," *Cancer*, 1985, 56(12):2756-61.

Vinorelbine-Cisplatin

Index Terms Cisplatin-Vinorelbine; VC

Use Lung cancer, nonsmall cell

Regimen NOTE: Multiple variations are listed.

Variation 1:
Cisplatin: I.V.: 50 mg/m²/day days 1 and 8
[total dose/cycle = 100 mg/m²]
Vinorelbine: I.V.: 25 mg/m²/day days 1, 8, 15, and 22
[total dose/cycle = 100 mg/m²]
Repeat cycle every 28 days for total of 4 cycles

Variation 2:
Vinorelbine: I.V.: 25 mg/m²/day days 1, 8, 15, and 22
[total dose/cycle = 100 mg/m²]
Cisplatin: I.V.: 100 mg/m² day 1
[total dose/cycle = 100 mg/m²]
Repeat cycle every 28 days

Variation 3:
Vinorelbine: I.V.: 30 mg/m² weekly
Cisplatin: I.V.: 120 mg/m²/day days 1 and 29, then once every 6 weeks

Variation 4:
Vinorelbine: I.V.: 30 mg/m²/day days 1, 8, and 15
[total dose/cycle = 90 mg/m²]
Cisplatin: I.V.: 80 mg/m² day 1
[total dose/cycle = 80 mg/m²]
Repeat cycle every 21 days for total of 4 cycles
Note: Vinorelbine treatment is discontinued after day 1 of cycle 4

Variation 5:
Vinorelbine: I.V.: 30 mg/m²/day days 1, 8, 15, and 22
[total dose/cycle = 120 mg/m²]
Cisplatin: I.V.: 100 mg/m² day 1
[total dose/cycle = 100 mg/m²]
Repeat cycle every 28 days for total of 3 or 4 cycles
Note: Vinorelbine treatment is discontinued after day 1 of last treatment cycle

References

Variation 1:
Winton T, Livingston R, Johnson D, et al, "Vinorelbine Plus Cisplatin Vs. Observation in Resected Non-Small-Cell Lung Cancer," *N Engl J Med*, 2005, 352(25):2589-97.

Variation 2:
Kelly K, Crowley J, Bunn PA Jr, et al, "Randomized Phase III Trial of Paclitaxel Plus Carboplatin Versus Vinorelbine Plus Cisplatin in the Treatment of Patients With Advanced Nonsmall-Cell Lung Cancer: A Southwest Oncology Group Trial," *J Clin Oncol*, 2001, 19(13):3210-8.

Wozniak AJ, Crowley JJ, Balcerzak SP, et al, "Randomized Trial Comparing Cisplatin With Cisplatin Plus Vinorelbine in the Treatment of Advanced Nonsmall-Cell Lung Cancer: A Southwest Oncology Group Study," *J Clin Oncol*, 1998, 16(7):2459-65.

Variation 3:
Le Chevalier T, Brisgand D, Douillard JY, et al, "Randomized Study of Vinorelbine and Cisplatin Versus Vindesine and Cisplatin Versus Vinorelbine Alone in Advanced Nonsmall-Cell Lung Cancer: Results of a European Multicenter Trial Including 612 Patients," *J Clin Oncol*, 1994, 12 (2):360-7.

Le Chevalier T, Pujol JL, Douillard JY, et al, "A Three-Arm Trial of Vinorelbine (Navelbine) Plus Cisplatin, Vindesine Plus Cisplatin, and Single-Agent Vinorelbine in the Treatment of Nonsmall Cell Lung Cancer: An Expanded Analysis," *Semin Oncol*, 1994, 21(5 Suppl 10):28-33; discussion 33-4.

Variations 4 and 5:
Arriagada R, Bergman B, Dunant A, et al, "Cisplatin-Based Adjuvant Chemotherapy in Patients With Completely Resected Non-Small-Cell Lung Cancer," *N Engl J Med*, 2004, 350(4):351-60.

Vinorelbine-FEC

Index Terms FEC-Vinorelbine

Use Breast cancer

Regimen

Cycles 1 and 2:

Vinorelbine: I.V.: 25 mg/m^2/day days 1, 8, and 15

[total dose/cycle = 75 mg/m^2]

Treatment cycle is 21 days

Cycle 3:

Vinorelbine: I.V.: 25 mg/m^2/day days 1 and 8

[total dose/cycle 3 = 50 mg/m^2]

Treatment cycle is 21 days

Cycles 4, 5, and 6 (FEC):

Fluorouracil: I.V.: 600 mg/m^2 day 1

[total dose/cycle = 600 mg/m^2]

Epirubicin: I.V.: 60 mg/m^2 day 1

[total dose/cycle = 60 mg/m^2]

Cyclophosphamide: I.V.: 600 mg/m^2 day 1

[total dose/cycle = 600 mg/m^2]

Repeat FEC cycle every 21 days for total of 3 cycles

References

Joensuu H, Kellokumpu-Lehtinen PL, Bono P, et al, "Adjuvant Docetaxel or Vinorelbine With or Without Trastuzumab for Breast Cancer," *N Engl J Med*, 2006, 354(8):809-20.

Vinorelbine-Gemcitabine

Use Lung cancer, nonsmall cell

Regimen

Vinorelbine: I.V.: 20 mg/m^2/day days 1, 8, and 15

[total dose/cycle = 60 mg/m^2]

Gemcitabine: I.V.: 800 mg/m^2/day days 1, 8, and 15

[total dose/cycle = 2400 mg/m^2]

Repeat cycle every 28 days

References

Chen YM, Perng RP, Yang KY, et al, "A Multicenter Phase II Trial of Vinorelbine Plus Gemcitabine in Previously Untreated Inoperable (Stage IIIB/IV) Nonsmall Cell Lung Cancer," *Chest*, 2000, 117 (6):1583-9.

♦ **Vinorelbine-Gemcitabine-Doxorubicin (Liposomal)** *see* Gemcitabine-Vinorelbine-Doxorubicin (Liposomal) *on page 1346*

Vinorelbine-Trastuzumab

Index Terms Trastuzumab-Vinorelbine

Use Breast cancer

Regimen

Week 1:

Trastuzumab: I.V.: 4 mg/kg (loading dose) day 1 week 1

[total dose/week 1 = 4 mg/kg]

Vinorelbine: I.V.: 25 mg/m^2 day 1

[total dose/week 1 = 25 mg/m^2]

Subsequent weeks:

Trastuzumab: I.V.: 2 mg/kg (loading dose) day 1

[total dose/week = 2 mg/kg]

◀ Vinorelbine: I.V.: 25 mg/m² day 1
[total dose/week = 25 mg/m²]
Repeat weekly

References
Burstein HJ, Kuter I, Campos SM, et al, "Clinical Activity of Trastuzumab and Vinorelbine in Women With HER2-Overexpressing Metastatic Breast Cancer," *J Clin Oncol*, 2001, 19(10):2722-30.

Vinorelbine-Trastuzumab-FEC

Index Terms Vinorelbine-Trastuzumab-FEC

Use Breast cancer

Regimen
Cycle 1:
Trastuzumab: I.V.: 4 mg/kg (loading dose) day 1 cycle 1
followed by I.V.: 2 mg/kg/day days 8 and 15 cycle 1
[total dose/cycle 1 = 8 mg/kg]
Vinorelbine: I.V.: 25 mg/m²/day days 1, 8, and 15
[total dose/cycle 1 = 75 mg/m²]
Treatment cycle is 21 days
Cycle 2:
Trastuzumab: I.V.: 2 mg/kg/day days 1, 8, and 15
[total dose/cycle = 6 mg/kg]
Vinorelbine: I.V.: 25 mg/m²/day days 1, 8, and 15
[total dose/cycle 2 = 75 mg/m²]
Treatment cycle is 21 days
Cycle 3:
Trastuzumab: I.V.: 2 mg/kg/day days 1, 8, and 15
[total dose/cycle = 6 mg/kg]
Vinorelbine: I.V.: 25 mg/m²/day days 1 and 8
[total dose/cycle 3 = 50 mg/m²]
Treatment cycle is 21 days
Cycles 4, 5, and 6 (FEC):
Fluorouracil: I.V.: 600 mg/m² day 1
[total dose/cycle = 600 mg/m²]
Epirubicin: I.V.: 60 mg/m² day 1
[total dose/cycle = 60 mg/m²]
Cyclophosphamide: I.V.: 600 mg/m² day 1
[total dose/cycle = 600 mg/m²]
Repeat FEC cycle every 21 days for total of 3 cycles

References
Joensuu H, Kellokumpu-Lehtinen PL, Bono P, et al, "Adjuvant Docetaxel or Vinorelbine With or Without Trastuzumab for Breast Cancer," *N Engl J Med*, 2006, 354(8):809-20.

◆ **Vinorelbine-Trastuzumab-FEC** *see* Vinorelbine-Trastuzumab-FEC *on page 1424*

VIP (Etoposide) (Testicular Cancer)

Use Testicular cancer

Regimen NOTE: Multiple variations are listed.
Variation 1:
Etoposide: I.V.: 75 mg/m²/day days 1 to 5
[total dose/cycle = 375 mg/m²]
Ifosfamide: I.V.: 1200 mg/m²/day days 1 to 5
[total dose/cycle = 6000 mg/m²]
Cisplatin: I.V.: 20 mg/m²/day days 1 to 5
[total dose/cycle = 100 mg/m²]

Mesna: I.V.: 400 mg day 1 only
followed by I.V.: 1200 mg/day continuous infusion days 1 to 5
[total dose/cycle = 6400 mg]
Repeat cycle every 21 days for 4 cycles
Variation 2:
Etoposide: I.V.: 100 mg/m^2/day days 1 to 5
[total dose/cycle = 500 mg/m^2]
Ifosfamide: I.V.: 1200 mg/m^2/day days 1 to 5
[total dose/cycle = 6000 mg/m^2]
Cisplatin: I.V.: 20 mg/m^2/day days 1 to 5
[total dose/cycle = 100 mg/m^2]
Mesna: I.V.: 200 mg/m^2 every 4 hours, for 3 doses each day, days 1, 2, and 3
[total dose/cycle = 1800 mg/m^2]
Repeat cycle every 21 days
Variation 3:
Ifosfamide: I.V.: 2500 mg/m^2/day days 1 and 2
[total dose/cycle = 5000 mg/m^2]
Mesna: I.V.: 2400 mg/m^2/day days 1 and 2
[total dose/cycle = 4800 mg/m^2]
Etoposide: I.V.: 100 mg/m^2/day days 3, 4, and 5
[total dose/cycle = 300 mg/m^2]
Cisplatin: I.V.: 40 mg/m^2/day days 3, 4, and 5
[total dose/cycle = 120 mg/m^2]
Repeat cycle every 21 days
Variation 4:
Etoposide: I.V.: 75 mg/m^2/day days 1 to 5
[total dose/cycle = 375 mg/m^2]
Ifosfamide: I.V.: 1200 mg/m^2/day days 1 to 5
[total dose/cycle = 6000 mg/m^2]
Cisplatin: I.V.: 20 mg/m^2/day days 1 to 5
[total dose/cycle = 100 mg/m^2]
Mesna: I.V.: 120 mg/m^2 day 1 only
followed by I.V.: 1200 mg/m^2/day continuous infusion days 1 to 5
[total dose/cycle = 6120 mg/m^2]
Repeat cycle every 21 days for 4 cycles

References

Variation 1:
Loehrer PJ Sr, Lauer R, Roth BJ, et al, "Salvage Therapy in Recurrent Germ Cell Cancer: Ifosfamide and Cisplatin Plus Either Vinblastine or Etoposide," *Ann Intern Med*, 1988, 109 (7):540-6.
Variation 2:
Harstrick A, Schmoll HJ, Wilke H, et al, "Cisplatin, Etoposide, and Ifosfamide Salvage Therapy for Refractory or Relapsing Germ Cell Carcinoma," *J Clin Oncol*, 1991, 9(9):1549-55.
Variation 3:
Pizzocaro G, Salvioni R, Piva L, et al, "Modified Cisplatin, Etoposide (or Vinblastine) and Ifosfamide Salvage Therapy for Male Germ-Cell Tumors. Long-Term Results," *Ann Oncol*, 1992, 3(3):211-6.
Variation 4:
Nichols CR, Catalano PJ, Crawford ED, et al, "Randomized Comparison of Cisplatin and Etoposide and Either Bleomycin or Ifosfamide in Treatment of Advanced Disseminated Germ Cell Tumors: An Eastern Cooperative Oncology Group, Southwest Oncology Group, and Cancer and Leukemia Group B Study," *J Clin Oncol*, 1998, 16(4):1287-93.

VIP (Small Cell Lung Cancer)

Use Lung cancer, small cell
Regimen
Etoposide: I.V.: 75 mg/m^2/day days 1 to 4
[total dose/cycle = 300 mg/m^2]

◀ Ifosfamide: I.V.: 1200 mg/m²/day days 1 to 4
  [total dose/cycle = 4800 mg/m²]
Cisplatin: I.V.: 20 mg/m²/day days 1 to 4
  [total dose/cycle = 80 mg/m²]
Mesna: I.V.: 300 mg/m² day 1 only
  followed by I.V.: 1200 mg/m²/day continuous infusion days 1 to 4
  [total dose/cycle = 5100 mg/m²]
Repeat cycle every 21 days

References

Loehrer PJ Sr, Ansari R, Gonin R, et al, "Cisplatin Plus Etoposide With and Without Ifosfamide in Extensive Small-Cell Lung Cancer: A Hoosier Oncology Group Study," *J Clin Oncol*, 1995, 13 (10):2594-9.

VIP (Vinblastine) (Testicular Cancer)

Use Testicular cancer

Regimen NOTE: Multiple variations are listed.

Variation 1:
  Vinblastine: I.V.: 0.11 mg/kg/day days 1 and 2
    [total dose/cycle = 0.22 mg/kg]
  Ifosfamide: I.V.: 1200 mg/m²/day days 1 to 5
    [total dose/cycle = 6000 mg/m²]
  Cisplatin: I.V.: 20 mg/m²/day days 1 to 5
    [total dose/cycle = 100 mg/m²]
  Mesna: I.V.: 400 mg day 1
    followed by I.V.: 1200 mg/day continuous infusion days 1 to 5
    [total dose/cycle = 6400 mg]
  Repeat cycle every 21 days for 4 cycles
Variation 2:
  Vinblastine: I.V.: 6 mg/m²/day days 1 and 2
    [total dose/cycle = 12 mg/m²]
  Ifosfamide: I.V.: 1500 mg/m²/day days 1 to 5
    [total dose/cycle = 7500 mg/m²]
  Cisplatin: I.V.: 20 mg/m²/day days 1 to 5
    [total dose/cycle = 100 mg/m²]
  Mesna: I.V.: 300 mg/m² 3 times/day days 1 to 5
    [total dose/cycle = 4500 mg/m²]
  Repeat cycle every 21 days for 4 cycles

References

Variation 1:
Loehrer PJ Sr, Lauer R, Roth BJ, et al, "Salvage Therapy in Recurrent Germ Cell Cancer: Ifosfamide and Cisplatin Plus Either Vinblastine or Etoposide," *Ann Intern Med*, 1988, 109 (7):540-6.
Variation 2:
Clemm C, Hartenstein R, Willich N, et al, "Vinblastine-Ifosfamide-Cisplatin Treatment of Bulky Seminoma," *Cancer*, 1986, 58(10):2203-7.

VM

Use Breast cancer

Regimen

Variation 1:
  Mitomycin: I.V.: 10 mg/m² days 1 and 28 for 2 cycles
    [total dose/cycle = 20 mg/m²]
    followed by I.V.: 10 mg/m² day 1 only for subsequent cycles
    [total dose/cycle = 10 mg/m²]

Vinblastine: I.V.: 5 mg/m^2/day days 1, 14, 28, and 42 for 2 cycles
[total dose/cycle = 20 mg/m^2]
followed by I.V.: 5 mg/m^2/day days 1 and 21
[total dose/cycle = 10 mg/m^2]
Repeat cycle every 6-8 weeks
Variation 2:
Mitomycin: I.V.: 10 mg/m^2/day days 1 and 28 for 2 cycles
[total dose/cycle = 20 mg/m^2]
followed by I.V.: 10 mg/m^2 day 1 only for subsequent cycles
[total dose/cycle = 10 mg/m^2]
Vindesine: I.V.: 2 mg/m^2/day days 1, 14, 28, and 42 for 2 cycles
[total dose/cycle = 8 mg/m^2]
followed by I.V.: 2 mg/m^2/ day days 1 and 21 for subsequent cycles
[total dose/cycle = 4 mg/m^2]
Repeat cycle every 6-8 weeks

References

Garewal HS, Brooks RJ, Jones SE, et al, "Treatment of Advanced Breast Cancer With Mitomycin C Combined With Vinblastine or Vindesine," *J Clin Oncol*, 1983, 1(12):772-5.

✦ **VMP** *see* Bortezomib-Melphalan-Prednisone *on page 1240*

✦ **VMPT** *see* Bortezomib-Melphalan-Prednisone-Thalidomide *on page 1241*

VP (Small Cell Lung Cancer)

Use Lung cancer, small cell
Regimen
Etoposide: I.V.: 100 mg/m^2/day days 1 to 4
[total dose/cycle = 400 mg/m^2]
Cisplatin: I.V.: 20 mg/m^2/day days 1 to 4
[total dose/cycle = 80 mg/m^2]
Repeat cycle every 21 days

References

Loehrer PJ Sr, Ansari R, Gonin R, et al, "Cisplatin Plus Etoposide With and Without Ifosfamide in Extensive Small Cell Lung Cancer: A Hoosier Oncology Group Study," *J Clin Oncol*, 1995, 13 (10):2594-9.

V-TAD

Use Leukemia, acute myeloid
Regimen Induction:
Etoposide: I.V.: 50 mg/m^2/day days 1, 2, and 3
[total dose/cycle = 150 mg/m^2]
Thioguanine: Oral: 75 mg/m^2/day every 12 hours days 1 to 5
[total dose/cycle = 750 mg/m^2]
Daunorubicin: I.V.: 20 mg/m^2/day days 1 and 2
[total dose/cycle = 40 mg/m^2]
Cytarabine: I.V.: 75 mg/m^2/day continuous infusion days 1 to 5
[total dose/cycle = 375 mg/m^2]
Up to 3 cycles may be given based on individual response; time between cycles not specified

References

Bigelow CL, Kopecky K, Files JC, et al, "Treatment of Acute Myelogenous Leukemia in Patients Over 50 Years of Age With V-TAD: A Southwest Oncology Group Study," *Am J Hematol*, 1995, 48 (4):228-32.

✦ **Xelox (Colorectal Cancer)** *see* CAPOX (Colorectal Cancer) *on page 1246*

SPECIAL TOPICS

FERTILITY AND CANCER THERAPY

Antineoplastic therapy (chemotherapy, radiation, surgery) or cancer itself can affect fertility and/or sexual function in both men and women. Temporary or permanent sequelae that impact pregnancy outcomes, neonatal development, pubertal development, and gonadal function are possible in cancer survivors. Factors influencing fertility and reproduction in cancer survivors include the type and intensity of therapy, duration of therapy, age, and gender.

Primary Antineoplastic Agents Associated With Sterility

Women	Men
Busulfan	Busulfan
Chlorambucil	Chlorambucil
Cyclophosphamide	Cyclophosphamide
Mechlorethamine	Mechlorethamine
Melphalan	Nitrosoureas
Procarbazine	Procarbazine
Other alkylating agents	Other alkylating agents
	Cisplatin

FEMALES

Antineoplastic drugs can stop the development of follicles (vesicles within ovarian that contain oocytes) or damage oocytes (female egg cells). Prepubertal gonads may be more resistant than postpubertal gonads, possibly due to a larger number of follicles as compared to ovaries in older patients. Gonadal destruction causes clinical findings associated with estrogen deficiency such as amenorrhea, endometrial hypoplasia, vaginal atrophy and dryness, and hot flashes. Follicle stimulating hormone (FSH) levels become elevated and estrogen levels decrease with impaired ovarian function. The onset and duration of symptoms is dose- and age-related. Younger patients are able to tolerate higher doses of chemotherapy before symptoms develop and have a higher likelihood of the return of menses when therapy is stopped.

The effect of radiation on fertility depends on the age of the patient, the number of remaining oocytes at the time of radiation, and the exposure dose and field. Childhood cancer survivors who have received a hypothalamic/pituitary radiation dose of 30 gray (Gy) (RR = 0.61) or more or an ovarian uterine radiation dose exceeding 5 Gy (RR = 0.56) are less likely to ever become pregnant than their female siblings.

In vitro fertilization with embryo cryopreservation is an option for circumventing the gonadotoxic effect of antineoplastic therapy. Ovarian stimulation for oocyte collection generally involves estrogenic therapy and may be risky in women with hormonally-responsive cancers. The investigational procedure of oocyte cryopreservation may be considered when *in vitro* fertilization is impractical for women without a partner to provide sperm. Ovarian cryopreservation with autotransplantation after completion of antineoplastic therapy is another investigational procedure that may provide an alternative option in the future.

Some women may choose to make use of a gestational surrogate to carry their child through pregnancy.

Gonadotropin releasing hormone (GnRH) agonists are under investigation as a tool to preserve female fertility throughout chemotherapy administration. GnRH agonists cause medical castration which may provide a gonadoprotective effect by decreasing the number of follicles entering the differentiation phase, the stage most sensitive to chemotherapy. In addition, decreased serum estrogen concentrations reduce ovarian perfusion, thereby reducing ovarian exposure to systemic chemotherapy. Additional proposed mechanisms of GnRh agonist gonadoprotection during chemotherapy administration include a direct effect of the GnRH on the ovary, indirect antiapoptotic effects, and protection of germ line cells. Women older than 36 years of age may not have an adequate follicular reserve to benefit from gonadoprotection from GnRh therapy during chemotherapy administration. One comparative trial evaluated return of spontaneous menstruation and ovulation in 80 women with breast cancer undergoing treatment with chemotherapy with or without goserelin. All women were younger than 40 years of age and received treatment with FAC (fluorouracil-doxorubicin-cyclophosphamide). Following completion of treatment, menses returned within 3-8 months for 90% of women in the cohort treated with chemotherapy and goserelin and 33% of women receiving chemotherapy alone. Ovulation returned for 69% of women in the goserelin cohort and 26% the control patients. This trial suggests a positive effect of GnRH agonist therapy for protection of female fertility during chemotherapy; however, continued research is required to substantiate these findings in a broader patient population and with longer follow-up. At present, most clinical evidence supporting use of a GnRh agonist to protect female fertility during chemotherapy is based on noncomparative phase II trials, case series, and case reports.

MALES

Antineoplastic drugs and radiation destroy epithelial germ cells in a dose-dependent fashion. This damage results in increased FSH levels, decreased testosterone levels, oligospermia, or azoospermia. Spermatogenesis is more susceptible than testosterone production; and postpubertal testes are more susceptible to damage than prepubertal testes. Azoospermia may or may not be reversible. When it does recover, return of spermatogenesis may take up to 49 months.

Effects of radiation therapy on the testes are dependent on the dose, stage of germ cell development, and pubertal stage of the patient. Spermatogonia (precursor cell for spermatocyte) are the most sensitive to radiation damage, followed in decreasing sensitivity by spermatocytes (produce spermatid by meiosis) and spermatids (precursor for spermatozoa that fertilize ovum). Prepubertal boys may have oligo- or azoospermia once they reach sexual maturation. They may also have delayed sexual maturation due to destruction of Leydig cells and thus decreased testosterone production. Prolonged azoospermia generally occurs following a cumulative radiation dose of 2.5 Gy to the testis.

Surgery can affect male sexuality and fertility. Surgery for testicular cancer includes orchiectomy (surgical castration) and retroperitoneal lymph node resection which can result in decreased semen volume, erectile dysfunction, and low sexual desire. Prostate cancer surgery can also produce erectile dysfunction and changes in semen volume or ejaculatory problems.

Impaired spermatogenesis is present at the time of diagnosis for 60% to 70% men with testicular cancer. Elevated serum levels of β-human chorionic gonadotropin (β-hCG), which is a finding in many cases of testicular cancer, is associated with inferior spermatogenesis relative to cases with normal β-hCG levels.

In men, cryopreservation of sperm is a viable alternative and should be offered. The clinical pregnancy success rate of cryopreserved sperm is 36% by intrauterine insemination and 50% with *in vitro* fertilization and intracytoplasmic sperm injection. During *in vitro* fertilization sperm fertilize ovum in a liquid medium. Intracytoplasmic sperm injection is a more advanced process that injects one sperm into one oocyte for fertilization.

OUTCOMES OF PREGNANCY

Improved survival for cancer patients introduces the concern of long term treatment- and disease-related sequelae, including pregnancy outcome. The Childhood Cancer Survivor Study is a collaborative effort involving 25 health care institutions in the United States and Canada to facilitate research pertaining to the long term health outcomes of childhood cancer survivors. Over 14,000 subjects surviving 5 years or more following the diagnosis of childhood cancer are participating in this project.

Analysis of data from the Childhood Cancer Survivor Study demonstrated that offspring of female cancer survivors were more likely to be born preterm (OR, 1.9; P<0.001) than offspring from their female siblings. Moreover, previous treatment with a cumulative radiation dose exceeding 0.5 Gy to the uterus was associated with preterm birth (OR, 3.5; P=0.003), low birth weight (<2.5 g) (OR, 6.8; P=0.001), and small for gestational age (OR, 4; P=0.003). Data from the Childhood Cancer Survivor Study was also evaluated to assess pregnancy outcome for the female partners of male cancer survivors. Pregnant partners of male cancer survivors were less likely to yield a live born infant (RR, 0.77) than the control group (P=0.007). This was particularly evident when anticancer treatment included radiation with the treatment field affecting the testicles with or without shielding. The offspring of male cancer survivors treated with non-alkylating chemotherapy were more likely to have low birth weight than offspring from the survivor's male siblings (RR, 3.03; P=0.025). Otherwise, there was no difference in birth weight between offspring of the male cancer survivors in comparison to the control group. The male:female ratio of offspring fathered by male cancer survivors was 1:1.03; whereas, the male:female ratio of offspring from the survivor's male siblings was 1.24:1.0 (P=0.016).

A British survey of 10,483 childhood cancer survivors examined pregnancy outcome and reported that women treated with radiation to the abdomen or brain produced markedly fewer offspring than expected. Women treated with abdominal radiation were threefold and twofold more likely to have preterm or low birth weight babies. In addition, the risk of miscarriage was slightly increased in this group.

The impact of malignant disease and antineoplastic treatment on pregnancy outcome is not fully defined. However, patients with cancer should be informed of the known risks and potential options for fertility and reproduction.

Selected Readings

Badawy A, Elnashar A, El-Ashry M, et al, "Gonadotropin-Releasing Hormone Agonists For Prevention of Chemotherapy-Induced Ovarian Damage: Prospective Randomized Study," *Fertil Steril*, 2009, 91(3):694-7.

Blumenfeld Z, "How to Preserve Fertility In Young Women Exposed to Chemotherapy? The Role of GnRH Agonist Cotreatment In Addition to Cryopreservation of Embrya, Oocytes, or Ovaries," *Oncologist*, 2007, 12(9):1044-54.

de Bruin D, de Jong IJ, Arts EG, et al, "Semen Quality in Men With Disseminated Testicular Cancer: Relation With Human Chorionic Gonadotropin Beta-Subunit and Pituitary Gonadal Hormones," *Fertil Steril*, 2009, 91(6):2481-6.

Green DM, Kawashima T, Stovall M, et al, "Fertility of Female Survivors of Childhood Cancer: A Report From the Childhood Cancer Survivor Study," *J Clin Oncol*, 2009, 27(16):2677-85.

Green DM, Whitton JA, Stovall M, et al, "Pregnancy Outcome of Partners of Male Survivors of Childhood Cancer: A Report From the Childhood Cancer Survivor Study," *J Clin Oncol*, 2003, 21 (4):716-21.

Krychman ML and King T, "Pregnancy After Breast Cancer: A Case Study Resolving the Reproductive Challenge With a Gestational Surrogate," *Breast J*, 2006, 12(4):363-5.

Neal MS, Nagel K, Duckworth J, et al, "Effectiveness of Sperm Banking In Adolescents and Young Adults With Cancer: A Regional Experience," *Cancer*, 2007, 110(5):1125-9.

Lee SJ, Schover LR, Partridge AH, et al, "American Society of Clinical Oncology Recommendations on Fertility Preservation in Cancer Patients," *J Clin Oncol*, 2006, 24 (18):2917-31.

Pentheroudakis G, Pavlidis N, and Castiglione M, "Cancer, Fertility and Pregnancy: ESMO Clinical Recommendations For Diagnosis, Treatment and Follow-Up," *Ann Oncol*, 2009, 20 (Suppl 4):178-81.

Reulen RC, Zeegers MP, Wallace WH, et al,"Pregnancy Outcomes Among Adult Survivors of Childhood Cancer In the British Childhood Cancer Survivor Study," *Cancer Epidemiol Biomarkers Prev*, 2009, 18(8):2239-47.

Robison LL, Mertens AC, Boice JD, et al, "Study Design and Cohort Characteristics of the Childhood Cancer Survivor Study: A Multi-Institutional Collaborative Project," *Med Pediatr Oncol*, 2002, 38(4):229-39.

Signorello LB, Cohen SS, Bosetti C, et al, "Female Survivors of Childhood Cancer: Preterm Birth and Low Birth Weight Among Their Children," *J Natl Cancer Inst*, 2006, 98(20):1453-61.

MANAGEMENT OF CHEMOTHERAPY-INDUCED NAUSEA AND VOMITING

> **Nausea:** The feeling or sensation of an imminent desire to vomit.
>
> **Vomiting:** The forceful upward expulsion of gastric contents.
>
> **Retching:** Rhythmic, labored, spasmodic respiratory movements involving the diaphragm, chest wall, and abdominal muscles.

Nausea and vomiting are common side effects of many antineoplastic agents. Studies, both prior to the advent of serotonin antagonists and after their introduction, have been conducted asking chemotherapy patients to rank the five most distressing symptoms in order from most to least severe. Nausea and vomiting remained among the top three most distressing symptoms, despite the use of serotonin antagonists for prevention or management of acute chemotherapy-induced nausea and vomiting. Uncontrolled nausea and vomiting can have a significant impact on a patient's overall attitude, quality of life, compliance, and response to treatment. Uncontrolled nausea and vomiting can result in dehydration, electrolyte imbalances, weight loss, and malnutrition. Prolonged vomiting and retching can cause esophageal and/or gastric ruptures (Mallory-Weiss tears, Boerhaave's syndrome) and bleeding. Even in the absence of actual emesis, patients may experience varying degrees of nausea, often accompanied by anorexia.

Table 1. Other Causes of Nausea or Vomiting

Abdominal Emergencies
  Appendicitis
  Cholecystitis
  GI obstruction
  Peritonitis
Acute Systemic Infections
  Bacterial
  Parasitic
  Viral
Cardiovascular Disorders
  Congestive heart failure
  Hypotension
  Myocardial infarction
  Syncope
Neurologic
  Increased intracranial pressure
  Mènière's disease
  Otitis interna
  Severe or chronic pain
  Anticipatory nausea and vomiting
  Vestibular dysfunction
Drugs
  Anesthetics
  Antibiotics
  Antineoplastics
  Aspirin
  Cardiac glycosides
  Ethanol
  Levodopa

Nonsteroidal anti-inflammatory
  agents
  Opiates
  Quinidine
  Steroids
  Theophylline
Endocrine Disorders
  Adrenal insufficiency
  Diabetes mellitus
Gastrointestinal Disorders
  Dyspepsia
  Gastric outlet obstruction
  Gastroparesis
  Heartburn
  Partial or complete bowel obstruction
  Constipation
  Hepatic metastases
Metabolic
  Hypercalcemia
  Hyperglycemia
  Hyponatremia
  Uremia
Pregnancy
Psychogenic Stimuli
Therapy-Related
  Postsurgical
  Radiation Therapy

Patterns of Drug-Induced Nausea / Vomiting

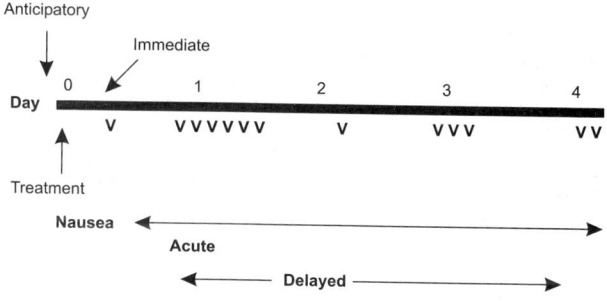

Table 2 describes the emetogenic potential of many of the antineoplastic agents. This table has been developed based on numerous guidelines and publications including: Multinational Association of Supportive Care in Cancer (MASCC), National Comprehensive Cancer Network (NCCN), and American Society of Clinical Oncology (ASCO). Several factors affect the emetic potential of these agents. For some drugs, such as cyclophosphamide or methotrexate, the dose administered has a significant effect on the drug's emetogenicity. Higher doses of these agents are much more emetogenic than low doses. The method of administration can also affect the incidence of nausea. Cytarabine, when given as a continuous infusion, is generally moderately emetogenic; however, higher cytarabine doses with short infusion times can produce a much higher incidence and severity of nausea and vomiting. Patient-related risk factors for nausea and vomiting include: Age, gender, prior experiences with chemotherapy, psychosocial factors (anxiety, depression), history of morning sickness with pregnancies, and history of motion sickness.

Table 2. Emetogenic Potential of Antineoplastic Agents

Highly Emetogenic Chemotherapy (Frequency of Emesis: >90%)

AC (either doxorubicin or epirubicin in combination with cyclophosphamide)
Altretamine
Carmustine >250 mg/m^2
Cisplatin ≥50 mg/m^2

Cyclophosphamide >1,500 mg/m^2
Dacarbazine
Mechlorethamine
Procarbazine (oral)
Streptozocin

Moderately Emetogenic Chemotherapy (Frequency of Emesis: 30% to 90%)

Aldesleukin >12-15 million units/m^2
Amifostine >300 mg/m^2
Arsenic trioxide
Azacitidine
Bendamustine
Busulfan ≥4 mg/day
Carboplatin
Carmustine ≤250 mg/m^2
Cisplatin <50 mg/m^2
Clofarabine

Cyclophosphamide ≤1,500 mg/m^2
Cyclophosphamide (oral)
Cytarabine >1,000 mg/m^2
Dactinomycin
Daunorubicin
Doxorubicin
Epirubicin
Etoposide (oral)
Idarubicin
Ifosfamide

Imatinib
Interferon alfa >10,000 units/m^2
Irinotecan
Lomustine
Melphalan >50 mg/m^2

Methotrexate 250->1,000 mg/m^2
Oxaliplatin
Temozolomide (I.V.)
Temozolomide (oral)
Vinorelbine (oral)

Low Emetogenic Chemotherapy (Frequency of Emesis: 10% to 30%)

Aldesleukin ≤12 million units/m^2
Amifostine ≤300 mg
Bexarotene
Bortezomib
Capecitabine
Cetuximab
Cytarabine 100-200 mg/m^2
Docetaxel
Doxorubicin, liposomal
Etoposide (I.V.)
Fludarabine (oral)
Fluorouracil
Gemcitabine
Interferon alfa >5000-<10,000 units/m^2
Ixabepilone

Lapatinib
Methotrexate >50-<250 mg/m^2
Mitomycin
Mitoxantrone
Nilotinib
Paclitaxel
Paclitaxel protein bound
Pemetrexed
Pentostatin
Topotecan
Trastuzumab
Tretinoin
UFT (oral)
Vorinostat

Minimal Emetogenic Chemotherapy (Frequency of Emesis: <10%)

Alemtuzumab
Asparaginase
Bevacizumab
Bleomycin
Busulfan <4 mg/day
Cetuximab
Chlorambucil
Cladribine
Cytarabine <100 mg/m^2
Dasatinib
Decitabine
Denileukin diftitox
Dexrazoxane
Erlotinib
Everolimus
Fludarabine (I.V.)
Gefitinib
Gemtuzumab ozogamicin
Hydroxyurea

Lapatinib
Lenalidamide
Melphalan (oral, low dose)
Mercaptopurine
Methotrexate ≤50 mg/m^2
Methotrexate (oral)
Nelarabine
Panitumumab
Pegaspargase
Rituximab
Sorafenib
Sunitinb
Temsirolimus
Thalidomide
Thioguanine (oral)
Valrubicin
Vinblastine
Vincristine
Vinorelbine (I.V.)

Nausea and vomiting caused by cytotoxic therapy generally falls into one of five categories: Acute, delayed, anticipatory, breakthrough, or refractory.

Acute nausea or vomiting is seen within the first 18-24 hours of drug administration, with the peak incidence seen at 4-6 hours. Acute nausea and vomiting tends to be responsive to drug therapy. Guidelines support the use of a neurokinin-1 receptor antagonist, serotonin antagonist, and dexamethasone combination for the prevention of acute nausea and vomiting in a patient receiving a highly emetogenic regimen. Patients receiving regimens classified as moderately emetogenic are recommended to be given a serotonin antagonist and dexamethasone.

Delayed nausea or vomiting usually begins after the first 18-24 hours of drug administration but may occur up to 5 days after chemotherapy, with the peak incidence in 2-3 days. The classic causative agent for delayed nausea and vomiting is cisplatin; however the phenomenon has also been described with cyclophosphamide, doxorubicin, carboplatin, and ifosfamide administration. The exact cause of this side effect is not clear; however, it is believed to have a separate mechanism from acute nausea or vomiting. Gastritis, tissue destruction, electrolyte fluctuations, or effects on the central or peripheral nervous system have all been postulated as possible mechanisms for delayed nausea and vomiting.

Delayed nausea and vomiting is not as responsive to drug therapy when compared to acute nausea and vomiting. The ASCO and MASCC guidelines recommend the use of dexamethasone and aprepitant for the prevention of delayed emesis associated with high emetic risk chemotherapy. For prevention of delayed emesis associated with moderate emetic risk chemotherapy, the ASCO guidelines recommend aprepitant as a single agent for cyclophosphamide and doxorubicin (AC) and single agent dexamethasone or a serotonin antagonist. The NCCN guidelines (v.4.2009) suggest that palonosetron may be of use in preventing delayed emesis.

While not drug-induced *per se*, anticipatory nausea and vomiting is also a relatively common complication of antineoplastic therapy. Anticipatory nausea and vomiting occurs due to inadequate control of nausea and vomiting in the past. Sights, smells, or sounds can also trigger anticipatory nausea and vomiting. This type of nausea and vomiting occurs before the administration of chemotherapy and has a variable response to drug therapy.

Breakthrough nausea and vomiting is defined as nausea and/or vomiting despite adequate prophylaxis therapy and requires rescue therapy. Refractory nausea and vomiting on the other hand occurs during subsequent cycles of chemotherapy when antiemetic prophylaxis or rescue therapy (or both) has failed in earlier cycles.

Before changing a patient's antiemetic regimen, it is important to determine when the patient experienced the nausea and vomiting. Basing the decision on the timing of the episode(s) will help guide the change(s) in the regimen. If the patient experienced nausea and vomiting within the first 24 hours, it would be appropriate to change the patient's acute regimen. If the patient had no episodes until day 2, it would be more appropriate to change the delayed regimen for the patient.

A number of possible alternatives exist when changing a patient's acute regimen, including switching to another serotonin antagonist, adding a neurokinin receptor antagonist (eg, aprepitant, fosaprepitant) to the previous serotonin antagonist/ steroid regimen, switching to a nonserotonin modulating antiemetic, or adding a benzodiazepine prophylactically. When changing the delayed regimen, there are numerous possibilities including: Adding a neurokinin receptor antagonist, dopamine antagonists, benzodiazepines, or cannabinoids, depending on the specific patient situation. Olanzapine is a thienobenzodiazepine antipsychotic that blocks multiple receptors associated with nausea or vomiting, including dopamine, histamine, muscarinic, and serotonin receptors. A few small trials have reported olanzapine effective (in combination with a steroid and serotonin antagonist) for prevention of delayed nausea and vomiting.

Table 3. Classification of Antiemetic Agents

Antihistamines	Diphenhydramine, hydroxyzine, promethazine
Anticholinergics	Scopolamine
Benzodiazepines	Diazepam, lorazepam
Butyrophenones	Droperidol, haloperidol
Cannabinoids	Dronabinol, nabilone
Corticosteroids	Dexamethasone, methylprednisolone
Neurokinin antagonists	Aprepitant, fosaprepitant
Phenothiazines	Chlorpromazine, perphenazine, prochlorperazine, thiethylperazine,[1] triflupromazine, (promethazine)
Serotonin antagonists	Dolasetron, granisetron, ondansetron, palonosetron, tropisetron[1]
Substituted benzamides	Metoclopramide, trimethobenzamide
Thienobenzodiazepines	Olanzapine

[1]Not commercially available in the United States

Table 4. Site of Action of Antiemetic Agents

Emetic center	Antihistamines, anticholinergics, serotonin antagonists, thienobenzodiazepines(?)
Chemoreceptor trigger zone (CTZ)	Benzamides, butyrophenones, phenothiazines, thienobenzodiazepines(?)
Cerebral cortex	Antihistamines, benzodiazepines, cannabinoids, (corticosteroids), neurokinin antagonists(?), thienobenzodiazepines(?)
Peripheral	Metoclopramide, neurokinin antagonists, serotonin antagonists, thienobenzodiazepines(?)
Unknown	Corticosteroids

Table 5. Equitherapeutic Serotonin Antagonist Doses

Drug	Oral	I.V.	Transdermal
Dolasetron	100-200 mg	1.8 mg/kg or 100 mg	
Granisetron	2 mg	10 mcg/kg or 1 mg	3.1 mg/24 h
Ondansetron	8-24 mg	8-10 mg	
Palonosetron	0.5 mg	0.25 mg	

Receptors for a large number of different neurotransmitters, including dopamine, serotonin, substance P, endocannabinoids, acetylcholine, histamine, opiates, and benzodiazepines, are involved in the vomiting reflex. Blockade of one or more of these receptors is the basic mechanism of action of most antiemetic agents.

Anticholinergics. Alkaloids (eg, atropine and scopolamine) exhibit some antiemetic activity, primarily postoperative nausea and vomiting, and motion sickness. The apparent mechanism of action is blockage of central muscarinic receptors. Toxicities, such as sedation, restlessness, blurred vision, and dry mouth, limit the systemic use of these agents. Transdermal application of scopolamine is is most useful in patients whose nausea is positional or due to motion. Scopolamine is also helpful as an adjunct in chemotherapy-induced delayed nausea or in treating prolonged mild nausea.

Antihistamines. The antihistamines block H_1 receptors both centrally and in the middle ear. A number of drugs in this class are effective against motion sickness and labyrinth disorders, but only diphenhydramine, hydroxyzine, and promethazine seem to have any activity against chemotherapy-induced nausea or vomiting. The major toxicities seen with these drugs are drowsiness, sedation, and dry mouth. These agents are most commonly used to enhance the efficacy of combination antiemetic regimens, although hydroxyzine or promethazine are occasionally used to treat mild-to-moderate nausea in patients who cannot tolerate, or are refractory to, other antiemetics. Diphenhydramine can be used in combination with dopamine antagonists to prevent extrapyramidal reactions seen with these agents at high doses.

Benzodiazepines. The exact antiemetic mechanism or location of action of the benzodiazepines is unclear. An inhibitory effect on the vomiting center, anxiolytic activity, and general CNS depression have all been postulated. Possible sites of action include the limbic system, vomiting center, cerebrum, and brain stem. The most common side effects include sedation, drowsiness, disinhibition, motor incoordination, and amnesia. In this setting, the anterograde amnesia induced by the benzodiazepine is usually considered a desired therapeutic effect rather than an adverse reaction. Benzodiazepines are commonly used as adjuncts to conventional antiemetics in the prophylaxis and treatment of chemotherapy-induced acute, breakthrough, and refractory nausea and vomiting. The benzodiazepines are also highly effective in the prevention of anticipatory nausea and vomiting. As single agents, the benzodiazepines have only mild antiemetic activity. Lorazepam is the most commonly used benzodiazepine for chemotherapy induced nausea and vomiting, but midazolam and diazepam have also been used.

Butyrophenones. A group of dopamine antagonists can be effective in treating chemotherapy-induced nausea and vomiting is the butyrophenones. Both haloperidol and droperidol have been reported to have antiemetic activity against highly, moderately, and mild emetogenic chemotherapy, although their use may be reserved for use in chemotherapy with low emetic potential. Droperidol has been associated with cardiovascular toxicities, particularly QT prolongation and torsade de points. These toxicities, some fatal, occurred in patients receiving recommended doses or lower and also in patients with no known risk factors, which has ultimately limited the use of this agent. However, one trial comparing ondansetron and droperidol found no difference in the incidence or severity of QT_c interval changes between the two drugs. As with most other antiemetics, the optimum response to the butyrophenones is seen in multidrug regimens. Like other dopamine blockers, extrapyramidal reactions, restlessness, sedation, and hypotension are relatively common side effects.

Cannabinoids. Proper evaluation of the antiemetic activity of cannabinoid derivatives has been hindered by social and political stigmas associated with marijuana use. Tetrahydrocannabinol, levonantradol, and nabilone are all reported to be effective in treating chemotherapy-induced nausea and vomiting. The specific site and mechanism of activity is unclear. Inhibition of endorphins in the emetic center, suppression of prostaglandin synthesis, and inhibition of medullary activity through an unspecified cortical action have all been postulated. Cannabinoids can inhibit buildup of cyclic adenosine monophosphate and cannabinoid receptors have been identified in the hippocampus, hypothalamus, and cortex. Cannabinoids used by the oral route seem to be most effective against mild-to-moderately emetogenic chemotherapy. Blurred vision, hypotension, and tachycardia, and a number of CNS complications, including euphoria, dysphoria, hallucinations, and sedation can be seen with cannabinoid therapy. Cannabinoids offer an alternative in patients unable to tolerate, or who are refractory to, other antiemetic agents.

Corticosteroids. The mechanism of antiemetic activity for the steroids is unknown, although alterations of cell permeability and inhibition of prostaglandin activity have been postulated. In spite of this uncertainty, corticosteroids, particularly dexamethasone, are frequent components of combination antiemetic regimens for high-to-moderately emetogenic chemotherapy. Studies have demonstrated a synergistic activity with metoclopramide and serotonin antagonists resulting in a 20% increase in effectiveness. For delayed nausea and vomiting, monotherapy dexamethasone appears to be more effective than, serotonin antagonists for delayed nausea and vomiting. Side effects from single or short term dosing of dexamethasone are infrequent, but may include euphoria, anxiety, insomnia, increased appetite, and hyperglycemia. For patients in whom a corticosteroid is not clearly contraindicated, these agents are an important component of antiemetic therapy.

Neurokinin-1 (NK$_1$) Receptor Antagonists. Neurokinin, or substance P, antagonists are the latest class of antiemetics. Substance P is a tachykinin (neurokinin) located in neurons of the central and peripheral nervous system. It is associated with a variety of functions, including emesis, depression, inflammatory pain and inflammatory/immune responses in asthma, and other diseases. Substance P's activity is mediated by the NK$_1$ receptor, a G-protein receptor coupled to the inositol phosphate signal pathway. Blocking this receptor is a mechanism to treat conditions mediated at least in part by substance P. Several neurokinin receptor antagonists, including aprepitant (MK-869, L-754030), its prodrug L-758298, ezlopitant (CJ-11974), fosaprepitant, vofopitant (GR-205171), and CP-122721 have been studied; aprepitant and fosaprepitant are approved for marketing.

NK$_1$ antagonists are effective in preventing cisplatin-induced nausea and vomiting, when used in conjunction with a serotonin antagonist and steroid. Addition of a neurokinin antagonist to a serotonin antagonist and steroid combination increases control of acute nausea by 10% to 15%, and control of delayed nausea by 20% to 30%. Most studies indicate the neurokinin receptors are less effective then serotonin antagonists, particularly for prevention of acute nausea within the first 8-12 hours. However, the neurokinin antagonists appear to be more effective than serotonin antagonists in preventing delayed nausea (days 2-5). Aprepitant has a very complex metabolism. Aprepitant is a substrate of 3A4 and when administered for 3 days is an inhibitor of 3A4, and an inducer of 3A4 and 2C9 if administered for more than 14 days. Caution should be used when administering with oral contraceptives, warfarin, dexamethasone, midazolam, and 3A4 inhibitors and inducers. Side effects, although similar to placebo, may include asthenia/fatigue, dizziness, hiccups, gastritis/heartburn, diarrhea, and mild and transient increase in LFTs. Current guidelines recommend aprepitant or fosaprepitant as initial therapy for highly emetogenic regimens (including high dose cisplatin) or moderately emetogenic regimens that contain both doxorubicin and cyclophosphamide.

Phenothiazines. Phenothiazines were the first class of drugs accepted as antiemetic therapy for antineoplastic chemotherapy. Blockade of dopamine (D$_2$) receptors in the area postrema (chemoreceptor trigger zone and vomiting center) appears to be their primary mechanism of action. A number of different drugs, including chlorpromazine, perphenazine, prochlorperazine, promethazine, and thiethylperazine (no longer marketed in the United States), have antiemetic activity. Common toxicities such as extrapyramidal reactions, restlessness, sedation, and hypotension limit the use of these drugs. Phenothiazines are most effective against mild-to-moderate nausea or vomiting, but have little impact on emesis from highly emetogenic agents such as dacarbazine or cisplatin. Higher doses of these agents may have increased activity, but the increased incidence and severity of side effects prohibits their use. Since the serotonin antagonists became available, use of the phenothiazines generally has been limited to prevention of nausea from mildly emetogenic chemotherapy, treatment of breakthrough nausea or vomiting in patients refractory to a serotonin blocker, or in association with dexamethasone to treat delayed nausea.

Serotonin (5-HT$_3$) Antagonists. A major advance in antiemetic therapy was the introduction of the serotonin (5-HT$_3$) antagonists. These agents have been shown to block serotonin in two ways: Peripheral antagonism by blocking release from enterochromaffin cells in the GI tract and central antagonism of receptors in the medulla. The high efficacy rate of these agents in preventing acute nausea and vomiting for highly and moderately emetogenic agents, coupled with their low incidence of side effects, has made them the standard of care in these settings.

Studies comparing serotonin antagonist plus dexamethasone with dexamethasone monotherapy or serotonin antagonist monotherapy have demonstrated that the combination regimen is significantly better than either agent alone. The addition of corticosteroids is synergistic and results in an increase in response of approximately 20%. Conversely, serotonin antagonists are not as efficacious as corticosteroids for delayed nausea and vomiting.

The major limitation to their use has historically been economic in nature. The high cost of serotonin antagonists has resulted in many institutions placing limitations on their use. Recently, generic versions of ondansetron have been approved by the FDA and are available for use at greatly reduced acquisition costs. Because the agents are therapeutically interchangeable, formulary decisions for these agents should be based on cost.

Recently two new formulations of serotonin antagonists have been approved: An oral formulation of palonosetron and a granisetron transdermal patch. Oral palonosetron 0.5 mg given 1 hour prior to moderately emetogenic chemotherapy was compared to 0.25 I.V. Efficacy was based on demonstrating noninferiority of oral palonosetron. The patch contains 34.3 mg of granisetron and releases 3.1 mg/day. The patch was approved based on a noninferiority study compared to oral granisetron in the setting of highly and moderately emetogenic chemotherapy. The patch is recommended to be applied 24-48 hours prior to chemotherapy.

The currently-available serotonin antagonists have relatively flat dose/response curves. Dose response studies have demonstrated that granisetron's efficacy seems to reach a plateau at 10 mcg/kg. There appears to be no difference in efficacy between granisetron doses of 10 mcg/kg and 40 mcg/kg. A few small studies suggest higher doses of granisetron (3 mg I.V. or 40-240 mcg/kg) may be effective in treating breakthrough nausea; however, none of these reports found the improvement to be statistically significant. A similar limitation exists for dolasetron, ondansetron, and palonosetron. A number of reports suggests that ondansetron doses between 20-32 mg have comparable efficacy in preventing nausea induced by a variety of antineoplastic drugs. Daily doses >32 mg seem to provide no increase in response. Data are also lacking on the value of using a different serotonin antagonist to treat nausea or vomiting resulting from the failure of the initial serotonin antagonist regimen.

Toxicities with these agents, including headache, constipation or diarrhea, and elevated transaminases, have been minimal. QT_c prolongation and/or ECG abnormalities have been observed with dolasetron, granisetron, ondansetron, and palonosetron.

Substituted Benzamides. Metoclopramide is the most commonly used antiemetic drug in this category. Prior to introduction of the serotonin antagonists, high-dose (1-3 mg/kg) metoclopramide was the preferred drug for prevention of nausea or vomiting from highly emetogenic chemotherapy. Metoclopramide's ability to block central and peripheral dopamine receptors was believed to be the mechanism of its antiemetic activity. Recognition that high doses also blocked peripheral serotonin receptors in the intestines led to the identification of the role serotonin inhibition has in preventing nausea or vomiting, and, ultimately, to development of the serotonin antagonists. Like the phenothiazines, use of metoclopramide is complicated by extrapyramidal reactions, restlessness, sedation, and hypotension. Diarrhea is also a significant side effect, especially with the high doses used for antiemetic therapy. Also like the phenothiazines, the current use of metoclopramide is generally limited to prevention of nausea from mild-to-moderately emetogenic chemotherapy and treatment of breakthrough nausea or vomiting.

Olanzapine is a thienobenzodiazepine antipsychotic that blocks multiple receptors associated with nausea or vomiting, including dopamine, histamine, muscarinic, and serotonin receptors. A few small trials have reported olanzapine effective (in combination with a steroid and 5-HT$_3$-antagonist) for prevention of delayed nausea and vomiting.

REPRESENTATIVE ANTIEMETIC REGIMENS

HIGHLY EMETOGENIC CHEMOTHERAPY

Aprepitant 125 mg orally or fosaprepitant 115 mg I.V. day 1 followed by aprepitant 80 mg orally days 2 and 3 **plus**

Dexamethasone 12 mg orally or I.V. days 1-4 or 12 mg followed by 8 mg once daily for 3-4 days or (if aprepitant/fosaprepitant are not included) 20 mg day 1 followed by 8 mg twice daily for 3-4 days **plus**

Serotonin antagonist as follows:

- Dolasetron 1.8 mg/kg or 100 mg I.V. or 100 mg orally day 1 **or**
- Granisetron 1-2 mg/day orally or 0.01 mg/kg (maximum: 1 mg) I.V. day 1 or 34.3 mg transdermal patch (3.1 mg/24 hours; maximum duration: 7 days) applied 24 hours prior to first chemotherapy dose **or**
- Ondansetron 16-24 mg orally or 8-12 mg I.V. or 0.15 mg/kg I.V. day 1 **or**
- Palonosetron 0.25 mg I.V. day 1

± Lorazepam 0.5-2 mg orally, I.V., or sublingual every 4-6 hours days 1-4, if needed

± H$_2$-blocker or proton pump inhibitor (PPI)

MODERATELY EMETOGENIC CHEMOTHERAPY

Day 1:

Aprepitant 125 mg orally or fosaprepitant 115 mg I.V. (in selected patients; eg, with AC) **plus**

Dexamethasone 12 mg orally or I.V. or 8 mg orally (if aprepitant/fosaprepitant nor included) **plus**

Serotonin antagonist as follows:

- Dolasetron 1.8 mg/kg or 100 mg I.V. or 100 mg orally **or**
- Granisetron 1-2 mg/day orally or 0.01 mg/kg (maximum: 1 mg) I.V. or 34.3 mg transdermal patch (3.1 mg/24 hours; maximum duration: 7 days) applied 24-48 hours prior to first chemotherapy dose **or**
- Ondansetron 16-24 mg orally or 8-12 mg I.V. or 0.15 mg/kg I.V. **or**
- Palonosetron 0.25 mg I.V.

± Lorazepam 0.5-2 mg orally, I.V., or sublingual every 4-6 hours days 1-4, if needed

± H_2 blocker or PPI

Day 2 (and beyond):

Aprepitant 80 mg orally days 2 and 3 (if aprepitant/fosaprepitant included day 1) **or**

± Dexamethasone 12 mg/day orally or I.V. for 2 days or 8 mg/day for 2-3 days **or**

Serotonin antagonist as follows:

- Dolasetron 1.8 mg/kg I.V. or 100 mg orally **or**
- Granisetron 1-2 mg/day orally or 0.01 mg/kg (maximum: 1 mg) I.V. **or**
- Ondansetron 16 mg/day orally or 8 mg I.V. or 0.15 mg/kg I.V.

± Lorazepam 0.5-2 mg orally, I.V., or sublingual every 4-6 hours days 1-4, if needed

± H_2 blocker or PPI

LOW EMETOGENIC CHEMOTHERAPY

Dexamethasone 12 mg orally or I.V. daily or 4-8 mg orally daily prior to chemotherapy **or**

Metoclopramide 10-40 mg orally or I.V. prior to chemotherapy and then every 4-6 hours if needed **or**

Prochlorperazine 10 mg orally or I.V. prior to chemotherapy and then every 4-6 hours if needed

± Lorazepam 0.5-2 mg orally, I.V., or sublingual every 4-6 hours days 1-4 if needed

± H_2 blocker or PPI

ORAL CHEMOTHERAPY

Antiemetic prophylaxis recommended:

Serotonin Antagonists (oral): Dolasetron 100 mg daily or granisetron 2 mg/day or ondansetron 16-24 mg daily

± Lorazepam 0.5-2 mg orally or sublingual every 4-6 hours days 1-4, if needed

± H_2 blocker or PPI

Requires only PRN antiemetic coverage (if experience nausea or emesis):

Metoclopramide 10-40 mg orally prior to chemotherapy and then every 4-6 hours **or**

Prochlorperazine 10 mg orally prior to chemotherapy and then every 4-6 hours

± Lorazepam 0.5-2 mg orally every 4-6 hours days 1-4, if needed

± H_2 blocker or PPI

BREAKTHROUGH TREATMENT OPTIONS

Prochlorperazine 25 mg rectally every 12 hours or 10 mg orally or I.V. every 4-6 hours **or**

Metoclopramide 10-40 mg orally or I.V. every 4-6 hours **or**

Promethazine 12.5-25 mg orally or I.V. every 4 hours **or**

Haloperidol 1-2 mg orally every 4-6 hours as needed **or**

Lorazepam 0.5-2 mg orally every 4-6 hours **or**

Dolasetron 1.8 mg/kg or 100 mg I.V. or 100 mg orally **or**

Granisetron 1-2 mg/day orally or 0.01 mg/kg (maximum: 1 mg) I.V. or 34.3 mg transdermal patch (3.1 mg/24 hours; maximum duration: 7 days) **or**

Ondansetron 16 mg/day orally or 8 mg I.V. daily **or**

Dronabinol 5-10 mg orally every 3-6 hours **or**

Nabilone 1-2 mg orally twice a day **or**

Dexamethasone 12 mg orally or I.V. daily **or**

Olanzapine 2.5-5 mg twice daily

GENERAL PRINCIPLES FOR MANAGING NAUSEA AND VOMITING

Key to prevention is aggressively prescribing the most effective antiemetic regimen during initial therapy.

A. **Prevention**

a. **Antiemetics are most effective when given prophylactically.**

b. Depending on the antiemetic agent(s) and route(s) of administration, pretreatment may range from 1 hour to 5 minutes prior to administration of the antineoplastic agent(s).

c. **Emetogenic potential is additive and may be different on different days of the regimen.**

d. **Provide patient with delayed nausea regimen and PRN antiemetics while at home.**

e. In most cases, **combination antiemetics are required for optimum control of nausea.** Two or more agents, from *different pharmacologic categories*, may be required to achieve optimal results.

f. **Avoid duplication of agents from the same pharmacologic category.**

g. **Doses and intervals of the antiemetic regimen need to be individualized for each patient.** "PRN" regimens should not be used. A fixed schedule of drug administration is preferable.

h. **If a patient has had no nausea for 24 hours** while on their scheduled antiemetic regimen, **it is usually possible to switch to a "PRN" regimen.** The patient should be advised to resume the fixed schedule *at the FIRST sign of recurrent nausea*, and continue it until they have had at least 24 hours without nausea.

i. **Titrate antiemetic dose to patient tolerance.**

j. **Anticipatory nausea and vomiting can often be minimized if the patient receives effective prophylaxis against nausea from the first cycle of therapy.**

k. **If anticipatory nausea does develop, an anxiolytic agent is usually the drug of choice.**

l. **"If it's not broken – DON'T fix it!"** Regardless of your own preferences, if the patient's current antiemetic regimen is working, don't change it.

B. **Antiemetics**

a. **The serotonin antagonists have a "ceiling" dose,** above which there is little or no added antiemetic effect.

b. **Serotonin antagonists are most effective within the first 24 hours.** Most studies of multiple day dosing show a sharp decline in the efficacy of the serotonin antagonists after the second or third day.

c. **Neurokinin antagonists are not very effective as single agents,** and should only be used in combination with a serotonin antagonist and steroid.

d. **Serotonin and neurokinin blockers are most effective in scheduled prophylactic regimens;** rather than in "PRN" regimens to chase existing vomiting.

e. **Serotonin and neurokinin antagonists have limited efficacy in stopping nausea or vomiting once it has begun.** A dopamine blocker may be more effective.

f. **Other antiemetics, such as cannabinoids, antihistamines, or anticholinergics) have limited use as initial therapy.** They are best used in combination with more effective agents (steroids, dopamine, or serotonin blockers); or, as second- or third-line therapy.

Selected References

Aapro M, "5-HT$_3$-Receptor Antagonists in the Management of Nausea and Vomiting in Cancer and Cancer Treatment," *Oncology*, 2005, 69(2):97-109.

Geling O and Eichler HG, "Should 5-Hydroxytryptamine-3 Receptor Antagonists Be Administered Beyond 24 Hours After Chemotherapy to Prevent Delayed Emesis? Systematic Re-evaluation of Clinical Evidence and Drug Cost Implications," *J Clin Oncol*, 2005, 23(6):1289-94.

Graves T, "Emesis as a Complication of Cancer Chemotherapy: Pathophysiology, Importance, and Treatment," *Pharmacotherapy*, 1992, 12(4):337-45.

Grunberg SM and Hesketh PJ, "Control of Chemotherapy-Induced Emesis," *N Engl J Med*, 1993, 329(24):1790-6.

Hesketh PJ, "Chemotherapy-Induced Nausea and Vomiting," *N Engl J Med*, 2008, 358 (23):2482-94.

Hesketh PJ, Kris MG, Grunberg SM, et al, "Proposal for Classifying the Acute Emetogenicity of Cancer Chemotherapy," *J Clin Oncol*, 1997, 15(1):103-9.

Hesketh PJ, Van Belle S, Aapro M, et al, "Differential Involvement of Neurotransmitters Through the Time Course of Cisplatin-Induced Emesis as Revealed by Therapy With Specific Receptor Antagonists," *Eur J Cancer*, 2003, 39(8):1074-80.

Holdsworth MT, "Ethical Issues Regarding Study Designs Used in Serotonin-Antagonist Drug Development," *Ann Pharmacother*, 1996, 30(10):1182-4.

Horiot JC, "Antiemetic Therapy in Cancer: An Update," *Expert Opin Pharmacother*, 2005, 6 (10):1713-23.

Jordan K, Schmoll HJ, and Aapro MS, "Comparative Activity of Antiemetic Drugs," *Crit Rev Oncol Hematol*, 2007, 61(2):162-75.

Kris MG, Hesketh PJ, Somerfield MR, et al, "American Society of Clinical Oncology Guideline for Antiemetics in Oncology: Update 2006," *J Clin Oncol*, 2006, 24(18)2932-47.

Multinational Association of Supportive Care in Cancer, "Antiemetic Consensus Guidelines." Available at http://www.mascc.org/media/Resource_centers/MASCC_Guidelines_Update.pdf. Accessed January 9, 2009.

National Comprehensive Cancer Network® (NCCN), "NCCN Clinical Practice Guidelines in Oncology™ - Antiemesis," V.4.2009. Available at http://www.nccn.org/professionals/physician _gls/PDF/antiemesis.pdf.

Navari RM, "Prevention of Emesis From Multiple-Day and High-Dose Chemotherapy Regimens," *J Natl Compr Canc Netw*, 2007, 5(1):51-9.

Oo TH and Hesketh PJ, "Drug Insight: New Antiemetics in the Management of Chemotherapy-Induced Nausea and Vomiting," *Nat Clin Pract Oncol*, 2005, 2(4):196-201.

MANAGEMENT OF DRUG EXTRAVASATIONS

Vesicant: An agent that has the potential to cause blistering, severe tissue injury, or tissue necrosis when extravasated.

Irritant: An agent that causes aching, tightness, and phlebitis with or without inflammation, but does not cause tissue necrosis.

Extravasation: Unintentional leakage (or instillation) of fluid out of a blood vessel into surrounding tissue.

Flare: Local, nonpainful, possibly allergic reaction often accompanied by reddening along the vein.

A potential complication of drug therapy is extravasation caused by leakage of the drug solution or instillation out of the vein. A variety of symptoms, including erythema, ulceration, pain, tissue sloughing, and necrosis are possible. This problem is not unique to antineoplastic therapy; a variety of drugs have been reported to cause tissue damage if extravasated. See table.

Vesicant Agents

Antineoplastic Agents	Nonantineoplastic Agents
Amsacrine[1]	Acyclovir (>7 mg/mL)
Cisplatin (>0.5 mg/mL)	Aminophylline
Dactinomycin	Calcium chloride (>10%)
Daunorubicin	Calcium gluconate
Doxorubicin	Calcium gluceptate
Epirubicin	Chlordiazepoxide
Idarubicin	Contrast media
Mechlorethamine	Crystalline amino acids (4.25%)
Mitomycin	Dextrose (>10%)
Mitoxantrone	Diazepam
Oxaliplatin	Digoxin
Streptozocin	Dobutamine
Vinblastine	Dopamine
Vincristine	Epinephrine
Vindesine[1]	Esmolol
Vinorelbine	Hydroxyzine
	Mannitol (>5%)
	Nafcillin
	Nitroglycerin
	Norepinephrine
	Phenylephrine
	Phenytoin
	Potassium acetate (>2 mEq/mL)
	Potassium chloride (>2 mEq/mL)
	Promethazine
	Propylene glycol
	Sodium bicarbonate (≥8.4%)
	Sodium chloride (>1%)
	Sodium thiopental
	Tromethamine
	Vasopressin

[1]Not commercially available in the U.S.

Antineoplastic Agents Associated With Irritation or Occasional Extravasation Reactions

Arsenic trioxide
Bleomycin
Bortezomib
Busulfan
Carboplatin
Carmustine
Cisplatin (< 5 mg/mL)
Cladribine
Cyclophosphamide
Cytarabine (liposomal)

Dacarbazine
Daunorubicin citrate
  (liposomal)
Docetaxel
Doxorubicin
  (liposomal)
Etoposide
Floxuridine
Fluorouracil
Gemcitabine

Ibritumomab
Ifosfamide
Irinotecan
Melphalan
Paclitaxel
Paclitaxel
  (protein bound)
Teniposide
Thiotepa
Topotecan

The actual incidence of drug extravasations is unknown. Some of the uncertainty stems from varying definitions of incidence. Incidence rates have been reported based on total number of drug doses administered, number of vesicant doses administered, number of treatments, number of patients treated with vesicants, and total number of patients treated. Most estimates place the incidence of extravasations with cytotoxic agents to be in the range of 1% to 7%.

The best management for extravasation is prevention, education, and close monitoring. Although it is not possible to prevent all accidents, a few simple precautions can minimize the risk to the patient. The vein used should be a large, intact vessel with good blood flow. Veins in the forearm (ie, basilic, cephalic, and median antebrachial) are usually good options for peripheral infusions. To minimize the risk of dislodging the catheter, veins in the hands, dorsum of the foot, and any joint space (eg, antecubital) should be avoided. It is also important to remember to not administer chemotherapy distal to a recent venipuncture.

A frequently recommended precaution against drug extravasation is the use of a central venous catheter. Use of a central line has several advantages, including high patient satisfaction, reliable venous access, high flow rates, and rapid dilution of the drug. Many institutions encourage or require use of a vascular access device for administration of vesicant agents. Despite their benefit, central lines are not an absolute solution. Vascular access devices are subject to a number of complications. Misplacement/migration of the catheter or improper placement of the needle in accessing injection ports, and cuts, punctures, or rupture of the catheter itself have all been reported.

Education of both the patient and practitioner is imperative. Educate the patient to immediately report any signs of pain, itching, tingling, burning, redness, or discomfort, all of which could be signs of extravasation. Ensure the health care team is informed of the risks and management strategies for both prevention and treatment of extravasations.

The nurse administering the chemotherapy agents needs to monitor the patient and I.V. site frequently. Prior to drug administration, the patency of the I.V. line should be verified. The line should be flushed with 5-10 mL of a saline or dextrose solution (depending on compatibility) and the drug(s) infused through the side of a free-flowing I.V. line over 2-5 minutes. If an extravasation occurs, it is important to monitor the site closely at 24 hours, 1 week, 2 weeks, and as necessary for any signs and symptoms of extravasation.

When a drug extravasation does occur, a number of immediate actions are recommended.

1. **Stop the infusion.** At the first suspicion of extravasation, the drug infusion and I.V. fluids should be stopped.

2. **Do NOT remove the catheter/needle.** The I.V. tubing should be disconnected, but the catheter/needle should not be removed. It should be left in place to facilitate aspiration of fluid from the extravasation site, and, if appropriate, administration of an antidote.

3. **Aspirate fluid.** To the extent possible, the extravasated drug solution should be removed from the subcutaneous tissues. It is important to avoid any friction or pressure to the area.

4. **Do NOT flush the line.** Flooding the infiltration site with saline or dextrose in an attempt to dilute the drug solution is not recommended.

5. **Remove the catheter/needle.** If an antidote is not going to be injected into the extravasation site, the catheter/needle should be removed. If an antidote is to be injected into the area, it should be injected through the catheter to ensure delivery of the antidote to the extravasation site. When this has been accomplished, the catheter should then be removed.

6. In addition, the affected extremity should be elevated, marked, and photographed if possible. Documentation of the event and follow up is also highly recommended.

Two issues for which there is less consensus are the application of heat or cold, and the use of various antidotes. A variety of recommendations exist for each of these concerns; however, there is no consensus concerning the proper approach.

Cold. Intermittent cooling of the area of extravasation results in vasoconstriction, potentially restricting the spread of the drug and decreasing the pain and inflammation in the area. Application of cold is usually recommended as immediate treatment for most drug extravasations, except the vinca alkaloids and epipodophyllotoxins.

Heat. Application of heat results in a localized vasodilation and increased blood flow. Increased circulation is believed to facilitate removal of the drug from the area of extravasation. Heat is generally recommended for treatment for vinca alkaloid and epipodophyllotoxins (eg, etoposide) extravasations. Most data are from animal studies with relatively few human case reports. Animal models indicate application of heat exacerbates the damage from anthracycline extravasations.

For some agents, such as cisplatin, epipodophyllotoxins, mechlorethamine, and paclitaxel, there are conflicting recommendations. Some reports recommend application of cold, others recommend heat. At least one report suggests neither cold nor heat is effective for paclitaxel extravasations.

EXTRAVASATION-SPECIFIC ANTIDOTES

A very wide variety of agents have been reported as possible antidotes for extravasated drugs, with no consensus on their proper use. For a number of reasons, evaluation of the various reports is difficult.

Agents Used as Antidotes

Dexrazoxane	Hyaluronidase
Dimethyl sulfoxide	Sodium thiosulfate

Dexrazoxane. Dexrazoxane, a derivative of EDTA, is an intracellular chelating agent used as a cardioprotective agent in patients receiving anthracycline therapy. It is believed that the cardioprotective effect of dexrazoxane is a result by chelating iron following intracellular hydrolysis. Dexrazoxane is not an effective chelator itself, but is hydrolyzed intracellularly to an open-ring chelator form, which complexes with iron, other heavy metals, and doxorubicin complexes to inhibit the generation of free radicals. It has been postulated that dexrazoxane's chelating effect, and its ability to stabilize topoisomerase II may be useful in preventing tissue damage from anthracycline extravasations.

Dexrazoxane was FDA approved in 2007 for the treatment of anthracycline-induced extravasations. Approval was based on two clinical trials including a total of 80 patients with anthracycline extravasations. Dexrazoxane was administered as 3 I.V. infusions over 1-2 hours through a different venous access location: 1,000 mg/m^2 within 6 hours, 1,000 mg/m^2 after 24 hours, and 500 mg/m^2 after 48 hours of the actual extravasation up to a maximum total dose of 2,000 mg on days 1 and 2 and 1,000 mg on day 3 respectively. Although localized cooling was permitted (except within 15 minutes of dexrazoxane infusion) in the trials, the number of patients in which this was used was not reported. Fifty-four of the 80 patients were evaluable. The primary endpoint was rate of surgical resection and necrosis. One patient (2%) required surgery and two patients (4%) developed tissue necrosis. Seventy-one percent of the patients were able to maintain chemotherapy appointments on schedule. Treatment has been associated with neutropenia, leukopenia, and thrombocytopenia. Hematological and liver function tests should be monitored. Other common yet reversible adverse events include: Nausea and vomiting, diarrhea, stomatitis, and infusion site burning. The proportion of toxicities that were attributable to dexrazoxane, or as a result of primary antineoplastic therapy was not clear. Prior to administering dexrazoxane, discontinue DMSO as studies suggest the single agent is more effective than when used in combinations with DMSO.

Dimethyl sulfoxide (DMSO). A number of case reports and small clinical trials have suggested application of DMSO is an effective treatment for chemotherapy extravasations. It is believed DMSO's protective effect is due to its ability to act as a free radical scavenger. DMSO may be considered as a treatment option for extravasations due to anthracyclines, mitomycin C, and actinomycin D. The optimal dose and duration is unknown. Common doses are to apply 1.5 mL of 50% DMSO topically with a saturated gauze pad every 6 hours for 7-14 days. Gently paint DMSO solution onto an area twice the size of the extravasation. Allow the site to dry. Do not cover with a dressing, as severe blistering may result. During application, DMSO may cause mild local burning, blistering, erythema, and itching.

There are a number of limitations for the use of DMSO. Results in animal models have been equivocal, with some reports indicating DMSO is beneficial, and some showing little or no effect. Clinical reports of its use are extremely difficult to interpret due to variations in DMSO concentration (50% to 99%), number of applications/day, duration of therapy, inclusion of nonvesicants in studies, and concomitant treatments. A number of different treatments, including cold, steroids, vitamin E, and sodium bicarbonate have been used in conjunction with DMSO. Also, most reports that suggest DMSO is effective in preventing tissue damage used DMSO concentrations >90% which is not available for clinical use in the United States. The product is only commercially available in the United States at a concentration 50% (vol/vol) solution in water; however, higher concentrations may be purchased at health food stores. And lastly, the only FDA approved indication is symptomatic relief interstitial cystitis (intravesicular administration). Based on these limitations many institutions, ONS, and the prescribing information do not include DMSO as a treatment option for anthracycline extravasations.

Hyaluronidase. Hyaluronidase is an enzyme that destroys hyaluronic acid, an essential component of connective tissue. This results in increased permeability of the tissue, facilitating diffusion and absorption of fluids. It is postulated that increasing the diffusion of extravasated fluids results in more rapid absorption, thereby limiting tissue damage. In individual case reports, hyaluronidase has been reported effective in preventing tissue damage from a wide variety of agents, including vinca alkaloids, epipodophyllotoxins, and taxanes. The recommended total dose is 1 mL (150 units) administered as 5 separate 0.2 mL SubQ injections via a 24-gauge or smaller needle. It is recommended to use a new syringe for each injection site.

Sodium thiosulfate. Sodium thiosulfate ($1/6$ molar) has been recommended for treatment of mechlorethamine, dacarbazine, and cisplatin extravasations. Sodium thiosulfate provides a substrate for alkylation by mechlorethamine, preventing the alkylation and subsequent destruction in subcutaneous tissue. The use of sodium thiosulfate to treat mechlorethamine extravasations is based almost exclusively on *in vitro* and animal data. A single case report of successful thiosulfate treatment of an accidental intramuscular mechlorethamine injection has been published. Thus far, no reports of thiosulfate treatment of mechlorethamine infiltrations have been published.

Preparation of a $1/6$ molar solution:

- Dilute 4 mL of a sodium thiosulfate 10% solution into a syringe with 6 mL of sterile water for injection resulting in 10 mL of $1/6$ molar solution or
- Dilute 1.6 mL of a sodium thiosulfate 25% solution with 8.4 mL of sterile water for injection resulting in 10 mL of $1/6$ molar solution.

Inject 1-5 mL of the $1/6$ molar solution subcutaneously around the edge of the extravasation site using a tuberculin syringe. The dose of sodium thiosulfate depends on the amount of drug extravasated. For mechlorethamine, administer 0.5-2 mL of sodium thiosulfate $1/6$ molar for every estimated 1 mg of mechlorethamine extravasated. For a cisplatin extravasation it is recommended to inject 2 mL of sodium thiosulfate for each estimated 100 mg of cisplatin extravasated. It is recommended to use a new syringe for each injection site.

Reported Treatment Regimens for Drug Extravasations

Treatment	Dose	Route	Duration	Concomitant Therapy	Used to Treat	Preparation	Administration
Cold	15 min 4 times/day	Topical	3-4 days	None	All agents except vinca alkaloids and epipodophyllotoxins	N/A	N/A
Heat	15 min on; 15 min off	Topical	1 day	None	Vinca alkaloids and epipodophyllotoxins	N/A	N/A
Dexrazoxane	1000 mg/m^2 500 mg/m^2	I.V.	Days 1 and 2 Day 3	Cold[1,3]	Anthracycline	1000 mL NS	I.V.
Dimethyl sulfoxide[2]	50%-99% every 6-8 hours	Topical	7-14 days		Anthracycline, mitomycin	N/A	Topical
Hyaluronidase	150 units (total)	SubQ	One time	Heat	Amino acid solutions, aminophylline, calcium, contrast media[3], dextrose, mannitol, nafcillin, phenytoin, potassium, vinca alkaloids	Reconstitute with 1 mL NS	5 injections (0.2 mL) into area of extravasation
Phentolamine	5 mg	SubQ	1 day	None	Vasopressors (dobutamine, dopamine, epinephrine, norepinephrine, phenylephrine)	Mix 5 mg with 9 mL NS	Inject a small amount into area of extravasation. Blanching should reverse immediately. If blanching should recur, additional injections may be needed.

Reported Treatment Regimens for Drug Extravasations *continued*

Treatment	Dose	Route	Duration	Concomitant Therapy	Used to Treat	Preparation	Administration
Sodium thiosulfate	$\frac{1}{6}$ M	I.V., SubQ	One time	Ice or heat	Mechlorethamine, cisplatin	Mix 4 mL of 10% sodium thiosulfate with 6 mL sterile water	Inject 2 mL for each 1 mg of mechlorethamine; inject locally for cisplatin infiltrates (>20 mL and >0.5 mg/mL)
Terbutaline	1 mg	SubQ			Vasopressors (dobutamine, dopamine, epinephrine, norepinephrine, phenylephrine)		

N/A = not applicable; I.V. = intravenous; SubQ = subcutaneous; I.D. = intradermal.

[1]Remove cooling 15 minutes prior to dexrazoxane infusion.

[2]DMSO concentrations >50% are not available for human use in the U.S.

[3]Large extravasations only.

Selected Readings

Bertelli G, "Prevention and Management of Extravasation of Cytotoxic Drugs," *Drug Saf*, 1995, 12 (4):245-55.

Boyle DM and Engelking C, "Vesicant Extravasation: Myths and Realities," *Oncol Nurs Forum*, 1995, 22(1):57-67.

Kurul S, Saip P, and Aydin T, "Totally Implantable Venous-Access Ports: Local Problems and Extravasation Injury," *Lancet Oncol*, 2002, 3(11):684-92.

Larson DL, "What Is the Appropriate Management of Tissue Extravasation by Antitumor Agents?" *Plast Reconstr Surg*, 1985, 75(3):397-405.

Larson DL, "Treatment of Tissue Extravasation by Antitumor Agents," *Cancer*, 1982, 49(9):1796-9.

Larson DL, "Alterations in Wound Healing Secondary to Infusion Injury," *Clin Plast Surg*, 1990, 17 (3):509-17.

MacCara ME, "Extravasation: A Hazard of Intravenous Therapy," *Drug Intell Clin Pharm*, 1983, 17 (10):713-7.

Mouridsen HT, Langer SW, Buter J, et al, "Treatment of Anthracycline Extravasation With Savene (Dexrazoxane): Results From Two Prospective Clinical Multicentre Studies," *Ann Oncol*, 2007, 18 (3):546-50.

Polovich M, Whitford JN and Olsen M, *Chemotherapy and Biotherapy Guidelines and Reccomendations for Practice*, 3rd ed, Pittsburgh, PA: Oncology Nursing Society, 2009.

Schrijvers DL, "Extravasation: A Dreaded Complication of Chemotherapy," *Ann Oncol*, 2003, 14 Suppl 3:iii26-30.

Schulmeister L and Camp-Sorrell D, "Chemotherapy Extravasation From Implanted Ports," *Oncol Nurs Forum*, 2000, 27(3):531-8.

MANAGEMENT OF INFECTIONS

Certain oncology patients are at increased risk of morbidity and mortality from infectious complications secondary to disease- or treatment-related loss of immunity (see table). Impaired immunity is generally associated with malignancies that arise from hematologic cells and lymphoid tissues. The most common iatrogenic reasons for impaired immunity are related to repeated courses of chemotherapy or radiation that are toxic to normal cells of the immune system or from a loss of innate barrier, such as mucositis, and central venous access device placement. Patients undergoing allogeneic hematopoietic stem cell (bone marrow) transplantation are at great risk for infectious complications because they generally have a hematologic malignancy, receive intensive chemotherapy prior to the bone marrow transplant, and require chronic immunosuppression to prevent graft-versus-host disease.

Disease-Related Risks for Infections

Cancer	Corresponding Normal Cell	Infectious Risk
Hodgkin's disease	Reed Sternberg cell (lymphocyte)	Encapsulated bacteria; *Pneumocystis jirovecii*; herpes simplex virus and varicella zoster virus; extensive chemotherapy/radiation
Non-Hodgkin's lymphoma	B cells (90%) T cells (10%)	*Pneumocystis jirovecii*; herpes simplex virus and varicella zoster virus; extensive chemotherapy/radiation
Acute lymphoblastic leukemia	B cells (90%) T cells (10%)	Extensive chemotherapy/radiation
Acute myeloid leukemia	Myeloid blood cell	Extensive chemotherapy/radiation
Chronic lymphocytic leukemia	B cells (90%) T cells (10%)	Atypical infections secondary to chronic immune impairment with protracted indolent course of disease

Neutropenia increases the risk of developing infection. The likelihood of morbidity or mortality from infection increases as the depth, rate of decline, and duration of neutropenia increase. The underlying cause of neutropenia is often anticancer treatment; however, it can also be secondary to the patient's malignant disease. It is important to distinguish the neutrophil count from the white blood cell count. The white blood cell count represents the sum of different types of white blood cells, including neutrophils, monocytes, lymphocytes, basophils, and mast cells. Patients with leukemias can present with a normal or markedly elevated white blood cell count, and at the same time, can be profoundly neutropenic because the vast majority of their circulating blood cells are blasts (malignant hematologic cells). An absolute neutrophil count (ANC) <500 cells/mm^3 blood increases the risk of infectious complications. In fact, patients are considered "high-risk" neutropenics when the ANC is ≤100 cells/mm^3 blood for ≥7 days. The ANC is calculated as follows.

ANC = WBC x [(% segmented neutrophils + % band neutrophils) / 100]

Most anticancer treatments reduce immunity by causing neutropenia and mucositis. However, some products also impair the adaptive arm of immunity, which includes cell mediated immunity and antibody production. Monoclonal antibodies that impair adaptive immunity include alemtuzumab, denileukin diftitox, and rituximab. Bortezomib and the cytotoxic purine nucleotides (eg, clofarabine, fludarabine, nelarabine) inhibit adaptive immunity. In addition, corticosteroids, such as dexamethasone and methylprednisolone, are used in the treatment of some lymphoid malignancies.

The most frequent source of opportunistic pathogens is the patient or close human contacts. Common causes of gram-positive bacterial infections include *Staphylococcus aureus*, *Staphylococcus epidermidis*, *Streptococcus pneumoniae*, *Streptococcus pyogenes*, *Streptococcus viridans*, *Enterococcus faecalis*, *Enterococcus faecium*, and *Corynebacterium* spp. Common causes of gram-negative bacterial infections include *Escherichia coli*, *Klebsiella pneumoniae*, and *Pseudomonas* spp. *Candida albicans* generally colonizes mucous membranes of the gastrointestinal and urogenital tract. Environmental sources of opportunistic pathogens include the surface of fresh fruits and vegetables (bacteria), dried foliage, tobacco, marijuana leaves (*Aspergillus* spp); recent construction or renovation (*Aspergillus* spp); and tap water (*Legionella* spp). Rarely, viruses can be transmitted by blood products (packed red blood cells, platelets, stem cells) or plasma-derived products (intravenous immune globulin).

Thorough and frequent handwashing reduces the risk of transmitting opportunistic pathogens to neutropenic patients. In addition, limitation of the number of visitations and personal contacts also reduces opportunity for transmission of opportunistic pathogens. Additional preventive measures which are generally implemented to reduce the risk of infection in patients at greatest risk (eg, allogeneic bone marrow transplant patients) include hospital room-specific instrumentation, HEPA filtration of patient rooms or nursing units, total room clean following discharge, low microbial diets, and diligent mouth care. HEPA filtration involves circulation of room air through a filter 8-12 times/hour to remove small airborne particles. Low microbial diets prohibit ingestion of fresh fruits and vegetables, or undercooked meat. Diligent mouth care requires swishing and expectoration of mouthwash 4-6 times daily. Mouthwashes may be 0.9% NaCl or dilute bicarbonate solution (sodium bicarbonate 50 mEq/L in sterile water), because the greatest utility of mouth care is to remove oral debris and thereby prohibit microbial growth. Chlorhexidine 0.12% may also be used as a mouthwash; however, this product can have a drying and irritating effect on damaged mucous membranes.

Selective gut decontamination using sulfamethoxazole-trimethoprim or a fluoroquinolone is used to reduce gram-negative colonization in patient undergoing intensive chemotherapy. Selective gut decontamination allows continued colonization of the lower gastrointestinal tract with anaerobic bacteria, which reduces the possibility of fungal overgrowth. High-risk patients undergoing treatment with intensive chemotherapy, such as allogeneic hematopoietic stem cell transplant recipients, or patients with acute myeloid leukemia undergoing induction chemotherapy, may also receive prophylactic acyclovir (or an equivalent antiviral) and fluconazole. Allogeneic bone marrow transplant recipients at risk for cytomegalovirus infection may receive prophylactic ganciclovir following engraftment. Sulfamethoxazole-trimethoprim is administered chronically to prevent *Pneumocystis jirovecii* pneumonia in some patients undergoing repeated chemotherapy treatments or alemtuzumab therapy for lymphoid malignancies.

The management of infections in cancer patients is directed by the nature and degree of immune compromise and the identified or suspected pathogen(s). Cancer patients without disease-related or treatment-related immune suppression are managed as appropriate for the type and severity of infection. A comprehensive discussion on all potential infections in cancer patients is outside of the scope of this chapter. For information on specific infections, such as pneumonia or cellulitis occurring in the cancer patient, the reader is referred to the National Comprehensive Cancer Network Clinical Practice Guidelines in Oncology™ "Prevention and Treatment of Cancer-Related Infections" (available at http://www.nccn.org).

Fever is frequently the only sign of infection in the neutropenic patient. Febrile neutropenic patients are empirically managed for presumed infection. Fever is defined as single oral temperature exceeding 38.3°C (101°F), or oral temperature 38°C (100.4°F) for at least 60 minutes. Evaluation of the febrile neutropenic patient should include history and physical examination, chest radiograph, blood cultures drawn from the central venous line (all ports), blood cultures drawn by peripheral venipuncture, specimens of urine and diarrheal stool, plus additional specimens as indicated by history and physical examination. Blood cultures must be drawn prior to initiation of antibiotics to increase the likelihood of acquiring a positive culture; although, blood cultures generally remain negative due to the small inoculum of microbes needed to cause infection in the neutropenic host and due to the early initiation of broad spectrum antibacterials. Empiric treatment with aggressive intravenous doses of broad spectrum, bactericidal antibiotics should be initiated as soon as possible after blood cultures have been collected. Choice of therapy greatly depends on the clinical status of the patient (ie, high vs. low risk), as well as the presumed origin of infection based on clinical presentation. Antibiotics should be infused through alternating central venous line ports.

Vancomycin is not recommended as a routine component of initial empiric therapy in the neutropenic patient due to concerns of emerging resistant organisms. Vancomycin should only be considered for patients considered high-risk for serious gram-positive infections. Criteria for use of vancomycin in the febrile neutropenia patient are listed in the table below. Vancomycin should be used in combination with a bactericidal agent that has activity against gram-negative organisms, including *Pseudomonas* spp (eg, cefepime, a carbapenem, or piperacillin/tazobactam). Aztreonam is a bactericidal alternative for the treatment of gram-negative microbes in patients who are allergic to penicillins, cephalosporins, or carbapenems. To minimize the development of resistant organisms, treatment with vancomycin should be discontinued in 2-3 days if resistant gram-positive organisms have not been identified. If history or cultures suggest vancomycin-resistant organisms (eg, enterococci), treatment options include daptomycin or linezolid. Monitor serum creatine kinase (CPK) levels at baseline and at least once weekly for patients receiving treatment with daptomycin. Myelosuppression is a reported side effect of linezolid. Use of this product in patients undergoing treatment with chemotherapy is reported in the medical literature; however, linezolid should be used with caution in any patients with additional risk factors for leukopenia, thrombocytopenia, or anemia.

Criteria for Use of Vancomycin in Febrile Neutropenia

- Clinically apparent, serious, catheter-related infection
- Positive blood cultures for gram positive bacterial prior to final identification and susceptibility testing
- Colonization with penicillin/cephalosporin-resistant pneumococci or methicillin resistant *Staphylococcus aureus*
- Clinically unstable (eg, hypotension, shock) without an identified pathogen
- Soft tissue infection

- Risk factors for viridans group streptococcal infections, such as prophylaxis with sulfamethoxazole/trimethoprim or fluoroquinolones anti-microbials, severe mucositis

When criteria for use of vancomycin is not met, the patient may receive monotherapy (eg, cefepime or carbapenem), or dual therapy (aminoglycoside or ciprofloxacin plus an antipseudomonal penicillin) should be initiated. The antipseudomonal beta lactam can be replaced with aztreonam for penicillin allergic patients. The choice for monotherapy versus dual therapy is determined by the patient's history and physical examination. The effect of antimicrobial therapy should be assessed in 72 hours or as indicated by the patient's clinical status.

The low-risk febrile neutropenic patient who defervesces within 72 hours following appropriate antibiotic therapy and is free of signs and symptoms of infection, may be converted to oral antibiotics (second generation cephalosporin or fluoroqui-nolone). Criteria for considering a patient high risk and continuing intravenous antibiotics include signs and symptoms of sepsis at presentation, additional signs of infection such as pneumonia or endocarditis, moderate-to-severe mucositis, dermal or mucosal loss of integrity, impending invasive procedure(s), or impending immunosuppressive therapy. If the patient remains febrile despite 72 hours of broad spectrum antibiotic coverage, the selection of antibiotics can be changed or additional antibiotics can be started. Vancomycin can be discontinued in patients who are clinically stable. Additional antibiotics should be added to patients who appear acutely ill from infection or are at high risk for infectious complications. The choice of antibiotic, which is dependent on current antimicrobial therapy in addition to the patient's history and physical examination, may include vancomycin, second gram-negative agent, antifungal with activity against invasive mold infections (voriconazole, caspofungin, an amphotericin product), or antianaerobic agent. Treatment with an antifungal should be started for patients with persistent fevers despite 5-7 days of appropriate empiric antibiotic therapy. Atypical pathogens, including *Legionella pneumoniae*, invasive molds (*Aspergillus* spp, *Fusarium* spp, mucormycoses), and viruses (cytomega-lovirus [CMV], adenovirus, herpes simplex), should be considered in the chronically immunosuppressed patient. Appropriate empiric treatment for suspected viral infection would include acyclovir, but valacyclovir or famciclovir are reasonable alternatives. Treatment with ganciclovir, valganciclovir, or foscarnet is recommended if there is concern for CMV. Ganciclovir plus intravenous immune globulin are administered for CMV pneumonitis. Positive cultures and antibiotic sensitivity reports may streamline therapy in the stable patient. However, the high-risk patient may continue receiving broad spectrum antibacterials because the finding of a specific pathogen does not exclude the possibility of additional infecting organisms in the neutropenic patient. Caspofungin or fluconazole are used for the treatment of mucocutaneous candidiasis in the neutropenic patient. Prolonged and persistent neutropenia is a risk factor for invasive aspergillosis. Initial antifungal therapy for presumed or microbiologically documented aspergillosis is voriconazole, or an amphotericin product, or caspofungin. Itraconazole has activity against antiaspergillus; however, characteristics of the formulation(s) make it a less attractive option. Central venous line removal is done judiciously due to the ongoing need for intravenous fluids, drugs, and blood products in the neutropenic and thrombocytopenic patient, and the risk of infection or bleeding with insertion of a new central venous line. Empiric antibiotics should be continued until the patient is afebrile and clinically stable. Empiric antibiotics can be discontinued after 7 days in the low-risk neutropenic patient. One may consider discontinuation of empiric antibiotics in the high-risk neutropenic patient following 5-7 days without fever. Although, antibiotics should be continued until the ANC is at least 500 cells/ mm^3 and severe mucositis, or signs and symptoms of sepsis have resolved. Four to 5 days following resolution of neutropenia, discontinuation of antibiotics may be considered in the low-risk, neutropenic, clinically stable patient with persistent fevers. With close observation and follow-up, antibiotics may be discontinued after 2 weeks of therapy in the clinically stable patient with persistent fever and persistent neutropenia.

Colony stimulating factors, which reduce the duration of neutropenia, are helpful in reducing hospital admission for neutropenic fevers in patients with a history of febrile neutropenia or prolonged neutropenia following outpatient chemotherapy.

Patients with chronic lymphocytic leukemia do not produce antibodies effectively and may require periodic administration of intravenous immune globulin to maintain normal serum immunoglobulin levels.

Selected Readings

Hughes WT, Armstrong D, Bodey GP, et al, "2002 Guidelines for the Use of Antimicrobial Agents in Neutropenic Patients With Cancer," *Clin Infect Dis*, 2002, 34(6):730-51.

Maki DG, Alvarado CJ, Hassemer CA, et al, "Relation of the Inanimate Hospital Environment to Endemic Nosocomial Infection," *N Engl J Med*, 1982, 307(25):1562-6.

National Comprehensive Cancer Network® (NCCN), "NCCN Clinical Practice Guidelines in Oncology™ - Prevention and Treatment of Cancer-Related Infections," V.2.2009. Available at http://www.nccn.org/professionals/physician_gls/PDF/infections.pdf.

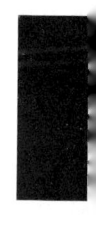

ORAL MUCOSITIS / STOMATITIS

Also known as mucosal barrier injury, mucositis and stomatitis are general terms for the erythema, edema, desquamation, and ulceration of the gastrointestinal tract caused by many antineoplastic drugs and external beam radiation therapy (radiotherapy). Stomatitis refers to the finding of mucositis in the mouth or oropharynx. Gastrointestinal complications of mucositis include pain, xerostomia, bloating, diarrhea, malabsorption, and dysmotility. Airway compromise can develop from severe tissue damage and inflammation. Mucositis is defined as severe (grade 3-4) when the pain and anatomic damage prevent adequate oral hydration and oral nutrition, or airway compromise is evident (Table 1). Severe mucositis increases the risk of infectious complications. Moreover, some opportunistic infections, such as herpesvirus, cause and exacerbate mucositis. In addition, severe and prolonged mucositis contributes to anticancer treatment dosage reductions and delays, and increases the cost of therapy.

Table 1. National Cancer Institute (NCI) Common Toxicity Criteria Grading for Mucositis

Grade 0	Grade 1	Grade 2	Grade 3	Grade 4
No signs or symptoms	Painless ulcers, erythema, or mild soreness in the absence of lesions	Painful erythema, edema, or ulcers, but can eat or swallow	Painful erythema, edema, or ulcers requiring I.V. hydration	Severe ulceration or requires parenteral or enteral nutritional support or prophylactic intubation

The severity of chemotherapy-associated mucositis is related to drug selection, increased dose, combination versus single agent chemotherapy, extended infusion of cell cycle-specific chemotherapy drugs, concurrent radiotherapy, and female gender. The frequency of severe mucositis for patients undergoing standard dose therapy and high dose therapy is 5% to 40% and 60% to 100%, respectively. Major organ impairment that prolongs the clearance of anticancer treatments can increase the likelihood and severity of mucositis. Patients with Down syndrome or carriers of the methylenetetrahydrofolate reductase *677 TT* genotype have an increased risk of severe mucositis following methotrexate administration. The severity of mucositis secondary to radiotherapy is related to the anatomic site of radiation exposure, radiation dose, and dosage fractionation. Grade 3-4 mucositis occurs in more than 50% of patients undergoing radiotherapy to the head and neck, abdomen, or pelvis. Table 2 lists various anticancer treatments associated with severe mucositis. The duration and severity of regimen-related mucositis can be increased by concurrent infections from opportunistic bacterial or viral pathogens affecting the gastrointestinal tract. Moreover, graft-versus-host disease can worsen regimen-related mucositis following allogeneic hematopoietic stem cell transplantation.

Table 2. Standard Dose Regimens Associated With Grade 3-4 Mucositis

Occurring in ≥30% of Patients	Occurring in ≥10% of Patients

Anthracycline + docetaxel + fluorouracil
Taxane + radiotherapy
Docetaxel + fluorouracil
Paclitaxel + fluorouracil + radiotherapy
Taxane + platinum + radiotherapy
Taxane + platinum + fluorouracil
Oxaliplatin + radiotherapy
Platinum + taxane + radiotherapy
Fluorouracil CIV[1] + platinum + radiotherapy
Fluorouracil + leucovorin + taxane
Irinotecan
Irinotecan + fluorouracil + radiotherapy
Irinotecan + fluorouracil + leucovorin
Irinotecan + fluorouracil + leucovorin +
  platinum
	Anthracycline + cyclophosphamide
	Anthracycline + taxane
	Anthracycline + cyclophosphamide +
	  docetaxel
	Anthracycline + cyclophosphamide +
	  paclitaxel
	Anthracycline + docetaxel + platinum
	Capecitabine + docetaxel
	Docetaxel
	Platinum + radiotherapy
	Platinum + gemcitabine + taxane
	Platinum + taxane + irinotecan
	Platinum + methotrexate + leucovorin
	Fluorouracil CIV[1]
	Fluorouracil CIV[1] + radiotherapy
	Fluorouracil CIV[1] + platinum
	Fluorouracil + leucovorin
	Fluorouracil + leucovorin + mitomycin
	Irinotecan + taxane

[1]CIV, continuous intravenous infusion; adapted from Sonis ST, Elting LS, Keefe D, et al,
"Perspectives on Cancer Therapy-Induced Mucosal Injury: Pathogenesis, Measurement,
Epidemiology, and Consequences for Patients," *Cancer*, 2004, 100(9 Suppl):1995-2025.

Mucositis Prevention and Treatment

Good oral hygiene is an essential constituent of routine supportive care for stomatitis and mucositis. Regular, gentle brushing with a soft toothbrush or cotton swab several times a day is helpful in removing dental plaque. Rinsing the mouth with a saline/bicarbonate solution helps remove debris and increases the pH, slowing the growth of oral flora. Use of mouthwashes containing alcohol may be painful or may dry the oral mucosa; phenol may promote mucosal ulceration.

Palifermin is a recombinant human keratinocyte growth factor that works in a receptor-mediated manner to reduce the duration and severity of mucositis by promoting epithelial cell proliferation, differentiation, and migration. Palifermin is indicated to decrease the incidence and duration of severe oral mucositis in patients with hematologic malignancies receiving myelotoxic therapy requiring hematopoietic stem cell support. The American Society of Clinical Oncology (ASCO) guidelines for the use of chemotherapy and radiotherapy protectants recommend palifermin to decrease the incidence of severe mucositis in patients undergoing autologous stem-cell transplantation with a total body irradiation (TBI) conditioning regimen. Additionally, palifermin may be considered in patients undergoing myeloablative allogeneic stem-cell transplantation with a TBI conditioning regimen. Data are insufficient however, for autologous and allogeneic transplant, to recommend palifermin when the conditioning regimen is chemotherapy only. Due to a lack of appropriate data, the ASCO guidelines also do not recommend palifermin use in non-stem-cell transplantation treatment regimens or for use when treating solid tumors. Palifermin is administered at 60 mcg/kg/day I.V. for 3 doses prior to myelotoxic therapy, with the 3rd dose given at least 24 hours before the chemotherapy and then 60 mcg/kg/day for 3 doses after myelotoxic therapy beginning on the same day as hematopoietic stem cell infusion (Hensley, 2009). Precautions from the manufacturer include the lack of safety and efficacy data in patients with solid tumors. The effect of palifermin on tumor growth in patients has not been established; however, palifermin promotes *in vitro* and *in vivo* epithelial tumor growth in experimental models.

Amifostine has been studied for reduction of chemotherapy-associated mucositis; however, the findings are equivocal. Due to insufficient data, the ASCO guidelines for the use of chemotherapy and radiotherapy protectants do not recommend amifostine to reduce the incidence of radiation therapy-induced mucositis associated with head and neck cancer or to prevent esophagitis due to concurrent chemoradiotherapy in patients with nonsmall cell lung cancer. Amifostine use to prevent xerostomia in patients with head and neck cancer receiving concurrent platinum-based chemotherapy is not supported; however, the guidelines suggest that the use of amifostine may be considered to reduce the incidence of xerostomia in patients with head and neck cancer undergoing radiation therapy alone (Hensley, 2009).

Supplementation with oral glutamine throughout chemotherapy administration may reduce the rate of clinically significant or severe mucositis. Regular gum chewing by pediatric patients to promote salivation as a means for preventing chemotherapy-induced mucositis did not reduce the rate of severe stomatitis following administration of intensive treatment regimens. However, the frequency of grades 1-4 stomatitis was significantly reduced with gum chewing five times daily with lower intensity chemotherapy regimens. In the multivariate analysis, the risk of oral mucositis was related only to the type of chemotherapy regimen used. Additional pharmaceutical agents and interventions that have been employed to reduce the duration and severity of mucositis, but lack sufficient evidence to support routine use, include allopurinol-cryotherapy, celecoxib, chlorhexidine, doxepin rinse, histamine gel, pilocarpine, sargramostim, vitamin E, and zinc sulfate.

Cryotherapy reduces oral mucositis associated with intravenous bolus administration of fluorouracil, methotrexate, and high-dose melphalan. Cryotherapy requires that the patient hold ice in their mouth for 30-60 minutes before and following chemotherapy administration. Cryotherapy purportedly reduces local oromucosal blood flow and consequently reduces chemotherapy exposure to the effected area. Patient tolerance limits the duration of cryotherapy treatments and reduces the utility of cryotherapy for chemotherapy with prolonged systemic clearance or drugs administered by protracted continuous infusion.

Therapy of stomatitis consists primarily of symptomatic support.

Pain control is a crucial part of stomatitis therapy. In addition to making the patient more comfortable, adequate pain control allows the patient to communicate and eat normally, thereby improving quality of life and reducing nutritional complications. Narcotic analgesia is frequently required for management of moderate-to-severe pain from mucositis. Topical application of local anesthetics is the most common approach to management of mild-to-moderate pain from stomatitis. Local application of cold sometimes provides adequate relief. Diphenhydramine has been used, but may cause drying of local tissues and sedation. Most products also contain significant amounts of alcohol which can exacerbate symptomatology. Local anesthetics (eg, benzocaine, lidocaine, tetracaine) are more potent than diphenhydramine, and are not associated with significant drying of local tissues. However, the numbing effect of these agents can impair swallowing. In addition, most of these products are unpalatable, and some are relatively expensive. The following table lists some of the commonly used agents.

Table 3. Various Mouth Care Products

Product	Concentration(s)	Dosage
Anesthetics		
Benzocaine	5% to 20%	1-5 mL; swish and expectorate q4-6h
Diphenhydramine	12.5 mg/5 mL	5 mL; swish and expectorate (or swallow) q4-6h
Lidocaine	1%	5 mL; swish and expectorate (or swallow) q2-3h
Antimicrobials		
Amphotericin B	100 mg/mL	1 mL qid; swish in mouth as long as possible; swallow or expectorate
Chlorhexidine gluconate	0.12%	15 mL q4-6h; swish and expectorate
Clotrimazole	10 mg	1 troche tid (prophylaxis) One 5 times/day for 14 days (treatment)
Nystatin	100,000 units/mL	5 mL; swish and expectorate (or swallow) q4-6h
	100,000 units (vaginal tablet)	1 q4-6h (dissolve in mouth)
Mouth Rinses		
Sodium bicarbonate (8.4 g/50 mEq/0.9% NaCl [1000 mL] mixture)	0.5 mEq/10 mL	5-15 mL q3-4h
Sodium chloride	0.9%	5-15 mL q3-4h

Many institutions and prescribers use locally compounded anesthetic formulations for treatment of stomatitis pain. Although the exact formulae may vary tremendously, the general rubric includes a local anesthetic to which one or more of the following are added: A second anesthetic, aluminum hydroxide/magnesium hydroxide suspension, diphenhydramine, hydrocortisone, kaolin/pectin suspension, sucralfate suspension, nystatin, tetracycline, and/or water. Controlled trials comparing various formulations with each other, or with the various individual ingredients are not available. However, these products often form the mainstay of symptomatic treatment for stomatitis. Examples of recipes for a few such formulations are found in Table 4.

Sucralfate is basic aluminum sucrose sulfate, a sulfate disaccharide, used primarily as an antiulcer agent. The activity of sucralfate appears to be local, rather than systemic. The drug forms a viscous material that adheres to the surface of gastric and duodenal ulcers, forming a protective barrier over the ulcer. Protected from the activity of gastric enzymes and acid, ulcers are able to heal naturally. This local activity stimulated investigation of sucralfate as a treatment for oral ulcers. A number of groups have studied sucralfate as a therapy for various oral ulcerative conditions with equivocal results. Although the results published to date do not demonstrate a real advantage to sucralfate therapy, some patients may benefit from its use. Sucralfate is commercially available as a tablet (1 g) or suspension (1 g/10 mL). When placed into water, the tablet readily absorbs the fluid and forms a gelatinous suspension.

Table 4. Examples of Extemporaneously Compounded Oral Stomatitis Products

Anesthetics

Diphenhydramine syrup 5 mL + lidocaine 2% 5-10 mL + aluminum/magnesium hydroxide suspension 5-15 mL (Maalox®/Mylanta®) (may also be referred to as "BMX"). **Note:** Avoid diphenhydramine products containing alcohol.

Lidocaine 2% 45 mL + diphenhydramine elixir 30 mL + sodium bicarbonate 8.4 g + 0.9% sodium chloride qs 1000 mL

Intubation: Nondepolarizing neuromuscular blockade should be used for the patient with severe mucositis requiring intubation to support the airway. One case report describes succinylcholine-induced hyperkalemia in a patient with severe mucositis following treatment chemotherapy.

Xerostomia

Xerostomia often accompanies stomatitis, particularly in patients who have received radiation to the neck and lower jaw. The condition can result in severe pain, dysphagia, malnutrition, and secondary infections. Subcutaneous or intravenous push administration of amifostine 200 mg/m^2 15-30 minutes prior to radiotherapy of the head and neck reduces acute and chronic xerostomia. The dose of amifostine for reduction of radiation-associated xerostomia and mucositis can be standardized to 500 mg in 0.9% sodium chloride 2.5 mL. Benzydamine oral rinse (not available in the United States), which has local anesthetic and anti-inflammatory properties, may be used for the prevention of radiation-induced mucositis in head and neck cancer patients. Artificial saliva substitutes can provide symptomatic relief from dry mouth and throat discomfort following chemotherapy and radiotherapy. Saliva substitutes, which generally contain a mixture of electrolytes, sugars(s), and carboxymethylcellulose, are available without a prescription.

Infections

In spite of good oral hygiene, some patients develop oral infections. This is particularly common in the patient with additional sources of immunosuppression, such as severe neutropenia, treatment with exogenous immunosuppressions, or disease-related immune impairment. One organism most commonly seen in such infections is *Candida albicans*. Topical treatment with nystatin or clotrimazole is usually sufficient to control these infections. Such treatments are usually well tolerated and produce minimal systemic effects. Nystatin 400,000-600,000 units (4-6 mL) four times a day, swished in the mouth for at least 2 minutes, then swallowed is recommended. Alternatively, nystatin vaginal tablets can be used orally. Clotrimazole 10 mg five times a day is another effective treatment for these infections. Troches are placed under the tongue or in a buccal cavity and allowed to dissolve. In some patients, clotrimazole used three times a day is an effective prophylaxis against oral *Candida* infections. Patients with significant xerostomia may have trouble dissolving the nystatin or clotrimazole tablets, and may require an artificial saliva product to moisten the mouth. Oral or intravenous administration of fluconazole 100-200 mg daily may be necessary for treatment of microbiologically documented or presumed oromucosal candidiasis in the patient with moderate-to-severe mucositis extending proximally beyond the mouth or the patient with additional sources of immune suppression. Fluconazole should be continued for at least 2 weeks, and until microbiologic and clinical evidence of infectious disease have resolved and the patient's immune recovery is considered adequate. Alternative systemic antifungal agents that can be considered for treatment of oromucosal and esophageal candidiasis include caspofungin, itraconazole, posaconazole, voriconazole, and amphotericin B products.

Herpes simplex virus is another common pathogen causing oral and other gastrointestinal infections in the patient with moderate-to-severe mucositis. The risk for oral Herpes simplex infection is greatest in patients with an additional source of immune compromise. Systemic treatment with acyclovir, famciclovir, or valacyclovir is required for oromucosal or gastrointestinal Herpes simplex infection. Alternative systemic antiviral agents for treatment of resistant Herpes simplex infections include ganciclovir, valganciclovir, and foscarnet.

Selected Readings

Aisa Y, Mori T, Kudo M, et al, "Oral Cryotherapy for the Prevention of High-Dose Melphalan-Induced Stomatitis in Allogeneic Hematopoietic Stem Cell Transplant Recipients," *Support Care Cancer*, 2005, 13(4):266-9.

Al-Khafaji AH, Dewhirst WE, Cornell CJ Jr, et al, "Succinylcholine-Induced Hyperkalemia in a Patient With Mucositis Secondary to Chemotherapy," *Crit Care Med*, 2001, 29(6):1274-6.

Alterio D, Jereczek-Fossa BA, Zuccotti GF, et al, "Tetracaine Oral Gel in Patients Treated With Radiotherapy for Head-and-Neck Cancer: Final Results of a Phase II Study," *Int J Radiat Oncol Biol Phys*, 2006, 64(2):392-5.

Aquino VM, Harvey AR, Garvin JH, et al, "A Double-Blind Randomized Placebo-Controlled Study of Oral Glutamine in the Prevention of Mucositis in Children Undergoing Hematopoietic Stem Cell Transplantation: A Pediatric Blood and Marrow Transplant Consortium Study," *Bone Marrow Transplant*, 2005, 36(7):611-6.

Awidi A, Homsi U, Kakail RI, et al, "Double-Blind, Placebo-Controlled Cross-Over Study of Oral Pilocarpine for the Prevention of Chemotherapy-Induced Oral Mucositis in Adult Patients With Cancer," *Eur J Cancer*, 2001, 37(16):2010-4.

Berger A, Henderson M, Nadoolman W, et al, "Oral Capsaicin Provides Temporary Relief for Oral Mucositis Pain Secondary to Chemotherapy/Radiation Therapy," *J Pain Symptom Manage*, 1995, 10(3):243-8.

Cerchietti LC, Navigante AH, Lutteral MA, et al, "Double-Blinded, Placebo-Controlled Trial on Intravenous L-Alanyl-L-Glutamine in the Incidence of Oral Mucositis Following Chemo-radiotherapy in Patients With Head-and-Neck Cancer," *Int J Radiat Oncol Biol Phys*, 2006, 65(5):1330-7.

Chan A and Ignoffo RJ, "Survey of Topical Oral Solutions for the Treatment of Chemo-Induced Oral Mucositis," *J Oncol Pharm Pract*, 2005, 11(4):139-43.

Chiara S, Nobile MT, Vincenti M, et al, "Sucralfate in the Treatment of Chemotherapy-Induced Stomatitis: A Double-Blind, Placebo-Controlled Pilot Study," *Anticancer Res*, 2001, 21(5):3707-10.

Choi K, Lee SS, Oh SJ, et al, "The Effect of Oral Glutamine on 5-Fluorouracil/Leucovorin-Induced Mucositis/Stomatitis Assessed by Intestinal Permeability Test," *Clin Nutr*, 2007, 26(1):57-62.

Dodd MJ, Miaskowski C, Greenspan D, et al, "Radiation-Induced Mucositis: A Randomized Clinical Trial of Micronized Sucralfate Versus Salt & Soda Mouthwashes," *Cancer Invest*, 2003, 21(1):21-33.

Elad S, Ackerstein A, Bitan M, et al, "A Prospective, Double-Blind Phase II Study Evaluating the Safety and Efficacy of a Topical Histamine Gel for the Prophylaxis of Oral Mucositis in Patients Post Hematopoietic Stem Cell Transplantation," *Bone Marrow Transplant*, 2006, 37(8):757-62.

El-Housseiny AA, Saleh SM, El-Masry AA, et al, "The Effectiveness of Vitamin "E" in the Treatment of Oral Mucositis in Children Receiving Chemotherapy," *J Clin Pediatr Dent*, 2007, 31(3):167-70.

Epstein JB, Epstein JD, Epstein MS, et al, "Oral Doxepin Rinse: The Analgesic Effect and Duration of Pain Reduction in Patients With Oral Mucositis Due to Cancer Therapy," *Anesth Analg*, 2006, 103(2):465-70.

Epstein JB, Silverman S Jr, Paggiarino DA, et al, "Benzydamine HCl for Prophylaxis of Radiation-Induced Oral Mucositis: Results From a Multicenter, Randomized, Double-Blind, Placebo-Controlled Clinical Trial," *Cancer*, 2001, 92(4):875-85.

Ertekin MV, Koc M, Karslioglu I, et al, "Zinc Sulfate in the Prevention of Radiation-Induced Oropharyngeal Mucositis: A Prospective, Placebo-Controlled, Randomized Study," *Int J Radiat Oncol Biol Phys*, 2004, 58(1):167-74.

Franzen L, Henriksson R, Littbrand B, et al, "Effects of Sucralfate on Mucositis During and Following Radiotherapy of Malignancies in the Head and Neck Region, A Double-Blind Placebo-Controlled Study" *Acta Oncol*, 1995, 34(2):219-23.

Gandemer V, Le Deley MC, Dollfus C, et al, "Multicenter Randomized Trial of Chewing Gum for Preventing Oral Mucositis in Children Receiving Chemotherapy," *J Pediatr Hematol Oncol*, 2007, 29(2):86-94.

Garre ML, Relling MV, Kalwinsky D, et al, "Pharmacokinetics and Toxicity of Methotrexate in Children With Down Syndrome and Acute Lymphocytic Leukemia," *J Pediatr*, 1987, 111 (4):606-12.

Gori E, Arpinati M, Bonifazi F, et al, "Cryotherapy in the Prevention of Oral Mucositis in Patients Receiving Low-Dose Methotrexate Following Myeloablative Allogeneic Stem Cell Transplantation: A Prospective Randomized Study of the Gruppo Italiano Trapianto Di Midollo Osseo Nurses Group," *Bone Marrow Transplant*, 2007, 39(6):347-52.

Hensley ML, Hagerty KL, Kewalramani T, et al, "American Society of Clinical Oncology 2008 Clinical Practice Guideline Update: Use of Chemotherapy and Radiotherapy Protectants," *J Clin Oncol*, 2009, 27(1): 127-45.

Huang EY, Leung SW, Wang CJ, et al, "Oral Glutamine to Alleviate Radiation-Induced Oral Mucositis: A Pilot Randomized Trial," *Int J Radiat Oncol Biol Phys*, 2000, 46(3):535-9.

Javle MM, Cao S, Durrani FA, et al, "Celecoxib and Mucosal Protection: Translation From an Animal Model to a Phase I Clinical Trial of Celecoxib, Irinotecan, and 5-Fluorouracil," *Clin Cancer Res*, 2007, 13(3):965-71.

Keefe DM, Schubert MM, Elting LS, et al, "Updated Clinical Practice Guidelines for the Prevention and Treatment of Mucositis," *Cancer*, 2007, 109(5):820-31.

Lilleby K, Garcia P, Gooley T, et al, "A Prospective, Randomized Study of Cryotherapy During Administration of High-Dose Melphalan to Decrease the Severity and Duration of Oral Mucositis in Patients With Multiple Myeloma Undergoing Autologous Peripheral Blood Stem Cell Transplantation," *Bone Marrow Transplant*, 2006, 37(11):1031-5.

Lin LC, Que J, Lin LK, et al, "Zinc Supplementation to Improve Mucositis and Dermatitis in Patients After Radiotherapy for Head-and-Neck Cancers: A Double-Blind, Randomized Study," *Int J Radiat Oncol Biol Phys*, 2006, 65(3):745-50.

Makkonen TA, Bostrom P, Vilja P, et al, "Sucralfate Mouth Washing in the Prevention of Radiation-Induced Mucositis: A Placebo-Controlled Double-Blind Randomized Study," *Int J Radiat Oncol Biol Phys*, 1994, 30:177-82.

McAleese JJ, Bishop KM, A'Hern R, et al, "Randomized Phase II Study of GM-CSF to Reduce Mucositis Caused by Accelerated Radiotherapy of Laryngeal Cancer," *Br J Radiol*, 2006, 79 (943):608-13.

Mori T, Yamazaki R, Aisa Y, et al, "Brief Oral Cryotherapy for the Prevention of High-Dose Melphalan-Induced Stomatitis in Allogeneic Hematopoietic Stem Cell Transplant Recipients," *Support Care Cancer*, 2006, 14(4):392-5.

"National Cancer Institute Common Terminology Criteria for Adverse Events (CTCAE) version 3," Available at: http://www.fda.gov/cder/cancer/toxicityframe.htm. Last accessed August 9, 2007.

Okuno SH, Woodhouse CO, Loprinzi CL, et al, "Phase III Controlled Evaluation of Glutamine for Decreasing Stomatitis in Patients Receiving Fluorouracil (5-FU)-Based Chemotherapy," *Am J Clin Oncol*, 1999, 22(3):258-61.

Peterson DE, Jones JB, and Petit RG 2nd, "Randomized, Placebo-Controlled Trial of Saforis for Prevention and Treatment of Oral Mucositis in Breast Cancer Patients Receiving Anthracycline-Based Chemotherapy," *Cancer*, 2007, 109(2):322-31.

Pfeiffer P, Madsen EL, Hansen O, et al, "Effect of Prophylactic Sucralfate Suspension on Stomatitis Induced by Cancer Chemotherapy: A Randomized, Double-Blind Cross-Over Study," *Acta Oncol*, 1990, 29(2):171-3.

Pitten FA, Kiefer T, Buth C, et al, "Do Cancer Patients With Chemotherapy-Induced Leukopenia Benefit From an Antiseptic Chlorhexidine-Based Oral Rinse? A Double-Blind, Block-Randomized, Controlled Study, " *J Hosp Infect*, 2003, 53(4):283-91.

Potting CM, Uitterhoeve R, Op Reimer WS, et al, "The Effectiveness of Commonly Used Mouthwashes for the Prevention of Chemotherapy-Induced Oral Mucositis: A Systematic Review," *Eur J Cancer Care (Engl)*, 2006, 15(5):431-9.

Quintiliani R, Owens NJ, Quercia RA, et al, "Treatment and Prevention of Oropharyngeal Candidiasis," *Am J Med*, 1984, 77(4D):44-8.

Rattan J, Schneider M, Arber N, et al, "Sucralfate Suspension as a Treatment of Recurrent Aphthous Stomatitis," *J Intern Med*, 1994, 236(3):341-3.

Rossi A, Rosati G, Colarusso D, et al, "Subcutaneous Granulocyte-Macrophage Colony-Stimulating Factor in Mucositis Induced by an Adjuvant 5-Fluorouracil Plus Leucovorin Regimen. A Phase II Study and Review of the Literature," *Oncology*, 2003, 64(4):353-60.

Ryu JK, Swann S, LeVeque F, et al, "The Impact of Concurrent Granulocyte Macrophage-Colony Stimulating Factor on Radiation-Induced Mucositis in Head and Neck Cancer Patients: A Double-Blind Placebo-Controlled Prospective Phase III Study by Radiation Therapy Oncology Group 9901," *Int J Radiat Oncol Biol Phys*, 2007, 67(3):643-50.

Saarilahti K, Kajanti M, Joensuu H, et al, "Comparison of Granulocyte-Macrophage Colony-Stimulating Factor and Sucralfate Mouthwashes in the Prevention of Radiation-Induced

Mucositis: A Double-Blind Prospective Randomized Phase III Study, " *Int J Radiat Oncol Biol Phys*, 2002, 54(2):479-85.

Scarantino C, LeVeque F, Swann RS, et al, "Effect of Pilocarpine During Radiation Therapy: Results of RTOG 97-09, a Phase III Randomized Study in Head and Neck Cancer Patients," *J Support Oncol*, 2006, 4(5):252-8.

Sonis ST, Elting LS, Keefe D, et al, "Perspectives on Cancer Therapy-Induced Mucosal Injury: Pathogenesis, Measurement, Epidemiology, and Consequences for Patients," *Cancer*, 2004, 100 (9 Suppl):1995-2025.

Stokman MA, Wachters FM, Koopmans P, et al, "Outcome of Local Application of Amifostine (WR-1065) on Epirubicin-Induced Oral Mucositis. A Phase II Study," *Anticancer Res*, 2004, 24 (5B):3263-7.

Sung L, Tomlinson GA, Greenberg ML, et al, "Serial Controlled N-of-1 Trials of Topical Vitamin E as Prophylaxis for Chemotherapy-Induced Oral Mucositis in Paediatric Patients," *Eur J Cancer*, 2007, 43(8):1269-75.

Ulrich CM, Yasui Y, Storb R, et al, "Pharmacogenetics of Methotrexate: Toxicity Among Marrow Transplantation Patients Varies With the Methylenetetrahydrofolate Reductase C677T Polymorphism," *Blood*, 2001, 98(1):231-4.

Vokurka S, Bystricka E, Koza V, et al, "Higher Incidence of Chemotherapy Induced Oral Mucositis in Females: A Supplement of Multivariate Analysis to a Randomized Multicentre Study," *Support Care Cancer*, 2006, 14(9):974-6.

Yokomizo H, Yoshimatsu K, Hashimoto M, et al, "Prophylactic Efficacy of Allopurinol Ice Ball for Leucovorin/5-Fluorouracil Therapy-Induced Stomatitis," *Anticancer Res*, 2004, 24(2C):1131-4.

TUMOR LYSIS SYNDROME

INTRODUCTION

Tumor lysis syndrome (TLS) is a potentially life threatening disorder that is characterized as an acute metabolic disturbance resulting from the rapid destruction of tumor cells. Cellular destruction releases cellular breakdown products (nucleic acids, anions, cations, peptides) that overwhelm the body's normal mechanisms for their utilization, excretion, and elimination. Signs and symptoms of TLS often develop within 72 hours of beginning cytotoxic chemotherapy in patients with newly diagnosed acute leukemias (acute lymphoblastic leukemia [ALL] and acute myeloid leukemia [AML]) or lymphoproliferative malignancies (Burkitt's and non-Burkitt's lymphomas). However, TLS can occur spontaneously in malignant diseases with vigorous cell turnover. Although most commonly reported in patients with hematologic and lymphoid malignancies, TLS has also been reported with solid tumors such as breast cancer, colon cancer, melanoma, ovarian cancer, prostate cancer, small cell lung cancer, and testicular cancer. Acute TLS attributed to administration of a corticosteroid, rituximab, and zoledronic acid in patients with treatment-sensitive tumors have been reported in the medical literature. Additional treatment and diagnostic procedures attributed with causing tumor lysis syndrome include total body irradiation, splenic irradiation, staging laparotomy, laparoscopic splenectomy preceded by splenic artery embolization, and radiofrequency interstitial thermal ablation of metastatic hepatic lesions. Metabolic abnormalities associated with acute TLS include hyperphosphatemia, hyperkalemia, hyperuricemia, azotemia, hypocalcemia, and metabolic acidosis. Cardiac arrhythmias, seizures, and major organ failure can occur in severe cases of TLS. Hyperkalemia, hyperuricemia, and hypocalcemia can produce cardiac arrhythmias, tetany, and sudden death. Acute renal failure can occur due to precipitation of uric acid and calcium phosphate in the renal tubules.

PREDISPOSING FACTORS

1. Bulky disease (>10 cm); leukemia with high white blood cell count (>25,000/mm^3)
2. Acute myelogenous leukemia with history of chronic myelomonocytic leukemia
3. Marked sensitivity of the tumor to a particular treatment modality
4. Male gender
5. Renal impairment, including pre-existing volume depletion
6. Elevated pretreatment lactic dehydrogenase serum levels (>2 times ULN)
7. Elevated pretreatment uric acid serum levels (>7.5 mg/dL) independent of renal impairment

CLINICAL FEATURES AND TREATMENT

General Principles

Prevention and early management of TLS are aimed at decreasing the risk of morbidity and mortality from cardiac arrhythmias, seizures, and organ failure. Vigorous hydration with intravenous 0.9% sodium chloride or crystalloid fluids (2-3 liters/m^2/24 hours) to maintain urine output of at least 80-100 mL/m^2/hour, with or without administration of loop or osmotic diuretics (avoid diuretic use in patient with hypovolemia or obstructive uropathy), is the cornerstone of the initial management for acute or potential TLS. Due to the tendency for calcium phosphate nephrocalcinosis and the potential for metabolic alkalosis, urinary alkalinization with sodium bicarbonate is no longer recommended for the treatment and prevention of TLS (Coiffier, 2008).

Allopurinol in doses of 100 mg/m^2 every 8 hours (maximum 800 mg/day) orally or 200-400 mg/m^2/day I.V. (in 1-3 divided doses; maximum 600 mg/day) should be administered to decrease endogenous uric acid production and to reduce associated urinary obstruction; dose reductions may be required for renal dysfunction (Coiffier, 2008). While allopurinol decreases uric acid production, it is ineffective in reducing high uric acid levels, may lead to urinary xanthine crystal precipitation which could lead to obstruction, and interacts with purine based drug therapy, such as mercaptopurine.

Rasburicase is administered for rapid reduction of uric acid levels. Rasburicase, which is a recombinant form of urate oxidase produced in *Saccharomyces cerevisiae*, catalyzes the degradation of uric acid to allantoin which is more soluble and readily excreted by the kidneys. Rasburicase is reserved for patients at risk for severe tumor lysis syndrome and patient's with elevated uric acid levels and signs of moderate-to-severe renal impairment or other major organ dysfunction. The major risks associated with administration of rasburicase include anaphylaxis, hypersensitivity reactions, methemoglobinemia, and hemolysis. This product is contraindicated in patients with glucose-6-phosphate dehydrogenase deficiency due to an elevated risk of hemolysis. An additional concern with rasburicase administration is the development of neutralizing antibodies. This phenomenon was observed in 64% of 28 normal, healthy volunteers studied; the effect of neutralizing antibodies on the efficacy of this product with repeated usage is unknown.

Rasburicase is approved for use in pediatric patients, with the labeled dose of 0.15-0.2 mg/kg/dose daily for a period of five days beginning 4-24 hours prior to the initiation of chemotherapy administration. However, due to the costs and risks of therapy plus the immediate and measurable effects of rasburicase, some centers administer a single dose which is repeated daily as warranted by plasma uric acid levels. The following dose levels (based on risk for TLS) with duration of treatment based on plasma uric acid levels have been recommended for children: 0.2 mg/kg once daily (duration based on plasma uric acid levels) for high risk patients, 0.15 mg/kg once daily (duration based on plasma uric acid levels) for intermediate risk, and 0.05-0.1 mg/kg once daily (duration based on clinical judgment) for low-risk patients (Coiffier, 2008). Although not approved for use in adults, weight- and risk-based dosing as detailed above has been reported. Fixed-dose rasburicase, ranging from 3-7.5 mg as a single dose (Hutcherson, 2006; McDonnell, 2006; Reeves, 2008; Trifilio, 2006) with doses (1.5-6 mg) repeated if needed (based on serum uric acid levels) has also been reported in adults.

Rasburicase will degrade uric acid *in vitro* when stored at room temperature. Consequently, to prevent artifactually low rasburicase levels, plasma samples must be collected in prechilled tubes, then immediately placed in an ice water bath until centrifuged at 4°C. Plasma must be analyzed within four hours of collection.

Clinical features and treatment for specific metabolic disorders are discussed in the following sections.

Hyperuricemia

Cytolysis during TLS releases purine and pyrimidine nucleotides into the bloodstream and extracellular tissues. Oxidation of the purines hypoxanthine and xanthine yields uric acid, which can precipitate in the renal tubules and cause oliguric renal failure. A high concentration of uric acid and an acidic urine pH promote uric acid crystallization and renotubular precipitation. Maintenance of urine flow and urinary alkalinization are utilized to reduce purine precipitation and preserve renal function. Allopurinol blocks the endogenous production of uric acid by inhibiting the enzyme xanthine oxidase, which oxidizes hypoxanthine and xanthine to uric acid. Allopurinol is used prophylactically during the early management of TLS. Rasburicase decreases existing uric acid concentrations by conversion of this molecule to the inactive and soluble metabolite allantoin, which is readily excreted by the kidneys.

Hyperkalemia

Potassium is primarily an intracellular ion that is released during massive cellular breakdown. Increasing levels of serum potassium can be dangerous, leading to cardiac arrhythmias or sudden death, especially in the presence of hypocalcemia (see following discussion). Standard treatments to remove potassium from the blood stream and extracellular fluids should be initiated as warranted by the patient's serum potassium level and electrocardiographic abnormalities. Other sources of potassium intake (including nutritional sources and medications and intravenous solutions) should be eliminated in patients at risk for or with TLS. Pharmaceutical measures routinely used to manage hyperkalemia in patients with TLS include volume expansion with forced diuresis, administration of glucose with insulin, and the cation exchange product sodium polystyrene sulfonate. Textbook algorithms for management of hyperkalemia include instructions for administration of calcium as a cardioprotective measure; however this is **not** a standard intervention in the setting of TLS. Calcium administration must be done judiciously in the patient with TLS because it can precipitate as calcium phosphate in highly perfused tissues.

Hyperphosphatemia and Hypocalcemia

The release of intracellular inorganic phosphate following massive cellular breakdown sets into motion several important clinical features. Serum phosphate levels will quickly exceed the threshold for normal renal excretion, with phosphate excretion becoming limited by the glomerular filtration rate. Any azotemia that develops during therapy will hinder phosphate excretion. Treatment includes the use of aluminum hydroxide for 1-2 days orally (or nasogastrically), or sevelamer, calcium carbonate, or lanthanum carbonate to reduce phosphate levels, and hemodialysis or hemofiltration, if necessary. High phosphate levels will also cause reciprocal hypocalcemia. Although generally asymptomatic, hypocalcemia may cause neuromuscular irritation, tetany, and cardiac dysrhythmias. Symptomatic patients may receive calcium gluconate 50-100 mg/kg intravenously (slowly, with ECG monitoring) to increase serum calcium levels. Unfortunately, despite hypocalcemia, the solubility product of calcium and phosphate may be exceeded in acute TLS, resulting in tissue calcification and organ failure.

Hemodialysis / Hemofiltration

Due to the unpredictability of TLS, intermittent hemodialysis, continuous arteriovenous hemodialysis, or continuous veno-venous hemodiafiltration may be needed and can be lifesaving. Hemodialysis or hemofiltration may be used to control and maintain fluid volume and/or to remove uric acid, phosphate, and potassium from serum. Intermittent hemodialysis, continuous arteriovenous hemodialysis, or continuous veno-venous hemodiafiltration should be considered as warranted by the severity of serum chemistry abnormalities, major organ dysfunction, and the patient's response to pharmaceutical treatments.

Selected Readings

Agha-Razii M, Amyot SL, Pichette V, et al, "Continuous Veno-Venous Hemodiafiltration for the Treatment of Spontaneous Tumor Lysis Syndrome Complicated by Acute Renal Failure and Severe Hyperuricemia," *Clin Nephrol*, 2000, 54(1):59-63.

Arnold TM, Reuter JP, Delman BS, et al, "Use of Single-Dose Rasburicase in an Obese Female," *Ann Pharmacother*, 2004, 38(9):1428-31.

Barry BD, Kell MR, and Redmond HP, "Tumor Lysis Syndrome Following Endoscopic Radiofrequency Interstitial Thermal Ablation of Colorectal Liver Metastases," *Surg Endosc*, 2002, 16(7):1109.

Cairo MS and Bishop M, "Tumour Lysis Syndrome: New Therapeutic Strategies and Classification," *Br J Haematol*, 2004, 127(1):3-11.

Chen SW, Hwang WS, Tsao CJ, et al, "Hydroxyurea and Splenic Irradiation-Induced Tumour Lysis Syndrome: A Case Report and Review of the Literature," *J Clin Pharm Ther*, 2005, 30(6):623-5.

Coiffier B, Altman A, Pui CH, et al, "Guidelines for the Management of Pediatric and Adult Tumor Lysis Syndrome: An Evidence-Based Review," *J Clin Oncol*, 2008, 26(16):2767-78.

Coiffier B, Mounier N, Bologna S, et al, "Efficacy and Safety of Rasburicase (Recombinant Urate Oxidase) for the Prevention and Treatment of Hyperuricemia During Induction Chemotherapy of Aggressive Non-Hodgkin's Lymphoma: Results of the GRAAL1 (Groupe d'Etude Des Lymphomes De l'Adulte Trial on Rasburicase Activity in Adult Lymphoma) Study," *J Clin Oncol*, 2003, 21(23):4402-6.

Duzova A, Cetin M, Gümrük F, et al, "Acute Tumour Lysis Syndrome Following a Single-Dose Corticosteroid in Children With Acute Lymphoblastic Leukaemia," *Eur J Haematol*, 2001, 66 (6):404-7.

Gemici C, "Tumour Lysis Syndrome in Solid Tumours," *Clin Oncol (R Coll Radiol)*, 2006, 18 (10):773-80.

Habib GS and Saliba WR, "Tumor Lysis Syndrome After Hydrocortisone Treatment in Metastatic Melanoma: A Case Report and Review of the Literature," *Am J Med Sci*, 2002, 323(3):155-7.

Hutcherson DA, Gammon DC, Bhatt MS, et al, "Reduced-Dose Rasburicase in the Treatment of Adults With Hyperuricemia Associated With Malignancy," *Pharmacotherapy*, 2006, 26(2):242-7.

Jabr FI, "Acute Tumor Lysis Syndrome Induced by Rituximab in Diffuse Large B-Cell Lymphoma," *Int J Hematol*, 2005, 82(4):312-4.

Kurt M, Onal IK, Elkiran T, et al, "Acute Tumor Lysis Syndrome Triggered by Zoledronic Acid in a Patient With Metastatic Lung Adenocarcinoma," *Med Oncol*, 2005, 22(2):203-6.

Lee MH, Cheng KI, Jang RC, et al, "Tumour Lysis Syndrome Developing During an Operation," *Anaesthesia*, 2003, 37(11):85-7.

Lee AC, Li CH, So KT, et al, "Treatment of Impending Tumor Lysis With Single-Dose Rasburicase," *Ann Pharmacother*, 2003, 37(11):1614-7.

Leibowitz AB, Adamsky C, Gabrilove J, et al, "Intraoperative Acute Tumor Lysis Syndrome During Laparoscopic Splenectomy Preceded by Splenic Artery Embolization," *Surg Laparosc Endosc Percutan Tech*, 2007, 17(3):210-1.

Lerza R, Botta M, Barsotti B, et al, "Dexamethazone-Induced Acute Tumor Lysis Syndrome in a T-Cell Malignant Lymphoma," *Leuk Lymphoma*, 2002, 43(5):1129-32.

Linck D, Basara N, Tran V, et al, "Peracute Onset of Severe Tumor Lysis Syndrome Immediately After 4 Gy Fractionated TBI as Part of Reduced Intensity Preparative Regimen in a Patient With T-ALL With High Tumor Burden," *Bone Marrow Transplant*, 2003, 31(10):935-7.

Liu CY, Sims-McCallum RP, and Schiffer CA, "A Single Dose of Rasburicase is Sufficient for the Treatment of Hyperuricemia in Patients Receiving Chemotherapy," *Leuk Res*, 2005, 29(4):463-5.

Mato AR, Riccio BE, Qin L, et al, "A Predictive Model for the Detection of Tumor Lysis Syndrome During AML Induction Therapy," *Leuk Lymphoma*, 2006, 47(5):877-83.

McDonnell AM, Lenz KL, Frei-Lahr DA, et al, "Single-Dose Rasburicase 6 Mg in the Management of Tumor Lysis Syndrome in Adults," *Pharmacotherapy*, 2006, 26(6):806-12.

Oztop I, Demirkan B, Yaren A, et al, "Rapid Tumor Lysis Syndrome in a Patient With Metastatic Colon Cancer as a Complication of Treatment With 5-Fluorouracil/Leucoverin and Irinotecan," *Tumori*, 2004, 90(5):514-6.

Reeves DJ and Bestul DJ, "Evaluation of a Single Fixed Dose of Rasburicase 7.5 mg for the Treatment of Hyperuricemia in Adults With Cancer," *Pharmacotherapy*, 2008, 28(6):685-90.

Riccio B, Mato A, Olson EM, et al, "Spontaneous Tumor Lysis Syndrome in Acute Myeloid Leukemia: Two Cases and a Review of the Literature," *Cancer Biol Ther*, 2006, 5(12):1614-7.

Rostom AY, El-Hussainy G, Kandil A, et al, "Tumor Lysis Syndrome Following Hemi-Body Irradiation for Metastatic Breast Cancer," *Ann Oncol*, 2000, 11(10):1349-51.

Schelling JR, Ghandour FZ, Strickland TJ, et al, "Management of Tumor Lysis Syndrome With Standard Continuous Arteriovenous Hemodialysis: Case Report and a Review of the Literature," *Ren Fail*, 1998, 20(4):635-44.

Sorscher SM, "Tumor Lysis Syndrome Following Docetaxel Therapy for Extensive Metastatic Prostate Cancer," *Cancer Chemother Pharmacol*, 2004, 54(2):191-2.

Theodorou D, Lagoudianakis E, Pattas M, et al, "Pretreatment Tumor Lysis Syndrome Associated With Bulky Retroperitoneal Tumors. Recognition is the Mainstay of Therapy," *Tumori*, 2006, 92 (6):540-1.

Tiu RV, Mountantonakis SE, Dunbar AJ, et al, "Tumor Lysis Syndrome," *Semin Thromb Hemost*, 2007, 33(4):397-407.

Trifilio S, Gordon L, Singhal S, et al, "Reduced-Dose Rasburicase (Recombinant Xanthine Oxidase) in Adult Cancer Patients With Hyperuricemia," *Bone Marrow Transplant*, 2006, 37 (11):997-1001.

Yahata T, Nishikawa N, Aoki Y, et al, "Tumor Lysis Syndrome Associated With Weekly Paclitaxel Treatment in a Case With Ovarian Cancer," *Gynecol Oncol*, 2006, 103(2):752-4.

Yim BT, Sims-McCallum RP, and Chong PH, "Rasburicase for the Treatment and Prevention of Hyperuricemia," *Ann Pharmacother*, 2003, 37(7-8):1047-54.

Zigrossi P, Brustia M, Bobbio F, et al, "Flare and Tumor Lysis Syndrome With Atypical Features After Letrozole Therapy in Advanced Breast Cancer. A Case Report," *Ann Ital Med Int*, 2001, 16 (2):112-7.

CHRONIC PAIN MANAGEMENT (CANCER)

DEFINITION AND INCIDENCE

Pain is defined by the International Society for the Study of Pain as "an unpleasant sensory and emotional experience associated with actual or potential tissue damage, or described in terms of such damage". The reported incidence of pain in cancer patients varies with the method used to determine the presence of pain, and the type and stage of cancer. It is estimated that 51% of patients with various stages of cancer experience pain, and patients with advanced disease are more likely to have severe pain. Pain in cancer patients may be due to the disease itself (eg, metastatic bone disease, visceral involvement); it may be secondary to some treatments (eg, painful neuropathy from vincristine or paclitaxel, or postoperative pain); it may result from complications associated with cancer (eg, postherpetic neuralgia); or it may have been present prior to the diagnosis of cancer and be unrelated to cancer (eg, arthritis). Most often, treatment guidelines and discussions are directed against chronic pain associated with progressive disease.

NONOPIOID ANALGESICS

The World Health Organization recommends a stepwise approach to the management of cancer pain (see figure).

WHO Three-Step Analgesic Ladder

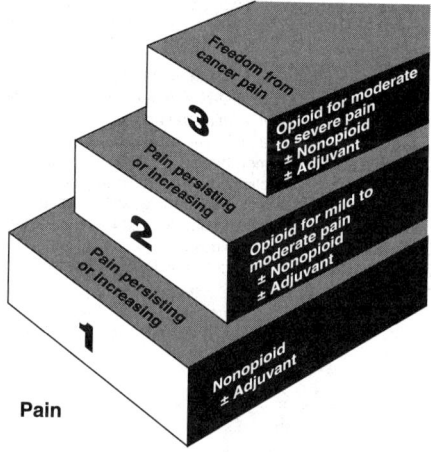

This approach recommends that the choice of therapy match the severity of pain (ie, strong opioids for moderate to severe pain). Nonopioids for (mild) cancer pain include acetaminophen, nonsteroidal anti-inflammatory drugs (NSAIDs), and aspirin. All of these have a ceiling above which increasing the dose will not enhance pain relief and will increase the likelihood of side effects. Although nonopioid analgesics are traditionally WHO step 1 products, they do have a role in the management of moderate-to-severe cancer pain. One blinded, placebo-controlled study reports that acetaminophen added to a strong opioid regimen in cancer patients improves pain control and well being.

Acetaminophen is commonly used for the management of mild-to-moderate pain. The manufacturer recommends a maximum daily dose of acetaminophen 4000 mg per 24-hours to reduce the risk of hepatotoxicity. Concerns regarding the use of NSAIDs in chronic cancer pain include the reversible inhibition of platelet aggregation, and the potential for gastropathy and nephrotoxicity. Aspirin is frequently avoided because of the potential for gastropathy and inhibition of platelet aggregation. Platelets exposed to aspirin become acetylated and permanently impaired. Celecoxib and nonacetylated salicylates, such as choline salicylate and magnesium salicylate, do not inhibit platelet aggregation.

OPIOID ANALGESICS

Opioid analgesic therapy should be initiated when adequate doses of nonopioid analgesics provide inadequate pain control or they are poorly tolerated.

Opioid analgesics for severe, persistent pain should be given "around-the-clock", not on an "as needed" or "PRN" basis. It is easier to prevent pain from recurring than to treat it once it has recurred. Titration of opioids to pain relief is easiest and safest using short-acting drugs (average duration of pain relief of 4 hours) or a continuous parenteral infusion. Once adequate pain relief is achieved, the 24-hour opioid dose can be given as a long-acting preparation (eg, sustained release morphine or oxycodone, transdermal fentanyl). In fact, opioid requirements can be increased in a similar manner for patients with worsening chronic pain daily. Medication for breakthrough pain, a transient worsening of otherwise stable pain in a patient taking an opioid, should always be available. Doses for breakthrough pain (ie, rescue doses) are commonly 5% to 15% of the 24-hour opioid dose, and may be administered every 1-2 hours as needed.

The oral route of administration for opioid analgesics is preferred whenever possible. All opioids undergo a high first-pass effect, which must be considered when converting from one route of administration to another. The parenteral to oral ratios for effectiveness of the different opioids vary from 1:2 to 1:6. The parenteral to oral dose ratio for morphine is 1:3 and 1:6 for the treatment of chronic pain and acute pain, respectively. Opioid equianalgesic doses are listed in the table that follows. Dose titration of opioid analgesics is based on pain control and patient tolerance. There is no maximum dosage for administration of opioid analgesics. Unlike the nonopioid analgesics, no ceiling on effectiveness of opioids has been identified and tolerance develops to most of the medication-related adverse effects.

Table 1. Opioid Analgesics

Drug	Route of Administration	Approx Equianalgesic Dose (mg)	Approx Duration[1] (h)
Codeine	I.M., I.V.	120	4-6
	Oral	200	
Fentanyl[2]	I.V.	0.1	0.5-2
Hydrocodone	Oral	20	4-6
Hydromorphone	I.M., I.V., SubQ	1.5	2-5
	Oral, rectal	7.5	
Meperidine	I.M., I.V., SubQ	75	2-4
	Oral	300	
Methadone	I.M., I.V., SubQ	5	6-12
	Oral	10	
Morphine	I.M., I.V., SubQ	10	3-4[3]
	Oral, rectal	30	
Oxycodone	Oral	20	4-6[3]

[1]Parenteral or immediate-release products.

[2]Transdermal fentanyl conversion presented in separate table that follows.

[3]Duration for sustained release dosage forms is 8-12 hours (MS Contin®, Oramorph SR®), 24 hours (Kadian®), 12 hours (Oxycontin®).

Meperidine is not recommended for chronic use. This is because of the potential for accumulation of a neurotoxic metabolite, normeperidine (see following information). Meperidine administration is best reserved for incident pain (ie, before a painful manipulation or procedure).

Tolerance is characterized by the requirement for a higher dose of opioid in order to produce the same effect previously seen with a lower dose. Tolerance develops to many side effects of opioids: respiratory depression, sedation, nausea, and vomiting. Tolerance does not usually develop to constipation. When a given dose of opioid is not effective, for whatever reason, and if side effects are tolerable, the dose can be increased. Physical dependence occurs with regular use of opioids, but is only of clinical importance if the opioid is abruptly discontinued or an opioid antagonist (eg, naloxone) administered, in which cases a withdrawal syndrome can be seen. Opioids should be tapered in patients whose pain improves. Signs and symptoms of withdrawal can be reduced by maintaining at least 25% of the previous day's opioid dose. The opioid can be discontinued when the total daily dose is the equivalent of 10-15 mg of intramuscular morphine. Psychological dependence is defined as a "pattern of compulsive drug use characterized by a continued craving for an opioid and the need to use the opioid for effects other than pain relief." Unlike tolerance and physical dependence, psychological dependence is a characteristic of the patient, and is a function of environmental, social, economic, and personality factors. Psychological dependence or addiction, can develop in patients requiring management of chronic pain; however, this is **not** a valid reason to undertreat pain.

The most troublesome side effect associated with chronic opioid use is constipation, and, as noted above, tolerance to constipation does not occur. Regular use of stimulant laxatives is often required.

Tolerance does develop to opioid-induced respiratory depression, allowing safe dose escalation. In the event of an acute overdose, or in the case of respiratory depression not responding to supportive measures, naloxone can be used. Naloxone administration is reserved for serious situations because it precipitates withdrawal symptoms and the prompt return of pain in patients physically dependent on opioids. Other side effects of naloxone administration include nausea, vomiting, sedation, sweating, itching, dry mouth, and tremulousness. Initiate naloxone therapy with low doses (0.1-0.2 mg) repeated and increased as warranted by respiratory rate and patient comfort. Nalmefene should be avoided due to the longer duration of action relative to that of naloxone, and the risk of prolonged rebound pain. Naltrexone is only available as an oral formulation, which limits its utility for acute reversal of opioid toxicity. Tolerance develops to nausea and vomiting, and these effects are more likely to occur when opioid therapy is initiated. Phenothiazines can be used to treat nausea and vomiting. Dimenhydrinate or meclizine can also be used to treat this side effect. Tolerance usually develops to sedation. For those patients in whom persistent or profound sedation limits opioid dose escalation and therefore pain relief, the use of stimulants (eg, dextroamphetamine, methylphenidate) should be considered. Sweating and itching are thought to be due to histamine release. Morphine and meperidine are notable for causing histamine release. Switching to another opioid should be considered for patients with intolerable sweating or itching. Seizures associated with opioids are generally attributed to accumulation of neurotoxic metabolites or large overdoses that presumably cause hypoxia. Normeperidine, a metabolite of meperidine that can accumulate with frequent repeated doses or in patients with renal insufficiency, is the most well known of these neurotoxic metabolites. Two weak opioid antagonists associated with seizures are tramadol and propoxyphene; these products are not recommended for management of chronic cancer pain. Distinct from seizures, myoclonic jerks may be seen with the use of high doses of opioids. Occasional reports indicate that they may also be seen with relatively lower doses. Benzodiazepines have been suggested to control this side effect.

Opioid-induced hyperalgesia (OIH) should be suspected when analgesic efficacy is inexplicably lost or when generalized or worsening pain develops during aggressive opioid titration. OIH is a rare consequence of opioid therapy in cancer patients, and most often seen with aggressive morphine titration. The underlying mechanism is thought to be related to inhibition of glycinergic activity at the level of the spinal cord by phenanthrene-type opioids that promotes a strychnine-like excitatory effect. Additional biochemical mechanisms implicated in OIH include upregulation of intracellular phosphokinase C which activates the NMDA receptor system, and intraspinal dynorphin-mediated substance P and glutamate release. In the scenario of OIH, continued dose escalation aggravates pain which then improves with dose reduction. Management of OIH includes dose reduction or interruption of treatment with the offending agent. Replacing a phenanthrene derivative to a piperidine-type opioid, such as fentanyl or methadone, is recommended.

As previously noted, the oral route of administration for opioids is generally preferred. When oral administration is not possible, several other routes are available (see Table 1). When patients suddenly become unable to take medication by mouth, opioids intended for oral administration have been administered rectally or vaginally. Morphine and hydromorphone are also available in rectal suppositories. The recommended rectal dose is the same as the oral dose. Continuous subcutaneous or intravenous infusions administered with an infusion control device are useful when oral administration is impossible. Continuous parenteral infusion of opioids provides more consistent pain relief and patient tolerance compared to intermittent injections which result in peaks and valleys of pain relief or side effects. Continuous infusions also allow for quick titration of opioid in patients with uncontrolled pain. Patient-controlled analgesia provides a continuous infusion of opioid with a capacity for patient-administered bolus injections for breakthrough pain. This is not unlike the concept of regularly scheduled sustained release oral opioid with immediate release tablets for breakthrough, as previously discussed. Assessment of the use of breakthrough doses, whether oral or parenteral, provides a basis for adjusting the dose/rate of the underlying opioid. Transdermal fentanyl is another alternative, long-acting, analgesic for patients unable to take oral opioids. Transdermal fentanyl should be avoided when initiating chronic analagia in opioid-naive patients to reduce the risk of profound respiratory depression. As is the case with sustained release oral opioids, it is preferable to titrate to pain relief using short-acting drugs, and then switch to transdermal fentanyl. The manufacturer recommends equianalgesic conversion to the fentanyl patch as presented in Table 2. This schema represents a conservative conversion from an oral or parenteral opioid to the fentanyl transdermal system, so the tabulated information should **not** be used to convert from fentanyl transdermal to an oral or parenteral opioid analgesic.

Table 2. Dosing Conversion Guidelines

Current Analgesic	Daily Dosage (mg/day)			
Morphine (oral)	60-134	135-224	225-314	315-404
Mophine (parenteral)	10-22	23-37	38-52	53-67
Hydromorphone (oral)	8-17	17.1-28	28.1-39	39.1-51
Hydromorphone (parenteral)	1.5-3.4	3.5-5.6	5.7-7.9	8-10
Oxycodone (oral)	30-67	67.5-112	112.5-157	157.5-202
Meperidine (parenteral)	75-165	166-278	279-390	391-503
Fentanyl transdermal recommended dose	**25 mcg/h**	**50 mcg/h**	**75 mcg/h**	**100 mcg/h**

One method for switching transdermal fentanyl and oral methadone is described by using the transdermal fentanyl:oral methadone conversion factor of 1:20 (daily dose:daily dose) to change patients (N=31) with inadequate pain control from one product to another (Mercandante, 2005). Oral methadone was administered in divided doses every eight hours. Fentanyl patches were removed when the first dose of methadone was administered. Conversely, for patients transitioning to transdermal fentanyl, the patch was applied with administration of the last methadone dose. This method was used successfully in 24 of 31 patients (78%) with improved pain control reported within 24 hours of product conversion and acceptable patient tolerance. Inadequate symptom control (6 patients) and adverse effects (1 patient) were the reasons for unsuccessful switching in seven patients. Using this conversion ratio, treatment with transdermal fentanyl 200 mcg/hour is switched to oral methadone 96 mg daily administered in divided doses as 30 mg every eight hours.

A similar method has been described which calculates the appropriate methadone dose using two steps (Benitez-Rosario, 2004). First, the patient's daily transdermal fentanyl dose is converted to the equivalent oral morphine dose using a ratio of fentanyl:oral morphine of 1:100. The resultant value is converted to the equivalent daily dose of oral methadone using the ratio of oral morphine: oral methadone ratio of 5:1 or 10:1. The calculated methadone dose is divided for administration every 8-12 hours beginning 8-24 hours following removal of the ▶

transdermal fentanyl system. Using this method, a patient with adequate pain control from transdermal fentanyl 100 mcg/hour would be receiving a daily dose of fentanyl 2.4 mg every 24 hours, which converts to oral morphine 240 mg per 24-hour, which converts to oral methadone 24-48 mg per 24 hours. So, 8-24 hours after removing the fentanyl patch, a dosage of oral methadone 15 mg administered every 8 or 12 hours can be started.

Intraspinal administration of opioids should be reserved for patients in whom systemic administration of opioids results in unacceptable or unmanageable toxicity. Epidural morphine is 5-10 times more potent than parenteral morphine, and intrathecal morphine is 10 times more potent than epidural morphine. Bupivacaine, clonidine, and ketamine have been added to epidural morphine infusions to enhance effectiveness.

Partial opioid agonists (eg, buprenorphine) or agonist-antagonists (eg, pentazocine, butorphanol, dezocine, nalbuphine) are generally not recommended for use in chronic cancer pain management. They have a ceiling for analgesic effectiveness, above which side effects are much more likely to increase, and they may precipitate withdrawal in patients receiving opioid agonists (eg, morphine). Naloxone may not be effective in reversing respiratory depression caused by buprenorphine.

Tramadol is a synthetic opioid that inhibits the neuronal reuptake of norepinephrine and serotonin. This product is indicated for the management of moderate pain. Its use is limited by the risk of seizures which have occurred in patients taking the usual and recommended dosage. Abrupt discontinuation of tramadol can precipitate withdrawal symptoms, such as tremors, sweating, diarrhea, upper respiratory symptoms, and rarely, hallucinations. Propoxyphene is another weak opioid not generally recommended for chronic cancer pain.

ADJUVANT ANALGESICS

Adjuvant analgesics are frequently used in addition to, rather than instead of, opioid analgesics. Adjuvants are often drugs that have primary indications other than pain, but may provide pain relief in certain situations. NSAIDs are commonly used for pain due to bone metastases (see individual NSAID monographs). Gabapentin and pregabalin are commonly used as adjunctive therapy for neuropathic pain. Additional drugs that have been used for this purpose include tricyclic antidepressants (eg, amitriptyline, nortriptyline), anticonvulsants (eg, carbamazepine), corticosteroids, and antiarrhythmics (eg, topical lidocaine). Methadone and ketamine are thought to improve neuropathic pain through blockade of the N-methyl-D-aspartate (NMDA) receptor. Neuropathic pain, often characterized by sharp, shooting, lancinating sensations, may result from nerve compression, infiltration, or destruction by tumor or from other associated conditions (eg, postherpetic neuralgia). Pain relief is usually not complete and, as is the case with NSAIDs in bone pain, these drugs are generally used in addition to opioids. Baclofen has also been used as an adjuvant analgesic for various types of neuropathic pain. Strontium-89 is a radiopharmaceutical that is reported to decrease the need for analgesics in patients with osteoblastic bone metastases. Prostate cancer is the most frequent malignancy associated with painful osteoblastic lesions. The bisphosphonates pamidronate and zoledronic acid are used to decrease pain and adverse skeletal events in patients with multiple myeloma and breast cancer. Calcitonin has also been used as an adjunct to analgesia in cancer pain. Capsaicin is a topically applied adjuvant analgesic that depletes substance P, a "painful" neurotransmitter. Capsaicin is recommended for use in postherpetic neuralgia and other painful neuropathies.

Selected Readings

American Pain Society, *Principles of Analgesic Use in the Treatment of Acute Pain and Chronic Cancer Pain*, 3rd ed, Skokie, IL: American Pain Society, 1992.

Axelrod DJ and Reville B, "Using Methadone to Treat Opioid-Induced Hyperalgesia and Refractory Pain," *J Opioid Manag*, 2007, 3(2):113-4.

Benitez-Rosario MA, Feria M, Salinas-Martín A, et al, "Opioid Switching From Transdermal Fentanyl to Oral Methadone in Patients With Cancer Pain," *Cancer*, 2004, 101(12):2866-73.

Benrath J, Scharbert G, Gustorff B, et al, "Long-Term Intrathecal S(+)-Ketamine in a Patient With Cancer-Related Neuropathic Pain," *Br J Anaesth*, 2005, 95(2):247-9.

Berenson JR, Lichtenstein A, Porter L, et al, "Efficacy of Pamidronate in Reducing Skeletal Events in Patients With Advanced Multiple Myeloma. Myeloma Aredia Study Group," *N Engl J Med*, 1996, 334(8):488-93.

Cordell GA and Araujo OE, "Capsaicin: Identification, Nomenclature, and Pharmacotherapy," *Ann Pharmacother*, 1993, 27(3):330-6.

Davis MP, Shaiova LA, and Angst MS, "When Opioids Cause Pain," *J Clin Oncol*, 2007, 25 (28):4497-8.

Elsner F, Radbruch L, Loick G, et al, "Intravenous Versus Subcutaneous Morphine Titration in Patients With Persisting Exacerbation of Cancer Pain," *J Palliat Med*, 2005, 8(4):743-50.

Foley KM, "The Treatment of Cancer Pain," *N Engl J Med*, 1985, 313(2):84-95.

Fromm GH, "Baclofen as an Adjuvant Analgesic," *J Pain Symptom Manage*, 1994, 9(8):500-9.

Højsted J and Sjøgren P, "Addiction to Opioids in Chronic Pain Patients: A Literature Review," *Eur J Pain*, 2007, 11(5):490-518.

Holdsworth MT, Adams VR, Chavez CM, et al, "Continuous Midazolam Infusion for the Management of Morphine-Induced Myoclonus," *Ann Pharmacother*, 1995, 29(1):25-9.

Jackson KC 2nd, "Pharmacotherapy for Neuropathic Pain," *Pain Pract*, 2006, 6(1):27-33.

Jacox A, Carr DB, Payne R, et al, "Management of Cancer Pain," *Clinical Practice Guideline No. 9*, AHCPR Publication No. 94-0592, Rockville, MD: Agency for Health Care Policy and Research, U.S. Department of Health and Human Services, Public Health Service, March 1994.

Laizure SC, "Considerations in Morphine Therapy," *Am J Hosp Pharm*, 1994, 51(16):2042-3.

Levy MH, "Pharmacologic Treatment of Cancer Pain," *N Engl J Med*, 1996, 335(15):1124-32.

Lossignol DA, Obiols-Portis M, and Body JJ, "Successful Use of Ketamine for Intractable Cancer Pain," *Support Care Cancer*, 2005, 13(3):188-93.

Mercadante SL, Berchovich M, Casuccio A, et al, "A Prospective Randomized Study of Corticosteroids as Adjuvant Drugs to Opioids in Advanced Cancer Patients," *Am J Hosp Palliat Care*, 2007, 24(1):13-9.

Mercadante S, Ferrera P, Villari P, et al, "Rapid Switching Between Transdermal Fentanyl and Methadone in Cancer Patients," *J Clin Oncol*, 2005, 23(22):5229-34.

Portenoy RK and Hagen NA, "Breakthrough Pain: Definition, Prevalence, and Characteristics," *Pain*, 1990, 41(3):273-81.

Potter JM, Reid DB, Shaw RJ, et al, "Myoclonus Associated With Treatment With High Doses of Morphine: The Role of Supplemental Drugs," *BMJ*, 1989, 299(6692):150-3.

Robinson RG, Preston DF, Baxter KG, et al, "Clinical Experience With Strontium-89 in Prostatic and Breast Cancer Patients," *Semin Oncol*, 1993, 20(3 Suppl 2):44-8.

Rodriguez RF, Castillo JM, Del Pilar Castillo M, et al, "Codeine/Acetaminophen and Hydrocodone/Acetaminophen Combination Tablets for the Management of Chronic Cancer Pain in Adults: A 23-Day, Prospective, Double-Blind, Randomized, Parallel-Group Study," *Clin Ther*, 2007, 29 (4):581-7.

Stearns L, Boortz-Marx R, Du Pen S, et al, "Intrathecal Drug Delivery for the Management of Cancer Pain: A Multidisciplinary Consensus of Best Clinical Practices," *J Support Oncol*, 2005, 3 (6):399-408.

Stockler M, Vardy J, Pillai A, et al, "Acetaminophen (Paracetamol) Improves Pain and Well-Being in People With Advanced Cancer Already Receiving a Strong Opioid Regimen: A Randomized, Double-Blind, Placebo-Controlled Cross-Over Trial," *J Clin Oncol*, 2004, 22(16):3389-94.

Szeto HH, Inturrisi CE, Houde R, et al, "Accumulation of Normeperidine, an Active Metabolite of Meperidine in Patients With Renal Failure of Cancer," *Ann Intern Med*, 1977, 86(6):738-41.

Tsavaris N, Kopterides P, Kosmas C, et al, "Analgesic Activity of High-Dose Intravenous Calcitonin in Cancer Patients With Bone Metastases," *Oncol Rep*, 2006, 16(4):871-5.

Vranken JH, van der Vegt MH, Kal JE, et al, "Treatment of Neuropathic Cancer Pain With Continuous Intrathecal Administration of S +-Ketamine," *Acta Anaesthesiol Scand*, 2004, 48 (2):249-52.

Wellington K and Goa KL, "Zoledronic Acid: A Review of Its Use in the Management of Bone Metastases and Hypercalcaemia of Malignancy," *Drugs*, 2003, 63(4):417-37.

Yucel A, Ozyalcin S, Koknel Talu G, et al, "The Effect of Venlafaxine on Ongoing and Experimentally Induced Pain in Neuropathic Pain Patients: A Double Blind, Placebo Controlled Study," *Eur J Pain*, 2005, 9(4):407-16.

COMMON TOXICITY CRITERIA

Selected Common Toxicity Criteria

Toxicity	Grade 0	Grade 1	Grade 2	Grade 3	Grade 4
Hematologic					
Leukocytes (WBC)	WNL	$3 \times 10^9/L$ to <LLN	2 to $<3 \times 10^9/L$	1 to $<2 \times 10^9/L$	$<1 \times 10^9/L$
Neutrophils (ANC)	WNL	$1.5 \times 10^9/L$ to <LLN	1 to $<1.5 \times 10^9/L$	0.5 to $<1 \times 10^9/L$	$<0.5 \times 10^9/L$
Lymphocytes	WNL	$0.8 \times 10^9/L$ to <LLN	0.5 to $<0.8 \times 10^9/L$	0.2 to $<0.5 \times 10^9/L$	$<0.2 \times 10^9/L$
Anemia (Hgb)	WNL	10 g/dL to <LLN	8 to <10 g/dL	6.5 to <8 g/dL	<6.5 g/dL
Platelets	WNL	$75 \times 10^9/L$ to <LLN	50 to $<75 \times 10^9/L$	25 to $<50 \times 10^9/L$	$<25 \times 10^9/L$
Hemorrhage	None	Mild, no transfusion		Transfusion indicated	Major intervention required
Cardiovascular					
Hypotension	None	Changes, no treatment required	Brief treatment required	Sustained treatment required, resolves	Shock
Hypertension	None	Increase by >20 mm Hg or to >150/100, treatment not required	Recurrent/persistent grade 1 level, minor treatment required	More intensive treatment required	Hypertensive crisis
Pericardial effusion	None	Asymptomatic effusion		Physiologic consequences	Life-threatening consequences
Syncope	Absent			Present	Life-threatening consequences
Thrombosis/embolism	None		DVT, intervention not indicated	DVT, intervention indicated	Pulmonary embolism/life threatening thrombus

Selected Common Toxicity Criteria *continued*

Toxicity	Grade 0	Grade 1	Grade 2	Grade 3	Grade 4
Dermatologic					
Rash (acne/acneiform)	None	Intervention not indicated	Intervention indicated	Pain, disfigurement, ulceration	
Rash (desquamation)	None	Macular or papular eruption	Erythema w/pruritus affecting <50% of BSA	Severe erythema/desquamation covering ≥50% of BSA	Generalized exfoliative or ulcerative dermatitis
Rash (erythema multiforme)	None		Scattered eruption	Severe eruption	Life-threatening eruption
Hand-foot syndrome	None	Minimal skin changes w/o pain	Skin changes or pain not interfering w/ADL	Skin changes/pain; interferes w/ADL	
Alopecia	None	Thinning/patchy	Complete		
Gastrointestinal					
Nausea	None	Loss of appetite/able to eat	Oral intake decreased/no weight loss	Inadequate intake/I.V. fluids required	Life-threatening consequences
Vomiting	None	1 episode/24 h	2-5 episodes/24 h	≥6 episodes/24 h, I.V. fluid required	Life-threatening consequences
Diarrhea	None	<4 stools/day increase over baseline	4-6 stools/day increase over baseline	≥7 stools/day increase/I.V. fluids required	Life-threatening consequences
Mucositis/stomatitis	None	Mucosal erythema	Patchy ulcerations	Confluent ulceration, bleeding	Tissue necrosis/bleeding; life-threatening
GI bleeding	None	Mild, intervention not indicated	Symptomatic, mild intervention indicated	Transfusion required, intervention indicated	Life-threatening consequences
Amylase elevation	None	>ULN to 1.5 x ULN	>1.5 to 2 x ULN	>2 to 5 x ULN	>5 x ULN
Lipase elevation	None	>ULN to 1.5 x ULN	>1.5 to 2 x ULN	>2 to 5 x ULN	>5 x ULN

Selected Common Toxicity Criteria *continued*

Toxicity	Grade 0	Grade 1	Grade 2	Grade 3	Grade 4
Hepatic					
Alkaline phosphatase elevation	WNL	>ULN to 2.5 x ULN	>2.5 to 5 x ULN	>5 to 20 x ULN	>20 x ULN
AST elevation	WNL	>ULN to 2.5 x ULN	>2.5 to 5 x ULN	>5 to 20 x ULN	>20 x ULN
ALT elevation	WNL	>ULN to 2.5 x ULN	>2.5 to 5 x ULN	>5 to 20 x ULN	>20 x ULN
Hyperbilirubinemia	WNL	>ULN to 1.5 x ULN	>1.5 to 3 x ULN	>3 to 10 x ULN	>10 x ULN
Ascites	None	Asymptomatic	Symptomatic, diuretics required	Symptomatic, procedure required	Life-threatening consequences
Veno-occlusive disease	None	Mild	Moderate	Severe	Life-threatening
Metabolic					
Hypercholesteremia	None	>ULN to 300 mg/dL	>300 to 400 mg/dL	>400 to 500 mg/dL	>500 mg/dL
Hyperglycemia	WNL	>ULN to 160 mg/dL	>160 to 250 mg/dL	>250 to 500 mg/dL	>500 mg/dL
Hypertriglyceridemia	None	>ULN to 2.5 x ULN	>2.5 to 5 x ULN	>5 to 10 x ULN	>10 x ULN
Hypoglycemia	WNL	55 to <LLN mg/dL	40 to <55 mg/dL	30 to <40 mg/dL	<30 mg/dL
Hypocalcemia	WNL	8 to <LLN mg/dL	7 to <8 mg/dL	6 to <7 mg/dL	<6 mg/dL
Hypokalemia	WNL	3 to <LLN mmol/L	–	2.5 to <3 mmol/L	<2.5 mmol/L
Hypomagnesemia	WNL	1.2 to <LLN mg/dL	0.9 to <1.2 mg/dL	0.7 to <0.9 mg/dL	<0.7 mg/dL
Hypophosphatemia	WNL	2.5 to <LLN mg/dL	2 to <2.5 mg/dL	1 to <2 mg/dL	<1 mg/dL

Selected Common Toxicity Criteria *continued*

Toxicity	Grade 0	Grade 1	Grade 2	Grade 3	Grade 4
Renal / Genitourinary					
Hematuria	None	Minimal or microscopic	Symptomatic, minor intervention required	Transfusion required, intervention indicated	Life-threatening consequences
Hypoalbuminemia	WNL	3 g/dL to <LLN	2 to <3 g/dL	<2 g/dL	
Serum creatinine elevation	WNL	>ULN to 1.5 x ULN	>1.5 to 3 x ULN	>3 to 6 x ULN	>6 x ULN
Respiratory					
Dyspnea	None	Mild dyspnea on exertion	Dyspnea on exertion	Dyspnea at ADL	Dyspnea at rest/ ventilator support indicated
Epistaxis	None	Mild, no transfusion	Symptomatic	Transfusion required, intervention indicated	Life-threatening consequences
Pleural effusion	None	Asymptomatic	Symptomatic, intervention required	Symptomatic, oxygen, or thoracentesis required	Life-threatening
CNS / Neurologic					
Fatigue/weakness	None	Mild fatigue over baseline	Moderate, some difficulty w/ADL	Severe, interferes w/ADL	Disabling
Neuropathy, motor	Normal	Asymptomatic, weakness on exam	Symptomatic weakness, mild difficulty w/function	Weakness, interferes w/ ADL	Life-threatening/disabling
Neuropathy, sensory	Normal	Paresthesia/deep tendon reflex loss	Paresthesia/sensory loss, interferes w/function	Sensory loss/ paresthesia; interferes w/ ADL	Disabling

Selected Common Toxicity Criteria *continued*

Toxicity	Grade 0	Grade 1	Grade 2	Grade 3	Grade 4
			Miscellaneous		
Allergy/hypersensitivity	None	Transient rash, drug fever <38°C	Urticaria, dyspnea, drug fever ≥38°C	Bronchospasm/parenteral treatment required	Anaphylaxis
Fever	None	38°C to 39°C (100.4°F to 102.2°F)	>39°C to 40°C (102.3°F to 104°F)	>40°C (104°F) for ≤24 h	>40°C (104°F) for >24 h
Infection w/o neutropenia	None		Localized, local intervention indicated	I.V. antimicrobials indicated	Life-threatening sepsis
Neutropenic fever	None			Present	Life-threatening sepsis

ADL = activities of daily living; WNL = within normal limits; LLN = lower limits of normal; ULN = upper limits of normal.

Adapted from the NCL Common Toxicity Criteria (http://ctep.cancer.gov/forms/CTCAEv3.pdf).

HOSPICE (END OF LIFE) CARE

Hospice care is provided to maintain comfort and control symptoms in the dying patient. Most patients receiving hospice care have a life expectancy of less than a few months. The pharmaceutical component of hospice care is one aspect pertaining to the quality of dying and death. The quality of dying and death entails the physical experience, psychological experience, social and cultural comprehension, spiritual or existential understanding, life closure and death preparation, and the circumstances of death. For cancer patients the type and stage of malignant disease and their health care experience impact the quality of dying and death.

Important communications between the patient and loved one or the patient and health care professional is best conducted early during hospice care rather than later. Many people are unable to effectively communicate within hours to days before death occurs. The percentage of patients who are awake, drowsy, or comatose one week prior to death is 56%, 44%, and zero, respectively. In comparison, 24 hours before death 26% of patients are awake, 62% of patients are drowsy, and 12% are comatose. And within 6 hours of death 8% of patients are awake, 42% of patients are drowsy, and 50% are comatose.

It is difficult to predict the expected time of impending death. Some patients become progressively less responsive until they die; whereas, other experience symptomatology portending death. Noisy respirations (also known as death rattle) occur when patients are obtunded or too weak to expectorate secretions. The noise is generated by secretions that accumulate in the hypopharynx and bronchial tree and oscillate with the movement of air during inspiration and exhalation. Noisy respirations generally develop within 2-3 days of death. Respiration with involuntary mandibular movement, cyanosis of the extremities, and loss of radial pulse occur approximately eight hours, five hours, and three hours, respectively, prior to death. Interestingly, the time from respiration with mandibular movement or cyanosis to death is markedly prolonged in patients with primary lung cancer or metastatic malignant disease affecting the lungs. Additional adverse events associated with dying include agitation or restlessness, delirium, dyspnea, incontinence of urine or stool, irregular breathing including gasping or 20-30 second interruptions in respiration, nausea, and swelling of the extremities.

It is important to provide safe and appropriate therapy relative to the expected outcome of therapy. Medications utilized in hospice care are often for off-label uses and are administered outside of the usual dosage range. In addition, many medications used for symptom control are prone to diversion for recreational use. In order to effectively deliver pharmacologic medication therapy for hospice care, it is important for institutions to develop policies and procedures governing the management and use of drugs for end of life care.

Noisy respirations are generally managed by placement of the patient in a semiprone position, reduction of parenteral hydration, explanation of the situation to family members and visitors, gentle nasopharyngeal or tracheal suctioning, and administration of anticholinergic medications. Transdermal scopolamine and parenteral glycopyrrolate are used in the management of noisy respirations. The commercially available patch delivers scopolamine 1 mg over 72 hours. A single patch may be sufficient for reduction of noisy respirations; however, additional patches can be applied without exceeding the daily dose of subcutaneous scopolamine administered to European hospice patients. Administration of scopolamine 1.2 mg per 24 hours by continuous subcutaneous infusion for reduction of noisy respirations is reported in the medical literature. Application of four patches is expected to deliver scopolamine 1.3 mg per 24 hours. Parenteral scopolamine is not licensed for use in the United States. Glycopyrrolate 0.2 mg can be administered by subcutaneous or intravenous bolus. Administration of glycopyrrolate 0.6 mg per 24 hours by continuous subcutaneous infusion for management of noisy respirations is reported in the medical literature. Administration of parenteral medications can be difficult for patients who are dying at home or outside of a hospital. In such circumstances, ipratropium bromide 0.03% nasal solution may provide an alternative to glycopyrrolate. Sublingual administration of ipratropium bromide 0.03% nasal solution two sprays 1-3 times daily is reportedly effective for reduction of drug induced sialorrhea. One drawback to sublingual administration may be erratic absorption for patients with excess secretions in the oral cavity. Atropine 1% ophthalmic drops are a suboptimal selection because each drop of solution delivers 0.5 mg of atropine, which is a pharmacologic dose that can modulate heart rate.

Opioid therapy is the cornerstone of treatment for pain and dyspnea in hospice care. Opioid requirements tend to increase in the dying patient. The proportion of dying patients requiring opioids expands from 42% one week before death to 78% during the final 48 hours of life. In addition, the daily opioid dose increases 2-3 fold during the same time frame. Increased opioid requirements are thought to be due to progression of the patient's underlying pathophysiologic problems instead of the development of tolerance. (Refer to Chronic Pain Management (Cancer) on page 1473 and Palliative Care Medication on page 1496.)

Pharmacologic sedation is often required for end of life restlessness and agitation. Normally the goal of sedation is to manage symptoms without appreciably reducing the patient's level of consciousness. Sedation during hospice care can include proportional palliative sedation (PPS) or, less commonly, palliative sedation to achieve unconsciousness (PSU). The goal of PPS is to provide an adequate amount of sedation for symptom control and maintain consciousness, as much as possible. Gradual titration of a benzodiazepine is commonly used for PPS. Two of the most commonly studied benzodiazepines for end of life sedation are midazolam and lorazepam. Additional drugs that have been utilized for end of life sedation are propofol and phenobarbital. Respiratory depression caused by phenobarbital should be considered when this product is administered. Limited information describes use of chlorpromazine and haloperidol for end of life restlessness and agitation. Chlorpromazine is suboptimal because it lowers the seizure threshold. Haloperidol should be reserved for use in patients with concurrent delirium. The potential for QT_c interval prolongation with haloperidol should be considered with use of this product. The goal of PSU is to induce unconsciousness. This is reserved for refractory cases with unbearable symptoms. PSU is generally accomplished by rapid titration of a benzodiazepine to the state of unconsciousness, with continuation of adequate doses to maintain unconsciousness.

Selected References

Back IN, Jenkins K, Blower A, et al, "A Study Comparing Hyoscine Hydrobromide and Glycopyrrolate in the Treatment of Death Rattle," *Palliat Med*, 2001, 15(4):329-36.

Hales S, Zimmermann C, and Rodin G, "The Quality of Dying and Death," *Arch Intern Med*, 2008, 168(9):912-8.

Hugel H, Ellershaw J, and Gambles M, "Respiratory Tract Secretions in the Dying Patient: A Comparison Between Glycopyrronium snd Hyoscine Hydrobromide," *J Palliat Med*, 2006, 9 (2):279-84.

Kåss RM and Ellershaw J, "Respiratory Tract Secretions in the Dying Patient: A Retrospective Study," *J Pain Symptom Manage*, 2003, 26(4):897-902.

Kehl KA, "Treatment of Terminal Restlessness: A Review of the Evidence," *J Pain Palliat Care Pharmacother*, 2004, 18(1):5-30.

Kintzel PE, Chase SL, Thomas W, et al, "Anticholinergic Medications for Managing Noisy Respirations in Adult Hospice Patients," *Am J Health Syst Pharm*, 2009, 66(5):458-64.

Morita T, Ichiki T, Tsunoda J, et al, "A Prospective Study on the Dying Process in Terminally Ill Cancer Patients," *Am J Hosp Palliat Care*, 1998, 15(4):217-22.

Pantilat SZ and Isaac M, "End-of-Life Care for the Hospitalized Patient," *Med Clin North Am*, 2008, 92(2):349-70.

Quill TE, Lo B, Brock DW, et al, "Last-Resort Options for Palliative Sedation," *Ann Intern Med*, 2009, 151(6):421-4.

HYPERCALCEMIA OF MALIGNANCY

INTRODUCTION

The most frequent causes of hypercalcemia are hyperparathyroidism and advanced malignant disease. In cancer patients, hypercalcemia affects 10% to 20% of patients with advanced disease and is the most frequently occurring life-threatening metabolic disorder. The incidence varies with the specific type of cancer; the highest incidence is seen in the hematologic malignancies multiple myeloma and human T-cell lymphotropic virus type 1 (HTLV-1)-associated T cell lymphoma, and the solid tumors lung cancer, breast cancer, and renal cell cancer. The median survival following the finding of hypercalcemia of malignancy is 64 days even with appropriate therapy. Poor prognostic indicators include corrected serum calcium exceeding 11.3 mg/dL [hazard ratio (HR): 2.21], serum albumin less than 3.6 g/dL (HR: 2.41), squamous cell carcinoma (HR: 2.64), and metastatic disease affecting the bone (HR: 1.44) or liver (HR: 2.22). Patients with breast cancer and multiple myeloma may have a better outcome from hypercalcemia relative to the prognosis of their cancer. Transient hypercalcemia can occur after initiation of tamoxifen therapy for breast cancer; this is considered to be evidence that the endocrine therapy is working effectively. In addition, women with metastatic breast cancer not affecting the central nervous system have a median survival of 14-25 months. Hypercalcemia is a manifestation of advanced multiple myeloma that does not in and of itself predict mortality in a median of 60 days.

The primary cause of hypercalcemia of malignancy is increased bone resorption secondary to osteoclast activation by way of complex interactions between tumor-derived factors and the patient's endogenous biologic environment. Although the underlying pathologic mechanism of this adverse event differs somewhat relative to whether the hypercalcemia is associated with a solid tumor without bone metastasis, or a solid tumor with bone metastasis, or a hematologic malignancy. Most cases involving solid tumors without bone metastasis are characterized by elevated serum levels of parathyroid hormone-related protein (PTHrP) that play a prominent role in augmented bone resorption. PTHrP initially stimulates osteoblasts to secrete receptor activator of nuclear factor-kappa ligand (RANKL). RANKL activates osteoclast precursors and subsequent osteolysis which promotes release of bone-derived growth factors, such as insulin-like growth factor-1 (IGF1) and transforming growth factor-beta (TGF-beta), in addition to increasing serum calcium levels. Subsequently, the bone-derived growth factors stimulate cancer cell proliferation and continued PTHrP production. PTHrP also promotes calcium reabsorption by the renal tubules. Additional factors produced by some tumors or the body's response to the tumor that contribute to hypercalcemia of malignancy include transforming growth factor-alpha, interleukin-1-alpha, and interleukin-6. Metastatic lesions from solid tumors that reside in the bone employ similar biochemical tools to promote bone resorption. However, hypercalcemia, secondary to osteolytic bone metastasis, is largely a paracrine process rather than the humorally-mediated event associated with solid tumors not affecting the bone. Hematologic cancers of lymphoid origin secret osteoclast activating factors to produce osteolytic bone lesions. Osteoclast activating factors are lymphokines, and include interleukin-1-alpha, interleukin-6, and lymphotoxin. Increased systemic levels of 1-25(OH)$_2$ vitamin D$_3$ contribute to hypercalcemia associated with T cell malignancies.

One early sign of hypercalcemia is polyuria, which develops as the body tries to eliminate excess ionized calcium from the serum. Polyuria causes intravascular volume depletion and dehydration, which signals the body to retain sodium. The ensuing renotubular reabsorption of sodium promotes concurrent reabsorption of calcium which fuels the hypercalcemia. Acute renal impairment can occur due to intravascular volume depletion and calcium-phosphate precipitation in the renal tubules. Neurologic adverse effects are generally the most serious sequelae of hypercalcemia. Confusion is common, and patients can progress to somnolence and coma. Malaise and muscle weakness occur. Gastrointestinal adverse effects include anorexia, constipation, ileus, nausea, and vomiting. Cardiac effects include bradycardia and other dysrhythmias. Symptom severity is related to the degree of hypercalcemia and the rate at which the serum calcium increased.

TREATMENT

The first treatment priority is reversal of dehydration to reduce the serum calcium concentration and preserve renal function. Once normovolemia is restored, furosemide is often added; however, the primary role of a loop diuretic in this situation is to prevent volume overload. First line therapies to reduce bone resorption include bisphosphonates and calcitonin. Second line therapies include corticosteroids for multiple myeloma and lymphoid malignancies, and gallium nitrate and plicamycin. Hemodialysis may be necessary in severe cases of hypercalcemia. For patients capable of ambulation, this should be encouraged to offset the negative calcium balance consequent to loss of weight bearing activities. Treatment of the underlying malignancy is also an option for reducing hypercalcemia of malignancy for some patients.

Treatment is based on symptomatology and the serum calcium level. The criteria for initiation of treatment are generally hypercalcemia with signs of toxicity (polyuria, mental status changes, renal dysfunction, cardiac dysrhythmias) attributed to hypercalcemia. A total calcium level exceeding 13 mg/dL is cited as criteria for initiation of therapy; although, it is unusual for hypercalcemia of malignancy to present without related symptomatology. Systemic calcium exists in equilibrium between an ionized and protein bound form. Adverse effects from hypercalcemia are due to elevated levels of ionized calcium in the serum. Most protein bound calcium is associated with albumin. Subsequently, patients with low serum albumin levels will have artifactually low total calcium levels. Laboratory monitoring can be done by directly measuring ionized calcium in addition to total (protein bound plus ionized) calcium, or by correcting the value for total calcium based on the patient's serum albumin level. Formulae used to correct serum total calcium for albumin [corrected Ca^{++} = measured Ca^{++} (mg/dL) + 0.8 mg/dL for each g albumin <4 g/dL, corrected Ca^{++} = measured Ca^{++} (mg/dL) - albumin (g/dL) + 4.0] may not yield accurate estimations of ionized calcium in all cases.

0.9% SODIUM CHLORIDE

The intravenous fluid used for rehydration is 0.9% sodium chloride because it effectively improves intravascular volume and promotes renal excretion of calcium. The rate of administration of sodium chloride depends on the degree of dehydration, the severity of hypercalcemia, and the cardiopulmonary status of the patient. Ideally, patients should receive 0.9% sodium chloride at a rate of 2-3 L/m^2 per 24 hours; however, this often must be attenuated relative to what the patient's cardiopulmonary status can accommodate. Hydration rates as high as 5 L/m^2 per 24 hours have been used in severe cases. Following rehydration, proximal tubular reabsorption of sodium, and therefore calcium, will decrease. Further, other treatments for hypercalcemia require prior volume replacement in order to minimize toxicities. Sodium chloride can lower serum calcium by approximately 2 mg/dL. Saline hydration has an immediate but transient effect. Even if normocalcemia is achieved, serum calcium will increase again unless additional treatments aimed at reducing bone resorption or treating the underlying malignancy are administered.

FUROSEMIDE

The major use of furosemide in the management of cancer-associated hypercalcemia is to prevent and manage fluid overload in order to facilitate the administration of sodium chloride for volume replacement. A usual starting dose of furosemide is 10-20 mg by intravenous push every 6-12 hours around the clock or as needed to maintain an acceptable rate of urine output. Loop diuretics are not effective agents for enhancing renal excretion of calcium. Loop diuretics should be used with caution to avoid intravascular volume depletion with exacerbation of hypercalcemia and renal impairment.

BISPHOSPHONATES

Bisphosphonates bind to hydroxyapatite in bone and inhibit osteoclastic bone resorption. Pamidronate and zoledronic acid are the most commonly used bisphosphonates for management of hypercalcemia of malignancy. Intravenous ibandronate is also a treatment option for this condition. In a randomized, double blind comparison with 275 of 287 subjects evaluable for efficacy zoledronic acid was superior to pamidronate for normalization of serum calcium by day 4 (50% versus 33% of patients) and day 10 (88% versus 70% of patients) of therapy. The median duration of normocalcemia was 32 days for zoledronic acid 4 mg and 18 days for pamidronate 90 mg. However, the frequency of renal impairment was greater in the zoledronic acid treatment arm. The dose of intravenous ibandronate used for hypercalcemia of malignancy in clinical trials is 2 mg or 4 mg.

Bisphosphonates should be used with caution in patients with severe renal impairment because these products are eliminated by the kidneys and can cause nephrotoxicity. Pamidronate has not been studied in patients with serum creatinine exceeding 3 mg/dL or creatinine clearance less than 30 mL/min. Renal dosage adjustment of zoledronic acid administered for the treatment of hypercalcemia of malignancy is not warranted when the serum creatinine is less than 4.5 mg/dL. The manufacturer of intravenous ibandronate recommends against use of this product for serum creatinine exceeding 2.3 mg/dL or creatinine clearance less than 30 mL/min.

Common side effects of bisphosphonates are mild and include fever and infusion site reactions, such as phlebitis. Avascular osteonecrosis of the jaw (ONJ) is an infrequent but serious adverse effect of bisphosphonate therapy. ONJ can be an extremely painful condition. Most reported cases of ONJ involve cancer patients receiving intravenous bisphosphonate therapy while undergoing dental procedures. Risk factors for ONJ during bisphosphonate therapy include cancer, chemotherapy, radiotherapy, corticosteroids, poor oral hygiene, pre-existing dental disease or infection, anemia, and coagulopathy. Patients should maintain good oral hygiene and have a dental examination with preventive dentistry prior to treatment with bisphosphonates. Another adverse effect identified in women receiving bisphosphonate therapy for postmenopausal osteoporosis is severe musculoskeletal pain that develops within days, weeks or months of beginning treatment. This condition may become debilitating and necessitate discontinuation of bisphosphonate therapy.

CALCITONIN

Calcitonin works in a receptor-mediated manner to inhibit bone resorption and enhance urinary excretion of calcium. It is the fastest acting of the agents used to treat hypercalcemia and may be given safely before rehydration is complete. The usual dose of calcitonin is 4 units/kg by subcutaneous injection every 12 hours. Side effects are mild and infrequent and include nausea, abdominal cramps, and flushing. Calcitonin lowers serum calcium by approximately 2 mg/dL. Resistance to the pharmacologic effects of calcitonin generally develops with a few days of therapy. In fact, this can become apparent clinically as rebound hypercalcemia.

CORTICOSTEROIDS

Corticosteroid administration is added to therapy when the underlying malignancy is a steroid-responsive disease, such as multiple myeloma, and lymphoma.

GALLIUM NITRATE

Gallium nitrate decreases serum calcium by adsorbing to hydroxyapatite and inhibiting bone resorption. It is given as a continuous intravenous infusion at a dose of 200 mg/m^2/day for 5 days. Most patients respond to gallium nitrate; however, its use is limited by the risk of nephrotoxicity and the cumbersome administration schedule. Gallium nitrate reduces serum calcium approximately 3 mg/dL after a complete 5-day course of therapy. Gallium nitrate was initially tested as an anticancer drug at higher daily doses than those used for hypercalcemia administered intravenously over 15-30 minutes. Dose limiting adverse effects were nephrotoxicity, neurotoxicity, and hypocalcemia. Nephrotoxicity attributed to gallium nitrate administration has been reported in patients treated for hypercalcemia. Nephrotoxicity may be potentiated by other nephrotoxic drugs. Gallium should not be used in patients with serum creatinine >2.5 mg/dL. Because of the potential for nephrotoxicity and the inconvenient dosing schedule relative to other agents, gallium should not be considered a first-line treatment for hypercalcemia.

PLICAMYCIN

Plicamycin is a specific osteoclast inhibitor and thus is effective in any hypercalcemic condition associated with accelerated osteoclast-mediated bone resorption. Treatment-related adverse effects limit the utility of plicamycin. Potential side effects include nephrotoxicity, hepatotoxicity, and platelet dysfunction.

OTHER

Treatment of the underlying malignancy is an option for some patients. However, the metabolic benefits of effective anticancer treatment may not be clinically evident for a period of weeks to months. And, unfortunately, many patients with hypercalcemia of malignancy have cancer that has progressed despite the standard anticancer therapies. Bortezomib has a dual anticancer and bone stabilizing effect. This product, which is used in the treatment of multiple myeloma and mantle cell lymphoma, stimulates osteoblast differentiation, and inhibits osteoclast formation and bone resorption independently of its anticancer effect. The investigational human monoclonal antibody denosumab targets the mediator of bone resorption RANKL. Denosumab is being tested for use in osteoporosis, treatment-induced bone loss, bone metastasis, multiple myeloma, and rheumatoid arthritis.

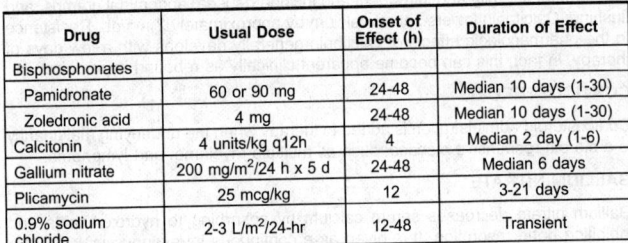

Drug	Usual Dose	Onset of Effect (h)	Duration of Effect
Bisphosphonates			
Pamidronate	60 or 90 mg	24-48	Median 10 days (1-30)
Zoledronic acid	4 mg	24-48	Median 10 days (1-30)
Calcitonin	4 units/kg q12h	4	Median 2 day (1-6)
Gallium nitrate	200 mg/m^2/24 h x 5 d	24-48	Median 6 days
Plicamycin	25 mcg/kg	12	3-21 days
0.9% sodium chloride	2-3 L/m^2/24-hr	12-48	Transient

Treatments are listed in alphabetical order. See text for guidance on priority and order of use.

Selected Readings

LeGrand SB, Leskuski D, and Zama I, "Narrative Review: Furosemide for Hypercalcemia: An Unproven Yet Common Practice," *Ann Intern Med*, 2008, 149(4):259-63.

Lumachi F, Brunello A, Roma A, et al, "Cancer-Induced Hypercalcemia," *Anticancer Res*, 2009, 29 (5):1551-5.

Major P, Lortholary A, Hon J, et al, "Zoledronic Acid Is Superior to Pamidronate in the Treatment of Hypercalcemia of Malignancy: A Pooled Analysis of Two Randomized, Controlled Clinical Trials," *J Clin Oncol*, 2001, 19(2):558-67.

Nussbaum SR, Younger J, Vandepol CJ, et al, "Single-Dose Intravenous Therapy With Pamidronate for the Treatment of Hypercalcemia of Malignancy: Comparison of 30-, 60-, and 90-mg Dosages," *Am J Med*, 1993, 95(3):297-304.

Penel N, Dewas S, Doutrelant P, et al, "Cancer-Associated Hypercalcemia Treated With Intravenous Diphosphonates: A Survival and Prognostic Factor Analysis," *Support Care Cancer*, 2008, 16(4):387-92.

Perlia CP, Gubisch NJ, Wolter J, et al, "Mithramycin Treatment of Hypercalcemia," *Cancer*, 1970, 25:389-94.

Shemerdiak WP, Kukreja SC, Lad TE, et al, "Evaluation of Routine Ionized Calcium Determination in Cancer Patients," *Clin Chem*, 1981, 27:1621-2.

Stewart AF, "Clinical Practice. Hypercalcemia Associated With Cancer, " *N Engl J Med*, 2005, 352 (4):373-9.

Warrell RP Jr, Israel R, Frisone M, et al, "Gallium Nitrate for Acute Treatment of Cancer-Related Hypercalcemia. A Randomized, Double-Blind Comparison to Calcitonin," *Ann Intern Med*, 1988, 108(5):699-74.

MALIGNANT EFFUSIONS

A malignant effusion is an accumulation of fluid in the pleural space separating the lung and the chest wall that generally occurs secondary to direct extension of a tumor or metastatic dissemination to the affected area. Carcinoma of the breast, carcinoma of the lung, and lymphomas account for two-thirds of malignant effusions but they are also found with gastric or ovarian carcinomas. A malignant effusion may be the presenting sign of cancer, but most often it is a complication of a previously diagnosed malignancy.

PATHOPHYSIOLOGY

The pleura is a thin membrane that covers the lungs and chest wall. It is composed of the visceral pleura (covering the surface of the lungs) and the parietal pleura (covering the thoracic cavity). The space between the visceral pleura and parietal pleura is the pleural space. Normally, pleural fluid production is <100 mL/day. Movement of fluid within the pleural space is governed by hydrostatic and oncotic pressures and follows Starling's law of transcapillary exchange. Hydrostatic pressure in the parietal capillaries is higher, causing a net movement into the pleural space. Reabsorption of the fluid occurs primarily through lymphatics on the parietal surface and less importantly via lymphatics on the visceral surface. Changes in pleural fluid production, reabsorption, or both produce a pleural effusion.

Malignancies can cause a fluid imbalance within the pleural space in several ways. Malignant cells within the pleural space can cause an inflammatory response that increases capillary permeability and increases the net filtration of fluid, proteins, and cells into the pleural space. In addition, malignant obstruction of lymphatic channels and changes in pleural fluid protein content can impair reabsorption and drainage of fluid from the pleural space. The resulting fluid accumulation is exudative and is characterized by an increased concentration of protein and cells, glucose levels less than that of the serum, and an absence of eosinophils. Normal pleural fluid is produced through a passive process; the ion content is similar to serum concentrations while the protein content is <2%.

CLINICAL SYMPTOMS

Patients with pleural effusions may be asymptomatic. The most common symptom is dyspnea, often in conjunction with cough, chest pain, and tachypnea. Symptoms are often related not to the amount of fluid present, but to the rate of fluid accumulation. A diagnosis often begins with a chest x-ray, which will demonstrate fluid accumulation on the posteroanterior (PA) and lateral decubitus film. Physical findings include dullness to percussion, decreased breath sounds, decreased diaphragmatic excursion, and possible contralateral tracheal deviation.

TREATMENT

The goal of treatment is to provide a cost-conscious, effective therapy that provides symptomatic relief with the least amount of discomfort to the patient. Not all patients with pleural effusions need to be treated. Some patients with effusions are asymptomatic and may not require treatment until symptoms develop. Patients with a life expectancy of less than 1 month might only require oxygen, opioids, and possibly thoracentesis. Patients with tumors that are sensitive to chemotherapy or radiation may have resolution of the effusion with appropriate treatment of the tumor.

◀ **LOCAL THERAPY**

Thoracentesis is the process of removing fluid from the pleural space using a specialized needle and syringe under local anesthetic. This procedure can be done at the bedside and is utilized frequently for symptomatic patients. Thoracentesis is ineffective for long-term control of the effusion. Recurrence is frequent, and repeated procedures carry a risk of increased complications such as pneumothorax. Ultrasound-guided thoracentesis can be performed to reduce the risk of pneumothorax.

Tube thoracostomy (chest tube) is effective in controlling a malignant effusion for a short period of time. Its 30-day success rate is approximately 70%. However, it is ineffective in the long-term control of effusions. It is most useful in draining the fluid from the pleural space prior to instilling a sclerosing agent.

Pleuroperitoneal shunts are used to manually pump fluid from the pleural space into the peritoneal cavity. The pumps must be manually operated daily and are prone to blockage by the high protein content of the fluid. Pleurectomy involves stripping the parietal and visceral pleura and it carries a high mortality and morbidity rate as compared to less invasive procedures.

PLEURODESIS

Pleurodesis, or sclerosis, should be considered in patients who experience symptomatic relief from thoracentesis with complete lung re-expansion and a life expectancy of weeks to months. The primary goals of pleurodesis are prevention of effusion reaccumulation and reduced hospitalizations for thoracentesis. Sclerosing agents act by causing an inflammatory response in the pleura, which resolves to cause adhesions of the visceral and parietal pleura, resulting in obliteration of the pleural space. Sclerosing agents are administered via a thoracostomy tube following adequate drainage (<100 mL/day). Factors affecting the success of the agent include uniform distribution in the pleural space, the presence of loculations that interfere with distribution, and the dose of the selected drug.

GENERAL METHOD OF ADMINISTRATION

Fluid is drained via a chest tube until the production is <100 mL/day. The patient is premedicated with systemic analgesia (usually a parenteral opioid), sedation, and intrapleural administration of a topical anesthetic (usually lidocaine 1%). The sclerosing agent is instilled through the chest tube and the tube is clamped for 30 minutes to 2 hours. Then the tube is unclamped, reconnected to water-seal suction until production is <100-150 mL/day, and the chest tube is removed. Some procedures include frequent repositioning of the patient during the time that the chest tube is clamped to facilitate uniform distribution of the sclerosing agent, although the efficacy of repositioning is untested and its use is controversial.

SCLEROSING AGENTS

Talc is one of the oldest and most effective treatments for malignant effusions. Meta-analysis infers that talc is a more effective sclerosing agent than bleomycin or tetracycline and tetracycline analogues. Pharmaceutical grade sterile asbestos-free talc is commercially available for use as a sclerosing agent. Talc powder is prepared as sterile slurry for administration through a chest tube. The usual dose of talc slurry is 5 g in 0.9% sodium chloride 50-100 mL. This can be done at the bedside. Powdered talc is also available in a pressurized spray canister for administration under video-assisted thoracic surgery (VATS, thoracoscopy) or open thoracotomy. The usual dose of aerosolized talc is

4-8 g. Aerosolized talc is available in single use 4 g canisters. Prior to availability of the commercial aerosolized product, talc administered by distribution of the powder throughout the intrapleural space during a surgical procedure was known as talc poudrage. Pain and fever are the most common acute side effect of pleurodesis. Rare serious adverse effects of pleurodesis using talc include adult respiratory distress syndrome (ARDS), pneumonia, empyema, hemoptysis, bronchopleural fistula, tachycardia, hypotension, and infection. Cases of ARDS have occurred in patients receiving instillations of talc slurry 10 g.

Bleomycin 1 mg/kg (1 unit/kg) in 100 mL of 0.9% sodium chloride has been studied and found to be an effective agent in controlling malignant effusions. The range of intrapleural bleomycin doses reported in the literature is 24-240 mg. However, due to a lack of increased efficacy at doses >60 mg, some authors have recommended limiting the dose to 60 mg or 1 mg/kg body weight. Common toxicities associated with intrapleural bleomycin include pain, fever, and gastrointestinal adverse effects (nausea, vomiting, diarrhea). Serious adverse effects are more common in patients with elderly age or reduced renal function.

Doxycycline and minocycline: Tetracycline was one of the most widely used sclerosing agents prior to its removal from the market in the mid-1990s. Doxycycline 500 mg mixed in 0.9% sodium chloride 50-100 mL effectively treats pleural effusions for 50% to 75% of patients; however, repeated instillations are generally required to achieve results similar to tetracycline. Intrapleural minocycline following VATS for spontaneous pneumothorax reduced prolonged postoperative air leaks, chest drainage, and hospital days for 313 patients relative to 51 consecutive historical controls. The author reported administration of minocycline 300-400 mg in 0.9% sodium chloride 20 mL through a chest tube. Due to a lack of stability information, this dose of minocycline should be prepared immediately before use. Chest pain was a common complaint after pleurodesis with minocycline.

Additional products that have been used as sclerosing agents for pleurodesis are iodopovidone, silver nitrate, quinacrine, *Corynebacterium parvum*, interferon-α, interferon-β, and various cytotoxic chemotherapy drugs.

COMPLICATIONS

Management of malignant effusions is associated with several complications. Pain from insertion of the chest tube or instillation of the sclerosing agent should be pretreated with parenteral opioids. Traction pneumothorax results from repeated attempts to re-expand the lung. Cough is caused by lung re-expansion and is self-limiting. Fluid loculation is associated with drainage and pleurodesis. Lysis of adhesions may be necessary prior to pleurodesis. Empyema (purulent fluid) formation from contamination or bronchopulmonary communication should be treated with appropriate antibiotics.

Selected Readings

Chen JS, Hsu HH, Kuo SW, et al, "Effects of Additional Minocycline Pleurodesis After Thoracoscopic Procedures For Primary Spontaneous Pneumothorax," *Chest*, 2004, 125(1):50-5.

Kvale PA, Selecky PA, and Prakash UB, "Palliative Care In Lung Cancer: ACCP Evidence-Based Clinical Practice Guidelines (2nd Edition)," *Chest*, 2007, 132(3 Suppl):368S-403S.

Shaw P and Agarwal R, "Pleurodesis For Malignant Pleural Effusions," *Cochrane Database Syst Rev*, 2004, (1):CD002916.

PALLIATIVE CARE MEDICINE

SCOPE OF PALLIATIVE CARE MEDICINE

The National Consensus Project for Quality Palliative Care states "The goal of palliative care is to prevent and relieve suffering and to support the best possible quality of life for patients and their families, regardless of the stage of the disease or the need for other therapies. Palliative care is both a philosophy of care and an organized, highly structured system for delivering care. Palliative care expands traditional disease-model medical treatments to include the goals of enhancing quality of life for patient and family, optimizing function, helping with decision making, and providing opportunities for personal growth. As such, it can be delivered concurrently with life-prolonging care or as the main focus of care." Palliative care addresses symptoms arising from serious life threatening diseases, and intractable symptoms from benign conditions that depreciate quality of life. Palliative care can be part of end of life (hospice) care; however, it is often used in the management of patients with life expectancies extending months, years, or decades.

Palliative care is provided most effectively by an interdisciplinary team specializing in this discipline of medicine. Clinical and regulatory challenges related to delivery of pharmaceutical products for palliative care impact the pharmacy department. One aspect of palliative care is symptom control for intractable situations following an adequate trial of the therapeutic standard of care. Subsequently, medications may be prescribed for off-label indications at doses outside of the norm, and for administration by atypical routes. Moreover, since palliative care medicine is an evolving field, the medical literature available supporting the safety and efficacy of certain interventions may be scant. Some medications used for symptom control are controlled substances or prone to diversion, so stringent methods of drug accountability must be adhered to. Pharmacy departments should formalize policies and procedures to support the delivery of palliative pharmaceutical care.

SYMPTOM MANAGEMENT

Pain

The management of pain should be optimized as per standard clinical practice. Refer to Chronic Pain Management (Cancer) on page 1473. Opioid and nonopioid analgesic therapy should be optimized. Nonsteroidal anti-inflammatory drugs, bisphosphonates, and radiotherapy should be used as appropriate for bone pain. External beam radiation can be helpful for tumor size reduction with pain relief in some cases. Nonsteroidal anti-inflammatory drugs or corticosteroids should be used as warranted for inflammatory pain. Gabapentin, pregabalin, and antidepressants can improve neuropathic pain.

High doses of opioid analgesia may be required for intractable pain. The oral route of administration is preferred whenever possible. Opioid administration by continuous subcutaneous or intravenous infusion with or without patient controlled PRN boluses is an option. Subcutaneous infusion of methadone should be avoided due to local irritation. Patients may require intraspinal opioid administration to achieve and tolerate adequate pain control.

Methadone can be administered by continuous intravenous infusion and patient controlled analgesia. However, this intervention is often reserved for select patients as a bridge to intraspinal therapy because methadone prolongs the QT_c

interval and there is discordance between the pharmacokinetics and pharmacodynamics of this drug. The risk of torsade de pointes is increased when the QT_c interval exceeds 500 milliseconds. Consensus guidelines (Shaiova, 2008) pertaining to intravenous administration of methadone recommend assessment of the QT_c interval at baseline, 24 hours and 4 days after initiation of methadone, and following any significant dose increase or at the discretion of the practitioner. More frequent monitoring of the QT_c interval should be considered for patients with a QT_c interval exceeding 450 milliseconds. Patients should be advised of the risk of dysrhythmias with methadone, so that they can make an informed decision about their therapy. Since the half-life of methadone exceeds the duration of analgesia, the consensus guidelines state that the initial rate titration must be done at least 12 hours after initiation of the infusion to allow evolution of side effects. Subsequent rate titrations should be done once daily. Liberal use of PRN boluses are recommended by the consensus guidelines before and between rate titration for methadone by continuous intravenous infusion. Due to incomplete cross tolerance between methadone and high dose morphine, the consensus guidelines recommend the following conversion factors (Shaiova, 2008). In addition, a 25% to 50% reduction in the calculated methadone dose at infusion initiation is recommended for patients requiring more than 50 mg/ hour of morphine.

| | | Methadone | |
Opioid	Basal Rate (mg/h)	Basal Rate (mg/h)	PRN Bolus Available Every 15 Minutes
Morphine	10	1	1
Hydromorphone	1.5	0.3	0.3
Fentanyl	0.25	1.25	1.25

Intravenous lidocaine is used for severe intractable neuropathic pain. The efficacy of lidocaine is greater in the treatment of peripheral sensory neuropathy versus symptoms caused by a central pain syndrome. Small studies report administration of intravenous lidocaine 1-5 mg/kg over a period of 30 minutes to 6 hours. Some centers use a set dose of 100-150 mg infused intravenously over a period of 30-60 minutes. Analgesia superior to placebo is reported in crossover design trials. The reported time to maximum analgesia is 1-6 hours, with the reported duration of analgesia ranging from hours to days to weeks. Common adverse effects include light headedness, vertical nystagmus, feeling drunk, and sedation. The rapid metabolism of lidocaine probably allows administration of 1-5 mg/kg over a period of 30 minutes to 6 hours without cardiac or central nervous system toxicity. Caution should be exercised when using intravenous lidocaine in patients who are elderly, debilitated, or have poor hepatic function. One case series of three patients with neuropathic cancer pain describes chronic administration of lidocaine 100-160 mg/hour by continuous subcutaneous infusion. Periodic assessment of serum lidocaine levels should be considered with administration by continuous infusion.

Ketamine is used as an adjunct to opioid therapy for intractable cancer pain and neuropathic pain. Ketamine can be administered orally, intravenously, and subcutaneously. Ketamine can be administered intramuscularly; however, this route is rarely used for repeated administration. The dose of oral ketamine is 20-60 mg 3-4 times daily plus PRN administration of ketamine 20 mg every 3 hours. Tapering the dose at a rate of 25% per 24 hours may reduce the likelihood of dysphoria when ketamine is being discontinued. Ketamine is commercially available as a parenteral formulation. The oral dose can be mixed in cola immediately prior to ingestion. To reduce the risk of drug diversion or inadvertent ingestion by a family member, some institutions have the nurse squirt the dose of ketamine from an oral syringe into the patient's mouth with cola or another beverage to follow. Intravenous ketamine is generally given as a continuous infusion starting at 1-2 mg/hour. Administration of intravenous ketamine 0.1-0.4 mg/kg as an intravenous bolus is reported in the literature. Ketamine can cause hallucinations, drowsiness, and confusion. At anesthetic doses (1-4.5 mg/kg intravenous bolus), ketamine causes hypertension and tachycardia.

Dyspnea

Opioid (usually morphine) administration is the cornerstone of medication therapy for reducing the sensation of chronic dyspnea in advanced cancer patients. The sensation of dyspnea is a complex disorder that is influenced by many pathophysiologic changes within and outside of the cardiopulmonary system. Morphine (or an equivalent opioid) can be administered to cancer patients with mild-to-severe dyspnea for symptom control without having a deleterious effect on SaO_2, $PaCO_2$, or heart rate. These findings are consistent when evaluated relative to whether the patient was hypoxic (SaO_2 <90%) at baseline or opioid-naïve. Opioid medications should always be used cautiously. However, medical literature supports the safety and efficacy of opioid administration for manage-ment of chronic dyspnea in patients with advanced cancer. For opioid naïve patients, morphine doses in the range of 1-3 mg by intravenous push or 5-10 mg orally every 4 hours as needed may be sufficient to improve dyspnea. Opioid tolerant patients will need higher doses to relieve dyspnea. There is no advantage to administration of morphine by nebulization versus use of the subcutaneous, intravenous, or oral routes.

Treatment of anxiety using lorazepam or another suitable product may improve the sensation of dyspnea. Addition of furosemide to therapy should be considered when heart failure may be contributing to the sensation of dyspnea. Long acting β-agonists improve dyspnea for patients with chronic obstructive pulmonary disease. The use of oxygen therapy is controversial due to conflicting information about its efficacy in the medical literature. Patients with chronic obstructive pulmonary disease are most likely to benefit from oxygen therapy.

Cough / Hiccups

Initial symptomatic treatment of persistent cough due to chronic disease affecting the lungs includes guaifenesin, dextromethorphan, and benzonatate. For intractable cough despite usual therapies, nebulized lidocaine may provide relief. Symptomatic relief occurs rapidly for responding patients. Common adverse effects include oropharyngeal numbness and an unpleasant taste. It is important to note that nebulized lidocaine causes a transient loss of gag reflex. Nebulized lidocaine for intractable cough is often administered as follows.

Nebulized Lidocaine for Intractable Cough Administration

Lidocaine 4% preservative free 2.5 mL

Administer by nebulization every 4 hours as needed

Note: Patient should have nothing by mouth for 30 minutes before and 2 hours after each dose.

Intractable hiccups, which are generally defined as hiccups lasting more than 1 month, impair the quality and activities of daily life. Hiccups are caused by repeated involuntary spasmodic contractions of the diaphragm followed by a sudden closure of the glottis which blocks the incoming air to produce the characteristic sounds. Hiccups can be secondary to gastric extension and diaphragmatic irritation. Drugs credited with causing intractable hiccups include aprepitant, dexamethasone, doxycycline, etoposide, megestrol acetate, and perphenazine. Interruption of therapy should be trialed when hiccups are thought to be medication-related. Nonpharmacologic methods for hiccup cessation should be attempted prior to drug therapy. Examples of nonpharmacologic therapy include holding one's breath, breathing inside of a paper (nonplastic) grocery bag, gasping with sudden fright, the Valsalva maneuver, hyperventilation, slowly drinking water, and drinking water from the "wrong side" of a glass.

Medications used for intractable hiccups include chlorpromazine, metoclopramide, baclofen, and gabapentin. Chlorpromazine 25-50 mg administered orally or by intravenous infusion 3-4 times daily as needed or around the clock can be used for control of hiccups. Chlorpromazine can also be administered intramuscularly; however, this route is seldom utilized for repeated administration. Metoclopramide 10 mg is generally administered 4 times daily for management of hiccups. Metoclopramide can be administered orally or intravenously. The dosage of baclofen for intractable hiccups is 5-10 mg by mouth 3-4 times daily. Gabapentin 300-400 mg 3 times daily by mouth for control of hiccups is reported in the medical literature. Gabapentin has a wide margin of safety and doses up to 3600 mg/day are well tolerated in patients with adequate renal function. Metoclopramide, baclofen, and gabapentin are administered on a scheduled basis around the clock (instead of PRN) for the management of intractable hiccups. Combination therapy using drugs with different pharmacologic mechanisms of action and nonoverlapping toxicity can be trialed for patients not responding to single agent therapy.

Hiccups that continue despite an adequate trial of chlorpromazine, metoclopramide, and baclofen may respond to nebulized lidocaine. The dosage, time to effect, and safety of nebulized lidocaine is described in the preceding section pertaining to management of intractable cough.

SELECTED REFERENCES

Attal N, Rouaud J, Brasseur L, et al, "Systemic Lidocaine in Pain Due to Peripheral Nerve Injury and Predictors of Response," *Neurology*, 2004, 62(2):218-25.

Brose WG and Cousins MJ, "Subcutaneous Lidocaine for Treatment of Neuropathic Cancer Pain," *Pain*, 1991, 45(2):145-8.

Clemens KE, Quednau I, and Klaschik E, "Use of Oxygen and Opioids in the Palliation of Dyspnoea in Hypoxic and Nonhypoxic Palliative Care Patients: A Prospective Study," *Support Care Cancer*, 2009, 17(4):367-77.

Clinical Practice Guidelines for Quality Palliative Care, 2nd ed, Pittsburgh, PA: National Consensus Project for Quality Palliative Care, 2009. Available at: http://www.nationalconsensusproject.org/guideline.pdf .

Dy SM, Lorenz KA, Naeim A, et al, "Evidence-Based Recommendations for Cancer Fatigue, Anorexia, Depression, and Dyspnea," *J Clin Oncol*, 2008, 26(23):3886-95.

Enarson MC, Hays H, and Woodroffe MA, "Clinical Experience With Oral Ketamine," *J Pain Symptom Manage*, 1999, 17(5):384-6.

Kannan TR, Saxena A, Bhatnagar S, et al, "Oral Ketamine as an Adjuvant to Oral Morphine for Neuropathic Pain in Cancer Patients," *J Pain Symptom Manage*, 2002, 23(1):60-5.

Midgren B, Hansson L, Karlsson JA, et al, "Capsaicin-Induced Cough in Humans," *Am Rev Respir Dis*, 1992, 146(2):347-51.

Neeno TA and Rosenow EC 3rd, "Intractable Hiccups. Consider Nebulized Lidocaine," *Chest*, 1996, 110(4):1129-30.

Qaseem A, Snow V, Shekelle P, et al, "Evidence-Based Interventions to Improve the Palliative Care of Pain, Dyspnea, and Depression at the End of Life: A Clinical Practice Guideline From the American College of Physicians," *Ann Intern Med*, 2008, 148(2):141-6.

Shaiova L, Berger A, Blinderman CD, et al, "Consensus Guideline on Parenteral Methadone Use in Pain and Palliative Care," *Palliat Support Care*, 2008, 6(2):165-76.

Tremont-Lukats IW, Hutson PR, and Backonja MM, "A Randomized, Double-Masked, Placebo-Controlled Pilot Trial of Extended I.V. Lidocaine Infusion for Relief of Ongoing Neuropathic Pain," *Clin J Pain*, 2006, 22(3):266-71.

HEMATOPOIETIC STEM CELL TRANSPLANTATION

Hematopoietic stem cell transplantation (SCT) involves the infusion of hematopoietic stem and progenitor cells into a patient in order to treat nonmalignant, hematologic, and immunologic diseases and a number of malignant diseases. Hematopoietic stem cells are immature cells that mature and differentiate into the various functional myeloid (eg, neutrophils, monocytes, macrophages, megakaryocytes, erythrocytes) and lymphoid cells (eg, T lymphocytes, B lymphocytes, natural killer cells) of the hematopoietic system. Hematopoietic stem cells are transplanted in order to replace diseased hematopoietic cells, reduce the duration of pancytopenia following administration of high dose chemotherapy, or to generate antitumor immunity in cancer patients. Allogeneic stem cell transplants require donation of stem cells from a healthy donor; whereas, autologous transplantation uses stem cells previously collected from the patient undergoing treatment. Allogeneic stem cell transplants are further classified as related transplants (donor and recipient are siblings), unrelated transplants (donor and recipient are not related), or syngeneic transplants (donor and recipient are identical twins). Immunologic likeness of the donor and recipient is determined by comparison of the genotype and phenotype of donor and recipient class I and class II major histocompatibility (MHC) antigens. MHC Class I antigens (HLA-A, HLA-B, HLA-C) are present on all nucleated cells in the body and provide a means for the immune system to differentiate self versus nonself. MHC Class II proteins (HLA-DP, HLA-DQ, HLA-DR) are present on antigen presenting cells, such as macrophages, dendritic cells, B lymphocytes, and activated endothelial cells, and are critical in initiation and maintenance of long-lasting immunity and tolerance.

Classification of stem cell transplants according to the intensity of the pretransplant preparative regimen differentiates myeloablative versus non-myeloablative regimens. Myeloablative chemotherapy regimens administer the highest possible dose of chemotherapy, with the doses limited by regimen-related nonhematologic toxicity. The goal of the myeloablative regimen is to achieve the maximum anticancer effect and complete immunosuppression through the effects of the high dose cytotoxic agents. The goal of the nonmyeloablative preparative regimen is to inhibit the recipient immune system adequately to allow engraftment of the donated hematopoietic cells. Complete donor engraftment following nonmyeloablative transplantation typically occurs after a period of mixed chimerism and is associated with antitumor effect mediated by donor immune cells. Less regimen-related morbidity occurs following treatment with non-myeloablative preparative regimens in comparison to myeloablative preparative regimens.

Terms that are synonymous with hematopoietic stem cell transplantation include stem cell transplantation, bone marrow transplantation, peripheral blood cell transplantation, and peripheral blood cell rescue. The following table lists clinical uses for allogeneic and autologous myeloablative hematopoietic stem cell transplantation.

Condition	Allogeneic	Autologous
Acute lymphocytic leukemia (ALL)	+	+
Acute myelogenous leukemia (AML)	+	+
Myelodysplastic syndrome	+	-
Chronic lymphocytic leukemia (CLL)	+	-
Chronic myelogenous leukemia (CML)	+	-
Non-Hodgkin's lymphoma (NHL)	+	+
Hodgkin's lymphoma	+	+
Multiple myeloma (MM)	+	+
Severe aplastic anemia (SAA)	+	-
Sickle cell disease (SCD)	+	-
Congenital immunodeficiency syndromes	+	-
Adult autoimmune disorders (eg, scleroderma, multiple sclerosis, rheumatoid arthritis)	-	+
Germ cell/testicular cancer	-	+
Neuroblastoma	-	+
Congenital hematopoietic disorders	+	-
Inborn errors of metabolism	+	-
Paroxysmal nocturnal hemoglobinuria	+	-
Thalassemia major	+	-
Wiskott-Aldrich syndrome	+	-

SOURCES, COLLECTION, AND PROCESSING OF HEMATOPOIETIC PROGENITOR CELLS

Peripheral blood is generally the site for obtaining the hematopoietic progenitor cells for transplantation. The hematopoietic stem and progenitor cells are removed via leukapheresis, which is easily done in an ambulatory setting and requires no anesthesia. Cells collected for autologous transplantation are processed and can be either used immediately or cryopreserved for future use. Cells collected for allogeneic transplantation are generally processed and infused immediately; however, cells for allogeneic transplantation have been frozen and stored prior to transplantation. Leukapheresis involves the processing of approximately 10 L of peripheral blood over a 2- to 6-hour period. The usual goal is a product containing at least 2×10^6/kg, ideally 5×10^6/kg of recipient weight of CD34$^+$ cells, which closely correlate with the content of stem and progenitor cells collected. This may be accomplished by 1 or several leukaphereses. Patients may require calcium supplementation during leukapheresis due to the citrate anticoagulant used during the procedure. Common medical risks to the allogeneic donor of peripheral hematopoietic stem cells include adverse effects from treatment with a colony-stimulating factor (bone pain) and adverse events associated with leukapheresis (acute hypocalcemia, catheter-related discomfort). Although no long-term toxicity has been reported in donors treated with colony-stimulating factors, rare serious toxicity such as splenic rupture can occur and the donor must be screened carefully prior to donation.

The peripheral blood concentration of hematopoietic stem cells and progenitor cells must be increased to facilitate successful collection. This process is known as peripheral progenitor cell mobilization. After administration of chemotherapy, colony-stimulating factors, or a combination of the two agents, the numbers of circulating early and late progenitor cells becomes greatly increased. A colony-stimulating factor, such as filgrastim or sargramostim, is used for this purpose in the healthy allogeneic donor. For the autologous donor, a colony-stimulating factor is administered alone or prescribed following chemotherapy. Mobilization of hematopoietic progenitor cells can be more difficult in patients with hematologic malignancies, or a history of extensive treatment with chemotherapy and radiation. The following table provides the dosage and schedule for some of the more commonly used mobilization regimens. Selection of the chemotherapy for mobilization in the autologous donor is primarily based on the type of cancer being treated. The CXCR4 analogue plerixafor (AMD3100) has been approved for use (in combination with filgrastim) in autologous transplantation.

Mobilization Agent	Dosage and Duration
Filgrastim (G-CSF)	10 mcg/kg/day SubQ for 5-7 days or until target WBC; dose escalation to 16-32 mcg/kg/day has been used to improve inadequate mobilization
Sargramostim (GM-CSF)	250 mg/m^2/day SubQ for 5-7 days or until target WBC
Etoposide (VP-16)	2 g/m^2 I.V. over 2 hours followed in 24 hours by G-CSF or GM-CSF until target WBC
Cyclophosphamide	4 g/m^2 (range of 1.5-7 g/m^2) I.V. over 2 hours followed at 24 hours by G-CSF 5-10 mcg/kg/day until target WBC; higher doses are also used (7 g/m^2)
Cytarabine plus etoposide	2 g/m^2 I.V. q12h x 8 doses + 40 mg/kg VP-16 over 4 days then G-CSF 10 mcg/kg/day from day 14 until cells collected
Plerixafor (in combination with filgrastim)	0.24 mg/kg SubQ once daily for up to 4 consecutive days beginning ~11 hours prior to apheresis; maximum dose: 40 mg/day

Historically, the bone marrow was the primary source of hematopoietic stem cells for transplantation and it still represents an equivalent, if not better stem cell source in the setting of allogeneic transplantation. The bone marrow contains populations of hematopoietic cells ranging from the pluripotent stem cell, early progenitor cells, and later, more differentiated progenitor cells that all exist within and are supported by the bone marrow stroma (matrix composed of connective tissue, reticuloendothelial cells, adipose cells). Compared to blood, the concentration of T lymphocytes is significantly lower in the marrow. Bone marrow can be harvested by removing an adequate volume of marrow (approximately 10 mL/kg) from the posterior iliac crests of the donor or patient. This is generally done in an operating room and requires general or local anesthesia. Bone marrow collected for autologous transplantation is processed in a cryopreservation laboratory and frozen until the day of transplantation. Common medical risks to the donor of bone marrow include the risks of undergoing anesthesia, and transient moderate pain in the area of cell harvesting. Severe anemia can also develop. The frequency of life-threatening complications, which have included thromboembolic disorders, aspiration pneumonia, and cardiac dysrhythmias, is ≤0.3%. Hematopoietic engraftment (normalization of the peripheral white blood cell count) occurs earlier following peripheral stem cell transplantation than following bone marrow transplantation. However, chronic graft-versus-host disease (GVHD) risk is lower with bone marrow.

Umbilical cord blood (UCB) is another source of hematopoietic progenitor cells. The product, which is harvested from the placenta and umbilical cord immediately after birth, can be processed and transplanted or frozen for future use. The product obtained from UCB contains a high proportion of pluripotent stem cells, and natural killer cells, and a low proportion of mature lymphocytes. The time to engraftment is generally longer following UCB transplantation than following hematopoietic stem cell transplantation when peripheral blood or bone marrow is harvested and infused. Moreover, UCB transplantation is generally reserved for children and small adults because the number of stem cells that can be collected from cord blood may be inadequate to support timely engraftment for larger patients. The risk for severe GVHD is lower with UCB even when HLA matching is not perfect. The process of harvesting UCB does not present a medical risk to the donor, because the actual collection of cells is done after the placenta is extruded as part of the birthing process.

The hematopoietic progenitor cells may be treated prior to transplantation to eradicate tumor cell contamination in the product following autologous donation or reduce the number of T lymphocytes that may promote graft-versus-host disease in an allogeneic recipient. The term purging refers to the removal of tumor cells by various techniques such as binding to specific monoclonal antibodies or incubation with cytotoxic drugs, such as 4-hydroperoxycyclophosphamide, that spare the immature stem cells. *Ex vivo* T lymphocyte reduction, also known as T cell depletion, is generally achieved using monoclonal antibodies directed against surface proteins expressed on T lymphocytes. An alternative to purging or T lymphocyte depletion is the application of positive selection techniques, which remove the $CD34^+$ cells (CD34 is a marker for the hematopoietic stem and progenitor cells) for use and discards the remaining cells. Engraftment is generally delayed following transplantation of hematopoietic progenitor cells that have undergone *ex vivo* purging, T cell depletion, or positive selection of $CD34^+$ cells.

AUTOLOGOUS MYELOABLATIVE TRANSPLANTATION

Chemotherapy selection for this type of SCT is based on three important principles:

1. Certain drugs such as alkylating agents and etoposide exhibit steep dose-response curves when used to treat susceptible malignancies. Therefore, when the dose-limiting adverse effect of these drugs is myelosuppression, high doses can be administered with hematopoietic stem cell rescue to achieve high response rates.

2. High doses of chemotherapy with nonoverlapping major organ toxicity can be combined without compromising dose.

3. Cryopreserved bone marrow and/or blood progenitor cells can rescue the patient from the myeloablative effects of the high-dose chemotherapy.

Administration of filgrastim or sargramostim following reinfusion of the autologous hematopoietic progenitor cells can significantly shorten the duration of neutropenia associated with myeloablative chemotherapy (refer to filgrastim or sargramostim monographs for dosing, etc). The hematopoietic recovery period following SCT is generally 1-2 weeks, which is shorter than that for bone marrow or UCB transplants which require 2-4 weeks. The monocytes and neutrophils engraft first followed by the platelets about a week later. The most common complications associated with autologous SCT are febrile neutropenia, serum electrolyte abnormalities, infection, bleeding, gastrointestinal toxicities (mucositis, nausea, vomiting, and diarrhea), and less commonly, other organ toxicities that are related to the specific chemotherapy administered. The following table lists commonly used chemotherapy agents with their dose-limiting toxicities in SCT.

Chemotherapy	Standard Dose	Maximum SCT Dose as Single Agent	Maximum SCT Dose in Combination	Dose-Limiting Toxicity
Busulfan (oral)	4 mg/d	16 mg/kg	16 mg/kg	GI, liver (VOD), CNS (seizure), pulmonary
Busulfan (I.V.)		12 mg/kg	12 mg/kg	GI, liver (VOD), CNS (seizure), pulmonary
Carboplatin	400 mg/m^2	2000 mg/m^2	1800 mg/m^2	Liver, renal
Carmustine	200 mg/m^2	800 mg/m^2	600 mg/m^2	Liver, pulmonary
Cisplatin	75-100 mg/m^2	180-200 mg/m^2	165-200 (in BEP) mg/m^2	Renal, neuropathy
Cyclophospha-mide	50 mg/kg or 600-1875 mg/m^2	200 mg/kg or 7.5 g/m^2	200 mg/kg or 7.5 g/m^2	Cardiac, hemorrhagic cystitis, liver (VOD)
Etoposide	360 mg/m^2	2400 mg/m^2	2400 mg/m^2	GI, hypotension
Melphalan	40 mg/m^2	220 mg/m^2	140-180 mg/m^2	GI
Mitoxantrone	12 mg/m^2/d x 3	90 mg/m^2	60-80 mg/m^2	GI, cardiac

ALLOGENEIC MYELOABLATIVE TRANSPLANTATION

The principle behind allogeneic myeloablative hematopoietic stem cell transplantation is that hematological disease can be cured by complete marrow ablation with profound immunosuppression so that the donor cells can engraft and successfully replace the patient's diseased hematopoietic system. Post-transplant immunosuppressive therapy is essential for successful engraftment of donor cells and prevention of graft-versus-host disease (GVHD). Preparative regimens for allogeneic transplantation are based on the need for both marrow ablation and immunosuppression. The most commonly used regimens are listed in the table on the next page.

Acronym	Chemotherapy Drugs (Total Dose)	Dosages and Scheduling
BuCy	Busulfan (12-16 mg/kg)	0.875-1 mg/kg/dose P.O. q6h x 16 doses; or 1 mg/kg/dose P.O. q6h x 12 doses; or 0.8 mg/kg I.V. q6h x 16 doses
	Cyclophosphamide (120 mg/kg)	60 mg/kg/dose I.V. q24h x 2 doses
FTBI/Cy, or CyTBI	Fractionated total body irradiation	1200-1500 cGy divided bid over 3-5 days
	Cyclophosphamide (120-200 mg/kg)	50 mg/kg/dose I.V. q24h x 4 doses or 60 mg/kg/dose I.V. q24h x 2 doses
Bu/Mel	Busulfan (16 mg/kg)	1 mg/kg/dose P.O. q6h x 16 doses
	Melphalan (135-140 mg/m^2)	45 mg/m^2/dose I.V. q24h x 3, or 140 mg/m^2 once
FTBI/Mel	Fractionated total body irradiation	1200-1500 cGy divided bid over 3-5 days
	Melphalan (135-140 mg/m^2)	45 mg/m^2/dose I.V. q24h x 2, or 70 mg/m^2/dose I.V. q24h x 2; or 140 mg/m^2 once
CyATG	Cyclophosphamide (200 mg/kg)	50 mg/kg/dose I.V. q24h x 4
	Lymphocyte immune globulin (90-160 mg/kg)	30-40 mg/kg/dose I.V. q24-48h x 3-4 doses

Lymphocyte immune globulin or antithymocyte globulin is included in the preparative regimen for patients with severe aplastic anemia. Lymphocyte immune globulin or antithymocyte globulin is often added to the preparative regimen for allogeneic transplants when the donor and recipient are immunologically mismatched or unrelated, and for umbilical cord blood transplants. This added immunosuppression improves engraftment and may decrease acute GVHD.

Graft versus host disease (GVHD) is an immune-mediated reaction initiated by donor T-cell recognition of recipient tissues as nonself. GVHD which occurs before 100 days post-transplant is called acute GVHD, and after this time it is called chronic GVHD. Acute GVHD primarily affects the skin, gastrointestinal tract, and liver. It is graded based on extent of organ involvement from grade I (mild) to grade IV (life-threatening). Chronic GVHD affects the skin, gastrointestinal tract, liver, and other organs and tissues including the lungs, lacrimal glands, and connective tissue. Chronic GVHD is generally graded as limited or extensive disease. Mortality from this toxicity ranges from 10% to 30%. There is a strong positive correlation between development of acute or chronic GVHD and decreased risk of malignancy recurrence due to associated graft vs malignancy effect.

Given the high morbidity and mortality associated with severe GVHD, post-transplant care is directed to prevent this complication. A combination of 2-3 immunosuppressants is used to prevent GVHD. The selection of prophylactic immunosuppressants used is based on the degree of risk for GVHD and the risk of malignant relapse. In general, as the depth and duration of immunosuppression increase so does the risk of malignant relapse, and infectious disease. Commonly used prophylactic immunosuppressants include cyclosporine or tacrolimus plus methotrexate, with addition of a methylprednisolone for patients at high risk for GVHD.

GVHD Prophylactic Agents	Usual Dose and Schedule
Cyclosporine	2.5-4 mg/kg/day I.V. continuous infusion or divided q12h over 2-6 hours. Dose adjust according to toxicity and blood concentrations. Convert to oral dose when appropriate.
Tacrolimus	0.03 mg/kg/day continuous infusion. Adjust dose according to toxicity and blood concentrations. Convert to oral dose when appropriate.
Methotrexate	15 mg/m^2/day on day + 1, 10 mg/m^2 on days +3, +6, and +11; give I.V. push, or "mini methotrexate" 5 mg/m^2/day IVP on days +1, +3, +6
Methylprednisolone	Variable; 0.5-1 mg/kg/day divided q6-12h then taper. May start +1 up to +7; increase dose for acute GVHD reactions.
Mycophenolate mofetil	1 g/dose I.V. or P.O. q12h; or 15 mg/kg/dose I.V. or P.O. q12h

Initial treatment of GVHD includes addition of a corticosteroid or a dosage increase of ongoing corticosteroid treatment. Additional agents used for the treatment of steroid-refractory acute GVHD include lymphocyte immune globulin or antithymocyte globulin, interleukin-2 receptor antagonists (basiliximab, daclizumab), tumor necrosis factor antagonists (etanercept, infliximab), sirolimus, pentostatin, and muromonab CD3. Additional agents used for the treatment of steroid-refractory chronic GVHD include thalidomide, pentostatin, PUVA (8-methoxypsoralen plus UV-A radiation), rituximab, and sirolimus.

Veno-occlusive disease (VOD) of the liver, also known as sinusoidal obstruction syndrome (SOS) may occur as a result of the pretransplant conditioning regimen. Patients with pre-existing liver disease, malignant involvement of the liver, and those previously treated with gemtuzumab ozogamicin are at increased risk for this complication. VOD, which usually presents within the first three weeks after transplant, results from obstruction of blood flow in the small hepatic veins. Signs and symptoms include right upper quadrant pain, hepatomegaly, weight gain, ascites, hyperbilirubinemia, and thrombocytopenia. Treatment options include supportive care, alteplase (has a high incidence of bleeding complications), antithrombin III, and defibrotide (an investigational antithrombotic agent with no system effect on coagulation). Low-dose heparin or ursodiol have been used for VOD prophylaxis.

Allogeneic stem cell transplantation is associated with a wide range of infectious complications that occur during identifiable time periods after the transplant. The early period of neutropenia is most commonly associated with bacterial infections, fungal infections (*Candida* species), and possibly herpes simplex virus (HSV) reactivation. *Pneumocystis pneumoniae* (PCP) risk increases with duration of immunosuppressive therapy. Other life-threatening infections typically occurring 2-3 months post-transplant include aspergillosis and CMV (disseminated or pneumonitis). Other serious atypical viral and fungal infections can also be seen at this later time.

Prophylaxis for certain infections is routine while others are treated when they are diagnosed. Trimethoprim-sulfamethoxazole is given during the preparative regimen as a selective gut decontaminant, and then restarted after hematopoietic recovery on a 2-3 times weekly schedule as PCP prophylaxis. The major concern with this drug is the myelosuppressive effect. Fluoroquinolones may be used as selective gut decontamination. Fungal prophylaxis is routinely given as well. This consists of either a daily low dose of amphotericin B (0.15-0.25 mg/kg) or fluconazole 100-400 mg daily. Inhalation amphotericin B can also be used to decrease risk of pulmonary aspergillosis. Acyclovir is routinely used to prevent

HSV reinfection. The role of acyclovir for prevention of CMV infection is controversial. Some centers routinely prescribe acyclovir immediately following the transplant for prevention of CMV or HSV infection. After cellular recovery, the patient may be switched to ganciclovir therapy. Ganciclovir is not used earlier due to the risk of graft failure. The role of antibacterial prophylaxis or gut decontamination varies with transplant centers but is often used in some form.

Hematopoietic growth factors (filgrastim or sargramostim) are usually administered after infusion of allogeneic donor blood cells. The doses range from 5-10 mcg/kg/day and administration is begun either on day 0 or +1 or may be delayed up to 6 days post cell infusion. The colony stimulating factors are discontinued when neutrophil recovery reaches some target number (5000-10,000/µL has been used).

NONMYELOABLATIVE TRANSPLANTS

Nonmyeloablative hematopoietic stem cell transplants are a new and largely investigational approach to the treatment of malignant and nonmalignant diseases. Clinical trials and case series describe use of nonmyeloablative hematopoietic stem cell transplantation for the following diseases: Congenital immunodeficiency syndromes, acute myelogenous leukemia, myelodysplastic syndrome, acute lymphocytic leukemia, multiple myeloma, non-Hodgkin's lymphoma, Hodgkin's disease, sickle cell disease, renal cell carcinoma, and various advanced solid tumors. Most of the published studies and case series report use of this procedure in patients with relapsed or refractory disease, elderly patients, or those unable to tolerate myeloablative preparative regimens.

The theory supporting nonmyeloablative transplantation is that nonmyeloablative, but sufficiently immunosuppressive conditioning regimens, can lead to a state of mixed chimerism in the recipient, which gradually converts to full donor chimerism. Even the chimeric engraftment will support a graft-versus-malignancy effect. The preparative regimens used for nonmyeloablative hematopoietic stem cell transplantation, which are termed "reduced-intensity preparative regimens", induce profound immunosuppression without total obliteration of the recipient's bone marrow. This supports chimeric engraftment, which involves engraftment of transplanted allogeneic hematopoietic progenitor cells in the presence of recipient hematopoietic cells. Complete donor engraftment, also known as 100% donor chimerism, occurs when all of the detectable hematopoietic cells are of donor origin. Complete donor chimerism occurring within 30-90 days following transplantation is generally associated with disease response. Because antitumor effects of nonmyeloablative allogeneic transplants appear somewhat late, 2-3 months after the procedure, patients with active or poorly controlled malignancies do not appear to be good candidates for this type of transplantation.

The preparative regimens used for nonmyeloablative hematopoietic stem cell transplantation are associated with less regimen-related toxicity than myeloablative preparative regimens. This provides the impetus for studying use of nonmyeloablative hematopoietic stem cell transplantation in patients unable to tolerate the myeloablative preparative regimens, such as the elderly, or patients with an extensive history of chemotherapy treatment, impaired major organ function, or comorbid conditions. Examples of reduced-intensity preparative regimens are listed in the following table.

Acronym	Chemotherapy Drugs (Total Dose)	Dosages and Scheduling
Flu/ATG	Lymphocyte immune globulin 40 mg/kg (Atgam®)	10 mg/kg/day I.V. on 4 consecutive days
	Antithymoglobulin 10 mg/kg (Thymoglobulin®)	2.5 mg/kg/day I.V. on 4 consecutive days
	Fludarabine 125 mg/m²	25 mg/m²/day I.V. on 5 consecutive days
FC-ATG	Fludarabine 125 mg/m²	25 mg/m²/day I.V. on days -6 to -2
	Cyclophosphamide 120 mg/kg	60 mg/kg/day I.V. on days -3 and -2
	Lymphocyte immune globulin 60 mg/kg (Atgam®)	20 mg/kg/day I.V. on 3 consecutive days
TBI/Flu	Total body irradiation 4 Gy	2 Gy/day on days -8 and -7
	Fludarabine 125 mg/m²	25 mg/m²/day I.V. on days -6 to -2
Flu/Mel/ATG	Fludarabine 125 mg/m²	25 mg/m²/day I.V. on days -6 to -2
	Melphalan 140-180 mg/m²	70-90 mg/m²/day I.V. on days -3 and -2
	Lymphocyte immune globulin 120 mg/kg (Atgam®)	30 mg/kg/day I.V. on days -4 to -1
Bu/Flu/ATG	Busulfan 8 mg/kg	1 mg/kg/dose P.O. q6h X8 doses on days -6 and -5
	Fludarabine 125 mg/m²	25 mg/m²/day I.V. on days -6 to -2
	Antithymocyte globulin (Fresinus) 10 mg/kg	2.5 mg/kg/day I.V. on 4 consecutive days
Cy/Flu/TBI	Cyclophosphamide 50 mg/kg	50 mg/kg I.V. on day -6
	Fludarabine 200 mg/m²	40 mg/m²/day I.V. on days -6 to -2
	TBI 200 cGy	TBI 200 cGy on day -1

GVHD prophylaxis generally includes cyclosporine or tacrolimus plus mycophenolate mofetil. Treatment of moderate-to-severe GVHD is similar to the approach taken for treatment of GVHD following myeloablative allogeneic hematopoietic stem cell transplantation. Most complications following nonmyeloablative hematopoietic stem cell transplantation are related to GVHD and the immunosuppression required for treatment of GVHD. Infectious complications from Cytomegalovirus, herpes virus, candidiasis, aspergillosis, and other atypical infections are common.

Selected Readings

Bacigalupo A, "Second EBMT Workshop on Reduced Intensity Allogeneic Hemopoietic Stem Cell Transplants (RI-HSCT)," *Bone Marrow Transplant*, 2002, 29:191-5.

Barker JN, Weisdorf DJ, DeFor TE, et al, "Rapid and Complete Donor Chimerism in Adult Recipients of Unrelated Donor Umbilical Cord Blood Transplantation After Reduced-Intensity Conditioning," *Blood*, 2003, 102(5):1915-9.

Cairo MS and Wagner JE, "Placental and/or Umbilical Cord Blood: An Alternative Source of Hematopoietic Stem Cells for Transplantation," *Blood*, 1997, 90:4665-78.

Champlin R, Khouri I, Anderlini P, et al, "Nonmyeloablative Preparative Regimens for Allogeneic Hematopoietic Transplantation," *Bone Marrow Transplant*, 2001, 27 Suppl 2:S13-22.

Copelan EA, "Hematopoietic Stem-Cell Transplantation," *N Engl J Med*, 2006, 354(17):1813-26.

DiPersio JF, Micallef IN, Stiff PJ, et al, "Phase III Prospective Randomized Double-Blind Placebo-Controlled Trial of Plerixafor Plus Granulocyte Colony-Stimulating Factor Compared With Placebo Plus Granulocyte Colony-Stimulating Factor for Autologous Stem-Cell Mobilization and Transplantation for Patients With Non-Hodgkin's Lymphoma," *J Clin Oncol*, 2009, 27 (28):4767-73.

DiPersio JF, Stadtmauer EA, Nademanee A, et al, "Plerixafor and G-CSF Versus Placebo and G-CSF to Mobilize Hematopoietic Stem Cells for Autologous Stem Cell Transplantation in Patients With Multiple Myeloma," *Blood*, 2009, 113(23):5720-6.

Ho VT and Soiffer RJ, "The History and Future of T-Cell Depletion as Graft-Versus-Host Disease Prophylaxis for Allogeneic Hematopoietic Stem Cell Transplantation," *Blood*, 2001, 98:3192-204.

Klingebiel T and Schlegel PG, "GVHD: Overview on Pathophysiology, Incidence, Clinical and Biological Features," *Bone Marrow Transplant*, 1998, 21 (Suppl 2):S45-9.

Kumar S, DeLeve LD, Kamath PS, et al, "Hepatic Veno-Occlusive Disease (Sinusoidal Obstruction Syndrome) After Hematopoietic Stem Cell Transplantation," *Mayo Clin Proc*, 2003, (78):589-98.

Mogul MJ, "Unrelated Cord Blood Transplantation Vs Matched Unrelated Donor Bone Marrow Transplantation: The Risks and Benefits of Each Choice," *Bone Marrow Transplant*, 2000, 25 (Suppl 2):S58-60.

Pegram AA and Kennedy LD, "Prevention and Treatment of Veno-Occlusive Disease," *Ann Pharmacother*, 2001, 35(7-8):935-42.

Rowe JM, Ciobanu N, Ascensao J, et al, "Recommended Guidelines for the Management of Autologous and Allogeneic Bone Marrow Transplantation. A Report From the Eastern Cooperative Oncology Group (ECOG)," *Ann Intern Med*, 1994, 120:143-58.

Stiff P, "Mucositis Associated With Stem Cell Transplantation: Current Status and Innovative Approaches to Management," *Bone Marrow Transplant* , 2001, 27 (Suppl 2):S3-S11.

Storb R, Deeg HJ, Whitehead J, et al, "Methotrexate and Cyclosporine Compared With Cyclosporine Alone for Prophylaxis of Acute Graft Versus Host Disease After Marrow Transplantation for Leukemia," *N Engl J Med*, 1986, 314:729-35.

Vogelsang GB and Arai S, "Mycophenolate Mofetil for the Prevention and Treatment of Graft-Versus-Host Disease Following Stem Cell Transplantation: Preliminary Findings," *Bone Marrow Transplant*, 2001, 27:1255-62.

DRUG DEVELOPMENT PROCESS

Drug development describes the process required to bring a drug from its original identity to becoming a commercially available product for use in human beings. The drug development process involves scientific, clinical, and regulatory activities. Bringing a new molecular entity or new active substance through the drug development process takes years of time and hundreds of millions to billions of dollars.

SCIENTIFIC CONTRIBUTION

The major scientific contribution is drug discovery and drug design. Candidates for drug development arise from biotechnologic or chemical synthesis and natural product extraction. Selection of drug candidates is often based on their ability *in vitro* to bind a molecular target or exert a biologic effect. This is an inefficient low-yield process despite the use of automated high throughput screening methods that can test thousands of drug candidates daily. A challenge of drug discovery is the myriad of factors that can abrogate the utility or efficacy of drug candidates as they proceed through preclinical and clinical testing.

Preclinical testing is done in several species of animals to evaluate toxicity, pharmacodynamics, and pharmacokinetics. Acute toxicity, chronic toxicity, fetotoxicity, teratogenicity, and carcinogenicity are tested in animals to identify common sites of toxicity and potentially use-limiting toxicity, such as neurologic adverse effects or carcinogenicity. Drug pharmacodynamics and pharmacokinetics are evaluated in animals to extrapolate a first in human (FIH) dose when the drug advances to clinical trials.

Additional scientific contributions to drug development include chemical characterization and pharmaceutical development of drug candidates.

REGULATORY PROCESS

In the United States, clinical trials administering drugs to human beings are regulated by the Food and Drug Administration (FDA). Regulation is directed and implemented through an application process required for various levels of clinical drug development. The Investigational New Drug (IND) application is required prior to testing a drug in human subjects or distributing it across state lines. The IND (Form 1571) contains preclinical data, proposed clinical protocol, investigator's brochure (if available), and manufacturing information. An Exploratory IND allows administration of subtherapeutic doses to a small number of subjects to assess whether the preclinically tested drug-target interaction occurs in humans. An Emergency IND allows distribution of an investigational drug on a patient-specific basis for management of a serious condition. Investigational drugs must have demonstrated a certain degree of efficacy and safety for an Emergency IND application to be granted. The New Drug Application (NDA) is reviewed by the FDA to determine whether drug testing is sufficient for product approval and consumer use. The NDA is a comprehensive document containing data supporting all of the chemical, pharmacologic, pharmaceutical, preclinical, therapeutic, safety, and pharmacokinetic information and claims required for product approval. Approval of generic equivalents can be achieved with an Abbreviated New Drug Application (ANDA). Generic drugs are reviewed using the ANDA because the efficacy and safety of these products was previously established by the original brand (innovator drug). Approval of a generic drug is based on scientific data demonstrating that the generic product is bioequivalent to the innovator product. Biologic products, such as monoclonal antibodies and vaccines, are approved for commercial use using a Biologic License Application (BLA).

The conduct of clinical trials is approved, monitored, and reviewed by an institutional review board (IRB), also known as human subjects committee, independent ethics committee, ethical review board, etc. The IRB is responsible for overseeing the conduct of biomedical and behavioral research involving human subjects. The IRB ensures that biomedical and behavioral research is ethical, informed consent is sufficient, and appropriate safeguards are established. The FDA Department of Health and Human Services Office for Human Research Protection empowers IRBs to approve, require modifications, or disapprove research conducted under their domain. Most IRBs are based at academic institutions or health care systems. However, independent commercial for profit IRBs exist that adhere to the same federal regulations as local committees.

CLINICAL TRIALS

Clinical trials include Phase 0, Phase I, Phase II, and Phase III analysis of a drug in humans. Phase 0 studies evaluate clinical drug-target interaction(s). Phase I testing is done to assess drug safety and pharmacokinetics. Phase 0 and Phase I clinical trials are FIH drug studies that are unlikely to provide any therapeutic benefit to the participating subjects. Phase II clinical trials test the efficacy of a drug in the management of a specific disease or pathophysiologic process. The purpose of Phase III clinical trials is to compare the investigational treatment to the standard of care. Phase IV testing (postmarketing surveillance) generally involves pharmacovigilance or additional pharmacokinetic or drug interaction characterization in FDA approved medications. Phase IV testing is often done independently by academic investigators or it may be a requirement imposed by the FDA.

ONCOLOGY AGENTS

Phase 0 clinical trials are an attempt to reduce the consumption of valuable time and resources that occur when promising preclinical candidates fail in Phase II clinical trials. Specifically, small doses of drug are administered to 15 or fewer subjects for a short period of time to evaluate whether the therapeutic drug-target interaction occurs in human beings. Drugs tested in Phase 0 clinical trials must have a wide margin of safety and a validated method for testing drug-target interaction(s).

Phase I clinical trials for anticancer treatments are used to identify the maximum tolerated dose (MTD) of cytotoxic chemotherapy. The FIH dose of cytotoxic chemotherapy is generally a small fraction (1/10th) of the preclinical dose that produced lethality in 10% of the most sensitive animal model. The dose is increased in a stepwise fashion until the dose-limiting toxicity (DLT) is reached in >33% of a patient cohort. The dose at which <33% of patients have DLT is utilized in Phase II studies. Dose calculation based on body surface area or weight is used as a tool to extrapolate clinical doses from those administered to animals in preclinical testing. Unlike Phase I clinical trials for nononcology medications conducted in normal human subjects, only patients with advanced cancer refractory to treatment and with normal organ function, are utilized for Phase I oncology studies. The dose of targeted anticancer treatments, such as monoclonal antibodies and tyrosine kinase inhibitors, that is designated for Phase II testing is generally based on receptor saturation or another surrogate marker of efficacy instead of MTD. Phase I methodology should be used when anticancer treatments with an established dose for single agent therapy or administered as combination therapy.

Phase II trials evaluate drug safety and efficacy in a group of patients with a disease the drug is intended to treat. Data is collected on adverse effects and response to the therapy. Phase II clinical trials may report efficacy based on tumor response (tumor shrinkage), which is a much less stringent measure of efficacy than survival.

Phase III studies involve a larger number of patients with a particular tumor. Patients are randomized to the new treatment or the current standard of care. A placebo arm is used for Phase III analysis of novel treatments for which there is no comparable standard of care. Primary endpoints for Phase III clinical trials evaluating anticancer treatments generally include disease response, duration of disease-free survival, duration of overall survival, and safety. As was the case with gemcitabine in pancreatic cancer, a clinical benefit response may be an endpoint that is measured.

COST(S)

Investigational new drugs are generally provided free of charge to the patient. However, there are cases when the manufacturer can seek FDA authorization to charge for use of an investigational new drug to recover costs necessary to continue drug development.

Selected Readings

Health and Human Services, Office for Human Research Protections (OHRP). Available at http://www.hhs.gov/ohrp.

"Drug Development and Approval Process." Available at http://www.fda.gov/Drugs/DevelopmentApprovalProcess/default.htm.

Egorin MJ, "Horseshoes, Hand Grenades, and Body-Surface Area-Based Dosing: Aiming For a Target," *J Clin Oncol*, 2003, 21(2):182-3.

Fojo T and Grady C, "How Much Is Life Worth: Cetuximab, Non-Small Cell Lung Cancer, and the $440 Billion Question," *J Natl Cancer Inst*, 2009, 101(15):1044-8.

Hamberg P and Verweij J, "Phase I Drug Combination Trial Design: Walking the Tightrope," *J Clin Oncol*, 2009 [epub ahead of print].

Mordenti J, Thomsen K, Licko V, et al, "Efficacy and Concentration-Response of Murine Anti-VEGF Monoclonal Antibody In Tumor-Bearing Mice and Extrapolation to Humans," *Toxicol Pathol*, 1999, 27(1):14-21.

Rowan K, "Oncology's First Phase 0 Trial," *J Natl Cancer Inst*, 2009, 101(14):978-9.

INVESTIGATIONAL DRUG SERVICE

An Investigational Drug Service (IDS) is an organized pharmacy-based service that controls the inventory, preparation, and dispensation of investigational drugs. Investigational drugs are administered only to patients who have, in an informed manner, signed a consent form to participate in the particular study using these investigational drugs. A patient formally enrolled to participate in a clinical study is known as a "subject." Investigational drugs used in this manner are frequently new drugs undergoing Phase I, Phase II, or Phase III evaluation prior to FDA approval for a medical purpose. In addition, investigational drugs can be commercially available drugs used under the direction of a protocol for a nonlabeled indication or as a supportive measure for a new drug. An IDS should be under the direction of an appropriately trained pharmacist with technical support as warranted by the workload.

A study protocol is the document describing the scientific background providing the basis for doing the study, specific study objectives and endpoints, treatments and tests done as part of the study, study drug information, statistical methodology, means for assurance of patient confidentiality, and the subject consent form. Some studies provide an Investigator's Drug Brochure, which presents very detailed and comprehensive study drug information. Each study is assigned a unique study number, eg, SWOG 9923, that is frequently a truncation of the year of study development and its position within a series of studies. Study protocols and Investigator's Drug Brochures are confidential, and frequently proprietary documents. Prior to study activation at an institution, it must be approved by the institutional investigational review board. All departments needed to provide personnel or resources for study implementation should review the protocol prior to study implementation to ensure that study activities can reasonably be supported with available resources. The IDS pharmacist should scrutinize each study protocol prior to study activation to determine the impact of study implementation on pharmacy department personnel and resources.

Investigational drug inventory must be stored at the appropriate conditions and separate from commercial drug inventory. An ongoing drug-specific inventory must be maintained for all investigational drugs housed within a pharmacy. Some studies will require lot number-specific, or subject-specific inventory for study drugs. Minimal inventory documentation should include study identification number, study drug dosage form and lot number, study drug expiration date or date of preparation, transaction date, transaction type (receipt, dispensation, return, waste), and current number of dosage forms available. Although it may be kept separately from individual study drug inventories, the pharmacy must maintain an ongoing refrigerator, freezer, and ambient temperature log for study drug storage facilities. All inventory records should be kept in a secure and accessible location by the pharmacy, even after study closure. In addition, study drug should be shipped directly to the Pharmacy Department rather than the Principal Investigator's office. This will ensure that the Pharmacy Department has shipping receipts and shipment invoices to verify receipt of the packaged contents. This will also reduce the possibility of prolonged study drug storage at inappropriate conditions, such as the institutional loading dock.

Study drug preparation should be described in the protocol or Investigator's Drug Brochure. Unfortunately, extensive admixture stability and compatibility information is not available for many injectable study drugs. Subsequently, these may have to be prepared on a dose-by-dose basis. Departmental inservices to acquaint professional and technical personnel with each new study are helpful tools for increasing staff familiarity with new studies and study drug preparation. Pharmacy department personnel should have 24-hour access to information about study drug preparation. Ideally, this is in the form of an easy-to-read and readily accessible fast facts sheet. Study protocols and Investigator's Drug Brochures should also be available to Pharmacy Department personnel around the clock for questions that arise outside of standard business hours. The Investigational Drug Service must develop a plan such that study drug doses are labeled in the manner directed by the study, are consistent with institutional policies and procedures, and are in accordance with state and federal regulations.

Study drug doses prepared for administration within a hospital or clinic should be dispensed directly to the study or institutional nurse for delivery to the patient's bedside for administration or placed directly into the subject's secured medication bin on the nursing unit. Generally, study drug doses should not be intermixed with standard medication doses transported via the routine intrainstitutional delivery system. Although the risk of inadvertent misplacement of a study drug dose may be low, the consequences can have ethical and legal implications. As an example, a study drug dose inadvertently transported to the wrong nursing unit may be mistakenly administered to a patient with a name similar to that of the actual study subject. In other words, the study drug dose could be administered to a person who did not consent to receive an investigational drug.

Pharmacy support of blinded studies can involve additional responsibilities and challenges. Pharmacy-related activities may include randomization (treatment assignment) of subjects when the Principal Investigator and other study personnel are blinded to the study treatment. Randomization for treatment assignment can be done for some studies by simply following a list of treatment assignments sequentially for consecutive subjects. However, randomization for large multicenter studies may require contacting a central randomization center with provision of patient-specific information. When pharmacy activities include randomization, it is important for the Investigational Drug Service to ensure that a workable plan is in place prior to study activation. Moreover, labeling of blinded study drug doses can be challenging since the traditional role of pharmacy labeling is to provide a completely clear description of the dosage form. In contrast, to maintain a study blind, the specific contents of a study dosage form must be omitted from the pharmacy label. Several approaches have been taken to balance study methods with institutional and legislative requirements. As an example, for a blinded study, protocol #9872, evaluating the efficacy of newazole 200 mg versus placebo (0.9% NaCl 100 mL), the following labeling techniques can be utilized to identify the dosage form: newazole 200 mg or placebo; newazole study drug; protocol #9872 study drug. Nursing personnel should be consulted regarding the proposed labeling of blinded study drug to ensure that the labeling used is compatible with medication administration records maintained by nursing staff.

The Investigational Drug Service determines fair charges for Pharmacy Department personnel time and resources utilized in the support of study activities. As a rule, routine pharmacy charges to the patient's bill, cannot be generated for investigational new drugs, or study drugs provided free-of-charge by the study sponsor. The Investigation Drug Service must charge the study funds. This is generally achieved at the institutional level by generating charges to the local Principal Investigator or Clinical Trials Office.

Additional information about handling investigational drugs is available from the National Cancer Institute Pharmaceutical Management Branch. Available at http://ctep.cancer.gov/branches/pmb/default.htm. Accessed September 20, 2009.

SAFE HANDLING OF HAZARDOUS DRUGS

Early concerns regarding the identification and exposure risk of hazardous drugs in healthcare setting were primarily focused on antineoplastic medications, but now have expanded to numerous other agents. While there is no strict agreement on the criteria for a hazardous drug, those agents considered carcinogenic, mutagenic, and causing reproductive and developmental toxicity are included in such a list. A number of agencies and organizations have developed definitions, created lists, and generated guidelines to minimize risk of exposure to products considered hazardous.

Hazardous drugs must be stored, transported, prepared, administered, and disposed of under conditions that protect the healthcare worker from either acute or chronic/low level exposure. Institutional policies or guidelines to minimize occupational exposure to hazardous drugs should include a focus on the following areas:

- Development and maintenance of a hazardous drugs list

  - Working definition/criteria of a hazardous drug
  - Volumes, forms, and frequency of hazardous drugs handled

    - Injection, oral (liquid, solid), topical

  Discussion points: Each institution or facility must create their own list of drugs deemed hazardous and in so doing should first have a working definition of hazardous drugs for their workplace. The Environmental Protection Agency (EPA), National Institute for Occupational Safety and Health (NIOSH), and American Society of Health-System Pharmacists (ASHP) have created definitions of hazardous agents (Table 1) which may be useful. Based on their definitions, these agencies developed lists of agents which are identified as hazardous drugs (Table 2). A 2009 NIOSH draft proposal of additions to and deletions from their previous list of hazardous drugs is currently under review. One specific hazardous drug criteria created by NIOSH and ASHP is the teratogenic risk of the agent. Table 3 provides a list of the FDA-assigned pregnancy categories D and X drugs in which studies in humans have demonstrated positive evidence of fetal risk. Until proven otherwise, most institutions consider investigational drugs to be hazardous and to be handled accordingly. Hazardous drug procedures must include all possible routes of administration.

- Identification of personnel and locations in the facility at risk for occupational exposure to hazardous drugs

  - Pharmacy

    - Storage and inventory
    - Dose preparation and dispensing
    - Drug waste disposal

  - Nursing Unit

    - Drug administration
    - Drug waste disposal
    - Patient waste disposal

- Other areas
  - Laboratory
  - Operating/procedure rooms
  - Veterinary department
  - Facility shipping/receiving

Discussion points: While the greatest risk of occupational exposure to hazardous drugs occurs during preparation and administration of these agents, it is important to recognize that a risk to exposure can occur throughout the facility from the moment of delivery through the disposal of product and contaminated human waste. Drug preparation and administration may occur in nontraditional areas of the institution including the operating room and in veterinary facilities. Procedures should address the importance of proper labeling and packaging and separation of hazardous vs nonhazardous inventories throughout the facility. Drug containers should be examined upon their arrival at the pharmacy. Containers that show signs of damage should be handled carefully and may require quarantine and decontamination before being placed in stock. Give consideration to routinely quarantining and decontaminating all hazardous drug containers as part of the inspection process before placing in stock.

- Mechanisms/routes of occupational exposure

  - Inhalation of dust or aerosolized droplets
  - Absorption through skin
  - Ingestion from contaminated food/drink
  - Accidental injection during preparation/administration/disposal

- Risk management

  - Use and maintenance of equipment designed to minimize exposure during handling

    - Biological safety cabinets, isolators
    - Closed system drug-transfer devices
    - Personal protective equipment
    - Deactivation, decontamination, and cleaning procedures

Discussion points: Barrier protection through the use of ventilation controls and personal protective equipment is the current standard to minimize exposure when handling hazardous drugs. NIOSH and ASHP recommend the use of Class II biological safety cabinets (type B2 preferred), but other options include the totally enclosed Class III biological safety cabinets and isolators. Self-contained or closed system devices have been recommended to minimize workplace contamination by preventing escape of drug or vapor out of the device. The PhaSeal® system is the prevalent device in the United States, but other systems (including ONGARD™, TEVADAPTOR™, and CLAVE® systems) are being evaluated. Not all hazardous drugs can be compounded with the PhaSeal® system due to limitations such as vial size, ampules, compatibility. Gloves, gowns, hair and shoe covers, and eye protection represent the core of personal protective equipment. Guidelines for choice of gowns and gloving, and the circumstances to employ this protection are published by ASHP, NIOSH, and in USP 797.

- Hazardous drug spill management
  - Size and location
  - Spill kit use
  - Worker contamination

  Discussion points: Procedures for handling spills throughout a facility are well described by ASHP and NIOSH. Institutional procedures should focus on location and size of the spill, how to handle a spill when a spill kit is not available, and how to respond to a worker contamination (emergent treatment, follow-up care).

- Personnel training in the handling of hazardous drugs
  - Prior to handling hazardous drugs
  - Periodic and ongoing testing

  Discussion points: Personnel throughout a facility must have training in the handling of hazardous drugs that are relevant to their job description. Pharmacy personnel who compound and dispense hazardous drugs must be fully trained in the storing, preparation, dispensing, and disposal of these agents. Such training should include didactic, as well as demonstrating hands-on technique, and such validation should be repeated on a regular schedule.

- Environmental and medical surveillance
  - Components of a comprehensive medical surveillance program
  - Potential use of environmental sampling techniques
  - Use of common marker hazardous drugs for assay purposes

  Discussion points: There is no current standard for environmental or medical surveillance of personnel handling hazardous drugs. It is recommended that some type of medical surveillance be employed by the facility, and may include the basic observation of employee symptom complaints or monitoring for changes in health status as part of routine checkups. Some programs follow the employee more closely, and procedures may include periodic blood counts, and a more detailed medical history and exposure history. Environmental sampling to look for surface contamination in hazardous drug preparation and administration areas may be considered, particularly in institutions with high volumes. Certain hazardous drugs serve as markers which allow for assay for measurable contamination, and can alert the facility for proper follow-up.

- Work practices regarding reproductive risks to health care workers
  - Alternative duty options

  Discussion points: Since hazardous drugs are associated with reproductive risks, policies and guidelines should address healthcare workers whom are pregnant, attempting to conceive or father a child, and whom are breast-feeding. Workers of reproductive capability should acknowledge in writing that they understand the risk of handling hazardous drugs, and be given the opportunity for reassignment or alternate work duty.

Table 1. Criteria for Defining Hazardous Agents

EPA	NIOSH	ASHP
Meets one of the following criteria: Ignitability: Create fire (under certain conditions) or are spontaneously combustible and have a flash point <60°C (140°F) Corrosivity: Acids or bases (pH ≤2 or ≥12.5) capable of corroding metal containers Reactivity: Unstable under "normal" conditions; may cause explosions, toxic fumes, gases, or vapors if heated, compressed, or mixed with water Toxicity: Harmful or fatal if ingested or absorbed; may leach from the waste and pollute ground water when disposed of on land	Manufacturer suggests use of special techniques in handling, administration, or disposal Genotoxic Carcinogenic Teratogenic, developmental toxicity, or reproductive toxicity	Genotoxic Carcinogenic Teratogenic or impairs fertility Causes serious organ or other toxic manifestation at low doses
OR	Toxic to an organ system at low doses	
Appears on one of the following lists: F: Wastes (nonspecific) from common or industrial manufacturing processes from nonspecific sources K: Specific (source) wastes from specific industries (eg, petroleum or pesticides) P or U: Wastes (unused form) from certain discarded commercial chemical products	New drugs with structural and toxicity profiles similar to existing hazardous drugs	

Table 2. Drugs Listed as Hazardous

EPA: Antineoplastic

Arsenic trioxide	Daunomycin	Streptozocin
Chlorambucil	Melphalan	Uracil mustard
Cyclophosphamide	Mitomycin	

EPA: Nonantineoplastic

Chloral hydrate	Mercury	Physostigmine salicylate
Chloroform	Nicotine	Reserpine
Dichlorodifluoromethane	Nitroglycerin	Resorcinol
Diethylstilbestrol	Paraldehyde	Saccharin
Epinephrine	Phenacetin	Selenium sulfide
Formaldehyde	Phenol	Trichloromonofluorome-thane
Hexachlorophene	Phenteramine	
Lindane	Physostigmine	Warfarin

NIOSH: Antineoplastic

Aldesleukin	Bleomycin	Dacarbazine
Alemtuzumab	Busulfan	Dactinomycin
Altretamine	Capecitabine	Daunorubicin HCl
Amsacrine	Carboplatin	Denileukin
Anastrozole	Carmustine	Docetaxel
Arsenic trioxide	Chlorambucil	Doxorubicin
Asparaginase	Cisplatin	Epirubicin
Azacitidine	Cladribine	Estramustine
Bexarotene	Cyclophosphamide	Etoposide
Bicalutamide	Cytarabine	Exemestane

1520

Floxuridine
Fludarabine
Fluorouracil
Flutamide
Fulvestrant
Gemcitabine
Gemtuzumab
  ozogamicin
Goserelin
Hydroxyurea
Ibritumomab
Idarubicin
Ifosfamide
Imatinib
Interferon alfa-2a
Interferon alfa-2b
Interferon alfa-n1
Interferon alfa-n3
Irinotecan
Letrozole
Leuprolide

Lomustine
Mechlorethamine
Melphalan
Mercaptopurine
Methotrexate
Mitomycin
Mitotane
Mitoxantrone
Nilutamide
Oxaliplatin
Paclitaxel
Pegaspargase
Pentostatin
Perphosphamide
Pipobroman
Piritrexim isethionate
Plicamycin
Prednimustine
Procarbazine
Raltitrexed

Streptozocin
Tamoxifen
Temozolomide
Teniposide
Thalidomide
Thioguanine
Thiotepa
Topotecan
Toremifene
Tositumomab
Trimetrexate
Triptorelin
Uracil mustard
Valrubicin
Vinblastine
Vincristine
Vindesine
Vinorelbine

NIOSH: Nonantineoplastic

Alitretinoin
Azathioprine
BCG vaccine
Cetrorelix acetate
Chloramphenicol
Choriogonadotropin alfa
Cidofovir
Colchicine
Cyclosporine
Dienestrol
Diethylstilbestrol
Dinoprostone
Dutasteride
Ergonovine/methyl-
  ergonovine
Estradiol

Estrogen-progestin
  combinations
Estrogens, conjugated
Estrogens, esterified
Estrone
Estropipate
Finasteride
Fluoxymesterone
Ganciclovir
Ganirelix acetate
Gonadotropin, chorionic
Leflunomide
Megestrol
Menotropins
Methyltestosterone
Mifepristone
Mycophenolate

Nafarelin
Oxytocin
Pentamidine
Podofilox
Podophyllum resin
Progesterone
Progestins
Raloxifene
Ribavirin
Tacrolimus
Testolactone
Testosterone
Tretinoin
Trifluridine
Valganciclovir
Vidarabine
Zidovudine

Product Labeling (not on EPA or NIOSH lists): Antineoplastic

Bendamustine
Bortezomib
Clofarabine
Cytarabine liposomal
Dasatinib
Daunorubicin citrate
  (liposomal)

Decitabine
Degarelix
Dexrazoxane
Doxorubicin liposomal
Ixabepilone
Nelarabine
Paclitaxel protein bound

Pemetrexed
Pralatrexate
Porfimer
Vorinostat

National Institute for Occupational Safety and Health (NIOSH), "Preventing Occupational Exposure to Antineoplastic and Other Hazardous Drugs in Health Care Settings," Available at: http://www.cdc.gov/niosh/docs/2004-165/ 2004-165d.html#o. Last accessed October 1, 2007

Table 3. Sample Listing of Teratogenic Agents

Pregnancy Risk Factor X: Antineoplastic

Abarelix
Anastrozole
Bexarotene
Bicalutamide

Degarelix
Goserelin
Lenalidomide
Leuprolide

Methotrexate
Sodium iodide I[131]
Thalidomide
Tositumomab

Pregnancy Risk Factor X: Nonantineoplastic

Acetohydroxamic acid
Acitretin
Alprostadil
Atorvastatin
Bosentan
Carboprost tromethamine
Cetrorelix
Chorionic gonadotropin
  (recombinant)
Clomiphene
Danazol
Dihydroergotamine
Dutasteride
Ergonovine
Ergotamine
Estazolam
Estradiol
Estrogens (conjugated
  A/synthetic)
Estrogens
  (conjugated/equine)

Estrogens (esterified)
Estropipate
Finasteride
Fluoxymesterone
Flurazepam
Fluvastatin
Follitropins
Ganirelix
Histrelin
Isotretinoin
Leflunomide
Levonorgestrel
Lovastatin
Lutropin alfa
Medroxyprogesterone
Megestrol
Menotropins
Methyltestosterone
Mifepristone
Miglustat
Misoprostol

Nafarelin
Nandrolone
Norethindrone
Norgestrel
Oxymetholone
Oxytocin
Podophyllum resin
Pravastatin
Quinine
Raloxifene
Ribavirin
Rosuvastatin
Simvastatin
Stanozolol
Tazarotene
Temazepam
Testosterone
Triazolam
Triptorelin
Warfarin

Pregnancy Risk Factor D: Antineoplastic

Alitretinoin
Altretamine
Aminoglutethimide
Arsenic trioxide
Azacitidine
Bleomycin
Bortezomib
Busulfan
Capecitabine
Carboplatin
Carmustine
Chlorambucil
Cisplatin
Cladribine
Clofarabine
Cyclophosphamide
Cytarabine
Cytarabine (liposomal)
Dactinomycin
Dasatinib
Daunorubicin citrate
  (liposomal)
Daunorubicin hydro-
  chloride

Decitabine
Dexrazoxane
Docetaxel
Doxorubicin
Doxorubicin (liposomal)
Epirubicin
Erlotinib
Etoposide
Etoposide phosphate
Everolimus
Exemestane
Floxuridine
Fludarabine
Fluorouracil
Flutamide
Fulvestrant
Gefitinib
Gemcitabine
Gemtuzumab ozogamicin
Hydroxyurea
Ibritumomab
Idarubicin
Ifosfamide
Imatinib

Irinotecan
Ixabepilone
Lapatinib
Letrozole
Lomustine
Mechlorethamine
Melphalan
Mercaptopurine
Mitomycin
Mitoxantrone
Nelarabine
Nilotinib
Oxaliplatin
Paclitaxel
Paclitaxel (protein bound)
Pemetrexed
Pentostatin
Pralatrexate
Procarbazine
Sorafenib
Streptozocin
Sunitinib
Tamoxifen
Temozolomide

Temsirolimus
Teniposide
Thioguanine
Thiotepa

Topotecan
Toremifene
Trastuzumab
Tretinoin

Vinblastine
Vincristine
Vinorelbine
Vorinostat

Pregnancy Risk Factor D: Nonantineoplastic

Alprazolam
Amiodarone
Amitriptyline & chlordiazepoxide
Amitriptyline & perphenazine
Amobarbital
Anthrax vaccine
Aspirin & codeine
Aspirin & dipyridamole
Aspirin & meprobamate
Atenolol
Atenolol & chlorthalidone
Azathioprine
Butabarbital
Clidinium & chlordiazepoxide

Demeclocycline
Doxycycline
Efavirenz
Fosphenytoin
Hydrocodone & aspirin
Meprobamate
Methimazole
Minocycline
Mycophenolate
Nicotine
Orphenadrine, aspirin, & caffeine
Oxycodone & aspirin
Pamidronate
Paroxetine
Penicillamine
Perindopril erbumine

Phenobarbital
Potassium iodide
Primidone
Propoxyphene
Propylthiouracil
Secobarbital
Streptomycin
Tetracycline
Tigecycline
Tolbutamide
Valproic acid & derivatives
Voriconazole
Zoledronic acid

Selected Readings

American Society of Hospital Pharmacists, "ASHP Guidelines on Handling Hazardous Drugs," 2006, 63(12):1172-93.

Baker ES and Connor TH, "Monitoring Occupational Exposure to Cancer Chemotherapy Drugs," *Am J Health Syst Pharm*, 1996, 53(22):2713-23.

Bos RP and Sessink PJ, "Biomonitoring of Occupational Exposures to Cytostatic Anticancer Drugs," *Rev Environ Health*, 1997, 12(1):43-58.

"Characteristic Wastes," Available at http://www.epa.gov/epawaste/hazard/wastetypes/characteristic.htm. Accessed June 26, 2009.

Connor TH, "Permeability of Nitrile Rubber, Latex, Polyurethane, and Neoprene Gloves to 18 Antineoplastic Drugs," *Am J Health Syst Pharm*, 1999, 56(23):2450-3.

Connor TH, Anderson RW, Sessink PJ, et al, "Surface Contamination With Antineoplastic Agents in Six Cancer Treatment Centers in Canada and the United States," *Am J Health Syst Pharm*, 1999, 62(5):475-84.

Connor TH and McDiarmid MA, "Preventing Occupational Exposures to Antineoplastic Drugs in Health Care Settings," *CA Cancer J Clin*, 2006, 56(6):354-65.

Connor TH, Sessink PJ, Harrison BR, et al, "Surface Contamination of Chemotherapy Drug Vials and Evaluation of New Vial-Cleaning Techniques: Results of Three Studies," *Am J Health Syst Pharm*, 2005, 62(5):475-84.

"Listed Wastes," Available at http://www.epa.gov/epawaste/hazard/wastetypes/listed.htm. Accessed June 26, 2009.

"Pharmaceutical Wastes in Healthcare Facilities," Available at http://www.hercenter.org/hazmat/pharma.cfm#comp. Accessed June 26, 2009.

Polovich M, Belcher C, Gkynn-Tucker EM, et al, *Safe Handling of Hazardous Drugs*, Pittsburgh, PA: Oncology Nursing Society, 2003.

"Preventing Occupational Exposure to Antineoplastic and Other Hazardous Drugs in Health Care Settings," Available at http://www.cdc.gov/niosh/docs/2004-165. Accessed February 6, 2005.

Sessink PJ, Anzion RB, Van den Broek PH, et al, "Detection of Contamination With Antineoplastic Agents in a Hospital Pharmacy Department," *Pharm Weekbl Sci*, 1992, 14(1):16-22.

Sessink PJ, Boer KA, Scheefhals AP, et al, "Occupational Exposure to Antineoplastic Agents at Several Departments in a Hospital. Environmental Contamination and Excretion of Cyclophosphamide and Ifosfamide in Urine of Exposed Workers," *Int Arch Occup Environ Health*, 1992, 64(2):105-12.

Sessink PJ and Bos RP, "Drugs Hazardous to Healthcare Workers. Evaluation of Methods for Monitoring Occupational Exposure to Cytostatic Drugs," *Drug Saf*, 1999, 20(4):347-59.

Solimando DA Jr and Wilson JP, "Demonstration of Skin Fluorescence Following Exposure to Doxorubicin," *Cancer Nurs*, 1983, 6(4):313-5.

Sorsa M and Anderson D, "Monitoring of Occupational Exposure to Cytostatic Anticancer Agents," *Mutat Res*, 1996, 355(1-2):253-61.

Wilson JP and Solimando DA Jr, "Aseptic Technique as a Safety Precaution in the Preparation of Antineoplastic Agents," *Hospital Pharmacy*, 1981, 16(11):575-81.

APPENDIX TABLE OF CONTENTS

MILLIEQUIVALENT AND MILLIMOLE CALCULATIONS AND CONVERSIONS

DEFINITIONS AND CALCULATIONS

Definitions

mole	=	gram molecular weight of a substance (aka molar weight)
millimole (mM)	=	milligram molecular weight of a substance (a millimole is 1/1000 of a mole)
equivalent weight	=	gram weight of a substance which will combine with or replace 1 gram (1 mole) of hydrogen; an equivalent weight can be determined by dividing the molar weight of a substance by its ionic valence
milliequivalent (mEq)	=	milligram weight of a substance which will combine with or replace 1 milligram (1 millimole) of hydrogen (a milliequivalent is 1/1000 of an equivalent)

Calculations

moles	=	$\dfrac{\text{weight of a substance (grams)}}{\text{molecular weight of that substance (grams)}}$
millimoles	=	$\dfrac{\text{weight of a substance (milligrams)}}{\text{molecular weight of that substance (milligrams)}}$
equivalents	=	moles x valence of ion
milliequivalents	=	millimoles x valence of ion
moles	=	$\dfrac{\text{equivalents}}{\text{valence of ion}}$
millimoles	=	$\dfrac{\text{milliequivalents}}{\text{valence of ion}}$
millimoles	=	moles x 1000
milliequivalents	=	equivalents x 1000

Note: Use of equivalents and milliequivalents is valid only for those substances which have fixed ionic valences (eg, sodium, potassium, calcium, chlorine, magnesium bromine, etc). For substances with variable ionic valences (eg, phosphorous), a reliable equivalent value cannot be determined. In these instances, one should calculate millimoles (which are fixed and reliable) rather than milliequivalents.

MILLIEQUIVALENT CONVERSIONS

To convert mg/100 mL to mEq/L the following formula may be used:

$$\frac{(\text{mg/100 mL}) \times 10 \times \text{valence}}{\text{atomic weight}} = \text{mEq/L}$$

To convert mEq/L to mg/100 mL the following formula may be used:

$$\frac{(\text{mEq/L}) \times \text{atomic weight}}{10 \times \text{valence}} = \text{mg/100 mL}$$

To convert mEq/L to volume of percent of a gas the following formula may be used:

$$\frac{(mEq/L) \times 22.4}{10} = \text{volume percent}$$

Valences and Atomic Weights of Selected Ions

Substance	Electrolyte	Valence	Molecular Wt
Calcium	Ca^{++}	2	40
Chloride	Cl^-	1	35.5
Magnesium	Mg^{++}	2	24
Phosphate	HPO_4^{--} (80%)	1.8	96[1]
pH = 7.4	$H_2PO_4^-$ (20%)	1.8	96[1]
Potassium	K^+	1	39
Sodium	Na^+	1	23
Sulfate	SO_4^{--}	2	96[1]

[1]The molecular weight of phosphorus only is 31, and sulfur only is 32.

Approximate Milliequivalents — Weights of Selected Ions

Salt	mEq/g Salt	mg Salt/mEq
Calcium carbonate [$CaCO_3$]	20	50
Calcium chloride [$CaCl_2 \cdot 2H_2O$]	14	74
Calcium gluceptate [$Ca(C_7H_{13}O_8)_2$]	4	245
Calcium gluconate [$Ca(C_6H_{11}O_7)_2 \cdot H_2O$]	5	224
Calcium lactate [$Ca(C_3H_5O_3)_2 \cdot 5H_2O$]	7	154
Magnesium gluconate [$Mg(C_6H_{11}O_7)_2 \cdot H_2O$]	5	216
Magnesium oxide [MgO]	50	20
Magnesium sulfate [$MgSO_4$]	17	60
Magnesium sulfate [$MgSO_4 \cdot 7H_2O$]	8	123
Potassium acetate [$K(C_2H_3O_2)$]	10	98
Potassium chloride [KCl]	13	75
Potassium citrate [$K_3(C_6H_5O_7) \cdot H_2O$]	9	108
Potassium iodide [KI]	6	166
Sodium acetate [$Na(C_2H_3O_2)$]	12	82
Sodium acetate [$Na(C_2H_3O_2) \cdot 3H_2O$]	7	136
Sodium bicarbonate [$NaHCO_3$]	12	84
Sodium chloride [$NaCl$]	17	58
Sodium citrate [$Na_3(C_6H_5O_7) \cdot 2H_2O$]	10	98
Sodium iodine [NaI]	7	150
Sodium lactate [$Na(C_3H_5O_3)$]	9	112
Zinc sulfate [$ZnSO_4 \cdot 7H_2O$]	7	144

CORRECTED SODIUM

Corrected Na^+ = measured Na^+ + [1.5 x (glucose – 150 divided by 100)]

Note: Do not correct for glucose <150.

WATER DEFICIT

Water deficit = 0.6 x body weight [1 – (140 divided by Na^+)]

Note: Body weight is estimated weight in kg when fully hydrated; **Na^+** is serum or plasma sodium. Use corrected Na^+ if necessary. Consult medical references for recommendations for replacement of deficit.

TOTAL SERUM CALCIUM CORRECTED FOR ALBUMIN LEVEL

[(Normal albumin – patient's albumin) x 0.8] + patient's measured total calcium

ACID-BASE ASSESSMENT

Henderson-Hasselbalch Equation

$pH = 6.1 + \log (HCO_3^- / (0.03) (pCO_2))$

Alveolar Gas Equation

$$PIO_2 = FiO_2 \text{ x (total atmospheric pressure – vapor pressure of } H_2O \text{ at } 37°C)$$

$$= FiO_2 \text{ x (760 mm Hg – 47 mm Hg)}$$

$$PAO_2 = PIO_2 – PACO_2 / R$$

Alveolar/arterial oxygen gradient = $PAO_2 – PaO_2$

Normal ranges:

Children	15-20 mm Hg
Adults	20-25 mm Hg

where:

PIO_2	=	Oxygen partial pressure of inspired gas (mm Hg) (150 mm Hg in room air at sea level)
FiO_2	=	Fractional pressure of oxygen in inspired gas (0.21 in room air)
PAO_2	=	Alveolar oxygen partial pressure
$PACO_2$	=	Alveolar carbon dioxide partial pressure
PaO_2	=	Arterial oxygen partial pressure
R	=	Respiratory exchange quotient (typically 0.8, increases with high carbohydrate diet, decreases with high fat diet)

Acid-Base Disorders

Acute metabolic acidosis:
$PaCO_2$ expected = 1.5 (HCO_3^-) + 8 ± 2 **or**
Expected decrease in $PaCO_2$ = 1.3 (1-1.5) x decrease in HCO_3^-

Acute metabolic alkalosis:
Expected increase in $PaCO_2$ = 0.6 (0.5-1) x increase in HCO_3^-

Acute respiratory acidosis (<6 h duration):
For every $PaCO_2$ increase of 10 mm Hg, HCO_3 increases by 1 mEq/L

Chronic respiratory acidosis (>6 h duration):
For every $PaCO_2$ increase of 10 mm Hg, HCO_3 increases by 4 mEq/L

Acute respiratory alkalosis (<6 h duration):
For every $PaCO_2$ decrease of 10 mm Hg, HCO_3 decreases by 2 mEq/L

Chronic respiratory alkalosis (>6 h duration):
For every $PaCO_2$ decrease of 10 mm Hg, HCO_3 increases by 5 mEq/L

ACID-BASE EQUATION

H^+ (in mEq/L) = (24 x $PaCO_2$) divided by HCO_3^-

Aa GRADIENT

Aa gradient $[(713)(FiO_2 - (PaCO_2 \text{ divided by } 0.8))] - PaO_2$

Aa gradient	=	alveolar-arterial oxygen gradient
FiO_2	=	inspired oxygen (expressed as a fraction)
$PaCO_2$	=	arterial partial pressure carbon dioxide (mm Hg)
PaO_2	=	arterial partial pressure oxygen (mm Hg)

OSMOLALITY

Definition: The summed concentrations of all osmotically active solute particles.

Predicted serum osmolality =

$$\text{mOsm/L} = (2 \times \text{serum Na}^{++}) + \frac{\text{serum glucose}}{18} + \frac{\text{BUN}}{2.8}$$

The normal range of serum osmolality is 285-295 mOsm/L.

Calculated Osm

Note: Osm is a term used to reconcile osmolality and osmolarity

Osmol gap = measured Osm − calculated Osm

0 to +10: Normal
>10: Abnormal
<0: Probable lab or calculation error

Drugs Causing Osmolar Gap
(by freezing-point depression, gap is >10 mOsm)

Ethanol
Ethylene glycol
Glycerol
Iodine (questionable)
Isopropanol (acetone)

Mannitol
Methanol
Sorbitol

BICARBONATE DEFICIT

HCO_3^- deficit = (0.4 x wt in kg) x (HCO_3^- desired – HCO_3^- measured)

Note: In clinical practice, the calculated quantity may differ markedly from the actual amount of bicarbonate needed or that which may be safely administered.

ANION GAP

Definition: The difference in concentration between unmeasured cation and anion equivalents in serum.

Anion gap = Na^+ – (Cl^- + HCO_3^-)
  (The normal anion gap is 10-14 mEq/L)

Differential Diagnosis of Increased Anion Gap Acidosis

Organic anions
  Lactate (sepsis, hypovolemia, seizures, large tumor burden)
  Pyruvate
  Uremia
  Ketoacidosis (β-hydroxybutyrate and acetoacetate)
  Amino acids and their metabolites
  Other organic acids

Inorganic anions
  Hyperphosphatemia
  Sulfates
  Nitrates

Differential Diagnosis of Decreased Anion Gap

Organic cations
  Hypergammaglobulinemia

Inorganic cations
  Hyperkalemia
  Hypercalcemia
  Hypermagnesemia

Medications and toxins
  Lithium

Hypoalbuminemia

RETICULOCYTE INDEX

(% retic divided by 2) x (patient's Hct divided by normal Hct) **or**
(% retic divided by 2) x (patient's Hgb divided by normal Hgb)

Normal index: 1.0
Good marrow response: 2.0-6.0

BODY SURFACE AREA

Body Surface Area (BSA) – Adults and Pediatric

$$BSA\ (m^2) = \frac{kg^{0.425} \times cm^{0.725} \times 71.84}{10,000}$$

or

$$\log BSA\ (m^2) = \frac{(\log kg \times 0.425) + (\log cm \times 0.725) + 1.8564}{10,000}$$

DuBois D and DuBois EF, "A Formula to Estimate the Approximate Surface Area if Height and Weight Be Known," *Arch Intern Med*, 1916, 17:863-71.

$$BSA\ (m^2) = \sqrt{\frac{ht\ (in) \times wt\ (lb)}{3131}} \quad or \quad BSA\ (m^2) = \sqrt{\frac{ht\ (cm) \times wt\ (kg)}{3600}}$$

Lam TK and Leung DT, "More on Simplified Calculation of Body-Surface Area," *N Engl J Med*, 1988, 318(17):1130 (letter).
Mosteller RD, "Simplified Calculation of Body Surface Area," *N Engl J Med*, 1987, 317:1098 (letter).

Ideal Body Weight

Men:	50 kg + 2.3 kg/inch >5 ft
Women:	45 kg + 2.3 kg/in >5 ft

Devine BJ, "Gentamicin Therapy," *Drug Intelligence and Clinical Pharmacy*, 1974, 8:650-5.

or

Men:	51.65 kg + 1.85 kg/in >5 ft
Women:	48.67 kg + 1.7 kg/in >5 ft

Robinson JD, Lupkiewicz SM, Palenik L, et al, "Determination of Ideal Body Weight for Drug Dosage Calculations," *Am J Hosp Pharm*, 1983, 40(6): 1016-9.

Adjusted Body Weight

Adjusted wt (kg) = actual weight (kg) – 0.4 [actual wt (kg) – ideal weight (kg)]
Notari EE, "Biopharmaceuticals and Clinical Pharmacokinetics," New York, Basel, 1987, 380.

Area Under the Curve (AUC) for Carboplatin Dosing

Carboplatin (mg) = desired AUC x (25 + GFR)

GFR = creatinine clearance (measured or estimated)
Calvert AH, Newell DR, Gumbrell LA, et al, "Carboplatin Dosage: Prospective Evaluation of a Simple Formula Based on Renal Function," *J Clin Oncol*, 1989, 7 (11):1748-56.

CREATININE CLEARANCE ESTIMATING METHODS IN PATIENTS WITH STABLE RENAL FUNCTION

These formulas provide an acceptable estimate of the patient's creatinine clearance **except** in the following instances.

- Patient's serum creatinine is changing rapidly (either increasing or decreasing).
- Patient is markedly emaciated.

In above situations, certain assumptions have to be made.

- In a patient with rapidly rising serum creatinine (ie, >0.5-0.7 mg/dL/day), it is best to assume that the patient's creatinine clearance is probably <10 mL/minute.
- In an emaciated patient, although their actual creatinine clearance is less than their calculated creatinine clearance (because of decreased creatinine production), it is not possible to easily predict how much less.

INFANTS

Estimation of creatinine clearance using serum creatinine and body length (to be used when an adequate timed specimen cannot be obtained). **Note:** This formula may not provide an accurate estimation of creatinine clearance for infants younger than 6 months of age and for patients with severe starvation or muscle wasting.

$$Cl_{cr} = K \times L/S_{cr}$$

where:

Cl_{cr} = creatinine clearance in mL/minute/1.73 m^2
K = constant of proportionality that is age specific

Age	K
Low birth weight ≤1 y	0.33
Full-term ≤1 y	0.45
2-12 y	0.55
13-21 y female	0.55
13-21 y male	0.70

L = length in cm
S_{cr} = serum creatinine concentration in mg/dL

Reference

Schwartz GJ, Brion LP, and Spitzer A, "The Use of Plasma Creatinine Concentration for Estimating Glomerular Filtration Rate in Infants, Children and Adolescents," *Pediatr Clin North Am*, 1987, 34 (3):571-90.

CHILDREN (1-18 years)

<u>Method 1</u>: (Traub SL and Johnson CE, *Am J Hosp Pharm*, 1980, 37(2):195-201)

$$Cl_{cr} = 0.48 \times (height) / S_{cr}$$

where:

Cl_{cr} = creatinine clearance in mL/min/1.73 m^2
S_{cr} = serum creatinine in mg/dL
Height = height in cm

<u>Method 2</u>: Nomogram (Traub SL and Johnson CE, *Am J Hosp Pharm*, 1980, 37 (2):195-201)

Children 1-18 Years

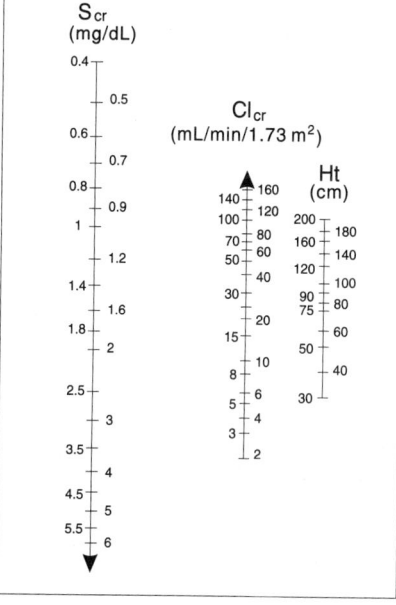

The nomogram below is for rapid evaluation of endogenous creatinine clearance (Cl_{cr}) in pediatric patients.

To predict Cl_{cr} connect the child's S_{cr} (serum creatinine) and Ht (height) with a ruler and read the Cl_{cr} where the ruler intersects the center line.

◀ **ADULTS (18 years and older)**

<u>Method 1</u>: (Cockroft DW and Gault MH, *Nephron*, 1976, 16:31-41)

Estimated creatinine clearance (Cl$_{cr}$) (mL/min):

Male = (140 − age) x BW (kg) / 72 x S$_{cr}$
Female = male x 0.85

Note: Use of actual body weight (BW) in obese patients (and possibly patients with ascites) may significantly overestimate creatinine clearance. Some clinicians prefer to use an adjusted ideal body weight (IBW) in such cases [eg, IBW + 0.4 (ABW-IBW)], especially when calculating dosages for aminoglycoside antibiotics.

<u>Method 2</u>: (Jelliffe RW, *Ann Intern Med*, 1973, 79:604)

Estimated creatinine clearance (Cl$_{cr}$) (mL/min/1.73 m^2):

Male = 98 − 0.8 (age − 20) / S$_{cr}$
Female = male x 0.90

RENAL FUNCTION TESTS

Endogenous Creatinine Clearance vs Age (timed collection)

Creatinine clearance (mL/min/1.73 m^2) = (Cr_uV/Cr_sT) (1.73/A)

where:

Cr_u	=	urine creatinine concentration (mg/dL)
V	=	total urine collected during sampling period (mL)
Cr_s	=	serum creatinine concentration (mg/dL)
T	=	duration of sampling period (min) (24 h = 1440 min)
A	=	body surface area (m^2)

Age-specific normal values

5-7 d		50.6 ± 5.8 mL/min/1.73 m^2
1-2 mo		64.6 ± 5.8 mL/min/1.73 m^2
5-8 mo		87.7 ± 11.9 mL/min/1.73 m^2
9-12 mo		86.9 ± 8.4 mL/min/1.73 m^2
≥18 mo		
	male	124 ± 26 mL/min/1.73 m^2
	female	109 ± 13.5 mL/min/1.73 m^2
Adults		
	male	105 ± 14 mL/min/1.73 m^2
	female	95 ± 18 mL/min/1.73 m^2

Note: In patients with renal failure (creatinine clearance <25 mL/min), creatinine clearance may be elevated over GFR because of tubular secretion of creatinine.

Calculation of Creatinine Clearance From a 24-Hour Urine Collection

Equation 1:

$$Cl_{cr} = \frac{U \times V}{P}$$

where:

Cl_{cr}	=	creatinine clearance
U	=	urine concentration of creatinine
V	=	total urine volume in the collection
P	=	plasma creatinine concentration

Equation 2:

$$Cl_{cr} = \frac{\text{(total urine volume [mL])} \times \text{(urine Cr concentration [mg/dL])}}{\text{(serum creatinine [mg/dL])} \times \text{(time of urine collection [minutes])}}$$

Occasionally, a patient will have a 12- or 24-hour urine collection done for direct calculation of creatinine clearance. Although a urine collection for 24 hours is best, it is difficult to do since many urine collections occur for a much shorter period. A 24-hour urine collection is the desired duration of urine collection

◀ because the urine excretion of creatinine is diurnal and thus the measured creatinine clearance will vary throughout the day as the creatinine in the urine varies. When the urine collection is less than 24 hours, the total excreted creatinine will be affected by the time of the day during which the collection is performed. A 24-hour urine collection is sufficient to be able to accurately average the diurnal creatinine excretion variations. If a patient has 24 hours of urine collected for creatinine clearance, equation 1 can be used for calculating the creatinine clearance. To use equation 1 to calculate the creatinine clearance, it will be necessary to know the duration of urine collection, the urine collection volume, the urine creatinine concentration, and the serum creatinine value that reflects the urine collection period. In most cases, a serum creatinine concentration is drawn anytime during the day, but it is best to have the value drawn halfway through the collection period.

Amylase:Creatinine Clearance Ratio

$$\frac{Amylase_u \times creatinine_p}{Amylase_p \times creatinine_u} \times 100$$

u = urine; p = plasma

Serum BUN:Serum Creatinine Ratio

Serum BUN (mg/dL:serum creatinine (mg/dL))

Normal BUN:creatinine ratio is 10-15

BUN:creatinine ratio >20 suggests prerenal azotemia (also seen with high urea-generation states such as GI bleeding)

BUN:creatinine ratio <5 may be seen with disorders affecting urea biosynthesis such as urea cycle enzyme deficiencies and with hepatitis.

Fractional Sodium Excretion

Fractional sodium secretion (FENa) = $Na_u Cr_s / Na_s Cr_u \times 100\%$

where:

$$Na_u = \text{urine sodium (mEq/L)}$$
$$Na_s = \text{serum sodium (mEq/L)}$$
$$Cr_u = \text{urine creatinine (mg/dL)}$$
$$Cr_s = \text{serum creatinine (mg/dL)}$$

FENa <1% suggests prerenal failure
FENa >2% suggest intrinsic renal failure (for newborns, normal FENa is approximately 2.5%)

Note: Disease states associated with a falsely elevated FENa include severe volume depletion (>10%), early acute tubular necrosis, and volume depletion in chronic renal disease. Disorders associated with a lowered FENa include acute glomerulonephritis, hemoglobinuric or myoglobinuric renal failure, nonoliguric acute tubular necrosis, and acute urinary tract obstruction. In addition, FENa may be <1% in patients with acute renal failure **and** a second condition predisposing to sodium retention (eg, burns, congestive heart failure, nephrotic syndrome).

Urine Calcium:Urine Creatinine Ratio (spot sample)

Urine calcium (mg/dL): urine creatinine (mg/dL)

Normal values <0.21 (mean values 0.08 males, 0.06 females)

Premature infants show wide variability of calcium:creatinine ratio, and tend to have lower thresholds for calcium loss than older children. Prematures without nephrolithiasis had mean Ca:Cr ratio of 0.75 ± 0.76. Infants with nephrolithiasis had mean Ca:Cr ratio of 1.32 ± 1.03 (Jacinto JS, Modanlou HD, Crade M, et al, "Renal Calcification Incidence in Very Low Birth Weight Infants," *Pediatrics*, 1988, 81:31.)

Urine Protein:Urine Creatinine Ratio (spot sample)

P_u/Cr_u	Total Protein Excretion (mg/m²/d)
0.1	80
1	800
10	8000

where:

P_u = urine protein concentration (mg/dL)
Cr_u = urine creatinine concentration (mg/dL)

INTRAVENOUS IMMUNE GLOBULIN

Brand Name	FDA-Approved Indications	Labeled Contraindications	IgA Content	Half-Life	pH	Osmolarity / Osmolality	Recommended Infusion Rates	Additional Comments
Carimune® NF	Primary immunodeficiency; ITP	IgA deficiency with IgA antibody; severe systemic reaction to human immune globulins	720 mcg/mL	3 weeks	6.4-6.8	3% solution in NS: 498 mOsmol/kg 6% solution in NS: 690 mOsmol/kg 9% solution in NS: 882 mOsmol/kg 12% solution in NS: 1074 mOsmol/kg 3% solution in D₅W: 444 mOsmol/kg 6% solution in D₅W: 636 mOsmol/kg 9% solution in D₅W: 828 mOsmol/kg 12% solution in D₅W: 1020 mOsmol/kg 3% solution in SWFI: 192 mOsmol/kg 6% solution in SWFI: 384 mOsmol/kg 9% solution in SWFI: 576 mOsmol/kg 12% solution in SWFI: 768 mOsmol/kg	Initial (3% solution): 0.5-1 mL/min Maximum (3% solution): 2 mg/kg/min	Contains sucrose
Flebo-gamma®	Primary immunodeficiency	IgA deficiency with IgA antibody; anaphylactic reactions to blood or blood derived products	<50 mcg/mL	30-45 days	5-6	240-350 mOsmol/L	Initial (5% solution): 0.01 mL/kg/min (0.5 mg/kg/min) Maximum (5% solution): 0.1 mL/kg/min (5 mg/kg/min) Maximum in patients with renal dysfunction (5% solution): 0.06 mL/kg/min (3 mg/kg/min)	Contains sorbitol

Brand Name	FDA-Approved Indications	Labeled Contraindications	IgA Content	Half-Life	pH	Osmolarity / Osmolality	Recommended Infusion Rates	Additional Comments
Gammagard Liquid	Primary immunodeficiency	IgA deficiency, history of anaphylaxis with immune globulin	37 mcg/mL	35 days	4.6 - 5.1	240-300 mOsmol/kg	Initial (10% solution): 0.5 mL/kg/h (0.8 mg/kg/min) Maximum (10% solution): 5 mL/kg/h (8.9 mg/kg/min); <2 mL/kg/h (3.3 mg/kg/min) in patients at risk for renal impairment or thrombosis	
Gammagard S/D	Primary immunodeficiency, ITP, CLL, Kawasaki syndrome	IgA deficiency	≤1 mcg/mL	~23-53 days	6.4 - 7.2		Initial (5% solution): 0.5 mL/kg/h Maximum (5% solution): 4 mL/kg/h Maximum concentration for infusion: 10%	Contains glucose
Gamunex®	Primary immunodeficiency, ITP, chronic inflammatory demyelinating polyneuropathy (CIDP)	IgA deficiency with IgA antibody; history of anaphylaxis with immune globulin	46 mcg/mL	35 days	4-4.5	258 mOsmol/kg	Initial (10% solution): 0.01 mL/kg/min Maximum (10% solution): 0.08 mL/kg/min Maximum concentration for infusion: 10%	

Brand Name	FDA-Approved Indications	Labeled Contraindications	IgA Content	Half-Life	pH	Osmolarity / Osmolality	Recommended Infusion Rates	Additional Comments
Octagam®	Primary immunodeficiency	IgA deficiency with IgA antibody	≤200 mcg/mL	Immunodeficiency: 40 days	5.1-6.0	310-380 mOsmol/kg	Initial: 30 mg/kg/h (0.01 mL/kg/min) Maximum: <200 mg/kg/h (<0.07 mL/kg/min) Maximum concentration for infusion: 5%	Contains maltose
Privigen™	Primary immunodeficiency, ITP	IgA deficiency; history of anaphylaxis with immune globulin; hyperprolinemia	≤25 mcg/mL	~37 days	4.6-5	240-440 mOsmol/kg	Initial: 0.5 mg/kg/min (0.005 mL/kg/min) Maximum primary immunodeficiency: 8 mg/kg/min (0.08 mL/kg/min; ITP- 4 mg/kg/min (0.04 mL/kg/min) Maximum concentration for solution: 10%	L-proline

Carimune® NF prescribing information, ZLB Behring LLC, Kankakee, IL, January 2005.

Flebogamma® 5% prescribing information, Grifols Biologicals, Inc, Los Angeles, CA, September 2004.

Gammagard Liquid prescribing information, Baxter Healthcare Corporation, Westlake Village, CA, April 2005.

Gammagard S/D prescribing information, Baxter Healthcare Corporation, Westlake Village, CA, March 2007.

Gamunex® prescribing information, Talecris Biotherapeutics, Inc, Research Triangle Park, NC, September 2008.

Octagam® prescribing information, Octapharma USA, Inc, Centreville, VA, March 2007.

Privigen™ prescribing information, CSL Behring, King of Prussia, PA, July 2007

REFERENCE VALUES FOR ADULTS

CHEMISTRY

Test	Values	Remarks
Serum / Plasma		
Acetone	Negative	
Albumin	3.2-5 g/dL	
Alcohol, ethyl	Negative	
Aldolase	1.2-7.6 IU/L	
Ammonia	20-70 mcg/dL	Specimen to be placed on ice as soon as collected.
Amylase	30-110 units/L	
Bilirubin, direct	0-0.3 mg/dL	
Bilirubin, total	0.1-1.2 mg/dL	
Calcium	8.6-10.3 mg/dL	
Calcium, ionized	2.24-2.46 mEq/L	
Chloride	95-108 mEq/L	
Cholesterol, total	≤200 mg/dL	Fasted blood required – normal value affected by dietary habits. This reference range is for a general adult population.
HDL cholesterol	40-60 mg/dL	Fasted blood required – normal value affected by dietary habits.
LDL cholesterol	<160 mg/dL	If triglyceride is >400 mg/dL, LDL cannot be calculated accurately (Friedewald equation). Target LDL-C depends on patient's risk factors.
CO_2	23-30 mEq/L	
Creatine kinase (CK) isoenzymes		
CK-BB	0%	
CK-MB (cardiac)	0%-3.9%	
CK-MM (muscle)	96%-100%	

CK-MB levels must be both ≥4% and 10 IU/L to meet diagnostic criteria for CK-MB positive result consistent with myocardial injury.

Creatine phosphokinase (CPK)	8-150 IU/L	
Creatinine	0.5-1.4 mg/dL	
Ferritin	13-300 ng/mL	
Folate	3.6-20 ng/dL	

▶

CHEMISTRY *(continued)*

Test	Values	Remarks
GGT (gamma-glutamyltranspeptidase)		
male	11-63 IU/L	
female	8-35 IU/L	
GLDH	To be determined	
Glucose (preprandial)	<115 mg/dL	Goals different for diabetics.
Glucose, fasting	60-110 mg/dL	Goals different for diabetics.
Glucose, nonfasting (2-h postprandial)	<120 mg/dL	Goals different for diabetics.
Hemoglobin A_{1c}	<8	
Hemoglobin, plasma free	<2.5 mg/100 mL	
Hemoglobin, total glycosolated (Hb A_1)	4%-8%	
Iron	65-150 mcg/dL	
Iron binding capacity, total (TIBC)	250-420 mcg/dL	
Lactic acid	0.7-2.1 mEq/L	Specimen to be kept on ice and sent to lab as soon as possible.
Lactate dehydrogenase (LDH)	56-194 IU/L	
Lactate dehydrogenase (LDH) isoenzymes		
LD_1	20%-34%	
LD_2	29%-41%	
LD_3	15%-25%	
LD_4	1%-12%	
LD_5	1%-15%	

Flipped LD_1/LD_2 ratios (>1 may be consistent with myocardial injury) particularly when considered in combination with a recent CK-MB positive result.

Test	Values	Remarks
Lipase	23-208 units/L	
Magnesium	1.6-2.5 mg/dL	Increased by slight hemolysis.
Osmolality	289-308 mOsm/kg	
Phosphatase, alkaline		
adults 25-60 y	33-131 IU/L	
adults ≥61 y	51-153 IU/L	
infancy-adolescence	Values range up to 3-5 times higher than adults	
Phosphate, inorganic	2.8-4.2 mg/dL	
Potassium	3.5-5.2 mEq/L	Increased by slight hemolysis.
Prealbumin	>15 mg/dL	

CHEMISTRY (continued)

Test	Values	Remarks
Protein, total	6.5-7.9 g/dL	
AST	<35 IU/L (20-48)	
ALT (10-35)	<35 IU/L	
Sodium	134-149 mEq/L	
Thyroid stimulating hormone (TSH)		
adults ≤20 y	0.7-6.4 mIU/L	
21-54 y	0.4-4.2 mIU/L	
55-87 y	0.5-8.9 mIU/L	
Transferrin	>200 mg/dL	
Triglycerides	45-155 mg/dL	Fasted blood required.
Troponin I	<1.5 ng/mL	
Urea nitrogen (BUN)	7-20 mg/dL	
Uric acid		
male	2-8 mg/dL	
female	2-7.5 mg/dL	
Cerebrospinal Fluid		
Glucose	50-70 mg/dL	
Protein	15-45 mg/dL	CSF obtained by lumbar puncture.

Note: Bloody specimen gives erroneously high value due to contamination with blood proteins

Urine
(24-hour specimen is required for all these tests unless specified)

Amylase	32-641 units/L	The value is in units/L and **not** calculated for total volume.
Amylase, fluid (random samples)		Interpretation of value left for physician, depends on the nature of fluid.
Calcium	Depends upon dietary intake	
Creatine		
male	150 mg/24 h	Higher value on children and during pregnancy.
female	250 mg/24 h	
Creatinine	1000-2000 mg/24 h	
Creatinine clearance (endogenous)		
male	85-125 mL/min	A blood sample must accompany urine specimen.
female	75-115 mL/min	
Glucose	1 g/24 h	

CHEMISTRY *(continued)*

Test	Values	Remarks
5-hydroxyindoleacetic acid	2-8 mg/24 h	
Iron	0.15 mg/24 h	Acid washed container required.
Magnesium	146-209 mg/24 h	
Osmolality	500-800 mOsm/kg	With normal fluid intake.
Oxalate	10-40 mg/24 h	
Phosphate	400-1300 mg/24 h	
Potassium	25-120 mEq/24 h	Varies with diet; the interpretation of urine electrolytes and osmolality should be left for the physician.
Sodium	40-220 mEq/24 h	
Porphobilinogen, qualitative	Negative	
Porphyrins, qualitative	Negative	
Proteins	0.05-0.1 g/24 h	
Salicylate	Negative	
Urea clearance	60-95 mL/min	A blood sample must accompany specimen.
Urea N	10-40 g/24 h	Dependent on protein intake.
Uric acid	250-750 mg/24 h	Dependent on diet and therapy.
Urobilinogen	0.5-3.5 mg/24 h	For qualitative determination on random urine, send sample to urinalysis section in Hematology Lab.
Xylose absorption test		
children	16%-33% of ingested xylose	

Feces

Test	Values	Remarks
Fat, 3-day collection	<5 g/d	Value depends on fat intake of 100 g/d for 3 days preceding and during collection.

Gastric Acidity

Test	Values	Remarks
Acidity, total, 12 h	10-60 mEq/L	Titrated at pH 7.

Blood Gases

	Arterial	Capillary	Venous
pH	7.35-7.45	7.35-7.45	7.32-7.42
pCO_2 (mm Hg)	35-45	35-45	38-52
pO_2 (mm Hg)	70-100	60-80	24-48
HCO_3 (mEq/L)	19-25	19-25	19-25
TCO_2 (mEq/L)	19-29	19-29	23-33
O_2 saturation (%)	90-95	90-95	40-70
Base excess (mEq/L)	-5 to +5	-5 to +5	-5 to +5

HEMATOLOGY

Complete Blood Count

Age	Hgb (g/dL)	Hct (%)	RBC (mill/mm³)	RDW
0-3 d	15.0-20.0	45-61	4.0-5.9	<18
1-2 wk	12.5-18.5	39-57	3.6-5.5	<17
1-6 mo	10.0-13.0	29-42	3.1-4.3	<16.5
7 mo to 2 y	10.5-13.0	33-38	3.7-4.9	<16
2-5 y	11.5-13.0	34-39	3.9-5.0	<15
5-8 y	11.5-14.5	35-42	4.0-4.9	<15
13-18 y	12.0-15.2	36-47	4.5-5.1	<14.5
Adult male	13.5-16.5	41-50	4.5-5.5	<14.5
Adult female	12.0-15.0	36-44	4.0-4.9	<14.5

Age	MCV (fL)	MCH (pg)	MCHC (%)	Plts (x 10³/mm³)
0-3 d	95-115	31-37	29-37	250-450
1-2 wk	86-110	28-36	28-38	250-450
1-6 mo	74-96	25-35	30-36	300-700
7 mo to 2 y	70-84	23-30	31-37	250-600
2-5 y	75-87	24-30	31-37	250-550
5-8 y	77-95	25-33	31-37	250-550
13-18 y	78-96	25-35	31-37	150-450
Adult male	80-100	26-34	31-37	150-450
Adult female	80-100	26-34	31-37	150-450

WBC and Differential

Age	WBC (x 10^3/mm^3)	Segs	Bands	Lymphs	Monos
0-3 d	9.0-35.0	32-62	10-18	19-29	5-7
1-2 wk	5.0-20.0	14-34	6-14	36-45	6-10
1-6 mo	6.0-17.5	13-33	4-12	41-71	4-7
7 mo to 2 y	6.0-17.0	15-35	5-11	45-76	3-6
2-5 y	5.5-15.5	23-45	5-11	35-65	3-6
5-8 y	5.0-14.5	32-54	5-11	28-48	3-6
13-18 y	4.5-13.0	34-64	5-11	25-45	3-6
Adults	4.5-11.0	35-66	5-11	24-44	3-6

Age	Eosinophils	Basophils	Atypical Lymphs	No. of NRBCs
0-3 d	0-2	0-1	0-8	0-2
1-2 wk	0-2	0-1	0-8	0
1-6 mo	0-3	0-1	0-8	0
7 mo to 2 y	0-3	0-1	0-8	0
2-5 y	0-3	0-1	0-8	0
5-8 y	0-3	0-1	0-8	0
13-18 y	0-3	0-1	0-8	0
Adults	0-3	0-1	0-8	0

Segs = segmented neutrophils.

Bands = band neutrophils.

Lymphs = lymphocytes.

Monos = monocytes.

Erythrocyte Sedimentation Rates and Reticulocyte Counts

Sedimentation rate, Westergren	Children	0-20 mm/h
	Adult male	0-15 mm/h
	Adult female	0-20 mm/h
Sedimentation rate, Wintrobe	Children	0-13 mm/h
	Adult male	0-10 mm/h
	Adult female	0-15 mm/h
Reticulocyte count	Newborns	2%-6%
	1-6 mo	0%-2.8%
	Adults	0.5%-1.5%

PHARMACOLOGIC CATEGORY INDEX